# ACP | MKSAP® 18
## Medical Knowledge Self-Assessment Program®

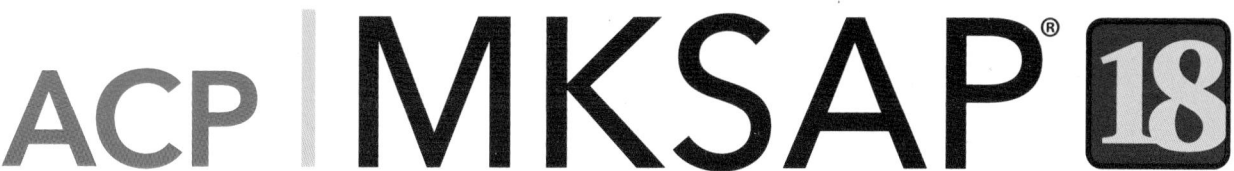

# Endocrinology and Metabolism

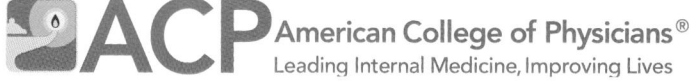

# Welcome to the Endocrinology and Metabolism Section of MKSAP 18!

In these pages, you will find updated information on disorders of glucose metabolism, disorders of the pituitary gland, disorders of the adrenal glands, disorders of the thyroid gland, reproduction disorders, transgender hormone therapy management, and calcium and bone disorders. All of these topics are uniquely focused on the needs of generalists and subspecialists *outside* of endocrinology.

The core content of MKSAP 18 has been developed as in previous editions–all essential information that is newly researched and written in 11 topic areas of internal medicine–created by dozens of leading generalists and subspecialists and guided by certification and recertification requirements, emerging knowledge in the field, and user feedback. MKSAP 18 also contains 1200 all-new peer-reviewed, psychometrically validated, multiple-choice questions (MCQs) for self-assessment and study, including 84 in Endocrinology and Metabolism. MKSAP 18 continues to include *High Value Care* (HVC) recommendations, based on the concept of balancing clinical benefit with costs and harms, with associated MCQs illustrating these principles and HVC Key Points called out in the text. Internists practicing in the hospital setting can easily find comprehensive *Hospitalist*-focused content and MCQs, specially designated in blue and with the 🄷 symbol.

If you purchased MKSAP 18 Complete, you also have access to MKSAP 18 Digital, with additional tools allowing you to customize your learning experience. MKSAP Digital includes regular text updates with new, practice-changing information, 200 new self-assessment questions, and enhanced custom-quiz options. MKSAP Complete also includes more than 1200 electronic, adaptive learning–enhanced flashcards for quick review of important concepts, as well as an updated and enhanced version of Virtual Dx, MKSAP's image-based self-assessment tool. As before, MKSAP 18 Digital is optimized for use on your mobile devices, with iOS- and Android-based apps allowing you to sync between your apps and online account and submit for CME credits and MOC points online.

Please visit us at the MKSAP Resource Site (mksap.acponline.org) to find out how we can help you study, earn CME credit and MOC points, and stay up to date.

On behalf of the many internists who have offered their time and expertise to create the content for MKSAP 18 and the editorial staff who work to bring this material to you in the best possible way, we are honored that you have chosen to use MKSAP 18 and appreciate any feedback about the program you may have. Please feel free to send any comments to mksap_editors@acponline.org.

Sincerely,

Patrick C. Alguire, MD, FACP
Editor-in-Chief
Senior Vice President Emeritus
Medical Education Division
American College of Physicians

# Endocrinology and Metabolism

## Committee

**Cynthia A. Burns, MD, FACP, Section Editor[1]**
Director of Undergraduate Medical Education in Internal
  Medicine
Internal Medicine Clerkship Director and Subspecialty
  Acting Internships Course Director
Associate Professor of Internal Medicine
Section of Endocrinology and Metabolism
Wake Forest School of Medicine
Winston-Salem, North Carolina

**Leigh M. Eck, MD, FACP[2]**
Program Director, Internal Medicine Residency Program
Associate Professor of Medicine
University of Kansas Health System
Kansas City, Kansas

**Kurt A. Kennel, MD[2]**
Assistant Professor of Medicine
Division of Endocrinology, Metabolism and Nutrition
Mayo Clinic College of Medicine and Science
Rochester, Minnesota

**Wanda C. Lakey, MD, MHS, FACP[2]**
Associate Professor of Medicine
Division of Endocrinology
Duke University Medical Center
Durham VA Medical Center
Durham, North Carolina

**Sarah E. Mayson, MD[2]**
Assistant Professor
Division of Endocrinology, Metabolism and Diabetes
University of Colorado School of Medicine
Aurora, Colorado

**Farah Morgan, MD[1]**
Assistant Professor
Cooper Medical School of Rowan University
Endocrine Fellowship Program Director
Cooper University Hospital
Camden, New Jersey

**Neena Natt, MD[1]**
Associate Professor, Endocrinology
Mayo Clinic College of Medicine and Science
Rochester, Minnesota

## Editor-in-Chief

**Patrick C. Alguire, MD, FACP[2]**
Senior Vice President Emeritus, Medical Education
American College of Physicians
Philadelphia, Pennsylvania

## Deputy Editor

**Denise M. Dupras, MD, PhD, FACP[1]**
Associate Program Director
Department of Internal Medicine
Associate Professor of Medicine
Mayo Clinic College of Medicine and Science
Rochester, Minnesota

## Endocrinology and Metabolism Reviewers

Karen Barnard, MBBCh[1]
Shankar S. Bettadahalli, MD, FACP[1]
Michelle L. Cordoba Kissee, MD[1]
Benjamin A. Dennis, MD[1]
Ruban Dhaliwal, MD[1]
Antonette Brigidi Frasch, MD, FACP[2]
Peter A. Goulden, MD[2]
Dona Leslie Gray, MD, FACP[2]
Airani Sathananthan, MD, FACP[2]
Sarah H. See, MD, FACP[1]
Michael H. Shanik, MD, FACP[2]

## Hospital Medicine Endocrinology and Metabolism Reviewers

Kyaw K. Soe, MD, FACP[1]
Scott M. Stevens, MD, FACP[2]

## Endocrinology and Metabolism ACP Editorial Staff

**Randy Hendrickson[1],** Production Administrator/Editor
**Julia Nawrocki[1],** Digital Content Associate/Editor
**Margaret Wells,** Director, Self-Assessment and Educational
  Programs
**Becky Krumm,** Managing Editor, Self-Assessment and
  Educational Programs

## ACP Principal Staff

**Davoren Chick, MD, FACP[2]**
*Senior Vice President, Medical Education*

**Patrick C. Alguire, MD, FACP[2]**
*Senior Vice President Emeritus, Medical Education*

**Sean McKinney[1]**
*Vice President, Medical Education*

**Margaret Wells**
*Director, Self-Assessment and Educational Programs*

**Becky Krumm[1]**
*Managing Editor*

**Valerie Dangovetsky[1]**
*Administrator*

**Ellen McDonald, PhD[1]**
*Senior Staff Editor*

**Megan Zborowski[1]**
*Senior Staff Editor*

**Jackie Twomey[1]**
*Senior Staff Editor*

**Randy Hendrickson[1]**
*Production Administrator/Editor*

**Julia Nawrocki[1]**
*Digital Content Associate/Editor*

**Linnea Donnarumma[1]**
*Staff Editor*

**Chuck Emig[1]**
*Staff Editor*

**Joysa Winter[1]**
*Staff Editor*

**Kimberly Kerns[1]**
*Administrative Coordinator*

---

1. Has no relationships with any entity producing, marketing, reselling, or distributing health care goods or services consumed by, or used on, patients.

2. Has disclosed relationship(s) with any entity producing, marketing, reselling, or distributing health care goods or services consumed by, or used on, patients.

**Disclosure of Relationships with any entity producing, marketing, reselling, or distributing health care goods or services consumed by, or used on, patients.**

**Patrick C. Alguire, MD, FACP**
*Royalties*
UpToDate

**Davoren Chick, MD, FACP**
*Royalties*
Wolters Kluwer Publishing
*Consultantship*
EBSCO Health's DynaMed Plus
*Other*
Owner and sole proprietor of Coding 101, LLC; Spouse: research consultant for Vedanta Biosciences

**Leigh M. Eck, MD, FACP**
*Consultantship*
NovoNordisk

**Antonette Brigidi Frasch, MD, FACP**
*Consultantship*
Medical Reviewers of America

**Peter A. Goulden, MD**
*Research Grants/Contracts*
NovoNordisk

**Dona Leslie Gray, MD, FACP**
*Speakers Bureau*
Janssen, Sanofi

**Kurt A. Kennel, MD**
*Consultantship*
Acupera
*Honoraria*
ACGME-I, American Association of Clinical Endocrinology

**Wanda C. Lakey, MD, MHS, FACP**
*Research Grants/Contracts*
Janssen, Regeneron, Amarin, Sanofi/Aventis

**Sarah E. Mayson, MD**
*Other:* Principal Investigator, Rosetta Genomics

**Airani Sathananthan, MD, FACP**
*Research Grants/Contracts*
Principal investigator for Western University for NovoNordisk/Sanofi

**Michael H. Shanik, MD, FACP**
*Research Grants/Contracts*
NovoNordisk, AstraZeneca, Boehringer Ingelheim, Eli Lilly, Amarin
*Speakers Bureau*
NovoNordisk, AstraZeneca, Boehringer Ingelheim, Eli Lilly, Amarin
*Consultantship*
NovoNordisk, Boehringer Ingelheim, Eli Lilly, Amarin

**Scott M. Stevens, MD, FACP**
*Research Grants/Contracts*
Bristol-Myers Squibb

## Acknowledgments

The American College of Physicians (ACP) gratefully acknowledges the special contributions to the development and production of the 18th edition of the Medical Knowledge Self-Assessment Program® (MKSAP® 18) made by the following people:

*Graphic Design:* Barry Moshinski (Director, Graphic Services), Michael Ripca (Graphics Technical Administrator), and Jennifer Gropper (Graphic Designer).

*Production/Systems:* Dan Hoffmann (Director, Information Technology), Scott Hurd (Manager, Content Systems), Neil Kohl (Senior Architect), and Chris Patterson (Senior Architect).

*MKSAP 18 Digital:* Under the direction of Steven Spadt (Senior Vice President, Technology), the digital version of MKSAP 18 was developed within the ACP's Digital Products and Services Department, led by Brian Sweigard (Director, Digital Products and Services). Other members of the team included Dan Barron (Senior Web Application Developer/ Architect), Chris Forrest (Senior Software Developer/Design Lead), Kathleen Hoover (Senior Web Developer), Kara Regis (Manager, User Interface Design and Development), Brad Lord (Senior Web Application Developer), and John McKnight (Senior Web Developer).

The College also wishes to acknowledge that many other persons, too numerous to mention, have contributed to the production of this program. Without their dedicated efforts, this program would not have been possible.

## MKSAP Resource Site (mksap.acponline.org)

The MKSAP Resource Site (mksap.acponline.org) is a continually updated site that provides links to MKSAP 18 online answer sheets for print subscribers; access to MKSAP 18 Digital; Board Basics® e-book access instructions; information on Continuing Medical Education (CME), Maintenance of Certification (MOC), and international Continuing Professional Development (CPD) and MOC; errata; and other new information.

## International MOC/CPD

For information and instructions on submission of international MOC/CPD, please go to the MKSAP Resource Site (mksap.acponline.org).

## Continuing Medical Education

The American College of Physicians is accredited by the Accreditation Council for Continuing Medical Education (ACCME) to provide continuing medical education for physicians.

The American College of Physicians designates this enduring material, MKSAP 18, for a maximum of 275 *AMA PRA Category 1 Credits*™. Physicians should claim only the credit commensurate with the extent of their participation in the activity.

Up to 19 *AMA PRA Category 1 Credits*™ are available from December 31, 2018, to December 31, 2021, for the MKSAP 18 Endocrinology and Metabolism section.

## Learning Objectives

The learning objectives of MKSAP 18 are to:

- Close gaps between actual care in your practice and preferred standards of care, based on best evidence
- Diagnose disease states that are less common and sometimes overlooked and confusing
- Improve management of comorbid conditions that can complicate patient care
- Determine when to refer patients for surgery or care by subspecialists
- Pass the ABIM Certification Examination
- Pass the ABIM Maintenance of Certification Examination

## Target Audience

- General internists and primary care physicians
- Subspecialists who need to remain up to date in internal medicine
- Residents preparing for the certifying examination in internal medicine
- Physicians preparing for maintenance of certification in internal medicine (recertification)

## ABIM Maintenance of Certification

Check the MKSAP Resource Site (mksap.acponline.org) for the latest information on how MKSAP tests can be used to apply to the American Board of Internal Medicine (ABIM) for Maintenance of Certification (MOC) points following completion of the CME activity.

Successful completion of the CME activity, which includes participation in the evaluation component, enables the participant to earn up to 275 medical knowledge MOC points in the ABIM's MOC program. It is the CME activity provider's responsibility to submit participant completion information to ACCME for the purpose of granting MOC credit.

## Earn Instantaneous CME Credits or MOC Points Online

Print subscribers can enter their answers online to earn instantaneous CME credits or MOC points. You can submit your answers using online answer sheets that are provided at mksap.acponline.org, where a record of your MKSAP 18 credits will be available. To earn CME credits or to apply for

MOC points, you need to answer all of the questions in a test and earn a score of at least 50% correct (number of correct answers divided by the total number of questions). Please note that if you are applying for MOC points, you must also enter your birth date and ABIM candidate number.

Take either of the following approaches:

1. Use the printed answer sheet at the back of this book to record your answers. Go to mksap.acponline.org, access the appropriate online answer sheet, transcribe your answers, and submit your test for instantaneous CME credits or MOC points. There is no additional fee for this service.

2. Go to mksap.acponline.org, access the appropriate online answer sheet, directly enter your answers, and submit your test for instantaneous CME credits or MOC points. There is no additional fee for this service.

## Earn CME Credits or MOC Points by Mail or Fax

Pay a $20 processing fee per answer sheet and submit the printed answer sheet at the back of this book by mail or fax, as instructed on the answer sheet. Make sure you calculate your score and enter your birth date and ABIM candidate number, and fax the answer sheet to 215-351-2799 or mail the answer sheet to Member and Customer Service, American College of Physicians, 190 N. Independence Mall West, Philadelphia, PA 19106-1572, using the courtesy envelope provided in your MKSAP 18 slipcase. You will need your 10-digit order number and 8-digit ACP ID number, which are printed on your packing slip. Please allow 4 to 6 weeks for your score report to be emailed back to you. Be sure to include your email address for a response.

If you do not have a 10-digit order number and 8-digit ACP ID number, or if you need help creating a user-name and password to access the MKSAP 18 online answer sheets, go to mksap.acponline.org or email custserv@ acponline.org.

## Disclosure Policy

It is the policy of the American College of Physicians (ACP) to ensure balance, independence, objectivity, and scientific rigor in all of its educational activities. To this end, and consistent with the policies of the ACP and the Accreditation Council for Continuing Medical Education (ACCME), contributors to all ACP continuing medical education activities are required to disclose all relevant financial relationships with any entity producing, marketing, re-selling, or distributing health care goods or services consumed by, or used on, patients. Contributors are required to use generic names in the discussion of therapeutic options and are required to identify any unapproved, off-label, or

investigative use of commercial products or devices. Where a trade name is used, all available trade names for the same product type are also included. If trade-name products manufactured by companies with whom contributors have relationships are discussed, contributors are asked to provide evidence-based citations in support of the discussion. The information is reviewed by the committee responsible for producing this text. If necessary, adjustments to topics or contributors' roles in content development are made to balance the discussion. Further, all readers of this text are asked to evaluate the content for evidence of commercial bias and send any relevant comments to mksap_editors@ acponline.org so that future decisions about content and contributors can be made in light of this information.

## Resolution of Conflicts

To resolve all conflicts of interest and influences of vested interests, ACP's content planners used best evidence and updated clinical care guidelines in developing content, when such evidence and guidelines were available. All content underwent review by peer reviewers not on the committee to ensure that the material was balanced and unbiased. Contributors' disclosure information can be found with the list of contributors' names and those of ACP principal staff listed in the beginning of this book.

## Hospital-Based Medicine

For the convenience of subscribers who provide care in hospital settings, content that is specific to the hospital setting has been highlighted in blue. Hospital icons (🄷) highlight where the hospital-only content begins, continues over more than one page, and ends.

## High Value Care Key Points

Key Points in the text that relate to High Value Care concepts (that is, concepts that discuss balancing clinical benefit with costs and harms) are designated by the HVC icon [HVC].

## Educational Disclaimer

The editors and publisher of MKSAP 18 recognize that the development of new material offers many opportunities for error. Despite our best efforts, some errors may persist in print. Drug dosage schedules are, we believe, accurate and in accordance with current standards. Readers are advised, however, to ensure that the recommended dosages in MKSAP 18 concur with the information provided in the product information material. This is especially important in cases of new, infrequently used, or highly toxic drugs. Application of the information in MKSAP 18 remains the professional responsibility of the practitioner.

The primary purpose of MKSAP 18 is educational. Information presented, as well as publications, technologies, products, and/or services discussed, is intended to inform subscribers about the knowledge, techniques, and experiences of the contributors. A diversity of professional opinion exists, and the views of the contributors are their own and not those of the ACP. Inclusion of any material in the program does not constitute endorsement or recommendation by the ACP. The ACP does not warrant the safety, reliability, accuracy, completeness, or usefulness of and disclaims any and all liability for damages and claims that may result from the use of information, publications, technologies, products, and/or services discussed in this program.

## Publisher's Information

## Disclaimer Regarding Direct Purchases from Online Retailers

CME and/or MOC for MKSAP 18 is available only if you purchase the program directly from ACP. CME credits and MOC points cannot be awarded to those purchasers who have purchased the program from non-authorized sellers such as Amazon, eBay, or any other such online retailer.

## Unauthorized Use of This Book Is Against the Law

MKSAP 18 ISBN: 978-1-938245-47-3
(Endocrinology and Metabolism) ISBN: 978-1-938245-54-1

Printed in the United States of America.

For order information in the U.S. or Canada call 800-ACP-1915. All other countries call 215-351-2600 (Monday to Friday, 9 AM – 5 PM ET). Fax inquiries to 215-351-2799 or email to custserv@acponline.org.

## Errata

Errata for MKSAP 18 will be available through the MKSAP Resource Site at mksap.acponline.org as new information becomes known to the editors.

# Table of Contents

# Endocrinology and Metabolism High Value Care Recommendations

The American College of Physicians, in collaboration with multiple other organizations, is engaged in a worldwide initiative to promote the practice of High Value Care (HVC). The goals of the HVC initiative are to improve health care outcomes by providing care of proven benefit and reducing costs by avoiding unnecessary and even harmful interventions. The initiative comprises several programs that integrate the important concept of health care value (balancing clinical benefit with costs and harms) for a given intervention into a broad range of educational materials to address the needs of trainees, practicing physicians, and patients.

HVC content has been integrated into MKSAP 18 in several important ways. MKSAP 18 includes HVC-identified key points in the text, HVC-focused multiple choice questions, and, for subscribers to MKSAP Digital, an HVC custom quiz. From the text and questions, we have generated the following list of HVC recommendations that meet the definition below of high value care and bring us closer to our goal of improving patient outcomes while conserving finite resources.

**High Value Care Recommendation:** A recommendation to choose diagnostic and management strategies for patients in specific clinical situations that balance clinical benefit with cost and harms with the goal of improving patient outcomes.

Below are the High Value Care Recommendations for the Endocrinology and Metabolism section of MKSAP 18.

- Tight inpatient glycemic control is not consistently associated with improved outcomes and may increase mortality.
- The sole use of "sliding-scale insulin" is not recommended since it leads to large glucose fluctuations.
- Treatment with an ACE inhibitor or angiotensin receptor blocker is not recommended for patients with diabetes who have a normal blood pressure, a urine albumin-creatinine ratio level less than 30 mg/g, and an estimated glomerular filtration rate (eGFR) greater than 60 mL/min/1.73 m$^2$.
- In the evaluation of fasting or postprandial hypoglycemia, specimens for C-peptide, insulin, proinsulin, β-hydroxybutyrate are obtained but are not sent for analysis unless a simultaneous glucose is less than 60 mg/dL (3.3 mmol/L).
- A history of normal menses rules out hypogonadotropic hypogonadism and additional testing is not required.
- Elevated plasma renin activity in patients taking an ACE inhibitor or angiotensin receptor blocker rules out hyperaldosteronism.
- Fine-needle aspiration biopsy is generally not needed for isolated subcentimeter thyroid nodules.
- Measurement of triiodothyronine in the setting of hypothyroidism is not needed.
- In the evaluation of Hashimoto thyroiditis, measurement of thyroid perioxidase (TPO) antibody titer is not necessary unless the diagnosis is unclear.
- Thyroid function should not be assessed in hospitalized patients unless there is a strong clinical suspicion of thyroid dysfunction.
- Before making the diagnosis of subclinical hypothyroidism, transient elevation of serum thyroid-stimulating hormone should be ruled out by repeating the measurement of thyroid-stimulating hormone in 2 to 3 months (see Item 65).
- Screening men with nonspecific symptoms of hypogonadism is not recommended.
- Testosterone therapy in men without biochemical evidence of deficiency is not beneficial and may be associated with significant harms.
- Routine screening for vitamin D deficiency is not recommended in healthy populations.
- For low-risk osteoporotic women, treatment with antiresorptive therapy for 5 years is sufficient (see Item 20).
- Screening for osteoporosis in premenopausal women is not indicated in the absence of risk factors (see Item 70).

# Endocrinology and Metabolism

## Disorders of Glucose Metabolism

Hyperglycemia results from abnormal carbohydrate metabolism secondary to insulin deficiency, peripheral resistance to insulin action, or a combination of both. Hyperglycemia that exceeds the normal glucose range but does not meet the diagnostic criteria for diabetes mellitus is defined as prediabetes, which increases the risk for the development of diabetes.

## Diabetes Mellitus

### Screening for Diabetes Mellitus

Screening for type 2 diabetes mellitus in the general adult population is indicated because: (1) type 2 diabetes is often preceded by a prolonged asymptomatic hyperglycemic period in which microvascular and macrovascular damage may occur; (2) lifestyle interventions and medications have demonstrated the ability to delay or prevent onset of type 2 diabetes in persons with prediabetes, and (3) early intensive glucose control and management of hyperlipidemia and hypertension may prevent or reduce the progression of microvascular and macrovascular cardiovascular disease (CVD).

The American Diabetes Association (ADA) and the U.S. Preventive Services Task Force (USPSTF) include age, BMI, race/ethnicity, and other risk factors as part of their criteria for screening recommendations for type 2 diabetes (**Table 1**). These risk factors are associated with a high risk of incident diabetes.

Screening for type 1 diabetes is not recommended. Antibody screening in a high-risk person with a relative with type 1 diabetes should occur within the context of a clinical trial (www.diabetestrialnet.org).

### Diagnostic Criteria for Diabetes Mellitus

Diabetes mellitus can be diagnosed by an abnormal result in one of three tests: hemoglobin $A_{1c}$, fasting plasma glucose (FPG), or 2-hour plasma glucose (2-hr PG) after a 75-gram carbohydrate challenge during an oral glucose tolerance test (OGTT) (**Table 2**). An abnormal result in asymptomatic persons should be confirmed with repeat testing. A single random plasma glucose value greater than or equal to 200 mg/dL (11.1 mmol/L) in the setting of symptomatic hyperglycemia is diagnostic of diabetes.

The results of testing for diabetes differ depending on which test is done, FPG, 2-hr PG, or hemoglobin $A_{1c}$. The 2-hr PG test has a higher sensitivity for the diagnosis of diabetes compared with FPG or hemoglobin $A_{1c}$. The advantages and disadvantages of the tests must be considered when determining the best screening option for a patient (**Table 3**). ▣

### KEY POINTS

- Diabetes mellitus can be diagnosed by an abnormal result in one of the following screening tests: hemoglobin $A_{1c}$, fasting plasma glucose, or 2-hour plasma glucose after a 75-gram carbohydrate challenge during an oral glucose tolerance test.

- An abnormal result in asymptomatic persons should be confirmed with repeat testing.

### Classification of Diabetes Mellitus

The underlying insulin abnormality, whether absolute or relative insulin deficiency, peripheral insulin resistance, or an overlap of both abnormalities, is important for classifying the type of diabetes mellitus and has implications for treatment options (**Table 4**).

### Insulin Deficiency

*Type 1 Diabetes Mellitus*
Type 1 diabetes mellitus is characterized by a state of insulin deficiency secondary to the destruction of the insulin-producing beta cells in the pancreas. The destruction may be secondary to autoimmunity, idiopathic, or acquired.

*Immune-Mediated Diabetes Mellitus*
Immune-mediated type 1 diabetes mellitus (type 1A) is the underlying cause in 5% to 10% of persons newly diagnosed with diabetes. The mechanism of the beta cell destruction is multifactorial and likely due to environmental factors in persons with genetic susceptibilities. Specific human leukocyte antigen (HLA) alleles demonstrate a strong association with immune-mediated type 1 diabetes. At diagnosis, one or more autoantibodies directed at the following targets are typically present: glutamic acid decarboxylase (GAD65), tyrosine phosphatases IA-2 and IA-2β, islet cells, insulin, and zinc transporter (Zn T-8). Owing to highly automated available assays, GAD65 and IA-2 autoantibodies are recommended for initial screening. GAD65 autoantibodies have a high prevalence (70%) at the time of diagnosis and may remain detectable for years.

Immune-mediated type 1 diabetes has a variable presentation that ranges from moderate hyperglycemia to life-threatening diabetic ketoacidosis (DKA). At the time of diagnosis, approximately 90% of the functioning beta cells have been destroyed. Initiating insulin at the time of diagnosis may decrease toxicity associated with extreme hyperglycemia allowing the beta cell

**TABLE 1.** Screening Guidelines for Type 2 Diabetes Mellitus in Asymptomatic Adults

| | ADA (2018)[a] | USPSTF (2015) |
|---|---|---|
| Screening criteria | Screen overweight adults (BMI ≥25 or ≥23 in Asian Americans) with at least one additional risk factor:<br><br>First-degree relative with diabetes<br><br>High-risk race/ethnicity (black, Hispanic/Latino, American Indian, Asian, Native Hawaiian/Pacific Islander)<br><br>History of gestational diabetes mellitus<br><br>History of cardiovascular disease<br><br>Physical inactivity<br><br>Hypertension (≥140/90 or on antihypertensive therapy)<br><br>HDL cholesterol <35 mg/dL (0.90 mmol/L) and/or triglyceride >250 mg/dL (2.82 mmol/L)<br><br>Polycystic ovary syndrome<br><br>Hemoglobin $A_{1c}$ ≥5.7% (39 mmol/mol), IGT, or IFG on previous testing<br><br>Other conditions associated with insulin resistance (severe obesity, acanthosis nigricans) | Screen adults aged 40 to 70 years who are overweight or obese as part of risk assessment for cardiovascular disease.<br><br>Other risk factors:<br><br>High percentage of abdominal fat<br><br>Hyperlipidemia<br><br>Hypertension<br><br>Physical inactivity<br><br>Smoking |
| Additional screening criteria | All adults age 45 years or older | — |
| Additional screening considerations | Consider screening patients on medications known to increase the risk of diabetes, such as glucocorticoids, thiazide diuretics, HIV medications, and atypical antipsychotics. | Diabetes may occur in younger patients or at a lower BMI. Consider screening earlier if one of the following risk factors is present:<br><br>Family history of diabetes<br><br>History of gestational diabetes<br><br>Polycystic ovary syndrome<br><br>High-risk race/ethnicity (black, Hispanic/Latino, Asian American, American Indian/Alaskan Native, Native Hawaiian/Pacific Islander) |
| Screening intervals | Rescreen every 3 years if results are normal. Yearly testing recommended if prediabetes is diagnosed (hemoglobin $A_{1c}$ between 5.7% and 6.4%, IGT, IFG). | Data supporting optimal screening intervals are limited. Rescreening every 3 years may be reasonable. |

ADA = American Diabetes Association; CVD = cardiovascular disease; IFG = impaired fasting glucose; IGT = impaired glucose tolerance; USPSTF = U.S. Preventive Services Task Force.

[a]An optional ADA screening tool for diabetes risk can be found at www.diabetes.org/are-you-at-risk/diabetes-risk-test/. Accessed May 16, 2018.

Recommendations from American Diabetes Association. 2. Classification and diagnosis of diabetes: standards of medical care in diabetes-2018. Diabetes Care. 2018;41:S13-S27. [PMID: 29222373]

Recommendations from Siu AL; U S Preventive Services Task Force. Screening for abnormal blood glucose and type 2 diabetes mellitus: U.S. Preventive Services Task Force Recommendation Statement. Ann Intern Med. 2015;163:861-8. [PMID: 26501513] doi:10. 7326/M15-2345.

to regain some ability to produce insulin. Although this "honeymoon period" can last several weeks to years, insulin use should be continued to decrease stress on the remaining functioning beta cells and prolong their lifespan. Insulin deficiency requires life-long use of insulin therapy.

Patients with immune-mediated type 1 diabetes also have an increased risk for other autoimmune disorders, including celiac disease, thyroid disorders, vitiligo, and autoimmune primary adrenal gland failure.

Late autoimmune diabetes in adults (LADA) is characterized by autoantibody development leading to beta cell destruction and ultimately insulin deficiency. Individuals with LADA are typically not insulin-dependent initially and are frequently misclassified as having type 2 diabetes. There

is a slow progression toward insulin dependence over months to years after diagnosis in the setting of positive autoantibodies.

**KEY POINT**

- Autoantibodies glutamic acid decarboxylase (GAD65) and tyrosine phosphatase IA-2 demonstrate a strong association with immune-mediated type 1 diabetes and should be measured at initial diagnosis to determine etiology.

*Idiopathic Type 1 Diabetes Mellitus*

Idiopathic type 1 diabetes (type 1B) is characterized by variable insulin deficiency due to beta cell destruction without the

| TABLE 2. | Diagnostic Criteria for Diabetes Mellitus[a] | | |
|---|---|---|---|
| Test | Normal Range | Increased Risk for Diabetes (Prediabetes) | Diabetes |
| Random plasma glucose | — | — | Hyperglycemic symptoms plus a random glucose ≥200 mg/dL (11.1 mmol/L) |
| Fasting plasma glucose[b] | <100 mg/dL (5.6 mmol/L) | 100-125 mg/dL (5.6-6.9 mmol/L) | ≥126 mg/dL (7.0 mmol/L) |
| 2-Hour plasma glucose during an OGTT[c] | <140 mg/dL (7.8 mmol/L) | 140-199 mg/dL (7.8-11.0 mmol/L) | ≥200 mg/dL (11.1 mmol/L) |
| Hemoglobin A$_{1c}$[d,e] | <5.7% (39 mmol/mol) | 5.7%-6.4% (39-46 mmol/mol) | ≥6.5% (48 mmol/mol) |

OGTT = oral glucose tolerance test.

[a]In the absence of hyperglycemic symptoms, an abnormal fasting plasma glucose, OGTT, or hemoglobin A$_{1c}$ should be confirmed by repeating the same test on a separate day. If two different tests demonstrate discordant results, the American Diabetes Association recommends repeating the test with the abnormal results.

[b]Fasting for at least 8 hours.

[c]An OGTT involves the consumption of a 75-g glucose load dissolved in water.

[d]The American Diabetes Association recommends a National Glychemoglobin Standardization Program (NGSP)-certified hemoglobin A$_{1c}$ assay that is standardized to the Diabetes Control and Complication Trial (DCCT) assay.

[e]The Veterans Affairs/Department of Defense guidelines recommend confirmation of diabetes based upon an elevated hemoglobin A$_{1c}$ value of 6.5% to 6.9% with an elevated fasting plasma glucose of ≥126 mg/dL (7.0 mmol/L) due to strong evidence supporting racial differences between glycemic control and hemoglobin A$_{1c}$ values for diagnosis and treatment.

Data from American Diabetes Association. 2. Classification and diagnosis of diabetes: Standards of Medical Care in Diabetes—2018. Diabetes Care. 2018;41 (Suppl. 1):S13-S27. [PMID: 29222373]

Data from U.S. Department of Veterans Affairs/U.S. Department of Defense. VA/DoD Clinical Practice Guidelines for the management of diabetes mellitus in primary care. 2017. www.healthquality.va.gov/guidelines/cd/diabetes. Accessed May 16, 2018.

presence of autoantibodies. Individuals with idiopathic type 1 diabetes may develop episodic DKA. There is typically a strong family history of type 2 diabetes in persons with idiopathic diabetes, and it is more common in Asian and African American patients, particularly with sub-Saharan African ancestry.

### Acquired Type 1 Diabetes Mellitus

Beta cell destruction may occur from diseases affecting the pancreas or from the effect of drugs or infections (see Table 4). This may result in impaired insulin production or secretion with the subsequent development of type 1 diabetes.

## Insulin Resistance

The ineffective use of insulin by the peripheral cells to utilize glucose and fatty acids characterizes insulin resistance. Blood glucose levels remain in the normal range as long as the beta cells can increase insulin production. Hyperglycemia results from a relative insulin deficiency when the pancreas can no longer produce enough insulin. Obesity increases the risk for insulin resistance, which is also a component of the metabolic syndrome and predisposes to the development of type 2 diabetes.

### Metabolic Syndrome

Metabolic syndrome comprises a constellation of risk factors for development of type 2 diabetes and CVD, which includes abdominal obesity, impaired glucose metabolism, hyperlipidemia, and hypertension. Multiple organizations define metabolic syndrome differently (Table 5). The Endocrine Society recommends screening patients with risk factors for metabolic syndrome every 3 years to evaluate fasting plasma glucose, fasting lipid panel, blood pressure, and waist circumference. Calculation of the 10-year cardiovascular risk, using either the Framingham Risk Score or the American College of Cardiology (ACC)/American Heart Association (AHA) risk calculator, is recommended for patients with metabolic syndrome.

### Type 2 Diabetes Mellitus

Most cases of diabetes (90% to 95%) meet the criteria for type 2 diabetes. Hyperglycemia accompanied by insulin resistance and/or relative insulin deficiency defines type 2 diabetes. The extent of beta cell dysfunction determines the degree of hyperglycemia, which may worsen over time with progressive decrease in insulin production. The pathogenesis of type 2 diabetes is multifactorial with influence from both genetic and environmental factors. Type 2 diabetes is commonly present in first-degree relatives of both individuals at high risk for or diagnosed with type 2 diabetes. There is also an increased risk in several ethnicities including: Hispanic/Latino, African American, American Indian, Asian American. Additional risk factors for diabetes risk include increasing age and decreased physical activity.

Type 2 diabetes classically presents in adults, although there is an increased incidence among children and adolescents as the rate of overweight/obesity increases in these populations. Type 2 diabetes has a gradual onset with most

**TABLE 3. Comparison of Screening Tests for Diabetes Mellitus**

| Test | Advantages | Disadvantages |
|---|---|---|
| Hemoglobin $A_{1c}$ | Convenient: Does not require fasting and no restrictions on collection time<br><br>Not altered by illness, stress, etc.<br><br>Measures blood glucose concentration over the prior 8-12 weeks<br><br>Minimal biological variability<br><br>Blood sample remains stable<br><br>Standardized assay<br><br>Test accuracy is monitored<br><br>Measurement correlates with microvascular and macrovascular outcomes | Lower sensitivity for diagnosis compared with FPG or 2-hr PG<br><br>Erroneous increases or decreases in hemoglobin $A_{1c}$ result secondary to factors affecting erythrocyte survival[a]:<br>  Iron deficiency anemia<br>  Blood loss/hemolysis<br>  Kidney disease<br>  Liver disease<br>  Pregnancy<br><br>Hemoglobin variants in individuals with African, Southeast Asian, and Mediterranean heritage[b]<br><br>Higher value in black compared with non-Hispanic white persons[c]<br><br>Affected by some glucose-6-phosphate dehydrogenase variants[d]<br><br>Unavailable in some areas of the world<br><br>Expensive |
| FPG | Inexpensive<br><br>Widely available<br><br>Automated assay | Inconvenient: ≥ 8 hour fasting required and restriction on time of collection<br><br>Affected by illness and stress<br><br>Measures single point in time<br><br>High biological variability within patient<br><br>Blood sample unstable after collection<br><br>Diurnal variation<br><br>Diabetes complications not as closely linked to FPG compared with hemoglobin $A_{1c}$<br><br>Sample source (capillary, venous, or arterial blood) alters the measurement<br><br>Assay standardization incomplete |
| 2-hr PG during an OGTT | Highly sensitive to detect risk of developing diabetes<br><br>Detects early abnormalities in glucose metabolism | Similar disadvantages as FPG test<br><br>Prolonged patient preparation<br><br>Risk of hypoglycemia at 4-6 hours in normal persons<br><br>Poor reproducibility<br><br>Expensive |

2-hr PG = 2-hour prandial glucose; FPG = fasting plasma glucose; OGTT = oral glucose tolerance test.

[a]Blood glucose tests should be used instead of hemoglobin $A_{1c}$ to screen for diabetes in the setting of altered red blood cell turnover.

[b]Some methods used to measure hemoglobin $A_{1c}$ can accurately measure hemoglobin $A_{1c}$ in individuals with hemoglobin variants who are heterozygous for HbS, HbE, HbC, HbD, and increased HbF. For individuals who are homozygous for HbS, HbC, or HbSC, blood glucose should be used instead of hemoglobin $A_{1c}$ for diagnostic purposes. Blacks who are heterozygous for HbS can have a hemoglobin $A_{1c}$ 0.3% lower than individuals without the trait for any level of mean glycemia.

[c]Hemoglobin $A_{1c}$ is higher in blacks compared with non-Hispanic whites in the setting of similar FPG and postprandial glucose values. Despite this, the risk of complications associated with $A_{1c}$ remains similar in blacks and non-Hispanic white persons.

[d]There is an association between a lower hemoglobin $A_{1c}$ and hemizygous men and homozygous women with X-linked glucose-6-phosphate dehydrogenase G202A by 0.8% and 0.7%, respectively.

Data from American Diabetes Association. 2. Classification and diagnosis of diabetes: Standards of Medical Care in Diabetes—2018. Diabetes Care. 2018;41:S13-S27. [PMID: 29222373]

Data from American Diabetes Association. 6. Glycemic targets: Standards of Medical Care in Diabetes—2018. Diabetes Care. 2018;41:S55-S64. [PMID: 29222377]

Data from Sacks DB. A1C versus glucose testing: a comparison. Diabetes Care. 2011;34:518-23. [PMID: 21270207]

Data from NGSP: Harmonizing Hemoglobin A1c Testing web site. www.ngsp.org. Accessed June 2018.

Data from National Institute of Diabetes and Digestive and Kidney Diseases. Comparing tests for diabetes and prediabetes. Mar. 2014. NIH Publication No. 14-7850. www.diabetes.niddk.nih.gov. Accessed June 2018.

| TABLE 4. | Classification of Diabetes Mellitus |
|---|---|

**Insulin Deficiency[a]**

Immune-mediated (type 1A)

  Type 1 diabetes

  LADA

  Rare forms: "stiff man" syndrome, anti-insulin receptor antibodies

Idiopathic (type 1B) (seronegative)

Acquired

  Diseases of the exocrine pancreas: pancreatitis, trauma/pancreatectomy, neoplasia, cystic fibrosis, hemochromatosis, fibrocalculous pancreatopathy

  Drug-related: Vacor (rat poison), intravenous pentamidine

  Infections: congenital rubella, enteroviruses

**Insulin Resistance**

Type 2 diabetes[b]

Ketosis-prone[c]

**Other or Rare Types**

Genetic defects in beta-cell function (including six distinct MODY syndromes)

Genetic defects in insulin action

Endocrinopathies:

  Acromegaly, Cushing syndrome, glucagonoma, pheochromocytoma, hyperthyroidism[d]

  Somatostatinoma, aldosteronoma[d]

Drug-related:

  Glucocorticoids, thiazides, β-blockers, diazoxide, tacrolimus, cyclosporine, niacin, HIV protease inhibitors, atypical antipsychotics (clozapine, olanzapine)[e]

Genetic syndromes:

  Down syndrome[f]

  Wolfram syndrome (DIDMOAD)[g]

  Klinefelter, Turner, and Prader-Willi syndromes; myotonic dystrophy[d]

DIDMOAD = diabetes insipidus, diabetes mellitus, optic atrophy, and deafness; LADA = late autoimmune diabetes in adults; MODY= maturity-onset diabetes of the young.

[a]Beta-cell destruction usually leading to absolute insulin deficiency.

[b]Insulin resistance with progressive relative insulin deficiency.

[c]More common in nonwhite persons who present with diabetic ketoacidosis but become non-insulin-dependent over time.

[d]Impaired insulin action.

[e]Impaired insulin secretion, impaired insulin action, or altered hepatic glucose metabolism.

[f]Insulin deficiency, immune-mediated.

[g]Insulin deficiency.

Data from American Diabetes Association. 2. Classification and diagnosis of diabetes: Standards of Medical Care—2018. Diabetes Care. 2018;41:S13-S27. [PMID: 29222373]

affected persons remaining asymptomatic for several years. At the time of diagnosis, these patients may already have microvascular and/or macrovascular CVD. Although the beta cell does not produce sufficient insulin to overcome insulin resistance and maintain euglycemia, there is adequate insulin production to suppress lipolysis and prevent DKA in type 2 diabetes. DKA in type 2 diabetes may rarely occur in the setting of extreme stress or illness.

The development of type 2 diabetes in high-risk individuals can be delayed or prevented with modifications to lifestyle (diet, exercise), pharmacologic intervention, or metabolic surgery. The goal of these interventions is weight loss and the reduction of insulin resistance. In the Diabetes Prevention Program (DPP), lifestyle modifications reduced the incidence of type 2 diabetes in persons with prediabetes by 58%. Thus, the ADA recommends the DPP goals of 7% weight loss over 6 months and at least 150 min/week of moderate-intensity exercise to reduce the risk of diabetes development. A diet rich in monounsaturated fat, whole grains, vegetables, whole fruits, and nuts is recommended.

Several pharmacologic interventions have demonstrated efficacy in diabetes risk reduction (**Table 6**). Safety data, cost, and long-term durability of each intervention must be considered for each individual patient. Metformin reduced the incidence of diabetes by 31% compared with placebo in the DPP. In addition metformin has long-term safety data. The ADA and the American Association of Clinical Endocrinologists (AACE) recommend metformin initially for diabetes risk prevention in individuals with prediabetes, particularly in those with increasing hemoglobin $A_{1c}$ values despite lifestyle modifications who are younger than 60 years of age, are obese, or have a history of gestational diabetes.

**KEY POINTS**

- According to the Diabetes Prevention Program, lifestyle modifications, including weight loss, healthy diet, and exercise, reduced the incidence of type 2 diabetes in persons with prediabetes by 58%.

- The American Diabetes Association (ADA) and the American Association of Clinical Endocrinologists (AACE) recommend metformin initially for diabetes risk prevention in individuals with prediabetes, particularly in those with increasing hemoglobin $A_{1c}$ values despite lifestyle modifications who are younger than 60 years of age, are obese, or have a history of gestational diabetes.

**Ketosis-Prone Diabetes Mellitus**

The term "ketosis-prone diabetes" (KPD) incorporates several glycemic syndromes also known as ketosis-prone type 2 diabetes, "Flatbush diabetes," type 1B diabetes, or atypical diabetes. These syndromes present with episodic DKA resulting from insulin deficiency but have variable periods of insulin dependence and independence.

For individuals with KPD, insulin therapy for the treatment of DKA is required until DKA has resolved and the beta cells are no longer impaired by glucose toxicity, if possible, and can produce sufficient amounts of insulin to suppress

**TABLE 5.** Criteria for the Definition of Metabolic Syndrome

| Qualifying Criteria | NCEP ATP III 2005 (Meets at Least 3 of 5 Criteria) | International Diabetes Federation (2006) (Required Central Obesity and at Least 2 of 4 Remaining Criteria) |
|---|---|---|
| Waist circumference | Men ≥40 in (102 cm)<br><br>Women ≥35 in (88 cm) | Europids<br>  Men ≥37 in (94 cm)<br>  Women ≥31 in (80 cm)<br>South Asians<br>  Men ≥35 in (90 cm)[a]<br>  Women ≥31 in (80 cm)<br>Chinese<br>  Men ≥35 in (90 cm)[a]<br>  Women ≥31 in (80 cm)<br>Japanese<br>  Men ≥35 in (90 cm)[a]<br>  Women ≥31 in (80 cm)<br>South/Central Americans<br>  Men ≥35 in (90 cm)[a]<br>  Women ≥31 in (80 cm)<br>Sub-Saharan Africans<br>  Men ≥37 in (94 cm)<br>  Women ≥31 in (80 cm)<br>Eastern Mediterranean and Middle East<br>  Men ≥37 in (94 cm)<br>  Women ≥31 in (80 cm) |
| Fasting TG | ≥150 mg/dL (1.7 mmol/L) or<br>Drug therapy treating increased TG | ≥150 mg/dL (1.7 mmol/L) or<br>Drug therapy treating increased TG |
| HDL cholesterol | Men <40 mg/dL (1.0 mmol/L)<br>Women <50 mg/dL (1.3 mmol/L) or<br>Drug therapy targeting decreased HDL cholesterol | Men <40 mg/dL (1.0 mmol/L)<br>Women <50 mg/dL (1.3 mmol/L) or<br>Drug therapy targeting decreased HDL cholesterol |
| Blood pressure | Systolic ≥130 mmHg<br>Diastolic ≥85 mmHg or<br>Drug therapy for hypertension | Systolic ≥130 mmHg<br>Diastolic ≥85 mmHg or<br>Drug therapy for hypertension |
| Fasting glucose | Blood glucose ≥100 mg/dL or<br>Drug therapy for increased glucose | Blood glucose ≥100 mg/dL or<br>Drug therapy for increased glucose |

HDL = high-density lipoprotein cholesterol; NCEP ACP III = National Cholesterol Education Program - Adult Treatment Panel III; TG = triglyceride.

[a]Waist circumference is 90 cm (35 inches) according to the International Diabetes Foundation and 88 cm (35 inches) according to the NCEP ATP III.

Data from Alberti KG, Eckel RH, Grundy SM, Zimmet PZ, Cleeman JI, Donato KA, et al; International Diabetes Federation Task Force on Epidemiology and Prevention. Harmonizing the metabolic syndrome: a joint interim statement of the International Diabetes Federation Task Force on Epidemiology and Prevention; National Heart, Lung, and Blood Institute; American Heart Association; World Heart Federation; International Atherosclerosis Society; and International Association for the Study of Obesity. Circulation. 2009;120:1640-5. [PMID: 19805654]

Data from International Diabetes Federation. The IDF consensus worldwide definition of the metabolic syndrome, 2006. www.idf.org/our-activities/advocacy-awareness/resources-and-tools/60:idfconsensus-worldwide-definitionof-the-metabolic-syndrome.html. Accessed June 2018.

CONT.

lipolysis. Given the variable clinical course exhibited with KPD, uncertainty prevails regarding the need for short-term and long-term insulin treatment regimens. Four classification systems have therefore been developed to provide predictive guidance on the length of insulin therapy. A longitudinal study demonstrated greater accuracy in predicting beta-cell reserve and insulin dependence 12 months after the initial episode of DKA with the Aβ system when compared to the other classification systems, with a sensitivity of 99% and specificity of 96%. With the Aβ system, autoantibody status (A) and

**TABLE 6. Strategies to Prevent or Delay Onset of Type 2 Diabetes Mellitus**

| Intervention | Effectiveness |
|---|---|
| Diet and exercise[a] | Shown to delay onset of diabetes by up to 10-20 years |
| Smoking cessation | Modestly effective as long as it does not cause weight gain, but is always recommended |
| Bariatric surgery | Effective if used in morbidly obese persons (BMI >40) |
| Metformin[a] | Shown to delay onset of diabetes by up to 10 years |
| Lipase inhibitors (orlistat) | Shown to delay onset of diabetes up to 4 years |
| α-Glucosidase inhibitors (acarbose, voglibose) | Shown to delay onset of diabetes up to 3 years |
| Thiazolidinediones (troglitazone, rosiglitazone, pioglitazone) | Shown to delay onset of diabetes up to 3 years |
| Glucagon-like peptide 1 (GLP-1) receptor agonists (exenatide, liraglutide) | Significant weight loss and improvements in glycemic control in high-risk persons in short-term studies |
| Insulin and insulin secretagogues (sulfonylureas, meglitinides) | Ineffective |
| ACE inhibitors and angiotensin receptor blockers | Ineffective |
| Estrogen-progestin | Modest effect only |

[a]Preferred.

Data from American Diabetes Association. 5. Prevention or delay of type 2 diabetes: Standards of Medical Care in Diabetes—2018. Diabetes Care. 2018;41:S51-S54. [PMID: 29222376]

Data from Garber AJ, Abrahamson MJ, Barzilay JI, Blonde L, Bloomgarden ZT, Bush MA, et al. Consensus statement by the American Association of Clinical Endocrinologists and American College of Endocrinology on the comprehensive type 2 diabetes management algorithm—2018 Executive Summary. Endocr Pract. 2018;24:91-120. [PMID: 29368965]

CONT.

beta-cell function (β) are key determinants affecting whether an individual will require long-term insulin. Longitudinal data from KPD cohorts indicate individuals without beta-cell reserve regardless of the antibody status (A⁺β⁻ and A⁻β⁻) are more likely to have poor glycemic control and develop long-term insulin dependence after the development of DKA compared to individuals with preserved beta-cell function. H

## Gestational Diabetes Mellitus

An increase in insulin resistance during the second and third trimester of pregnancy is a normal physiologic phenomenon driven by placental hormones. With impaired beta-cell function, insulin production will be inadequate to overcome the insulin resistance with subsequent development of hyperglycemia.

Gestational diabetes is defined as hyperglycemia during the second or third trimester in women without a prepregnancy diagnosis of type 1 or type 2 diabetes. Risk factors include age over 25 years, overweight/obesity, family history of type 2 diabetes,

and high-risk racial/ethnic groups (blacks, Hispanic/Latino Americans, South or East Asians, Pacific Islanders, and American Indians). Adverse maternal and neonatal outcomes related to gestational diabetes increase with worsening hyperglycemia. Complications include macrosomia, labor and delivery complications, preeclampsia, fetal defects, neonatal hypoglycemia, spontaneous abortion, and intrauterine fetal demise.

Given the increased prevalence of undiagnosed type 2 diabetes in the general population, the ADA recommends standard screening for any pregnant woman with diabetes risk factors at the initial prenatal visit. Women with hyperglycemia identified during the first trimester are classified as having type 2 diabetes instead of gestational diabetes. For all other pregnant women without a prior diabetes diagnosis, gestational diabetes screening should occur between gestation weeks 24 and 28. The screening method recommended varies among expert groups. The "one-step" OGTT involves blood glucose measurements at baseline (fasting) and 1 and 2 hours after a 75-g oral glucose load. One abnormal value above the cut-point is diagnostic of gestational diabetes. The "two-step" OGTT involves an initial blood glucose measurement 1 hour after a 50-g OGTT. If the blood glucose is abnormal, the second step is initiated. Glucose is measured at baseline (fasting) and 1, 2, and 3 hours after a 100-g oral glucose load. Two abnormal blood glucose values after the 100-g load are diagnostic for gestational diabetes.

Most women with gestational diabetes have glucose normalization after pregnancy, but they are at an increased risk for development of recurrent gestational diabetes and type 2 diabetes. The ADA recommends a 75-g OGTT 4 to 12 weeks postpartum to confirm resolution of hyperglycemia. If the initial postpartum screen is normal, life-long screening should continue every 1 to 3 years with a 75-g OGTT, hemoglobin $A_{1c}$, or fasting plasma glucose.

## Uncommon Types of Diabetes Mellitus

Genetic defects impairing either insulin secretion or insulin action are rare forms of diabetes mellitus (see Table 4). Maturity-onset diabetes of the young (MODY) is characterized as an autosomal dominant monogenetic defect on different chromosomal loci resulting in six subtypes defined by the specific gene affected. Although insulin action remains normal in MODY, glucose sensing and insulin secretion are altered. Autoantibodies are absent. Individuals with MODY present with a clinical course that is frequently atypical of type 1 or type 2 diabetes. The onset of symptoms occurs before 25 years of age, and there is typically a strong family history of atypical diabetes in nonobese patients.

Excess hormone production associated with several endocrinopathies can also impair insulin secretion or insulin action-inducing hyperglycemia (see Table 4).

## Management of Diabetes Mellitus

Effective diabetes management is best achieved through a patient-centered approach with patients and their caregivers developing individualized goals and treatment plans compatible with patient preferences, lifestyle requirements, comorbidities, and safety. Management should also incorporate patient education, self-monitoring of blood glucose, lifestyle modifications, and pharmacologic therapies.

- Effective diabetes management requires a patient-centered approach that individualizes goals and treatment plans, taking into consideration unique characteristics of the patient and patient preferences.

## Patient Education

Diabetes self-management education and support (DSMES) provides the knowledge and skills for patients to perform diabetes-related self-care and develop effective problem-solving strategies. The ADA recommends consideration of referral for DSMES at several critical periods in care: at time of diagnosis, annually to reassess needs during care transitions, and when self-management skills are impacted by health status changes. DSMES has been shown to improve outcomes, such as hemoglobin $A_{1c}$ and quality of life, and also reduce costs, as patients are able to reduce utilization of acute care and inpatient facilities for diabetes management.

## Self-Monitoring of Blood Glucose

Self-monitoring of blood glucose (SMBG) is recommended for patients on intensive insulin regimens (multiple-dose insulin regimens or insulin pump therapy). Specific regimens for SMBG monitoring are individualized and may include prior to meals, at bedtime, before and after exercise, and before operation of machinery. SMBG may be used to detect and correct hypoglycemia. SMBG may be informative when preprandial blood glucose values are at the target goal, but the hemoglobin $A_{1c}$ is above goal. Measuring postprandial blood glucose levels may identify undetected hyperglycemia.

In motivated patients on nonintensive insulin regimens, SMBG can be considered; however, the optimal testing frequency has not been determined in these patients.

Hemoglobin $A_{1c}$ generally correlates with average 3-month blood glucose level in patients without hemoglobinopathies or increased erythrocyte turnover; therefore, treatment efficacy can be measured by combining SMBG and hemoglobin $A_{1c}$ data (**Table 7** and **Table 8**).

Another option is a continuous glucose monitoring system (CGMS), which can alert the user to retrospective and current trends of hypoglycemia and hyperglycemia. In addition, the FDA has approved a CGMS for real-time insulin dosing as well as monitoring. The goals in using a CGMS are to improve diabetes care by lowering hemoglobin $A_{1c}$ and avoiding hypoglycemia, which is critical for those with hypoglycemic unawareness. The ADA endorses CGMS use in adults (≥18 years of age) with type 1 diabetes who are not meeting glycemic targets. The Endocrine Society endorses the use of CGMS in patients with type 1 diabetes with an elevated hemoglobin $A_{1c}$ or an $A_{1c}$ level at goal when worn daily, since data

demonstrate improved glycemic control with longer duration of CGMS use. In the future, CGMS may be indicated for patients with type 2 diabetes on intensive insulin regimens as well.

- Self-monitoring of blood glucose or a continuous glucose monitoring system is recommended for patients on intensive insulin regimens (multiple-dose insulin regimens or insulin pump therapy).

## Recommended Vaccinations and Screening

Persons with diabetes should receive age-appropriate vaccinations as recommended by the Advisory Committee on Immunization Practices guidelines. Additionally, patients with diabetes should receive influenza vaccinations annually, the pneumococcal polysaccharide vaccine (PPVS23), and the series of hepatitis B vaccinations. The CDC's recommended immunization schedule can be reviewed at: https://www.cdc.gov/vaccines/schedules/hcp/imz/adult.html.

## Nonpharmacologic Approaches to Diabetes Management

Lifestyle changes are essential for the long-term management of diabetes and prevention of cardiovascular complications. While they should be individualized, diet and physical activity are critical components for patients with type 1 and type 2 diabetes.

Medical nutrition therapy with a registered dietitian provides individualized diabetes-specific education to promote healthy diet choices to achieve glycemic goals and weight management and has also been associated with reductions in hemoglobin $A_{1c}$ in patients with type 1 and type 2 diabetes. The ADA does not recommend a specific diet; however, in overweight and obese patients with type 2 diabetes, a goal of at least 5% weight loss is recommended and has been shown to improve glycemic control.

Physical activity recommendations are the same as those of the DPP program: moderate to vigorous intensity aerobic activity for 150 minutes/week, vigorous-intensity aerobic activity for 75 minutes/week, or a combination of both. This has been shown to reduce hemoglobin $A_{1c}$, decrease weight, improve a sense of wellbeing, and improve CAD risk factors. Resistance training is recommended two or more times per week. Older adults with diabetes should engage in flexibility and balance training two to three times per week, if possible. Prolonged sedentary behavior should be interrupted at 30-minute intervals with light activity or standing.

Weight loss medications or metabolic surgery are alternative options to consider if medical nutrition therapy and physical activity are unsuccessful (see MKSAP 18 General Internal Medicine). Metabolic surgery should be considered in obese persons with type 2 diabetes. Significant weight loss and improvements in glycemic control, including diabetes remission, can occur postoperatively.

Additional factors to consider and address in patients with diabetes mellitus include anxiety, depression, and

| State of Health | Characteristics of Patients | Hemoglobin $A_{1c}$[a] | Preprandial Capillary Glucose | Postprandial Capillary Glucose (1-2 Hours After Meal)[c] | Bedtime Capillary Glucose |
|---|---|---|---|---|---|
| | **TABLE 7.** American Diabetes Association Recommended Outpatient Glycemic Goals for Adults with Diabetes Mellitus | | | | |
| Healthy | Early in disease course | <7.0% | 80-130 mg/dL | <180 mg/dL[c] | |
| | Few comorbidities | <6.5% for select patients[b] | (4.4-7.2 mmol/L) | (10.0 mmol/L) | |
| | Preconception | | | | |
| | Patient preference | | | | |
| | Life expectancy >10 years | | | | |
| Complex health issues | Significant comorbidities including advanced atherosclerosis or microvascular complications | <8.0% | | | |
| | Longer duration of diabetes with difficulty achieving glycemic goals despite appropriate management | | | | |
| | Frequent hypoglycemia | | | | |
| | Hypoglycemia unawareness | | | | |
| | Life expectancy <10 years | | | | |
| Older adults | Healthy | <7.5% | 90-130 mg/dL (5.0-7.2 mmol/L) | | 90-150 mg/dL (5.0-8.3 mmol/L) |
| | Few comorbidities | | | | |
| | Extended life expectancy | | | | |
| | No impairment of cognition or function | | | | |
| | Complex/Intermediate | <8.0% | 90-150 mg/dL (5.0-8.3 mmol/L) | | 100-180 mg/dL (5.6-10.0 mmol/L) |
| | Multiple comorbidities | | | | |
| | Hypoglycemia risk | | | | |
| | Fall risk | | | | |
| | Multiple instrumental ADL impairments | | | | |
| | Mild-to-moderate impairment in cognition | | | | |
| | Very complex/poor health | <8.5% | 100-180 mg/dL (5.6-10.0 mmol/L) | | 110-200 mg/dL (6.1-11.1 mmol/L) |
| | Chronic comorbidities with end-stage disease | | | | |
| | Long-term care placement | | | | |
| | Moderate-to-severe impairment in cognition | | | | |
| | Multiple ADL dependencies | | | | |
| | Limited life expectancy | | | | |
| Pregnant women[d] | Preexisting type 1 diabetes, preexisting type 2 diabetes, or gestational diabetes | 6.0-6.5% without severe hypoglycemia[e] (<6.0% may be optimal as pregnancy progresses) | Fasting ≤95 mg/dL (5.3 mmol/L) | 1-hour postprandial ≤140 mg/dL (7.8 mmol/L) or 2-hour postprandial ≤120 mg/dL (6.7 mmol/L) | |

ADL = activities of daily living.

[a]Recommended if goal can be met without severe recurrent hypoglycemia. If severe recurrent hypoglycemia is present, there is no recommended hemoglobin $A_{1c}$ goal, as modification of the patient's diabetes regimen to resolve severe recurrent hypoglycemia should take precedence. When severe recurrent hypoglycemia has resolved, a hemoglobin $A_{1c}$ goal can be chosen, and treatment decisions can again be made based on that individualized goal without frequent hypoglycemia. Hemoglobin $A_{1c}$ should be measured at diagnosis followed by 3-month intervals as changes to lifestyle modifications and/or pharmacologic therapies occur. Hemoglobin $A_{1c}$ measurements can be reduced to every 6 months once glycemic targets are achieved.

[b]This can be considered for patients with an early diagnosis of diabetes mellitus, no significant cardiovascular disease, long life expectancy, or managed with lifestyle modifications or metformin.

[c]When the hemoglobin $A_{1c}$ is not at goal despite meeting preprandial glucose goals, the postprandial glucose values should be targeted. Elevated postprandial glucose values have a greater impact on $A_{1c}$ values near 7%.

[d]Both preprandial and postprandial glucose monitoring are recommended in pregnant women.

[e]Preprandial and postprandial glucose measurements should be the primary evaluation of glycemic control, as hemoglobin $A_{1c}$ values decrease with increased red blood cell turnover associated with pregnancy.

Recommendations from American Diabetes Association. 6. Glycemic targets: Standards of Medical Care in Diabetes—2018. Diabetes Care. 2018;41(Suppl. 1):S55-S64. [PMID: 29222377]

Recommendations from American Diabetes Association. 11. Older adults: Standards of Medical Care in Diabetes—2018. Diabetes Care. 2018;41(Suppl. 1):S119-S125. [PMID: 29222382]

Recommendations from American Diabetes Association. 13. Management of diabetes in pregnancy: Standards of Medical Care in Diabetes—2018. Diabetes Care. 2018;41:S137-S143. [PMID: 29222384]

**TABLE 8.** Comparison of Hemoglobin A₁c Value and Estimated Plasma Glucose Level

| Hemoglobin A$_{1c}$ | Estimated Average Plasma Glucose Level | Estimated Average Plasma Glucose Level |
|---|---|---|
| (%) | mg/dL (95% CI) | mmol/L (95% CI) |
| 6 | 126 (100-152) | 7.0 (5.5-8.5) |
| 7 | 154 (123-185) | 8.6 (6.8-10.3) |
| 8 | 183 (147-217) | 10.2 (8.1-12.1) |
| 9 | 212 (170-249) | 11.8 (9.4-13.9) |
| 10 | 240 (193-282) | 13.4 (10.7-15.7) |
| 11 | 269 (217-314) | 14.9 (12.0-17.5) |
| 12 | 298 (240-347) | 16.5 (13.3-19.3) |

Data from American Diabetes Association. 6. Glycemic targets: Standards of Medical Care in Diabetes—2018. Diabetes Care. 2018;41:S55-S64. [PMID: 29222377]

diabetes-related distress. Screening for psychosocial issues and behavioral health conditions should occur at the time of diabetes diagnosis and periodically. These conditions can adversely affect glycemic control directly and through challenges with patient adherence to management plans.

**Pharmacologic Therapy**

Pharmacologic therapy should be individualized taking into consideration a person's age, state of health, weight, the pathophysiology of his/her hyperglycemia, specific risks/benefits of a potential therapeutic agent, medication cost, and the person's lifestyle and personal treatment goals. The hemoglobin A$_{1c}$ goals are generally not stringent in patients with significant comorbid conditions, macrovascular CVD, short life expectancy, long duration of diabetes, limited resources and social support, low health literacy/numeracy, nonadherence, and at high risk for complications from hypoglycemia. Most clinical practice guidelines, including the ADA, recommend target hemoglobin A$_{1c}$ thresholds based on a patient's state of health (see Table 7). In contrast, the VA/DoD guidelines for the management of type 2 diabetes recommend a hemoglobin A$_{1c}$ target range instead of a target threshold. The VA/DoD guidelines attempt to avoid intensification of pharmacologic therapy based solely upon marginal changes in hemoglobin A$_{1c}$ caused by known patient characteristics and laboratory limitations that could potentially cause greater harm than benefit in individuals with major comorbidities, microvascular complications, or advancing age.

The American College of Physicians (ACP) recommends a hemoglobin A$_{1c}$ level between 7% and 8% in most patients with type 2 diabetes, and clinicians should consider deintensifying pharmacologic therapy in patients who achieve hemoglobin A$_{1c}$ levels less than 6.5%. The rationale for these targets is based on evidence that collectively shows treating to targets of less than 7% compared with targets around 8% did not reduce death or macrovascular events over about 5 to 10 years of treatment but did result in substantial harms. More stringent

targets may be appropriate for patients who have a long life expectancy (>15 years) and are interested in more intensive glycemic control with pharmacologic therapy despite the risk for harms, including but not limited to hypoglycemia, patient burden, and pharmacologic costs. ACP also recommends avoiding targeting an hemoglobin A$_{1c}$ level in patients with a life expectancy less than 10 years due to advanced age (80 years or older), residence in a nursing home, or chronic medical conditions because the harms outweigh the benefits in this population.

Several landmark studies provide guidance on glycemic goals and CVD risk reduction. Intensive glycemic control compared with standard control significantly reduces the incidence and progression of microvascular complications in patients with type 1 and type 2 diabetes, as demonstrated by the Diabetes Control and Complications Trial (DCCT) and the UK Prospective Diabetes Study (UKPDS). Long-term follow-up demonstrated continued reductions in microvascular complications despite convergence in glycemic control between the study arms. Action to Control Cardiovascular Risk in Diabetes (ACCORD), Action in Diabetes and Vascular Disease: Preterax and Diamicron MR Controlled Evaluation (ADVANCE), and the Veterans Affairs Diabetes Trial (VADT) further reinforced the association of reduced microvascular complications with tight glycemic control, but also highlighted that patients and providers must balance the risks/benefits of a labor-intensive regimen with the potential morbidity and mortality in specific populations.

Long-term follow-up evaluation of participants in the intensive insulin arms of the DCCT and UKPDS trials who were early in the course of diabetes demonstrated a significant reduction in CVD and mortality. In contrast, ACCORD, ADVANCE, and VADT evaluated tight glycemic control in older persons with more advanced type 2 diabetes and preexisting CVD or CVD risk factors. CVD was not significantly reduced in the ACCORD and ADVANCE trials. VADT demonstrated a significant reduction in cardiovascular events, but no change in cardiovascular or overall mortality.

Recently, the EMPA-REG Outcome trial, a randomized controlled trial (RCT), found that in patients with established CVD, empagliflozin, a sodium-glucose cotransporter 2 (SGLT2) inhibitor, reduced the composite outcome (cardiovascular death, nonfatal myocardial infarction, or nonfatal stroke); it was primarily driven by a significant relative risk reduction in rates of cardiovascular death by 38%. There was also a significant reduction in all-cause mortality by 32% and hospitalization for heart failure by 35%. As a result of this trial, empagliflozin received FDA approval for reduction of cardiovascular death in adults with type 2 diabetes and CVD. Another SGLT2 inhibitor, canagliflozin, also demonstrated a reduction in cardiovascular events, but not cardiovascular death, in patients with type 2 diabetes at high risk for cardiovascular disease when compared to placebo in the CANVAS (Canagliflozin Cardiovascular Assessment Study) Program.

The Liraglutide Effect and Action in Diabetes: Evaluation of Cardiovascular Outcome Results (LEADER) RCT included subjects at risk for CVD and found that liraglutide, a glucagon-like peptide 1 (GLP-1) analogue, significantly reduced the primary composite outcome (cardiovascular death, nonfatal MI, or nonfatal stroke) by 13% compared with placebo (relative risk reduction). Liraglutide also significantly reduced cardiovascular death (22%) and all-cause mortality (15%) relative to placebo. Based on the LEADER data, the FDA approved liraglutide for the reduction of major cardiovascular events and cardiovascular deaths in adults with type 2 diabetes and CVD. ⊞

**KEY POINT**

HVC • Pharmacologic therapy should be individualized taking into consideration a person's age, state of health, weight, the pathophysiology of his/her hyperglycemia, specific risks/benefits of a potential therapeutic agent, medication cost, and the person's lifestyle and personal treatment goals.

*Therapy for Type 1 Diabetes Mellitus*
Due to destruction of the beta cells and subsequent insulin deficiency, life-long insulin therapy is required for persons with type 1 diabetes mellitus. Ideally, an intensive insulin regimen should be prescribed, which includes multiple daily doses of insulin (MDI) to mimic the physiologic action of the pancreas. The insulin regimen should include basal coverage to maintain glycemic control while fasting and between meals, prandial coverage, and supplemental insulin for correction of hyperglycemia. This can be accomplished with subcutaneous insulin injections, inhaled insulin preparations, or continuous subcutaneous insulin infusions (CSII) with an insulin pump.

Initial total daily insulin dosing ranges from 0.4 to 1.0 U/kg/day in patients with type 1 diabetes. Basal insulin typically encompasses approximately 50% of the total daily dose of insulin, with prandial insulin covering the remaining 50%. The available insulin formulations and their activity profiles are summarized in **Table 9**.

The timing and mode of prandial insulin delivery varies based on patient needs/preferences and dietary habits. MDI prandial dosing can be accomplished with fixed-dosing, carbohydrate counting, or modified carbohydrate counting. In general, 1 unit of insulin covers 10 to 20 grams of carbohydrates consumed. A modified carbohydrate counting method can be used when the grams of carbohydrates consumed cannot be accurately counted. With this method, regular or analogue insulin doses can be adjusted by 50% based on the portion of food consumed. For example, the dose for the size of the meal would be as follows: small (50%), regular (100%), large (150%). MDI should also incorporate supplemental insulin to correct hyperglycemia. A common method to calculate the correction dose of insulin is to give an additional 1 unit of regular or analogue insulin at the time of the premeal measurement for every glucose value 50 mg/dL (2.8 mmol/L) above the target glucose value in insulin-sensitive individuals and

| TABLE 9. Pharmacokinetic Properties of Insulin Products[a] | | | |
|---|---|---|---|
| **Insulin Type** | **Onset** | **Peak** | **Duration** |
| Rapid-acting analogues | | | |
| Lispro, aspart, glulisine | 5-15 min | 45-90 min | 2-4 h |
| Inhaled insulin | 5-15 min | 50 min | 2-3 h |
| Concentrated rapid-acting analogue | | | |
| Lispro (200 U/mL) | 5-15 min | 45-90 min | 2-4 h |
| Short-acting | | | |
| Human regular | 0.5 h | 2-5 h | 4-8 h |
| Intermediate-acting | | | |
| NPH insulin | 1-3 h | 4-10 h | 10-18 h |
| Concentrated human regular | | | |
| Human regular U-500 (500 U/mL) | 0.5 h | 2-5 h | 13-24 h |
| Long-acting basal analogues | | | |
| Detemir | 1-2 h | None[b] | 12-24 h[c] |
| Glargine | 2-3 h | None[b] | 20-24+ h |
| Degludec | 1-3 h | None | 24-42 h |
| Concentrated basal analogue (ultra long-acting) | | | |
| Glargine (300 U/mL) | 6 h | None | 24-36 h |
| Degludec (200 U/mL) | 1-3 h | None | 24-42 h |
| Premixed insulins[d] | | | |
| 70% NPH/30% regular | 0.5-1 h | 2-10 h | 10-18 h |
| 75% NPL/25% lispro | 10-20 min | 1-6 h | 10-18 h |
| 50% NPL/50% lispro | 10-20 min | 1-6 h | 10-18 h |
| 70% NPA/30% aspart | 10-20 min | 1-6 h | 10-18 h |
| 70% degludec/30% aspart | 10-30 min | 0.5-2 h | 24+ h |

NPA = neutral protamine aspart; NPH = neutral protamine Hagedorn; NPL = neutral protamine lispro.

[a]The time course of each insulin varies significantly between persons and within the same person on different days. Therefore, the time periods listed should be considered general guidelines only.

[b]Both detemir insulin and glargine insulin can produce a peak effect in some persons, especially at higher doses.

[c]The duration of action for detemir insulin varies depending on the dose given.

[d]Premixed insulins containing a larger proportion of rapid- or short-acting insulin tend to have larger peaks occurring at an earlier time than mixtures containing smaller proportions of rapid- and short-acting insulin.

1 unit for every 25 mg/dL (1.4 mmol/L) in insulin-resistant individuals. The supplemental insulin can be given with the prandial insulin in one injection. For example, an additional 3 units of insulin would be given with the prandial insulin if the target glucose was 120 mg/dL (6.7 mmol/L) and the current glucose was 270 mg/dL (15.0 mmol/L) in someone with type 1 diabetes.

CONT.

Premixed insulin formulations combine intermediate-acting or long-acting basal insulin and rapid-acting or short-acting insulin in fixed concentrations. These formulations are typically administered twice daily and should be considered for those who are unable or unwilling to perform more frequent daily insulin injections. Premixed formulations can increase glycemic excursions, including hypoglycemia, since this is a nonphysiologic regimen.

Inhaled insulin is a rapid-acting formulation for prandial dosing. The availability of inhaled insulin in cartridges with preset doses of insulin (4, 8, and 12 units) limits the flexibility of insulin dosing. Pulmonary function should be assessed at baseline and monitored because lung function may decline with use of inhaled insulin.

CSII provides continuous delivery of basal insulin and uses a bolus calculator programmed to achieve individual glycemic goals to calculate prandial and bolus correction doses. The Endocrine Society recommends CSII over MDI for all adults with type 1 diabetes who have not attained their hemoglobin $A_{1c}$ goal and for those who have attained their $A_{1c}$ goal but have large glycemic variability, severe hypoglycemia, or hypoglycemia unawareness. Additional considerations include a need for flexibility in insulin delivery, early morning hyperglycemia ("dawn phenomenon"), active lifestyle, or patient preference. There are CSII systems that will decrease or stop delivery of insulin if glucose levels fall below a threshold value that is set within the CSII system and will increase delivery if glucose levels are above a threshold value. Insulin delivery will be reinitiated or increased/decreased back to baseline when the threshold is no longer met.

Hypoglycemia and weight gain are risks associated with insulin use. The risk of hypoglycemia is lower with analogue insulin compared with regular insulin due to a shorter duration of action. Hypoglycemia caused by insulin stacking occurs when insulin dosing is too frequent and overlaps with the duration of action of a prior insulin injection. This can be avoided by allowing at least 3 to 4 hours between sequential injections of analogue insulin.

An adjunctive therapy approved for use with insulin in type 1 diabetes is pramlintide, an amylin analogue. Pramlintide can lead to improved glycemic control, decreased insulin doses, and weight loss through delayed gastric emptying, increased satiety, and decreased glucagon secretion.

**KEY POINTS**

- Life-long insulin therapy is required for persons with type 1 diabetes mellitus.
- The Endocrine Society recommends continuous subcutaneous insulin infusions over multiple daily doses of insulin for all adults with type 1 diabetes who have not attained their hemoglobin $A_{1c}$ goal and for those who have attained their $A_{1c}$ goal but have large glycemic variability, severe hypoglycemia, or hypoglycemia unawareness.

*Therapy for Type 2 Diabetes Mellitus*

As beta cell function declines, pharmacologic therapies must often be combined with lifestyle modifications to obtain glycemic control. Therapeutic options may include monotherapy or a combination of oral agents with injectable agents (**Table 10**).

The ADA recommends initiation of monotherapy if the $A_{1c}$ is less than 8% at the time of diagnosis. Metformin is the recommended first-line oral agent for newly diagnosed type 2 diabetes due to known effectiveness and low hypoglycemia risk. Gastrointestinal side effects of metformin are common and may be reduced by slow titration of doses, administration with food, and/or use of an extended release formulation. Lactic acidosis is a rare, potential risk associated with metformin use. Heart failure requiring pharmacologic treatment and hepatic dysfunction may increase the risk. An estimated glomerular filtration rate (eGFR) greater than 45 mL/min/ 1.73 $m^2$ is recommended for metformin initiation to avoid potential lactic acidosis with kidney dysfunction. Clinicians should assess benefits and risks of continuing therapy in patients whose eGFR falls below 45 mL/min/1.73 $m^2$ during therapy. Metformin is contraindicated at eGFR less than 30 mL/min/1.73 $m^2$.

If an iodinated contrast agent is administered with an eGFR between 30 and 60 mL/min/1.73 $m^2$, metformin should be held until kidney function is stable for 48 hours. Metformin should also be held in situations that may induce dehydration, such as vomiting or diarrhea. A reduction in vitamin $B_{12}$ intestinal absorption occurs in up to 30% of patients on metformin whereas 5% to 10% develop vitamin $B_{12}$ deficiency. Periodic monitoring may be warranted, particularly in the setting of anemia or peripheral neuropathy.

Glycemic control should be assessed every 3 months with adjustments to therapy until the glycemic target is achieved, and every 6 months if at goal. There are limited data on comparative effectiveness to guide the addition of additional agents when glycemic goals are not met with metformin and lifestyle modifications; thus, many guidelines are based on expert opinion. If the hemoglobin $A_{1c}$ level is 9% or higher at the time of diagnosis or after 3 months of metformin therapy, the ADA recommends advancing to dual therapy defined as metformin combined with another therapeutic agent (see Table 9 and Table 10). For individuals with CVD, therapeutic agents that have been shown to reduce major adverse cardiovascular events (canagliflozin, empagliflozin, and liraglutide) and cardiovascular mortality (empagliflozin and liraglutide) should be considered for dual therapy. AACE/ACE recommends initiation of metformin if the hemoglobin $A_{1c}$ level is less than 7.5% at diagnosis.

Dual therapy should be initiated if the hemoglobin $A_{1c}$ level is 7.5% or higher at diagnosis or after 3 months of monotherapy. The ADA and AACE/ACE both recommend advancement to triple therapy if dual therapy fails to meet glycemic goals after 3 months. Triple therapy should be advanced to combination injectable therapy if glycemic goals are still

**TABLE 10.** Pharmacologic Agents Used to Lower Blood Glucose Levels in Type 2 Diabetes Mellitus[a,b]

| Class | Mechanism of Action | Effect on Weight | Disadvantages | Long-Term Studies on Definitive Outcomes |
|---|---|---|---|---|
| Insulin | Decreases hepatic glucose production<br><br>Increases peripheral glucose uptake<br><br>Suppresses ketogenesis | Increase | Hypoglycemia, weight gain, training required, injectable forms, pulmonary toxicity with inhaled insulin | Decrease in microvascular events (UKPDS)[c,d] |
| Sulfonylureas (tolbutamide, chlorpropamide, glipizide, glyburide, gliclazide, glimepiride) | Stimulates insulin secretion | Increase | Hypoglycemia (especially in drugs with long half-lives or in older populations); weight gain; lacks glucose-lowering durability | Decrease in microvascular events (UKPDS)[c]; possible increase in CVD events |
| Biguanides (metformin) | Decreases hepatic glucose production<br><br>Increases insulin-mediated uptake of glucose in muscles | Neutral | Diarrhea and abdominal discomfort, vitamin $B_{12}$ deficiency, lactic acidosis (rare).<br><br>Contraindicated with progressive liver, kidney, or cardiac failure. | Decrease in CVD events (UKPDS)[d] |
| α-Glucosidase inhibitors (acarbose, miglitol) | Inhibits polysaccharide absorption | Neutral | Flatulence, abdominal discomfort | Possible decrease in CVD events in prediabetes (STOP-NIDDM)[e] |
| Thiazolidinediones (rosiglitazone, pioglitazone) | Increases peripheral uptake of glucose | Increase | Fluid retention, heart failure, edema, fractures, possible increased risk of bladder cancer with pioglitazone | Possible decrease in CVD events with pioglitazone (PROactive)[f] |
| Meglitinides (repaglinide, nateglinide) | Stimulates insulin release | Increase | Hypoglycemia, weight gain, frequent dosing | None |
| Amylin mimetic (pramlintide) | Slows gastric emptying<br><br>Suppresses glucagon secretion<br><br>Increases satiety | Decrease | Nausea, vomiting, exacerbates gastroparesis, increased hypoglycemia risk with concomitant use of insulin, training required, injectable, frequent dosing | None |
| GLP-1 receptor agonists (exenatide, exenatide extended release, liraglutide, albiglutide, lixisenatide, dulaglutide, semaglutide) | Glucose-dependent increase in insulin secretion<br><br>Slows gastric emptying<br><br>Glucose-dependent suppression of glucagon secretion<br><br>Increases satiety | Decrease | Hypoglycemia when used in combination with sulfonylureas, nausea, vomiting, diarrhea, exacerbates gastroparesis, increased heart rate, possible pancreatitis, animal studies demonstrate C-cell hyperplasia and medullary thyroid tumors, training required, injectable | Decrease in CVD events and mortality in high-risk individuals with type 2 diabetes with liraglutide (LEADER)[g] |
| DPP-4 inhibitors (sitagliptin, saxagliptin, linagliptin, alogliptin) | Glucose-dependent increase in insulin secretion<br><br>Glucose-dependent suppression of glucagon secretion | Neutral | Hypoglycemia when used in combination with sulfonylureas, increased risk of infections, possible increased risk of pancreatitis, dermatologic reactions, requires dose adjustments for decreasing kidney function except for linagliptin | Increased heart failure hospitalizations [saxagliptin (SAVOR-TIMI 53)][h] |

*(Continued on the next page)*

**TABLE 10.** Pharmacologic Agents Used to Lower Blood Glucose Levels in Type 2 Diabetes Mellitus[a,b] *(Continued)*

| Class | Mechanism of Action | Effect on Weight | Disadvantages | Long-Term Studies on Definitive Outcomes |
|---|---|---|---|---|
| SGLT2 inhibitors (canagliflozin, dapagliflozin, empagliflozin, ertugliflozin) | Increases kidney excretion of glucose | Decrease | Hypoglycemia with insulin secretagogues, dehydration/hypotension, acute kidney injury (canagliflozin, dapagliflozin), hypersensitivity reactions, increased candida infections and urinary tract infections, "euglycemic" DKA, possible increase in amputations (canagliflozin), hyperkalemia (canagliflozin), fractures (canagliflozin), bladder cancer (dapagliflozin) | Decrease in CVD events and mortality in high-risk individuals with type 2 diabetes with empagliflozin (EMPA-REG OUTCOME)[i]<br><br>Decreases incident or worsening nephropathy in high CVD risk individuals with type 2 diabetes (EMPA-REG OUTCOME)[i]<br><br>Decrease in CVD events in high-risk individuals with type 2 diabetes with canagliflozin (CANVAS Program)[j] |
| Bile acid sequestrants (colesevelam) | Incompletely understood:<br><br>Possible decrease in hepatic glucose production<br><br>Possible increase in incretin levels | Neutral | Constipation, dyspepsia, increased triglycerides, possible interference with absorption of other medications | None |
| Dopamine-2 agonists (bromocriptine quick release) | Increases insulin sensitivity<br><br>Alters metabolism via hypothalamus | Neutral | Nausea, orthostasis, fatigue | Possible decrease in CVD events (Cycloset Safety Trial)[k] |

CVD = cardiovascular disease; DKA = diabetic ketoacidosis; DPP-4 = dipeptidyl peptidase-4; GLP-1 = glucagon-like peptide-1; SGLT2 = sodium-glucose cotransporter-2.

[a]Data from American Diabetes Association. 8. Pharmacologic approaches to glycemic treatment: Standards of Medical Care in Diabetes—2018. Diabetes Care. 2018;419Suppl. 1):S73-S85. [PMID: 29222379 ]

[b]Recommendations from Garber AJ, Abrahamson MJ, Barzilay JI, Blonde L, Bloomgarden ZT, Bush MA, et al; American Association of Clinical Endocrinologists (AACE). Consensus Statement by the American Association of Clinical Endocrinologists and American College of Endocrinology on the Comprehensive Type 2 Diabetes Management Algorithm—2018 Executive Summary. Endocr Pract. 2018;24:91-120. [PMID: 29368965]

[c]Data from Intensive blood-glucose control with sulfonylureas or insulin compared with conventional treatment and risk of complications in patients with type 2 diabetes (UKPDS 33). UK Prospective Diabetes Study (UKPDS) Group. Lancet. 1998;352:837-53. [PMID: 9742976]

[d]Data from Effect of intensive blood-glucose control with metformin on complications in overweight patients with type 2 diabetes (UKPDS 34). UK Prospective Diabetes Study (UKPDS) Group. Lancet. 1998;352:854-65. [PMID: 9742977]

[e]Data from Chiasson JL, Josse RG, Gomis R, Hanefeld M, Karasik A, Laakso M; STOP-NIDDM Trial Research Group. Acarbose treatment and the risk of cardiovascular disease and hypertension in patients with impaired glucose tolerance: the STOP-NIDDM trial. JAMA. 2003;290:486-94. [PMID: 12876091]

[f]Data from Dormandy JA, Charbonnel B, Eckland DJ, Erdmann E, Massi-Benedetti M, Moules IK, et al; PROactive Investigators. Secondary prevention of macrovascular events in patients with type 2 diabetes in the PROactive Study (PROspective pioglitAzone Clinical Trial In macroVascular Events): a randomised controlled trial. Lancet. 2005;366:1279-89. [PMID: 16214598]

[g]Data from Marso SP, Daniels GH, Brown-Frandsen K, Kristensen P, Mann JF, Nauck MA, et al; LEADER Steering Committee. Liraglutide and cardiovascular outcomes in type 2 diabetes. N Engl J Med. 2016;375:311-22. [PMID: 27295427]

[h]Data from Scirica BM, Bhatt DL, Braunwald E, Steg PG, Davidson J, Hirshberg B, et al; SAVOR-TIMI 53 Steering Committee and Investigators. Saxagliptin and cardiovascular outcomes in patients with type 2 diabetes mellitus. N Engl J Med. 2013;369:1317-26. [PMID: 23992601]

[i]Data from Zinman B, Wanner C, Lachin JM, Fitchett D, Bluhmki E, Hantel S, et al; EMPA-REG OUTCOME investigators. Empagliflozin, cardiovascular outcomes, and mortality in type 2 diabetes. N Engl J Med. 2015;373:2117-28. [PMID: 26378978]

[j]Data from Neal B, Perkovic V, Mahaffey KW, de Zeeuw D, Fulcher G, Erondu N, et al; CANVAS Program Collaborative Group. Canagliflozin and cardiovascular and renal events in type 2 diabetes. N Engl J Med. 2017;377:644-657. [PMID: 28605608]i

[k]Data from Gaziano JM, Cincotta AH, O'Connor CM, Ezrokhi M, Rutty D, Ma ZJ, et al. Randomized clinical trial of quick-release bromocriptine among patients with type 2 diabetes on overall safety and cardiovascular outcomes. Diabetes Care. 2010;33:1503-8. [PMID: 20332352]

unmet. This includes continued metformin and initiation of a GLP-1 receptor agonist or basal insulin if not already prescribed, initiation of basal insulin on background GLP-1 receptor agonist therapy, or initiation of a GLP-1 receptor agonist or prandial insulin on optimized background basal insulin.

Algorithms from the ADA and AACE/ACE provide guidance on initiation and dosing of basal and prandial insulin

regimens (**Table 11**). The ADA recommends combination injectable therapy initially in the setting of symptomatic hyperglycemia (polydipsia, polyuria), hemoglobin $A_{1c}$ 10% or higher, or a glucose level of 300 mg/dL (16.6 mmol/L) or higher.

AACE/ACE recommends initiating insulin therapy with other agents if the initial hemoglobin $A_{1c}$ is more than 9% in a

**TABLE 11.** Comparison of Insulin Dosing Algorithms from the ADA and AACE/ACE

| Insulin Initiation or Modification | ADA | AACE/ACE |
|---|---|---|
| Basal insulin | Starting dose:<br><br>10 U/d or 0.1-0.2 U/kg/d | Starting dose:<br><br>If A$_{1c}$ <8%: 0.1-0.2 U/kg/d<br><br>If A$_{1c}$ >8%: 0.2-0.3 U/kg/d |
| Basal insulin dose titration | For hyperglycemia:<br><br>Increase dose 1-2 times/week until glycemic goal met<br><br>Increase dose by:<br><br>10%-15% or 2-4 U | For hyperglycemia:<br><br>Increase dose every 2-3 days until glycemic goal met<br><br>Increase dose by:<br><br>2 U or<br><br>20% if FBG >180 mg/dL (10 mmol/L)<br><br>10% if FBG 140-180 mg/dL (7.8-9.9 mmol/L)<br><br>1 U if FBG is 110-139 mg/dL (6.1-7.7 mmol/L) |
| | For hypoglycemia:<br><br>Decrease dose by: 10%-20% or 4 U | For hypoglycemia:<br><br>Decrease dose by:<br><br>10%-20% if FBG <70 mg/dL (3/9 mmol/L)<br><br>20%-40% if FBG <40 mg/dL (2.2 mmol/L) |
| Prandial insulin plus basal insulin<br><br>(1 meal) | Initiate prandial insulin at largest meal<br><br>Starting dose:<br><br>4 U, 10% of basal dose, or 0.1 U/kg<br><br>To avoid hypoglycemia, consider decreasing basal dose by same amount if A$_{1c}$ <8%. | Initiate prandial insulin at largest meal<br><br>Starting dose:<br><br>5 U or 10% of basal dose |
| Basal-bolus insulin regimen<br><br>(≥ 2 or more meals) | Prandial insulin starting dose:<br><br>4 U, 10% of basal dose, or 0.1 U/kg/meal<br><br>To avoid hypoglycemia, consider decreasing basal dose by same amount if A$_{1c}$ <8%. | Prandial insulin starting dose:<br><br>0.3-0.5 U/kg = TDD<br><br>50% of TDD = basal insulin<br><br>50% of TDD = prandial insulin<br><br>Each meal-time dose = 1/3 prandial insulin dose |
| Prandial insulin dose titration | For hyperglycemia:<br><br>Increase dose 1-2 days/week until glycemic goal met<br><br>Increase dose by:<br><br>10%-15% or 1-2 U<br><br>If hyperglycemia persists at other meals, add additional meal-time insulin doses (basal-bolus) | For hyperglycemia:<br><br>Increase dose every 2-3 days until glycemic goal met<br><br>Increase dose by:<br><br>10% or 1-2 U if BG >140 mg/dL (7.8 mmol/L) 2 hours after meal or at next meal.<br><br>If hyperglycemia persists at other meals, add additional meal-time insulin doses (basal-bolus). |
| | For hypoglycemia:<br><br>Decrease dose by:<br><br>10%-20% or 2-4 U | For hypoglycemia:<br><br>Decrease TDD dose (basal and/or prandial) by:<br><br>10%-20% if BG <70 mg/dL (3.9 mmol/L)<br><br>20%-40% if BG <40 mg/dL (2.2 mmol/L) |
| Premixed insulin 2× daily | Starting dose:<br><br>Current basal dose given at breakfast and dinner distributed as 2/3 AM and 1/3 PM or 1/2 AM and 1/2 PM | |
| Premixed analog insulin 3× daily | Add additional insulin dose at lunch | |
| Premixed insulin dose titration | For hyperglycemia:<br><br>Increase dose 1-2 days/week until glycemic goal met<br><br>Increase dose by:<br><br>10%-15% or 1-2 U<br><br>For hypoglycemia:<br><br>Decrease dose by:<br><br>10%-20% or 2-4 U | |

ADA = American Diabetes Association; AACE = American Association of Clinical Endocrinologists; ACE = American College of Endocrinology; BG = blood glucose; FBG = fasting blood glucose; TDD = total daily dose.

Data from American Diabetes Association. 8. Pharmacologic approaches to glycemic treatment: Standards of Medical Care in Diabetes—2018. Diabetes Care. 2018;40(Suppl. 1): S73-S85. [PMID: 2922379]

Data from Garber AJ, Abrahamson MJ, Barzilay JI, Blonde L, Bloomgarden ZT, Bush MA, et al; American Association of Clinical Endocrinologists (AACE). Consensus statement by the American Association of Clinical Endocrinologists and American College of Endocrinology on the comprehensive type 2 diabetes management algorithm—2018 Executive Summary. Endocr Pract. 2018;24:91-120. [PMID: 29368965]

CONT.

symptomatic individual. After optimizing the basal insulin dose, prandial insulin should be added prior to the largest meal if hyperglycemia persists. A basal-bolus insulin regimen, with prandial insulin prior to two or more meals, should be employed for continued hyperglycemia.

Ultralong-acting basal analogue insulins may be advantageous compared with long-acting basal analogue insulins due to a prolonged action profile (>24 hours), peakless insulin delivery, and decreased variability in action between and within individuals. The pharmacodynamic profile may decrease hypoglycemia in high-risk patients, improve glycemic fluctuations, and allow for flexibility in dosing beyond 24-hour time periods.

In patients with type 2 diabetes not at glycemic goal despite adherence to glucose monitoring and multiple treatment modalities, CSII may be considered.

**KEY POINTS**

- Metformin is the recommended first-line oral agent for newly diagnosed type 2 diabetes due to known effectiveness and low hypoglycemia risk.

- Glycemic control should be assessed every 3 months with subsequent adjustments to therapeutic agents until the glycemic target is achieved, and every 6 months if at goal.

*Therapy for Gestational Diabetes Mellitus*
Pharmacologic therapy should be prescribed for patients with gestational diabetes to improve perinatal outcomes if lifestyle interventions do not achieve glycemic targets. Insulin is the recommended therapy. While metformin or sulfonylurea therapy may be considered, both therapies cross the placenta, and there is no long-term safety data for their use during pregnancy. Additionally, sulfonylurea therapy has been associated with higher rates of neonatal macrosomia and hypoglycemia.

# Drug-Induced Hyperglycemia

Several drugs can induce hyperglycemia through multiple mechanisms: increased hepatic glucose production, impaired insulin action, or decreased insulin secretion (**Table 12**). Whereas hyperglycemia with temporary drug therapies may resolve after discontinuation, many of these drugs are used indefinitely for chronic medical conditions. Persons at risk for hyperglycemia and the development of diabetes due to medications should be monitored periodically.

#  Inpatient Management of Hyperglycemia

Tight inpatient glycemic control (80-110 mg/dL [4.4-6.1 mmol/L]) is not consistently associated with improved outcomes and may increase mortality. As a result, current inpatient glycemic

goals strive to avoid complications from severe hypoglycemia and hyperglycemia, such as electrolyte abnormalities and dehydration.

Modifications to diet are necessary with consistent values above 140 mg/dL (7.8 mmol/L). If hyperglycemia persists, therapy should be initiated. Clinical status changes may increase the risk of adverse events associated with noninsulin therapies. Insulin is therefore preferred for inpatient management of hyperglycemia 180 mg/dL (10.0 mmol/L) and higher and adjusted to maintain a glucose level between 140 and 180 mg/dL (7.8-10.0 mmol/L) for most patients. Glucose values less than 140 mg/dL (7.8 mmol/L) may be reasonable in select noncritically ill patients if hypoglycemia is avoided, according to the ADA and AACE. In contrast, the American College of Physicians (ACP) does not recommend glucose values less than 140 mg/dL (7.8 mmol/L) due to increased hypoglycemia risk. Several factors may lead to inpatient hypoglycemia: altered mental status, fasting (expected or unexpected), illness, insulin–meal timing mismatch, poor oral intake, and alterations in hyperglycemia-inducing therapies.

**KEY POINT**

- Tight inpatient glycemic control (80-110 mg/dL [4.4-6.1 mmol/L]) is not consistently associated with improved outcomes and may increase mortality.

**HVC**

## Hospitalized Patients with Diabetes Mellitus

In critically ill patients with type 1 and type 2 diabetes mellitus, intravenous insulin therapy is recommended. Intravenous insulin dose adjustments should be based on a validated algorithm that incorporates point-of-care (POC) monitoring every 1 to 2 hours.

For noncritically ill patients, subcutaneous insulin is appropriate. Persons with type 1 diabetes require continuous insulin therapy. Basal insulin must be provided to avoid development of DKA. Persons with type 2 diabetes with glucose values 180 mg/dL (10.0 mmol/L) or higher should also receive insulin therapy.

If the patient is eating, the ideal insulin regimen is a basal-bolus regimen with prandial coverage and correction boluses for premeal hyperglycemia. POC measurements and prandial insulin injections should occur prior to meal consumption. Postprandial insulin administration may be appropriate to allow for dose reduction with decreased oral intake for some persons or those with delayed gastric emptying. Overnight POC measurements are warranted if there are concerns for undetected hypoglycemia; otherwise glucose checks overnight should be avoided due to sleep disruption and increased risk of insulin stacking. The sole use of correction insulin ("sliding-scale insulin") is not recommended since it is a reactive, nonphysiologic approach that leads to large glucose fluctuations.

Continuation of outpatient CSII therapy may be appropriate for those patients with normal mental status who can

| TABLE 12. Drug-Induced Hyperglycemia | | |
|---|---|---|
| **Drug Category** | **Drug** | **Mechanism of Hyperglycemia** |
| Glucocorticoid | All systemic glucocorticoids | Decreased insulin production |
| | | Increased peripheral insulin resistance |
| | | Increased hepatic glucose production |
| Immunosuppressants | Calcineurin inhibitors | Decreased insulin production and release |
| | Sirolimus | |
| | Tacrolimus | |
| | Cyclosporine | |
| Antiretrovirals | Protease inhibitors | Increased peripheral insulin resistance |
| | NRTIs | Pancreatic damage through drug-induced pancreatitis (didanosine) |
| Cardiovascular medications | Niacin | Increased hepatic glucose production |
| | Statins | Impaired pancreatic beta-cell function |
| | | Increased peripheral resistance |
| | β-blockers | Decreased insulin release |
| | Atenolol | Increased peripheral insulin resistance |
| | Metoprolol | Carvedilol (α-blocking) has a neutral effect on glucose |
| | Propranolol | |
| | Thiazides | Decreased insulin secretion secondary to hypokalemia |
| | Hydrochlorothiazide | Increased insulin resistance |
| | Chlorthalidone | |
| | Chlorothiazide | |
| | Indapamide | |
| | Vasopressors | Decreased insulin secretion |
| | Epinephrine | Increased glycogenolysis |
| | Norepinephrine | Increased hepatic glucose production |
| | | Stimulation of glucagon and cortisol |
| Hormonal medications | Oral contraceptives | Abnormal hepatic glucose metabolism |
| | Combined estrogen-progestin | Increased peripheral insulin resistance |
| | Progestin only | Decreased risk of hyperglycemia with low-dose pills containing ≤35 µg ethinyl estradiol |
| | Progestin | Increased peripheral insulin resistance |
| | Megestrol acetate | |
| | Growth hormone | Increased peripheral insulin resistance |
| Atypical antipsychotics (second generation) | Clozapine | Unclear |
| | Olanzapine | Possible increased peripheral insulin resistance |
| | Ziprasidone | |
| | Quetiapine | |
| | Risperidone | |
| | Iloperidone | |
| | Paliperidone | |
| Antibiotics | Moxifloxacin | Altered insulin secretion |
| | Gatifloxacin | |

NRTI = nucleoside reverse transcriptase inhibitors.

Data from Fathallah N, Slim R, Larif S, Hmouda H, Ben Salem C. Drug-induced hyperglycaemia and diabetes. Drug Saf. 2015;38:1153-68. [PMID: 26370106]

Data from Thomas Z, Bandali F, McCowen K, Malhotra A. Drug-induced endocrine disorders in the intensive care unit. Crit Care Med. 2010;38:S219-30. [PMID: 20502175]

CONT.

manage the device under the supervision of health care providers proficient in this technology. If a hospitalized patient becomes unable to safely manage CSII therapy, it should be discontinued and replaced with either a subcutaneous insulin regimen or intravenous insulin.

Continuation of outpatient oral or noninsulin injectable agents is not recommended when patients are admitted due to potential hemodynamic and/or nutritional changes that may occur. Insulin therapy should be initiated for glycemic management. As a patient nears hospital discharge with stability in nutritional status and hemodynamics, reinitiation of these agents may be considered if organ function has returned to baseline. H

### KEY POINTS

- Critically ill patients with type 1 and type 2 diabetes mellitus require intravenous insulin therapy with dosing based on a validated algorithm incorporating point-of-care monitoring every 1 to 2 hours.

- Noncritically ill persons with type 1 diabetes require basal insulin in addition to prandial insulin therapy; persons with type 2 diabetes with glucose values 180 mg/dL (10.0 mmol/L) or higher should also receive insulin therapy.

**HVC**
- The sole use of correction insulin ("sliding-scale insulin") is not recommended since it is a reactive, nonphysiologic approach that leads to large glucose fluctuations.

## Hospitalized Patients Without Diabetes Mellitus

Stress associated with acute illness, enteral/parenteral nutrition, and hyperglycemia-inducing medications in the inpatient setting may induce glucose abnormalities in persons without diabetes.

Hyperglycemia management should follow the same guidelines as hospitalized patients with diabetes.

It is important to recognize that inpatient hyperglycemia may occur in the setting of previously unrecognized diabetes. An inpatient hemoglobin $A_{1c}$ measurement of 6.5% or higher is indicative of glucose abnormalities prior to the hospitalization, and these patients require discharge planning for management of newly diagnosed diabetes.

# Acute Complications of Diabetes Mellitus

## Diabetic Ketoacidosis/Hyperglycemic Hyperosmolar Syndrome

Diabetic ketoacidosis (DKA) and hyperglycemic hyperosmolar syndrome (HHS) occur with extreme hyperglycemia and must be treated early and aggressively to avoid life-threatening consequences from dehydration and electrolyte abnormalities. Severe hyperglycemia is a consequence of insufficient insulin levels coupled with an increase in counterregulatory hormones. This impairs efficient glucose utilization and subsequently drives glycogenolysis and gluconeogenesis for fuel production.

DKA typically occurs in individuals with type 1 diabetes younger than 65 years of age. It is a relative or absolute insulin deficiency state resulting in unsuppressed lipolysis. Fatty acid oxidation occurs with subsequent ketone body production and development of metabolic acidosis. HHS typically occurs in individuals with type 2 diabetes who are older than 65 years of age. It is associated with a higher mortality rate compared with DKA. It is characterized as a partial insulin deficiency that is able to suppress lipolysis and prevent ketone body production, but unable to correct hyperglycemia or prevent the subsequent dehydration and electrolyte abnormalities. Younger patients with type 1 diabetes have a higher glomerular filtration rate, which allows a higher level of glucosuria compared with those with type 2 diabetes. As a result, HHS is associated with more extreme hyperglycemia compared to DKA (**Figure 1**).

Inciting factors for the development of DKA or HHS include infection, myocardial infarction, accidental or deliberate nonadherence to diabetes therapy, stress, trauma, and confounding medications (atypical antipsychotics, glucocorticoids, and SGLT2 inhibitors). DKA or HHS may be the initial presentation of a person with undiagnosed diabetes.

DKA and HHS may present with a multitude of symptoms and plasma glucose levels that can be normal to very high. Symptoms from DKA typically occur within 24 hours of onset, whereas symptoms from HHS may not appear for several days. DKA and HHS symptoms may include abdominal pain, nausea, polyuria, polydipsia, vomiting, weight loss, or shortness of breath. Extreme glucosuria causes an osmotic diuresis and severe volume depletion, which may be exacerbated by gastrointestinal losses of volume and electrolytes. The condition may progress to lethargy, obtundation, and death if the hyperglycemia, dehydration, and electrolyte abnormalities are not treated aggressively and early.

Initial evaluation includes the measurement of serum glucose levels, serum electrolytes, serum ketones, blood urea nitrogen and serum creatinine, plasma osmolality, complete blood count, arterial blood gases, urinalysis, and urine ketones. An electrocardiogram should also be reviewed. Cultures (blood, sputum, urine) and a chest radiograph may be obtained if an infection is suspected after a history is gathered and examination performed.

Multiple laboratory abnormalities are present with DKA and HHS. An increased anion gap metabolic acidosis is present in DKA secondary to production of acetoacetic acid and β-hydroxybutyrate. Although some patients with HHS may have an increased anion gap, typically with glucose levels above 400 to 600 mg/dL (22.2-33.3 mmol/L), they do not develop significant ketoacidosis as seen in DKA.

A moderate to severe reduction in serum bicarbonate levels is present in DKA, but levels may remain normal or mildly reduced (>20 mEq/L [20 mmol/L]) in HHS. Serum pH is typically

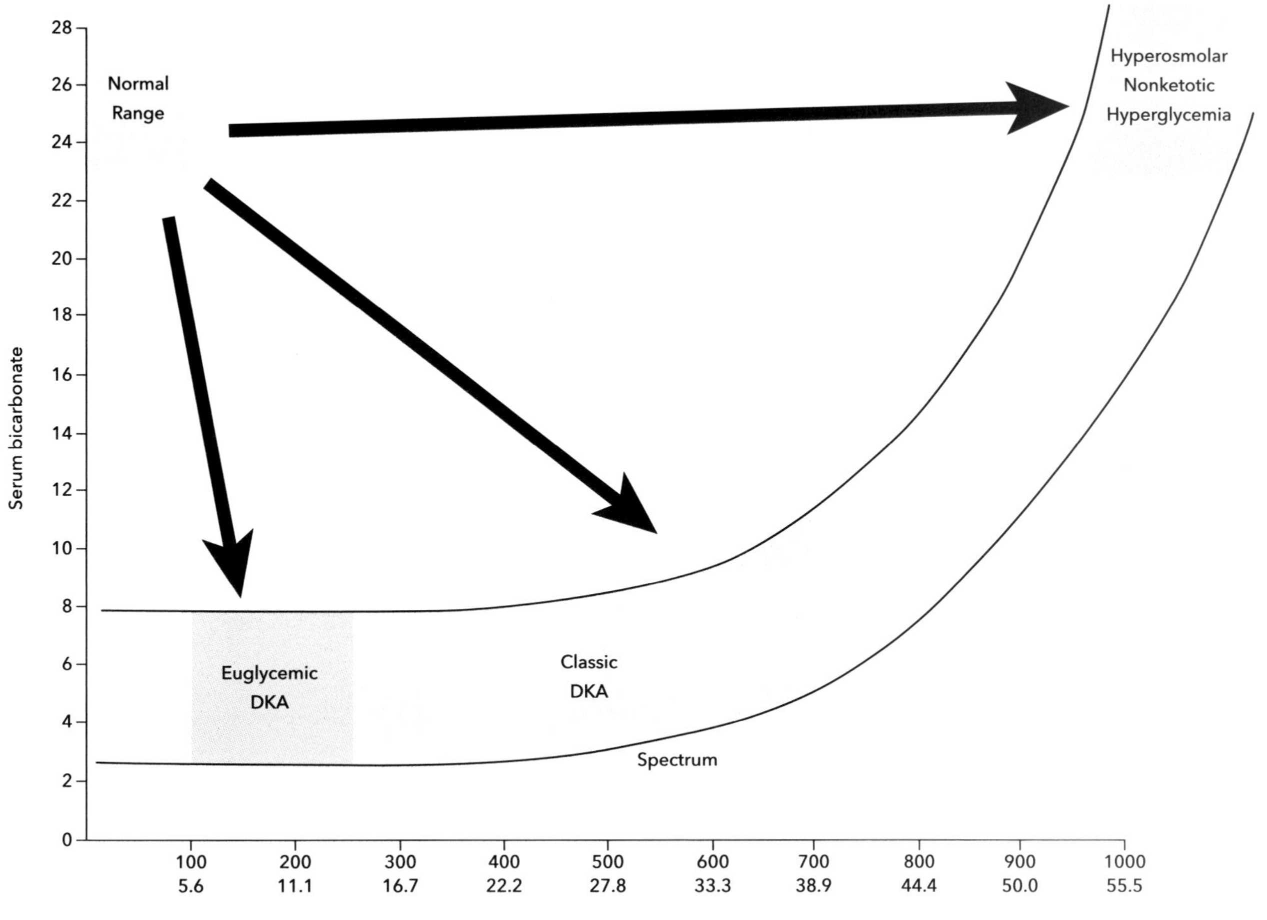

**FIGURE 1.** Spectrum of metabolic decompensation that occurs in diabetic ketoacidosis. DKA = diabetic ketoacidosis.

greater than 7.3 in HHS. Pseudohyponatremia may occur in DKA and HHS with extreme hyperglycemia and osmotic shifts of water from intracellular to extracellular compartments. A normal or elevated sodium level indicates severe dehydration. Increased osmolality, frequently greater than 320 mOsm/kg $H_2O$, is often present in HHS secondary to more severe hyperglycemia and water loss from osmotic diuresis compared with type 1 diabetes. Serum potassium levels may be elevated due to shifts from the intracellular to extracellular spaces due to ketoacidosis and the absence of sufficient insulin. Normal or low serum potassium levels indicate a depletion of body stores and require supplementation prior to insulin therapy to avoid cardiac arrhythmias. Stress may induce mild leukocytosis, but higher levels may indicate an infectious cause for DKA or HHS.

A multi-pronged approach is required to treat DKA and HHS (**Table 13**). Intravenous hydration is necessary for volume repletion. Electrolyte deficits, such as potassium, should be repleted. Hyperglycemia should be corrected preferably with intravenous insulin with hourly glucose measurements to guide dose adjustments. Frequent electrolyte measurements are necessary to guide repletion as hydration and insulin therapy continues. Most patients with DKA or HHS are managed in the ICU due to the high complexity of care required. Other conditions that contributed to the development of DKA or HHS, such as infection, should be treated.

**KEY POINTS**

- Diabetic ketoacidosis and hyperglycemic hyperosmolar syndrome occur with extreme hyperglycemia and must be treated early and aggressively to avoid life-threatening consequences from dehydration and electrolyte abnormalities.

- Inciting factors for the development of diabetic ketoacidosis and hyperglycemic hyperosmolar syndrome include infection, myocardial infarction, accidental or deliberate nonadherence to diabetes therapy, stress, trauma, and confounding medications (SGLT2 inhibitors, atypical antipsychotics, and glucocorticoids).

- Treatment of diabetic ketoacidosis and hyperglycemic hyperosmolar syndrome requires correction of hyperglycemia, intravenous hydration, electrolyte repletion, and treatment of suspected infections.

| TABLE 13. | Management of Hyperglycemic Crisis: Diabetic Ketoacidosis and Hyperglycemic Hyperosmolar Syndrome | | |
|---|---|---|---|
| **Fluids** | **Insulin (Regular)** | **Potassium** | **Correction of Acidosis** |
| Assess for volume status, then give 0.9% saline IV at 1 L/h initially in all patients, and continue if patient is severely hypovolemic. Switch to 0.45% normal saline at 250-500 mL/h if corrected serum sodium level becomes normal or high.

When the plasma glucose level reaches 200 mg/dL (11.1 mmol/L) in patients with DKA or 300 mg/dL (16.7 mmol/L) in HHS in the setting of continued IV insulin, switch to 5% dextrose with 0.45% normal saline at 150-250 mL/h to maintain the blood glucose and avoid hypoglycemia. | Give regular insulin, 0.1 U/kg, as an IV bolus followed by 0.1 U/kg/h as an IV infusion.

If the plasma glucose level does not decrease by 10% in the first hour, give an additional bolus of 0.14 U/kg and resume previous infusion rate.

When the plasma glucose level reaches 200 mg/dL (11.1 mmol/L) in DKA and 300 mg/dL (16.7 mmol/L) in HHS, reduce to 0.02-0.05 U/kg/h, and maintain the plasma glucose level between 150-200 mg/dL (8.3-11.1 mmol/L) until anion gap acidosis is resolved in DKA.

The plasma glucose should be maintained between 250-300 mg/dL in HHS until the patient is alert and the hyperosmolar state resolves. | Assess for adequate kidney function, with adequate urine output (approximately 50 mL/h).

If serum potassium is <3.3 mEq/L (3.3 mmol/L), do not start insulin but instead give IV potassium chloride, 20-30 mEq/h, through a central line catheter until the serum potassium level is >3.3 mEq/L (3.3 mmol/L). Then add 20-30 mEq of potassium chloride to each liter of IV fluids to keep the serum potassium level in the 4.0-5.0 mEq/L (4.0-5.0 mmol/L) range.

If the serum potassium level is >5.2 mEq/L (5.2 mmol/L), do not give potassium chloride, but instead start insulin and IV fluids, and check the serum potassium level every 2 hours. | If pH is <6.9, consider sodium bicarbonate, 100 mmol in 400 mL of water, and potassium chloride, 20 mEq, infused over 2 hours.

If pH is 6.9 or greater, do not give sodium bicarbonate. |

DKA = diabetic ketoacidosis; HHS = hyperglycemic hyperosmolar syndrome; IV = intravenous.

Recommendations from Kitabchi AE, Umpierrez GE, Miles JM, Fisher JN. Hyperglycemic crises in adult patients with diabetes. Diabetes Care. 2009;32:1335-43. [PMID: 19564476]

# Chronic Complications of Diabetes Mellitus

##  Cardiovascular Morbidity

A major cause of morbidity and mortality in persons with diabetes mellitus is cardiovascular disease (CVD). Diabetes is an independent risk factor for CVD. Other significant risk factors for CVD include hypertension, dyslipidemia, tobacco use, family history, and albuminuria. Simultaneous management of CVD risk factors is recommended to decrease morbidity and mortality. Screening interval guidelines for risk factors are listed in **Table 14**.

Hypertension contributes to the development of macrovascular and microvascular complications. The American Diabetes Association (ADA) defines hypertension as sustained blood pressures 140/90 mm Hg or higher. Citing concerns for increased treatment complications with a lower blood pressure target below 130/80 mm Hg, the ADA treatment goal for most persons is below 140/90 mm Hg. Those persons at high risk for CVD may aim for lower blood pressure targets if this can be achieved safely. In contrast, guidelines from the American Association of Clinical Endocrinologists/American College of Endocrinology (AACE/ACE) and the American College of Cardiology/American Heart Association (ACC/AHA) and nine other organizations advocate for a treatment target below 130/80 mm Hg for most patients with diabetes. ADA recommended treatment strategies include lifestyle modifications (for blood pressure >120/80 mm Hg) and pharmacologic therapies (for blood pressure >140/90 mm Hg). Initial recommended antihypertensive regimens include ACE inhibitors, angiotensin receptor blockers (ARBs), dihydropyridine calcium channel blockers, and thiazide diuretics. Multiple agents are frequently required to reach the blood pressure target. Underlying comorbidities should guide selection of therapeutic agents, such as the use of an ACE inhibitor or ARB in the presence of microalbuminuria.

Lipid management in diabetes frequently requires a combination of lifestyle modifications and pharmacologic agents. The ACC/AHA risk calculator can determine the 10-year atherosclerotic cardiovascular disease (ASCVD) risk to guide therapeutic management. Statin therapy is the recommended initial pharmacologic treatment for all qualifying persons with diabetes (see MKSAP 18 General Internal Medicine).

Antiplatelet therapy with aspirin (75-162 mg/day) is recommended by the ADA for secondary prevention in those persons with diabetes and ASCVD. Aspirin therapy for primary prevention of ASCVD in persons with type 1 and type 2 diabetes may not provide universal benefit, so aspirin therapy (75-162 mg/day) may be considered in persons 50 years of age and older with at least one additional ASCVD risk factor. The ADA does not recommend aspirin therapy for persons younger than 50 years of age at low risk for ASCVD.

**TABLE 14.** Screening Recommendations for Chronic Complications of Diabetes Mellitus

| Chronic Complication | Clinical Situation | When to Start Screening | Screening Frequency | Preferred Screening Test |
|---|---|---|---|---|
| Retinopathy | Type 1 diabetes | At 5 years after diagnosis | Annually[a] | Dilated and comprehensive eye examination[b] |
| | Type 2 diabetes | At diagnosis | Annually[a] | Dilated and comprehensive eye examination[b] |
| | In pregnant women with either type of diabetes | First trimester | Every trimester and then closely for 1 year postpartum | Dilated and comprehensive eye examination[b] |
| | In women with either type of diabetes planning to conceive | During preconception planning | Same as recommendations for pregnant women once conception occurs | Dilated and comprehensive eye examination[b] |
| Nephropathy | Type 1 diabetes | At 5 years after diagnosis | Annually[c] | Albumin-creatinine ratio on random spot urine, eGFR |
| | Type 2 diabetes | At diagnosis | Annually[c] | Albumin-creatinine ratio on random spot urine, eGFR |
| Neuropathy (distal symmetric polyneuropathy)[d] | Type 1 diabetes | At 5 years after diagnosis | Annually | Skin assessment, evaluate for foot deformities, lower extremity pulse assessment, neurologic assessment (10-g monofilament plus 128-Hz tuning fork, ankle reflexes, pinprick, or temperature) |
| | Type 2 diabetes | At diagnosis | Annually | Skin assessment, evaluate for foot deformities, lower extremity pulse assessment, neurologic assessment (10-g monofilament plus 128-Hz tuning fork, ankle reflexes, pinprick, or temperature) |
| Cardiovascular disease | Hypertension | At diagnosis | Every visit | Blood pressure measurement |
| | Dyslipidemia | At diagnosis and prior to initiating statin therapy | Annually[e] | Lipid profile |

eGFR = estimated glomerular filtration rate.

[a]It is reasonable to screen every 1 to 2 years if no diabetic retinopathy is present and to screen more often than annually if diabetic retinopathy is advanced or progressing rapidly.

[b]Retinal photography is a possible alternative means of screening for diabetic retinopathy that may improve access to care and reduce costs. Retinal photography, when interpreted by eye care specialists, can detect most clinically significant diabetic retinopathy.

[c]The American Diabetes Association guidelines state that it is reasonable to assess progression of disease and response to therapeutic interventions with continued monitoring of urinary albumin-creatinine excretion.

[d]Although diabetes commonly causes peripheral neuropathy, other differential diagnoses to consider during the screening process include vitamin $B_{12}$ deficiency, alcoholism, hypothyroidism, renal disease, malignancy and chemotherapies, vasculitis, and inherited neuropathies.

[e]Annual or periodic screening to monitor therapeutic response after initiation of statin therapy. May screen every 5 years if not on statin therapy.

Recommendations from American Diabetes Association. 9. Cardiovascular disease and risk management: Standards of Medical Care in Diabetes—2018. Diabetes Care. 2018;41(Suppl. 1):S86-S104. [PMID: 29222380]

Recommendations from American Diabetes Association. 10. Microvascular complications and foot care: Standards of Medical Care in Diabetes—2018. Diabetes Care. 2018; 41 (Suppl. 1):S105-S118. [PMID: 29222381]

Recommendations from Garber AJ, Abrahamson MJ, Barzilay JI, Blonde L, Bloomgarden ZT, Bush MA, et al; American Association of Clinical Endocrinologists (AACE). Consensus Statement by the American Association of Clinical Endocrinologists and American College of Endocrinology on the comprehensive type 2 diabetes management algorithm—2018 executive summary. Endocr Pract. 2018;24:91-120. [PMID: 29368965]

**KEY POINTS**

- The American Diabetes Association (ADA) recommends a blood pressure treatment goal below 140/90 mm Hg or lower for persons at high risk for CVD if this can be achieved safely; the American Association of Clinical Endocrinologists/American College of Endocrinology (AACE/ACE) and the American College of Cardiology/American Heart Association (ACC/AHA) and nine other organizations recommend a target below 130/80 mm Hg for most patients with diabetes.

*(Continued)*

**KEY POINTS** *(continued)*

- Lipid management in diabetes frequently requires a combination of lifestyle modifications and pharmacologic agents; statin therapy is the recommended initial pharmacologic treatment for all qualifying persons with diabetes.

- The American Diabetes Association (ADA) does not recommend aspirin therapy for persons younger than 50 years of age at low risk for atherosclerotic cardiovascular disease.

**HVC**

## Diabetic Retinopathy

Retinopathy is the leading cause of preventable blindness among persons with diabetes between 20 and 74 years of age in developed countries. Risk factors for retinopathy include duration of diabetes, degree of hyperglycemia, hypertension, albuminuria, and dyslipidemia.

Diabetic retinopathy changes are classified as nonproliferative (occurs within the retina) or proliferative (occurs in the vitreous or retinal inner surface). Nonproliferative retinopathy findings may include microaneurysms, dot and blot hemorrhages, hard exudates (lipid deposition), soft exudates or cotton-wool spots (ischemic superficial nerve fibers), venous bleeding, and intraretinal microvascular abnormalities. Neovascularization due to chronic ischemia characterizes proliferative retinopathy, which may cause intraocular hemorrhage, retinal detachment, and vision loss.

Macular edema may occur with nonproliferative and proliferative retinopathy.

Screening guidelines were developed for early detection of asymptomatic abnormalities to allow for treatment interventions to prevent vision loss (see Table 14).

Optimal control of blood pressure, glucose, and lipid parameters can prevent and delay the progression of retinopathy. Panretinal laser photocoagulation can treat high-risk proliferative diabetic retinopathy and severe nonproliferative retinopathy. In addition, intravitreal injections with anti-vascular endothelial growth factor (anti-VEGF) to reduce vision loss associated with proliferative retinopathy is not inferior to panretinal laser photocoagulation. Retinopathy may develop or accelerate during pregnancy or with rapid glycemic improvements, and may require laser photocoagulation to decrease the risk of vision loss. Macular edema is preferentially treated with anti-VEGF intravitreal injections to improve vision loss. Anti-VEGF injections require monthly injections for at least 12 months followed by intermittent injections to prevent recurrent macular edema.

### KEY POINTS

- Patients with type 2 diabetes should have an eye examination at the time of diagnosis.

- Optimal control of glucose, blood pressure, and lipid parameters can prevent and delay the progression of retinopathy.

- Panretinal laser photocoagulation or intravitreal injections of anti-vascular endothelial growth factor can treat high-risk proliferative diabetic retinopathy and severe nonproliferative retinopathy.

## Diabetic Nephropathy

Diabetic nephropathy is the leading cause of end-stage kidney disease (ESKD). Diabetes is typically present for 5 to 10 years prior to the development of nephropathy. Individuals with a first-degree relative with ESKD due to diabetic nephropathy have increased risk of progressing to ESKD themselves.

Measurement of estimated glomerular filtration rate (eGFR) and screening for the presence of microalbuminuria is recommended for early detection of kidney disease (see Table 14). Urinary albumin excretion can be determined from a random urine collection as an albumin-creatinine ratio (UACR). An elevated UACR level (≥30 mg/g creatinine) should be confirmed by multiple measurements over 3 to 6 months due to possible temporary elevations from biological variability, illness, hyperglycemia, heart failure, hypertension, exercise, and menstruation. Annual measurements of eGFR and UACR may identify progression of nephropathy and guide therapeutic decisions. More frequent assessments may be necessary with worsening kidney function. An eGFR less than 30 mL/min/1.73 m$^2$ warrants a referral to a nephrologist.

Uncontrolled hyperglycemia and hypertension are risk factors for diabetic nephropathy; thus treatment to attain glucose and blood pressure goals is recommended. The ADA recommends an ACE inhibitor or an angiotensin receptor blocker (ARB) as first-line therapy to slow progression of nephropathy and prevent CVD in nonpregnant persons with diabetes, hypertension, a reduced eGFR (<60 mL/min/1.73 m$^2$), and an elevated UACR (≥300 mg/g creatinine). An ACE inhibitor or an ARB is also recommended for treatment of an elevated UACR between 30 and 299 mg/g creatinine in nonpregnant persons with hypertension. Treatment with an ACE inhibitor or ARB is not recommended for patients with diabetes who have a normal blood pressure, a UACR level less than 30 mg/g creatinine, and an eGFR level greater than 60 mL/min/1.73 m$^2$.

### KEY POINTS

- Measurement of estimated glomerular filtration rate and screening for the presence of microalbuminuria are recommended for early detection of kidney disease.

- The American Diabetes Association recommends an ACE inhibitor or an angiotensin receptor blocker as first-line therapy to slow progression of nephropathy and prevent cardiovascular disease in nonpregnant persons with diabetes, hypertension, a reduced estimated glomerular filtration rate (<60 mL/min/1.73 m$^2$), and an elevated urine albumin-creatinine ratio (≥300 mg/g creatinine).

- Treatment with an ACE inhibitor or angiotensin receptor **HVC** blocker is not recommended for patients with diabetes who have a normal blood pressure, a urine albumin-to-creatinine ratio level less than 30 mg/g creatinine, and an estimated glomerular filtration rate level greater than 60 mL/min/1.73 m$^2$.

## Diabetic Neuropathy

CONT.

Diabetic neuropathy involves damage to nerves or nerve roots due to hyperglycemia. Symptoms are dependent on the affected nerve(s) and may be focal or diffuse in nature. Neuropathy may occur peripherally and/or affect the autonomic nervous system. Glycemic control may prevent peripheral neuropathy and cardiac autonomic neuropathy in individuals with type 1 diabetes and can delay progression of neuropathy in type 2 diabetes.

Diabetic peripheral neuropathy (distal symmetric polyneuropathy) typically has an ascending presentation with a "stocking and glove" distribution. It may involve damage to both small and large nerve fibers. Symptoms from small nerve fiber damage include pain, burning, and tingling. Small nerve fiber abnormalities can be detected on examination by assessment of pinprick and temperature sensations. Abnormalities in position sense, vibration, and light touch are indicative of large nerve fiber damage and convey an increased risk for foot ulcerations. Assessment of large nerve fiber damage can be achieved by assessing ankle reflexes and with a 128-Hz tuning fork and a 10-g monofilament. Since diabetic peripheral neuropathy may be asymptomatic, screening should occur for early detection to prevent limb loss (see Table 14).

Autonomic neuropathy may affect one or multiple organs with symptoms varying based on the affected organ. Symptoms may include hypoglycemia unawareness, gastroparesis, constipation, diarrhea, erectile dysfunction, and bladder dysfunction. Symptoms from cardiac autonomic dysfunction may include orthostatic hypotension, resting sinus tachycardia, and exercise intolerance. Cardiac autonomic neuropathy is an independent risk factor for sudden death.

The goal of treatment of diabetic neuropathy is symptom control. Two FDA-approved medications, pregabalin or duloxetine, are recommended as initial therapy. Other agents may provide symptom relief but are not FDA approved and include tricyclic antidepressants, venlafaxine, carbamazepine, capsaicin, and gabapentin. The primary treatment of orthostatic hypotension is nonpharmacologic and includes diet, use of compression stockings, and changing positions slowly. Medications that cause or worsen the orthostatic changes should be discontinued and other agents (fludrocortisone, midodrine, or droxidopa) added for refractory symptoms. Small and frequent low-fat, low-fiber meals may improve symptoms of gastroparesis. Metoclopramide is the only prokinetic agent approved by the FDA for the treatment of gastroparesis. Given the risk of side effects, including dystonia, careful assessment of risks and benefits should be undertaken before prescribing (see MKSAP 18 Gastroenterology and Hepatology).

Diabetic amyotrophy is a rare condition affecting the lumbosacral plexus that may occur secondary to infarction or immune vasculopathy. Presentation is acute and associated with severe asymmetric pain or proximal weakness in a leg with associated muscle wasting. Partial remission may occur over many months. Treatment is supportive.

Mononeuropathies and nerve compression syndromes (carpal tunnel syndrome, peroneal palsy) can occur in patients with diabetes. Mononeuropathies frequently resolve without intervention within a few months. Compression syndromes may respond to conservative management, or surgery may be necessary for symptom relief.

### KEY POINTS

- Diabetic peripheral neuropathy (distal symmetric polyneuropathy) presents with a "stocking and glove" distribution, involving damage to both small and large nerve fibers; symptoms include pain, burning, and tingling.
- Glycemic control can delay progression of neuropathy in type 2 diabetes.

## Diabetic Foot Ulcers

Significant morbidity and mortality are associated with lower extremity ulcers and amputations (see MKSAP 18 Infectious Disease). Lower extremities should be inspected at every visit and a comprehensive foot examination, including 10-g monofilament testing, should be performed at least annually. Risk factors for ulcer include: hyperglycemia, peripheral artery disease, history of foot ulcer or amputation, foot deformity, peripheral neuropathy, impaired vision, tobacco use, and diabetic nephropathy. Vascular assessment should occur in persons with absent pedal pulses or symptoms concerning for claudication. Foot care specialists should be involved in the care of high-risk individuals. Patients should be educated on the importance of daily foot inspections and properly fitting footwear.

# Hypoglycemia

Hypoglycemia is defined as a glucose value less than 70 mg/dL (3.9 mmol/L). Glucose values less than 54 mg/dL (3.0 mmol/L) are serious and clinically significant. Severe hypoglycemia is any glucose value at which a person requires external assistance to correct the glucose.

Hyperadrenergic symptoms (sweating, tremors, anxiety, tachycardia) are the normal physiologic response to the development of hypoglycemia. Counterregulatory hormones (glucagon, epinephrine, norepinephrine, cortisol, and growth hormone) are subsequently released by the body to correct hypoglycemia. Neuroglycopenic signs (altered mental status, dysarthria, confusion) are associated with severe hypoglycemia. Obtundation, seizures, and death may occur if severe hypoglycemia is not corrected rapidly.

## Hypoglycemia in Patients with Diabetes Mellitus

Hypoglycemia can become a rate-limiting step in achieving glycemic goals for many persons. Severe recurrent hypoglycemia is

CONT.

associated with acquired cognitive deficits and can lead to dementia. Therapies must be adjusted to eliminate hypoglycemia, and glycemic goals should be individualized to accommodate targets that can be safely achieved.

Several factors contribute to hypoglycemia including a mismatch of food consumption and insulin delivery, increased physical exertion, weight loss, worsening kidney impairment, abnormalities in gastrointestinal motility and absorption, and accidental/intentional overdose of insulin. Older adults are also at an increased risk for hypoglycemia.

Hypoglycemia can also occur with the use of oral antidiabetic agents due to incorrect dosages, drug-drug interactions, and intercurrent illnesses that alter the metabolism or excretion of drugs.

Hypoglycemia treatment in an alert person includes consumption of 15 to 20 grams of a fast-acting carbohydrate followed by a self-monitored blood glucose (SMBG) measurement 15 to 20 minutes later. If the glucose has not improved, repeat treatment with 15 grams of carbohydrates should occur. After glucose normalization (>70 mg/dL [3.9 mmol/L]), a meal or snack should be consumed to avoid recurrent hypoglycemia. Glucagon should be provided to those persons at risk for developing clinically significant hypoglycemia (<54 mg/dL [3.0 mmol/L]) and used intramuscularly by close contacts if the person is not able to safely consume carbohydrates to correct hypoglycemia.

Relative hypoglycemia characterizes symptoms of hypoglycemia in the setting of plasma glucose values greater than 70 mg/dL (3.9 mmol/L). This may occur with a large, rapid decrease in glucose or rapid normalization of glucose with treatment intensification in an individual with prolonged plasma glucose values above 200 mg/dL (11.1 mmol/L). Relative hypoglycemia can be prevented by avoiding large glycemic excursions and by slow correction of long-standing hyperglycemia to goal to allow a longer adjustment period. **H**

**KEY POINTS**

- Hypoglycemia is defined as a glucose value less than 70 mg/dL (3.9 mmol/L) and serious hypoglycemia as less than 54 mg/dL (3.0 mmol/L).

- Initial treatment of hypoglycemia requires oral consumption of carbohydrates or administration of glucagon with a goal of increasing the glucose to greater than 70 mg/dL (3.9 mmol/L).

- Relative hypoglycemia can be prevented by avoiding large glycemic excursions and by slow correction of long-standing hyperglycemia to goal to allow a longer adjustment period.

## Hypoglycemia in Patients Without Diabetes Mellitus

Hypoglycemia without concomitant diabetes is uncommon and warrants further assessment. A hypoglycemia evaluation should commence if the criteria for Whipple triad are met: neuroglycopenic symptoms, hypoglycemia at or below 55 mg/dL (3.1 mmol/L), and resolution of symptoms with glucose ingestion. Laboratory measurement of glucose must confirm true hypoglycemia, as point-of-contact (POC) glucose values are not reliable in this scenario. Hypoglycemia in persons without diabetes may be attributable to the following causes: drugs, alcohol, illness, organ dysfunction (kidney or liver), hormonal deficiencies (adrenal insufficiency), malnutrition, and pancreatogenous insulinoma or noninsulinoma (endogenous hyperinsulinemic hypoglycemia that is not caused by an insulinoma).

Although there may be overlap in presentation, hypoglycemia typically occurs in the fasting or in the postprandial state. Diagnostic blood and urine studies should be obtained during a hypoglycemic episode in which Whipple triad has been demonstrated. If a spontaneous episode is not witnessed, measures should be implemented to recreate circumstances that normally induce hypoglycemia (fasting or ingestion of a typical meal that causes an episode in that particular patient). Imaging studies for tumor localization should only occur after confirmation of endogenous hyperinsulinism from the diagnostic blood and urine studies. **H**

**KEY POINT**

- Imaging studies for tumor localization should only occur after confirmation of endogenous hyperinsulinism from the diagnostic blood and urine studies.

**HVC**

### Fasting Hypoglycemia

A prolonged fast, up to 72 hours, should be initiated if the hypoglycemia typically occurs while fasting.

Five blood specimens are drawn simultaneously every 6 hours: glucose, C-peptide, insulin, proinsulin, $\beta$-hydroxybutyrate. Insulin antibodies and an oral hypoglycemic agent screen should also be measured at the beginning of the fast. Blood specimen collection should increase to every 1 to 2 hours when the glucose measurement is less than 60 mg/dL (3.3 mmol/L).

Testing is complete when one of the following parameters is met: plasma glucose 45 mg/dL (2.5 mmol/L) or below with neuroglycopenia, or plasma glucose less than 55 mg/dL (3.1 mmol/L) if Whipple triad was documented previously. POC glucose values and hyperadrenergic symptoms should not be used to determine the end of the fast. Blood specimens should be collected again at the end of the 72-hour time period if neither of the above criteria has been met.

The interpretation of the diagnostic testing results is found in **Table 15**. To decrease the cost of this procedure, the plasma glucose should be sent to the laboratory as soon as possible, and if it is less than 60 mg/dL (3.3 mmol/L), the other four blood samples should be sent. **H**

**TABLE 15.** Differential Diagnosis of Spontaneous Fasting Hypoglycemia[a] in a Person Without Diabetes Mellitus

| Diagnosis | Serum Insulin | Plasma C-Peptide[b] | Plasma Proinsulin[b] | Serum β-hydroxybutyrate[c] | Serum Insulin Antibodies | Urine or Blood Metabolites of Sulfonylureas or Meglitinides |
|---|---|---|---|---|---|---|
| Insulinoma[d, e] | ↑ | ↑ | ↑ | ↓ | Negative | Negative |
| Surreptitious use of sulfonylureas or meglitinides | ↑ | ↑ | ↑ | ↓ | Negative | Positive |
| Surreptitious use of insulin | ↑ | ↓ | ↓ | ↓ | Negative | Negative |
| Insulin autoimmune hypoglycemia | ↑ | ↑ | ↑ | ↓ | Positive | Negative |
| IGF-II[f] | ↓ | ↓ | ↓ | ↓ | Negative | Negative |

[a]Symptomatic hypoglycemia, fasting plasma glucose 55 mg/dL (3.1 mmol/L) or lower, and prompt symptomatic relief with correction of hypoglycemia (Whipple triad).

[b]C-peptide and proinsulin are indicative of endogenous insulin production.

[c]β-hydroxybutyrate will be suppressed in the presence of insulin, but elevated with hypoglycemia that is not mediated by insulin.

[d]Blood specimens should be collected at the end of testing and glucagon should be administered followed by serial glucose measurements over 30 minutes. Insulin suppresses glycogenolysis and preserves glycogen stores. In the setting of an insulinoma, glucose will increase in response to glucagon as the glycogen stores are utilized.

[e]Similar results can also be seen with non-insulinoma pancreatogenous hypoglycemia syndrome or post-gastric bypass hypoglycemia.

[f]Insulin-like growth factor (IGF)-II or its precursors may be produced by tumors and induce hypoglycemia by stimulating the insulin receptors with subsequent increases in glucose use.

Data from Cryer PE, Axelrod L, Grossman AB, Heller SR, Montori VM, Seaquist ER, et al; Endocrine Society. Evaluation and management of adult hypoglycemic disorders: an Endocrine Society Clinical Practice Guideline. Clin Endocrinol Metab. 2009;94:709-28. [PMID: 19088155]

**KEY POINT**

HVC
- For fasting hypoglycemia, five blood specimens are drawn simultaneously every 6 hours: glucose, C-peptide, insulin, proinsulin, β-hydroxybutyrate; to decrease the cost of this procedure, the plasma glucose should be sent to the laboratory as soon as possible, and if it is less than 60 mg/dL (3.3 mmol/L), the other four blood samples should be sent.

## Postprandial Hypoglycemia

Postprandial hypoglycemia typically occurs within 5 hours of the last meal. Altered gastrointestinal anatomy, as occurs after Roux-en-Y gastric bypass surgery, is frequently the cause of the postprandial hypoglycemia. Meals consisting of simple carbohydrates (pancakes, syrup, juice) are frequently the culprit. A mixed-meal test consisting of the types of food that normally induce the hypoglycemia should be performed to determine the cause. Baseline laboratory studies including glucose, C-peptide, insulin, and proinsulin should be obtained prior to meal consumption. These tests should be repeated every 30 minutes for 5 hours. If neuroglycopenia occurs, the tests should be repeated prior to administration of carbohydrates. To decrease the cost of this procedure, the plasma glucose should be sent to the laboratory as soon as possible, and if it is less than 60 mg/dL (3.3 mmol/L), the other three blood samples should be sent.

Screening should also occur for insulin antibodies and oral hypoglycemic agents if symptomatic hypoglycemia occurs. Interpretation of the results is similar to those obtained during fasting hypoglycemia (see Table 15).

Treatment generally consists of small frequent mixed meals with a balance of protein, fat, and carbohydrates.

**KEY POINT**

- For postprandial hypoglycemia, baseline laboratory studies including glucose, C-peptide, insulin, and proinsulin should be obtained prior to meal consumption; to decrease the cost of this procedure, the plasma glucose should be sent to the laboratory as soon as possible, and if it is less than 60 mg/dL (3.3 mmol/L), the other three blood samples should be sent.

HVC

## Hypoglycemia Unawareness

Hypoglycemia unawareness is characterized by insufficient release of counterregulatory hormones and an inadequate autonomic response to hypoglycemia. Prior episodes of hypoglycemia increase the risk of developing hypoglycemia unawareness. Treatment involves relaxation of glycemic targets and modifications of hypoglycemia-inducing diabetes therapies to avoid continued hypoglycemia. Avoidance of hypoglycemia for several weeks may reverse hypoglycemia unawareness in some persons and result in the return of adrenergic symptoms with glucose levels less than 70 mg/dL (3.9 mmol/L). A continuous glucose monitoring system may be beneficial in appropriate individuals to provide early detection of impending severe hypoglycemia for early intervention.

# Disorders of the Pituitary Gland

## Hypothalamic and Pituitary Anatomy and Physiology

The pituitary gland is located in the sella turcica posterior to the sphenoid sinus. The optic chiasm is located superior to the pituitary gland, and the carotid arteries are lateral (**Figure 2**). The gland is composed of the anterior pituitary (adenohypophysis), which is glandular tissue, and the posterior pituitary gland (neurohypophysis), which arises from neural tissue. A rich portal vascular network connects the hypothalamus to the anterior pituitary, whereas the posterior pituitary gland consists of nerve endings projected from neurons in the supraoptic and paraventricular nuclei in the hypothalamus. Both the portal network and hypothalamic neurons travel from the hypothalamus to the pituitary through the pituitary stalk. The carotid arteries provide blood to the pituitary through the hypophysial arteries, and venous drainage occurs by means of the petrosal sinuses to the jugular vein.

Stimulatory and inhibitory hormones, secreted into the portal blood by the hypothalamus, regulate the anterior pituitary, and the posterior pituitary hormones are synthesized in the hypothalamic nuclei and travel through neurons to be released by the posterior pituitary gland.

The anterior pituitary secretes six pituitary hormones: luteinizing hormone (LH), follicle-stimulating hormone (FSH), adrenocorticotrophic hormone (ACTH), prolactin, thyroid-stimulating hormone (TSH), and growth hormone (GH). Gonadotropin-releasing hormone (GnRH) is released from the hypothalamus in pulses, which in turn control the release of LH and FSH. LH and FSH regulate male and female reproduction including stimulation of the gonads to produce testosterone and estrogen, as well as stimulation of ovarian follicles and spermatogenesis (see Reproductive Disorders). Corticotropin-releasing hormone (CRH), produced in the hypothalamus, stimulates the production of ACTH in the pituitary, which then stimulates cortisol production from the adrenal glands. Prolactin is synthesized in the lactotroph cells. Its synthesis and secretion is suppressed by hypothalamic dopamine, which traverses the pituitary stalk through the portal circulation. TSH is released in response to stimulation from thyrotropin-releasing hormone (TRH) produced in the hypothalamus. TSH binds to receptors on the thyroid, resulting in synthesis and secretion of thyroid hormone. GH release is regulated by two hypothalamic hormones, growth hormone-releasing hormone (GHRH), which stimulates GH release, and somatostatin, which inhibits GH release.

The posterior pituitary gland secretes oxytocin, necessary for parturition and lactation, and antidiuretic hormone (ADH), which maintains water balance.

**Table 16** lists the pituitary hormones and the initial evaluation for suspected pituitary excess or deficiency of each hormone.

## Pituitary Abnormalities
### Incidentally Noted Pituitary Masses

When a pituitary lesion is discovered incidentally on imaging obtained for an unrelated reason, the lesion is termed a "pituitary incidentaloma." Small incidentally noted pituitary lesions are quite common. In patients undergoing MRI for nonpituitary reasons, microadenomas are found in 10% to 38%, whereas incidental macroadenomas are seen in 0.2%. Most pituitary incidentalomas are benign nonfunctional pituitary adenomas; however, a small percentage may be Rathke cleft cysts, craniopharyngiomas, or meningiomas. In patients with a history of malignancy, metastatic disease should be considered. Pituitary adenomas measuring 1 cm or larger are

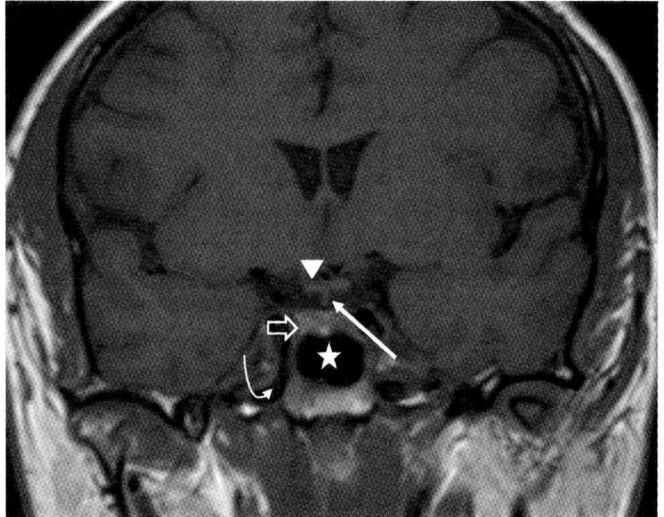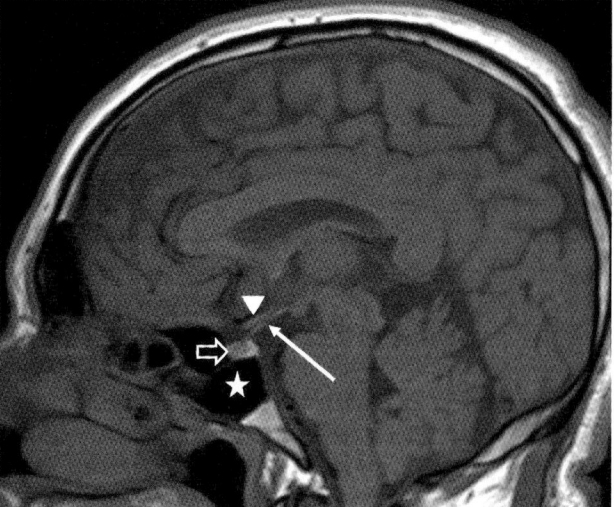

**FIGURE 2.** A coronal MRI (*left*) and sagittal MRI (*right*) showing the pituitary gland (*open arrow*), pituitary stalk (*thin arrow*), optic chiasm (*arrowhead*), sphenoid sinus (*star*), and carotid artery (*curved arrow*).

**TABLE 16.** Initial Testing for Pituitary Hormone Deficiency and Excess

| | | **Pituitary Hormone Excess** | |
|---|---|---|---|
| **Pituitary Hormone** | **Peripheral Hormone** | **Initial Test(s)** | |
| ACTH | Cortisol | 24-Hour urine free cortisol (×2) OR nocturnal salivary cortisol (×2) OR overnight low-dose dexamethasone test | |
| ADH | ADH | Simultaneous serum sodium, serum osmolality, urine sodium, and urine osmolality | |
| GH | IGF-1 | IGF-1 | |
| TSH | Thyroxine, triiodothyronine | TSH, free (or total) thyroxine | |
| PRL | Prolactin | Serum prolactin | |
| | | **Pituitary Hormone Deficiency** | |
| **Pituitary Hormone** | **Peripheral Hormone** | **Initial Test(s)** | **Confirmatory Test[a]** |
| ACTH | Cortisol | Simultaneous ACTH, cortisol | ACTH stimulation test |
| ADH | ADH | Simultaneous serum sodium, urine and serum osmolality | Water deprivation test |
| LH and FSH[b] | Testosterone or estradiol | Simultaneous LH, FSH, total testosterone (male), estradiol (female) | |
| TSH | Thyroxine, triiodothyronine | Simultaneous TSH, free (or total) thyroxine | |
| GH | IGF-1 | IGF-1 | GHRH-arginine test Insulin-tolerance test |

ACTH = adrenocorticotropic hormone; ADH = antidiuretic hormone; FSH = follicle-stimulating hormone; GH = growth hormone; GHRH = growth hormone-releasing hormone; IGF-1 = insulin-like growth factor 1; LH = luteinizing hormone; PRL = prolactin; TSH = thyroid-stimulating hormone.

[a]See Table 18 for additional information on confirmatory testing for pituitary dysfunction.

[b]Routine testing for deficiency is not recommended without specific signs of deficiency, such as amenorrhea, gynecomastia, or impotence.

macroadenomas; those measuring less than 1 cm are microadenomas (see Evaluation of Pituitary Tumors).

**KEY POINT**

- Most incidentally noted pituitary masses are benign nonfunctional pituitary adenomas; however, a small percentage may be Rathke cleft cysts, craniopharyngiomas, or meningiomas.

## Empty Sella

Empty sella is also typically an incidental finding on imaging done for a nonpituitary-related reason. It is a radiologic finding, rather than a medical condition. This term is used when the sella turcica is enlarged and not entirely filled with pituitary tissue. No gland may be visualized, or it is inordinately small. Primary empty sella is the result of herniation of subarachnoid space into the sella, compressing the normal pituitary gland. Primary empty sella is caused by incompetence of the sellar diaphragm, increased intracranial pressure, or volumetric changes in the pituitary gland (as can occur in pregnancy, particularly in multiparous women). Secondary empty sella can be related to infarction of a pituitary tumor or other causes including infection, autoimmune disease, trauma, or radiotherapy.

Patients with an empty sella usually have normal pituitary function because there is gland present, but it is lining the enlarged sella, like the rind of an orange. All patients with empty sella should have clinical assessment for signs and symptoms of pituitary deficiencies. Hyperprolactinemia, the most common pituitary abnormality in empty sella, can be treated with dopamine agonist therapy when needed. Asymptomatic patients should be screened with 8 AM cortisol level measurement, as well as TSH and free $T_4$ measurement. Additional testing should be targeted to the pituitary axes if there are signs or symptoms of deficiency.

Patients with no initial abnormalities are unlikely to develop hormonal or radiologic changes. Because of the theoretical risk of progression, however, it is recommended that asymptomatic patients with empty sella have repeat endocrine, radiologic, and ophthalmologic evaluation in 24 to 36 months. If no progression, further evaluation can be limited to those who require it clinically.

**KEY POINT**

- Empty sella is diagnosed when the sella turcica is enlarged and not entirely filled with pituitary tissue; all patients with empty sella should have clinical assessment for signs and symptoms of pituitary deficiencies.

## Other Abnormalities

The pituitary gland can also be affected by other pathologic processes, such as autoimmune disease, infection, infiltrative diseases, metastatic disease, or infarction (**Table 17**).

## Drug-Induced Abnormalities

There are a number of drugs that can affect pituitary gland function. Any hormone administered exogenously provides negative feedback to the normal cells in the pituitary gland. Exogenous estrogen or testosterone will suppress the gonadotropins, LH and FSH, whereas excess exogenous thyroid hormone will suppress TSH. Likewise, physiologic and supraphysiologic doses of glucocorticoids will suppress ACTH. Opiates have a number of effects. Most notably, chronic opioid use suppresses gonadotroph function, resulting in hypogonadotropic hypogonadism, and is increasingly recognized as a cause of ACTH deficiency.

A relatively new class of drugs, checkpoint-blocking antibodies, has been associated with pituitary abnormalities related to hypophysitis. These drugs, including nivolumab, ipilimumab, tremelimumab, and pembrolizumab, are used to treat metastatic melanoma, renal cell carcinoma, non–small cell lung cancer, and head and neck cancers. Hypophysitis occurs in 0.5% to 5% of patients and often presents with headache and fatigue. Endocrine evaluation usually reveals secondary adrenal insufficiency (ACTH deficiency) and secondary hypothyroidism (TSH deficiency), as well as low levels of LH, GH, and prolactin. Imaging demonstrates enhancement and/or enlargement of the pituitary gland with thickening of the pituitary stalk. Diabetes insipidus is uncommon. Treatment includes replacement of the hormone deficiencies along with high-dose glucocorticoids to treat the inflammatory process. Despite resolution of the inflammation, hormone deficiencies often persist.

## Mass Effects of Pituitary Tumors

Mass effects of pituitary tumors most commonly include compression of the pituitary gland resulting in hormone deficiencies or compression of the optic chiasm most commonly resulting in bitemporal hemianopsia; other patterns of visual loss can also occur. Stalk compression can lead to hyperprolactinemia. Headaches can be a symptom of pituitary tumors but do not correlate well with tumor size. Headache alone is not an indication for surgery.

Pituitary deficiencies related to compression of the gland can vary from an isolated hormone deficiency, most often gonadotropin deficiency, to panhypopituitarism (deficiency of all anterior pituitary hormones).

Similarly, pituitary tumors can have variable effects on compression of surrounding structures. A rapidly growing

**TABLE 17.** Other Pituitary Abnormalities

| Pathology | Cause | Mass Effect | Hormone Abnormalities | Clinical Context |
|---|---|---|---|---|
| **Inflammation** | | | | |
| Lymphocytic hypophysitis | Autoimmune | Possible | Most common is ACTH deficiency | Pregnancy, postpartum |
| **Malignancy** | | | | |
| Pituitary metastasis | Metastasis of malignant tumor to pituitary gland | Optic nerve dysfunction occurs in 24% Can also have cranial nerve palsies and headache | Diabetes insipidus most common Also can have anterior pituitary deficits | Patients with the following primary malignancies: breast (most common), lung, lymphoma, renal cell |
| Pituitary carcinoma (rare) 0.1% of all pituitary tumors | Malignant pituitary tumor | Often present initially as macroadenoma | Most often there is some pituitary hypersecretion rather than deficiency | Patients found to have pituitary adenoma with significant cavernous sinus invasion or suprasellar extension |
| **Infiltrative** | | | | |
| Sarcoidosis | Pituitary infiltration | Possible | Combination of anterior and posterior pituitary abnormalities | Occurs in up to 10% of patients with sarcoidosis |
| Hemochromatosis | Iron deposition | No | Gonadotropin deficiency | *HFE* gene mutation |
| Langerhans cell histiocytosis | Deposition of Langerhans cells within the pituitary gland | No | Diabetes insipidus Less likely anterior pituitary deficiencies | Rarely occur in adults |

ACTH = adrenocorticotropic hormone.

CONT.

pituitary tumor or rapid expansion due to pituitary apoplexy (sudden hemorrhage or infarction of a pituitary adenoma) causing compression of the optic chiasm may result in complete bitemporal hemianopsia or even blindness. Pituitary apoplexy may even result in cranial nerve (CN) palsies of CNs III, IV, and VI, whereas a slowly growing pituitary tumor that abuts the optic chiasm may cause minimal or no loss in peripheral vision. All patients with pituitary tumors that abut or compress the optic chiasm should have an evaluation by an ophthalmologist (preferentially a neuro-ophthalmologist). Any abnormality on visual examination is an indication for surgery, unless the tumor is a prolactinoma.

Pituitary tumors can invade the cavernous sinus but rarely cause mass effect on brain tissue or narrowing of the carotid within the cavernous sinus.

**KEY POINT**

- Mass effects of pituitary tumors most commonly include compression of the pituitary gland resulting in hormone deficiencies or compression of the optic chiasm most commonly resulting in bitemporal hemianopsia; stalk compression can lead to hyperprolactinemia.

### Evaluation of Pituitary Tumors

In patients with a pituitary tumor on CT imaging, a dedicated pituitary MRI with and without contrast with dynamic cuts through the sella should be obtained. A formal visual field examination is required for any tumor that abuts or compresses the optic chiasm.

Pituitary hypersecretion should be ruled out by measurement of prolactin and insulin-like growth factor 1 (IGF-1). Evaluation for Cushing disease is not necessary in patients without signs or symptoms of cortisol excess.

Pituitary tumors can also cause hypopituitarism. Screening for hypopituitarism is recommended in all pituitary tumors regardless of symptoms with measurement of FSH, LH, cortisol, TSH, free thyroxine ($T_4$), and additionally total testosterone in men. Hypogonadotropic hypogonadism can be assessed in premenopausal women through menstrual history. A history of oligomenorrhea or amenorrhea would raise concern for hypogonadotropic hypogonadism and require further hormone testing, whereas a history of normal menses would essentially rule out hypogonadotropic hypogonadism. Abnormal baseline testing may prompt further stimulatory testing to confirm hypopituitarism (**Table 18**), and referral to an endocrinologist is recommended.

If a patient does not require surgical intervention for mass effect or pituitary hypersecretion, repeat pituitary hormone assessment and imaging is performed in 6 months for macroadenomas and then yearly if no change.

Microadenomas should be reassessed with imaging in 1 year and then every 1 to 2 years thereafter. Repeat evaluation of pituitary function is not necessary in microadenomas if initial testing is normal and there has been no change clinically or in the pituitary MRI.

After 3 years of imaging follow up for a pituitary tumor (both microadenomas and macroadenomas), imaging can be performed less frequently, as long as clinical status of the patient remains stable.

**KEY POINTS**

- Pituitary hypersecretion should be ruled out by measurement of prolactin and insulin-like growth factor 1; evaluation for Cushing disease is not necessary in patients without signs or symptoms of cortisol excess. **HVC**

- A history of oligomenorrhea or amenorrhea would raise concern for hypogonadotropic hypogonadism and require further hormone testing, whereas a history of normal menses would essentially rule out hypogonadotropic hypogonadism. **HVC**

### Treatment of Clinically Nonfunctioning Pituitary Tumors

Patients with a nonfunctioning pituitary tumor should be referred for neurosurgical evaluation if any of the following are present: visual deficits related to the tumor, a lesion abuts or compresses the chiasm or optic nerves on pituitary MRI, or pituitary apoplexy with visual disturbance. Surgery should also be considered for a tumor with clinically significant growth, such as growth toward the optic chiasm, and for patients with new loss of endocrine function. Women with a macroadenoma close to the optic chiasm who are planning pregnancy may benefit from surgical decompression of the pituitary tumor due to the risk of enlargement during pregnancy. Microadenomas rarely increase in size during pregnancy. The most common surgical approach for these tumors is transsphenoidal through the nares or mouth. Occasionally, craniotomy is needed for very large tumors. Most nonfunctioning macroadenomas will have immunocytochemistry consistent with a gonadotroph adenoma and are clinically "silent" (without hypersecretion of functional gonadotropins).

**KEY POINTS**

- Patients with a nonfunctioning pituitary tumor should be referred for neurosurgical evaluation if there are visual deficits related to the tumor, a lesion abuts or compresses the chiasm or optic nerves on pituitary MRI, or pituitary apoplexy with visual disturbance is present.

- Surgery should be considered for a tumor with clinically significant growth, such as growth potentially affecting vision, and for patients with new loss of endocrine function.

## Pituitary Hormone Deficiency

Hypopituitarism is defined as one or more pituitary hormone deficiencies. It can occur as a result of compression of the normal pituitary cells by a tumor or as a complication of cranial surgery or radiation therapy. Somatotrophs and gonadotrophs

**TABLE 18.** Dynamic Testing for Pituitary Dysfunction

| Indication | Test | Technique | Interpretation |
|---|---|---|---|
| ACTH (cortisol) deficiency | ACTH stimulation test | Measure baseline serum cortisol level. <br><br> Administer 250 µg of synthetic ACTH IM or IV. <br><br> Measure cortisol levels at 30 and 60 minutes. | Serum cortisol level >18 µg/dL (496.8 nmol/L) at any measurement indicates a normal response. |
| ADH deficiency (DI) | Water deprivation test, followed by desmopressin challenge, if indicated | Patient empties bladder, and baseline weight is measured. <br><br> Measure urine volume and osmolality hourly. <br><br> Measure serum sodium, osmolality, and weight every 2 h. <br><br> *The test is stopped when one of the following occurs:* <br><br> Urine osmolality/plasma osmolality is >2 <br><br> Patient has lost >3% of body weight <br><br> Urine osmolality is stable for 2-3 h while serum osmolality rises <br><br> Plasma osmolality >295 mOsm/kg $H_2O$ <br><br> Serum sodium >145 mEq/L (145 mmol/L) <br><br> *Desmopressin challenge:* <br><br> If final urine osmolality <600 mOsm/kg, serum osmolality >295 mOsm/kg $H_2O$, or serum sodium >145 mEq/L (145 mmol/L): give desmopressin 2 µg subcutaneously. <br><br> Measure urine osmolality and urine volume hourly for 4 hours after desmopressin. | *Water deprivation test interpretation:* <br><br> Urine osmolality >750-800 mOsm/kg $H_2O$ is a normal response to water deprivation, indicating ADH production and peripheral effect are intact. <br><br> Serum osmolality >295 mOsm/kg $H_2O$ and/or serum sodium >145 mEq/L (145 mmol/L) with inappropriately dilute urine (urine osmolality/plasma osmolality <2) is diagnostic of DI. <br><br><br> *Desmopressin challenge interpretation:* <br><br> Urine osmolality >800 mOsm/kg after desmopressin is consistent with complete central DI. <br><br> No increase in urine osmolality (remains <300 mOsm/kg) is diagnostic of complete nephrogenic DI. <br><br> Urine osmolality between 300 and 800 mOsm is consistent with partial DI |
| Growth hormone excess (acromegaly) | Glucose tolerance test | 75-g oral glucose tolerance test. Measure glucose and GH at 0, 30, 60, 90, 120, and 150 minutes. | GH <0.2 ng/mL (0.2 µg/L) is a normal response. GH nadir ≥1.0 ng/mL (1.0 µg/L) (or ≥0.3 ng/mL [0.3 µg/L] on an ultrasensitive assay) is diagnostic of acromegaly. |

ACTH = adrenocorticotropic hormone; ADH = antidiuretic hormone; DI = diabetes insipidus; GH = growth hormone.

appear to be the most sensitive to injury, so GH as well as LH and FSH are the most common pituitary deficiencies. ACTH and TSH deficiency are less common, but more serious.

Pituitary apoplexy and Sheehan syndrome (pituitary infarction associated with postpartum hemorrhage) can cause acute life-threatening hypopituitarism due to ACTH deficiency.

A full list of causes of hypopituitarism can be found in **Table 19**.

## Panhypopituitarism

Panhypopituitarism occurs when a patient lacks adequate production of all anterior pituitary hormones, usually due to a large tumor or complications of pituitary surgery. These patients require daily replacement of thyroxine and cortisol. Replacement of sex steroids and GH is individualized, based on the clinical situation and evaluation of risks and benefits of treatment. Patients with panhypopituitarism should wear

medical alert identification as a deficiency of glucocorticoids can be life threatening.

## Adrenocorticotropic Hormone Deficiency (Secondary Cortisol Deficiency)

The most common cause of adrenocorticotropic hormone (ACTH) deficiency is iatrogenic following administration of exogenous glucocorticoids and suppression of ACTH production. Oral, injectable (intraarticular, intramuscular), and even occasionally topical glucocorticoids can suppress ACTH. Inhaled glucocorticoids attenuate the recovery of endogenous ACTH production but rarely cause suppression of ACTH production directly. Patients with iatrogenic adrenal insufficiency have intact renin-aldosterone systems; they are at lower risk for hypotension and adrenal crisis.

Glucocorticoids prescribed in supraphysiologic doses for 3 weeks or longer should be tapered off to allow recovery of the pituitary-adrenal axis. Once the glucocorticoid dose is

| TABLE 19. | Causes of Hypopituitarism |
|---|---|
| **Neoplastic** | |
| Pituitary adenoma | |
| Meningioma | |
| Craniopharyngioma | |
| Metastatic cancer | |
| Lymphoma | |
| **Infiltrative Disease** | |
| Sarcoidosis | |
| Hemochromatosis | |
| Langerhan cell histiocytosis | |
| **Inflammation** | |
| Lymphocytic hypophysitis | |
| **Iatrogenic** | |
| Surgery | |
| Radiation | |
| **Congenital Deficiencies** | |
| **Vascular** | |
| Pituitary infarction | |
| Pituitary apoplexy | |
| **Empty Sella** | |
| **Hypothalamic Disease** | |
| **Traumatic Brain Injury** | |
| **Medications** | |
| Opiates | |
| Checkpoint inhibitors (nivolumab, ipilimumab, tremelimumab, pembrolizumab) | |

close to physiologic (equivalent of 15-20 mg hydrocortisone), hydrocortisone should be substituted. The dose can then be reduced by 5 mg every 1 to 2 weeks as tolerated. AM-only dosing may facilitate recovery of the adrenal axis.

Once on physiologic AM-only hydrocortisone, the adrenal axis can then be tested for recovery. An 8 AM cortisol level higher than 10 μg/dL (276 nmol/L) after withholding glucocorticoids for 24 hours suggests recovery of the pituitary-adrenal axis. This should be confirmed with an ACTH stimulation test. Despite recovery of the pituitary-adrenal axis, patients may take longer to recover their ability to respond to stress and may require stress-dose or sick-day dosing of glucocorticoids in the setting of an illness for up to a year.

ACTH deficiency can also occur in the setting of damage to the pituitary gland. Symptoms of secondary cortisol deficiency can include fatigue, malaise, weight loss, nausea, vomiting, asymptomatic hypoglycemia, dizziness, and hyponatremia. Because only cortisol production is affected (mineralocorticoid

production is intact), patients do not develop hyperkalemia and are less likely to have hypotension. Furthermore, patients with secondary adrenal insufficiency do not develop hyperpigmentation. Nonetheless, patients with secondary adrenal insufficiency do require physiologic glucocorticoid replacement and stress dosing during illness.

Morning cortisol levels less than 3 μg/dL (82.8 nmol/L) are diagnostic of cortisol deficiency; however, a morning cortisol level greater than 15 μg/dL (414 nmol/L) likely rules it out. Patients with cortisol levels between 3 and 15 μg/dL (82.8-414 nmol/L) should undergo an ACTH stimulation test (see Table 18). A peak cortisol level greater than or equal to 18 μg/dL (496.8 nmol/L) at 0, 30, or 60 minutes rules out cortisol deficiency. Once diagnosed, secondary adrenal insufficiency should be treated with hydrocortisone 15 to 20 mg in two divided doses, such as 10 to 15 mg in the morning and 5 mg in the afternoon. In the setting of an emergency such as pituitary apoplexy, an immediate intravenous dose of 100 mg hydrocortisone should be administered.

Glucocorticoid dosing must be adjusted in the setting of physiologic stress or acute illness. Administering two to three times the baseline dose of cortisol replacement for 2 to 3 days is usually sufficient for minor to moderate illness including minor or moderate surgery. In patients with major physiologic stress including major surgery or active labor, 100 mg hydrocortisone should be administered by intravenous injection followed by a continuous infusion of 200 mg every 24 hours or 50 mg intravenous injection every 6 hours (see Disorders of the Adrenal Glands).

**KEY POINTS**

- The most common cause of adrenocorticotropic hormone deficiency is iatrogenic following administration of exogenous glucocorticoids and suppression of adrenocorticotropic hormone production.  **HVC**

- Glucocorticoids prescribed in greater than physiologic doses for 3 weeks or longer should be tapered off to allow recovery of the pituitary-adrenal axis.

- Glucocorticoid dosing must be adjusted in the setting of physiologic stress or acute illness.

## Thyroid-Stimulating Hormone Deficiency

Deficiency of thyroid-stimulating hormone (TSH) results in the inability of the thyroid gland to produce thyroxine ($T_4$). The result is insufficient $T_4$ production with low or inappropriately normal TSH. The clinical symptoms of secondary hypothyroidism are the same as seen with primary hypothyroidism.

The treatment is daily administration of levothyroxine. TSH cannot be used to monitor therapy and should not be measured. Dosing based on TSH level can lead to underdosing. Free $T_4$ should be used to monitor dose adequacy and should be maintained in the mid to upper half of the normal range. While it takes 6 to 8 weeks for TSH to accurately reflect thyroid hormone status in primary hypothyroidism, free T$_4$ levels can be checked 2 to 3 weeks after a dose change to assess for adequacy in secondary hypothyroidism.

**KEY POINT**

- Treatment of thyroid-stimulating hormone deficiency is daily administration of levothyroxine; only free thyroxine can be used to monitor dose adequacy, and free thyroxine should be maintained in the mid to upper half of the normal range.

## Gonadotropin Deficiency

Gonadotropin deficiency can be a result of pituitary disease or a result of gonadotropin-releasing hormone (GnRH) deficiency as is seen in Kallmann syndrome and hypothalamic amenorrhea. Certain drugs, including opiates, can also suppress GnRH. Deficiency of gonadotropins, LH and FSH, results in deficiency of male and female sex hormones. The combination of low or inappropriately normal LH and FSH with low sex steroids is termed "central" or "hypogonadotropic" hypogonadism.

Treatment of hypogonadotropic hypogonadism can usually be achieved by replacing sex steroids in those with no contraindication and who do not desire fertility; testosterone treatment in men and combined estrogen-progesterone treatment in premenopausal women are used. While oral contraceptive pills may be more acceptable in young women for this purpose, other forms of estrogen and progesterone (such as estradiol patch with cycled oral progesterone) may be preferred in certain cases. In men and women who desire fertility, replacement of gonadotropins is necessary because exogenous testosterone and estrogen suppresses spermatogenesis in men and ovulation in women, respectively.

## Growth Hormone Deficiency

Growth hormone (GH) is necessary for linear growth. Deficiency of GH in children causes short stature. Symptoms of growth hormone deficiency in adults are more subtle and include fatigue, loss of muscle mass, and increased ratio of fatty tissue to lean mass.

While isolated GH deficiency can occur in children, idiopathic isolated GH deficiency in adults is quite rare. Only patients with a history of hypothalamic or pituitary disease, surgery or radiation to these areas, head trauma, or other pituitary hormone deficiencies should be considered for evaluation of adult-onset isolated GH deficiency.

Owing to the pulsatile nature of GH, direct measurement is uninterpretable and GH deficiency should be assessed through measurement of insulin-like growth factor 1 (IGF-1). An IGF-1 level below the normal range for gender and age is highly suggestive of GH deficiency, whereas a normal IGF-1 level does not completely rule out growth hormone deficiency if pretest suspicion is high. Provocative tests such as an insulin tolerance test or GnRH-arginine test can be performed in consultation with an endocrinologist to establish the diagnosis of adult GH deficiency.

Benefits of treatment in those with GH deficiency include improvement in exercise capacity, body composition, and bone density. The decision to start growth hormone replacement should be individualized. It is contraindicated in the setting of malignancy or with an untreated pituitary tumor because of the potential for stimulation of tumor growth. Additionally, caution should be used in those with diabetes mellitus as it may worsen hyperglycemia. When therapy is indicated in adults, GH can be replaced with a low-dose daily injection titrated to a normal IGF-1 level and clinical assessment.

**KEY POINT**

- Idiopathic isolated growth hormone deficiency in adults is rare; only adults with a history of hypothalamic or pituitary disease, surgery or radiation to these areas, head trauma, or other pituitary hormone deficiencies should be evaluated.    **HVC**

## Central Diabetes Insipidus

Inability of the posterior pituitary gland to produce adequate antidiuretic hormone (ADH) results in central diabetes insipidus (DI). Absent antidiuretic hormone (ADH) (complete DI) and reduced ADH (partial DI) prevent the reabsorption of water in the kidneys resulting in polyuria and polydipsia. Although significant hypernatremia is rare in patients with an intact thirst mechanism and free access to water, it can be severe if patients cannot drink to thirst.

An inappropriately low urine osmolality in the setting of an elevated serum osmolality and hypernatremia in a patient with polyuria (>50 mL/kg/24 hours in the absence of glucosuria) is diagnostic of DI. A water deprivation test can be performed when the diagnosis is uncertain (see Table 18).

DI is treated with desmopressin (DDAVP) administered intranasally, orally, or subcutaneously. Bioavailability of oral DDAVP is much lower and doses are considerably higher than with intranasal and subcutaneous routes. Despite this, oral preparations may be preferred in certain circumstances as intranasal absorption of DDAVP may be altered by changes in nasal mucosa. Doses are usually administered once nightly to prevent nocturia and ensure uninterrupted sleep, or twice daily if symptoms interfere with daily function. Caution should be taken to avoid overreplacement as this can result in hyponatremia, water intoxication, and volume overload.

**KEY POINTS**

- An inappropriately low urine osmolality in the setting of an elevated serum osmolality and hypernatremia in a patient with polyuria (>50 mL/kg/24 hours in the absence of glucosuria) is diagnostic of diabetes insipidus.

- Diabetes insipidus is treated with desmopressin administered intranasally, orally, or subcutaneously; caution should be taken to avoid overreplacement as this can result in hyponatremia, water intoxication, and volume overload.

# Pituitary Hormone Excess

Pituitary tumors are considered functional when they secrete pituitary hormones in excess. The most common functional pituitary tumors are prolactinomas. Although pituitary tumors that produce ACTH or GH are less common, they are important to recognize because of the clinical consequences. TSH-secreting adenomas are a very rare cause of hyperthyroidism. Pituitary tumors rarely cosecrete more than one excess hormone. Cosecretion most commonly occurs with GH and prolactin.

## Hyperprolactinemia and Prolactinoma

The most common cause of hyperprolactinemia is physiologic, related to pregnancy and lactation. Physiologic stress, coitus, sleep, and nipple stimulation are other nonpathologic causes of mild hyperprolactinemia. A comprehensive list of causes of hyperprolactinemia is provided in **Table 20**. Symptoms of hyperprolactinemia include amenorrhea, and sometimes galactorrhea, in premenopausal women. Men often present later with symptoms of mass effect or hypogonadism, such as decreased libido or difficulty with erections; less commonly, they experience gynecomastia and breast tenderness.

The most common cause of pathologic non–tumor-related hyperprolactinemia is medications. Of patients taking typical antipsychotics (see Table 20), 40% to 90% will have hyperprolactinemia caused by the dopamine antagonist effect of these medications. While medication-induced hyperprolactinemia most often results in prolactin levels of 25 to 100 ng/mL (25-100 µg/L), drugs such as metoclopramide, risperidone, and phenothiazines can lead to prolactin levels above 200 ng/mL (200 µg/L). Confirming that the hyperprolactinemia is related to medication can be challenging. If possible, the offending medication should be withheld for 3 days to determine whether prolactin levels return to normal.

Discontinuation of any psychotropic drug should be done only in consultation with the patient's psychiatrist. If the medication cannot be withheld and the prolactin elevation cannot be correlated to the timing of the drug initiation, a pituitary MRI should be performed to rule out prolactinoma. Antipsychotic medication-induced hyperprolactinemia is best treated in consultation with the patient's psychiatrist by switching to a drug that is less likely to cause hyperprolactinemia. While asymptomatic hyperprolactinemia related to medication does not require treatment, patients with hypogonadism should be treated with estrogen or testosterone to preserve bone mass. Treating medication-induced hyperprolactinemia with a dopamine agonist (cabergoline or bromocriptine) is controversial as it can exacerbate psychosis.

An MRI of the pituitary is indicated in all patients with unexplained hyperprolactinemia. Assessment and treatment decisions are then based on the prolactin level and MRI findings.

A prolactin level above 500 ng/mL (500 µg/L) is diagnostic of a macroprolactinoma. While levels greater than 250 ng/mL (250 µg/L) are suggestive of a macroprolactinoma, there are some medications that can raise prolactin to this level. Prolactin levels generally correlate with tumor size. Therefore when a macroadenoma is present with a prolactin level below 100 ng/mL (100 µg/L), pituitary stalk compression from a nonfunctioning tumor should be suspected for the cause of the hyperprolactinemia, rather than prolactinoma.

Patients with asymptomatic microadenomas do not require treatment. Women with hypogonadism related to a microadenoma can be treated with a combined oral contraceptive if they do not desire fertility or with a dopamine agonist if they do. Postmenopausal women with microadenomas do not require treatment.

In patients with macroadenomas, dopamine agonist therapy is recommended to lower prolactin, reduce tumor size, and restore gonadal function. Cabergoline is the preferred agent because of its superior efficacy in lowering prolactin and

| TABLE 20. | Causes of Hyperprolactinemia | |
|---|---|---|
| **Physiologic** | **Medication** | **Other** |
| Coitus | Antipsychotics | Chest wall trauma |
| Exercise | Typical antipsychotics | Chronic kidney disease |
| Lactation | Chlorpromazine | |
| Nipple stimulation | Fluphenazine | Cirrhosis |
| | Haloperidol | Cocaine |
| Pregnancy | Prochlorperazine | Empty sella syndrome |
| Sleep | Atypical antipsychotics | Herpes zoster |
| Stress | Amisulpride | Polycystic ovary syndrome |
| | Olanzapine (rarely) | |
| | Paliperidone | Prolactinoma |
| | Risperidone | Seizures |
| | Ziprasidone (rarely) | Severe hypothyroidism |
| | SSRIs | Stalk compression |
| | Citalopram | |
| | Escitalopram | |
| | Fluoxetine | |
| | Paroxetine | |
| | Sertraline | |
| | Antihypertensives | |
| | Methyldopa | |
| | Verapamil | |
| | Other | |
| | Cimetidine | |
| | Domperidone | |
| | Estrogen | |
| | Metoclopramide | |
| | Opiates | |

SSRI = selective serotonin reuptake inhibitor.

tumor shrinkage compared with bromocriptine. In addition, cabergoline dosing is twice per week compared with 1 to 3 times daily for bromocriptine. Prolactin can be monitored 2 to 4 weeks after initiation of therapy and then every 3 to 4 months once stable. MRI should be repeated for a microadenoma in 1 year. If both the tumor and prolactin are stable at 1 year follow up, no further imaging is needed. A macroadenoma should be reimaged 3 months after medical therapy and then every 6 to 12 months until stability is confirmed. Reimaging should be performed if the prolactin level rises despite therapy.

Surgery is not first-line therapy because up to 50% of prolactinomas recur after resection. Surgery should only be considered for prolactinomas in symptomatic patients who cannot tolerate dopamine agonist therapy or whose tumors do not shrink or even grow while on dopamine agonist therapy.

**KEY POINTS**

- HVC • The most common cause of hyperprolactinemia is physiologic, related to pregnancy and lactation.

- HVC • The most common cause of pathologic non–tumor-related hyperprolactinemia is medications.

- HVC • Patients with asymptomatic microadenomas do not require treatment; for patients with macroadenomas, dopamine agonist therapy is recommended to lower prolactin, reduce tumor size, and restore gonadal function.

- HVC • Surgery is not first-line therapy because up to 50% of prolactinomas recur after resection.

## Prolactinomas and Pregnancy

Due to lactotroph hyperplasia in pregnancy, there is concern for enlargement of prolactinomas in pregnancy. Because microadenomas are not likely to enlarge during pregnancy, dopamine agonist therapy should be discontinued when pregnancy is discovered. However, patients who have macroadenomas without prior surgical or radiation therapy have a significant risk of tumor growth. Surgical tumor debulking prior to pregnancy or dopamine agonist therapy throughout pregnancy may be required in these patients. Bromocriptine is the preferred agent in pregnancy.

Patients with macroadenomas should be monitored with visual field testing each trimester while those with microadenomas can be monitored clinically. Headaches or visual field changes should prompt a noncontrast pituitary MRI.

## Acromegaly

Acromegaly is caused by excess secretion of GH from a pituitary tumor in 95% of patients. In fewer than 5% of patients with GH excess, a growth hormone-releasing hormone (GHRH)-secreting tumor or neuroendocrine tumor is the cause of acromegaly. When GH-secreting pituitary tumors are present in children prior to puberty, the result is increased longitudinal growth resulting in gigantism. While gigantism is easily recognized in children, features of excess growth hormone are more subtle in adults, often not recognized for many years. A list of clinical features of acromegaly can be found in **Table 21**.

An IGF-1 level should be obtained to screen for suspected acromegaly. In those with an elevated level, an oral glucose tolerance test should be performed to confirm the diagnosis (see Table 18). A level above 1 ng/mL (1 μg/L) confirms the diagnosis of acromegaly. Once GH excess is demonstrated, a pituitary MRI should be obtained.

Transsphenoidal resection (TSR) of the GH-secreting tumor is the mainstay of therapy. Those who do not achieve remission with surgery can be treated with medical therapy and/or stereotactic radiation. Somatostatin analogues are the medications of choice as they result in reduction of tumor size as well as reduction in GH levels. Pegvisomant, a GH receptor antagonist, can be used in combination with a somatostatin analogue when needed; cabergoline can sometimes be used as well. Stereotactic radiotherapy (gamma knife) is used in certain cases. Once remission is achieved, MRI and IGF-1 levels are followed annually.

Patients with acromegaly can have increased mortality due to heart disease, sleep apnea, and cancer, but risk returns to baseline when IGF-1 is kept in the normal range. Appropriate screening and treatment for comorbidities are as important as managing the IGF-1 level.

| TABLE 21. Features of Acromegaly |
|---|
| **Clinical Signs and Symptoms** |
| Prognathism |
| Macroglossia |
| Wide-spaced teeth (typically the first sign of growth hormone excess) |
| Wide nose |
| Enlarged and swollen hands and feet |
| Increased sweating |
| Skin tags |
| Joint pain |
| Headache |
| **Disease Associations** |
| Sleep apnea |
| Hypertension |
| Insulin resistance |
| Hypertrophic cardiomyopathy |
| Colon polyps and colon cancer |
| Thyroid nodules and thyroid cancer |
| Valvular heart disease |
| Arthropathy |
| Carpal tunnel syndrome |

- An insulin-like growth factor 1 level should be obtained to screen for suspected acromegaly; in those with an elevated level, an oral glucose tolerance test should be performed to confirm the diagnosis followed by a pituitary MRI.
- Transsphenoidal resection of the growth hormone-secreting tumor is the mainstay of therapy; however, somatostatin analogues reduce the tumor size as well as growth hormone levels in those who do not achieve remission with surgery.

## Thyroid-Stimulating Hormone-Secreting Tumors

Thyroid-stimulating hormone (TSH)-secreting pituitary tumors are extremely rare. Signs and symptoms of a TSH-secreting adenoma are those seen in hyperthyroidism, although laboratory evaluation reveals elevated $T_4$ and $T_3$ levels with an inappropriately normal or elevated TSH level. Once other causes of the laboratory abnormalities have been excluded (thyroid assay interference, thyroid hormone resistance, or familial dysalbuminemic hyperthyroxinemia), a pituitary MRI should be performed. TSR of the TSH-producing tumor is the treatment of choice. Medical therapy with somatostatin analogues can be used to control hyperthyroidism prior to surgery and following surgery in those who do not achieve remission.

## Excess Antidiuretic Hormone Secretion

The syndrome of inappropriate antidiuretic hormone secretion (SIADH) results in water retention with resultant hyponatremia, often severe. CNS disorders (trauma, stroke, brain metastases, infection) drugs, pulmonary disease, and pituitary surgery (3-7 days postoperatively) can result in excess release of ADH. SIADH is a diagnosis of exclusion. Treatment involves correcting the underlying pathology, fluid restriction, vasopressin receptor antagonists, and hypertonic saline in severe hyponatremia. If hypertonic saline is being considered, consultation with an endocrinologist or nephrologist is recommended (see MKSAP 18 Nephrology).

## Excess Adrenocorticotropic Hormone from Pituitary Source (Cushing Disease)

Cushing syndrome is a term used to describe hypercortisolism regardless of the cause; Cushing disease (the most common cause of endogenous Cushing syndrome) is the term used to describe hypercortisolism as a result of excess ACTH secretion from a pituitary tumor. Symptoms and signs of Cushing syndrome are listed in **Table 22**.

The diagnosis of Cushing syndrome is made by first establishing evidence of hypercortisolism (see Disorders of Adrenal Glands). Measuring ACTH establishes whether it is ACTH-dependent or ACTH-independent.

Once diagnosis of ACTH-dependent Cushing syndrome is established, a pituitary MRI should be performed for

| TABLE 22. Symptoms and Signs of Cushing Syndrome |
|---|
| **Symptoms** |
| Depression |
| Fatigue |
| Rapid weight gain |
| Decreased libido |
| Menstrual abnormalities |
| **Signs** |
| Striae (especially if reddish purple and >1 cm in width)[a] |
| Easy bruising[a] |
| Facial plethora[a] |
| Muscle weakness (proximal myopathy) |
| Abdominal obesity |
| Skin tears (secondary to thinning of the epidermis) |
| Acne |
| Hirsutism |
| Dorsocervical fat pad (buffalo hump)[a] |
| Supraclavicular fad pad[a] |
| Hypokalemia |
| Hypertension |
| Diabetes |

[a]Features that best discriminate Cushing syndrome from the general population.

confirmation. If no pituitary tumor is seen or if the tumor is less than 6 mm, a high-dose 8-mg dexamethasone suppression test (DST) is done to evaluate for the presence of an ectopic ACTH-producing tumor (lung, pancreas, thymus carcinoma most commonly), which is highly resistant to dexamethasone suppression. Inferior petrosal sinus sampling (IPSS) is often recommended prior to TSR to confirm a pituitary source of ACTH excess due to low sensitivity and specificity of the high-dose DST.

The treatment of choice is TSR of the pituitary adenoma. Remission is generally defined by a morning serum cortisol level less than 5 µg/dL (138 nmol/L) within 7 days of surgery. Patients require glucocorticoid replacement postoperatively until the normal corticotroph cells recover from prolonged cortisol suppression. Recovery can take up to a year, and occasionally there is no recovery and the patient will require life-long cortisol replacement therapy.

If remission is not achieved following surgery, radiation or medical therapy (**Table 23**) may be required. Rarely, bilateral adrenalectomy is needed in patients unresponsive to all other therapies; these patients will require life-long glucocorticoid and mineralocorticoid replacement for acquired primary adrenal insufficiency. In addition, there is the risk of pituitary tumor enlargement following adrenalectomy (Nelson syndrome) due to unfettered stimulation of ACTH production.

Patients with Cushing disease require imaging and biochemical follow-up (urine free cortisol or late-night salivary

**TABLE 23.** Medication Management for Treatment of Cushing Syndrome

| Steroidogenesis Inhibitors (Inhibits Cortisol Synthesis) | Pituitary Directed (Inhibits ACTH Secretion) | Glucocorticoid Receptor Antagonist (Inhibits Cortisol Action) |
|---|---|---|
| Ketoconazole | Pasireotide | Mifepristone |
| Metyrapone | Cabergoline | |
| Mitotane | | |
| Etomidate | | |

ACTH = adrenocorticotropic hormone.

cortisol measurement) every year for several years, and then on a less frequent basis. The first biochemical sign of recurrence is often elevated late-night salivary cortisol levels. Recurrences are managed by repeat TSR, radiation, and/or medical therapy.

**KEY POINTS**

- The diagnosis of Cushing syndrome is made by first establishing evidence of hypercortisolism; once adrenocorticotropic hormone–dependent Cushing disease is confirmed, a pituitary MRI should be performed.
- The treatment of choice for adrenocorticotropic hormone–dependent Cushing disease is transsphenoidal resection of the pituitary adenoma, followed by glucocorticoid replacement until the normal corticotroph cells recover from cortisol suppression.

# Disorders of the Adrenal Glands

## Adrenal Anatomy and Physiology

Although considered one organ, the adrenal glands have two functionally distinct regions: an outer cortex and an inner medulla. The cortex secretes hormones that are classified as mineralocorticoid (aldosterone), glucocorticoid (cortisol), and androgen (dehydroepiandrosterone [DHEA]). The medulla secretes catecholamines.

The adrenal cortex is composed of three zones: the zona glomerulosa (outer), zona fasciculate (middle), and zona reticularis (inner). Aldosterone production in the zona glomerulosa is regulated by the renin-angiotensin system and promotes sodium reabsorption and potassium excretion across the distal tubule of the kidney. The resultant expansion of extracellular volume increases blood pressure. Aldosterone also has direct inflammatory and fibrotic effects on other organs that are independent of its effects on blood pressure. Major stimuli to aldosterone secretion include hypotension, hypovolemia, and hyperkalemia.

Cortisol production in the zona fasciculata is regulated by release of adrenocorticotropic hormone (ACTH) from the pituitary gland. Cortisol exhibits a distinct diurnal rhythm characterized by peak levels on awakening that decrease to very low levels by bedtime. Superimposed on this diurnal rhythm are small oscillations of cortisol secretion while awake. Most cortisol circulates in the blood attached to cortisol-binding protein, with only a small fraction circulating as biologically active, free hormone. Cortisol is crucial to the body's adaptive response to physiologic stress, and levels increase in response to psychological stress, as well as physical illness. Cortisol actions are diverse and include immune, vascular, anti-inflammatory, and metabolic effects.

DHEA, produced in the zona reticularis, and its sulfate DHEAS, are weak adrenal androgens that mediate their effects through peripheral conversion to testosterone. In women the adrenal gland is a significant contributor to circulating androgen levels. In men the adrenal contribution to androgen effect is negligible.

The adrenal medulla secretes the catecholamines norepinephrine and epinephrine in response to hypotension, hypoglycemia, fear, anxiety, acute illness, and other causes of psychological and physical stress. Catecholamines interact with α- and β-adrenergic receptors to increase pulse and blood pressure, relax smooth muscle, dilate bronchioles, and increase metabolic rate. A small fraction of norepinephrine and epinephrine is excreted in the urine as free hormone; the rest is degraded in the liver to metanephrine and normetanephrine prior to urinary excretion.

## Adrenal Hormone Excess
### Cortisol Excess (Cushing Syndrome Due to Adrenal Mass)

Cortisol-secreting adrenal adenomas and, rarely, carcinomas account for 20% of endogenous causes of Cushing syndrome. Excess cortisol secretion from these tumors suppresses ACTH production from the pituitary gland, resulting in a form of Cushing syndrome classified as ACTH-independent. ACTH-dependent Cushing syndrome is more common and is most commonly caused by pituitary adenomas (see Disorders of the Pituitary Gland). While many of the symptoms and signs of Cushing syndrome are common in the general population, some, including supraclavicular fat pads, proximal muscle weakness, facial plethora, and wide violaceous striae (**Figure 3**), are considered more discriminatory (see Disorders of the Pituitary Gland). Diagnosis of Cushing syndrome is challenging because patients present along a spectrum ranging from mild disease with subtle findings to severe, life-threatening disease. In addition, hypercortisolemia from psychological stress and physical illness can also occur in the absence of Cushing syndrome. In severe stress states such as major depression, anxiety, psychosis, poorly controlled diabetes mellitus, and severe visceral obesity, a pseudo-Cushing state may occur in which

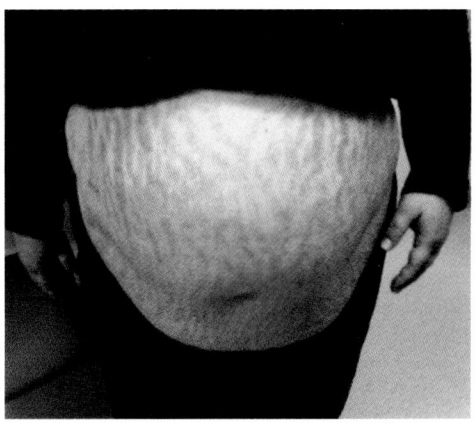

**FIGURE 3.** Wide violaceous striae are seen on the abdomen of a patient with Cushing syndrome. Striae larger than 1 cm in width are highly specific for hypercortisolism.

hypercortisolemia and nonspecific clinical features of Cushing syndrome coexist.

Evaluation for Cushing syndrome in patients without specific signs of Cushing syndrome is not recommended.

The evaluation of Cushing syndrome involves (1) initial testing followed by confirmatory testing for Cushing syndrome; (2) determining Cushing syndrome as ACTH-independent or -dependent; and (3) localizing the source of ACTH in ACTH-dependent disease or confirming the presence of adrenal mass (or masses) in ACTH-independent disease. It is imperative that biochemical Cushing syndrome be confirmed with certainty prior to looking for the source, as misdiagnosis may lead to unnecessary testing and treatment.

The diagnosis of Cushing syndrome necessitates a combination and repetition of tests (**Figure 4**). Measurement of morning or random serum cortisol is unreliable, due to

overlap of serum cortisol levels among normal patients, those with Cushing syndrome, and those with mild hypercortisolism/pseudo-Cushing state in the absence of Cushing syndrome. In addition, total cortisol levels are unreliable when binding proteins are affected by oral estrogen, acute illness, and low protein states.

Initial tests for Cushing syndrome have similar diagnostic accuracy and include measurement of 24-hour urine free cortisol, serial late night salivary cortisols, and the 1-mg overnight dexamethasone suppression test. When suspicion for Cushing syndrome is low, a single test, if negative, makes Cushing syndrome unlikely. When there is a higher index of suspicion for Cushing syndrome, two different initial tests are recommended.

Urine free cortisol and late night salivary cortisol represent the serum free cortisol fraction and avoid pitfalls in interpretation related to changes in cortisol-binding proteins. Spurious elevation of urine free cortisol can result from hypercortisolemia not related to Cushing syndrome/pseudo-Cushing state or when significant polyuria (>5 L/d) is present. False-negative results can occur in advanced kidney disease or in patients with variable secretory rates of cortisol.

Late-night salivary cortisol is collected at home by the patient between 11 PM and midnight on at least two different nights. This test assesses for the normal diurnal rhythm of cortisol, which is lost in Cushing syndrome, and the cortisol level will not be low as expected. This test is not recommended in patients who do shift work or have an inconsistent sleep pattern. Recent cigarette smoking or contamination of the sample by topical glucocorticoids can falsely increase results.

The 1-mg (low-dose) dexamethasone suppression test depends on the principle that autonomous cortisol secretion is not subject to feedback suppression with exogenous glucocorticoids. Dexamethasone is taken at 11 PM and serum total cortisol is measured at 8 AM the following morning.

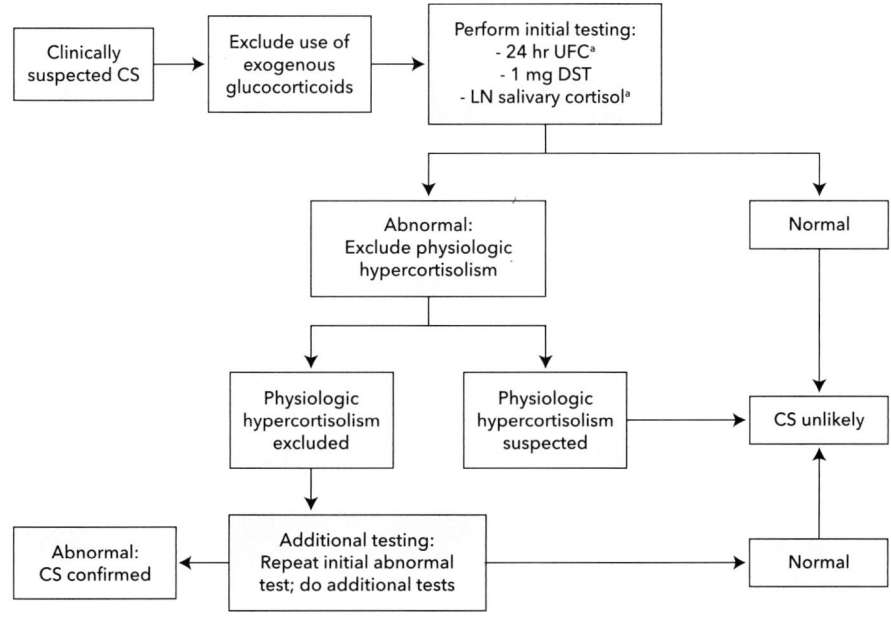

**FIGURE 4.** Algorithm to confirm or rule out the diagnosis of Cushing syndrome. CS = Cushing syndrome; DST = dexamethasone suppression test; LN salivary cortisol = late-night salivary cortisol; UFC = urine free cortisol.

ªMust be performed at least twice.

A post-dexamethasone cortisol level of greater than 5 μg/dL (138 nmol/L) is considered a positive test. A lower cut-off cortisol value of greater than 1.8 μg/dL (49.7 nmol/L) has been advocated to improve test sensitivity, but this occurs at the expense of reduced specificity. False-positive results may occur with concomitant use of medications (carbamazepine, phenytoin, and pioglitazone) that induce hepatic CYP3A4 enzymes and accelerate dexamethasone metabolism. Simultaneous measurement of serum dexamethasone can confirm patient adherence or altered dexamethasone metabolism.

Many factors can raise cortisol levels in the absence of Cushing syndrome, so test interpretation should incorporate the pretest probability of Cushing syndrome. A urine free cortisol level greater than 3 times the upper normal range in the setting of clinical manifestations of Cushing syndrome is considered diagnostic of the disorder, whereas a positive test in the setting of low suspicion for Cushing syndrome does not support the diagnosis. If initial testing is positive, confirmation and further evaluation should involve consultation with an endocrinologist. Once the diagnosis of Cushing syndrome is established, the next step is measurement of ACTH; if suppressed (<5 pg/mL [1.1 pmol/L]) indicating an ACTH-independent cause of Cushing syndrome, a dedicated adrenal CT or MRI is indicated. If adrenal glands appear normal on imaging, the diagnosis of Cushing syndrome should be questioned.

Surgical resection is the definitive treatment for benign and malignant cortisol-secreting adrenal tumors.

Following adrenalectomy, patients require daily hydrocortisone therapy to allow recovery from prolonged ACTH suppression due to hypercortisolism. Recovery of adrenal fasciculate function may take up to 1 year or longer depending on the severity of Cushing syndrome (see Disorders of the Pituitary Gland).

### KEY POINTS

- The evaluation of Cushing syndrome involves (1) initial testing followed by confirmatory testing for Cushing syndrome; (2) determining Cushing syndrome as adrenocorticotropic hormone (ACTH)-independent or -dependent; and (3) localizing the source of ACTH in ACTH-dependent disease or confirming the presence of adrenal mass (or masses) in ACTH-independent disease.

- Initial tests for Cushing syndrome have similar diagnostic accuracy and include measurement of 24-hour urine free cortisol, serial late-night salivary cortisols, and the 1-mg overnight dexamethasone suppression test.

**HVC** - Evaluation for Cushing syndrome in patients without specific signs of Cushing syndrome is not recommended.

## Primary Aldosteronism

Primary aldosteronism (PA) is a common cause of secondary hypertension. Traditionally, hypokalemia was considered to be a biochemical prerequisite for the diagnosis of PA, but it is now recognized that more than 60% of patients have normal potassium levels. As hypertension is often the only sign of primary aldosteronism, the condition frequently goes undiagnosed. Identification of patients with primary aldosteronism is important because aldosterone has deleterious effects on the cardiovascular system and treatment prevents progression and can sometimes reverse changes. Higher cardiovascular morbidity and mortality have been noted in patients with primary aldosteronism compared to those with primary hypertension with similar blood pressure control. The potential health impact of untreated primary aldosteronism and the importance of recognizing primary aldosteronism is reflected in updated guidelines on case-detection testing for primary aldosteronism (**Table 24**).

Primary aldosteronism is caused by hyperplasia of both adrenal glands (idiopathic hyperaldosteronism) in two-thirds of cases, and a unilateral aldosterone-producing adenoma (APA) in one-third of cases. The diagnosis of primary aldosteronism involves performing stepwise case detection, as well as confirmatory and localization studies. The most reliable case-detection test is calculation of an plasma aldosterone-plasma renin ratio (ARR) by measuring plasma aldosterone concentration and plasma renin activity (or

**TABLE 24.** Case Detection Indications for Primary Aldosteronism and Pheochromocytoma

**Primary Aldosteronism**

Untreated hypertension with sustained BP >150/100 mm Hg

Hypertension (>140/90 mm Hg) on three-drug therapy

Hypertension and an incidentally discovered adrenal mass

Hypertension associated with spontaneous or diuretic-induced hypokalemia

Hypertension in the setting of a first-degree relative with PA

Hypertension in the setting of family history of hypertension onset age <40 years

**Pheochromocytoma**

Adrenergic-type spells (headache, sweating, and tachycardia) with or without hypertension

Incidentally discovered adrenal mass with or without hypertension

Hypertension (>140/90 mm Hg) on three-drug therapy

Hypertension with onset age <20 years

Idiopathic cardiomyopathy

Hypertensive episode induced by anesthesia, surgery, or angiography

Paraganglioma

Familial syndromes that predispose to pheochromocytoma: VHL, NF-1, and MEN 2

Family history of pheochromocytoma or paraganglioma

BP = blood pressure; MEN 2 = multiple endocrine neoplasia type 2; NF-1 = neurofibromatosis type 1; PA = primary aldosteronism; VHL = von Hippel-Lindau.

direct renin concentration) in a mid-morning seated sample. In patients taking an ACE inhibitor or an angiotensin receptor blocker, renin should be elevated, so in these patients, a simple initial test is plasma renin activity measurement. If the plasma renin activity is suppressed, the likelihood of primary aldosteronism is high and an ARR should be performed; if not, hyperaldosterone state is ruled out. Mineralocorticoid receptor antagonists (spironolactone and eplerenone) and high-dose amiloride can significantly interfere with interpretation of ARR and should be discontinued 6 weeks prior to evaluation.

Other antihypertensive agents can be continued, but because some may have minor effects on aldosterone and/or renin levels (**Table 25**), the results of the ARR should be interpreted with these effects in mind. Hydralazine, a selective α-adrenergic receptor blocker, and slow-release verapamil have minimal effects on aldosterone and renin secretion, and they can be substituted when feasible for other agents if the ARR is equivocal. An ARR greater than 20 with a plasma aldosterone concentration of at least 15 ng/dL (414 pmol/L) is considered a positive result, and patients should be referred to an endocrinologist, who may perform additional testing to confirm inappropriate aldosterone secretion in a salt-replete state.

The localization study of choice for primary aldosteronism is a dedicated adrenal CT. Findings may include normal adrenal glands or unilateral or bilateral adenoma(s)/hyperplasia. In one third of patients, the CT may not identify the cause of primary aldosteronism because some APAs are too small to see or there is an incidental adrenal mass unrelated to primary aldosteronism. Consequently, most patients with confirmed primary aldosteronism should undergo adrenal vein sampling to confirm the source of the hyperaldosteronism.

Medical therapy with an aldosterone receptor antagonist (spironolactone or eplerenone) is the treatment of choice for primary aldosteronism due to idiopathic hyperaldosteronism, or when patients with APA are not candidates for, or do not wish to undergo, surgery. Spironolactone is often preferred over eplerenone because it is less expensive and more potent. However, patients on spironolactone are more likely to develop dose-dependent side effects of gynecomastia and erectile dysfunction in men and menstrual irregularities in women. Hypokalemia almost always resolves with treatment, but blood pressure control may require additional agents. No studies clearly show superiority of adrenalectomy compared to medical therapy for APA, but surgery may be more cost-effective in the long term.

Laparoscopic adrenalectomy is effective for unilateral disease and reduces plasma aldosterone and its attendant increased risk of cardiovascular disease. Hypertension is improved in most patients and cured in about 40% of patients. Persistent hypertension following adrenalectomy may be due to vascular changes caused by chronic hypertension or coexistent primary hypertension. Patients are more likely to achieve resolution of hypertension if they were taking fewer than three antihypertensive agents preoperatively, and if they have one or fewer first-degree relatives with hypertension. Serum potassium should be monitored weekly for the first month postoperatively, and patients should be instructed to eat a high-salt diet due to risk of hyperkalemia from transient reduction in aldosterone production in the remaining adrenal gland due to chronic suppression of the renin-angiotensin system during the period of hyperaldosteronism. Short-term mineralocorticoid replacement is required in those patients who develop hyperkalemia.

**KEY POINTS**

- The most reliable case-detection test for primary aldosteronism is calculation of a plasma aldosterone-plasma renin ratio by measuring plasma aldosterone concentration and plasma renin activity (or direct renin concentration) in a mid-morning seated sample; if the plasma renin activity is suppressed, the likelihood of primary aldosteronism is high.

- In patients taking an ACE inhibitor or an angiotensin receptor blocker, renin should be elevated, so in these patients, a simple initial test is a plasma renin activity measurement; if the plasma renin activity is suppressed, the likelihood of primary aldosteronism is high and a plasma aldosterone-plasma renin ratio should be performed; if not, hyperaldosterone state is ruled out.  **HVC**

*(Continued)*

| TABLE 25. The Effect of Commonly Prescribed Medications on Measurements of Plasma Renin Activity and Plasma Aldosterone Concentration | | | | |
|---|---|---|---|---|
| **Effect on Test Results** | **Medication Class** | **PRA** | **PAC** | **PAC/ PRA** |
| False-Positive | α$_2$-Adrenoceptor agonist | ↓↓ | ↓ | ↑ |
| | β-Adrenoceptor blocker | ↓↓ | ↓ | ↑ |
| | Direct renin inhibitor | ↓ | ↓ | ↑ |
| | NSAID | ↓↓ | ↓ | ↑ |
| False-Negative | ACE inhibitor/ARB | ↑↑ | ↓ | ↓ |
| | Dihydropyridine CCB | ↑ | ↓ | ↓ |
| | Diuretic[a] | ↑↑ | ↑ | ↓ |
| | Mineralocorticoid receptor antagonist | ↑↑ | ↑ | ↓ |
| | SSRI | | ↑ | ↓ |

ARB = angiotensin receptor antagonist; CCB = calcium channel blocker; PAC = plasma aldosterone concentration; PRA = plasma renin activity; SSRI = selective serotonin reuptake inhibitor.

[a]Both potassium-sparing (amiloride) and potassium-wasting (hydrochlorothiazide) diuretics.

- Laparoscopic adrenalectomy for unilateral disease results in reduction of plasma aldosterone; medical therapy with an aldosterone receptor antagonist (spironolactone or eplerenone) is the treatment of choice for primary aldosteronism due to idiopathic hyperaldosteronism, or when patients with aldosterone-producing adenoma are not candidates for, or do not wish to undergo, surgery.

## Pheochromocytoma and Paraganglioma

Pheochromocytomas and paragangliomas are catecholamine-secreting tumors that arise from chromaffin cells of the adrenal medulla (80%) and extra-adrenal (mostly abdominal) sympathetic ganglia, respectively. Tumors can also arise from parasympathetic ganglia in the head and neck, but these rarely secrete catecholamines.

At least one-third of pheochromocytomas/paragangliomas are associated with a germline mutation. Pheochromocytomas may occur in familial syndromes including multiple endocrine neoplasia type 2, von Hippel-Lindau syndrome, and neurofibromatosis type 2 (**Table 26**). All patients with catecholamine-secreting tumors should, therefore, be offered genetic counseling.

Hypertension associated with pheochromocytoma/paraganglioma can show a sustained pattern, with or without paroxysms, or occur as paroxysms only. Some patients (10% to 15%) remain normotensive. The classic triad of palpitations, headache, and diaphoresis is seen in fewer than 50% of patients with pheochromocytoma. Multiple symptoms related to catecholamine excess can occur including abdominal pain, skin pallor, blurred vision, or polyuria. Rarely, patients can present with acute myocardial infarction, cardiomyopathy, or stroke.

Indications for testing for pheochromocytoma are shown in Table 24. Initial tests for pheochromocytoma include measurement of plasma-free metanephrine collected in a supine position or 24-hour urine fractionated metanephrine and catecholamine levels. Elevation in catecholamines can occur in patients under psychological or physical stress. Medications can affect results (**Table 27**) and should be discontinued at least 2 weeks prior to testing. Accurate diagnosis is further confounded by the fact that patients with or without hypertension may have adrenergic-type spells in the absence of a catecholamine-secreting tumor. Interpretation of the test results must consider the extent of metanephrine elevation rather than whether the result is normal or abnormal. Mild elevations may require repeat testing. Levels more than four times the upper limit of normal, in the absence of acute stress or illness, are consistent with a catecholamine-secreting tumor. The plasma-free metanephrine is highly sensitive (96% to 100%). The specificity is 85% to 89%. Urine fractionated metanephrine and catecholamines have higher specificity (98%) and high sensitivity (up to 97%). Neither test is superior, so clinicians can use an estimate of pretest probability to select the initial test. When there is a high index of suspicion, plasma-free metanephrine is chosen, and when suspicion is low, urine fractionated metanephrine and catecholamines may be a better option.

The search for a tumor should begin when a biochemical diagnosis of pheochromocytoma/paraganglioma is supported by laboratory results, to avoid misdiagnosing an incidental nonfunctioning adrenal mass as a pheochromocytoma. It is difficult to determine clinical relevance of significantly elevated metanephrine levels in hospitalized patients. The imaging modality of choice is an abdominal and pelvic contrast-enhanced CT as 85% of catecholamine-secreting tumors are intra-adrenal (and 95% reside in the abdomen or pelvis). Typical imaging features of pheochromocytomas are shown in **Table 28**. The average size of a symptomatic pheochromocytoma at diagnosis is 4 cm. If the CT is negative, reconsidering the diagnosis is the first step; however, if suspicion of a catecholamine-secreting tumor is high, the

| TABLE 26. | Multiple Endocrine Neoplasm Syndromes | | |
|---|---|---|---|
| **Type** | **Mutation** | **Most Common Feature** | **Associated Features** |
| 1 | *MEN1*<br><br>(inheritance of one mutated allele with somatic mutation in other allele leads to neoplasia) | Parathyroid adenoma (often multiple) | Pancreatic islet cell and enteric tumors (gastrinoma, insulinoma most common)<br><br>Pituitary adenoma<br><br>Other (carcinoid tumors, adrenocortical adenoma) |
| 2A | *RET*<br><br>(exon 11, codon 634[a]) | Medullary thyroid carcinoma | Pheochromocytoma (often multifocal)<br><br>Parathyroid hyperplasia |
| 2B | *RET*<br><br>(exon 16, codon 918[a]) | Medullary thyroid carcinoma | Pheochromocytoma (often multifocal)<br><br>Mucosal neuroma<br><br>Gastrointestinal ganglioneuroma<br><br>Marfanoid body habitus |
| [a]Most common mutation observed. | | | |

**TABLE 27. Substances Associated with False-Positive Biochemical Testing for Pheochromocytoma**

| Drug Class | Medication/Substance |
|---|---|
| Analgesics | Acetaminophen |
| Antiemetics | Prochlorperazine |
| Antihypertensives | Phenoxybenzamine[a] |
| Psychiatric medications | Antipsychotics |
| | Buspirone |
| | Monoamine oxidase inhibitors |
| | Serotonin norepinephrine reuptake inhibitors (SNRIs) |
| | Tricyclic antidepressants[a] |
| Stimulants | Amphetamines |
| | Methylphenidate |
| | Cocaine |
| | Caffeine |
| Other agents | Levodopa |
| | Decongestants (pseudoephedrine) |
| | Reserpine |
| Withdrawal | Clonidine |
| | Ethanol |
| | Illicit drugs |

[a]Most likely to cause false-positive results.

next step is iodine 123 ($^{123}$I)-metaiodobenzylguanidine scanning. This test may also be indicated in patients with very large pheochromocytomas (>10 cm) to detect metastatic disease or paragangliomas to detect multiple tumors. Fludeoxyglucose-position emission tomography is more sensitive for detection of metastatic disease, but its use is generally reserved for those patients with established malignant tumors.

The definitive treatment for pheochromocytoma/paraganglioma is surgical resection. Preoperative β-receptor blockade with phenoxybenzamine for 10 to 14 days before surgery is essential to prevent hypertensive crises during surgery. The dose is progressively increased to achieve a blood pressure of 130/80 mm Hg or less and pulse of 60 to 70/min seated, and systolic pressure of 90 mm Hg or higher with pulse of 70 to 80/min standing. Side effects include dizziness, nasal congestion, and fatigue. To facilitate dose escalation and mitigate the volume contraction effects of α-receptor blockade, patients are instructed to liberalize their salt and fluid intake. A β-blocker is added once α-blockade is achieved to manage reflex tachycardia, but it should never be started prior to adequate α-blockade because unopposed α-adrenergic vasoconstriction can result in a hypertensive crisis.

For large pheochromocytomas with a high hormone secretion rate, other agents such as a calcium channel blocker and/or metyrosine are added to the treatment regimen. Calcium channel blockers can also be used in patients who develop significant hypotension on small doses of α-blocker. Selective α-1 receptor blockers such as doxazosin can be used as an alternative to phenoxybenzamine if availability or lack of insurance coverage of the latter is a problem. Postoperatively, patients can have significant hypotension, and most require fluid and vasopressor support at least briefly in the

**TABLE 28. Typical Imaging Characteristics of Adrenal Masses**

| Adrenal Mass | Overall | CT | MRI Signal Intensity[a] |
|---|---|---|---|
| Adrenal adenoma | Diameter <4 cm<br>Homogeneous enhancement[b]<br>Round, clear margins | Density <10 HU<br>Contrast washout >50% (10 min) | Isointense on T2-weighted images |
| Adrenocortical carcinoma | Usually >4 cm<br>Heterogeneous enhancement[b]<br>Irregular margins<br>Calcifications, necrosis | Density >10 HU<br>Contrast washout <50% (10 min) | Hyperintense on T2-weighted images |
| Pheochromocytoma | Variable size<br>Heterogeneous enhancement[b], cystic areas<br>Round, clear margins<br>Can be bilateral | Density >10 HU<br>Contrast washout <50% (10 min) | Hyperintense on T2-weighted images |
| Metastases | Variable margins<br>Can be bilateral | Density >10 HU<br>Contrast washout <50% (10 min) | Hyperintense on T2-weighted images |

HU = Hounsfield units (measure of radiodensity compared with water).

[a]Signal intensity as compared with liver.

[b]Enhancement following intravenous contrast administration.

**CONT.**

postoperative period. Patients with pheochromocytoma may have impaired fasting glucose or type 2 diabetes related to insulin resistance induced by catecholamine excess. This can improve or reverse following adrenalectomy. **H**

Approximately 83% of pheochromocytomas/paragangliomas are benign. Pathologic findings do not predict which tumors will become malignant and develop metastases. Since metastases can occur decades after the initial diagnosis, patients should undergo long-term annual biochemical screening, typically with plasma-free metanephrine.

**KEY POINTS**

- Initial tests for pheochromocytoma include measurement of plasma free metanephrine levels or 24-hour urine fractionated metanephrine and catecholamine levels; certain medications can affect results and need to be discontinued at least 2 weeks prior to testing.

- The search for a tumor should begin when a biochemical diagnosis of pheochromocytoma/paraganglioma is clear in laboratory results, to avoid misdiagnosing an incidental nonfunctioning adrenal mass as a pheochromocytoma.

- The definitive treatment for pheochromocytoma/paraganglioma is surgical resection; preoperative α-blockade with phenoxybenzamine is essential to prevent hypertensive crises during surgery.

**HVC**
- Selective α-1 receptor blockers such as doxazosin can be used as an alternative to phenoxybenzamine if availability or lack of insurance coverage of the latter is a problem.

## Androgen-Producing Adrenal Tumors

Androgen-producing adrenal tumors are rare and lead to menstrual irregularities and virilization in women including hirsutism, voice-deepening, increased muscle mass, increased libido, and clitoromegaly. Tumors secrete DHEA/DHEAS and androstenedione, which are subsequently converted to testosterone in the periphery. DHEAS-secreting tumors of the adrenal gland are readily visible on CT imaging, and adrenal vein sampling to localize the tumor is rarely required. Approximately 50% are benign, and the treatment of choice is resection.

# Adrenal Hormone Deficiency
## Primary Adrenal Insufficiency
### Causes and Clinical Features

Primary adrenal insufficiency (AI) is a life-threatening disorder that often presents with insidious onset of symptoms making diagnosis a challenge (**Table 29**). It may also present as adrenal crisis, often precipitated by an acute illness or the initiation of thyroid hormone replacement in a patient with unrecognized chronic AI. Although skin hyperpigmentation from stimulation of melanocytes by high ACTH levels is considered a hallmark of primary adrenal insufficiency, it is not present in approximately 5% patients. The most common cause of primary adrenal insufficiency is autoimmune destruction of all layers of the adrenal cortex leading to progressive mineralocorticoid, glucocorticoid, and adrenal androgen deficiency. Most patients have positive 21-hydroxylase antibodies, and approximately 50% will develop another autoimmune

| **TABLE 29.** Clinical and Laboratory Manifestations of Primary Adrenal Failure | | | |
|---|---|---|---|
| **Hormone Deficiency** | **Symptoms** | **Signs** | **Laboratory Findings** |
| Cortisol | Fatigue | Hyperpigmentation[b] (palmar creases, extensor surfaces, buccal mucosa) | ↓ Serum cortisol |
| | Weakness | Decrease in BP | ↑ Plasma ACTH |
| | Low-grade fever | | ↓ Serum sodium[c] |
| | Weight loss | | ↓ Plasma glucose[d] |
| | Anorexia | | |
| | Nausea/vomiting | | |
| | Abdominal pain | | |
| | Arthralgia | | |
| | Myalgia | | |
| Aldosterone | Salt craving | Orthostasis | ↑ PRA |
| | Dizziness | Hypotension | ↓ Serum sodium |
| | | | ↑ Serum potassium |
| DHEAS | Reduced libido[a] | Decreased axillary or pubic hair[a] | ↓ Serum DHEAS |

ACTH = adrenocorticotropic hormone; BP = blood pressure; DHEAS = dehydroepiandrosterone sulfate; PRA = plasma renin activity.

[a]Women only.

[b]Occurs exclusively in primary adrenal failure.

[c]Cortisol inhibits the secretion of antidiuretic hormone (ADH), so hypocortisolemia will lead to increased secretion of ADH and hyponatremia.

[d]Rare in adults.

endocrine disorder in their lifetime (primary hypothyroidism, primary ovarian insufficiency, celiac disease, hypoparathyroidism, or type 1 diabetes mellitus).

Primary adrenal insufficiency can also be caused by infiltrative disorders such as infection (tuberculosis, fungal infections), sarcoidosis, and lymphoma, which result in bilateral adrenal gland enlargement. Metastatic disease involving the adrenals, most commonly from lung cancer, renal cell carcinoma, and melanoma rarely leads to adrenal insufficiency even if both adrenal glands are involved.

Bilateral adrenal hemorrhage can present as acute adrenal insufficiency and should be considered if unexpected hypotension develops. Risk factors for bilateral adrenal hemorrhage include protein C deficiency, anticoagulation, disseminated intravascular coagulopathy, and sepsis.

### Diagnosis

An algorithm for the diagnosis of adrenal insufficiency is outlined in **Figure 5**. Initial evaluation includes the measurement of morning serum total cortisol and ACTH levels. Primary adrenal insufficiency is confirmed by the combination of low serum cortisol and elevated serum ACTH levels. Important considerations in the interpretation of the results are shown in Figure 5 and often require referral to an endocrinologist. Additional evaluation may include measurement of 21-hydroxylase antibodies; positive 21-hydroxylase antibodies are found in approximately 90% of autoimmune adrenalitis cases. If negative, CT scan of the adrenal glands should be obtained.

### Treatment

Both glucocorticoid and mineralocorticoid therapy is required for treatment of primary AI. The preferred glucocorticoid is hydrocortisone taken 2 or 3 times daily. Adherence to multiple daily doses can be challenging so prednisone can be used as an alternative (**Table 30**). The principle of replacement is to administer a higher dose in the morning and to avoid replacement in the evening. Despite this attempt to mimic diurnal variation, patients with primary AI report a decrease in health-related quality of life. It is imperative to avoid overreplacement with glucocorticoid, to avoid iatrogenic Cushing syndrome with its risk of obesity, type 2 diabetes mellitus, hypertension, hyperlipidemia, bone loss, and cardiovascular disease. Some patients "feel better" at higher than physiologic replacement doses, but the risks outweigh the benefits of supraphysiologic doses. Mineralocorticoid replacement is achieved with daily fludrocortisone. DHEAS replacement is controversial in women due to lack of robust data for benefit and concerns regarding the safety and quality of U.S. preparations, which are supplements and not regulated as drugs.

Patients cannot mount an appropriate increase in cortisol  with illness, and therefore, instruction in "sick day" rules is essential to prevent adrenal crisis (**Table 31**). For minor physiologic stress states such as respiratory infection, fever, or minor surgery under local anesthesia, patients should double or triple their baseline glucocorticoid dose for 2 to 3 days. Higher doses of glucocorticoid are required during moderate or major physiologic stress. Patients who present with adrenal

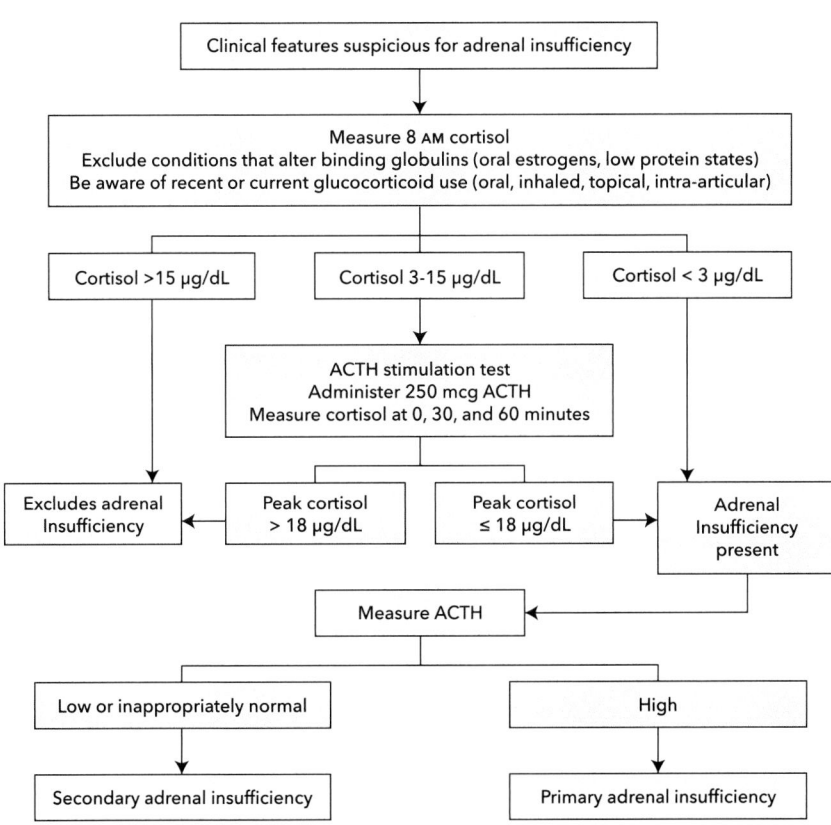

**FIGURE 5.** Algorithm for the diagnosis of adrenal insufficiency. ACTH = adrenocorticotropic hormone.

**TABLE 30.** Dose Equivalence and Relative Potencies of Common Synthetic Oral Glucocorticoids

| Synthetic Glucocorticoid | Equivalent Dose (mg) | Biologic Half-Life (hours) | Relative Anti-Inflammatory Potency[a] | Relative Mineralocorticoid Potency[b] |
|---|---|---|---|---|
| Hydrocortisone | 20 | 8-12 | 1 | 1/125 |
| Prednisolone/ prednisone | 5 | 18-36 | 4 | 1/150 |
| Methylprednisolone | 4 | 18-36 | 5 | 0 |
| Dexamethasone | 0.75 | 36-54 | 25-50 | 0 |

[a]Anti-inflammatory potency relative to hydrocortisone.

[b]Mineralocorticoid potency relative to fludrocortisone.

**TABLE 31.** Chronic Medical Treatment of Primary Adrenal Failure

| Medication | Basal Dose | Considerations |
|---|---|---|
| Glucocorticoid[a] | | *"Sick day rules":* |
| Hydrocortisone | Usually 15-25 mg/d, divided into 2-3 doses over the day | Patient follows at home. |
| Prednisone | Prednisone 5 mg once daily | *For minor physiologic stress (upper respiratory infection, fever, minor surgery under local anesthesia):* |
| | *How to dose:* | 2-3 times basal dose for 2-3 days |
| | Titrate to clinical response with goal of no signs or symptoms of cortisol deficiency or excess (increase dose if symptoms of cortisol deficiency remain; decrease if CS signs and symptoms are present) | *Stress dosing*: Health care providers follow while patient is in the hospital. *For moderate physiologic stress (minor or moderate surgery with general anesthesia):* Hydrocortisone 25-75 mg/d orally or IV for 1-2 days *For major physiologic stress (major surgery, trauma, critical illness, or childbirth):* Hydrocortisone 100 mg IV followed by 50 mg every 6 h IV; rapid tapering and switch to oral regimen depending on clinical state |
| Mineralocorticoid | | |
| Fludrocortisone | 0.05-0.2 mg once daily in the morning | Fludrocortisone is not required if hydrocortisone dose is >40 mg/d. |
| | *How to dose:* Titrate to: 1. Normal BP 2. Normal serum Na, K | |
| Adrenal androgen | | |
| DHEA | 25-50 mg once daily | Consider DHEA for women with impaired mood or sense of well-being when glucocorticoid replacement has been optimized. |

BP = blood pressure; CS = Cushing syndrome; DHEA = dehydroepiandrosterone; IV = intravenous; Na = sodium; K = potassium.

[a]Shorter-acting glucocorticoids are preferred over longer-acting agents due to lower risk of glucocorticoid excess. Longer-acting preparations have the advantage of once-daily dosing.

CONT.

crisis should receive fluid resuscitation and an initial immediate dose of intravenous hydrocortisone (100 mg), followed by intravenous hydrocortisone (100 mg) every 8 hours for the next 24 hours, with subsequent dosing governed by clinical status. Patients with concomitant untreated adrenal insufficiency and hypothyroidism should always receive glucocorticoid replacement therapy first to prevent precipitation of adrenal crisis by thyroid hormone replacement. Patients should also be counselled to wear a medic-alert identification at all times. No increase in mineralocorticoid dose is necessary with illness. 

The term "adrenal fatigue" is used by some alternative medicine providers to represent a constellation of symptoms purported to occur in patients who experience chronic emotional or physical stress that are claimed to be caused by simultaneous hyper- and hypocortisolism. There is no scientific evidence to support such a condition. Patients may undergo salivary cortisol testing, but interpretation of the results is often unreliable. Some patients labeled with "adrenal fatigue" are given hydrocortisone therapy or animal-derived adrenal gland extract that may contain active glucocorticoid, leading to exogenous suppression of ACTH production and iatrogenic Cushing syndrome. Sudden discontinuation of these products can lead to acute adrenal insufficiency. Patients with "adrenal fatigue" should be carefully tapered off any glucocorticoid therapy and other potential causes for their symptoms explored.

### KEY POINTS

- The most common cause of primary adrenal insufficiency is autoimmune destruction of all layers of the adrenal cortex leading to progressive mineralocorticoid, glucocorticoid, and adrenal androgen deficiency.

- Both glucocorticoid and mineralocorticoid therapy is required for treatment of primary adrenal insufficiency.

- Patients cannot mount an appropriate increase in cortisol with illness, and therefore, instruction in "sick day" rules regarding glucocorticoid dosing is essential to prevent adrenal crisis.

## Adrenal Function During Critical Illness

During times of physiologic stress, the hypothalamic-pituitary-adrenal axis is stimulated to produce increased levels of cortisol. In some patients, the increase in cortisol secretion is thought to be suboptimal and termed "relative AI." There is debate, however, as to whether the entity of relative adrenal insufficiency is a true disease. Cortisol-binding globulin and albumin decrease in critical illness, lowering the measured total cortisol. There is no agreement on a set of diagnostic criteria for relative AI despite the ability to measure free cortisol, calculated free cortisol, and basal and ACTH-stimulated total cortisol level in critically ill patients. Studies to date do not show improved survival in patients with relative AI treated with high-dose glucocorticoid therapy. Reversal of shock, however, may be improved, and hence it is currently recommended that stress-dose hydrocortisone be administered to patients with shock that is resistant to standard fluid and vasopressor therapy. ☐

## Adrenal Mass

### Incidentally Noted Adrenal Masses

An adrenal incidentaloma is defined as an adrenal mass greater than 1 cm in diameter that is detected on imaging performed for purposes other than suspicion of adrenal disease. The prevalence of adrenal incidentaloma increases with age and is estimated to be approximately 10% in those 70 years of age or older. Most lesions are benign, nonfunctioning adenomas, and approximately 10% to 15% secrete excess hormones. Other causes include metastases (probability increases if known

primary malignancy), myelolipoma, cysts, and adrenocortical carcinoma.

The finding of an incidental adrenal mass prompts two main questions: (1) Is it secreting excess hormone (aldosterone, cortisol, or catecholamines)? and (2) Is it benign or malignant? Patients with hypertension or with hypokalemia require testing for primary aldosteronism. Biochemical testing for pheochromocytoma, such as a 24-hour urine total metanephrine measurement, should be undertaken in all patients, even in the absence of typical symptoms or hypertension.

All patients should also be evaluated for subclinical Cushing syndrome, a condition characterized by ACTH-independent cortisol secretion that may result in metabolic (hyperglycemia and hypertension) and bone (osteoporosis) effects of hypercortisolism, but not the more specific clinical features of Cushing syndrome, such as supraclavicular fat pads, wide violaceous striae, facial plethora, and proximal muscle weakness. Initial testing for subclinical Cushing syndrome is achieved with a 1-mg overnight dexamethasone suppression test, with a cortisol level greater than 5 µg/dL (138 nmol/L) considered a positive test. Following a positive result, further tests are required to confirm cortisol autonomy and may include measurement of ACTH (suppressed), DHEAS (low), 24-hour urine free cortisol, and an 8-mg overnight dexamethasone suppression test; referral to an endocrinologist is recommended at this point. The decision whether to proceed to adrenalectomy should take into account the risks versus benefits of surgery. Studies to date have not been robust enough to show clear postoperative improvement in clinically important outcomes but suggest improved glucose, lipid, blood pressure, and bone density measurements.

Imaging findings can help differentiate between a benign and a malignant adrenal mass (see Table 28). Most adrenocortical carcinomas measure more than 4 cm at the time of discovery. Approximately 75% of benign adrenal masses, however, are also in this size range. Approximately 66% of benign adenomas are lipid-rich and exhibit low attenuation (<10 HU) on CT imaging. Benign adrenal adenomas also exhibit rapid washout (>50%) of contrast material compared to non-benign lesions. Adrenal biopsy has a limited role in evaluation of incidentalomas and is reserved for lesions suspicious for metastases or an infiltrative process such as lymphoma or infection. Pheochromocytomas should be ruled out prior to biopsy to avoid the possibility of a hypertensive crisis. Biopsy should not be performed when there is suspicion for primary adrenocortical carcinoma because, without review of the whole specimen, pathology cannot reliably distinguish this from a benign cortical adenoma, and tumor seeding is possible. If the former is suspected, the diagnosis should be established by adrenalectomy.

An algorithm for management of adrenal incidentaloma, including monitoring of lesions that do not require adrenalectomy, is shown in **Figure 6**.

**KEY POINTS**

- All patients with adrenal incidentaloma should be evaluated for pheochromocytoma; those with hypertension or hypokalemia should also be evaluated for primary aldosteronism, and all patients should be evaluated for subclinical Cushing syndrome.
- Imaging findings can help differentiate between a benign and malignant adrenal mass.

## Adrenocortical Carcinoma

Adrenocortical carcinoma (ACC) is a rare, aggressive tumor that often secretes excess cortisol and/or androgens. Patients may present with rapid onset of Cushing syndrome, with or without virilization and/or symptoms from mass effect, such as increased abdominal girth and lower extremity edema. Fifty percent of ACCs secrete cortisol; 20% secrete multiple hormones, including cortisol and aldosterone precursors; and less than 10% secrete aldosterone. Some ACCs are discovered as an incidental adrenal mass that is either indeterminate or suspicious for ACC (see Table 28). Lesions are often large (>4 cm), and disease is at an advanced stage at the time of diagnosis. For localized disease, first-line therapy includes open resection. Debulking surgery, radiation therapy, and/or chemotherapy may also be options for palliation in advanced ACC.

Mitotane is an adrenolytic agent commonly used as adjuvant therapy that has been shown to be associated with longer recurrence-free survival. Mitotane causes primary AI, and daily glucocorticoid replacement therapy is required, often in supraphysiologic doses, due to mitotane-induced accelerated metabolism of glucocorticoids. Some patients also develop aldosterone deficiency manifested by hyponatremia, hyperkalemia, elevated renin levels, and postural hypotension, requiring fludrocortisone replacement. Five-year survival rates range from 62% to 82% for those with disease confined to the adrenal gland and 13% for tumors associated with distant metastases.

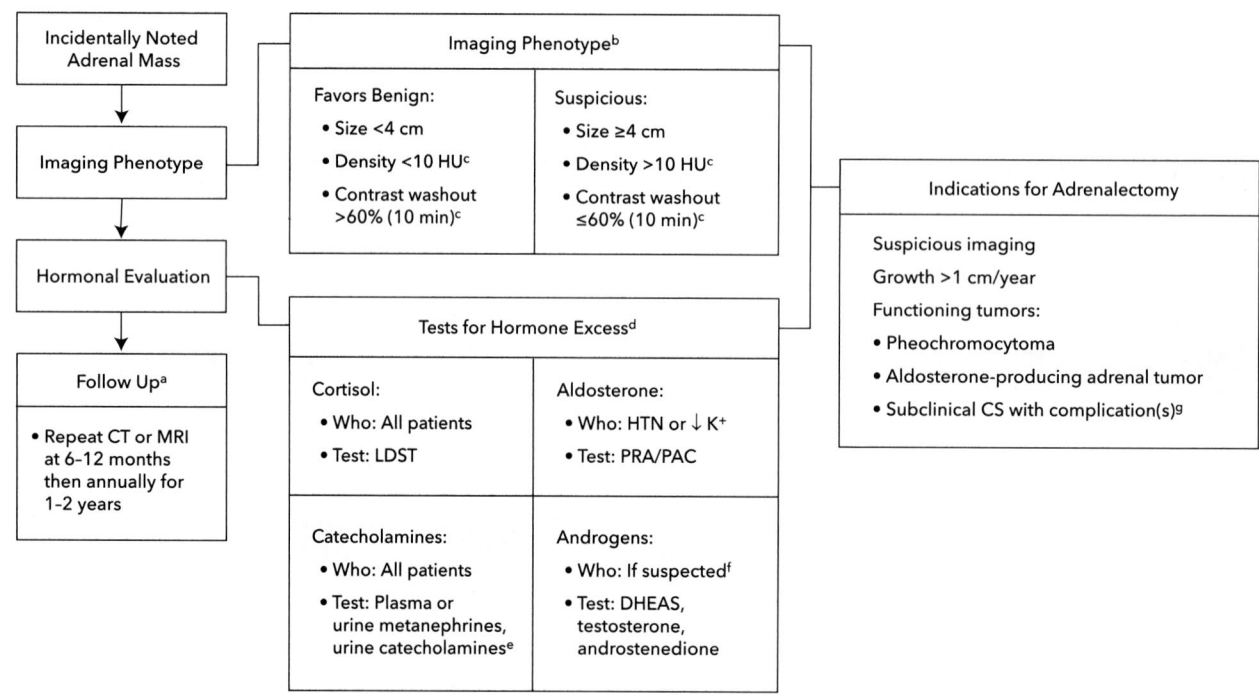

**FIGURE 6.** Algorithm for the initial diagnostic evaluation and follow up of an incidentally noted adrenal mass. CS = Cushing syndrome; DHEAS = dehydroepiandrosterone sulfate; HTN = hypertension; HU = Hounsfield units; K = potassium; LDST = low-dose (1-mg) dexamethasone suppression test; PAC = plasma aldosterone concentration; PRA = plasma renin activity.

[a]Repeat imaging is indicated for adrenal masses not meeting criteria for surgery at initial diagnosis.

[b]Refer to Table 28 for more CT and MRI findings. If imaging is suspicious in a patient with known malignancy, biopsy should be considered to confirm adrenal metastasis after screening for pheochromocytoma is completed.

[c]CT scan findings.

[d]Positive screening tests usually require further biochemical evaluation to confirm the diagnosis (see text).

[e]Measure plasma metanephrines if radiographic appearance is typical for a pheochromocytoma; otherwise measure 24-hour urine metanephrines and catecholamines.

[f]Hormonal evaluation for an androgen-producing adrenal tumor is indicated only if clinically suspected based on the presence of hirsutism, virilization, or menstrual irregularities in women.

[g]Adrenalectomy is considered for confirmed cases of subclinical CS associated with recent onset of diabetes, hypertension, obesity, or low bone mass.

- Adrenocortical carcinoma is a rare, aggressive tumor that often secretes excess cortisol and/or androgens and hormonal precursors causing hypertension and Cushing syndrome; patients may present with rapid onset of Cushing syndrome with or without virilization and/or symptoms from mass effect, such as increased abdominal girth and lower extremity edema.

- For localized disease, first-line therapy includes open resection; debulking surgery, radiation therapy, and/or chemotherapy may also be options for palliation in advanced adrenocortical carcinoma.

- Mitotane is an adrenolytic agent, commonly used as adjuvant therapy, that has been associated with longer recurrence-free survival.

# Disorders of the Thyroid Gland

## Thyroid Anatomy and Physiology

The thyroid gland is the largest dedicated endocrine organ. The usual anatomic location of the isthmus is just anterior to the second to fourth tracheal rings. The parathyroid glands are often located posterior to the superior and middle portions of each thyroid lobe. The recurrent laryngeal nerves, which innervate most of the intrinsic muscles of the larynx, course behind the thyroid gland. Thyroid pathology may cause compressive symptoms including shortness of breath, cough, dysphagia, and voice changes due to the close proximity of the thyroid to the trachea, esophagus, and recurrent laryngeal nerves.

The thyroid gland contains thyroid follicular cells and parafollicular cells (c-cells). Calcitonin is produced by the parafollicular cells and inhibits bone resorption; however, it plays a minor role in bone physiology. Follicular cells produce the thyroid hormones, thyroxine ($T_4$) and triiodothyronine ($T_3$). The synthesis and secretion of thyroid hormones is tightly regulated by the hypothalamic-pituitary-thyroid axis. Thyrotropin-releasing hormone (TRH) from the hypothalamus triggers the pulsatile release of thyroid-stimulating hormone (TSH) from thyrotrope cells in the anterior pituitary gland. TSH, through activation of the TSH-receptor, stimulates thyroid cell growth, iodide metabolism, and thyroid hormone synthesis and secretion. $T_4$ and $T_3$ exert negative feedback on the hypothalamus and pituitary gland to moderate further hormone synthesis.

Iodine is an essential dietary micronutrient and a key structural component of $T_4$ and $T_3$.

The thyroid gland is the exclusive source of $T_4$, whereas approximately 80% of $T_3$ is the result of removing one iodine molecule from $T_4$, through deiodinase activity in peripheral tissues. This occurs primarily in the liver and kidney. Most of $T_4$ (99.96%) and $T_3$ (99.6%) are bound to proteins in serum. Approximately 70% of $T_4$ and $T_3$ are bound to thyroxine-binding globulin. Albumin, transthyretin, and lipoproteins carry a smaller proportion. Only the tiny amount of free $T_4$ and $T_3$ is biologically active. While $T_4$ largely serves as a prohormone, $T_3$ binds with high affinity to thyroid hormone nuclear receptors affecting gene transcription in target tissues and mediating its physiologic effects. It has positive inotropic and chronotropic effects in the heart and enhances myocardial adrenergic sensitivity. It also increases the rate of myocardial diastolic relaxation, augments intravascular volume, and lowers peripheral vascular resistance. It increases gastrointestinal motility, bone turnover, and regulates heat generation and energy expenditure.

## Thyroid Examination

The thyroid gland is located in the neck midway between the sternal notch and thyroid cartilage. It attaches to the trachea posteriorly and elevates with swallowing. Examination involves both visualization and palpation while the patient swallows liquid. It can be palpated with the examiner behind the patient with circumferential hand positioning to allow focus on palpation or with the examiner facing the patient, which allows the examiner to see the thyroid during palpation. The anterior approach is preferred with necks of larger diameter.

## Structural Disorders of the Thyroid Gland

### Thyroid Nodules

Thyroid nodules are discrete structural lesions, distinct from the background gland parenchyma on ultrasound. They are most commonly detected as incidental findings on imaging studies performed for other reasons. The prevalence of nodules palpated on examination is 5% in women and 1% in men. They are detected on ultrasound in 40% of the U.S. population and are more common with increasing age. Thyroid nodules can result from multiple pathologic processes, ranging from benign cysts and inflammatory nodules, to malignancies including primary thyroid, lymphoma, or metastatic lesions. Non-thyroidal lesions, such as parathyroid adenomas, can also present as nodules. Primary thyroid neoplasms are clonal in origin and include follicular adenomas and thyroid cancer.

The initial evaluation of a thyroid nodule begins with measuring serum TSH (**Figure 7**). TSH suppression may indicate the presence of autonomously functioning or "hot" nodules, which account for 5% to 10% of palpable thyroid nodules. Autonomous nodules may cause hyperthyroidism and are associated with a very low risk of malignancy. They do not require fine-needle aspiration biopsy (FNAB). Patients with thyroid nodules and a suppressed TSH are evaluated with thyroid scintigraphy. A radioactive isotope, preferably iodine

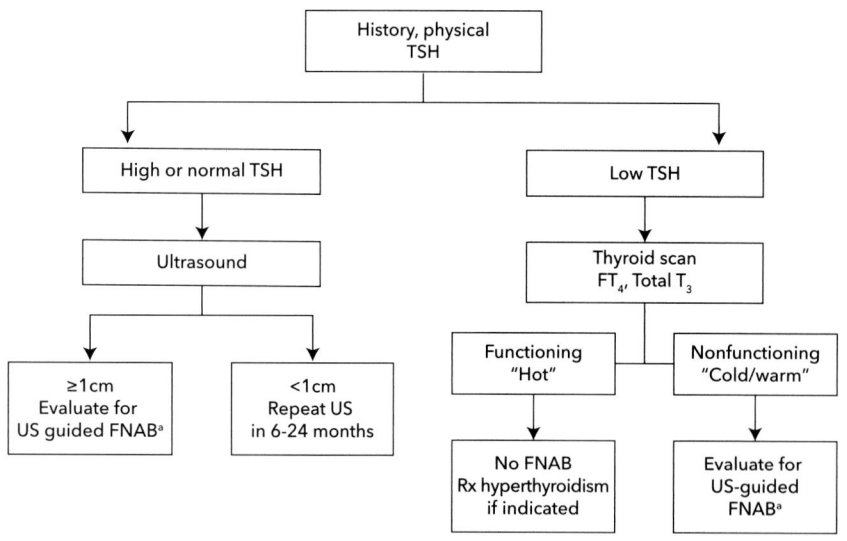

**FIGURE 7.** Initial evaluation of a thyroid nodule. There are size thresholds for FNAB based on US appearance. A less suspicious lesion may not need FNAB until it is larger than 2 cm, suspicious nodules if larger than 1 cm. FNAB = fine-needle aspiration biopsy; $FT_3$ = free triiodothyronine; $FT_4$ = free thyroxine; TSH = thyroid-stimulating hormone; US = ultrasound.

ªNeed for US-guided FNAB depends on clinical risk factors for thyroid cancer, nodule size, and US appearance.

123 ($^{123}$I), is administered, the percentage taken up by the thyroid is calculated (radioactive iodine uptake [RAIU]), and an image is obtained (thyroid scan). Hot nodules concentrate radioactive iodine to a greater extent than normal thyroid tissue.

Thyroid/neck ultrasound is performed in patients with a normal or elevated TSH to confirm the presence of thyroid nodules. The management of nonfunctioning thyroid nodules is determined by the ultrasound results and presence of symptoms. The 2015 American Thyroid Association guidelines classify thyroid nodules into five sonographic patterns based on echogenicity, whether they are solid, cystic, or both, and features of malignancy (**Table 32**). Hyperechoic nodules are brighter, isoechoic nodules are equally bright, and hypoechoic nodules are darker than the background parenchyma. Ultrasound can determine the size of the nodule. FNAB is not recommended for subcentimeter nodules unless associated with symptoms, pathologic lymphadenopathy, or extrathyroidal extension.

Thyroid nodule FNAB should be performed under ultrasound guidance when possible because of improved accuracy compared with palpation biopsy. Thyroid cytopathology is usually interpreted and classified according to criteria developed at the National Cancer Institute Thyroid Fine Needle Aspiration State of the Science Conference (Bethesda Conference). The Bethesda classification system is summarized in **Table 33**. Thyroid FNAB cytology can be nondiagnostic in up to 5% to 10% of specimens. Approximately 60% to 70% of biopsied nodules have benign cytology, 20% are indeterminate, and 5% to 10% have evidence of malignancy.

The management of cytologically indeterminate thyroid nodules (Bethesda III-V) can be challenging, and referral to an endocrinologist is recommended. Clinical monitoring is indicated for all thyroid nodules and should include measurement of serum TSH, as structurally abnormal thyroid glands are at increased risk for thyroid dysfunction (see Disorders of Thyroid Function). American Thyroid Association sonographic

pattern and clinical context guide the timing of initial ultrasound follow up for benign nodules and those not evaluated with FNAB. Repeat ultrasound should be performed in 6 to 12 months for all high suspicion nodules, 12 to 24 months for intermediate and low suspicion nodules, and 24 months or longer for very low suspicion nodules. Repeat FNAB is indicated for all high suspicion nodules, nodules with concerning new sonographic findings, and intermediate or low suspicion nodules that increase significantly in size, which is defined as a 20% increase in at least two dimensions or an increase in nodule volume of more than 50%. Repeat FNAB is not recommended for nodules that have had two negative biopsies.

**KEY POINTS**

- The initial evaluation of a thyroid nodule begins with measuring serum thyroid-stimulating hormone.
- Patients with a suppressed thyroid-stimulating hormone level are evaluated with thyroid scintigraphy; those patients with normal or elevated thyroid-stimulating hormone are evaluated with ultrasonography.
- Patients with nodules 1 cm or larger should be evaluated with fine-needle aspiration biopsy.
- Fine-needle aspiration biopsy is not recommended for subcentimeter nodules unless associated with symptoms, pathologic lymphadenopathy, or extrathyroidal extension. **HVC**

## Goiters

The term "goiter" denotes an enlarged thyroid gland. Goiters can be seen in the setting of normal thyroid function, hypothyroidism, or hyperthyroidism. The most common cause worldwide is endemic goiter due to severe iodine deficiency. Patients presenting with goiter should be questioned about iodine intake, rate of change in size, and risk factors for thyroid cancer (see Thyroid Cancer). Clinical history should focus on

**TABLE 32.** Summary of 2015 American Thyroid Association Guidelines: Sonographic Patterns and Recommendations for Fine-Needle Aspiration Biopsy

| Sonographic Pattern | Representative Image | Description | Estimated Risk of Malignancy | Size Threshold for Fine-Needle Aspiration Biopsy |
|---|---|---|---|---|
| Benign | | Pure cyst (anechoic with no internal blood flow) | <1% | Fine-needle aspiration biopsy not recommended |
| Very low suspicion | | Some mixed cystic and solid nodules (spongiform nodules)[a] | <3% | 2 cm[c] |
| Low suspicion | | Isoechoic/hyperechoic solid nodules; some mixed cystic and solid nodules | 5%-10% | 1.5 cm |
| Intermediate suspicion | | Hypoechoic solid nodules | 10%-20% | 1 cm |
| High suspicion | | Hypoechoic solid nodules with one or more suspicious feature[b] | >70%-90% | 1 cm |

[a]Microcystic spaces occupying more than 50% of the nodule volume is highly correlated with benign cytology.

[b]Microcalcifications, shape taller than wide in the transverse plane, irregular margins, extrathyroidal extension or pathologic lymph nodes (image shows hypoechoic solid nodule with irregular margins).

[c]Clinical observation is an acceptable alternative.

Reprinted and adapted from: Haugen Bryan R., Alexander Erik K., Bible Keith C., Doherty Gerard M., Mandel Susan J., Nikiforov Yuri E., Pacini Furio, Randolph Gregory W., Sawka Anna M., Schlumberger Martin, Schuff Kathryn G., Sherman Steven I., Sosa Julie Ann, Steward David L., Tuttle R. Michael, and Wartofsky Leonard. Thyroid. Jan 2016. ahead of print http://doi.org/10.1089/thy.2015.0020 Published in Volume: 26 Issue 1: January 12, 2016; Online Ahead of Editing: October 14, 2015.

symptoms suggestive of thyroid hormone excess or deficiency and compression. Compressive symptoms include shortness of breath, cough, dysphagia, and voice changes and are evident in 10% to 20% of patients with goiter, most of whom also have clinically apparent thyromegaly. On examination tracheal deviation should be assessed and the size, symmetry, and consistency of the thyroid and presence of nodules should be noted. Possible venous obstruction should be assessed by having the patient raise the arms above the head. The findings of jugular venous distension, facial plethora, and flushing indicate possible thoracic outlet obstruction with reduced venous return (Pemberton sign) (**Figure 8**). Serum TSH level should be assessed in patients with goiter. If low, free $T_4$ and total $T_3$ should be measured and thyroid scintigraphy performed. If normal or elevated, thyroid/neck ultrasound is indicated in patients with risk factors for thyroid cancer, palpable thyroid nodules, gland asymmetry, large goiters, rapid growth pattern, or compressive symptoms. Patients with signs or symptoms of compression require additional testing as outlined below, and surgery may be needed for symptomatic

**TABLE 33.** Diagnoses Obtained by Fine-Needle Aspiration Biopsy of Thyroid Nodules and Risk for Malignancy

| Fine-Needle Aspiration Biopsy Diagnosis | Risk for Malignancy[a] | Management |
|---|---|---|
| Benign | 0%-3% | Repeat ultrasound in 6-24 months[b] |
| Atypia of uncertain significance/follicular lesion of uncertain significance | 10%-30% | Repeat FNAB in 3 months[c] |
| Suspicious for follicular neoplasm | 25%-40% | Lobectomy[b] |
| Suspicious for malignancy | 50%-70% | Lobectomy or total thyroidectomy |
| Malignant | 97%-99% | Lobectomy or total thyroidectomy |
| Nondiagnostic | 5%-10% | Repeat FNAB |
| | | If two nondiagnostic FNABs, surgery |

FNAB = fine-needle aspiration biopsy.

[a]Risk for malignancy by cytology diagnosis includes noninvasive follicular thyroid neoplasm with papillary-like nuclear features (NIFTP), a "pre-cancerous" lesion. If counted as benign, the risk of malignancy is reduced for all Bethesda categories except nondiagnostic and benign readings. Data from Cibas ES, Ali SZ. The 2017 Bethesda System for reporting thyroid cytopathology. Thyroid. 2017 Nov;27(11):1341-1346. doi: 10.1089/thy.2017.0500. PubMed PMID: 29091573.

[b]If American Thyroid Association "high suspicion" pattern, repeat ultrasound and FNAB in 6 to 12 months.

[c]Supplementary management strategies include molecular genetic testing of the nodule and selective use of thyroid scintigraphy (when serum thyroid-stimulation hormone level is low-normal).

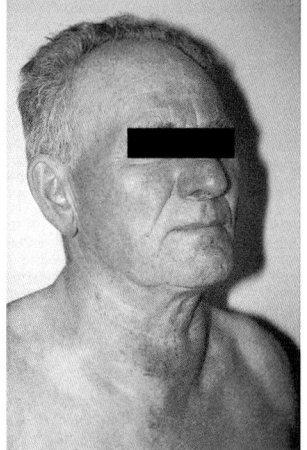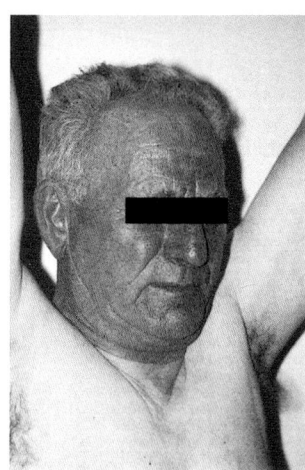

**FIGURE 8.** The Pemberton sign. Head and neck with arms down (*left*) and arms elevated (*right*).

management. Treatment of hypothyroid and hyperthyroid conditions in the setting of goiter is discussed below.

**KEY POINTS**

- The most common worldwide cause of goiter is severe iodine deficiency.
- Patients with goiter should be questioned about iodine intake, rate of change in size, assessed for signs and symptoms of compression, and evaluated for clinical manifestations of thyroid hormone excess or deficiency.
- Serum thyroid-stimulating hormone should be assessed in patients with goiter; if low, free thyroxine ($T_4$) and total triiodothyronine ($T_3$) should be measured and thyroid scintigraphy performed; if $T_4$ and $T_3$ are normal or elevated, a thyroid/neck ultrasound is indicated in the presence of risk factors for thyroid cancer, palpable thyroid nodules, gland asymmetry, large goiters, rapid growth pattern, or compressive symptoms.

## Multinodular Goiter

Multinodular goiter is the most common cause of goiter in older adults in the United States. Evaluation includes measurement of serum TSH and, when TSH is not suppressed, thyroid/

neck ultrasound should be performed and discrete nodules evaluated as discussed previously (see Thyroid Nodules). The frequency of thyroid malignancy in patients with multinodular goiter is similar to those with solitary thyroid nodules. Signs and symptoms of compression or suspected substernal extension require additional testing. CT or MRI of the neck and chest (when substernal goiter is suspected) can define anatomic relationships and assess for tracheal narrowing. The administration of iodinated contrast should be avoided when possible to avoid precipitating iodine-induced hyperthyroidism (Jod-Basedow phenomenon). A flow-volume loop study is indicated in patients with symptoms of airway compression or when the tracheal lumen measures less than 1 cm in diameter on CT or MR (see MKSAP 18 Pulmonary and Critical Care Medicine). Endoscopy or a swallowing study can assess for extrinsic compression of the esophagus in patients with cervical dysphagia. Consultation with an otolaryngologist is indicated to confirm clinically suspected vocal cord paralysis. Surgery is indicated for significant compression or suspected malignancy.

## Diffuse Goiter

The most common cause of diffuse goiter is autoimmune thyroid disease associated with thyroid dysfunction (Hashimoto thyroiditis and Graves disease). Infiltrative disorders, such as Riedel (IgG4-related) thyroiditis, are rare causes of diffuse goiter. Diffuse goiter may also occur in euthyroid patients in the absence of predisposing inflammatory or neoplastic processes. Genetic predisposition, iodine insufficiency, and cigarette smoking are contributing factors. Thyroid/neck ultrasound is indicated in euthyroid patients with diffuse goiter. It is recommended for patients with Graves disease or Hashimoto thyroiditis when there is thyroid gland asymmetry or nodules on examination. As discussed previously, additional testing is indicated if compressive signs or symptoms are present. Thyroid surgery is considered in the setting of significant compression.

## Thyroid Cancer

Thyroid cancer is diagnosed in 13.9 per 100,000 people per year in the United States. The incidence of thyroid cancer has increased over the last four decades and now is the fifth most common cancer in women. Much of this change is attributable to a rise in the diagnosis of small noninvasive cancers, initially detected incidentally on imaging done for other reasons (carotid Doppler studies, neck/chest CT, PET scan). Mortality rates have remained stable with an overall 5-year survival rate of 98.1%. Papillary thyroid carcinoma and follicular thyroid carcinoma, collectively known as differentiated thyroid cancer, account for the most thyroid cancer diagnoses in the United States. Papillary thyroid carcinoma commonly spreads to cervical lymph nodes but is associated with a low risk of distant metastases; whereas lymph node metastases are rare in follicular thyroid carcinoma, metastases to lung, bone, and other sites can be seen. The types and frequency of thyroid cancer are shown in **Figure 9**.

Thyroid cancer is often identified incidentally; however, it may be detected on neck examination. Risk factors for thyroid cancer include a personal history of ionizing radiation exposure with a higher prevalence of papillary thyroid carcinoma in persons exposed to ionizing radiation (>10 rads), with the highest risk seen following childhood exposures, such as with nuclear accidents (Chernobyl), and a personal or family history of thyroid malignancy. Additional risk factors for thyroid cancer include extremes of age (younger than 30 or older than 60) and male gender. Findings suggestive of malignancy include rapid nodule growth, a hard fixed nodule, dysphagia, vocal cord paralysis (hoarseness), and cervical lymphadenopathy. The diagnosis is confirmed by fine-needle aspiration biopsy.

Surgery is the mainstay of thyroid cancer treatment. Either total thyroidectomy or hemithyroidectomy is acceptable for unilateral differentiated thyroid cancers measuring 1 to 4 cm, as long as locoregional spread is not suspected. Total thyroidectomy is otherwise indicated. Unique risks of

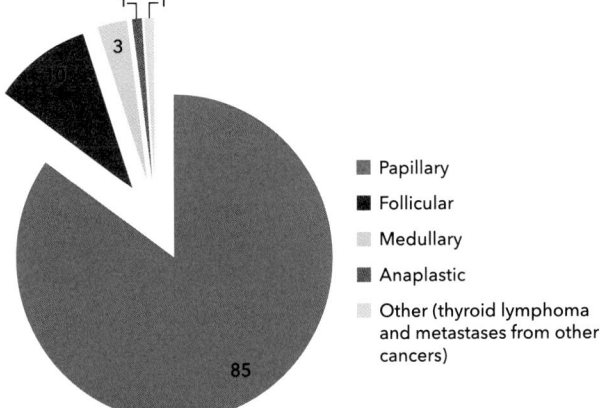

**FIGURE 9.** Relative frequency of the types of thyroid cancer.

Papillary
Follicular
Medullary
Anaplastic
Other (thyroid lymphoma and metastases from other cancers)

Data from Hundahl SA, Fleming ID, Fremgen AM, Menck HR. A National Cancer Data Base report on 53,856 cases of thyroid carcinoma treated in the U.S., 1985-1995. Cancer. 1998 Dec 15;83(12):2638-48. [PMID: 9874472]

thyroid surgery include hypocalcemia as a result of removal or devascularization of the parathyroid glands and difficulty breathing or voice changes from recurrent laryngeal nerve injury. Referral to a high-volume thyroid surgeon (>90 cases per year) is preferred due to a lower risk of postoperative complications.

Postoperative radioactive iodine ($^{131}$I) should be considered for the dual purposes of thyroid remnant ablation and adjuvant therapy for patients with differentiated thyroid cancer and an intermediate to high risk of recurrence, such as with extrathyroidal extension, lymphovascular invasion, poorly differentiated/more aggressive histology, or metastatic disease. TSH stimulation, achieved either by withdrawal of thyroid hormone (levothyroxine) replacement or administration of recombinant human TSH (rhTSH), is required to promote $^{131}$I uptake by thyroid follicular cells. Following $^{131}$I therapy, patients undergo whole-body scanning to identify areas of $^{131}$I uptake corresponding to metastatic disease. Uptake is expected in the postsurgical thyroid bed but not elsewhere. $^{131}$I therapy is also used to treat thyroid cancer recurrences not amenable to surgical resection.

After initial cancer treatment, serum thyroglobulin (Tg), a sensitive marker for the detection of persistent or recurrent disease, and thyroglobulin antibody (TgAb) titers are monitored. When TgAb is present, Tg levels are uninterpretable because TgAb can falsely lower Tg measurement. In this case, the TgAb level serves as a surrogate marker. A falling TgAb titer over time correlates with a favorable prognosis, whereas a rising titer is suspicious for persistent or recurrent disease.

Neck ultrasound is regularly performed in routine thyroid cancer surveillance, usually 6 to 12 months after the initial cancer treatment. In patients at high risk of recurrent disease, diagnostic radioactive iodine ($^{123}$I or $^{131}$I) whole-body scanning with TSH-stimulated Tg measurement can be performed. If residual or recurrent thyroid cancer is suspected, such as when serum Tg is persistently elevated or rising over time but not identified by neck ultrasound or radioactive iodine whole-body scanning, adjunctive imaging tests including CT, MRI, bone scan, or PET/CT can be useful in disease localization.

Treatment of intermediate to high-risk differentiated thyroid cancer includes TSH suppression with daily levothyroxine. Thyroid follicular cells are TSH responsive, as are most well-differentiated thyroid cancers. To reduce cancer recurrence, a sufficient dose of levothyroxine is administered to suppress the serum TSH below normal with the specific goal individualized. A serum TSH level less than or equal to 2 but at or above the lower limit of the reference range can be targeted in patients with low risk thyroid cancer. Monitoring and dose adjustment by internists is appropriate in conjunction with the endocrinologist. Metastatic thyroid cancer is managed with active surveillance, additional surgery, or $^{131}$I therapy, followed by external beam radiation therapy and/or chemotherapy (tyrosine kinase inhibitors).

Anaplastic thyroid cancer is a rare but aggressive thyroid malignancy that can occur in patients with preexisting differentiated thyroid cancer or de novo. It carries a dismal prognosis with median survival of 5 months. Anaplastic thyroid cancer presents with a rapidly enlarging neck mass and may be unresectable at the time of diagnosis. Treatment is palliative in most cases with surgery, external beam radiation therapy, and chemotherapy.

Medullary thyroid cancer arises from parafollicular cells. Germline *RET* oncogene mutations occur with familial medullary thyroid cancer and multiple endocrine neoplasia (MEN) 2A and 2B. MEN should be ruled out with genetic testing prior to surgery, given its association with pheochromocytoma. Medullary thyroid cancer is treated with total thyroidectomy and central neck lymph node dissection. Levothyroxine is indicated to treat postoperative hypothyroidism in patients with medullary thyroid cancer with a goal serum TSH level within the reference range. Serum calcitonin, serum carcinoembryonic antigen levels, and neck ultrasound are part of routine cancer surveillance.

Low-risk papillary thyroid cancer, confined to the thyroid gland, that has been completely resected, has not metastasized, and does not demonstrate aggressive pathologic features (lymphovascular invasion or tall cell variant), requires no additional treatment. The risk of disease-related death is less than 1%, and the risk of structural disease recurrence is 1% to 2% for low-risk unifocal papillary microcarcinomas. Patients receiving either lobectomy or thyroidectomy have similarly excellent outcomes.

### KEY POINTS

- Thyroid cancer is often detected incidentally but can be detected when a thyroid nodule or abnormal lymph node is noted on neck examination.

- Surgery is the mainstay of thyroid cancer treatment; either hemithyroidectomy or total thyroidectomy is acceptable for unilateral differentiated thyroid cancers measuring 1 to 4 cm, as long as locoregional spread is not suspected, while total thyroidectomy is preferred in all other cases.

- In addition to surgery, patients with differentiated thyroid cancer and an intermediate to high risk of recurrence are treated with radioactive iodine therapy ($^{131}$I) and thyroid-stimulating hormone suppression with levothyroxine.

# Evaluation of Thyroid Function

Serum TSH is the most sensitive and recommended initial test of thyroid function. It is used to determine euthyroidism, hypothyroidism or hyperthyroidism. If TSH is suppressed, free $T_4$ and total $T_3$ should be assessed to detect overt or subclinical hyperthyroidism, and if TSH is elevated, free $T_4$ should be assessed to detect overt or subclinical hypothyroidism.

Measuring serum TSH alone is sufficient except in certain circumstances, such as suspected central hypothyroidism, where free $T_4$ measurement is also indicated (see Disorders of the Pituitary Gland).

Total and free $T_4$ and total $T_3$ concentrations can be assessed with a variety of assays and can be accurately measured in most patients with overt thyroid dysfunction. Commercially available free $T_3$ assays are less reliable. Perturbations in thyroxine-binding globulin and other binding proteins can occur with physiologic changes (pregnancy), certain disease states (nephrotic syndrome), and as a result of medications (oral estrogen therapy). Levels of total $T_4$ and $T_3$ will vary based on increasing or decreasing binding proteins and do not reflect actual thyroid function. Measurement of free $T_4$, the unbound fraction of $T_4$ in serum, is most commonly determined using widely available immunometric assays. These tests are accurate in most clinical settings, including in patients with mild binding protein derangements; however, they can be inaccurate with more significant perturbations (familial dysalbuminemic hyperthyroxinemia). Measuring free $T_4$ by equilibrium dialysis is highly accurate, but expensive, not widely available, and rarely necessary.

Patients taking more than 5 to 10 mg/day of biotin should be counseled to discontinue ingestion for 2 days prior to the laboratory assessment of thyroid function. Biotin is a water-soluble vitamin that is commonly found in over-the-counter dietary supplements. High circulating levels of biotin have been shown to interfere with laboratory assays that utilize streptavidin–biotin as an immobilizing system. Biotin interference causes falsely high results with competitive immunoassays used to measure small molecules (free $T_4$, free $T_3$, total $T_4$, and total $T_3$) and causes falsely low results with sandwich assays used to measure large molecules (TSH).

Measurement of $T_3$ is recommended in three settings: (1) in the evaluation of thyrotoxicosis to identify isolated $T_3$ toxicosis, (2) to assess the severity of hyperthyroidism and response to therapy, and (3) potentially, to differentiate hyperthyroidism from destructive thyroiditis. In $T_3$ toxicosis, the $T_3$:$T_4$ ratio is often greater than 20 due to preferential secretion of $T_3$. Multiple drugs can affect thyroid function and replacement (**Table 34**).

Measurement of $T_3$ in the setting of hypothyroidism is not necessary or recommended; normal levels are maintained unless hypothyroidism is severe. TSH will become elevated in hypothyroidism first, followed by abnormalities in $T_4$ level.

There is no clinical indication to assess reverse $T_3$ levels, and thus it is not recommended.

### KEY POINT

- Measurement of triiodothyronine in the setting of hypothyroidism is not necessary or recommended; normal levels are maintained unless hypothyroidism is severe. **HVC**

**TABLE 34.** Medications that Affect Thyroid Function or Replacement

| Mechanism of Action | Drugs | Comments |
|---|---|---|
| Decreased absorption or enterohepatic circulation of levothyroxine | Calcium | Recommend that levothyroxine administration be separated from these medications by several hours |
| | Proton pump inhibitors | |
| | Iron | |
| | Cholestyramine | |
| | Aluminum hydroxide | |
| | Soybean oil | |
| | Sucralfate | |
| | Psyllium | |
| Increased metabolism of levothyroxine | Phenytoin | Higher levothyroxine doses may be required to maintain TSH in the normal range |
| | Carbamazepine | |
| | Rifampin | |
| | Phenobarbital | |
| | Sertraline | |
| Thyroiditis | Amiodarone | May cause hypo- or hyperthyroidism |
| | Lithium | |
| | Interferon alfa | |
| | Interleukin-2 | |
| | Tyrosine kinase inhibitors | Sunitinib |
| | Immune checkpoint inhibitors | Nivolumab, pembrolizumab |
| De novo development of antithyroid antibodies | Interferon alfa | May develop Hashimoto thyroiditis, Graves disease, or painless thyroiditis |
| Inhibition of TSH synthesis or release | Glucocorticoids | Leads to TSH suppression; TSH should be rechecked 6-8 weeks after these medications are stopped to assess for return to normal. |
| | Dopamine | |
| | Dobutamine | |
| | Octreotide | |
| Increased thyroxine-binding globulin | Estrogen | False elevation of total $T_3$ and $T_4$ levels; free $T_3$ and $T_4$ are a more accurate reflection of hormone levels |
| | Tamoxifen | |
| | Methadone | |
| Decreased thyroxine-binding globulin | Androgen therapy | False lowering of total $T_3$ and $T_4$ levels; free $T_3$ and $T_4$ are a more accurate reflection of hormone levels |
| | Glucocorticoids | |
| | Niacin | |

$T_3$ = triiodothyronine; $T_4$ = thyroxine; TSH = thyroid-stimulating hormone.

# Disorders of Thyroid Function

## Thyroid Hormone Excess (Hyperthyroidism and Thyrotoxicosis)

The term *thyrotoxicosis* describes the exposure of tissues to high levels of circulating thyroid hormones ($T_4$ and/or $T_3$) from any cause. Hyperthyroidism is thyrotoxicosis caused by excessive endogenous production of thyroid hormones. The overall prevalence of hyperthyroidism in the United States is 1.3%. In primary hyperthyroidism, the thyroid gland is the anatomic site of dysfunction. Increased secretion of TSH is a rare secondary cause of hyperthyroidism.

## Clinical Features and Diagnosis

**Table 35** lists signs and symptoms of thyroid hormone excess. In elderly patients hyperthyroidism may be apathetic instead of presenting with classic symptoms. Lid lag (eyelid retraction) can be seen in thyrotoxicosis of any cause and results from increased adrenergic tone. The diagnosis of hyperthyroidism is based on biochemical testing demonstrating a low-serum TSH level and elevated concentrations of free $T_4$ and/or total $T_3$. Thyroid scintigraphy with radioactive iodine uptake (RAIU) can verify the cause. RAIU is high (above 30%) or inappropriately normal in hyperthyroidism and low (less than 10%) in other causes of thyrotoxicosis.

**TABLE 35.** Clinical Manifestations of Thyrotoxicosis and Thyroid Hormone Deficiency[a]

| Sign or Symptom | Thyrotoxicosis | Thyroid Hormone Deficiency |
|---|---|---|
| General | Fatigue, weight loss,[b] heat intolerance | Fatigue, weight gain, cold intolerance |
| Neuropsychiatric | Decreased concentration, anxiety, irritability, insomnia | Decreased concentration, depression, psychomotor retardation, hypersomnolence |
| | Hyperreflexia, tremor, lid lag | Delayed relaxation of DTRs |
| Cardiovascular | Palpitations, tachycardia, systolic hypertension, high output heart failure | Bradycardia, diastolic hypertension |
| Gastrointestinal | Hyperphagia, increased frequency of bowel movements, loose stools, diarrhea | Constipation |
| Genitourinary | Menstrual disturbance (oligomenorrhea, amenorrhea) | Menstrual disturbance (menorrhagia) |
| Musculoskeletal | Muscle weakness | Myalgia, arthralgia |
| Cutaneous | Hair loss, increased sweating, increased oil production/acne; periorbital edema | Hair loss, dry skin, brittle nails, periorbital edema, lateral truncation of the eyebrows, myxedematous skin changes |

DTRs = deep tendon reflexes.

[a]Goiter may be present in thyrotoxicosis or thyroid hormone deficiency. See text for physical findings characteristic of Graves disease.

[b]Mild weight gain can occur with subclinical hyperthyroidism (thyroid-stimulating hormone suppression without $T_4$ or $T_3$ elevation) due to appetite stimulation.

Additional testing can be done when the clinical diagnosis is not clear; when RAIU is unavailable or unreliable (patients on amiodarone, lithium, or exposed to recent iodinated contrast material); or when scintigraphy is contraindicated (pregnancy and lactation). Tests include measurement of thyroid-stimulating immunoglobulin (TSI) or thyrotropin (TSH) receptor antibodies (TRAb) if Graves disease is suspected but the diagnosis remains clinically unclear, and thyroid ultrasound to assess for patterns of vascularity.

**KEY POINTS**

- The diagnosis of hyperthyroidism is based on biochemical testing demonstrating a low serum thyroid-stimulating hormone level and elevated concentrations of free thyroxine and/or total triiodothyronine.
- Thyroid scintigraphy with determination of radioactive iodine uptake can verify the cause of hyperthyroidism.

## Causes

Causes of thyrotoxicosis are listed in **Table 36**. Graves disease, toxic multinodular goiter, and toxic adenoma are the most common causes of hyperthyroidism.

### Graves Disease

Graves disease is a multisystem disease and can affect the thyroid, ocular muscles, and skin. It causes 80% of hyperthyroidism in iodine-sufficient areas. It is an autoimmune thyroid disorder predominantly affecting women with a peak incidence among patients aged 30 to 60 years. Graves disease is also more common in patients with other autoimmune disorders or a family history of thyroid autoimmunity. T lymphocytes become sensitized to thyroid antigens and

**TABLE 36.** Causes of Thyrotoxicosis

| Disorder | Comments |
|---|---|
| Graves disease | Common; TRAb mediated activation of TSHR |
| Toxic multinodular goiter | Common; autonomously functioning thyroid tissue |
| Toxic adenoma | Common; autonomously functioning thyroid tissue |
| Thyroiditis (acute, subacute, painless) | Common; thyroid inflammation resulting in release of stored thyroid hormones |
| Medication induced | Common; amiodarone, lithium, interferon alfa, interleukin-2, tyrosine kinase inhibitors, immune checkpoint inhibitors |
| Thyrotoxicosis factitia | Common; administration of exogenous thyroid hormone; ingestion of contaminated pork or beef products |
| HCG-mediated (Pregnancy, trophoblastic disease, germ cell tumor) | Common in pregnancy, other forms rare; indiscriminant binding of HCG to TSHR due to common alpha subunit shared by TSH and HCG. |
| Struma ovarii | Rare; autonomously functioning thyroid tissue in an ovarian teratoma accounting for >50% of the tumor |
| Follicular thyroid cancer metastases | Rare; autonomously functioning follicular thyroid carcinoma metastases |
| Thyrotrope adenoma | Rare; TSH-secreting pituitary adenoma |

HCG = human chorionic growth hormone; TSH = thyroid-stimulating hormone; TRAb = thyrotropin (TSH) receptor antibodies; TSHR = TSH receptor.

stimulate B lymphocytes to produce antibodies against the TSH receptor (TSI or TRAb). The thyroid is diffusely enlarged, may have a bruit, and has a firm, smooth texture on examination; cervical lymphadenopathy can occur. Systolic hypertension, tachycardia, hyperreflexia, and warm moist skin are often present.

Graves ophthalmopathy affects 25% of patients. Cigarette smoking is a risk factor. Clinical manifestations include periorbital edema, chemosis (conjunctival edema), proptosis (protrusion of the globe), diplopia (due to oculomotor paresis), and vision loss. Graves ophthalmopathy does not respond to the treatment of hyperthyroidism and often requires glucocorticoids or surgery.

Pretibial myxedema is a rare infiltrative dermopathy of Graves disease that affects 2% to 3% of patients; it is a nonpitting edema that is indurated, with a peau d'orange appearance, typically on the shins (see MKSAP 18 Dermatology).

### KEY POINTS

- In Graves disease, the thyroid is diffusely enlarged, may have a bruit, and has a firm, smooth texture on examination; cervical lymphadenopathy can also occur.
- Graves ophthalmopathy does not respond to the treatment of hyperthyroidism and often requires glucocorticoids or surgery.

### Toxic Adenoma and Multinodular Goiter
Toxic adenoma and multinodular goiter typically affect older adults as the prevalence of thyroid nodules increases with age. Thyroid nodules synthesize and secrete thyroid hormones independent of TSH stimulation. Exposure to iodinated contrast can precipitate conversion from nontoxic to toxic adenoma(s), such as with contrasted CT scanning and cardiac catheterization.

### Destructive Thyroiditis
Thyrotoxicosis occurs in destructive thyroiditis as a result of unregulated release of preformed thyroid hormone from thyroid follicles damaged by inflammation. Causes are listed in **Table 37**. Thyroiditis typically has three phases: thyrotoxic, hypothyroid, and return to euthyroidism. The first two phases can last up to 3 months each. A person has increased risk of additional bouts of thyroiditis once the initial thyroiditis has resolved.

### Management
Most thyrotoxic patients benefit from β-blockers (atenolol, metoprolol, propranolol) to reduce adrenergic symptoms rapidly. Propranolol decreases the peripheral conversion of $T_4$ to $T_3$, but is non-cardioselective and requires twice or three times daily dosing. Atenolol and metoprolol are preferred owing to once-daily dosing that increases adherence and their cardioselective nature that decreases central nervous system side effects.

There are three treatment modalities for hyperthyroidism: thioamides (methimazole and propylthiouracil [PTU]),

**TABLE 37.** Causes of Destructive Thyroiditis

| Disorder | Comments |
|---|---|
| Painless (silent) thyroiditis | Seen with underlying autoimmune thyroid disease (Hashimoto thyroiditis) |
| Postpartum thyroiditis | Painless thyroiditis occurring postpartum; permanent hypothyroidism occurs in 20% |
| Medication-induced thyroiditis | Painless thyroiditis; amiodarone, lithium, interferon alfa, interleukin-2, tyrosine kinase inhibitors, immune checkpoint inhibitors |
| Subacute thyroiditis (de Quervain or subacute granulomatous) | Painful thyroiditis; follows a viral upper respiratory tract infection |
| Infectious (suppurative) | Painful thyroiditis; *Staphylococcus* or *Streptococcus* species infection usually seen in immunocompromised patients |
| Radiation-induced thyroiditis | Painful thyroiditis; occurs after radioactive iodine therapy or neck external beam radiation therapy |

radioactive iodine ($^{131}$I) ablative therapy, and thyroidectomy. The choice of treatment is predicated on the cause of the hyperthyroidism and patient preference. Short-term use of methimazole to normalize thyroid function prior to $^{131}$I therapy or thyroidectomy is recommended for patients 65 years of age or older or who have prevalent cardiovascular disease or multiple comorbidities. Referral to an endocrinologist is recommended.

### Graves Disease
Antithyroid drugs (thionamides) are often used in the initial treatment of Graves hyperthyroidism because up to 50% will have spontaneous remission of hyperthyroidism within 24 months, especially if the goiter is small and only low doses of thioamide are required to achieve euthyroidism. Recurrent hyperthyroidism is likely if TRAb levels remain elevated at the time of drug discontinuation. If Graves hyperthyroidism recurs, definitive treatment is recommended.

Agranulocytosis and liver dysfunction are two rare but serious side effects of thioamides. Prior to treatment, baseline CBC with differential and liver profile should be assessed. Agranulocytosis should be suspected and the patient's neutrophil count assessed in the setting of fever or pharyngitis. Liver function should be assessed in any patient with symptoms or signs of hepatic dysfunction (jaundice, icterus). Methimazole is the antithyroid drug of choice, except in the first trimester of pregnancy, because PTU has been associated with fatal hepatonecrosis.

The goal of $^{131}$I ablative therapy in Graves disease is to render the patient hypothyroid. Women receiving $^{131}$I therapy must avoid pregnancy for 6 to 12 months after treatment. In patients with Graves ophthalmopathy, there is an acute escalation of thyroid autoantibody titers following radioiodine therapy that may exacerbate ocular symptoms. Pretreatment of

Graves ophthalmopathy or selection of alternative treatments depends on the severity of the eye disease.

Thyroidectomy in Graves hyperthyroidism is most appropriate when there is a large goiter with compressive symptoms, moderate to severe Graves ophthalmopathy, and/or with coexistent thyroid cancer or primary hyperparathyroidism.

### Other Causes

First-line therapy for a toxic adenoma or toxic multinodular goiter is either $^{131}$I therapy or thyroid surgery. Choice is determined by patient preference, presence of compressive symptoms, and access to a high-volume thyroid surgeon.

Destructive thyroiditis is managed expectantly with β-blockers to control adrenergic symptoms and NSAIDs, followed by high-dose glucocorticoid therapy, for pain control in painful thyroiditis.

**KEY POINTS**

- Most thyrotoxic patients benefit from β-blockers to reduce adrenergic symptoms.
- The three treatment modalities for hyperthyroidism are thionamides (methimazole and propylthiouracil), radioactive iodine ($^{131}$I) ablative therapy, and thyroidectomy; the choice of treatment is predicated on the cause of the hyperthyroidism and patient preference.
- Antithyroid drugs (thionamides) are associated with up to a 50% spontaneous remission rate within 24 months; agranulocytosis and liver dysfunction are two rare but serious side effects.

### Subclinical Hyperthyroidism

Subclinical hyperthyroidism diagnosis is based on suppression of the serum TSH, with normal $T_4$ and $T_3$ levels. Subclinical hyperthyroidism affects 0.7% of the U.S. population. Approximately 0.5% to 7% progress to overt hyperthyroidism per year and 5% to 12% revert to normal thyroid function. The most common cause is toxic multinodular goiter.

Subclinical hyperthyroidism has been associated with an increased risk of atrial fibrillation and cardiovascular events. A recent large prospective cohort study demonstrated higher rates of hip fracture with subclinical hyperthyroidism (7% in subclinical hyperthyroidism vs. 4.5% in euthyroid patients); however, it is unknown whether treatment reduces fracture risk.

The TSH will normalize at 6 weeks in more than 25% of patients with subclinical hyperthyroidism. Therefore, observation and rechecking thyroid function prior to the initiation of treatment is reasonable unless the risk of complications is high, such as in patients with cardiac disease. Higher risk of cardiovascular and skeletal complications is seen with serum TSH level under 0.1 µU/mL (0.1 mU/L). Treatment of subclinical hyperthyroidism is recommended for patients with serum TSH levels below 0.1 µU/mL (0.1 mU/L) and with symptoms, cardiac risk factors, heart disease, or osteoporosis, as well as for postmenopausal women not taking estrogen therapy or bisphosphonates.

**KEY POINTS**

- Subclinical hyperthyroidism is diagnosed based on suppression of the serum thyroid-stimulating hormone, but normal thyroxine and triiodothyronine levels.
- Treatment of subclinical hyperthyroidism is recommended for patients with serum thyroid-stimulating levels below 0.1 µU/mL (0.1 mU/L) and symptoms, cardiac risk factors, heart disease, or osteoporosis, as well as for postmenopausal women not taking estrogen therapy or bisphosphonates.

## Thyroid Hormone Deficiency

Thyroid hormone deficiency affects more than 10 million Americans. It is 10 times more common in women than men.

### Clinical Features and Diagnosis

Signs and symptoms of thyroid hormone deficiency are listed in Table 35. Thyroid hormone deficiency is also associated with laboratory abnormalities including anemia, elevated LDL cholesterol, and hyponatremia.

The diagnosis of primary hypothyroidism is made by measuring serum TSH, and if elevated, measuring free $T_4$, which can be added on in most laboratories. Serum TSH is elevated in both overt and subclinical hypothyroidism, but free $T_4$ is normal when subclinical and low in overt hypothyroidism. Thyroid autoantibodies [thyroid perioxidase (TPO) antibodies] are present in most patients with Hashimoto thyroiditis; however, measurement of TPO antibody titer is not necessary unless the diagnosis is unclear. The diagnosis of hypothyroidism is discussed elsewhere (see Disorders of the Pituitary Gland).

**KEY POINTS**

- The diagnosis of hypothyroidism is made by measuring serum thyroid-stimulating hormone, and if elevated, then measuring free thyroxine.
- Serum thyroid-stimulating hormone is elevated in both overt and subclinical hypothyroidism, but free thyroxine is normal in subclinical hypothyroidism and low in overt hypothyroidism.
- Thyroid autoantibodies [thyroid perioxidase (TPO) antibodies] are present in most patients with Hashimoto thyroiditis; however, measurement of TPO antibody titer is not necessary unless the diagnosis is unclear. **HVC**

### Causes

Causes of hypothyroidism are listed in **Table 38**. The most common cause in the United States is autoimmune thyroid gland failure (due to Hashimoto thyroiditis), while iodine deficiency, which affects 2 billion people worldwide, is the most common cause globally. Iodide deficiency is uncommon in the

**TABLE 38.** Causes of Thyroid Hormone Deficiency

| Disorder | Comments |
|----------|----------|
| Hashimoto thyroiditis | Autoimmune thyroid disorder associated with anti-TPO antibodies |
| Post-thyroidectomy | Treatment of Graves disease, goiter, thyroid nodules, or thyroid cancer |
| Post-radioactive iodine therapy | Treatment of Graves disease or toxic adenoma/multinodular goiter |
| External beam radiation to the neck | Treatment of Hodgkin lymphoma and head/neck malignancies |
| Thyroiditis (acute, subacute, suppurative) | Typically a transient hypothyroidism prior to recovery of euthyroid state |
| Central hypothyroidism | TSH deficiency from hypothalamic or pituitary disease; TSH should not be used to assess for replacement dose adequacy; $T_4$ level should be used for dosing |
| Congenital hypothyroidism | Universal neonatal screening in the United States where the incidence is 1 in 3500 |
| Iodide deficiency | Common worldwide in developing countries with severe iodine deficiency |
| Drug-induced | Amiodarone, lithium, interferon-alpha, interleukin-2, iodine, thionamides (methimazole), ethionamide, tyrosine kinase inhibitors (sunitinib), immune checkpoint inhibitors (ipilimumab) |

Anti-TPO = anti-thyroid peroxidase; TSH = thyroid-stimulating hormone; $T_4$ = thyroxine.

United States as a result of efforts to fortify food (iodized salt). Central hypothyroidism is also uncommon.

### Primary Hypothyroidism

Hashimoto thyroiditis (chronic lymphocytic thyroiditis) is an autoimmune thyroid disorder characterized by diffuse infiltration of the thyroid gland by lymphocytes and plasma cells with subsequent follicular atrophy and scarring. It is more common in patients with other autoimmune disorders or a family history of thyroid autoimmunity. Diffuse goiter can be seen most commonly in younger patients. Most patients (90%) have TPO antibodies, and the risk of developing hypothyroidism is four times higher in euthyroid patients with TPO antibodies.

Hypothyroidism occurs in all patients after thyroidectomy and 20% of patients after thyroid lobectomy. Postablative hypothyroidism occurs after [131]I therapy in 90% of patients with Graves disease within 1 year of radioactive iodine therapy, and in 60% of patients with toxic multinodular goiter, although onset of hypothyroidism may be delayed for many years in the latter case. External beam radiation to the neck also can cause hypothyroidism, as with Hodgkin lymphoma and head/neck malignancies.

Drug-induced hypothyroidism is another cause of primary hypothyroidism (see Table 38).

**KEY POINTS**

- The most common cause of primary hypothyroidism is autoimmune thyroid gland failure due to Hashimoto thyroiditis, typically associated with thyroid perioxidase antibodies.

- In addition to Hashimoto thyroiditis, common causes of hypothyroidism include thyroid surgery and postablative hypothyroidism following [131]I therapy for treatment of Graves disease or toxic multinodular goiter.

### Subclinical Hypothyroidism

Subclinical hypothyroidism is typically asymptomatic and diagnosed by a serum TSH level above the upper limit of the reference range and a normal free $T_4$ level. It affects 5% to 10% of the general population. Transient elevation of serum TSH should be ruled out by repeating the measurement in 6 to 8 weeks. The rate of progression from subclinical to overt hypothyroidism is 2% to 4% per year, while one-third of patients spontaneously revert to normal thyroid function. The normal range for TSH increases with age, and a TSH level of up to 10 µU/mL (10 mU/L) is within the normal range for persons 80 years of age and older.

Subclinical hypothyroidism with TSH above 10 µU/mL (10 mU/L) may be a risk factor for coronary artery disease and heart failure. There is no evidence that treating subclinical hypothyroidism improves quality of life, cognitive function, blood pressure, or weight, but in patients with elevated LDL cholesterol, normalization of the TSH will lower LDL cholesterol.

### Management

Thyroid hormone replacement with levothyroxine is the treatment of choice for thyroid hormone deficiency. Goals of treatment are to normalize serum TSH (in primary hypothyroidism) or free $T_4$ (in central hypothyroidism) and to resolve signs and symptoms of hypothyroidism. Beginning a full replacement dose (1.6 µg/kg lean body weight) is appropriate for most patients with overt hypothyroidism, except in older adults and patients with cardiovascular disease for whom lower initial doses (25-50 µg/day) are recommended. Assessment of the adequacy of treatment should be done with a repeat serum TSH level at least 6 weeks after initiation or change in dose with a goal of a normal TSH.

$T_3$-containing compounds are not recommended in the treatment of hypothyroidism due to its short half-life, which results in spikes in $T_3$ levels. Studies have failed to show that $T_3$ alone or in combination with $T_4$ has clear benefit in treatment of hypothyroidism.

Subclinical hypothyroidism with a serum TSH value above 10 µU/mL (10 mU/L) should be treated. Initial treatment is 25 to 50 µg of levothyroxine per day. There is unclear benefit and potential for harm in treating mild subclinical hypothyroidism

(TSH > 5-10 µU/mL [5-10 mU/L]). Overtreatment is seen in more than one-third of patients over 65, which may increase risk for dysrhythmia and bone loss.

Oral levothyroxine is absorbed in the jejunum and ileum. Ideally it should be taken on an empty stomach (60 minutes before breakfast or coffee are consumed). If the patient is having difficulty adhering to morning administration, then it can be taken before bed. Missed doses can be taken the following day in younger patients struggling with daily adherence. The absorption of an orally administered dose is 70% to 80% under optimum fasting conditions. Gastrointestinal disorders (such as celiac disease) may impact absorption and result in higher than expected levothyroxine dose requirements. Medications can also interfere with the absorption or metabolism of levothyroxine (see Table 34).

**KEY POINTS**

- Levothyroxine is the treatment of choice for thyroid hormone deficiency; it should be taken on an empty stomach 60 minutes before eating breakfast or consuming coffee.

HVC
- Triiodothyronine-containing compounds are not recommended in the treatment of hypothyroidism due to its short half-life, which results in spikes in triiodothyronine levels.

HVC
- Overtreatment of subclinical hypothyroidism is common, especially in patients older than 65 years of age, and should be avoided.

### Drug-Induced Thyroid Dysfunction

Many medications can affect thyroid function and are listed in Table 34.

Amiodarone is an antiarrhythmic medication with high iodine content (37%) and prolonged half-life of approximately 60 days. Thyroid dysfunction occurs in approximately 25% of amiodarone-treated patients and can present as hypothyroidism, hyperthyroidism, painless thyroiditis, or goiter. Hypothyroidism, seen in 20% of affected patients, is usually seen in the setting of Hashimoto thyroiditis. All patients can have a transient rise in TSH levels in the first few months of amiodarone therapy due to the Wolff-Chaikoff effect (temporary decrease in thyroid production due to iodine load), but most regain normal thyroid function.

Thyrotoxicosis affects 5% of patients treated with amiodarone. Type 1 (hyperthyroidism) amiodarone-induced thyrotoxicosis occurs in patients with Graves disease or thyroid nodules. It is a form of iodine-induced hyperthyroidism (Jod-Basedow phenomenon). It is treated with thioamides, typically methimazole. Type 2 (destructive thyroiditis) amiodarone-induced thyrotoxicosis is more common and occurs in patients without underlying thyroid disease. It is usually self-limiting but sometimes requires treatment with moderate- to high-dose glucocorticoids. The decision to discontinue amiodarone

depends on the patient's cardiac condition and type of thyrotoxicosis (type 1 or 2).

**KEY POINT**

- Thyroid dysfunction occurs in approximately 25% of patients taking amiodarone and can present as hypothyroidism, hyperthyroidism, painless thyroiditis, or goiter.

## Thyroid Function and Dysfunction in Pregnancy

Thyroid hormones are essential for normal fetal development. The size of the maternal thyroid gland can increase up to 40% during pregnancy. Production of $T_4$ and $T_3$ increases up to 50% to compensate for the increased thyroxine-binding globulin production associated with pregnancy-related increase in estrogen. Iodine requirements also increase up to 50%. Pregnant and lactating women should therefore be counseled to supplement their dietary iodine intake with a daily oral supplement containing 150 µg of iodine, which is included in some but not all over-the-counter and prescription prenatal vitamins. Universal screening of TSH in pregnant women is not recommended. However, those at increased risk of thyroid dysfunction should be screened, which includes those 30 years of age and older; with known hypothyroidism and/or a strong family history of thyroid dysfunction; prior head/neck irradiation; prior neck surgery; positive TPO, TSI, or TRAb status; or other autoimmune disorders.

Changes in thyroid function tests are depicted in **Figure 10**. Placental human chorionic gonadotropin (hCG) stimulates

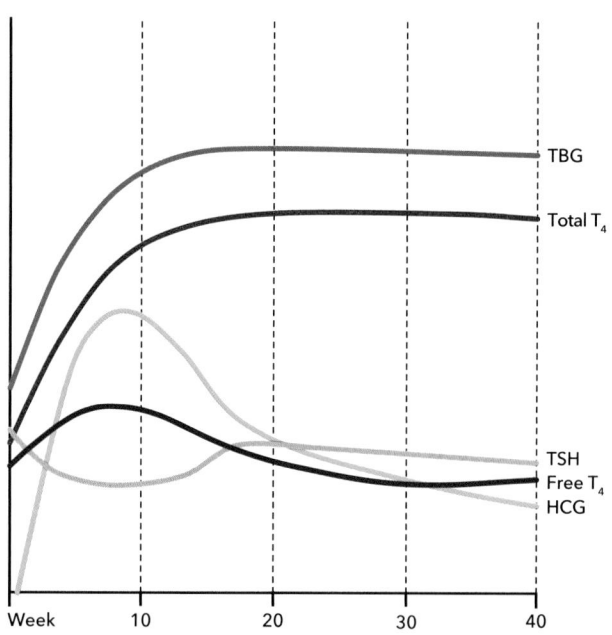

**FIGURE 10.** Changes in thyroid function tests in pregnancy. HCG = human chorionic gonadotropin; $T_4$ = thyroxine; TBG = thyroid-binding globulin; TSH = thyroid-stimulating hormone.

thyroid hormone secretion and TSH may be mildly suppressed as a result. In the late first trimester (weeks 7-12) the lower limit of the TSH reference range decreases by 0.4 µU/mL (0.4 mU/L) and upper limit by 0.5 µU/mL (0.5 mU/L). Serum TSH gradually returns to the nonpregnant reference range in the second and third trimester.

Measured total $T_4$ concentrations increase linearly during pregnancy. After week 16, the upper limit of the total $T_4$ reference range can be estimated by multiplying the nonpregnant upper limit by 1.5. Free $T_4$ measured by indirect analogue immunoassays are inaccurate in pregnancy unless method and trimester-specific reference ranges are applied.

Consultation with an endocrinologist is indicated for management of thyrotoxicosis during pregnancy. Gestational thyrotoxicosis from high human chorionic gonadotropin levels is the most common cause of transient TSH suppression. If serum total or free $T_4$ remains within the trimester-specific reference range, treatment is not needed. Women with moderate to severe hyperthyroidism in early pregnancy should be treated with PTU because potential teratogenic effects are less severe than with methimazole. After the first trimester, women can be transitioned to methimazole. Thyroid function should be followed closely and the serum total or free $T_4$ should be maintained at or just above the trimester-specific reference range to avoid fetal hypothyroidism.

Graves disease affects 0.2% of pregnant women and can be confirmed by classic physical findings or elevated TSI or TRAb. Women with Graves disease are considered high-risk pregnancies and should be followed by maternal fetal specialists throughout the pregnancy.

Hypothyroidism in pregnancy is associated with increases in miscarriage, premature birth, low birth weight, and decreased infant neurocognitive function. Levothyroxine is the treatment of choice.

For women with preexisting hypothyroidism, levothyroxine dosing can be empirically increased by 30% when pregnancy is confirmed. In treatment-naïve pregnant women with positive TPO antibodies, levothyroxine is started if TSH level is ≥2.5 µU/mL (2.5 mU/L). Treatment is indicated for TPO-negative pregnant women if TSH is above the pregnancy-specific reference range. TSH should be measured every 4 weeks for the first half of pregnancy and around 30 weeks in all hypothyroid women and in those at risk for hypothyroidism (antibody positive or history of hemithyroidectomy or [131]I therapy). A TSH level less than 2.5 µU/mL (2.5 mU/L) should be targeted in treated hypothyroid women both preconception and during pregnancy.

Thyroid nodules detected in pregnant women should be evaluated as in nonpregnant patients. The timing of FNAB, whether during or after pregnancy, is determined by the likelihood of cancer and patient preference. Consultation with an endocrinologist is indicated for management of thyroid cancer

detected during pregnancy. Pregnant women with a history of thyroid cancer should be managed as when not pregnant.

**KEY POINTS**

- For women with preexisting hypothyroidism, levothyroxine dosing can be empirically increased by 30% when pregnancy is confirmed.

- In treatment-naïve pregnant women with positive thyroid peroxidase (TPO) antibodies, levothyroxine is started if thyroid-stimulating hormone level is 2.5 µU/mL (2.5 mU/L) or higher; and treatment is indicated for TPO-negative pregnant women if the thyroid-stimulating hormone level is above the pregnancy-specific reference range.

# Nonthyroidal Illness Syndrome (Euthyroid Sick Syndrome)

Nonthyroidal illness syndrome (NTIS) commonly occurs in patients who are hospitalized and critically ill. Up to 75% of hospitalized patients have thyroid function test abnormalities. Nonthyroidal illness suppresses thyrotropin-releasing hormone, which typically results in suppressed but detectable TSH. An undetectable TSH is not consistent with NTIS. Infrequently, TSH can be mildly elevated in NTIS, but a TSH level of 20 µU/mL (20 mU/L) or greater is not consistent with NTIS. $T_4$ is typically normal, but due to decreased deiodinase activity in $T_4$ metabolism, $T_3$ decreases and reverse $T_3$ increases (biologically inactive). Thyroid-binding globulin decreases in illness, lowering the total $T_4$ and $T_3$ levels. NTIS can be interpreted as an adaptive response to systemic illness and macronutrient restriction.

Treatment of NTIS is not recommended due to lack of significant clinical benefit. In general, thyroid function should not be assessed in hospitalized patients unless there is a strong clinical suspicion of thyroid dysfunction. If NTIS is diagnosed, TSH should be rechecked approximately 6 weeks after the patient has recovered from their nonthyroidal illness to assess for return to normal.

**KEY POINTS**

- Treatment of nonthyroidal illness syndrome is not recommended due to lack of significant clinical benefit. **HVC**

- Thyroid function should not be assessed in hospitalized patients unless there is a strong clinical suspicion of thyroid dysfunction. **HVC**

# Thyroid Emergencies
### Thyroid Storm

Thyroid storm is a rare disorder with high mortality (up to 30%) characterized by severe thyrotoxicosis (suppressed TSH, elevated free $T_4$ and/or total $T_3$) and systemic hemodynamic decompensation (shock). Serum thyroid hormone concentrations do not

CONT.

differentiate thyroid storm from severe thyrotoxicosis. It is the presence of shock that makes the diagnosis of thyroid storm.

Presentation often follows discontinuation of antithyroid drug therapy, systemic illness, labor and delivery, surgery, or trauma. Patients with Graves disease are at higher risk. Clinical manifestations include high fever, tachycardia, altered mental status, and cardiac and hepatic dysfunction. A scoring system, such as the Burch and Wartofsky Point Scale (Table 39), can support the diagnosis, but thyroid storm is diagnosed clinically.

Management includes ICU-level care, treatment of any precipitant illness, thyrotoxicosis-directed therapy, and supportive measures. Thyrotoxicosis is treated with intravenous β-blockers (esmolol infusion), thioamide (typically PTU, transitioning to methimazole when more stable), intravenous high-dose glucocorticoids, and potassium iodide. Iodide should be administered more than 1 hour after antithyroid drugs to avoid providing substrate to the gland. Glucocorticoid therapy is a potent inhibitor of peripheral $T_4$ to $T_3$ conversion. Bile acid sequestrants can be used to decrease $T_4$ and $T_3$ levels, especially in patients unable to take thioamides. Plasmapheresis or emergent thyroidectomy is used in patients who respond poorly to medical therapy. Definitive treatment with thyroidectomy or [131]I therapy is indicated in patients who survive thyroid storm. 

### KEY POINTS

- Thyroid storm is a rare disorder with high mortality (up to 30%) characterized by severe thyrotoxicosis and systemic hemodynamic decompensation.
- Thyroid storm often occurs with discontinuation of antithyroid drug therapy, systemic illness, labor and delivery, surgery, or trauma.
- ICU-level care; treating any precipitating illness; and the use of intravenous β-blockers, thioamide, intravenous high-dose glucocorticoids, and potassium iodide are all used to manage thyroid storm.

##  Myxedema Coma

Myxedema coma is a life-threatening presentation of severe hypothyroidism with hemodynamic compromise that affects 0.22 people per million per year. Mortality is high (up to 40%), and ICU-level care is required. Risk factors for myxedema coma are female gender, advanced age, cold exposure, or a precipitant event in patients with undiagnosed hypothyroidism, such as myocardial infarction, sepsis, trauma, or stroke. Mental status changes ranging from lethargy to coma to psychosis, coupled with hypothermia (temperature below 34.4 °C (94.0 °F) are the most common clinical manifestations. Bradycardia, hypotension, or decreased respiration rate with resultant hypoxia and hypercapnia are also frequently present. Careful examination of the neck for thyroidectomy scar is critical. Free $T_4$ is low in myxedema coma. TSH is typically elevated, but without an overtly low free $T_4$, myxedema coma

| Criteria | Points |
|---|---|
| **Thermoregulatory Dysfunction** | |
| Temperature °F (°C) | |
| 99-99.9 (37.2-37.7) | 5 |
| 100-100.9 (37.8-38.2) | 10 |
| 101-101.9 (38.3-38.8) | 15 |
| 102-102.9 (38.9-39.3) | 20 |
| 103-103.9 (39.4-39.9) | 25 |
| ≥104 (40) | 30 |
| **Cardiovascular** | |
| Tachycardia (bpm) | |
| 100-109 | 5 |
| 110-119 | 10 |
| 120-129 | 15 |
| 130-139 | 20 |
| ≥140 | 25 |
| Atrial fibrillation | |
| Absent | 0 |
| Present | 10 |
| Congestive heart failure | |
| Absent | 0 |
| Mild | 5 |
| Moderate | 10 |
| Severe | 20 |
| **Gastrointestinal-Hepatic Dysfunction** | |
| Absent | 0 |
| Moderate (diarrhea, abdominal pain, nausea, vomiting) | 10 |
| Severe (jaundice) | 20 |
| **Central Nervous System Disturbance** | |
| Absent | 0 |
| Mild (agitation) | 10 |
| Moderate (delirium, psychosis, extreme lethargy) | 20 |
| Severe (seizure, coma) | 30 |
| **Precipitant History** | |
| Absent | 0 |
| Present | 10 |
| **Scores Totaled** | |
| <25 | Thyroid storm is unlikely |
| 25-45 | Impending thyroid storm |
| >45 | Thyroid storm is likely |

**TABLE 39.** Burch and Wartofsky Point Scale to Support the Diagnosis of Thyroid Storm[a]

[a]Thyroid storm is diagnosed clinically in the presence of hemodynamic compromise.

From Burch HB, Wartofsky L. Life-threatening thyrotoxicosis: thyroid storm. Endocrinol Metab Clin North Am. 1993 Jun;22(2):263-77. Review. PMID: 8325286.

CONT.

is unlikely regardless of how high the TSH. Other metabolic derangements include hyponatremia and hypoglycemia. Cortisol should be drawn with initial laboratory studies to assess for concomitant cortisol deficiency.

Aggressive supportive measures include fluids, vasopressors if necessary, ventilator support, and passive warming rather than active warming to avoid vasodilation, which can worsen hypotension. Stress-dose glucocorticoids (100 mg intravenous hydrocortisone every 8 hours) are administered empirically before thyroid hormone is initiated to treat possible concomitant adrenal insufficiency. If random cortisol level is above 18 mg/dL (496.8 nmol/L), hydrocortisone can be discontinued. Replacement of thyroid hormone requires consideration of the need to normalize the thyroid hormone level rapidly and the risk of a fatal cardiac event caused by thyroid hormone administration. Initial treatment is intravenous levothyroxine with loading dose of 200 to 400 µg, followed by a daily oral dose of 1.6 µg/kg. The dose should be reduced to 75% if administered intravenously. Lower levothyroxine doses are recommended with advanced age and/or cardiac disease. Goals of treatment are improved mental status, metabolic parameters, and cardiopulmonary function. When the patient is stable, transition to oral levothyroxine is the goal.

### KEY POINTS

- Myxedema coma is a life-threatening presentation of severe hypothyroidism with hemodynamic compromise; it most often occurs when a systemic illness is superimposed on previously undiagnosed hypothyroidism.

- In addition to aggressive supportive measures, stress-dose glucocorticoids (100 mg intravenous hydrocortisone every 8 hours) are administered empirically before thyroid hormone is initiated to treat possible concomitant adrenal insufficiency.

# Reproductive Disorders
## Physiology of Female Reproduction

Coordinated actions of the hypothalamus, pituitary gland, and ovaries (known as the hypothalamic-pituitary-ovarian axis) give rise to ovulatory cycles in women. The pulsatile release of gonadotropin-releasing hormone (GnRH) drives the anterior pituitary cells to secrete follicle-stimulating hormone (FSH) and luteinizing hormone (LH) (**Figure 11**). FSH regulates estradiol production and follicle growth in the follicular phase of the menstrual cycle. A sudden rise in LH levels causes release of an ovum midcycle, signaling the start of the luteal phase, which is a constant 14 days. Endometrial sloughing follows decreased estrogen or progesterone levels if a fertilized embryo does not implant. Menses occur every 25 to 35 days; menstrual cycles shorter than 25 days or longer than 35 days in women

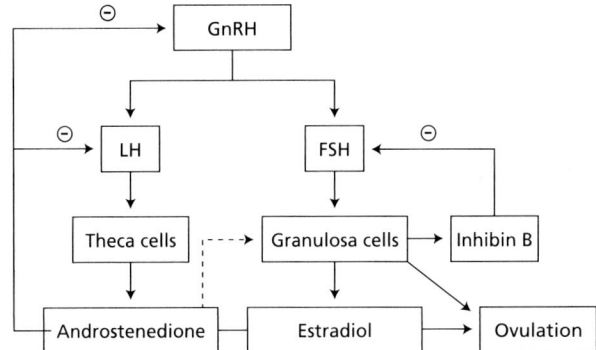

**FIGURE 11.** Female reproductive axis. Pulses of GnRH drive LH and FSH production. LH acts on theca cells to stimulate androgen (principally androstenedione) production. Androstenedione is metabolized to estradiol in granulosa cells. FSH acts on granulosa cells to enhance follicle maturation. Granulosa cells produce inhibin B as a feedback regulator of FSH production. FSH = follicle-stimulating hormone; GnRH = gonadotropin-releasing hormone; LH = luteinizing hormone; – (circled) = negative feedback.

younger than age 40 years are likely anovulatory, resulting in abnormal uterine bleeding or oligomenorrhea. Before puberty, ovaries are quiescent due to immaturity of the hypothalamus. After menopause, all reproductive function and most endocrine function of the ovaries ceases.

### KEY POINT

- In women younger than age 40 years, menstrual cycles shorter than 25 days or longer than 35 days are likely anovulatory.

## Amenorrhea

Amenorrhea, the absence of menses, can be intermittent or permanent. It may result from hypothalamic, pituitary, ovarian, uterine, or outflow tract disorders.

### Clinical Features
#### Primary Amenorrhea
Primary amenorrhea is defined as absence of menses at age 15 years in the presence of normal growth and secondary sexual characteristics. Primary amenorrhea is most commonly caused by a genetic (50%) or anatomic (15%) abnormality. Most causes of secondary amenorrhea can also present as primary amenorrhea.

The most common cause of primary amenorrhea is gonadal dysgenesis, most commonly with Turner syndrome (45,X0). Turner syndrome is caused by loss of part or all of an X chromosome. It occurs in 1 in 2500 live female births. It is associated with short stature and primary ovarian insufficiency (POI); primary amenorrhea is seen in approximately 90% of patients with Turner syndrome.

Anatomic abnormalities that can cause primary amenorrhea include an intact hymen, transverse vaginal septum, and vaginal agenesis. Vaginal agenesis (also known as müllerian agenesis or Mayer-Rokitansky-Küster-Hauser syndrome) is the second most common cause of primary amenorrhea, with an incidence of 1 in 5000 live female births. Women with vaginal agenesis have a normal female karyotype and ovarian function, and thus, normal external genitalia and secondary sexual characteristics.

## Secondary Amenorrhea

Secondary amenorrhea is defined as absence of menses for more than 3 months in women who previously had regular menstrual cycles or for 6 months in women who have irregular menses. In women with oligomenorrhea, defined as fewer than nine menstrual cycles per year or cycle length longer than 35 days, the evaluation is the same as for secondary amenorrhea.

Functional hypothalamic amenorrhea (FHA) is caused by a disruption of the hypothalamic-pituitary-ovarian axis and is the most common cause of secondary amenorrhea after pregnancy. Disruption of the pulsatile release of hypothalamic GnRH may occur due to stress, weight loss, or exercise. In many cases, all three factors are present. FHA is a diagnosis of exclusion; history and physical examination, biochemical testing, and, imaging, when appropriate, should be undertaken to rule out other causes of secondary amenorrhea including intracranial tumor, infiltrative or destructive disorders such as lymphocytic hypophysitis, histiocytosis X, sarcoidosis, Sheehan syndrome, and acute or chronic systemic illness.

Premenopausal women with hyperprolactinemia present more often with oligomenorrhea or amenorrhea than galactorrhea. Hyperprolactinemia accounts for 10% to 20% of non-pregnancy-mediated amenorrhea. Menstrual dysfunction in hyperprolactinemia results from inhibition of GnRH.

Menstrual dysfunction is common in women with thyroid disorders; while heavy bleeding is typical with hypothyroidism, secondary amenorrhea can also occur.

Hyperandrogenic disorders are associated with amenorrhea, with polycystic ovary syndrome by far the most common hyperandrogenic cause.

Spontaneous primary ovarian insufficiency (POI) can be diagnosed in women younger than age 40 years with menstrual dysfunction in association with two serum FSH levels in the menopausal range. POI affects 1 in 100 women. In addition to disordered menses, affected women may develop symptoms related to estrogen deficiency, such as vasomotor symptoms, sleep disturbance, and dyspareunia related to vaginal dryness. Most cases are sporadic, but a first-degree relative with POI suggests a familial etiology, whereas a personal history of autoimmune disorders can suggest an autoimmune polyglandular syndrome. Women with POI have increased risk for development of autoimmune adrenal insufficiency.

Intrauterine adhesions are the only uterine cause of secondary amenorrhea. Amenorrhea results from the development of scar tissue within the uterine cavity preventing build up and shedding of endometrial cells. Adhesions develop following uterine instrumentation, most commonly associated with uterine curettage for pregnancy complications (Asherman syndrome).

## Evaluation of Amenorrhea

A thorough history and physical examination is the first step in evaluating amenorrhea. Important data include medication and illicit drug exposure, changes in weight, exercise history, psychosocial stressors, and family history related to menarche. Symptoms can include headaches or visual changes suggesting pituitary pathology, symptoms of thyroid excess or deficiency, galactorrhea suggesting hyperprolactinemia, or vasomotor symptoms associated with estrogen deficiency.

Physical examination should include a pelvic examination to evaluate the vagina, cervix, and uterus for abnormalities. Imaging may be necessary to confirm a normal uterus. Physical examination should also include evaluation for features of Turner syndrome, such as a low hairline, webbed neck, shield chest, and widely spaced nipples.

In patients with primary or secondary amenorrhea, measurement of height, weight, and BMI is important. A low BMI (<18.5) may suggest FHA due to an eating disorder, excessive exercise, or systemic illness. A high BMI (≥30) is frequently seen in women with polycystic ovary syndrome (PCOS). Additional physical examination findings suggestive of PCOS include acne and hirsutism. Hypercortisolism is associated with acne and hirsutism, as well as abnormal fat pad distribution, centripetal obesity, facial plethora, proximal muscle weakness, and wide (>1 cm) violaceous striae. Vitiligo or other signs of autoimmune disease increase the likelihood of autoimmune POI. Breast examination should include assessment for expressible galactorrhea. Vulvovaginal atrophy suggests estrogen deficiency.

After ruling out pregnancy, initial laboratory testing in both primary and secondary amenorrhea should include measurement of FSH, thyroid-stimulating hormone (TSH), free thyroxine, and prolactin levels. Next steps are guided by these laboratory results (**Figure 12**).

If the TSH level is abnormal, evaluation and management of thyroid dysfunction should occur (see Disorders of the Thyroid Gland).

If the prolactin level is elevated, repeat prolactin testing is needed to confirm the diagnosis. A careful review of medications is essential because many drugs can cause hyperprolactinemia. Kidney and liver function testing is also required (see Disorders of the Pituitary Gland).

If the FSH level is elevated, testing should be repeated in 1 month with simultaneous serum estradiol testing. If the FSH

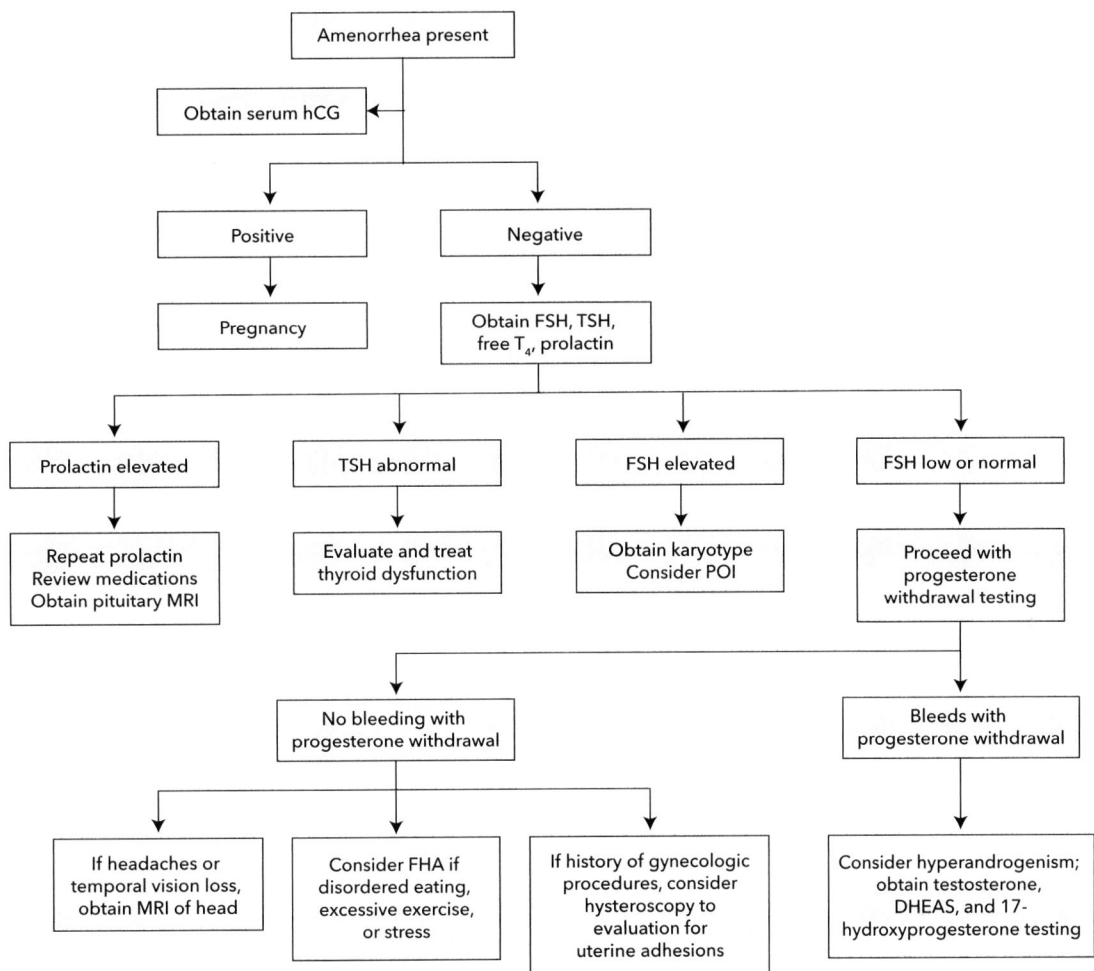

**FIGURE 12.** Algorithm for evaluating amenorrhea. FHA = functional hypothalamic amenorrhea; FSH = follicle-stimulating hormone; DHEAS = dehydroepiandrosterone sulfate; hCG = human chorionic gonadotropin; POI = primary ovarian insufficiency; T$_4$ = thyroxine; TSH = thyroid-stimulating hormone.

level is elevated on repeat testing and estradiol level is low, karyotype analysis is indicated to evaluate for Turner syndrome. POI and menopause also cause elevated FSH levels.

In women with normal or low FSH levels, the history and physical examination findings determine next steps. Further assessment of estrogen status can be determined by a progestin withdrawal test. If a normal estrogen state is confirmed (bleeding within a week of stopping progesterone), hyperandrogenism should be considered. Laboratory evaluation for hyperandrogenism includes measurement of total testosterone and sex hormone-binding globulin (SHBG) levels. PCOS is the most likely cause of menstrual dysfunction in women with hyperandrogenism; however, other hyperandrogenic disorders must be excluded before diagnosing PCOS. If no bleeding occurs, a low-estrogen state due to hypothalamic hypogonadism is most likely.

Imaging studies that can be utilized in the evaluation of amenorrhea include MRI of the sellar region (to evaluate for structural integrity of the pituitary), pelvic ultrasound (to assess for anatomic abnormalities of uterus, vagina, and ovaries), hysterosalpingogram and hysteroscopy (to assess for

uterine outflow obstructions). Choice of imaging study, as well as necessity of imaging at all, is predicated on prior biochemical test results indicating the cause of the amenorrhea.

**KEY POINT**

- After ruling out pregnancy, initial laboratory testing in both primary and secondary amenorrhea should include measurement of follicle-stimulating hormone, thyroid-stimulating hormone, free thyroxine, and prolactin.

## Treatment of Amenorrhea

Almost all women with Turner syndrome will need exogenous estrogen therapy with cyclic progestin to prevent endometrial hyperplasia. Estrogen-progestin therapy is continued until age 51 years, the average age of menopause.

Treatment for FHA includes less-restrictive eating patterns, weight gain, or a reduction in strenuous exercise to restore menses. Additionally, it is important to treat conditions associated with FHA, including low bone mass, eating disorders, anxiety, and other mood disorders.

Amenorrhea due to hyperprolactinemia with a lactotroph adenoma is managed with dopamine agonist therapy if fertility is desired, or with estrogen/progestin if not, to prevent bone loss. If hyperprolactinemia-induced amenorrhea is related to medications that cannot be stopped (such as antipsychotic agents), estrogen/progestin therapy is indicated.

Treatment of POI includes estrogen/progestin therapy until approximately age 51 years. Psychosocial support is important due to higher scores on depression, anxiety, and negative affect scales in patients with POI; subspecialty consultation to discuss fertility options is also indicated.

Treatment of vaginal agenesis includes nonsurgical vaginal dilation; surgical options can be considered if nonsurgical therapy fails.

# Hyperandrogenism Syndromes

## Hirsutism and Polycystic Ovary Syndrome

Elevated serum concentrations of androgens in women most commonly manifest with hirsutism and may also present with acne, androgenetic alopecia, and/or virilization. Hirsutism is the presence of excessive terminal hair in male-pattern growth distribution; it affects approximately 10% of women. Virilization (voice deepening, clitoromegaly, male pattern baldness, severe acne) occurs only in severe hyperandrogenism and raises concern for ovarian hyperthecosis or an androgen-producing ovarian or adrenal tumor. Onset of hirsutism in a woman older than age 30 years also raises concern for an androgen-producing tumor. Although androgen-secreting ovarian tumors are rare, they should be considered in patients with abrupt, rapidly progressive hirsutism or severe hyperandrogenemia as well as in women with marked hyperandrogenemia (total testosterone >150 ng/dL [5.2 nmol/L]).

Women with chronic hirsutism and menstrual cycles every 25 to 35 days most likely have idiopathic hirsutism or PCOS. Fifteen to 40% of women with hyperandrogenism and menses every 21 to 35 days have ovulatory dysfunction. PCOS is the most common cause of hirsutism, accounting for 95% of cases.

PCOS is a disorder characterized by hyperandrogenism and ovulatory dysfunction. PCOS affects 6% to 10% of women and is the most common cause of anovulatory infertility in women. It is associated with rapid GnRH pulses, an excess of LH, and insufficient FSH secretion, resulting in excessive ovarian androgen production and ovulatory dysfunction. It is accompanied by insulin resistance. Elevated insulin levels in PCOS further enhance ovarian and adrenal androgen production, as well as increase bioavailability of androgens related to a reduction in SHBG. PCOS is associated with increased incidence of metabolic syndrome, prediabetes, type 2 diabetes mellitus, hypercholesterolemia, and obesity.

There are a variety of diagnostic criteria for PCOS (**Table 40**). It is important to remember that PCOS is a diagnosis of exclusion; other causes of oligo-/anovulation must be considered including thyroid dysfunction, nonclassical congenital adrenal hyperplasia, hyperprolactinemia, and androgen-secreting tumors.

**KEY POINTS**

- Polycystic ovary syndrome is a disorder characterized by hyperandrogenism and ovulatory dysfunction affecting 6% to 10% of women.

- Polycystic ovary syndrome is a diagnosis of exclusion; other causes of oligo-/anovulation must be considered including thyroid dysfunction, nonclassical congenital adrenal hyperplasia, hyperprolactinemia, and androgen-secreting tumors.

### Evaluation of Hyperandrogenism

The history and physical examination should include details about the onset of hirsutism and other symptoms/signs of hyperandrogenism, menstrual history, family history of hyperandrogenism, signs of insulin resistance (obesity, acanthosis nigricans, skin tags), distribution of terminal hair growth, and hair loss. Exposure to exogenous testosterone (topical, oral, or injected) should be assessed as a possible cause of hyperandrogenism and virilization.

Women with hirsutism should have total testosterone with SHBG measured, as well as morning 17-hydroxyprogesterone to screen for congenital adrenal hyperplasia. Laboratory evaluation for oligomenorrhea or amenorrhea (human chorionic gonadotropin [hCG], prolactin, FSH, TSH, free thyroxine) is also indicated. Serum dehydroepiandrosterone sulfate (DHEAS) measurement should be obtained in cases of recent onset of rapidly progressive hirsutism and/or virilization.

Markedly high DHEAS and/or testosterone levels are not consistent with PCOS. Patients with total testosterone levels

| TABLE 40. Diagnostic Criteria for Polycystic Ovary Syndrome | | |
|---|---|---|
| **NIH Consensus Criteria 1990 (All Required)** | **Rotterdam Criteria 2003 (Two of Three Required)** | **Androgen Excess and Polycystic Ovary Syndrome Society Criteria (All Required)** |
| Menstrual irregularity due to oligo-/anovulation | Oligo-/anovulation | Clinical and/or biochemical signs of hyperandrogenism |
| Clinical and/or biochemical signs of hyperandrogenism | Clinical and/or biochemical signs of hyperandrogenism | Ovarian dysfunction – oligo-/anovulation and/or polycystic ovaries on ultrasound |
| Exclusion of other disorders | Polycystic ovaries on ultrasound | Exclusion of other androgen excess or ovulatory disorders |

greater than 200 ng/dL (6.9 nmol/L) or DHEAS values greater than 7.0 µg/mL (18.9 µmol/L) require imaging to assess for adrenal tumor (adrenal CT or MRI) or ovarian tumor (transvaginal ultrasound).

## Management of Hyperandrogenism

Mechanical hair removal (threading, depilatories, electrolysis, laser) may be adequate for cosmesis in women with idiopathic hirsutism. First-line pharmacologic management of hirsutism is combined hormonal (estrogen-progestin) oral contraceptive agents; these agents suppress gonadotropin secretion and ovarian androgen production, as well as increase SHBG levels. Antiandrogen therapy (spironolactone) can be added for a better cosmetic response; concomitant contraception is mandatory with this therapy due to teratogenesis in male fetuses. Topical eflornithine is also approved for treatment of unwanted hair growth.

In PCOS, weight loss is a first-line intervention in patients with BMI of 25 or greater. Sustained weight loss of 5% to 10% improves androgen levels, menstrual function, and possibly fertility. Oral contraceptive agents are first-line pharmacologic therapy for hirsutism and menstrual dysfunction unless fertility is desired. An antiandrogen agent is added after 6 months if cosmesis is suboptimal with oral contraceptive agents. If fertility is desired, clomiphene citrate or letrozole can be used to correct oligo-/anovulation. Metformin reduces hyperinsulinemia and androgen levels but has minimal impact on hirsutism and ovulation.

Patients with PCOS should be screened for prediabetes/diabetes mellitus, hypercholesterolemia, obesity, hypertension, and obstructive sleep apnea due to increased risk for these conditions. Metformin is indicated when impaired glucose tolerance, prediabetes, or type 2 diabetes mellitus does not respond adequately to lifestyle modification.

### KEY POINTS

- Oral contraceptive agents are first-line drug therapy for hirsutism and menstrual dysfunction; an antiandrogen agent may be added for better cosmetic response.
- Patients with polycystic ovary syndrome should be screened for prediabetes/diabetes mellitus, hypercholesterolemia, obesity, hypertension, and obstructive sleep apnea.

## Female Infertility

Infertility evaluation is appropriate after 1 year of unprotected intercourse, on average twice weekly, in women younger than age 35 years and after 6 months in women age 35 years or older. Treatment of infertility is typically managed by a reproductive endocrinologist. Both partners should be evaluated concurrently; often, multiple factors are present (see Male Infertility).

History and physical examination findings may suggest the cause of infertility. Key factors include menstrual history (to determine ovulatory status) and assessment for thyroid dysfunction, galactorrhea, hirsutism, pelvic pain, dysmenorrhea, and dyspareunia. History of previous pregnancies, cancer therapy, substance use disorder, sexually transmitted infections, pelvic inflammatory disease, and gynecologic procedures should be explored. Frequency of coitus is important information. Physical examination should include BMI and assessment for signs of hyperandrogenism, estrogen deficiency, hyperprolactinemia, and thyroid dysfunction.

Assessment of ovulatory function is the first step in evaluation. Women with menses approximately every 28 days with molimina symptoms (breast tenderness, abdominal bloating, ovulatory pain) are likely ovulatory. In women without such cycles, assessment of ovulatory status is assessed with a midluteal phase serum progesterone level (obtained 1 week before the expected menses); a progesterone level greater than 3 ng/mL (9.5 nmol/L) is evidence of recent ovulation. If anovulatory cycles are suspected, the initial evaluation includes prolactin, TSH, and FSH measurements, with subsequent assessment for PCOS.

Hysterosalpingogram is used to assess for tubal occlusion and to evaluate the uterine cavity. Exploratory laparoscopy may be used if endometriosis or pelvic adhesions are suspected. If no abnormalities are found, fertility treatments will be offered under the direction of a reproductive endocrinologist, possibly including ovarian stimulation with clomiphene citrate or letrozole, intrauterine insemination, and in vitro fertilization, which may be offered to women age 40 years or older as first-line therapy.

### KEY POINTS

- Infertility evaluation is appropriate after 1 year of unprotected intercourse in women younger than age 35 years and after 6 months in women age 35 years or older.
- Both partners should be evaluated concurrently; often, **HVC** multiple factors are present.
- Assessment of ovulatory function is the first step in evaluation for female infertility.

## Physiology of Male Reproduction

The testes contain two anatomical units: the spermatogenic tubules composed of germ cells and Sertoli cells, and the interstitium containing Leydig cells. The three steroids of primary importance in male reproduction are testosterone, dihydrotestosterone, and estradiol. It is the pulsatile secretion of gonadotropin-releasing hormone (GnRH) by the hypothalamus that elicits pulsatile secretion of luteinizing hormone (LH) and follicle-stimulating hormone (FSH) by the gonadotroph cells of the anterior pituitary.

LH regulates testosterone synthesis in Leydig cells in a diurnal pattern; LH secretion is regulated by negative feedback of testosterone and estradiol. FSH regulates Sertoli cell spermatogenesis. Inhibin B is an important peptide inhibitor of pituitary FSH secretion (**Figure 13**). The hypothalamic-pituitary-testicular axis is sensitive to stressors, including acute and chronic illness, fasting, and strenuous exercise, all of which can lower testosterone levels.

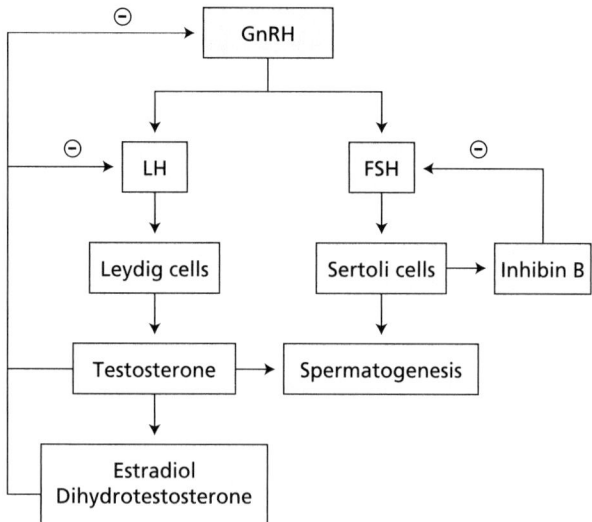

**FIGURE 13.** Male reproductive axis. Pulses of GnRH elicit pulses of LH and FSH. FSH acts on Sertoli cells, which assist sperm maturation and produce inhibin B, the major negative regulator of basal FSH production. The Leydig cells produce testosterone, which feeds back to inhibit GnRH and LH release. Some testosterone is irreversibly converted to dihydrotestosterone or estradiol, which are both more potent than testosterone in suppressing GnRH and LH. FSH = follicle-stimulating hormone; GnRH = gonadotropin-releasing hormone; LH = luteinizing hormone; − (circled) = negative feedback.

# Hypogonadism

## Causes

Male hypogonadism is a clinical syndrome that results from failure of the testes to produce physiologic levels of testosterone and a normal number of spermatozoa due to disruption of the hypothalamic-pituitary-testicular axis.

Primary hypogonadism is caused by testicular abnormalities. Common causes of acquired primary hypogonadism in adults include mumps orchitis, sequelae of radiation treatment, antineoplastic agents or toxins, testicular trauma or torsion, and acute and chronic systemic illnesses. Klinefelter syndrome (47,XXY) is the most common congenital cause of primary hypogonadism and is associated with tall stature, small testes, developmental delay, and socialization difficulties.

Secondary hypogonadism reflects a hypothalamic (GnRH) and/or pituitary (LH/FSH) deficiency. There are rare congenital causes, such as Kallmann syndrome, which are associated with anosmia. Common causes of acquired hypogonadotrophic hypogonadism are hyperprolactinemia, medications, critical illness, untreated sleep disorders, obesity, liver and kidney disease, alcoholism, marijuana use, and disordered eating. Tumors, trauma, thalassemias, and infiltrative diseases that cause disruption of gonadotropin production (such as sarcoidosis and hemochromatosis) are uncommon causes.

**KEY POINT**

- Primary hypogonadism is caused by testicular abnormalities; secondary hypogonadism reflects hypothalamic and/or pituitary dysfunction.

## Clinical Features

Specific symptoms of hypogonadism in the adult male include decreased morning and spontaneous erections, decreased libido, mastodynia, gynecomastia, decreased need for shaving, and/or decreased axillary and genital hair. Hot flashes, decreased bone mass, and low-trauma fractures are associated with profound and/or longstanding testosterone deficiency. Nonspecific symptoms include decreased mood, energy, concentration, muscle strength and bulk, and stamina, as well as poor sleep and memory. Infertility is more likely to occur with primary than secondary hypogonadism.

Men who develop hypogonadism before puberty have small testes and phallus and lack secondary sexual characteristics. With onset after puberty, there may be some regression of secondary sexual characteristics. A decrease in testes and/or phallus size and development of gynecomastia in adults is more likely due to a primary cause.

## Evaluation

Screening men with nonspecific symptoms of hypogonadism is not recommended. In men with specific signs and symptoms, measuring an 8 AM total testosterone level is indicated. If the testosterone level is low, a second 8 AM testosterone level is measured. The diagnosis is made with two low serum testosterone measurements. Measurement of free testosterone is appropriate in obese men because obesity lowers SHBG, leading to a falsely low measured total testosterone level. If testosterone is low, a serum LH measurement is indicated.

An elevated LH level reflects primary hypogonadism and further evaluation should be directed toward identifying the cause.

A low or normal LH level with simultaneous low testosterone reflects secondary hypogonadism. Medications including GnRH analogues (prostate therapy treatment), gonadal steroids (such as anabolic steroid use or megestrol for appetite stimulation), high-dose glucocorticoid treatment, and chronic opiate use can all suppress gonadotropins, resulting in secondary hypogonadism. Additional evaluation includes measurement of serum prolactin and screening for hemochromatosis. Assessment for other pituitary hormone deficiencies is indicated if signs or symptoms are present. Dedicated pituitary MRI should be performed if hyperprolactinemia is present, other pituitary hormone abnormalities are identified, testosterone level is less than 150 mg/dL (5.2 nmol/L), or if there are signs or symptoms of mass effect (**Figure 14**).

**KEY POINTS**

- Screening men with nonspecific symptoms of hypogonadism is not recommended. **HVC**

- The diagnosis of male hypogonadism is made with two 8 AM low serum total testosterone measurements.

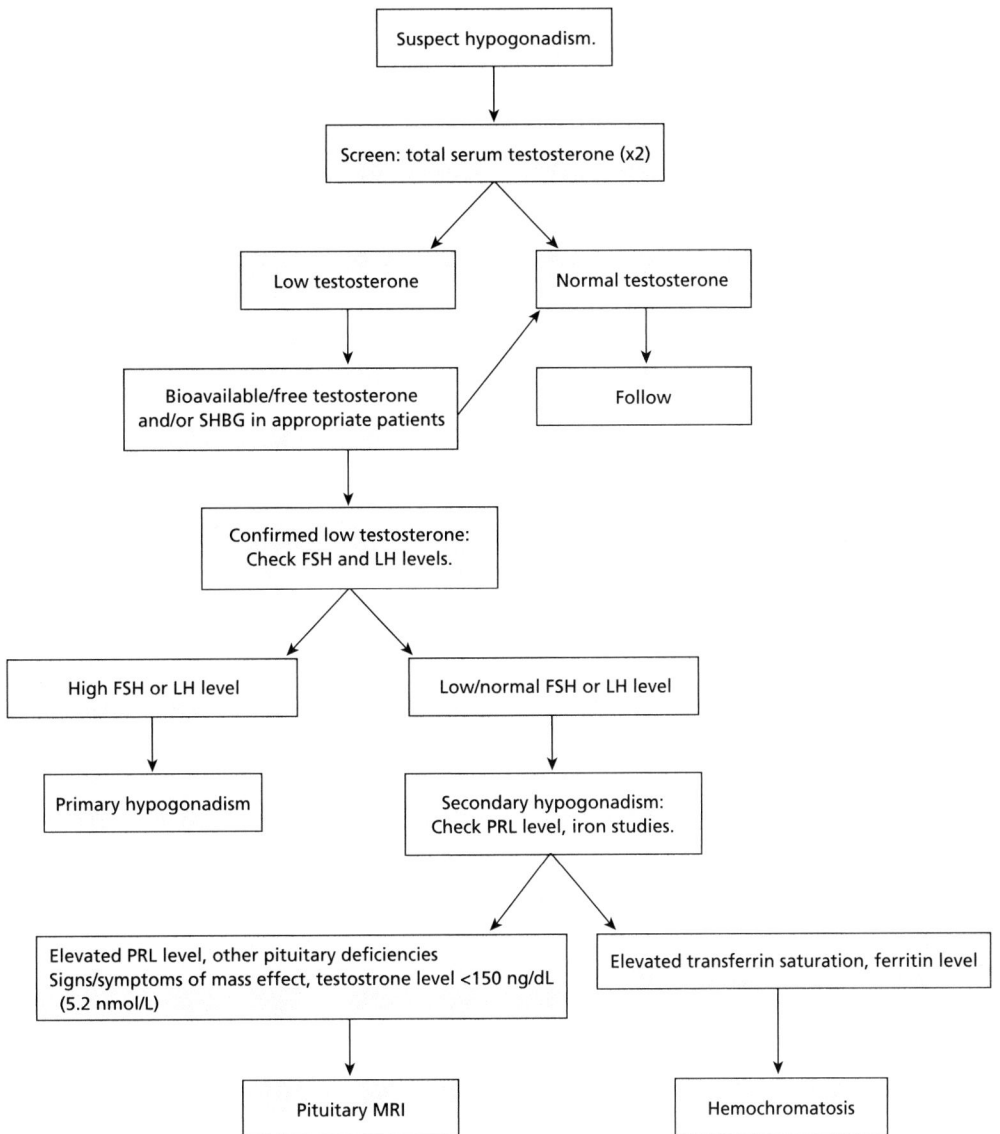

**FIGURE 14.** Algorithm for evaluating male hypogonadism. FSH = follicle-stimulating hormone; LH = luteinizing hormone; PRL = prolactin; SHBG = sex hormone-binding globulin; ×2 = two separate measurements.

## Management

In men with biochemically proven hypogonadism, testosterone therapy can be initiated, after the etiology is determined. There are a variety of testosterone replacement preparations available (**Table 41**). The goal is to replace testosterone so that the measured total testosterone value is in the mid-normal range.

Clinical benefits of testosterone therapy include an increase in libido, lean muscle mass, fat free mass, bone density, and secondary sexual characteristics. Potential adverse effects include acne, impact on prostate tissue, obstructive sleep apnea, thrombophilia, and erythrocytosis (**Table 42**).

Testosterone therapy is only indicated for treatment of testosterone deficiency; it is not used for impaired

spermatogenesis, and in fact further impairs spermatogenesis by suppressing pituitary FSH secretion. Patients should be counselled on the decreased fertility associated with exogenous testosterone therapy.

**KEY POINTS**

- After the etiology of hypogonadism is determined, testosterone therapy should be initiated with a goal of achieving a mid-normal range total testosterone measurement.
- Testosterone therapy is only indicated for treatment of **HVC** testosterone deficiency; it is not used for impaired spermatogenesis.

**TABLE 41.** Recommended Testosterone Replacement Therapy

| Route of Administration | Preparation | Typical Dosing Pattern | Timing of Initial Monitoring | Advantages; *Disadvantages* |
|---|---|---|---|---|
| Intramuscular injection | Testosterone cypionate | 100-200 mg every 2 weeks | Testosterone midway between injections | Low cost; *fluctuation in testosterone level* |
| Intramuscular injection | Testosterone enanthate | 100-200 mg every 2 weeks | Testosterone midway between injections | Low cost; *fluctuation in testosterone level* |
| Transdermal patch | Testosterone transdermal 24-hour patch | 2-6 mg/day | Morning testosterone ~14 days after starting therapy | Stable levels; *skin rash/ poor adherence to skin* |
| Transdermal gel | AndroGel 1% | 50-100 mg daily | Morning testosterone ~14 days after starting therapy | Stable levels; *potential for skin transfer to others* |
| Transdermal gel | AndroGel 1.62% | 20.25-81 mg daily | Morning testosterone 14-28 days after starting therapy | Stable levels; *potential for skin transfer to others* |
| Transdermal gel | Fortesta | 10-70 mg daily | 2 hours after application ~14 days after starting therapy | Stable levels; *potential for skin transfer to others* |
| Transdermal gel | Testim | 50-100 mg daily | Morning testosterone ~14 days after starting therapy | Stable levels; *potential for skin transfer to others* |
| Transdermal gel | Vogelxo | 50-100 mg daily | Morning testosterone ~14 days after starting therapy, prior to application | Stable levels; *potential for skin transfer to others* |
| Transdermal solution | Axiron | 30-120 mg daily | 2-8 hours after application ~14 days after starting therapy | Stable levels; *potential for skin transfer to others* |
| Subcutaneous implants | Testosterone implant pellets | 150-450 mg every 3-6 months | Measure at the end of the dosing interval | Infrequent dosing/Incision required for insertion; *risk of recurrent symptomatic hypogonadism as the duration of action is widely variable* |

**TABLE 42.** Endocrine Society Clinical Guidelines for Monitoring Adverse Effects of Testosterone Replacement Therapy

| Parameter | Recommended Screening Schedule | Alerts |
|---|---|---|
| Hematocrit | Value obtained at baseline and then at 3 months and 6 months after therapy initiation, followed by yearly measurements. | Value >54% |
| PSA level | For patients >40 years of age with a baseline value >0.6 ng/mL (0.6 µg/L), DRE and PSA level (determined at 3 and 6 months after therapy initiation followed by regular screening). | Increase >1.4 ng/ mL (1.4 µg/L) in 1 year or >0.4 ng/mL (0.4 µg/L) after 6 months of use; abnormal results on DRE; AUA prostate symptoms score/ IPSS >19 |

AUA = American Urological Association; DRE = digital rectal examination; IPSS = International Prostate Symptom Score; PSA = prostate-specific antigen.

Data from Bhasin S, Cunningham GR, Hayes FJ, Matsumoto AM, Snyder PJ, Swerdloff RS, et al; Task Force, Endocrine Society. Testosterone therapy in men with androgen deficiency syndromes: an Endocrine Society clinical practice guideline. J Clin Endocrinol Metab. 2010;95:2536-59. [PMID: 20525905]

# Anabolic Steroid Abuse in Men

Abuse of anabolic steroids is a serious public health concern that goes beyond the professional athlete. The prevalence of anabolic steroids use in men approaches 7%. Steroids are often purchased on the internet and dosing patterns vary. Labile mood, acne, excessive muscle bulk, and small testes may indicate anabolic steroid abuse. Reproductive side effects of anabolic steroid abuse include gynecomastia (due to peripheral conversion of testosterone to estradiol), testicular atrophy, diminished spermatogenesis and fertility, and iatrogenic hypogonadotropic hypogonadism, which may be permanent. Laboratory evidence suggestive of anabolic steroid abuse includes elevated hematocrit, undetectable or low LH level, low SHBG level, and low total testosterone level with elevated testosterone precursor(s), such as androstenedione.

**KEY POINTS**

- Labile mood, acne, excessive muscle bulk, and small testes may indicate anabolic steroid abuse.

- Side effects of anabolic steroid abuse include gynecomastia, testicular atrophy, diminished spermatogenesis and fertility, and iatrogenic hypogonadotropic hypogonadism, which may be permanent.

# Testosterone Changes in the Aging Man

With aging, total testosterone and free testosterone levels in men decline and SHBG increases, which results from testicular and hypothalamic-pituitary dysfunction. While serum testosterone levels decline 1% to 2% per year, most men do not become hypogonadal. Sperm production does not change significantly with age. The consequences of "andropause" are not fully elucidated, but adverse effects may include a negative impact on sexual function, muscle mass, erythropoiesis, and bone health.

The Endocrine Society supports treating older men with biochemically confirmed testosterone deficiency. The goal is replacement to a low-normal range of testosterone. Prior to initiation of treatment, some recommend shared decision making with the patient and discussion of the uncertainty of harms and benefits of testosterone therapy. This strategy is controversial.

Testosterone therapy in men without biochemical evidence of deficiency has not been shown to be beneficial, and studies have shown increased risk for cardiovascular disease and death, venous thromboembolism, and prostate cancer with use of testosterone therapy.

**KEY POINTS**

- Testosterone changes in men associated with aging do not result in symptomatic hypogonadism in most men.

HVC
- Testosterone therapy in men without biochemical evidence of deficiency has not been shown to be beneficial, and studies have shown increased risk for cardiovascular disease and death, venous thromboembolism, and prostate cancer with use of testosterone therapy.

# Male Infertility

In couples with infertility, assessment of male infertility should be undertaken concurrently with female assessment. A comprehensive history should focus on potential causes of infertility: developmental history, chronic illness, infection, surgery, drugs and environmental exposures, sexual history, and prior fertility. Physical examination should focus on evidence of androgen deficiency, with careful examination of the external genitals. If testicular examination is abnormal, consider referral to a urologist. Semen analysis is the initial laboratory assessment; collection should occur after 2 to 3 days of sexual abstinence, but no longer to avoid decreased sperm motility. If semen analysis is abnormal, it should be repeated at least 2 weeks later, and if results are abnormal, referral to a reproductive endocrinologist is recommended.

**KEY POINT**

- Semen analysis is the initial laboratory assessment for male infertility; if results are abnormal, testing should be repeated at least 2 weeks later, with referral to a reproductive endocrinologist if results are abnormal again.

# Gynecomastia

Gynecomastia, a benign proliferation of breast glandular tissue due to an increased action of estrogen relative to androgens, occurs in one- to two-thirds of older men. A thorough history and careful review of medications is necessary. Antiandrogen agents, such as spironolactone, cimetidine, and protease inhibitors, have a clear association with gynecomastia. Other identified causes include substance use disorder, malnutrition, cirrhosis, hypogonadism, testicular germ cell tumors, hyperthyroidism, and chronic kidney disease.

On physical examination, gynecomastia presents as a rubbery, concentric, subareolar mass. It is typically bilateral and may be tender if early in its course of development. Unilateral, nontender, and/or fixed breast masses should prompt an evaluation for breast cancer with a mammogram. Pseudogynecomastia is characterized by increased subareolar fat without glandular enlargement.

In a male presenting with painful gynecomastia, measurement of human chorionic gonadotropin, LH, morning total testosterone, and estradiol levels should be obtained if no clear cause is identified on history and physical examination.

Treatment of a specific cause of gynecomastia during the active proliferative phase may result in regression. If gynecomastia is longstanding, regression (spontaneously or with medical therapy) is unlikely due to fibrotic changes. In this scenario, plastic surgery referral may be the best option for cosmetic improvement.

**KEY POINT**

- Treatment of a specific cause of gynecomastia during the active proliferative phase may result in regression; if gynecomastia is longstanding, regression is unlikely due to fibrotic changes.

# Transgender Hormone Therapy Management

Transgender medicine involves the care of persons whose gender identity differs from their sexual assignment at birth. Gender incongruence is persistent incongruence between gender identity and external sexual anatomy at birth not arising from a confounding mental disorder; gender dysphoria is discomfort arising from incongruence between a person's gender identity and their external sexual anatomy at birth. A transgender man is someone with a male gender identity and a female birth-assigned sex; a transgender woman is someone with a female gender identity and a male birth-assigned sex.

Transgender people may avoid health care because of discriminatory or disrespectful interactions in prior health care encounters. Providing a safe environment is critical to ensure that transgender people establish and continue primary and gendering-affirming care. It is important for providers to understand basic terminology used by the trans community, which varies regionally.

Psychological and medical care must be provided in an environment that avoids preconceptions, and proper environmental signage, terminology, and staff training is essential (see WPATH Standards of Care). Accurate collection of gender identity information is also important; many organizations use a "two-step" method to collect these data: (1) gender identity and (2) sex listed on the original birth certificate, thus avoiding invisibility of transgender status.

Prior to a physical examination, history taking is necessary to understand an individual's anatomic changes associated with gender-affirming hormone therapy (GAHT) and surgical intervention. Secondary sex characteristics present on a wide spectrum of development in transgender patients. Providers should offer appropriate health maintenance and cancer screening based on an individual's anatomy.

GAHT is the most common medical intervention sought by transgender people and does not require subspecialty care. Primary care providers, gynecologists, and endocrinologists may prescribe this therapy. Treatment includes medications for hirsutism (spironolactone), contraception (estradiol/progestin), abnormal uterine bleeding (estradiol/progestins), menopause (estradiol/progestin), testosterone deficiency (testosterone), and benign prostatic hyperplasia (5-α reductase inhibitors).

GAHT must be patient-centered and individualized to the patient's goals. A discussion of the risks/benefits associated with treatment and informed consent are essential before beginning treatment. Criteria to consider before initiating GAHT include persistent, well-documented gender dysphoria, capacity to make a fully informed decision, age of majority in a given country, and if present, control of significant medical or psychological conditions. GAHT limits fertility, thus reproductive options should be discussed with patients prior to initiation of GAHT. Endocrine Society Clinical Practice Guidelines for GAHT are available. With GAHT, most physical changes occur over the course of 2 years, but the exact timeline of change is highly variable.

Feminizing hormone therapy is typically estradiol in combination with an androgen blocker. Goals are breast development; fat redistribution; and reductions in muscle mass, body hair, erectile function, sperm count, and testicular size. Estrogen therapy increases risk of deep venous thrombosis (DVT) and, to a lesser extent based on cohort study results, ischemic stroke and myocardial infarction; contraindications to estrogen therapy include a history of DVT, estrogen-sensitive neoplasm, and end-stage liver disease. Tobacco cessation should be encouraged prior to initiation of estrogen therapy due to increased risk of DVT. Anti-androgen therapy, such as spironolactone, diminishes secondary male sex characteristics and minimizes the estrogen dose needed, thus reducing risks associated with high-dose exogenous estrogen therapy.

Monitoring testosterone and estradiol levels for adequate response to therapy is necessary for the first year.

Masculinizing hormone therapy is achieved using topical or injected testosterone with a goal of cessation of menses, facial hair growth, voice deepening, fat redistribution, increased muscle mass and body hair, and clitoral growth. Contraindications to testosterone therapy include pregnancy, unstable coronary artery disease, and polycythemia. Monitoring testosterone and estradiol levels for adequate response to therapy should occur for the first year. Hemoglobin also should be monitored.

Gender confirmation surgery is often the last intervention in transgender persons. Many transgender persons do not pursue surgery, but it is essential for alleviation of gender dysphoria in others. For transgender women, surgical procedures may include augmentation mammoplasty, genital surgery (penectomy, orchiectomy, vaginoplasty, clitoroplasty, vulvoplasty), and non-genital, non-breast surgery (facial feminization, voice surgery, thyroid cartilage reduction). For transgender men, surgical procedures may include mastectomy, hysterectomy with oophorectomy, phalloplasty, vaginectomy, scrotoplasty, and implantation of penile and/or testicular prostheses.

Stringent criteria must be met prior to undergoing irreversible gender reassignment surgery.

**KEY POINTS**

- Gender-affirming hormone therapy is the most common medical intervention sought by transgender people and does not require subspecialty care; criteria for gender-affirming hormone therapy include persistent, well-documented gender dysphoria, capacity to make a fully informed decision, age of majority in a given country, and if present, control of significant medical or psychological conditions.

- Screening and preventive medicine in transgender patients should be based on the individual's anatomy.

# Calcium and Bone Disorders
## Calcium Homeostasis and Bone Physiology

Regulation of serum calcium level is complex and dependent on the actions of vitamin D and parathyroid hormone (PTH). The primary effect of vitamin D is to enhance the absorption of calcium within the intestinal tract, whereas the effects of PTH are primarily mediated through regulation of calcium retention and excretion in the kidney (**Figure 15**). Measured calcium levels depend on the amount bound to albumin, which can be affected by nutrition and acid-base status. Hypoalbuminemia of any cause, such as cirrhosis or

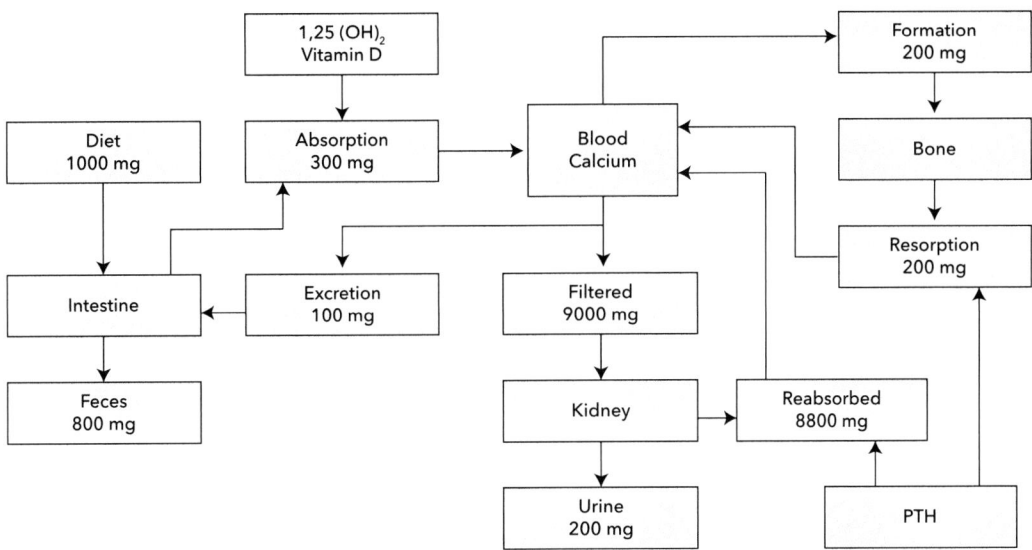

**FIGURE 15.** Neutral flux of calcium between bone and blood in adults is coordinated by parathyroid hormone (PTH). While most calcium filtered into urine is reabsorbed independent of PTH, PTH further increases retention of calcium from the urine. PTH indirectly augments calcium absorption in the gut by increasing production of 1,25 $(OH)_2$ vitamin D. Both effects of PTH are increasingly important at lower intakes of calcium and as blood levels of calcium decline. Amounts of calcium shown illustrate relative contribution of each organ to calcium homeostasis in a healthy adult.

malignancy-related cachexia, will cause low total calcium levels. When albumin concentration is low, measurement of ionized calcium or calculation of corrected total calcium is required to accurately assess calcium levels.

The level of vitamin D is determined by both production in the skin in response to sunlight and by ingestion, either from food or supplements. While vitamin $D_2$ (ergocalciferol) and vitamin $D_3$ (cholecalciferol) are available as supplements, the latter may be more efficacious due to greater potency, longer half-life, and being identical to that formed from ultraviolet light exposure. Activation of vitamins $D_2$ and $D_3$ requires hydroxylation initially by the liver and subsequently by the kidney, resulting in the active form of vitamin D, 1,25-dihydroxyvitamin D, calcitriol. 25-Hydroxyvitamin D is the storage form of vitamin D in the body, and measurement of 25-hydroxyvitamin D is the most appropriate test for assessing vitamin stores.

The initial response to a decline in serum calcium is an increase in PTH secretion, which decreases renal calcium excretion and increases calcium resorption from the bones to raise the serum calcium level. PTH also induces increased renal conversion of 25-hydroxyvitamin D to the active metabolite 1,25-dihydroxyvitamin D, which improves the efficiency of intestinal calcium absorption. Continued PTH-mediated mobilization of calcium from bone over months to years in response to chronic negative calcium balance can lead to metabolic bone disease. In contrast, the skeleton, gut, and vitamin D metabolism do not significantly contribute to the correction of hypercalcemia. Instead, an increased filtered load and suppression of PTH secretion leads to robust excretion of calcium by the kidneys provided that effective circulating volume is adequate.

In addition to its role in mineral metabolism, the adult skeleton provides a reservoir of calcium, structural support for mobility, muscle attachment, and protection of vital organs. Bone remodeling allows for continuous skeletal adaptation and repair. Osteocytes coordinate bone remodeling, which is initiated by osteoclastic resorption then followed by much slower osteoblastic bone formation and mineralization of a collagen/protein matrix. The entire skeleton is remodeled approximately every 10 years.

**KEY POINTS**

- The primary effect of vitamin D is to enhance the absorption of calcium within the intestinal tract, whereas the effects of parathyroid hormone are primarily mediated through regulation of calcium retention and excretion in the kidney.

- Measurement of 25-hydroxyvitamin D is the most appropriate test for vitamin D deficiency.

# Hypercalcemia

## Clinical Features of Hypercalcemia

Hypercalcemia is diagnosed when the calcium level exceeds normal levels, typically 10.5 mg/dL (2.6 mmol/L). Incidental finding of asymptomatic hypercalcemia on routine or screening blood tests is common.

Classic symptoms of hypercalcemia include polyuria, polydipsia, and nocturia. Additional symptoms may include anorexia, nausea, abdominal pain, constipation, and mental status changes. At higher levels, patients may become obtunded. Symptoms do not correlate linearly with serum calcium or PTH levels.

Severe hypercalcemia and hypercalciuria can lead to volume depletion and acute kidney injury, nephrolithiasis, or nephrocalcinosis. Skeletal manifestations reflect the underlying cause of hypercalcemia. Primary hyperparathyroidism may present as osteoporosis with fragility fractures and low bone density. Severe hyperparathyroidism from parathyroid carcinoma or secondary hyperparathyroidism due to kidney disease may be associated with bone pain and osteitis fibrosa cystica (a radiographic diagnosis). Hypercalcemia associated with lytic bone lesions is often the result of multiple myeloma or breast cancer.

**KEY POINT**

- Symptoms of hypercalcemia are variable but may include polyuria, polydipsia, nocturia, anorexia, nausea, abdominal pain, constipation, and mental status changes, and they may be associated with acute kidney injury, nephrolithiasis, nephrocalcinosis, and skeletal changes.

## Causes and Diagnosis of Hypercalcemia

Clues to the underlying cause of hypercalcemia include the severity, acuity of illness, and patient factors including concurrent illnesses. Hypercalcemia is categorized as mild (<12 mg/dL [3 mmol/L]), moderate (12-14 mg/dL [3–3.5 mmol/L]), or (severe >14 mg/dL [3.5 mmol/L]). When hypercalcemia is incidentally noted, repeat measurement is indicated. If hypercalcemia is confirmed, simultaneous measurement of serum calcium and PTH is a critical first step in diagnosing the cause and categorizing PTH-mediated and non–PTH-mediated hypercalcemia. Ionized calcium measurement is not helpful when the serum albumin level is normal or when there are no acute acid-base disorders. A thorough history and physical examination, as well as careful review of all medications including supplements, should be done in all patients with hypercalcemia.

**KEY POINT**

- Initial diagnostic testing for hypercalcemia requires simultaneous measurement of serum calcium and parathyroid hormone (PTH), which allows classification as PTH-related and non–PTH-related disease.

## Medications Causing Hypercalcemia

Thiazide diuretics may cause mild hypercalcemia, especially in the setting of previously unrecognized, mild primary hyperparathyroidism. Hypercalcemia associated with lithium therapy is due to altered PTH secretion and may occur years after initiation of therapy. If possible, stopping the medication and rechecking calcium levels is a reasonable first step in management. If the calcium returns to normal, this suggests the medication was responsible.

## Parathyroid Hormone–Mediated Hypercalcemia

PTH secretion decreases abruptly in response to a rise in serum calcium concentration. Therefore, an elevated or inappropriately normal (usually in the upper half of the reference range) PTH level in a patient with hypercalcemia is diagnostic of PTH-mediated hypercalcemia (**Figure 16**). Patients with an elevated PTH level but normal levels of calcium and vitamin D (normocalcemic primary hyperparathyroidism) may be managed similarly to those with asymptomatic primary hyperparathyroidism.

### Primary Hyperparathyroidism

Primary hyperparathyroidism is typically caused by a solitary parathyroid adenoma. Women are more often affected than men, with a peak incidence in the seventh decade of life. Hypercalcemia is usually mild (within 1 mg/dL [0.25 mmol/L] of the upper limits of normal) and may be intermittently normal. Hypercalciuria is present in up to 30% of patients. Since

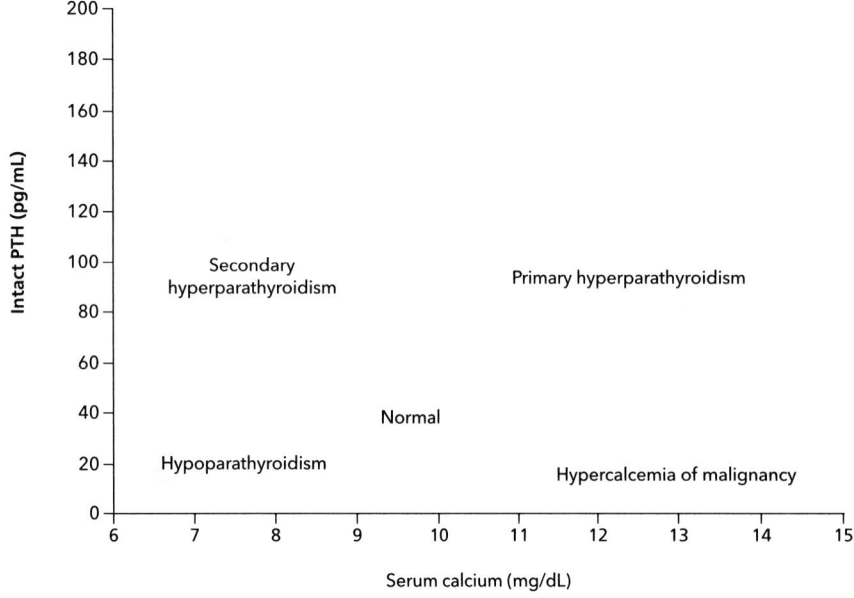

**FIGURE 16.** Relationship of calcium and parathyroid hormone (PTH) in normal conditions and in several diseases.

PTH enhances kidney phosphate excretion, low or low-normal serum phosphorus concentrations support the diagnosis. Assessment of bone mineral density (BMD) with dual-energy x-ray absorptiometry (DEXA) should include the nondominant forearm, which can be particularly affected in patients with hyperparathyroidism. Although parathyroid imaging with sestamibi or neck ultrasound may localize an adenoma, the presence of an adenoma does not influence the decision to proceed with surgery in the setting of primary hyperparathyroidism. Imaging may be beneficial to the surgeon for planning surgical intervention. In the absence of a history of calcium nephrolithiasis, kidney imaging may be indicated to exclude occult stones if this finding would change management.

Dietary calcium intake should be approximately 1000 mg/d to avoid further increases in urine calcium excretion and PTH secretion. Measurement of 25-hydroxyvitamin D and cautious correction of vitamin D deficiency is important. Repletion is recommended in patients whose levels are below 30 ng/dL (75 nmol/L) with careful attention to urine calcium excretion and serum calcium once vitamin D values are greater than 30 ng/dL (75 nmol/L).

Changes in specific endpoints during monitoring that lead to a recommendation for parathyroid surgery are outlined in **Table 43**. Surgery results in a 95% cure rate and less than 1% rate of complications with an experienced surgeon using minimally invasive techniques. Preoperative correction of vitamin D deficiency is important to avoid postoperative hypocalcemia, which is the result of relative hypoparathyroidism and reduced PTH-mediated production of 1,25-dihydroxyvitamin D culminating in a rapid flux of calcium into bone (hungry bone syndrome). Patients with mild primary hyperparathyroidism commonly require calcium supplementation for up to

1 week after parathyroidectomy until residual parathyroid tissue normalizes serum calcium concentrations. Reassessment of BMD 1 year after parathyroidectomy may show improvement in BMD, especially at the spine.

Approximately one in three patients with asymptomatic primary hyperparathyroidism who initially defer surgery will develop indications for surgery during 10 to 15 years of observation. In those not deemed eligible or who elect not to undergo surgery, evaluation should include annual measurement of serum calcium, creatinine, and glomerular filtration rate (GFR). If kidney stones are suspected, imaging and 24-hour urine collection for biochemical stone profile should be considered. BMD should be obtained every 2 years, and spine imaging should be considered if the patient has significant loss of height or back pain in the setting of a normal BMD.

**KEY POINT**

- Measurement of 25-hydroxyvitamin D and cautious correction of vitamin D deficiency is important in patients with primary hyperparathyroidism.

## Parathyroid Carcinoma
Parathyroid carcinoma is very rare, but may present with symptoms of severe hypercalcemia, with serum levels greater than 14 mg/dL (3.5 mmol/L) and markedly high PTH concentrations. Imaging is not useful and fine-needle aspiration is not recommended due to concerns of tumor seeding. The primary treatment is surgical resection. Unfortunately, 50% of patients may have residual or recurrent disease. Severe hypercalcemia in parathyroid carcinoma that is not amenable to surgery can be treated chronically with cinacalcet. Medical management options are limited, and patients are most likely to die from complications of hypercalcemia.

## Tertiary Hyperparathyroidism
In patients with end-stage kidney disease, multigland hyperplasia results from chronic stimulus of PTH (a sequela of long-standing secondary hyperparathyroidism) due to poorly controlled hypocalcemia and hyperphosphatemia. In some cases of secondary hyperparathyroidism, the serum calcium can normalize if the hyperplasia and associated PTH secretion is robust. Chronic stimulation of the parathyroid glands can lead to autonomous production of PTH by all four glands, resulting in hypercalcemia. Tertiary hyperparathyroidism is most commonly recognized after kidney transplantation. Although historically treated with subtotal multigland parathyroidectomy, the hypercalcemia can be resolved in most patients by treatment with paricalcitol or cinacalcet.

## Genetic Causes of Hypercalcemia
### Familial Hypocalciuric Hypercalcemia
Familial hypocalciuric hypercalcemia (FHH) is an autosomal dominant condition and the most common type of familial hypercalcemia. Patients are asymptomatic. The parathyroid glands and kidney detect serum calcium concentrations

**TABLE 43.** Indications for Parathyroid Surgery During Monitoring

| Assessment | Indication[a] |
|---|---|
| Serum calcium (>upper limit of normal) | >1 mg/dL (>0.25 mmol/L) |
| Skeletal | T-score <−2.5 at lumbar spine, total hip, femoral neck, or distal 1/3 radius; or a significant reduction in BMD[a] |
| | Vertebral fracture by x-ray, CT, MRI, or VFA |
| Renal | CrCl <60 mL/min |
| | Clinical development of a kidney stone or by imaging (x-ray, ultrasound, or CT) |

CrCl = creatinine clearance; MRI = magnetic resonance imaging; VFA = vertebral fracture assessment.

[a]A significant change is defined by a reduction that is greater than the least significant change as defined by the International Society for Clinical Densitometry.

From Bilezikian JP, Brandi ML, Eastell R, Silverberg SJ, Udelsman R, Marcocci C, et al. Guidelines for the Management of Asymptomatic Primary Hyperparathyroidism: Summary Statement from the Fourth International Workshop. J Clin Endocrinol Metab. 2014;99:3561-9. [PMID: 25162665]

through the calcium-sensing receptor (CaSR). In FHH, inactivating mutation of the CaSR gene causes the parathyroid gland to perceive serum calcium concentrations as low, resulting in increased PTH secretion and a higher serum calcium level. Simultaneously, the mutated CaSR in the kidney increases kidney reabsorption of calcium, leading to paradoxical hypocalciuria in the setting of hypercalcemia.

Although these patients appear to have primary hyperparathyroidism, FHH is a benign condition that is not treated with parathyroidectomy. Hypercalcemia will not resolve with surgery. Patients do not have sequelae of hypercalcemia, such as stones or osteoporosis. Signs suggestive of FHH include: mild hypercalcemia since childhood; low 24-hour urine calcium excretion, especially if calcium-creatinine clearance ratio is below 0.01; and/or family history of parathyroidectomy without resolution of hypercalcemia. If clinically ambiguous, the diagnosis can be confirmed by CaSR genetic testing.

**KEY POINT**

- The distinction between primary hyperparathyroidism and familial hypocalciuric hypercalcemia can be made by a 24-hour urine collection for calcium and creatinine, which will establish the amount of kidney calcium excretion and will allow evaluation of the calcium-creatinine clearance ratio.

### Multiple Endocrine Neoplasia Syndrome

Primary hyperparathyroidism in adolescents and young adults may be the first sign of multiple endocrine neoplasia syndrome (MEN). Primary hyperparathyroidism is associated with MEN1 and MEN2A syndromes. If the family history reveals primary hyperparathyroidism, pituitary tumor, Zollinger-Ellison syndrome, early death from pancreatic neoplasm, pheochromocytoma, or medullary thyroid cancer, MEN is more likely and screening should be considered. In contrast to sporadic primary hyperparathyroidism, MEN syndromes have recurrence of hyperparathyroidism due to ongoing hyperplasia in the remaining parathyroid tissue after parathyroidectomy. MEN1 is associated with mutation of the tumor suppressor *MEN1* gene, and MEN2A is associated with mutation of the *RET* gene. This is best managed in conjunction with or by an endocrinologist.

### Non–Parathyroid Hormone-Mediated Hypercalcemia

The differential diagnosis of hypercalcemia with suppressed PTH is broad. In patients with severe hypercalcemia, the history, symptoms, and findings may suggest the underlying cause. Treatment should commence without delay while awaiting results of laboratory testing. In PTH-independent hypercalcemic states, hypercalciuria can be severe and may precede hypercalcemia. PTH is usually undetectable but may be very low (<20 pg/mL [20 ng/L]) if hypercalcemia is mild.

### Malignancy-Associated Hypercalcemia

The most common cause of non–parathyroid hormone-mediated hypercalcemia is malignancy, and it is typically severe (>14 mg/dL [3.5 mmol/L]). It is often the result of tumor-produced PTH-related protein (PTHrP) leading to extensive resorption of bone. Renal cell carcinoma, breast cancer, and squamous cell cancers are associated with PTHrP-related hypercalcemia. Rarely, locally mediated osteolysis from extensive skeletal metastases, typically in multiple myeloma and breast cancer, may cause efflux of calcium from bone resulting in significant hypercalcemia. For more information, see MKSAP 18 Hematology and Oncology.

### Vitamin D–Dependent Hypercalcemia

Vitamin D–dependent hypercalcemia is associated with normal to elevated serum phosphorus levels because vitamin D enhances intestinal absorption of phosphorus and suppressed PTH secretion reduces kidney phosphorus excretion.

Unregulated conversion of 25-hydroxyvitamin D to 1,25-dihydroxyvitamin D may occur in granulomatous tissue associated with fungal infection, tuberculosis, sarcoidosis, and lymphoma, leading to increased intestinal absorption of calcium. These conditions are associated with an inappropriately normal or frankly elevated 1,25-dihydroxyvitamin D level and suppressed PTH. Decreased serum and urine calcium after intake of calcium and vitamin D is restricted or a rapid decrease in calcium after glucocorticoid therapy (which inhibits the hydroxylation of 25-hydroxyvitamin D) is consistent with these disorders.

Vitamin D intoxication from chronic high-dose ingestion of vitamin D (typically >50,000 units daily in patients without malabsorptive conditions) and increased storage in fat causes protracted hypercalciuria, nephrolithiasis, impaired kidney function, and elevated 25-hydroxyvitamin D levels.

### Other Causes

Ingestion of large amounts of calcium typically from antacid use (for example, calcium carbonate), especially with coexistent chronic kidney disease, causes milk-alkali syndrome.

Glucocorticoid and mineralocorticoid replacement and volume repletion resolve the mild hypercalcemia sometimes associated with Addisonian crisis.

Severe thyrotoxicosis occasionally causes hypercalcemia or hypercalciuria by increasing bone resorption.

Acute prolonged immobilization, as seen in spinal cord injuries, can cause large efflux of calcium from the skeleton through uncoupled bone remodeling with decreased osteoblastic activity despite increased osteoclastic activity. Patients with primary hyperparathyroidism or skeletal metastases are predisposed to hypercalcemia due to immobilization as are young patients where increased bone remodeling is normal.

### Management of Hypercalcemia

Management is dependent on the severity of the hypercalcemia. If mild (<12 mg/dL [3 mmol/L]), treatment of the underlying disorder (for example, parathyroidectomy in primary hyperparathyroidism) is sufficient. Hospitalization

CONT.
may be needed in patients with acute kidney injury, mental status changes, or calcium levels above 12 mg/dL (3 mmol/L). Initial treatment of severe hypercalcemia is aggressive hydration to replete volume loss and increase kidney excretion of calcium. Loop diuretics are not recommended unless kidney failure or heart failure is present, in which case volume expansion should precede the administration of loop diuretics to avoid hypotension and further kidney injury. For the acutely symptomatic patient, subcutaneous calcitonin can be used; however, the drug effect wanes after 48 hours. Long-term management of hypercalcemia may require intravenous bisphosphonate therapy to prevent mobilization of calcium from the skeleton, but requires adequate kidney function. Glucocorticoids and restriction of calcium and vitamin D intake are uniquely beneficial in vitamin D–dependent hypercalcemia. Hemodialysis is reserved for the treatment of severe hypercalcemia in oliguric patients.

**KEY POINT**

- Initial treatment of moderate to severe hypercalcemia is aggressive hydration to replete volume loss and increase kidney excretion of calcium; loop diuretics are not recommended unless kidney failure or heart failure is present, in which case volume expansion should precede the administration of loop diuretics to avoid hypotension and further kidney injury.

# Hypocalcemia
## Clinical Features of Hypocalcemia

Signs and symptoms of hypocalcemia reflect its severity and acuity. Hypocalcemic disorders in outpatients are typically detected on screening blood tests and are mild, with serum calcium 7.5 to 8.9 mg/dL (1.9-2.2 mmol/L). It may also be detected during evaluation for low-intensity traumatic fractures or low bone mass. Most patients will be asymptomatic or report symptoms of intermittent paresthesia of the hands and feet or perioral numbness. Hypocalcemia due to chronic hypoparathyroidism can also be associated with cataract formation, basal ganglia calcification, papilledema, and dental enamel hypoplasia.

Patients with severe hypocalcemia may present with neuromuscular symptoms and signs. Carpopedal spasm with characteristic hand posture (flexion at metacarpophalangeal joints and extension at interphalangeal joints) may be spontaneous or triggered by transient distal limb ischemia during blood pressure assessment (Trousseau sign). Facial nerve hyperirritability and muscle spasm can be demonstrated by percussion of the facial nerve just anterior to the ear (Chvostek sign). Importantly, laryngospasm, seizure, myocardial dysfunction, and QT-interval prolongation leading to sudden cardiac death due to severe hypocalcemia (<7.5 mg/dL [1.9 mmol/L]) can occur without prodromal paresthesia or muscle cramping.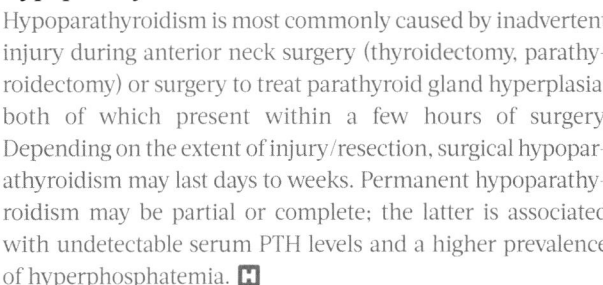

**KEY POINT**

- Laryngospasm, seizure, myocardial dysfunction, and QT-interval prolongation leading to sudden cardiac death due to severe hypocalcemia (<7.5 mg/dL [1.9 mmol/L]) can occur without prodromal paresthesia or muscle cramping.

## Causes and Diagnosis of Hypocalcemia

Hypocalcemia should be confirmed with a second measurement, which requires assessment of and correction for serum albumin concentrations. Ionized calcium measurement is indicated in the setting of fluctuating acid/base status. Simultaneous measurement of serum calcium, phosphorus, creatinine, and PTH is the next step. PTH should be elevated in the setting of hypocalcemia (see Figure 16).

### Hypoparathyroidism

Hypoparathyroidism is most commonly caused by inadvertent injury during anterior neck surgery (thyroidectomy, parathyroidectomy) or surgery to treat parathyroid gland hyperplasia, both of which present within a few hours of surgery. Depending on the extent of injury/resection, surgical hypoparathyroidism may last days to weeks. Permanent hypoparathyroidism may be partial or complete; the latter is associated with undetectable serum PTH levels and a higher prevalence of hyperphosphatemia.

Inappropriately normal PTH levels with concurrent hypocalcemia represents the former. Other causes of hypocalcemia due to insufficient PTH secretion include infiltrative disorders (hemochromatosis or Wilson disease), radiation, autoimmunity, and congenital disorders (such as 22q11.2 deletion syndrome). Chronic hypocalcemia with inappropriately normal PTH occurring within a family may represent an activating mutation of the CaSR gene. Hypomagnesemia, seen in the settings of malnutrition, alcoholism, and with use of loop diuretics and chronic proton pump inhibitor therapy, causes functional, reversible parathyroid hypofunction and must be excluded before a low or inappropriately normal PTH level is attributed to hypoparathyroidism. PTH resistance (pseudohypoparathyroidism) is a rare genetic cause of hypocalcemia.

**KEY POINT**

- Hypomagnesemia causes functional, reversible parathyroid hypofunction and must be excluded before a low or inappropriately normal parathyroid hormone level is attributed to hypoparathyroidism.

### Other Causes of Hypocalcemia

Malnutrition and/or malabsorption of either or both vitamin D and calcium may be suspected based on clinical history (bariatric surgery, celiac disease) and confirmed by low serum 25-hydroxyvitamin D level or low 24-hour urine calcium excretion (a proxy indicator of calcium intake and absorption). The most common cause of acquired hypocalcemia is chronic kidney failure due to impaired production of 1,25-dihydroxy-vitamin D and hyperphosphatemia. Hypercalciuria is most often idiopathic, but can also be due to chronic loop diuretic use. Rhabdomyolysis and tumor lysis syndrome increase serum phosphorus and calcium phosphate binding in the vascular space, causing low ionized calcium.

Hungry bone syndrome (rapid flux of calcium into bone after parathyroidectomy for severe primary hyperparathyroidism) and widespread osteoblastic metastases (prostate cancer, breast cancer) can cause hypocalcemia, as can saponification of calcium (and magnesium) in necrotic fat in acute pancreatitis.

Potent antiresorptive drugs, such as intravenous bisphosphonates and denosumab, can cause severe and protracted hypocalcemia by impairing physiologic efflux of calcium from the skeleton in patients with vitamin D deficiency. Therefore, it is important to assess vitamin D levels and correct deficiency before beginning treatment with an antiresorptive drug.

## Management of Hypocalcemia

 Because severe neuromuscular complications of hypocalcemia can occur in the absence of prodromal muscle tetany, severe hypocalcemia (<7.5 mg/dL [1.9 mmol/L]) requires urgent treatment with intravenous calcium. Slow administration through central intravenous access with electrocardiographic monitoring is preferred. Alternatively, teriparatide 20 µg twice per day rapidly eliminates hypocalcemic symptoms in acute postsurgical hypoparathyroidism (off-label indication).

Vitamin D supplementation 1000 to 4000 IU/d and oral calcium carbonate or calcium citrate at doses of 1 to 3 g/d in divided doses may normalize or sufficiently treat mild or chronic hypocalcemia. Calcitriol is needed in the setting of hypoparathyroidism with undetectable PTH and kidney failure because 1,25-dihydroxyvitamin D activation requires both PTH and sufficient kidney function.

In chronic hypoparathyroidism, goals of therapy are to eliminate symptoms while avoiding complications of therapy. A reasonable goal for most patients is a serum calcium concentration at or just below the reference range without hypercalciuria. Monitoring of urine calcium excretion is mandatory because hypercalciuria often limits therapy. Correction of coexisting hypomagnesemia is also required. Thiazide diuretics are commonly used because they decrease urine calcium excretion.

Initial treatment of hyperphosphatemia is reduction of dietary phosphorus but occasionally requires the addition of oral phosphate binders if serum phosphorus exceeds the normal range. Recombinant human PTH is available for patients who do not meet treatment goals with calcium and calcitriol therapy alone.

### KEY POINT

- A reasonable goal for most patients with hypoparathyroidism is a serum calcium concentration at or just below the reference range without hypercalciuria.

# Metabolic Bone Disease

## Low Bone Mass and Osteoporosis

Bone mass, mineral content, and macro- and microarchitecture determine bone strength. Bone mineral density (BMD) reflects bone mass and mineral content and, in older adults, predicts deterioration of microarchitecture. This relationship and epidemiologic data underpin the use of BMD determined by dual-energy x-ray absorptiometry (DEXA) to diagnose low bone mass and refine fracture risk assessment in older adults. Fragility fractures (those occurring with minimal trauma, equivalent or less than a fall from a standing height) after age 50 indicate low bone strength and define clinical osteoporosis regardless of BMD. Skull, feet, and hand fractures cannot, by definition, be fragility fractures.

### Pathophysiology

Low bone mass in adults may represent poor bone formation, bone loss, or both. Factors that can affect peak bone mass formation include genetic conditions, lifestyle factors, and poor health, especially in the second decade of life. Net loss of bone mass can occur in adults when osteoclastic bone remodeling is faster than osteoblastic bone formation. The list of risk factors for low bone mass and osteoporosis is extensive and is included in **Table 44** and **Table 45**. Some patients, however, have osteoporosis caused by secondary causes. Testing for secondary causes is summarized in **Table 46**.

### Screening for Osteoporosis

Current guidelines recommend screening average risk postmenopausal women beginning at age 65. Guidelines vary in their recommendations for routine screening for osteoporosis in men. The American College of Rheumatology recommends BMD testing within 6 months of starting long-term glucocorticoid therapy in adults 40 years of age and older and in adults under 40 years of age with risk factors for osteoporosis or a history of fragility fractures.

Patients with risk factors for low bone mass or osteoporosis, fragility fractures of the femur, vertebra (**Figure 17**), pelvis, humerus or radius, height loss of 4 cm (1.6 in) or more, or kyphosis, should have BMD testing earlier than standard screening recommendations. BMD may also be indicated if the risk of fractures is elevated based on the results of risk assessment tools such as the Simple Calculated Osteoporosis Risk Estimate (SCORE), Osteoporosis Self-Assessment Tool (OST), the Osteoporosis Risk Assessment Instrument (ORAI), and Fracture Risk Assessment Tool (FRAX). **Table 47** lists recommendations for BMD testing and vertebral imaging.

Screening of younger women may be indicated if one or more risk factors for osteoporosis are present. In premenopausal women without risk factors, assessment of BMD for fracture risk is not advised or validated. However, if testing is done in an otherwise healthy person, results that are below age- and gender-matched averages (Z-score <0) generally do not require further evaluation or serial monitoring.

**TABLE 44. Risk Factors for Low Bone Density and Osteoporosis**

| Lifestyle/Modifiable | Non-Modifiable | Medications/Supplements |
|---|---|---|
| Alcohol use | Race/Ethnicity | Anticonvulsants |
| Immobilization | Age | Antiretroviral therapy (tenofovir) |
| BMI <17 | Gender | Aromatase inhibitors |
| Low calcium intake | First-degree relative with low BMD | Calcineurin inhibitors |
| Smoking | Genetic | Depo-medroxyprogesterone |
| Vitamin D deficiency | Cystic fibrosis | Glucocorticoids (≥5 mg/day prednisone or equivalent for ≥3 months) |
| Weight loss | Hypophosphatasia | Heparin |
| Recurrent falls | Ehlers-Danlos | GnRH agonists |
| | Osteogenesis imperfecta | Proton pump inhibitors |
| | | Thiazolidinediones |
| | | Lithium |
| | | Androgen deprivation therapy |

BMD = bone mineral density; GnRH = gonadotropin-releasing hormone.

**TABLE 45. Conditions and Comorbidities Associated with Increased Risk for Low Bone Mass and Osteoporosis**

| Endocrine | Gastrointestinal | Hematologic | Rheumatologic | Neurologic | Other |
|---|---|---|---|---|---|
| Anorexia nervosa | Bariatric surgery | Amyloidosis | Ankylosing spondylitis | Multiple sclerosis | AIDS/HIV |
| Cushing syndrome | Celiac disease | Leukemia and lymphoma | Rheumatoid arthritis | Muscular dystrophy | Chronic obstructive lung disease |
| Diabetes mellitus | Inflammatory bowel disease | Monoclonal gammopathies | Systemic lupus | Spinal cord injury with paralysis | End-stage kidney disease |
| Hyperparathyroidism | Malabsorption | Multiple myeloma | | | Idiopathic hypercalciuria |
| Hypogonadism | Primary biliary | Amyloidosis | | | |
| Thyrotoxicosis | | | | | |
| Turner syndrome | | | | | |

**TABLE 46. Diagnostic Studies to Evaluate for Secondary Causes of Osteoporosis**

| Blood Testing |
|---|
| Complete blood count |
| Calcium, phosphorus, and magnesium |
| Kidney function tests |
| Liver function tests |
| Thyroid-stimulating hormone |
| 25-hydroxyvitamin D |
| Total testosterone (younger men) |
| Tryptase |
| **Urine Testing** |
| 24-h urinary calcium |
| Urinary free cortisol level |

Extent of testing should be influenced by clinical suspicion and severity of osteoporosis.

**KEY POINT**

- Current guidelines recommend screening average risk postmenopausal women beginning at age 65; screening recommendations for men vary by organization.

## Diagnosis

In postmenopausal women and men over 50 years of age, the diagnosis of osteopenia is determined by BMD testing (T-score between −1 and −2.5) alone, whereas osteoporosis can be diagnosed clinically based on the presence of fragility fractures, hip fracture, vertebral compression fracture, or by DEXA. Without secondary causes of low BMD or a fragility fracture, osteoporosis is diagnosed when the femur neck, total hip, nondominant radius, or composite (two or more consecutive diagnostic vertebrae) lumbar spine T-score is −2.5 or less, as defined by the World Health Organization. If hip or spine cannot be accurately measured by BMD, DEXA of the distal third of the radius can be used.

Diagnosis of osteoporosis in premenopausal women and men under 50 years can be made with diagnosis of a fragility fracture or low bone mass on DEXA defined by a Z-score less than −2, which indicates "low bone mass for age."

BMD assessment using quantitative calcaneal ultrasonography may be used to screen for osteoporosis, but abnormal results require confirmation by DEXA. Quantitative CT provides a DEXA equivalent T-score, is not hindered by degenerative changes in the lumbar spine, and is highly sensitive for detection of vertebral compression fractures, but its cost and

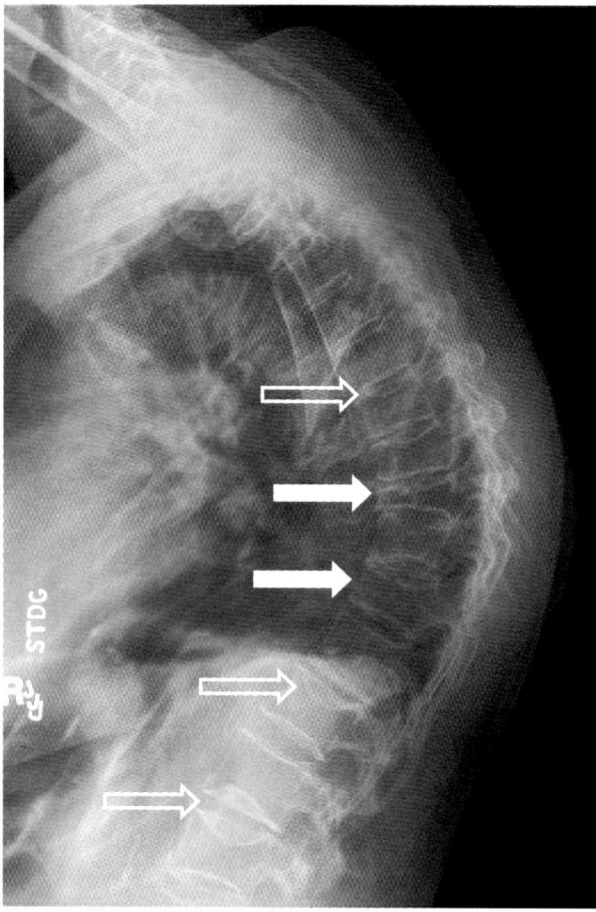

**FIGURE 17.** Asymptomatic vertebral compression fractures detected by spine radiograph in a patient with height loss and kyphosis. Depicted is vertebral endplate depression without loss of vertebral height in upper lumbar vertebrae (*empty arrows*) and severe wedging and height loss of multiple mid-thoracic vertebral bodies (*solid arrows*).

| TABLE 47. Recommendations for Measurement of Bone Mineral Density and Vertebral Imaging |
| --- |
| **Bone Mineral Density Testing[a]** |
| Women age 65 and older |
| For men, evidence is insufficient to assess the benefits/harms of screening for osteoporosis[b] |
| Postmenopausal women and men age 50 to 69, based on risk-factor profile |
| Those who have had a fracture, to determine degree of disease severity |
| Radiographic findings suggestive of osteoporosis or vertebral deformity |
| Glucocorticoid therapy for more than 3 months |
| Primary hyperparathyroidism |
| **Vertebral Imaging[c]** |
| Women ≥70 and men ≥80 if T-score at the spine, total hip, or femoral neck is ≤ −1.0 |
| Women aged 65-69 and men aged 75-79 if T-score at the spine, total hip, or femoral neck is ≤1.5 |
| In postmenopausal women age 50-64 and men aged 50-69 with the following risk factors: |
|     Low-trauma fractures |
|     Historic height loss of 1.5 in or more (4 cm) |
|     Height loss of 0.8 inches or more (2 cm) |
|     Recent or ongoing long-term glucocorticoid treatment |

[a]BMD testing should be performed at DEXA facilities using accepted quality assurance measures.

[b]The National Osteoporosis Foundation recommends screening men 70 and older, and the Endocrine Society recommends screening men 70 and older and men aged 50-69 who have risk factors such as low body weight, prior fracture as an adult, or smoking.

[c]Vertebral imaging should be repeated when a new loss of height is noted or new back pain is reported.

radiation exposure are greater and is not recommended for osteoporosis screening.

**KEY POINTS**

- Osteoporosis can be diagnosed clinically based on fragility fractures, hip fracture, vertebral compression fracture, or a bone mineral density measurement of ≤−2.5.

**HVC**
- Quantitative CT provides a dual-energy x-ray absorptiometry equivalent T-score, is not hindered by degenerative changes in the lumbar spine, and is highly sensitive for detection of vertebral compression fractures, but its cost and radiation exposure are greater and is not recommended for osteoporosis screening.

### Evaluation of Secondary Causes of Low Bone Mass

Non-modifiable factors are the most common cause of low bone mass, but there are many other causes (see Table 44 and Table 45). Low bone mass may be the presentation for conditions such as idiopathic hypercalciuria or celiac disease. All patients should have a thorough history and physical examination and additional testing based on findings (see Table 46). Although BMD may not be required in all patients to make the diagnosis of osteoporosis, it may be helpful to determine if additional testing is needed and to guide treatment.

### Osteomalacia

Osteomalacia is most commonly caused by severe and prolonged vitamin D deficiency, which results in inadequate concentrations of calcium and/or phosphate in the bone, which in turn prevents mineralization of newly formed bone matrix. Unlike osteoporosis, osteomalacia does not result in permanent loss of bone structure. A period of months to years of disordered mineralization is required before bone strength is compromised.

Symptoms of osteomalacia include diffuse bone pain, bone tenderness to palpation (tibial plateau and sternum), and proximal muscle weakness; however, early osteomalacia may present only with low bone mass on DEXA and can be indistinguishable from osteoporosis without further testing. Very low BMD (Z-score ≤-2), low or low-normal serum calcium and phosphorus levels, very low 25-hydroxyvitamin D (<10 ng/mL [25 nmol/L]) level, and secondary hyperparathyroidism distinguishes osteomalacia from osteoporosis. Elevated serum alkaline phosphatase level is particularly suggestive of osteomalacia, although mild elevation can be seen with recent osteoporotic fracture. Radiographs may display an unusual distribution of fractures in severe osteomalacia (**Figure 18**). When bone pain is not explained by conventional radiographic findings in the setting of suspected osteomalacia, imaging with radionuclide bone scan or MRI may reveal fractures.

The goal of treatment is to optimize conditions for bone mineralization using supplementation to normalize serum 25-hydroxyvitamin D (>30 ng/mL [75 nmol/L]), calcium, and phosphorus concentrations. The skeletal response to treatment is reflected by gradual normalization of alkaline phosphatase level and symptom relief. Resolution of osteomalacia may take as long as 12 months; subsequent BMD testing will show significant increases and/or normalization of BMD.

### Other Causes

Low bone mass and fragility fractures in young and middle-aged adults may result from genetic disorders (see Table 45). Patients with mild (type 1) osteogenesis imperfecta may present with a history of childhood fractures that decrease in frequency as adults. Hypermobility raises suspicion for Ehlers-Danlos and related syndromes. Hypophosphatasia should be suspected in middle-aged patients with fractures and serum alkaline phosphatase levels well below the reference range.

### Nonpharmacologic Management

Exercise involving weight-bearing, resistance, and balance is important for bone health and may reduce fracture risk at any age, but especially in patients over 65 years. Although the

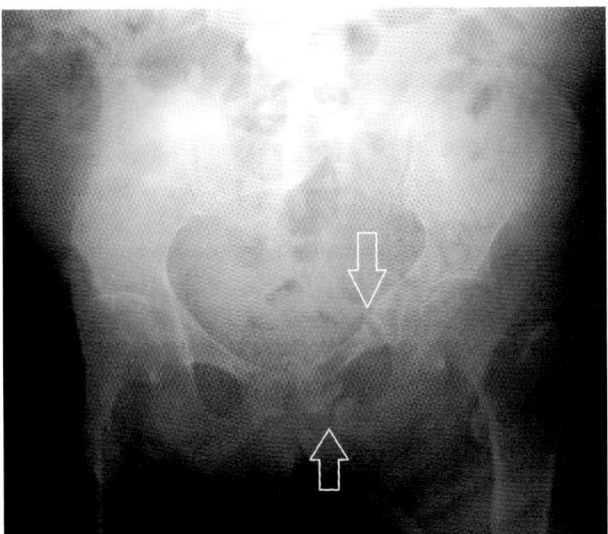

**FIGURE 18.** Pseudofractures appear as radiolucent areas perpendicular to the bone surface and are typically bilateral and/or symmetrical. The pubic rami (shown here), medial aspect of the proximal femur, proximal fibula, and metatarsals are common sites.

measurable treatment effect may be small, calcium and vitamin D were universally supplemented in osteoporosis pharmacotherapy trials; the National Academy of Medicine recommends calcium intake of 1000 to 1200 mg/d, ideally from dietary sources. A calcium supplement may be used for patients whose diets are insufficient, but should not be recommended independent of dietary assessment and intervention. As many osteoporosis clinical trials, including those testing pharmacotherapy, sought to achieve 25-hydroxyvitamin D levels of at least 30 ng/mL (75 nmol/L), a vitamin D supplement of 1000 to 2000 IU/d may be appropriate in the context of osteoporosis care.

### Pharmacologic Management

The goal of treatment is reduce risk of fractures in patients with osteoporosis or those at increased risk of fracture (primary prevention). The U.S. National Osteoporosis Foundation recommends pharmacologic treatment for patients with osteoporosis-related hip or spine fractures, those with a BMD T-score of −2.5 or less, and those with a BMD T-score between −1 and −2.5 with a 10-year risk of 3% or greater for hip fracture or risk of 20% or greater for major osteoporosis-related fracture as estimated by the Fracture Risk Assessment Tool (FRAX). Some studies suggest that different thresholds for initiation of treatment should be considered in other at-risk populations. The American College of Rheumatology recommends treatment for glucocorticoid-induced osteoporosis based on age, gender, and fracture risk.

Pharmacotherapy may also be used to prevent loss of BMD in postmenopausal women at risk of osteoporosis and to prevent or treat glucocorticoid-induced osteoporosis. Although estrogen therapy may be considered for management of vasomotor symptoms in postmenopausal women, it is no longer considered first-line therapy for prevention of osteoporosis. The FDA has recently approved a combination pill, bazedoxifene and conjugated estrogen, for prevention of postmenopausal osteoporosis. FDA-approved drugs for treatment of osteoporosis and options for prevention are listed in **Table 48**.

### Bisphosphonates

Oral bisphosphonates, alendronate and risedronate, are antiresorptive agents and are generally first-line treatment in postmenopausal women and men over 50 years of age. They have been shown to reduce the risk for spine, hip, and non-vertebral fractures. Another bisphosphonate, ibandronate, has only shown efficacy in reducing vertebral fractures. In glucocorticoid-induced osteoporosis with moderate to high fracture risk, oral bisphosphonates are recommended as first-line therapy in adult men and women regardless of age. Intravenous zoledronic acid once a year is an option if patients experience upper gastrointestinal symptoms or have difficulty taking the medication as directed. An acute-phase response reaction including pyrexia and myalgia may occur after first administration in as many as one in three patients, but does not occur typically with subsequent administrations. Bisphosphonates

**TABLE 48.** FDA-Approved Medications for Treatment and Prevention of Osteoporosis and Skeletal Sites of Proven Fracture Prevention When Used to Treat Osteoporosis

| | Prevention | | Documented Fracture Prevention | | | |
|---|---|---|---|---|---|---|
| | PMO | GIO | Recurrent | Hip | Vertebral | Non-Vertebral |
| Bisphosphonates | | | | | | |
| Alendronate | √ | | | √ | √ | √ |
| Risedronate | √ | √ | | √ | √ | √ |
| Ibandronate | √ | | | | √ | |
| Zoledronic acid (IV) | √ | √ | √ | √ | √ | √ |
| Denosumab | | | | √ | √ | √ |
| Raloxifene | √ | | | | √ | |
| Anabolic | | | | | | |
| Abaloparatide | | | | | √ | √ |
| Teriparatide | | | | | √ | √ |

GIO = glucocorticoid-induced osteoporosis; PMO = postmenopausal osteoporosis.

are contraindicated in patients with reduced kidney function (glomerular filtration rate [GFR] <35 mL/min/1.73 m$^2$) and should not be given until vitamin D deficiency and hypocalcemia are treated, if present.

Rare side effects of antiresorptive agents are osteonecrosis of the jaw and atypical femur fracture. Osteonecrosis of the jaw may occur at any point in therapy; whereas the risk for atypical femur fracture appears to increase with duration of therapy. For most patients, the benefits in reduction of osteoporosis fractures far outweigh the risk of these uncommon side effects. A drug holiday can be considered in women who are not at high fracture risk after 3 years (intravenous) to 5 years (oral) of bisphosphonate treatment. In postmenopausal women at high risk due to a T-score -3.5 or below, previous osteoporotic fracture, or who sustain a fracture while on therapy, continuation of treatment for up to 10 years (oral) or 6 years (intravenous) should be considered. While there are no data to guide the duration of the drug holiday, factors taken into consideration include the bisphosphonate used and whether BMD is maintained on DEXA.

### KEY POINTS

- Bisphosphonates are generally the first-line treatment of osteoporosis; only alendronate and risedronate reduce the risk for spine, hip, and nonvertebral fractures.

- A drug holiday can be considered in postmenopausal women who are not at high fracture risk after 3 years (intravenous) to 5 years (oral) of bisphosphonate treatment.

### Receptor Activator of Nuclear Factor KB (RANK) Ligand Inhibitors

Denosumab is a monoclonal antibody that inhibits osteoclast activation. When administered subcutaneously twice yearly, denosumab suppresses bone resorption, increases bone density, and reduces the incidence of osteoporotic fractures in men and women. The effects of denosumab are not sustained when treatment is stopped. Denosumab may be preferred in patients with stage 4 chronic kidney disease and in those intolerant of or incompletely responding to bisphosphonate therapy. Adverse effects include hypocalcemia, especially in older patients with vitamin D deficiency, and an increased rate of cellulitis and bronchitis. Medication-related osteonecrosis of the jaw and atypical femur fracture have been reported with denosumab use as well.

### Anabolic Agents

Teriparatide, rhPTH (1-34), is approved for use in postmenopausal women and men or women with glucocorticoid-induced osteoporosis who are at high risk of osteoporotic fracture. It is also used to improve bone mass in men with primary or hypogonadism-related osteoporosis at high risk of fracture. Abaloparatide, rhPTHrP (1-34), is approved for the treatment of postmenopausal women with osteoporosis at high risk for fracture. Both agents stimulate bone formation and require daily subcutaneous injection. Treatment should be limited to 2 years. Improvement in BMD is most evident at the spine. To prevent the loss of newly formed bone, sequential therapy with an antiresorptive agent must begin within 1 month of completing the course of anabolic treatment.

### Follow-up of Patients with Low Bone Mass

Routine serial DEXA measurements of BMD are not indicated for follow-up of low-risk patients who do not have osteoporosis. Subsequent BMD testing depends on baseline BMD. Repeating after 15 years may be reasonable if the hip T-score is normal (>-1), while retesting at 2 years may be considered if the hip T-score is -2 to -2.4.

The primary reason for repeating BMD testing in patients taking antiresorptive agents is to detect treatment failure. Declining BMD, indicated by a statistically significant percent drop in g/cm$^2$ of bone (not declining T-scores in subsequent DEXA scans) or a fracture while on treatment, raises concern for an unrecognized secondary cause, nonadherence, or insufficient response that necessitates reevaluation. The American College of Physicians recommends against monitoring of bone mineral density during treatment because data from several studies showed that women treated with antiresorptive treatment benefited from reduced fractures even if BMD did not increase. Instead follow-up management should include review of indication for treatment, monitoring of adherence to treatment, and reinforcement of lifestyle measures to prevent fractures, minimize bone loss, and avoid frailty. Drug holiday from antiresorptive therapy usually involves measurement of BMD to establish a baseline and repeated measurement in 2 to 3 years. Although this approach would ostensibly inform subsequent treatment decisions, it has not been validated.

## Vitamin D Deficiency

The most appropriate test to assess adequacy of vitamin D is measurement of serum 25-hydroxyvitamin D, which reflects dietary and skin-derived vitamin D. At least 20 ng/mL (50 nmol/L) is recommended to prevent metabolic bone disease in otherwise healthy populations and generally can be met with an intake of 600 to 800 IU/d.

Routine screening for vitamin D deficiency is not recommended in healthy populations; however, testing for deficiency is appropriate in groups at high risk or in patients presenting with low bone mass, fractures, hypocalcemia, or hyperparathyroidism. In patients with bone, parathyroid, or calcium disorders, to raise blood levels consistently above 30 ng/dL (75 nmol/L) may require 1000 to 2000 U/d. Patients with malabsorption, chronic lack of sun exposure, BMI greater than 40, advanced liver disease, and medications interfering with vitamin D metabolism, such as phenytoin and phenobarbital, may require 2000 to 4000 U/d for repletion and maintenance of vitamin D stores as guided by 25 hydroxyvitamin D levels obtained 3 months after initiation of treatment.

Loading doses using 50,000 U/d of either vitamin D$_2$ (ergocalciferol) or vitamin D$_3$ (cholecalciferol) once weekly for 8 weeks is appropriate in severe deficiency especially in the setting of malabsorption. Candidates for loading doses include: undetectable 25-hydroxyvitamin D, hypocalcemia, and osteomalacia due to vitamin D deficiency. Maintenance therapy of 1000 to 4000 U/d is recommended to maintain sufficiency after a loading dose.

Widespread public interest and a proliferation of scientific publications regarding vitamin D stem from established autocrine and paracrine effects in most tissues as well as extensive observational data associating 25-hydroxyvitamin D levels with extraskeletal health outcomes. However, intervention trials have not convincingly demonstrated a benefit of vitamin D supplementation on most disease outcomes,

suggesting that low 25-hydroxyvitamin D levels may be a marker rather than a cause of ill health.

- Routine screening for vitamin D deficiency is not recommended in healthy populations; however, testing for deficiency is appropriate in groups at high risk or patients presenting with low bone mass, fractures, hypocalcemia, or hyperparathyroidism.

**HVC**

## Paget Disease of Bone

Although Paget disease of bone may present with localized symptoms, it is most commonly diagnosed in asymptomatic older patients presenting with elevated alkaline phosphatase levels or incidental radiographic findings. Commonly affected bones include the skull, spine, sacrum, pelvis, femur, and tibia. The skeletal site and extent of involvement including rate of bone turnover determine clinical features. Involvement of weight-bearing bones of the lower extremity may result in bone pain, deformity, or fracture. Involvement of a bone approximating a joint can contribute to degenerative joint disease (**Figure 19**). Expansion of Pagetic bone of the upper spine or skull base may cause spinal cord or cranial nerve compression.

Diagnosis is based on radiographic findings of thickening of cortical bone, coarsened trabecular markings, and distortion and expansion of involved bone. Biopsy is rarely needed. Serum alkaline phosphatase, a marker of increased bone turnover, is generally elevated but may not be elevated in some patients with longstanding disease that has become metabolically inactive. Alkaline phosphatase may be elevated in other

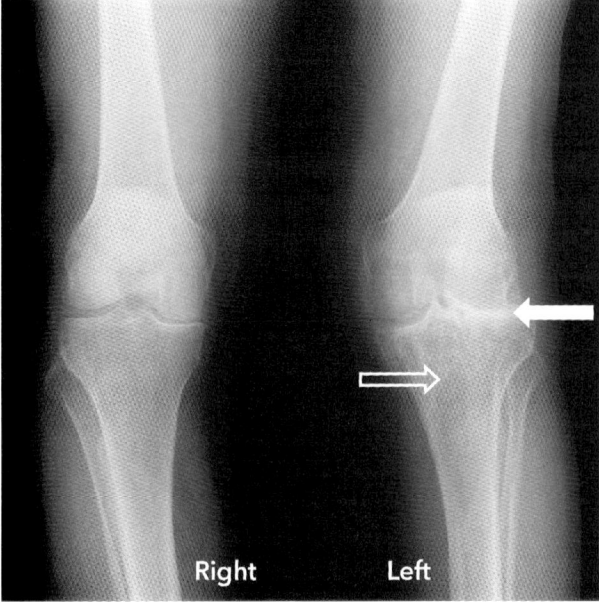

**FIGURE 19.** Coarsening of trabecular structures (*empty arrow*) without cortical deformity is diagnostic of Paget disease of bone in the proximal left tibia. Also shown is advanced degenerative arthritis in the adjacent left knee (*solid arrow*).

conditions, including vitamin D deficiency, other metabolic bone disease (such as osteomalacia), or recent fracture. Therefore, all patients with suspected Paget disease of bone require assessment of serum calcium, 25-hydroxyvitamin D, and a whole-body radionuclide bone scan. If the bone scan reveals other skeletal sites suspicious for Paget disease of bone, radiography of those sites is required for further evaluation.

Management of Paget disease is based on symptoms, location of involvement, and disease activity. Indications for treatment include: bone pain; risk for fracture and progressive deformity that could compromise bone, joint, or neurologic function; and elevated alkaline phosphatase concentrations. Bisphosphonates, particularly a one-time dose of 5 mg of intravenous zoledronic acid, often achieve the treatment goal of reducing pain and normalizing of alkaline phosphatase for up to 5 years. Oral bisphosphonates may also be used, but duration of treatment is variable.

Annual alkaline phosphatase levels should be monitored. Retreatment is indicated if previously normalized levels of alkaline phosphatase exceed normal levels. Imaging is required if there is a dramatic rise in alkaline phosphatase levels or acceleration in symptoms, which raises a concern for the rare sarcomatous transformation of Pagetic bone.

### KEY POINTS

- Although Paget disease of bone may present with localized symptoms, it is most commonly diagnosed in asymptomatic older patients presenting with elevated alkaline phosphatase levels or incidental radiographic findings.

- Indications for treatment of Paget disease include bone pain; risk for fracture and progressive deformity that could compromise bone, joint, or neurologic function; and alkaline phosphatase concentrations.

- A one-time dose of intravenous zoledronic acid will often achieve the treatment goal of reducing pain and normalizing of alkaline phosphatase in patients with Paget disease of bone.

## Bibliography

**Disorders of Glucose Metabolism**

American Diabetes Association. Standards of medical care in diabetes—2018. 2018; 41(Suppl 1): S1-S159.

Bergenstal RM, Klonoff DC, Garg SK, Bode BW, Meredith M, Slover RH, et al; ASPIRE In-Home Study Group. Threshold-based insulin-pump interruption for reduction of hypoglycemia. N Engl J Med. 2013;369:224-32. [PMID: 23789889] doi:10.1056/NEJMoa1303576

Cryer PE, Axelrod L, Grossman AB, et al. Evaluation and management of adult hypoglycemic disorders: an Endocrine Society Clinical Practice Guideline. J Clin Endocrinol Metabl. 2009; 94:709-28. [PMID: 19088155]

Duckworth W, Abraira C, Moritz T, Reda D, Emanuele N, Reaven PD, et al; VADT Investigators. Glucose control and vascular complications in veterans with type 2 diabetes. N Engl J Med. 2009;360:129-39. [PMID: 19092145] doi:10.1056/NEJMoa0808431

Garber AJ, Abrahamson MJ, Barzilay JI, et al. Consensus statement by the American Association of Clinical Endocrinologists and American College of Endocrinology on the comprehensive type 2 diabetes management algorithm-2018 executive summary. Endoc Pract. 2018; 24:91-120. [PMID: 29368965]

Hayward RA, Reaven PD, Wiitala WL, Bahn GD, Reda DJ, Ge L, et al; VADT investigators. Follow-up of glycemic control and cardiovascular outcomes in type 2 diabetes. N Engl J Med. 2015;372:2197-206. [PMID: 26039600] doi:10.1056/NEJMoa1414266

Holman RR, Paul SK, Bethel MA, Matthews DR, Neil HA. 10-year follow-up of intensive glucose control in type 2 diabetes. N Engl J Med. 2008;359:1577-89. [PMID: 18784090] doi:10.1056/NEJMoa0806470

Ismail-Beigi F, Craven T, Banerji MA, Basile J, Calles J, Cohen RM, et al; ACCORD trial group. Effect of intensive treatment of hyperglycaemia on microvascular outcomes in type 2 diabetes: an analysis of the ACCORD randomised trial. Lancet. 2010;376:419-30. [PMID: 20594588] doi:10.1016/S0140-6736(10)60576-4

Knowler WC, Barrett-Connor E, Fowler SE, Hamman RF, Lachin JM, Walker EA, et al; Diabetes Prevention Program Research Group. Reduction in the incidence of type 2 diabetes with lifestyle intervention or metformin. N Engl J Med. 2002;346:393-403. [PMID: 11832527]

Maldonado M, Hampe CS, Gaur LK, et al. Ketosis-prone diabetes: dissection of a heterogeneous syndrome using an immunogenetic and β-cell functional classification, prospective analysis, and clinical outcomes. J Clin Endocrinol Metab 2003;88:5090-98. [PMID: 14602731]

Marso SP, Daniels GH, Brown-Frandsen K, et al. Liraglutide and cardiovascular outcomes in type 2 diabetes. N Engl J Med. 2016; 375:311-322. [PMID:27295427]

Nathan DM, Cleary PA, Backlund JY, Genuth SM, Lachin JM, Orchard TJ, et al; Diabetes Control and Complications Trial/Epidemiology of Diabetes Interventions and Complications (DCCT/EDIC) Study Research Group. Intensive diabetes treatment and cardiovascular disease in patients with type 1 diabetes. N Engl J Med. 2005;353:2643-53. [PMID: 16371630]

Nathan DM, Zinman B, Cleary PA, Backlund JY, Genuth S, Miller R, et al; Diabetes Control and Complications Trial/Epidemiology of Diabetes Interventions and Complications (DCCT/EDIC) Research Group. Modern-day clinical course of type 1 diabetes mellitus after 30 years' duration: the diabetes control and complications trial/epidemiology of diabetes interventions and complications and Pittsburgh epidemiology of diabetes complications experience (1983-2005). Arch Intern Med. 2009;169:1307-16. [PMID: 19636033] doi:10.1001/archinternmed.2009.193

Neal B, Perkovic V, Mahaffey KW, de Zeeuw D, Fulcher G, Erondu N, et al; Canagliflozin and cardiovascular and renal events in type 2 diabetes. N Engl J Med. 2017;377:644-57. [PMID: 28605608]

Patel A, MacMahon S, Chalmers J, Neal B, Billot L, Woodward M, et al; ADVANCE Collaborative Group. Intensive blood glucose control and vascular outcomes in patients with type 2 diabetes. N Engl J Med. 2008;358:2560-72. [PMID: 18539916] doi:10.1056/NEJMoa0802987

Peters AL, Ahmann AJ, Battelino T, Evert A, Hirsch IB, Murad MH, et al. Diabetes technology-continuous subcutaneous insulin infusion therapy and continuous glucose monitoring in adults: an Endocrine Society Clinical Practice Guideline. J Clin Endocrinol Metab. 2016;101:3922-3937. [PMID: 27588440]

Qaseem A, Wilt TJ, Kansagara D, Horwitch C, Barry MJ, Forciea MA; Clinical Guidelines Committee of the American College of Physicians. Hemoglobin A1c targets for glycemic control with pharmacologic therapy for nonpregnant adults with type 2 diabetes mellitus: a guidance statement update from the American College of Physicians. Ann Intern Med. 2018 Mar 6. doi: 10.7326/M17-0939. [Epub ahead of print] PubMed PMID: 29507945.

Siu AL; U.S. Preventive Services Task Force. Screening for abnormal blood glucose and type 2 diabetes mellitus: U.S. Preventive Services Task Force recommendation statement. Ann Intern Med. 2015;163:861-868. [PMID: 26501513]

U.S. Department of Veterans Affairs/U.S. Department of Defense. VA/DoD Clinical Practice Guidelines for the management of diabetes mellitus in primary care. 2017. www.healthquality.va.gov/guidelines/cd/diabetes. Accessed May 16, 2018.

Whelton PK, Carey RM, Aronow WS, Casey DE Jr, Collins KJ, Dennison Himmelfarb C, et al; 2017 ACC/AHA/AAPA/ABC/ACPM/AGS/APhA/ASH/ASPC/NMA/PCNA guidelines for the prevention, detection, evaluation, and management of high blood pressure in adults: a report of the American College of Cardiology/American Heart Association Task Force on Clinical Practice Guidelines. J Am Coll Cardiol. 2017; doi: 10.1016/j.jacc.2017.11.006.

Zinman B, Wanner C, Lachin JM, et al. Empagliflozin, cardiovascular outcomes, and mortality in type 2 diabetes. N Engl J Med. 2015; 373: 2117-2128. [PMID: 26378978]

**Disorders of the Pituitary Gland**

Corsello SM, Barnabei A, Marchetti P, De Vecchis L, Salvatori R, Torino F. Endocrine side effects induced by immune checkpoint inhibitors. J Clin Endocrinol Metab. 2013;98:1361-75. [PMID: 23471977] doi:10.1210/jc.2012-4075

Fleseriu M, Hashim IA, Karavitaki N, Melmed S, Murad MH, Salvatori R, et al. Hormonal replacement in hypopituitarism in adults: an Endocrine Society Clinical Practice Guideline. J Clin Endocrinol Metab. 2016;101:3888-3921. [PMID: 27736313]

Freda PU, Beckers AM, Katznelson L, Molitch ME, Montori VM, Post KD, et al; Endocrine Society. Pituitary incidentaloma: an Endocrine Society Clinical Practice Guideline. J Clin Endocrinol Metab. 2011;96:894-904. [PMID: 21474686] doi:10.1210/jc.2010-1048

Guielman M, Basavilbaso, NG, Vitale M et al. Primary empty sella (PES). Pituitary. 2013;16:270-274. [PMID: 22875743]

Katznelson L, Laws ER Jr, Melmed S, Molitch ME, Murad MH, Utz A, et al; Endocrine Society. Acromegaly: an Endocrine Society Clinical Practice Guideline. J Clin Endocrinol Metab. 2014;99:3933-51. [PMID: 25356808] doi:10.1210/jc.2014-2700

Melmed S, Casanueva FF, Hoffman AR, Kleinberg DL, Montori VM, Schlechte JA, et al; Endocrine Society. Diagnosis and treatment of hyperprolactinemia: an Endocrine Society Clinical Practice Guideline. J Clin Endocrinol Metab. 2011;96:273-88. [PMID: 21296991] doi:10.1210/jc.2010-1692

Molitch ME, Clemmons DR, Malozowski S, Merriam GR, Vance ML; Endocrine Society. Evaluation and treatment of adult growth hormone deficiency: an Endocrine Society Clinical Practice Guideline. J Clin Endocrinol Metab. 2011;96:1587-609. [PMID: 21602453] doi:10.1210/jc.2011-0179

Nieman LK, Biller BM, Findling JW, Murad MH, Newell-Price J, Savage MO, et al; Endocrine Society. Treatment of Cushing's syndrome: an Endocrine Society Clinical Practice Guideline. J Clin Endocrinol Metab. 2015;100:2807-31. [PMID: 26222757] doi:10.1210/jc.2015-1818

Nieman LK, Biller BM, Findling JW, Newell-Price J, Savage MO, Stewart PM, et al. The diagnosis of Cushing's syndrome: an Endocrine Society Clinical Practice Guideline. J Clin Endocrinol Metab. 2008;93:1526-40. [PMID: 18334580] doi:10.1210/jc.2008-0125

**Disorders of the Adrenal Glands**

Bornstein SR, Allolio B, Arlt W, Barthel A, Don-Wauchope A, Hammer GD, et al. Diagnosis and treatment of primary adrenal insufficiency: an Endocrine Society Clinical Practice Guideline. J Clin Endocrinol Metab. 2016;101:364-89. [PMID: 26760044] doi:10.1210/jc.2015-1710

Fassnacht M, Arlt W, Bancos I, Dralle H, Newell-Price J, Sahdev A, et al. Management of adrenal incidentalomas: European Society of Endocrinology Clinical Practice Guideline in collaboration with the European Network for the Study of Adrenal Tumors. Eur J Endocrinol. 2016;175:G1-G34. [PMID: 27390021] doi:10.1530/EJE-16-0467

Funder JW, Carey RM, Mantero F, Murad MH, Reincke M, Shibata H, et al. The management of primary aldosteronism: case detection, diagnosis, and treatment: an Endocrine Society Clinical Practice Guideline. J Clin Endocrinol Metab. 2016;101:1889-916. [PMID: 26934393] doi:10.1210/jc.2015-4061

Lacroix A, Feelders RA, Stratakis CA, Nieman LK. Cushing's syndrome. Lancet. 2015 Aug 29;386(9996):913-27. doi: 10.1016/S0140-6736(14)61375-1. Epub 2015 May 21. Review. PubMed PMID: 26004339.

Lenders JW, Duh QY, Eisenhofer G, Gimenez-Roqueplo AP, Grebe SK, Murad MH, et al; Endocrine Society. Pheochromocytoma and paraganglioma: an Endocrine Society Clinical Practice Guideline. J Clin Endocrinol Metab. 2014;99:1915-42. [PMID: 24893135] doi:10.1210/jc.2014-1498

Libé R. Adrenocortical carcinoma (ACC): diagnosis, prognosis, and treatment. Front Cell Dev Biol. 2015;3:45. [PMID: 26191527] doi:10.3389/fcell.2015.00045

Nieman LK, Biller BM, Findling JW, Newell-Price J, Savage MO, Stewart PM, et al. The diagnosis of Cushing's syndrome: an Endocrine Society Clinical Practice Guideline. J Clin Endocrinol Metab. 2008;93:1526-40. [PMID: 18334580] doi:10.1210/jc.2008-0125

Rossi GP, Cesari M, Cuspidi C, Maiolino G, Cicala MV, Bisogni V, et al. Long-term control of arterial hypertension and regression of left ventricular hypertrophy with treatment of primary aldosteronism. Hypertension. 2013;62:62-9. [PMID: 23648698] doi:10.1161/HYPERTENSIONAHA.113.01316

**Disorders of the Thyroid Gland**

Alexander EK, Pearce EN, Brent GA, Brown RS, Chen H, Dosiou C, et al. 2017 Guidelines of the American Thyroid Association for the diagnosis and management of thyroid disease during pregnancy and the postpartum. Thyroid. 2017;27:315-389. [PMID: 28056690] doi:10.1089/thy.2016.0457

Burch HB, Cooper DS. Management of Graves disease: a review. JAMA. 2015;314:2544-54. [PMID: 26670972] doi:10.1001/jama.2015.16535

Cohen-Lehman J, Dahl P, Danzi S, Klein I. Effects of amiodarone therapy on thyroid function. Nat Rev Endocrinol. 2010;6:34-41. [PMID: 19935743] doi:10.1038/nrendo.2009.225

Cooper DS, Biondi B. Subclinical thyroid disease. Lancet. 2012;379:1142-54. [PMID: 22273398] doi:10.1016/S0140-6736(11)60276-6

De Leo S, Lee SY, Braverman LE. Hyperthyroidism. Lancet. 2016;388:906-18. [PMID: 27038492] doi:10.1016/S0140-6736(16)00278-6

Demers LM, Spencer CA. Laboratory medicine practice guidelines: laboratory support for the diagnosis and monitoring of thyroid disease. Clin Endocrinol (Oxf). 2003;58:138-40. [PMID: 12580927].

Fliers E, Bianco AC, Langouche L, Boelen A. Thyroid function in critically ill patients. Lancet Diabetes Endocrinol. 2015;3:816-25. [PMID: 26071885] doi:10.1016/S2213-8587(15)00225-9

Haugen BR, Alexander EK, Bible KC, Doherty GM, Mandel SJ, Nikiforov YE, et al. 2015 American Thyroid Association management guidelines for adult patients with thyroid nodules and differentiated thyroid cancer: the American Thyroid Association Guidelines Task Force on Thyroid Nodules and Differentiated Thyroid Cancer. Thyroid. 2016;26:1-133. [PMID: 26462967] doi:10.1089/thy.2015.0020

Hennessey JV. The emergence of levothyroxine as a treatment for hypothyroidism. Endocrine. 2017;55:6-18. [PMID: 27981511] doi:10.1007/s12020-016-1199-8

Kundra P, Burman KD. The effect of medications on thyroid function tests. Med Clin North Am. 2012;96:283-95. [PMID: 22443976] doi:10.1016/j.mcna.2012.02.001

Ross DS, Burch HB, Cooper DS, Greenlee MC, Laurberg P, Maia AL, et al. 2016 American Thyroid Association guidelines for diagnosis and management of hyperthyroidism and other causes of thyrotoxicosis. Thyroid. 2016;26:1343-1421. [PMID: 27521067]

**Reproductive Disorders**

Bhasin S, Brito JP, Cunningham GR, Hayes FJ, Hodis HN, Matsumoto AM, Snyder PJ, Swerdloff RS, Wu FC, Yialamas MA. Testosterone therapy in men with hypogonadism: an Endocrine Society Clinical Practice Guideline. J Clin Endocrinol Metab. 2018 May 1;103(5):1715-1744. [PMID: 29562364] doi: 10.1210/jc.2018-00229.

Bhasin S, Cunningham GR, Hayes FJ, Matsumoto AM, Snyder PJ, Swerdloff RS, et al; Task Force, Endocrine Society. Testosterone therapy in men with androgen deficiency syndromes: an Endocrine Society Clinical Practice Guideline. J Clin Endocrinol Metab. 2010;95:2536-59. [PMID: 20525905] doi:10.1210/jc.2009-2354

Bondy CA; Turner Syndrome Study Group. Care of girls and women with Turner syndrome: a guideline of the Turner Syndrome Study Group. J Clin Endocrinol Metab. 2007;92:10-25. [PMID: 17047017]

Brennan MJ. The effect of opioid therapy on endocrine function. Am J Med. 2013;126:S12-8. [PMID: 23414717] doi:10.1016/j.amjmed.2012.12.001

Fourman LT, Fazeli PK. Neuroendocrine causes of amenorrhea—an update. J Clin Endocrinol Metab. 2015;100:812-24. [PMID: 25581597] doi:10.1210/jc.2014-3344

Gordon CM. Clinical practice. Functional hypothalamic amenorrhea. N Engl J Med. 2010;363:365-71. [PMID: 20660404] doi:10.1056/NEJMcp0912024

Legro RS, Arslanian SA, Ehrmann DA, Hoeger KM, Murad MH, Pasquali R, et al; Endocrine Society. Diagnosis and treatment of polycystic ovary syndrome: an Endocrine Society Clinical Practice Guideline. J Clin Endocrinol Metab. 2013;98:4565-92. [PMID: 24151290] doi:10.1210/jc.2013-2350

Lindsay TJ, Vitrikas KR. Evaluation and treatment of infertility. Am Fam Physician. 2015;91:308-14. [PMID: 25822387]

Pope HG Jr, Wood RI, Rogol A, Nyberg F, Bowers L, Bhasin S. Adverse health consequences of performance-enhancing drugs: an Endocrine Society scientific statement. Endocr Rev. 2014;35:341-75. [PMID: 24423981] doi:10.1210/er.2013-1058

**Transgender Hormone Therapy Management**

American Psychological Association. Guidelines for psychological practice with transgender and gender nonconforming people. Am Psychol. 2015 Dec;70(9):832-64. doi: 10.1037/a0039906. PubMed PMID: 26653312. www.apa.org/practice/guidelines/transgender.pdf. Accessed May 15, 2018.

Center for Excellence for Transgender Health website. www.transhealth.ucsf.edu/trans?page=guidelines-home. Accessed May 15, 2018.

Coleman E, Bockting W, Botzer M, et al. Standards of care for the health of transsexual, transgender, and gender-nonconforming people, version 7. Int J Transgend. 2012;13:165.

Getahun D, Nash R, Flanders WD, Baird TC, Becerra-Culqui TA, Cromwell L, et al. Cross-sex hormones and acute cardiovascular events in transgender persons: a cohort study. Ann Intern Med. 2018 Jul 10. doi: 10.7326/M17-2785. [Epub ahead of print] PubMed PMID: 29987313.

Hembree WC, Cohen-Kettenis P, Delemarre-van de Waal HA, Gooren LJ, Meyer WJ 3rd, Spack NP, et al; Endocrine Society. Endocrine treatment of transsexual persons: an Endocrine Society Clinical Practice Guideline. J Clin Endocrinol Metab. 2009;94:3132-54. [PMID: 19509099] doi:10.1210/jc.2009-0345

Wylie K, Knudson G, Khan SI, Bonierbale M, Watanyusakul S, Baral S. Serving transgender people: clinical care considerations and service delivery models in transgender health. Lancet. 2016;388:401-11. [PMID: 27323926] doi:10.1016/S0140-6736(16)00682-6

**Calcium and Bone Disorders**

Adler RA, El-Hajj Fuleihan G, Bauer DC, Camacho PM, Clarke BL, Clines GA, et al. Managing osteoporosis in patients on long-term bisphosphonate treatment: report of a task force of the American Society for Bone and Mineral Research. J Bone Miner Res. 2016;31:1910. [PMID: 27759931] doi:10.1002/jbmr.2918

Bilezikian JP, Brandi ML, Eastell R, Silverberg SJ, Udelsman R, Marcocci C, et al. Guidelines for the management of asymptomatic primary hyperparathyroidism: summary statement from the Fourth International Workshop. J Clin Endocrinol Metab. 2014;99:3561-9. [PMID: 25162665] doi:10.1210/jc.2014-1413

Black DM, Rosen CJ. Postmenopausal osteoporosis [Letter]. N Engl J Med. 2016;374:2096-7. [PMID: 27223157] doi:10.1056/NEJMc1602599

Brandi ML, Bilezikian JP, Shoback D, Bouillon R, Clarke BL, Thakker RV, et al. Management of hypoparathyroidism: summary statement and guidelines. J Clin Endocrinol Metab. 2016;101:2273-83. [PMID: 26943719] doi:10.1210/jc.2015-3907

Buckley L, Guyatt G, Fink HA, Cannon M, Grossman J, Hansen KE, et al. 2017 American College of Rheumatology Guideline for the Prevention and Treatment of Glucocorticoid-Induced Osteoporosis. Arthritis & Rheumatology. 2017;69(8):1521-37.[PMID: 28585373] doi:10.1002/art.40137

Camacho PM, Petak SM, Binkley N, Clarke BL, Harris ST, Hurley DL, et al. American Association of Clinical Endocrinologist and American College of Endocrinology Clinical Practice Guidelines for the Diagnosis and Treatment of Postmenopausal Osteoporosis - 2016. Endocrine Practice. 2016;22(9):1111-8. [PMID 27643923] doi: 10.4158/EP161435.ESGL

Cosman F, de Beur SJ, LeBoff MS, Lewiecki EM, Tanner B, Randall S, et al; National Osteoporosis Foundation. Clinician's guide to prevention and treatment of osteoporosis. Osteoporos Int. 2014;25:2359-81. [PMID: 25182228] doi:10.1007/s00198-014-2794-2

Manson JE, Brannon PM, Rosen CJ, Taylor CL. Vitamin D deficiency - is there really a pandemic? N Engl J Med. 2016;375:1817-1820. [PMID: 27959647]

Singer FR, Bone HG 3rd, Hosking DJ, Lyles KW, Murad MH, Reid IR, et al; Endocrine Society. Paget's disease of bone: an Endocrine Society Clinical Practice Guideline. J Clin Endocrinol Metab. 2014;99:4408-22. [PMID: 25406796] doi:10.1210/jc.2014-2910

# Endocrinology and Metabolism Self-Assessment Test

This self-assessment test contains one-best-answer multiple-choice questions. Please read these directions carefully before answering the questions. Answers, critiques, and bibliographies immediately follow these multiple-choice questions. The American College of Physicians (ACP) is accredited by the Accreditation Council for Continuing Medical Education (ACCME) to provide continuing medical education for physicians.

The American College of Physicians designates MKSAP 18 Endocrinology and Metabolism for a maximum of 19 *AMA PRA Category 1 Credits*™. Physicians should claim only the credit commensurate with the extent of their participation in the activity.

Successful completion of the CME activity, which includes participation in the evaluation component, enables the participant to earn up to 19 medical knowledge MOC points in the American Board of Internal Medicine's Maintenance of Certification (MOC) program. It is the CME activity provider's responsibility to submit participant completion information to ACCME for the purpose of granting MOC credit.

## Earn Instantaneous CME Credits or MOC Points Online

Print subscribers can enter their answers online to earn instantaneous CME credits or MOC points. You can submit your answers using online answer sheets that are provided at mksap.acponline.org, where a record of your MKSAP 18 credits will be available. To earn CME credits or to apply for MOC points, you need to answer all of the questions in a test and earn a score of at least 50% correct (number of correct answers divided by the total number of questions). Please note that if you are applying for MOC points, you must also enter your birth date and ABIM candidate number.

Take either of the following approaches:

- Use the printed answer sheet at the back of this book to record your answers. Go to mksap.acponline.org, access the appropriate online answer sheet, transcribe your answers, and submit your test for instantaneous CME credits or MOC points. There is no additional fee for this service.

- Go to mksap.acponline.org, access the appropriate online answer sheet, directly enter your answers, and submit your test for instantaneous CME credits or MOC points. There is no additional fee for this service.

## Earn CME Credits or MOC Points by Mail or Fax

Pay a $20 processing fee per answer sheet and submit the printed answer sheet at the back of this book by mail or fax, as instructed on the answer sheet. Make sure you calculate your score and enter your birth date and ABIM candidate number, and fax the answer sheet to 215-351-2799 or mail the answer sheet to Member and Customer Service, American College of Physicians, 190 N. Independence Mall West, Philadelphia, PA 19106-1572, using the courtesy envelope provided in your MKSAP 18 slipcase. You will need your 10-digit order number and 8-digit ACP ID number, which are printed on your packing slip. Please allow 4 to 6 weeks for your score report to be emailed back to you. Be sure to include your email address for a response.

If you do not have a 10-digit order number and 8-digit ACP ID number, or if you need help creating a username and password to access the MKSAP 18 online answer sheets, go to mksap.acponline.org or email custserv@acponline.org.

CME credits and MOC points are available from the publication date of December 31, 2018, until December 31, 2021. You may submit your answer sheet or enter your answers online at any time during this period.

## Item 1

A 32-year-old woman is seen for follow-up evaluation of thyroid nodules. At her visit 2 weeks ago, a 3-cm right thyroid nodule and 2-cm right lateral neck mass were palpated on examination. The patient is asymptomatic. At age 12 she was treated with combination chemotherapy plus involved-field radiation for Hodgkin lymphoma. There is no family history of thyroid disease.

Laboratory studies show a serum thyroid-stimulating hormone level of 3.0 µU/mL (3.0 mU/L). Results of other laboratory studies are normal.

Thyroid ultrasound demonstrates a 3.1 × 2.8 × 1.6-cm hypoechoic solid right thyroid nodule with irregular margins. Right cervical lymphadenopathy was confirmed on ultrasonography.

**Which of the following is the most likely diagnosis?**

(A) Benign follicular thyroid nodule
(B) Follicular thyroid cancer
(C) Medullary thyroid cancer
(D) Papillary thyroid cancer

## Item 2

A 45-year-old woman is evaluated for management of type 2 diabetes mellitus diagnosed 3 months ago. She was asymptomatic at diagnosis with an initial hemoglobin $A_{1c}$ value of 9.7%. Her initial interventions included lifestyle modifications with weight loss and metformin. She is motivated to continue to lose weight. Medical history is significant for hypertension, hyperlipidemia, and frequent vulvovaginal candidiasis. She has no family history of thyroid or pancreatic malignancy. Medications are metformin, lisinopril, and atorvastatin.

On physical examination, vital signs are normal. BMI is 30. The remainder of the examination is unremarkable.

Results of laboratory studies show a hemoglobin $A_{1c}$ level of 9.1%. Chemistry panel and creatinine levels are normal.

**Which of the following is the most appropriate management for this patient's diabetes?**

(A) Initiate empagliflozin
(B) Initiate glipizide
(C) Initiate insulin glargine
(D) Initiate liraglutide

## Item 3

A 33-year-old man is evaluated for fatigue, headache, loss of appetite, and nausea for 6 months' duration. He has lost 9.1 kg (20 lb). Medical history is unremarkable, and he takes no medications.

On physical examination, temperature is normal, blood pressure is 118/70 mm Hg sitting and 98/68 mm Hg standing, pulse rate is 88/min sitting and 106/min standing, and respiration rate is 18/min. BMI is 19. The remainder of the physical examination is normal.

**Laboratory studies:**

| | |
|---|---|
| Potassium | 5.6 mEq/L (5.6 mmol/L) |
| Sodium | 136 mEq/L (136 mmol/L) |
| Adrenocorticotropic hormone (ACTH) | 450 pg/mL (99 pmol/L) |
| Cortisol, 8 AM | 2.6 µg/dL (71.8 nmol/L) |

**Which of the following is the most appropriate next test?**

(A) Cosyntropin stimulation test
(B) 21-Hydroxylase antibody measurement
(C) Pituitary MRI
(D) Serum aldosterone measurement

## Item 4

A 23-year-old woman is seen in follow-up for evaluation of amenorrhea of 4 months' duration. Her only other medical problem is schizophrenia treated with risperidone.

On physical examination, vital signs and physical examination are normal.

**Laboratory studies:**

| | |
|---|---|
| Prolactin | 220 ng/mL (220 µg/L) |
| Thyroid-stimulating hormone | 2.2 µU/mL (2.2 mU/L) |
| Thyroxine ($T_4$), free | 1.2 ng/dL (15.5 pmol/L) |
| Urine human chorionic gonadotropin | Negative |

**Which of the following is the most appropriate next step?**

(A) Obtain a pituitary MRI
(B) Start cabergoline
(C) Start an oral contraceptive
(D) Stop risperidone

## Item 5

A 22-year-old woman is evaluated for loss of appetite and fatigue and 4.5-kg (10-lb) weight loss over the past 6 months. Medical history is otherwise unremarkable, and she takes no medications.

On physical examination, blood pressure is 100/70 mm Hg and pulse rate is 94/min. Other vital signs are normal. BMI is 22. The patient looks tanned, even in areas not exposed to the sun, and has buccal and palmar hyperpigmentation.

**Laboratory studies:**

| | |
|---|---|
| Potassium | 5.3 mEq/L (5.3 mmol/L) |
| Sodium | 134 mEq/L (134 mmol/L) |
| Adrenocorticotropic hormone (ACTH) | 650 pg/mL (143 pmol/L) |
| Cortisol | 2.8 µg/dL (77.3 nmol/L) |

**Which of the following is the most appropriate treatment?**

(A) Dexamethasone twice daily
(B) Hydrocortisone twice daily
(C) Hydrocortisone twice daily and fludrocortisone once daily
(D) Prednisone twice daily
(E) Prednisone twice daily and fludrocortisone once daily

## Item 6

A 72-year-old man is evaluated during a follow-up office visit. Medical history is significant for prostate cancer managed with active surveillance since the age of 69 years. His only symptom is new-onset upper back pain. He takes no medication.

On physical examination, vital signs are normal. The upper spine is tender to palpation.

Laboratory studies show a serum calcium level of 9.9 mg/dL (2.5 mmol/L), serum creatinine level of 1.2 mg/dL (106.1 μmol/L), and prostate-specific antigen less than 4 ng/mL (4 μg/L).

Whole body radionuclide bone scan shows focal increased uptake at T7. There are no other abnormalities. Spine radiograph shows coarsening of trabeculae and expansion of body of T7 without cortical disruption consistent with Paget disease of bone.

**Which of the following is the most appropriate management?**

(A) Alkaline phosphatase measurement
(B) Bone mineral density testing
(C) Thoracic spine CT scan
(D) Zoledronic acid therapy

## Item 7

A 25-year-old woman is evaluated for anterior neck pain, fatigue, exercise intolerance, excessive sweating, and tremors that began 6 weeks ago. Other than an upper respiratory infection 2 months ago, she has been healthy. Medical history is otherwise unremarkable, and she takes no medications.

On physical examination, pulse rate is 105/min. Other vital signs are normal. The patient's thyroid gland is tender to palpation and is without discrete nodules. No thyroid bruit is auscultated. Bilateral lid lag is noted, but there is no proptosis, conjunctival injection, or chemosis. There is a fine tremor of her outstretched hands. Deep tendon reflexes are brisk.

Laboratory studies show a serum thyroid-stimulating hormone (TSH) level less than 0.01 μU/mL (0.01 mU/L), a serum free thyroxine ($T_4$) level of 2.8 ng/dL (36.1 pmol/L), and a serum total triiodothyronine ($T_3$) level of 190 ng/dL (2.9 nmol/L). Urine pregnancy test is negative.

**Which of the following is the most likely diagnosis?**

(A) Graves disease
(B) Molar pregnancy
(C) Subacute thyroiditis
(D) Toxic multinodular goiter

## Item 8

A 24-year-old woman is evaluated for management of type 1 diabetes mellitus. She was first diagnosed at 13 years of age. Having recently completed nursing school, the patient is motivated to gain control of diabetes to prevent complications, particularly diabetic neuropathy. Her only medication is insulin lispro, delivered through continuous subcutaneous insulin infusion pump therapy.

On physical examination, blood pressure is 142/92 mm Hg; the remainder of the vital signs is normal. BMI is 26. A comprehensive foot examination is normal.

Laboratory studies show hemoglobin $A_{1c}$ level of 8.7% and an LDL cholesterol level of 110 mg/dL (2.8 mmol/L).

**Which of the following is the most appropriate measure to reduce the risk of diabetic neuropathy?**

(A) Improve blood pressure control
(B) Improve glycemic control
(C) Improve lipid control
(D) Initiate pregabalin
(E) Weight loss

## Item 9

A 77-year-old woman is evaluated in the emergency department for new-onset generalized weakness and myalgia 2 days after receiving zoledronic acid for a recent diagnosis of osteoporosis. Medical history is significant for rheumatoid arthritis. She is mainly sedentary and uses a walker for ambulation. She lives alone and prepares her own meals. Her medications are zoledronic acid, methotrexate, prednisone, folic acid, and tramadol.

On physical examination, vital signs are normal; however, she develops hand spasm during the blood pressure measurement. BMI is 18. The patient is frail appearing. There is ulnar deviation at the metacarpophalangeal joints of both hands, but no signs of active synovitis.

Laboratory studies show a calcium level of 7.5 mg/dL (1.9 mmol/L).

**Which of the following is the most likely diagnosis?**

(A) Hungry bone syndrome
(B) Hyperphosphatemia
(C) Hypoparathyroidism
(D) Hypovitaminosis D

## Item 10

A 65-year-old woman is evaluated for a 6-month history of increased facial and body hair and loss of scalp hair. Her voice has become deeper. Medical history is otherwise unremarkable, and she takes no medications. She has been menopausal since age 52 years.

On physical examination, blood pressure is 140/95 mm Hg and pulse rate is 82/min. Other vital signs are normal. BMI is 28. There are coarse dark hairs on the upper lip, chin, chest, and abdomen. She also has a deep voice, frontal hair loss, and clitoromegaly.

Laboratory studies show a total testosterone level of 89 ng/dL (3.1 nmol/L) and a dehydroepiandrosterone sulfate (DHEAS) level of 890 μg/dL (24.0 μmol/L) (normal <50-450 μg/dL [1.35-12.2 μmol/L]).

**Which of the following is the most appropriate diagnostic test to perform next?**

(A) Abdominal CT
(B) Adrenal vein sampling
(C) Pelvic MRI
(D) Pelvic ultrasound

## Item 11

A 70-year-old man was admitted to the hospital 3 days ago with an ST-elevation myocardial infarction complicated by pulmonary edema and atrial fibrillation. He underwent emergency cardiac catheterization and left anterior descending (LAD) artery stent placement. Today the patient is feeling much better with complete resolution of his initial presenting symptoms.

Medications are aspirin, atorvastatin, clopidogrel, lisinopril, metoprolol, and low-molecular-weight heparin.

On physical examination, pulse rate is 92/min. Other vital signs are normal.

Cardiac examination reveals new findings of an irregularly irregular rhythm and an $S_4$. His physical examination is otherwise normal.

**Laboratory studies obtained at the time of cardiac catheterization:**

| | |
|---|---|
| Thyroid-stimulating hormone (TSH) | 0.2 µU/mL (0.2 mU/L) |
| Thyroxine ($T_4$), total | 6.5 µg/dL (83.8 nmol/L) |
| Thyroxine ($T_4$), free | 1.0 ng/dL (12.9 pmol/L) |
| Triiodothyronine ($T_3$), total | 60 ng/dL (0.9 nmol/L) |

**Which of the following is the most likely diagnosis?**

(A) Central hypothyroidism
(B) Heparin-induced thyroid function test abnormality
(C) Nonthyroidal illness syndrome
(D) Subclinical hyperthyroidism

## Item 12

A 27-year-old woman was diagnosed with a 2-cm left cortisol-producing adrenal adenoma. She is admitted to the hospital for an adrenalectomy. Medical history is otherwise unremarkable, and she takes no medications.

On physical examination, blood pressure is 152/88 mm Hg; the remainder of the vital signs is normal. Centripetal obesity, facial plethora, fat deposition in the supraclavicular areas, and wide violaceous striae are present.

**Which of the following is the most appropriate management following adrenalectomy?**

(A) Epinephrine
(B) Fludrocortisone
(C) Hydrocortisone
(D) Phenoxybenzamine

## Item 13

A 47-year-old man is evaluated during a follow-up visit to manage fatigue and decreased libido. Medical history is significant for hypertension and dyslipidemia. Medications are hydrochlorothiazide and atorvastatin.

On physical examination, vital signs are normal. He has normal hair distribution, no gynecomastia, and normal testicular examination.

Laboratory studies obtained at 3 PM revealed a total testosterone level of 275 ng/dL (9.5 nmol/L) and a luteinizing hormone level of 5 mU/mL (5 U/L).

**Which of the following is the most appropriate management?**

(A) Initiate testosterone replacement therapy
(B) Measure serum iron and total iron binding capacity
(C) Measure testosterone at 8 AM
(D) Obtain pituitary MRI

## Item 14

A 58-year-old woman is evaluated during a follow-up visit 6 months after thyroidectomy for differentiated papillary thyroid cancer. She developed symptomatic hypocalcemia following surgery but is currently asymptomatic. Medications are calcium citrate, calcitriol, and levothyroxine.

Vital signs and physical examination are normal.

**Laboratory studies:**

| | |
|---|---|
| Calcium | 9.5 mg/dL (2.4 mmol/L) |
| Creatinine | 1.0 mg/dL (88.4 µmol/L) |
| Phosphorus | 4.5 mg/dL (1.5 mmol/L) |
| Magnesium | 2.3 mg/dL (0.95 mmol/L) |
| Parathyroid hormone | <10 pg/mL (10 ng/L) |

**Which additional measurement is appropriate now?**

(A) Bone mineral density
(B) 1,25-Dihydroxyvitamin D
(C) 24-Hour urine calcium
(D) 25-Hydroxyvitamin D
(E) Ionized calcium

## Item 15

A 52-year-old woman is evaluated for a 1-year history of a 6.8-kg (15-lb) weight gain, easy bruising, hypertension, and worsening diabetes control. Medical history is also significant for a history of depression and anxiety. Medications are metformin and lisinopril.

On physical examination, blood pressure is 155/97 mm Hg and pulse rate is 82/min. Other vital signs are normal. BMI is 33. The patient has central obesity, supraclavicular and dorsocervical fat pads, and facial hirsutism. There are a few bruises on her arms and no abdominal striae.

Laboratory studies show a 24-hour urine free cortisol level of 205 µg/24 h, (564.9 nmol/24 h), midnight salivary cortisol of 298 ng/mL (821.2 nmol/L)(normal <100 ng/mL [275.6 nmol/L]), and adrenocorticotropic hormone (ACTH) less than 5 pg/mL (1.1 pmol/L).

**Which of the following is the most likely cause of this patient's hypercortisolism?**

(A) Adrenal tumor
(B) Bronchial carcinoid
(C) Pituitary tumor
(D) Psychiatric illness

## Item 16

A 27-year-old man is evaluated for decreased libido. He is a professional body builder and reports longstanding use of anabolic steroids to improve physical appearance and muscular performance. His medical history is otherwise unremarkable, and he currently takes no medications other than anabolic steroids.

On physical examination, vital signs are normal. He has a muscular build, acne, bilateral symmetric gynecomastia, and small testes.

**Laboratory studies:**

| | |
|---|---|
| Hematocrit | 52% |
| Follicle-stimulating hormone | 2 mU/mL (2 U/L) |
| Luteinizing hormone | 3 mU/mL (3 U/L) |
| Testosterone, total (8 AM) | 170 ng/dL (5.9 nmol/L) |

Liver enzyme testing is normal.

**Which of the following is the most appropriate management?**

(A) Anastrozole

(B) Cessation of anabolic steroid use

(C) Clomiphene citrate

(D) Human chorionic gonadotropin

(E) Testosterone replacement

## Item 17

A 25-year-old woman comes to the office to establish care. She is 5 weeks pregnant. She has hypothyroidism due to Hashimoto thyroiditis that was diagnosed 4 years ago. She is asymptomatic. Her only medications are levothyroxine and folic acid.

On physical examination, vital signs are normal. The patient's thyroid gland is nontender and diffusely enlarged without nodules. Pregnancy test is positive.

Serum thyroid-stimulating hormone level measured 4 months ago was 2.2 µU/mL (2.2 mU/L).

**Which of the following is the most appropriate management of this patient's hypothyroidism?**

(A) Check serum thyroid-stimulating hormone in 2 months

(B) Decrease levothyroxine dose by 30%

(C) Increase levothyroxine dose by 30%

(D) Stop levothyroxine and start liothyronine

## Item 18

A 34-year-old transgender woman is evaluated during a routine examination. She desires gender-affirming hormone therapy. Her gender incongruence diagnosis has been made and confirmed by qualified medical providers. She smokes one pack of cigarettes per day, with a 15-pack-year history. Medical history is otherwise unremarkable. She takes no medications.

On physical examination, vital signs are normal. She has male hair distribution. Normal male genitalia are present. There are no evident inguinal hernias.

**In addition to advising smoking cessation, which of the following is the most appropriate next step in management?**

(A) Initiation of an androgen blocker

(B) Initiation of estradiol therapy

(C) Refer for gender confirmation surgery consultation

(D) Refer for discussion on fertility preservation options

(E) Return for treatment 1 year after living in desired gender role

## Item 19

A 54-year-old woman is evaluated for flushing of the face of 1 year's duration. These episodes occur two or three times per week and last about 30 minutes. She went through menopause at age 50 and is on estrogen and progesterone hormone therapy. She also experiences episodes of anxiety, diaphoresis, and tachycardia. Medical history is significant for increasingly frequent migraine headaches, difficult to control hypertension, and gastroesophageal reflux disease. Medications are amitriptyline, chlorthalidone, metoprolol, conjugated estrogens, progesterone, and omeprazole.

On physical examination, blood pressure is 156/92 mm Hg; the remainder of the vital signs is normal. BMI is 32. The remainder of the examination is unremarkable.

**Which of the following medications should be discontinued prior to screening for secondary causes of hypertension?**

(A) Amitriptyline

(B) Chlorthalidone

(C) Metoprolol

(D) Omeprazole

(E) Progesterone

## Item 20

A 74-year-old woman is seen in follow-up for osteoporosis diagnosed 5 years ago. She has been taking alendronate (70 mg weekly) without adverse effect for 5 years. Medical history is otherwise unremarkable. Alendronate is her only medication.

On physical examination, vital signs are normal. She has no kyphosis or height loss, and the remainder of her examination is also normal.

Her recent bone mineral density by dual-energy x-ray absorptiometry (DEXA) scan showed a lumbar spine T-score of –2.2 and femoral neck T-score of –2.4.

**Which of the following is the most appropriate management?**

(A) C-terminal peptide of type 1 collagen (CTx) measurement

(B) Continue alendronate for 5 additional years

(C) Decrease alendronate dose

(D) Discontinue alendronate

## Item 21

A 67-year-old woman is evaluated for management of her type 2 diabetes mellitus. Medical history is significant for type 2 diabetes diagnosed 15 years ago, hypertension, hyperlipidemia, and obesity. She also has diabetic complications including nephropathy, retinopathy, and neuropathy. She does not have hypoglycemia. Medications are enalapril, atorvastatin, insulin glargine, insulin aspart, and metformin.

On physical examination, vital signs are normal. BMI is 31. Ophthalmoscopic examination reveals nonproliferative diabetic retinopathy. A foot examination reveals an insensate foot with intact skin. Vibratory sense is absent in the toes and ankle. The remainder of the physical examination is unremarkable.

Laboratory studies show a hemoglobin $A_{1c}$ level of 7.7% and serum creatinine level of 1.4 mg/dL (123.8 µmol/L). She has had a gradual decline in her estimated glomerular filtration rate (eGFR) from 50 to 39 mL/min/1.73 m² over the last 5 years.

**Which of the following is the most appropriate management?**

(A) Continue current regimen
(B) Discontinue metformin dose
(C) Increase insulin glargine dose
(D) Increase glipizide dose

## Item 22

A 19-year-old woman is evaluated for irregular menstrual cycles since menarche at 12 years of age, increasing amount of coarse facial hair, and acne. Symptoms have worsened since she stopped playing high school sports and subsequently gained weight. She is most concerned about the hair growth and acne. Medical history is otherwise unremarkable, and she takes no medications.

On physical examination, vital signs are normal. BMI is 31. She has coarse terminal hair on the upper lip and chin, acne on the face and back, and non-discolored striae on the abdomen. There is no galactorrhea and no other evidence of virilization such as deepening of the voice, clitoromegaly, or male pattern balding.

Laboratory studies show a total testosterone level of 73 ng/dL (2.5 nmol/L), dehydroepiandrosterone sulfate level of 1.8 µg/mL (4.9 µmol/L), and hemoglobin $A_{1c}$ of 5.4%. Other laboratory results are normal. Serum pregnancy test is negative.

**In addition to exercise and weight loss, which of the following is the most appropriate next step in management?**

(A) Combined oral contraceptive therapy
(B) Metformin
(C) Pelvic ultrasound
(D) Spironolactone

## Item 23

A 43-year-old man is evaluated for a change in his usual migraine headache. The headaches are now more frequent and respond poorly to his previously effective migraine headache medications. His medical history is otherwise unremarkable. Medications include ibuprofen and sumatriptan.

On physical examination, vital signs are normal. Physical examination including funduscopic examination is normal.

MRI reveals a 1-cm pituitary adenoma with suprasellar extension with no compression or abutment of the optic chiasm or optic nerves.

Laboratory studies show a cortisol level of 17 µg/dL (469.2 nmol/L), thyroid-stimulating hormone level of 2.6 µU/mL (2.6 mU/L), and thyroxine ($T_4$) level of 1.2 ng/dL (15.5 pmol/L).

**Which of the following is the most appropriate diagnostic test to perform next?**

(A) Measurement of prolactin and insulin-like growth factor 1 (IGF-1)
(B) Measurement of urine free cortisol
(C) Visual field examination
(D) No further evaluation is needed

## Item 24

A 42-year-old woman is evaluated prior to surgery following a diagnosis of pheochromocytoma. Her symptoms are palpitations, hypertension, and sweating for 8 months' duration. Medications are lisinopril and hydralazine.

On physical examination, blood pressure is 155/98 mm Hg. Other vital signs and the remainder of the examination are normal.

**Which of the following is the most appropriate next step in management?**

(A) Increase hydralazine
(B) Increase lisinopril
(C) Start chlorthalidone
(D) Start metoprolol
(E) Start phenoxybenzamine

## Item 25

A 60-year-old man is evaluated during a routine office visit. He was diagnosed with type 2 diabetes mellitus 6 years ago. Medical history is significant for coronary artery disease, hypertension, hyperlipidemia, and biliary pancreatitis. Medications are lisinopril, metoprolol, metformin, aspirin, and atorvastatin.

On physical examination, other than a blood pressure of 152/91 mm Hg, the vital signs are normal. BMI is 27. The remainder of the examination is normal.

Laboratory studies show a hemoglobin $A_{1c}$ level of 8.2%.

**Which of the following is the most appropriate treatment for this patient?**

(A) Empagliflozin
(B) Glipizide
(C) Liraglutide
(D) Sitagliptin

## Item 26

A 24-year-old woman is evaluated for a 6-month history of amenorrhea. Previously, menstrual cycles were regular. She also notes vaginal dryness. She reports no acne, stretch marks, breast discharge, or changes in weight. Medical history is otherwise unremarkable, and she takes no medications.

On physical examination vital signs are normal. BMI is 26. Vulvovaginal atrophy is noted on pelvic examination. The remainder of the examination is unremarkable.

Laboratory studies show undetectable beta-human chorionic gonadotropin. Prolactin and thyroid-stimulating hormone levels are within normal limits.

**Which of the following is the most appropriate next diagnostic test?**

(A) Dehydroepiandrosterone sulfate (DHEAS) measurement

(B) Follicle-stimulating hormone measurement

(C) Pelvic MRI

(D) Testosterone measurement

(E) Transvaginal ultrasound

## Item 27

A 66-year-old woman was admitted to the hospital 24 hours ago with community-acquired pneumonia. Since admission, she has been confused and her oral intake has been poor. Appropriate antibiotics, intravenous fluids, and oxygen have been initiated. She has no other known medical problems.

On physical examination, temperature is 39 °C (102.2 °F), blood pressure is 142/88 mm Hg, pulse rate is 98/min, and respiration rate is 20/min. Oxygen saturation is 98% on oxygen, 2 L/min by nasal cannula. Crackles are evident in the right posterior thorax.

Laboratory studies show glucose values of 185 to 215 mg/dL (10.3-11.9 mmol/L) and a hemoglobin $A_{1c}$ level is 5.5%.

A chest radiograph demonstrates a right lower lobe infiltrate.

**Which of the following is the most appropriate management of this patient's hyperglycemia?**

(A) Empagliflozin and sliding-scale insulin

(B) Metformin and sliding-scale insulin

(C) Scheduled basal insulin and correction insulin

(D) Sliding-scale insulin only

## Item 28

A 45-year-old man is evaluated for anorexia, dizziness, and weakness. He was discharged from the hospital 5 days ago after transsphenoidal pituitary surgery for a pituitary macroadenoma abutting the optic chiasm. His postoperative course was uneventful, and his postoperative hormone evaluation was normal; he did not require any hormone replacement. He denies any polyuria or increase in thirst. He takes no medications.

On physical examination, vital signs and physical examination are normal.

**Which of the following is the most appropriate diagnostic test to perform next?**

(A) Antidiuretic hormone testing

(B) MRI of the pituitary

(C) Serum sodium measurement

(D) Thyroid-stimulating hormone measurement

## Item 29

A 34-year-old woman is evaluated for new onset headaches of 4 months' duration. Her menstrual periods have been irregular for the last year. She has been trying to conceive for the last 6 months. Her last menstrual period was 7 weeks ago. She is otherwise healthy and takes no medications.

On physical examination, vital signs are normal. Visual field examination is normal. Examination of the optic discs and cranial nerve examination are normal. The remainder of the physical examination is noncontributory.

MRI obtained to evaluate her headaches reveals a partially empty sella with no evidence of pituitary tumor or other masses.

**Laboratory studies:**

| | |
|---|---|
| Cortisol (8:00 AM) | 15 µg/dL (414 nmol/L) |
| Estradiol | 20 pg/mL (73.4 pmol/L) |
| Follicle-stimulating hormone | 5 mU/mL (5 U/L) |
| Human chorionic gonadotropin, serum | Negative |
| Luteinizing hormone | 4 mU/mL (4 U/L) |
| Prolactin | 62 ng/mL (62 µg/L) |
| Thyroid-stimulating hormone | 2.4 µU/mL (2.4 mU/L) |
| Thyroxine ($T_4$), free | 1.3 ng/dL (16.8 pmol/L) |
| Serum human chorionic gonadotropin | Negative |

**Which of the following is the most appropriate management?**

(A) Dopamine agonist therapy

(B) Neurosurgery consultation

(C) Oral contraceptive pill

(D) No treatment necessary

## Item 30

A 21-year-old woman is seen in the office following parathyroidectomy for hyperparathyroidism. The pathology of three resected enlarged parathyroid glands showed hyperplasia. Her medical history is significant for oligomenorrhea. Family history is notable for hypercalcemia and kidney stones in her father, who died at age 49 from pancreatic cancer, and a pituitary tumor in her sister at age 16.

Her vital signs are normal. Skin findings include dermatofibroma. Her physical examination is normal with the exception of the surgical scar on her neck.

**Which of the following is the most likely diagnosis?**

(A) Familial hypocalciuric hypercalcemia

(B) Multiple endocrine neoplasia type 1 (MEN1)

(C) Parathyroid carcinoma

(D) Secondary hyperparathyroidism

(E) Tertiary hyperparathyroidism

## Item 31

A 57-year-old woman is evaluated for cough, exertional dyspnea, and fatigue for 12 months' duration. Medical history is otherwise unremarkable, and she takes no medications.

On physical examination, temperature is 38.1 °C (100.6 °F), blood pressure is 132/78 mm Hg, pulse rate is 84/min, respiratory rate is 18/min; oxygen saturation is 95% breathing ambient air. The cardiac examination is normal. There are no wheezes or crackles on pulmonary examination. The remainder of the examination is unremarkable.

**Laboratory studies:**

| | |
|---|---|
| Calcium | 11.1 mg/dL (2.8 mmol/L) |
| Creatinine | 1.2 mg/dL (106.1 µmol/L) |
| Phosphorus | 4.7 mg/dL (1.5 mmol/L) |
| Parathyroid hormone | <10 pg/mL (10 ng/L) |

Chest radiograph is shown.

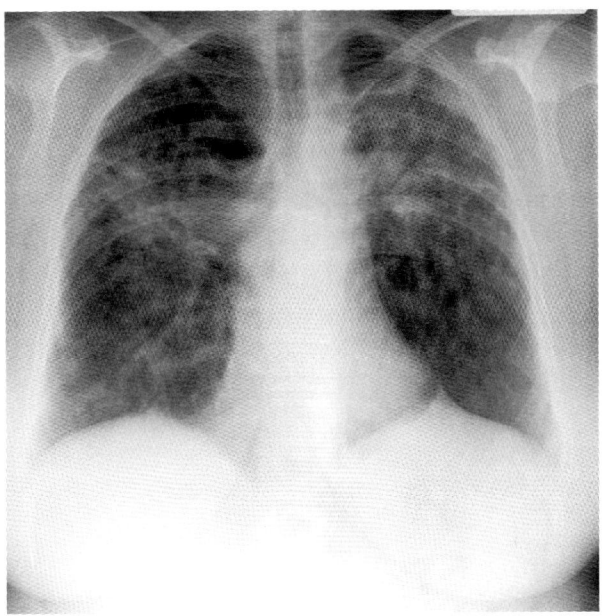

A tuberculin skin test is normal.

**Which of the following is the most appropriate laboratory test to perform next?**

(A) Alkaline phosphatase level
(B) Cortisol level
(C) 1,25-Dihydroxyvitamin D level
(D) Parathyroid hormone–related protein level

## Item 32

A 28-year-old woman is evaluated for preconception counseling. She desires to achieve pregnancy in the next 6 months. Medical history is significant for type 1 diabetes mellitus diagnosed at 12 years of age. She has no known microvascular or macrovascular complications of diabetes. She is up to date on screening for microvascular complications with her last eye examination performed 11 months prior and a normal creatinine level, urine albumin-creatinine ratio, lipid panel, and foot examination 9 months prior. Thyroid-stimulating hormone level was 0.5 µU/mL (0.5 mU/L) 3 months ago. She is currently using a condom for contraception. Medical history also includes autoimmune thyroid disease. Medications are insulin lispro delivered through continuous subcutaneous insulin infusion and levothyroxine.

On physical examination, vital signs are normal. Nondilated retinal examination, thyroid examination, and monofilament testing are all normal.

Laboratory studies reveal that hemoglobin A$_{1c}$ level is currently 6.7%, improved from 9% 3 months ago.

**Which of the following is the most appropriate preconception management to perform next?**

(A) Dilated eye examination
(B) Fasting lipid profile
(C) Nephrology referral
(D) Thyroid-stimulating hormone measurement
(E) Urine albumin-creatinine ratio

## Item 33

A 38-year-old woman presents for first assessment of bone health 4 months into prednisone therapy. Medical history is significant for treatment of antiphospholipid syndrome with recurrent diffuse alveolar hemorrhage and secondary diabetes mellitus. She is not sexually active. She has had no fractures. Medications are prednisone, cyclophosphamide, neutral protamine Hagedorn (NPH) insulin, calcium citrate/vitamin D$_3$, sulfamethoxazole-trimethoprim, and omeprazole. She is expected to continue prednisone therapy, 7.5 mg or more, for at least the next 6 months.

On physical examination, vital signs are normal. BMI is 37. The remainder of the examination is normal.

Bone mineral density by dual-energy x-ray absorptiometry shows a lumbar spine Z-score of –2.1 and total hip Z-score of –3.1. Radiograph of the spine shows no vertebral compression.

**Which of the following is the most appropriate treatment?**

(A) Alendronate
(B) Teriparatide
(C) Zoledronic acid
(D) No additional therapy

## Item 34

A 29-year-old woman is seen in follow-up for evaluation of abnormal thyroid laboratory results. She is currently 26 weeks pregnant. She was originally evaluated 1 week ago for concerns about lack of weight gain during pregnancy, palpitations, anxiety, and insomnia. There is no family history of thyroid or autoimmune disease. Medical history is unremarkable, and her only medication is a prenatal vitamin.

On physical examination, other than a pulse rate of 98/min, vital signs are normal. The patient is a thin, gravid woman with a mild tremor of the outstretched hands, lid lag, and small goiter. There is no exophthalmus.

Laboratory studies obtained last week show a thyroid-stimulating hormone level of 6.5 µU/mL (6.5 mU/mL) and a free thyroxine (T$_4$) level of 2.6 ng/dL (33.5 pmol/L).

**Which of the following is the most likely diagnosis?**

(A) Gestational thyrotoxicosis
(B) Graves disease
(C) Hypothyroidism
(D) Thyroid-stimulating hormone–secreting adenoma

## Item 35

A 31-year-old woman is evaluated for amenorrhea. She stopped taking her oral contraceptive pill (OCP) 6 months ago with the goal of becoming pregnant. She has not had a menstrual cycle since stopping her OCP. Her cycles were regular prior to starting an OCP 6 years ago and while on the OCP. She notes a small amount of breast discharge with nipple stimulation; this has been a noted issue for approximately 3 months. Medical history is otherwise unremarkable. Her only medication is a folic acid supplement.

On physical examination, vital signs are normal. There is an elicitable milky discharge from the nipples bilaterally. Thyroid and skin examinations are normal. Visual field testing is normal.

Laboratory studies show a prolactin level of 75 ng/mL (75 µg/L). Serum pregnancy test is negative, and thyroid-stimulating hormone level, kidney function tests, and liver chemistry tests are normal.

MRI of the brain with and without contrast with fine cuts through pituitary reveals a 7-mm pituitary microadenoma.

**Which of the following is the most appropriate management?**

(A) Clomiphene citrate therapy
(B) Dopamine agonist therapy
(C) Pituitary surgery
(D) Resume oral contraceptive pill

## Item 36

A 19-year-old man is evaluated during a follow-up evaluation of his type 1 diabetes mellitus. He was diagnosed 4 months ago with symptoms of hyperglycemia. His hemoglobin $A_{1c}$ level at diagnosis was 11.1%, and antibodies to glutamic acid decarboxylase (GAD65) were positive. He was begun on prandial and basal insulin. He now reports progressive improvement in his glycemic control over the last 8 weeks without changes to his diet, activity level, or insulin doses. Data from his glucometer demonstrates an average fasting, preprandial, and bedtime blood glucose level of 80 mg/dL (4.4 mmol/L). He has several postprandial blood glucose values of approximately 60 mg/dL (3.3 mmol/L) associated with hypoglycemic symptoms. His current hemoglobin $A_{1c}$ level is 5.0%. Medications are insulin glargine (8 U) and insulin aspart (2 U before meals).

His physical examination is notable for an increase in BMI from 18 at the time of his diabetes diagnosis, to now at 20. Vital signs and the remainder of the physical examination are normal.

**Which of the following is the most appropriate management of this patient's diabetes?**

(A) Continue insulin glargine dose, decrease insulin aspart dose
(B) Decrease insulin glargine dose, discontinue insulin aspart
(C) Discontinue insulin glargine, discontinue insulin aspart
(D) Discontinue insulin glargine, discontinue insulin aspart, add sliding-scale insulin regimen

## Item 37

A 63-year-old woman was diagnosed with osteoporosis 6 years ago. Initial treatment with an oral bisphosphonate resulted in upper gastrointestinal symptoms, so subcutaneous denosumab twice yearly was prescribed. The patient has now completed 5 years of denosumab therapy. Medical history is otherwise unremarkable. Denosumab was last administered 6 months ago.

Vital signs and the remainder of the physical examination are normal.

**Which of the following is the most appropriate management?**

(A) Continue denosumab
(B) Dual-energy x-ray absorptiometry (DEXA) scan
(C) Osteoporosis drug holiday
(D) Switch to zoledronic acid

## Item 38

A 55-year-old man with type 1 diabetes mellitus was admitted to the hospital for management of a non–ST-elevation myocardial infarction. He is clinically stable and eating well. He will begin fasting at midnight in preparation for a cardiac catheterization tomorrow. His current fasting blood glucose values range from 70 to 80 mg/dL (3.9-4.4 mmol/L), and his premeal blood glucose values range from 140 to 160 mg/dL (7.8-8.9 mmol/L) on his home doses of basal insulin glargine and prandial insulin aspart. His last hemoglobin $A_{1c}$ value was 7.2%.

**In addition to holding prandial insulin, which of the following is the most appropriate management for this patient's diabetes?**

(A) Continue basal insulin dose
(B) Continue basal insulin dose and add correction insulin regimen
(C) Decrease basal insulin dose and add correction insulin regimen
(D) Hold basal insulin and add sliding-scale insulin regimen

## Item 39

A 38-year-old woman is seen in follow-up to discuss the findings of an abdominal and pelvic CT scan done to evaluate renal colic, which has since resolved. The abdominal CT scan showed two small nonobstructing renal calculi in the right kidney and a 1.6-cm left adrenal mass with a density of 21 Hounsfield units (indeterminate for adrenal adenoma). Other than nephrolithiasis, the remainder of the medical history is unremarkable, and she takes no medications.

On physical examination, vital signs and the remainder of the examination are unremarkable.

Laboratory studies show normal serum electrolytes.

**Which of the following is the most appropriate test to perform next?**

(A) 24-Hour urine free cortisol measurement
(B) 24-Hour urine total metanephrine measurement
(C) Plasma aldosterone-plasma renin ratio (ARR) measurement
(D) Serum dehydroepiandrosterone sulfate (DHEAS) measurement

## Item 40

A 57-year-old woman is evaluated during hospitalization following surgical fixation of a right femur neck pathologic fracture. Pathology of the femur shows a neoplasm containing numerous giant cells consistent with brown tumor.

On physical examination, vital signs are normal. There is a palpable mass on the lower left side of the right neck. There is an incision with surgical staples on the right hip. The remainder of the examination is unremarkable.

Laboratory studies:

| | |
|---|---|
| Alkaline phosphatase | 260 U/L |
| Calcium | 13.2 mg/dL (3.3 mmol/L) |
| Creatinine | 1.6 mg/dL (141.4 µmol/L) |
| Phosphorus | 1.9 mg/dL (0.6 mmol/L) |
| Parathyroid hormone | 1142 pg/mL (1142 ng/L) |

Neck ultrasound shows a solid hypervascular mass (6 × 2.9 × 3 cm) posterior to the left lobe of the thyroid, with compression and displacement of the trachea. A parathyroidectomy is planned.

Which of the following is the most appropriate test to perform next?

(A) 1,25-Dihydroxyvitamin D level
(B) 24-Hour urine calcium level
(C) 25-Hydroxyvitamin D level
(D) Ionized calcium level

## Item 41

A 51-year-old woman underwent CT scan of the abdomen following a motor vehicle accident. This revealed a 2.5-cm right adrenal mass with a density of 6 Hounsfield units (compatible with adrenal adenoma). Medical history is significant for hypertension diagnosed 2 years ago. She is perimenopausal and has been experiencing sweating and hot flushes. Medications are hydrochlorothiazide and doxazosin.

On physical examination, blood pressure is 142/90 mm Hg, pulse rate is 90/min. Other vital signs are normal. BMI is 33. There are no supraclavicular fats pads or abdominal striae.

Laboratory studies show a cortisol level following a 1-mg overnight dexamethasone suppression test of 8 µg/dL (220.8 nmol/L), plasma aldosterone-plasma renin ratio (ARR) of 13, and plasma fractionated free metanephrines 32 pg/mL (0.17 nmol/L).

Which of the following is the most likely diagnosis?

(A) Non-hormone–secreting adrenal adenoma
(B) Pheochromocytoma
(C) Primary aldosteronism
(D) Subclinical Cushing syndrome

## Item 42

A 48-year-old woman is evaluated for a 1-year history of 11.3-kg (25-lb) weight gain, fatigue, easy bruising, and difficulty remembering things. She works the night shift at a hotel reception desk. Medical history is significant for hypertension, type 2 diabetes mellitus, and menopausal hot flushes. Medications are lisinopril, estradiol, aspirin, and metformin.

On physical examination, blood pressure is 142/88 mm Hg. Other vital signs are normal. BMI is 34. The patient has central obesity and a dorsocervical fat pad is present. There are no abdominal striae, no proximal muscle weakness, and no supraclavicular fat pads.

Which of the following is the most appropriate next step in evaluation of this patient?

(A) 1-mg overnight dexamethasone suppression test
(B) 24-Hour urine free cortisol measurement
(C) Late night salivary cortisol measurement
(D) Morning serum total cortisol measurement

## Item 43

A 52-year-old man is evaluated for gradual-onset breast tenderness and enlargement over the past 6 months. Medical history is significant for hypertension and symptomatic heart failure with reduced ejection fraction diagnosed 1 year ago. His medications are metoprolol, lisinopril, and spironolactone. He has noticed no change in his sexual function over the past year and reports the presence of morning erections.

On physical examination, vital signs are normal. BMI is 31. There is notable bilateral breast tenderness with rubbery concentric masses noted bilaterally at the areolae. There is no thyroid enlargement, hepatomegaly, or testicular abnormalities including atrophy or mass.

Which of the following is the most likely diagnosis?

(A) Breast cancer
(B) Germ cell tumor
(C) Hypogonadal-associated gynecomastia
(D) Pseudogynecomastia
(E) Spironolactone-induced gynecomastia

## Item 44

A 24-year-old man is seen for follow-up management of hypothyroidism. He was diagnosed with hypothyroidism due to Hashimoto thyroiditis 8 years ago. Until 6 months ago, he had been euthyroid on the same dose of levothyroxine. More recently he has required escalating doses of levothyroxine to maintain euthyroidism. He reports that he is still taking levothyroxine as he always has–first thing in the morning on an empty stomach at least 1 hour before eating breakfast. At present, the patient admits to hypothyroid symptoms and intermittent crampy abdominal pain. He has an unintentional weight loss of 2.3 kg (5 lb) over the last 2 months and a new, very pruritic rash on his knees and elbows. His only medication is levothyroxine.

On physical examination, vital signs are normal. The patient's thyroid gland is normal to palpation without nodules. He has papules and excoriated blisters on his elbows, knees, and buttocks.

Laboratory studies show a serum thyroid-stimulating hormone level of 14 µU/mL (14 mU/L) and a free thyroxine (T$_4$) level of 0.9 ng/dL (11.6 pmol/L).

**Which of the following is the most likely diagnosis?**

(A) Celiac disease

(B) Medication noncompliance

(C) Primary adrenal insufficiency

(D) Thyroid hormone resistance

## Item 45

A 37-year-old woman is unable to achieve pregnancy despite 7 months of unprotected intercourse. Her menstrual cycles are normal, occurring every 28 days with associated breast tenderness and bloating. There have been no prior pregnancies or attempts to achieve pregnancy by either the patient or her male partner. There is no history of previous sexually transmitted infections. She is otherwise healthy.

Medical history is significant for appendicitis at age 26 for which she had an uncomplicated appendectomy. Her only medication is a prenatal vitamin.

On physical examination, vital signs are normal. She has a well-healed abdominal scar. Thyroid, skin, and pelvic examinations are all unremarkable. There is no elicitable breast discharge, no signs of hyperandrogenism, and no visual field cuts.

**Which of the following is the most appropriate management?**

(A) Obtain midluteal phase serum progesterone level

(B) Obtain semen analysis

(C) Recommend an additional 5 months of unprotected intercourse

(D) Refer for laparoscopy

## Item 46

A 55-year-old man is referred for evaluation of fatigue, weight gain, decreased libido, and difficulty maintaining an erection. Sexual functioning was normal until 6 months ago, and he has fathered two children. Medical history is significant for polysubstance abuse that is being managed with daily methadone. His medical history is otherwise unremarkable, and his only medication is methadone.

On physical examination, vital signs are normal. Neurological, genitalia, and the remainder of the physical examination are normal.

**Laboratory studies:**

| | |
|---|---|
| Follicle-stimulating hormone | 5 mU/mL (5 U/L) |
| Luteinizing hormone | 4 mU/ml (4 U/L) |
| Prolactin | 12 ng/mL (12 µg/L) |
| Testosterone | 185 ng/dL (6.4 nmol/L) |
| Thyroid-stimulating hormone | 2.4 µU/mL (2.4 mU/L) |
| Thyroxine ($T_4$), free | 1.3 ng/dL (16.8 pmol/L) |

**Which of the following is the most likely cause of this patient's hypogonadism?**

(A) Age-related decline in gonadal function

(B) Chronic opioid therapy

(C) Pituitary tumor

(D) Primary gonadal failure

## Item 47

An 18-year-old woman is evaluated for absence of menarche. She has undergone some breast development (Tanner stage II). Medical history is unremarkable, and she takes no medications.

On physical examination, her height is 150 cm (59 in) and weight is 47 kg (103.6 lb). BMI is 21. Vital signs and the remainder of the physical examination, including pelvic examination, are normal.

Laboratory studies show a follicle-stimulating hormone level of 74 mU/mL (74 U/L). Serum beta-human chorionic gonadotropin level is undetectable. Thyroid-stimulating hormone and prolactin levels are normal.

On pelvic ultrasound, a uterus is present, but ovaries are difficult to visualize.

**Which of the following is the most likely diagnosis?**

(A) Functional hypothalamic amenorrhea

(B) Primary ovarian insufficiency

(C) Turner syndrome

(D) Vaginal agenesis

## Item 48

A 47-year-old man is evaluated for intermittent episodes of anxiety, diaphoresis, and palpitations. These episodes occur approximately 4 hours after a meal. His first episode occurred while at work. A fingerstick blood glucose reading performed by the employee health nurse was 48 mg/dL (2.7 mmol/L). His symptoms resolved with juice. He has had three similar episodes over the last month. He has increased his consumption of snacks between meals in an attempt to avoid repeat episodes. He denies use of over-the counter supplements or illicit drug use. He does not consume alcohol. He is asymptomatic today. Medical history is significant for Roux-en-Y gastric bypass surgery 3 years ago. He takes no glucose-lowering medications.

On physical examination, vital signs are normal. BMI is 31. The remainder of his examination is normal.

His fingerstick blood glucose level is 85 mg/dL (4.7 mmol/L). Laboratory studies show a hemoglobin $A_{1c}$ level of 5%. All other laboratory results are normal.

**Which of the following is the most appropriate diagnostic test to perform next?**

(A) 72-Hour fast

(B) Mixed-meal testing

(C) Oral glucose tolerance test

(D) Pancreatic imaging

## Item 49

A 65-year-old woman is admitted to the hospital for fatigue and weakness over the last 1 to 2 weeks. Medical history is significant for hypertension, type 2 diabetes mellitus, and rheumatoid arthritis. For the past 3 months, the patient's rheumatoid arthritis has been treated with methotrexate and prednisone. Because of inadequate control, etanercept was added 2 weeks ago. At that time, the patient decided to discontinue prednisone due to increased bruising of her skin.

**CONT.**

Current medications are methotrexate, etanercept, amlodipine, folic acid, metformin, and aspirin.

On physical examination, blood pressure is 110/68 mm Hg sitting and 90/64 mm Hg standing, and pulse rate is 102/min sitting and 110/min standing. Symmetrical synovial bogginess is noted in the metacarpophalangeal joints and wrists bilaterally.

Laboratory studies show an 8 AM cortisol level of 2 µg/dL (55.2 nmol/L).

**Which of the following is the most appropriate management?**

(A) Initiation of hydrocortisone

(B) Initiation of hydrocortisone and fludrocortisone

(C) Performance of an adrenocorticotropic hormone (ACTH) stimulation test

(D) Performance of an ACTH stimulation test after administration of dexamethasone

## Item 50

A 45-year-old woman comes to the office to review her thyroid function test results. Thyroid function testing was ordered in response to a recent diagnosis of hypercholesterolemia. The patient is otherwise well, and she takes no medications.

On physical examination, vital signs are normal. Her physical examination is normal with the exception of slowed relaxation phase of deep tendon reflexes.

Laboratory studies show a serum thyroid-stimulating hormone (TSH) level of 24 µU/mL (24 mU/L) and a free thyroxine (T$_4$) level of 0.65 ng/dL (8.4 pmol/L).

**Which of the following is the most appropriate treatment?**

(A) Desiccated thyroid extract

(B) Low-dose (25-µg) levothyroxine

(C) Weight-based replacement dose of levothyroxine

(D) No treatment

## Item 51

A 24-year-old woman is evaluated for 6 months of amenorrhea, weight gain, and depressed mood. Medical history is otherwise unremarkable, and she takes no medications.

On physical examination, blood pressure is 134/86 mm Hg and pulse rate is 82/min. BMI is 31. Other vital signs are normal. The patient has facial plethora. Skin examination reveals multiple ecchymoses. There are wide pigmented striae on the abdomen as well as a dorsocervical fat pad.

**Laboratory studies:**

Cortisol, free, urine
Initial measurement          120 µg/24 h (330.7 nmol/24 h)
Repeat measurement           240 µg/24 h (661.3 nmol/24 h)
Cortisol after 1 mg          6.0 µg/dL (165.6 nmol/L)
dexamethasone test

**Which of the following is the most appropriate diagnostic test to perform next?**

(A) Adrenocorticotropic hormone (ACTH) level

(B) 8-mg Dexamethasone suppression test

(C) Inferior petrosal sinus sampling for ACTH

(D) Pituitary MRI

## Item 52

A 56-year-old man is evaluated for palpitations and difficulty sleeping over the past month. His past medical history is significant for hypothyroidism following subtotal thyroidectomy 6 months ago for management of compressive symptoms from a multinodular goiter. Two months ago, he was diagnosed with hypogonadism and was prescribed intramuscular testosterone. He takes his levothyroxine on an empty stomach with a cup of coffee every morning. His medications are levothyroxine, testosterone enanthate, calcium carbonate, and omeprazole for gastroesophageal reflux disease.

On physical examination, his vital signs are normal. He has a well-healed anterior neck scar. There is a fine tremor of his outstretched hands. The remainder of the examination is normal.

**Laboratory studies:**

|  | 2 Months Ago | Today |
|---|---|---|
| Serum thyroid-stimulating hormone | 1.5 µU/mL (1.5 mU/L) | 0.08 µU/mL (0.08 mU/L) |
| Thyroxine (T$_4$), free | 1.1 ng/dL (14.2 pmol/L) | 1.4 ng/dL (18.1 pmol/L) |

**Which of the following is the most likely explanation for the thyroid function test results?**

(A) Calcium carbonate

(B) Levothyroxine with coffee

(C) Omeprazole

(D) Testosterone

## Item 53

A 74-year-old woman is evaluated for back pain after a fall occurring 2 weeks ago. Medical history is significant for deep venous thrombosis 3 years ago following a 12-hour airplane flight. Medications are acetaminophen as needed for back pain and calcium carbonate with vitamin D.

On physical examination, vital signs are normal. She has minimal pain to percussion over T8. Her examination is otherwise normal.

**Laboratory studies:**

| Alkaline phosphatase | 82 U/L |
|---|---|
| Calcium, serum | 9.9 mg/dL (2.5 mmol/L) |
| Creatinine, serum | 1.1 mg/dL (97.2 µmol/L) |
| 25-Hydroxyvitamin D | 40 ng/mL (99.8 nmol/L) |

Lateral spine radiograph shows 30% compression of T8, not present on prior radiographs. Bone mineral density by DEXA shows a lumbar spine T-score of –3.0 and femur neck T-score of –2.8.

**Which of the following is the most appropriate treatment?**

(A) Alendronate

(B) Calcitonin

(C) Denosumab

(D) Raloxifene

(E) Teriparatide

## Item 54

A 78-year-old man with type 2 diabetes mellitus is evaluated during a routine follow-up examination. He reports hypoglycemia occurring approximately twice per week before dinner. It is worse if he plays golf in the afternoon. He has had three episodes in the last 3 months in which he required assistance from his wife. Medical history is significant for dyslipidemia, hypertension, and obesity. Medications are aspirin, atorvastatin, glyburide, lisinopril, and metformin.

On physical examination, vital signs are normal. BMI is 32. The remainder of the examination is normal.

Laboratory studies show a hemoglobin $A_{1c}$ level of 6.5% and an estimated glomerular filtration rate (eGFR) of 50 mL/min/1.73 m$^2$.

**Which of the following is the most appropriate management of hypoglycemia?**

(A) Increase carbohydrate intake with the noon meal
(B) Prescribe glucagon
(C) Stop glyburide therapy
(D) Stop metformin therapy

## Item 55

A 58-year-old man is evaluated for resistant hypertension. He was first diagnosed with hypertension 10 years ago, and his blood pressure has been increasingly difficult to control. Testing for secondary causes of hypertension will be undertaken. Medical history is otherwise unremarkable. Medications are lisinopril, spironolactone, hydrochlorothiazide, and metoprolol.

On physical examination, blood pressure is 149/93 mm Hg. Other vital signs are normal. BMI is 29. The remainder of the physical examination is unremarkable.

**Which of the following should be discontinued prior to screening for secondary causes of hypertension?**

(A) Hydrochlorothiazide
(B) Lisinopril
(C) Metoprolol
(D) Spironolactone

## Item 56

A 75-year old man is evaluated for ongoing management of his type 2 diabetes mellitus. He was diagnosed with diabetes 11 years ago. In addition to diabetes, medical history is significant for hypertension, hyperlipidemia, and chronic kidney disease stage G3b. He had a myocardial infarction 6 months ago with subsequent placement of two drug-eluting stents. His hemoglobin $A_{1c}$ level has decreased from 8.7% to 7.8% with adherence to lifestyle modifications and his basal and prandial insulin regimen. Medications are rosuvastatin, lisinopril, metoprolol, chlorthalidone, low-dose aspirin, and clopidogrel.

On physical examination, vital signs are normal. BMI is 29. Other than an S4, the cardiac examination and the remainder of the physical examination are normal.

**According to the American Diabetes Association, which of the following is the most appropriate hemoglobin $A_{1c}$ goal for this patient?**

(A) Less than 7%
(B) 7% to less than 7.5%
(C) 7.5% to less than 8%
(D) 8% to less than 9%

## Item 57

A 67-year-old man is evaluated for headache, fatigue, and weakness for the past several weeks. Medical history is significant for metastatic melanoma that is being treated with ipilimumab, which is his only medication.

On physical examination, vital signs are normal. There is a well-healed excisional scar on his posterior right shoulder. The remainder of the physical examination is normal.

MRI shows enlarged pituitary with homogeneous enhancement. There is no compression of the optic chiasm.

**Laboratory studies:**

| | |
|---|---|
| Cortisol (8 AM) | 3 µg/dL (82.8 nmol/L) |
| Prolactin | 12 ng/mL (12 µg/L) |
| Thyroid-stimulating hormone | 0.2 µU/mL (0.2 mU/L) |
| Thyroxine ($T_4$), free | 0.6 ng/dL (7.7 pmol/L) |

**Which of the following is the most likely cause of this patient's findings?**

(A) Ipilimumab-induced hypophysitis
(B) Lymphocytic hypophysitis
(C) Pituitary adenoma
(D) Primary hypothyroidism

## Item 58

A 45-year-old man underwent abdominal CT imaging for evaluation of bloating and constipation. The CT scan shows a 5-cm right adrenal mass with a density of 42 Hounsfield units and absolute contrast washout of 38% at 10 minutes. Testing for pheochromocytoma and subclinical Cushing syndrome was negative. Medical history is otherwise unremarkable, and he takes no medications.

On physical examination, vital signs and the remainder of the physical examination are normal.

**Which of the following is the most appropriate next step in management?**

(A) Adrenal biopsy
(B) Adrenalectomy
(C) Mitotane therapy
(D) Repeat CT at 6 months

## Item 59

A 55-year-old woman returns to the emergency department for persistent weakness, shakiness, and intermittent hand spasms. Three days ago, she was diagnosed with hypocalcemia, and vitamin D and calcium were initiated at that time.

CONT.

Medical history is significant for metastatic ovarian cancer, currently treated with cisplatin and etoposide chemotherapy. Additional medications are calcium carbonate and vitamin $D_3$.

On physical examination, vital signs are normal. Tetany of the hand is noted during blood pressure assessment. Chvostek sign is positive.

**Laboratory studies:**

| | |
|---|---|
| Albumin | 3.5 g/dL (35 g/L) |
| Calcium | 7.6 mg/dL (1.9 mmol/L) |
| Creatinine | 1.0 mg/dL (88.4 µmol/L) |
| Parathyroid hormone | 19 pg/mL (19 ng/L) |
| Potassium | 4.2 mEq/L (4.2 mmol/L) |

The laboratory results are similar to those obtained 3 days ago.

Electrocardiography shows a prolonged QTc interval.

**Which of the following measurements is most appropriate to perform next?**

(A) Bicarbonate

(B) Ionized calcium

(C) Magnesium

(D) Phosphorus

## Item 60

A 60-year-old man is evaluated for management of type 2 diabetes mellitus. Three months ago he was diagnosed with type 2 diabetes mellitus and chronic kidney disease. At that time, he received diabetes education and began lifestyle modifications. Medical history is significant for chronic kidney disease, hypertension, and hyperlipidemia. His medications are lisinopril and atorvastatin.

On physical examination, his blood pressure is 146/88 mm Hg. BMI is 28.5. The remainder of his vital signs and physical examination are normal.

Laboratory studies show a hemoglobin $A_{1c}$ level of 8.3%, serum creatinine level of 1.5 mg/dL (132.6 µmol/L), and estimated glomerular filtration rate of 48 mL/min/1.73 m².

**Which of the following is the most appropriate treatment of this patient's diabetes?**

(A) Empagliflozin

(B) Glipizide

(C) Metformin

(D) Saxagliptin

## Item 61

A 55-year-old woman is seen during a follow-up evaluation for hyperthyroidism that was diagnosed 1 week ago. Thyroid examination revealed a palpable right thyroid nodule.

Thyroid-stimulating hormone (TSH) was less than 0.01 µU/mL (0.01 mU/L), free thyroxine ($T_4$) and total triiodothyronine ($T_3$) were 2.1 ng/dL (27.1 pmol/L) and 210 ng/dL (3.2 nmol/L), respectively. Atenolol was prescribed, and thyroid scintigraphy with determination of radioactive iodine uptake was ordered.

On physical examination, vital signs are normal. The neck and corresponding thyroid technetium-99 scan is shown.

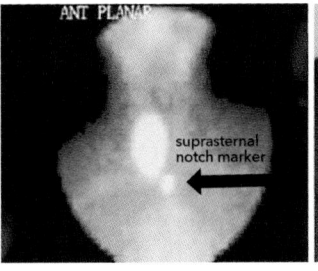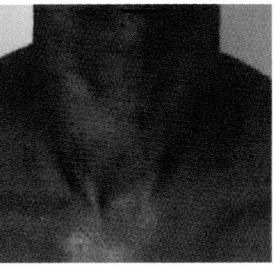

Uptake at 24 hours is 30% (normal 14% to 30%).

**Which of the following is the most appropriate management?**

(A) Fine-needle aspiration biopsy of the thyroid nodule

(B) Increase atenolol dosage

(C) Methimazole

(D) Radioactive iodine ($^{131}I$) therapy

## Item 62

A 55-year-old man is evaluated during a follow-up visit after he was diagnosed with type 2 diabetes mellitus based on two hemoglobin $A_{1c}$ measurements of 7.8%. His medical history is significant for dyslipidemia and hypertension. Medications are aspirin, atorvastatin, and lisinopril.

On physical examination, vital signs are normal. BMI is 33. The general physical examination, including nondilated eye examination, is normal.

The patient will initiate therapeutic lifestyle modifications, and metformin will be started.

**In addition to spot urine albumin-creatinine ratio testing, which of the following screening tests should be done now?**

(A) Comprehensive foot examination and dilated eye examination

(B) Fasting plasma glucose and 2-hour 75-g oral glucose tolerance test

(C) Serum $B_{12}$ and folate concentrations

(D) 24-Hour urine protein and creatinine measurement

## Item 63

A 45-year-man is seen in routine follow-up for his type 2 diabetes mellitus. He was diagnosed 5 years ago, and he does not have any diabetes-related complications. His current treatment includes insulin detemir, prandial insulin lispro, and metformin. His hemoglobin $A_{1c}$ level has decreased to 7.4%. His fasting and preprandial blood glucose measurements range from 110 to 130 mg/dL (6.1-7.2 mmol/L). He has had no hypoglycemia. Medical history is significant for obesity. He wishes to reduce his hemoglobin $A_{1c}$ level to below 7%, but he is reluctant to add another injectable medication to his regimen. Medications are insulin detemir, insulin lispro, and metformin.

On physical examination, vital signs are normal. BMI is 33. The remainder of the physical examination is unremarkable.

**Which of the following is the most appropriate management of this patient's diabetes?**

(A) Add liraglutide
(B) Continue current regimen
(C) Increase insulin detemir dose
(D) Measure postprandial blood glucose level

## Item 64

A 65-year-old woman is evaluated for hypercalcemia that was incidentally discovered on routine blood testing for a new life insurance policy. She has no symptoms. Medical history is unremarkable. Her only medication is calcium carbonate taken as needed for occasional heartburn.

On physical examination, vital signs are normal. Height is unchanged from prior measurements. The remainder of her examination is normal.

**Laboratory studies:**

| | |
|---|---|
| Estimate glomerular filtration rate | Greater than 60 mL/min/1.73 m² |
| Calcium | 10.6 mg/dL (2.6 mmol/L) |
| Phosphorus | 3.1 mg/dL (1.0 mmol/L) |
| Parathyroid hormone | 72 pg/mL (72 ng/L) |
| 25-Hydroxyvitamin D | 35 ng/mL (87.4 nmol/L) |
| 24-Hour urine calcium | 240 mg/24 h (6 mmol/24 h) |

Kidney-urinary-bladder radiograph is negative for kidney stones. Dual-energy x-ray absorptiometry (DEXA) bone mineral density scan shows femur neck T-score of –1.4, lumbar spine T-score of –1.4, and one-third radius T-score of –1.7.

**Which of the following is the most appropriate management?**

(A) Parathyroid sestamibi scan
(B) Reevaluate in 6 months
(C) Start alendronate
(D) Start cinacalcet

## Item 65

A 45-year-old man is seen for follow-up evaluation for depression and to review the results of laboratory testing. He was seen 1 month ago for a 6-month history of depressed mood, difficulty sleeping, decreased appetite, 2.3-kg (5-lb) weight loss, and fatigue. Major depressive disorder was diagnosed, and escitalopram was prescribed. Today the patient reports a significant improvement in his mood, appetite, and the quality of his sleep since starting treatment.

On physical examination, vital signs and physical examination are normal. Screening laboratory studies from 1 month ago show a thyroid-stimulating hormone (TSH) level of 7 µU/mL (7 mU/L) and a free thyroxine (T₄) level of 1.0 ng/dL (12.9 pmol/L).

**Which of the following is the most appropriate management?**

(A) Measure thyroid peroxidase antibodies
(B) Measure thyrotropin receptor antibodies
(C) Measure serum triiodothyronine (T₃) level
(D) Prescribe levothyroxine
(E) Repeat serum TSH testing in 2 months

## Item 66

A 52-year-old man is evaluated for difficult-to-control hypertension. Biochemical evaluation confirms a diagnosis of primary aldosteronism. Medications are amlodipine, losartan, and metoprolol.

On physical examination, blood pressure is 149/98 mm Hg and pulse rate is 75/min. The remainder of the vital signs and physical examination are unremarkable.

CT scan shows a 0.8-cm right adrenal mass with a density of 13 Hounsfield units.

**Which of the following is the most appropriate management?**

(A) Adrenal vein sampling
(B) Increase metoprolol
(C) Increase losartan
(D) Right adrenalectomy

## Item 67

A 65-year-old woman comes to the office to establish care. Her medical history is notable for hypothyroidism due to Hashimoto thyroiditis treated with levothyroxine. She does not have any symptoms at this time. There is no history of head or neck radiation exposure.

On physical examination, vital signs are normal. The patient's thyroid gland is enlarged. The right lobe is larger than the left, and a mobile 2-cm nodule is palpable in the lower pole. There is no palpable cervical adenopathy.

Laboratory studies show a serum thyroid-stimulating hormone level of 2.0 µU/mL (2.0 mU/L).

**Which of the following is the most appropriate diagnostic test to perform next?**

(A) CT scan of the neck
(B) Fine-needle aspiration biopsy of the thyroid nodule
(C) Thyroid uptake and ¹³¹I scan
(D) Ultrasound of the neck

## Item 68

A 59-year-old woman is evaluated for fatigue and weight gain over the past 2 months. Her medical history is significant for a pituitary tumor, treated with surgery followed by radiation therapy, at age 54. She has recently self-initiated calcium and vitamin D and a multivitamin. Her only other medication is levothyroxine.

On physical examination, vital signs are normal. BMI is 31. The remainder of the physical examination is normal.

**Which of the following is the most appropriate next step in management?**

(A) Increase the levothyroxine dose

(B) Measure free thyroxine ($T_4$) level

(C) Measure thyroid-stimulating hormone level

(D) MRI of the brain

## Item 69

A 53-year-old man returns for a follow-up visit for management of his type 2 diabetes mellitus. He was diagnosed with diabetes 10 years ago. In addition to diabetes, his medical history is significant for hypertension. Medications are enalapril and insulin glargine at bedtime and aspart insulin at meals.

On physical examination, blood pressure is 142/84 mm Hg. BMI is 27. The remainder of the vital signs and physical examination are unremarkable.

His fasting blood glucose level ranges from 150 to 180 mg/dL (8.3-10.0 mmol/L). His remaining premeal and bedtime blood glucose levels range from 110 to 130 mg/dL (6.1-7.2 mmol/L). He has intermittent episodes of hypoglycemia with recorded values ranging from 30 to 65 mg/dL (1.7-3.6 mmol/L). These occur once per week without a clear cause or pattern. For many episodes of hypoglycemia he experiences no symptoms, but he is able to detect hypoglycemia at blood glucose values less than 40 mg/dL (2.2 mmol/L). His most recent hemoglobin $A_{1c}$ level is 8.2%. He desires a hemoglobin $A_{1c}$ level less than 7%.

**Which of the following is the most appropriate treatment of this patient's diabetes?**

(A) Decrease all insulin doses

(B) Increase glargine insulin dose

(C) Initiate empagliflozin

(D) Initiate metformin

## Item 70

A 42-year-old woman is evaluated in the office for osteoporosis because she was told her heel ultrasound screening test was abnormal at a health fair. She has no history of fractures. Family history is significant for osteoporosis in her mother, diagnosed at age 68 years; she has no history of fracture. Her only medication is a combination estradiol-levonorgestrel oral contraceptive pill.

On physical examination, vital signs are normal. BMI is 19. The remainder of her physical examination is normal.

Report of the quantitative heel ultrasound shows a Z-score of –0.5.

**Which of the following is the most appropriate management?**

(A) Lifestyle counseling for osteoporosis prevention

(B) Dual-energy x-ray absorptiometry (DEXA) scan

(C) Evaluation of secondary causes of bone loss

(D) Serial quantitative heel ultrasound testing

## Item 71

A 27-year-old woman is seen in a follow-up visit for hyperthyroidism. Three months ago she was diagnosed with Graves disease, and methimazole was initiated. Today the patient reports an overall improvement in hyperthyroid symptoms, but over the past week she has developed a fever, sore throat, and painful swallowing. She reports no cough. Medications are methimazole and propranolol.

On physical examination, temperature is 38.7 °C (101.6 °F), blood pressure is 112/78 mm Hg, pulse rate is 98/min, and respiration rate is 18/min. The patient's posterior oropharynx is erythematous without exudates. Her examination is otherwise normal.

**Which of the following is the most appropriate management?**

(A) Begin empiric oral penicillin V

(B) Obtain a rapid antigen detection test for Group A streptococcus

(C) Obtain a throat culture

(D) Stop methimazole and obtain complete blood count with differential

## Item 72

A 66-year-old man recently diagnosed with type 2 diabetes mellitus is evaluated in the emergency department for nausea, vomiting, and fatigue. He was diagnosed with type 2 diabetes 18 months ago. In the past month metformin was discontinued due to severe diarrhea, and glipizide and empagliflozin were initiated. In addition to type 2 diabetes, medical history is significant for coronary artery disease, hypertension, and dyslipidemia. Medications are aspirin, lisinopril, metoprolol, atorvastatin, glipizide, and empagliflozin.

On physical examination, temperature is normal, blood pressure is 90/60 mm Hg, pulse rate is 120/min, and respiration rate is 22/min. Dry mucous membranes are noted. There is diffuse abdominal tenderness to palpation without guarding. Other than tachycardia, the remainder of the examination is normal.

Laboratory studies:

| | |
|---|---|
| Sodium | 133 mEq/L (133 mmol/L) |
| Bicarbonate | 10 mEq/L (10 mmol/L) |
| Glucose | 150 mg/dL (8.3 mmol/L) |
| Anion gap | 17 mEq/L (17 mmol/L) |
| β-hydroxybutyrate | Elevated |

**Which of the following is most likely responsible for the patient's findings?**

(A) Atorvastatin

(B) Discontinuation of metformin

(C) Empagliflozin

(D) Glipizide

(E) Lisinopril

## Item 73

A 32-year-old man is evaluated for decreased libido and fatigue. His symptoms have increased over the last 6 months.

His medical history is otherwise unremarkable, and he takes no medications.

On physical examination, vital signs are normal. BMI is 26. He has gynecomastia. Visual field acuity testing and testicular examination are normal. Smell is intact.

**Laboratory studies:**

| | |
|---|---|
| Follicle-stimulating hormone | 4 mU/mL (4 U/L) |
| Luteinizing hormone | 5 mU/mL (5 U/L) |
| Prolactin | 100 ng/mL (100 µg/L) |
| Testosterone | 110 ng/dL (3.8 nmol/L) |

**Which of the following is the most appropriate diagnostic test to perform next?**

(A) Karyotype analysis
(B) Pituitary MRI
(C) Screening for anabolic steroid abuse
(D) Serum ferritin measurement
(E) Sex hormone-binding globulin measurement

## Item 74

A 74-year-old woman is evaluated in the emergency department for decreased responsiveness. She has become progressively confused and lethargic. She lives alone and stopped taking her medications at some time unknown. She was brought to the emergency department by a family member.

The patient had a near-total thyroidectomy for multinodular goiter 3 years ago.

On physical examination, temperature is 36.1 °C (97.0 °F), blood pressure is 80/45 mm Hg, pulse rate is 46/min, respiration rate is 10/min, and oxygen saturation is 92% breathing ambient air. BMI is 28. The patient is arousable with painful stimuli. She has a well-healed anterior neck scar. The patient's skin is cool and dry. She has periorbital edema and bipedal edema. Other than bradycardia, the cardiac examination is normal. The relaxation phase of her deep tendon reflexes is delayed.

Laboratory results show a sodium level of 129 mEq/L (129 mmol/L). Intravenous fluids are initiated.

**Which of the following is the essential initial step in the management of this patient?**

(A) Administer intravenous hydrocortisone
(B) Administer intravenous levothyroxine and liothyronine
(C) Administer norepinephrine
(D) Administer oral levothyroxine

## Item 75

A 35-year-old woman is seen in follow-up evaluation for her type 2 diabetes mellitus. She was diagnosed 3 years ago. She checks her fasting and 2-hour postprandial blood glucose values several times per week. Her fasting blood glucose levels range from 100 to 110 mg/dL (5.5-6.1 mmol/L) and her 2-hour postprandial values are 120 to 165 mg/dL (6.7-9.1 mmol/L). Her review of symptoms is positive for chronic heavy menses. Medications are metformin and liraglutide.

On physical examination, blood pressure is 123/74 mm Hg and pulse rate is 76/min. BMI is 31.2. The examination is otherwise unremarkable.

**Laboratory studies:**

| | |
|---|---|
| Hematocrit | 33% |
| Iron studies | |
| Ferritin | 11 ng/mL (11 µg/L) |
| Iron | 40 µg/dL (7.2 µmol/L) |
| Iron-binding capacity, total | 600 µg/dL (107.4 µmol/L) |
| Hemoglobin A$_{1c}$ | 7.3% |

**Which of the following is the most appropriate management of the elevated hemoglobin A$_{1c}$ level?**

(A) Basal insulin
(B) Empagliflozin
(C) Ferrous sulfate
(D) Hemoglobin electrophoresis

## Item 76

A 69-year-old woman is seen in the office following a left thyroid lobectomy and isthmusectomy 1 week ago for management of compressive symptoms related to a large left thyroid nodule. The preoperative thyroid/neck ultrasound showed the nodule without suspicious features and no abnormal cervical lymph nodes. The pathology report describes a 4.5-cm left adenomatous nodule in a background of multinodular hyperplasia. There is a single focus of papillary thyroid carcinoma measuring 0.5 cm in the greatest dimension. No lymphovascular or extrathyroidal invasion is noted. Surgical margins are negative.

The patient is currently feeling well and reports complete resolution of her prior symptoms. Her medical history is otherwise unremarkable, and she takes no medications.

On physical examination, vital signs are normal. There is a well-healed anterior neck scar. Laboratory studies show a serum thyroid-stimulating hormone (TSH) level of 1.8 µU/mL (1.8 mU/L).

**Which of the following is the most appropriate treatment?**

(A) Levothyroxine to suppress serum TSH
(B) Radioactive iodine ($^{131}$I) therapy
(C) Resection of the remaining thyroid lobe
(D) No additional treatment

## Item 77

A 37-year-old man is evaluated in the hospital for polyuria 1 day after transsphenoidal pituitary surgery for a craniopharyngioma. The patient reports increased thirst overnight. Urine output is currently 300 mL/hour for the last 12 hours. He takes no medications.

On physical examination, vital signs are normal. He has dry mucous membranes.

Laboratory studies show a sodium level of 146 mEq/L (146 mmol/L).

**Which of the following is the most appropriate diagnostic test to perform next?**

(A) Desmopressin challenge
(B) Urine and serum osmolality
(C) Urine electrolytes
(D) Water deprivation test

## Item 78

A 22-year-old woman is evaluated for tachycardia, fever, agitation, and confusion 3 days following laparoscopic cholecystectomy for acute cholecystitis.

Medical history is significant for type 1 diabetes mellitus well controlled on basal-bolus insulin and Graves disease previously treated with methimazole. Methimazole was discontinued 6 months ago when she was considered to be in remission. Medications are insulin glargine and insulin aspart.

On physical examination, temperature is 39.0 °C (102.2 °F), blood pressure is 95/50 mm Hg, pulse rate is 132/min and irregular, and respiration rate is 24/min. The patient is confused and appears flushed and diaphoretic. Lid lag is noted. The thyroid gland is diffusely enlarged with an audible bruit. Her deep tendon reflexes are brisk. There is a fine tremor of her hands. Her examination is otherwise normal.

**Which of the following is the most likely diagnosis?**

(A) Adrenal crisis

(B) Malignant hyperthermia

(C) Myxedema coma

(D) Thyroid storm

## Item 79

A 54-year-old man is evaluated at a follow-up visit after being diagnosed with type 2 diabetes mellitus 3 months ago. His initial hemoglobin $A_{1c}$ level was 8.5%. He opted for lifestyle modifications initially. He has lost 4.5 kg (10 lb) in the interim after making significant changes to his diet and increasing his activity level. His average blood glucose level currently is 180 mg/dL (10 mmol/L). Medical history is otherwise unremarkable.

On physical examination, blood pressure is 130/74 mm Hg and pulse is 70/min. BMI is 27. The examination is otherwise unremarkable.

His repeat hemoglobin $A_{1c}$ level today is 7.9%, but he would like it lower. Results of other laboratory studies are within normal ranges.

**Which of the following is the most appropriate management?**

(A) Continue current management

(B) Initiate empagliflozin

(C) Initiate liraglutide

(D) Initiate metformin

## Item 80

A 22-year-old man was admitted to the intensive care unit 24 hours ago with nausea, vomiting, and lethargy of 2 days' duration. Medical history is unremarkable, and he takes no medications. His admission laboratory values were consistent with diabetic ketoacidosis, and he was initiated on intravenous fluids and intravenous insulin therapy. After 24 hours, he is currently receiving 0.45% normal saline at 250 mL/h with 20 mEq (20 mmol) of potassium chloride per liter and an insulin drip at 5 U/h. His nausea continues, but his vomiting has ceased. He is unable to eat.

On physical examination, vital signs are normal. He is alert and oriented, and the remainder of his physical examination is unremarkable.

**Laboratory studies:**

Electrolytes

| | |
|---|---|
| Sodium | 141 mEq/L (141 mmol/L) |
| Potassium | 4.0 mEq/L (4.0 mmol/L) |
| Chloride | 104 mEq/L (104 mmol/L) |
| Bicarbonate | 20 mEq/L (20 mmol/L) |
| Glucose | 180 mg/dL (10 mmol/L) |
| pH | 7.32 |

**Which of the following is the most appropriate management?**

(A) Continue current insulin drip rate

(B) Decrease insulin drip rate and add intravenous dextrose

(C) Discontinue intravenous potassium

(D) Transition insulin drip to subcutaneous insulin regimen

## Item 81

A 68-year-old man is evaluated in the office for increasing shortness of breath, palpitations, difficulty sleeping, fatigue, generalized weakness, and 4.5-kg (10-lb) weight loss over the past month. His medical history is significant for heart failure and atrial fibrillation. For the past 2 years his medications have been metoprolol, lisinopril, amiodarone, and dabigatran.

On physical examination, the patient is afebrile, blood pressure is 140/80 mm Hg, pulse is 102/min, and respiration rate is 24/min. Deep tendon reflexes are brisk and symmetric. A fine tremor of his outstretched hands, bilateral lid lag, and an irregularly irregular heart rhythm are noted. Examination of the thyroid gland and remainder of the physical examination are normal.

Laboratory studies show a serum thyroid-stimulating hormone (TSH) level less than 0.01 µU/mL (0.01 mU/L), a free thyroxine ($T_4$) level of 3.1 ng/dL (40 pmol/L), and a serum total triiodothyronine ($T_3$) level of 190 ng/dL (2.9 nmol/L). TSH receptor antibodies are undetectable. Other laboratory studies are normal.

On thyroid ultrasound, the thyroid lobes and isthmus are normal in size. No thyroid nodules are seen. The background thyroid parenchyma demonstrates no demonstrable vascularity on color flow Doppler. Chest radiograph is normal.

**In addition to increasing the metoprolol dose, which of the following is the most appropriate initial management?**

(A) Discontinue amiodarone

(B) Begin methimazole

(C) Begin prednisone

(D) Thyroid scintigraphy with radioactive iodine uptake

## Item 82

A 36-year-old woman is evaluated for new-onset hirsutism noted on the face, chest, and abdomen. Hirsute hair growth has rapidly progressed over the last 6 months. Additionally, she notes frontal hair loss. Menstrual cycles have become irregular over the same time course. Medical history is otherwise unremarkable, and she takes no medications.

On physical examination, her blood pressure is 142/88 mm Hg; the remainder of the vital signs is normal. BMI is 26. On skin examination, acne is noted. Dark terminal hair appears on the face, chest, and abdomen. The patient has diffuse hair thinning on top of the head. The remainder of the physical examination is noncontributory.

**Laboratory studies:**

| | |
|---|---|
| Estradiol | 68 pg/mL (249.6 pmol/L) |
| Follicle-stimulating hormone | 12 mU/mL (12 U/L) |
| Human chorionic gonadotropin, serum | Negative |
| Prolactin | Normal |
| Testosterone, total | 220 ng/dL (7.6 nmol/L) |
| Thyroid-stimulating hormone | Normal |

**Which of the following is the most appropriate management?**

(A) Adrenal vein sampling for cortisol and androgens

(B) 24-Hour urine free cortisol

(C) Oral contraceptive therapy

(D) Pelvic ultrasound

## Item 83

A 62-year-old woman is evaluated for management of her type 2 diabetes mellitus. She was diagnosed 2 years ago, and treatment was advanced to include lifestyle modifications, metformin, liraglutide, and empagliflozin, but it was not successful in reaching her hemoglobin $A_{1c}$ goal. Her current regimen includes metformin and basal and prandial insulins. Her fasting and preprandial blood glucose values range from 150 to 200 mg/dL (8.3-11.1 mmol/L) with intermittent episodes of hypoglycemia. She has had a weight gain of 2.3 kg (5 lb) over the last 3 months. Medical history is also significant for hypertension, hyperlipidemia, and osteoarthritis. Medications are detemir insulin, lispro insulin, metformin, lisinopril, and atorvastatin.

On physical examination, blood pressure is 142/90 mm Hg and pulse rate is 63/min. BMI is 36. The remainder of the physical examination is unremarkable. Laboratory studies show a hemoglobin $A_{1c}$ level of 8.8%.

**Which of the following is the most appropriate management of this patient's diabetes?**

(A) Add sitagliptin

(B) Add pioglitazone

(C) Increase insulin

(D) Metabolic surgery referral

## Item 84

A 57-year-old woman is evaluated for progressive right upper leg pain for the past 2 years. The pain is worse with weight bearing. She is postmenopausal and otherwise in good health. She has no family history of fractures. She takes no medications.

On physical examination, vital signs are normal. BMI is 36. She has difficulty bearing weight and limps when walking. She has discomfort on palpation over the anterior tibia. The remainder of the physical examination is normal.

**Laboratory studies:**

| | |
|---|---|
| Alkaline phosphatase | 150 U/L |
| Calcium | 8.2 mg/dL (2.0 mmol/L) |
| Creatinine | 0.8 mg/dL (70.7 µmol/L) |
| Phosphorus | 2.4 mg/dL (0.8 mmol/L) |
| Parathyroid hormone | 176 pg/mL (176 ng/L) |
| 25-Hydroxyvitamin D | <6 ng/mL (15.0 nmol/L) |

**Which of the following is the most likely diagnosis?**

(A) Osteitis fibrosa cystica

(B) Osteogenesis imperfecta

(C) Osteomalacia

(D) Postmenopausal osteoporosis

# Answers and Critiques

## Item 1    Answer:  D

**Educational Objective:** Diagnose radiation-induced papillary thyroid cancer.

The most likely diagnosis is papillary thyroid cancer. Radiation exposure of the thyroid during childhood is the strongest environmental risk factor for thyroid cancer. Patients under the age of 15, especially those younger than 5 years, have the highest risk of subsequently developing papillary thyroid cancer following a significant radiation exposure (>10 rads).

A benign follicular nodule is not the most likely diagnosis due to the history of radiation exposure in childhood, ultrasound findings (hypoechoic solid nodule with irregular margins), and cervical lymphadenopathy. Fine-needle aspiration biopsy (FNAB) of both the thyroid nodule and abnormal lymph nodes should be pursued to confirm the suspected diagnosis and inform surgical management. In addition to thyroidectomy, patients with thyroid cancer that has metastasized to cervical lymph nodes require dissection of the affected compartment (central neck dissection for central lymph node metastases, and central and lateral neck dissection for lateral metastases). Abnormal findings on sonography vary considerably in their specificity for predicting malignant lymph node involvement (range 43% to 100%). For this reason, FNAB of the thyroid nodule and any abnormal lymph nodes are usually performed simultaneously. The false-negative rate for lymph node FNAB is 6% to 8% overall, but increases to 20% for samples with inadequate cellularity. Inadequate cellularity is common for metastatic lymph nodes that have undergone cystic degeneration, which is common in papillary thyroid cancer. Measuring thyroglobulin in the aspirate can significantly improve diagnostic sensitivity of lymph node FNAB.

While radiation exposure is a risk factor for follicular thyroid cancer, this is a less likely diagnosis than papillary thyroid cancer. Follicular thyroid cancer is less common than papillary thyroid cancer, it tends to occur in older persons, and it rarely metastasizes to lymph nodes.

Medullary thyroid cancer is an unlikely diagnosis because it is the least common of the thyroid malignancies, representing about 1% to 2% of all thyroid cancers. Approximately 25% of medullary thyroid cancers are hereditary; all patients with medullary thyroid cancer should be screened with *RET* proto-oncogene sequencing. Medullary thyroid cancer may be associated with several syndromes, including multiple endocrine neoplasia type 2A (MEN2A) (which may include pheochromocytoma and hyperparathyroidism), MEN2B (marfanoid habitus and mucosal ganglioneuromas), or familial medullary thyroid cancer (medullary thyroid cancer alone).

### KEY POINT

- Radiation exposure of the thyroid during childhood is the strongest environmental risk factor for thyroid cancer, most commonly papillary cancer.

### Bibliography

Haugen BR, Alexander EK, Bible KC, Doherty GM, Mandel SJ, Nikiforov YE, et al. 2015 American Thyroid Association management guidelines for adult patients with thyroid nodules and differentiated thyroid cancer: The American Thyroid Association Guidelines Task Force on Thyroid Nodules and Differentiated Thyroid Cancer. Thyroid. 2016;26:1-133. [PMID: 26462967] doi:10.1089/thy.2015.0020

## Item 2    Answer:  D

**Educational Objective:** Treat type 2 diabetes mellitus in an obese patient.

According to the American Diabetes Association (ADA), this patient's goal hemoglobin $A_{1c}$ level is less than 7% given that she is healthy and early in the disease course. The American College of Physicians (ACP) recommends a target hemoglobin $A_{1c}$ level between 7% and 8% for most patients with type 2 diabetes. The ACP notes that more stringent targets may be appropriate for patients who have a long life expectancy (>15 years) and are interested in more intensive glycemic control despite the risk for harms, including but not limited to hypoglycemia, patient burden, and pharmacologic costs. Her hemoglobin $A_{1c}$ level remains above goal despite 3 months of lifestyle modifications and metformin. The ADA recommends advancing to dual-therapy if the hemoglobin $A_{1c}$ remains at 9% or above after 3 months of metformin therapy. Sequential therapeutic agents added to metformin should be selected based on the degree of hyperglycemia, comorbidities, weight, side effect profiles, cost, and patient preferences. Liraglutide, a glucagon-like peptide-1 (GLP-1) receptor agonist, is an appropriate adjunctive agent with metformin in this patient as it will improve glycemic control and contribute to desired weight loss. There are potential concerns for development of pancreatitis and medullary thyroid carcinoma with GLP-1 receptor agonists. The patient does not have a personal or family history of these abnormalities to preclude use of liraglutide.

Empagliflozin, a sodium-glucose transporter-2 (SGLT2) inhibitor, may be added to metformin when the hemoglobin $A_{1c}$ remains above goal. SGLT2 inhibitor use improves glycemic control and induces weight loss, but it also increases the risk of genital mycotic infections. Empagliflozin should not be used in this patient because it may exacerbate her frequent vulvovaginal candidiasis infections.

Glipizide, a sulfonylurea, may also be added to metformin when the hemoglobin $A_{1c}$ remains above goal. Glipizide will improve glycemic control, but it is associated with

CONT.

weight gain that is not in concordance with the patient's desire for continued weight loss.

Basal insulin coverage can be provided with one to two daily injections of insulin detemir, glargine, or neutral protamine Hagedorn (NPH) insulin. Basal insulin may be added to metformin when the hemoglobin $A_{1c}$ level remains above goal. Basal insulin will improve glycemic control, but it is associated with weight gain that is not in concordance with the patient's desire for continued weight loss.

**KEY POINT**

- Liraglutide is an add-on therapy to metformin to achieve improvement in hemoglobin $A_{1c}$ level and weight loss.

**Bibliography**

American Diabetes Association. 8. Pharmacologic approaches to glycemic treatment: Standards of Medical Care in Diabetes-2018. Diabetes Care. 2018;41(Suppl 1):S73-S85. doi: 10.2337/dc18-S008. [PMID: 29222379]

**Item 3          Answer:     B**

**Educational Objective:** Diagnose the cause of primary adrenal insufficiency.

The most appropriate next test is measurement of 21-hydroxylase antibodies. This patient has primary adrenal insufficiency as confirmed by the combination of low serum cortisol and elevated serum adrenocorticotropic hormone (ACTH). The most common cause of primary adrenal insufficiency in the United States is autoimmune adrenalitis, and positive 21-hydroxylase antibodies are found in approximately 90% of those cases.

Patients with autoimmune adrenalitis are at risk for the development of other autoimmune disorders including primary hypothyroidism, primary ovarian insufficiency, type 1 diabetes mellitus, celiac disease, and autoimmune gastritis. If 21-hydroxylase antibody measurement is negative, abdominal CT imaging should be performed. In autoimmune disease, the adrenal glands often appear atrophic, although normal-sized adrenal glands do not rule out this diagnosis. Other causes of primary adrenal insufficiency typically cause enlargement of the adrenal glands. These include infiltrative disorders such as lymphoma, sarcoidosis, histoplasmosis, or tuberculosis (the latter can be associated with normal-sized adrenal glands). Bilateral adrenal enlargement is also seen in primary adrenal insufficiency caused by bilateral adrenal hemorrhage. Metastatic disease to the adrenal glands rarely causes adrenal insufficiency.

Cosyntropin stimulation testing is used to diagnose the presence of adrenal insufficiency, but it will not help determine the underlying cause. In this patient, the diagnosis of primary adrenal insufficiency is confirmed by the presence of a serum cortisol level of less than 3 µg/dL (82.8 nmol/L) in combination with an elevated serum ACTH level. Hence, cosyntropin stimulation testing will not add further to the diagnosis or management.

MRI of the pituitary gland is not indicated in this patient with primary adrenal insufficiency, but it is the imaging modality of choice for investigation of secondary adrenal insufficiency. The latter is characterized by low serum cortisol in the setting of low or inappropriately normal serum ACTH levels.

Measurement of serum aldosterone would not help determine the underlying cause of this patient's primary adrenal insufficiency. Low or inappropriately normal serum aldosterone levels (associated with elevated plasma renin activity) are present in most patients with primary adrenal insufficiency due to destruction of the layers of the adrenal cortex by the underlying disease process. Aldosterone deficiency results in hyperkalemia, as noted in this patient, and hyponatremia may also be present.

**KEY POINT**

- The most common cause of primary adrenal insufficiency in the United States is autoimmune adrenalitis, and positive 21-hydroxylase antibodies are found in approximately 90% of those cases.

**Bibliography**

Bancos I, Hahner S, Tomlinson J, Arlt W. Diagnosis and management of adrenal insufficiency. Lancet Diabetes Endocrinol. 2015;3:216-26. [PMID: 25098712] doi:10.1016/S2213-8587(14)70142-1

**Item 4          Answer:     A**

**Educational Objective:** Diagnose the cause of hyperprolactinemia.

The most appropriate next step in managing this patient is to obtain a pituitary MRI. The most common cause of hyperprolactinemia is physiologic; prolactin is released during pregnancy and postpartum to cause lactation. Another common cause of hyperprolactinemia is primary hypothyroidism. Hypothyroidism can cause diffuse hypertrophy of the pituitary gland that may resemble enlargement due to a pituitary adenoma on imaging. Nonfunctioning pituitary adenomas can also cause hyperprolactinemia by compressing the pituitary stalk and decreasing dopamine inhibition of prolactin secretion. Medications are a common cause of hyperprolactinemia. Antipsychotic agents cause hyperprolactinemia due to their antidopaminergic effect that interrupts the inhibition of prolactin by dopamine. Agents such as risperidone may raise the prolactin level above 200 ng/mL (200 µg/L). Evaluation for pituitary hypersecretion when a patient is taking a medication known to raise the prolactin level is difficult. When the prolactin level is only mildly elevated (<50 ng/mL [50 µg/L]), it may be reasonable to assume that hyperprolactinemia is a medication side effect. When significantly elevated (>100 ng/mL [100 µg/L]), either the medication needs to be withheld to further assess or a pituitary MRI obtained to evaluate for prolactinoma. Caution is warranted when discontinuation of an antipsychotic agent is being considered, and consultation with a psychiatrist is recommended prior to discontinuation. If the medication cannot be discontinued, a pituitary MRI is required to exclude the diagnosis of pituitary tumor.

Prolactinomas are treated with dopamine agonists. The two FDA-approved dopamine agonists are bromocriptine and cabergoline. Dopamine agonists typically decrease the size and hormone production of prolactinomas rapidly. Decreasing serum prolactin usually correlates with decreasing size of the tumor. Dopamine agonist therapy is not warranted without first diagnosing a prolactinoma with an MRI. Furthermore, addition of dopamine agonist therapy could worsen this patient's psychiatric disease.

Starting an oral contraceptive pill is inappropriate at this time since this patient needs a pituitary MRI to rule out a pituitary tumor prior to making a treatment decision. Once a pituitary tumor is ruled out, she can be started on an oral contraceptive pill to treat her estrogen deficiency caused by the hyperprolactinemia.

While stopping risperidone, or any psychiatric medication, may lead to decreased prolactin, this requires consultation and coordination of care with the patient's psychiatrist.

### KEY POINT

- Antipsychotic agents cause hyperprolactinemia due to their antidopaminergic effect, which interrupts the inhibition of prolactin by dopamine; risperidone may raise the prolactin level above 200 ng/mL (200 µg/L).

### Bibliography

Peuskens J, Pani L, Detraux J, De Hert M. The effects of novel and newly approved antipsychotics on serum prolactin levels: a comprehensive review. CNS Drugs. 2014;28:421-53. doi: 10.1007/s40263-014-0157-3. [PMID: 24677189]

## Item 5    Answer:    C

**Educational Objective:** Treat primary adrenal insufficiency.

This most appropriate treatment for this patient is hydrocortisone twice daily and fludrocortisone once daily. She has primary adrenal insufficiency, which affects all layers of the adrenal cortex, and therefore she requires both glucocorticoid and mineralocorticoid (aldosterone) therapy. Primary adrenal insufficiency is confirmed in this patient by the combination of low serum cortisol level and elevated serum adrenocorticotropic hormone (ACTH) level. Manifestations of aldosterone deficiency are hyponatremia and hyperkalemia. Some patients with primary adrenal insufficiency have normal serum electrolytes and therefore require measurement of plasma renin activity (high) and serum aldosterone (low or inappropriately normal) to confirm mineralocorticoid deficiency. The preferred glucocorticoid for treatment of adrenal insufficiency is hydrocortisone which, because of its shorter duration of action, can be prescribed two or three times daily to better mimic the circadian rhythm of endogenous cortisol secretion. The total daily recommended dose of hydrocortisone ranges from 15 to 25 mg. A higher dose of hydrocortisone (~15 mg) is given in the morning with the remaining dose (~5 mg) given in the afternoon (or in a thrice daily regimen, the second dose of hydrocortisone is given at noon with the

third, smaller dose taken later in the afternoon). For patients who have difficulty adhering to a twice-daily medication regimen, prednisone once daily in the morning may be substituted.

Dexamethasone has a long duration of action with the potential to cause comorbidities from excess glucocorticoid exposure and therefore should not be used long-term to treat adrenal insufficiency.

There are no adequate trial data to direct optimal dose and timing of glucocorticoid replacement. Measurement of serum cortisol and/or ACTH is not helpful. Glucocorticoid dosing is guided by patient symptoms. Administration of doses of glucocorticoid in excess of physiologic replacement can be associated with decreased bone mineral density and features of Cushing syndrome, with increased risk of metabolic syndrome, type 2 diabetes mellitus, hypertension, hyperlipidemia, obesity, and cardiovascular disease. Adequate mineralocorticoid replacement is indicated by normal blood pressure without orthostasis, absence of edema, and normal serum electrolytes.

Only glucocorticoid therapy is required in the treatment of secondary adrenal insufficiency. Fludrocortisone replacement is not required as aldosterone secretion is not under the control of ACTH. Hence, patients with secondary adrenal insufficiency do not develop hyperkalemia. Hyponatremia may be present in secondary adrenal insufficiency due to inappropriate antidiuretic hormone secretion and action, with resultant inability to excrete free water.

### KEY POINT

- Patients with primary adrenal failure require both glucocorticoid and mineralocorticoid replacement therapy.

### Bibliography

Bancos I, Hahner S, Tomlinson J, Arlt W. Diagnosis and management of adrenal insufficiency. Lancet Diabetes Endocrinol. 2015;3:216-26. [PMID: 25098712] doi:10.1016/S2213-8587(14)70142-1

## Item 6    Answer:    A

**Educational Objective:** Evaluate Paget disease of bone.

The laboratory results and findings on radiographs are most consistent with Paget disease of bone. Measurement of serum total alkaline phosphatase is the next step after radiographic diagnosis and delineation of which bones are affected. It reflects the metabolic activity of Paget disease of bone at diagnosis and is used in follow-up evaluation whether treatment is given or not. Occasionally, total alkaline phosphatase may be normal in newly diagnosed patients with radiographic and radionuclide bone scan evidence of Paget disease. This quiescent or "burnt-out" stage of the disease does not require treatment.

Many patients with Paget disease are older and may have risk factors for osteoporosis. These two conditions, however, are unrelated, have different treatment endpoints, and different bisphosphonate dosing. If bone mineral density were to be ordered, it would be for reasons independent of the evaluation and treatment of Paget disease.

CT imaging of bones provides greater resolution and is superior to conventional radiographs in detecting and characterizing some metabolic bone disorders. With the exception of clarifying the extent of basilar skull involvement and risk for cranial nerve impingement, clinically relevant Paget disease is readily detected and diagnosed by conventional radiographs and radionuclide bone scans.

Bisphosphonates, particularly intravenous zoledronic acid, are highly effective, often requiring a single dose to normalize alkaline phosphatase for several years in patients with Paget disease. Given the risk for spinal cord compression or compression fracture, involvement of T7 with Paget disease would be an indication for treatment unless the disease were metabolically inactive. Therefore, zoledronic acid would not be given prior to assessment of serum total alkaline phosphatase.

**KEY POINT**

- Serum alkaline phosphatase, a marker of increased bone turnover, should be measured after radiographic diagnosis of Paget disease of bone.

**Bibliography**

Singer FR, Bone HG 3rd, Hosking DJ, Lyles KW, Murad MH, Reid IR, et al; Endocrine Society. Paget's disease of bone: an Endocrine Society Clinical Practice Guideline. J Clin Endocrinol Metab. 2014;99:4408-22. [PMID: 25406796] doi:10.1210/jc.2014-2910

## Item 7    Answer:    C

**Educational Objective:** Diagnose subacute thyroiditis.

The most likely diagnosis is subacute thyroiditis. Subacute thyroiditis is an uncommon cause of thyrotoxicosis that presents following a viral upper respiratory tract infection and is distinguished by a tender or painful thyroid. This is a form of destructive thyroiditis resulting from the leakage of stored thyroid hormone from damaged thyroid follicles. The diagnosis can be confirmed by determining radioactive iodine uptake, which would be low (<10%). Management is aimed at controlling symptoms. This includes treatment with β-blockers and pain control with NSAIDs or, less commonly, glucocorticoids. In most cases, thyrotoxicosis typically lasts 2 to 6 weeks. It is followed by a hypothyroid phase after stored thyroid hormone is depleted, typically lasting 6 to 12 weeks. The patient may become clinically hypothyroid and require temporary levothyroxine therapy. Most patients with thyroiditis eventually recover to a euthyroid state.

Graves disease is the most common cause of thyrotoxicosis in the United States and most frequently affects young women. This patient does not have pathognomic features of Graves disease (thyroid bruit, eye disease, or dermopathy), making this an unlikely diagnosis.

Molar pregnancy is a rare cause of hyperthyroidism resulting from the binding of human chorionic gonadotropin (HCG) to the thyroid-stimulating hormone (TSH) receptor in the setting of very high HCG levels. The negative pregnancy test excludes this diagnosis.

Nodular thyroid disease (toxic adenoma and multinodular goiter) is the next most common cause of thyrotoxicosis after Graves disease and is more commonly seen in older adults. This patient lacks palpable thyroid nodules on examination, which is usually seen with hyperthyroidism from nodular thyroid disease. In addition, neither Graves disease nor nodular thyroid disease cause thyroid pain.

**KEY POINT**

- Subacute thyroiditis is an uncommon cause of thyrotoxicosis that presents following a viral upper respiratory tract infection and is distinguished by a tender or painful thyroid, suppressed thyroid-stimulating hormone, and elevated serum free thyroxine.

**Bibliography**

De Leo S, Lee SY, Braverman LE. Hyperthyroidism. Lancet. 2016;388:906-18. [PMID: 27038492] doi:10.1016/S0140-6736(16)00278-6

## Item 8    Answer:    B

**Educational Objective:** Reduce the risk of diabetic neuropathy in a patient with type 1 diabetes mellitus.

According to high-quality evidence, enhanced glucose control significantly prevents the development of clinical neuropathy and reduces nerve conduction and vibration threshold abnormalities in type 1 diabetes mellitus. Glycemic control can delay progression of neuropathy in type 2 diabetes. Other than glucose control, no other preventive strategies are available for diabetic neuropathy. Hemoglobin $A_{1c}$ goals in patients with diabetes should be individually tailored taking into account the demonstrated benefits with regard to prevention and delay in microvascular complications with the risk of hypoglycemia. A reasonable goal of therapy might be a hemoglobin $A_{1c}$ value less than or equal to 7% for most patients, with higher targets for older adult patients and those with comorbidities or a limited life expectancy and more stringent control for those patients with type 1 diabetes and during pregnancy.

The American Diabetes Association advocates for a target systolic blood pressure between 125 and 130 mm Hg in select patients (young, long life expectancy, increased risk of stroke), if this can be accomplished safely. While this patient will benefit from improved blood pressure control by reducing the risk of cardiovascular disease, it will have no impact on her risk for the development of diabetic neuropathy.

While lifestyle intervention to improve the lipid profile should be undertaken in all patients with diabetes, for patients without cardiovascular disease and under age 40 years, statin therapy should be considered only in those with multiple cardiovascular disease risk factors; the American College of Cardiology/American Heart Association risk calculator can determine the 10-year atherosclerotic cardiovascular disease risk to guide therapeutic management. Improved lipid control, while indicated and beneficial for the prevention of cardiovascular disease, does not assist in the prevention of diabetic neuropathy.

Although pregabalin is indicated to treat painful diabetic neuropathy, it does not prevent diabetic neuropathy.

Although weight loss should be discussed as part of a therapeutic lifestyle plan, there is no data to suggest weight loss prevents the development of diabetic neuropathy.

**KEY POINT**

- Enhanced glucose control significantly prevents the development of clinical neuropathy and reduces nerve conduction and vibration threshold abnormalities in type 1 diabetes mellitus.

**Bibliography**

Callaghan BC, Little AA, Feldman EL, Hughes RA. Enhanced glucose control for preventing and treating diabetic neuropathy. Cochrane Database Syst Rev. 2012:CD007543. [PMID: 22696371] doi:10.1002/14651858.CD007543. pub2

## Item 9     Answer:   D

**Educational Objective:** Identify vitamin D deficiency as a cause of hypocalcemia after antiresorptive therapy for osteoporosis.

The most likely diagnosis is vitamin D deficiency. Special populations will have lower levels of vitamin D owing to medical conditions or medication side effects. Obesity has been correlated with lower vitamin D levels possibly related to fat sequestration. Phenobarbital and phenytoin may increase the metabolism of vitamin D to inactive forms. Glucocorticoids can decrease vitamin D metabolism to active forms. Agents that decrease absorption such as orlistat can decrease vitamin D absorption. Malabsorption disorders, including celiac disease and bariatric surgery, can also result in vitamin D deficiency. This patient has multiple risk factors for vitamin D deficiency including age, possible malnutrition, glucocorticoid use, and being home bound. In the face of ongoing vitamin D deficiency, normocalcemia is maintained through increased bone resorption through increased osteoclastic activity. Antiresorptive drugs, especially the first dose of intravenous bisphosphonates and denosumab, rapidly suppress osteoclastic bone resorption and can precipitate hypocalcemia in these patients. Vitamin D sufficiency should be assessed prior to initiating antiresorptive drugs, especially those administered parenterally.

High baseline bone turnover and abrupt alteration in calcium flux between blood and bone are also features of hungry bone syndrome. However, this syndrome specifically occurs after parathyroidectomy for primary hyperparathyroidism. It is caused by rapid influx of calcium from the blood into the skeleton. In the absence of parathyroidectomy, hungry bone syndrome cannot explain this patient's findings.

Acute hyperphosphatemia from tumor lysis syndrome or phosphorus-containing bowel preparations may cause acute hypocalcemia. Chronic hyperphosphatemia associated with chronic kidney disease can also result in hypocalcemia. However, these conditions are not present and, in the case of chronic kidney disease, cannot account for the patient's rapid clinical deterioration.

In contrast to surgery, hypoparathyroidism due to autoimmunity, radiation, or infiltrative processes develops slowly and serum calcium declines gradually over months to years, which is not consistent with the precipitous drop seen in this patient over 2 days.

**KEY POINT**

- Potent antiresorptive drugs can cause severe hypocalcemia by impairing efflux of calcium from the skeleton in patients with vitamin D deficiency; it is important to assess vitamin D levels and correct deficiency before beginning treatment with an antiresorptive drug.

**Bibliography**

Kaur U, Chakrabarti SS, Gambhir IS. Zoledronic acid-induced hypocalcemia and hypophosphatemia in osteoporosis: a cause of concern. Curr Drug Saf. 2016;11:267-9. [PMID: 27113952]

## Item 10     Answer:   A

**Educational Objective:** Diagnose an androgen-producing adrenal tumor.

The most appropriate test to perform next is a CT scan of the abdomen. This postmenopausal woman has new-onset hyperandrogenism associated with significant elevation of serum dehydroepiandrosterone sulfate (DHEAS). The clinical picture of rapid-onset hirsutism and signs of virilization indicate an androgen-secreting tumor. Signs of virilization are deepening of the voice, clitoromegaly, hirsutism, and temporal hair loss. Under normal conditions, androgen production in women occurs in both the adrenal glands and ovaries, as well as by peripheral conversion. The major source of DHEAS is the adrenal gland, and an abdominal CT is recommended when serum DHEAS value is above 700 µg/dL (18.9 µmol/L).

DHEAS-secreting tumors of the adrenal gland are readily visible on CT imaging and adrenal vein sampling to localize the tumor is rarely required.

Pelvic MRI may be more sensitive at detecting small ovarian tumors and is often considered as second-line imaging when pelvic ultrasound is negative. If both pelvic ultrasound and MRI imaging are negative in the setting of suspicion for a testosterone-secreting ovarian tumor, ovarian vein sampling may be required to reveal the location of the tumor. Ovarian vein sampling is reserved for premenopausal women. Postmenopausal women can forego this invasive procedure and proceed directly to bilateral oophorectomy. Significant testosterone secretion can also be due to a non-tumorous condition called ovarian hyperthecosis. Hyperandrogenic symptoms are typically (but not always) of slower onset compared with that seen with androgen-secreting tumors.

A pelvic ultrasound is recommended as the first imaging study if testosterone is above 150 ng/dL (5.2 nmol/L). This patient's testosterone level was only mildly elevated, but the DHEAS was quite elevated making a testosterone-producing ovarian tumor less likely than an adrenal tumor.

> **KEY POINT**
>
> - Signs of androgen excess such as progressive hirsutism and virilization over a short period of time in female patients suggest the diagnosis of an androgen-producing adrenal or ovarian tumor.

### Bibliography

Markopoulos MC, Kassi E, Alexandraki KI, Mastorakos G, Kaltsas G. Hyperandrogenism after menopause. Eur J Endocrinol. 2015;172:R79-91. [PMID: 25225480] doi:10.1530/EJE-14-0468

## Item 11    Answer:    C

**Educational Objective:**  Diagnose nonthyroidal illness syndrome.

The most likely diagnosis is nonthyroidal illness syndrome (euthyroid sick syndrome), which is most often seen in critically ill hospitalized patients and is characterized by a reduced serum triiodothyronine ($T_3$) level, low or low-normal serum thyroxine ($T_4$) level, and normal or low (but detectable) serum thyroid-stimulating hormone (TSH) level. These findings result from changes in the peripheral uptake of thyroid hormones, reduced levels of thyroid hormone-binding proteins, and alterations in the expression and activity of deiodinases. Very low serum $T_4$ levels are associated with poor overall outcome. Treatment with levothyroxine or liothyronine is not indicated due to lack of evidence of benefit.

Central hypothyroidism is not the most likely diagnosis. The patient described here has no signs or symptoms suggestive of hypothyroidism. Characteristic biochemical findings in central hypothyroidism include low or inappropriately normal serum TSH in the setting of low total and free $T_4$ levels and reduced or low-normal serum $T_3$. In contrast to nonthyroidal illness, in which the $T_3$ to $T_4$ ratio is low, a high serum $T_3$ to $T_4$ ratio is seen in central hypothyroidism because conversion of $T_4$ to $T_3$ in peripheral tissues is maintained.

Heparin-induced thyroid function test abnormality is also incorrect. A single intravenous heparin injection may increase serum free $T_4$ up to 5 times the baseline value within minutes. This spurious laboratory finding is related to heparin-induced stimulation of lipoprotein lipase and generation of free fatty acids, which displace $T_4$ from binding proteins. Heparin has no effect on serum TSH, total $T_4$, or total $T_3$ values.

Subclinical hyperthyroidism is also not the most likely diagnosis. This patient has atrial fibrillation, but no other clinical findings suggestive of thyroid hormone excess. Although the low serum TSH level is consistent with this diagnosis, the total and free $T_4$ levels are near the lower limit of the normal range and total $T_3$ is reduced.

> **KEY POINT**
>
> - Nonthyroidal illness syndrome (euthyroid sick syndrome) is characterized by reduced serum $T_3$, low or low-normal serum $T_4$, and normal or low (but detectable) serum TSH levels.

### Bibliography

Fliers E, Bianco AC, Langouche L, Boelen A. Thyroid function in critically ill patients. Lancet Diabetes Endocrinol. 2015;3:816-25. [PMID: 26071885] doi:10.1016/S2213-8587(15)00225-9

## Item 12    Answer:    C

**Educational Objective:**  Manage Cushing syndrome with glucocorticoid therapy following adrenalectomy.

The most appropriate management of this patient following adrenalectomy for treatment of Cushing syndrome is hydrocortisone therapy. Patients who have undergone adrenalectomy for Cushing syndrome are at risk of secondary adrenal insufficiency due to hypercortisolism-induced suppression of the hypothalamic (corticotropin-releasing hormone [CRH]) and pituitary (adrenocorticotropic [ACTH] hormone) axis. Subsequent recovery of the hypothalamic-pituitary axis following removal of the source of excess cortisol secretion can take time, and hence endogenous cortisol production is impaired. In addition, cortisol-producing cells from the contralateral adrenal gland may have undergone atrophy due to lack of ACTH stimulation. Patients often require higher than physiologic doses of glucocorticoid therapy to prevent "glucocorticoid withdrawal syndrome," an ill-defined complex of symptoms of fatigue, loss of appetite, nausea, and/or myalgia. There is no agreed upon glucocorticoid regimen following adrenalectomy and treatment of Cushing syndrome. The process of tapering and eventual discontinuation of glucocorticoid therapy is guided by patient symptoms and can be a lengthy process, taking up to 1 year or longer for the remaining adrenal gland to produce adequate cortisol.

ACTH-dependent causes of Cushing syndrome also lead to suppression of endogenous CRH and ACTH production, and hence patients with these disorders also require glucocorticoid therapy following successful treatment of Cushing syndrome.

Epinephrine is also not under ACTH control, and therefore epinephrine replacement is not required after adrenalectomy. In addition, epinephrine replacement is not required following bilateral adrenalectomy, as lack of epinephrine is not known to be associated with clinical disease.

Likewise, fludrocortisone therapy is not required following adrenalectomy as mineralocorticoid secretion is not under ACTH control. Therefore, aldosterone secretion from the contralateral adrenal gland is not impacted by Cushing syndrome. Fludrocortisone therapy is required following bilateral adrenalectomy.

Phenoxybenzamine is used as a preoperative $\alpha$-receptor blockade for 10 to 14 days before surgery for pheochromocytomas and paragangliomas to prevent hypertensive crises

CONT.

during surgery and is not indicated following adrenalectomy for Cushing syndrome.

**KEY POINT**

- Following adrenalectomy for Cushing syndrome, patients require daily glucocorticoid replacement therapy to allow recovery from prolonged suppression due to hypercortisolism; recovery of adrenal function may take up to 1 year or longer depending on the severity of Cushing syndrome.

**Bibliography**
Hochberg Z, Pacak K, Chrousos GP. Endocrine withdrawal syndromes. Endocr Rev. 2003;24:523-38. [PMID: 12920153]

## Item 13      Answer:    C

**Educational Objective: Diagnose male hypogonadism.**

The most appropriate management is to repeat testosterone measurement at 8 AM. The clinical diagnosis of hypogonadism is made on the basis of signs and symptoms consistent with androgen deficiency with the finding of low morning testosterone concentrations on at least two occasions. Timing of initial laboratory assessment is important due to the diurnal variation of testosterone. Additionally, assessment of hypogonadism should not be undertaken during acute illness. The next step in management of this patient would be to obtain a morning testosterone concentration; if low, testing should be confirmed with a repeat morning measurement. After the initial diagnosis, determination of primary or secondary hypogonadism is established by measurement of luteinizing hormone (LH) and follicle-stimulating hormone (FSH) levels. Elevated gonadotropin levels are seen in primary hypogonadism with LH and FSH levels low or inappropriately normal in secondary hypogonadism.

Based on Endocrine Society guidelines, men with hypogonadism should be treated with exogenous testosterone when they have consistent signs and symptoms of hypogonadism and low serum testosterone levels. Patients requiring testosterone replacement therapy should have testosterone levels monitored at 3 and 6 months after initiation and annually thereafter; the goal total testosterone level should be in the mid-normal range. Monitoring of the prostate specific antigen and hematocrit level should follow Endocrine Society guidelines. Before initiating testosterone therapy in this patient, the diagnosis of hypogonadism needs to be confirmed with two appropriately timed testosterone measurements.

The most sensitive and cost-effective initial diagnostic study in patients with suspected hemochromatosis is measurement of the fasting serum transferrin saturation (calculated as [serum iron/total iron binding capacity] ×100). Serum ferritin level measurement is indicated in patients with elevated transferrin saturation. Evaluation for hemochromatosis is only appropriate after the diagnosis of hypogonadism is established. The first diagnostic step for this patient is the collection of two properly collected serum testosterone levels to establish the diagnosis of hypogonadism.

If subsequent evaluation of the patient confirms the presence of hypogonadotrophic hypogonadism (low testosterone and low LH and FSH levels), MRI of the pituitary to detect a pituitary adenoma or other mass would be appropriate. A pituitary MRI would be premature at this point.

**KEY POINT**

- In men with specific signs and symptoms of hypogonadism, measuring an 8 AM total testosterone level is indicated; if the testosterone level is low, a second 8 AM confirmatory testosterone level is measured.

**Bibliography**
Basaria S. Male hypogonadism. Lancet. 2014;383:1250-63. [PMID: 24119423] doi:10.1016/S0140-6736(13)61126-5

## Item 14      Answer:    C

**Educational Objective: Prevent complications of management of chronic hypoparathyroidism.**

The most appropriate test to perform now is measurement of 24-hour urine calcium. In chronic hypoparathyroidism, goals of therapy are to eliminate symptoms while avoiding complications of therapy; monitoring of urine calcium excretion is mandatory because hypercalciuria often limits therapy. Without parathyroid hormone (PTH), urinary calcium excretion is higher than normal for any given serum calcium level. Complications of prolonged hypercalciuria include nephrolithiasis and impaired glomerular filtration rate. Serum calcium, magnesium, creatinine, and urine calcium levels should be assessed on a regular basis. The goal calcium levels should be low-normal without hypercalciuria. The magnesium level should ideally be greater than 2 mg/dL (0.83 mmol/L), and creatinine levels should remain in the normal range. If the urine calcium level is greater than 300 mg/24 h (hypercalciuria), calcium and/or vitamin D replacement needs to be decreased. Calcium is usually decreased first if the 25-hydroxyvitamin D level is within the normal sufficiency range (≥30 ng/mL [75 nmol/L]). Thiazide diuretics reduce urine calcium excretion and thus may permit sufficient calcium and vitamin D therapy to achieve goal calcium levels.

Hypoparathyroidism slows bone metabolism and is relatively protective against the development of postmenopausal osteoporosis. Further, osteoporosis medications would rarely be indicated in these patients. Therefore, bone mineral density testing is not indicated.

The dose of calcitriol administered is titrated by the serum calcium and/or phosphorus level rather than the serum 1,25-dihydroxyvitamin D level.

If serum PTH is not detectable 6 months after the onset of surgical hypoparathyroidism, it can be considered chronic. Without PTH, vitamin D activation, specifically the conversion of 25-hydroxyvitamin D to 1,25-dihydroxyvitamin D (calcitriol) in the kidney, is severely impaired. Although vitamin D nutritional status as assessed by 25-hydroxyvitamin D may be relevant for other health conditions, its measurement in not useful in the setting of chronic hypoparathyroidism unless residual PTH production remains.

Ionized calcium, rather than total calcium, is the relevant calcium fraction in the blood. However, in an otherwise healthy person in whom serum albumin concentrations are presumed to be normal, measurement of ionized calcium does not contribute to the management of hypoparathyroidism.

### KEY POINT

- In chronic hypoparathyroidism, the goals of therapy are to eliminate symptoms while avoiding complications of therapy; monitoring urine calcium excretion is mandatory because hypercalciuria often limits therapy.

### Bibliography

Brandi ML, Bilezikian JP, Shoback D, Bouillon R, Clarke BL, Thakker RV, Khan AA, Potts JT Jr. Management of hypoparathyroidism: summary statement and guidelines. J Clin Endocrinol Metab. 2016;101:2273-83. doi:10.1210/jc.2015-3907. [PMID: 26943719]

### Item 15          Answer:     A

**Educational Objective:** Diagnose adrenocorticotropic hormone (ACTH)-independent Cushing syndrome.

The most likely cause of this patient's hypercortisolism is adrenocorticotropic hormone (ACTH)-independent Cushing syndrome caused by an adrenal tumor. The diagnosis of Cushing syndrome is confirmed by the combination of clinical features (central obesity, dorsocervical and supraclavicular fat pads, new onset hypertension, and worsening diabetes control), in the setting of two positive diagnostic tests for Cushing syndrome: elevated 24-hour urine free cortisol level and elevated midnight salivary cortisol level. A 24-hour urine free cortisol that is three times the upper limit of the normal range (as in this patient) is considered to be confirmatory for Cushing syndrome if compatible clinical features are also present. Once Cushing syndrome is confirmed, the next step in the diagnosis is to categorize Cushing syndrome into ACTH-dependent and ACTH-independent types, which in turn governs subsequent localization tests. A low serum ACTH level, as in this patient, indicates ACTH-independent Cushing syndrome. Excluding glucocorticoid administration, the most common cause of ACTH-independent Cushing syndrome is a cortisol-secreting adrenal tumor. ACTH is suppressed in this situation due to elevated cortisol levels causing negative feedback at the level of the hypothalamus and pituitary gland, which inhibits ACTH production.

Cushing syndrome in the presence of a detectable or elevated serum ACTH indicates ACTH-dependent disease. Causes of ACTH-dependent Cushing syndrome include ACTH secretion from a pituitary tumor (most commonly) or from an ectopic source such as a bronchial carcinoid tumor.

Hypercortisolism in the absence of Cushing syndrome can occur with psychiatric illness. The mechanism of hypercortisolism associated with psychiatric illness is activation of the hypothalamic-pituitary axis; in this situation ACTH

production is not suppressed. In addition, patients do not manifest clinical features of Cushing syndrome. This patient's suppressed serum ACTH rules out psychiatric illness as the primary cause of her hypercortisolism.

### KEY POINT

- Excluding glucocorticoid administration, the most common cause of adrenocorticotropic hormone (ACTH)-independent Cushing syndrome is an adrenal tumor.

### Bibliography

Loriaux DL. Diagnosis and differential diagnosis of Cushing's syndrome. N Engl J Med. 2017;376:1451-1459. doi: 10.1056/NEJMra1505550. [PMID: 28402781]

### Item 16          Answer:     B

**Educational Objective:** Manage anabolic steroid-induced hypogonadism.

Cessation of anabolic steroid use is the appropriate management plan at this time. This patient presents with symptoms and signs suggestive of anabolic steroid-induced hypogonadism including decreased libido, acne, gynecomastia, small testes, and suppressed gonadotropins with resultant hypogonadism. Extratesticular effects may also be noted, including low HDL cholesterol level, hepatotoxicity, erythrocytosis, and increased risk of obstructive sleep apnea. Mood disorders are common in anabolic steroid users. He will remain hypogonadal for an undetermined amount of time after stopping exogenous androgens before recovery of his hypothalamic-pituitary-gonadal axis.

Anastrozole is an aromatase inhibitor. It blocks the conversion of androgens to estrogens leading to increased serum testosterone levels. Clomiphene is a selective estrogen receptor modulator that stimulates pituitary gonadotropins and consequently testosterone production. Human chorionic gonadotropin (HCG) binds to the luteinizing hormone (LH) receptor resulting in stimulation of testosterone secretion by Leydig cells. While all of these agents may be requested by patients to mitigate the effects of anabolic steroid-induced hypogonadism, there is no strong evidence supporting their effectiveness and safety for management of anabolic steroid-induced hypogonadism.

Testosterone therapy has been associated with increased hemoglobin and hematocrit levels, worsened obstructive sleep apnea, and decreased HDL cholesterol levels. Since this patient's hemoglobin level is already significantly elevated, testosterone replacement therapy might be potentially harmful. Also, testosterone replacement therapy would not resolve his acne, gynecomastia, or small testes. Furthermore, initiation of testosterone replacement therapy would delay resolution of the expected hypogonadism seen following the discontinuation of anabolic steroids.

### KEY POINT

- Cessation of anabolic steroid use is the most appropriate management of steroid-induced hypogonadism.

## Bibliography

Karavolos S, Reynolds M, Panagiotopoulou N, McEleny K, Scally M, Quinton R. Male central hypogonadism secondary to exogenous androgens: a review of the drugs and protocols highlighted by the online community of users for prevention and/or mitigation of adverse effects. Clin Endocrinol (Oxf). 2015;82:624-32. [PMID: 25333666] doi:10.1111/cen.12641

## Item 17     Answer:   C

**Educational Objective:** Treat hypothyroidism in pregnancy.

For women with hypothyroidism adequately treated with levothyroxine before pregnancy, dosing can be empirically increased by 30% when pregnancy is confirmed. Levothyroxine is the treatment of choice for the management of hypothyroidism during pregnancy. Patients can be counseled to start taking an additional two tablets of their prepregnancy levothyroxine dose per week, which is roughly equivalent to a 30% increase. In euthyroid women without thyroid disease, the total body thyroxine ($T_4$) pool increases by 40% to 50% during pregnancy. This is mediated by the stimulatory effects of thyroid-stimulating hormone (TSH) and placental human chorionic gonadotropin. Pregnant women with hypothyroidism are unable to augment thyroidal production of $T_4$ and triiodothyronine ($T_3$). The levothyroxine dose of hypothyroid women must therefore be adjusted to maintain a euthyroid state. Because $T_4$ requirements may begin to increase as early as 4 to 6 weeks of pregnancy, women with hypothyroidism should increase their levothyroxine dose or serum TSH should be measured as soon as pregnancy is confirmed. TSH should be measured every 4 weeks for the first half of pregnancy and around 30 weeks of gestation in all women with hypothyroidism. A TSH value in the lower half of the reference range should be targeted (equivalent to a TSH level below 2.5 µU/mL [2.5 mU/L]) both in preconception planning and during pregnancy.

Continuing the patient on her current dose of levothyroxine and checking serum TSH in 2 months or decreasing the patient's levothyroxine dose are both inappropriate management and could precipitate maternal or fetal hypothyroidism. The use of liothyronine or $T_3$-containing preparations including desiccated thyroid is contraindicated in pregnancy because the fetal central nervous system is relatively impermeable to $T_3$. Thyroid hormone is essential for normal fetal development and is especially critical for the fetal brain.

### KEY POINT

- For women with hypothyroidism adequately treated with levothyroxine before pregnancy, dosing can be empirically increased by 30% when pregnancy is confirmed.

## Bibliography

Alexander EK, Pearce EN, Brent GA, Brown RS, Chen H, Dosiou C, et al. 2017 Guidelines of the American Thyroid Association for the Diagnosis and Management of Thyroid Disease During Pregnancy and the Postpartum. Thyroid. 2017;27:315-389. [PMID: 28056690] doi:10.1089/thy.2016.0457

## Item 18     Answer:   D

**Educational Objective:** Understand risks associated with gender-affirming therapy.

Transgender medicine is the care of persons whose gender identity differs from the sex that was assigned at birth. Gender incongruence is persistent incongruence between gender identity and external sexual anatomy at birth absent of a confounding mental disorder. A transgender man is someone with a male gender identity and a female birth assigned sex; a transgender woman (as in this patient) is someone with a female gender identity and a male birth assigned sex.

The most appropriate next step in management is to refer the patient for discussion on fertility preservation options. Gender-affirming hormone therapy is the primary medical intervention sought by transgender people. Criteria for hormone therapy include persistent, well-documented gender dysphoria; capacity to make a fully informed decision; age of majority in a given country; and if present, control of significant medical or psychological conditions. Gender-affirmation hormone therapy limits fertility, thus reproductive options should be discussed with patients prior to initiation of hormone therapy.

While feminizing hormone therapy is typically estradiol with an androgen blocker, it would not be appropriate to initiate therapy without first considering its impact on fertility. Additionally, due to the risk of thromboembolic disease with estrogen therapy, smoking cessation must first be undertaken. Gender confirmation surgery is often the last step in the treatment process for gender dysphoria. It is recommended that individuals undergoing irreversible gender-affirming surgery, which affects fertility, engage in at least 1 year of satisfactory social role change as well as consistent and compliant hormone treatment, unless hormone therapy is not desired or medically contraindicated.

### KEY POINT

- Because gender-affirming hormone therapy limits fertility, reproductive options should be discussed with patients prior to initiation.

## Bibliography

Hembree WC, Cohen-Kettenis PT, Gooren L, et al. Endocrine treatment of gender-dysphoric/gender-incongruent persons: an Endocrine Society Clinical Practice Guideline. J Clin Endocrinol Metab 2017; 102:3869. [PMID: 28945902]

## Item 19     Answer:   A

**Educational Objective:** Recognize medications that can cause falsely elevated plasma free metanephrine levels.

Amitriptyline can cause falsely elevated normetanephrine levels and should be discontinued prior to screening for pheochromocytoma. Most pheochromocytomas secrete norepinephrine, resulting in episodic or sustained hypertension. Orthostatic hypotension can also be seen and likely reflects low plasma volume. In addition to the classic triad of diaphoresis, headache, and tachycardia, common symptoms include palpitations, tremor, pallor, and anxiety. Screening for pheochromocytoma is appropriate in this patient, following discontinuation of amitriptyline. Amitriptyline acts by inhibiting norepinephrine uptake into nerve terminals, with subsequent elevation of its metabolite, normetanephrine. False-positive elevation of plasma free normetanephrine levels can occur with other tricyclic medications such as nortriptyline or combination serotonin/norepinephrine uptake inhibitors such as venlafaxine or duloxetine. False-positive elevation of plasma normetanephrine and metanephrine levels can also occur with other medications including levodopa (a substrate for catecholamine synthesis); psychoactive medications such as buspirone, prochlorperazine, amphetamines; and over-the-counter decongestant medications that contain adrenergic receptor agonists. Plasma free metanephrines can also be elevated during acute or stressful medical situations including psychiatric illness. Therefore, unless there is significant suspicion for pheochromocytoma, testing should be delayed until the acute illness has passed. Medications that can interfere with catecholamine metabolism should be discontinued (with tapering if indicated) at least 2 weeks prior to testing for pheochromocytoma.

Omeprazole, chlorthalidone, metoprolol, and progesterone do not impact catecholamine metabolism and, therefore, can be continued during screening for pheochromocytoma.

### KEY POINT

- Many medications cause falsely high levels of catecholamines or metanephrines including certain antidepressants that inhibit norepinephrine uptake; therefore discontinuation of these agents at least 2 weeks prior to testing for pheochromocytoma is recommended.

### Bibliography

van Berkel A, Lenders JW, Timmers HJ. Diagnosis of endocrine disease: biochemical diagnosis of phaeochromocytoma and paraganglioma. Eur J Endocrinol. 2014;170:R109-19. [PMID: 24347425] doi:10.1530/EJE-13-0882

### Item 20        Answer:    D

**Educational Objective:** Manage a patient who has completed 5 years of oral bisphosphonate therapy.

The most appropriate management of this patient is to discontinue alendronate. The Fracture Intervention Trial Long-term Extension (FLEX) trial showed that continuing alendronate treatment for 10 years compared with stopping after 5 years resulted in a small decrease in the incidence of clinical vertebral fractures but not nonvertebral fractures. Subject characteristics most predictive of incident fracture after alendronate discontinuation were age older than 76 years, current femur neck T-score below –2.5, and prior osteoporotic fracture. Importantly, women with femur neck T-score below –3.5 or who fractured during the initial 5 years of alendronate therapy were not included in the FLEX trial. The authors concluded that patients at high risk of fracture may benefit

from continuing alendronate therapy for up to 10 years. There is inconsistency among expert groups regarding the need to monitor bone mineral density during osteoporosis therapy and at 5 years to inform decision making about discontinuation of therapy. Contrary to other groups, the American College of Physicians recommends against monitoring because data from several studies showed that women treated with antiresorptive treatment benefit from reduced fractures even if BMD did not increase.

The antiresorptive effect of alendronate can be assessed by bone turnover markers including serum C-terminal peptide of type 1 collagen (CTx). However, neither CTx levels on alendronate nor change with discontinuation predict which patients will fracture if alendronate is discontinued. Furthermore, serum CTx levels in patients taking alendronate vary widely and cannot be reliably interpreted without pretreatment values.

The FLEX trial included postmenopausal women who had taken 5 years of alendronate 5 mg daily (equivalent to 35 mg weekly) or 10 mg daily (equivalent to 70 mg weekly). There was no difference in outcomes based on alendronate dose. Therefore, the management decision to be made after 5 years of alendronate therapy is to continue or discontinue rather than to modify the dose.

### KEY POINT

- For low-risk osteoporotic women, treatment with antiresorptive therapy for 5 years is sufficient.

### Bibliography

Qaseem A, Forciea MA, McLean RM, Denberg TD; Clinical Guidelines Committee of the American College of Physicians. Treatment of low bone density or osteoporosis to prevent fractures in men and women: a Clinical Practice Guideline Update from the American College of Physicians. Ann Intern Med. 2017;166:818-839. doi: 10.7326/M15-1361. Epub 2017 May 9. [PMID: 28492856]

### Item 21        Answer:    A

**Educational Objective:** Manage type 2 diabetes mellitus in a patient with decreasing kidney function.

The most appropriate management of this patient's diabetes mellitus is to continue the current regimen. This is an older patient with multiple comorbidities. She is at her goal hemoglobin $A_{1c}$ level of less than 8% per the American Diabetes Association guidelines with her current regimen. In contrast, the American College of Physicians recommends that clinicians should avoid targeting an hemoglobin $A_{1c}$ level in patients with a life expectancy less than 10 years due to advanced age (80 years or older), residence in a nursing home, or chronic conditions (such as end-stage kidney disease) because the harms outweigh the benefits in this population.

The FDA previously considered serum creatinine levels of 1.4 mg/dL (123.8 µmol/L) or higher in women and 1.5 mg/dL (132.6 µmol/L) or higher in men a contraindication to metformin use due to concerns for development of lactic acidosis. After further review of safety data from multiple studies, the criteria for continued safe use of metformin have been revised by the FDA. The use of serum creatinine for determining safe use of metformin was replaced by estimated glomerular filtration rate (eGFR) to better estimate kidney function. Patients who have a decrease in eGFR to 30 to 45 mL/min/1.73 m² while treated with metformin may continue use after consideration of risks and benefits. If metformin is continued, frequent monitoring of kidney function (every 3 months) is recommended. Metformin should be discontinued if the eGFR falls below 30 mL/min/1.73 m².

Because she is at her goal hemoglobin $A_{1c}$ level of less than 8%, intensifying her therapy with either insulin glargine or glipizide is unnecessary, In addition, increasing the insulin glargine or glipizide dose in the setting of worsening kidney function could increase the risk for hypoglycemia. Additional weight gain may also occur with an increased insulin glargine or glipizide dose.

### KEY POINT

- Metformin may be continued in patients with an estimated glomerular filtration rate to 30 to 45 mL/min/1.73 m² after consideration of risks and benefits; if metformin is continued, frequent monitoring of kidney function (every 3 months) is recommended.

### Bibliography

American Diabetes Association. 8. Pharmacologic approaches to glycemic treatment: Standards of Medical Care in Diabetes-2018. Diabetes Care. 2018;41(Suppl 1):S73-S85. doi: 10.2337/dc18-S008. [PMID: 29222379]

## Item 22    Answer:    A

### Educational Objective:  Treat polycystic ovary syndrome.

This patient has ovulatory dysfunction with clinical and biochemical evidence of hyperandrogenism. While this is suggestive of polycystic ovary syndrome, this is a diagnosis of exclusion. The prolonged clinical course and absence of the more concerning findings of virilization also support the diagnosis of polycystic ovary syndrome. Given that this patient is most concerned about hirsutism and acne, oral contraceptive therapy is the first-line therapeutic agent. Oral contraceptive therapy suppresses gonadotropin secretion and resultant ovarian androgen production. Additionally, the estrogen component increases sex hormone-binding globulin resulting in less androgen bioavailability. Oral contraceptives that contain 30 to 35 μg of ethinyl estradiol appear to be more effective in managing hirsutism than formulations containing less ethinyl estradiol. Furthermore, oral contraceptive therapy reduces new terminal hair growth, improves acne, and regulates menses to prevent endometrial hyperplasia.

Metformin minimally effects hirsutism and is not recommended for this indication. In patients with polycystic ovary syndrome, metformin could be considered for off-label treatment of prediabetes or treatment of type 2 diabetes, in addition to lifestyle modification.

Pelvic ultrasound and adrenal CT should be performed to exclude an ovarian or adrenal neoplasm if the serum total testosterone level is greater than 150 ng/dL (5.2 nmol/L), and adrenal CT is necessary to exclude an adrenal cortisol-secreting and/or androgen-secreting neoplasm if the plasma dehydroepiandrosterone sulfate (DHEAS) level is greater than 7.0 μg/mL (18.9 μmol/L). Pelvic ultrasound and adrenal CT are not indicated in this patient as her testosterone and DHEAS levels are not elevated to the degree that ovarian tumor is a consideration.

While spironolactone can reduce the growth of terminal hair, it is used as an add-on treatment to oral contraceptive therapy. This antiandrogen medication may disrupt organogenesis in a male fetus; thus, concomitant reliable contraception is mandated when initiating this treatment.

### KEY POINT

- Oral contraceptive agents are first-line pharmacologic therapy for hirsutism, acne, and menstrual dysfunction unless fertility is desired in a patient with polycystic ovary syndrome.

### Bibliography

McCartney CR, Marshall JC. Clinical practice: polycystic ovary syndrome. N Engl J Med. 2016;375:54-64. [PMID: 27406348] doi:10.1056/NEJMcp1514916

## Item 23    Answer:    A

### Educational Objective:  Evaluate a pituitary tumor for hypersecretion.

Measurement of prolactin and insulin-like growth factor 1 (IGF-1) is recommended for the evaluation of possible hypersecretion of an incidentally discovered pituitary tumor. When a pituitary tumor is incidentally noted, investigation must determine (1) whether it is causing a mass effect, (2) whether it is secreting excess hormones, and (3) whether it has a propensity to grow and cause problems in the future. After a thorough history and physical examination, biochemical testing can be undertaken in a targeted fashion based on the patient's clinical signs and symptoms. Although not generally useful in the differential diagnosis of a pituitary mass, all patients should be evaluated for hormone hyposecretion in order to identify and replace hormone deficiencies. Initial tests to evaluate for hormone deficiency should include measurement of 8 AM cortisol, thyroid-stimulating hormone (TSH), free (or total) thyroxine ($T_4$), follicle stimulating hormone (FSH), testosterone in men and menstrual history in women (normal menstrual cycles eliminates the need to measure hormone levels). Prolactin and IGF-1 are measured to rule out pituitary hormone hypersecretion. Screening for growth hormone excess in pituitary incidentalomas may allow early detection of a growth hormone secreting tumor therefore increasing the chance of a surgical cure. If the tumor is not causing mass effect and there is no evidence of hormone excess, a pituitary MRI should be repeated in 6 months for a macroadenoma (≥1 cm) and 12 months for a microadenoma (<1 cm) to assess for growth. If no growth occurs, MRIs should be repeated every 1 to 2 years for the next 3 years and then intermittently thereafter.

Measurement of urine free cortisol is not necessary in every patient with a pituitary tumor. This should be measured only when Cushing disease is suspected based on clinical history and physical examination findings. This patient has no physical features suspicious for Cushing disease nor does he have diseases associated with Cushing disease such as diabetes or hypertension.

Visual field examination is absolutely necessary in all patients with a macroadenoma that abuts or compresses the optic chiasm, but it is not necessary in patients with no evidence of involvement of the optic chiasm on MRI. This patient's tumor does not abut or compress the optic chiasm or optic nerves.

No further evaluation is inappropriate as pituitary hypersecretion should be evaluated in all pituitary tumors.

### KEY POINT

- In patients with pituitary tumors, pituitary hypersecretion should be ruled out by biochemical testing.

### Bibliography

Freda PU, Beckers AM, Katznelson L, Molitch ME, Montori VM, Post KD, et al; Endocrine Society. Pituitary incidentaloma: an Endocrine Society Clinical Practice Guideline. J Clin Endocrinol Metab. 2011;96:894-904. [PMID: 21474686] doi:10.1210/jc.2010-1048.

## Item 24    Answer:    E

**Educational Objective:** Manage a patient with pheochromocytoma prior to surgery.

The most appropriate preoperative management in this patient with a pheochromocytoma is an α-adrenergic blocking agent. An α-receptor blockade is required prior to adrenalectomy to prevent potential hypertensive crisis caused by catecholamine release during anesthesia induction and/or manipulation of the tumor. Phenoxybenzamine is started approximately 10 to 14 days prior to surgery, and the dose progressively increased to achieve a desired blood pressure of 130/80 mm Hg or lower when seated, and systolic pressure of 90 mm Hg or higher when standing. Because phenoxybenzamine causes vasodilation, an expected consequence of therapy is postural hypotension. To counteract this and allow appropriate dose escalation of phenoxybenzamine, patients are advised to drink plenty of fluids, eat high salt-containing foods, and to make liberal use of the salt shaker at meal times. If blood pressure is not adequately controlled with an α-receptor blockade (or prohibitive side effects occur with required higher doses), a calcium-channel blocker such as amlodipine can be added. A short-acting, selective α-blocker such as prazosin, doxazosin, or terazosin, can be considered alternatives to phenoxybenzamine, based on decreased cost and limited data suggesting similar patient outcomes.

Hydralazine or lisinopril do not provide the needed α-receptor blockade, and therefore increasing the dose of these medications would not be helpful before surgery.

Diuretics, such as chlorthalidone, should be avoided in patients with pheochromocytoma. These patients may have diminished intravascular volume secondary to intense vasoconstriction and further diuretic-induced volume depletion may lead to severe hypotension. Finally, diuretic treatment will not prevent hypertensive crisis during adrenalectomy.

Metoprolol or other β-blockers should never be started prior to adequate α-receptor blockade in patients with pheochromocytoma, as unopposed α-receptor stimulation can precipitate a hypertensive crisis. Once adequate α-receptor blockade has been achieved, however, a β-blocker is typically added to the medication regimen 2 to 3 days prior to surgery to counteract vasodilation-induced tachycardia.

In the case of very large tumors and/or significant metanephrine elevation, the catecholamine synthesis inhibitor metyrosine may also be added to the medication regimen. Metyrosine is not given routinely in the preoperative management of pheochromocytoma due to significant side effects associated with body-wide catecholamine deficiency.

### KEY POINT

- An α-receptor blockade with phenoxybenzamine or another α-blocker is required prior to adrenalectomy for pheochromocytoma to prevent potential hypertensive crisis during anesthesia induction and/or manipulation of the tumor.

### Bibliography

Lenders JW, Duh QY, Eisenhofer G, et al; Endocrine Society. Pheochromocytoma and paraganglioma: an Endocrine Society Clinical Practice Guideline. J Clin Endocrinol Metab. 2014 Jun;99(6):1915-42. doi: 10.1210/jc.2014-1498. PubMed PMID: 24893135.

## Item 25    Answer:    A

**Educational Objective:** Treat type 2 diabetes mellitus in a patient with cardiovascular disease.

The patient has uncontrolled diabetes in the setting of coronary artery disease, and empagliflozin is the most appropriate treatment. Empagliflozin increases excretion of glucose by the kidneys through inhibition of the sodium-glucose transporter-2 (SGLT2) receptors. Empagliflozin received approval from the FDA for patients with type 2 diabetes and established cardiovascular disease based upon the results of the Empagliflozin Cardiovascular Outcome Event Trial in Type 2 Diabetes Mellitus Patients (EMPA-REG OUTCOME). This study demonstrated a reduction in the primary composite outcome (cardiovascular-related death, nonfatal myocardial infarction, nonfatal stroke) and all-cause mortality when empagliflozin was added to standard care versus placebo. Empagliflozin has the additional potential benefit of inducing weight loss and blood pressure lowering in this overweight patient with uncontrolled hypertension.

Although the sulfonylurea, glipizide, could improve the patient's glycemic control, it has the potential side effect of weight gain; the combination of metformin plus an SGLT2 inhibitor is superior to metformin plus a sulfonylurea (mean between-group difference, 4.7 kg [CI, 4.4 to 5.0 kg]). The combination of metformin and an SGLT2 inhibitor reduces systolic blood pressure more than that of metformin and a sulfonylurea (between-group difference, 5.1 mm Hg [CI, 4.2 to 6.0 mm Hg]).

In patients with type 2 diabetes and cardiovascular risk factors, a significant reduction in the primary composite outcome (cardiovascular death, nonfatal myocardial infarction, or nonfatal stroke) and rates of cardiovascular death and all-cause mortality has also been associated with liraglutide. There have been postmarketing reports of fatal and nonfatal acute pancreatitis associated with liraglutide. While it is not known if liraglutide increases risk for development of pancreatitis in patients with a history of pancreatitis, many experts avoid its use in this patient population.

The dipeptidyl peptidase-4 (DPP-4) inhibitor, sitagliptin, could improve the patient's glycemic control; however, the combination of metformin and an SGLT2 inhibitor reduces systolic blood pressure more than metformin and a DPP-4 inhibitor (pooled between-group difference, 4.1 mm Hg [CI, 3.6 to 4.6 mm Hg]) and SGLT2 inhibitors reduced weight more than DPP-4 inhibitors (between group difference, 2.5 to 2.7 kg). There have been postmarketing reports of fatal and nonfatal acute pancreatitis associated with sitagliptin. While no causal relationship has been established, FDA labeling guidelines recommend that sitagliptin be used with caution in patients with a history of pancreatitis and some experts recommend against its use entirely in this population.

**KEY POINT**

- Empagliflozin has been shown to reduce cardiovascular-related events and all-cause mortality in patients with type 2 diabetes mellitus and cardiovascular disease.

**Bibliography**

Barry MJ, Humphrey LL, Qaseem A. Oral pharmacologic treatment of type 2 diabetes mellitus. Ann Intern Med. 2017;167:75-76. doi:10.7326/L17-0234. [PMID: 28672387]

## Item 26      Answer:    B

**Educational Objective:** Evaluate secondary amenorrhea.

This patient presents with secondary amenorrhea, defined as absence of menses for more than 3 months in women who previously had regular menstrual cycles. After ruling out pregnancy, the initial laboratory evaluation in secondary amenorrhea includes measurement of follicle-stimulating hormone (FSH), thyroid-stimulating hormone (TSH), and prolactin levels. Given negative pregnancy testing and normal TSH and prolactin levels in this patient, FSH testing is the remaining initial laboratory data point that has yet to be explored. If the FSH level is elevated, testing should be repeated in 1 month and accompanied by serum estradiol testing. If the FSH level is elevated on repeat testing and estradiol level is low, karyotype analysis is indicated to evaluate for Turner syndrome. Primary ovarian insufficiency is also associated with an elevated FSH and low estradiol levels. In women with normal or low FSH levels, the evaluation is typically directed by history and physical examination findings.

For example, a high BMI (≥30) and acne are frequently seen in women with polycystic ovary syndrome. In addition, a progestin withdrawal test can be performed to further assess the estrogen status of the patient. If a normal estrogen state is confirmed (bleeding within a week of stopping progesterone), hyperandrogenism should be considered.

Testosterone and dehydroepiandrosterone sulfate (DHEAS) are measured in patients with suspected hyperandrogenism as the cause of amenorrhea based on history, physical examination, and following initial laboratory evaluation (serum human chorionic gonadotropin, FSH, TSH, and prolactin).

Primary amenorrhea is the absence of menses by age 16 years accompanied by normal sexual hair pattern and normal breast development. Approximately 15% of patients presenting with primary amenorrhea may have an anatomic abnormality of the uterus, cervix, or vagina such as müllerian agenesis, transverse vaginal septum, or imperforate hymen. Digital vaginal examination, transvaginal ultrasound, or pelvic MRI may help to identify outflow tract anomalies. Because this patient has secondary amenorrhea, evaluation for anatomic abnormalities with transvaginal ultrasound or pelvic MRI is not indicated.

**KEY POINT**

- After ruling out pregnancy, the initial laboratory evaluation in secondary amenorrhea includes measurement of follicle-stimulating hormone, thyroid-stimulating hormone, and prolactin levels.

**Bibliography**

Klein DA, Poth MA. Amenorrhea: an approach to diagnosis and management. Am Fam Physician. 2013;87:781-8. [PMID: 23939500]

## Item 27      Answer:    C    H

**Educational Objective:** Manage hyperglycemia in the hospital.

The most appropriate management of this patient's hyperglycemia is to initiate scheduled basal insulin and correction insulin. Inpatient hyperglycemia, defined as consistently elevated plasma glucose values above 140 mg/dL (7.8 mmol/L), is associated with poor outcomes. Attempts to decrease morbidity and mortality with tight glycemic control (80-110 mg/dL [4.4-6.1 mmol/L]) have not consistently demonstrated improvements in adverse outcomes and, in some settings, have shown increased rates of severe hypoglycemic events and mortality. As a result, revised inpatient glycemic targets are less stringent than outpatient glucose targets to avoid both hypoglycemia and severe hyperglycemia that can lead to volume depletion and electrolyte abnormalities. Dietary modifications should be made once glucose levels exceed 140 mg/dL (7.8 mmol/L). At persistent glucose levels of 180 mg/dL (10.0 mmol/L) and higher, the American Diabetes Association recommends initiation of scheduled insulin with a blood glucose target of 140 to 180 mg/dL (7.8-10.0 mmol/L) for most critically ill and noncritically ill patients to decrease

CONT.

the risk of adverse outcomes. Scheduled basal insulin or basal insulin plus correction insulin is appropriate for patients who are fasting or who have poor oral intake, such as this patient, with frequent bedside point-of-care monitoring every 4 to 6 hours for insulin adjustments. Scheduled basal and prandial insulin plus correction insulin are appropriate for patients who are eating.

The safety of oral antihyperglycemic agents, including empagliflozin, in the hospital setting has not been fully studied or established. In addition, sodium-glucose transporter-2 (SGLT2) inhibitors have been associated with diabetic ketoacidosis and should be avoided in situations that may produce ketone bodies, such as severe illness or prolonged fasting. Scheduled insulin therapy is the recommended treatment regimen for hyperglycemia in the hospital setting.

The safety of oral antihyperglycemic agents, including metformin, in the hospital setting has not been fully studied or established. Scheduled insulin therapy is the recommended treatment regimen for hyperglycemia in the hospital setting.

The sole use of correction insulin for the management of hyperglycemia is not recommended. It is a reactive approach to hyperglycemia that can lead to large fluctuations in glucose levels coupled with the near universal lag time between measurement of glucose and injection of insulin that occurs in most hospitals.

### KEY POINT

- To manage in-patient hyperglycemia, scheduled basal insulin or basal insulin plus correction insulin is appropriate for patients who are fasting or who have poor oral intake.

### Bibliography

American Diabetes Association. 14. Diabetes care in the hospital: Standards of Medical Care in Diabetes-2018. Diabetes Care. 2018;41(Suppl 1):S144-S151.doi: 10.2337/dc18-S014. [PMID: 29222385]

### Item 28    Answer:    C

**Educational Objective:** Diagnose syndrome of inappropriate antidiuretic hormone secretion (SIADH) following transsphenoidal pituitary surgery.

Serum sodium level should be measured in this patient. Sodium and water imbalance are common after pituitary surgery. Patients may exhibit findings of diabetes insipidus (DI) (polyuria, elevated or high normal serum sodium, and dilute urine) followed by syndrome of inappropriate antidiuretic hormone secretion (SIADH) followed again by DI. Central DI may be transient, lasting only a few weeks, or permanent. There is great variability in the presentation of these disorders; some patients manifest all phases, whereas others may manifest only DI or SIADH. During the postoperative hospital recovery, patients are assessed for hormone deficiency that may have occurred as the result of surgery and are then monitored by measuring fluid intake and output, serum sodium,

and urine osmolality. Following discharge, most experts measure serum sodium 1 week postoperatively to screen for SIADH. This patient denies any polyuria or polydipsia so it is unlikely that he has DI, but he is at risk for SIADH given the time frame of presentation. SIADH can occur 3 to 7 days after pituitary surgery. It is important to diagnose SIADH as treatment with fluid restriction will prevent further reduction in sodium levels.

Hyponatremia, defined as a serum sodium concentration less than 136 mEq/L (136 mmol/L), most often results from an increase in circulating antidiuretic hormone (ADH) in response to a true or sensed reduction in effective arterial blood volume with resulting fluid retention. Hyponatremia may also be caused by elevated ADH levels associated with SIADH. The first step in diagnosis of suspected SIADH is measurement of the serum sodium. The initial evaluation of patients with confirmed hyponatremia is measurement of plasma and urine osmolality and urine sodium as well as a careful assessment of the volume status. Measurement of antidiuretic hormone is not part of the diagnostic algorithm as ADH measurement is not quickly available, and results are difficult to interpret.

Pituitary MRI is unnecessary since the patient has no focal findings (cranial nerve deficit or fever) to suggest intracranial pathology or infection.

Measuring thyroid-stimulating hormone is incorrect as the result could be misleading in this patient following pituitary surgery. Measuring the free thyroxine ($T_4$) level would be more appropriate. In addition, given the long half-life of free $T_4$, testing is more appropriate 4 weeks after pituitary surgery to assess for secondary hypothyroidism. Symptoms occurring 5 days after pituitary surgery are not likely due to thyroid deficiency.

### KEY POINT

- Syndrome of inappropriate antidiuretic hormone secretion (SIADH) is a common complication of pituitary surgery that may occur 3 to 7 days following surgery; treatment with fluid restriction will prevent further reduction in sodium levels.

### Bibliography

Kiran Z, Sheikh A, Momin SN, Majeed I, Awan S, Rashid O, et al. Sodium and water imbalance after sellar, suprasellar, and parasellar surgery. Endocr Pract. 2017;23:309-317. [PMID: 27967227] doi:10.4158/EP161616.OR

### Item 29    Answer:    A

**Educational Objective:** Manage hypogonadotropic hypogonadism due to hyperprolactinemia.

The patient has hypogonadism due to hyperprolactinemia, and the most appropriate management is dopamine agonist therapy. Empty sella is diagnosed when the normal pituitary gland is not visualized or is excessively small on MRI. The pituitary sella is said to be "empty" because normal tissue is not seen. The finding may be primarily due to increased cerebrospinal fluid entering and enlarging the sella, or it may be secondary to a tumor, previous pituitary surgery, radiation, or infarction. When empty sella is found incidentally on imaging, an evaluation should be completed to determine if there is a known cause for secondary empty sella and if the patient has signs or symptoms of pituitary hormone deficiency. A patient without signs or symptoms should be screened for cortisol deficiency and hypothyroidism. The most common pituitary abnormality in empty sella is hyperprolactinemia. Hyperprolactinemia should be treated with dopamine agonist therapy in a woman with irregular menstrual periods who is trying to conceive. This normalizes the prolactin level and allows recovery of the gonadal axis.

Neurosurgical consultation is not necessary in the absence of signs/symptoms of increased intracranial pressure or visual deficit. Although this patient's original MRI was done for headache, she has no current signs of increased intracranial pressure or visual deficit on examination.

An oral contraceptive pill could be used for treatment if she were not trying to conceive. This is appropriate treatment for hypogonadism related to hyperprolactinemia in empty sella or in women with hyperprolactinemia secondary to a pituitary microadenoma to reduce her risk of developing osteoporosis.

Providing no treatment at this time is inappropriate given the patient's menstrual irregularity. In her case, she requires dopamine agonist therapy to treat her hypogonadism as she is trying to conceive; however, even if she were not trying to conceive, she would require treatment with either dopamine agonist therapy or an oral contraceptive pill to treat her hypogonadism and reduce her risk of developing osteoporosis.

### KEY POINT

- Dopamine agonist therapy should be used to treat hyperprolactinemia in women with irregular periods who are trying to conceive.

### Bibliography

Guitelman M, Garcia Basavilbaso N, Vitale M, Chervin A, Katz D, Miragaya K, et al. Primary empty sella (PES): a review of 175 cases. Pituitary. 2013;16:270-4. [PMID: 22875743] doi:10.1007/s11102-012-0416-6

### Item 30    Answer:    B

**Educational Objective:** Diagnose multiple endocrine neoplasia type 1 (MEN1).

Multigland hyperplasia causing primary hyperparathyroidism should lead to further investigation for an underlying disorder, especially in younger persons and those with a family history of primary hyperparathyroidism. Although there are several familial hyperparathyroidism syndromes, multiple endocrine neoplasia type 1 (MEN1) is the most common. In addition to genetic testing, MEN1 can be discriminated from other disorders by personal or family history of recurrent primary hyperparathyroidism and neoplasia in other endocrine tissues, most prominently neuroendocrine tumors arising from the pancreas and tumors of the pituitary gland.

In contrast, familial hypocalciuric hypercalcemia (FHH) presents as mild, stable hypercalcemia with normal parathyroid hormone (PTH) level and relatively low urine calcium excretion. PTH may be elevated in a small percentage of patients with coexistence of vitamin D deficiency. Kidney health is unaffected. A family history of persistent hypercalcemia despite parathyroidectomy is suggestive. Genetic testing may help to discriminate FHH from primary hyperparathyroidism prior to surgical exploration.

Parathyroid carcinoma is rare. Rapidly worsening or severe hypercalcemia accompanied by very high PTH levels, increased alkaline phosphatase, and locally invasive tumor arising from a single parathyroid gland are diagnostic.

Secondary hyperparathyroidism is a response to hypocalcemia often related to vitamin D deficiency or chronic kidney disease-related hyperphosphatemia. Left untreated, a chronic stimulus to PTH secretion may lead to parathyroid gland hyperplasia. Tertiary hyperparathyroidism is the result of long-standing secondary hyperparathyroidism in which the hyperplastic parathyroid glands exhibit autonomous function even after correction of underlying disease (for example, following kidney transplantation). Although the biochemical profile is similar to primary hyperparathyroidism, a history of preexisting and long-standing hypocalcemia or hyperphosphatemia is evident.

### KEY POINT

- Primary hyperparathyroidism may be the first sign of multiple endocrine neoplasia syndrome 1 (MEN1) in persons with a family history of recurrent primary hyperparathyroidism and neuroendocrine tumors arising from the pancreas and tumors of the pituitary gland.

### Bibliography

Thakker RV, Newey PJ, Walls GV, Bilezikian J, Dralle H, Ebeling PR, et al; Endocrine Society. Clinical Practice Guidelines for Multiple Endocrine Neoplasia Type 1 (MEN1). J Clin Endocrinol Metab. 2012;97:2990-3011. [PMID: 22723327] doi:10.1210/jc.2012-1230

### Item 31    Answer:    C

**Educational Objective:** Diagnose vitamin D-dependent hypercalcemia.

The most likely diagnosis is vitamin D-dependent hypercalcemia, and 1,25-dihydroxyvitamin D level should be measured. Vitamin D-dependent hypercalcemia is most commonly due to disorders associated with granulomatous inflammation. The patient's chest radiograph shows extensive infiltrates that are most prominent in the upper lung zones and are associated with hilar enlargement, highly suggestive of pulmonary sarcoidosis. Sarcoidosis is a multisystem granulomatous disease of unclear cause with a predilection for the lung; pulmonary involvement occurs in more than 90% of patients. Macrophages within granulomas convert 25-hydroxyvitamin D to 1,25-dihydroxyvitamin D without regulation by parathyroid hormone in contrast to renal conversion of vitamin D. An elevated 1,25-dihydroxyvitamin D level and suppressed parathyroid hormone is diagnostic of vitamin D-dependent hypercalcemia. As vitamin D enhances absorption of both calcium and phosphorus, concurrent elevation of serum calcium and phosphorus is also suggestive of vitamin D-dependent hypercalcemia.

There are two mechanisms of hypercalcemia of malignancy: local osteolytic and humoral. When lytic bone metastases are present, hypercalcemia is the result of increased mobilization of calcium from the bone. In these cases, the serum alkaline phosphatase level is typically elevated. Humoral hypercalcemia is less common and occurs when the tumor itself produces parathyroid-related protein (PTHrP) that binds to and activates the parathyroid receptor, raising serum calcium levels. Squamous cell carcinomas, breast cancers, and renal cell carcinomas are the tumors most commonly associated with hypercalcemia of malignancy. These diagnoses cannot explain the patient's prolonged clinical course, pulmonary infiltrates, and hilar lymphadenopathy.

When hypercalcemia is due to adrenal insufficiency, it is in the setting of adrenal crisis which is characterized by hypotension, fever, nausea, vomiting, abdominal pain, tachycardia, and even death. The patient's clinical course is not compatible with acute adrenal insufficiency.

### KEY POINT

- An elevated 1,25-dihydroxyvitamin D level and suppressed parathyroid hormone is diagnostic of vitamin D-dependent hypercalcemia.

### Bibliography

Donovan PJ, Sundac L, Pretorius CJ, d'Emden MC, McLeod DS. Calcitriol-mediated hypercalcemia: causes and course in 101 patients. J Clin Endocrinol Metab. 2013;98:4023-9. [PMID: 23979953] doi:10.1210/jc.2013-2016

## Item 32    Answer:    A

**Educational Objective:** Screen for diabetic retinopathy in a woman of childbearing age.

The most appropriate preconception management for this patient is a dilated eye examination. Women with type 1 or type 2 diabetes mellitus who are planning pregnancy should be counseled on the risk of development or progression of diabetic retinopathy. Additionally, rapid improvement in glycemic control in the setting of retinopathy is associated with temporary worsening of retinopathy. Given tight glycemic targets in pregnancy, this is often a time of intensified glycemic control for women placing them at greater risk for this complication. Dilated eye examinations should occur before pregnancy or in first trimester if not done prior to pregnancy. Patients should be monitored every trimester and then closely for 1 year postpartum as indicated by the degree of retinopathy.

This patient is up to date on lipid screening and additional screening as part of preconception management is not necessary.

Thyroid-stimulating hormone (TSH) levels should be monitored closely in pregnancy due to increased level of thyroid-binding globulin in pregnancy resulting in increased levothyroxine needs. This patient has had a TSH measurement with normal results 3 months ago. The dose of levothyroxine may need to be increased on average by 30% to 50% during pregnancy, and patients should have their TSH level checked as soon as a pregnancy test is positive.

A referral to a physician experienced in the care of kidney disease should be undertaken in patients with advanced kidney disease, which is not present in this patient as her most recent serum creatinine and urine albumin-creatinine ratio were normal.

### KEY POINT

- Women with type 1 or type 2 diabetes mellitus who are planning pregnancy should be counseled on the risk of development or progression of diabetic retinopathy; rapid improvements in glycemic levels during pregnancy can temporarily worsen preexisting retinopathy.

### Bibliography

American Diabetes Association. 10. Microvascular complications and foot care: Standards of Medical Care in Diabetes-2018. Diabetes Care. 2018;41(Suppl 1):S105-S118. doi: 10.2337/dc18-S010. [PMID: 29222381]

## Item 33    Answer:    A

**Educational Objective:** Treat glucocorticoid-induced osteoporosis.

The most appropriate treatment is alendronate. The American College of Rheumatology recommends that in all adults and children, an initial clinical fracture risk assessment for glucocorticoid-induced osteoporosis should be performed as soon as possible, but at least within 6 months of the initiation of long-term glucocorticoid treatment. Patients are categorized according to fracture risk. High fracture risk in patients younger than 40 years is defined as by a previous osteoporotic fracture. Moderate fracture risk is defined as hip or spine bone mineral density Z score less than −3 or rapid bone loss (>10% at the hip or spine over 1 year) and continuing glucocorticoid treatment at >7.5 mg/day for >6 months. Low risk is defined as no osteoporotic risk factors other than glucocorticoid use. Other criteria are used for defining low, moderate, and high fracture risk in patients age 40 years and older. Oral bisphosphonates are recommended as first-line therapy for patients with moderate to high fracture risk, such as this woman, regardless of age. This includes women of childbearing potential provided they are not planning a pregnancy during the period of bisphosphonate treatment.

Optimized calcium and vitamin D intake, lifestyle modifications, and reassessment of fracture risk including bone mineral density testing every 2 to 3 years is recommended over osteoporosis medications for patients younger than 40 at low risk of fracture. However, this patient is not low risk, and treatment with an oral bisphosphonate is indicated.

Teriparatide is indicated for the treatment of men and women with osteoporosis associated with sustained systemic glucocorticoid therapy at high risk for fracture. Although it increases bone mineral density at the spine and hip more than oral bisphosphonate therapy, it is less desirable due to expense and the requirement of daily injections.

Zoledronic acid is indicated for the treatment and prevention of glucocorticoid-induced osteoporosis in patients who cannot tolerate oral bisphosphonates. Due to uncertain impact on pregnancy outcomes, it is considered a third-line agent in younger women.

### KEY POINT

- Oral bisphosphonates are recommended as first-line therapy in adult men and women on chronic glucocorticoid therapy with moderate to high fracture risk regardless of age.

### Bibliography

Buckley L, Guyatt G, Fink HA, Cannon M, Grossman J, Hansen KE, Humphrey MB, Lane NE, Magrey M, Miller M, Morrison L, Rao M, Byun Robinson A, Saha S, Wolver S, Bannuru RR, Vaysbrot E, Osani M, Turgunbaev M, Miller AS, McAlindon T. 2017 American College of Rheumatology Guideline for the Prevention and Treatment of Glucocorticoid-Induced Osteoporosis. Arthritis Care Res (Hoboken). 2017;69:1095-1110. doi: 10.1002/acr.23279. Epub 2017 Jun 6. [PMID: 28585410]

## Item 34      Answer:     D

**Educational Objective:** Diagnose thyroid-stimulating hormone-secreting adenoma.

This patient most likely has a thyroid-stimulating hormone (TSH)-secreting adenoma. The initial evaluation based on clinical signs and/or symptoms of thyrotoxicosis should be measurement of serum TSH alone, followed by measurement of thyroxine ($T_4$) and triiodothyronine ($T_3$) levels if TSH is suppressed because the typical pattern of hyperthyroidism is TSH suppression with an elevated $T_4$ and/or $T_3$. However, this patient has signs and symptoms of hyperthyroidism with elevated TSH and free $T_4$ levels, which is concerning for a TSH-secreting adenoma. These tumors are extremely rare and are managed differently from other causes of thyrotoxicosis. Before this diagnosis is made, other causes of the laboratory abnormalities must be excluded (thyroid hormone resistance and familial dysalbuminemic hyperthyroxinemia). If there is no other explanation for elevated TSH and $T_4$ levels, a pituitary MRI should be performed. The patient's symptoms of hyperthyroidism and lack of family history of thyroid disease make a TSH-secreting adenoma more likely.

Serum TSH and human chorionic gonadotropin have a common α-subunit, allowing cross-reactivity at the TSH receptor. Gestational thyrotoxicosis typically occurs in the first trimester secondary to human chorionic gonadotropin (HCG) stimulation of the TSH receptor. Laboratory results would look similar to hyperthyroidism with suppressed TSH and elevated free $T_4$.

The clinical manifestations of hypothyroidism include fatigue, cold intolerance, constipation, heavy menses, weight gain, impaired concentration, dry skin, edema, depression, mood changes, muscle cramps, myalgia, and reduced fertility. Hypothyroidism is unlikely as her symptoms are not compatible and her TSH levels would be elevated with a normal or low free $T_4$ level.

The symptoms of thyrotoxicosis include heat intolerance, palpitations, dyspnea, tremulousness, menstrual irregularities, hyperdefecation, weight loss, increased appetite, proximal muscle weakness, fatigue, insomnia, and mood disturbances. The most common causes of hyperthyroidism are Graves disease and toxic adenoma(s). While the patient has thyrotoxicosis-related symptoms, hyperthyroidism due to Graves disease results in a suppressed TSH level with an elevated free $T_4$ level, which is not found in this case.

### KEY POINT

- Signs and symptoms of a thyroid-stimulating hormone-secreting adenoma are those seen in hyperthyroidism, although laboratory evaluation reveals an elevated free thyroxine ($T_4$) level with an inappropriately normal or elevated thyroid-stimulating hormone level.

### Bibliography

Amlashi FG, Tritos NA. Thyrotropin-secreting pituitary adenomas: epidemiology, diagnosis, and management. Endocrine. 2016;52:427-40. [PMID: 26792794] doi:10.1007/s12020-016-0863-3

## Item 35      Answer:     B

**Educational Objective:** Manage secondary amenorrhea due to a prolactinoma.

This patient has a prolactinoma resulting in amenorrhea and infertility due to the inhibitory effect of the elevated prolactin level on gonadotropin secretion. Prolactinomas are treated with dopamine agonists. The two FDA-approved dopamine agonists are bromocriptine and cabergoline. Cabergoline is much better tolerated and more effective at normalizing prolactin and tumor shrinkage, so it is typically the initial therapy chosen but is more expensive than bromocriptine. Dopamine agonists typically decrease the size and hormone production of prolactinomas rapidly. Response to therapy can be monitored by checking serum prolactin levels 1 month after initiating therapy and then every 3 to 4 months. Decreasing serum prolactin usually correlates with decreasing the size of the tumor. Normalization of prolactin concentrations with dopamine agonist therapy to allow spontaneous ovulation is the goal of management in women with microadenomas (<1 cm in size) considering pregnancy. Dopamine agonist therapy is effective at lowering prolactin levels, decreasing tumor size, and restoring gonadal function.

For women who do not ovulate with dopamine agonist therapy, clomiphene citrate therapy is sometimes added.

Unlike other pituitary tumors, medication rather than surgery is first-line therapy for prolactinomas. Even patients with severe mass effect such as vision loss are treated with medical therapy initially. Rarely, very large tumors or more invasive prolactinomas do not shrink with medical therapy and, also rarely, continue to grow. In these patients, surgery should be considered, followed by radiotherapy if growth recurs or continues. After being debulked, the prolactinoma may respond better to medical therapy.

Resuming an oral contraceptive pill will not correct the underlying disorder and would not assist this patient in becoming pregnant.

### KEY POINT

- Symptomatic prolactinomas are treated with dopamine agonists.

### Bibliography

Melmed S, Casanueva FF, Hoffman AR, Kleinberg DL, Montori VM, Schlechte JA, et al; Endocrine Society. Diagnosis and treatment of hyperprolactinemia: an Endocrine Society Clinical Practice Guideline. J Clin Endocrinol Metab. 2011;96:273-88. [PMID: 21296991] doi:10.1210/jc.2010-1692

## Item 36　　Answer:　B

**Educational Objective:** Manage the "honeymoon phase" of type 1 diabetes mellitus.

The most appropriate management of this patient's diabetes is to decrease the insulin glargine dose and discontinue insulin aspart. The drastic reduction in endogenous insulin production secondary to pancreatic beta cell destruction in type 1 diabetes creates a glucose toxicity that induces a functional impairment of the remaining beta cells. As exogenous insulin therapy improves glycemic control, the remaining beta cells experience less metabolic stress, resulting in an improvement in the ability to produce insulin. This "honeymoon phase" may occur shortly after the diagnosis of diabetes and may last months to years. It is characterized by drastic improvements in glycemic control and reductions in insulin requirements, as seen in this patient. To prevent rapid return of glucose toxicity and to preserve the remaining beta cells as long as possible, insulin therapy should be continued during the "honeymoon phase" if possible without causing hypoglycemia. It is appropriate to decrease this patient's basal glargine insulin dose to improve his fasting hypoglycemia while also maintaining continuous insulin therapy. Given the symptomatic postprandial hypoglycemia he is experiencing on low doses of prandial insulin, it is appropriate to discontinue it at this time with close monitoring for postprandial hyperglycemia at the end of the "honeymoon phase."

Sole use of a sliding-scale insulin regimen is not recommended for glycemic control as it is reactionary in nature to elevated glucose values only. Using this strategy, it would be possible that the patient may not receive daily insulin during the "honeymoon phase," which would accelerate the risk of developing glucose toxicity again.

### KEY POINT

- Continuing insulin, even at low doses, is recommended during the "honeymoon phase" of type 1 diabetes mellitus to reduce metabolic stress on functioning beta cells and preserve any residual function for as long as possible.

### Bibliography

DeWitt DE, Hirsch IB. Outpatient insulin therapy in type 1 and type 2 diabetes mellitus: scientific review. JAMA. 2003;289:2254-64. [PMID: 12734137]

## Item 37　　Answer:　A

**Educational Objective:** Manage postmenopausal osteoporosis in patients taking denosumab.

The most appropriate management for this patient is to continue denosumab. Denosumab, a monoclonal antibody against the receptor activator of nuclear factor κB ligand (RANKL), reduces bone resorption by inhibiting the development of osteoclasts. It circulates in the blood for up to 9 months after subcutaneous injection, but once cleared from the circulation, bone resorption transiently but dramatically increases, resulting in an abrupt decline in bone mineral density and, in some cases, vertebral fractures. Once initiated, there is no defined endpoint for cessation of denosumab therapy.

Although bone mineral density increases in response to denosumab therapy, it does not impact management with respect to dose and duration of treatment. Therefore, a DEXA scan is not necessary.

In the pharmacologic management of osteoporosis, drug holidays are considered during the course of bisphosphonate therapy. Due to their binding to bone tissue, bisphosphonates have durable effects on bone remodeling and fracture risk after discontinuation. After 5 years of treatment, patients at low risk for fracture can be considered for a bisphosphonate drug holiday. One study showed no cumulative difference in the risk for nonvertebral fractures in women continuing alendronate therapy for 5 versus 10 years. Post hoc analysis of this study showed that women with femoral neck T scores of –2.5 or worse and baseline prevalent vertebral fracture had reduced fracture risk by continuing alendronate therapy for 10 years versus stopping after 5 years compared with placebo.

Zoledronic acid is an intravenous bisphosphonate indicated for the treatment of osteoporosis especially in patients intolerant to oral bisphosphonates. Patients switched from zoledronic acid to denosumab experience further gains in bone mineral density suggesting additive benefit from this sequence of therapy. However, in patients receiving long-term denosumab, switching to zoledronic acid attenuated but did prevent loss of bone mineral density suggesting that denosumab therapy should be continued once initiated.

### KEY POINT

- When administered subcutaneously twice yearly, denosumab suppresses bone resorption, increases bone density, and reduces the incidence of osteoporotic fractures in men and women; the effects of denosumab are not sustained when treatment is stopped.

### Bibliography

Anastasilakis AD, Polyzos SA, Makras P, Aubry-Rozier B, Kaouri S, Lamy O. Clinical features of 24 patients with rebound-associated vertebral fractures after denosumab discontinuation: systematic review and additional cases. J Bone Miner Res. 2017;32:1291-1296. [PMID: 28240371] doi:10.1002/jbmr.3110

## Item 38        Answer:    C

**Educational Objective:  Manage type 1 diabetes mellitus in a hospitalized patient.**

The most appropriate management of this patient's type 1 diabetes mellitus is to decrease basal insulin dose by 10% to 20% and add correction insulin regimen. This patient's fasting blood glucose values were already low on his home basal insulin doses, thus it is most appropriate to continue his basal insulin but at a reduced dose to avoid diabetic ketoacidosis and hypoglycemia. Correction insulin with basal insulin will treat hyperglycemia while he is fasting. Patients with type 1 diabetes must have continuous insulin therapy, particularly basal insulin, to avoid the development of DKA. Because of the requirement of continuous insulin, prolonged fasting in a patient with type 1 diabetes can be complicated by hypoglycemia. Proactive adjustments to insulin doses are required to avoid extreme fluctuations in glycemic control while in the fasting state.

This patient's fasting blood glucose value of 70 mg/dL (3.9 mmol/L) on the current basal insulin dose meets the American Diabetes Association's threshold value for downward titration of insulin doses to avoid hypoglycemia. The basal insulin dose should be decreased in addition to holding the prandial insulin in the fasting state. A sliding-scale insulin regimen should also be added to the basal insulin to help manage hyperglycemia that may occur while fasting.

Efficient glucose utilization is impaired when continuous insulin therapy, such as basal insulin, is held in type 1 diabetes. This may cause the development of diabetic ketoacidosis as a result of increased glycogenolysis and gluconeogenesis for fuel production. A sliding-scale insulin regimen alone is not physiologic and may cause large fluctuations in the blood glucose levels owing to the inherent reactive nature of its dosing, coupled with the near universal lag time between measurement of glucose and injection of insulin that occurs in most hospitals.

### KEY POINT

- In fasting hospitalized patients with type 1 diabetes mellitus, the basal insulin dose should be decreased, the prandial insulin held to avoid hypoglycemia, and a correction insulin regimen should be added to help manage hyperglycemia.

### Bibliography

Chiang JL, Kirkman MS, Laffel LM, Peters AL; Type 1 diabetes sourcebook authors. Type 1 diabetes through the life span: a position statement of the American Diabetes Association. Diabetes Care. 2014;37:2034-54. [PMID: 24935775] doi:10.2337/dc14-1140

## Item 39        Answer:    B

**Educational Objective:  Screen for adrenal hyperfunction in an incidentally noted adrenal mass.**

The most appropriate next test to perform is a 24-hour urine total metanephrine measurement to screen for pheochromocytoma. Even though this patient does not have hypertension, she should be screened for pheochromocytoma, as

these tumors may exist in the absence of typical symptoms or hypertension. Approximately 50% of pheochromocytomas are now first discovered as an incidental adrenal mass. An alternative screening test for pheochromocytoma is measuring the fractionated free plasma metanephrine level. This test has a false-positive rate of approximately 11%, and, therefore, may be considered more useful when suspicion for pheochromocytoma is high. This patient should also be screened for subclinical Cushing syndrome with a 1-mg overnight dexamethasone suppression test. The prevalence of incidentally noted adrenal masses increases with age and is estimated to be about 10% in the elderly. Most lesions are benign, nonfunctioning adenomas, and approximately 10% to 15% secrete excess hormones.

The 24-hour urine free cortisol test is not sensitive enough to diagnose subclinical autonomous cortisol secretion from an adrenal mass. The 24-hour urine free cortisol levels are usually within the normal range in subclinical Cushing syndrome.

The patient does not require screening for primary aldosteronism with a plasma aldosterone-plasma renin ratio (ARR) as she does not have hypertension. Only patients with an incidental adrenal mass and hypertension require screening for primary aldosteronism. Hypokalemia, traditionally thought to be a key feature of primary aldosteronism, is no longer a prerequisite for diagnosis because many patients with this disorder have normal potassium levels.

In women, rapid onset of hirsutism, menstrual irregularities, and virilization should raise suspicion for tumoral hyperandrogenism. Measurement of dehydroepiandrosterone sulfate (DHEAS) is not indicated in this patient, as she did not show signs of hyperandrogenism (hirsutism, deep voice, male pattern balding, clitoromegaly). Serum DHEAS may be measured if signs of significant hyperandrogenism are present in the setting of an adrenal mass that has radiologic features suspicious for malignancy (size >4 cm, heterogeneous enhancement with contrast administration, irregular margins, presence of calcifications or necrosis).

### KEY POINT

- Biochemical testing for pheochromocytoma should be undertaken in all patients with an adrenal mass, even in the absence of typical symptoms or hypertension.

### Bibliography

Fassnacht M, Arlt W, Bancos I, Dralle H, Newell-Price J, Sahdev A, et al. Management of adrenal incidentalomas: European Society of Endocrinology Clinical Practice Guideline in collaboration with the European Network for the Study of Adrenal Tumors. Eur J Endocrinol. 2016;175:G1-G34. [PMID: 27390021] doi:10.1530/EJE-16-0467

## Item 40        Answer:    C

**Educational Objective:  Manage a patient with severe primary hyperparathyroidism who is to undergo parathyroidectomy.**

The most appropriate test to perform next for this patient is measurement of her 25-hydroxyvitamin D level. Vitamin D

CONT.

deficiency is common in patients with primary hyperparathyroidism (HPT) due to increased conversion of 25-hydroxyvitamin D to 1,25-dihydroxyvitamin D. Supplementation of vitamin D in patients with HPT has been shown to reduce parathyroid hormone levels, decrease bone turnover, and improve bone mineral density. Identifying and treating vitamin D deficiency perioperatively helps manage transient hypocalcemia, which routinely occurs after parathyroidectomy and especially in severe HPT where high bone turnover (as evidence by an elevated alkaline phosphatase) portends hungry bone syndrome.

Due to increased conversion, 1,25-dihydroxyvitamin D levels are frankly elevated in most instances of hyperparathyroidism and even in patients who are vitamin D deficient. It is not a useful test to identify and manage vitamin D deficiency in any circumstance and could be falsely reassuring in patients with HPT.

Given kidney excretion of calcium is the dominant mechanism by which hypercalcemia is corrected, urine calcium excretion can be assumed to be high in severe hypercalcemia with the exception of patients with severe acute kidney injury. Although guidelines suggest routine assessment of 24-hour urine calcium in the evaluation of HPT to exclude familial hypocalciuric hypercalcemia, the need for such screening primarily occurs when parathyroid hormone and calcium levels are mildly elevated. Additionally, a clinical diagnosis has already been established for this patient making 24-hour urine calcium measurement unnecessary.

Ionized calcium is the best test to assess the state of calcium homeostasis and is recommended by some experts when managing HPT. However, it is primarily of use when evaluating and managing hypocalcemia, especially when assumptions cannot be made regarding serum protein concentrations and blood pH.

**KEY POINT**

- In patients with primary hyperparathyroidism who are undergoing parathyroidectomy surgery, identifying and correcting vitamin D deficiency is important to avoid postoperative hypocalcemia, which occurs due to rapid flux of serum calcium into bone (hungry bone syndrome).

**Bibliography**

Kaderli RM, Riss P, Dunkler D, Pietschmann P, Selberherr A, Scheuba C, Niederle B. The impact of vitamin D status on hungry bone syndrome after surgery for primary hyperparathyroidism. Eur J Endocrinol. 2017 Sep 6. pii: EJE-17-0416. doi: 10.1530/EJE-17-0416. [Epub ahead of print] [PMID: 28877925]

## Item 41    Answer:    D

**Educational Objective:** Diagnose subclinical Cushing syndrome in a patient with an incidentally noted adrenal mass.

The most likely diagnosis in this patient with an incidentally discovered adrenal mass is subclinical Cushing syndrome. All patients with an incidental adrenal mass should be screened for subclinical Cushing syndrome (SCS), a condition characterized by adrenocorticotropic hormone (ACTH)-independent cortisol secretion that may result in metabolic (hyperglycemia and hypertension) and bone (osteoporosis) effects of hypercortisolism, but not the more specific features of Cushing syndrome (centripetal obesity, facial plethora, abnormal fat deposition in the supraclavicular or dorsocervical areas, and wide violaceous striae). The preferred diagnostic test for SCS is a 1-mg overnight dexamethasone suppression test, with a morning cortisol level greater than 5 µg/dL (138 nmol/L) considered positive. Following a positive result for SCS, measurement of ACTH, dehydroepiandrosterone sulfate (DHEAS), urine free cortisol, and an 8-mg overnight dexamethasone suppression test are often required to confirm autonomous cortisol secretion. If SCS is confirmed, the risks and benefits of surgery need to be considered. Surgery for SCS has been associated with improvements in bone density and glucose, lipid, and blood pressure control.

This patient's serum cortisol level did not suppress to less than 5 µg/dL (138 nmol/L) following dexamethasone administration. Under normal conditions, exposure to dexamethasone results in suppression of ACTH secretion and hence suppression of adrenal cortisol secretion. In the setting of autonomous cortisol secretion from an adrenal mass, cortisol suppression following dexamethasone administration would not occur, as tumor production of cortisol is not under normal physiologic feedback control.

The patient's plasma free metanephrine levels were within the normal range. This test has excellent sensitivity, and a normal result rules out pheochromocytoma.

Primary aldosteronism is also unlikely based on a calculated plasma aldosterone-plasma renin ratio (ARR) of less than 20. Her blood pressure medications, hydrochlorothiazide and doxazosin, have minimal or mild effects on the ARR, and therefore the result can be reliably interpreted.

**KEY POINT**

- Initial testing for subclinical Cushing syndrome is a 1-mg overnight dexamethasone suppression test; a cortisol level greater than 5 µg/dL (138 nmol/L) is considered a positive test.

**Bibliography**

Fassnacht M, Wiebke A, Bancos I, Dralle H, Newell-Price J, Sahdev A, Tabarin A, Terzolo M, Tsagarakis S, Dekkers OM. Management of adrenal incidentalomas: European Society of Endocrinology Clinical Practice Guideline in collaboration with the European Network for the Study of Adrenal Tumors. Eur J Endocrinol. 2016;175(2):G1–G34. PMID: 27390021.

## Item 42    Answer:    B

**Educational Objective:** Screen for Cushing syndrome in a patient with an alternate sleep schedule.

This patient should be screened for Cushing syndrome, and the best screening test in this patient is measurement of 24-hour urine free cortisol to quantify total daily cortisol secretion. Biochemical testing is used to establish the diagnosis of Cushing syndrome. It is critical that the biochemical diagnosis is firmly established prior to any imaging studies due to the relatively high prevalence of clinically insignificant pituitary and adrenal masses. Initial tests include the 1-mg overnight dexamethasone suppression test, 24-hour urine free cortisol, and late-night salivary cortisol. While the 1-mg overnight dexamethasone test and the late-night salivary cortisol test may be more convenient, they are likely to be less accurate in this patient because of her shift work and estrogen use. Measurement of 24-hour urine free cortisol is not impacted by estrogen therapy or sleeping patterns. A threefold or greater increase over normal values is diagnostic of Cushing syndrome if compatible clinical features are present (centripetal obesity, facial plethora, abnormal fat deposition in the supraclavicular or dorsocervical areas, and wide violaceous striae); if this increase is present, test results should be repeated to confirm the abnormal result.

The 1-mg overnight dexamethasone suppression test is also not reliable in this patient because it relies on serum cortisol measurement.

The late night salivary cortisol test is not a reliable screening test in this patient because she works a night shift and therefore her diurnal cortisol secretion will be reversed.

Measurement of morning serum cortisol is unreliable as a screening test for Cushing syndrome because normal secretion of cortisol is pulsatile and the normal range is broad. Hence, there is considerable overlap between serum cortisol levels seen in normal people, those with Cushing syndrome, and those with hypercortisolism due to psychological or medical stressors.

In addition, serum cortisol measurement is unreliable in this patient as she is on oral estrogen, which leads to an increase in cortisol binding proteins and subsequent elevation of serum total cortisol levels without impacting free cortisol levels.

### KEY POINT

- The 24-hour urine free cortisol test for Cushing syndrome is not impacted by either estrogen therapy or sleeping patterns.

### Bibliography
Loriaux DL. Diagnosis and differential diagnosis of Cushing's syndrome. N Engl J Med. 2017;376:1451-1459. doi: 10.1056/NEJMra1505550. [PMID:28402781]

### Item 43    Answer:    E

**Educational Objective:** Diagnose medication-induced male gynecomastia.

This patient most likely has spironolactone-induced gynecomastia. Gynecomastia occurs due to an imbalance between free estrogen and free androgen actions in breast tissue. Spironolactone is a known cause of gynecomastia. Spironolactone can increase the aromatization of testosterone to estradiol, decrease the testosterone production by the testes, and displace testosterone from sex hormone-binding globulin,

thereby increasing its metabolic clearance rate. Additionally, spironolactone also acts as an antiandrogen by binding to androgen receptors and displacing binding of testosterone and dihydrotestosterone to their receptors. Other recognized drug-related causes of gynecomastia include marijuana, alcohol, 5α-reductase inhibitors, $H_2$-receptor antagonists, digoxin, ketoconazole, calcium channel blockers, ACE inhibitors, antiretroviral agents, tricyclic antidepressants, and selective serotonin reuptake inhibitors.

Breast cancers are typically unilateral and nontender with a discrete fixed mass displaced from the nipple-areolar complex, whereas gynecomastia presents as a rubbery, concentric, subareolar mass. Gynecomastia is typically bilateral and often associated with breast tenderness.

Germ cell tumors account for 95% of testicular neoplasms with 6% of patients presenting with gynecomastia at time of diagnosis. The temporal association of gynecomastia with the initiation of a medication known to cause gynecomastia and a normal testicular examination makes germ cell tumor a much less likely diagnosis.

Hypogonadism, primary more so than secondary, is associated with gynecomastia due to an increase in estradiol relative to testosterone secretion. With primary hypogonadism, a rise in luteinizing hormone results in increased aromatization of testosterone to estradiol; this elevated luteinizing hormone is absent in secondary hypogonadism thus making gynecomastia a less prominent sign. This patient has unchanged sexual functioning, morning erections, and no evidence of testicular atrophy making hypogonadism an unlikely diagnosis.

Pseudogynecomastia is often seen in obese men. It occurs due to an increase in breast fat without any proliferation of glandular tissue. Gynecomastia and pseudogynecomastia are differentiated by examination. Pseudogynecomastia is characterized by the presence of subareolar adipose tissue, without glandular proliferation. True gynecomastia typically distorts the normally flat contour of the male nipple, causing it to protrude owing to the mass of glandular tissue beneath it. In pseudogynecomastia, the nipple is typically still flat but soft, and nondescript subcutaneous fat tissue is present in the breast area.

### KEY POINT

- Gynecomastia can be an adverse effect of medications; spironolactone causes an imbalance between free estrogen and free androgen resulting in glandular breast tissue enlargement.

### Bibliography
Dickson G. Gynecomastia. Am Fam Physician. 2012;85:716-22. [PMID:22534349]

### Item 44    Answer:    A

**Educational Objective:** Diagnose celiac disease as a cause of thyroxine malabsorption.

The most likely diagnosis is celiac disease. The patient had been taking the same dose of levothyroxine for many years, but recently has required increasing doses to maintain euthyroidism. Despite his levothyroxine dose being increased, his serum thyroid-stimulating hormone (TSH) level remains elevated, his free thyroxine (T$_4$) is at the lower limit of the normal reference range, and he continues to have symptoms of thyroid hormone deficiency. Rising levothyroxine requirements in the absence of obvious medication noncompliance or inappropriate administration should alert the treating physician about possible malabsorption. Since levothyroxine is principally absorbed in the jejunum and ileum, any disease process affecting the small bowel can affect the fraction of an orally administered dose that is absorbed. The patient reports diarrhea, abdominal pain, and weight loss, and a rash that is characteristic of dermatitis herpetiformis, a finding that is unique to celiac disease. Patients with celiac disease frequently experience malabsorption of medications, vitamins, and other nutrients.

Medication noncompliance is a less likely explanation for this patient's escalating levothyroxine requirements given his prior history of being easily maintained on a stable dose of levothyroxine and self-reported adherence to his prescribed regimen. Medication noncompliance would not explain his associated symptoms of abdominal cramping, skin rash, and unintentional weight loss.

Autoimmune primary adrenal insufficiency occurs more commonly in patients with other autoimmune disorders, and this patient does report gastrointestinal symptoms and weight loss; however, he does not demonstrate hyperpigmentation or hypotension. Moreover, adrenal insufficiency would not provide an explanation for his rising levothyroxine dose requirements or skin rash.

Thyroid hormone resistance is also unlikely. The patient would not be expected to have had normal thyroid function test results previously, and his free T$_4$ would be elevated.

**KEY POINT**

• Malabsorptive disorders may decrease levothyroxine absorption resulting in higher than expected levothyroxine dose requirements.

**Bibliography**
Centanni M, Benvenga S, Sachmechi I. Diagnosis and management of treatment-refractory hypothyroidism: an expert consensus report. J Endocrinol Invest. 2017 Jul 10. doi: 10.1007/s40618-017-0706-y. [Epub ahead of print] [PMID: 28695483]

## Item 45    Answer:   B
**Educational Objective:** Manage infertility.

When evaluating infertility, both female and male factors should be considered concurrently. Thus, semen analysis is part of the initial diagnostic evaluation. Collection should occur after 2 to 3 days of sexual abstinence, but no longer to avoid decreased sperm motility. If semen analysis is abnormal, it should be repeated at least 2 weeks later, and if results are abnormal, referral to a reproductive endocrinologist is recommended.

Given that this patient has regular menses every 28 days with molimina symptoms (breast pain and bloating), her cycles appear to be ovulatory. Thus, laboratory assessment of ovulatory function is not needed at this time. In patients who do not have normal menstrual cycles with ovulation, laboratory assessment should be performed. A midluteal phase serum progesterone level, obtained approximately 1 week before the expected menses, is an effective way to assess ovulatory status. A progesterone level above 3 ng/mL (9.5 nmol/L) is evidence of recent ovulation. Measurement of serum thyroid stimulating hormone and prolactin levels is appropriate to exclude thyroid disease and hyperprolactinemia as causes of oligo-ovulation.

In women over the age of 35 years, an infertility evaluation is initiated after 6 months of unprotected intercourse; in women under the age of 35, an infertility evaluation is initiated after 1 year of regular unprotected intercourse. Recommending an additional 5 months of unprotected intercourse is unnecessary for this 37-year-old woman.

Laparoscopy for evaluation of pelvic adhesions or mild endometriosis may be warranted in patients with dysmenorrhea, history of sexually transmitted infections, or previous pelvic surgery. While assessment of tubal patency may be indicated in this patient given her prior history of appendicitis and abdominal surgery (putting her at risk for adhesions), laparoscopy is not indicated at this immediate time prior to moving forward with an initial noninvasive diagnostic evaluation.

**KEY POINT**

• When evaluating infertility, both female and male factors should be considered concurrently; semen analysis is part of the initial diagnostic evaluation.

**Bibliography**
Marshburn PB. Counseling and diagnostic evaluation for the infertile couple. Obstet Gynecol Clin North Am. 2015;42:1-14. [PMID: 25681836] doi:10.1016/j.ogc.2014.10.001

## Item 46    Answer:   B
**Educational Objective:** Recognize the effect of opioids on pituitary function.

This patient's opioid use is most likely responsible for his sexual dysfunction. Secondary hypogonadism is typically a result of insufficient gonadotropin-releasing hormone production by the hypothalamus or deficient luteinizing hormone (LH)/follicle-stimulating hormone (FSH) secretion by the anterior pituitary. This patient has symptoms of hypogonadism and a low testosterone level. Low or inappropriately normal FSH and LH levels in the presence of simultaneous low testosterone levels are diagnostic of secondary hypogonadism (hypogonadotropic hypogonadism). Untreated sleep apnea, exogenous testosterone administration, and obesity are common causes of secondary hypogonadism. Other acquired causes include hyperprolactinemia, chronic opioid use, glucocorticoid use, or infiltrative disease (lymphoma or hemochromatosis). Chronic opioid therapy is a well-established cause of hypogonadotropic hypogonadism. The mechanism of opioid-induced hypogonadism is thought to be central hypogonadism, with downregulation of gonadotropin-releasing hormone and subsequently LH and FSH. This, in turn, results in decreased testosterone production.

This patient's decline in gonadal function is not a result of his age. Although testosterone levels may decline with age, this patient's testosterone level of 185 ng/dL (6.4 nmol/L) is well below the normal range and below what would be expected for age-related decline in testosterone.

Although a pituitary tumor isn't completely ruled out without an MRI, the most likely cause of this patient's hypogonadism is the chronic opioid therapy. Testosterone levels greater than 150 ng/dL (5.2 nmol/L) are less likely to be related to a pituitary tumor. Patients with hypogonadotropic hypogonadism and testosterone levels less than 150 ng/dL (5.2 nmol/L) should have an MRI to evaluate for a pituitary tumor. The normal TSH and prolactin levels also argue against a pituitary or hypothalamic tumor.

In primary gonadal failure, there would be elevated FSH and LH levels with a low testosterone level. A low testosterone level with inappropriately normal or low FSH and LH levels is consistent with hypogonadotropic hypogonadism.

**KEY POINT**

- Chronic opioid use suppresses gonadotroph function, resulting in hypogonadotropic hypogonadism, which is increasingly recognized as a cause of secondary hypogonadism.

**Bibliography**
O'Rourke TK Jr, Wosnitzer MS. Opioid-induced androgen deficiency (opiad): diagnosis, management, and literature review. Curr Urol Rep. 2016;17:76. [PMID: 27586511] doi:10.1007/s11934-016-0634-y.

## Item 47    Answer:    C
**Educational Objective:** Diagnose Turner syndrome.

The most common cause of primary amenorrhea is gonadal dysgenesis caused by chromosomal abnormalities, most commonly those associated with Turner syndrome (TS). TS is caused by loss of part or all of an X chromosome (45,X0) occurring in 1 in 2500 live female births. In some studies, more than 20% of patients are diagnosed after 12 years of age; primary amenorrhea may be the presenting sign. The most consistent physical finding is short stature, as seen in this patient. Other findings may include neck webbing, hearing loss, aortic coarctation, and bicuspid aortic valve. Primary amenorrhea is seen in approximately 90% of women with TS. TS should be considered in women with primary or secondary amenorrhea, particularly those of short stature. Diagnosis is made by karyotype analysis.

Functional hypothalamic amenorrhea is caused by a functional disruption of the hypothalamic-pituitary-ovarian axis in which no anatomic or organic disease is identified. Disruption of the pulsatile release of hypothalamic gonad-otropin-releasing hormone may occur due to stress, weight loss, or exercise; follicle-stimulating hormone (FSH) levels are not elevated in functional hypothalamic amenorrhea.

Primary ovarian insufficiency is considered when a woman younger than 40 years of age develops secondary amenorrhea with two serum FSH levels in the menopausal range (>35 mU/mL [35 U/L]). This condition impacts 1 in 100 women by the age of 40 years. If during the evaluation of secondary amenorrhea, an elevated FSH is found, it should be repeated in 1 month, along with a serum estradiol measurement. In young women, karyotype analysis is also indicated to rule out Turner syndrome.

Vaginal agenesis is the second most common cause of primary amenorrhea with an incidence of 1 in 5000. Vaginal agenesis is characterized by congenital absence of the vagina with variable uterine development. These women have a normal female karyotype and ovarian function, thus develop normal secondary sexual characteristics. Presentation is typically after age 15 years due to primary amenorrhea. Examination reveals normal external genitalia with a dimple or small pouch replacing the vagina. On laboratory testing, gonadotropins are unremarkable. This patient's normal pelvic examination eliminates this vaginal agenesis as a cause of primary amenorrhea.

**KEY POINT**

- The most common cause of primary amenorrhea is gonadal dysgenesis, most commonly associated with Turner syndrome (45,X0).

**Bibliography**
Pinsker JE. Clinical review: Turner syndrome: updating the paradigm of clinical care. J Clin Endocrinol Metab. 2012;97:E994-1003. [PMID: 22472565] doi:10.1210/jc.2012-1245

## Item 48    Answer:    B
**Educational Objective:** Evaluate postprandial hypoglycemia in a patient without diabetes.

The most appropriate diagnostic test to perform next is mixed-meal testing. Hypoglycemia in persons without diabetes is extremely rare and requires additional investigation. Causes of hypoglycemia in adults without diabetes include drug or alcohol use, critical illness, hormonal deficiency, non-islet cell tumor, endogenous hyperinsulinism, accidental or intentional hypoglycemia, and prior Roux-en-Y gastric bypass surgery. Postprandial hypoglycemia can develop 2 to 3 years after Roux-en-Y gastric bypass surgery. The patient either denies or does not have clinical evidence for the presence of many of these causes. The timing of the hypoglycemia can guide the appropriate next diagnostic test.

This patient is experiencing postprandial symptoms consistent with an increase in sympathetic activity within 5 hours of a meal. He meets two out of three criteria for a hypoglycemic disorder as defined by the Whipple triad: symptoms that can be attributed to hypoglycemia and resolution of symptoms with food consumption. He does not have documented hypoglycemia at the time of symptoms from a reliable laboratory method to meet the third criteria of the Whipple triad. Point-of-care fingerstick measurements lack precision to confirm hypoglycemia. An attempt should be made to recreate the scenario that is likely to cause the symptoms. Since his symptoms occur in the postprandial state, a mixed-meal test should be performed. The mixed-meal consists of food types that have induced the onset of symptoms in the past. The patient should have the following hypoglycemic laboratory tests measured at baseline and every 30 minutes for 5 hours after consuming the mixed-meal: plasma glucose, insulin, C-peptide, β-hydroxybutyrate (low in the presence of insulin), and proinsulin. He should also repeat these tests at the time of symptomatic hypoglycemia (<60 mg/dL [3.3 mmol/L]) before administering carbohydrates. If symptomatic hypoglycemia is documented during the mixed-meal testing, the patient should also be screened for insulin secretagogues (sulfonylureas and meglitinides) and insulin antibodies.

A 72-hour fast involves prolonged fasting while measuring the hypoglycemic laboratory test (plasma glucose, insulin, C-peptide, β-hydroxybutyrate, and proinsulin) every 6 hours, followed by every 1 to 2 hours once the glucose is less than 60 mg/dL (3.3 mmol/L) or the patient becomes symptomatic. Given that the patient is experiencing postprandial symptoms, the 72-hour fast would likely not induce hypoglycemia.

An oral glucose tolerance test (OGTT) consists of liquid caloric consumption that is usually not similar to the type of food that induces symptomatic postprandial hypoglycemia. The OGTT can produce unreliable results, particularly in those patients with altered gastric anatomy or gastric motility.

Pancreatic imaging should only occur after biochemical confirmation of endogenous hyperinsulinism.

### KEY POINT

- A mixed-meal test consisting of the types of food that normally induce the hypoglycemia should be performed to determine the cause of postprandial hypoglycemia.

### Bibliography

Cryer PE, Axelrod L, Grossman AB, Heller SR, Montori VM, Seaquist ER, et al; Endocrine Society. Evaluation and management of adult hypoglycemic disorders: an Endocrine Society Clinical Practice Guideline. J Clin Endocrinol Metab. 2009;94:709-28. [PMID: 19088155] doi:10.1210/jc.2008-1410

### Item 49    Answer:    A

**Educational Objective:** Treat secondary adrenal insufficiency.

This patient has secondary adrenal insufficiency, and hydrocortisone is the most appropriate treatment. Oral, injectable (including joint injections), and occasionally even topical glucocorticoids are able to suppress adrenocorticotropic hormone (ACTH) secretion. Glucocorticoids prescribed at doses above physiologic replacement for longer than 3 weeks should be tapered when discontinued allowing recovery of the pituitary-adrenal axis; if therapy has lasted less than 3 weeks, no taper is required for pituitary-adrenal axis recovery. The diagnosis of adrenal insufficiency is based on demonstrating inappropriately low serum cortisol levels. Because most assays measure total cortisol, abnormalities in cortisol-binding protein or albumin can trigger spurious results. An early morning (8 AM) serum cortisol of less than 3 µg/dL (82.8 nmol/L) is consistent with cortisol deficiency, whereas values greater than 15 to 18 µg/dL (414.0-496.8 nmol/L) exclude the diagnosis when binding protein abnormalities and synthetic glucocorticoid exposure are excluded.

Fludrocortisone in addition to hydrocortisone is unwarranted as fludrocortisone is needed only in primary adrenal insufficiency. There is no mineralocorticoid deficiency in secondary adrenal insufficiency.

An ACTH stimulation test is not necessary in this patient since the cortisol level less than 3 µg/dL (82.8 nmol/L) is diagnostic of adrenal insufficiency. If an ACTH stimulation test were necessary, dexamethasone can be given prior to the ACTH stimulation test since dexamethasone is not measureable in the cortisol assay. That is unnecessary given this patient's cortisol level.

### KEY POINT

- Oral, injectable (including joint injections), and even topical glucocorticoids are able to suppress adrenocorticotropic hormone (ACTH) secretion and result in secondary adrenal insufficiency.

### Bibliography

Pazderska A, Pearce SH. Adrenal insufficiency - recognition and management. Clin Med (Lond). 2017;17:258-262. doi: 0.7861/clinmedicine.17-3-258. [PMID: 28572228]

### Item 50    Answer:    C

**Educational Objective:** Treat hypothyroidism with weight-based dosing of levothyroxine.

This patient has hypothyroidism, and the most appropriate treatment is to prescribe a weight-based replacement dose of levothyroxine (1.6 µg/kg lean body weight). For patients with high body mass index values, an estimate of lean mass should be determined. Levothyroxine is the treatment of choice for thyroid hormone deficiency. Goals of therapy are to resolve signs and symptoms of hypothyroidism, normalize serum thyroid-stimulating hormone (TSH), and avoid overtreatment.

Although some patients express a preference for treatment with desiccated thyroid hormone (thyroid extract), there are potential safety concerns and lack of data on long-term outcomes. The physiologic ratio of thyroxine ($T_4$) to triiodothyronine ($T_3$) secreted by the human thyroid is approximately 15:1, whereas desiccated thyroid hormone, as originally derived from animal thyroid glands, contains supraphysiologic $T_3$ ($T_4$ to $T_3$ ratio 4:1). Patients taking desiccated thyroid hormone frequently experience low serum $T_4$

and supraphysiologic $T_3$ levels despite having a serum TSH within the reference range.

Although a full replacement dose of levothyroxine can be administered to most patients with overt hypothyroidism, older adults (age 65 years and older) and patients with cardiovascular disease should be prescribed a lower initial dose (25-50 µg/day) due to the effects of thyroid hormone on myocardial oxygen demand. The dose should be titrated based on TSH levels measured 6 to 8 weeks after any dose change. The patient described here is an otherwise healthy woman in her fifth decade of life. Prescribing a low initial dose of levothyroxine would unnecessarily delay correction of hypothyroidism.

Not prescribing treatment is also inappropriate. Although the patient does not currently report symptoms of thyroid hormone deficiency, she has overt hypothyroidism with physical findings consistent with this diagnosis (slowed reflexes) and evidence of metabolic complications (hypercholesterolemia). Hypothyroidism causes hypercholesterolemia through reduced cholesterol metabolism and contributes to the development cardiovascular disease. Treatment of patients with overt hypothyroidism and all nonpregnant adults with subclinical hypothyroidism and a serum TSH level above 10 µU/mL (10 mU/L) is indicated to ameliorate the risk of these complications.

### KEY POINT

- Levothyroxine is the treatment of choice for thyroid hormone deficiency; for most younger adults without cardiac disease, a weight-based replacement dose of levothyroxine (1.6 µg/kg lean body weight) is recommended.

### Bibliography
Hennessey JV. The emergence of levothyroxine as a treatment for hypothyroidism. Endocrine. 2017;55:6-18. [PMID: 27981511] doi:10.1007/s12020-016-1199-8

## Item 51    Answer:    A

**Educational Objective:** Diagnose the cause of Cushing syndrome.

The most appropriate diagnostic test for this patient is measurement of the adrenocorticotropic hormone (ACTH) level. Cushing disease is the term used to indicate excess cortisol production due to an ACTH-secreting pituitary adenoma. Cushing syndrome refers to hypercortisolism from any cause, exogenous or endogenous, ACTH-dependent or not. The most common cause of endogenous Cushing syndrome is Cushing disease. The initial step in evaluation for Cushing disease is to seek biochemical evidence of hypercortisolism. At least two first-line tests should be diagnostically abnormal before the diagnosis is confirmed. Initial tests include the overnight low-dose dexamethasone suppression test, 24-hour urine free cortisol, and late-night salivary cortisol. The 24-hour urine free cortisol and late night salivary cortisol tests should be performed at least twice to ensure reproducibility of results.

The abnormal dexamethasone suppression test and elevated urine free cortisol levels establish the diagnosis of Cushing syndrome in this patient. An ACTH measurement should be obtained once the diagnosis of Cushing syndrome is established to determine if it is ACTH dependent or ACTH independent.

Once ACTH-dependent Cushing syndrome is confirmed biochemically, a pituitary MRI should be obtained. If no pituitary tumor or a tumor less than 6 mm is visualized on MRI, an 8-mg dexamethasone suppression test is used to differentiate Cushing disease from an ectopic source of ACTH. Dexamethasone is administered at 11 PM, and cortisol is tested at 8 AM. A pituitary source of ACTH will respond to negative feedback from high doses of dexamethasone, suppressing plasma cortisol at 8 AM by more than 50%, whereas an ectopic source of ACTH will not have suppressible cortisol. However, this test has low sensitivity (88%) and specificity (57%) for Cushing disease, so inferior petrosal sinus sampling (IPSS) is often recommended before exploratory pituitary surgery. In IPSS, ACTH levels in the petrosal sinus are compared with those in the periphery after the administration of corticotropin-releasing hormone (CRH). A central to peripheral gradient greater than 2.0 before CRH or greater than 3.0 after CRH is diagnostic of Cushing disease.

An 8-mg dexamethasone suppression test, inferior petrosal sinus sampling, and pituitary MRI should follow, if necessary, ACTH testing. Their inclusion in the diagnostic algorithm at this point is premature and possibly unnecessary.

### KEY POINT

- An adrenocorticotropic hormone (ACTH) measurement should be obtained once the diagnosis of Cushing syndrome is established to determine if it is ACTH dependent or ACTH independent.

### Bibliography
Loriaux DL. Diagnosis and differential diagnosis of Cushing's syndrome. N Engl J Med. 2017;376:1451-1459. doi: 10.1056/NEJMra1505550. [PMID:28402781]

## Item 52    Answer:    D

**Educational Objective:** Diagnose testosterone-induced change in thyroxine-binding globulin.

The most likely explanation for the observed change in this patient's thyroid function test results is the initiation of testosterone. The administration of androgens and anabolic steroids leads to a reduction in thyroxine-binding globulin, which consequently increases the proportion of metabolically active free thyroxine that is available. Consequently, a reduction in levothyroxine dosing may be needed to prevent iatrogenic thyrotoxicosis. Conversely, higher levothyroxine doses are often required after the initiation of estrogen or selective estrogen receptor modulating therapies (tamoxifen and raloxifene) due to an increase in serum thyroxine-binding globulin concentrations.

Administering levothyroxine with coffee or calcium carbonate and treatment with omeprazole all decrease the absorption of thyroxine, resulting in reduced levels of free thyroxine ($T_4$) and elevated levels of thyroid-stimulating hormone. Calcium carbonate reduces the maximum absorption of levothyroxine by 25%. Because calcium and ferrous sulfate can bind levothyroxine, the ingestion of either medication, even as a component of a multivitamin, should be separated from levothyroxine by 4 hours. Administering levothyroxine with coffee, whether caffeinated or not, has been shown to reduce the absorption of levothyroxine. Ideally, levothyroxine should be taken 60 minutes before food or coffee is consumed. Oral levothyroxine is absorbed in the jejunum and ileum. The absorption of an orally administered dose is 70% to 80% under optimum fasting conditions, and an acidic gastric pH is important. Chronic therapy with omeprazole and other proton pump inhibitors impairs levothyroxine absorption by increasing gastric pH.

**KEY POINT**

- In patients receiving thyroxine replacement therapy, initiation of estrogen or raloxifene increases thyroxine-binding globulin levels whereas testosterone reduces thyroxine-binding globulin levels; in either situation a change in thyroxine dosage may be required.

**Bibliography**

Tahboub R, Arafah BM. Sex steroids and the thyroid. Best Pract Res Clin Endocrinol Metab. 2009 Dec;23(6):769-80. doi: 10.1016/j.beem.2009.06.005. [PMID: 19942152]

## Item 53    Answer:    A

**Educational Objective:** Treat postmenopausal osteoporosis.

The most appropriate treatment for this patient is alendronate. The American College of Physicians (ACP) recommends that clinicians offer pharmacologic treatment with alendronate, risedronate, zoledronic acid, or denosumab to reduce the risk for hip and vertebral fractures in women who have known osteoporosis. Individual patient factors and cost help decide which agent is initially used. Bisphosphonates are the most commonly prescribed first-line therapy as they have been shown to reduce the risk of fractures in large, randomized, placebo-controlled trials, and are generally well tolerated with low risk for serious adverse effects.

Although calcitonin increases spine bone mineral density in clinical trials, its anti-fracture efficacy is inconsistent at the spine. The availability of intravenous bisphosphonates and denosumab negates the argument for calcitonin in patients who cannot tolerate oral osteoporosis medications.

Denosumab is effective for prevention of vertebral fracture in postmenopausal women, yet it is expensive and, once started, should be continued indefinitely. Even if followed by intravenous bisphosphonate therapy, discontinuation results in loss of bone mineral density and has been associated with an increased risk of vertebral fracture. Denosumab may be

used safely in the setting of compromised kidney function (KDIGO stage G3b and G4). It may also be preferred in patients with poor adherence or tolerance of oral bisphosphonates.

Raloxifene is approved in postmenopausal women for the prevention and treatment of osteoporosis and the prevention of invasive breast cancer in those at high risk. However, raloxifene is contraindicated in those at increased risk of venous thromboembolism. ACP recommends against raloxifene for the treatment of osteoporosis in women.

Teriparatide and abaloparatide are anabolic therapies that reduce the risk of vertebral fracture in postmenopausal osteoporosis. Each increases bone mass and strength of the spine more than antiresorptive drugs and may be preferred if spine bone mineral density is severely low (T-score ≤ –3.5), in patients who fail bisphosphonate therapy, and in glucocorticoid-induced osteoporosis. Neither drug should be prescribed for patients who are at increased risk for osteosarcoma including those with a history of radiation therapy.

**KEY POINT**

- Alendronate, risedronate, zoledronic acid, and denosumab have been shown to reduce the risk for spine, hip, and nonvertebral fractures, and are generally well tolerated with low risk for serious adverse effects.

**Bibliography**

Qaseem A, Forciea MA, McLean RM, Denberg TD; Clinical Guidelines Committee of the American College of Physicians. Treatment of low bone density or osteoporosis to prevent fractures in men and women: A Clinical Practice Guideline Update From the American College of Physicians. Ann Intern Med. 2017;166:818-839. [PMID: 28492856] doi:10.7326/M15-1361

## Item 54    Answer:    C

**Educational Objective:** Manage medication-related hypoglycemia.

The most appropriate management of hypoglycemia for this patient is to stop glyburide therapy. Hypoglycemia can become a rate-limiting step in achieving glycemic goals for many persons. Clinicians should consider de-intensifying pharmacologic therapy in patients with type 2 diabetes who achieve hemoglobin $A_{1c}$ levels less than 6.5%; furthermore, benefits of targeting a specific hemoglobin $A_{1c}$ target level in patients with a life expectancy less than 10 years due to advanced age should be considered carefully because the harms outweigh the benefits in this population. Therapies must be adjusted to eliminate hypoglycemia, and glycemic goals should be individualized to accommodate targets that can be safely achieved. Several factors contribute to hypoglycemia including a mismatch of food consumption and insulin delivery, increased physical exertion, weight loss, worsening kidney impairment, abnormalities in gastrointestinal motility and absorption, and accidental/intentional overdose of insulin or other hypoglycemic agents such as sulfonylureas. Older adults are also at an increased risk for hypoglycemia. Sulfonylureas stimulate insulin secretion regardless of glycemic status. Thus, they pose risk for hypoglycemia, especially in drugs with long half-lives, such as glyburide, or in older persons. In light of this patient's age, kidney impairment, and frequency of hypoglycemia, glyburide should be stopped.

Immediate carbohydrate intake is the appropriate management of hypoglycemia in the alert individual; consumption of 15 grams of a fast-acting carbohydrate followed by a self-monitored blood glucose measurement 15 minutes later with repeat treatment if glucose is not improved. In this obese male, increased carbohydrate intake is not the appropriate way to manage this situation on a long-term basis as it can lead to further weight gain and increased insulin resistance.

If this patient was to remain on therapy that can induce hypoglycemia, glucagon should be prescribed. Glucagon should be provided to patients at risk for developing hypoglycemia and used intramuscularly by close contacts if the individual is not able to safely consume carbohydrates to correct hypoglycemia.

Metformin is the recommended first-line oral agent for type 2 diabetes due to known effectiveness and decreased hypoglycemia risk. Although this patient has a degree of kidney impairment, it is not such that metformin needs to be discontinued. After consideration of the risk and benefits, cautious continuation of metformin in kidney impairment may occur with an estimated glomerular filtration rate (eGFR) between 30 and 45 mL/min/1.73 m². Metformin should be discontinued if the eGFR falls below 30 mL/min/1.73 m².

### KEY POINT

- Sulfonylureas stimulate insulin secretion, and they pose risk for hypoglycemia, especially drugs with long half-lives, such as glyburide, or in older persons.

### Bibliography

Qaseem A, Wilt TJ, Kansagara D, Horwitch C, Barry MJ, Forciea MA, et al. Hemoglobin A$_{1c}$ targets for glycemic control with pharmacologic therapy for nonpregnant adults with type 2 diabetes mellitus: a guidance statement update from tthe American College of Physicians. Ann Intern Med. [Epub ahead of print 6 March 2018]:. doi: 10.7326/M17-0939

### Item 55    Answer:    D

**Educational Objective:** Recognize medications that interfere with screening for primary aldosteronism.

Spironolactone can significantly interfere with interpretation of the plasma aldosterone-plasma renin ratio (ARR) and therefore should be discontinued approximately 6 weeks prior to screening for primary aldosteronism. Treatment-resistant hypertension is defined as blood pressure that remains above goal despite concurrent use of three antihypertensive agents of different classes, one of which is a diuretic. Possible situations in which screening for secondary causes of hypertension include: severe or resistant hypertension; young age of onset (in childhood or adolescence), especially in the absence of family history; abrupt worsening of blood pressure in a previously well-controlled patient; or clinical

features of an underlying disorder associated with hypertension (for example, cushingoid features). Hyperaldosteronism, usually from an aldosterone-producing adenoma or bilateral idiopathic hyperaldosteronism, may be present in up to 10% of patients with hypertension. Testing for primary aldosteronism should be considered in all patients with difficult to control hypertension. It should also be performed in patients with hypertension and an incidentally noted adrenal mass or spontaneous or diuretic-induced hypokalemia. Spironolactone and eplerenone cause elevation of renin levels and hence can result in a false-negative ARR. On stopping a mineralocorticoid antagonist, the patient may develop hypokalemia if the underlying diagnosis is primary aldosteronism. Potassium should be replaced accordingly prior to screening for primary aldosteronism, as hypokalemia results in lowering of aldosterone levels and hence impacts the ARR.

In general, most antihypertensive agents can be continued during screening for primary aldosteronism except for spironolactone, eplerenone, and high-dose amiloride therapy. Specifically, verapamil, doxazosin, and hydralazine have minimal impact on the ARR and, therefore, can be continued during screening for primary aldosteronism.

Other antihypertensive agents that have minor effects on the ARR can also be continued during screening for primary aldosteronism as long as the results of the ARR are interpreted with these effects in mind. The hallmark of primary aldosteronism is a suppressed renin level. Any medication that increases renin can result in a false-negative result. On the other hand, a suppressed renin in the presence of a medication that usually would raise renin (an ACE inhibitor) raises the suspicion for primary aldosteronism.

### KEY POINT

- Spironolactone and eplerenone can significantly interfere with interpretation of the plasma aldosterone-plasma renin ratio (ARR) and therefore should be discontinued approximately 6 weeks prior to screening for primary aldosteronism.

### Bibliography

Funder JW, Carey RM, Mantero F, Murad MH, Reincke M, Shibata H, et al. The management of primary aldosteronism: case detection, diagnosis, and treatment: an Endocrine Society Clinical Practice Guideline. J Clin Endocrinol Metab. 2016;101:1889-916. [PMID: 26934393] doi:10.1210/jc.2015-4061

### Item 56    Answer:    C

**Educational Objective:** Manage type 2 diabetes mellitus by individualizing glycemic targets.

This patient is an older adult with a complex/intermediate medical history. The American Diabetes Association (ADA) defines complex/intermediate medical history as the presence of at least three coexisting chronic illnesses serious enough to require medications or lifestyle management and may include arthritis, cancer, heart failure, depression, emphysema, falls, hypertension, incontinence, stage 3 or worse chronic kidney disease, myocardial infarction, and stroke. These patients are expected to have "intermediate life-expectancy," high treatment burden, hypoglycemia vulnerability, and fall risk. The ADA's recommended hemoglobin $A_{1c}$ goal for a patient with similar characteristics and health status is 7.5% to 8%, if this can be achieved without significant hypoglycemia. Tighter glycemic control in this scenario would likely require an escalation in treatment burden with a subsequent increase in risks that may outweigh any potential long-term benefits. Additionally, the patient's reduced kidney function increases his hypoglycemia risk with more intense glycemic goals. The American College of Physicians (ACP) recommends that clinicians avoid targeting an hemoglobin $A_{1c}$ level in patients with a life expectancy less than 10 years due to advanced age (80 years or older), residence in a nursing home, or chronic conditions (such as dementia, cancer, end-stage kidney disease, severe chronic obstructive pulmonary disease, or heart failure) because the harms outweigh the benefits in this population.

Intensive glycemic control early in the disease course in patients with type 2 diabetes may decrease the incidence of long-term cardiovascular events, as suggested from the 10-year follow-up from the UK Prospective Diabetes Study (UKPDS). Similar reductions in cardiovascular disease did not occur when tight glycemic control was applied to older adults with long-standing type 2 diabetes with prior cardiovascular events or cardiovascular risk factors in three landmark studies: Action to Control Cardiovascular Risk on Diabetes (ACCORD), Action in Diabetes and Vascular Disease: Preterax and Diamicron Modified Release Controlled Evaluation (ADVANCE), and Veterans Affairs Diabetes Trial (VADT). In addition, subjects in the intensive treatment arms had increased rates of hypoglycemia in all three studies and a higher rate of death in the ACCORD trial.

In an older healthy adult with little comorbidity, intact cognitive and functional status, the ADA recommends a hemoglobin $A_{1c}$ goal of less than 7.5% given the expected longer life expectancy for that person. This patient does not meet these criteria. In contrast, the ACP recommends hemoglobin $A_{1c}$ level between 7% and 8% in most patients with type 2 diabetes based on lack of mortality benefit for death or macrovascular events over 5 to 10 years and risk in substantial harms.

In patients with complex or poor health, a hemoglobin $A_{1c}$ level less than 8.5% is recommended by the ADA, if it can be achieved without significant hypoglycemia. The ADA defines very complex or poor health requiring residence in a long-term care facility or end-stage chronic illnesses (stage 3–4 heart failure, oxygen-dependent lung disease, chronic kidney disease requiring dialysis, or uncontrolled metastatic cancer), moderate to severe cognitive impairment, or two or more activity of daily living dependencies.

Hemoglobin $A_{1c}$ targets greater than 8.5% are generally not recommended due to an increased risk for hyperglycemia-related complications, such as dehydration from glycosuria, infections, and hyperglycemic hyperosmolar syndrome.

**KEY POINT**

- A hemoglobin $A_{1c}$ goal of 7.5% to 8% is recommended for older adults with complex medical history and significant comorbidities.

**Bibliography**

American Diabetes Association. 11. Older adults: Standards of Medical Care in Diabetes-2018. Diabetes Care. 2018;41(Suppl 1):S119–S125. doi:10.2337/dc18-S011. [PMID: 29222382]

## Item 57          Answer:    A

**Educational Objective:** Diagnose ipilimumab-induced hypophysitis.

In this patient, the most likely cause of pituitary enlargement and evidence of hypopituitarism is drug-induced hypophysitis. Ipilimumab is a checkpoint inhibitor that has been repeatedly associated with the development of hypophysitis in up to 17% of treated patients. Most patients present with the combination of headache, pituitary enlargement, and hypopituitarism occurring during the early phase of therapy, typically within 10 weeks. While the pituitary enlargement often resolves spontaneously, the panhypopituitarism appears to be permanent.

Lymphocytic hypophysitis is an autoimmune disease most commonly occurring in women during pregnancy and postpartum. It leads to pituitary enlargement, possible mass effect, and often deficiency of adrenocorticotropic hormone (ACTH). While the imaging and laboratory characteristics described could be consistent with lymphocytic hypophysitis, the patient's exposure to a drug known to cause hypophysitis and other aspects of the clinical history are not consistent with this diagnosis.

A pituitary adenoma is less likely given the homogeneous enhancement on MRI. Pituitary adenomas are usually evident on MRI after contrast administration. They appear as a relatively nonenhancing lesion within a homogeneously enhancing pituitary gland. This patient's MRI is not consistent with a pituitary adenoma.

Untreated primary hypothyroidism can cause pituitary enlargement due to thyrotroph hyperplasia and can mimic a pituitary adenoma. This patient's low thyroid-stimulating hormone and free thyroxine levels do not support a diagnosis of primary hypothyroidism.

**KEY POINT**

- Checkpoint inhibitors such as nivolumab, ipilimumab, and pembrolizumab have been associated with the development of hypophysitis with most patients presenting with the combination of headache, pituitary enlargement, and hypopituitarism.

**Bibliography**

Byun DJ, Wolchok JD, Rosenberg LM, Girotra M. Cancer immunotherapy - immune checkpoint blockade and associated endocrinopathies. Nat Rev Endocrinol. 2017;13:195–207. [PMID: 28106152] doi:10.1038/nrendo.2016.205

## Item 58      Answer:      B

**Educational Objective:** Treat a large, indeterminate adrenal mass.

The most appropriate next step in management is adrenalectomy. The patient presented with an incidental adrenal mass with radiologic features that are indeterminate for adenoma and may indicate an adrenal malignancy (size >4 cm, density ≥10 Hounsfield units, and absolute contrast washout <50% at 10 minutes). Benign adrenal adenomas tend to be small (<4 cm), often have an intracytoplasmic fat content and appear less dense on noncontrast CT scan (<10 Hounsfield units), and exhibit rapid contrast washout during delayed contrast imaging (>50% at 10 minutes). These radiologic features are not diagnostic of malignancy, as one-third of benign adrenal masses are lipid poor (≥10 Hounsfield units) and many are larger than 4 cm. However, because adrenal carcinoma is an aggressive tumor and data indicate that prognosis may be more favorable when the disease is diagnosed and treated at an earlier stage, adrenalectomy is usually recommended.

Adrenal biopsy is not routinely indicated in the diagnostic evaluation of an incidentally discovered adrenal mass, even if the suspected diagnosis is primary adrenal malignancy, because adrenocortical carcinoma can be missed due to sampling error. Adrenal biopsy may be indicated when adrenal metastasis or an infiltrative disorder such as infection or lymphoma is suspected. Screening for pheochromocytoma should be performed prior to adrenal biopsy to avoid potential hypertensive crisis during the procedure.

Mitotane, an adrenolytic drug, may be used as adjuvant therapy following primary resection. Adrenalectomy is the first-line treatment of choice for patients with suspected adrenocortical carcinoma.

Repeat abdominal CT imaging at 6 months is suggested for adrenal masses that are small (<4 cm) and have benign radiologic features. The optimal time to repeat CT imaging in the radiologically benign-appearing, or even indeterminate-appearing, incidentally noted adrenal mass, is controversial. Repeat CT imaging is not indicated in this patient with high-risk features for adrenal carcinoma.

### KEY POINT

- Adrenalectomy is recommended for incidental adrenal masses with radiologic features that suggest increased risk of an adrenal malignancy (size >4 cm, density ≥10 Hounsfield units, and absolute contrast washout <50% at 10 minutes).

### Bibliography

Fassnacht M, Arlt W, Bancos I, Dralle H, Newell-Price J, Sahdev A, et al. Management of adrenal incidentalomas: European Society of Endocrinology Clinical Practice Guideline in collaboration with the European Network for the Study of Adrenal Tumors. Eur J Endocrinol. 2016;175:G1-G34. [PMID: 27390021] doi:10.1530/EJE-16-0467

## Item 59      Answer:      C

**Educational Objective:** Diagnose hypomagnesemia as the cause of hypocalcemia.

The most appropriate test to perform next is measurement of magnesium. Hypocalcemia is likely the result of hypoparathyroidism, which is most commonly caused by surgical injury. Autoimmune, infiltrative (hemochromatosis, Wilson disease, granulomas), and radiation-related injury can also cause acquired hypoparathyroidism. Other, less common causes of hypocalcemia include poor calcium intake, activating mutations in the calcium-sensing receptor (*CASR*) gene, parathyroid hormone (PTH) resistance, increased phosphate binding in vascular space (rhabdomyolysis or tumor lysis syndrome), increased citrate chelation with large volume blood transfusions, sepsis, vitamin D deficiency, and hypomagnesemia. Low levels of magnesium (due to medications, alcohol abuse, or malnutrition) activate G-proteins that stimulate calcium-sensing receptors and decrease PTH secretion. Functional hypoparathyroidism due to hypomagnesemia must be excluded before other diagnoses are pursued. Hypomagnesemia to the extent required to cause hypoparathyroidism is most commonly due to medications impairing renal handling of magnesium including platinum-based chemotherapeutic agents. Prompt resolution of hypocalcemia following correction of hypomagnesemia confirms the diagnosis.

Measurement of serum bicarbonate would allow assessment of acid-base derangements. Acute respiratory alkalosis causes transient symptomatic hypocalcemia due to a rapid increase in the fraction of intravascular calcium bound to albumin. However, changes in blood pH due to metabolic alkalosis are relatively small and gradual, allowing prevention of hypocalcemia by an increase in parathyroid hormone. This patient has a more compelling reason for persistent hypocalcemia, and measurement of serum bicarbonate is not necessary.

Approximately 40% to 45% of the calcium in serum is bound to protein, principally albumin, although the physiologically active form of calcium is in an ionized (or free) state. In most patients with relatively normal serum albumin levels, the total calcium usually accurately reflects the ionized calcium fraction. In this case, the patient's albumin level is normal and the patient's symptoms correspond to the measured calcium level, therefore measurement of ionized calcium is not needed.

Given phosphorus homeostasis and calcium homeostasis are closely linked, changes in serum phosphorus concentration should be routinely explored when evaluating hypocalcemia. Even so, hyperparathyroidism rather than hypoparathyroidism would be present if the primary cause of hypocalcemia was due to hyperphosphatemia.

### KEY POINT

- Hypomagnesemia causes functional, reversible parathyroid hypofunction and must be excluded before a low or inappropriately normal parathyroid level is attributed to hypoparathyroidism.

**Bibliography**

Brandi ML, Bilezikian JP, Shoback D, Bouillon R, Clarke BL, Thakker RV, Khan AA, Potts JT Jr. Management of hypoparathyroidism: summary statement and guidelines. J Clin Endocrinol Metab. 2016;101:2273-83. doi:10.1210/jc.2015-3907. [PMID: 26943719]

## Item 60          Answer:     C

**Educational Objective:** Treat type 2 diabetes mellitus in a patient with chronic kidney disease.

The most appropriate treatment of this patient's diabetes mellitus is to initiate metformin. This patient's hemoglobin $A_{1c}$ is above goal despite lifestyle modifications, and his treatment plan should be intensified. The first-line therapy recommended by the American Diabetes Association in conjunction with lifestyle modifications for treatment of type 2 diabetes is metformin. Previously, metformin use was contraindicated at serum creatinine levels of 1.4 mg/dL (123.8 μmol/L) or higher in women and 1.5 mg/dL (132.6 μmol/L) or higher in men. However, in a recent update the FDA concluded that metformin is considered to be safe in those with an estimated glomerular filtration rate (eGFR) greater than 45 mL/min/1.73 m² and is contraindicated in those with an eGFR less than 30 mL/min/1.73 m². The FDA recommends not initiating metformin for patients with eGFR greater than 30 mL/min/1.73 m² to less than 45 mL/min/1.73 m², or alternately, initiating metformin at a reduced dose (50%) with frequent monitoring of kidney function (every 3 months). The patient qualifies metformin therapy and frequent monitoring with his current kidney function.

Empagliflozin, a sodium-glucose transporter-2 (SGLT2) inhibitor, is a second-line agent after metformin initiation. In addition, SGLT2 inhibitors may cause hypotension due to intravascular volume depletion, especially in patients with kidney impairment, and acute kidney injury has been reported with its use. The FDA advises that risk factors for acute kidney injury (hypovolemia, chronic kidney disease, heart failure, and use of diuretics, ACE inhibitors, angiotensin receptor blockers, or NSAIDs) be considered before initiating this class of drugs.

The sulfonylurea, glipizide, is a second-line agent after metformin initiation. Glipizide could be considered as part of dual therapy if the glycemic goal is not reached with metformin. While sulfonylureas are the least expensive oral agent to add to metformin, they are associated with an increased risk for hypoglycemia as well as weight gain as compared with other potential combination therapies.

Saxagliptin, a dipeptidyl peptidase-4 (DPP-4) inhibitor, is a second-line agent after metformin initiation. Saxagliptin could be considered as part of dual therapy if the glycemic goal is not reached with metformin. However, the FDA has warned that the DPP-4 inhibitors saxagliptin and alogliptin may increase the risk for heart failure, especially in patients who already have heart or kidney disease.

**KEY POINT**

- Metformin is considered to be safe in those with an estimate glomerular filtration rate (eGFR) greater than 45 mL/minute/1.73 m² and is contraindicated in those with an eGFR less than 30 mL/min/1.73 m².

**Bibliography**

Barry MJ, Humphrey LL, Qaseem A. Oral pharmacologic treatment of type 2 diabetes mellitus. Ann Intern Med. 2017;167:75-76. doi:10.7326/L17-0234. [PMID: 28672387]

## Item 61          Answer:     D

**Educational Objective:** Treat toxic adenoma with radioactive iodine.

The most appropriate management is radioactive iodine ($^{131}$I) therapy. The patient's examination findings and thyroid scintigraphy results are consistent with a diagnosis of toxic adenoma. Toxic adenoma and multinodular goiter are the second most common cause of hyperthyroidism overall and are most frequently seen in older adults. These autonomously functioning nodules synthesize and secrete thyroid hormones independent of thyroid-stimulating hormone (TSH) stimulation as a result of activating mutations of the TSH receptor or $G_{s\alpha}$. They are usually large and can be easily palpated on examination. First-line treatment options include radioactive iodine therapy or surgery. Radioactive iodine is the most commonly used first-line treatment. The radioisotope $^{131}$I emits both gamma and beta radiation. Gamma radiation can be detected by the camera to determine radioactive iodine uptake and create an image of the thyroid gland during thyroid scintigraphy, whereas beta radiation yields the therapeutic effect by triggering thyroid follicular cell death. If a patient has a particularly large goiter with compressive symptoms or if there is concern for malignancy, surgery is recommended as first-line therapy.

Autonomous nodules are associated with a very low risk of malignancy (<1%), and fine-needle aspiration biopsy is not indicated. If biopsy is performed, it frequently yields indeterminate cytology results, such as suspicion for follicular neoplasm, and generates inappropriate concern and unnecessary recommendations for follow-up examinations and biopsies.

Increasing the atenolol dosage and prescribing methimazole are also not the best management options. While β-blockers ameliorate adrenergic symptoms, they do not address the underlying cause. This patient has a normal heart rate and blood pressure on her current dose of atenolol, so increasing this further is not indicated.

Antithyroid drugs (methimazole) are not first line for managing hyperthyroidism because spontaneous remission does not occur and treatment would have to be continued indefinitely.

**KEY POINT**

- First-line therapy for toxic adenoma is radioactive iodine ($^{131}$I) therapy or surgery.

## Bibliography

Haugen BR, Alexander EK, Bible KC, Doherty GM, Mandel SJ, Nikiforov YE, Pacini F, Randolph GW, Sawka AM, Schlumberger M, Schuff KG, Sherman SI, Sosa JA, Steward DL, Tuttle RM, Wartofsky L. 2015 American Thyroid Association Management Guidelines for Adult Patients with Thyroid Nodules and Differentiated Thyroid Cancer: The American Thyroid Association Guidelines Task Force on Thyroid Nodules and Differentiated Thyroid Cancer. Thyroid. 2016;26:1-133. doi:10.1089/thy.2015.0020. [PMID: 26462967]

## Item 62          Answer:    A

**Educational Objective:** Screen for neuropathy and retinopathy in type 2 diabetes mellitus.

This patient requires a comprehensive foot examination and dilated eye examination. Patients with diabetes mellitus require monitoring for complications. A thorough foot examination should be done annually in patients with type 2 diabetes. Although this patient had an unremarkable visual foot inspection, he has not yet had a comprehensive foot examination, which is indicated at the time of diagnosis of type 2 diabetes and then annually thereafter. A comprehensive foot examination includes inspection of the skin, assessment of foot deformities, neurologic assessment (10-g monofilament testing with at least one other nerve assessment–pinprick, temperature, vibration, or ankle reflexes), and vascular assessment including pulses in the legs and feet. In patients with type 1 diabetes mellitus, a dilated comprehensive eye examination 5 years after diagnosis is appropriate; however, in patients with type 2 diabetes, a dilated comprehensive eye examination is indicated at time of diagnosis.

Prediabetes and diabetes can be diagnosed based on the elevated results from one of the following screening tests repeated on two separate occasions: fasting plasma glucose, 2-hour postprandial glucose during an oral glucose tolerance test, or hemoglobin $A_{1c}$. This patient has two abnormal hemoglobin $A_{1c}$ measurements and additional testing with a fasting plasma glucose test and oral glucose tolerance test for the purposes of diagnosis is not warranted.

Although long-term use of metformin may be associated with vitamin $B_{12}$ deficiency and periodic measurement of vitamin $B_{12}$ levels should be considered in metformin treatment patients, $B_{12}$ and folate measurements are not recommended at time of initiation of metformin therapy.

Annual screening for albuminuria in patients with type 2 diabetes should be undertaken starting at the time of diagnosis; this is done on a random spot urine sample as planned in this patient, not a 24-hour urine collection for protein and creatinine.

### KEY POINT

- Screening for dyslipidemia, hypertension, a dilated eye examination, spot urine albumin–creatinine ratio, and a comprehensive foot examination should be performed at the time of diagnosis of type 2 diabetes.

## Bibliography

American Diabetes Association. 10. Microvascular complications and foot care: Standards of Medical Care in Diabetes-2018. Diabetes Care. 2018;41(Suppl 1):S105-S118. doi: 10.2337/dc18-S010. [PMID: 29222381]

## Item 63          Answer:    D

**Educational Objective:** Diagnose hyperglycemia in a patient meeting preprandial glycemic targets.

Measuring postprandial blood glucose level is the most appropriate management of this patient's diabetes. This patient is healthy with few comorbidities. His preprandial blood glucose target is 80 to 130 mg/dL (4.4-7.2 mmol/L). Despite meeting his preprandial glycemic targets, his hemoglobin $A_{1c}$ level remains above his goal of less than 7%. Postprandial hyperglycemia has a greater effect on hemoglobin $A_{1c}$ when it is near 7%. Measuring postprandial blood glucose levels in this patient may identify undetected hyperglycemia that could be treated with an increase in his prandial insulin lispro dose.

Liraglutide is an injectable glucagon-like peptide-1 (GLP-1) receptor agonist with several mechanisms of action: slows gastric emptying, glucose-dependent increase in insulin secretion, and glucose-dependent suppression of glucagon secretion. Although liraglutide has the potential to aid with weight loss in this obese patient and improve his hemoglobin $A_{1c}$ to goal, adding another injectable agent to the regimen of a patient who is reluctant to do this does not take into consideration patient preferences. In addition, liraglutide has not been approved by the FDA for combination use with prandial insulin.

Continuing his current regimen will not allow him to achieve his target hemoglobin $A_{1c}$ goal. The American Diabetes Association recommends a hemoglobin $A_{1c}$ goal of less than 6.5% to 7% for healthy persons with type 2 diabetes mellitus with few comorbidities to decrease the incidence of diabetes-related complications in the future. The American College of Physicians (ACP) recommends a target hemoglobin $A_{1c}$ level between 7% and 8% for most patients with type 2 diabetes. ACP notes that more stringent targets may be appropriate for patients who have a long life expectancy (>15 years) and are interested in more intensive glycemic control despite the risk for harms.

The patient has reached the recommended preprandial glycemic goal of 80 to 130 mg/dL (4.4-7.2 mmol/L). Increasing his insulin detemir dose may increase his risk of developing hypoglycemia and would not adequately treat postprandial hyperglycemia that may be contributing to the elevated hemoglobin $A_{1c}$.

### KEY POINT

- Measuring postprandial blood glucose levels may identify undetected hyperglycemia when preprandial blood glucose values are at target goal, but the hemoglobin $A_{1c}$ is above goal.

**Bibliography**

American Diabetes Association. 6. Glycemic targets: Standards of Medical Care in Diabetes-2018. Diabetes Care. 2018;41(Suppl 1):S55–S64. doi:10.2337/dc18-S006. [PMID: 29222377]

## Item 64    Answer:    B

**Educational Objective:** Manage a patient with asymptomatic primary hyperparathyroidism.

The most appropriate management for this patient is to reassess the patient in 6 to 12 months. Guideline-recommended indications for parathyroidectomy include increase in serum calcium level ≥1 mg/dL (0.25 mmol/L) above upper limit of normal; creatinine clearance <60 mL/min, 24-hour urine calcium >400 mg/day (>10 mmol/day), or increased stone risk by biochemical stone risk analysis; presence of nephrolithiasis or nephrocalcinosis by radiograph, ultrasound, or CT; T-score (on DEXA scan) of less than or equal to -2.5 at any site or evidence of vertebral fracture; and age younger than 50 years. Parathyroidectomy is also indicated in patients in whom medical surveillance is neither desired nor possible, and those with complications of hyperparathyroidism including significant bone, kidney, gastrointestinal, or neuromuscular symptoms. Patients without indications for parathyroidectomy require periodic reassessment that includes serum calcium and creatinine every 6 to 12 months and bone mineral density of the lumbar spine, hip, and distal radius every 2 years.

Although imaging tests such as parathyroid sestamibi scan may be performed as part of evaluation of primary hyperparathyroidism, it is most appropriate once surgery is indicated. The results of imaging do not influence the management of nonsurgical patients.

Primary hyperparathyroidism is associated with increased bone turnover and decreased bone strength. Although alendronate suppresses bone resorption and improves bone mineral density at the lumbar spine in patients with primary hyperparathyroidism, it has not been shown to reduce fracture risk or to reduce serum calcium levels. Patients at high risk of fracture (T-score ≤-2.5 and/or prevalent fragility fracture) at presentation or during monitoring should undergo parathyroidectomy.

Cinacalcet is indicated to treat symptomatic, severe hypercalcemia in adults with primary hyperparathyroidism for whom parathyroidectomy cannot be performed. Although it may be used chronically, cinacalcet is more commonly used until surgery is feasible.

### KEY POINT

- Patients with primary hyperparathyroidism who do not undergo surgery require monitoring of serum calcium and creatinine every 6 to 12 months and bone mineral density of the lumbar spine, hip, and distal radius every 2 years.

**Bibliography**

Bilezikian JP, Brandi ML, Eastell R, Silverberg SJ, Udelsman R, Marcocci C, et al. Guidelines for the management of asymptomatic primary hyperparathyroidism: summary statement from the Fourth International Workshop. J Clin Endocrinol Metab. 2014;99:3561-9. [PMID: 25162665] doi:10.1210/jc.2014-1413

## Item 65    Answer:    E

**Educational Objective:** Manage subclinical hypothyroidism.

This patient has subclinical hypothyroidism, and the most appropriate management is to repeat serum thyroid-stimulating hormone (TSH) testing in 2 months. Free thyroxine ($T_4$) and thyroid peroxide antibodies could also be measured at that time. Subclinical hypothyroidism is an early form of primary hypothyroidism affecting up to 10% of the population and is characterized by a serum TSH level above the upper limit of the reference range and normal free $T_4$ level. Before making this diagnosis; however, transient elevation of serum TSH levels should be ruled out by repeating the measurement of TSH in 2 to 3 months.

Thyroid peroxidase (TPO) antibodies are frequently seen in the setting of Hashimoto thyroiditis, the most common cause of hypothyroidism in the United States. TPO antibody positivity would support a diagnosis of primary hypothyroidism, predict risk of progression to overt hypothyroidism, and may impact treatment decisions accordingly. However, the most appropriate next step in the management of this patient is to confirm the diagnosis of subclinical hypothyroidism by documenting persistent serum TSH elevation.

Thyrotropin receptor antibodies would be more consistent with Graves disease and testing for these antibodies would not be appropriate in this setting.

Measurement of serum triiodothyronine ($T_3$) in patients with known or suspected primary hypothyroidism is generally not indicated. Elevation of serum TSH is the earliest biochemical change observed in the setting of primary hypothyroidism. Reductions in serum $T_3$ are not usually seen until after free $T_4$ levels are low. Measuring serum $T_3$ has little to no impact on diagnosis or management decisions.

More severe subclinical hypothyroidism, serum TSH greater than 10 µU/mL (10 mU/L), may increase the risk of coronary artery disease and heart failure, whereas serum TSH levels below 7 to 10 µU/mL (7–10 mU/L) are not associated with increased morbidity or mortality. Treatment with levothyroxine would be considered if the patient's serum TSH is similar or higher on reassessment, but this is not the most appropriate next step in management.

### KEY POINT

- Subclinical hypothyroidism is characterized by a serum thyroid-stimulating hormone (TSH) level above the upper limit of the reference range and normal free thyroxine ($T_4$) level; before making this diagnosis, however, transient elevation of serum TSH should be ruled out by repeating the measurement of TSH in 2 to 3 months.

**Bibliography**

Peeters RP. Subclinical hypothyroidism. N Engl J Med. 2017 Jun 29; 376(26):2556–2565. doi: 10.1056/NEJMcp1611144. [PMID: 28657873]

## Item 66      Answer:      A

**Educational Objective:** **Diagnose the cause of primary aldosteronism.**

The next step in this patient's management is adrenal vein sampling. Once the diagnosis of primary aldosteronism has been confirmed biochemically, radiographic localization with abdominal CT is indicated. CT is recommended over MRI in most cases due to similar efficacy and lower cost. Adrenal hyperplasia and adenomas secreting excess aldosterone, however, may not always be visualized. Adrenal vein sampling is, therefore, needed in most patients to determine the source of aldosterone secretion when imaging is unrevealing and to confirm lateralization when imaging demonstrates an adrenal adenoma, such as in this case. Adrenal vein sampling is especially important in older patients because of a higher frequency of nonfunctioning adrenal incidentalomas. Patients with an aldosterone-secreting adenoma are usually offered adrenalectomy, whereas those with primary aldosteronism due to bilateral adrenal hyperplasia are treated medically. Omission of adrenal vein sampling can lead to misdiagnosis in approximately 25% of cases, and subsequent unnecessary adrenalectomy, or medical therapy when adrenalectomy could be offered. Right adrenalectomy should not be performed in this patient without further confirmation of the source of primary aldosteronism.

Aldosterone likely exerts direct toxic effects on cardiac cells as evidenced by a higher prevalence of left ventricular hypertrophy and decreased left ventricular function when compared with matched control patients with similar levels of hypertension. These deleterious effects are likely mediated by mineralocorticoid receptors in the heart, coronary arteries, aorta, and other blood vessels. Increasing this patient's losartan or metoprolol dose may lead to better control of his hypertension, but neither of these medications blocks the aldosterone receptor. Therefore, the patient would still be subject to the deleterious effects of excess stimulation of aldosterone receptors, which may lead to cardiac disease.

**KEY POINT**

• Most patients with biochemically confirmed primary aldosteronism should undergo adrenal vein sampling to confirm the source of the hyperaldosteronism.

**Bibliography**

Rossi GP, Auchus RJ, Brown M, Lenders JW, Naruse M, Plouin PF, et al. An expert consensus statement on use of adrenal vein sampling for the subtyping of primary aldosteronism. Hypertension. 2014;63:151–60. [PMID: 24218436] doi:10.1161/HYPERTENSIONAHA.113.02097

## Item 67      Answer:      D

**Educational Objective:** **Evaluate a thyroid nodule with neck ultrasonography.**

The most appropriate diagnostic test to perform next is ultrasound of the neck. Ultrasound can confirm the presence of thyroid nodules palpated on examination and those detected on other imaging studies. Ultrasound must be performed prior to fine-needle aspiration biopsy (FNAB) to confirm the presence of a nodule, determine that biopsy is indicated, ensure that there are no additional nonpalpable nodules that warrant FNAB, and assess the cervical lymph nodes. In patients with solitary palpable nodules, 15% will have no corresponding nodule on ultrasound, and a similar proportion will have an additional nodule measuring 1 cm or larger.

Performing a CT scan of the neck is a more costly test, exposes the patient to unnecessary radiation, and is inferior to ultrasound at assessing the thyroid gland.

FNAB should not be performed prior to thyroid/neck ultrasound. Whether or not FNAB is indicated depends on the size and sonographic appearance of the nodule, clinical risk factors for malignancy, and presence of pathologic lymph nodes. Nodules that are predominantly cystic or posteriorly located within the thyroid gland are prone to sampling error.

Measurement of serum thyroid-stimulating hormone (TSH) is also part of the initial evaluation of a thyroid nodule. The purpose of measuring TSH is to evaluate for the presence of autonomously functioning or "hot" nodules, which account for 5% to 10% of palpable thyroid nodules. Autonomous nodules may cause hyperthyroidism and are associated with a very low risk of malignancy. Autonomous nodules can be confirmed by performing a thyroid uptake and scan. They concentrate radioactive iodine to a greater extent than normal thyroid tissue, which shows absent or diminished uptake. The TSH in this patient is normal, which does not support a diagnosis of an autonomously functioning thyroid nodule; therefore performing a thyroid uptake and $^{131}$I scan is not indicated.

**KEY POINT**

• Ultrasound can confirm the presence of thyroid nodules palpated on examination and based on findings can help to determine if fine-needle aspiration is needed to assess for malignancy.

**Bibliography**

Haugen BR, Alexander EK, Bible KC, Doherty GM, Mandel SJ, Nikiforov YE, et al. 2015 American Thyroid Association Management Guidelines for Adult Patients with Thyroid Nodules and Differentiated Thyroid Cancer: The American Thyroid Association Guidelines Task Force on Thyroid Nodules and Differentiated Thyroid Cancer. Thyroid. 2016;26:1–133. [PMID: 26462967] doi:10.1089/thy.2015.0020

## Item 68      Answer:      B

**Educational Objective:** **Manage secondary hypothyroidism.**

The most appropriate next step in management is measurement of the free thyroxine ($T_4$) level. Thyroid-stimulating hormone (TSH) deficiency leads to secondary or central hypothyroidism. Secondary hypothyroidism symptoms are clinically identical to primary hypothyroidism symptoms. Secondary hypothyroidism is diagnosed by demonstrating a simultaneously inappropriately normal or low TSH and low $T_4$ (free or total). Patients are treated with levothyroxine replacement in the same manner as primary hypothyroidism; however, the serum TSH cannot be used to monitor and assess for adequacy of thyroid hormone replacement dosing. Instead, the levothyroxine dose is adjusted based on free $T_4$ levels with the goal of obtaining a value within the normal reference range. The patient's recent symptoms of fatigue and weight gain may be due to hypothyroidism resulting from impaired absorption of levothyroxine after recently starting a calcium supplement. A low $T_4$ level will confirm the diagnosis. In general the therapeutic goal is to keep the free $T_4$ in the upper half of the normal range. To improve gastrointestinal absorption, levothyroxine should be taken on an empty stomach, 1 hour before or 3 hours after ingestion of food. Medications that would interfere with absorption, such as calcium- or iron-containing supplements should be separated by 4 hours.

Increasing the levothyroxine would not be appropriate without first documenting the presence of hypothyroidism by measuring the $T_4$ level. In addition, the preferred initial therapy may simply be to discontinue the calcium, if not warranted, or to separate ingestion of calcium and levothyroxine by at least 2 to 3 hours.

The patient has no symptoms suggestive of a pituitary mass effect or other indication to recommend pituitary imaging.

### KEY POINT

- Serum thyroid-stimulating hormone level cannot be used to monitor and assess for adequacy of thyroid hormone replacement dosing in secondary hypothyroidism; the levothyroxine dose is adjusted based on free thyroxine ($T_4$) levels with the goal of obtaining a value within the upper half of the normal reference range.

### Bibliography

Beck-Peccoz P, Rodari G, Giavoli C, Lania A. Central hypothyroidism - a neglected thyroid disorder. Nat Rev Endocrinol. 2017;13:588-598. doi:10.1038/nrendo.2017.47. Epub 2017 May 26. [PMID: 28549061]

### Item 69     Answer:    A

**Educational Objective:** Treat hypoglycemic unawareness.

The most appropriate treatment of this patient's diabetes is to decrease all insulin doses. He is having hypoglycemia at least once per week with some of these events qualifying as clinically significant per the American Diabetes Association with glucose values less than 54 mg/dL (3.0 mmol/L). He is developing hypoglycemia unawareness as evidenced by his inability to detect decreases in his blood glucose until it is less than 40 mg/dL (2.2 mmol/L). This is secondary to an ineffective response of the autonomic system to hypoglycemia, in addition to an inadequate release of counterregulatory hormones to correct hypoglycemia. Blood glucose targets should be relaxed, and insulin dosing should be decreased in the setting of hypoglycemia unawareness. Avoidance of hypoglycemia for

several weeks may restore the ability to detect hypoglycemia in some patients. Since the hypoglycemia is intermittent and without a pattern for this patient, all insulin doses should be decreased to avoid hypoglycemia.

The patient has fasting hyperglycemia and a hemoglobin $A_{1c}$ level above goal. Increasing the dose of his glargine insulin could lower his glucose values, but it may potentially exacerbate his hypoglycemia.

Empagliflozin could improve this patient's hyperglycemia while also improving his blood pressure control and inducing weight loss; however, it may also exacerbate the hypoglycemia when used in conjunction with insulin.

Metformin could improve hyperglycemia for this patient, particularly fasting hyperglycemia secondary to hepatic gluconeogenesis. Given the clinically significant hypoglycemia experienced by this patient, that should be addressed first by relaxing his glycemic goals.

### KEY POINT

- Treatment for hypoglycemic unawareness is to reduce the insulin dose and avoid hypoglycemia in order to provide the body an opportunity to restore the ability to detect hypoglycemia.

### Bibliography

American Diabetes Association. 6. Glycemic targets: Standards of Medical Care in Diabetes-2018. Diabetes Care. 2018;41(Suppl 1):S55-S64. doi:10.2337/dc18-S006. [PMID: 29222377]

### Item 70     Answer:    A

**Educational Objective:** Avoid inappropriate screening for osteoporosis.

The most appropriate management for this patient is lifestyle counseling for osteoporosis prevention. Lifestyle measures include adequate calcium and vitamin D, exercise, smoking cessation, counseling on fall prevention, and avoidance of heavy alcohol use.

Most guidelines recommend screening for osteoporosis with dual-energy x-ray absorptiometry (DEXA) scan in women 65 years of age and older. Screening of younger women may be indicated if one or more risk factors for osteoporosis are present. In premenopausal women without risk factors, assessment of bone mineral density (BMD) for fracture risk is not advised or validated. However, if testing is done in an otherwise healthy person, such as this patient, results that are below age- and gender-matched averages (Z-score <0) generally do not require further evaluation or serial monitoring. The discovery of below average BMD could lead to a discussion regarding osteoporosis prevention with lifestyle modification and assessment of BMD after menopause, but prior to age 65, when screening might otherwise occur.

Testing for secondary causes of bone loss is unnecessary when BMD is normal for age. Below average BMD in adults may in fact represent below average peak bone mass rather than loss of bone.

Although BMD measured by quantitative heel ultrasound is predictive of osteoporotic fracture in older women and men, BMD measurement by DEXA scan remains the gold standard for diagnosis of osteoporosis and fracture risk assessment. Therefore, abnormal ultrasound results in these populations should be confirmed by DEXA scan. Even so, a DEXA scan should not be performed in this patient given that screening is not indicated and the heel ultrasound result is within the normal range.

**KEY POINT**

- Screening for osteoporosis in premenopausal women is not indicated in the absence of risk factors.

**Bibliography**

Cosman F, de Beur SJ, LeBoff MS, Lewiecki EM, Tanner B, Randall S, et al; National Osteoporosis Foundation. Clinician's guide to prevention and treatment of osteoporosis. Osteoporos Int. 2014;25:2359-81. [PMID: 25182228] doi:10.1007/s00198-014-2794-2

## Item 71      Answer:   D

**Educational Objective:** Diagnose methimazole-induced agranulocytosis.

The most appropriate management is to stop methimazole and order a complete blood count with differential. The patient has been receiving methimazole for treatment of Graves hyperthyroidism over the past 3 months. She has both a sore throat and a fever, which can be seen in patients with methimazole-induced agranulocytosis. Agranulocytosis affects between one in 300 and one in 500 patients taking antithyroid drug therapy. Agranulocytosis from methimazole usually occurs within the first several months of initiating therapy but generally is not seen with doses below 20 mg per day. Suspected agranulocytosis should be managed with cessation of the offending drug and assessment of the patient's neutrophil count. An absolute neutrophil count below 500/μL $(0.5 \times 10^9/L)$ confirms the diagnosis. Management of agranulocytosis may include hospitalization, broad-spectrum antibiotics, and hematopoietic growth factor therapy. Patients should be counseled regarding agranulocytosis as a potential side effect at the initiation of therapy and instructed to contact the prescribing physician immediately with occurrence of any suggestive symptoms.

Diagnosis and treatment of patients with Group A streptococcus (GAS) pharyngitis has traditionally been aided by the four-point Centor criteria: (1) fever, (2) absence of cough, (3) tonsillar exudates, and (4) tender anterior cervical lymphadenopathy. The Centor criteria have a low positive predictive value for GAS infection; according to the Infectious Disease Society of America, these criteria may be used to determine which patients have a low likelihood of GAS pharyngitis and require no further testing. No additional testing or treatment is needed for patients who meet fewer than three criteria. Patients who meet three or more criteria should have a confirmatory test (either a rapid antigen detection test for GAS or throat culture). Penicillin or amoxicillin is first-line

treatment for GAS pharyngitis. However, the clinical situation of most immediate concern is the possibility of methimazole-induced agranulocytosis, a potentially fatal condition. The most appropriate management is to stop the drug and measure the neutrophil count.

**KEY POINT**

- Antithyroid drug-related agranulocytosis affects between one in 300 and one in 500 patients taking therapy and may present with fever and sore throat; initial management includes stopping the drug and assessment of the neutrophil count.

**Bibliography**

Vicente N, Cardoso L, Barros L, Carrilho F. Antithyroid drug-induced agranulocytosis: state of the art on diagnosis and management. Drugs R D. 2017;17:91-96. doi: 10.1007/s40268-017-0172-1. [PMID: 28105610]

## Item 72      Answer:   C

**Educational Objective:** Diagnose diabetic ketoacidosis associated with a sodium-glucose cotransporter 2 (SGLT2) inhibitor.

Sodium-glucose cotransporter 2 (SGLT2) inhibitors (canagliflozin, dapagliflozin, and empagliflozin) improve glycemia by increasing excretion of glucose by the kidney. SGLT2 is expressed in the proximal tubule and mediates reabsorption of approximately 90% of the filtered glucose load. SGLT2 inhibitors promote excretion of glucose by the kidneys and thereby modestly lower elevated blood glucose levels in patients with type 2 diabetes. Euglycemic diabetic ketoacidosis has been reported in patients with type 2 diabetes taking SGLT2 inhibitors. Because of this, the FDA issued a Drug Safety Communication that warns of an increased risk of diabetic ketoacidosis with uncharacteristically mild to moderate glucose elevations (euglycemic diabetic ketoacidosis) associated with the use of all the approved SGLT2 inhibitors. SGLT2 inhibitors should be discontinued in patients who develop acidosis on these agents.

Statins may cause myopathy and liver aminotransferase elevations and are associated with an increased risk of diabetes and, possibly, cognitive dysfunction. The incidence of these adverse effects ranges from 1% to 10%, but permanent disability related to statin intolerance is rare. Statin therapy is not associated with ketoacidosis.

According to labeling guidelines, initiation of metformin therapy is not recommended if the estimated glomerular filtration rate (eGFR) is between 30 and 45 mL/min/1.73 m² and is contraindicated if the eGFR is less than 30 mL/min/1.73 m² due to the risk of lactic acidosis. Metformin should be used cautiously in patients with heart failure or hepatic impairment. The discontinuation of metformin is not associated with the development of lactic acidosis or ketoacidosis.

Glipizide is a sulfonylurea. Sulfonylurea agents work by stimulating insulin secretion. Sulfonylurea agents are associated with weight gain, and they can cause hypoglycemia.

CONT.

They are not, however, associated with the development of ketoacidosis in patients with type 2 diabetes.

A common adverse effect of ACE inhibitors is a dry, non-productive cough. Other common adverse effects include hyperkalemia and, occasionally, worsening kidney function. ACE inhibitors can cause life-threatening angioedema but not ketoacidosis.

**KEY POINT**

- An increased risk of diabetic ketoacidosis with mild to moderate glucose elevations has been associated with the use of all the approved sodium-glucose transporter-2 (SGLT2) inhibitors (canagliflozin, dapagliflozin, and empagliflozin).

**Bibliography**

FDA Drug Safety Communication. FDA warns that SGLT2 inhibitors for diabetes may result in a serious condition of too much acid in the blood. May 15, 2015 https://www.fda.gov/downloads/drugs/drugsafety/ucm446954.pdf. Accessed March 1, 2018.

## Item 73    Answer:    B

**Educational Objective:** Evaluate secondary hypogonadism.

The most appropriate test for this patient is a pituitary MRI. With a low testosterone level and low serum luteinizing hormone (LH) and follicle-stimulating hormone (FSH) concentrations, this patient has secondary hypogonadism. Hyperprolactinemia is the most likely cause of his hypogonadism; hyperprolactinemia leads to secondary hypogonadism through suppression of gonadotropin-releasing hormone synthesis and secretion. This patient is on no medications that might cause hyperprolactinemia. In the absence of a culprit drug, the most likely cause of his hyperprolactinemia is a lactotroph adenoma; therefore a pituitary MRI is indicated.

A karyotype analysis is not indicated in the evaluation of secondary hypogonadism; however, it should be considered in men and women who have primary hypogonadism.

Anabolic steroid use will result in low or normal gonadotropin levels, a low testosterone level, and clinical evidence of hyperandrogenism such as excessive muscle bulk, acne, gynecomastia, and decreased testicular volume. Anabolic steroid abuse, however, would not cause hyperprolactinemia as seen in this patient.

Most patients with hereditary hemochromatosis are diagnosed in the presymptomatic phase when iron test results are abnormal. In patients with symptoms, clinical presentation varies and often includes nonspecific findings such as chronic fatigue, weakness, nonspecific abdominal pain, arthralgia, and elevated liver enzymes. Endocrine organs are commonly affected, and diabetes mellitus, hypothyroidism, and gonadal failure may occur. Laboratory evaluation of hemochromatosis-related gonadal failure most commonly demonstrates a hypogonadotropic state (low LH and FSH levels). While this patient is hypogonadotrophic, he has an elevated prolactin level, and a pituitary MRI is the best next diagnostic test.

Obesity results in decreased concentrations of sex hormone-binding globulin (SHBG); if SHBG is low, free testosterone should be measured in patients with low total testosterone concentrations. This patient is not obese and has evidence of secondary hypogonadism (low testosterone level and low serum LH and FSH concentrations), making determination of SHBG concentration unnecessary.

**KEY POINT**

- Secondary hypogonadism is characterized by low testosterone level and low or inappropriately normal serum luteinizing hormone and follicle-stimulating hormone concentrations; MRI of the pituitary is typically performed to evaluate secondary hypogonadism in the absence of obvious reversible causes such as drugs.

**Bibliography**

Basaria S. Male hypogonadism. Lancet. 2014;383:1250-63. [PMID: 24119423] doi:10.1016/S0140-6736(13)61126-5.

## Item 74    Answer:    A

**Educational Objective:** Treat myxedema coma.

The most appropriate next step in the management of this patient is to administer intravenous hydrocortisone. This patient has myxedema coma, which has a very high mortality rate if there is a delay in treatment. Myxedema coma is more common in elderly women; it may occur in those with a history of hypothyroidism or no antecedent illness. Myocardial infarction, infection, stroke, trauma, and gastrointestinal bleeding are common precipitating events. Mental status changes and hypothermia are the most common clinical manifestations. Ventilatory drive is decreased, resulting in hypoxemia and hypercapnia. Additional signs include bradycardia, hypoglycemia, hyponatremia, and/or hypotension. This patient's condition was likely precipitated by recent nonadherence with her prescribed medications. The serum cortisol level should be checked as soon as possible to evaluate for concomitant adrenal insufficiency prior to initiation of thyroid hormone replacement. While awaiting the results of the serum cortisol measurement, it is advisable to empirically initiate high-dose hydrocortisone. This therapy may be discontinued if the serum cortisol level is found to be normal or high. In patients with adrenal insufficiency, administering thyroid hormone prior to glucocorticoids could precipitate an adrenal crisis by augmenting cortisol metabolism.

Following the administration of glucocorticoids, intravenous thyroid hormone replacement should be initiated. Treatment with levothyroxine is universally recommended. Although controversial, some experts suggest administering liothyronine concomitantly. Once clinically improved, the patient can be transitioned to oral levothyroxine.

Hypotension can generally be resolved over a matter of hours with the administration of fluids and treatment of the hypothyroidism. Persistent hypotension can be treated

CONT.

with a vasopressor drug. The initiation of norepinephrine is premature in this patient.

**KEY POINT**

- In patients with myxedema coma, intravenous hydrocortisone should be administered before thyroid hormones to treat possible adrenal insufficiency.

**Bibliography**

Ono Y, Ono S, Yasunaga H, Matsui H, Fushimi K, Tanaka Y. Clinical characteristics and outcomes of myxedema coma: analysis of a national inpatient database in Japan. J Epidemiol. 2017 Mar;27(3):117-122. Epub 2017 Jan 5. PMID: 28142035.

## Item 75     Answer:     C

**Educational Objective:** Recognize limitations of hemoglobin $A_{1c}$ measurements.

The most appropriate management for this patient is to initiate ferrous sulfate. This patient has iron-deficiency anemia, a hypoproliferative anemia, which has been shown to erroneously increase the hemoglobin $A_{1c}$ level due to an increase in the proportion of older erythrocytes. Hemoglobin $A_{1c}$ testing measures hemoglobin glycation as a consequence of glucose exposure over the preceding 8 to 12 weeks. Given the patient's age and relatively few comorbidities, her goal hemoglobin $A_{1c}$ level should be less than 6.5% to 7%. Her hemoglobin $A_{1c}$ level is above this goal, but her fingerstick blood glucose data are within her fasting goal of 80 to 130 mg/dL (4.4-7.2 mmol/L) and within her 2-hour postprandial goal of less than 180 mg/dL (10 mmol/L) per the American Diabetes Association (ADA) guidelines. Initiating iron supplementation to correct her iron deficiency anemia will increase erythrocyte turnover and shift the proportion toward younger cells, thus allowing a more accurate measurement of glycemic exposure by the hemoglobin $A_{1c}$ to guide therapeutic decisions.

The patient's fasting blood glucose values are within her goal range of 80 to 130 mg/dL (4.4-7.2 mmol/L) per the ADA guidelines. Initiating basal insulin based solely on the elevated hemoglobin $A_{1c}$ value with her current fasting blood sugars will increase her risk of hypoglycemia. Similarly, the risk of hypoglycemia is increased by initiating empagliflozen. Increasing the accuracy of the hemoglobin $A_{1c}$ measurement by correcting her iron deficiency anemia should be addressed before considering other drug therapy.

Hemoglobin $A_{1c}$ measurements may be unreliable not only in the setting of anemia, but also in the presence of certain hemoglobinopathies or kidney or liver disease. For example, hemoglobin $A_{1c}$ values may be falsely elevated in patients with hemoglobin F or low with hemoglobin S. However, this patient has an explanation for the discordant hemoglobin $A_{1c}$ and blood glucose results, and the iron deficiency anemia should be the focus of management. Additionally, newer methods of measuring $A_{1c}$ are not altered by the presence of the most common hemoglobinopathies. Therefore, a hemoglobin electrophoresis is not indicated at this time.

**KEY POINT**

- Iron-deficiency anemia can erroneously increase the hemoglobin $A_{1c}$ level due to an increase in the proportion of older erythrocytes.

**Bibliography**

Sacks DB. A1C versus glucose testing: a comparison. Diabetes Care. 2011;34:518-23. [PMID: 21270207] doi:10.2337/dc10-1546

## Item 76     Answer:     D

**Educational Objective:** Treat low-risk papillary thyroid cancer.

No additional treatment is needed. The incidence of thyroid cancer has increased over the last four decades with much of this change attributable to a rise in the diagnosis of small noninvasive papillary thyroid carcinomas. The incidence of papillary microcarcinoma (<1 cm) is 5% to 15% in the United States based on autopsy series. Low-risk papillary thyroid cancer is that which is confined to the thyroid gland, completely resected at surgery, does not demonstrate aggressive pathologic features (lymphovascular invasion or tall cell variant), and has not metastasized. The risk of disease-related death is less than 1%, and the risk of structural disease recurrence is 1% to 2% for low-risk unifocal papillary microcarcinomas. Patients receiving either lobectomy or thyroidectomy have similarly excellent outcomes. Therefore, resection of the remaining thyroid lobe would not be required for this patient.

Suppression of thyroid-stimulating hormone (TSH) with levothyroxine therapy may also be used to improve morbidity and reduce mortality, particularly in patients with persistent disease or distant metastases. The necessary degree of TSH suppression varies according to the risk of cancer progression and comorbidities of the patient. Patients with persistent disease typically require lowering of their TSH level to less than 0.1 µU/mL (0.1 mU/L), whereas patients who are disease-free with a low risk of recurrence should maintain a TSH level of 0.3 to 2.0 µU/mL (0.3-2.0 mU/L). This is typically accomplished without the use of thyroxine suppressive therapy.

Patients with distant metastases have improved survival with successful radioiodine therapy, whereas administration of radioactive iodine may decrease the likelihood of recurrent disease in those patients with nodal metastases. Radioactive iodine ($^{131}$I) therapy offers this patient no appreciable benefit since her prognosis is already excellent and such therapy would result in substantial unnecessary costs and radiation exposure.

**KEY POINT**

- Lobectomy is the treatment of choice for low-risk papillary thyroid cancer that is confined to the thyroid gland, completely resected at surgery, does not demonstrate aggressive pathologic features (lymphovascular invasion or tall cell variant), and has not metastasized.

## Bibliography

Vaccarella S, Franceschi S, Bray F, Wild CP, Plummer M, Dal Maso L. Worldwide thyroid-cancer epidemic? The increasing impact of overdiagnosis. N Engl J Med. 2016 Aug 18;375(7):614-7. doi: 10.1056/NEJMp1604412. [PMID: 27532827]

## Item 77          Answer:     B

**Educational Objective:** Diagnose diabetes insipidus.

The most appropriate diagnostic test for this patient is urine and serum osmolality measurement. Central diabetes insipidus (DI) results from inadequate production of antidiuretic hormone (ADH) by the posterior pituitary gland. In the presence of ADH, aquaporin water channels are inserted in the collecting tubules and allow water to be reabsorbed. In the absence of ADH, excessive water is excreted by the kidneys. Excretion of more than 3 liters of urine per day is considered polyuric. Frank hypernatremia is unusual because patients develop extreme thirst and polydipsia, and with free access to water, can maintain serum sodium in the high normal range. When patients do not drink enough to replace the water lost in the urine, due to poor or absent thirst drive or lack of free access to water, they develop hypernatremia. A low urine osmolality in the setting of a high serum osmolality and high serum sodium in a patient with polyuria is diagnostic of DI. Patients with craniopharyngiomas are at higher risk of developing central DI.

Desmopressin challenge is not appropriate at this time. Prior to initiating desmopressin, one must confirm the diagnosis of DI by measuring urine and serum osmolality. Once confirmed, desmopressin can be administered and urine osmolality remeasured to assure that administration of desmopressin resulted in an increase in urine osmolality. After desmopressin is given. urine concentrates to more than 800 mOsm/kg in central DI, less than 300 mOsm/kg in nephrogenic DI, and between 300 and 800 mOsm/kg in partial DI.

Measurement of urine electrolytes is not helpful in the diagnosis of DI.

A water deprivation test should not be performed in this patient. He already has hypernatremia so further water deprivation could result in serious hypernatremia. In the setting of hypernatremia, a urine and serum osmolality are the best tests to confirm the diagnosis of DI. A water deprivation test can be pursued when the diagnosis is unclear. Urine osmolality above 800 mOsm/kg $H_2O$ is a normal response to water deprivation, indicating ADH production and peripheral effect are intact. A serum osmolality above 295 mOsm/kg with inappropriately hypotonic urine (urine osmolality-serum osmolality ratio <2) during fluid deprivation confirms DI.

### KEY POINT

- A low urine osmolality in the setting of a high serum osmolality and high serum sodium in a patient with polyuria is diagnostic of diabetes insipidus.

## Bibliography

Prete A, Corsello SM, Salvatori R. Current best practice in the management of patients after pituitary surgery. Ther Adv Endocrinol Metab. 2017;8:33-48. [PMID: 28377801] doi:10.1177/2042018816687240

## Item 78          Answer:     D

**Educational Objective:** Diagnose thyroid storm.

The most likely diagnosis is thyroid storm. Thyroid storm is characterized by severe thyrotoxicosis associated with systemic decompensation. Presentation often follows a precipitating event, such as non-thyroid surgery as in this patient's case. Clinical manifestations include high fever, altered mental status and seizures, tachycardia, atrial fibrillation and heart failure, and hepatic dysfunction. A diagnostic system, such as the Burch and Wartofsky Point Scale, can support the diagnosis with scores greater than or equal to 45 being highly suggestive. The patient's thyroid function tests should be assessed to confirm recurrent hyperthyroidism and aggressive treatment should be initiated in the ICU. Management includes treatment of any precipitant illness, supportive care, and thyrotoxicosis-directed therapy including β-adrenergic blockers (esmolol infusion), antithyroid drug therapy, intravenous glucocorticoids, and potassium iodide. Plasmapheresis and emergent thyroidectomy are utilized in patients who cannot be sufficiently managed with medical therapy alone.

Adrenal crisis is not the most likely diagnosis. Although autoimmune primary adrenal failure occurs more commonly in patients with other autoimmune disorders, patients with adrenal crisis usually present with hypotension, hyponatremia, and hyperkalemia, in addition to gastrointestinal manifestations. This diagnosis cannot explain the patient's hyperthermia, lid lag, thyromegaly, brisk reflexes, or tremor.

Malignant hyperthermia is an uncommon cause of severe hyperthermia that occurs in genetically susceptible individuals upon exposure to a volatile anesthetic such as halothane or isoflurane. Symptoms begin intraoperatively or in postoperative recovery, not 3 days following surgery. Features include mixed respiratory and metabolic acidosis, muscle rigidity, hyperkalemia, and rhabdomyolysis. This diagnosis does not explain the patient's thyrotoxicosis-related findings. Finally, the patient lacks muscle rigidity, a pathognomonic finding in malignant hyperthermia.

Myxedema coma is also unlikely. Although patients with myxedema coma may experience cardiac dysfunction and mental status changes, this patient is presenting with signs and symptoms of thyroid hormone excess, not deficiency. She has a history of Graves disease in remission after treatment with antithyroid drug therapy. She has not received radioactive iodine or thyroidectomy and thus the development of hypothyroidism at this point would be unusual.

### KEY POINT

- Thyroid storm is a severe manifestation of thyrotoxicosis with life-threatening secondary systemic decompensation; it occurs most commonly with underlying Graves disease coupled with a precipitating factor such as surgery.

## Bibliography

De Leo S, Lee SY, Braverman LE. Hyperthyroidism. Lancet. 2016;388:906-18. [PMID: 27038492] doi:10.1016/S0140-6736(16)00278-6

## Item 79      Answer:    D

**Educational Objective:** Manage early type 2 diabetes mellitus with metformin monotherapy.

The American Diabetes Association (ADA) recommends a hemoglobin $A_{1c}$ goal of less than 6.5% to 7% in patients who are early in the disease course and with few comorbidities. This patient meets these criteria and should aim for tighter glycemic control than he is currently achieving with 3 months of lifestyle modifications alone. Pharmacologic therapy should now be added to his lifestyle modifications. The American College of Physicians recommends a hemoglobin $A_{1c}$ level between 7% and 8% in most patients with type 2 diabetes. More stringent targets may be appropriate for patients who have a long life expectancy (>15 years) and are interested in more intensive glycemic control with pharmacologic therapy despite the risk for harms, including but not limited to hypoglycemia, patient burden, and pharmacologic costs. The ADA and the American College of Physicians (ACP) recommend metformin as first-line therapy for all patients with type 2 diabetes without contraindications. This recommendation is based on data from multiple studies demonstrating the effectiveness and safety of metformin. In addition, metformin is inexpensive.

The patient has had a reduction in his weight and hemoglobin $A_{1c}$ with lifestyle modifications alone over a 3-month period. Despite this, he remains above his hemoglobin $A_{1c}$ goal of less than 6.5% to 7%. Therefore, continuing his current management protocol would not be appropriate. Achieving glucose goals early in the disease course can reduce the risk of developing microvascular and possibly macrovascular complications in the future. He will require the addition of pharmacologic agents at this time to reach his glycemic target.

Empagliflozin has the ability to improve glycemic control while also reducing blood pressure and weight. Empagliflozin is considered second-line therapy after metformin by ADA and ACP.

Liraglutide also has the ability to improve glycemic control while also reducing weight. There are studies also demonstrating a reduction in blood pressure with liraglutide use. Liraglutide is considered second-line therapy after metformin by the ADA and ACP.

If the patient does not achieve his hemoglobin $A_{1c}$ target after 3 months of lifestyle modifications and metformin, dual therapy with metformin and liraglutide or metformin and empagliflozin could be considered.

### KEY POINT

- Metformin is first-line therapy for all patients with type 2 diabetes without contraindications.

## Bibliography

Barry MJ, Humphrey LL, Qaseem A. Oral pharmacologic treatment of type 2 diabetes mellitus. Ann Intern Med. 2017;167:75-76.doi:10.7326/L17-0234. [PMID: 28672387]

## Item 80      Answer:    B

**Educational Objective:** Manage diabetic ketoacidosis.

The most appropriate management for this patient is to decrease the insulin drip rate and add intravenous (IV) dextrose. This patient continues to have anion gap acidosis and should remain on IV insulin therapy to suppress ketogenesis until this resolves. His current blood glucose level below 200 to 250 mg/dL (11.1-13.9 mmol/L) increases his risk for hypoglycemia with continued IV insulin therapy. This risk can be mitigated by transitioning his IV fluids to 5% dextrose with 0.45% normal saline at 150 to 250 mL/h to maintain his glucose between 150 and 200 mg/dL (8.3-11.1 mmol/L) until his diabetic ketoacidosis resolves. Reducing the insulin drip rate to maintain his blood glucose between 150 and 200 mg/dL (8.3-11.1 mmol/L) will also decrease the risk of hypoglycemia while still suppressing ketogenesis.

If he continues at the current insulin drip rate or if he does not have the addition of IV dextrose, he has an increased risk of developing hypoglycemia now that his blood glucose is less than 200 mg/dL (11.1 mmol/L).

Insulin deficiency and urinary potassium losses induce shifts in potassium from the intracellular to extracellular compartments. This can result in low or normal serum potassium levels in the setting of depleted potassium stores. Potassium shifts back from the extracellular to intracellular compartments with resultant hypokalemia as insulin administration corrects the hyperglycemia, anion gap acidosis, and hyperosmolality associated with diabetic ketoacidosis. To avoid cardiac complications, serum potassium must be greater than 3.3 mEq/L (3.3. mmol/L) before initiating IV insulin. Once potassium is 3.3 mEq/L (3.3 mmol/L) or higher and IV insulin has been initiated, 20 to 30 mEq (20-30 mmol/L) of potassium chloride will usually need to be added to each liter of IV fluid to maintain a serum potassium level of 4.0 to 5.0 mEq/L (4.0-5.0 mmol/L). He is at risk of developing hypokalemia if his potassium supplementation is discontinued at this time.

Although subcutaneous insulin would provide insulin to suppress ketogenesis, the IV insulin drip provides greater flexibility in dose adjustments than subcutaneous insulin. Once the patient's anion gap acidosis has resolved, transitioning from the insulin drip to a subcutaneous insulin regimen should occur.

### KEY POINT

- In patients with diabetic ketoacidosis, intravenous insulin therapy should be continued until complete resolution of the anion gap acidosis; as acidosis improves, it may be necessary to reduce the insulin infusion rate and add intravenous dextrose to prevent hypoglycemia.

## Bibliography

Fayfman M, Pasquel FJ, Umpierrez GE. Management of hyperglycemic crises: diabetic ketoacidosis and hyperglycemic hyperosmolar state. Med Clin North Am. 2017;101:587-606. doi: 10.1016/j.mcna.2016.12.011. [PMID:28372715]

## Item 81     Answer:    C

**Educational Objective:** Treat type-2 amiodarone-induced thyrotoxicosis.

The most appropriate initial management for this patient is to prescribe prednisone. Amiodarone is an antiarrhythmic medication with high iodine content and prolonged half-life of approximately 40 days. Thyrotoxicosis affects 5% of patients taking amiodarone and can occur at any time during or up to 9 months after treatment. Type 1 (hyperthyroidism) amiodarone-induced thyrotoxicosis occurs in patients with underlying multinodular goiter or latent Graves disease and is associated with increased vascularity on color flow Doppler ultrasonography. Type 2 (destructive thyroiditis) usually affects those without thyroid disease and is not associated with increased vascularity on color flow Doppler. Mixed forms can also be seen and making the correct diagnosis can be difficult. The patient's clinical presentation is most consistent with type 2 amiodarone-induced thyrotoxicosis given the absence of structural thyroid disease (no nodules or goiter), absent thyroid-stimulating hormone (TSH) receptor antibody, and absent parenchymal flow seen on Doppler ultrasound. Moderate- to high-dose prednisone is an effective treatment that can be gradually tapered over 1 to 3 months.

Discontinuation of amiodarone would not yield any immediate clinical benefit due to its prolonged half-life elimination. The decision to discontinue amiodarone depends on the patient's cardiac status, availability of effective alternatives, and type of thyrotoxicosis, with treatment cessation being more important in type 1 than type 2.

Methimazole is most effective in treating type 1 (hyperthyroidism) amiodarone-induced thyrotoxicosis, which occurs in patients with Graves disease or thyroid nodules. Since this patient's presentation is most consistent with type 2 amiodarone-induced thyrotoxicosis (destructive thyroiditis), prednisone is the preferred treatment.

Performing thyroid scintigraphy with radioactive iodine uptake is not indicated. Amiodarone has a very high iodine content, which results in high serum iodine levels. This iodine competes with the radioactive isotope used for the test ($^{123}$I or $^{131}$I) resulting in very low radioactive iodine uptake (<1%) in most patients. This test does not discriminate well between type 1 and 2 amiodarone-induced thyrotoxicosis and is not clinically useful.

### KEY POINT

- Type 2 amiodarone-induced thyrotoxicosis (destructive thyroiditis) can be treated with moderate- to high-dose prednisone that can be gradually tapered over 1 to 3 months.

### Bibliography

Danzi S, Klein I. Amiodarone-induced thyroid dysfunction. J Intensive Care Med. 2015;30:179–85. doi: 10.1177/0885066613503278. Epub 2013 Sep 24. [PMID: 24067547]

## Item 82     Answer:    D

**Educational Objective:** Diagnose the cause of rapid-onset hirsutism.

A pelvic ultrasound is the most appropriate management for this patient. Although androgen-secreting ovarian tumors are rare, they should be considered in patients with abrupt, rapidly progressive, or severe hyperandrogenism as well as in women with marked hyperandrogenemia (total testosterone >150 ng/dL [5.2 nmol/L]). Given this patient's rapid onset of hirsutism coupled with significantly elevated total testosterone level, a pelvic ultrasound is the best next step in evaluation to assess for a possible ovarian tumor.

Adrenal vein sampling is a procedure used to confirm whether autonomous adrenal hormone production is unilateral or bilateral. It is most commonly performed in the evaluation of primary aldosteronism. Adrenal vein sampling is needed in most patients to determine the source of aldosterone secretion when imaging is unrevealing and to confirm lateralization when imaging demonstrates an adrenal adenoma. For this patient, adrenal CT is more appropriate to exclude an adrenal cortisol-secreting and/or androgen-secreting neoplasm and may be appropriate if the pelvic ultrasound is unrevealing. There is no indication for this procedure at this time in this patient.

Cushing syndrome (CS) results from elevated levels of cortisol. Clinical findings that are highly specific for CS include centripetal obesity, facial plethora, abnormal fat deposition in the supraclavicular or dorsocervical ("buffalo hump") areas, and wide (>1 cm) violaceous striae. Evaluation for CS is most appropriate in patients who have specific signs and symptoms of CS, rather than in patients who are diffusely obese, have nonpathologic striae, and are having trouble losing weight because endogenous CS is such a rare condition with a costly evaluation algorithm. At least two first-line tests should be abnormal before the diagnosis is confirmed. Initial tests include the overnight low-dose dexamethasone suppression test, 24-hour urine free cortisol, and late-night salivary cortisol. Since the patient has none of the specific findings of CS, a 24-hour urine cortisol test is not indicated.

In addition to weight loss, combined hormonal oral contraceptives are first-line agents for treatment of polycystic ovary syndrome. Polycystic ovary syndrome is a diagnosis of exclusion; given this patient's rapid onset of hirsutism coupled with degree of her total testosterone elevation, an androgen-secreting tumor must be considered.

### KEY POINT

- An androgen-secreting ovarian tumor should be considered in patients with abrupt, rapidly progressive, or severe hyperandrogenism as well as in women with marked hyperandrogenemia (total testosterone >150 ng/dL [5.2 nmol/L]).

### Bibliography

Mihailidis J, Dermesropian R, Taxel P, Luthra P, Grant-Kels JM. Endocrine evaluation of hirsutism. Int J Womens Dermatol. 2017;3(1 Suppl):S6–S10. doi: 10.1016/j.ijwd.2017.02.007. eCollection 2017 Mar. [PMID:28492032]

## Item 83    Answer:    D

**Educational Objective:** Treat type 2 diabetes mellitus with metabolic surgery in an obese patient.

This patient should be referred for metabolic surgery. The gastrointestinal tract plays an important role in glucose homeostasis and serves as an important physiologic target for improving glycemic control. Short- and mid-term data from randomized controlled trials of metabolic surgery demonstrated greater improvements in glycemic control and cardiovascular risk factors compared with optimized medical therapy and lifestyle modifications. Retrospective cohort studies and prospective observational studies suggest a reduction in cardiovascular deaths and lower incidence of cardiovascular events in patients undergoing metabolic surgery. Metabolic surgery should be recommended to patients with type 2 diabetes who have class III obesity (BMI ≥ 40) independent of glycemic control and diabetes treatment regimen and to patients with type 2 diabetes with class II obesity (BMI 35.0-39.9) who fail to meet their glycemic goals despite optimizing medical therapies and lifestyle modifications. In addition, patients with class I obesity (BMI 30.0-34.9) who do not meet their glycemic goals despite optimizing medical therapy should be considered for metabolic surgery. The patient has class II obesity with an inability to meet her hemoglobin $A_{1c}$ goal of less than 7% on her current medical regimen. Further modifications to her current regimen may either exacerbate hypoglycemia and accelerate weight gain or not reach her glycemic goal.

Although sitagliptin, a dipeptidyl peptidase (DPP)-4-inhibitor, is a weight neutral oral agent that could potentially improve her hemoglobin $A_{1c}$ level by 0.95% to 1.1%, it would not achieve her target hemoglobin $A_{1c}$ of less than 7%.

Pioglitazone, a thiazolidinedione (TZD), improves insulin sensitivity and hemoglobin $A_{1c}$ by 0.9% to 1.1%. The addition of pioglitazone in this patient would likely not achieve her target hemoglobin $A_{1c}$ goal and could potentially induce additional weight gain, a known side effect of this drug class.

Increasing the patient's insulin doses may improve her hemoglobin $A_{1c}$ to goal, but it will exacerbate her hypoglycemia and promote additional weight gain.

### KEY POINT

- Metabolic surgery demonstrates greater improvements in glycemic control and cardiovascular risk factors compared with optimized medical therapy and lifestyle modifications.

### Bibliography

Rubino F, Nathan DM, Eckel RH, Schauer PR, Alberti KG, Zimmet PZ, et al; Delegates of the 2nd Diabetes Surgery Summit. Metabolic surgery in the treatment algorithm for type 2 diabetes: a joint statement by International Diabetes Organizations. Diabetes Care. 2016;39:861-77. [PMID: 27222544] doi:10.2337/dc16-0236

## Item 84    Answer:    C

**Educational Objective:** Diagnose osteomalacia.

The most likely diagnosis in this patient is osteomalacia causing bone pain or fracture of the pelvis or proximal right lower extremity. An insidious, protracted course involving enigmatic pain is typical of osteomalacia, which may be dismissed by patients or symptomatically treated by health care providers. Chronically low levels of vitamin D can lead to rickets in children and osteomalacia in adults. Vitamin D deficiency is caused by factors such as intestinal malabsorption due to gastrointestinal disorders or restricted access to sunlight. In promoting absorption from the gut, vitamin D enables proper bone mineralization by maintenance of calcium and phosphorus levels. Vitamin D also modulates the actions of osteoblasts and osteoclasts to ensure proper bone growth and remodeling. The more common forms of osteomalacia related to malabsorption or dietary factors are characterized by low 25-hydroxyvitamin D (calcidiol), low calcium and phosphate, and elevated parathyroid hormone (PTH) (secondary hyperparathyroidism) and alkaline phosphatase levels. Depending on the duration and severity of vitamin D deficiency, the serum concentration of 1,25-dihydroxyvitamin D may be normal, low, or high and is not helpful in the diagnosis of most forms of osteomalacia.

Osteitis fibrosa cystica is due to abnormally high bone turnover that can occur after prolonged exposure of bone to sustained high levels of PTH in hyperparathyroidism. It is associated with very high bone turnover, expansion of osteoid surfaces, and exuberant bone resorption resulting in an increased risk of fracture. Patients can be asymptomatic, or they may have bone pain. Classic skeletal changes on radiograph may include subperiosteal resorption of bone, most prominently at the phalanges of the hands. Osteitis fibrosa cystica is most commonly seen in patients with chronic kidney failure and is rarely associated with severe primary hyperparathyroidism.

Osteogenesis imperfecta (OI) comprises four genetic syndromes characterized by autosomal dominant or recessive mutations in *COL* genes, leading to abnormalities in the structure of type I collagen. OI is associated with bone fractures, short stature, body deformity, hearing loss, and dental deformity. A classic feature of OI is blue sclerae (reflecting visibility of the underlying choroid), but it is not sensitive or specific to OI. The biochemical profile is usually normal in OI.

Postmenopausal osteoporosis is a diagnosis of exclusion, made only after having evaluated and eliminated other causes of low bone mineral density such as osteomalacia. Patients with osteoporosis have a normal biochemical profile.

### KEY POINT

- Osteomalacia related to malabsorption or dietary factors is characterized by low 25-hydroxyvitamin D, calcium, and phosphate levels and elevated parathyroid hormone and alkaline phosphatase levels.

### Bibliography

Uday S, Högler W. Nutritional rickets and osteomalacia in the twenty-first century: revised concepts, public health, and prevention strategies. Curr Osteoporos Rep. 2017 Aug;15(4):293-302. doi: 10.1007/s11914-017-0383-y. Erratum in: Curr Osteoporos Rep. 2017 Aug 14; [PMID: 28612338]

# Index

**A** | **NAME AND ADDRESS (Please complete.)**

_____
Last Name                    First Name          Middle Initial

_____
Address

_____
Address cont.

_____
City                         State               ZIP Code

_____
Country

_____
Email address

**ACP®**
American College of Physicians
Leading Internal Medicine, Improving Lives

**Medical Knowledge Self-Assessment Program® 18**

**TO EARN *CME Credits and/or MOC Points* YOU MUST:**

1. Answer all questions.
2. Score a minimum of 50% correct.

===========================================

**TO EARN *FREE* INSTANTANEOUS *CME Credits and/or MOC Points* ONLINE:**

1. Answer all of your questions.
2. Go to **mksap.acponline.org** and enter your ACP Online username and password to access an online answer sheet.
3. Enter your answers.
4. You can also enter your answers directly at **mksap.acponline.org** without first using this answer sheet.

**To Submit Your Answer Sheet by Mail or FAX for a $20 Administrative Fee per Answer Sheet:**

1. Answer all of your questions and calculate your score.
2. Complete boxes A-H.
3. Complete payment information.
4. Send the answer sheet and payment information to ACP, using the FAX number/address listed below.

**B** | **Order Number**
(Use the 10-digit Order Number on your MKSAP materials packing slip.)

**C** | **ACP ID Number**
(Refer to packing slip in your MKSAP materials for your 8-digit ACP ID Number.)

**D** | **Required Submission Information if Applying for MOC**

Birth Month and Day
M M  D D

ABIM Candidate Number

**COMPLETE FORM BELOW ONLY IF YOU SUBMIT BY MAIL OR FAX**

Last Name | First Name | MI

**Payment Information. Must remit in US funds, drawn on a US bank.**
**The processing fee for each paper answer sheet is $20.**

☐ Check, made payable to ACP, enclosed

Charge to  ☐ **VISA**  ☐ **MasterCard**  ☐ **AMERICAN EXPRESS**  ☐ **DISCOVER**

Card Number _____

Expiration Date _____ / _____     Security code (3 or 4 digit #s) _____
                MM            YY

Signature _____

**Fax to:** 215-351-2799

**Mail to:**
Member and Customer Service
American College of Physicians
190 N. Independence Mall West
Philadelphia, PA 19106-1572

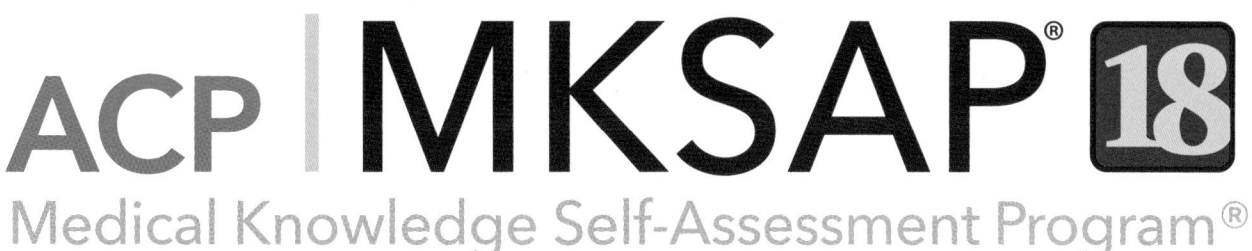

# Infectious Disease

![ACP logo] **ACP** American College of Physicians®
Leading Internal Medicine, Improving Lives

# Welcome to the Infectious Disease Section of MKSAP 18!

In these pages, you will find updated information on central nervous system infections, skin and soft tissue infections, community-acquired pneumonia, tick-borne diseases, urinary tract infections, *Mycobacterium tuberculosis* and nontuberculous mycobacterial infections, sexually transmitted infections, bioterrorism, travel medicine, infectious gastrointestinal syndromes, transplant-associated infections, HIV and AIDS, health care–associated infections, and other clinical challenges. All of these topics are uniquely focused on the needs of generalists and subspecialists *outside* of infectious disease.

The core content of MKSAP 18 has been developed as in previous editions—all essential information that is newly researched and written in 11 topic areas of internal medicine—created by dozens of leading generalists and subspecialists and guided by certification and recertification requirements, emerging knowledge in the field, and user feedback. MKSAP 18 also contains 1200 all-new peer-reviewed, psychometrically validated, multiple-choice questions (MCQs) for self-assessment and study, including 108 in Infectious Disease. MKSAP 18 continues to include *High Value Care* (HVC) recommendations, based on the concept of balancing clinical benefit with costs and harms, with associated MCQs illustrating these principles and HVC Key Points called out in the text. Internists practicing in the hospital setting can easily find comprehensive *Hospitalist*-focused content and MCQs, specially designated in blue and with the ◫ symbol.

If you purchased MKSAP 18 Complete, you also have access to MKSAP 18 Digital, with additional tools allowing you to customize your learning experience. MKSAP Digital includes regular text updates with new, practice-changing information, 200 new self-assessment questions, and enhanced custom-quiz options. MKSAP Complete also includes more than 1200 electronic, adaptive learning–enhanced flashcards for quick review of important concepts, as well as an updated and enhanced version of Virtual Dx, MKSAP's image-based self-assessment tool. As before, MKSAP 18 Digital is optimized for use on your mobile devices, with iOS- and Android-based apps allowing you to sync between your apps and online account and submit for CME credits and MOC points online.

Please visit us at the MKSAP Resource Site (mksap.acponline.org) to find out how we can help you study, earn CME credit and MOC points, and stay up to date.

On behalf of the many internists who have offered their time and expertise to create the content for MKSAP 18 and the editorial staff who work to bring this material to you in the best possible way, we are honored that you have chosen to use MKSAP 18 and appreciate any feedback about the program you may have. Please feel free to send any comments to mksap_editors@acponline.org.

Sincerely,

Patrick Alguire

Patrick C. Alguire, MD, FACP
Editor-in-Chief
Senior Vice President Emeritus
Medical Education Division
American College of Physicians

# Infectious Disease

## Committee

**Patricia D. Brown, MD, FACP, Section Editor[1]**
Professor of Medicine
Wayne State University School of Medicine
Associate Chief of Staff for Medicine
John D. Dingell VA Medical Center
Detroit, Michigan

**Karen C. Bloch, MD, MPH, FACP[1]**
Associate Professor
Department of Medicine and Health Policy
Division of Infectious Diseases
Vanderbilt University Medical Center
Nashville, Tennessee

**Larry M. Bush, MD, FACP[2]**
Affiliated Professor of Biomedical Sciences
Charles E. Schmidt College of Medicine
Florida Atlantic University
Boca Raton, Florida
Affiliated Associate Professor of Medicine
University of Miami-Miller School of Medicine
JFK Medical Center
Palm Beach County, Florida

**Louise M. Dembry, MD, MS, MBA, FACP[2]**
Professor of Medicine
Infectious Diseases and Epidemiology
Yale University School of Medicine
New Haven, Connecticut

**Michael Frank, MD, FACP[1]**
Professor of Medicine
Chief, Division of Infectious Diseases
Vice Chair for Education
Department of Medicine
Medical College of Wisconsin
Milwaukee, Wisconsin

**Rodrigo Hasbun, MD, MPH[2]**
Professor of Medicine
Department of Infectious Diseases
UT Health-McGovern Medical School
Houston, Texas

**Fred A. Lopez, MD, MACP[2]**
Richard Vial Professor
Vice Chair for Education
Department of Medicine
Louisiana State University Health Sciences Center
New Orleans, Louisiana

**Jose A. Vazquez, MD, FACP[2]**
Chief, Division of Infectious Diseases
Professor, Department of Medicine
Medical College of Georgia at Augusta University
Augusta, Georgia

## Editor-in-Chief

**Patrick C. Alguire, MD, FACP[2]**
Senior Vice President Emeritus, Medical Education
American College of Physicians
Philadelphia, Pennsylvania

## Deputy Editor

**Davoren Chick, MD, FACP[2]**
Senior Vice President, Medical Education
American College of Physicians
Philadelphia, Pennsylvania

**Infectious Disease Reviewers**
Susan C. Bleasdale, MD, FACP[2]
Beata C. Casanas, DO, FACP[2]
Manjit S. Dhillon, MBBS, FACP[1]
Dimitri M. Drekonja, MD, FACP[1]
Lisa A. Grohskopf, MD[1]
Muhammad Umar Khan, MBBS, FACP[1]
Felicia M. Lewis, MD, FACP[1]
Maricar F. Malinis, MD, FACP[2]
Zaw Min, MD, FACP[1]
George Samuel, MD[1]

## Hospital Medicine Infectious Disease Reviewers

Ji Hoon Baang, MD, FACP[2]
Jeana Benwill, MD[1]

## Infectious Disease ACP Editorial Staff

**Linnea Donnarumma[1]**, Staff Editor
**Margaret Wells[1]**, Director, Self-Assessment and Educational
  Programs
**Becky Krumm[1]**, Managing Editor, Self-Assessment and
  Educational Programs

## ACP Principal Staff

**Davoren Chick, MD FACP[2]**
*Senior Vice President, Medical Education*

## Acknowledgments

The American College of Physicians (ACP) gratefully acknowledges the special contributions to the development and production of the 18th edition of the Medical Knowledge Self-Assessment Program® (MKSAP® 18) made by the following people:

*Graphic Design:* Barry Moshinski (Director, Graphic Services), Michael Ripca (Graphics Technical Administrator), and Jennifer Gropper (Graphic Designer).

*Production/Systems:* Dan Hoffmann (Director, Information Technology), Scott Hurd (Manager, Content Systems), Neil Kohl (Senior Architect), and Chris Patterson (Senior Architect).

*MKSAP 18 Digital:* Under the direction of Steven Spadt (Senior Vice President, Technology), the digital version of MKSAP 18 was developed within the ACP's Digital Products and Services Department, led by Brian Sweigard (Director, Digital Products and Services). Other members of the team included Dan Barron (Senior Web Application Developer/ Architect), Chris Forrest (Senior Software Developer/Design Lead), Kathleen Hoover (Senior Web Developer), Kara Regis (Manager, User Interface Design and Development), Brad Lord (Senior Web Application Developer), and John McKnight (Senior Web Developer).

The College also wishes to acknowledge that many other persons, too numerous to mention, have contributed to the production of this program. Without their dedicated efforts, this program would not have been possible.

## MKSAP Resource Site (mksap.acponline.org)

The MKSAP Resource Site (mksap.acponline.org) is a continually updated site that provides links to MKSAP 18 online answer sheets for print subscribers; access to MKSAP 18 Digital; Board Basics® e-book access instructions; information on Continuing Medical Education (CME), Maintenance of Certification (MOC), and international Continuing Professional Development (CPD) and MOC; errata; and other new information.

## International MOC/CPD

For information and instructions on submission of international MOC/CPD, please go to the MKSAP Resource Site (mksap.acponline.org).

## Continuing Medical Education

The American College of Physicians is accredited by the Accreditation Council for Continuing Medical Education (ACCME) to provide continuing medical education for physicians.

The American College of Physicians designates this enduring material, MKSAP 18, for a maximum of 275 *AMA PRA Category 1 Credits*™. Physicians should claim only the credit commensurate with the extent of their participation in the activity.

Up to 25 *AMA PRA Category 1 Credits*™ are available from December 31, 2018, to December 31, 2021, for the MKSAP 18 Infectious Disease section.

## Learning Objectives

The learning objectives of MKSAP 18 are to:

- Close gaps between actual care in your practice and preferred standards of care, based on best evidence
- Diagnose disease states that are less common and sometimes overlooked and confusing
- Improve management of comorbid conditions that can complicate patient care
- Determine when to refer patients for surgery or care by subspecialists
- Pass the ABIM Certification Examination
- Pass the ABIM Maintenance of Certification Examination

## Target Audience

- General internists and primary care physicians
- Subspecialists who need to remain up to date in internal medicine
- Residents preparing for the certifying examination in internal medicine
- Physicians preparing for maintenance of certification in internal medicine (recertification)

## ABIM Maintenance of Certification

Check the MKSAP Resource Site (mksap.acponline.org) for the latest information on how MKSAP tests can be used to apply to the American Board of Internal Medicine (ABIM) for Maintenance of Certification (MOC) points following completion of the CME activity.

Successful completion of the CME activity, which includes participation in the evaluation component, enables the participant to earn up to 275 medical knowledge MOC points in the ABIM's MOC program. It is the CME activity provider's responsibility to submit participant completion information to ACCME for the purpose of granting MOC credit.

## Earn Instantaneous CME Credits or MOC Points Online

Print subscribers can enter their answers online to earn instantaneous CME credits or MOC points. You can submit your answers using online answer sheets that are provided at mksap.acponline.org, where a record of your MKSAP 18 credits will be available. To earn CME credits or to apply for MOC points, you need to answer all of the questions in a test and earn a score of at least 50% correct (number of correct answers divided by the total number of questions). Please note that if you are applying for MOC points, you must also enter your birth date and ABIM candidate number.

Take either of the following approaches:

1. Use the printed answer sheet at the back of this book to record your answers. Go to mksap.acponline.org, access the appropriate online answer sheet, transcribe your answers, and submit your test for instantaneous CME credits or MOC points. There is no additional fee for this service.

2. Go to mksap.acponline.org, access the appropriate online answer sheet, directly enter your answers, and submit your test for instantaneous CME credits or MOC points. There is no additional fee for this service.

## Earn CME Credits or MOC Points by Mail or Fax

Pay a $20 processing fee per answer sheet and submit the printed answer sheet at the back of this book by mail or fax, as instructed on the answer sheet. Make sure you calculate your score and enter your birth date and ABIM candidate number, and fax the answer sheet to 215-351-2799 or mail the answer sheet to Member and Customer Service, American College of Physicians, 190 N. Independence Mall West, Philadelphia, PA 19106-1572, using the courtesy envelope provided in your MKSAP 18 slipcase. You will need your 10-digit order number and 8-digit ACP ID number, which are printed on your packing slip. Please allow 4 to 6 weeks for your score report to be emailed back to you. Be sure to include your email address for a response.

If you do not have a 10-digit order number and 8-digit ACP ID number, or if you need help creating a user-name and password to access the MKSAP 18 online answer sheets, go to mksap.acponline.org or email custserv@acponline.org.

## Disclosure Policy

It is the policy of the American College of Physicians (ACP) to ensure balance, independence, objectivity, and scientific rigor in all of its educational activities. To this end, and consistent with the policies of the ACP and the Accreditation Council for Continuing Medical Education (ACCME), contributors to all ACP continuing medical education activities are required to disclose all relevant financial relationships with any entity producing, marketing, re-selling, or distributing health care goods or services consumed by, or used on, patients. Contributors are required to use generic names in the discussion of therapeutic options and are required to identify any unapproved, off-label, or investigative use of commercial products or devices. Where a trade name is used, all available

trade names for the same product type are also included. If trade-name products manufactured by companies with whom contributors have relationships are discussed, contributors are asked to provide evidence-based citations in support of the discussion. The information is reviewed by the committee responsible for producing this text. If necessary, adjustments to topics or contributors' roles in content development are made to balance the discussion. Further, all readers of this text are asked to evaluate the content for evidence of commercial bias and send any relevant comments to mksap_editors@acponline.org so that future decisions about content and contributors can be made in light of this information.

## Resolution of Conflicts

To resolve all conflicts of interest and influences of vested interests, ACP's content planners used best evidence and updated clinical care guidelines in developing content, when such evidence and guidelines were available. All content underwent review by peer reviewers not on the committee to ensure that the material was balanced and unbiased. Contributors' disclosure information can be found with the list of contributors' names and those of ACP principal staff listed in the beginning of this book.

## Hospital-Based Medicine

For the convenience of subscribers who provide care in hospital settings, content that is specific to the hospital setting has been highlighted in blue. Hospital icons (H) highlight where the hospital-only content begins, continues over more than one page, and ends.

## High Value Care Key Points

Key Points in the text that relate to High Value Care concepts (that is, concepts that discuss balancing clinical benefit with costs and harms) are designated by the HVC icon [HVC].

## Educational Disclaimer

The editors and publisher of MKSAP 18 recognize that the development of new material offers many opportunities for error. Despite our best efforts, some errors may persist in print. Drug dosage schedules are, we believe, accurate and in accordance with current standards. Readers are advised, however, to ensure that the recommended dosages in MKSAP 18 concur with the information provided in the product information material. This is especially important in cases of new, infrequently used, or highly toxic drugs. Application of the information in MKSAP 18 remains the professional responsibility of the practitioner.

The primary purpose of MKSAP 18 is educational. Information presented, as well as publications, technologies, products, and/or services discussed, is intended to inform subscribers about the knowledge, techniques, and experiences of the contributors. A diversity of professional opinion exists, and the views of the contributors are their own and not those of the ACP. Inclusion of any material in the program does not constitute endorsement or recommendation by the ACP. The ACP does not warrant the safety, reliability, accuracy, completeness, or usefulness of and disclaims any and all liability for damages and claims that may result from the use of information, publications, technologies, products, and/or services discussed in this program.

## Publisher's Information

## Disclaimer Regarding Direct Purchases from Online Retailers

CME and/or MOC for MKSAP 18 is available only if you purchase the program directly from ACP. CME credits and MOC points cannot be awarded to those purchasers who have purchased the program from non-authorized sellers such as Amazon, eBay, or any other such online retailer.

## Unauthorized Use of This Book Is Against the Law

MKSAP 18 ISBN: 978-1-938245-47-3
(Infectious Disease) ISBN: 978-1-938245-56-5

Printed in the United States of America.

For order information in the U.S. or Canada call 800-ACP-1915. All other countries call 215-351-2600, (Monday to Friday, 9 AM – 5 PM ET). Fax inquiries to 215-351-2799 or email to custserv@acponline.org.

## Errata

Errata for MKSAP 18 will be available through the MKSAP Resource Site at mksap.acponline.org as new information becomes known to the editors.

# Table of Contents

# Infectious Disease High Value Care Recommendations

The American College of Physicians, in collaboration with multiple other organizations, is engaged in a worldwide initiative to promote the practice of High Value Care (HVC). The goals of the HVC initiative are to improve health care outcomes by providing care of proven benefit and reducing costs by avoiding unnecessary and even harmful interventions. The initiative comprises several programs that integrate the important concept of health care value (balancing clinical benefit with costs and harms) for a given intervention into a broad range of educational materials to address the needs of trainees, practicing physicians, and patients.

HVC content has been integrated into MKSAP 18 in several important ways. MKSAP 18 includes HVC-identified key points in the text, HVC-focused multiple choice questions, and, for subscribers to MKSAP Digital, an HVC custom quiz. From the text and questions, we have generated the following list of HVC recommendations that meet the definition below of high value care and bring us closer to our goal of improving patient outcomes while conserving finite resources.

**High Value Care Recommendation**: A recommendation to choose diagnostic and management strategies for patients in specific clinical situations that balance clinical benefit with cost and harms with the goal of improving patient outcomes.

Below are the High Value Care Recommendations for the Infectious Disease section of MKSAP 18.

- Blood cultures are not routinely indicated in patients with erysipelas and cellulitis.
- Primary treatment for abscesses, furuncles, and carbuncles is incision and drainage; mild infections do not require antibiotic therapy.
- Uninfected diabetic foot wounds should not be cultured or treated with antibiotics.
- Diagnostic studies to identify a causative organism are not routinely indicated in outpatients with community-acquired pneumonia.
- Patients with erythema migrans and a compatible exposure history do not require confirmatory laboratory testing for Lyme disease and should receive oral antibiotic therapy.

- No treatment is indicated for asymptomatic bacteriuria in otherwise healthy, nonpregnant patients (see Item 100).
- Urine culture is not recommended in women with uncomplicated cystitis.
- Indications for screening for and possibly treating asymptomatic bacteriuria include pregnancy and before an invasive urologic procedure (see Item 12).
- Follow-up urine cultures for acute pyelonephritis are only indicated in pregnant women.
- Acute, uncomplicated pyelonephritis can usually be managed with oral outpatient antimicrobial therapy (see Item 14).
- *Candida* isolated from the respiratory tract and urinary tract usually represents colonization; treatment is not indicated unless clinical infection is suspected.
- Test of cure is not recommended for *Chlamydia trachomatis* infection except in pregnancy.
- Test of cure in patients with *Neisseria gonorrhoeae* infection is recommended only when pharyngeal gonorrhea is treated with an alternate antibiotic regimen.
- The specificity of plain radiographs can confirm the diagnosis of osteomyelitis in most patients.
- Fluid replacement is the mainstay of treatment for travelers' diarrhea.
- Most healthy patients with watery diarrhea of less than 3 days' duration can be treated with supportive care and no antibiotic therapy or microscopic assessment.
- Most uncomplicated *Salmonella* infections in adults younger than 50 years resolve within 1 week and require only supportive care.
- Enterotoxigenic *Escherichia coli* infection is usually a self-limiting illness that resolves without treatment after approximately 4 days.
- Hand hygiene is the foundation of infection prevention.
- Catheter-associated asymptomatic bacteriuria generally does not require treatment.
- Antimicrobial- or antiseptic-coated catheters have not shown benefit for short-term or long-term bladder catheterization.
- Central venous catheters should be assessed daily for continued necessity and removed promptly when they are no longer needed (see Item 41).

# Infectious Disease

## Central Nervous System Infections

### Meningitis

A positive Gram stain result for bacteria or yeast is seen in only 5% of patients with community-acquired meningitis. Meningitis with a negative Gram stain result is a diagnostic and management challenge because the differential diagnosis includes urgent treatable causes, such as bacterial or fungal meningitis. Bacterial cultures of cerebrospinal fluid (CSF) or blood are needed for antimicrobial sensitivity studies in suspected bacterial meningitis, but results are insufficiently timely to differentiate bacterial from viral meningitis. In situations of clinical uncertainty, rapid diagnostic techniques such as polymerase chain reaction (PCR) for common viruses and arboviral serologies can reduce use of clinically unhelpful cranial imaging, hospitalization, and antimicrobial therapy.

### Viral Meningitis

Enteroviruses are the most common cause of viral meningitis, usually presenting between May and November in the Western Hemisphere, with symptoms including headache, fever, nuchal rigidity, photophobia, nausea, vomiting, myalgias, pharyngitis, maculopapular rash, and cough. Lymphocytic pleocytosis of the CSF with a normal glucose level and mildly elevated protein level is typical (**Table 1**). The diagnosis is confirmed by enterovirus PCR. Treatment is supportive with a benign clinical course.

Herpesviruses can cause meningitis year round and include herpes simplex virus (HSV) types 1 and 2, varicella-zoster virus (VZV), cytomegalovirus, Epstein-Barr virus, and human herpesvirus 6. Of the herpesviruses, HSV-2 is the most common cause of viral meningitis that can sometimes recur (recurrent benign lymphocytic meningitis, also called Mollaret meningitis). The CSF findings resemble enteroviral meningitis. Outcomes for HSV-2 meningitis are generally favorable without the need for acyclovir therapy.

VZV can cause encephalitis, aseptic meningitis, myelitis, and a vasculitis presenting as a stroke. Vesicular lesions are a clue to the diagnosis but may be absent (zoster sine herpete). VZV encephalitis and vasculitis may present with a hemorrhagic CSF. VZV may be present in the CSF without meningitis or encephalitis, and patients with primary varicella or zoster do not require lumbar puncture unless they have clinical signs of central nervous system (CNS) involvement. Immunocompromised and older adult patients are at higher risk of VZV meningitis and encephalitis. The diagnosis is confirmed by VZV PCR of the CSF, and therapy is parenteral acyclovir.

**TABLE 1.** Typical CSF Findings in Patients with Viral and Bacterial Meningitis

| CSF Parameter | Viral Meningitis[a] | Bacterial Meningitis |
|---|---|---|
| Opening pressure | $\leq$250 mm $H_2O$ | 200-500[b] mm $H_2O$ |
| Leukocyte count | 50-1000/µL (50-1000 × 10$^6$/L) | 1000-5000/µL (1000-5000 × 10$^6$/L)[c] |
| Leukocyte predominance | Lymphocytes[d] | Neutrophils |
| Glucose level | >45 mg/dL (2.5 mmol/L)[e] | <40 mg/dL (2.2 mmol/L)[f] |
| Protein level | <200 mg/dL (2000 mg/L) | 100-500 mg/dL (1000-5000 mg/L) |
| Gram stain | Negative | Positive in 60%-90%[g] |
| Culture | Negative | Positive in 70%-85%[h] |

CSF = cerebrospinal fluid.

[a]Primarily nonpolio enteroviruses (echoviruses and coxsackieviruses) and West Nile virus between June and October; herpes simplex type 2 year round.

[b]Values exceeding 600 mm $H_2O$ suggest the presence of cerebral edema, intracranial suppurative foci, or communicating hydrocephalus.

[c]Range may be <100/µL (100 × 10$^6$/L) to >10,000/µL (10,000 × 10$^6$/L).

[d]Neutrophil predominance occurs in 25% of viral meningitis cases, usually early in infection and more likely in young children with enteroviral infection.

[e]A mild hypoglycorrhachia (30-45 mg/dL [1.7-2.5 mmol/L]) can be seen in viral infections such as herpes simplex virus and West Nile virus.

[f]The CSF-to-plasma glucose ratio is $\leq$0.40 in most patients.

[g]The likelihood of a positive Gram stain correlates with the number of bacteria in the CSF.

[h]The yield of positive results is significantly reduced by previous administration of antimicrobial therapy.

CONT.

Mosquito-borne viruses such as West Nile virus (WNV), St. Louis encephalitis, and California encephalitis can cause meningitis or encephalitis between June and October in the Western Hemisphere. Neuroinvasive WNV may present with acute flaccid paralysis, which may lead to persistent weakness or death. The CSF formula resembles enteroviral meningitis. The diagnosis is made by serum or CSF serology (WNV IgM); WNV PCR of the CSF is insensitive. Treatment is supportive.

Acute HIV infection can present as aseptic meningitis associated with a mononucleosis-like syndrome with fever, rash, and myalgias.

Less common viral causes include mumps, lymphocytic choriomeningitis virus, parainfluenza, adenoviruses, influenza A and B, measles, rubella, poliovirus, rotavirus, and parvovirus B19.

### KEY POINTS

- Enteroviruses are the most common cause of viral meningitis, usually presenting with symptoms of headache, fever, nuchal rigidity, photophobia, nausea, vomiting, myalgias, pharyngitis, maculopapular rash, and cough between May and November.
- Herpesviruses can cause meningitis year round; herpes simplex virus 2 is the most common cause and can recur.
- Neuroinvasive West Nile virus may present with acute flaccid paralysis, which may lead to persistent weakness or death.

## Bacterial Meningitis

Bacterial meningitis usually presents with acute meningeal signs (fever, nuchal rigidity) and altered mental status. Since the introduction of conjugate vaccines, *Haemophilus influenzae* and *Neisseria meningitides* meningitis incidence has decreased, making *Streptococcus pneumoniae* the most common cause of community-acquired bacterial meningitis. *N. meningitides* serogroup B accounts for 40% of infections in the United States because the quadrivalent conjugate vaccine (ACYW-135) does not include serogroup B. Two FDA-approved vaccines that target serogroup B are available in the United States. *Streptococcus agalactiae* is now the third most common cause of bacterial meningitis in adults. *Listeria monocytogenes* is an uncommon cause of meningitis in adults; however, the risk increases in older adults and those with altered cell-mediated immunity.

Bacterial endocarditis caused by *S. pneumoniae* and *Staphylococcus aureus* can present as purulent meningitis. Clinical clues include a history of valvular disease, a new regurgitant murmur, embolic phenomena, or other stigmata of endocarditis. Injection drug use and hemodialysis are risk factors for *S. aureus*, and alcoholism is a risk factor for *S. pneumoniae* endocarditis. Patients may also present with stroke symptoms secondary to embolic infarction.

Lyme disease, caused by *Borrelia burgdorferi*, can present with a lymphocytic meningitis approximately 2 to 10 weeks after development of erythema migrans. Common clinical features include headache, photophobia, nausea, history of erythema migrans, tick bite in an endemic area, and facial paralysis, which can be unilateral or bilateral. Because the CSF formula resembles enteroviral meningitis, the "rule of 7s" was derived and validated to accurately classify a patient at low risk of having Lyme disease (headache duration <7 days, <70% CSF mononuclear cells, and absence of a seventh facial nerve palsy).

*Treponema pallidum* meningitis can occur in the secondary or tertiary phase of syphilis. Headache and meningismus are common, and the CSF usually shows a lymphocytic pleocytosis with an elevated protein level. In tertiary syphilis, neurosyphilis can be asymptomatic or symptomatic. Symptomatic neurosyphilis can present with primarily meningovascular (stroke presentation) or parenchymatous (tabes dorsalis, general paresis) features.

Leptospiral meningitis develops in the immune or second phase of the illness and is classically associated with uveitis, rash, conjunctival suffusion, lymphadenopathy, and hepatosplenomegaly. The CSF formula resembles enteroviral meningitis, and the diagnosis is established by CSF or urine culture or by serology.

### Evaluation

All patients with suspected meningitis should undergo lumbar puncture. CSF findings characteristic of bacterial meningitis are provided in Table 1. A negative CSF Gram stain result is more common in patients with previous antibiotic therapy or in patients with *L. monocytogenes* or gram-negative bacilli (sensitivity <50%) infections. CSF latex agglutination tests for detecting bacterial antigens are no longer recommended because of low sensitivity (70%) and specificity, although they may play a role in patients with previous antibiotic therapy or culture-negative meningitis. Multiplex PCR assay for detection of *S. pneumoniae*, *N. meningitidis*, *H. influenzae*, and *L. monocytogenes* has high sensitivity (100%) and specificity (98%) and is increasingly available. If a head CT is indicated before lumbar puncture (focal neurologic findings, altered mental status, papilledema, new seizure, history of CNS disease, or immunocompromise), imaging should not delay empiric antibiotic therapy, which should be started after promptly obtaining blood cultures. See **Figure 1** for management of suspected bacterial meningitis.

### Management

Intravenous antibiotic therapy should be started as soon as possible. If the CSF Gram stain result is negative, initial empiric antibiotic selection is based on age, local epidemiologic patterns of pneumococcal resistance, and the necessity for ampicillin coverage for *L. monocytogenes* (**Table 2**). Despite antibiotic therapy, mortality for bacterial meningitis remains approximately 25%. Adjunctive dexamethasone (10 mg every 6 hours for 4 days)

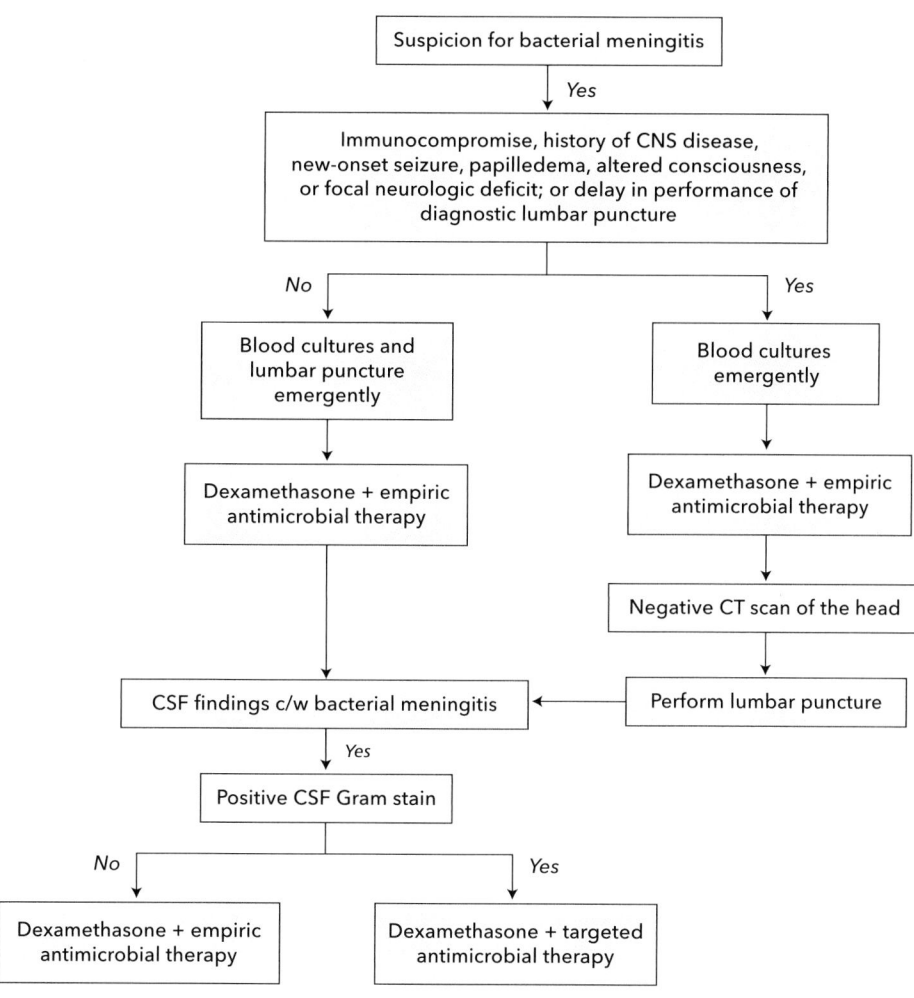

**FIGURE 1.** Management algorithm for adults suspected of having bacterial meningitis. CNS = central nervous system; c/w = consistent with; CSF = cerebrospinal fluid.

Adapted with permission from Tunkel AR, Hartman BJ, Kaplan SL, Kaufman BA, Roos KL, Scheld WM, et al. Practice guidelines for the management of bacterial meningitis. Clin Infect Dis. 2004;39:1267-84. [PMID: 15494903] Copyright 2004 Oxford University Press.

| TABLE 2. | Antibiotic Management of Bacterial Meningitis |
| --- | --- |
| **Clinical Characteristics** | **Empiric Antibiotic Regimen** |
| Immunocompetent host age <50 y with community-acquired bacterial meningitis | IV ceftriaxone or cefotaxime plus IV vancomycin |
| Patient age >50 y or those with altered cell-mediated immunity | IV ampicillin (Listeria coverage) plus IV ceftriaxone or cefotaxime plus IV vancomycin |
| Allergies to β-lactams | IV moxifloxacin instead of cephalosporin |
| | IV trimethoprim-sulfamethoxazole instead of ampicillin |
| Hospital-acquired bacterial meningitis | IV vancomycin plus either IV ceftazidime, cefepime, or meropenem |
| Neurosurgical procedures | IV vancomycin plus either IV ceftazidime, cefepime, or meropenem |

IV = intravenous.

reduces morbidity and mortality in adults with pneumococcal meningitis and reduces the risk of neurologic sequelae in bacterial meningitis in developed countries; it should be given concomitantly with the first dose of antibiotic therapy.  CONT.

**KEY POINTS**

- For diagnosis of bacterial meningitis, the cerebrospinal fluid Gram stain result is positive in 60% to 90% of infections; latex agglutination testing for bacterial antigens is not recommended because of low sensitivity and specificity.

- Intravenous antibiotic therapy and dexamethasone should be started as soon as possible when bacterial meningitis is suspected; selection of initial empiric antibiotics is based on age, local epidemiologic patterns of pneumococcal resistance, and the necessity for ampicillin coverage for *Listeria monocytogenes*.

- Adjunctive dexamethasone reduces morbidity and mortality in adults with pneumococcal meningitis and reduces the risk of neurologic sequelae in bacterial meningitis in developed countries.

## Subacute and Chronic Meningitis

Subacute and chronic meningitis are defined by symptom duration between 5 and 30 days and more than 30 days, respectively. The most common infectious causes are *Mycobacterium tuberculosis* and fungi.

### Tuberculous Meningitis

Mycobacterial tuberculosis meningitis classically presents as basilar meningitis with cranial neuropathies (particularly of cranial nerve VI), mental status changes, and the syndrome of inappropriate secretion of antidiuretic hormone. A history of tuberculosis exposure, an abnormal chest radiograph, a positive tuberculin skin test result, and a positive interferon-γ release assay result are suggestive but can be absent. CSF examination shows a lymphocytic pleocytosis (leukocyte count of 100-500/µL [100-500 × 10$^6$/L]), elevated protein level, and hypoglycorrhachia. CSF acid-fast bacilli smear is insensitive, and culture results are positive in only 38% to 88% of patients. Culture sensitivity increases when lumbar punctures are performed serially for at least 3 days. Nucleic acid amplification testing should be performed when possible, especially when the acid-fast bacilli stain result is negative and suspicion is high, because it might increase diagnostic yield. Antituberculous therapy should be administered for 1 year, and adjunctive glucocorticoids should be given initially because of their association with improved outcomes.

### Fungal Meningitis

Fungal pathogens, including *Cryptococcus neoformans*, *Coccidioides immitis*, *Histoplasma capsulatum*, and endemic mycoses, are a significant cause of subacute or chronic meningitis syndromes. Fungal meningitis is discussed in the Fungal Infections chapter.

### Neurobrucellosis

Neurobrucellosis occurs in 4% to 11% of patients with brucellosis, which is endemic to countries in the Mediterranean, Middle East, and Central America. It may present with meningitis, meningoencephalitis, cranial neuropathies, myelopathy, radiculopathy, or stroke or as a brain abscess. The diagnosis is made by a positive culture or serologic test result for brucellosis in the CSF or blood. Treatment consists of combination antimicrobial therapy (such as ceftriaxone, rifampin, and doxycycline) for at least 6 months.

### Parasitic Meningitis

Acute primary amebic meningoencephalitis caused by *Naegleria*, *Balamuthia*, and *Acanthamoeba* species is a fatal infection that clinically resembles bacterial meningitis. Freshwater exposure is a key historical clue. Examination of a fresh CSF sample can reveal motile trophozoites, but the Centers for Disease Control and Prevention should perform confirmatory testing by PCR. Treatment should include miltefosine.

Helminth infections causing eosinophilic meningitis include *Angiostrongylus cantonensis*, *Baylisascaris procyonis*, *Taenia solium* (neurocysticercosis), *Schistosoma* species (schistosomiasis), and *Gnathostoma*. Neurocysticercosis is endemic in Mexico, South America, and Asia. It most commonly presents with seizures or hydrocephalus, and CT scan of the head shows multiple cysts or calcified lesions.

### Noninfectious Causes

Medications such as NSAIDS, antibiotics, and intravenous immune globulin can occasionally cause aseptic meningitis. Meningeal involvement of leukemia, lymphoma, and metastatic carcinoma can also present as aseptic meningitis, with the CSF cytology showing atypical or immature cells and severe hypoglycorrhachia (<10 mg/dL [0.6 mmol/L]). Systemic lupus erythematosus, Behçet disease (recurrent oral and genital ulcers with iridocyclitis), Vogt-Koyanagi-Harada syndrome (uveomeningoencephalitis), and neurosarcoidosis can all present with aseptic meningitis. Finally, chemical meningitis can be seen after intrathecal injections, neurosurgical procedures, or spinal anesthesia.

**KEY POINTS**

- Tuberculous meningitis classically presents as basilar meningitis with cranial neuropathies, mental status changes, and the syndrome of inappropriate secretion of antidiuretic hormone; it should be treated with antituberculous therapy for 1 year along with initial adjunctive glucocorticoids.

- Freshwater exposure is a key historical clue in suspected acute primary amebic meningoencephalitis.

- Medications such as NSAIDS, antibiotics, and intravenous immune globulin can occasionally cause aseptic meningitis.

## Health Care–Associated Meningitis and Ventriculitis

Health care–associated meningitis and ventriculitis, or nosocomial meningitis, can occur after head trauma or a neurosurgical procedure (craniotomy, lumbar puncture) or secondary to a device infection (for example, CSF shunt or drain, intrathecal pump, deep brain stimulator). Normal or abnormal CSF cell count, glucose level, and protein level do not reliably confirm or rule out infection in these patients. *Staphylococcus* species and enteric gram-negative bacteria are the most common causes, but up to 50% of infections can have negative culture results. The use of β-D-glucan and galactomannan CSF assays may aid in the diagnosis of health care–related fungal ventriculitis and meningitis. Empiric antimicrobial therapy is outlined in Table 2 and should be accompanied by device removal if present.

**KEY POINT**

- *Staphylococcus* species and enteric gram-negative bacteria are the most common causes of health care–associated meningitis and ventriculitis, but up to 50% of infections can have negative culture results.

# Focal Central Nervous System Infections

## Brain Abscesses

Brain abscesses can occur in immunocompetent or immunosuppressed persons and are most commonly seen in men. Predisposing conditions in immunocompetent patients can be seen in **Table 3**. Brain abscesses are most commonly caused by anaerobes, aerobic and microaerophilic streptococci, and Enterobacteriaceae. Initial empiric therapy is guided by the likely predisposing condition and is outlined in **Table 4**. Aspiration of the brain abscess for culture is preferred for definitive diagnosis; surgical or stereotactic drainage should be

performed if the abscess is large (>2.5 cm). Antibiotic therapy should be given for 4 to 8 weeks with follow-up cranial imaging to ensure resolution of the infection.

Immunosuppressed patients (those with HIV or AIDS, patients undergoing solid organ or bone marrow transplantation) are at risk for development of brain abscesses from several opportunistic infections. See HIV/AIDS and Infections in Transplant Recipients for further discussion.

### KEY POINT

- Brain abscesses in immunocompetent patients are treated empirically based on the likely predisposing factor with surgical or stereotactic drainage of abscesses greater than 2.5 cm.

## Cranial Abscess

Cranial epidural and subdural abscesses can arise from underlying osteomyelitis complicating paranasal sinusitis (Pott puffy tumor) or otitis media or after neurosurgical procedures or head trauma. Rarely, they may arise as a complication of bacterial meningitis. Cranial epidural abscesses are usually slow growing, presenting with subacute to chronic symptoms of headache, localized bone pain, and focal neurologic signs. In contrast, subdural empyema is a rapidly progressive infection

**TABLE 3.** Predisposing Conditions for Brain Abscess

| Condition | Incidence |
|---|---|
| Contiguous foci of infection such as sinusitis (frontal lobe) and otitis media (temporal lobe or cerebellum) | ~50% |
| Hematogenous, sometimes with multiple abscesses (odontogenic resulting from viridans streptococci, endocarditis, injection drug use) | 25% |
| Cryptogenic (most likely odontogenic) | 15% |
| Neurosurgery or penetrating head trauma | 10% |

**TABLE 4.** Predisposing Conditions, Causative Agents, and Empiric Antimicrobial Therapy in Patients with Bacterial Brain Abscess

| Predisposing Condition | Usual Causative Agents | Empiric Antimicrobial Therapy |
|---|---|---|
| Otitis media or mastoiditis | Streptococci (aerobic or anaerobic), *Bacteroides* species, *Prevotella* species, Enterobacteriaceae | Metronidazole plus a third-generation cephalosporin[a] |
| Sinusitis | Streptococci, *Bacteroides* species, Enterobacteriaceae, *Staphylococcus aureus*, *Haemophilus* species | Metronidazole plus a third-generation cephalosporin[a,b] |
| Dental sepsis | Mixed *Fusobacterium, Prevotella,* and *Bacteroides* species; streptococci | Penicillin plus metronidazole |
| Penetrating trauma or after neurosurgery | *S. aureus*, streptococci, Enterobacteriaceae, *Clostridium* species | Vancomycin plus a third-generation cephalosporin[a,c] |
| Lung abscess, empyema, bronchiectasis | *Fusobacterium, Actinomyces, Bacteroides,* and *Prevotella* species; streptococci; *Nocardia* species | Penicillin plus metronidazole plus a sulfonamide[d] |
| Endocarditis | *S. aureus*, streptococci | Vancomycin plus gentamicin |
| Hematogenous spread from pelvic, intra-abdominal, or gynecologic infections | Enteric gram-negative bacteria, anaerobic bacteria | Metronidazole plus a third-generation cephalosporin[a,b,c] |
| Immunocompromised patients / HIV-infected patients | *Listeria* species, fungal organisms (*Cryptococcus neoformans*), or parasitic or protozoal organisms (*Toxoplasma gondii*); *Aspergillus, Coccidioides,* and *Nocardia* species | Metronidazole plus a third-generation cephalosporin[a,b,c,d,e]; antifungal or antiparasitic agent |

[a]Cefotaxime or ceftriaxone; the fourth-generation cephalosporin cefepime may also be used.

[b]Add vancomycin if infection caused by methicillin-resistant *Staphylococcus aureus* is suspected. Vancomycin can then be transitioned to antistaphylococcal β-lactam (oxacillin-nafcillin)-penicillin if methicillin-sensitive *S. aureus* is confirmed.

[c]Use ceftazidime or cefepime if infection caused by *Pseudomonas aeruginosa* is suspected. Meropenem can also be used for antipseudomonal coverage.

[d]Use trimethoprim-sulfamethoxazole if infection caused by *Nocardia* species is suspected.

[e]Use ampicillin if infection caused by *Listeria* species is suspected.

NOTE: If predisposing condition is unknown, empiric treatment should include vancomycin plus metronidazole and a third-generation cephalosporin.

with high mortality that represents a neurosurgical emergency. The CSF formula in both parameningeal infections shows neutrophilic pleocytosis and a very high protein level, frequently with negative Gram stain and culture results. Pathogen identification is best achieved by culture of the abscess obtained during surgical drainage.

**KEY POINT**

- In cranial epidural and subdural abscess, pathogen identification is best achieved by culture of the abscess obtained during surgical drainage.

## Spinal Epidural Abscess

Spinal epidural abscess most commonly results from hematogenous dissemination, with *S. aureus* accounting for approximately 50% of infections; streptococcus and gram-negative bacilli such as *Escherichia coli* are also implicated. Predisposing factors for bacteremia include endocarditis, injection drug use, long-term intravenous catheters (hemodialysis catheters, central lines), and urinary tract infection. Spinal epidural abscess can also occur after neurosurgical procedures (spinal fusion, epidural catheter placement) or paraspinal injection. Patients usually develop localized pain at the site of infection that later radiates down the spine. MRI is the imaging modality of choice to identify location and extent of the abscess. All patients should undergo a baseline laboratory evaluation, including erythrocyte sedimentation rate and C-reactive protein. Blood cultures should be obtained before starting antibiotics. Although the duration of antibiotic therapy lacks robust supporting data and must be determined on a case-by-case basis, at least 6 weeks of effective antimicrobial therapy is reasonable. Surgical drainage is indicated in patients with neurologic symptoms or signs (lower extremity weakness, numbness, bladder and bowel dysfunction). Follow-up MRI is not indicated unless the patient has persistent elevation of inflammatory markers, lack of clinical response, or new neurologic symptoms or signs. Tuberculosis (Pott disease) and brucellosis should be considered in patients with negative culture results and appropriate travel history and risk factors.

**KEY POINT**

- MRI is the imaging modality of choice to identify location and extent of a spinal epidural abscess, and blood cultures should be obtained before starting antibiotic therapy.

# Encephalitis

Encephalitis is inflammation of the brain parenchyma. Possible encephalitis is defined by the presence of one major (altered consciousness for more than 24 hours) and two minor (fever, new-onset seizure, new-onset focal neurologic findings, CSF pleocytosis, and abnormal MRI or electroencephalographic findings) criteria from the International Encephalitis Consortium; probable or confirmed encephalitis requires one

major and at least three minor criteria. The causative agent is unknown in 37% to 70% of infections, depending on whether viral PCR is used and autoimmune causes are investigated. The most common known causes are viral (herpes simplex virus types 1 and 6, varicella-zoster virus, and West Nile virus) and autoimmune diseases.

## Viral Encephalitis
### Herpes Simplex Encephalitis

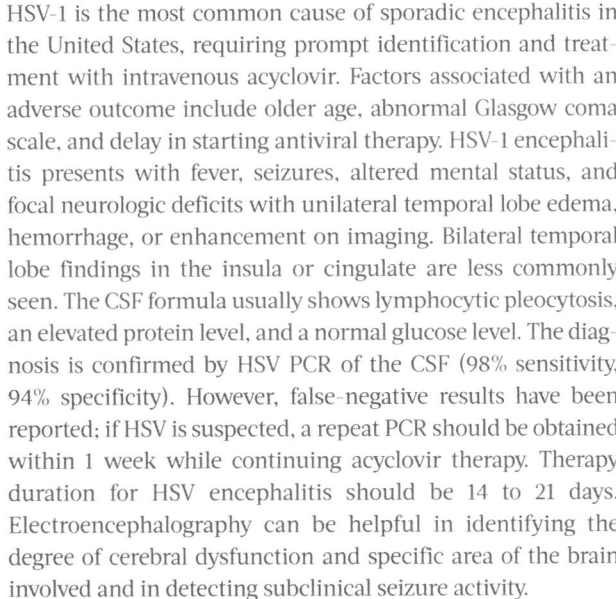

HSV-1 is the most common cause of sporadic encephalitis in the United States, requiring prompt identification and treatment with intravenous acyclovir. Factors associated with an adverse outcome include older age, abnormal Glasgow coma scale, and delay in starting antiviral therapy. HSV-1 encephalitis presents with fever, seizures, altered mental status, and focal neurologic deficits with unilateral temporal lobe edema, hemorrhage, or enhancement on imaging. Bilateral temporal lobe findings in the insula or cingulate are less commonly seen. The CSF formula usually shows lymphocytic pleocytosis, an elevated protein level, and a normal glucose level. The diagnosis is confirmed by HSV PCR of the CSF (98% sensitivity, 94% specificity). However, false-negative results have been reported; if HSV is suspected, a repeat PCR should be obtained within 1 week while continuing acyclovir therapy. Therapy duration for HSV encephalitis should be 14 to 21 days. Electroencephalography can be helpful in identifying the degree of cerebral dysfunction and specific area of the brain involved and in detecting subclinical seizure activity.

Human herpesvirus 6 can cause severe encephalitis in transplant recipients. Cytomegalovirus can cause encephalitis with periventricular enhancement on imaging in immunosuppressed patients (those with AIDS or after transplantation). Diagnosis is by PCR of the CSF for cytomegalovirus, and treatment is parenteral ganciclovir. Cytomegalovirus and Epstein-Barr virus can cause meningoencephalitis in young, immunocompetent patients presenting with infectious mononucleosis syndromes.

### Varicella-Zoster Virus Encephalitis

Varicella-zoster virus (VZV) is a commonly underdiagnosed, treatable cause of encephalitis in adults. VZV can present with vasculopathy with a stroke, encephalitis, meningitis, radiculopathy, or myelitis. Patients can present without a vesicular rash, so a PCR of the CSF or a serum-to-CSF anti-VZV IgG should be ordered in all patients with encephalitis. Treatment with intravenous acyclovir for 10 to 14 days is recommended.

### Arboviruses

Arboviral CNS infections in the United States are most commonly seen in summer or fall and include West Nile (WNV), Eastern and Western equine encephalitis, St. Louis encephalitis, Powassan, and La Crosse viruses. WNV is the most common cause of epidemic viral encephalitis in the United States. WNV can cause meningitis, encephalitis, acute flaccid paralysis (similar to poliomyelitis), neuropathy, and retinopathy.

CONT.

Older patients and those who have undergone transplantation or are immunosuppressed have a higher risk of death. WNV affects the thalamus and the basal ganglia; patients present with facial or arm tremors, parkinsonism, and myoclonus. Hypodense lesions or enhancements may be seen in the thalamus, basal ganglia, and midbrain on MRI of the brain. Diagnosis is confirmed by a positive WNV IgM in the CSF or serum; treatment is supportive.

HIV encephalitis is the cause of HIV-associated dementia in later stages of the untreated illness; it can also present as CD8 encephalitis, consisting of perivascular inflammation resulting from infiltration of CD8+ lymphocytes, which may occur as part of an immune reconstitution syndrome, in some cases associated with viral escape (low levels of detectable HIV RNA in CSF).

**KEY POINTS**

- Herpes simplex virus 1 is the most common cause of sporadic encephalitis in the United States, presenting with fever, seizures, altered mental status, and focal neurologic deficits; prompt identification and treatment with intravenous acyclovir improves outcomes.
- Varicella-zoster virus (VZV) is a treatable form of encephalitis and may present without vesicular rash, so polymerase chain reaction of the cerebrospinal fluid (CSF) or a serum-to-CSF anti-VZV IgG should be ordered in all patients with encephalitis.
- West Nile virus is the most common cause of epidemic viral encephalitis in the United States.

### Autoimmune Encephalitis

Autoimmune neurologic diseases can manifest as encephalitis, cerebellitis, dystonia, status epilepticus, cranial neuropathies, and myoclonus. Anti-N-methyl-D-aspartate receptor encephalitis is most common; it was initially described as a paraneoplastic syndrome affecting young women with ovarian teratomas, but it can be associated with other tumors (sex cord stromal tumors, small cell lung cancer) or occur without a tumor. Young women (<35 years) often present after viral-like illness with behavioral changes, headaches, and fever followed by altered mental status, seizures, abnormal movements, and autonomic instability. Treatment includes intravenous glucocorticoids, intravenous immune globulin, tumor removal (if present), and, in some cases, plasmapheresis and rituximab.

# Prion Diseases of the Central Nervous System

Prions cause rare but relentlessly progressive and rapidly fatal neurodegenerative diseases characterized by dementia and ataxia. The cause of disease is an abnormally folded prion protein. In humans, prion diseases occur by three mechanisms: sporadic (spontaneous), familial (genetic), and acquired

(infectious or transmissible). In patients of any age presenting with otherwise unexplained rapidly progressive dementia and ataxia, diagnosis of a prion disease should be considered (**Table 5**); the infectious forms are now rare (**Table 6**). Prion diseases have no known therapy.

## Sporadic Creutzfeldt-Jakob Disease

Spontaneous (sporadic) disease is the most common form of Creutzfeldt-Jakob disease (CJD), with an incidence of 1 per million worldwide. No environmental risk factors are known. Clinical manifestations include rapidly progressive dementia, usually over 4 to 6 months. Ataxia, myoclonus, and pyramidal and extrapyramidal signs may be observed. Loss of vision is not uncommon, and patients become comatose before dying.

**TABLE 5.** Criteria for Diagnosis of Probable Prion Disease[a,b]

**University of California, San Francisco Criteria (2007)[b]**

Rapid cognitive decline

Two of the following signs or symptoms:
  Myoclonus
  Pyramidal/extrapyramidal dysfunction
  Visual dysfunction
  Cerebellar dysfunction
  Akinetic mutism
  Focal cortical signs (for example, neglect, aphasia, acalculia, apraxia)

Typical EEG and/or MRI

Other investigations should not suggest an alternative diagnosis

**European MRI-CJD Consortium Criteria (2009)[b]**

Progressive dementia

One of the following signs or symptoms:
  Myoclonus
  Pyramidal/extrapyramidal symptoms
  Visual/cerebellar dysfunction
  Akinetic mutism

AND

Either
  Typical EEG
  Elevated CSF protein 14-3-3 (with total disease duration <2 years)
  OR
  Typical MRI

Routine investigations should not suggest an alternative diagnosis

CJD = Creutzfeldt-Jakob disease; CSF = cerebrospinal fluid; EEG = electroencephalography.

[a]Definitive diagnosis requires neuropathologic confirmation.

[b]Fulfilling one criterion in all categories signifies a probable diagnosis.

**TABLE 6.** Human Transmissible Spongiform Encephalopathies

| Disease Classification | Presentation |
|---|---|
| Acquired | |
| Idiopathic only (not environmental) | Sporadic fatal familial insomnia |
| | Sporadic CJD |
| Idiopathic/transmissible | Variant CJD (from BSE) |
| | Kuru |
| Inherited | Familial CJD |
| | GSS |
| | Fatal familial insomnia |

BSE = bovine spongiform encephalopathy; CJD = Creutzfeldt-Jakob disease; GSS = Gerstmann-Sträussler-Scheinker syndrome.

The diagnosis can be made by clinical history and MRI; a cerebrospinal fluid analysis positive for either total Tau or 14-3-3 protein may also be useful.

## Transmissible Prion Diseases

Variant CJD (vCJD) is the human form of bovine spongiform encephalopathy. It generally affects younger persons (age 15-50 years), frequently presenting with rapidly progressive neuropsychiatric manifestations (depression, withdrawal) and peripheral neuropathy, followed by cerebellar ataxia, involuntary movements, and cognitive decline over a 12-month period. Because vCJD can be transmitted through blood products and tissue, it is a serious public health concern worldwide. Probable vCJD is diagnosed by typical MRI findings ("hockey stick sign" in the posterior thalamus) and tonsil biopsy to detect scrapie-associated prion protein in a patient with a compatible clinical presentation (see Table 5).

Iatrogenic CJD is exceedingly rare, but transmission has been documented with contaminated cadaveric pituitary-derived human growth hormone and gonadotropin, dura mater, stereotactic electroencephalography needles, neurosurgical instruments, corneal transplants, medical instruments, implanted electroencephalography electrodes, and blood transfusions.

## Familial Prion Disease

Many mutations have been associated with the prion protein gene. All are autosomally dominant. These include the gradually progressive Gerstmann-Sträussler-Scheinker syndrome and the rapidly progressive fatal familial insomnia.

### KEY POINTS

- Prion disease should be included in the differential diagnosis of a patient of any age presenting with otherwise unexplained rapidly progressive dementia and ataxia.
- Spontaneous Creutzfeldt-Jakob disease is the most common form of prion disease and has no known risk factors.

# Skin and Soft Tissue Infections

## Introduction

Skin infections usually result from epidermal compromise that allows skin colonizers such as *Staphylococcus aureus* and *Streptococcus pyogenes* to become pathogenic. Predisposing conditions include vascular disease, immunodeficiency, neuropathy, previous cellulitis, obesity, skin trauma, tinea pedis, and lymphedema. Infections can be characterized by anatomic involvement and presence or absence of pus. Nonpurulent spreading skin infections include erysipelas, cellulitis, and necrotizing soft tissue infection; purulent skin infections refer to abscesses (**Figure 2**), furuncles, and carbuncles. Purulent skin infections are generally caused by staphylococci, including methicillin-resistant *Staphylococcus aureus* (MRSA); nonpurulent skin infections are usually caused by β-hemolytic streptococci. **Table 7** includes other skin pathogens and their associated risk factors for less common causes of skin infection. Complications of infections include systemic inflammatory response (as in severe cellulitis) or systemic toxin release (as in toxic shock syndrome).

## Erysipelas and Cellulitis

Erysipelas refers to infection of the epidermis, upper dermis, and superficial lymphatics. Usually involving the face or lower extremities, this infection is brightly erythematous with distinct elevated borders and associated fever, lymphangitis, and regional lymphadenopathy (see MKSAP 18 Dermatology). Cellulitis refers to infection involving the deeper dermis and subcutaneous fat tissue. Inflammatory signs of infection are similar to erysipelas, but the area of involvement is less well demarcated.

Although the diagnosis of erysipelas or cellulitis is usually established clinically, approximately one third of patients are

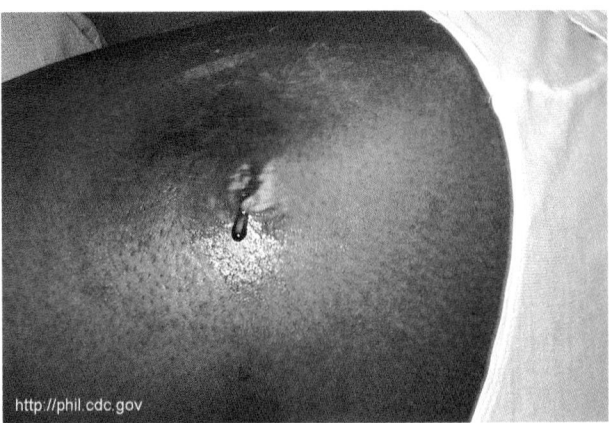
http://phil.cdc.gov

**FIGURE 2.** A cutaneous abscess draining purulent material is shown; it is caused by methicillin-resistant *Staphylococcus aureus* bacteria.

Image credit to the Centers for Disease Control and Prevention/Bruno Coignard, MD; Jeff Hageman, MHS.

| TABLE 7. | Skin Pathogens and Associated Risk Factors | |
| --- | --- | --- |
| Pathogen | Risk Factor | Comment |
| *Aeromonas hydrophila* | Contact with freshwater lakes, streams, rivers (including brackish water)<br><br>Contact with leeches | Cellulitis nonspecific in clinical appearance; minor trauma to skin usually leads to inoculation of organism |
| *Vibrio vulnificus, Vibrio parahaemolyticus* | Contact with salt water or brackish water | Cellulitis through direct inoculation into skin |
| | Contact with drippings from raw seafood | Ingestion leads to bacteremia with secondary skin infection |
| | Consumption of undercooked shellfish (particularly oysters) | Hallmark is hemorrhagic bullae in area of cellulitis lesion(s) |
| | Liver cirrhosis or chronic liver disease | |
| *Erysipelothrix rhusiopathiae* | Contact with saltwater marine life (can also infect freshwater fish) | Cellulitis usually involves the hand or arm, especially in those handling fish, shellfish, or, occasionally, poultry or meat contaminated with bacterium<br><br>Causes erysipeloid disease |
| *Pasteurella multocida* | Contact primarily with cats and dogs | Cellulitis occurs as a result of cat scratch or bite |
| *Capnocytophaga canimorsus* | Contact primarily with dogs | Cellulitis and sepsis are present, particularly in patients with hyposplenism |
| *Bacillus anthracis* | Contact with infected animals or animal products. May be the result of bioterrorism | Edematous pruritic lesion with central eschar; spore-forming organism |
| *Francisella tularensis* | Contact with or bite from infected animal (particularly cats); arthropod bites (particularly ticks) | Ulceroglandular syndrome characterized by ulcerative lesion with central eschar and localized tender lymphadenopathy; constitutional symptoms often present |
| *Burkholderia mallei* | Contact with tissues or bodily fluids of infected mules or horses | Pustules with suppurative localized lymph nodes or ulcerative nodules at site of inoculation |
| *Clostridium perfringens* | Surgery or other significant trauma | Necrotizing infection, often referred to as clostridial myonecrosis or gas gangrene |
| *Mycobacterium marinum* | Contact with fresh water or salt water, including fish tanks and swimming pools | Lesion is often trauma associated and often involves the upper extremity; papular lesions become ulcerative at site of inoculation; ascending lymphatic spread can be seen ("sporotrichoid" appearance); systemic toxicity usually absent |
| *Mycobacterium fortuitum* | Exposure to freshwater footbaths/pedicures at nail salons, particularly after razor shaving; surgery | Furuncle(s); postoperative wound infection |

CONT.

misdiagnosed. Clinical mimics include contact or stasis dermatitis, lymphedema, erythema nodosum, deep venous thrombosis, thrombophlebitis, lipodermatosclerosis, erythromelalgia, trauma-related inflammation, and hypersensitivity reactions (see MKSAP 18 Dermatology). Blood culture results are positive in approximately 5% of patients with erysipelas and cellulitis and are not routinely indicated; however, cultures should be performed for those who are immunocompromised, exhibit severe sepsis, or have unusual precipitating circumstances, including immersion injury or animal bites. Culture of skin tissue aspirate or biopsy should also be considered for these patients. Radiographic imaging is not helpful for the diagnosis of erysipelas or cellulitis but may be helpful when a deeper necrotizing infection is suspected.

For immunocompetent patients with cellulitis or erysipelas who have no systemic signs or symptoms (mild infection),

empiric oral therapy directed against streptococci is recommended as outlined in **Table 8** (see MKSAP 18 Dermatology). Treatment duration for uncomplicated infection can be as short as 5 days but should be extended as necessary until the infection improves. In patients with systemic signs (moderate infection), intravenous treatment is recommended (see Table 8). Treating predisposing factors (such as tinea pedis, edema, and primary skin disorders) may decrease the risk for recurrent infection. Prophylactic antibiotics such as penicillin or erythromycin can be considered in patients with more than three episodes of cellulitis annually.

Patients who are immunocompromised, who have systemic inflammatory response syndrome and hypotension, or who have evidence of deeper necrotizing infection such as bullae and desquamation (severe infection) should receive urgent surgical evaluation for debridement. Initial empiric

**TABLE 8.** Treatment of Skin Infections

| Infection | Treatment |
| --- | --- |
| Erysipelas or cellulitis | Mild: Oral penicillin, amoxicillin, cephalexin, dicloxacillin, clindamycin |
| | Moderate: Intravenous penicillin, ceftriaxone, cefazolin, clindamycin |
| | Severe: Surgical assessment for possible necrotizing component and empiric intravenous vancomycin plus piperacillin-tazobactam, imipenem, or meropenem |
| Necrotizing fasciitis | Polymicrobial infection: Surgical assessment/debridement and combination therapy such as vancomycin plus piperacillin-tazobactam or imipenem or meropenem |
| | *Streptococcus pyogenes* or *Clostridium perfringens*: Surgical assessment/debridement and penicillin plus clindamycin |
| | *Aeromonas hydrophila*: Surgical assessment/debridement and ciprofloxacin plus doxycycline |
| | *Vibrio vulnificus*: Surgical assessment/debridement and ceftazidime, ceftriaxone, or cefotaxime plus doxycycline |
| Furuncle, carbuncle, or abscess | Mild: Incision and drainage |
| | Moderate: Incision and drainage plus empiric trimethoprim-sulfamethoxazole or doxycycline pending culture and susceptibilities |
| | Severe: Incision and drainage plus empiric vancomycin, daptomycin, linezolid, telavancin, or ceftaroline pending culture and susceptibilities |

broad-spectrum antibiotic therapy should be started (see Table 8); then treatment may be adjusted based on culture and sensitivity results from lesion-associated specimens. H

**KEY POINTS**

HVC
- Blood cultures are positive in approximately 5% of patients with erysipelas and cellulitis and are not routinely indicated; however, cultures should be performed for those who are immunocompromised, exhibit severe sepsis, or have unusual precipitating circumstances, including immersion injury or animal bites.

- Patients with evidence of deeper necrotizing infection such as bullae and desquamation (severe infection) should receive urgent surgical evaluation for debridement and empiric broad-spectrum antibiotic therapy.

## Necrotizing Fasciitis

Necrotizing soft tissue infections, which involve subdermal compartments including fascia and possibly muscle, are uncommon but potentially life threatening. In necrotizing fasciitis (NF), infection usually spreads along the superficial fascia. These infections may be monomicrobial or polymicrobial, consisting of a mixture of aerobic and anaerobic bacteria, and are often associated with the production of toxins. In monomicrobial infection, the classically associated pathogen is *Streptococcus pyogenes*; other potential organisms include *Staphylococcus aureus*, *Streptococcus agalactiae*, *Aeromonas hydrophila*, *Vibrio vulnificus*, and *Clostridium perfringens*.

NF characteristically occurs in the setting of previous skin trauma or infection and most commonly affects the extremities. Risk factors include diabetes mellitus, injection drug use, malignancy, immunosuppression, and liver disease. Patients with liver disease are at particular risk for infection with

*V. vulnificus* (**Figure 3**). Patients with diabetes are at risk for NF of the perineum, a polymicrobial infection known as Fournier gangrene that usually results from antecedent genitourinary, traumatic, or anorectal infection.

The initial presentation of NF resembles cellulitis before potentially rapid progression with edema, severe pain, hemorrhagic bullous lesions, skin necrosis, and local crepitus. Systemic toxicity manifests with fever, hypotension, tachycardia, mental status changes, and tachypnea. A hallmark of infection is "woody" induration appreciated by palpation of involved subcutaneous tissues. Necrosis of local nerves may result in anesthesia.

Laboratory study results are individually nonspecific. The Laboratory Risk Indicator for Necrotizing Fasciitis (LRINEC) score is derived from six variables that, when added together, are associated with an increased likelihood of necrotizing skin

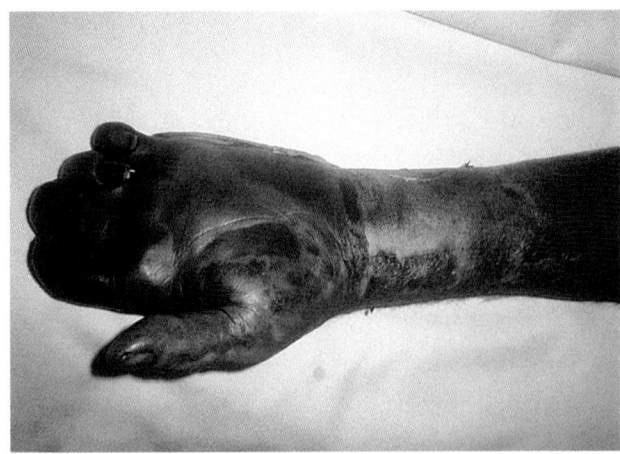

**FIGURE 3.** Bullous cellulitis characteristic of *Vibrio vulnificus* infection is shown in a patient with cirrhosis; cutaneous necrosis is also evident, most likely associated with disseminated intravascular coagulation.

CONT.

infection: C-reactive protein level (>15 mg/dL [150 mg/L]), total leukocyte count (>15,000-25,000/μL [15-25 × 10⁹/L]), hemoglobin level (<11-13.5 g/dL [110-135 g/L]), sodium level (<135 mEq/L [135 mmol/L]), creatinine level (>1.6 mg/dL [141 μmol/L]), and glucose level (>180 mg/dL [10 mmol/L]). This tool was developed to improve diagnostic accuracy; the reported positive and negative predictive values are 92% and 96%, respectively. However, use of the score has not been prospectively validated in all clinical settings, so operative debridement should be pursued in patients with a high index of clinical suspicion for NF.

Plain radiographs and CT scans may demonstrate gas in soft tissues, but MRI with contrast is more sensitive and can help delineate anatomic involvement. Surgical exploration can confirm the diagnosis of NF. Blood culture(s) obtained before surgery and antibiotic administration or deep intraoperative specimen culture can establish the microbiologic cause.

In confirmed cases of NF, repeated surgical debridement is typically required. Pending culture results, empiric antibiotic treatment includes broad-spectrum coverage for aerobic and anaerobic organisms (including MRSA) and consists of vancomycin, daptomycin, or linezolid plus piperacillin-tazobactam, a carbapenem, ceftriaxone plus metronidazole, or a fluoroquinolone plus metronidazole. Some experts also recommend adding empiric clindamycin because of its suppression of toxin production by staphylococci and streptococci. See Table 8 for treatment of NF caused by *S. pyogenes*, *V. vulnificus*, *A. hydrophila*, or clostridial species. Antimicrobial discontinuation can be considered when the patient is afebrile and clinically stable, and surgical debridement is no longer required. **H**

**KEY POINTS**

- Necrotizing fasciitis initially resembles cellulitis before rapid progression of subdermal infection manifesting with clinical signs of edema, "woody" induration, severe pain, hemorrhagic bullous lesions, skin necrosis, local crepitus, fever, hypotension, tachycardia, mental status changes, and tachypnea; necrosis of local nerves may result in anesthesia.

- In patients with suspected necrotizing fasciitis, MRI with contrast is more sensitive than plain radiography or CT and can help delineate anatomic involvement.

## Purulent Skin Infections

Abscesses are erythematous, nodular, localized collections of pus within the dermis and subcutaneous fat. Furuncles (boils) are hair follicle–associated abscesses that extend into the dermis and subcutaneous tissue. These inflammatory nodules are typically seen on the face, neck, and axilla. Infection that extends subcutaneously to involve several furuncles is known as a carbuncle. This coalescence of abscesses can result in systemic signs of infection.

Primary treatment for abscesses, furuncles, and carbuncles is incision and drainage. Gram stain and culture should be obtained from the purulent drainage when antibiotic administration is planned. Mild lesions without systemic symptoms do not require antibiotic therapy after drainage. For patients with moderate infections who have systemic signs of infection, empiric treatment is recommended (see Table 8). Empiric treatment with parenteral therapy is also recommended in immunocompromised patients, patients with hypotension and systemic inflammatory response syndrome (severe infection), or patients in whom incision and drainage plus oral antibiotics fail. Treatment is adjusted based on sensitivities from culture of the purulent drainage.

If MRSA is the cause of multiple recurrences of purulent skin infection, decolonization with topical intranasal mupirocin and chlorhexidine washes should be considered. Other diagnoses such as hidradenitis suppurativa, pilonidal cysts, or a foreign body should be considered when no microbial cause is identified.

Newer antibiotics for skin and soft tissue infections caused by *Streptococcus* and *Staphylococcus* species (including MRSA) include tedizolid, oritavancin, and dalbavancin. Use of these antibiotics is recommended in consultation with infectious disease specialists. **H**

**KEY POINTS**

- Primary treatment for abscesses, furuncles, and carbuncles is incision and drainage; mild infections (without systemic symptoms) do not require antibiotic therapy.

**HVC**

- For moderate and severe purulent infections associated with systemic symptoms, Gram stain and culture should be performed on the purulent drainage followed by empiric oral antibiotic treatment for moderate infections and empiric intravenous antibiotics for severe infections.

## Animal Bites

Bites from cats and dogs represent approximately 1% of emergency department visits in the United States; most wounds (about 80%) will not become infected. Cat bites are more likely to become infected because of deeper puncture wounds created by cats' sharp, slender teeth. The microbiology of infection depends on the microbiota of the animal's mouth and of the patient's skin. Mixed aerobes and anaerobes, including staphylococci, streptococci, *Bacteroides* species, *Porphyromonas* species, *Fusobacterium* species, and *Pasteurella* species, typically compose the bacteria in bite wounds. *Capnocytophaga canimorsus* is a common constituent of canine microbiota and can cause severe infections in patients with asplenia.

Wound management includes irrigation with sterile normal saline. Irrigation also allows for characterization of wound extent and dimensions; signs of inflammation and infection, including edema, erythema, pain, necrosis, lymphangitis, and pus; and local neurovascular involvement. Surgical evaluation for possible debridement and removal of foreign bodies is particularly important with hand bites. Culture of deep intraoperative tissue and antibiotic susceptibilities of isolated organisms allows for pathogen-directed therapy. Radiographs may demonstrate fracture, other bony involvement, or foreign bodies. Assessment for tetanus and rabies prophylaxis is essential. With the exception of facial wounds, primary wound closure is not generally pursued.

The decision to begin early antibiotic prophylaxis in the absence of clinical signs of infection is based on the severity of the wound and the immune status of the patient. Because of its activity against pathogens associated with animal bite wounds, a 3- to 5-day course of amoxicillin-clavulanate is recommended for patients who are immunosuppressed, including patients with cirrhosis and asplenia. Pre-emptive antibiotic therapy is also recommended for wounds with associated edema or lymphatic or venous insufficiency; crush injury; wounds involving a joint or bone; deep puncture wounds; or moderate to severe injuries, especially involving the face, genitalia, or hand. If a patient is allergic to penicillin, a combination of trimethoprim-sulfamethoxazole, or a fluoroquinolone, or doxycycline plus clindamycin or metronidazole can be used.

For clinically infected bite wounds, antibiotics are recommended after tissue wound cultures (and blood cultures, if systemic signs of infection are present) are obtained. For outpatient management of mildly infected wounds, oral antibiotics are recommended. The duration of antibiotic therapy is usually less than 2 weeks unless bone or joint involvement dictates a more prolonged course. Intravenous therapy is indicated for severe infections with systemic involvement, including sepsis; severe injuries, particularly those associated with tendon, nerve, vascular, or crush injuries; and hand infections. Intravenous antibiotic options include β-lactam or β-lactamase inhibitors (ampicillin-sulbactam, piperacillin-tazobactam), carbapenems (imipenem, meropenem, ertapenem), or ceftriaxone or a fluoroquinolone plus clindamycin or metronidazole. Empiric MRSA coverage may be included in patients with risk factors for MRSA infection (MRSA nasal colonization, recent hospitalization, recent antibiotic use, previous MRSA infection). Surgical consultation is usually obtained.

**KEY POINTS**

- Bite wound management includes irrigation with sterile normal saline; with the exception of facial wounds, primary closure is not generally pursued.

- Assessment for tetanus and rabies prophylaxis is essential in patients with animal bite wounds.

- Pre-emptive amoxicillin-clavulanate is recommended for patients who are immunosuppressed; wounds with associated edema or lymphatic or venous insufficiency; crush injury; wounds involving a joint or bone; deep puncture wounds; or moderate to severe injuries, especially involving the face, genitalia, or hand.

## Human Bites

Intentional biting of others, self-inflicted wounds such as those occurring from fingernail biting, and clenched-fist injuries after a punch to another person's mouth are the most common causes of human bite wounds. These wounds are at risk for infection with human skin and mouth organisms. These organisms comprise aerobic organisms, including staphylococci, streptococci, and *Eikenella corrodens*, and anaerobic organisms, including *Peptostreptococcus, Fusobacterium,* and *Prevotella* species. Short-course prophylactic antibiotic therapy with amoxicillin-clavulanate is recommended for all human bites. The management of infected wounds is similar to that for animal bites, including empiric MRSA coverage in patients at increased risk for MRSA infection. Hand involvement warrants surgical evaluation. In addition to assessment for tetanus prophylaxis, evaluation for potential exposure to hepatitis B and C viruses, HIV, and other bodily fluid–transmitted pathogens is warranted.

**KEY POINTS**

- Short-course prophylactic antibiotic therapy with amoxicillin-clavulanate is recommended for all human bites.

- In addition to assessment for tetanus prophylaxis, evaluation of human bites for potential exposure to hepatitis B and C viruses, HIV, and other bodily fluid–transmitted pathogens is warranted.

## Diabetic Foot Infections

Diabetic foot infections typically result after trauma in persons with vasculopathy, neuropathy, suboptimal glucose control, and immunologic deficits. Additional risk factors for infection include presence of an ulcer for greater than 1 month, recurrent ulcers, lower extremity amputation, kidney function impairment, walking barefoot, and a positive probe-to-bone test in the wound. Infection is diagnosed when pus or two or more inflammatory signs (warmth, induration, erythema, pain, and tenderness) are present.

Following debridement of overlying callous or necrotic tissue as necessary, infections should be classified according to severity and extent. Mild infections involve only skin and subcutaneous tissue with erythema confined to 2 cm beyond the ulcer. Moderate infections extend deeper than subcutaneous tissue (for example, abscess, fasciitis, and osteomyelitis), or the erythema is more extensive. Severe infections are associated with systemic signs such as fever, tachycardia, tachypnea, leukocytosis, and hypotension or metabolic complications such as acidosis, worsening kidney function, and hyperglycemia. The affected foot or limb should also be assessed for arterial ischemia, venous insufficiency, neuropathy, and biomechanical abnormalities such as Charcot arthropathy or hammer toe. Evidence of critical ischemia can be considered a proxy for severe infection.

Uninfected wounds should not be cultured or treated with antibiotics. Mild infections are typically caused by aerobic

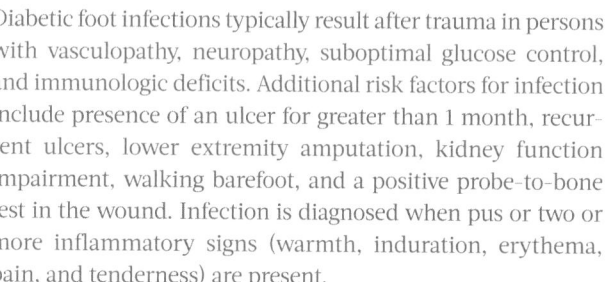

CONT.

staphylococci (non-MRSA) and streptococci and can be empirically treated with a short course (7-14 days) of oral antibiotics, such as cephalexin, clindamycin, amoxicillin-clavulanate, or dicloxacillin. For mild infections with pus or MRSA risk factors (previous MRSA infection or colonization within the last year or high local prevalence), wound cultures should be obtained by curettage or biopsy of deep tissue before initiating antibiotics. Doxycycline or trimethoprim-sulfamethoxazole can also be used with a β-lactam antibiotic. For moderate and severe infections, polymicrobial coverage of staphylococci (including MRSA), streptococci, aerobic gram-negative bacilli, and anaerobes is recommended. Following deep-tissue culture, initial antibiotic regimens include β-lactam or β-lactamase inhibitors, carbapenems, or metronidazole plus a fluoroquinolone or third-generation cephalosporin in addition to an anti-MRSA agent (vancomycin, daptomycin, linezolid). Antibiotic choices are guided by culture results. Moderate to severe infections are usually treated with a longer course of antibiotics (2-4 weeks); if osteomyelitis is present, approximately 6 weeks of antibiotic therapy is administered after surgical debridement.

A positive probe-to-bone test in a diabetic foot wound is associated with increased risk for osteomyelitis. Surgical consultation is often pursued to evaluate the need for debridement, resection, amputation, or revascularization. Plain imaging is recommended for all patients with new foot infections to assess for soft tissue gas, foreign body, and bony involvement; additional imaging with ultrasonography (for abscess) or MRI (for bone involvement) is recommended when clinically indicated. CT with intravenous contrast or a labeled leukocyte scan combined with a radionuclide bone scan can be considered when MRI is not possible. Wound care, glycemic control, and off-loading areas of biomechanical stress are essential.

---

**KEY POINTS**

- Diabetic foot infection is diagnosed when pus or two or more inflammatory signs (warmth, induration, erythema, pain, and tenderness) are present.

**HVC** • Uninfected diabetic foot wounds should not be cultured or treated with antibiotics.

- Deep-tissue culture (curettage or biopsy) is indicated before antibiotic therapy for moderate or severe infections and complicated mild infections (presence of pus or MRSA risk factors).

- Plain imaging is recommended for all patients with new diabetic foot infections; additional imaging with ultrasonography or MRI is recommended when abscess or bone involvement is suspected.

## Toxic Shock Syndrome

S. aureus- and S. pyogenes-associated exotoxins result in cytokine production that can result in toxic shock syndrome (TSS) (**Table 9** and **Table 10**). Staphylococcal TSS is associated with tampon use, nasal packings, surgical wounds, skin ulcers,

---

**TABLE 9.** Diagnostic Criteria for Staphylococcal Toxic Shock Syndrome[a]

Fever >38.9 °C (102.0 °F)

Systolic blood pressure <90 mm Hg

Diffuse macular rash with subsequent desquamation, especially on palms and soles

Involvement of three or more of the following organ systems:

    Gastrointestinal (nausea, vomiting, diarrhea)

    Muscular (severe myalgia or fivefold or greater increase in serum creatine kinase level)

    Mucous membrane (hyperemia of the vagina, conjunctivae, or pharynx)

    Kidney (blood urea nitrogen or serum creatinine level at least twice the upper limit of normal)

    Liver (bilirubin, aspartate aminotransferase, or alanine aminotransferase concentration twice the upper limit of normal)

    Blood (platelet count <100,000/μL [100 × 10⁹/L])

    Central nervous system (disorientation without focal neurologic signs)

Negative results on serologic testing for Rocky Mountain spotted fever, leptospirosis, and measles; negative cerebrospinal fluid cultures for organisms other than *Staphylococcus aureus*

[a]Diagnosis is considered confirmed when fever, hypotension, and rash with involvement of three or more organ systems listed and negative serologic and cerebrospinal fluid results listed are all present.

Adapted with permission from Moreillon P, Que YA, Glauser MP. *Staphylococcus aureus*. In: Mandell GL, Dolin R, Bennett JE, eds. Principles and practice of infectious disease. 6th ed. Philadelphia, PA: Churchill Livingstone; 2005:2331. Copyright 2005, Elsevier.

---

**TABLE 10.** Diagnostic Criteria for Streptococcal Toxic Shock Syndrome[a]

Definite case

    Isolation of GABHS from a sterile site (blood, cerebrospinal fluid, operative wound)

Probable case

    Isolation of GABHS from a nonsterile site (throat, vagina, skin lesion)

Hypotension (systolic pressure ≤90 mm Hg)

The presence of ≥2 of the following findings:

    Kidney (acute kidney injury or failure)

    Liver (elevated aminotransferase concentrations)

    Skin (erythematous macular rash, soft tissue necrosis)

    Blood (coagulopathy, including thrombocytopenia and disseminated intravascular coagulation)

    Pulmonary (acute respiratory distress syndrome)

GABHS = group A β-hemolytic streptococci.

[a]A definite case is defined by the isolation of GABHS from a sterile site; hypotension with systolic blood pressure ≤90 mm Hg; plus the presence of two or more of the clinical findings listed.

burns, catheters, and injection drug use. Streptococcal TSS is associated with skin and soft tissue infection, particularly NF. Bacteremia and mortality rates are higher with streptococcal than staphylococcal TSS. Source control typically requires surgical debridement. Antibiotics for streptococcal TSS consist of penicillin plus clindamycin, the latter added to eradicate the high inoculum of bacteria present and to suppress toxin production. If methicillin-susceptible *S. aureus* is the cause, nafcillin and clindamycin are recommended; for MRSA, vancomycin plus clindamycin or linezolid monotherapy is preferred. More studies are needed to establish the exact role of intravenous immune globulin in this setting, and it is not recommended in the most recent guidelines by the Infectious Diseases Society of America.

### KEY POINTS

- Source control for toxic shock syndrome typically requires surgical debridement.
- Streptococcal toxic shock syndrome is treated with penicillin and clindamycin.
- Infection with methicillin-susceptible *Staphylococcus aureus* is treated with nafcillin and clindamycin; linezolid monotherapy or vancomycin plus clindamycin is preferred for infection with methicillin-resistant *S. aureus*.

# Community-Acquired Pneumonia

## Epidemiology

Community-acquired pneumonia (CAP) is a leading cause of infection and hospitalization in the United States, associated with more than $10 billion annually in health care expenditures. The spectrum of illness due to CAP ranges from mild disease, with approximately 50% of patients managed in the ambulatory setting, to fatal infections. Rates of hospitalization increase with advanced age; the incidence of hospitalization for CAP among adults 80 years or older is 25 times higher than in adults younger than 50 years.

The definition of CAP has recently expanded to include some patients previously categorized as having health care–associated pneumonia (HCAP). This change was made because the microbiology and treatment of patients with CAP in long-term care facilities or who were hospitalized in the preceding 3 months do not differ substantially from that of community-dwelling patients with similar comorbidities. Practically, elimination of the HCAP classification simplifies treatment and has antibiotic stewardship implications, leading to a decrease in the use of unnecessarily broad antibiotics. Differentiating CAP from true hospital-acquired pneumonia (HAP) remains clinically meaningful (see Health Care–Associated Infections for HAP discussion).

## Microbiology

CAP is usually caused by infection with a viral or bacterial pathogen; fungal or mycobacterial infections occur much less frequently. The probability of infection with a specific organism varies based on age, comorbidities, seasonality, and geography. Epidemiologic risk factors or conditions associated with specific pathogens are listed in **Table 11**. Because causative organisms have variable virulence, severity of illness, which influences site of care, is used to guide empiric antibiotic therapy (**Table 12**).

*Streptococcus pneumoniae,* previously considered the leading cause of CAP, accounts for only 5% to 15% of hospitalized cases in recent studies. This decrease in incidence at least partially results from the success of vaccination strategies. Conversely, rates of CAP caused by *Staphylococcus aureus* and Enterobacteriaceae are rising, even among patients without identifiable health care exposure. The CDC-EPIC trial, a recent multicenter study that performed prospective microbiologic and molecular testing on patients hospitalized with CAP, more frequently identified a single or multiple viruses rather than a bacterial pathogen in CAP infections requiring hospitalization (**Figure 4**). *S. pneumoniae* was the most common bacterial cause, although rhinovirus (9%) and influenza virus (6%) were higher in incidence. The significance of viral detection in CAP is unclear; an antecedent mild respiratory viral infection may increase the risk for a secondary bacterial infection. This phenomenon is well documented for postinfluenza CAP caused by *S. aureus*, *S. pneumoniae*, and *Streptococcus pyogenes*. Despite extensive laboratory investigation, no causative organism was identified in 62% of patients in the CDC-EPIC trial.

Atypical pneumonia refers to CAP caused by organisms not cultivatable on standard bacterial media, including viruses and fastidious bacteria such as *Legionella* species, *Mycoplasma*

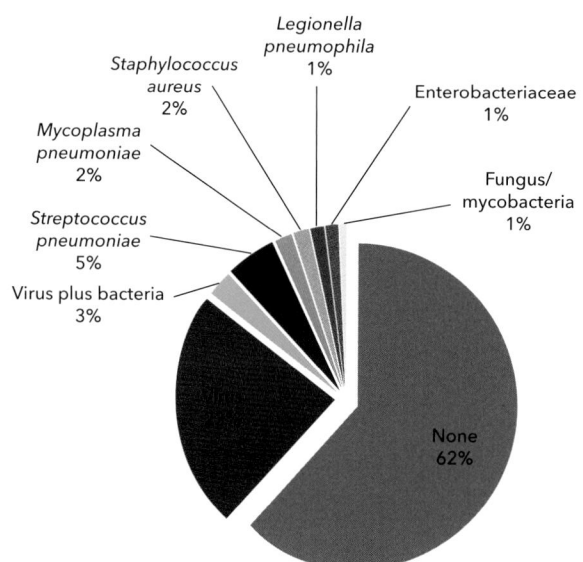

**FIGURE 4.** The chart depicts percentages of pathogens detected among hospitalized patients with community-acquired pneumonia in the CDC-EPIC Study.

Data from Jain S, Self WH, Wunderink RG, et al. Community-acquired pneumonia requiring hospitalization among U.S. adults. N Engl J Med. 2015;373:415-27.

**TABLE 11.** Risk Factors for Pathogens Causing Community-Acquired Pneumonia

| Risk Factor | Common Pathogens |
|---|---|
| Heavy alcohol use | *Streptococcus pneumoniae*, oral flora (aspiration), *Klebsiella pneumoniae* |
| COPD | *Haemophilus influenzae*, *S. pneumoniae*, *Moraxella catarrhalis*, *Legionella pneumophila*, *Pseudomonas aeruginosa* |
| Structural lung disease (bronchiectasis, cystic fibrosis) | *P. aeruginosa*, *Burkholderia cepacia*, *Stenotrophomonas maltophilia*, *Staphylococcus aureus* |
| Aspiration (seizures, neurologic impairment, loss of consciousness) | Oral anaerobes, Enterobacteriaceae |
| Age >65 years | Influenza virus, *S. pneumoniae*, rhinovirus |
| Post-viral illness | *S. aureus*, *Streptococcus pyogenes*, *S. pneumoniae* |
| Animal exposure | |
| Birds | *Chlamydophila psittaci*, *Histoplasma capsulatum*, *Cryptococcus neoformans* |
| Dogs | *Bordetella bronchiseptica* |
| Cats | *Pasteurella multocida* |
| Farm animals or domesticated pregnant animals | *Coxiella burnetii*, *Brucella* species |
| Horses | *Rhodococcus equi* |
| Rodent droppings | Hantavirus |
| Rabbits | *Francisella tularensis* |
| Hot tub exposure | *Legionella pneumoniae*, atypical mycobacteria (causing a hypersensitivity pneumonitis) |
| Geographic | |
| Eastern United States | *Histoplasma capsulatum*, *Blastomyces dermatitidis* |
| Southwest United States | Coccidioides |
| Southeast Asia | *Burkholderia pseudomallei*, SARS, avian influenza |
| Middle East | MERS |
| Late fall, winter, early spring (Western hemisphere) | Influenza virus, parainfluenza virus, rhinovirus |

MERS = Middle East respiratory syndrome; SARS = severe acute respiratory syndrome.

*pneumoniae*, and *Chlamydophila pneumoniae*. Respiratory viruses account for nearly all viral pneumonia infections, but less common pathogens include varicella-zoster virus or Hantavirus. *Legionella pneumophila* is a recognized cause of CAP requiring hospitalization or ICU admission. Legionellosis is associated with water exposure, including hot tubs and air conditioning units; however, infection may occur without an obvious source. A history of travel has been reported in approximately 10% of *Legionella* cases reported to the CDC.

CAP caused by anaerobic bacteria is uncommon, is primarily seen with aspiration, and is caused by microaerophilic oropharyngeal flora. Risk factors for aspiration pneumonia include decreased consciousness (alcohol or illicit substance use, seizures, stroke), poor dentition, gastroesophageal reflux, and vomiting. Zoonotic causes of CAP include *Coxiella burnetii* and *Francisella tularensis*. Mycobacterial or fungal causes of CAP should be considered in patients with immunocompromising conditions, epidemiologic risk factors for infection (such as incarceration, certain hobbies or occupations, and pertinent regional or foreign travel), or subacute presentations and in those who do not respond to conventional antibacterial treatment.

**KEY POINTS**

- The definition of community-acquired pneumonia (CAP) has recently expanded to include some patients previously categorized as having health care–associated pneumonia because the microbiology and treatment of patients with CAP in long-term care facilities or who were hospitalized in the preceding 3 months do not differ substantially from that of community-dwelling patients with similar comorbidities.

- *Streptococcus pneumoniae* accounts for only 5% to 15% of community-acquired pneumonia (CAP) infections requiring hospitalization, whereas rates of CAP caused by *Staphylococcus aureus* and Enterobacteriaceae are rising, even among patients without identifiable health care exposure.

- The significance of viral detection in community-acquired pneumonia is unclear; however, an antecedent mild respiratory viral infection may increase the risk for a secondary bacterial infection.

| TABLE 12. | IDSA/ATS Recommendations for Empiric Antibiotics in Community-Acquired Pneumonia | | |
|---|---|---|---|
| **Site of Treatment** | **Patient or Epidemiologic Considerations** | **Most Common Organisms** | **Regimens(s)** |
| Outpatient | Healthy patient without antibiotics in preceding 3 months | *Streptococcus pneumoniae* <br> *Mycoplasma* <br> *Chlamydophila* <br> Respiratory viruses | Macrolide <br> OR <br> Doxycycline |
| | Healthy patient from region with >25% macrolide resistance among *S. pneumoniae* | Same as above | Respiratory quinolone <br> OR <br> β-lactam plus a macrolide |
| | Comorbidities[a] or antibiotic use in preceding 3 months | Same as inpatient, non-ICU | Respiratory quinolone <br> OR <br> β-lactam plus a macrolide |
| Inpatient, non-ICU | | *S. pneumoniae* <br> *Mycoplasma* <br> *Chlamydophila* <br> *Haemophilus influenzae* <br> *Legionella* <br> Oral anaerobes <br> Respiratory viruses | β-lactam plus a macrolide <br> OR <br> Respiratory quinolone |
| ICU treatment | | *S. pneumoniae* <br> *Staphylococcus aureus* <br> *H. influenzae* <br> *Legionella* <br> Gram-negative bacilli | Parenteral β-lactam plus either azithromycin or a respiratory quinolone <br> OR <br> If penicillin allergic, a respiratory quinolone plus aztreonam |
| Any | Risk factor for *Pseudomonas* (see text) | | Antipseudomonal β-lactam plus an antipseudomonal quinolone <br> OR <br> If penicillin allergic, a respiratory quinolone plus aztreonam |
| Any | Risk factor for CA-MRSA (see text) | | Standard therapy PLUS vancomycin <br> OR <br> linezolid |

CA-MRSA = community-acquired methicillin-resistant *Staphylococcus aureus*.

[a]Comorbidities include chronic heart, lung, liver, or kidney disease; diabetes mellitus; alcoholism; asplenia; malignancies; and immunosuppression.

Adapted with permission from Mandell LA, Wunderink RG, Anzueto A, Bartlett JG, Campbell GD, Dean NC, Dowell SF, File TM Jr, Musher DM, Niederman MS, Torres A, Whitney CG; Infectious Diseases Society of America; American Thoracic Society. Infectious Diseases Society of America/American Thoracic Society consensus guidelines on the management of community-acquired pneumonia in adults. Clin Infect Dis. 2007 Mar 1;44 Suppl 2:S27-72. [PMID: 17278083]

# Diagnostic Evaluation

CAP should be suspected and chest imaging performed in any patient presenting with fever associated with cough, dyspnea, or chest pain. Symptoms may be subtle or absent in older adults or immunosuppressed patients, and clinicians should maintain a low threshold for pursuing radiographic studies in these populations. Posteroanterior and lateral chest radiography is recommended. In addition to confirming the diagnosis, radiographic patterns may provide clues to particular pathogens (**Table 13**) and guide clinical decisions regarding appropriate site of care. When plain radiographs are normal but suspicion for CAP remains high, chest radiography may be repeated after 24 hours; for patients at high risk (febrile neutropenia, risk for anthrax, or acute respiratory distress syndrome requiring intervention) with normal radiographs, chest CT should be pursued.

Routine laboratory studies are indicated to ascertain the severity of infection, determine the optimal site of care, and ensure appropriate antimicrobial dosing. HIV testing should

**TABLE 13.** Radiographic Patterns Associated with Specific Causes of Community-Acquired Pneumonia

| Radiographic Appearance | Common Pathogens |
| --- | --- |
| Lobar pneumonia | *Streptococcus pneumoniae* |
| Right lower lobe pneumonia | Oral anaerobes (aspiration) |
| Lung abscess/cavitary lesion | Oral anaerobes, *Staphylococcus aureus*, *Klebsiella pneumoniae*, *Nocardia*, *Actinomyces*, *Rhodococcus*, mycobacteria, endemic fungi |
| Interstitial infiltrate | Atypical pathogens (*Legionella*, *Mycoplasma*, *Chlamydophila*), viruses |
| Pleural effusion/empyema | Oral anaerobes, anginosus-constellatus group streptococci, *S. aureus*, *S. pneumoniae* |

**CONT.**

be performed if indicated; a positive result expands the spectrum of potentially causative organisms. Procalcitonin level, if available as a point-of-care test, is insufficiently sensitive or specific to independently diagnosis CAP or a microbiologic cause but may support a diagnosis along with other clinical findings. Rapid testing for influenza virus may assist in identifying patients who would benefit from oseltamivir and who require droplet precautions at hospital admission, but a positive test result does not exclude a concomitant bacterial pathogen.

Diagnostic studies to identify a causative organism are not routinely indicated in outpatients with CAP but should be considered in non-ICU hospitalized patients when this information would change therapy or allow treatment de-escalation. All patients with CAP who require admission to the ICU should undergo diagnostic evaluation in an attempt to confirm a microbial cause. Interpretation of sputum Gram stain and culture is hampered by the presence of oropharyngeal colonization, and growth may reflect nonpathogenic organisms. A good-quality sputum culture obtained before antibiotic initiation is suggestive or diagnostic in up to 80% of cases of pneumococcal pneumonia; sensitivity decreases after antibiotic therapy. Sputum Gram stain and culture are appropriate for patients admitted to the ICU, patients who did not respond to outpatient antibiotic therapy, patients with cavitary lung lesions, and patients with underlying structural lung disease. In these cases, consideration for mycobacterial or fungal causes may be necessary.

Blood culture results are positive in 20% to 25% of patients with pneumococcal pneumonia; fewer culture results are positive in patients with other bacterial causes. Pneumococcal urinary antigen testing is more than 70% sensitive, and results are not affected by antibiotic administration. *Legionella* urinary antigen test results are positive in most patients with *L. pneumophila* serotype 1 infection. However, the test does not detect other strains, and results can remain positive for prolonged periods after infection. Rapid antigen testing for

influenza virus on nasal swabs offers the advantage of point-of-care diagnosis but is less sensitive than polymerase chain reaction–based techniques. Respiratory viral panel results using nucleic acid amplification are positive in up to 40% of patients hospitalized with CAP; however, a positive result may reflect viral coinfection or antecedent predisposing infection rather than current clinical illness. Although these panels are less helpful in guiding decisions about discontinuing antibiotic therapy, a positive respiratory viral panel might have significant infection control implications among patients admitted to the hospital.

Additional testing is indicated only in select patients based on epidemiologic risk factors (see Table 11), clinical findings, or radiographic patterns (see Table 13). Fungal and acid-fast bacilli stains of sputum or fungal antigen testing can be performed. Serology for *Coxiella burnetii*, *Francisella tularensis*, *Legionella*, *Mycoplasma*, and *Chlamydophila*, using acute and convalescent sera, can document seroconversion or a fourfold increase in titers.

Patients with pleural effusions of unknown cause or those thicker than 1 cm should undergo thoracentesis to exclude concomitant empyema requiring drainage (see MKSAP 18 Pulmonary and Critical Care Medicine). Bronchoscopy with transbronchial biopsy should be considered in patients with an unrevealing noninvasive evaluation who do not respond to empiric therapy.

### KEY POINTS

- Diagnostic studies to identify a causative organism are not routinely indicated in outpatients with community-acquired pneumonia (CAP) but should be considered in non-ICU hospitalized patients when this information would change management; diagnostic studies should be performed in all patients admitted to the ICU with CAP.   **HVC**

- For patients with pneumococcal pneumonia, a good-quality sputum culture obtained before antibiotic initiation is suggestive or diagnostic in up to 80% of cases; blood culture results are positive in 20% to 25% of cases; pneumococcal urinary antigen testing is more than 70% sensitive, and results are not affected by antibiotic administration.

- *Legionella* urinary antigen test results are positive in most patients with *L. pneumophila* serotype 1 infection, but it does not detect other strains, and results can remain positive for prolonged periods after infection.

## Management

### Site of Care

Ambulatory management is adequate for many patients with CAP. Multiple clinical prediction models are available to identify patients who would most benefit from hospital or ICU admission (**Table 14**), but complexity and lack of consensus limit their use. Although prediction rules may aid in

**TABLE 14.** Community-Acquired Pneumonia Clinical Decision Support Scoring Systems for Site of Care

| Variable | PSI[a] | CURB-65[b] | IDSA/ATS Criteria[c] |
|---|---|---|---|
| Age | >50 years | ≥65 years | |
| Comorbidities | Malignancy | | |
| | Congestive heart failure | | |
| | Cerebrovascular disease | | |
| | Kidney disease | | |
| | Liver disease | | |
| Vital signs | Heart rate ≥125/min | | |
| | Respiration rate ≥30/min | Respiration rate ≥30/min | Respiration rate ≥30/min |
| | Temperature <35 °C (95 °F) or ≥40 °C (104 °F) | | Temperature <36 °C (96.8 °F) |
| | SBP <90 mm Hg | SBP <90 mm Hg or DBP ≤60 mm Hg | Hypotension requiring aggressive fluid resuscitation |
| Physical examination | Altered mentation | Confusion | Confusion or disorientation |
| Laboratory findings | | BUN >20 mg/dL (7.1 mmol/L) | BUN ≥20 mg/dL (≥7.1 mmol/L) |
| | | | Leukocyte count <4000/µL (4 × 10$^9$/L) |
| | | | Platelet count <100,000/µL (100 × 10$^9$/L) |
| | | | P$o_2$/F$io_2$ ratio ≤250 |
| Radiographic findings | | | Multilobar infiltrate |

ATS = American Thoracic Society; BUN = blood urea nitrogen; CURB = Confusion, Urea, Respiration rate, Blood pressure; DBP = diastolic blood pressure; IDSA = Infectious Diseases Society of America; PSI = Pneumonia Severity Index; SBP = systolic blood pressure.

[a]PSI Step 1 Screen: If no factors are present, patient is assigned risk class I and can likely be managed as an outpatient. Patients with at least one risk factor are stratified by a more complex Step 2 scale (not shown) into risk class II-V.

[b]CURB-65 Score: Each variable present is assigned one point. Patients with a cumulative score of 0-1 are usually appropriate for outpatient treatment.

[c]IDSA/ATS ICU admission scale: Patients with a major criterion (either need for mechanical ventilation or septic shock requiring vasopressors) or ≥3 of the minor criteria are best managed in the ICU.

CONT.

site-of-care decisions, scores should not supersede clinical judgment.

The Pneumonia Severity Index (PSI) is a validated predictor of all-cause mortality at 30 days. The initial assessment determines the presence of 11 variables associated with adverse outcomes (see Table 14). Patients with no risk factors (severity risk class I) can typically be managed as outpatients. Those with at least one risk factor are stratified using a second scoring system into a risk classification between II and V based on a more complex point system that includes residence in a nursing home, abnormal laboratory test results, and radiographic findings.

The CURB-65 (Confusion, blood Urea nitrogen [BUN], Respiratory rate, Blood pressure, and age ≥65 years) score is a simplified, albeit slightly less predictive, tool for identifying patients at low risk. Thirty-day mortality among patients with a CURB-65 score of 0 or 1 was less than 3%, so ambulatory treatment is appropriate for most patients with scores less than 2. The modified CRB-65 omits BUN measurement and supports ambulatory clinical assessment; patients with a score of 1 or more warrant consideration for hospitalization.

Consensus guidelines by the Infectious Diseases Society of America and American Thoracic Society (IDSA/ATS) provide criteria to identify patients best managed in the ICU. The need for mechanical ventilation or vasopressor support to maintain blood pressure was considered a major criterion and mandated ICU admission. Minor criteria are listed in Table 14; the presence of three or more criteria suggests a higher mortality rate and necessitates ICU admission.

**KEY POINT**

- A clinical prediction model (the Pneumonia Severity Index, CURB-65 or CRB-65, or Infectious Diseases Society of America/American Thoracic Society criteria) can be used to identify patients with community-acquired pneumonia who may require hospital or ICU admission.

## Antimicrobial Therapy

IDSA/ATS guidelines for CAP treatment balance the need to effectively treat infection, often in the absence of an identified pathogen, with the competing imperative for judicious antibiotic use. Treatment recommendations are stratified by site of care (see Table 12). Since publication of these guidelines, studies have documented the changing microbiology of CAP in the United States and questioned the importance of empiric treatment for atypical bacteria. Updated CAP guidelines, which are scheduled to be published in 2018, are anticipated to address these issues.

Ambulatory empiric therapy for CAP is directed against *S. pneumoniae, Haemophilus influenzae*, and atypical bacteria, even though a significant proportion of patients with CAP infected with viral pathogens do not benefit from antibiotic therapy. In otherwise healthy patients, regimens include monotherapy with doxycycline or a macrolide (either azithromycin or clarithromycin). If local *S. pneumoniae* macrolide resistance is greater than 25%, a β-lactam plus a macrolide or a respiratory quinolone could be used instead. Respiratory quinolones include levofloxacin and moxifloxacin, which are active against *S. pneumoniae*; ciprofloxacin is not a respiratory quinolone because its activity against streptococcal species is limited.

For patients with significant comorbidities treated as outpatients, a respiratory quinolone or a β-lactam plus a macrolide is recommended. Options for oral β-lactams include high-dose amoxicillin; a second-generation cephalosporin is an alternative for patients allergic to penicillin. The risk of infection with drug-resistant *S. pneumoniae* is increased with antibiotic use in the preceding 3 months; these patients should be treated similarly to outpatients with comorbidities using an agent from a different class. Macrolides and quinolones may rarely induce fatal arrhythmias, and care should be used when these antibiotics are prescribed in conjunction with other medications that prolong the QTc interval. When macrolides and quinolones are contraindicated, doxycycline can be substituted for a macrolide and given in conjunction with a β-lactam.

Patients with more severe infections requiring hospitalization may be infected with a broader spectrum of bacterial pathogens, reflecting host susceptibility and organism virulence. Patients with CAP who warrant non-ICU hospital admission are most commonly infected with the organisms shown in Figure 1. Recommended empiric regimens include a parenteral β-lactam agent (a third-generation cephalosporin or ampicillin-sulbactam) plus a macrolide or a respiratory fluoroquinolone. Use of ampicillin-sulbactam or other penicillin-based antibiotics offers the advantage of increased anaerobic spectrum and should be considered when aspiration pneumonia is a concern. For patients allergic to β-lactams or those treated with a component of this regimen in the preceding 3 months, monotherapy with a respiratory quinolone is appropriate.

An area of controversy is whether empiric therapy for atypical bacterial infection confers an outcome advantage among hospitalized patients with CAP who do not require ICU care. The CAP-START study, a randomized controlled trial published in 2015, evaluated the two currently recommended regimens (a β-lactam plus a macrolide or a respiratory quinolone) compared with β-lactam monotherapy in this

population and found no significant difference in outcomes among the three groups. This result was not replicated in a second randomized trial or in several observational studies that found excess mortality associated with β-lactam monotherapy compared with standard therapy. Furthermore, several studies have shown a survival benefit for patients with bacteremic CAP caused by *S. pneumoniae* treated with combination β-lactam plus macrolide therapy; whether this benefit reflects a direct antimicrobial effect or the anti-inflammatory properties of azithromycin is uncertain.

The microbiology among patients with CAP requiring ICU care is shown in Table 12. In this population, monotherapy with a respiratory quinolone is contraindicated. Suggested regimens include coadministration of a parenteral β-lactam active against *S. pneumoniae* and a second agent active against *Legionella* species (either azithromycin or a quinolone). For patients with a history of immediate hypersensitivity reaction to β-lactam antibiotics, aztreonam, which is purely active against gram-negative bacteria, is an acceptable alternative if given with a respiratory quinolone to treat *S. pneumoniae* and atypical organisms.

Methicillin-resistant *S. aureus* (MRSA) is not adequately treated by the previously discussed empiric regimens, yet is increasingly recognized as causing CAP, particularly in critically ill patients. CAP caused by MRSA is associated with preceding influenza infection and injection drug use, although it may present in patients without any identifiable risk factors. Empiric therapy for MRSA should be considered in patients with one of these risk factors, a suspicious Gram stain (gram-positive cocci in clusters), conventional therapy failure, pleural-based lung nodules (suggesting septic pulmonary emboli), or cavitary lung lesions. Optimal treatment for MRSA CAP has not been defined, but options include vancomycin, linezolid, and ceftaroline. Notably, daptomycin binds to surfactant, resulting in negligible alveolar levels, and is therefore not effective in pulmonary infections.

*Pseudomonas aeruginosa*, a significant cause of HAP, can also cause CAP and is not adequately treated by standard empiric regimens. *Pseudomonas* should be considered in immunocompromised patients and in patients with underlying structural lung disease (bronchiectasis or cystic fibrosis) or medical conditions requiring repeated courses of antibiotics. When clinical concern for *Pseudomonas* is present, initial empiric therapy with two active agents is indicated. Options include an antipseudomonal β-lactam (piperacillin-tazobactam, cefepime, or meropenem) in conjunction with either a quinolone (levofloxacin or ciprofloxacin) or an aminoglycoside. If an aminoglycoside is chosen, a macrolide should be added for empiric coverage of atypical bacteria. Moxifloxacin, a respiratory quinolone with activity against *S. pneumoniae*, is relatively ineffective against *Pseudomonas* and should not be used for treatment when *Pseudomonas* is a concern. Inclusion of a quinolone in the empiric regimen is relatively contraindicated in patients who did not respond to previous courses of this drug.

Controversy exists over optimal management of hospitalized patients with CAP and a positive rapid viral test result.

**CONT.**

Although respiratory viruses may cause severe CAP, a viral cause does not exclude a bacterial coinfection. *S. aureus*, *S. pneumoniae*, and *Streptococcus pyogenes* have all been associated with postinfluenza necrotizing CAP. Therefore, many authorities recommend continuing antibiotics for CAP even when a viral pathogen is identified.

For patients with uncomplicated CAP who demonstrate rapid defervescence and clinical improvement over the first 3 days, a 5-day course of therapy is adequate for cure. Exceptions include patients with cavitary disease or lung abscess, empyema, concomitant bacteremia, extrapulmonary infection, or ongoing instability, defined as persistent fever, abnormal vital signs, or hypoxia. Many authorities also recommend prolonged duration of antibiotics (at least 14 days) for CAP caused by *S. aureus* or Enterobacteriaceae; fungal or mycobacterial lung infections may require a more prolonged course of treatment. **H**

**KEY POINTS**

- Ambulatory empiric therapy for community-acquired pneumonia in otherwise healthy patients includes monotherapy with doxycycline or a macrolide (either azithromycin or clarithromycin); if local *Streptococcus pneumoniae* macrolide resistance is greater than 25%, a β-lactam plus a macrolide or a respiratory quinolone could be used instead.

- Recommended empiric regimens for hospitalized non-ICU patients include a parenteral β-lactam agent (a third-generation cephalosporin or ampicillin–sulbactam) plus a macrolide; for patients allergic to β-lactams or those treated with a component of this regimen in the preceding 3 months, monotherapy with a respiratory quinolone is appropriate.

*(Continued)*

**KEY POINTS** *(continued)*

- Treatment regimens for patients with community-acquired pneumonia requiring ICU care include coadministration of a parenteral β-lactam active against *Streptococcus pneumoniae* and a second agent active against *Legionella* species.

## Complications

CAP has a mortality rate of 10% to 12% among hospitalized patients. Survivors may experience significant morbidity, including prolonged hospitalization, protracted convalescence, and high rates of hospital readmission. Related complications include localized lung inflammation, secondary spread of infection, and toxicity related to treatment (**Table 15**).

Lack of response to antimicrobials raises consideration of a resistant or atypical organism, loculated infection (such as empyema), or an infection mimic (tumor, vasculitis, pulmonary embolism). Patients with significant pleural fluid collections should undergo diagnostic thoracentesis; chest tube drainage is indicated for empyema.

Severe CAP is often associated with a vigorous immune response resulting in acute respiratory distress syndrome. A recent meta-analysis found that for patients hospitalized for CAP, glucocorticoid administration was associated with significantly reduced mortality, reduced mechanical ventilation needs, and shorter hospital stay. Whether this glucocorticoid benefit extends to all hospitalized patients with CAP or is restricted to a subset at highest risk for acute respiratory distress syndrome has not been established; therefore, adjunctive glucocorticoids should not be routinely administered to all patients with severe CAP. **H**

| TABLE 15. | Complications of Community-Acquired Pneumonia | |
|---|---|---|
| **Organ System** | **Syndrome** | **Comments** |
| Pulmonary | Nonresolving pneumonia | Consider resistant infections, noninfectious causes |
| | Lung abscess | Prolonged course of antimicrobial treatment |
| | Empyema | Chest tube drainage of infected pleural fluid |
| | ARDS | Lung protective ventilation strategy indicated; glucocorticoids may decrease this complication |
| Neurologic | Delirium | May reflect hypoxemia, hypercarbia, or ICU stay |
| Hematologic | Leukopenia | May be related to sepsis, medication effect |
| | Thrombocytopenia | May be related to sepsis, medication effect |
| Cardiac | Acute coronary syndrome | Seen in 5%-10% of hospitalized patients |
| | Cardiac arrhythmias | Most commonly atrial fibrillation |
| Kidney | Acute kidney injury | May be related to hypoperfusion or medication effect |
| Endocrine | Adrenal insufficiency | Waterhouse-Friderichsen syndrome (acute adrenal necrosis), occurring in the setting of overwhelming bacterial infection/septic shock |

ARDS = acute respiratory distress syndrome.

- Lack of response to antimicrobials in patients with community-acquired pneumonia raises consideration of a resistant or atypical organism, loculated infection, an infection mimic, or empyema.

- Patients hospitalized with community-acquired pneumonia experience significant morbidity and are at high risk for readmission.

## Follow-up

For patients who do not require hospitalization, additional evaluation is only necessary in those who do not respond to empiric therapy within 3 days (of a standard 5-day course) or who develop new symptoms.

In contrast, readmission rates among hospitalized patients approach 20%. This population should have close outpatient follow-up to ensure clinical stability after therapy completion. Radiographic clearance often lags behind clinical response, so repeat imaging should be deferred at initial follow-up unless clinical improvement is slow or new symptoms have developed. Postobstructive pneumonia may be the presenting symptom of bronchial carcinoma, and repeat chest radiography in 2 to 3 months is recommended in patients at high risk (age >50 years or those with a significant smoking history) to document resolution.

**HVC**

- For patients who do not require hospitalization for community-acquired pneumonia, additional evaluation is only necessary in those who do not respond to empiric therapy within 3 days (of a 5-day course) or who develop new symptoms.

# Tick-Borne Diseases

## Lyme Disease

Lyme disease is the most common vector-borne infection in the United States. More than 30,000 new infections are reported annually, which likely represent only 10% of actual infections. More than 95% of infections in the United States occur in the northeastern, mid-Atlantic, and upper Midwest regions (**Figure 5**). These areas are endemic for the vector, *Ixodes scapularis* (the black-legged deer tick). The causative spirochete, *Borrelia burgdorferi*, is transmitted intradermally when a tick ingests a blood meal. In Europe, *Borrelia garinii* and *Borellia afzelii* cause Lyme disease, with *Ixodes ricinus* as the tick vector.

After a tick bite by *I. scapularis*, administration of a single dose (200 mg) of doxycycline may decrease the risk of subsequent Lyme disease development but should be considered only if (1) the tick is reliably identified as a black-legged deer tick; (2) attachment lasts 36 hours or longer; (3) antibiotics can

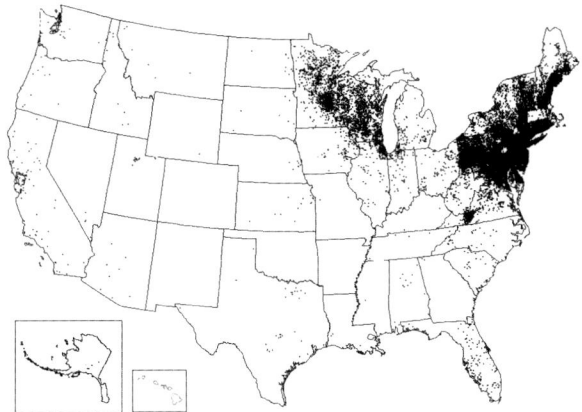

**FIGURE 5.** Lyme disease cases reported during 2016. Each dot represents the county of residence (not necessarily acquisition) for a confirmed case.

Reprinted with permission from "Reported Cases of Lyme Disease—United States 2016" (Washington, D.C.: Department of Health and Human Services, 2016), https://www.cdc.gov/lyme/resources/reportedcasesoflyme disease_2016.pdf.

be started less than 72 hours after tick removal; (4) prevalence of *B. burgdorferi* infection of ticks in the region exceeds 20%; and (5) doxycycline treatment is not contraindicated. Except for these selected situations, observation is recommended, with treatment given if suggestive symptoms occur.

The clinical manifestations, diagnostic testing, and treatment of Lyme disease vary according to the stage of infection (**Table 16**).

### Early Localized Disease

Early localized disease presents within 4 weeks of infection. Most infected persons (70% to 80%) develop erythema migrans (EM), an annular skin lesion that often presents with central clearing (**Figure 6**). Systemic symptoms are variably present.

EM lesions are typically painless, nonpruritic, and circumferentially enlarging. Atypical presentations of EM, with confluent erythroderma, ulceration, or vesiculation, may confound the diagnosis. Local cutaneous reactions due to hypersensitivity to tick saliva may resemble EM but tend to occur earlier, are pruritic, and do not enlarge significantly after onset.

A patient with EM and a compatible exposure history does not require confirmatory laboratory testing. In fact, antibody testing in early localized disease is insensitive because seroconversion may be delayed for several weeks after onset of an EM lesion. Treatment is with an oral agent. Doxycycline offers the advantage of treating incubating *Anaplasma phagocytophilum*, which also is spread by black-legged ticks and can coinfect patients with Lyme disease.

### Early Disseminated Disease

In the absence of treatment, hematogenous dissemination occurs in up to 60% of patients. Symptoms of early disseminated disease present weeks to months after infection. The most common manifestation is a flu-like illness characterized by fevers, arthralgia, myalgia, and lymphadenopathy and often

**TABLE 16.** Clinical Manifestations, Diagnostic Testing, and Treatment of Lyme Disease by Stage of Infection

| Lyme Stage | Onset after Infection | Clinical Findings | Laboratory Confirmation | Treatment[a] |
|---|---|---|---|---|
| Early localized | ≤4 wk | EM at site of tick attachment, fever, lymphadenopathy, myalgia | Not needed if EM present | Doxycycline, 100 mg PO BID × 10-21 d (first-line therapy) *or* Amoxicillin, 500 mg PO TID × 14-21 d *or* Cefuroxime axetil, 500 mg PO BID × 14-21 d |
| Early disseminated | 2 wk-6 mo | Multiple sites of EM, flu-like syndrome, heart block, myocarditis, facial nerve palsy, meningitis, radiculitis | Not needed if EM is present; otherwise, two-tier serologic testing CSF testing for intrathecal antibody production if CNS involvement is a concern | 1. First-degree block with PR interval ≥300 msec, second- or third-degree AV nodal block, myocarditis: IV penicillin or IV ceftriaxone × 28 d 2. First-degree AV block with PR interval <300 msec: oral treatment same as for early localized disease × 14-28 d 3. Meningitis: IV penicillin or IV ceftriaxone × 28 d 4. Other manifestations (including facial palsy): oral treatment the same as for early localized disease × 14-28 d |
| Late disseminated | ≥6 mo | Recurrent large joint arthritis; neurologic symptoms (peripheral neuropathy, encephalopathy), or dermatologic symptoms (acrodermatitis chronica atrophicans) | Two-tier serologic testing | Initial rheumatologic treatment: same as for early localized but × 30 d Recurrent arthritis after initial treatment: IV ceftriaxone Neurologic disease: IV ceftriaxone × 28 d |

AV = atrioventricular; BID = twice daily; CSF = cerebrospinal fluid; CNS = central nervous system; EM = erythema migrans; IV = intravenous; PO = by mouth; TID = three times daily.

[a]Doses are for adults with normal kidney function.

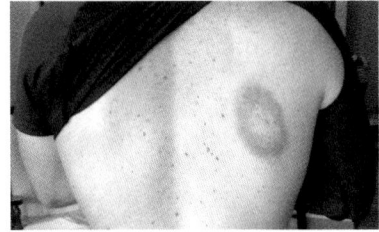

**FIGURE 6.** Erythema migrans lesion at site of tick attachment.

Figure courtesy of Dr. Karen Bloch.

associated with multiple concurrent EM lesions at sites distant from the original tick attachment.

Infection of cardiac tissue results in injury to the conduction system and atrioventricular (AV) nodal block. Progression to complete heart block can occur rapidly despite antibiotic treatment, so hospitalization is indicated for close monitoring of patients with severe cardiac involvement: symptomatic patients with dizziness, syncope, or dyspnea; asymptomatic patients with first-degree AV block

and a PR interval of 300 milliseconds or greater; and patients with a higher-degree AV block. Permanent pacemaker placement is not necessary because the heart block is reversible.

Infection of neurologic tissue occurs in approximately 15% of untreated patients. Aseptic meningitis, facial palsy (unilateral or bilateral), and radiculopathy may be present in isolation or associated with skin, musculoskeletal, or cardiac findings. Lumbar puncture is indicated when central nervous system infection (such as neuroborreliosis) is suspected; cerebrospinal fluid lymphocytic pleocytosis supports the diagnosis (see Central Nervous System Infection).

When EM lesions are present, laboratory confirmation is unnecessary. In the absence of diagnostic skin findings, serologic diagnosis should be pursued through a two-tiered approach (**Figure 7**); the initial enzyme-linked immunosorbent assay (ELISA) is highly sensitive but lacks specificity and must be confirmed by a Western blot test. The C6 ELISA test detects antibody against a highly conserved bacterial epitope and may be more sensitive than traditional whole-cell sonicate ELISA, especially for the

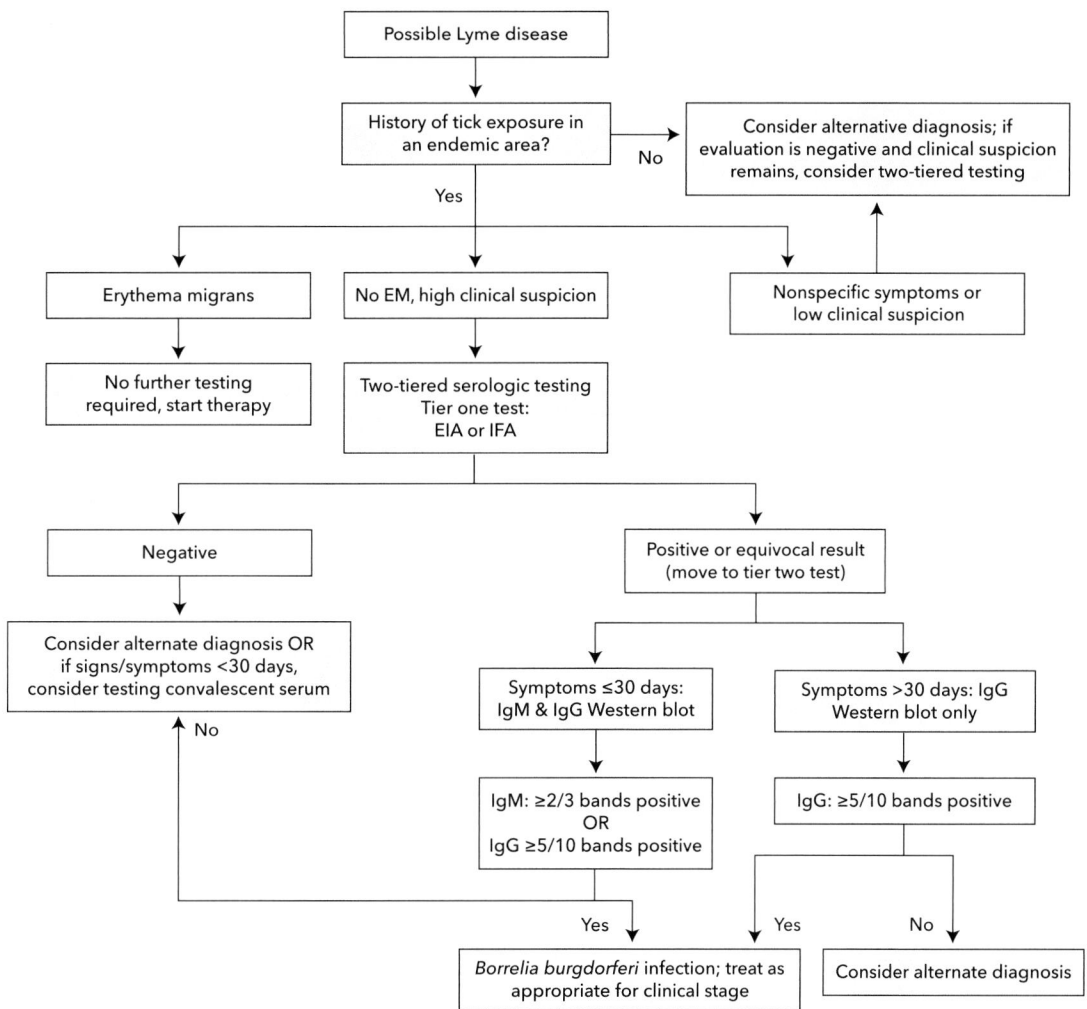

**FIGURE 7.** Serologic testing for Lyme disease. EIA = enzyme-linked immunosorbent assay; EM = erythema migrans; IFA = immunofluorescent antibody assay.

Adapted with permission from Moore A, Nelson C, Molins C, Mead P, Schriefer M. Current guidelines, common clinical pitfalls, and future directions for laboratory diagnosis of Lyme disease, United States. Emerg Infect Dis. 2016;22:1169. [PMID: 27314832] doi:10.3201/eid2207.151694

European strains *B. garinii* and *B. afzelii*, but, because of insufficient specificity, confirmatory Western blot testing is still required.

IgM antibody is detectable before IgG antibody in early infection; however, IgG antibody should be detectable after 30 days of symptoms. Because isolated IgM positivity is likely to be a false positive after the first month of symptoms, testing for IgM is not recommended after this time period. Antibodies may remain for years despite treatment; therefore, serial titers are not useful.

### Late Disseminated Disease

Approximately 60% of untreated patients with Lyme disease develop a monoarticular or oligoarticular inflammatory arthritis as a late complication. The knee and other large joints are disproportionally affected. Even without antibiotic treatment, inflammation typically resolves over weeks to months but can have a relapsing-remitting pattern. In approximately 10% of untreated patients, arthritis persists (see MKSAP 18 Rheumatology). Late neurologic or skin findings (acrodermatitis chronica atrophicans and borrelial lymphocytoma) are rare in the United States but more frequent in European infections. Diagnosis is made with the two-tier serologic test. Treatment requires prolonged oral antibiotics; parenteral therapy is used when oral therapy is unsuccessful (see Table 16).

### Post-Lyme Disease Syndrome

Post–Lyme disease syndrome has been reported in approximately 10% of patients after treatment of EM (**Table 17**). Although often erroneously called "chronic Lyme disease," studies have found no microbiologic evidence of chronic or latent infection after appropriate treatment. Symptoms include fatigue, arthralgia, myalgia, and impairment of memory or cognition that can last for years after treatment of the acute infection. Clinical trials have shown no benefit of prolonged antibiotic treatment for post–Lyme disease syndrome.

**TABLE 17.** Definition of Post-Lyme Disease Syndrome

**Inclusion Criteria**

Diagnosis of Lyme disease based on CDC case criteria (EM or positive serologic finding)

Resolution or stabilization of the objective manifestations of Lyme disease after standard treatment

Onset of at least one of the following within 6 months of Lyme disease diagnosis, with persistence for at least 6 months after antibiotic treatment, that is of sufficient severity to result in decreased level of functioning:

1. Fatigue

2. Widespread musculoskeletal pain

3. Cognitive impairment

**Exclusion Criteria**

An untreated tick-borne coinfection (such as babesiosis)

Ongoing symptoms attributable to Lyme disease (such as antibiotic-refractory Lyme arthritis)

Symptoms of fatigue or musculoskeletal pains or a diagnosis of fibromyalgia or chronic fatigue syndrome predating the onset of Lyme disease

An alternative diagnosis accounting for the symptoms

CDC = Centers for Disease Control and Prevention; EM = erythema migrans.

Source: Wormser GP, Dattwyler RJ, Shapiro ED, Halperin JJ, Steere AC, Klempner MS, et al. The clinical assessment, treatment, and prevention of Lyme disease, human granulocytic anaplasmosis, and babesiosis: clinical practice guidelines by the Infectious Diseases Society of America. Clin Infect Dis. 2006;43:1089-134. [PMID: 17029130]

Evaluation for coinfection with another tick-borne pathogen or for a noninfectious cause is indicated; when no alternative diagnosis is found, treatment is symptomatic.

**KEY POINTS**

- The causative spirochete of Lyme disease may be transmitted when an infected *Ixodes scapularis* tick attaches for at least 36 hours.

**HVC**
- Early localized Lyme disease usually presents within 4 weeks of infection and is characterized by erythema migrans (EM) at the site of tick attachment; patients with EM and a compatible exposure history do not require confirmatory laboratory testing and should receive oral antibiotic therapy.

- Early disseminated Lyme disease can affect the cardiovascular and neurologic systems; the diagnosis should be confirmed through an enzyme-linked immunosorbent assay followed by confirmatory Western blot testing, with presumptive treatment depending on disease severity.

- Post–Lyme disease syndrome (fatigue, arthralgia, myalgia, and impairment of memory or cognition) can last for years, even after treatment of the acute infection; there is no role for prolonged antibiotics for this condition.

# Babesiosis

Babesiosis is caused by the intraerythrocytic protozoan *Babesia microti*, which is spread by the black-legged deer tick. Because of the common vector, babesiosis occurs in areas of Lyme endemicity (see Figure 5), most frequently during summer months. In Europe, babesiosis is caused by several different *Babesia* species and is spread by the *I. ricinus* tick. Transfusion of infected blood products and rare congenital transmission also allows for year-round infection, which may occur outside endemic regions.

Clinical findings range from asymptomatic presentations (approximately 20%) to fatal disease (10%). Risk factors for severe disease include age older than 50 years, immunocompromise, or asplenia. Symptoms begin within 1 month after tick bite and within 6 months after transfusion of infected blood products. Symptoms are nonspecific and include fever (89%), fatigue (82%), chills (67%), headache (47%), myalgia (43%), and cough (28%). Physical examination may reveal jaundice, hepatomegaly, and splenomegaly, which rarely progresses to splenic rupture. The hallmark of babesiosis is hemolysis, with anemia almost invariably present. With severe disease, thrombocytopenia, elevated liver enzyme levels, and acute kidney injury are possible.

Babesiosis is diagnosed by visualization of the causative organism on thin blood smears, manifesting as intraerythrocytic ring forms similar to those seen in malaria or as tetrads resembling a Maltese cross (**Figure 8**). With low-level parasitemia, multiple smears may need to be examined, and the sensitivity of microscopy is low. Therefore, polymerase chain reaction or serology should be pursued if smear findings are negative but clinical suspicion of babesiosis is high.

Treatment depends on disease severity (**Table 18**). After treatment, patients should be monitored closely for relapse; if relapse occurs, prolonged therapy extending more than 2 weeks after clearance of parasitemia is necessary for cure.

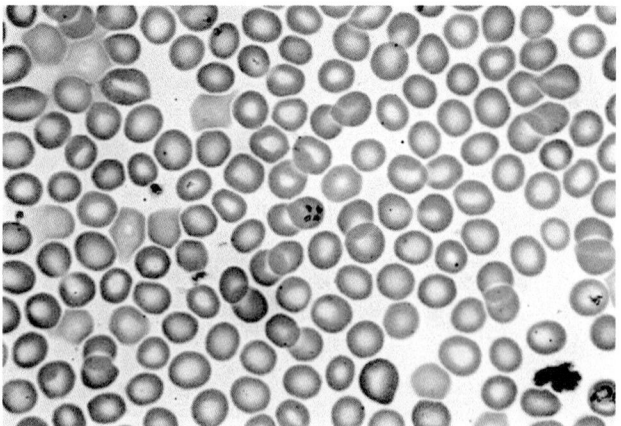

**FIGURE 8.** Peripheral blood smear showing babesiosis. The diagnosis of babesiosis is typically established by evaluation of a peripheral blood smear showing intraerythrocytic parasites. Occasionally, merozoites are arranged in tetrads, resembling a Maltese cross.

**TABLE 18.** Treatment for Babesiosis

| Severity | Regimen |
|---|---|
| Asymptomatic, ≤3 months of parasitemia | Monitor for clearance; no treatment indicated |
| Asymptomatic, >3 months of parasitemia | Atovaquone plus azithromycin |
| Mild to moderate disease | Atovaquone plus azithromycin |
| Severe disease requiring ICU admission | Clindamycin plus quinine |
| Severe disease with >10% parasitemia, hemoglobin level <10 g/dL (100 g/L), ARDS, liver failure or kidney failure | Clindamycin plus quinine *and* Exchange transfusion |

ARDS = acute respiratory distress syndrome.

**KEY POINTS**

- Babesiosis, an infection caused by an intraerythrocytic protozoan, presents with clinical findings ranging from asymptomatic infection to fatal disease; symptoms are usually nonspecific, but hemolytic anemia is a hallmark of disease.

- Diagnosis of babesiosis is by visualization of the organism on blood smear, serology, or polymerase chain reaction.

- Treatment of babesiosis depends on disease severity; atovaquone plus azithromycin are most appropriate for mild disease, whereas clindamycin plus quinine remains the regimen of choice for severe disease.

## Southern Tick-Associated Rash Illness

Southern tick–associated rash illness (STARI) presents with EM lesions identical to those seen in Lyme disease but without clinical progression or complications. STARI is associated with *Amblyomma americanum*, also known as the Lone Star tick, and occurs in the southeastern, south-central, and eastern United States. No infectious cause has been confirmed. Therefore, diagnosis is based on clinical and geographic features. Because STARI and early-stage Lyme disease may be clinically indistinguishable, treatment with doxycycline is recommended.

**KEY POINT**

- Southern tick–associated rash illness may be clinically indistinguishable from early-stage Lyme disease, and thus treatment with doxycycline is recommended.

## Human Monocytic Ehrlichiosis and Granulocytic Anaplasmosis

Human monocytic ehrlichiosis (HME) and human granulocytic anaplasmosis (HGA) are clinically similar illnesses spread by different tick vectors and caused by distinct bacterial pathogens. HME is caused by *Ehrlichia chaffeensis*, which is transmitted by the Lone Star tick, and occurs most commonly in the southeastern and south-central United States. HGA is caused by *Anaplasma phagocytophilum*, which is transmitted by *Ixodes* ticks, and occurs in areas of Lyme endemicity (see Figure 5).

These syndromes typically begin with a nonspecific febrile illness 1 to 2 weeks after a tick bite (**Table 19**). Rash is uncommon in contrast to Rocky Mountain spotted fever. Laboratory study abnormalities, including leukopenia, thrombocytopenia, and increased serum aminotransferase levels, are nonspecific.

The organisms causing HME and HGA replicate inside leukocytes and cause hallmark basophilic inclusion bodies called morulae (**Figure 9**). Serologic findings often are negative in acute illness; testing of a convalescent specimen 2 to 4 weeks after onset of symptoms is usually confirmatory. Polymerase chain reaction of whole blood at the time of acute illness may be diagnostic, particularly if performed before therapy. Doxycycline is the recommended treatment for both HME and HGA. Because delay in treatment is associated with increased mortality, empiric therapy should be started even in the absence of confirmatory testing.

**KEY POINTS**

- Human monocytic ehrlichiosis and human granulocytic anaplasmosis cause a nonspecific febrile illness beginning 1 to 2 weeks after a tick bite.

- Acute serologic findings are often negative in both human monocytic ehrlichiosis and human granulocytic anaplasmosis; polymerase chain reaction of whole blood at the time of acute illness may be diagnostic.

- Doxycycline is recommended for both human monocytic ehrlichiosis and human granulocytic anaplasmosis; empiric therapy should be started without awaiting results of confirmatory testing.

## Rocky Mountain Spotted Fever

Rocky Mountain spotted fever (RMSF) is caused by *Rickettsia rickettsii* and transmitted by multiple tick vectors. It has been reported throughout the continental United States but occurs most frequently in the "RMSF belt" extending from North Carolina to Oklahoma.

Clinically, RMSF presents with nonspecific symptoms similar to those of HME and HGA (Table 19) but can progress to aseptic meningoencephalitis. The hallmark feature is a macular eruption around the ankles or wrists, with central spread and progression to petechiae or purpura (**Figure 10**). Lesions are found on the palms and soles in as many as 50% of patients; the face is generally spared. Purpura fulminans may occur and result in loss of digits or limbs. Although skin findings are ultimately noted in greater than 90% of patients with RMSF, the earliest macular rash occurs a median of 3 days after onset

**TABLE 19.** Comparison of Epidemiologic and Clinical Features of Human Monocytic Ehrlichiosis, Human Granulocytic Anaplasmosis, and Rocky Mountain Spotted Fever

| Feature | HME | HGA | RMSF |
|---|---|---|---|
| Vector | Lone Star tick | Black-legged deer tick | American dog tick, brown dog tick, Rocky Mountain wood tick |
| Geography | Southeastern, mid-Atlantic, and south-central United States | Northeastern and upper Midwest United States | Throughout the United States[a] |
| Coinfection | Not reported; potential for coinfection with STARI or Heartland virus because of common vector | Lyme disease, babesiosis, Powassan virus, *Borrelia miyamotoi* | None |
| Incubation period | 5-14 days | 5-14 days | 3-12 days |
| Presenting signs and symptoms | Fever, headache, myalgias, nausea, vomiting, diarrhea, conjunctival injection | Fever, headache, myalgias, chills | Fever, headache, chills, mylagia, nausea, abdominal pain, photophobia, aseptic meningitis |
| Cutaneous signs | Nonspecific rash in <30% of adults, with median onset 5 days after fever | Rash rare (<10%) | Maculopapular eruption in >90% of patients, progressing to petechia with involvement of palms and soles, edema; onset, median of 3 days after fever |
| Laboratory study abnormalities | Leukopenia, thrombocytopenia, increased serum aminotransferase levels, mild anemia | Leukopenia, thrombocytopenia, increased serum aminotransferase levels, mild anemia | Thrombocytopenia, increased serum aminotransferase levels, normal or slightly increased leukocyte count, hyponatremia |
| Diagnosis | Morulae in monocytes (<30%), acute and convalescent serologies, whole-blood PCR | Morulae in neutrophils (~50%), acute and convalescent serologies, whole-blood PCR | Acute and convalescent serologies, biopsy of skin with immunohistochemical analysis |
| Treatment | Doxycycline | Doxycycline | Doxycycline |
| Fatality | 3% | <1% | 5%-10% |

HGA = human granulocytic anaplasmosis; HME = human monocytic ehrlichiosis; PCR = polymerase chain reaction; RMSF = Rocky Mountain spotted fever; STARI = Southern tick-associated rash illness.

[a]Two thirds of all patients with RMSF are infected in Arkansas, Missouri, North Carolina, Oklahoma, and Tennessee.

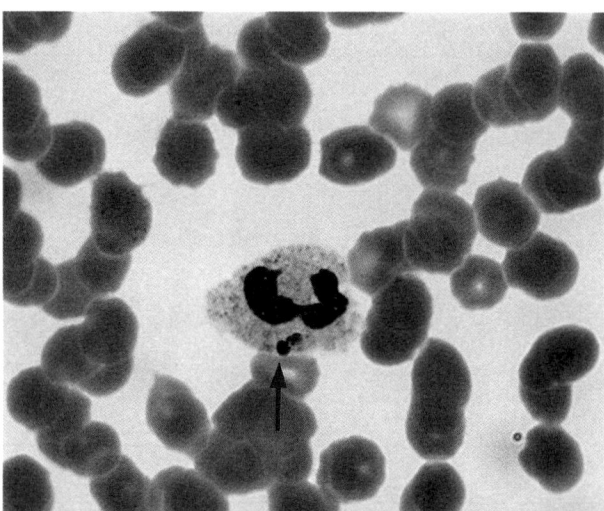

**FIGURE 9.** Morulae (*arrow*) appearing as basophilic inclusion bodies in leukocytes of a patient with ehrlichiosis.

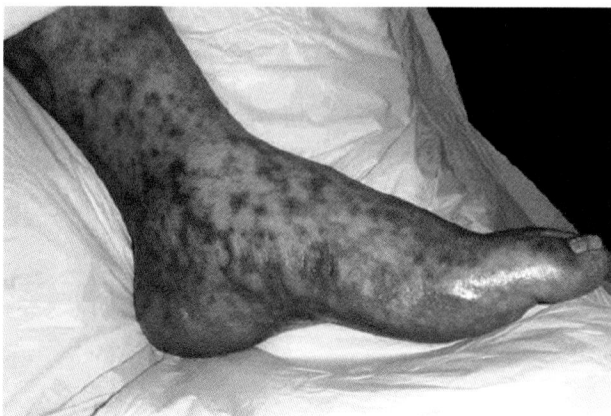

**FIGURE 10.** Petechial and purpuric skin eruption in a patient with late-stage Rocky Mountain spotted fever.

Reprinted with permission from Biggs HM, Behravesh CB, Bradley KK, Dahlgren FS, Drexler NA, Dumler JS, et al. Diagnosis and management of tickborne rickettsial diseases: Rocky Mountain spotted fever and other spotted fever group rickettsioses, ehrlichioses, and anaplasmosis - United States. MMWR Recomm Rep. 2016;65:1-44. [PMID: 27172113] doi:10.15585/mmwr.rr6502a1

of fever and thus may not be found at the first clinical presentation.

Immunohistochemical analysis of skin biopsy samples may be diagnostic. As with HME and HGA, acute serology is not sensitive, although testing convalescent serum may provide a retrospective diagnosis. Doxycycline should be given empirically when RMSF is clinically suspected because treatment delay is associated with more severe disease and increased mortality.

- Rocky Mountain spotted fever (RMSF) presents similarly to both human monocytic ehrlichiosis and human granulocytic anaplasmosis; the major differentiating feature of RMSF is the presence of a rash, but the rash may not appear until 3 days after onset of fever.
- Doxycycline should be given empirically when Rocky Mountain spotted fever is clinically suspected.

# Urinary Tract Infections

## H Epidemiology and Microbiology

Community-acquired urinary tract infections (UTIs) account for approximately 8 million ambulatory visits and 1 million hospitalizations each year in the United States, making them one of the most common infections for which an antibiotic is prescribed in clinical practice. Another 1 million nosocomial UTIs are diagnosed annually, primarily indwelling urinary catheter–associated UTIs, accounting for an estimated 40% of all health care–associated infections (see Health Care–Associated Infections). Approximately half of all women experience a UTI by age 30 years; sexual activity is a major risk factor. Approximately 5% of otherwise healthy women who experience a UTI are at greater risk of developing future infections. Other UTI risk factors include structural and functional abnormalities, use of spermicidal agents and diaphragms, pregnancy, diabetes mellitus, obesity, urethral catheterization (or other urinary tract instrumentation), immunosuppression, and genetic factors.

UTIs are classified based on anatomic location as lower (cystitis), upper (pyelonephritis, perinephric abscess), or prostatitis. The term *uncomplicated* UTI refers to infections in nonpregnant women without structural or neurologic abnormalities or comorbidities. UTIs in men, pregnant women, and persons with foreign bodies (for example, indwelling catheters, calculi), kidney disease, immunocompromise, obstruction, urinary retention from neurologic disorders, health care–associated infections, or recent antibiotic use are considered to be *complicated*. Advanced age in the presence of other major comorbidities or with significant frailty may be considered a complicating factor in UTI, although age alone does not define a complicated versus uncomplicated infection. Designating an infection as complicated influences the choice and duration of antimicrobial therapy and extent of investigation. Nevertheless, the potential for uncomplicated UTIs to evolve into clinically severe disease should not be underestimated, nor should the urgency or seriousness of complicated UTIs be overstated.

Most infections occur by the ascending route. In 95% of these cases, UTIs are caused by a single bacterial species, mainly gram-negative aerobic bacilli originating from the bowel. Uropathogenic *Escherichia coli* accounts for 75% to 95% of UTIs in women. Less common urinary pathogens include other members of the Enterobacteriaceae family,

streptococci (in particular *Streptococcus agalactiae*), enterococci, and staphylococci (most often *Staphylococcus saprophyticus*). UTIs occurring in hospitals and long-term care facilities frequently involve a more varied group of organisms (such as *Enterobacter*, *Providencia*, *Morganella*, *Citrobacter*, *Serratia*, and *Pseudomonas*). Isolation of *Staphylococcus aureus* from the urine may be related to instrumentation but should suggest the possibility of a hematogenous infection from a source outside the urinary tract. H

- The term *uncomplicated* urinary tract infection refers to infections in nonpregnant women without structural or neurologic abnormalities or comorbidities.
- Designating an infection as complicated influences the choice and duration of antimicrobial therapy and extent of investigation.
- Urinary tract infections in men, pregnant women, and persons with foreign bodies, kidney disease, immunocompromise, obstruction, urinary retention from neurologic disorders, health care–associated infections, or recent antibiotic use are considered to be *complicated*.

## Diagnosis H

In persons with symptoms of UTI, diagnosis in the outpatient setting is based on a combination of clinical features, determining if the presumed infectious process is in the lower or upper urinary tract, and the findings of significant pyuria (≥10 leukocytes/µL) and bacteriuria (bacteria in the urine). Pyuria can be detected by urine dipstick, which relies on the presence of leukocyte esterase. Although the sensitivity and specificity of dipstick testing are high (about 75% and 85%, respectively), pyuria may result from urinary tract disorders other than infection. The presence of leukocyte casts supports a diagnosis of pyelonephritis. Microscopic or gross hematuria may be present with a UTI but may also be encountered with nephrolithiasis and tumors. A positive nitrite test result signifies the presence of gram-negative bacteria capable of converting nitrates into nitrites but is negative in UTI caused by nonconverting organisms (*Enterococcus*, *Staphylococcus*, or *Streptococcus* species).

Quantitative cultures of a midstream, clean-void urine sample are the most accurate way to demonstrate bacteriuria in patients with suspected UTI. Because the microbiology is predictable and treatment courses are short, culture is not recommended in women with uncomplicated cystitis. Urine cultures are indicated in pyelonephritis, complicated cystitis, and recurrent UTIs; additionally, they are recommended in patients with histories of multiple antibiotic allergies and in those in whom the presence of a resistant organism is suspected (such as recent antibiotic treatment, health care–associated infection, previous multidrug-resistant UTI). The growth of $10^5$ colony-forming units (CFU)/mL of urine is considered significant bacteriuria; however, lower CFU counts support a diagnosis in those with UTI symptoms.

CONT.

In most adults, imaging studies are not required for diagnosis or treatment of UTIs. Imaging may be indicated when the diagnosis is unclear, when a structural abnormality or complication is suspected, or in patients with severe illness, immunocompromise, or lack of response to appropriate therapy. Ultrasonography can detect obstruction, whereas non-contrast helical CT is recommended for visualizing kidney stones. Although less sensitive than CT, kidney ultrasonography is less expensive, requires less radiation exposure, and can be used in pregnant women or if CT is unavailable. Contrast-enhanced CT (CT urography) is recommended when intrarenal or perinephric abscess is suspected.

**KEY POINTS**

- Quantitative cultures of a midstream, clean-void urine sample are the most accurate way to demonstrate bacteriuria in patients with suspected urinary tract infection.

HVC
- Urine culture is not recommended in women with uncomplicated cystitis but is indicated in pyelonephritis, complicated cystitis, recurrent urinary tract infections, patients with multiple antibiotic allergies, and in patients in whom a resistant organism is suspected.

# Management

## Asymptomatic Bacteriuria

Asymptomatic bacteriuria is defined as the presence of at least $10^5$ CFU/mL of a uropathogen from two consecutive voided urine specimens in women or one specimen in men, or more than $10^2$ CFU/mL of one bacterial species from a catheterized urine specimen in women or men, in all cases without local or systemic signs or symptoms of active infection. The prevalence of asymptomatic bacteriuria is as low as 1% to 5% in healthy premenopausal women (2%-10% in pregnant women) and nearly 100% in patients with long-term indwelling urinary catheters.

The presence of pyuria accompanying asymptomatic bacteriuria is not an indication for antimicrobial treatment. Although bacteriuria increases the risk of symptomatic UTI, treatment of asymptomatic bacteriuria neither decreases the frequency of symptomatic infections nor improves other outcomes. Inappropriate treatment of asymptomatic bacteriuria is a major driver of antimicrobial resistance, particularly in health care facilities. Treatment of asymptomatic bacteriuria is, however, indicated in pregnant women and in patients scheduled to undergo an invasive procedure involving the urinary tract.

**KEY POINTS**

HVC
- Inappropriate treatment of asymptomatic bacteriuria is a major driver of antimicrobial resistance, particularly in health care facilities.

- Treatment of asymptomatic bacteriuria is indicated in pregnant women and in patients scheduled to undergo an invasive procedure involving the urinary tract.

## Cystitis

Recommended first-line antibiotic regimens for uncomplicated cystitis (urinary frequency and urgency, dysuria, and suprapubic discomfort) should consider the increased rate of antimicrobial resistance of *E. coli*, the efficacy and advantages of short-course therapies, and the potential adverse effects (of the ecology and on patients). Preferred agents include nitrofurantoin (5 days), trimethoprim-sulfamethoxazole (3 days), and fosfomycin (1 dose, but expensive and less efficacious).

In geographic areas where trimethoprim-sulfamethoxazole resistance exceeds 20%, an alternative agent should be selected. The FDA recently indicated that fluoroquinolones should be reserved for other serious bacterial infections; however, fluoroquinolones (3 days) and β-lactam agents (including amoxicillin-clavulanate, cefdinir, cefaclor, and cefpodoxime-proxetil, each 3-7 days) are considered acceptable alternative second-line therapies. β-Lactams are not preferred if other recommended agents are available because they are less effective in eradicating infection. During pregnancy, the safest antibiotics are amoxicillin-clavulanate, cephalosporins, and nitrofurantoin. Tetracyclines and fluoroquinolones are contraindicated, and trimethoprim-sulfamethoxazole can only be used safely during the second trimester. Extended-spectrum β-lactamase–producing strains of Enterobacteriaceae causing cystitis have increased in frequency, especially in patients with recent antimicrobial or health care–facility exposure. Because of the greater risk of resistant and polymicrobial infections, urine culture and susceptibility testing are indicated in all patients with complicated cystitis. Fluoroquinolones are the preferred choice pending results, although fosfomycin and nitrofurantoin are reasonable options. The recommended treatment duration is 7 to 10 days rather than a 3-day, short-course regimen but is much less well defined. Other than in pregnant women, test of cure is not indicated in those reporting resolution of symptoms.

**KEY POINT**

- Preferred agents for uncomplicated cystitis include nitrofurantoin (5 days), trimethoprim-sulfamethoxazole (3 days), and fosfomycin (1 day, but least preferred); fluoroquinolones should not be used as first-line therapy in cystitis.

## Acute Pyelonephritis

Lower urinary tract symptoms (frequency, urgency, and dysuria) often precede the onset of fever, chills, flank pain, and at times nausea and vomiting, which characterize acute pyelonephritis. Infection can usually be managed in the outpatient setting with oral antibiotics. Hospitalization is advised for patients with hemodynamic instability, obstructive disease, pregnancy, complicating comorbidities, known pathogen resistance requiring parenteral antibiotic therapy, inability to tolerate oral medications, or lack of reliable home supervision and clinical follow-up.

CONT.

Every patient requires a urine culture with susceptibility testing obtained before initiation of empiric therapy. Fluoroquinolones (ciprofloxacin for 7 days or levofloxacin for 5 days for uncomplicated infections, 10-14 days in complicated infections) are the only oral agents recommended for empiric outpatient treatment, but an initial dose of a long-acting parenteral antibiotic (such as ceftriaxone, 1 g, or a once-daily aminoglycoside) should replace fluoroquinolones when local resistance rates exceed 10%. When a fluoroquinolone is contraindicated, trimethoprim-sulfamethoxazole twice daily for 14 days may be used after the pathogen is proven to be susceptible; trimethoprim-sulfamethoxazole should be avoided as initial empiric therapy because of the high level of *E. coli* resistance to this antibiotic in the community.

Depending on the risk of antimicrobial resistance and on recent antibiotic use, inpatient parenteral antimicrobial options include a fluoroquinolone, extended-spectrum cephalosporins (ceftriaxone or cefepime) or penicillins (piperacillin-tazobactam), or a carbapenem (meropenem, imipenem, or ertapenem). Again, fluoroquinolones are avoided for empiric therapy in severely ill patients with complicated pyelonephritis because of the increasing potential for resistance in *E. coli* and other aerobic gram-negative bacilli.

Therapy can be completed with active oral agents when an adequate clinical response has been observed. Patients with bacteremia do not require longer courses of treatment and may be converted to appropriate oral therapy when clinically stable.

Imaging studies are only necessary in patients with prolonged fever (>72 hours) or persistent bacteremia, in which complications such as obstruction or perinephric and intrarenal abscesses must be excluded. Routine follow-up urine cultures are only indicated in pregnant women.

**KEY POINTS**

HVC
- Every patient with acute pyelonephritis requires a urine culture with susceptibility testing obtained before initiation of empiric therapy; follow-up urine cultures are only indicated in pregnant women.

- It is prudent to avoid choosing a fluoroquinolone in severely ill patients with complicated pyelonephritis because of the increasing potential for resistance in *Escherichia coli* as well as other aerobic gram-negative bacilli.

## Recurrent Urinary Tract Infections in Women

An estimated 25% to 30% of patients experience a second episode of infection within 6 months of their first UTI. *Relapsed* infections are those that recur within 2 weeks of completing antimicrobial therapy (5%-10% of cases) with the same organism (determined by repeat culture). Relapse suggests infection with a resistant strain of bacteria, incomplete treatment of an infection of the upper urinary tract, or a structural abnormality, including renal calculi. *Reinfection*, the most common type of recurrent UTI, is generally caused by a bacterial strain

separate from the original infection and presents more than 2 weeks after cessation of treatment for the previous infection. Symptomatic relapsed infection requires a urine culture. Assuming the organism is sensitive, patients are treated for infection of the upper urinary tract for 7 to 10 days with the same antibiotic as prescribed for the previous infection or, if bacterial resistance is discovered, an alternative agent. Likewise, the same first-line antimicrobial agent can be given for reinfections, although an alternative antibiotic should be used if the recurrence occurs within 6 months, particularly if the original agent was trimethoprim-sulfamethoxazole, because of the increased chance of resistance.

Strategies to prevent infection recurrence include avoidance of spermicide contraceptives, urination soon after intercourse, topical vaginal estrogens, ascorbic acid (vitamin C), and methenamine salts. Cranberry products have not been proven effective in controlled trials. Prophylactic daily antimicrobial agents have been found to reduce the risk of recurrences by nearly 95%; they are an option in women who have had three or more UTIs in the previous 12 months, or two or more in the previous 6 months, and have received no benefit from other prevention efforts. Prophylactic therapy should be considered in pregnant patients who have required treatment for cystitis or asymptomatic bacteriuria to prevent recurrence during pregnancy. Antibiotic complications and potential emergence of resistance must be considered. Approximately 50% of patients revert to previous recurrence patterns within 6 months of prophylaxis discontinuation. Recommended prophylactic antibiotics include nitrofurantoin, trimethoprim-sulfamethoxazole, trimethoprim, cephalexin, or fosfomycin. Fluoroquinolones are very effective but not recommended. Other options include postcoital antimicrobial prophylaxis and self-diagnosis with self-treatment.

**KEY POINTS**

- Reinfection is generally caused by a bacterial strain separate from the original infection and presents more than 2 weeks after cessation of treatment for the previous infection.

- Prophylactic daily antimicrobial therapy is an option in women who have had three or more urinary tract infections in the previous 12 months or two or more in the previous 6 months; other options include postcoital antimicrobial prophylaxis and self-diagnosis with self-treatment.

## Acute Bacterial Prostatitis

Benign prostatic hyperplasia resulting in urinary obstruction and altered urine flow is the most common reason for the increased incidence of UTIs in men older than 60 years. Other risk factors include unprotected sexual intercourse, chronic indwelling urinary catheters, and transrectal prostate biopsy. Approximately 5% of men develop chronic prostatitis after acute infection.

CONT.

Presenting symptoms include sudden onset of fever, pelvic or perineal pain, urinary frequency and dysuria, and increasing obstructive symptoms. Acute bacterial prostatitis frequently presents as a severe systemic infection and is the most common cause of bacteremia in older men. Cautious digital rectal examination of the prostate reveals a boggy and tender gland. Urinalysis and culture are required to confirm the diagnosis. Although pyuria may be present for reasons other than infection, its absence strongly indicates no infection. Prostate-specific antigen test results may be elevated because of inflammation of the gland and should be avoided in the setting of presumed infection.

Hospitalized patients and those with severe infection require blood cultures. Gram-negative uropathogens account for about 80% of infections, two thirds of which are *E. coli*; *Proteus, Enterobacter, Serratia, Klebsiella*, and sometimes *Pseudomonas* and enterococcal species compose most of the other pathogens. In men 35 years or younger, sexually transmitted infections, including *Neisseria gonorrhoeae* and *Chlamydia trachomatis*, must be considered.

Fluoroquinolone antibiotics (ciprofloxacin, levofloxacin) are the preferred oral agents for treating acute bacterial prostatitis but should not be used if recent genitourinary instrumentation was performed, especially transrectal prostate biopsies, because most *E. coli* strains are now resistant to fluoroquinolones. Treatment duration is typically 4 weeks. Hospitalized patients should initially receive a broad-spectrum parenteral antibiotic, such as an extended-spectrum penicillin or cephalosporin, with the possible addition of an aminoglycoside. Imaging studies are not recommended unless a prostatic abscess is suspected clinically.

**KEY POINTS**

- Gram-negative uropathogens account for about 80% of acute prostatitis infections; in men 35 years or younger, sexually transmitted infections, including *Neisseria gonorrhoeae* and *Chlamydia trachomatis*, must be considered.

- Fluoroquinolone antibiotics are the preferred oral agents for treating acute bacterial prostatitis but should not be used if recent genitourinary instrumentation was performed because most *E. coli* strains are now resistant to fluoroquinolones.

# *Mycobacterium tuberculosis* Infection

## Epidemiology

Tuberculosis is one of the oldest and most prevalent infectious diseases in the world. It remains one of the most common causes of death from an infectious disease worldwide. Although rates of *Mycobacterium tuberculosis* infection remain relatively low in North America, approximately one third of the world's population is infected with the bacteria. As of 2015, approximately 10 million new cases are reported each year throughout the world, and approximately 2 million deaths are documented each year, including 360,000 in persons infected with HIV. More than 60% of infections are reported from Southeast Asia, India, China, Micronesia, Russia, and sub-Saharan Africa. Multidrug-resistant tuberculosis (MDR-TB) accounts for 3.3% of new infections and 20% of relapsed infections. Extremely drug-resistant tuberculosis now accounts for approximately 10% of all MDR-TB infections worldwide. In 2015, 9557 tuberculosis infections were reported in the United States (3.0 per 100,000 persons). Most infections in the United States occur in foreign-born persons; however, other persons at high risk include those with alcoholism, urban poor, homeless persons, injection drug users, prison inmates, persons living in shelters, HIV-positive persons, and older adults.

Despite great strides worldwide in controlling *M. tuberculosis*, it remains a major global health concern. The burden of disease throughout the world and rapid travel from country to country ensures a steady stream of active tuberculosis cases in the United States.

**KEY POINTS**

- Most *Mycobacterium tuberculosis* infections in the United States occur in foreign-born persons; however, other persons at high risk include those with alcoholism, urban poor, homeless persons, injection drug users, prison inmates, persons living in shelters, HIV-positive persons, and older adults.

- Multidrug-resistant tuberculosis (MDR-TB) accounts for 3.3% of new infections and 20% of relapsed infections; extremely drug-resistant tuberculosis now accounts for approximately 10% of all MDR-TB infections worldwide.

## Pathophysiology

Humans are the only known reservoir for *M. tuberculosis*, which is most commonly transmitted from person to person by aerosolized droplets. Although the droplets dry rapidly, the smallest droplets may remain suspended in the air for several hours. Persons who have visible acid-fast bacilli (AFB) on microscopy are the most likely to transmit infection. The most contagious patients are those with cavitary or laryngeal tuberculosis and those whose sputum contains a high bacterial load. After deposition in the respiratory tract, tubercular bacilli are ingested by alveolar macrophages that initiate an immunologic cascade eventually resulting in the development of classic caseating granulomas.

Most persons (>90%) who become infected with *M. tuberculosis* remain asymptomatic and develop latent tuberculosis. The risk of developing disease after infection depends primarily on endogenous factors such as the person's innate immune system, nonimmunologic defenses (alveolar macrophages, phagosome formation, phagocytosis), and the function of cell-mediated immunity. Specific risk factors for developing active tuberculosis among infected persons are shown in **Table 20**. The risk for developing active infection is approximately 5% in the first 2 years after infection and then 5% for the remainder of their life, assuming no cause of immunosuppression is present (see Table 20).

**KEY POINTS**

- Most persons who become infected with *Mycobacterium tuberculosis* remain asymptomatic and develop latent tuberculosis.

- Risk factors for developing active tuberculosis include immunosuppression, tumor necrosis factor-α inhibitors, injection drug use, silicosis, chronic kidney disease, diabetes mellitus, recent infection, and malnutrition.

# Clinical Manifestations

Tuberculosis is classified as pulmonary, extrapulmonary, or both; the two main forms are primary and secondary tuberculosis. Primary tuberculosis occurs soon after the initial infection, most frequently in children and immunosuppressed persons. Often, the lesions heal spontaneously. Secondary or reactivation tuberculosis results from endogenous reactivation of a latent infection. Most cases of active tuberculosis are caused by reactivation of latent tuberculosis in the setting of immunosuppression. Seventy-five percent of secondary infections are pulmonary, except in those infected with HIV, in whom two thirds of patients have pulmonary and extrapulmonary infection.

Frequent manifestations include fever, weight loss, productive cough (occasionally blood tinged), anorexia, malaise, and pleuritic chest pain. Patients may have a normal lung

**TABLE 20. Risk Factors for Acquiring *Mycobacterium tuberculosis***

Recent infection (<1 year)

Pulmonary fibrotic lesions

Malnutrition

Comorbidities

    HIV infection

    Silicosis

    Chronic kidney disease

    Diabetes mellitus

    Injection drug use

    Immunosuppressive therapy

    Jejunoileal bypass

    Solid organ transplantation

    Tumor necrosis factor-α inhibitors

    Head and neck cancer

examination or have crackles, rhonchi, or dullness to percussion. Hemoptysis occurs in 10% to 20% of patients with positive AFB smear results. In immunosuppressed patients, the infection may also disseminate into the bloodstream, producing miliary (disseminated) tuberculosis, which can result in a systemic inflammatory response syndrome, septic shock, and ultimately death if not diagnosed and treated early. Additionally, patients with disseminated infection may present with atypical clinical manifestations and chest radiographs. Extrapulmonary disease may be the result of hematogenous dissemination, can be seen in up to 30% of patients with active tuberculosis, and may involve almost any organ or organ system, including the pleura, lymph nodes, central nervous system, skeletal system, pericardium, larynx, peritoneum, and genitourinary system. ⬛

**KEY POINTS**

- Clinical manifestations of tuberculosis include fever, weight loss, productive cough (occasionally blood tinged), anorexia, malaise, and pleuritic chest pain.

- In immunosuppressed patients, tuberculosis infection may disseminate to the bloodstream, which can result in a systemic inflammatory response syndrome, septic shock, and ultimately death if not treated early.

# Diagnosis

The key to the diagnosis of tuberculosis is a high index of suspicion in patients at high risk.

## Diagnosis of Latent Tuberculosis Infection

The goal of diagnosing latent tuberculosis infection (LTBI) is to identify and treat persons at increased risk for reactivation tuberculosis. Testing methods include interferon-γ release assay (IGRA) performed on a blood sample or tuberculin skin testing (TST). LTBI is diagnosed when an asymptomatic patient has a positive TST result or an IGRA with no clinical or radiographic manifestations of active tuberculosis.

The Centers for Disease Control and Prevention (CDC) recommends performing an IGRA rather than a TST in persons 5 years or older who are likely to have *M. tuberculosis* infection, have a low or intermediate risk of disease progression, have a history of bacillus Calmette-Guérin (BCG) vaccination, or are unlikely to return to have their TST result interpreted. IGRAs are in vitro assays that measure T-cell release of interferon-γ in response to stimulation with highly tuberculosis-specific antigens ESAT-6 and CFP-10 (QuantiFERON-TB Gold In-Tube and T-SPOT TB test). IGRAs are more specific than TST because they have less cross-reactivity resulting from BCG vaccination and sensitization by nontuberculous mycobacteria. Although not used to diagnose active tuberculosis, IGRAs appear to be at least as sensitive as the TST in patients with active tuberculosis.

TST has become the alternative diagnostic test if IGRA is not feasible or available. The purified protein derivative is injected intradermally and interpreted after 48 to 72 hours by measuring the transverse diameter of induration, not erythema. A positive result indicates delayed-type hypersensitivity response. The criteria for a positive TST result are based on the patient's risk factors for tuberculosis (**Table 21**). A false-negative TST result may occur in patients with recent tuberculosis infection, overwhelming active tuberculosis infection, recent viral infections, or severe immunocompromise (AIDS) and in those younger than 6 years. Patients with remote exposure to *M. tuberculosis* may initially have a negative TST result that can become positive several weeks later after a second TST, known as the "booster effect." The second test is recommended in health care workers 7 to 21 days after initial testing and should be performed on the opposite forearm; it is not required if IGRA is used. IGRAs are recommended in nearly all clinical settings in which TST is recommended; one exception is children younger than 5 years, for whom experts recommend both tests to increase specificity.

### KEY POINTS

**HVC** • The Centers for Disease Control and Prevention recommends performing an interferon-γ release assay instead of tuberculin skin testing in persons 5 years or older who are likely to have *Mycobacterium tuberculosis* infection, have a low or intermediate risk of disease progression, have a history of bacillus Calmette-Guérin vaccination, or are unlikely to return to have their tuberculin skin test interpreted.

• Latent tuberculosis infection is diagnosed when an asymptomatic patient has a positive tuberculin skin test or interferon-γ release assay result with no clinical or radiographic manifestations of active tuberculosis.

### Diagnosis of Active Tuberculosis Infection

The CDC recommends AFB smear microscopy in all patients suspected of having active pulmonary tuberculosis. In vitro fluorescence microscopy of sputum is the preferred methodology. Testing three specimens is highly recommended because false-negative results from a single specimen are not uncommon. However, false-positive results are also not uncommon, thus a positive smear result requires mycobacterial culture confirmation. At least 3 mL of sputum should be submitted, although 5 to 10 mL is preferred. Serial specimens must be obtained at least 8 hours apart, and one must be an early morning specimen. Sputum induction is preferable to bronchoscopy as the sample methodology because of its greater sensitivity in patients who are unable to expectorate sputum.

The gold standard for diagnosis of active *M. tuberculosis* infection remains the mycobacterial culture. Whether AFB staining results are positive or negative, liquid and solid cultures should be performed for every specimen obtained. Liquid culture allows for faster growth and more rapid identification of organisms (2-4 weeks).

When a sputum smear result is positive for AFB, nucleic acid amplification testing (NAAT) is highly recommended to verify the organism. The positive predictive value of a NAAT on a smear-positive sputum sample is 95%. In patients with an intermediate to high level of suspicion for active disease who have a negative smear, the NAAT result will be positive in 65% of cases. If available, a NAAT assay that also detects for rifampin resistance is recommended for timely detection of rifampin resistance. Although the NAAT assays are quick and sensitive, mycobacterial cultures are still recommended for performance of in vitro susceptibilities to all antimicrobial agents. It is important to note that a negative NAAT result cannot be used to exclude pulmonary tuberculosis; NAAT can rapidly confirm the presence of *M. tuberculosis* in 50% to 80% of AFB smear-negative, culture-positive specimens. Moreover, NAAT can facilitate earlier decision making regarding whether to initiate tuberculosis therapy.

If signs of extrapulmonary infection are present, samples from those areas should be obtained and sent for AFB stain, mycobacterial culture, and histopathology. Histopathology may be beneficial by demonstrating caseating granulomas, which are suggestive for but not exclusive to or diagnostic of tuberculosis. In disseminated tuberculosis, blood cultures for mycobacteria using isolator methodology are helpful. ▪

| **TABLE 21.** Interpretation of Tuberculin Skin Test Results | | |
|---|---|---|
| **Criteria for Tuberculin Positivity by Risk Group** | | |
| **≥5 mm Induration** | **≥10 mm Induration** | **≥15 mm Induration** |
| HIV-positive persons | Recent (<5 years) arrivals from high-prevalence countries | All others with no risk factors for TB |
| Recent contacts of persons with active TB | Injection drug users | |
| Persons with fibrotic changes on chest radiograph consistent with old TB | Residents or employees of high-risk congregate settings: prisons and jails, nursing homes and other long-term facilities for the elderly, hospitals and other health care facilities, residential facilities for patients with AIDS, homeless shelters | |
| Patients with organ transplants and other immunosuppressive conditions (receiving the equivalent of ≥15 mg/d of prednisone for >4 weeks) | Mycobacteriology laboratory personnel; persons with clinical conditions that put them at high risk for active disease (silicosis, diabetes mellitus, severe kidney disease, certain types of cancer, some intestinal conditions); children aged <4 years or exposed to adults in high-risk categories | |
| TB = tuberculosis infection. | | |

## KEY POINTS

- The gold standard for the diagnosis of active *Mycobacterium tuberculosis* infection remains the mycobacterial culture; when a sputum smear result is positive for acid-fast bacilli, nucleic acid amplification testing is highly recommended to verify the organism.

- If signs of extrapulmonary tuberculosis infection are present, samples from those areas should be obtained and sent for acid-fast bacilli staining, mycobacterial culture, and histopathology.

## Radiographic Procedures

The classic radiographic finding in pulmonary tuberculosis is that of upper lobe disease with air space disease and cavities. However, any radiographic pattern can be seen, from a "normal chest radiograph" or a solitary pulmonary nodule to diffuse alveolar infiltrates with acute respiratory distress syndrome.

## Management

The primary goals of therapy include preventing additional morbidity, preventing mortality, and disrupting transmission of *M. tuberculosis* by eradicating the infection. When suitable antimicrobial therapy is administered and taken appropriately, clinical trials demonstrate clinical and microbiologic cure rates of approximately 95%. Therapy depends on several factors, including the classification of infection (latent versus active), pulmonary versus extrapulmonary infection, and patient adherence.

### Treatment of Latent Tuberculosis

Patients who have a positive IGRA or a positive TST result should be evaluated for active disease with a full medical history, physical examination, and chest radiography. If no sign of active infection is present, all patients should be offered treatment for LTBI. CDC guidelines recommend four different treatment regimens (**Table 22**). Pyridoxine is recommended in

**TABLE 22.** Treatment Regimens for Latent Tuberculosis Infection

| Drugs[a] | Duration | Dose[b] | Frequency | Total Doses |
|---|---|---|---|---|
| Isoniazid | 9 months | 5 mg/kg<br>Maximum dose: 300 mg | Daily | 270 |
| | | 15 mg/kg<br>Maximum dose: 900 mg | Twice weekly[c] | 76 |
| | 6 months | 5 mg/kg<br>Maximum dose: 300 mg | Daily | 180 |
| | | 15 mg/kg<br>Maximum dose: 900 mg | Twice weekly[c] | 52 |
| Isoniazid and rifapentine | 3 months | Isoniazid[d]: 15 mg/kg rounded up to the nearest 50 or 100 mg; 900 mg maximum<br>Rifapentine[d]:<br>10.0-14.0 kg: 300 mg<br>14.1-25.0 kg: 450 mg<br>25.1-32.0 kg: 600 mg<br>32.1-49.9 kg: 750 mg<br>≥50.0 kg: 900 mg maximum | Once weekly[e] | 12 |
| Rifampin | 4 months | 10 mg/kg<br>Maximum dose: 600 mg | Daily | 120 |

[a]Isoniazid is the preferred regimen, with therapy for 9 months preferable in patients with HIV and therapy for 6 months for patients without HIV and pulmonary lesions. CDC recommendations include isoniazid plus rifapentine in adults, in children aged 2-17 years, and in persons with HIV/AIDS taking antiretroviral therapy that does not interact with rifapentine. Rifampin is an option if other regimens cannot be used.

[b]Doses listed are for adults.

[c]Therapy may be either directly observed therapy (DOT) or self-administered therapy (SAT) in patients ≥2 years of age.

[d]Isoniazid is formulated in 100-mg and 300-mg tablets. Rifapentine is formulated in 150-mg tablets in blister packs that should be kept sealed until use.

[e]May be provided by DOT or SAT. Factors that should be considered when choosing between DOT and SAT include local practice, patient attributes and preferences, and risk of progression to severe disease. Use of concomitant latent tuberculosis infection treatment and antiretroviral agents should be guided by clinicians experienced in the management of both conditions.

Recommendations from the Centers for Disease Control and Prevention. Latent tuberculosis infection: a guide for primary health care providers. Treatment of latent TB infection. Table 2. Choosing the most effective LTBI treatment regimen. www.cdc.gov/tb/publications/ltbi/treatment.htm#2. Accessed October 15, 2017; and Borisov AS, Bamrah Morris S, Njie GJ, Winston CA, Burton D, Goldberg S, et al. Update of recommendations for use of once-weekly isoniazid-rifapentine regimen to treat latent mycobacterium tuberculosis infection. MMWR Morb Mortal Wkly Rep. 2018;67:723-726. [PMID: 29953429] doi:10.15585/mmwr.mm6725a5

patients who will receive isoniazid and are at risk for peripheral neuropathy (diabetes mellitus, chronic kidney disease, malnutrition, HIV, and alcoholism). Baseline and monthly monitoring of liver chemistry tests are not routinely required unless patients are at risk for hepatotoxicity (HIV infection, chronic hepatitis B or C, alcohol abuse, pregnancy, concurrent hepatotoxic drugs, or underlying liver disease).

In pregnant women with LTBI, a 6- to 9-month regimen of isoniazid plus pyridoxine may be offered; however, some experts prefer to defer therapy until after delivery, unless the patient is at high risk of developing active infection owing to immunocompromise, including HIV infection.

### KEY POINTS

- Patients with a positive interferon-γ release assay or tuberculin skin test result should be evaluated for active disease; if no sign of active infection is present, patients should be offered treatment for latent tuberculosis infection.
- Recommended treatment regimens for latent tuberculosis infection are isoniazid (daily or twice weekly) for 9 or 6 months, isoniazid plus rifapentine weekly for 3 months, or rifampin daily for 4 months.

### Treatment of Active Tuberculosis

When active tuberculosis is verified, in vitro susceptibility testing of the initial isolate should be done for the first-line agents (isoniazid, rifampin, pyrazinamide, and ethambutol). This becomes increasingly important because of the advent of multidrug-resistant and extensively drug-resistant tuberculosis. If rifampin resistance has been detected during NAAT assessment, in vitro susceptibilities to first-line and second-line agents should be performed (**Table 23**).

The American Thoracic Society/CDC guidelines published in 2016 recommend 6 to 9 months of treatment in patients with drug-susceptible active tuberculosis. A four-drug regimen is given daily for 2 months, followed by a continuation phase of isoniazid plus rifampin daily, usually for 4 months (**Table 24**).

Directly observed therapy, generally through the local health department, is recommended for the treatment of active tuberculosis. Sputum specimens should be evaluated at 1- and 2-month intervals to assess for efficacy. In addition, clinical assessment and laboratory testing (complete blood count, liver chemistry testing, hepatitis serology) should be performed before initiating therapy.

It is essential to advise the patient of the possible adverse effect profiles of the various medications (see Table 23). In several studies, approximately 15% to 25% of patients receiving the four-drug regimen experienced some type of adverse effect. Most adverse effects are mild, and therapy may be continued; up to 15% are severe enough that therapy must be discontinued temporarily. If a hypersensitivity reaction is observed, then all four drugs should be discontinued and rechallenged sequentially to determine the cause.

### KEY POINTS

- Directly observed therapy is recommended for the treatment of active tuberculosis.
- American Thoracic Society/Centers for Disease Control and Prevention guidelines recommend 6 to 9 months of treatment in patients with drug-susceptible active tuberculosis; a four-drug regimen is given daily for 2 months, followed by a continuation phase of isoniazid plus rifampin daily, usually for 4 months.

### Drug-Resistant Tuberculosis

*M. tuberculosis* resistance to individual drugs arises by spontaneous point mutations. Depending on the resistance, the regimen must be altered. In isoniazid-resistant tuberculosis, the regimen of isoniazid, rifampin, and ethambutol can be safely administered for 6 months, although some experts would add a fluoroquinolone. In those with isoniazid- and rifampin-resistant tuberculosis (MDR-TB), experts agree that a five-drug regimen depending on the susceptibility of the isolate should be provided for 4 months, followed by a four-drug regimen for an additional 12 to 18 months (see Table 23). Consultation with an expert in the event of MDR-TB is required.

Tuberculosis in patients with HIV infection may be complicated by immune reconstitution inflammatory syndrome. Although the general recommendations for treatment are the same, antiretroviral therapy should be initiated within 2 weeks for patients with a CD4 cell count less than 50/µL and by 8 to 12 weeks for those with CD4 cell counts of 50/µL or more. An exception is HIV-positive patients with tuberculous meningitis, in whom antiretroviral therapy should not be initiated during the first 8 weeks of tuberculosis therapy regardless of the CD4 cell count to avoid increased morbidity because of immune reconstitution inflammatory syndrome.

### KEY POINTS

- In patients with multidrug-resistant tuberculosis, experts agree that a five-drug regimen should be provided for 4 months, followed by a four-drug regimen for an additional 12 to 18 months.
- Tuberculosis in patients with HIV infection may be complicated by immune reconstitution inflammatory syndrome, and antiretroviral therapy initiation should be delayed to prevent this occurrence.

### Tumor Necrosis Factor Antagonist and Tuberculosis

Patients being treated with a tumor necrosis factor inhibitor (such as infliximab, etanercept, adalimumab, or certolizumab) have been reported to have an increased risk of reactivation to active infection or death from disseminated disease. It is recommended that these patients be evaluated for active or latent tuberculosis by performing chest radiography and simultaneous TST or IGRA. All patients should receive treatment for LTBI if identified, although LTBI treatment does not completely

**TABLE 23.** Antituberculous Drugs

| Agent | Adverse Effects | Notes |
|---|---|---|
| **First-Line Medications** | | |
| Isoniazid | Rash; liver enzyme elevation; hepatitis; peripheral neuropathy; lupus-like syndrome | Hepatitis risk increases with age and alcohol consumption. Pyridoxine may prevent peripheral neuropathy. Adjust for kidney injury. |
| Pyrazinamide | Hepatitis; rash; GI upset; hyperuricemia | May make glucose control more difficult in patients with diabetes. Adjust for kidney injury. |
| Rifampin | Hepatitis; rash; GI upset | Contraindicated or should be used with caution when administered with protease inhibitors and nonnucleoside reverse transcriptase inhibitors. Do not administer to patients also taking saquinavir/ritonavir. Colors body fluids orange. |
| Rifabutin | Rash; hepatitis; thrombocytopenia; severe arthralgia; uveitis; leukopenia | Dose adjustment required if taken with protease inhibitors or nonnucleoside reverse transcriptase inhibitors. Monitor for decreased antiretroviral activity and for rifabutin toxicity. |
| Rifapentine | Similar to rifampin | Contraindicated in patients who are HIV positive (unacceptable rate of failure/relapse). |
| Ethambutol | Optic neuritis; rash | Baseline and periodic tests of visual acuity and color vision. Patients are advised to call immediately if visual acuity or color vision changes. Adjust for kidney injury. |
| **Second-Line Medications**[a] | | |
| Streptomycin | Auditory, vestibular, and kidney toxicity | Avoid or reduce dose in adults >59 years. Monitor hearing and kidney function test results. Adjust for kidney injury. |
| Cycloserine | Psychosis; convulsions; depression; headaches; rash; drug interactions | Pyridoxine may decrease CNS adverse effects. Measure drug serum levels. |
| Capreomycin | Kidney, vestibular, and auditory toxicity | Monitor hearing and kidney function test results. Adjust for kidney injury. |
| Ethionamide | GI upset; hepatotoxicity; hypersensitivity | May cause hypothyroidism. |
| Kanamycin and amikacin | Auditory, vestibular, and kidney toxicity | Not approved by the FDA for TB treatment. Monitor vestibular, hearing, and kidney function. |
| Levofloxacin, moxifloxacin | GI upset; dizziness; hypersensitivity; drug interactions | Not approved by the FDA for TB treatment. Should not be used in children. |
| Para-aminosalicylic acid | GI upset; hypersensitivity; hepatotoxicity | May cause hypothyroidism, especially if used with ethionamide. Measure liver enzyme levels. |
| Bedaquiline | Nausea, joint pain, headache, elevated aminotransferase levels, hemoptysis, prolonged QT interval | FDA-approved oral agent for MDR pulmonary TB treatment indicated for combination therapy when other alternatives are not available. Novel mechanism of action inhibits mycobacterial adenosine triphosphate synthase. Should be given as directly observed therapy. |

CNS = central nervous system; GI = gastrointestinal; MDR = multidrug resistant; TB = tuberculosis.

[a]Use these drugs in consultation with a clinician experienced in the management of drug-resistant TB.

eliminate risk for active mycobacterial infection in this population.

**KEY POINT**

- All patients diagnosed with latent tuberculosis who are being treated with a tumor necrosis factor inhibitor should receive treatment to reduce risk of reactivation and death from disseminated disease.

## Prevention

From the public health perspective, the best way to prevent tuberculosis is to diagnose, isolate, and treat infection rapidly until patients are considered noncontagious and the disease is cured. In the hospital, this means having a high index of suspicion for *M. tuberculosis* in high-risk groups and initiating immediate airborne isolation in negative pressure rooms (airborne infection isolation rooms) until the diagnosis can be excluded.

Recent CDC guidelines recommend criteria to determine that a patient is no longer contagious and a possible public health threat. These include appropriate antimicrobial therapy for at least 2 weeks, clinical improvement of signs and symptoms, and three negative sputum smears collected at least 8 hours apart, with one being an early-morning specimen. Patients with negative smear results are less contagious, although they may still have tuberculosis.

**TABLE 24.** Preferred Treatment Regimens for Active Tuberculosis

| Treatment Phase | Regimen | Comments |
|---|---|---|
| Initial | Daily INH, RIF, PZA, and EMB[a] for 56 doses (8 wk) *or* | Alternative regimens available at https://www.cdc.gov/tb/topic/treatment/tbdisease.htm |
| | DOT 5 d/wk for 90 doses (18 wk) | DOT should be used when medications are administered less than 7 d/wk |
| | | Pyridoxine 25-50 mg/d is given to all patients at risk for neuropathy[b]; 100 mg/d for patients with peripheral neuropathy |
| Continuation | INH and RIF 7 d/wk for 126 doses (18 wk) *or* | Based on expert opinion, patients with cavitation on the initial chest radiograph and positive cultures at completion of 2 months of therapy should receive a 7-month (31-wk) continuation phase |
| | DOT 5 d/wk for 90 doses (18 wk) | |

DOT = directly observed therapy; EMB = ethambutol; INH = isoniazid; PZA = pyrazinamide; RIF = rifampin.

[a]EMB can be discontinued if drug susceptibility studies demonstrate susceptibility to first-line drugs.

[b]Pregnant women; breastfeeding infants; persons with HIV; patients with diabetes, alcoholism, malnutrition, or chronic kidney disease; patients of advanced age.

Recommendations from the Centers for Disease Control and Prevention. Tuberculosis. Treatment for TB disease. Table 1. Basic TB disease treatment regimens. Available at www.cdc.gov/tb/topic/treatment/tbdisease.htm. Accessed August 27, 2014.

The BCG vaccination is a live-attenuated vaccine derived from an attenuated strain of *Mycobacterium bovis*. It has been in use for more than 90 years throughout the world, although it is not routinely used in the United States. It is recommended for use at birth in countries with high rates of *M. tuberculosis*. In several international studies, the BCG vaccine has been shown to be effective in preventing severe infection, including meningitis in children. However, the efficacy in adults has not been established. CDC guidelines do not recommend the vaccine in the United States; however, the World Health Organization still recommends its use in high-prevalence areas.

**KEY POINT**

- Guidelines for determining a patient with tuberculosis is no longer contagious include appropriate antimicrobial therapy for at least 2 weeks, clinical improvement in signs and symptoms, and three negative sputum smears collected at least 8 hours apart.

**TABLE 25.** Classification of Common Nontuberculous Mycobacteria

| Slow-growing Mycobacteria |
|---|
| *M. kansasii* |
| *M. marinum* |
| *M. gordonae* |
| *M. scrofulaceum* |
| *M. avium* complex |
| *M. ulcerans* |
| *M. xenopi* |

| Rapidly Growing Mycobacteria |
|---|
| *M. abscessus* |
| *M. chelonae* |
| *M. fortuitum* |

# Nontuberculous Mycobacterial Infections

Nontuberculous mycobacteria (NTM) comprise species other than *Mycobacterium tuberculosis* complex and *Mycobacterium leprae*. NTM are often divided into slow and rapid growers (**Table 25**). These organisms are found in surface water, soil, domestic and wild animals, milk, and food products. Additionally, they can be colonizers, particularly in the airways of persons with chronic lung disease. They can cause a spectrum of infections (**Table 26**).

Risk factors for NTM infections include immunocompromise, chronic lung disease, and postoperative status. Health care–associated *Mycobacterium chimaera* infections have been documented worldwide in association with heater-cooler units used during cardiac surgery.

NTM diagnosis is difficult because a positive culture result from a nonsterile site (such as the lung) without other evidence of disease may reflect colonization rather than infection. However, when recovered from a normally sterile site, active infection is very likely. Because antibiotic susceptibility of species vary, it is important to identify organisms to species level. American Thoracic Society (ATS) guidelines recommend fulfillment of clinical, radiologic, and microbiologic criteria to diagnose an NTM pulmonary infection. Most NTM infections require treatment with two to four antimicrobials; ATS guidelines should be used to guide therapy.

| TABLE 26. | Diseases Caused by Nontuberculous Mycobacteria | | | |
|---|---|---|---|
| **Clinical Disease** | **More Common** | **Less Common** | **Infection Risks** |
| Pulmonary | MAC<br><br>*M. kansasii*<br><br>*M. abscessus* | *M. fortuitum*<br><br>*M. xenopi*<br><br>*M. malmoense*<br><br>*M. szulgai*<br><br>*M. simiae*<br><br>*M. asiaticum* | Older persons with or without underlying lung disease; cystic fibrosis |
| Lymphadenitis | MAC | *M. abscessus*<br><br>*M. fortuitum*<br><br>*M. scrofulaceum*<br><br>*M. malmoense* | Children |
| Skin and soft tissue | *M. marinum*<br><br>*M. ulcerans*<br><br>*M. abscessus* | MAC<br><br>*M. kansasii* | Direct inoculation |
| Catheter-related bloodstream infections | Rapidly growing mycobacteria | MAC<br><br>*M. kansasii* | Long-term catheterization |
| Disseminated | MAC<br><br>*M. kansasii* (in persons with AIDS and CD4 cell count <100/µL) | Rapidly growing mycobacteria | Immunocompromise, especially persons with AIDS or those taking tumor necrosis factor-α inhibitors |

MAC = *Mycobacterium avium* complex.

- Risk factors for nontuberculous mycobacteria infections include immunocompromise, chronic lung disease, and postoperative status; additionally, health care–associated *Mycobacterium chimaera* infections have been documented in association with heater-cooler units used during cardiac surgery.

- Because antibiotic susceptibility of nontuberculous mycobacteria species varies, it is important to identify organisms to species level.

## *Mycobacterium avium* Complex Infection

*Mycobacterium avium* complex is the most common cause of chronic lung infection worldwide. Cavitary lung disease is seen classically in white, middle-aged, or older adult men, especially those with underlying lung disease, such as COPD, cystic fibrosis, or interstitial lung disease. Disseminated infection is seen predominantly in patients with HIV with CD4 cell counts less than 50/µL. The clinical presentation often consists of fever, night sweats, weight loss, and gastrointestinal symptoms.

## *Mycobacterium kansasii*

*M. kansasii* infection mimics pulmonary tuberculosis with cavitary lung disease. Predisposing conditions include underlying lung disease, alcoholism, cancer, and immunocompromised status.

## Rapidly Growing Mycobacteria

Rapidly growing NTM have been implicated in NTM outbreaks. The most common rapidly growing mycobacterial species include *M. abscessus*, *M. chelonae*, and *M. fortuitum*. Of these, *M. abscessus* is most frequently identified and one of the most difficult to treat. These mycobacteria are associated with chronic, nonhealing ulcers unresponsive to appropriate empiric antibiotic therapy for typical skin and soft tissue infections.

- *Mycobacterium avium* complex is the most common cause of chronic lung infection worldwide, causing cavitary lung disease.

- *Mycobacterium abscessus*, *Mycobacterium chelonae*, and *Mycobacterium fortuitum* can produce lung disease, adenitis, skin and soft tissue infections, surgical site infections, and prosthetic device infections.

# Fungal Infections

The incidence of fungal infection is increasing because of the increased recognition of these infections and an increase in the population at risk worldwide. According to a recent analysis by the Prospective Antifungal Therapy Alliance, the most commonly encountered infections in North America were caused by *Candida* species (73%) followed by *Aspergillus* species (14.8%), other yeast (such as *Cryptococcus* species; 6.2%), and mucormycetes (including *Rhizopus* species and *Mucor* species; 1.7%).

## Systemic Candidiasis

*Candida* species are the fourth most commonly isolated organisms in bloodstream infections and are associated with a mortality rate of 30% to 40%. Risk factors for systemic candidiasis are listed in **Table 27**.

Manifestations of candidiasis depend on the organ involved. Candidemia can present as an isolated fever or septic shock. Signs and symptoms of focal infection depend on the site involved (abscess or peritonitis in the peritoneum, empyema in the pleural cavity, or pyelonephritis in the kidneys). Other forms of invasive infection include meningitis, osteomyelitis, septic arthritis, and endocarditis. Although often found in the respiratory tract, *Candida* species rarely cause infections there and are likely the result of colonization. The presence of yeast in the urinary tract (for example, because of the presence of an indwelling catheter) may represent colonization (most commonly) or true infection.

Diagnosis of invasive candidiasis is challenging because only 40% to 60% of patients with infection have positive blood culture results, and cultures can take days to demonstrate growth. Recognizing risk factors (see Table 27) for candidiasis is thus essential to avoid delays in initiating antifungal therapy and resultant increased mortality. The T2 magnetic resonance assay of whole blood provides rapid (within hours) diagnosis of culture-negative invasive candidal infections and can be performed on blood samples even after initiation of antifungal therapy. The $\beta$-D-glucan assay also can be used to diagnose invasive candidiasis in patients with negative blood culture

results. These assays should be obtained when a patient at high risk (see Table 27) receiving antimicrobial agents is not responding to therapy.

When the *Candida* genus is identified from a sterile site (blood or tissue), specific species identification is necessary. Although more than 160 species of *Candida* are known, fewer than 15 produce disease in humans. Additionally, several species (such as *C. glabrata* and *C. krusei*) have intrinsic resistance to antifungal agents, especially the azoles, and their proper identification guides therapy.

Treatment of candidemia and invasive candidiasis should include an echinocandin (caspofungin, micafungin, or anidulafungin) and removal of intravascular devices (if possible). However, because of poor penetration of echinocandins into the central nervous system (CNS) and the eye, patients with these infections should be treated with an azole or amphotericin B. Additional treatment of candidal endophthalmitis varies depending on the extent of disease (chorioretinitis with or without macular involvement, vitreous involvement). All patients initially given amphotericin B or an echinocandin may be de-escalated to an oral azole (fluconazole or voriconazole) if the *Candida* species is susceptible and the gastrointestinal tract is functional. Duration of antifungal therapy for candidemia should be 14 days from the first negative blood culture result in patients with uncomplicated candidemia or 14 to 42 days in patients with invasive candidal infections.

**KEY POINTS**

- *Candida* species are the fourth most commonly isolated organisms in bloodstream infections and are associated with a 30% to 40% mortality rate.

- Because only 40% to 60% of patients with invasive candidal infection have positive blood culture results, recognizing risk factors of candidiasis is essential to avoid delays in initiating effective antifungal therapy.

- The T2 magnetic resonance assay of whole blood may provide a rapid diagnosis of culture-negative invasive candidal infections.

- *Candida* species isolated from the respiratory tract and from the urinary tract usually represent colonization; treatment is not indicated unless clinical infection is suspected. **HVC**

- Treatment of candidemia and invasive candidiasis should include an echinocandin (caspofungin, micafungin, or anidulafungin) and removal of intravascular devices (if possible); central nervous system and ocular infections require amphotericin B or an azole.

| TABLE 27. | Risk Factors for Systemic Candidiasis |
|---|---|
| Central venous catheters | |
| Broad-spectrum antimicrobial agents | |
| Neutropenia | |
| ICU stay for more than 3 days | |
| Total parenteral nutrition | |
| General surgery (especially of the gastrointestinal tract) | |
| Burns | |
| Trauma | |
| Mechanical ventilation for more than 3 days | |
| Transplantation (bone marrow/solid organ) | |
| Hemodialysis-associated catheters | |
| Severe acute pancreatitis | |

## Aspergillosis and Aspergilloma

*Aspergillus* is ubiquitous in the environment. The most common species are *A. fumigatus*, *A. flavus*, *A. niger*, and the amphotericin-resistant *A. terreus*. *Aspergillus* produces disease after inhalation of airborne spores (90%) and only occasionally by traumatic skin inoculation. Of all the fungi, *Aspergillus* is notable for the diverse settings in which it can occur and the various clinical manifestations it can produce.

Invasive pulmonary aspergillosis, the most serious form of *Aspergillus* infection, most often occurs in immunosuppressed patients who are neutropenic or are hematopoietic stem cell transplant recipients (**Table 28**). This type of aspergillosis usually begins in the respiratory tract and then enters the circulatory system (angioinvasion). This is followed by the formation of a fungus-septic emboli complex with subsequent hematogenous dissemination. The most common manifestation of angioinvasive disease is pulmonary aspergillosis (60%), but sinusitis, brain abscess, endocarditis, disseminated infection, and osteomyelitis also may occur. Timely diagnosis of invasive aspergillosis is essential to decrease morbidity and mortality, but symptoms and signs are nonspecific (**Table 29**), and blood

culture results are generally negative. Therefore, bronchoscopy, bronchoalveolar lavage, and, if possible, tissue biopsy are often necessary to establish a definitive diagnosis. Early CT of the chest in patients with suspected invasive pulmonary aspergillosis—with typical findings suggestive of septic emboli (nodules, often with a "halo sign") (**Figure 11**), thromboembolic pulmonary infarction (wedge-shaped peripheral densities), or necrosis with cavitation and a crescent sign—and the serum galactomannan assay can be useful in establishing a presumptive diagnosis of invasive infection, especially in neutropenic patients and hematopoietic stem cell transplant recipients, in whom the assay has a sensitivity of approximately 80%. First-line treatment of invasive aspergillosis is with a triazole (voriconazole, posaconazole, or isavuconazole); amphotericin B deoxycholate or liposomal amphotericin B can be used for amphotericin-sensitive *Aspergillus* species if triazoles are not available. When possible, reversal of immunosuppression improves treatment response.

Other forms of *Aspergillus* infection occur in different clinical settings. Chronic necrotizing aspergillosis is a semi-invasive indolent form of infection that does not disseminate and occurs in patients who have lesser degrees of immunosuppression (such as those who take chronic glucocorticoids or those who have intrinsic immune defects) or chronic pulmonary disease. Treatment is similar to that for invasive pulmonary aspergillosis.

Allergic bronchopulmonary aspergillosis results from a  hypersensitivity overreaction to *Aspergillus* species colonizing the respiratory tract; this disorder is seen primarily in patients with cystic fibrosis and occasionally in those with asthma (see MKSAP 18 Pulmonary and Critical Care Medicine for more information). Because allergic bronchopulmonary aspergillosis represents a hypersensitivity response, systemic glucocorticoids are the mainstay of treatment (sometimes supplemented by antifungal therapy with an azole).

**TABLE 28.** Risk Factors for Invasive Aspergillosis

| Major | Minor |
|---|---|
| Neutropenia | COPD treated with glucocorticoids |
| Graft-versus-host disease | Cirrhosis |
| Cytomegalovirus infection/reactivation | Burns |
| Hematopoietic stem cell transplantation | Solid organ malignancies |
| Solid organ transplantation | Immunosuppressants |
| Systemic glucocorticoids (>1 mg/kg/d) or inhaled steroids | Cyclosporine |
| Hematologic malignancies | Methotrexate |
| | Azathioprine |
| | Cyclophosphamide |
| | Advanced HIV with CD4 cell count <50/µL (50 × 10^6/L) |
| | Injection drug use (rare) |
| | Gram-negative bacterial pneumonia |

**TABLE 29.** Clinical Features of Invasive Aspergillosis

Fever[a]

Pulmonary findings

    Pleuritic chest pain, pleural rub

    Dry cough

    Dyspnea

    Hemoptysis: usually minor but occasionally catastrophic

Chest radiograph: potentially normal in early disease; infiltrates, infarction, nodules, and cavitation in late disease

Focal neurologic deficits

Multiorgan dysfunction

Hemorrhagic skin lesions

[a]Frequently the only feature present.

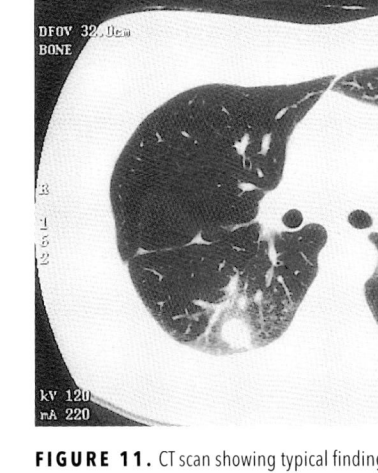

**FIGURE 11.** CT scan showing typical findings suggestive of septic emboli. Note the nodule with a "halo sign," which is a surrounding area of low attenuation that reflects hemorrhage into the tissues surrounding the fungus.

Pulmonary aspergillomas (fungus balls consisting of hyphae, mucus, and cellular debris) may form in patients with pre-existing cavities, such as old tuberculosis cavities and in bullae of patients with COPD; the presence of significant hemoptysis is a potential complication. In the absence of associated symptoms or hemoptysis, pulmonary aspergillomas may not require therapy; however, in the setting of significant bleeding, surgical resection or embolization may be necessary. Antifungal therapy is typically not effective against pulmonary aspergillomas, and its role in aspergilloma treatment is unclear.

**KEY POINTS**

- *Aspergillus* species produce disease after inhalation of airborne spores (90% of affected patients).

- *Aspergillus* infection can manifest in various ways, including invasive pulmonary aspergillosis, chronic necrotizing pulmonary aspergillosis, allergic bronchopulmonary aspergillosis, and aspergillomas.

- Tissue biopsy is frequently necessary to establish a definitive diagnosis of invasive aspergillosis; however, early chest CT and the serum galactomannan assay can be useful in establishing a presumptive diagnosis in patients at high risk of infection.

- First-line treatment of invasive or chronic pulmonary *Aspergillus* infection is with a triazole, such as voriconazole, posaconazole, or isavuconazole; liposomal amphotericin B can be used as an alternative in sensitive species and if triazoles are not available.

## Cryptococcosis

*Cryptococcus* is an encapsulated yeast that is ubiquitous in the environment. Although cryptococcal infection can occur in healthy persons, most infected patients have advanced immune suppression, such as AIDS, neutropenia, or organ transplantation. *C. neoformans* is the most commonly identified species, but *C. gattii* is seen with increased frequency in the Pacific Northwest region of North America and has been associated with severe and recalcitrant infection. Pathogenesis of cryptococcosis involves inhalation of spores into the respiratory tract, followed by dissemination into susceptible tissues, especially the CNS.

 Cryptococcal infection most commonly manifests in the CNS, and cryptococcosis is the most common cause of fungal meningitis worldwide. Clinical manifestations are listed in **Table 30**, and indicators of a poor prognosis in cryptococcal meningitis are provided in **Table 31**. Because patients with cryptococcosis-related increased intracranial pressure (ICP) may develop sudden blindness, deafness, or coma, initial opening pressure should be documented during lumbar puncture. Cerebrospinal fluid analysis is essential to diagnose CNS involvement; classic findings include an increased leukocyte count (mainly lymphocytes), an increased protein

| TABLE 30. | Clinical Features of Cryptococcosis |
|---|---|
| **Signs and Symptoms of Meningeal Infection (% Affected)** | |
| Fever (60%-90%) | |
| Headache (80%-90%) | |
| Nausea/vomiting (~50%) | |
| Meningism (30%) | |
| Altered mental status (20%-30%) | |
| **Extrameningeal Infection Sites** | |
| Lung | |
| Bone marrow | |
| Skin | |
| Prostate (cryptic source) | |

| TABLE 31. | Indicators of Poor Prognosis in Cryptococcal Meningitis |
|---|---|
| Altered mental state | |
| Visual abnormalities | |
| CSF leukocyte count less than 20/µL (20 × 10⁶/L) | |
| CSF cryptococcal antigen assay greater than 1:10,000 | |
| No previous antiretroviral therapy in those with HIV infection | |
| CSF = cerebrospinal fluid. | |

level, a low to normal glucose level, and the presence of cryptococcal antigen. Serum cryptococcal antigen also is positive in greater than 95% of infected patients; occasionally, blood culture results are positive and thus indicate disseminated disease. 

Many symptoms of increased ICP may be improved by cerebrospinal fluid removal through daily lumbar puncture or insertion of a shunt. Aggressive reduction of ICP reduces early morbidity and mortality. Amphotericin B plus flucytosine is the treatment of choice and is effective in more than 90% of patients. HIV-infected patients require maintenance antifungal therapy until they have maintained their CD4 cell counts above 100/µL (100 × 10⁶/L) for a minimum of 3 months and have a suppressed viral load.

**KEY POINTS**

- In patients with suspected cryptococcal infection, cerebrospinal fluid (CSF) analysis is necessary, as is documentation of the CSF opening pressure; CSF and serum cryptococcal antigen are both highly sensitive for identifying infection.

- Amphotericin B plus flucytosine is effective in more than 90% of patients; for those with elevated intracranial pressure (ICP), cerebrospinal fluid removal through daily lumbar puncture or insertion of a shunt can reduce ICP and thus early morbidity and mortality.

# Histoplasmosis

*Histoplasma capsulatum* is responsible for one of the most common endemic mycoses in the world. Acquired by inhalation of airborne conidia, this organism primarily produces asymptomatic pulmonary infection. It is distributed along the Mississippi River Valley (Ohio, Missouri, Indiana, Mississippi) in the United States, in Central and South America, in the Caribbean, and in regions of Africa, Australia, and India.

Histoplasmosis most commonly presents with acute respiratory symptoms. Other presentations, in declining order of frequency, include asymptomatic infection, disseminated infection, chronic pulmonary symptoms, rheumatologic symptoms, pericarditis, and sclerosing mediastinitis.

The *Histoplasma* urinary antigen assay has a sensitivity and specificity of greater than 85% in acute and disseminated infection but less than 50% in chronic infection. Identification of the fungus by tissue culture can be a lengthy process but is indicated for clinically suspected cases in which the urinary antigen assay result is negative.

Asymptomatic and mild pulmonary histoplasmosis typically resolves without treatment. Antifungal therapy is recommended for more severe or disseminated disease. Itraconazole is the agent of choice; duration of therapy is 6 to 12 weeks for acute infection and as long as 12 months for chronic cavitary pulmonary infection. For severe lung disease and disseminated infection, liposomal amphotericin B should be used initially, followed by de-escalation to oral itraconazole for an additional 12 weeks.

**KEY POINTS**

- *Histoplasma* urinary antigen assay has a sensitivity and specificity of greater than 85% in acute and disseminated infection but less than 50% in chronic infection.
- Itraconazole is the antifungal agent of choice for most patients with histoplasmosis; liposomal amphotericin B should be used initially for those with severe lung disease and disseminated infection.

# Coccidioidomycosis

*Coccidioides* is a dimorphic fungus that exists as a mold in the environment. There are two species: *C. immitis* refers to isolates from California, and *C. posadasii* refers to isolates from all other endemic areas, including Arizona, New Mexico, western Texas, northern Mexico, and parts of Central and South America. In endemic areas, the annual risk of infection is approximately 3% for most persons, although the risk of infection (and dissemination) is greater in those who are pregnant, younger than 5 years or older than 50 years, or of African, Filipino (and possibly other Asian), and Native American ancestry.

Infection is usually acquired by inhalation of aerosolized arthroconidia. Once inhaled, the fungus begins its dimorphic change in the lungs and becomes a yeast cell. Several clinical syndromes are seen in coccidioidomycosis and may manifest as acute or chronic pulmonary infection, as cutaneous infection (~40%), as meningitis (~33%), or as musculoskeletal infection.

Diagnosis is straightforward in endemic areas and usually is based on clinical manifestations and confirmatory testing by a mycologic culture of affected tissue, histopathologic evaluation of tissue, serology for *Coccidioides* antibodies, or urinary antigen testing.

Fluconazole is the first-line treatment for symptomatic infection. In patients with meningitis, fluconazole is continued for life. In patients who do not respond to azoles, intrathecal amphotericin B may be an alternative.

**KEY POINTS**

- The diagnosis of coccidioidomycosis should be suspected clinically in endemic areas and may be confirmed by a mycologic culture of affected tissues, histopathologic evaluation of tissue, serology for *Coccidioides* antibodies, or urinary antigen testing.
- Fluconazole is first-line treatment for symptomatic coccidioidomycosis infection.

# Blastomycosis

*Blastomyces dermatitidis* is a dimorphic, round, budding yeast; daughter cells form a bud with a broad base. Blastomycosis affects immunocompetent hosts. In the United States, blastomycosis is found primarily along the Mississippi and Ohio River valleys but can be found as far north as Wisconsin and Minnesota and as far south as Florida. As with most dimorphic yeast, infection occurs by inhalation of conidia and manifests initially as a primary pulmonary infection (acute or chronic pneumonia). Occasionally, a chest radiograph shows a spiculated nodular appearance that may be mistaken for lung cancer. Rarely, dissemination occurs and produces extrapulmonary disease (osteomyelitis, genitourinary infection, or CNS infection).

Diagnosis of blastomycosis can be made by direct fungal stain of clinical specimens (sputum, tissue, or purulent material) and confirmed by culture or serology for *Blastomyces* antibodies. Urinary antigen testing is also available. The preferred treatment for mild to moderate infection is itraconazole for 6 to 12 months. Liposomal amphotericin B is recommended for CNS, severe pulmonary, and disseminated infections.

**KEY POINTS**

- Blastomycosis occurs by inhalation of *Blastomyces dermatitidis* conidia and manifests initially as a primary pulmonary infection; diagnosis is made by direct fungal stain of clinical specimens and confirmed by culture, urinary antigen testing, or serology for *Blastomyces* antibodies.
- The preferred treatment for mild to moderate infection is itraconazole, with liposomal amphotericin B used for central nervous system and disseminated infection.

## Sporotrichosis

*Sporothrix schenckii* is a dimorphic fungus found most often in soil, living plants, or plant debris. Although found worldwide, most reported infections are from North and South America and Japan. Infection can occur after direct contact with plants, such as roses and sphagnum moss. Direct inoculation of the organism into the skin or subcutaneous tissue manifests as fixed, "plaque-like" cutaneous sporotrichosis or as lymphocutaneous sporotrichosis presenting as papular lesions along lymphatic channels proximal to the inoculation site. Extracutaneous infection (osteoarticular, pulmonary, ocular, or disseminated) can occur in immunocompromised hosts.

Diagnosis requires culture of the organism from affected tissues. Treatment is with itraconazole and should extend for 2 to 4 weeks after lesions have resolved.

### KEY POINTS

- Sporotrichosis is an infection of cutaneous and lymphocutaneous tissues and usually is caused by direct contact with plants; extracutaneous infection can occur in immunocompromised hosts.
- Itraconazole is the preferred treatment for cutaneous and lymphocutaneous sporotrichosis.

## Mucormycosis

Mucormycosis (formerly zygomycosis) is the third most frequent cause of invasive fungal infections in immunocompromised hosts but is rarely seen in immunocompetent hosts. Particularly at risk are patients with neutropenia, diabetes mellitus, and acidosis. The most common mucormycetes are *Rhizopus arrhizus* and *Mucor* species. These fungi are commonly found in the environment on decaying organic debris, including fruit, bread, and soil.

Infection is acute and rapidly fatal, even with early diagnosis and treatment. Major blood vessels are invaded, with ensuing ischemia, necrosis, and infarction of adjacent tissues. Mucormycosis has five major clinical forms: (1) rhinocerebral; (2) pulmonary; (3) abdominal, pelvic, gastric, gastrointestinal; (4) primary cutaneous; and (5) disseminated.

Because laboratory studies are nonspecific, diagnosis relies on a high index of suspicion in a host with appropriate risk factors and evidence of tissue invasion, including the characteristic appearance of broad, nonseptate hyphae with acute-angle branches. Serologic tests and blood cultures offer no diagnostic benefit.

Treatment requires reversal of any predisposing condition, extensive surgical removal of affected tissue, and early antifungal therapy. Initial treatment is high-dose liposomal amphotericin B, with later de-escalation to posaconazole or isavuconazole. If amphotericin B is not tolerated, initial therapy with one of the azoles is warranted. Mortality rates remain as high as 60% to 80%, even with therapy.

### KEY POINTS

- Mucormycosis is acute and rapidly fatal, even with early diagnosis and treatment.
- Because laboratory studies are nonspecific, diagnosis relies on a high index of suspicion; serologic tests and blood cultures offer no diagnostic benefit.
- Treatment requires reversal of any predisposing condition, extensive surgical removal of affected tissue, and initial antifungal therapy with high-dose liposomal amphotericin B.

# Sexually Transmitted Infections

## Introduction

Sexually transmitted infections (STIs) occur most commonly in adolescents, young adults, and men who have sex with men (MSM), but STIs affect all demographics. Most infections are asymptomatic, so it is imperative that a detailed sexual history, including sexual practices, be obtained to understand individual risk. STI risk factors include a new partner, more than one current partner, a partner with an STI, or a partner who has concurrent partners. Particularly high-risk populations include persons attending STI clinics and MSM.

Unrecognized or inadequately treated upper genitourinary tract infection is a preventable cause of infertility in women. Evidence-based guidelines for the evaluation and management of STIs are available from the World Health Organization and the Centers for Disease Control and Prevention (CDC); the CDC guidelines are recommended for use in the United States. Any patient diagnosed with an STI should be evaluated for other STIs, including HIV, and receive risk reduction counseling.

## *Chlamydia trachomatis* Infection

*Chlamydia trachomatis* is the most commonly reported bacterial STI in the United States, and incidence has increased steadily over the past two decades. Screening of all sexually active women younger than 25 years is recommended. Women aged 25 years and older should be screened if they have STI risk factors. The U.S. Preventive Services Task Force (USPSTF) concluded that evidence is insufficient to support routine screening in men; the CDC recommends screening men in settings or populations with high prevalence or burden of disease (MSM, STI clinics).

Nucleic acid amplification testing (NAAT) is preferred for screening and diagnosis. First-catch urine (for men and women) and endocervical (for women) or urethral (for men) swabs can be used. NAAT of urine samples for *C. trachomatis* and *Neisseria gonorrhoeae* has been shown to have a sensitivity and specificity nearly identical to tests obtained from urethral and endocervical samples. In addition to cervicitis and urethritis, chlamydia may cause oropharyngeal and rectal infection, and these sites should be evaluated based on history of sexual practices. Although commercially available, NAAT may not be FDA cleared for testing extragenital sites; laboratories can provide this testing if they have confirmed internal criteria for validity of test results.

Treatment of clinical syndromes caused by *C. trachomatis* is outlined in **Table 32**. Test of cure is not recommended,

**TABLE 32.** Treatment of *Chlamydia trachomatis* and *Neisseria gonorrhoeae* Infections and Their Complications

| Clinical Syndrome | Preferred Regimen | Alternate Regimen |
|---|---|---|
| Cervicitis and urethritis (empiric therapy) | Ceftriaxone, 250 mg IM single dose, plus azithromycin, 1 g PO single dose (preferred), *or* doxycycline[a], 100 mg PO twice daily for 7 d (only if azithromycin cannot be used) | Cefixime, 400 mg PO single dose, plus azithromycin, 1 g PO single dose (preferred), *or* doxycycline, 100 mg PO twice daily for 7 d |
| *Chlamydia* cervicitis, urethritis, or proctitis | Azithromycin, 1 g PO single dose, *or* doxycycline, 100 mg PO twice daily for 7 d (21 d if *C. trachomatis* LGV serovars suspected or confirmed) | Erythromycin base, 500 mg PO four times daily, *or* erythromycin ethylsuccinate, 800 mg PO four times daily, *or* levofloxacin, 500 mg PO daily, *or* ofloxacin, 300 mg PO twice daily for 7 d |
| Gonococcal cervicitis, urethritis, or proctitis and pharyngeal infection[b] | Ceftriaxone, 250 mg IM single dose, plus azithromycin, 1 g PO single dose (preferred), *or* doxycycline, 100 mg PO twice daily for 7 d (only if azithromycin cannot be used) | Cefixime[c], 400 mg PO single dose, plus azithromycin, 1 g PO single dose (preferred), *or* doxycycline, 100 mg PO twice daily for 7 d<br><br>Test of cure 2 weeks after treatment for pharyngeal gonorrhea treated with an alternate regimen |
| Disseminated gonococcal infection[d] | Ceftriaxone, 1 g IM or IV every 24 h, plus azithromycin, 1 g PO single dose | Cefotaxime, 1 g IV every 8 h, *or* ceftizoxime[e], 1 g IV every 8 h, plus azithromycin, 1 g PO single dose |
| Pelvic inflammatory disease | | |
|    Parenteral therapy[f] | Cefotetan, 2 g IV every 12 h, or cefoxitin, 2 g IV every 6 h, plus doxycycline, 100 mg IV or PO every 12 h<br><br>OR<br><br>Clindamycin, 900 mg IV every 8 h, plus gentamicin, 2 mg/kg IV loading dose followed by 1.5 mg/kg IV every 8 hours or a single daily dose of 3-5 mg/kg/d | Ampicillin-sulbactam, 3 g IV every 6 h, plus doxycycline, 100 mg IV or PO every 12 h |
|    Oral/IM therapy | Ceftriaxone, 250 mg IM single dose, plus doxycycline, 100 mg PO twice daily for 14 d, with or without metronidazole, 500 mg PO twice daily for 14 d, *or* cefoxitin, 2 g IM single dose, with probenecid, 1 g PO, plus doxycycline, 100 mg PO every 12 h for 14 d, with or without metronidazole, 500 mg PO twice daily for 14 d | |
| Epididymitis | Ceftriaxone, 250 mg IM single dose, plus doxycycline, 100 mg PO twice daily for 10 d if infection most likely due to chlamydia/gonorrhea<br><br>Ceftriaxone, 250 mg IM single dose, plus levofloxacin, 500 mg PO once daily, or ofloxacin, 300 mg PO twice daily for 10 d if infection might be caused by chlamydia/gonorrhea and enteric organisms (insertive anal intercourse)<br><br>Levofloxacin, 500 mg PO once daily, or ofloxacin, 300 mg PO twice daily, for 10 d if infection most likely caused by enteric organisms | |

IM = intramuscularly; IV = intravenously; LGV = lymphogranuloma venereum; PO = orally.

[a]Doxycyline should be avoided or used with caution in pregnant patients.

[b]Treatment for possible chlamydial infection is recommended for all patients diagnosed with gonorrhea. Currently recommended treatment regimens for gonorrhea provide this coverage.

[c]Cefixime should be used only if ceftriaxone is unavailable because oral cephalosporin resistance to *N. gonorrhoeae* has been increasingly reported.

[d]For arthritis-dermatitis syndrome, parenteral therapy should be used until 24 to 48 hours after substantial clinical improvement and then switched to an oral therapy based on susceptibility results for a total of 7 to 10 days of treatment. Parenteral therapy is required for the entire course of treatment for meningitis (10 to 14 days) and endocarditis (at least 28 days).

[e]Not available in the United States.

[f]Patients can be switched to oral therapy within 24 to 48 hours of clinical improvement using doxycycline, 100 mg PO twice daily, with or without metronidazole, 500 mg PO twice daily, to complete a total of 14 days of therapy.

except in pregnancy. Because of the high risk of repeat infection, men and women should be retested after 3 months or the next time they are seen for medical care.

**KEY POINTS**

- First-catch urine (or genital swab) nucleic acid amplification testing is the preferred screening and diagnostic method for *Chlamydia trachomatis* infection.

**HVC** • Test of cure is not recommended in patients with *Chlamydia trachomatis* infection except in pregnancy; however, patients should be retested for possible repeat infection after 3 months or at their next medical visit.

# *Neisseria gonorrhoeae* Infection

The incidence of *N. gonorrhoeae* infection has been increasing since 2013, with rates of infection increasing more rapidly among men than women. Persons aged 20 to 24 years are at highest risk. In addition to cervicitis, urethritis, pharyngitis, and rectal infection, disseminated gonococcal infection (presenting as arthritis-dermatitis syndrome) can occur (see MKSAP 18 Rheumatology). Infection can be asymptomatic, especially in women, so screening is recommended for women younger than 25 years and those 25 years and older with STI risk factors. The USPSTF does not recommend screening for men; the CDC recommends screening men at high risk, as for *C. trachomatis*.

 For screening and diagnosis, NAAT is preferred. Men and women can be screened using a first-catch urine sample; endocervical and urethral swabs may also be used. NAAT availability for samples from extragenital sites is limited, and physicians should determine what testing is available from their preferred laboratory. In patients with disseminated gonococcal infection (arthritis-dermatitis, endocarditis, or meningitis), all *N. gonorrhoeae* isolates should be tested for antimicrobial susceptibility. Patients with suspected disseminated gonococcal infection should have cultures performed on blood, joint fluid (if arthritis is present), purulent skin lesions (if present), and cerebrospinal fluid (if meningitis is suspected); however, culture yield is not high, so NAAT from all potential sites of exposure (genital, pharyngeal, rectal) should be obtained.

Treatment of *N. gonorrhoeae* is outlined in Table 32. Because of the increasing prevalence of antimicrobial resistance among *N. gonorrhoeae* isolates in the United States, cephalosporins are the only antimicrobial class recommended. Previously, the rationale for combination therapy was to treat concomitant *C. trachomatis* infection; the current rationale is based on increased efficacy of combination therapy. In the United States, *N. gonorrhoeae* isolates are more likely to be susceptible to azithromycin than doxycycline, and azithromycin can be given as a single dose. Doxycycline should only be used in the setting of macrolide allergy. In patients with an allergy precluding use of cephalosporins, oral gemifloxacin or parenteral gentamicin plus oral azithromycin is an option;

however, the dose of azithromycin is higher, which is associated with a high incidence of gastrointestinal intolerance.

Test of cure is only recommended 2 weeks after therapy when pharyngeal gonorrhea is treated with an alternate antibiotic regimen. Patients with infections caused by *N. gonorrhoeae* who do not respond to treatment should have repeat testing with NAAT and culture so that susceptibility data can be obtained; consultation with an expert in the management of these infections should be sought.

**KEY POINTS**

- Screening for *Neisseria gonorrhoeae* infection is recommended for women younger than 25 years and those 25 years and older with risk factors (new partner, more than one partner, a partner with an STI, or a partner who has concurrent partners).

- First-catch urine (or genital swab) sample nucleic acid amplification testing is the preferred screening and diagnostic method for *Neisseria gonorrhoeae* infection.

- Parenteral ceftriaxone with oral azithromycin is the preferred regimen for the treatment of *Neisseria gonorrhoeae* infection.

- Test of cure in patients with *Neisseria gonorrhoeae* **HVC** infection is recommended 2 weeks after therapy only when pharyngeal gonorrhea is treated with an alternate antibiotic regimen.

# Clinical Syndromes
## Cervicitis

Women with cervicitis may present with vaginal discharge and intermenstrual bleeding, but many are asymptomatic. The major diagnostic criteria are (1) visualization of mucopurulent discharge from the cervical os or on a swab obtained from the endocervical canal and (2) eliciting bleeding by passing a swab into the cervical os; cervicitis should be considered in women with either of these findings. *N. gonorrhoeae* and *C. trachomatis* are the most commonly isolated pathogens; however, many cases are enigmatic. The role of *Mycoplasma genitalium* is still unclear; herpes simplex virus is occasionally implicated. Noninfectious causes (for example, chemical irritation from douching) should be sought. Patients should be tested for *N. gonorrhoeae* and *C. trachomatis* with NAAT; evaluation for bacterial vaginosis and trichomoniasis should also be performed (see MKSAP 18 General Internal Medicine).

## Pelvic Inflammatory Disease

Unrecognized pelvic inflammatory disease (PID) may result in long-term sequelae, including infertility, chronic pelvic pain, and ectopic pregnancy. Symptoms include lower abdominal pain, vaginal discharge, intermenstrual bleeding or bleeding after intercourse, and dyspareunia. Some women have fever and other signs of systemic toxicity, but this is uncommon.

The diagnostic accuracy of clinical examination is poor; however, because of the potential consequences of untreated infection, clinical findings with a high sensitivity for PID should be used. The presence of uterine tenderness, adnexal tenderness, or cervical motion tenderness is sufficient to make a clinical diagnosis of PID, especially if accompanied by mucopurulent cervical discharge.

PID is believed to be polymicrobial; however, testing only for *N. gonorrhoeae* and *C. trachomatis* is indicated. Most women can be managed in the ambulatory setting with oral antibiotics (see Table 32). Indications for hospitalization include inability to exclude a surgical emergency such as appendicitis, pregnancy, severe systemic toxicity, tubo-ovarian abscess, inability to tolerate oral antibiotics, and failure of initial outpatient management.

## Urethritis

Men with urethritis present with dysuria, urethral pruritus, and discharge. Mucopurulent discharge may be the only symptom and is clinically diagnostic. *N. gonorrhoeae, C. trachomatis*, and *M. genitalium* are common causes of urethritis; *Trichomonas* may also be causative. The role of other *Mycoplasma* and *Ureaplasma* species is uncertain at present. A first-catch urine sample should be tested for *N. gonorrhoeae* and *C. trachomatis* by NAAT for diagnosis and for public reporting purposes; FDA-approved tests for *M. genitalium* are not yet available. Microscopic examination of a urethral sample that reveals more than 2 leukocytes per high-powered field has a high positive predictive value for infectious urethritis, but the negative predictive value is poor. A positive leukocyte esterase test result or a microscopic examination with 10 or more leukocytes on a first-void urine specimen is also diagnostic for infectious urethritis. This testing is not required if mucoid, mucopurulent, or purulent urethral discharge is demonstrated on examination. **H**

## Epididymitis

Men with epididymitis present with unilateral pain and swelling in the epididymis; the testes may also be inflamed (epididymo-orchitis). Testicular torsion must be excluded in men with symptoms of sudden onset. *N. gonorrhoeae* and *C. trachomatis* are likely causes in younger, sexually active men. Older men and men who practice insertive anal intercourse may be infected with enteric gram-negative organisms such as *Escherichia coli*. NAAT for STI pathogens should be performed on first-catch urine, and a urine culture should be obtained. See MKSAP 18 General Internal Medicine for further information.

## Anorectal Infections

Patients who present with anorectal pain, rectal discharge, or tenesmus should be questioned regarding sexual practices. In addition to receptive anal intercourse, infection may occur in women as a result of autoinoculation from vaginal discharge. Causes include *C. trachomatis, N.*

gonorrhoeae, syphilis, and herpes simplex virus (HSV). Infections caused by the lymphogranuloma venereum (LGV) serovars (L1, L2, or L3) of *C. trachomatis* had previously been rarely described in the United States, but they are increasingly reported as a cause of proctitis and proctocolitis, mainly among MSM.

Diagnostic evaluation should include NAAT for *C. trachomatis, N. gonorrhoeae*, and HSV as well as serologic testing for syphilis (dark-field examination should be performed if available). Additional molecular testing is required to identify LGV serovars of *C. trachomatis*, but it is not widely available commercially; LGV serovars of *C. trachomatis* will be detected by currently available NAATs.

### KEY POINTS

- *Chlamydia trachomatis* and *Neisseria gonorrhoeae* are the primary causative organisms in cervicitis, pelvic inflammatory disease, urethritis, epididymitis, and anorectal infections, although other organisms may also be implicated.
- The two major diagnostic criteria of cervicitis are visualization of mucopurulent discharge from the cervical os or on a swab obtained from the endocervical canal or eliciting bleeding by passing a swab into the cervical os.
- The presence of uterine tenderness, adnexal tenderness, or cervical motion tenderness is sufficient to make a clinical diagnosis of pelvic inflammatory disease, especially if accompanied by mucopurulent cervical discharge.
- *Neisseria gonorrhoeae* and *Chlamydia trachomatis* are likely causes of epididymitis in younger, sexually active men; older men and men who practice insertive anal intercourse may be infected with enteric gram-negative organisms such as *Escherichia coli*.

## Treatment

Treatment of the clinical syndromes discussed previously is outlined in Table 32. Symptomatic patients evaluated in urgent care centers or emergency departments and others who may not be able to return for follow-up should be treated empirically based on clinical syndrome. Diagnostic testing should still be obtained because STIs are reportable and test results will be informative if the infection fails to respond to empiric therapy.

Patients should abstain from sexual contact for 7 days after completion of therapy and until all sexual partners have been treated. Sexual partners in the previous 60 days, or the most recent partner if greater than 60 days, should be referred for evaluation and treatment. Although independent evaluation and testing of sexual partners is preferred, most states have provisions for providing empiric antibiotic therapy prescriptions to the patient for their partners (expedited partner therapy, or EPT).

- Diagnostic testing should be performed even if empiric therapy will be provided to patients unlikely to return for follow-up care, because *Neisseria gonorrhoeae* and *Chlamydia trachomatis* infections are reportable, and because test results will be informative if the infection fails to respond to therapy.
- Most states have provisions for providing empiric antibiotic therapy prescriptions for sexual partners (expedited partner therapy, or EPT).

# Genital Ulcers

## Herpes Simplex Virus

The epidemiology of HSV genital ulcer disease is changing; in some populations, such as young heterosexual women and MSM, HSV-1 is now a more common cause of symptomatic primary infection than HSV-2. Although the clinical manifestations of primary infection by HSV-1 and HSV-2 are indistinguishable, HSV-1 is less likely than HSV-2 to cause symptomatic recurrent ulcers and subclinical shedding. Differentiation between the two viral subtypes is important in counseling patients regarding the natural history of their infection.

Primary infection presents as multiple painful lesions that begin as erythematous papules, progress to vesicles, then ulcerate, crust, and eventually heal within 2 to 3 weeks (**Figure 12**). Primary infection is often accompanied by significant systemic symptoms. Tender inguinal lymphadenopathy may be present.

Although the clinical manifestations of primary infection are quite characteristic, the viral cause and HSV subtype should be confirmed. NAAT, such as polymerase chain reaction, for HSV-1 and HSV-2 is preferred; other methodologies are far less sensitive. Testing is performed by obtaining a swab from the ulcer base; if only vesicles are present, a vesicle must be unroofed to obtain cells from the ulcer base. The swab must be placed in viral transport medium, so the appropriate sample collection kit must be used. Type-specific serologic testing is not advised for the diagnosis of symptomatic ulcer disease

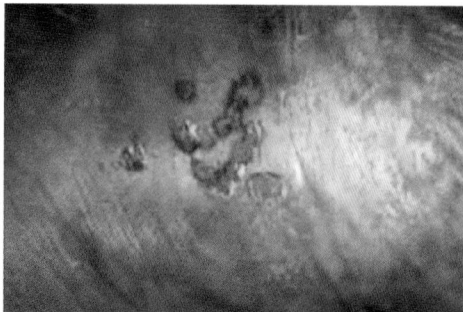

**FIGURE 12.** Penile lesions seen in herpes simplex virus (HSV) type 2. Patients with genital HSV infection initially have painful lesions that begin as vesicles and progress to ulcers on an erythematous base.

because patients can be seropositive for HSV-1 or HSV-2 yet have genital ulcers from another cause. Potential roles for serologic testing include testing a sexual partner when evaluating the potential benefits of long-term suppressive therapy because a partner who is already infected would not be at risk for transmission. The CDC recommends considering HSV serologic testing in persons who present for STI evaluation, MSM, and persons with HIV infection. Serologic screening in the general population is not recommended.

Antiviral therapy for primary infection has been shown to decrease time to resolution of symptoms, lesion healing, and viral shedding. Antiviral regimens appropriate for treatment of primary infection are outlined in **Table 33**.

Recurrent genital HSV infections are less severe, and symptom duration, time to lesion healing, and duration of viral shedding are reduced. Many patients will experience prodromal itching, burning, or tingling before ulcers appear. Atypical presentations such as fissures and excoriations may occur. Recurrent infection can be managed with either episodic self-start therapy (initiated within 24 hours of symptoms) or long-term suppressive therapy (see Table 33). Long-term suppressive therapy should be considered for persons with frequent recurrences and should be discussed with all patients because this strategy has been shown to decrease the risk of transmission to sexual partners. Laboratory monitoring is not required for patients undergoing long-term suppressive therapy; however, the continued need for therapy should be reviewed annually. Length of time since last recurrence and potential benefits of continued suppression in preventing

| TABLE 33. | Treatment of Herpes Simplex Virus Genital Infections |
|---|---|
| **Clinical Syndrome** | **Recommended Regimen[a]** |
| Primary infection[b] | Acyclovir, 400 mg three times daily, *or* acyclovir, 200 mg five times daily, *or* famciclovir, 250 mg three times daily, *or* valacyclovir, 1 g twice daily; all regimens for 7-10 days |
| Recurrent infection | Acyclovir, 400 mg three times daily for 5 days, *or* acyclovir, 800 mg twice daily for 5 days, *or* acyclovir, 800 mg three times daily for 2 days, *or* famciclovir, 125 mg twice daily for 5 days, *or* famciclovir, 1 g twice daily for 1 day, *or* famciclovir, 500 mg once followed by 250 mg twice daily for 2 days, *or* valacyclovir, 500 mg twice daily for 3 days, *or* valacyclovir, 1 g once daily for 5 days |
| Suppressive therapy | Acyclovir, 400 mg twice daily, *or* famciclovir, 250 mg twice daily, *or* valacyclovir, 500 mg daily[c], *or* valacyclovir, 1 g daily |

[a]All regimens are given orally; topical preparations are not recommended for treatment of genital herpes simplex virus.

[b]Therapy can be extended if healing is incomplete after 10 days of treatment.

[c]The 500-mg dose of valacyclovir may be less effective than the 1-g dose in patients who have very frequent recurrences (≥10 episodes per year).

CONT.

transmission to sexual partners are factors that can inform the decision to stop suppressive therapy.

Patients should be counseled regarding the natural history of infection and informed that asymptomatic viral shedding is the most common source of HSV transmission to sexual partners. Condoms and abstinence from sexual activity when lesions are present can reduce the risk of transmission. Suppressive therapy to reduce risk of transmission should be discussed. Men and women should be counseled about the risks of neonatal HSV infection. Women should be advised to inform their obstetric provider and pediatrician of HSV infection in themselves or their sexual partner if they become pregnant. ▣

**KEY POINTS**

- Viral cause and herpes simplex virus subtype in primary infection should be confirmed by nucleic acid amplification testing, such as polymerase chain reaction, using a swab obtained from the ulcer base.

- The Centers for Disease Control and Prevention recommend considering herpes simplex virus serologic testing in persons who present for sexually transmitted infection evaluation, men who have sex with men, and persons with HIV infection; screening in the general population is not recommended.

- Long-term suppressive therapy of recurrent herpes simplex virus infection may be preferred over self-start episodic therapy because of decreased risk of transmission to sexual partners.

## Syphilis

The incidence of primary and secondary syphilis has been increasing in the United States since 2000. The USPSTF recommends screening nonpregnant adolescents and adults at high risk of infection. Persons at risk include MSM and commercial sex workers and those with HIV infection, multiple sex partners, and previous syphilis. In 2015, the CDC issued a clinical advisory regarding the increasing incidence of ocular syphilis.

Primary syphilis presents as a painless genital ulcer (chancre) with a raised regular border that demonstrates firm induration on palpation (**Figure 13**). Several chancres may be present and may occur in the oral cavity. Regional lymphadenopathy may be present. The diagnosis of primary syphilis can be made on the basis of dark-field examination of material from a suspect lesion. Serologic test results may be negative in early primary infection. Even in the absence of treatment, lesions heal spontaneously in 3 to 6 weeks.

The most common manifestation of secondary syphilis is rash. Various morphologies are described; involvement of the palms and soles is characteristic. In intertriginous areas, papules may coalesce to form condyloma lata (plaque-like lesions). Mucous patches (superficial erosions on mucosal surfaces) may occur in the oral cavity and moist genital regions and are

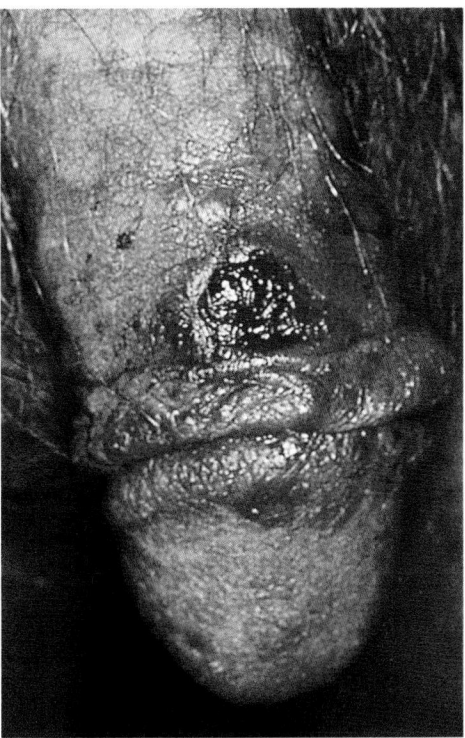

**FIGURE 13.** The primary ulcerative lesion (chancre) in patients with syphilis develops approximately 3 weeks after infection occurs, has a clean appearance with heaped-up borders, and is indurated and usually painless. It is often unrecognized.

highly infectious. Prominent systemic symptoms and generalized lymphadenopathy are common. Uveitis and neurosyphilis (meningitis) can occur. Secondary syphilis manifestations can also resolve without treatment, followed by latent infection (a positive serologic test result without clinical manifestations). If latent infection is of less than 12 months' duration, it is termed early latent; if greater than 12 months' duration, it is late latent. Practically, these determinations can be made only if past serology results are available. Otherwise, patients are considered to have syphilis of unknown duration.

Tertiary syphilis is rarely seen in the United States, although neurologic disease still occurs. Spinal fluid examination should be sought in any patient with unexplained neurologic symptoms and serologic evidence of syphilis as well as in those who do not demonstrate an appropriate serologic response to syphilis treatment.

Diagnosis of secondary and tertiary syphilis relies on serologic testing. Many laboratories use the "reverse" serologic testing strategy, starting with an automated enzyme immunoassay followed by a nonspecific test (rapid plasma reagin or Venereal Disease Research Lab test). Patients with a positive enzyme immunoassay result but negative rapid plasma reagin or Venereal Disease Research Lab test result should have a second specific treponemal antibody test to confirm the result. Those with a confirmed positive result and no history of syphilis treatment should be offered treatment for syphilis of unknown duration.

CONT.

Syphilis treatment is outlined in **Table 34**. Sexual partners of those with primary, secondary, or early latent syphilis exposed in the preceding 90 days should be treated regardless of serologic results. ▪

### KEY POINTS

- Primary syphilis presents as a painless genital ulcer (chancre) with a raised regular border that demonstrates firm induration on palpation; lesions heal spontaneously in 3 to 6 weeks even without treatment.

- The most common manifestation of secondary syphilis is rash, with characteristic involvement of the palms and soles; in intertriginous areas, papules may coalesce to form condyloma lata (plaque-like lesions), and mucous patches (superficial erosions on mucosal surfaces) may occur in the oral cavity and moist genital regions and are highly infectious.

- Diagnosis of secondary and tertiary syphilis relies on serologic testing; patients with a positive enzyme immunoassay result and positive rapid plasma reagin or Venereal Disease Research Lab test result and no history of syphilis treatment should be offered treatment for syphilis of unknown duration.

## Chancroid and Lymphogranuloma Venereum

With the exception of proctitis or proctocolitis caused by the LGV serovars of *C. trachomatis*, these two STIs are rarely seen in the United States. The clinical presentation and evaluation are outlined in **Table 35**, and treatment is outlined in **Table 36**.

## Genital Warts

Genital warts have a variety of appearances, including papular or pedunculated lesions (**Figure 14**). Larger, verrucous, exophytic lesions can occur. Most are asymptomatic; however, large lesions may cause irritation or pain depending on their location. Nononcogenic types of human papillomavirus (HPV) are responsible for most lesions. Oncogenic subtypes less commonly cause genital warts. HPV infection can be diagnosed based on the presence of lesions with a consistent morphologic appearance. Specific testing for HPV is not recommended for diagnosis.

Warts will often resolve without therapy, but treatment is indicated for symptomatic warts or if the cosmetic appearance of the warts is causing psychological distress. Patients should be counseled that successful treatment may not eliminate the risk of transmission. Therapy includes patient-applied

| TABLE 34. | Treatment of Syphilis | |
|---|---|---|
| **Stage** | **Recommended Regimen[a]** | **Alternate Regimen for Penicillin-Allergic Patients** |
| Primary and secondary | Benzathine penicillin G, 2.4 million units IM single dose | Doxycycline, 100 mg PO twice daily, *or* tetracycline, 500 mg PO four times daily, for 14 days |
| Early latent | Benzathine penicillin G, 2.4 million units IM single dose | Doxycycline, 100 mg PO twice daily, *or* tetracycline, 500 mg PO four times daily, for 14 days |
| Late latent or syphilis of unknown duration | Benzathine penicillin G, 2.4 million units IM at 1-week intervals for 3 doses | Doxycycline, 100 mg PO twice daily, *or* tetracycline, 500 mg PO four times daily, for 28 days |
| Neurosyphilis | Aqueous crystalline penicillin G, 18-24 million units daily given as 3-4 million units IV every 4 hours or by continuous infusion for 10-14 days, *or* procaine penicillin, 2.4 million units IM daily, plus probenecid, 500 mg PO four times daily, both for 10-14 days | Ceftriaxone, 2 g IM or IV daily for 10-14 days[b] |

IM = intramuscularly; IV = intravenously; PO = orally.

[a]Penicillin is the only effective antimicrobial agent for treatment of syphilis at any stage in pregnancy; therefore, pregnant penicillin-allergic patients should be desensitized and treated with the appropriate penicillin regimen as outlined above.

[b]Limited data are available to support the use of this alternate regimen, and the possibility of cross-reaction in penicillin-allergic patients must be considered. In patients who cannot take ceftriaxone, penicillin desensitization is recommended.

| TABLE 35. | Clinical Presentation and Diagnosis of Chancroid and Lymphogranuloma Venereum | | |
|---|---|---|---|
| **Clinical Entity** | **Causative Agent** | **Presentation** | **Diagnosis** |
| Chancroid | *Haemophilus ducreyi* | Painful genital ulcer; tender inguinal lymph nodes, which often suppurate | Culture is difficult; consider diagnosis if painful ulcer with tender and suppurative regional lymphadenopathy, no evidence of syphilis by dark-field examination or serology, and negative HSV PCR or HSV culture |
| LGV | L1, L2, and L3 serovars of *Chlamydia trachomatis* | Painless genital papule or ulcer with unilateral tender inguinal lymphadenopathy | NAAT for *C. trachomatis*; does not distinguish the serovars, so diagnosis is made based on clinical and epidemiologic findings |

HSV = herpes simplex virus; LGV = lymphogranuloma venereum; NAAT = nucleic acid amplification test; PCR = polymerase chain reaction.

| TABLE 36. | Treatment of Chancroid and Lymphogranuloma Venereum |
|---|---|
| **Clinical Entity** | **Recommended Regimen** |
| Chancroid | Azithromycin, 1 g PO single dose, *or* ceftriaxone, 250 mg IM single dose, *or* ciprofloxacin, 500 mg PO twice daily for 3 days, *or* erythromycin base, 500 mg PO three times daily for 7 days |
| Lymphogranuloma venereum | Doxycycline[a], 100 mg PO twice daily for 21 days (preferred), *or* erythromycin base, 500 mg PO four times daily for 21 days (alternate) |

IM = intramuscularly; PO = orally.

[a]Doxycyline should be avoided or used with caution in pregnant patients.

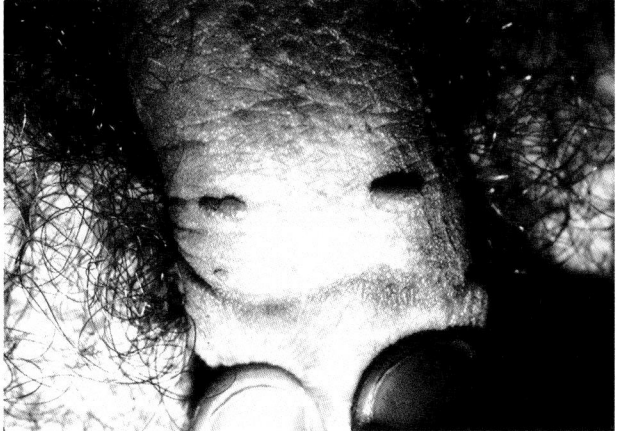

**FIGURE 14.** Genital warts caused by human papillomavirus infection are typically flesh colored and exophytic; pedunculated lesions often occur.

or physician-administered modalities. Patient-applied therapies include imiquimod, podofilox, and sinecatechins; provider-administered therapies include trichloroacetic acid or bichloroacetic acid, cryotherapy with liquid nitrogen or cryoprobe, or surgical removal. The modality chosen depends on size, number, and location of warts; patient preference; and provider experience. No evidence indicates superiority of any of the modalities recommended. Ulcerated or pigmented warts and those that fail to respond to or worsen after therapy should be biopsied to exclude a cancerous lesion.

**KEY POINT**

- Nononcogenic types of human papillomavirus are responsible for most genital warts, which often resolve without therapy.

#  Osteomyelitis

Osteomyelitis occurs as a result of hematogenous dissemination or contiguous spread of bacteria. Hematogenous osteomyelitis in adults most commonly affects vertebral bodies,

although involvement of other sites has been described, particularly in persons who inject drugs. Contiguous-spread osteomyelitis may arise from direct contamination (fracture, joint replacement, orthopedic implant), wounds (pressure sores, diabetic foot ulcers), or adjacent soft tissue infection. Population-based studies suggest that the incidence of osteomyelitis among adults is increasing in the United States, most likely because of the increasing prevalence of diabetes mellitus. Osteomyelitis can be difficult to diagnose, can cause indolent infections that persist for prolonged periods, and requires long-term antibiotic treatment; thus, the economic impact of this infection is substantial.

## Clinical Manifestations

Osteomyelitis frequently presents as subacute or chronic pain over the affected region of bone. If osteomyelitis has resulted from direct contamination of a wound, the wound may fail to heal or may reopen after healing. Spontaneously opening wounds accompanied by drainage (sinus tracts) are a late manifestation of infection. Underlying osteomyelitis should be considered when chronic wounds, such as pressure ulcers, do not respond to appropriate therapy. Fever and other systemic manifestations of infection are not common but are more likely in patients with acute hematogenously disseminated infection. Clinical findings in patients with diabetes-associated foot ulcer osteomyelitis and vertebral osteomyelitis are discussed separately.

**KEY POINTS**

- Osteomyelitis frequently presents as subacute to chronic pain over the affected region of bone; fever and other systemic manifestations of infection are uncommon.
- Underlying osteomyelitis should be considered when chronic wounds, such as pressure ulcers, do not respond to appropriate therapy.

## Diagnosis

### Laboratory and Imaging Studies

Laboratory studies are nondiagnostic for osteomyelitis. Elevated inflammatory markers, such as erythrocyte sedimentation rate or C-reactive protein level, increase the pretest probability of infection and can be useful in monitoring therapeutic response; normal inflammatory markers alone are insufficient to exclude the diagnosis. Except in acute hematogenous osteomyelitis, leukocytosis is uncommon; in chronic osteomyelitis, anemia may be present. Blood culture results are rarely positive, except in patients with hematogenous osteomyelitis (such as vertebral osteomyelitis). Blood cultures should be obtained when hematogenous osteomyelitis is suspected or in patients with systemic manifestations of sepsis.

Plain radiography is not adequately sensitive to exclude a diagnosis of osteomyelitis, but it is recommended during

CONT.

initial evaluation because of the relatively low cost. The specificity of plain radiography is sufficient to confirm the diagnosis in most patients. If a plain radiograph is not diagnostic, MRI, with and without intravenous contrast, is preferred. If MRI cannot be obtained because of specific contraindications, CT with intravenous contrast is an alternative. Nuclear medicine studies are less sensitive and specific for osteomyelitis but can be used when neither CT with contrast nor MRI are possible after review with the consulting radiologist.

**KEY POINTS**

- Laboratory studies are nondiagnostic for osteomyelitis; blood culture results are rarely positive, except in patients with hematogenous osteomyelitis.

HVC
- The specificity of plain radiographs is sufficient to confirm the diagnosis in most patients; if plain radiographs do not positively identify osteomyelitis, MRI, with and without intravenous contrast, is the preferred imaging modality.

### Bone Biopsy

Obtaining biopsy material for culture and pathologic examination is essential to the evaluation of suspected osteomyelitis. Confirming the presence of a pathogen maximizes the chance that the chosen antibiotic therapy will be successful. Specimens may be obtained at surgery or by image-guided biopsy. A bone biopsy is generally not required in persons with positive blood culture results. A possible exception is injection drug users because they have frequent bacteremias, and the organism in the blood culture may not represent the pathogen in the bone. In culture-negative disease, additional testing of biopsy material with nucleic acid amplification techniques, such as broad-range 16S ribosomal RNA gene amplification, may yield the causative organism, although these techniques will not provide information regarding antimicrobial susceptibilities.

**KEY POINT**

- Obtaining biopsy material for culture and pathologic examination is essential to the evaluation of suspected osteomyelitis.

### Treatment

Antibiotic therapy for osteomyelitis should be based on results of susceptibility testing from bone or blood culture isolates and knowledge of antibiotic levels achievable in bone for the selected agent. Unless systemic signs of sepsis or concomitant soft tissue infection or bacteremia are present, empiric antibiotics should be withheld until a bone biopsy is obtained. Surgical debridement is indicated if bone necrosis is extensive. Orthopedic hardware should be removed, if possible, to increase the chance of therapeutic success. Parenteral antimicrobial agents are usually chosen initially, but highly bioavailable oral agents with good bone penetration, such as

fluoroquinolones, may be considered. Rifampin should be used in combination with another antistaphylococcal agent to manage *Staphylococcus aureus* infections in the setting of orthopedic hardware if the hardware cannot be removed. Little evidence is available to guide recommendations on duration of therapy; 4 to 6 weeks of antibiotics is considered sufficient for acute infections, whereas longer courses may be required for chronic infections. In some circumstances, especially when hardware cannot be removed, indefinite suppressive therapy may be required. Patients should be informed about the risk of relapse and told that relapse can occur many years after therapy completion.

**KEY POINTS**

- Unless systemic signs of sepsis or concomitant soft tissue infection or bacteremia are present, empiric antibiotics should be withheld in suspected osteomyelitis until a bone biopsy is obtained.

- Surgical debridement is indicated for osteomyelitis if bone necrosis is extensive.

- Generally, 4 to 6 weeks of antibiotic therapy is sufficient for acute osteomyelitis; longer courses are required for chronic infections.

## Evaluation and Management of Osteomyelitis in Diabetic Foot Ulcers

The incidence of diabetic foot infection is increasing with the increasing prevalence of diabetes mellitus both in the United States and worldwide (see MKSAP 18 Dermatology). These infections are the most frequent diabetes-related complication necessitating hospitalization, cause significant morbidity (especially limb amputation), and are associated with increased mortality. Nonhealing ulcers become colonized with bacteria, after which infection may develop with contiguous spread to bone.

A diagnosis of osteomyelitis should be considered when a diabetic foot ulcer is deep (presence of exposed bone), large (>2 cm in diameter), or chronic (nonhealing after 6 weeks of standard care). Up to two thirds of affected patients do not have leukocytosis or elevated inflammatory markers. A probe-to-bone test (sterile probe inserted into the ulcer base to evaluate for contact with a hard or gritty surface representing bone or joint capsule) should be performed. In a clinically infected ulcer (presence of pus), the positive predictive value of the probe-to-bone test is high; in a noninfected ulcer, the negative predictive value is high. Imaging options are as described for other causes of osteomyelitis. All patients with a new diabetic foot infection should have plain radiography to assess for bony abnormalities, soft tissue gas, and foreign bodies.

Bone samples for histologic confirmation of diagnosis and for culture can be obtained during bone debridement; if debridement is not required, a bone biopsy should be

CONT.

obtained. *S. aureus* and streptococcal species account for most osteomyelitis complicating diabetic foot ulcers; gram-negative organisms are found in as many as 25% of infections. Anaerobes are much less common. Infections may be polymicrobial.

Although deep sinus-tract tissue cultures can be obtained, the correlation with bone biopsy samples is variable, and bone biopsy remains the recommended modality for microbiologic diagnosis. Recent evidence shows that patients treated with antibiotics chosen on the basis of bone culture results have a better outcome than those treated without these results. If infected but viable bone is present, a 4- to 6-week course of parenteral or oral antibiotic therapy is recommended, as it is for other forms of osteomyelitis. Prolonged oral therapy is indicated if there is residual necrotic bone.

Indications for amputation include persistent sepsis, inability to tolerate antibiotic therapy, progressive bone destruction despite appropriate therapy, or bone destruction that compromises the mechanical integrity of the foot. The patient may also choose amputation over prolonged antibiotic therapy. Hyperbaric oxygen therapy, growth factors, and topical negative-pressure therapy have insufficient evidence of benefit to recommend their use. However, limb salvage may be possible far more often than previously thought when treatment is directed by a dedicated multidisciplinary team consisting of a foot surgeon, a vascular surgeon, an internist, an infectious diseases specialist, nurses, and a physical therapist.

### KEY POINTS

- Osteomyelitis should be considered when a diabetic foot ulcer is deep (presence of exposed bone), large (>2 cm in diameter), or chronic (nonhealing after 6 weeks of standard care).

- Bone samples for diagnosis and guidance of antimicrobial therapy should be obtained in patients with osteomyelitis during bone debridement or by bone biopsy.

- If infected but viable bone is present in patients with diabetes mellitus–associated osteomyelitis, a 4- to 6-week course of antibiotic therapy is recommended; prolonged oral therapy is indicated for patients with residual necrotic bone.

##  Evaluation and Management of Vertebral Osteomyelitis

Except when resulting from surgical instrumentation, vertebral osteomyelitis is almost exclusively secondary to hematogenous dissemination. Risk factors for vertebral osteomyelitis include older age, immunocompromise, indwelling catheters, hemodialysis, and injection drug use. Infection occurs in the intervertebral disk space and then spreads to the adjacent vertebral bodies (spondylodiskitis). The lumbar spine is most frequently involved, followed by the thoracic and then the

cervical spine. Most infections are due to *S. aureus*, but *S. lugdunensis* is increasingly implicated. Persistent bacteremia with other coagulase-negative staphylococci in patients treated with hemodialysis and those with intravascular devices may obviate the need for biopsy. Enterobacteriaceae, *Pseudomonas aeruginosa* (especially in persons who inject drugs), and *Candida* species also may cause vertebral osteomyelitis.

New-onset back or neck pain or progressive worsening of chronic pain that is unresponsive to conservative management should raise concern for vertebral osteomyelitis, especially when accompanied by elevated levels of inflammatory markers, neurologic findings, or unexplained fever. Neurologic findings can include sensory loss, weakness, or radiculopathy and are reported in up to one third of patients. Point tenderness is present in as few as one third of patients. Delay in diagnosis is common; in a third of patients, pain is initially attributed to degenerative disease.

As with other forms of osteomyelitis, MRI is the preferred imaging modality. Blood cultures should be performed in all patients. Testing for *Mycobacterium tuberculosis* infection (with tuberculin skin testing or an interferon-γ release assay), fungal blood cultures, and serologic tests for *Brucella* species are appropriate for patients at risk for these pathogens (see *Mycobacterium tuberculosis* Infection, Fungal Infections, and Travel Medicine). A positive *Brucella* serologic result in the correct epidemiologic setting is considered diagnostic, and biopsy is not needed. Otherwise, image-guided biopsy has a diagnostic yield of approximately 60% and should be used in patients with negative blood culture results. A second biopsy should be obtained if the first is not diagnostic. Nucleic acid amplification techniques can increase biopsy yield; specimens should also be sent for pathologic examination. Open biopsy or percutaneous endoscopic diskectomy and drainage may be considered if the microbiologic diagnosis remains elusive after a second image-guided biopsy attempt.

Patients with neurologic compromise or evidence of spinal instability should undergo evaluation for immediate surgical intervention. Patients with complications, such as severe sepsis, progressive neurologic deficit, spinal instability, or epidural abscess, should receive empiric antibiotic therapy. Otherwise, initiation of antibiotic therapy for uncomplicated vertebral osteomyelitis is based on culture results. Parenteral therapy is generally recommended, especially for *S. aureus*. However, oral agents with high bioavailability and good bone penetration (such as fluoroquinolones) may be used, especially for Enterobacteriaceae. The duration of antibiotic therapy for vertebral osteomyelitis is typically 6 weeks. Patients should be followed clinically for improvement in symptoms, and inflammatory markers can be monitored. Repeat imaging, especially MRI, should be reserved for patients who do not respond clinically; worsening of imaging findings in patients with a satisfactory clinical response is well described.

- New-onset back or neck pain or progressive worsening of chronic pain that is unresponsive to conservative management should raise concern for vertebral osteomyelitis, especially when accompanied by elevated inflammatory markers, neurologic findings, or unexplained fever.

- The diagnostic evaluation of vertebral osteomyelitis should include blood cultures for all patients; testing for *Mycobacterium tuberculosis* infection, fungal blood cultures, and serologic tests for *Brucella* species are appropriate for patients at risk for these pathogens.

- Parenteral antibiotic therapy chosen on the basis of culture results is recommended for uncomplicated vertebral osteomyelitis, although oral agents with high bioavailability and good bone penetration also can be used; duration of treatment is 6 weeks.

# Fever of Unknown Origin

## Introduction

The classic definition of fever of unknown origin (FUO) has changed over time (including removing the requirement for in-hospital evaluation), and three categories have been added: health care–associated, neutropenic, and HIV-associated (**Table 37**). Diagnostic advances have revealed a spectrum of diseases causing FUO, with origins more rapidly identifiable for many cases.

## Causes

The differential diagnosis of FUO includes more than 200 diseases, although most adult cases are attributed to one of several dozen causes. Common causes of FUO include infections, neoplasm or malignancy, rheumatologic or inflammatory disorders, and miscellaneous causes (see Table 37).

## Evaluation

Many FUO occurrences are atypical presentations of common diseases. A careful history and physical examination should be performed and repeated intermittently during the period of evaluation. The history should include procedures, surgeries, presence of foreign bodies or implants, immunosuppression, travel, animal and other exposures (including hobbies), dietary habits, and medications (including over-the-counter medications). The degree and pattern of fever is not specific and not diagnostic in most instances.

**TABLE 37. Categories and Common Causes of Fever of Unknown Origin**

| Category | Definition | Common Causes |
|---|---|---|
| Classic | Temperature >38.3 °C (100.9 °F) for at least 3 weeks with at least 1 week of in-hospital investigation[a]<br><br>*or*<br><br>Temperature >38.3 °C (100.9 °F) for at least 3 weeks that remains undiagnosed after 2 visits in the ambulatory setting[b] or 3 days in the hospital | Infection (endocarditis, tuberculosis [extrapulmonary/disseminated], abscess, endemic mycoses), neoplasm (leukemia, lymphoma, renal cell carcinoma, hepatocellular carcinoma), connective tissue disease (adult-onset Still disease, polymyalgia rheumatica, vasculitis, systemic lupus erythematosus, giant cell arteritis), endocrine disorder (hyperthyroidism, subacute thyroiditis), genetic (familial Mediterranean fever), or miscellaneous (drug fever, factitious fever) |
| Health care–associated | Temperature >38.3 °C (100.9 °F) in patients hospitalized ≥3 days (without fever or evidence of potential infection at the time of admission) and negative evaluation for at least 3 days | Drug fever, septic thrombophlebitis, deep venous thrombosis/pulmonary embolism, sinusitis in the setting of a nasogastric tube, chronic sinusitis without a nasogastric tube, postoperative abscess, *Clostridium difficile* infection, device- or procedure-related endocarditis |
| Neutropenic | Temperature >38.3 °C (100.9 °F) and neutrophil count <500/µL (0.5 × 10⁹/L) for >3 days and negative evaluation after 48 hours | Bacteremia, opportunistic fungal infections (aspergillosis, candidiasis; more common than bacteremia after 7 days), drug fever, deep venous thrombosis/pulmonary embolism, underlying malignancy, allograft rejection in transplant; undocumented in 40%-60% of cases |
| HIV-associated | Temperature >38.3 °C (100.9 °F) for >3 weeks (outpatients) or >3 days (inpatients) in patients with confirmed HIV infection | Primary HIV infection, opportunistic infections (cytomegalovirus, cryptococcosis, tuberculosis, atypical mycobacteria, toxoplasmosis, *Pneumocystis jirovecii* pneumonia), lymphoma, immune reconstitution inflammatory syndrome |

[a]Original definition of fever of unknown origin.

[b]Ambulatory setting is the preferred venue for evaluation and treatment.

Initial testing for the evaluation of classic FUO includes complete blood count with differential, electrolyte levels, kidney and liver function tests (hepatitis serology if results are abnormal), lactate dehydrogenase level, urinalysis or microscopy and urine culture, erythrocyte sedimentation rate, C-reactive protein, antinuclear antibodies, rheumatoid factor, HIV testing, cytomegalovirus polymerase chain reaction testing, blood cultures (three sets, each set obtained at least several hours apart), tuberculosis testing, and chest radiography (or chest CT). Q-fever serology should be considered if risk factors exist, and mycobacterial blood cultures should be obtained in HIV-positive patients with CD4 cell counts of 50/μL or less.

If initial tests do not suggest a cause, abdominal or pelvic CT may be considered to evaluate for intra-abdominal abscess or lymphoproliferative disorders. Liver, lymph node, and temporal artery biopsies have a diagnostic yield of about 35%, particularly when performed when infection is unlikely. Posterior cervical, supraclavicular, infraclavicular, epitrochlear, hilar, mediastinal, and mesenteric lymph node biopsies are more likely to provide a diagnosis than that of other lymph nodes. Bone marrow biopsy can be helpful when leukopenia or thrombocytopenia is present.

A definitive diagnosis is lacking in up to half of patients after extensive evaluation. FUO lasting more than 1 year is unlikely to be caused by infection or malignancy. Undiagnosed FUO is generally associated with a benign long-term course, particularly when fever is not associated with weight loss or other signs of underlying serious disease.

**KEY POINTS**

- The classic definition of fever of unknown origin no longer requires inpatient evaluation and has been expanded to include health care–associated, neutropenic, and HIV-associated designations.

- In patients with fever of unknown origin, a careful history and physical examination should be performed, including past procedures or surgeries, presence of foreign bodies or implants, immunosuppression, travel, animal or other exposures, dietary habits, and medications.

- A definitive diagnosis is lacking in up to half of patients with fever of unknown origin after extensive evaluation, but duration of more than 1 year is unlikely to be caused by infection or malignancy.

# Primary Immunodeficiencies
## Introduction

Primary immunodeficiency disorders often present during childhood, but milder heritable forms may not manifest until adulthood. Primary immunodeficiency should be considered when patients present with frequent infections or infections with unusual organisms. The specific microbiology is often a clue to which arm of the immune system is affected (**Table 38**).

**TABLE 38.** Properties of Selected Primary Immunodeficiency Disorders

| | Common Infections and Pathogens | Diagnostic Testing | Treatment |
|---|---|---|---|
| Selective IgA deficiency | Sinopulmonary infections: *Streptococcus pneumoniae* *Haemophilus influenzae* <br><br> Diarrhea/malabsorption: *Giardia lamblia* | Undetectable (severe deficiency) or low (partial deficiency) IgA level with normal IgG and IgM levels | Vaccination against *S. pneumoniae* <br><br> Prophylactic antibiotics are controversial |
| Common variable immunodeficiency | Sinopulmonary infections: *S. pneumoniae* *H. influenzae* *Mycoplasma pneumoniae* <br><br> Respiratory viruses <br><br> Diarrhea: Norovirus *Campylobacter* *G. lamblia* <br><br> Urethritis: *Mycoplasma* *Ureaplasma* | IgG level and either IgA or IgM ≤2 standard deviations below the mean PLUS impaired humoral response to vaccination | Immune globulin replacement therapy <br><br> Immunization with inactivated vaccines <br><br> Prophylactic antibiotics are controversial |
| Complement deficiency | Early components (C2-C4): Similar to CVID <br><br> Late components (C5-C9): Recurrent infections with *Neisseria gonorrhoeae* or *Neisseria meningitidis* | Decreased level of total hemolytic complement (CH$_{50}$) | Same as CVID for C2-C4 complement deficiency <br><br> Quadrivalent meningococcal conjugate and serogroup B meningococcal vaccines for C5-C9 complement deficiency |

CVID = common variable immunodeficiency.

Diagnosis of primary immunodeficiency allows directed therapy, targeted immunization, and optimized empiric treatment of secondary infections.

## Selective IgA Deficiency

Although most patients with selective IgA deficiency (SIgAD) remain asymptomatic, it is the most common primary antibody deficiency. IgA provides mucosal immunity; therefore, patients with SIgAD are susceptible to infections of the respiratory tract and, less frequently, gastrointestinal tract. Sinopulmonary infections are the most common presenting manifestation, particularly with encapsulated bacteria (see Table 38). Anaphylaxis to blood products may occur because of the presence of anti-IgA antibodies. Testing for anti-IgA antibodies should be considered in patients with severe SIgAD or history of reaction to blood products or intravenous immune globulin infusion.

**KEY POINT**

- Patients with selective IgA deficiency may be asymptomatic, present with sinopulmonary or gastrointestinal tract infections, or experience anaphylaxis to blood products.

## Common Variable Immunodeficiency

Common variable immunodeficiency (CVID) is a heterogenous syndrome associated with decreased quantitative immunoglobulin levels and impaired humoral response to antigens. Impaired humoral response can be tested by measuring specific antibody production before and after immunization with tetanus and pneumococcal polysaccharide vaccines. Diagnosis is usually delayed until adolescence or adulthood, although a history of recurrent infection throughout childhood may often be elicited.

CVID increases risk of infections of the upper and lower respiratory tracts caused by encapsulated bacteria, *Mycoplasma* species, and respiratory viruses. Gastrointestinal infections typically present with acute diarrhea caused by common enteropathogenic viruses or bacteria. Chronic diarrhea with malabsorption suggests giardiasis or chronic norovirus infection, an increasingly recognized pathogen in this population. Additionally, patients with CVID are at increased risk of autoimmune disease, inflammatory bowel disease, granulomatous disease (noncaseating granulomas in the lymphoid or solid organs), bronchiectasis, and malignancy.

Pooled immune globulin replacement therapy for CVID is performed through intravenous infusions or subcutaneous injections. Passive replacement is associated with lower rates of infections and hospitalizations. Immunization is only partially effective because of impaired vaccination response; live vaccines should be avoided. The role of prophylactic antibiotics is controversial because they can predispose patients to infection with more resistant organisms.

**KEY POINTS**

- Patients with common variable immunodeficiency can experience recurrent infections and are at increased risk of noninfectious complications, including autoimmune disease, inflammatory bowel disease, granulomatous disease, bronchiectasis, and malignancy.
- Live vaccines should be avoided in persons with common variable immunodeficiency.

## Abnormalities in the Complement System

Infections and other antigenic stimuli trigger an inflammatory reaction through the classical, alternative, or lectin pathway of the complement cascade system. The result is formation of the membrane attack complex, which adheres to pathogens to facilitate immune detection and destruction.

Complement deficiencies can be divided into deficiencies in early or activating components (C2, C3, C4) and late or terminal components (C5-C9). Early component deficiency, especially C4, is associated with increased rates of systemic lupus erythematosus and increased risk of infection with encapsulated organisms. Patients with early complement deficiency present similarly to patients with CVID, with recurrent sinopulmonary infections. Terminal complement protein defects lead to an inability to form the membrane attack complex and typically present with recurrent infections of *Neisseria* species, particularly meningococcal meningitis. *N. meningitidis* infection in this population tends to be less severe than in immunocompetent persons, perhaps owing to uncommon serogroups. A personal or family history of recurrent *Neisseria* infections is an indication to test the total hemolytic complement ($CH_{50}$) level because any defect in the classical complement pathway will result in a low total level.

**KEY POINTS**

- Early component complement deficiency is associated with an increased rate of systemic lupus erythematosus and risk of infection with encapsulated organisms; terminal complement defects can result in recurrent *Neisseria* infections.
- Any defect in the classical complement pathway will result in low total hemolytic complement ($CH_{50}$) level.

# Bioterrorism
## Introduction

Unusually severe illness, rapid increase in disease incidence, atypical clinical presentation, and uncommon geographic, temporal, or demographic clustering of disease outbreaks suggest a bioterrorism attack. Bioterrorism agents are classified (**Table 39**) according to ease of dissemination, mortality rate, potential for public panic and social disruption, and need for special action for public health preparedness.

## Anthrax

Anthrax infection is caused by *Bacillus anthracis* spores (**Figure 15** panel A and Figure 15 panel B). Spores may be spread by aerosolization or in the mail, with infection following inhalation; any case of inhalation anthrax must be considered potential bioterrorism. Infection may also occur by cutaneous contact, with a characteristic black eschar forming (Figure 15 panel C), or by ingestion. Person-to-person transmission does not occur.

The clinical presentation of inhalational anthrax includes malaise, myalgia, fever, cough, dyspnea, and substernal chest discomfort. Meningitis occurs in up to 50% of persons. Rapid clinical deterioration leads to shock and death. Diagnosis is made by culture or polymerase chain reaction (PCR) of blood, tissues, or fluid samples. Radiographic imaging reveals a widened mediastinum (Figure 15 panel D).

Treatment is outlined in **Table 40**. Toxin-neutralizing human monoclonal antibodies and anthrax immune globulin are approved for treatment and prevention of inhalation anthrax in conjunction with antibiotics. Postexposure prophylaxis consists of a fluoroquinolone or doxycycline in conjunction with vaccination.

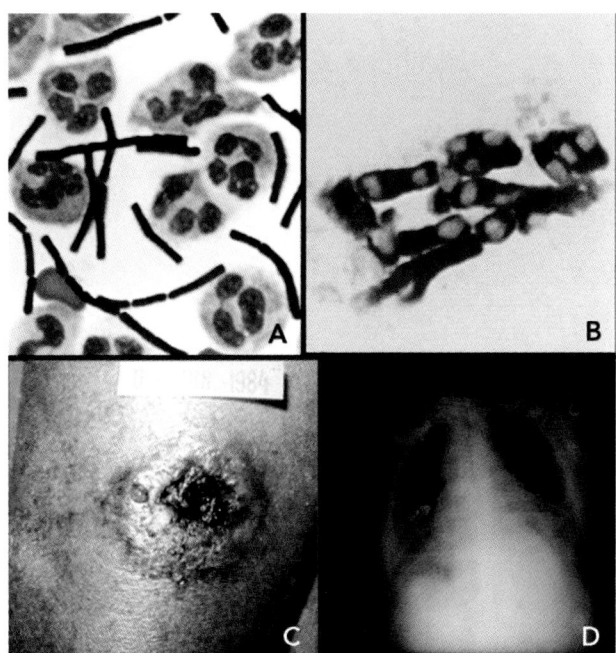

**FIGURE 15.** *A*, "box-car"-shaped, gram-positive *Bacillus anthracis* bacilli in the cerebrospinal fluid of the index case of inhalational anthrax resulting from bioterrorism in the United States; *B*, terminal and subterminal spores of *B. anthracis*; *C*, black eschar lesion of cutaneous anthrax; *D*, chest radiograph of a patient with anthrax showing a widened mediastinum caused by hemorrhagic lymphadenopathy.

### KEY POINTS

- Any case of inhalation anthrax should be considered potential bioterrorism.
- Patients with inhalational anthrax infection present with malaise, myalgia, fever, cough, dyspnea, and substernal chest discomfort; radiographic imaging reveals a widened mediastinum.

## Smallpox (Variola)

Routine smallpox vaccination ceased in 1980, after the World Health Organization declared the disease eradicated, leaving much of the world's population without immunity. Following inhalation, multiplication in regional lymph nodes results in viremia.

Secondary viremia occurs 1 week later, accompanied by fever, systemic symptoms, and rash, beginning with lesions on the oral mucosa and face and then the arms, legs, hands and feet, and to a lesser extent the trunk. Lesions evolve synchronously (same stage of maturation on any one area of the body) from macules to papules to vesicles to pustules before eventually crusting (**Figure 16**). Patients remain contagious until all scabs and crusts are shed. Mortality ranges from 15% to 50%.

Treatment is listed in Table 40. The oral antiviral agent tecovirimat was approved in 2018 for the treatment of smallpox in the event of a potential outbreak. Vaccination within

| TABLE 39. | Potential Agents of Bioterrorism | |
|---|---|---|
| **Class A**[a] | **Class B**[b] | **Class C**[c] |
| Anthrax | Q fever | Emerging infectious diseases |
| Botulism | Brucellosis | |
| Plague | Glanders | Nipah virus |
| Smallpox | Melioidosis | Hantavirus |
| Tularemia | Viral encephalitis | |
| Viral hemorrhagic fever | Typhus fever | |
| | Ricin toxin | |
| | Staphylococcal enterotoxin B | |
| | Psittacosis | |
| | Foodborne illness | |
| | Waterborne illness | |

[a]Greatest potential for use in an attack, easy dissemination, high mortality, and profound public health implications.

[b]Less easily spread, fewer illnesses and deaths, fewer public health preparation measures required.

[c]Potential to be engineered for future mass dissemination and significant mortality.

**TABLE 40.** Class A Bioterrorism Agents

| Disease—Agent | Incubation Period | Clinical Features | Treatment | Prophylaxis |
|---|---|---|---|---|
| Anthrax—*Bacillus anthracis* | 1-60 days | Inhalational: febrile respiratory distress<br><br>Cutaneous: necrotic eschar<br><br>Gastrointestinal: distention, peritonitis | Ciprofloxacin, levofloxacin, moxifloxacin, or doxycycline plus one or two additional agents[a] for 60 days<br><br>Consider raxibacumab, obiltoxaximab, or intravenous anthrax immune globulin | Ciprofloxacin, levofloxacin, moxifloxacin, or doxycycline<br><br>Amoxicillin if penicillin-sensitive strain |
| Smallpox virus—variola virus | 7-17 days | Fever followed by pustular cutaneous rash (face, followed by upper extremities, lower extremities, and trunk) | Tecovirimat | Vaccine if exposure occurred in the previous 7 days |
| Plague—*Yersinia pestis* | 1-6 days | Fulminant pneumonia and sepsis | Streptomycin or gentamicin for 7 to 10 days<br><br>Alternatives: doxycycline or levofloxacin if aminoglycosides contraindicated | Doxycycline or levofloxacin for 7 days |
| Botulism—*Clostridium botulinum* | 2 hours to 8 days | Cranial nerve palsies and descending flaccid paralysis | Antitoxin and supportive care | Antibotulinum antitoxin (equine serum heptavalent botulism toxin) |
| Tularemia—*Francisella tularensis* | 3-5 days | Fever, respiratory distress, and sepsis | Streptomycin or gentamicin (severe disease) for 7 to 14 days<br><br>Doxycycline or ciprofloxacin (nonsevere disease) for 14 days | Doxycycline or ciprofloxacin |
| Viral hemorrhagic fevers— Ebola and Marburg viruses | Variable | Hemorrhage and multiorgan failure | Supportive care | None available |

[a]Penicillin, ampicillin, imipenem, meropenem, clindamycin, linezolid, rifampin, vancomycin, or clarithromycin.

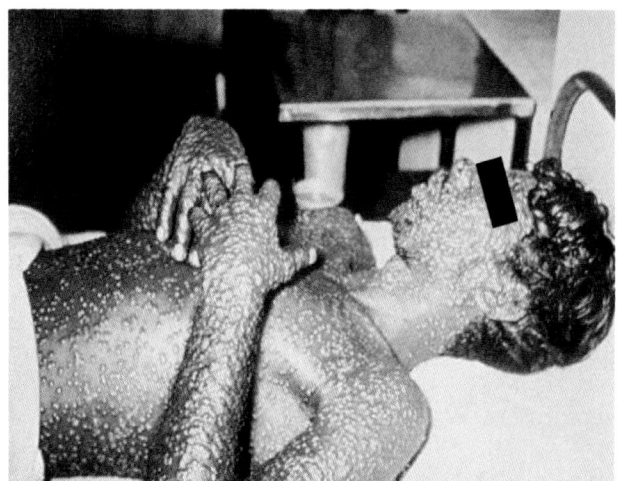

**FIGURE 16.** Diffuse synchronous skin lesions of smallpox.

7 days of potential exposure is effective in preventing or lessening disease severity and should be provided to close contacts. Intravenous vaccinia immune globulin is indicated in certain vaccinia-related complications or when vaccination is contraindicated.

**KEY POINT**

• Smallpox viremia results in fever and systemic symptoms, followed by lesions on the oral mucosa, then the face, and then the arms, legs, hands and feet, and to a lesser extent the trunk.

## Plague

Primary pneumonic plague occurs after *Yersinia pestis* (**Figure 17**) exposure through infectious aerosols and person-to-person transmission through respiratory droplets, which are likely scenarios for bioterrorism. Patients with suspected pneumonic plague require droplet precautions.

Bubonic plague is characterized by lymphadenopathy (buboes), fever, rigors, and headache. Chest radiographs are nonspecific. Gram stain and cultures of sputum and blood (performed using the highest level biosafety procedures) are often diagnostic.

Untreated, pneumonic plague is uniformly fatal. Treatment is outlined in Table 40. Asymptomatic persons exposed to aerosolized *Y. pestis* and close contacts of infected patients within the previous 7 days warrant postexposure

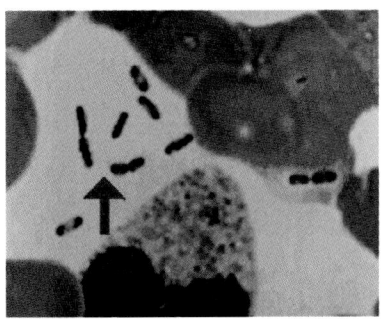

**FIGURE 17.** This Wright-Giemsa stain shows *Yersinia pestis*, a gram-negative coccobacillus with a "safety-pin" appearance (bipolar staining pattern).

prophylaxis. The available vaccine is ineffective at protecting against pneumonic plague. A live attenuated vaccine with protection from respiratory challenge is under investigation.

**KEY POINTS**

- Primary pneumonic plague occurs after *Yersinia pestis* exposure through infectious aerosols and person-to-person transmission through respiratory droplets, which are likely scenarios for bioterrorism.

- Asymptomatic persons exposed to aerosolized *Yersinia pestis* and close contacts of infected patients within the previous 7 days warrant postexposure prophylaxis with levofloxacin or doxycycline.

## Botulism

Botulism may spread in a bioterrorism attack through inhalation or ingestion of botulinum neurotoxin after deliberate aerosol release or purposeful food contamination. Patients present with symmetric, descending flaccid paralysis with prominent bulbar signs (the "4 Ds": diplopia, dysarthria, dysphonia, and dysphagia), which may progress to respiratory failure. Patients remain afebrile and mental status remains normal, but nausea, abdominal pain, and dry mouth often accompany the paralysis. Autonomic dysfunction may also occur.

Diagnosis depends on identifying the toxin from serum, vomitus, stool, gastric contents, or foods. Organism isolation is rare. Treatment is supportive (see Table 40). Antitoxin should be obtained from the Centers for Disease Control and Prevention and administered promptly but will not reverse existent paralysis. Antibiotics are not useful.

**KEY POINT**

- Botulism treatment includes supportive care and early administration of antitoxin, although this will not reverse existent paralysis.

## Tularemia

*Francisella tularensis* transmission to humans occurs by vectors, direct animal contact, and inhalation; person-to-person

spread does not occur. Abrupt onset of fever and respiratory symptoms follow inhalation of even a small inoculum of organisms. Chest radiographs demonstrate infiltrates, hilar lymphadenopathy, and pleural effusions.

Rapid diagnosis relies on serologic, immunohistochemical, and PCR testing; culture of tissues and fluids is low yield and potentially dangerous to laboratory personnel. Treatment is noted in Table 40. Death occurs in less than 4% of treated patients, with mortality rates reaching 30% in untreated pneumonic or typhoidal tularemia. No vaccine is available.

**KEY POINT**

- Patients with tularemia experience abrupt onset of fever and respiratory symptoms, and chest radiographs demonstrate infiltrates, hilar lymphadenopathy, and pleural effusions.

## Viral Hemorrhagic Fever

The Ebola and Marburg viruses are the most likely to be used as biologic weapons. In endemic areas, spread to humans occurs by vectors, contact with bodily fluids, or fomites. Aerosolization is a likely mode of terrorist dissemination. Symptoms of fever, headache, myalgia, abdominal pain, diarrhea, and unexplained bleeding and bruising appear 2 to 21 days after exposure. Disease progression results in maculopapular rash, hemorrhagic diathesis, shock, and multiorgan failure. Mortality rates can reach 90%. Persons are contagious only after symptom onset, but virus may spread by sexual contact in semen for weeks to months after recovery.

Depending on the stage of infection, diagnosis may be confirmed by virus detection in blood or other bodily fluids and tissues, antigen and antibody assays, and PCR. Exposed persons are monitored during the 21-day incubation period, with prompt isolation if symptoms develop. Treatment is supportive (see Table 40). Vaccine and antiviral medications are under development.

**KEY POINT**

- Symptoms of viral hemorrhagic fever include fever, headache, myalgia, abdominal pain, diarrhea, and unexplained bleeding and bruising, appearing 2 to 21 days after exposure; disease progression results in maculopapular rash, hemorrhagic diathesis, shock, and multiorgan failure.

# Travel Medicine

## Introduction

Pretravel consultation should occur no less than 4 to 6 weeks before departure. Regularly updated information by country is available on the Centers for Disease Control and Prevention (CDC) and World Health Organization (WHO) websites (http://www.cdc.gov/travel and http://www.who.int/ith).

Travel-related illnesses (mostly febrile, diarrheal, respiratory, and cutaneous infections) are reported in 20% to 60% of returning travelers; many of these are vaccine preventable. Required and recommended pretravel immunizations are listed in **Table 41**. Potentially severe travel-associated infections are listed in **Table 42**, the most significant of which are reviewed here.

# Malaria

Malaria is transmitted to humans by the female *Anopheles* mosquito. It is the most common cause of febrile illness in returning travelers, particularly from sub-Saharan Africa and large parts of Asia. Preventive measures include limiting outdoor exposure between dusk and dawn, using insecticide-impregnated bed nets and insect repellents containing 20% N-diethyl-3-methylbensamide (DEET), and using antimalarial chemoprophylaxis.

Incubation periods vary by species and range from 1 week to 3 months in semi-immune persons or those taking inadequate prophylaxis. Symptoms include fever (characteristically paroxysms in 48- or 72-hour cycles), headache, myalgia, and gastrointestinal symptoms. More severe disease occurs with hyperparasitemia (5%-10% parasitized erythrocytes) leading to adherence in small blood vessels causing infarcts, capillary leakage, and multiorgan system dysfunction. Serious disease primarily occurs with *Plasmodium falciparum*; manifestations include mental status alterations, seizures, hepatic failure, disseminated intravascular coagulation, brisk intravascular hemolysis, metabolic acidosis, kidney disease, hemoglobinuria, and hypoglycemia. Subsequently, patients may develop anemia, thrombocytopenia, splenomegaly, and elevated aminotransferase levels. See **Table 43** for specific features of the five *Plasmodium* species.

Diagnosis is made by identification of malarial parasites on the peripheral blood smear. Morphologic features help determine the specific species. Rapid tests that detect malaria antigens are available but may lack sensitivity and specificity. Polymerase chain reaction (PCR) and serologic assays exist, although each has limitations.

It is critical to identify *P. falciparum* and *P. knowlesi* because of their potential for severe infection. The onset of malarial symptoms shortly after returning from travel to endemic zones, such as Africa, and recognition of a high level of parasitemia and distinctive morphologic characteristics (**Figure 18**) should raise suspicion for *P. falciparum* infection. *P. knowlesi* is an emerging human pathogen found in South and Southeast Asia; high levels of parasitemia may occur, and examination of the peripheral blood smear reveals all stages of the parasite.

Malarial chemoprophylaxis and treatment depend on possible drug resistance and individual contraindications to specific medications (**Table 44** on page 61 and **Table 45** on page 62). Additional detailed information about malaria is provided in the CDC Yellow Book (https://wwwnc.cdc.gov/travel/yellowbook/2018/infectious-diseases-related-to-travel/malaria) or by calling the CDC malaria hotline (855-856-4713).

**KEY POINTS**

- Malaria is the most common cause of febrile illness in returning travelers; symptoms include fever, headache, myalgia, and gastrointestinal symptoms.

- The onset of malarial symptoms shortly after returning from travel to endemic zones, such as Africa, and recognition of a high level of parasitemia and distinctive morphologic characteristics should raise suspicion for *Plasmodium falciparum* infection.

# Typhoid (Enteric) Fever

*Salmonella typhi* and *Salmonella paratyphi* (A, B, and C) cause prolonged febrile and often serious infection (typhoid fever). Infection is acquired by consuming food or water contaminated by organisms shed in the stool of infected humans.

| TABLE 41. | Immunizations for Travel[a] |
|---|---|
| **Recommended According to Destination, Itinerary, and Purpose of Travel** | |
| Hepatitis A[b]: 1 month before travel, booster at 6-18 months | |
| Hepatitis B[b]: 0, 1 month, 6 months; accelerated schedule: 0, 1 week, 3 weeks, and 12 months (combination vaccine with hepatitis A available) | |
| Typhoid[c]: Live-attenuated oral vaccine (Ty21a); 0, 2 days, 4 days, 6 days; capsular Vi polysaccharide intramuscular vaccine; 1 dose (preferred for immunocompromised persons) | |
| Cholera: Live oral, 10 days before travel; killed oral, whole-cell-B subunit; 0, 1 week (available outside the United States) | |
| Rabies: Inactivated; 0, 7 days, 21-28 days | |
| Japanese encephalitis: Inactivated; 0, 28 days | |
| Tick-borne encephalitis: Inactivated; 0, 1-3 months, 9-12 months (not available in the United States) | |
| **Required for Certain Destinations** | |
| Yellow fever: Live attenuated; 1 dose | |
| Meningococcal: Quadrivalent conjugate (MenACWY) or polysaccharide (MPSV4); 1 dose; travel to Saudi Arabia during the Hajj | |
| Meningococcal B (MenB); 2 or 3 doses; high-risk groups | |

[a]All patients being evaluated for travel should receive or be up to date with all scheduled immunizations, including influenza, pneumococcal, tetanus-diphtheria-pertussis, polio, varicella, and zoster vaccines. See MKSAP 18 General Internal Medicine for routine adult immunization recommendations.

[b]If not received as part of routine scheduled immunizations. If the vaccine series was completed as part of scheduled immunization, repeat immunization is not required.

[c]Oral vaccine should not be administered within 24 hours of the antimalarial drug mefloquine because of the potential to decrease the vaccine's immunogenicity; patients must not take any antibiotic for at least 72 hours before receiving the vaccine.

Data from the Centers for Disease Control and Prevention. CDC Yellow Book 2018: Health Information for International Travel. New York: Oxford University Press; 2017. Available online at https://wwwnc.cdc.gov/travel/yellowbook/2018/.

**TABLE 42.** Travel-Associated Infections

| Condition | Clinical Clues |
|---|---|
| **Febrile Illnesses** | |
| Malaria | Paroxysmal fever (every 48 or 72 hours, depending on the species and may be continuous with *Plasmodium falciparum*), intraerythrocytic parasites, thrombocytopenia |
| Dengue fever | Acute onset of fever with chills, biphasic fever pattern ("saddleback"), frontal headache, lumbosacral pain, extensor surface petechiae |
| Chikungunya fever | Fever (abrupt onset up to 40 °C [104 °F] with rigors with recrudescent episodes), rash, and small joint polyarthritis |
| Zika virus | Mosquito exposure in endemic areas; nonspecific symptoms of fever, rash, joint pain, and/or conjunctivitis (asymptomatic in up to 80% of persons) |
| Typhoid fever | Prolonged fever, pulse-temperature dissociation, diarrhea or constipation, faint salmon-colored macules on the abdomen and trunk ("rose spots") |
| Rickettsial infection | Tick or flea exposure, maculopapular or petechial rash, eschar, lymphadenopathy, fever |
| *Coxiella* infection (Q fever) | Animal contact, self-limited febrile illness common, atypical pneumonia, elevated aminotransferase levels |
| Yellow fever | Abrupt fever with periods of remission, bradycardia, jaundice, kidney injury, hemorrhage |
| Viral hepatitis | High fever initially, then low-grade fever, fatigue and anorexia, hepatomegaly, dark urine, clay-colored stools |
| Mononucleosis syndrome (cytomegalovirus and Epstein-Barr virus) | Sore throat, fever, cervical lymphadenopathy, splenomegaly, atypical lymphocytes, elevated aminotransferase levels |
| Brucellosis | Zoonotic exposure, waxing and waning (undulant) fever, arthralgia, hepatosplenomegaly, depression |
| Leptospirosis | Conjunctival suffusion (erythema without inflammatory exudates), calf and lumbar spine muscle tenderness, aseptic meningitis, jaundice, kidney failure, acute high remittent fever in initial septicemic phase with brief decline before second immune phase |
| Lyme disease | Flu-like syndrome, target skin lesions (erythema migrans) may be accompanied by fever, arthralgias, bilateral Bell palsy |
| Histoplasmosis | Nonproductive cough, chest pain, fever |
| Legionellosis | Pneumonia, diarrhea, dry cough, progressive dyspnea, lymphopenia, thrombocytopenia, elevated aminotransferase and lactate dehydrogenase levels |
| Novel coronaviruses (severe acute respiratory syndrome [SARS], Middle East respiratory syndrome [MERS-CoV]) | Flu-like syndrome prodrome, diarrhea, dry cough with progressive dyspnea, lymphopenia, thrombocytopenia, elevated lactate dehydrogenase levels |
| Japanese encephalitis | High fever, altered mentation, cranial nerve palsies |
| Hemorrhagic fever viruses (Ebola, Marburg, and Lassa) | Fever, malaise, myalgia, vomiting, diarrhea, coagulation disorders, and bleeding |
| Rabies | Paresthesias or pain at wound site, fever, nausea and vomiting, hydrophobia, delirium, agitation |
| **Travelers' Diarrhea** | |
| Bacterial agents: *Escherichia coli*, *Campylobacter* species, *Salmonella* species, *Vibrio* species, *Shigella* species | Abrupt onset, crampy diarrhea, blood in stools |
| Viral agents: rotavirus, norovirus | Closed setting (such as cruise ship or classroom) acquisition, vomiting, diarrhea, short duration |
| Protozoa: *Cryptosporidium* species, microsporidia, *Giardia* species, *Entamoeba histolytica*, and *Isospora* species | Gradual onset, progressive and prolonged diarrhea, foul-smelling and greasy stools, mucus or visible blood in stools |

Travel to South, East, and Southeast Asia (Indian subcontinent) and portions of sub-Saharan Africa pose the greatest risk of infection. Unlike other nontyphoidal *Salmonella* (see Infectious Gastrointestinal Syndromes), the causative agents of enteric fever are human–only pathogens. Oral and parenteral vaccines (see Table 41) afford temporary protective immunity in 50% to 80% of recipients.

The gradual onset of fever with headache, arthralgia, myalgia, pharyngitis, and anorexia follows a 1- to 2-week incubation period. Abdominal pain and tenderness can be

| TABLE 43. | Characteristics of *Plasmodium* Species | | | | |
|---|---|---|---|---|---|
| Characteristics | *P. vivax* | *P. ovale* | *P. malariae* | *P. falciparum* | *P. knowlesi* |
| Incubation period | 10-30 days | 10-20 days | 15-35 days | 8-25 days | Indeterminate |
| Geographic distribution | Tropical and temperate zones | West Africa and Southeast Asia | Tropical zones | Tropical and temperate zones | South and Southeast Asia |
| Parasitemia | Low | Low | Very low | High | Can be high |
| Risk for disease severity | Low risk | Low risk | Very low risk | High risk | High risk |
| Disease relapse risk | Yes | Yes | Yes | No | No |
| Chloroquine resistance | Yes | No | Rare | Yes | No |

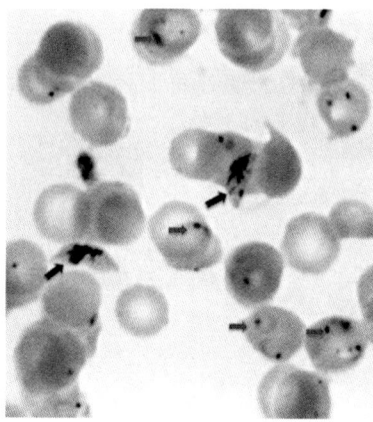

**FIGURE 18.** Thin, often multiple rings (*blue arrows*) on the inner surface of young and old erythrocytes as well as banana-shaped gametocytes (*black arrows*) are distinctive morphologic characteristics of *Plasmodium falciparum* species.

accompanied by early-onset diarrhea, which may spontaneously resolve or become severe late in disease. One fifth of patients have constipation at diagnosis. In untreated illness, temperature progressively increases and may remain elevated (up to 40 °C [104 °F]) for 4 to 8 weeks. A pulse-temperature dissociation (relative bradycardia) and prostration are common. During the second week of illness, discrete, blanching, 1- to 4-mm salmon-colored macules, known as rose spots (**Figure 19**, on page 63) develop in crops on the chest and abdomen in about 20% of patients. Moderate hepatosplenomegaly, leukopenia, anemia, thrombocytopenia, and elevated aminotransferase levels are common. Secondary bacteremia may cause pyogenic complications such as empyema, muscle abscess, and endovascular infections. Intestinal hemorrhage or perforation may occur 2 to 3 weeks after infection onset. Encephalopathy occurs in more severe cases.

Invasion of the gallbladder by typhoid bacilli may result in a long-term carrier state with shedding of organisms in the stool for more than 1 year. Those with gallstones and chronic biliary disease are at greatest risk.

Diagnosis is made through isolation of *S. typhi* or *S. paratyphi* from blood, stool, urine, or bone marrow; isolation success declines after the first week of illness. Rapid serologic tests are available to distinguish *Salmonella enterica* serotype *typhi* antibodies.

Antibiotic treatment decreases mortality and shortens the duration of fever. The emergence of antibiotic resistance in many geographic areas necessitates that in vitro susceptibility testing be performed on all clinical isolates. Ceftriaxone, fluoroquinolones, and azithromycin are preferred treatments. Dexamethasone has been shown to decrease mortality in severe illness, such as in patients with shock and encephalopathy. A 28-day course of ciprofloxacin is effective in eradicating chronic carriage, although cholecystectomy may be needed in cases of cholelithiasis.

**KEY POINTS**

- Typhoid fever commonly presents with fever, headache, arthralgia, myalgia, pharyngitis, anorexia, abdominal pain with early-onset diarrhea, pulse-temperature dissociation (relative bradycardia), and prostration.

- Ceftriaxone, fluoroquinolones, and azithromycin are preferred treatments for typhoid fever; dexamethasone decreases mortality in severe disease, such as patients with shock and encephalopathy.

## Travelers' Diarrhea

The most common travel-associated infection is diarrhea, defined by the sudden onset of three or more loose or watery stools per day with at least one additional gastrointestinal or systemic clinical sign or symptom (fever, cramps, nausea, abdominal pain, or blood in the stools). Risk factors, including geographic location (greatest in South and Southeast Asia, sub-Saharan Africa, the Middle East, and Latin America), type and duration of travel, and host characteristics, contribute to the 30% to 60% occurrence rate.

Most travelers' diarrhea episodes occur within the first 2 weeks of travel. Episodes are usually self-limited, lasting approximately 4 days; however, life-threatening volume depletion or severe colitis with systemic manifestations can occur. Some travelers develop chronic diarrhea or a postinfective irritable bowel syndrome.

**TABLE 44.** Antimalarial Chemoprophylaxis Regimens

| Drug | Dose | Time of Prophylaxis Initiation (before Travel) | Time of Prophylaxis Discontinuation (after Returning) |
|------|------|-----------------------------------------------|------------------------------------------------------|
| **For endemic areas with chloroquine-resistant *Plasmodium falciparum*** | | | |
| Atovaquone/proguanil[a] | 250 mg/100 mg once daily | 1-2 days | 7 days |
| Mefloquine | 250 mg once weekly | 1-2 weeks | 4 weeks |
| Doxycycline[a] | 100 mg once daily | 1-2 days | 4 weeks |
| **For endemic areas with chloroquine and mefloquine-resistant *P. falciparum*[b]** | | | |
| Atovaquone/proguanil | 250 mg/100 mg once daily | 1-2 days | 7 days |
| Doxycycline | 100 mg once daily | 1-2 days | 4 weeks |
| **For endemic areas with chloroquine-sensitive *P. falciparum*** | | | |
| Chloroquine | 500 mg once weekly | 1-2 weeks | 4 weeks |
| Hydroxychloroquine | 400 mg once weekly | 1-2 weeks | 4 weeks |
| Atovaquone/proguanil | 250/100 mg once daily | 1-2 days | 7 days |
| Mefloquine | 250 mg once weekly | 2 weeks | 4 weeks |
| Doxycycline | 100 mg once daily | 1-2 days | 4 weeks |
| Primaquine | 26.3 mg once daily | 1-2 days | 1 week |
| **For endemic areas with *Plasmodium vivax*** | | | |
| Primaquine[c] | 52.6 mg once daily | 1-2 days | 1 week |
| Chloroquine | 500 mg once weekly | 1-2 days | 4 weeks |
| Hydroxychloroquine | 400 mg once weekly | 1-2 days | 4 weeks |
| Atovaquone/proguanil | 250/100 mg once daily | 1-2 days | 7 days |
| Mefloquine | 250 mg once weekly | 2 weeks | 4 weeks |
| Doxycycline | 100 mg once daily | 1-2 days | 4 weeks |
| **Prophylaxis for relapse due to *P. vivax* or *Plasmodium ovale*** | | | |
| Primaquine | 52.6 mg once daily | As soon as possible | 2 weeks |

[a]Should not be used in pregnant women.

[b]Borders of Thailand with Cambodia and Myanmar (Burma).

[c]Contraindicated in persons with severe forms of glucose-6-phosphate dehydrogenase deficiency or methemoglobin reductase deficiency; should not be administered to pregnant women.

Recommendations from the Centers for Disease Control and Prevention. CDC Yellow Book 2018: Health Information for International Travel. New York: Oxford University Press; 2017. Available online at https://wwwnc.cdc.gov/travel/yellowbook/2018/infectious-diseases-related-to-travel/malaria.

Enterotoxigenic *Escherichia coli* is the most common causative agent (see Table 42). Younger age, use of gastric acid–reducing medications, abnormal gastrointestinal motility or altered anatomy, O blood type, and other genetic factors increase risk. Immunocompromised travelers may experience more serious and protracted illness with typical pathogens and are more prone to infection with opportunistic infectious agents. Chronic gastrointestinal conditions (such as inflammatory bowel disease) do not increase risk of infection but do predispose travelers to more severe symptoms.

Pretravel advice includes avoiding consumption of tap water (through drinks, ice, or when brushing teeth), undercooked meats, unpasteurized dairy products, and fruits that are not peeled just before eating. Water disinfection can be accomplished by boiling for 3 minutes or by chemical means using chlorine and iodine. Two drops of sodium hypochlorite (bleach) or five drops of tincture of iodine per liter of water are equally effective. Commercial water filters are not as dependable.

Antimicrobial prophylaxis for travelers' diarrhea is effective but is generally not recommended because of the potential for adverse effects. Prophylaxis should be considered in persons with coexisting inflammatory bowel disease, immunocompromised states (including advanced HIV), and comorbidities that would be adversely affected by significant dehydration. Bismuth subsalicylate can be used to prevent diarrhea, but the doses required are inconvenient and can lead to salicylate toxicity. Probiotics have not been proven

| TABLE 45. Malaria Treatment Regimens[a] | |
|---|---|
| **Drug** | **Dose and Duration** |
| **Non-*falciparum* Species[b]** | |
| Chloroquine phosphate (500 mg) | 1000 mg, then 500 mg at 6, 24, and 48 h |
| Hydroxychloroquine (400 mg) | 800 mg, then 400 mg at 6, 24, and 48 h |
| ***Plasmodium falciparum* or Species Not Identified** | |
| **Acquired in chloroquine-sensitive area** | |
| Chloroquine phosphate (500 mg) or Hydroxychloroquine (400 mg) | Same as for non-*falciparum* species |
| **Acquired in chloroquine-resistant area** | |
| Atovaquone-proguanil (250 mg/100 mg) | 4 tabs daily (or 2 tabs twice/d) for 3 d |
| Artemether-lumefantrine[c] (20 mg/120 mg) | 4 tabs at 0, 8, 24, 36, 48, and 60 h |
| Quinine sulfate (325 mg) plus one of the following: | 2 tabs (650 mg) three times/d for 3 or 7 d[d] |
| Doxycycline (100 mg) | 100 mg twice/d for 7 d |
| Tetracycline (250 mg) | 250 mg four times/d for 7 d |
| Clindamycin (300 mg) | 20 mg base/kg/d divided three times/d for 7 d |
| Mefloquine[e] (250 mg) | 3 tabs (750 mg), then 2 tabs (500 mg) in 6-12 h |
| **Acquired in mefloquine-resistant area[f]** | |
| Atovaquone-proguanil or Quinine sulfate plus doxycycline or tetracycline or clindamycin | Same as above |
| **Relapse prevention (infection with *Plasmodium vivax* or *Plasmodium ovale*)** | |
| Primaquine phosphate[g] (15 mg) | 2 tabs daily for 14 d |
| **Treatment in pregnant women** | |
| Chloroquine-sensitive species: Chloroquine phosphate (500 mg) | Same as above |
| *P. vivax* and *P. ovale* relapse prevention: Chloroquine phosphate (500 mg) | Once weekly until after delivery |
| Chloroquine-resistant *P. falciparum*[h]: Quinine sulfate plus clindamycin or mefloquine | Same as above |
| **Treatment of severe disease (acquired in all malarial areas)** | |
| Quinidine gluconate | Initial 10 mg/kg IV over 1-2 h, then 0.02 mg/kg/min continuous IV for at least 24 h until parasitemia ≤1% and oral medications can be tolerated |
| Artesunate[i] (parenteral) | 2.4 mg/kg IV at 0, 12, 24, and 48 h |

IV = intravenous.

[a]Patients who develop malaria while receiving prophylaxis should be treated with a different drug regimen.

[b]*P. vivax* acquired in Papua New Guinea or Indonesia should be considered chloroquine resistant.

[c]Artemisin-based combination therapies (ACTs) are the most rapid and effective therapies and active against all malarial species. Artemether-lumefantrine is the only approved ACT in the United States.

[d]Seven-day duration is indicated if infection was acquired in Southeast Asia.

[e]Increased risk of neuropsychiatric reactions; not recommended for *P. falciparum* infection acquired in Southeast Asia because of drug resistance.

[f]Found on the eastern border of Myanmar (Burma) and adjacent parts of China, Laos, and Thailand; western border of Thailand and adjacent parts of Cambodia and Laos; and southern Vietnam.

[g]Confirm absence of glucose-6-phosphate dehydrogenase deficiency in patient. Not indicated in pregnant women.

[h]Atovaquone-proguanil and artemether-lumefantrine are generally not recommended for use in pregnant women. Doxycycline and tetracycline are not indicated in pregnancy.

[i]Available in the United States from the CDC under an investigational new drug protocol; www.CDC.gov/malaria (call 770-448-7100).

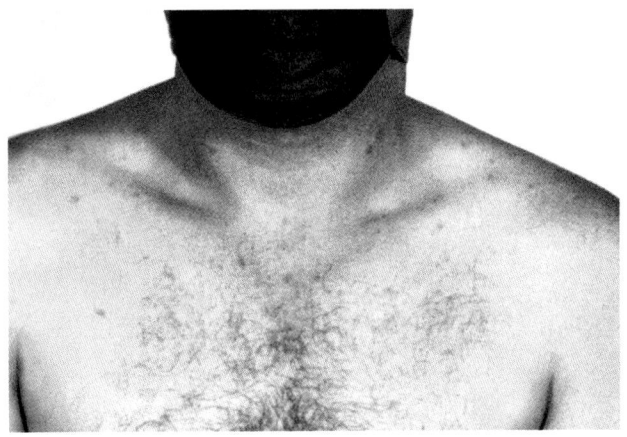

**FIGURE 19.** Rose spots on the chest of a patient with typhoid fever caused by the bacterium *Salmonella typhi*.

Reproduced from the CDC Public Health Image Library.

effective in the prevention of travelers' diarrhea and are not recommended.

Fluid replacement is the mainstay of treatment. Antimicrobials reduce the duration of diarrhea by 1 to 2 days but are recommended only in severe disease (**Table 46**). Self-treatment with a fluoroquinolone, azithromycin (preferred in South and Southeast Asia), or rifaximin is usually sufficient. Bismuth subsalicylate in large doses can be beneficial in decreasing the frequency and duration of diarrhea in milder cases. Antimotility drugs such as loperamide and diphenoxylate should only be given in conjunction with antimicrobial

**TABLE 46.** Oral Treatment and Prophylaxis for Travelers' Diarrhea

| Agent | Regimen |
|---|---|
| **Treatment** | |
| Bismuth subsalicylate | 1 oz every 30 min for 8 doses |
| Norfloxacin | 400 mg twice daily for 3 d |
| Ciprofloxacin | 500 mg twice daily for 3 d |
| Ofloxacin | 200 mg twice daily for 3 d |
| Levofloxacin | 500 mg once daily for 3 d |
| Azithromycin | 1000 mg, single dose |
| Rifaximin | 200 mg three times daily for 3 d |
| **Prophylaxis** | |
| Bismuth subsalicylate | Two tablets chewed 4 times daily |
| Norfloxacin | 400 mg daily[a] |
| Ciprofloxacin | 500 mg daily[a] |
| Rifaximin | 200 mg once or twice daily[a] |

[a]Chemoprophylaxis is recommended for no more than 2 to 3 weeks (the duration studied in trials and a period short enough to minimize the risk for antimicrobial-associated adverse effects).

Source: Hill DR, Ericsson CD, Pearson RD, Keystone JS, Freedman DO, Kozarsky PE, et al; Infectious Diseases Society of America. The practice of travel medicine: guidelines by the Infectious Diseases Society of America. Clin Infect Dis. 2006;43: 1499-539. [PMID: 17109284]

therapy but should not be used in cases of dysentery or bloody diarrhea because of increased risk of colitis and colonic perforation.

**KEY POINTS**

- Fluid replacement is the mainstay of treatment for travelers' diarrhea; fluoroquinolones, azithromycin (preferred in South and Southeast Asia), and rifaximin reduce the duration of diarrhea by 1 to 2 days but are recommended only in severe disease.    **HVC**

- Antimicrobial prophylaxis for travelers' diarrhea is generally not recommended; however, prophylaxis should be considered in persons with coexisting inflammatory bowel disease, immunocompromised states (including advanced HIV), and comorbidities that would be adversely affected by significant dehydration.

# Dengue Fever, Chikungunya, and Zika

Arboviruses are spread by arthropod vectors. Mosquitoes spread most travel-related arboviral diseases. Some arboviruses, such as yellow fever, are endemic throughout the tropics, and several countries require proof of vaccination before allowing entry by travelers. Other viruses, such as Japanese encephalitis, have more restricted geographic areas. The dengue fever, chikungunya, and Zika arboviruses are all spread by *Aedes* species mosquitoes and will be discussed here (**Table 47**).

Dengue fever is the most prevalent arthropod-borne viral infection in the world. Endemic areas include Southeast Asia, the South Pacific, South and Central America, and the Caribbean. The incubation period is 4 to 7 days. Patients may be asymptomatic or present with an acute febrile illness associated with frontal headache, retro-orbital pain, myalgia, and arthralgia, with or without minor spontaneous bleeding. Gastrointestinal or respiratory symptoms may predominate. Severe lumbosacral pain is characteristic. As the fever abates, a macular or

**TABLE 47.** Important Clinical Distinguishing Features of Arbovirus Infection

| Clinical Finding | Dengue | Chikungunya | Zika |
|---|---|---|---|
| Fever | +++ | +++ | ++ |
| Myalgia | ++ | + | + |
| Arthralgia | + | +++ | ++ |
| Headache | ++ | ++ | + |
| Conjunctivitis | − | − | ++ |
| Rash | + | ++ | +++ |
| Bleeding | ++ | − | − |
| Shock | + | − | − |

+++ = always; ++ = common; + = rare; − = almost never

scarlatiniform rash, which spares the palms and soles, may develop and evolve into areas of petechiae on extensor surfaces (**Figure 20**). Fever resolves after 5 to 7 days; however, some patients experience a second febrile period (saddleback pattern). A prolonged period of severe fatigue may follow. In patients with severe infection, life-threatening hemorrhage (dengue hemorrhagic fever) or shock may ensue, with liver failure, encephalopathy, and myocardial damage. This syndrome appears to be related to previous infection of a different serotype and is unlikely in travelers who have not had dengue fever previously. Abnormal laboratory findings include leukopenia, thrombocytopenia, and elevated serum aminotransferase levels.

Diagnosis of dengue fever is based on clinical suspicion in a patient who traveled to an endemic area and presents with fever and other typical signs, symptoms, and abnormal laboratory findings. Diagnosis is confirmed by serology (IgM and IgG) or reverse transcriptase PCR. Therapy is supportive. No licensed dengue vaccine is available in the United States, although clinical trials are ongoing. A live attenuated tetravalent vaccine, CYD-TDV, which is recommended for use only in persons previously infected by dengue virus, is available in several countries outside the United States.

Historically, chikungunya virus was limited to Southeast Asia and Africa but has recently emerged in the Americas, with outbreaks in Central and South America and the Caribbean. No vaccine is available. Symptoms resemble dengue fever, including abrupt onset of fever (≥39.0 °C [102.2 °F]) and severe bilateral and symmetrical polyarthralgia, often involving the hands and feet. A maculopapular rash on the limbs and trunk is common. Rarely, central nervous system, ophthalmologic, hepatic, and kidney manifestations are present. Abnormal laboratory findings include lymphopenia, thrombocytopenia, and elevated aminotransferase levels. Definitive diagnosis relies on serologic assays or detection of viral RNA by reverse transcriptase PCR testing. Disease is generally self-limited, resolving in 7 to 10 days. However, some patients may experience relapsing and chronic rheumatologic

symptoms for months or even years. Symptomatic treatment includes NSAIDs and aspirin avoidance (risk of bleeding complications and potential risk of Reye syndrome in children).

Before the 2015 Zika virus epidemic in Central and South America, human infection occurred chiefly in Africa, Southeast Asia, and the Pacific Islands. More than 5600 infections have been reported in the United States since the epidemic, of which greater than 225 are presumed to be from local transmission (Florida and Texas) and 55 acquired by sexual or laboratory transmission. This flavivirus is closely related to dengue, yellow fever, and Japanese encephalitis viruses. Intrauterine and perinatal maternal-fetal spread and sexual transmission from an infected male partner are other less common modes of transmission. An estimated 18% of those infected demonstrate clinical symptoms, which are similar to dengue and chikungunya virus infections, with the additional finding of conjunctivitis in most Zika infections. Most patients recover uneventfully after a mild illness lasting about 1 week, but some develop Guillain-Barré syndrome. Of most concern are risks to fetal development in pregnant women infected with Zika, including microcephaly, other severe brain and eye defects, and impaired growth and fetal loss. Women who are pregnant must be advised against travel to areas where Zika virus is known to be present. Likewise, women and men who are planning to conceive in the near future should consider avoiding nonessential travel to areas with risk of Zika infection; it is recommended couples wait to conceive until at least 3 months (for men) or 8 weeks (for women) after the last possible Zika virus exposure or from the onset of symptoms or diagnosis. Those not planning to conceive should use condoms for all forms of sexual activity together with their chosen birth control method or abstain from sex if Zika virus transmission is a concern. All pregnant women should be assessed for possible Zika exposure, and those who return from areas with outbreaks should be screened for evidence of infection. Reverse transcriptase PCR testing on serum and urine is used for diagnostic evaluation during the initial 2 weeks after illness onset. Thereafter, IgM antibody detection is used. Virus-specific plaque reduction neutralization tests can discriminate between Zika virus and cross-reacting antibodies against related flaviviruses. Because the epidemiology of Zika infection in the United States is still evolving, women who are pregnant and those who are planning to conceive should consult the CDC website for the most updated information when considering travel. No specific medications are available for treating Zika virus. Active vaccine development is ongoing.

### KEY POINTS

- Dengue fever typically presents with acute febrile illness, frontal headache, retro-orbital pain, myalgia, and arthralgia, with or without minor spontaneous bleeding; gastrointestinal or respiratory symptoms may predominate, and severe lumbosacral pain is characteristic.

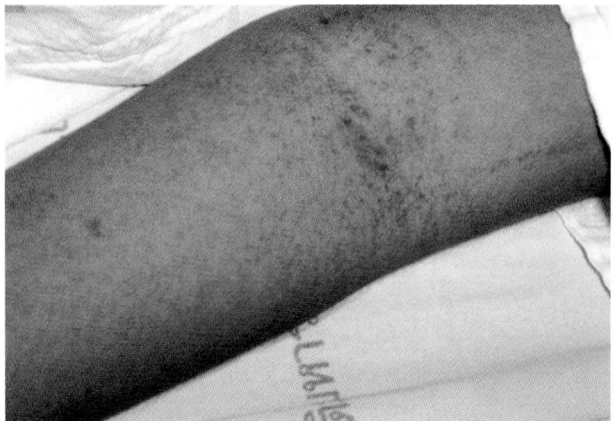

**FIGURE 20.** Petechial rash following application of blood pressure cuff constituting a positive "tourniquet test" that supports the presence of microvascular fragility compatible with dengue fever.

*(Continued)*

- Symptoms of chikungunya resemble dengue fever, including abrupt onset of fever (≥39.0 °C [102.2 °F]) and severe bilateral and symmetrical polyarthralgia, often involving the hands and feet; a maculopapular rash on the limbs and trunk is common.

- Of most concern in Zika virus infection is the risk to fetal development in infected pregnant women, including microcephaly, other severe brain and eye defects, impaired growth, and fetal loss.

# Hepatitis Virus Infections

Hepatitis A virus (HAV) infection is acquired through ingestion of food and water contaminated with fecal waste from another infected human in geographic areas with poor sanitation practices. Travel to Central and South America, Mexico, South Asia, and Africa poses the greatest risk of infection (for further information, see MKSAP 18 Gastroenterology and Hepatology).

Hepatitis A vaccination is recommended for persons traveling to developing countries who are not already immune (see Table 41). Protective antibody titers develop within 2 to 4 weeks in almost 100% of healthy recipients. A booster dose is given 6 to 12 months after the initial injection and provides protection for at least 10 years. Serum immune globulin is indicated for persons aged 12 months or younger and for those who decline vaccination or are allergic to its components. It has also been recommended for immunocompromised persons (who are less responsive to hepatitis A vaccine) and patients with chronic liver disease. Concurrent administration of hepatitis A vaccine and immune globulin is no longer recommended for those planning to depart within 2 weeks.

The risk for travel-associated acquisition of hepatitis B virus (HBV) is low. Previously unvaccinated persons traveling as health care workers, seeking medical care, or likely to engage in sexual activity with local residents in countries where HBV is prevalent warrant pretravel vaccination. Persons with insufficient time before travel to receive the standard three-dose/6-month vaccination series can complete an accelerated vaccination schedule (0, 7, and 21-30 days); these persons require a booster dose at 12 months to ensure long-term protection. A combined hepatitis A/B vaccine is also available for this rapid three-dose schedule.

No vaccine prevents hepatitis C virus infection, and immune globulin offers no protection (see MKSAP 18 Gastroenterology and Hepatology).

- Protective hepatitis A antibody titers develop within 2 to 4 weeks following vaccination in almost 100% of healthy recipients; concurrent administration of hepatitis A vaccine and immune globulin is no longer recommended for those planning to depart within 2 weeks.

*(Continued)*

- Persons with insufficient time before travel to receive the standard three-dose/6-month hepatitis B vaccination series can complete an accelerated vaccination schedule (0, 7, and 21-30 days), which is also available in a combined hepatitis A/B vaccine; these persons require a booster dose at 12 months to ensure long-term protection.

# Rickettsial Infection

Rickettsial infections occur worldwide. They usually belong to the typhus or spotted fever groups and are transmitted by small vectors (fleas, lice, mites, and ticks). Outbreaks have been associated with war and natural disasters and are promoted by suboptimal hygiene conditions and tick infestation. *Rickettsia typhi* is prevalent in tropical and subtropical areas. *Rickettsia prowazeki* is the only rickettsial species transmitted by human body lice and has a worldwide distribution.

Fever is the most common presenting symptom; African tick typhus (*Rickettsia africae*) is second only to malaria as the cause of febrile illness in those who have journeyed to Africa, especially South Africa. Clinical presentation also includes headache, malaise, conjunctivitis, and pharyngitis often accompanied by a maculopapular, vesicular, or petechial rash. Following the bite of an infected tick or mite, an eschar with regional lymphadenopathy develops at the site of inoculation with *R. africae*, *Rickettsia conorii*, and *Orientia tsutsugamushi*. Endothelial damage in the microcirculation leads to increased vascular permeability and is the hallmark of rickettsial infections, with extensive vasculitic-appearing lesions. Severe complications may include shock, meningoencephalitis, and significant damage to the kidneys, lungs, liver, and gastrointestinal tract. Recrudescent attacks designated Brill-Zinsser disease are known to occur months and even years later.

Diagnosis is confirmed by PCR, immunohistochemical analysis of tissue samples, or culture during the acute stage of illness before antibiotics are initiated. Confirmatory serologic assays often do not detect antibodies until the convalescent phase of illness, limiting their utility with acute disease. When clinical suspicion is high, empiric therapy is warranted. The treatment of choice for all rickettsial infections is doxycycline for 7 to 10 days.

- Rickettsial infections occur worldwide, with clinical presentation including fever, headache, malaise, conjunctivitis, and pharyngitis often accompanied by a maculopapular, vesicular, or petechial rash.

- The treatment of choice for all rickettsial infections is doxycycline for 7 to 10 days.

# Brucellosis

Human brucellosis may follow ingestion of unpasteurized dairy products or undercooked meat, by direct contact with fluids from infected animals through skin wounds or mucous membranes, or by inhalation of contaminated aerosols. *Brucella* is present in animal reservoirs worldwide, but the highest prevalence is found in the Mediterranean countries, Balkans, Persian Gulf, Middle East, and Central and South America. *Brucella melitensis* (from sheep and goats) has the highest pathogenicity and is the leading cause of human brucellosis.

After a variable incubation period, patients develop fever, myalgia, arthralgia, fatigue, headache, and night sweats. Focal infection may occur, commonly affecting the central nervous system and osteoarticular, cardiovascular, and genitourinary systems. Depression is frequent. Hepatosplenomegaly and lymphadenopathy may be apparent on physical examination with granuloma formation in reticuloendothelial tissues and organs. Disease relapse and chronic infection may occur owing to persistent foci of infection or inadequate antibiotic treatment.

Diagnosis relies on isolating the organism from cultures of blood, bone marrow, other body fluids, or tissue. The serum agglutination test is the most widely used available serologic test. An initial elevated titer of 1:160 or greater or demonstration of a fourfold increase from acute to convalescent titers is considered diagnostic. The Rose Bengal slide agglutination test, if available, is a convenient, simple, rapid, and sensitive point-of-care screening test.

The treatment of choice for uncomplicated brucellosis is a combination of doxycycline, rifampin, and streptomycin (or gentamicin), often given for several weeks. Neurobrucellosis requires several months of combined ceftriaxone, doxycycline, and rifampin.

**KEY POINT**

- The treatment of choice for uncomplicated brucellosis is a combination of doxycycline, rifampin, and streptomycin (or gentamicin), often given for several weeks; neurobrucellosis requires several months of combined ceftriaxone, doxycycline, and rifampin.

# Infectious Gastrointestinal Syndromes

## Overview

Diarrhea, defined as three or more unformed stools daily or a quantity greater than 250 grams daily, is a major public health concern. Diarrhea lasting less than 14 days is considered acute, 14 to 30 days is persistent, and longer than 30 days is chronic. Acute infectious diarrheal presentations include acute gastroenteritis, with associated fever, nausea, vomiting, flatulence, tenesmus, and crampy abdominal pain. Chronic infectious diarrhea is most likely due to parasites. Not all diarrheal presentations are infectious, such as inflammatory bowel disease, endocrine disorders, celiac disease, irritable bowel syndrome, and medication-induced diarrhea.

Patients with mucoid or bloody diarrhea, fever, significant abdominal cramping, or suspected sepsis and those who are immunocompromised or require hospitalization should have diagnostic assessment of their stool to guide antimicrobial use. Additional areas of concern include symptoms that persist for longer than 1 week or outbreak settings where day-care participants, institutional residents, health care providers, or food handlers are involved. Increasingly more available, rapid multiplex molecular gastrointestinal assays that identify common bacterial, parasitic, and viral pathogens from a single stool sample are generally more sensitive than historical stool culture and microscopy with special stains. (**Table 48**). Isolates from culture, however, can provide antibiotic susceptibilities and strain-typing information in outbreak situations that are not available from culture-independent diagnostic assays.

Most healthy patients with watery diarrhea of less than 3 days' duration can be treated with supportive care and no antibiotic therapy or diagnostic assessment. When acute diarrhea is debilitating (moderate or severe) and associated with travel, antibiotic therapy with a fluoroquinolone, azithromycin, or rifaximin is recommended. If a patient has dysentery with visible mucus or blood in the stool and a temperature less than 37.8 °C (100 °F), then microbiologic assessment is recommended to guide therapy. When severe debilitating disease is present with temperatures of 38.4 °C (101.1 °F) or greater, microbiologic assessment should be considered, followed by empiric azithromycin treatment (see Table 48). Antimotility agents, such as loperamide, are discouraged in patients with inflammatory diarrhea (fever, abdominal pain, bloody stools) or *Clostridium difficile*-associated infection.

**KEY POINTS**

- Patients with mucoid or bloody diarrhea, fever, significant abdominal cramping, or suspected sepsis and those who are immunocompromised or require hospitalization should have diagnostic assessment of their stool to guide antimicrobial use; rapid multiplex molecular gastrointestinal assays that identify common bacterial, parasitic, and viral pathogens in stool specimens are generally more sensitive than historical stool culture and microscopy with special stains.

- Most healthy patients with watery diarrhea of less than **HVC** 3 days' duration can be treated with supportive care and no antibiotic therapy or microscopic assessment; when the illness is debilitating and associated with travel, antibiotic therapy with a fluoroquinolone, azithromycin, or rifaximin is recommended.

**TABLE 48.** Causative Agents, Clinical Presentation, and Management of Infectious Diarrhea

| Agent | Clinical Findings | Diagnosis[a] | Antimicrobial Treatment[b] |
|---|---|---|---|
| **Bacterial Agent** | | | |
| Campylobacter | Fevers, chills, diarrhea (watery or bloody), crampy abdominal pain; postinfection Guillain-Barré syndrome, IBS, or reactive arthritis | Standard stool culture or NAAT | Azithromycin; ciprofloxacin (alternative) |
| Shigella | Dysentery (fevers, abdominal cramps, tenesmus, bloody/mucous-filled stools); postinfection HUS, reactive arthritis or IBS | Routine stool culture or NAAT; blood cultures (with severe disease) | Fluoroquinolone (ciprofloxacin) or azithromycin or ceftriaxone |
| Salmonella | Fever, chills, diarrhea (watery or bloody), cramps, myalgia; bacteremia in 10%-25% of patients; postinfection reactive arthritis | Routine stool culture or NAAT; blood cultures (moderate to severe disease); bone marrow and duodenal fluid cultures may also be helpful when enteric fever suspected | Mild: none<br><br>Underlying disease or severe illness: fluoroquinolone (ciprofloxacin) and/or parenteral third-generation cephalosporin |
| EHEC/STEC, including Escherichia coli O157:H7 | Bloody stools in >80% of patients; fever often absent or low grade; may be associated with HUS | Stool culture with specialized media and immunoassay for Shiga toxin or NAAT | None |
| ETEC (travelers' diarrhea) | Nonbloody, watery stools; constitutional symptoms rare | None—usually a clinical diagnosis | Fluoroquinolone, azithromycin, or rifaximin |
| Yersinia | Fever, diarrhea, right lower quadrant pain (may mimic appendicitis); pharyngitis; postinfection reactive arthritis and erythema nodosum | Stool culture with specialized media (or culture of other involved sites); NAAT | Trimethoprim-sulfamethoxazole<br><br>Alternatives: a fluoroquinolone (ciprofloxacin) or a third-generation cephalosporin (such as cefotaxime or ceftriaxone)<br><br>Severe extraintestinal disease: requires a longer treatment duration, including intravenous agents (such as a third-generation cephalosporin) |
| Vibrio (not V. cholerae) | Bloody stools (>25% of patients), fever, vomiting (>50% of patients) | Stool culture with specialized media (blood culture with suspected invasive disease) | Usually no treatment unless invasive<br><br>Fluoroquinolone (ciprofloxacin), azithromycin, or doxycycline if treating gastrointestinal illness<br><br>Doxycycline plus ceftriaxone for invasive infection |
| Clostridium difficile | Diarrhea, fever, abdominal pain/cramping, colonic distention (including toxic megacolon in severe disease), leukocytosis, sepsis; gross blood uncommon | Stool NAAT alone or stool EIA toxin test as part of stepwise approach, including NAAT plus toxin, or GDH plus toxin, or GDH plus toxin followed by NAAT when results are discordant | Nonsevere: oral vancomycin or oral fidaxomicin; if neither is available, oral metronidazole<br><br>Severe: oral vancomycin or fidaxomicin<br><br>Fulminant: oral vancomycin, IV metronidazole, and (possibly) vancomycin enema |
| **Viral** | | | |
| Norovirus | Watery, noninflammatory diarrhea and fever; vomiting in >50% of patients; short incubation period and high attack rate | NAAT, particularly for outbreak investigations | None |
| **Parasitic** | | | |
| Giardia | Watery diarrhea, abdominal cramping, nausea, steatorrhea, flatulence, weight loss; fever uncommon; postinfection lactose intolerance | EIA or NAAT preferred; stool microscopy for ova and parasites | Tinidazole, nitazoxanide, or metronidazole |
| Cryptosporidium | Watery diarrhea; abdominal cramping; malaise; weight loss | Modified acid-fast stain; immunoassays; NAAT | Nitazoxanide<br><br>Effective antiretroviral therapy in patients with HIV infection |
| Amebiasis | Dysentery, abdominal pain, fever, weight loss | Stool microscopy for ova and parasites; stool antigen immunoassay; NAAT; serologic antibodies | Tinidazole or metronidazole followed by paromomycin or diloxanide |
| Cyclospora | Watery diarrhea, bloating, flatulence, weight loss, nausea, anorexia | Modified acid-fast stain; fluorescence microscopy; NAAT | Trimethoprim-sulfamethoxazole |

EHEC = enterohemorrhagic E. coli; EIA = enzyme immunoassay; ETEC = enterotoxigenic E. coli; GDH = glutamate dehydrogenase; HUS = hemolytic uremic syndrome; IBS = irritable bowel syndrome; IV = intravenous; NAAT = nucleic acid amplification test; STEC = Shiga toxin–producing E. coli.

[a]Multiplex molecular assays are becoming increasingly available for identification of bacterial, parasitic, and viral gastrointestinal pathogens.

[b]Empiric treatment, with the final choice of the antimicrobial agent to use guided by in vitro susceptibility testing.

## *Campylobacter* Infection

*Campylobacter* species–associated gastroenteritis is usually foodborne, often secondary to consumption of inadequately cooked poultry. The incubation period is several days, and symptoms typically include diarrhea (visibly bloody in <15% of patients), crampy abdominal pain, and fever. Stool culture can confirm the diagnosis, and blood cultures can identify extraintestinal disease. Diarrhea usually resolves spontaneously without antibiotics. Patients who have severe disease (bloody stools, bacteremia, high fever, or prolonged [>1 week] symptoms) or are immunocompromised should receive antibiotic therapy. When indicated, macrolide therapy is preferred empirically because of increasing fluoroquinolone resistance. Possible post–*Campylobacter* infection complications include irritable bowel syndrome, reactive arthritis, and Guillain-Barré syndrome.

**KEY POINT**

- *Campylobacter* infection–associated diarrhea usually resolves spontaneously without antibiotic therapy; macrolides are the preferred empiric treatment for those who have severe disease or are immunocompromised.

## *Shigella* Infection

*Shigella* infection is more commonly spread from person to person than by consumption of contaminated food or water. Fewer than 100 bacteria can cause infection, and the incubation period is approximately 3 days. Patients typically present with crampy abdominal pain, tenesmus, small-volume bloody and/or mucoid diarrhea, high fever, and (possibly) vomiting. More serious complications include bacteremia, seizures, and intestinal obstruction and perforation. Potential postinfectious sequelae include hemolytic uremic syndrome, reactive arthritis, and irritable bowel syndrome. Routine stool culture or molecular testing will establish the diagnosis. Invasive disease in patients with severe infection can also be established with blood cultures. Treatment with antibiotic agents is recommended for those with severe illness (that is, those who require hospitalization, have invasive disease, or have complications of infection) and those who are immunocompromised. Public health officials may also recommend treatment when outbreaks occur. Antibiotic susceptibilities should be obtained to determine treatment because of increasing resistance rates against the quinolones.

**KEY POINT**

- In patients with *Shigella* infection, treatment with antibiotic agents is recommended for those with severe illness (that is, those who require hospitalization, have invasive disease, or have complications of infection) and those who are immunocompromised.

## *Salmonella* Infection

*Salmonella* infection can be typhoidal (serotypes Paratyphi or Typhi) or nontyphoidal. The typhoidal types cause enteric fever, a syndrome consisting of fever, abdominal pain, rash, hepatosplenomegaly, and relative bradycardia. This type of infection is uncommon in the United States, with most affected persons traveling to endemic areas and ingesting contaminated water or food. In contrast, nontyphoidal *Salmonella* serotypes are the most common bacterial cause of foodborne illness in the United States.

Nontyphoidal *Salmonella* infection usually results from ingesting fecally contaminated water or food of animal origin, including poultry, beef, eggs, and milk. Contact with infected animals (including pet reptiles, turtles, and snakes; farm animals; amphibians; and rodents) is a much less common mode of transmission. The incubation period is usually less than 3 days, and symptoms typically include crampy abdominal pain, fever, diarrhea (not usually visibly bloody), headache, nausea, and vomiting. Diagnosis can be made by stool culture or molecular testing. Illness is usually self-limited, although bacteremia with extraintestinal infection (involving vascular endothelium, joints, or meninges) may occur; *Salmonella* osteomyelitis also can occur and is classically associated with sickle cell disease. Severe invasive disease is more likely in infants, older adults, patients with cell-mediated immunodeficiency, and patients with hypochlorhydria. Reactive arthritis is a potential postinfection complication.

Most uncomplicated *Salmonella* infections in adults younger than 50 years resolve within 1 week and require only supportive care. Antibiotic agents are typically reserved for patients with more serious illness (including severe diarrhea requiring hospitalization, bacteremia, or high fever or sepsis) and those at high risk for severe complicated invasive disease (including infants, patients 50 years and older, or those with prosthetic materials, significant atherosclerotic disease, or immunocompromising conditions [such as HIV infection]). When empiric treatment is indicated, fluoroquinolones (such as levofloxacin or ciprofloxacin) are most likely to be effective, but azithromycin, trimethoprim-sulfamethoxazole, and amoxicillin also are potentially active agents. A fluoroquinolone, third-generation cephalosporin (such as ceftriaxone), or both are often initiated as empiric therapy for patients with severe disease requiring hospitalization. Local antibiotic susceptibilities of *Salmonella* should dictate choice of empiric therapy.

**KEY POINTS**

- Nontyphoidal *Salmonella* serotypes are the most common bacterial cause of foodborne illness in the United States; diagnosis is made by stool culture or molecular testing, and the illness is usually self-limited, although bacteremia with extraintestinal infection may occur.

*(Continued)*

- Most uncomplicated *Salmonella* infections in adults younger than 50 years resolve within 1 week and require only supportive care; when empiric treatment is indicated for those with more severe or invasive disease, fluoroquinolones (such as levofloxacin or ciprofloxacin) are most likely to be effective.

## *Escherichia coli* Infection

Although *Escherichia coli* are normal inhabitants of the intestinal microbiome, some strains become enteropathogenic by using different mechanisms of infection (**Table 49**).

Enterotoxigenic *E. coli* infection (ETEC) is the most common cause of travelers' diarrhea. ETEC results from ingestion of water or food contaminated with stool and has an incubation period of 1 to 3 days. Enterotoxins cause watery diarrhea with associated abdominal cramping, nausea, and low-grade or no fever. Usually self-limiting, the illness resolves after approximately 4 days. Hydration and empiric antibiotic therapy with fluoroquinolones, azithromycin, or rifaximin are recommended in travelers with ETEC when symptoms restrict activities.

Enterohemorrhagic *E. coli* (EHEC) strains, such as -0157:H7 and -0104:H4, produce a Shiga-like toxin that can cause hemorrhagic colitis. EHEC bacteria are found in cow intestines and are transmitted by ingestion of undercooked hamburgers or fecally contaminated food (such as spinach, lettuce, fruit, milk, and flour) and water;

fecal-oral transmission through exposure to infected animals at petting zoos is also possible. The incubation period is 3 to 4 days, and patients typically have visibly bloody diarrhea, crampy abdominal pain, and no fever, the latter a distinguishing feature from other causes of bloody diarrhea. Alerting the laboratory about the symptoms is recommended so that appropriate media, antigen testing, and Shiga toxin assays can be performed. Hemolytic uremic syndrome is found in less than 10% of patients infected with EHEC and manifests as microangiopathic hemolytic anemia, thrombocytopenia, and kidney injury. Treatment of EHEC infection is primarily supportive; antibiotics and antimotility agents may increase the risk of developing hemolytic uremic syndrome and do not appear to shorten the duration of infection.

- Enterotoxigenic *Escherichia coli* infection is usually a self-limiting illness that resolves without treatment after approximately 4 days; hydration and empiric antibiotic therapy with fluoroquinolones, azithromycin, or rifaximin are recommended in travelers when symptoms restrict activities. **HVC**

- Enterohemorrhagic *Escherichia coli* strains produce a Shiga-like toxin that can cause hemorrhagic colitis; treatment is primarily supportive because antibiotics and antimotility agents may increase the risk of developing hemolytic uremic syndrome and do not appear to shorten the duration of infection. **HVC**

## *Yersinia* Infection

Most diarrheal illness due to *Yersinia* species is caused by *Yersinia enterocolitica*, usually after ingestion of contaminated food, particularly undercooked pork. Patients with iron overload states, including hemochromatosis, are at increased risk for infection (including bacteremia) owing to the siderophilic characteristics of *Yersinia* species. The incubation period is approximately 5 days, and patients typically have fever, abdominal pain, diarrhea (possibly bloody), and (sometimes) nausea and emesis at presentation. The organism has tropism for lymphoid tissue (including tonsillar tissue and mesenteric lymph nodes), which results in pharyngitis or right lower-quadrant pain mimicking appendicitis. Postinfection complications include erythema nodosum and reactive arthritis. The diagnosis is confirmed by molecular testing of stool or by culture of stool, blood, a throat swab, or infected tissue; the testing laboratory should be alerted when *Yersinia enterocolitica* infection is suspected so that optimal media and enrichment conditions are applied. When treatment is indicated, trimethoprim-sulfamethoxazole (first choice) or a fluoroquinolone (such as ciprofloxacin) or a third-generation cephalosporin is recommended.

| TABLE 49. Diarrheagenic Strains of *Escherichia coli* | | |
|---|---|---|
| **Strain** | **Epidemiology** | **Clinical Findings** |
| Enteroaggregative *E. coli* (EAEC) | Diarrhea in travelers, young children, and patients with HIV infection | Watery diarrhea, fever typically absent |
| Enteroinvasive *E. coli* (EIEC) | All ages, primarily in developing countries | Inflammatory diarrhea (dysentery) with fever, abdominal pain |
| Enteropathogenic *E. coli* (EPEC) | Sporadic, occasionally persistent diarrhea in young children | Nausea, vomiting, malnutrition (when chronic) |
| Enterotoxigenic *E. coli* (ETEC) | Diarrhea in travelers, foodborne outbreaks | Watery diarrhea, fever typically absent or low grade |
| Shiga toxin-producing *E. coli* (STEC) | Foodborne outbreaks (associated with beef and other contaminated food), person-to-person, and zoonotic transmission | Bloody stools, progression to hemolytic uremic syndrome, fever typically absent |

- Most diarrheal illness due to *Yersinia* species is caused by *Yersinia enterocolitica*, usually after ingestion of contaminated food, particularly undercooked pork; the diagnosis is confirmed by molecular testing of stool or by culture of stool, blood, a throat swab, or infected tissue.

- When treatment is indicated, trimethoprim-sulfamethoxazole (first choice) or either a fluoroquinolone (such as ciprofloxacin) or a third-generation cephalosporin is recommended.

# *Vibrio* Infection

In the United States, *Vibrio parahaemolyticus* is the most common *Vibrio* species to cause gastrointestinal illness, usually after consumption of contaminated or undercooked oysters and other shellfish. The incubation period is approximately 1 day; infected patients typically report diarrhea (not commonly bloody), fever, nausea or emesis, and crampy abdominal pain at presentation. *V. parahaemolyticus* can cause septicemia in patients who have liver disease, which may lead to secondary necrotizing skin infections. Severe noninvasive gastrointestinal illness can be treated with doxycycline, although fluoroquinolones and macrolides also can be used. Patients with septicemia require more aggressive combination therapy, typically with doxycycline plus ceftriaxone.

- *Vibrio parahaemolyticus* can cause septicemia and necrotizing skin infections in patients who have liver disease.

- Severe noninvasive *Vibrio parahaemolyticus* gastrointestinal illness is treated with doxycycline, although fluoroquinolones and macrolides also can be used.

# H *Clostridium difficile* Infection

*Clostridium difficile* is the leading cause of hospital-acquired infectious diarrhea and results from fecal-oral transmission. The number of these infections reported in the United States has increased significantly since the year 2000, owing in large part to the emergence of a hypervirulent strain. Risk factors for infection include exposure to antibiotic and chemotherapeutic agents, older age, presence of inflammatory bowel disease, gastrointestinal surgery, and (possibly) gastric acid suppression with proton pump inhibitors. Antibiotic stewardship is paramount in reducing incidence of infection, and hand washing with soap and water is the gold standard for infection control; alcohol-based gels do not eliminate spores.

Asymptomatic colonization can occur; for those with pathologic infection, the incubation period can be as long as 6 weeks after perturbation of the intestinal flora with antibiotic agents. Community-acquired infections without previous exposure to health care settings, antibiotic agents, or both have been increasingly reported.

*Clostridium difficile* produces both an enterotoxin (toxin A) and a cytotoxin (toxin B) that are pathogenic. Symptomatic patients typically have watery diarrhea (rarely bloody), crampy abdominal pain, malaise, and sometimes nausea and fever. Abnormal laboratory study findings are nonspecific but can include leukocytosis, an elevated creatinine level, and hypoalbuminemia. Radiographic imaging, also nonspecific, may demonstrate colonic wall thickening, mucosal edema, fat stranding, and megacolon. Colonoscopy, although not a routine diagnostic modality, may visualize pseudomembranes associated with infection.

Diagnosis is usually established by testing unformed stools from persons not taking laxatives who have unexplained new-onset diarrhea occurring three or more times daily. Although highly specific and rapid, enzyme immunoassay (EIA) testing for presence of toxin A or B lacks sensitivity. EIA testing for presence of glutamate dehydrogenase, an antigenic protein present in all *C. difficile* isolates, is quite sensitive but lacks specificity. Nucleic acid amplification testing (NAAT) for *C. difficile* toxin genes is rapid, highly sensitive, and specific. If NAAT is not used as a stand-alone technique, then combining EIA tests for glutamate dehydrogenase plus toxin (discordant results require polymerase chain reaction testing for resolution) or NAAT plus toxin can be performed.

In all infected patients, the antibiotic agent associated with the infection should be stopped if possible. Treatment is otherwise dictated by severity of disease (**Table 50**). Severe disease is supported clinically by a leukocyte count of 15,000/μL ($15 \times 10^9$/L) or greater or a serum creatinine level greater than 1.5 mg/dL (133 μmol/L). Oral vancomycin or fidaxomicin for 10 days is recommended. Fulminant disease is defined as severe *C. difficile* infection with associated shock, ileus, toxic megacolon, ICU admission, elevated serum lactate level, hypotension, altered mental status, or organ failure. Higher-dose oral or nasogastric vancomycin, intravenous metronidazole, and (possibly) vancomycin enema (when ileus is present) are recommended. Patients with

| TABLE 50. | Treatment of *Clostridium difficile* Infection[a] |
|---|---|
| **Severity of Disease** | **Treatment** |
| Nonsevere | Vancomycin, 125 mg four times daily PO × 10 d *or* |
| | Fidaxomicin, 200 mg twice daily PO × 10 d |
| | If neither of these agents is available, metronidazole, 500 mg three times daily PO × 10 d |
| Severe | Vancomycin, 125 mg four times daily PO × 10 d *or* |
| | Fidaxomicin, 200 mg twice daily PO × 10 d |
| Fulminant | Vancomycin, 500 mg four times daily PO *or* |
| | NGT plus metronidazole, 500 mg every 8 h IV |
| | When ileus is present, consideration of vancomycin PR |

IV = intravenously; NGT = by nasogastric tube; PO = by mouth; PR = per rectum.

[a]Initial presentation.

CONT.

fulminant disease warrant surgical evaluation. For nonsevere disease, defined as *C. difficile* infection that is neither severe nor fulminant, oral vancomycin or fidaxomicin for 10 days is recommended. If neither of these agents is available, oral metronidazole for 10 days can be used.

Recurrent infection is reported in as many as 25% of patients, and treatment recommendations are found in **Table 51**. Studies have shown that fecal microbiota transplantation is effective in the management of patients with multiple recurrences. Retesting stool for *C. difficile* after treatment for evidence of cure in patients who have no symptoms is not recommended. [H]

### KEY POINTS

**HVC**

- *Clostridium difficile* is the leading cause of hospital-acquired infectious diarrhea; antibiotic stewardship is paramount in reducing incidence of infection, and hand washing with soap and water is important to eliminate spores.

- Testing unformed stools usually establishes the diagnosis; nucleic acid amplification testing for *Clostridium difficile* toxin genes is rapid, highly sensitive, and specific; enzyme immunoassay testing for presence of toxin A or B is highly specific and rapid but lacks sensitivity, and enzyme immunoassay testing for presence of glutamate dehydrogenase is quite sensitive but lacks specificity.

- Treatment of an initial *Clostridium difficile* infection is dictated by severity of disease, with nonsevere disease treated with oral vancomycin or fidaxomicin (or with oral metronidazole if neither of these drugs is available), severe disease treated with oral vancomycin or fidaxomicin, and fulminant disease treated with higher-dose oral vancomycin, intravenous metronidazole, and (when ileus is present) vancomycin enema.

| TABLE 51. | Treatment of Recurrent *Clostridium difficile* Infection |
|---|---|
| First recurrence | Vancomycin, 125 mg four times daily PO × 10 d, if metronidazole used for initial episode *or* |
| | Prolonged tapered and pulsed vancomycin if standard regimen was used for initial episode (that is, vancomycin, 125 mg four times daily PO × 10 d, then 125 mg twice daily PO × 7 d, then 125 mg every 2 or 3 d PO for 2-8 wk) *or* |
| | Fidaxomicin, 200 mg twice daily PO × 10 d, if vancomycin was used for the initial episode |
| Second or subsequent recurrence | Prolonged tapered and pulsed vancomycin PO (see above) *or* |
| | Vancomycin, 125 mg four times daily PO × 10 d, followed by rifaximin, 400 mg three times daily PO × 20 d *or* |
| | Fidaxomicin, 200 mg twice daily PO × 10 d *or* |
| | Fecal microbiota transplantation (after two recurrences treated with appropriate antibiotics) |

PO = by mouth.

## Viral Gastroenteritis

Viruses are responsible for acute gastroenteritis in most patients. Rotavirus infects young children, and noroviruses, which are estimated to cause more than 50% of foodborne gastroenteritis in the United States, affect all ages. Norovirus outbreaks on cruise ships and in schools and other institution-alized settings are well documented. Transmission from person to person is primarily fecal-oral. Highly contagious infection can develop after ingestion of fewer than 100 viral particles. The incubation period is typically less than 2 days, and infected patients typically have watery diarrhea, nausea, vomiting, and fever at presentation. Infection is usually self-limited and requires supportive care because of the lack of effective antiviral agents. Diagnostic molecular testing is available. Viral shedding persists for as long as 2 weeks after symptom resolution, which contributes to its high infectivity.

### KEY POINT

- Noroviruses cause more than 50% of foodborne gastro-enteritis in the United States; the incubation period is typically less than 2 days; viral shedding persists as long as 2 weeks after symptom resolution, which contributes to high infectivity.

## Parasitic Infection

Parasitic infection should be considered in patients with persistent or chronic diarrhea. Immunosuppressed persons are at increased risk for more chronic and severe infection.

### *Giardia lamblia* Infection

*Giardia lamblia* is the most common parasitic pathogen in the United States. Cysts from infected animals are excreted in stool into reservoirs of natural fresh water, and subsequent ingestion of contaminated water (or food) can lead to human infection. Secondary spread from person to person via fecal-oral transmission is also possible because cysts may be excreted for many months. Persons at risk for infection include international outdoor travelers, children in day-care centers, immunocompromised hosts (particularly those with humoral immunodeficiency), and persons engaged in sexual activity that includes oral-anal contact. The incubation period ranges from 1 to 3 weeks. More than half of infected patients are asymptomatic. Symptomatic patients typically report watery diarrhea that is fatty and foul smelling, flatulence, bloating, nausea, and crampy abdominal pain; fever is uncommon. Symptoms can last for several weeks until spontaneously resolving; chronic infection may develop, particularly in persons with hypogammaglobulinemia. EIA and molecular testing of stool is more sensitive than stool microscopy for confirming the diagnosis. Treatment is recommended for symptomatic patients; metronidazole, tinidazole, or nitazoxanide can be used. Postinfection lactose intolerance is common and may be mistaken for recurrent or resistant *Giardia* infection.

- More than half of patients infected with *Giardia lamblia* are asymptomatic; treatment with metronidazole, tinidazole, or nitazoxanide can be used.
- Postinfection lactose intolerance is common and may be mistaken for recurrent or resistant *Giardia* infection.

## *Cryptosporidium* Infection

*Cryptosporidium* species can infect humans and other mammals. Infection occurs through consumption of fecally contaminated water or food or through close person-to-person or animal-to-person transmission. Municipal water supplies and swimming pools can be a source of infection because the thick-walled oocysts are chlorine resistant and can evade filtration. This parasite is highly infectious; ingestion of fewer than 50 oocysts may result in infection. The incubation period is 7 days. Although some infected patients will be asymptomatic, symptomatic patients typically report watery diarrhea, crampy abdominal pain, nausea, vomiting, malaise, fever, dehydration, and weight loss. Symptoms usually last less than 2 weeks before spontaneously resolving in immunocompetent hosts. Immunocompromised patients, in particular patients with AIDS, can develop serious and prolonged infection. Diagnosis can be established microscopically by visualization of oocysts with modified acid-fast staining, molecular testing, and enzyme or direct fluorescent immunoassay testing. Treatment for immunocompetent patients usually consists of supportive care. When antimicrobial agents are considered for severe or prolonged infection, nitazoxanide is recommended. In HIV-infected patients, antiretroviral therapy is most effective in resolving infection. Nitazoxanide also can be considered when supportive care does not result in symptom resolution.

- The diagnosis of *Cryptosporidium* infection can be established microscopically by visualization of oocysts using modified acid-fast staining, polymerase chain reaction testing, and enzyme immunoassay or direct fluorescent antibody testing.
- Treatment of *Cryptosporidium* infection consists of supportive care for most immunocompetent hosts; nitazoxanide is recommended for severe or prolonged infection or if supportive care does not resolve symptoms; antiretroviral therapy is most effective in resolving infection in HIV-infected patients.

## Amebiasis

*Entamoeba histolytica* is the parasitic organism responsible for amebiasis. In the United States, most infections are diagnosed in travelers returning from visits to unsanitary tropical or developing countries, immigrants from these areas, persons in institutionalized settings, or those who practice oral-anal sex. Amebiasis is highly infectious, with ingestion of only a small number of infective cysts in contaminated water or food needed for infection. The incubation period is 2 to 4 weeks. Most infections are asymptomatic, but some patients develop diarrhea with visible blood, mucus, or both and associated abdominal pain, fever, and weight loss. Colonic perforation, peritonitis, and death may complicate more fulminant infections. Risk factors for severe infection in adults include immunodeficiency. Diagnosis can be established microscopically by visualization of cysts or trophozoites, immunoassay testing, molecular testing, and serologic antibody testing, although the latter technique does not distinguish current from remote infection. Treatment is recommended for all infected patients. In symptomatic patients, treatment with metronidazole or tinidazole is recommended initially for parasitic clearance followed by an intraluminal amebicide, such as paromomycin or diloxanide, for cyst clearance. In asymptomatic infections, an intraluminal agent for eradication of cysts is recommended.

- Treatment is recommended for all patients with amebiasis; for symptomatic patients, treatment with metronidazole or tinidazole is recommended initially for parasitic clearance followed by an intraluminal amebicide for cyst clearance, and for asymptomatic patients, an intraluminal agent for eradication of cysts is recommended.

## *Cyclospora* Infection

*Cyclospora* infections are typically acquired after consumption of food or water that is fecally contaminated with *Cyclospora* oocysts. In the United States, most of these infections have been traced to imported fresh produce from tropical areas or have occurred in persons who have traveled to areas of endemicity. The incubation period is approximately 1 week. Infected patients typically report watery diarrhea, decreased appetite, weight loss, crampy abdominal pain, bloating, flatulence, nausea, fatigue, and (sometimes) fever. Symptoms can last for several weeks and may be more pronounced in HIV-infected patients. Diagnosis is typically established microscopically by visualization of oocysts with modified acid-fast staining, microscopy with ultraviolet fluorescence, or molecular testing. Trimethoprim-sulfamethoxazole is recommended for treatment of symptomatic infection.

- *Cyclospora* infection is typically diagnosed microscopically by visualization of oocysts with modified acid-fast staining, microscopy with ultraviolet fluorescence, or molecular testing; trimethoprim-sulfamethoxazole is recommended for treatment of symptomatic infection.

# Infections in Transplant Recipients

## Introduction

Despite improvements in immunosuppression and antimicrobial therapy, infection remains a significant cause of morbidity and mortality after solid organ transplantation (SOT) and hematopoietic stem cell transplantation (HSCT). Infection is the most common cause of death in the first year after SOT. Additionally, the interaction of the immune system and infection goes both ways; although immune suppression to prevent rejection increases risk of infection, infection also raises the risk of rejection.

The occurrence of SOT and HSCT procedures continues to increase, as do long-term survival rates owing to improved management of rejection and decreased complications. With more patients living longer after transplantation, awareness of principles involved in the recognition and prevention of infection in transplant recipients remains important for physicians who are not transplant specialists.

## Antirejection Drugs in Transplant Recipients

Success after transplantation depends on modulating the immune system to prevent organ rejection in SOT and to minimize graft-versus-host disease (GVHD) in allogeneic HSCT. Antirejection regimens involve multiple agents (**Table 52**) with

**TABLE 52.** Immunosuppressive Agents Used in Transplantation

| Class | Agents |
|---|---|
| Glucocorticoids | Prednisone, others |
| Cytotoxic agents (DNA synthesis inhibitors, antimetabolites) | Mycophenolate mofetil |
| | Mycophenolate sodium |
| | Azathioprine |
| | Methotrexate |
| | Cyclophosphamide |
| Calcineurin pathway inhibitors | Cyclosporine |
| | Tacrolimus |
| mTOR inhibitors | Sirolimus (rapamycin) |
| | Everolimus |
| Lymphocyte-depleting antibodies | |
| Polyclonal | Antithymocyte globulins |
| Monoclonal | Muromonab (anti-CD3) |
| | Basiliximab (anti-IL-2 receptor) |
| | Daclizumab (anti-IL-2 receptor) |
| | Rituximab (anti-CD20) |
| | Alemtuzumab (anti-CD52) |

IL-2 = interleukin-2; mTOR = mammalian target of rapamycin.

different mechanisms of action, which are chosen to minimize overlapping toxicities. After SOT, an induction and maintenance strategy is applied; immunosuppression is most intensive in the early period after transplantation and often includes lymphocyte depletion therapy. Immunosuppression may require intensification later for episodes of rejection, and this may again increase the risk of infection.

Glucocorticoids have historically been the cornerstone of antirejection therapy, but steroid-sparing or minimizing regimens are increasingly being used to avoid the toxicities of long-term therapy. Tacrolimus, cyclosporine, or sirolimus are the cornerstones, usually with mycophenolate or, less commonly, azathioprine. Drug interactions are common with these agents, and many drugs can affect antirejection medication levels. Monitoring is important to balance adequate immunosuppression with toxicity.

**KEY POINT**

- Glucocorticoid-sparing or minimizing regimens (with tacrolimus, cyclosporine, or sirolimus) are increasingly used to avoid the toxicities of long-term steroid therapy.

## Posttransplantation Infections

### Timeline and Type of Transplant

Infection may occur at any time after transplantation, but periods of highest immunosuppression, usually within the first few months after transplantation, carry the highest likelihood. Risk for infection is also affected by pre-existing conditions (such as diabetes mellitus, cirrhosis, or neutropenia) and by colonization with resistant organisms (such as *Burkholderia* in cystic fibrosis).

The risk of specific infections varies depending on the time frame after transplantation. **Table 53** shows the typical timeline of risk for specific infections after SOT. However, the timeline restarts when treating episodes of rejection, and infection risk in the late period depends on the level of immunosuppression required. Knowledge of the risk timeline and effect of the immunosuppression level can be helpful in recognizing likely infections and in preventing infections through targeted prophylaxis. In the first month after SOT, infections are similar to those seen in other hospitalized postsurgical patients, including a risk of resistant bacteria, and most often involve the lungs, urinary tract, and surgical sites. The middle period usually encompasses the most intensive immunosuppression, with significant risk for viral (such as cytomegalovirus) and fungal (such as *Pneumocystis*) infections owing to defects in cell-mediated immunity. If immunosuppression can be de-escalated during the late period, risk for opportunistic infections decreases overall, but patients remain at risk for certain viral infections and have increased risk for community-acquired bacterial infections.

Additional general considerations include the higher likelihood of infections to disseminate after transplantation and the subtle or atypical presentation of infection because of

**TABLE 53.** Timeline of Common Infections after Solid Organ Transplantation

| Early Period (<1 Month after Transplantation) | Middle Period (1-6 Months after Transplantation) | Late Period (>6 Months after Transplantation)[a] |
|---|---|---|
| *Staphylococcus aureus* infection (including methicillin-resistant) | Cytomegalovirus infection | Epstein-Barr virus (including PTLD) infection |
| Nosocomial gram-negative bacterial infection | Epstein-Barr virus (including PTLD) infection | Varicella-zoster virus infection |
| *Clostridium difficile* colitis | Herpes simplex virus infection | Community-acquired pneumonia |
| *Candida* infection | Varicella-zoster virus infection | Urinary tract infections |
| *Aspergillus* infection | Polyoma BK virus infection | Polyoma BK virus infection |
| Surgical site infections | *Pneumocystis jirovecii* infection | Cytomegalovirus infection |
| Nosocomial pneumonia | *Toxoplasma, Trypanosoma, Strongyloides* | |
| Catheter-related bacteremia | *Listeria* infection | |
| Urinary tract infections | *Nocardia* infection | |
| | Tuberculosis reactivation | |
| | Fungal infections, including *Cryptococcus* | |

PTLD = posttransplant lymphoproliferative disorder.

[a]For opportunistic infections in the late period, risk depends on level of immunosuppression. Infections such as *Pneumocystis* and other fungi, *Listeria*, and *Nocardia* can be seen in the late period in patients with higher immunosuppression.

changed anatomy after transplantation. Immunosuppressive drugs may also contribute to altered presentation because of reduction in fever and other inflammatory responses making the usual signs and symptoms of infection less prominent. Noninfectious complications such as GVHD or malignancy may also be confused with infection. For some infections, the risk strongly depends on donor and recipient characteristics. Standard donor and recipient pretransplantation testing includes serologies for cytomegalovirus; Epstein-Barr virus; varicella-zoster virus; HIV; hepatitis B, C, and E viruses; syphilis; toxoplasmosis; and *Strongyloides, Leishmania,* and *Trypanosoma* if from an endemic area and interferon-γ release assay for latent tuberculosis infection.

Risk after HSCT is much greater for allogeneic than autologous transplantation because of the myeloablative conditioning regimen. After allogeneic HSCT, patients undergo a prolonged period of intense neutropenia, putting them at risk for bacterial infections, *Candida* and mold infections, and herpes simplex and other virus reactivation. This is followed by a prolonged period of impaired cell-mediated and humoral immunity because of immunosuppression to reduce GVHD.

Development of chronic GVHD can also increase risk for infections caused by immune system effects and breakdowns in mucosal and other barriers. Infections in this later period are similar to those in the later period after SOT. **Figure 21** shows the timeline of risk for specific infection after allogeneic HSCT.

**KEY POINTS**

- Infection may occur at any time after transplantation but is most likely at periods of highest immunosuppression; the risk for specific organisms varies depending on the time frame after transplantation.
- Infection risk is much greater after allogeneic than autologous hematopoietic stem cell transplantation because of myeloablative conditioning with a prolonged period of neutropenia and immunosuppression given to reduce graft-versus-host disease.

## Specific Posttransplantation Infections
### Viral Infections

Cytomegalovirus is the most significant viral infection after transplantation, with risk for infection depending on donor and recipient serology. After SOT, the risk for cytomegalovirus is highest (>50%) for donor-positive/recipient-negative, intermediate (15%-20%) for recipient-positive, and lowest for donor-negative/recipient-negative transplantations. Risk is also significantly increased with use of lymphocyte-depleting agents. Comparatively, after allogeneic HSCT, the risk of cytomegalovirus is highest for donor-negative/recipient-positive transplantations. Cytomegalovirus is an immunomodulatory virus, and active cytomegalovirus infection after transplantation is associated with increased rates of rejection and GVHD, as well as increases in other opportunistic infections and posttransplant lymphoproliferative disorder (PTLD). Cytomegalovirus often presents as a nonspecific viral syndrome with fever and cytopenias. Specific organ disease owing to cytomegalovirus includes pneumonitis (more common in HSCT than SOT), encephalitis, hepatitis, and other gastrointestinal sites. Although cytomegalovirus can cause disease anywhere in the gastrointestinal tract, colitis is the most common gastrointestinal disease after SOT, whereas esophagitis is more common after HSCT. Definitive diagnosis of organ disease depends on demonstration of cytomegalovirus in biopsy, although presumptive diagnosis can be made based on cytomegalovirus viremia, demonstrated by quantitative nucleic acid amplification testing, in the appropriate clinical setting.

Epstein-Barr virus is most significant for its relationship to PTLD resulting from B-cell proliferation; PTLD should be suspected in any patient in the middle or late period presenting with lymphadenopathy or an extranodal mass, often with fever. Treatment of PTLD involves rituximab and decreasing immunosuppression. Reactivation of herpes simplex virus is especially common after HSCT and can be reduced with acyclovir prophylaxis (if the patient is not already receiving an agent for cytomegalovirus). Patients with chronic hepatitis B

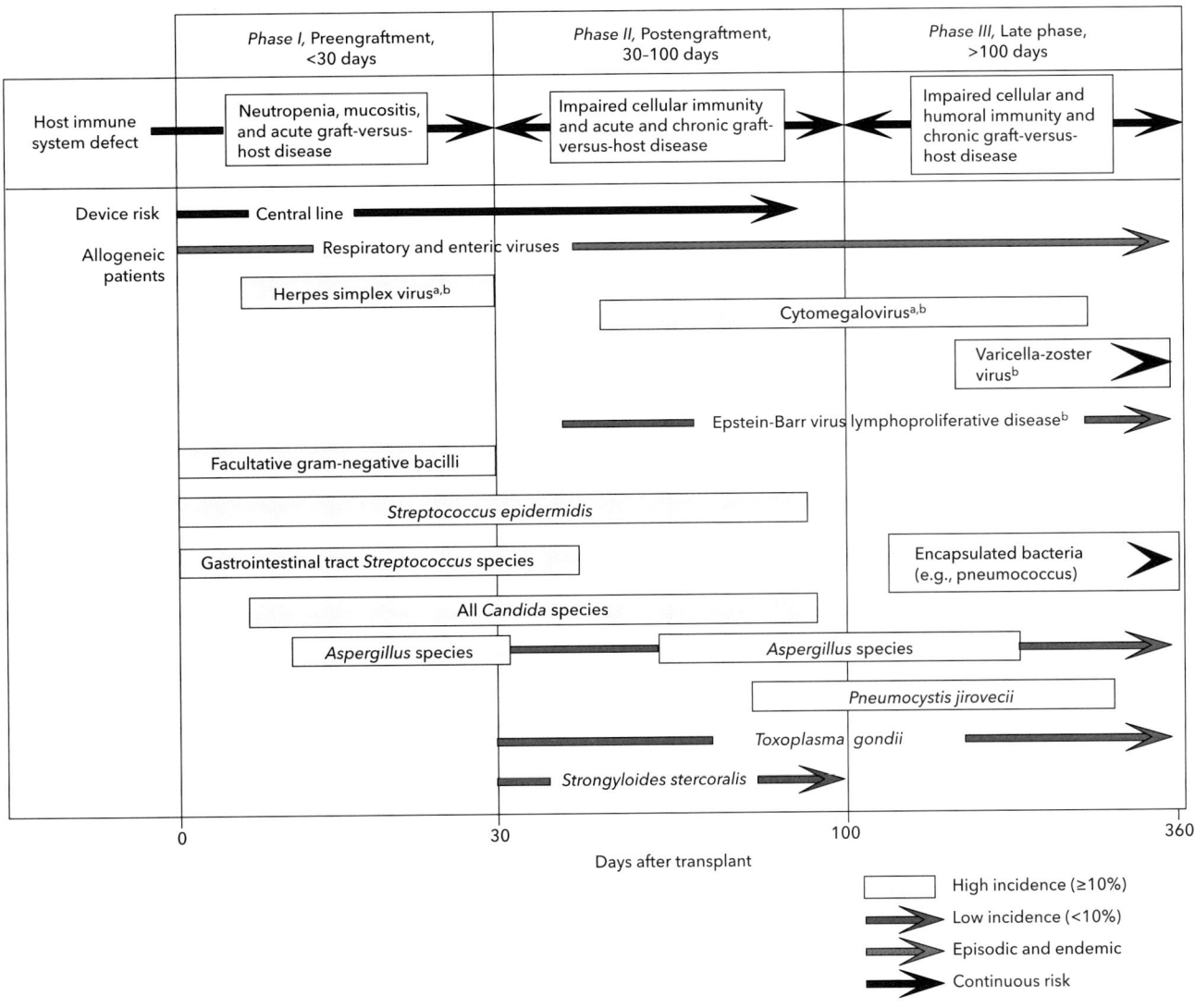

**FIGURE 21.** Phases of opportunistic infections in allogeneic hematopoietic stem cell transplant recipients.

[a]Without standard prophylaxis.

[b]Primarily among persons who are seropositive before transplantation.

Reprinted with permission from CDC, Infectious Diseases Society of America, and the American Society of Blood and Marrow Transplantation. Guidelines for preventing opportunistic infections among hematopoietic stem cell transplant recipients. Recommendations of CDC, the Infectious Diseases Society of America, and the American Society of Blood and Marrow Transplantation. Cytotherapy. 2001;3(1):41-54. PMID: 12028843

can have flares of disease if not taking suppressive therapy. Polyoma BK virus can cause a nephropathy in the middle or late period after transplantation.

## Bacterial Infections

Bacterial infections are common in the early period after SOT and during neutropenia after HSCT. These are often typical nosocomial infections, including resistant organisms such as methicillin-resistant staphylococci, vancomycin-resistant enterococci, and multidrug-resistant gram-negative organisms. *Clostridium difficile* colitis is common, especially with the extensive antibiotic use that accompanies transplantation. *Mycobacterium tuberculosis* can reactivate with the immunosuppression of transplantation and may present with an

atypical pattern on chest radiography or with extrapulmonary disease. Related to persistently low antibody levels, encapsulated organisms such as *Streptococcus pneumoniae* remain common even late after HSCT. ▣

## Fungal Infections

Fungal infections are most common in the middle period after SOT but may also occur late, especially in the setting of rejection or cytomegalovirus infection. The most common fungal infection without prophylaxis is *Pneumocystis* pneumonia, which is typically a more aggressive pneumonia in patients after transplantation than in those with AIDS. Cryptococcosis usually presents as subacute meningitis with fever, headache, mental status changes, and lymphocytic pleocytosis in cerebrospinal fluid, although skin and other organ involvement may also occur; cryptococcal antigen testing is key to diagnosis. Histoplasmosis may also occur in geographically endemic areas and is more likely to present with disseminated disease after transplantation. Mucocutaneous candidiasis is common after SOT and HSCT. Invasive *Candida* infections and candidemia can be seen, especially in the neutropenic phase after HSCT, as can aspergillosis and other invasive molds, such as *Mucor*. The risk for invasive fungal infection after HSCT is also increased in later periods by the use of immunosuppressive agents for GVHD. In SOT, pulmonary aspergillosis is most common after lung transplantation.

### Protozoa and Helminths

*Toxoplasma gondii* is a protozoan that can reactivate with immunosuppression after transplantation, usually causing encephalitis with fever, headache, and focal neurologic deficits and with multiple ring-enhancing brain lesions on imaging. *Strongyloides* can cause a hyperinfection syndrome with significant immunosuppression (especially glucocorticoid use), often with secondary pneumonia and gram-negative bacteremia. Reactivation of *Trypanosoma* or *Leishmania* can also occur after transplantation, if the recipient or donor were from an endemic area.

**KEY POINTS**

- Cytomegalovirus is the most significant viral infection after transplantation and may present as a nonspecific viral syndrome with fever and cytopenias or with specific organ disease, including pneumonitis, encephalitis, esophagitis, and colitis.

- *Clostridium difficile* colitis is common after transplantation, complicating the extensive antibiotic use that accompanies transplantation.

- *Mycobacterium tuberculosis* can reactivate with the immunosuppression of transplantation and may present with an atypical pattern on chest radiography or with extrapulmonary disease.

- *Pneumocystis* pneumonia is the most common fungal infection without prophylaxis; it is typically a more aggressive pneumonia in patients after transplantation than in those with AIDS.

## Prevention of Infections in Transplant Recipients

Prevention is preferred over treatment strategies for most common infections after transplantation because most opportunistic infections have devastating effects and the cost and toxicity of prophylaxis and immunization are relatively low. Recommended immunizations for SOT and HSCT are shown in **Table 54**. Most immunizations are safe in patients after transplantation except for live virus vaccines, which should be avoided after transplantation.

Trimethoprim-sulfamethoxazole is one of the most important prophylactic medications after transplantation. Used to prevent *Pneumocystis*, it may also reduce toxoplasmosis and certain bacteria, including *Listeria* and agents causing urinary tract infections. Trimethoprim-sulfamethoxazole is usually given up to 1 year after transplantation and often longer if immunosuppression cannot be adequately reduced.

Antifungal prophylaxis is indicated during the early months after HSCT and may need to be extended in the setting of GVHD. Coverage should include *Candida* and *Aspergillus*, typically with posaconazole or voriconazole.

Strategies to reduce the effects of cytomegalovirus remain important and include primary prophylaxis, usually with valganciclovir, or regular monitoring for active cytomegalovirus replication by quantitative nucleic acid amplification testing and institution of pre-emptive therapy based on results. Monitoring and pre-emptive therapy is more often used after HSCT, partially because of increased concerns for neutropenia as an adverse effect of prophylaxis and because prophylaxis was not found to be superior to pre-emptive therapy in a randomized controlled trial. The potential role of letermovir, a new antiviral agent without the hematologic toxicity of ganciclovir, is being studied for cytomegalovirus prophylaxis. For SOT, prophylaxis with valganciclovir is preferred for patients at high risk (donor-positive/recipient-negative, those receiving lymphocyte-depleting agents, lung transplants) and is usually given for at least 3 to 6 months.

**KEY POINTS**

- Prophylaxis and immunization are preferred over treating active infections after transplantation; live virus vaccines should not be given after transplantation. **HVC**

- Monitoring by quantitative nucleic acid amplification testing for active cytomegalovirus replication and institution of pre-emptive therapy based on results is preferred to ganciclovir primary prophylaxis of cytomegalovirus infection after hematopoietic stem cell transplantation.

# Health Care-Associated Infections

## Epidemiology

Health care–associated infections (HCAI) have been linked to indwelling medical devices, prosthetic devices and materials, surgery, invasive procedures, transmission of organisms between patients and health care personnel, and environmental factors. Four percent of hospitalized patients acquire at least one HCAI, costing the U.S. health care system an estimated $28 billion to $45 billion annually. HCAIs include pneumonia and surgical site infections (21.8% each), gastrointestinal infections (17.1%), urinary tract infections (12.9%; 67.7%

**TABLE 54.** Immunization Recommendations for Adult Recipients of Transplants[a]

| Immunization | Recommendations for Solid Organ Transplantation | Recommendations for Hematopoietic Stem Cell Transplantation[b] |
|---|---|---|
| Pneumococcal | Before transplantation: PCV13 followed 8 weeks later by PPSV23 | 3-6 months after transplantation: 3-4 doses of PCV13 |
| | After transplantation: PCV13 (if not administered pretransplantation) 2-6 months after transplantation; 1 dose PPSV23 at least 8 weeks after PCV13 and 5 years after any previous PPSV23 | 12 months after transplantation: 1 dose of PPSV23 |
| Influenza (inactivated only) | Annually | Annually |
| Tdap | Before transplantation: complete series, including Tdap booster | 6 months after transplantation: 3 doses Tdap |
| MMR | Contraindicated after transplantation | 24 months after transplantation: 1-2 doses, only if no GVHD or immune suppression |
| Inactivated polio | Before transplantation: complete series | 6-12 months after transplantation: 3 doses |
| *Haemophilus influenzae* type B | No recommendation | 6-12 months after transplantation: 3 doses |
| Meningococcal | Per recommendations for nontransplant patients | 6 months after transplantation: both quadrivalent conjugate vaccine and serogroup B vaccine |
| Hepatitis B | Before transplantation: complete series if not already immune | 6-12 months after transplantation: 3 doses if indications for nontransplant patients are met |
| Hepatitis A | Before transplantation: complete series if not already immune | Per recommendations for nontransplant patients |
| Varicella-zoster virus | | |
|     Live attenuated vaccine | >4 weeks before transplantation: varicella if not immune | >4 weeks before transplantation: varicella if not immune |
| | >4 weeks before transplantation: zoster if same indications as nontransplant patients are met | 24 months after transplantation: 2 doses varicella if seronegative and only if no GVHD or immunosuppression |
| | Both contraindicated after transplantation | |
|     Recombinant adjuvanted zoster vaccine | Theoretically safe, but data in severely immunocompromised patients not yet available; no recommendations after transplantation | Theoretically safe, but data in severely immunocompromised patients not yet available; no recommendations after transplantation |
| | Should be given before transplantation if possible | Should be given before transplantation if possible |
| Human papillomavirus | Before transplantation: per recommendations for nontransplant patients | Per recommendations for nontransplant patients |

GVHD = graft-versus-host disease; MMR = measles, mumps, and rubella vaccine; PCV13 = 13-valent pneumococcal conjugate vaccine; PPSV23 = 23-valent pneumococcal polysaccharide vaccine; Tdap = tetanus, diphtheria, and acellular pertussis vaccine.

[a]See MKSAP 18 General Internal Medicine for more information on vaccination recommendations and schedules.

[b]For multiple-dose immunizations, the time period between doses is generally 1-2 months.

CONT.

associated with catheters), and primary bloodstream infection (9.9%; 84% associated with central venous catheters).

Elimination of HCAIs remains important for the U.S. health care system. Sixty-five percent to 70% of catheter-associated bloodstream and urinary tract infections and 55% of ventilator-associated pneumonias and surgical site infections are preventable. Progress toward elimination varies by type of infection. Central line–associated bloodstream infections decreased by 50% and surgical site infections by 17% between 2008 and 2014; rates of catheter-associated urinary tract infections showed little change between 2009 and 2014.

**KEY POINT**

- Approximately 65% to 70% of catheter-associated bloodstream and urinary tract infections and 55% of ventilator-associated pneumonias and surgical site infections are preventable.

## Prevention

Hand hygiene is the foundation of infection prevention, but adherence has been reported as less than 50%. Most facilities have improved in the last decade, with some facilities showing

**CONT.** sustained improvement to 90% adherence. Hand hygiene should be performed at least before and after every patient contact. The World Health Organization's five key hand hygiene moments are commonly used to define hand hygiene opportunities: before touching a patient, before clean or aseptic procedures, after body fluid exposure risk, after touching a patient, and after touching patient surroundings. Hand hygiene should include all surfaces of the hands up to the wrists, between fingers, and the fingertips. Alcohol-based hand rubs are generally preferred to soap and water hand disinfection, except when hands are visibly soiled, when personnel come in direct contact with blood or body fluids, or after contact with a patient with *Clostridium difficile* infection or his or her environment.

Standard precautions should be practiced for every patient to protect health care personnel from exposure to bloodborne pathogens. Blood and all body fluids except sweat are potentially infectious, regardless of the patient's presumed or known infection status. Personal protective equipment (gloves, gown, mask, and eye protection) are barriers protecting health care personnel from exposure to blood and body fluids. Protective equipment should be removed in the following order: 1) gloves, careful not to contaminate hands; 2) goggles/face shields; 3) gown, pull away from neck and shoulders, turn inside out to discard; 4) mask/respirator by grasping bottom then top ties/elastic. This process should be followed by hand hygiene. Transmission-based precautions (airborne, contact, droplet) are performed in addition to standard precautions to prevent transmission of epidemiologically significant organisms (**Table 55**).

Additional preventive measures include careful and judicious device use, safe injection practices (one needle, one syringe, only one time), aseptic technique for invasive procedures and surgery, and a clean environment and patient equipment. HCAI prevention "bundles" comprise three to five evidence-based processes of care that, when performed together, consistently have a greater impact on decreasing HCAIs than individual components performed inconsistently. **H**

**KEY POINT**

- Hand hygiene is the foundation of infection prevention; the World Health Organization has identified five key hand hygiene moments (before touching a patient, before clean or aseptic procedure, after body fluid exposure risk, after touching a patient, and after touching patient surroundings).

## Catheter-Associated Urinary Tract Infections

Catheter-associated urinary tract infections (CAUTIs) are the most common device-associated HCAI, and 17% to 69% may be preventable. Urinary catheters are used in 15% to 25% of hospitalized patients in the United States, compelling efforts to establish appropriateness criteria for catheter use. Adverse outcomes related to CAUTI include pyelonephritis, perinephric abscess, and bacteremia (<5%). *Escherichia coli* is the most common CAUTI pathogen, followed by *Pseudomonas aeruginosa*, *Klebsiella pneumoniae/Klebsiella oxytoca*, *Candida* species, and *Enterococcus* species; antibiotic resistance among these pathogens is increasing.

Duration of catheterization is the primary modifiable risk factor for CAUTI; each day of catheterization increases the risk of CAUTI. Nonadherence to aseptic technique (for example, opening a closed system) and insertion by a less experienced operator also increase the risk. Other risk factors for CAUTI include female sex, age older than 50 years, diabetes mellitus, severe or nonsurgical underlying illness, and serum creatinine level greater than 2.0 mg/dL (176.8 μmol/L). Appropriate indications for indwelling urinary catheters are listed in **Table 56**. Management of urinary incontinence using external catheters is preferred when feasible. Provision of care in the ICU is not itself an indication for a catheter.

### Diagnosis

Patients with an indwelling urethral or suprapubic catheter (or catheter removed in the 48 hours before symptom onset) or

| **Precaution Type** | **Indications** | **Precaution** | **Examples** |
|---|---|---|---|
| Airborne | Organisms transmitted from respiratory tract by small droplet nuclei (≤5 microns) that travel long distances on air currents | Airborne infection isolation room (negative-pressure room); HCP wear fit-tested N95 respirator | Chickenpox (plus contact precautions), tuberculosis, measles |
| Contact | Organisms transmitted by direct or indirect contact | Single room; gloves and gown for HCP entering room | Multidrug-resistant organisms (such as MRSA, VRE, ESBL-producing gram-negative organisms), *Clostridium difficile*, rotavirus |
| Droplet | Organisms transmitted from respiratory tract by large droplet nuclei (>5 microns) that travel less than 3 feet on air currents | Single room; HCP wear face or surgical mask when within 3 feet of patient | Influenza, *Bordetella pertussis*, *Neisseria meningitidis* for first 24 hours of therapy, mumps |

**TABLE 55.** Transmission-Based Precautions[a]

ESBL = extended-spectrum β-lactamase; HCP = health care personnel; MRSA = methicillin-resistant *Staphylococcus aureus*; VRE = vancomycin-resistant enterococci.

[a]Some organisms and infections require a combination of transmission-based precautions (adenovirus: contact and droplet; disseminated varicella-zoster virus: airborne and contact).

**TABLE 56.** Appropriate Indications for Use of Indwelling Urinary Catheters

| Indication |
| --- |
| Management of acute urinary retention without bladder outlet obstruction |
| Management of acute urinary retention with bladder outlet obstruction not related to infection or trauma |
| Management of chronic urinary retention with bladder outlet obstruction when ISC is not feasible |
| Management of stage III or IV or unstageable pressure ulcers that cannot be kept clear of urinary incontinence despite other urinary management strategies (e.g., barrier creams, absorbent pads, prompted toileting, non-indwelling catheters) |
| Hourly measurement of urine volume required to provide treatment |
| Daily measurement of urine volume required to provide treatment when it cannot be assessed by other volume (e.g., daily weighing, physical examination) and urine collection (e.g., urinal, bedside commode, bedpan, external catheter, ISC) strategies |
| Collection of a single 24-hour urine sample needed for diagnostic test that cannot be obtained by other urine collection strategies |
| Reduction in instances of acute, severe pain with movement when other urine management strategies are difficult |
| Improvement in comfort when urine collection by catheter addresses patient and family goals in a dying patient |
| Management of gross hematuria with blood clots in urine |
| Management of clinical condition for which ISC or external catheter is appropriate but placement is difficult or bladder emptying is inadequate for the patient with non-indwelling strategies |

ISC = intermittent straight catheterization.

CONT.

using intermittent catheterization who have signs and symptoms compatible with urinary tract infection (UTI; see Urinary Tract Infections for information), no other identifiable infection source, and ≥10³ colony-forming units/mL of one or more bacterial species in a urine specimen are diagnosed with a CAUTI. Catheter-associated asymptomatic bacteriuria (≥10³ colony-forming units/mL without urinary tract signs or symptoms) is common and generally does not require treatment. [H]

### KEY POINT

HVC
- Catheter-associated asymptomatic bacteriuria (≥10³ colony-forming units/mL without urinary tract signs or symptoms) is common and generally does not require treatment.

### Treatment

A urinalysis and urine culture should always be obtained before initiating antimicrobial treatment to determine if antimicrobial resistance is present and to guide definitive therapy. CAUTI management includes removing the urinary catheter (and only replacing if still needed). Removal is strongly recommended for catheters in place for 2 or more weeks because

biofilm on the catheter makes it difficult to eradicate bacteriuria or funguria and may lead to antimicrobial resistance. Therapy should always be adjusted to the narrowest coverage spectrum possible based on culture results. Treatment is given for 7 days if symptoms resolve promptly and longer (10-14 days) for patients with delayed response. Candiduria in a patient with a catheter almost always represents colonization and rarely requires treatment. *Candida* CAUTI is considered when significant candiduria persists despite catheter removal or replacement and the patient is symptomatic. CAUTIs caused by *Candida* species requiring treatment should be treated for 14 days. [H]

### KEY POINTS

- Catheter-associated urinary tract infection management includes catheter removal, with replacement only if still necessary. **HVC**
- Candiduria in a patient with a catheter almost always represents colonization and rarely requires treatment. **HVC**

### Prevention

Key prevention strategies include appropriately limiting urinary catheter use (see Table 56) and considering other options associated with lower infection risk (intermittent straight catheterization, external catheters) when urine collection is necessary (**Table 57**). Most studies have not shown definitive benefit of antimicrobial- or antiseptic-coated catheters for short- (<14 days) or long-term catheterization; these catheters are more expensive and, in some cases (such as nitrofurazone-coated catheters), cause more patient discomfort. [H]

### KEY POINT

- Antimicrobial- or antiseptic-coated catheters have not shown benefit for short-term or long-term catheterization, are more expensive, and, in some cases, cause more patient discomfort. **HVC**

## Surgical Site Infections

Surgical site infections (SSIs) account for 23% of HCAIs. The overall risk of developing an SSI after surgery is 1.9%. Wound class affects the risk of infection, with clean wounds having less than a 2% risk of infection, clean contaminated wounds having less than a 10% risk, and contaminated wounds having a 20% risk. Most infections occur within 30 days after surgery or within 90 days after surgery with implants; however, infections can manifest beyond these ranges. Risk factors include patient-related, procedure-related, and postoperative factors (**Table 58**). The patient's skin and gastrointestinal or female genital tracts are major sources of organisms causing infection, depending on the type of surgery. The time during which the surgical site is open represents the period of greatest risk. Common SSI pathogens are *Staphylococcus aureus* (23%), coagulase-negative staphylococci (17%), enterococci (7%), *Escherichia coli* (5%), and

**TABLE 57.** Prevention of Catheter-Associated Urinary Tract Infection

| Period | Preventive Measures |
|---|---|
| Before catheterization | Avoid catheterization whenever possible |
| | Insert catheter only for appropriate indications |
| | Consider alternatives, such as condom catheters and intermittent catheterization |
| At time of catheter insertion | Ensure that only properly trained persons insert and maintain catheters |
| | Adhere to hand hygiene practices and standard (or appropriate isolation) precautions according to CDC HICPAC/WHO guidelines |
| | Use proper aseptic techniques and sterile equipment when inserting the catheter (acute care setting) |
| After catheter insertion | Promote early catheter removal whenever possible |
| | Secure the catheter |
| | Use aseptic technique when handling the catheter, including for sample collection from the designated port (not collecting bag) |
| | Maintain a closed drainage system |
| | Avoid unnecessary system disconnections |
| | Maintain unobstructed urine flow |
| | Keep the collecting bag below the level of the bladder and off the floor |
| | Empty the collecting bag regularly, using a separate collecting container for each patient |

CDC = Centers for Disease Control and Prevention; HICPAC = Healthcare Infection Control Practices Advisory Committee; WHO = World Health Organization.

**TABLE 58.** Mitigation of Risk Factors for Surgical Site Infection

| Risk Factor | Intervention |
|---|---|
| Hyperglycemia | Maintain blood glucose level ≤180 mg/dL (10 mmol/L) during first 48 hours after surgery |
| Immunosuppression | Reduce doses of immunosuppressive agents |
| Tobacco use | Cease 30 days before surgery |
| Obesity | Weight loss |
| Malnutrition | Optimize nutritional status before surgery |
| S. aureus nasal carriage | For cardiovascular and orthopedic surgeries, test for nasal carriage 1-2 weeks before |
| | If positive, decolonize using intranasal 2% mupirocin ointment with or without chlorhexidine body wash |
| Skin preparation | Shower the night before (soap or an antiseptic) |
| | Use an alcohol-based chlorhexidine scrub at incision site |
| Hair removal | Do not shave site of incision |
| | If hair must be removed, it should be clipped as close to time of incision as possible |
| Hypothermia and hypovolemia | Maintain perioperative normothermia (temperature >36 °C [96.8 °F]) and adequate volume replacement to ensure maximum tissue oxygen delivery |
| | 2 °C (3.6 °F) decrease in body temperature associated with threefold increase in surgical site infection |
| Incision dressing | Primarily closed incision covered with sterile dressing for 24-48 hours |

*Pseudomonas aeruginosa* (5%). Exogenous sources of organisms (surgical personnel, surgical instruments, environment) are less common causes of SSIs, usually identified when a cluster of infections is present. ⊞

**KEY POINT**

- Most surgical site infections occur within 30 days after surgery or within 90 days after surgery with implants.

## Diagnosis

Clinical signs and symptoms vary by site and type of infection as well as by implicated organism (for example, some are more likely to cause purulence). Inflammatory changes at the surgical site (pain or tenderness, warmth, swelling, erythema) and purulent drainage suggest a superficial incisional infection. Deep incisional SSIs have more extensive tenderness expanding outside the area of erythema and more systemic signs, such as fever and leukocytosis. Wound dehiscence suggests a deep incisional SSI unless the wound or drainage is culture negative. Organ and deep-space SSIs are associated with more systemic signs and local symptoms related to a deep abscess or infected fluid collection. In cases of suspected organ or deep-space SSIs, CT is helpful to localize the infection and determine the best approach to drainage of the fluid or abscess for culture and treatment. When an SSI is suspected, drainage, purulent fluid, and infected tissue should be obtained for culture. Deep-tissue or wound cultures are preferable to superficial wound swab cultures that are likely to reflect skin or wound colonization and not necessarily yield the causative pathogen. ⊞

**KEY POINT**

- Deep tissue, drainage, and purulent fluid should be obtained for culture in surgical site infections; superficial wound swab cultures are likely to reflect skin or wound colonization rather than the causative pathogen.

## Treatment

SSI treatment requires debridement of necrotic tissue, drainage of abscesses or infected fluid, and specific antimicrobial therapy

CONT.

for organ or deep-space and deep incisional infections. Repeat debridement or drainage may be required to control and resolve the infection even with appropriate antimicrobial therapy. When an SSI involves an implant, removal of the implant is preferred, followed by a prolonged course of antibiotics (6-8 weeks). Superficial incisional infections can usually be managed with oral antibiotics without tissue debridement. The choice of antimicrobial agent is guided by culture results; duration of treatment varies by anatomic site and by depth of infection. **H**

**KEY POINT**

- Surgical site infection treatment requires debridement of necrotic tissue, drainage of abscesses or infected fluid, and specific antimicrobial therapy for organ or deep-space and deep incisional infections.

## Prevention

Prevention is divided into preoperative, intraoperative, and postoperative measures (see Table 58). Modifiable host factors should be optimized before surgery. If antibiotic prophylaxis is indicated, select the correct agent, dose, and time for administration (60 minutes before incision, 2 hours before incision for vancomycin or fluoroquinolones), and redose during surgery based on surgery duration and antibiotic half-life. Continuing antibiotics postoperatively does not decrease SSI incidence, even in cases of intraoperative spillage of gastrointestinal contents or presence of wound drains. **H**

**KEY POINT**

- Optimizing modifiable risk factors before surgery (hyperglycemia control, reduction of immunosuppressive agents, cessation of tobacco use, weight loss) can help prevent surgical site infections.

## Central Line-Associated Bloodstream Infections

Central line-associated bloodstream infections (CLABSIs), associated with all types of central venous catheters (CVCs), are the most preventable HCAI. In the United States, CVC rates are 55% in ICU patients and 24% in non-ICU patients. Pathogens associated with CLABSIs include coagulase-negative staphylococci (20.5%), *S. aureus* (12.3%), *Enterococcus faecalis* (8.8%), non-albicans *Candida* species (8.1%), *Klebsiella pneumoniae* or *oxytoca* (7.9%), *Enterococcus faecium* (7%), and *Candida albicans* (6.5%). Antimicrobial resistance is a problem for many of these pathogens. CLABSI risk factors include prolonged hospitalization before catheterization, neutropenia, and reduced nurse-to-patient ratio in the ICU. Additional risk factors (modifiable) are shown in **Table 59**.

### Diagnosis

CLABSI is suspected when a patient with a CVC has bacteremia not resulting from infection at another site. Two

**TABLE 59.** Mitigation of Risk Factors for Central Line-Associated Bloodstream Infections

| Modifiable (Extrinsic) Risk Factor | Intervention |
|---|---|
| Prolonged catheterization | Daily review of continued need for CVC |
| | Discontinue as soon as practical |
| Multiple CVCs (increases risk 3.4-fold) | Minimize the number of CVCs as much as practical |
| Multilumen CVC | Use a catheter with the minimum number of lumens needed |
| Femoral vein catheterization; particularly in obese patients | Use subclavian site when possible |
| | Use ultrasonographic guidance for internal jugular catheter insertion |
| | Remove femoral vein CVCs as soon as practical, relocate to another site (e.g., subclavian, internal jugular vein) when possible |
| Heavy microbial colonization at insertion site and catheter hub | Chlorhexidine skin antisepsis at time of insertion |
| | Chlorhexidine-impregnated dressing |
| | Daily chlorhexidine bathing of patients in ICU |
| | Minimize catheter access |
| | Hand hygiene before manipulation of IV system; use aseptic technique for all IV access |
| | Disinfect catheter hub and needleless connectors ("scrub the hub") before accessing |
| Lack of maximal sterile barriers for insertion and breaks in aseptic technique | Follow CVC insertion bundle |
| Emergent insertion | When adherence to aseptic technique cannot be ensured, replace CVC as soon as possible (at least within 48 hours) to a new site |
| Total parenteral nutrition | Consider other options for delivering nutrition when possible |

CVC = central venous catheter; IV = intravenous.

sets of peripheral blood cultures (20 mL blood/set) should be obtained from different sites before starting antibiotics. Blood cultures drawn directly from CVCs have a higher rate of false positivity and should be avoided; they may falsely identify a CLABSI and lead to unnecessary antibiotic therapy. **H**

**KEY POINT**

- A central line-associated bloodstream infection should be suspected when a patient with a central venous catheter has bacteremia not resulting from infection at another site.

### Treatment

Infected CVCs should be removed. CVC removal is particularly important for *S. aureus*, *P. aeruginosa*, and *Candida* species infections. The duration of therapy for most cases of uncomplicated non–*S. aureus* CLABSI is 7 to 14 days (**Table 60**). *S. aureus* CLABSI is usually treated for at least 4 weeks; however, shorter-term therapy may be considered in select patients who have immediate catheter removal with resolution of fever and bacteremia within 72 hours of starting appropriate therapy and who have no implanted prosthetic devices, no evidence of endocarditis by echocardiography (preferably transesophageal), no evidence of suppurative thrombophlebitis, no evidence of metastatic infection, and neither diabetes mellitus nor immunosuppression. Bacteremia clearance should be confirmed with follow-up blood cultures. If bacteremia persists after CVC removal and appropriate antimicrobial therapy, evaluation for a deeper source of infection, including endocarditis, should be performed. All patients with candidemia should be evaluated by an ophthalmologist to rule out the presence of candida endophthalmitis within 1 to 2 weeks. **H**

**KEY POINT**

- The duration of therapy for most cases of uncomplicated non–*Staphylococcus aureus* central line–associated bloodstream infection is 7 to 14 days, although *S. aureus* infection is usually treated for at least 4 weeks.

### Prevention

CVCs should be inserted only by experienced personnel using the insertion bundle of hand hygiene, chlorhexidine skin antisepsis of the insertion site using recommended application methods and contact time, maximal barrier precautions (mask, cap, gown, sterile gloves, large sterile drape covering patient), and optimal catheter site selection (subclavian site preferred, avoid femoral site). See Table 59 for further modifiable factors to prevent CLABSI. Insertion bundles, checklists, and staff education have significantly reduced CLABSIs. If CLABSI rates remain high despite adherence to these strategies, patient chlorhexidine bathing and antimicrobial-impregnated catheters (silver–sulfadiazine–chlorhexidine, minocycline-rifampin) may be considered. Routine CVC exchange or replacement or administration of systemic antimicrobial prophylaxis at time of insertion or during CVC use should be avoided.

## *Staphylococcus aureus* Bacteremia

*S. aureus* is a leading cause of hospital-acquired bacteremia. Endocarditis and vertebral osteomyelitis are two important complications of *S. aureus* bacteremia, although they are less likely when the infection is hospital acquired. The source of bacteremia and possible metastatic infection should be determined, starting with a detailed history and examination. All patients should undergo evaluation for endocarditis with echocardiography, preferably transesophageal. Source control with removal or drainage of any focus of infection is important for treatment success. Blood cultures should be repeated every 2 to 4 days until results are negative to document clearance.

Bacteremia caused by methicillin-sensitive *S. aureus* (MSSA) should be treated with a penicillinase-resistant semisynthetic penicillin (such as oxacillin) or first-generation cephalosporin (such as cefazolin) at maximal doses. Vancomycin should be avoided in patients with MSSA who are not allergic to β-lactam antibiotics. Vancomycin is associated with higher rates of relapse and microbiologic failure in the treatment of MSSA bacteremia.

For methicillin-resistant *S. aureus* (MRSA) bacteremia, vancomycin and daptomycin are the preferred antibiotics. Vancomycin trough concentrations of 15 to 20 μg/mL are recommended; however, these concentrations increase the risk of nephrotoxicity, and kidney function should be closely monitored. Patients with concomitant *S. aureus* pneumonia should not receive daptomycin because it is inactivated by surfactant. The clinical and microbiologic response (clearance of bacteremia) determines whether to continue vancomycin or change to daptomycin when the MRSA isolate has a vancomycin

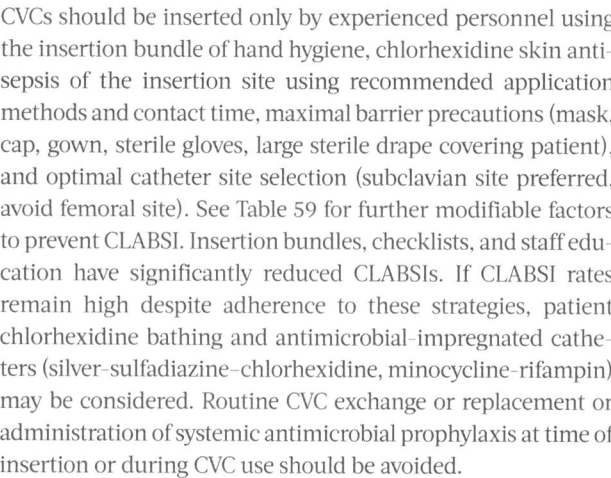

**TABLE 60.** Management of Central Venous Catheter-Related Bloodstream Infection Based on Pathogen[a]

| Organism | Treatment |
|---|---|
| **Uncomplicated**[b] | |
| Coagulase-negative staphylococci | Remove catheter, antimicrobial therapy for 5-7 days |
| | If catheter is not removed, systemic antimicrobials and antimicrobial lock treatment[c] for 10-14 days |
| *Staphylococcus aureus* (no active malignancy or immunosuppression) | Remove catheter, antimicrobials for ≥14 days (usually 4 weeks) |
| *Enterococcus* species | Remove catheter, antimicrobials for 7-14 days |
| Gram-negative bacilli | Remove catheter, antimicrobials for 7-14 days |
| *Candida* species | Remove catheter, antifungal agent for 14 additional days after first negative blood culture |
| **Complicated** | |
| Suppurative thrombophlebitis, endocarditis, osteomyelitis, other site of metastatic or deep-seated infection | Remove catheter, antimicrobials for 4-6 weeks (6-8 weeks for osteomyelitis) |

[a]Short-term catheters.

[b]Bloodstream infection and fever resolve in 72 hours, no intravascular hardware, no endocarditis or suppurative thrombophlebitis.

[c]Antimicrobial solution (such as vancomycin) instilled into the lumen of a catheter and removed after a specified period of time.

CONT.

minimum inhibitory concentration of ≤2 µg/mL. Persistent bacteremia may be the result of slow bactericidal activity of vancomycin, inadequate dosing, poor tissue penetration, or inadequate source control. Higher-dose daptomycin (8-10 mg/kg/d) is sometimes used if bacteremia persists despite adequate source control. Vancomycin should not be used when the isolate has a minimum inhibitory concentration greater than 2 µg/mL; daptomycin is an acceptable alternative if the isolate is susceptible. The median time to clearance of MRSA bacteremia is 7 to 9 days.

Bacteremia that persists beyond 72 hours of starting appropriate antibiotic treatment suggests a complicated *S. aureus* infection and requires additional evaluation and a longer course of antibiotics (4-6 weeks). Management of persistent MSSA and MRSA bacteremia also includes a thorough search for and removal of all foci of infection, including surgical debridement of infected wounds and abscess drainage. A new focus of infection may develop with persistent bacteremia and should always be considered in the evaluation of persistent bacteremia. Combination antimicrobial agents (for example, a β-lactam and aminoglycoside, vancomycin and rifampin) have not been shown to improve outcomes and should not be used. H

**KEY POINTS**

- Bacteremia caused by methicillin-sensitive *Staphylococcus aureus* (MSSA) should be treated with a penicillinase-resistant semisynthetic penicillin or first-generation cephalosporin at maximal doses; vancomycin should be avoided in patients who are not allergic to β-lactam antibiotics because it is associated with higher rates of relapse and microbiologic failure in the treatment of MSSA bacteremia.

- Vancomycin and daptomycin are the preferred antibiotics for methicillin-resistant *Staphylococcus aureus* bacteremia, although patients with concomitant *S. aureus* pneumonia should not receive daptomycin because it is inactivated by surfactant.

# Hospital-Acquired Pneumonia and Ventilator-Associated Pneumonia

Hospital-acquired pneumonia (HAP) is pneumonia developing more than 48 hours after hospitalization. Ventilator-associated pneumonia (VAP) is pneumonia developing 48 hours after endotracheal intubation; it occurs in 10% of patients undergoing ventilation. Half of patients with HAP develop serious complications, including respiratory failure, pleural effusion, septic shock, empyema, and kidney injury. Mechanical ventilation increases the risk of pneumonia 6-fold to 21-fold. HAP and VAP risk factors include age older than 70 years, recent abdominal or thoracic surgery, immunosuppression, and underlying chronic lung disease. Modifiable risk factors are listed in **Table 61**.

**TABLE 61.** Mitigation of Risk Factors for Ventilator-Associated Pneumonia

| Risk Factor | Intervention |
|---|---|
| Mechanical ventilation | Consider noninvasive, positive-pressure ventilation |
| Sedation | Minimize |
| | Intermittent infusions or daily interruption and daily assessment of readiness for extubation |
| Supine position | Risk highest for patients receiving enteral nutrition |
| | Elevate head of bed 30°-45° |
| Oropharyngeal colonization | Daily oral care; oral care with chlorhexidine may be beneficial in some patients |
| Physical conditioning | Facilitate early mobility (speeds extubation) |
| Reintubation | Consider noninvasive, positive-pressure ventilation |

HAP and VAP are most commonly caused by bacteria, but viral and fungal pathogens should be considered in immunocompromised patients. The main risk factor for MRSA, antibiotic-resistant *Pseudomonas*, or other antibiotic-resistant pathogens is intravenous antibiotic use within the past 90 days. Additional risk factors for multidrug-resistant pathogens associated with VAP are septic shock at the time of VAP, acute respiratory distress syndrome preceding VAP, 5 or more days of hospitalization before VAP, and acute kidney replacement therapy before VAP.

## Diagnosis

Diagnosis relies on a combination of clinical, radiographic, and microbiologic findings. A new lung infiltrate on imaging plus clinical findings, including new-onset fever (temperature >38 °C [100.4 °F]), leukocytosis or leukopenia, purulent sputum, and decline in oxygenation, suggest pneumonia. Noninvasive sampling (endotracheal aspiration) with semi-quantitative sputum cultures (heavy, moderate, light, and no growth) are suggested for diagnosing VAP. Clinical findings without radiographic support suggest tracheobronchitis, which does not require antibiotic treatment. H

**KEY POINT**

- The diagnosis of hospital-acquired and ventilator-associated pneumonia are suggested by a new lung infiltrate on imaging plus clinical findings, including new-onset fever, leukocytosis or leukopenia, purulent sputum, and decline in oxygenation.

## Treatment

Therapy for suspected HAP should be based on respiratory sample culture results; a specimen from the lower respiratory tract should be obtained before starting antimicrobial therapy. However, inability to obtain a specimen should not delay therapy initiation for VAP, and empiric antimicrobial therapy

CONT.

should be instituted for patients with VAP pending results of noninvasive sampling with semiquantitative cultures and based on local VAP antibiograms, if available.

Empiric VAP regimens should include coverage for *S. aureus*, *P. aeruginosa*, and other gram-negative bacilli. An agent active against MRSA (vancomycin, linezolid) should be included for patients with MRSA risk factors or those in a unit with MRSA prevalence greater than 10% to 20% or unknown. Two antipseudomonal agents of different classes are recommended for empiric regimens only for patients with risk factors for resistance, with structural lung disease (bronchiectasis, cystic fibrosis), or in a unit with greater than 10% resistance to an agent being considered for monotherapy. Similar regimens are recommended for patients with HAP who are treated empirically. Antimicrobial coverage for oral anaerobes may be considered in patients with witnessed aspiration events or recent surgery. Cephalosporins should be avoided as monotherapy in settings where extended-spectrum β-lactamase (ESBL)–producing gram-negative organisms (such as *Klebsiella pneumoniae*) are prevalent; consider a carbapenem instead. VAP caused by gram-negative organisms sensitive only to aminoglycosides or colistin may be treated with a combination of systemic and aerosolized antibiotics.

Microbiologic results should be reviewed at 48 to 72 hours, and all patients should be re-evaluated for clinical improvement. Antimicrobial therapy should be de-escalated (to narrow-spectrum or oral therapy) based on microbiologic results and clinical stabilization or discontinued if the diagnosis of pneumonia is in doubt. Patients who do not improve within 72 hours of appropriate therapy should undergo investigation for infectious complications, an alternate diagnosis, or another site of infection. HAP and VAP should be treated for 7 days or less.

### KEY POINT

- Empiric ventilator-associated pneumonia regimens should include coverage for *Staphylococcus aureus*, *Pseudomonas aeruginosa*, and other gram-negative bacilli; an agent active against methicillin-resistant *S. aureus* (MRSA) should be included for patients with MRSA risk factors or where MRSA prevalence exceeds 10% (or is unknown); similar regimens are recommended for empiric hospital-acquired pneumonia treatment.

### Prevention

Commonly used ventilator bundles include subglottic suctioning, peptic ulcer disease and deep venous thrombosis prophylaxis, and avoiding gastric overdistention. Use of ventilator bundles has been shown to decrease VAP rates by 71%. Additional interventions are listed in Table 61.

### KEY POINT

**HVC**  
- In patients receiving mechanical ventilation, the head of the bed should be elevated 30° to 45°; a supine position, particularly in patients receiving enteral nutrition, increases the risk for developing ventilator-associated pneumonia.

## Hospital-Acquired Infections Caused by Multidrug-Resistant Organisms

Antimicrobial resistance has been noted in nearly all bacterial pathogens. Multidrug-resistant organisms (MDROs) are most prevalent in health care settings (highest incidence in long-term acute care hospitals) but are also observed in the community. Seven of the 15 MDROs deemed urgent threats are predominantly health care associated. Nearly half of *S. aureus* HCAIs in the United States are methicillin resistant, 30% of enterococci are vancomycin resistant, 18% of Enterobacteriaceae produce ESBL and are resistant to all β-lactam antibiotics, 4% of Enterobacteriaceae are resistant to carbapenems, and 16% of *P. aeruginosa* and about half of *Acinetobacter* species are multidrug resistant. *Clostridium difficile* is not technically an MDRO, but it is a problematic pathogen in health care settings.

MDRO infections are difficult to treat, with mortality rates up to four times higher than infections caused by antibiotic-sensitive strains. Limiting transmission of MDROs in health care settings requires full adherence to hand hygiene protocols, contact precautions, and cleaning and disinfecting of the environment and patient care equipment. More than half of hospitalized patients receive antibiotics, a major risk for acquiring an antibiotic-resistant organism and *C. difficile* infection. Judicious use of antimicrobial agents is increasingly important to combat the rise of MDROs and emergence of untreatable infections.

### KEY POINTS

- Multidrug-resistant organisms (MDROs) are most prevalent in health care settings (highest incidence in long-term acute care hospitals) but are also observed in the community.
- Limiting emergence and transmission of multidrug-resistant organisms in health care settings requires full adherence to hand hygiene protocols, contact precautions, cleaning and disinfecting of the environment and equipment, and judicious use of antimicrobial agents.

**HVC**

# HIV/AIDS

HIV is a retrovirus that infects CD4 lymphocytes, among other cell types. Depletion of CD4 T-helper cells results in impairment of cell-mediated immunity and increasing risk for opportunistic infections. This chapter will focus on HIV-1. Infection with HIV-2 primarily occurs in parts of Africa and remains rare in the United States; HIV-2 generally is a less progressive disease with less immunocompromise and lower risk of opportunistic infections. Current testing for HIV infection detects HIV-1 and HIV-2 antibodies (see Screening and Diagnosis).

# Epidemiology and Prevention

HIV infection remains a significant global health concern despite being a treatable disease. Many persons living with HIV infection are not aware of their status because they have never been tested; others have been diagnosed but are not receiving care. Those with undiagnosed or untreated infection are responsible for most new infections. Diagnosis and successful treatment are crucial for personal and public health.

HIV transmission occurs through sexual contact or exposure to other body fluids (**Table 62**). Reducing transmission can be accomplished by using barrier methods, such as condoms during sexual contact, and through clean syringe services programs (needle exchange programs) for injection drug users. Universal blood donor testing has all but eliminated infection through blood transfusion in the United States, with current risk estimated to be one in 2 million.

HIV treatment has extraordinary potential to reduce new infections in addition to benefiting the treated person. Successful treatment is associated with significant reductions in HIV transmission. Although reducing viral load to an undetectable level in blood does not prove absence of virus in semen or vaginal fluid, the rate of transmission from a sexual partner with undetectable blood viral load has been demonstrated to be close to zero, at a level the Centers for Disease Control and Prevention (CDC) called "effectively no risk" in a September 2017 statement, leading to the slogan "Undetectable = Untransmissable" ("U=U"). In what is known as the "treatment cascade," steps of medical care necessary to achieve successful viral suppression consist of testing and diagnosing infected persons, linking them to health care for counseling and treatment, keeping them in a treatment program, and ensuring antiretroviral and other treatment adherence. Each step along this continuum of care is a potential obstacle to successful management of HIV on a personal and public health level. Even high-income countries, such as the United States, have poor rates of retention in care and adherence to medication. One study estimated that the undiagnosed and not-in-care groups with HIV infection were responsible for 91.5% of HIV transmissions in the United States in 2009.

In 2014, the Joint United Nations Programme on HIV/AIDS (UNAIDS) launched its "90-90-90" program of ambitious goals for reducing new HIV infection worldwide. These goals include that by 2020, 90% of HIV-infected persons will have been diagnosed, 90% of those diagnosed will be receiving treatment, and 90% of those receiving treatment will have successful viral suppression. Achieving such goals will require considerable resource commitment but, if achieved, will also dramatically reduce transmission and new HIV infections.

Postexposure prophylaxis antiretroviral therapy has been used successfully for many years in uninfected persons to prevent infection after occupational and nonoccupational HIV exposure. Prophylaxis should be started as soon as possible after exposure; it is not recommended if more than 72 hours have passed. A three-drug regimen is given for 4 weeks; the preferred regimen is tenofovir disoproxil fumarate and emtricitabine plus either raltegravir or dolutegravir. HIV testing of the exposed person should be conducted at baseline and at 4 to 6 weeks and 3 months after exposure. **Figure 22** shows an algorithm for evaluation of possible HIV exposure.

Pre-exposure prophylaxis (PrEP) with antiretroviral medication is recommended in select persons at high risk for exposure to HIV to reduce the risk of infection. A two-drug combination of tenofovir disoproxil fumarate and emtricitabine, taken once daily, is FDA approved for HIV PrEP; it has been shown to be effective in reducing infection in heterosexual couples, men who have sex with men, and injection drug users. Effectiveness is greater than 90% in those with proven adherence. Patients should also be counseled on the need to continue barrier precautions, on medication toxicity, and on continued risk for other sexually transmitted infections (STIs). Testing should be performed for HIV, hepatitis B virus (HBV), kidney function, and pregnancy before PrEP initiation; monitoring for HIV, other STIs, and pregnancy every 3 months and performing kidney function assessment every 6 months are also recommended during PrEP therapy. Persons taking PrEP who test positive for HIV should have a third drug (either ritonavir-boosted darunavir or dolutegravir) added to the two-drug PrEP regimen pending results of HIV RNA and viral resistance testing. The evidence is conflicting concerning potentially increased high-risk behavior and incidence of other STIs in PrEP users during therapy. PrEP has also been calculated to have favorable cost effectiveness, well below that for other accepted preventive health measures.

**TABLE 62.** Risk of HIV-1 Transmission per Single Exposure

| Exposure | Risk (%) |
| --- | --- |
| Occupational—needlestick | 0.23 |
| Occupational—mucous membrane | 0.09 |
| Needle-sharing injection drug use | 0.63 |
| Receptive anal intercourse | 1.4 |
| Receptive vaginal intercourse | 0.08 |
| Insertive anal intercourse | 0.11 |
| Insertive vaginal intercourse | 0.04 |
| Oral sex | 0.01 |

**KEY POINTS**

- Although reducing viral load to an undetectable level in blood does not equal absence of virus in semen or vaginal fluid, the rate of transmission from a sexual partner with undetectable blood viral load is exceedingly low, with reductions in risk greater than 95%.

- Postexposure prophylaxis with a three-drug regimen (tenofovir disoproxil fumarate and emtricitabine plus either raltegravir or dolutegravir) should be started as soon as possible after HIV exposure; it is not recommended if more than 72 hours have passed.

*(Continued)*

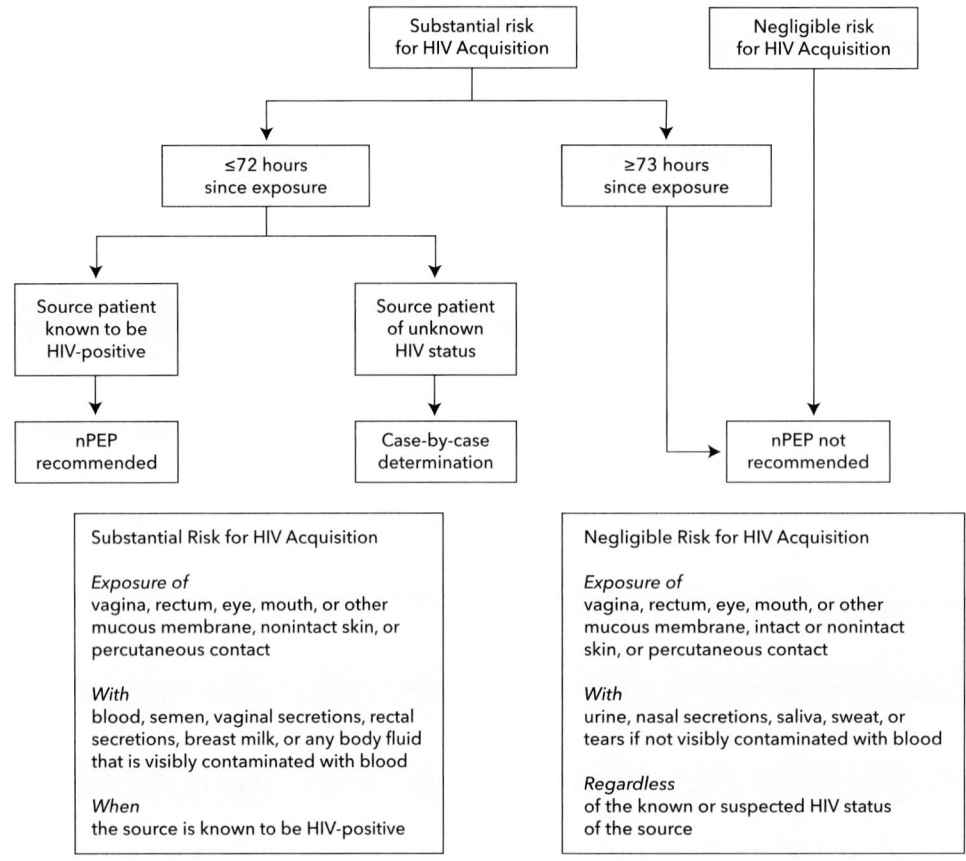

**FIGURE 22.** Algorithm for evaluation and treatment of possible HIV exposure. nPEP = nonoccupational postexposure prophylaxis.

**KEY POINTS** *(continued)*

- Pre-exposure prophylaxis with two antiretroviral medications (tenofovir disoproxil fumarate and emtricitabine) is recommended in select persons at high risk for exposure to HIV to reduce the risk of infection.

# Pathophysiology and Natural History

## Acute Retroviral Syndrome

Most persons with acute HIV infection are symptomatic; however, because symptoms are nonspecific and self-limited, most acute infections are not diagnosed accurately. The frequency of signs and symptoms at presentation is shown in **Table 63**. The differential diagnosis includes Epstein-Barr virus infection, cytomegalovirus infection, and secondary syphilis. During symptomatic acute infection, HIV antibody may not yet be detectable, and diagnosis depends on demonstration of p24 antigen or HIV RNA. Currently recommended HIV testing includes p24 antigen testing as part of the initial evaluation (see Screening and Diagnosis). Persons with acute HIV infection should be immediately linked to care for prompt initiation of treatment.

**TABLE 63.** Signs and Symptoms of Acute HIV Infection (Acute Retroviral Syndrome)

| Sign/Symptom | Frequency (%) |
|---|---|
| Fever | 75 |
| Fatigue | 68 |
| Myalgia | 49 |
| Rash | 48 |
| Headache | 45 |
| Pharyngitis | 40 |
| Lymphadenopathy | 39 |
| Arthralgia | 30 |
| Night sweats | 28 |
| Diarrhea | 27 |

**KEY POINT**

- Most persons with acute HIV infection are symptomatic; however, because symptoms are nonspecific and self-limited, most acute infections are not diagnosed accurately.

## Chronic HIV Infection and AIDS

Patients with chronic HIV infection may present with opportunistic infections, especially when CD4 counts are less than 200/µL, meeting the definition for AIDS (see Opportunistic Infections). Even before progression to AIDS, patients with HIV infection may present with recurrent or severe episodes of infections that do not qualify as opportunistic, such as bacterial pneumonia, herpes zoster, herpes simplex virus, or vaginal candidiasis. Other symptoms can result from chronic HIV infection itself, including lymphadenopathy, fever, night sweats, fatigue, weight loss, chronic diarrhea, and various oral and skin conditions (see MKSAP 18 Dermatology). HIV should also be considered in patients with unexplained cytopenias or nephropathy.

### KEY POINTS

- Before progression to AIDS, patients with chronic HIV infection may present with recurrent or severe episodes of infections that do not qualify as opportunistic, such as bacterial pneumonia, herpes zoster, herpes simplex virus, or vaginal candidiasis.
- Symptoms that can result from chronic HIV infection itself include lymphadenopathy, fever, night sweats, fatigue, weight loss, chronic diarrhea, and various oral and skin conditions.

## Screening and Diagnosis

Although any of the presenting symptoms described previously should prompt HIV testing, testing only symptomatic persons neglects numerous persons who are infected. Thus, the CDC, American College of Physicians, Infectious Diseases Society of America, and U.S. Preventive Services Task Force (USPSTF) recommend universal screening for HIV in all adults at least once. The USPSTF suggests those at higher risk (injection drug users and their sexual partners, people who exchange sex for money or drugs, sexual partners of HIV-infected persons, and those with more than one sexual partner since their most recent HIV test) should undergo repeat HIV testing at least annually. In 2017, the CDC reaffirmed its support for this recommendation but noted that clinicians can consider the potential benefits of more frequent HIV screening (for example, every 3 or 6 months) for some asymptomatic sexually active men who have sex with men based on their individual risk factors, local HIV epidemiology, and local policies.

Current (fourth generation) HIV testing uses a combination assay for HIV antibody and HIV p24 antigen, which detects acute infection at least 1 week earlier than older assays. A positive result on the combination assay leads to testing with an HIV-1/HIV-2 antibody differentiation immunoassay, which, if positive, confirms infection. Specimens that test positive on the initial combination assay but negative for HIV antibody are tested for HIV RNA by nucleic acid amplification testing; if positive, acute HIV infection is confirmed (**Figure 23**). Although the initial combination assay has a 99.6% specificity, testing in low prevalence populations (such as general screening) can still result in false positives, so waiting for the results of the confirmatory antibody differentiation immunoassay and nucleic acid amplification testing is important for a definitive diagnosis.

### KEY POINTS

- It is recommended that all adults be tested for HIV infection at least once.
- A combination assay for HIV antibody and HIV p24 antigen now detects acute infection at least 1 week earlier than older assays; a positive HIV-1/HIV-2 antibody immunoassay result confirms infection, or a positive HIV RNA nucleic acid amplification test result confirms acute HIV infection.

## Initiation of Care

### Initial Evaluation and Laboratory Testing

All persons who test positive for HIV should be immediately referred to a health care provider with HIV infection management expertise. Initial evaluation should include complete history (including social and sexual) and examination for signs and symptoms of opportunistic infection or other complications. Patient education and counseling should include information on transmission and prevention. Initial laboratory tests include baseline organ function and evaluation for other infections with higher prevalence in persons with HIV (**Table 64**). A baseline CD4 cell count guides opportunistic infection prophylaxis, and a baseline viral load supports monitoring antiretroviral therapy effectiveness (see Management of HIV Infection).

### Immunizations and Prophylaxis for Opportunistic Infections

Numerous immunizations are recommended for all persons with HIV, starting with the 13-valent pneumococcal conjugate and 23-valent pneumococcal polysaccharide vaccines, respectively, at least 8 weeks apart; a 23-valent polysaccharide vaccine booster is also recommended after 5 years. Patients who are not already immune or infected with HBV should receive the hepatitis B vaccine series. Influenza, tetanus-diphtheria-pertussis, hepatitis A, and human papillomavirus vaccinations are indicated as for the general population. Measles-mumps-rubella and varicella vaccines can be given as long as the CD4 cell count is greater than 200/µL. Although the recombinant zoster vaccine is considered safe in immunocompromised persons because it does not contain live virus, safety and efficacy data in patients with HIV are not yet available to inform recommendations. The Advisory Committee on Immunization Practices recommends that all persons with HIV infection be vaccinated for meningococcal disease with the quadrivalent meningococcal vaccine, including boosters every 5 years.

Prophylaxis for opportunistic infections depends on the patient's CD4 cell count (**Table 65**). Before beginning

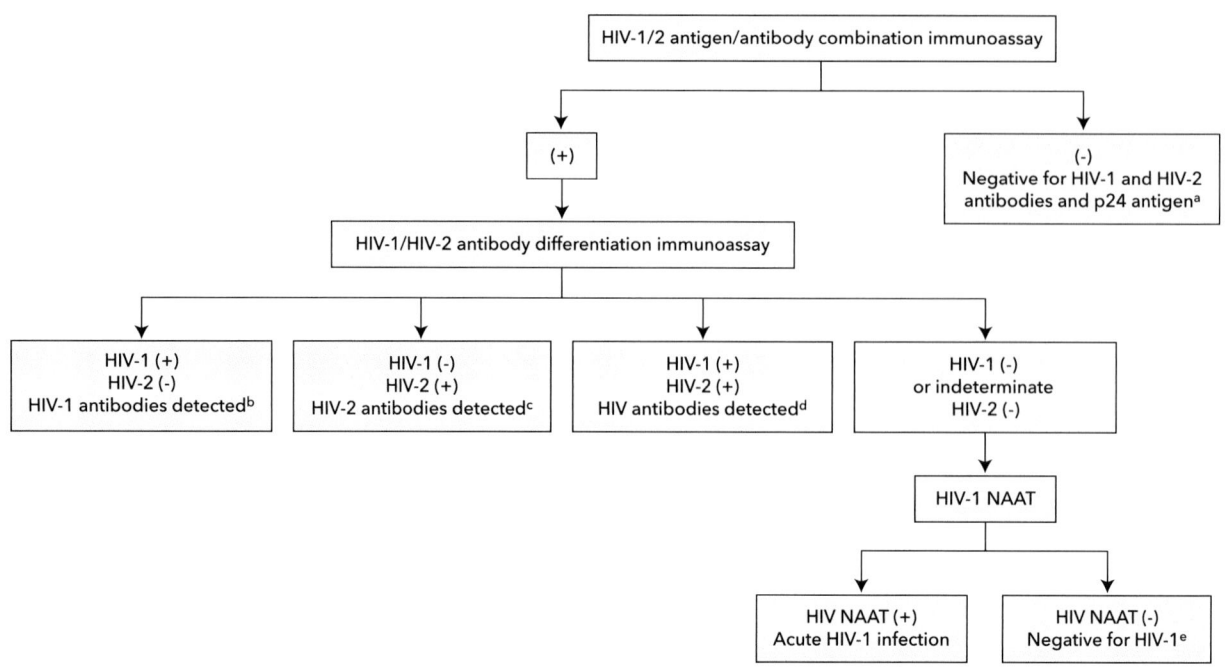

**FIGURE 23.** CDC-recommended algorithm for laboratory HIV testing. NAAT = nucleic acid amplification test. (+) indicates reactive test result. (−) indicates nonreactive test result.

[a] No evidence of HIV infection.

[b] HIV-1 infection.

[c] HIV-2 infection.

[d] HIV-1 and HIV-2 infection.

[e] HIV-1/2 antigen/antibody combination immunoassay result was a false positive.

Centers for Disease Control and Prevention; Association of Public Health Laboratories. Laboratory testing for the diagnosis of HIV infection: updated recommendations. January 2018. Available at https://stacks.cdc.gov/view/cdc/50872.

**TABLE 64. Laboratory Testing as Part of the Evaluation of HIV Infection**

Repeat HIV antibody testing if no documentation

Viral resistance testing at baseline and for treatment failure

Quantitative HIV RNA assay (viral load)

T-cell subsets (CD4 cell count)

Complete blood count with differential

Chemistries, including kidney function studies and fasting plasma glucose level

Liver chemistry studies/liver enzyme levels

Fasting serum lipid profile

Urinalysis or quantitative measure of proteinuria

Tuberculin skin test or interferon-γ release assay

Serologic testing for hepatitis A, B, and C virus infection

Serologic testing for syphilis; testing for other sexually transmitted infections

Serologic testing for toxoplasmosis

Cervical Pap test

**TABLE 65. Prophylaxis against Opportunistic Infections in HIV/AIDS**

| Opportunistic Infection | Indication | Preferred Drug |
|---|---|---|
| *Pneumocystis jirovecii* | CD4 cell count <200/μL[a] | TMP-SMX, double-strength or single-strength tablet once daily |
| Toxoplasmosis | CD4 cell count <100/μL and positive serologic results[a] | TMP-SMX, double-strength tablet once daily |
| *Mycobacterium avium* complex | CD4 cell count <50/μL | Azithromycin, 1200 mg once weekly or 600 mg twice weekly; clarithromycin, 500 mg twice daily |
| Latent tuberculosis | TST >5 mm or positive IGRA results | Isoniazid, 300 mg once daily for 9 months or 900 mg twice weekly, both with pyridoxine, 25 mg once daily |

IGRA = interferon-γ release assay; TMP-SMX = trimethoprim-sulfamethoxazole; TST = tuberculin skin test.

[a] Prophylaxis may be discontinued in patients with suppressed viral load and CD4 cell count ≥200/μL for ≥3 months.

prophylaxis, active infection should be ruled out clinically and with any indicated testing to avoid undertreatment and selection for resistance, especially for tuberculosis and disseminated *Mycobacterium avium* complex.

- All persons with HIV should receive the 13-valent pneumococcal conjugate and 23-valent polysaccharide vaccines, hepatitis B vaccine series (in those not already infected or immune), and meningococcal vaccine; influenza, tetanus-diphtheria-pertussis, hepatitis A, and human papillomavirus vaccines are indicated as for the general population.
- Active infection should be ruled out before initiation of prophylaxis for opportunistic infections.

# Complications of HIV Infection in the Antiretroviral Therapy Era

## Metabolic, Kidney, and Liver Disorders

As HIV has become a treatable illness and persons with HIV age, metabolic disorders and specific organ diseases have become increasingly significant. HIV infection itself may be associated with manifestations of accelerated aging, and neurocognitive impairment can be exacerbated by HIV. Age-associated comorbidities and declines in kidney and liver function can also complicate management through drug interactions and increased toxicity.

HIV infection itself and some antiretrovirals affect lipids and can worsen hyperlipidemia; this is especially true for boosted protease inhibitor–based regimens, which can also worsen insulin resistance. Fasting glucose or hemoglobin $A_{1c}$ and lipid levels should be checked at baseline and 3 months after initiating or changing antiretrovirals.

Chronic kidney disease is increasingly common in HIV infection, although, with effective antiretroviral therapy, it is less often attributed to HIV nephropathy. It is recommended that kidney function be assessed at least every 6 months in patients with HIV. Tenofovir, a very commonly used nucleoside analogue, is associated with risk for tubular nephrotoxicity, which usually manifests as proteinuria. Patients using a regimen containing tenofovir should undergo urinalysis or quantitative measurement of urine protein twice per year.

Bone mineral density is reduced in HIV, and tenofovir is also associated with possible worsening of bone density. Dual-energy x-ray absorptiometry scanning is recommended in men older than 50 years, postmenopausal women, patients with a history of fragility fracture, those with chronic glucocorticoid use, and those at high risk for falls. A newer prodrug of tenofovir, tenofovir alafenamide (TAF), achieves high intracellular levels of active drug with much lower dosing and lower systemic levels compared with the older formulation, tenofovir disoproxil fumarate (TDF). Compared with TDF, TAF has equal antiviral efficacy with reduced kidney and bone

toxicity and should be used preferentially over TDF in patients with or at risk for bone or kidney disease.

Liver disease is also increased in HIV infection, often because of coinfection with hepatitis B or C virus. All patients with HIV should be screened for hepatitis B and C viruses. Patients should be immunized if they are HBV negative. If coinfected with HIV and HBV, patients should receive treatment with a tenofovir (either TDF or TAF) plus emtricitabine or lamivudine-based regimen, which treats both viruses. Patients coinfected with hepatitis C virus should be given a course of curative direct-acting antiviral treatment, although attention must be paid to drug interactions between the antiviral regimens (see MKSAP 18 Gastroenterology and Hepatology).

- Fasting glucose or hemoglobin $A_{1c}$ and lipid levels should be checked at baseline and 3 months after initiating or changing antiretroviral therapy.
- Tenofovir disoproxil fumarate (TDF), a very commonly used nucleoside analogue in HIV therapy, is associated with increased risks of tubular nephrotoxicity and worsening of bone mineral density; tenofovir alafenamide should be used preferentially over TDF in patients with or at risk for bone or kidney disease.

## Cardiovascular Disease

Rates of cardiovascular disease, including myocardial infarction and stroke, are higher in persons with HIV infection; this association remains after correction for increased risk factors such as smoking. Some of the increase may result from hyperlipidemia, but evidence indicates that the increase partially results from HIV infection being a chronic inflammatory state. It is clear that patients with untreated HIV infection have a higher risk of cardiovascular events compared with patients taking effective antiretroviral therapy, regardless of any worsening of lipid levels from the antiretroviral therapy. Attention to traditional risk factors such as smoking, lipid levels, and hypertension is crucial in patients with HIV, as is use of statin therapy (with attention to drug interactions between some statins and some antiretrovirals) based on current risk calculations. An international multicenter trial is addressing whether patients with HIV should be treated with statins even with a 10-year risk less than 7.5%.

- Rates of cardiovascular disease, including myocardial infarction and stroke, are higher in persons with HIV infection; control of cardiovascular risk factors (smoking, lipid levels, and hypertension) is essential, including statin therapy based on clinical risk calculations.

## Immune Reconstitution Inflammatory Syndrome

Immune reconstitution inflammatory syndrome (IRIS) is a disorder associated either with worsening of a pre-existing infectious process (paradoxical IRIS) or with revelation of a previously unrecognized pre-existing infection (unmasking IRIS). It has also been reported with noninfectious complications, such as lymphoma. IRIS usually occurs within a few months of initiating effective antiretroviral therapy in patients with low pretreatment CD4 cell counts (<100/µL). Management of IRIS includes continuing antiretroviral therapy while treating the opportunistic infection. In select patients, NSAIDs or glucocorticoids may be useful in mitigating inflammatory symptoms.

**KEY POINT**

- Immune reconstitution inflammatory syndrome is caused by an inflammatory response to a pre-existing infectious process; it usually occurs within a few months of initiating effective antiretroviral therapy and presents with a wide variety of infections and noninfectious complications.

## Opportunistic Infections

Mucocutaneous *Candida* infections can occur in HIV-infected patients at relatively preserved CD4 cell counts. HIV-infected patients do not usually develop invasive *Candida* infection unless they have other risk factors, such as neutropenia. Oral candidiasis usually presents as thrush, with mucosal whitish plaques, and can be treated topically (for example, with clotrimazole troches) or with a short course of oral fluconazole. Swallowing symptoms suggest esophageal disease, which requires systemic treatment, such as fluconazole, for a longer course; a lack of treatment response is an indication for endoscopy.

Reactivation of latent tuberculosis is also significantly increased in HIV infection, even without a decreased CD4 cell count. Tuberculosis is also more likely to present in extrapulmonary sites or with an atypical chest radiograph. Tuberculosis treatment in HIV must consider interactions of rifamycins with many antiretrovirals.

Infections with other opportunistic organisms usually occur at CD4 cell counts less than 200/µL. *Pneumocystis jirovecii* pneumonia usually presents as a subacute illness with fever, dyspnea, and dry cough in a patient with a CD4 cell count less than 200/µL who is not receiving prophylaxis. Chest radiographs most often show bilateral interstitial infiltrates; cavitation or pleural effusion is unusual and suggests another diagnosis. A normal chest radiograph does not exclude the diagnosis, and chest CT is more sensitive, demonstrating patchy "ground-glass" opacities. Normal lactate dehydrogenase levels and stable exercise oxygen saturation have a high negative predictive value, but elevated lactate dehydrogenase levels and oxygen desaturation with exercise are nonspecific. Diagnosis depends on demonstration of causative organisms and often requires bronchoscopy. The treatment of choice is high-dose trimethoprim-sulfamethoxazole; patients who are hypoxic at presentation should be given adjunctive glucocorticoids to prevent the worsening that may accompany initiation of treatment.

*Cryptococcus* infection usually presents as subacute meningitis with headache, mental status changes, and fever.  Because it often involves the basilar area, cranial nerve deficits may also be seen. The diagnosis can be made most swiftly by antigen testing of cerebrospinal fluid and blood. Management includes antifungal therapy and attention to increased intracranial pressure, which is usually responsible for the morbidity and mortality associated with cryptococcal meningitis (see Fungal Infections). **H**

*Toxoplasma gondii* infection in AIDS usually presents in patients with CD4 cell counts less than 100/µL. Because it is a reactivation disease, patients are usually serology positive. Clinical presentation includes headache, fever, and focal neurologic deficits. Imaging by CT or MRI (which is more sensitive) reveals multiple ring-enhancing lesions. The differential diagnosis includes primary central nervous system lymphoma, which most often appears as a single lesion on imaging, and progressive multifocal leukoencephalopathy, which is usually nonenhancing. Diagnosis of central nervous system toxoplasmosis is usually presumptive based on presentation, imaging, and response to empiric treatment.

*Mycobacterium avium* complex infection usually presents as disseminated disease in patients with CD4 cell counts less than 50/µL; symptoms and signs include fever, sweats, weight loss, hepatosplenomegaly, lymphadenopathy, and cytopenias. Blood cultures for acid-fast bacilli will usually grow *Mycobacterium avium* complex, but it may also be found on lymph node or liver biopsy when necessary.

Cytomegalovirus most commonly presents with CD4 cell counts less than 50/µL. Cytomegalovirus retinitis, presenting with vision changes or floaters, is much more likely in AIDS than in other immunocompromised conditions, such as after transplantation. Gastrointestinal cytomegalovirus disease is also common, most often as esophagitis or colitis.

Patients with AIDS are also more likely to develop certain malignancies, especially those related to viruses. Non–Hodgkin lymphoma, especially primary central nervous system lymphoma related to Epstein-Barr virus, is significantly increased compared with age-matched controls. Kaposi sarcoma is caused by human herpes virus type 8 and presents as dark red, brown, or violaceous lesions of the skin or mucous membranes (**Figure 24**); human herpes virus type 8 can also cause primary effusion lymphoma and Castleman disease (giant lymph node hyperplasia). Human papillomavirus–related malignancies are significantly increased in HIV, including cervical and anal cancers, and regular guideline-based screening is important.

**KEY POINTS**

- *Pneumocystis jirovecii* pneumonia usually presents as a subacute illness with fever, dyspnea, and dry cough; although chest radiographs most often show bilateral interstitial infiltrates, a normal chest radiograph does not exclude the diagnosis.

*(Continued)*

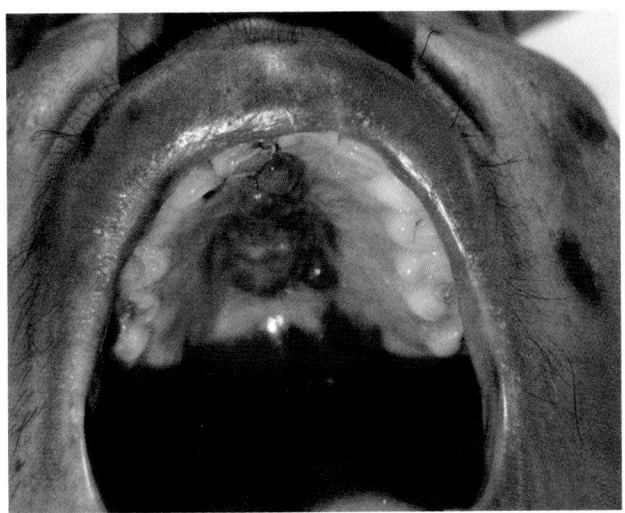

**FIGURE 24.** Kaposi sarcoma, presenting as firm purple nodules on the face and purple palatal nodules, is seen in a patient with AIDS.

**KEY POINTS** *(continued)*

- Successful management of *Cryptococcus* infection in patients with HIV includes antifungal therapy and attention to increased intracranial pressure, which is usually responsible for the morbidity and mortality associated with cryptococcal meningitis.

- *Toxoplasma gondii* infection in patients with HIV presents as multifocal central nervous system abscesses; MRI is more sensitive than CT in revealing characteristic ring-enhancing lesions.

- *Mycobacterium avium* complex and cytomegalovirus infections usually present in patients with HIV with CD4 cell counts less than 50/µL.

- Patients with AIDS are more likely to develop certain malignancies, including non-Hodgkin lymphoma, Kaposi sarcoma, and human papillomavirus–related malignancies (cervical and anal cancers).

# Management of HIV Infection

## When to Initiate Treatment

All persons with HIV infection should begin antiretroviral therapy as soon as they are ready, regardless of CD4 cell count. Previous controversy over whether to start antiretroviral treatment in asymptomatic patients with normal CD4 cell counts has been resolved with demonstration of clear clinical benefit in a large prospective, randomized clinical trial.

## Antiretroviral Regimens

Antiretroviral agents used in the United States are shown in **Table 66**. Standards for effective antiretroviral regimens include use of three drugs from two different classes, preferably combining two nucleoside reverse transcriptase inhibitors with an integrase strand transfer inhibitor. Preferred regimens

also feature a high barrier to resistance, good tolerability and safety, and combination pills with once-daily dosing to facilitate adherence (**Table 67**).

Patients with or at risk for reduced kidney function or osteopenia should not be given TDF. Patients who are prescribed abacavir must first undergo testing to show they are HLA-B*5701 negative to reduce the risk of hypersensitivity. Many antiretrovirals have interactions with other drugs, and potential drug interactions must always be assessed when beginning HIV therapy or beginning any drug for someone already taking antiretroviral therapy. Such assessment is especially necessary when pharmacokinetic boosters (ritonavir or cobicistat) are used specifically to inhibit drug metabolism and raise levels of antiretrovirals.

Viral load levels and CD4 cell counts are monitored to ensure effectiveness and to assess for immune recovery. With optimal therapy, HIV RNA in blood should become and stay undetectable. CD4 cell counts will increase, although cell counts may take time to improve and may not show full recovery, especially in those who are older or who have other factors affecting lymphocytes. Patients taking antiretroviral therapy who are stable with a CD4 cell count of 500/µL or more for more than 2 years can stop T-cell monitoring as long as viral load remains undetectable.

## Resistance Testing

Viral resistance testing should be performed at baseline to ensure selection of a fully active regimen and should be repeated if the viral load increases during antiretroviral treatment. The most common reason for breakthrough viremia is poor medication adherence. In general, plasma levels of HIV RNA must be greater than 500 copies/mL to provide enough virus for resistance testing. Viral resistance testing can be genotypic (looking for mutations associated with drug resistance) or phenotypic (assessing whether virus can replicate in the presence of the drug). Genotypic testing is faster and cheaper, but phenotypic testing may be better in the presence of multiple mutations or for drugs such as protease inhibitors in which the correlation of specific mutations and resistance is less straightforward. Resistance testing results are used to guide selection of a new regimen in the event resistant virus develops, but previous resistance testing results as well as previous regimens and responses must also be considered. Resistance testing may not be reliable if performed while the patient is not taking an antiretroviral regimen because resistance may not be detectable without the selective pressure of the antiretrovirals. Once selected for, previous mutations are generally archived in the viral population and may re-emerge even if resistance testing does not demonstrate the mutation. A regimen may also be switched because of adverse effects or to ease adherence or avoid drug interactions. Laboratory monitoring tests should be repeated 1 month after switching regimens to assess effectiveness and toxicity.

**TABLE 66.** Antiretroviral Agents Used in the United States to Treat HIV Infection

| Class | Agent[a] | Adverse Effects |
|---|---|---|
| Nucleoside RTIs | Abacavir | Hypersensitivity[b] (exclude HLA-B*5701 before prescribing) |
| | Emtricitabine | Minimal toxicity; has activity against HBV, and exacerbations have occurred with discontinuation of therapy |
| | Lamivudine | Minimal toxicity; has HBV activity, but dosing differs for HIV and HBV treatment |
| | TDF | Nausea, kidney disease, Fanconi syndrome, decreased bone density; has activity against HBV, and exacerbations have occurred with discontinuation of therapy |
| | TAF | Nausea; less kidney and bone toxicity than TDF |
| | Zidovudine | Nausea, headache, anemia[b], leukopenia[b], lactic acidosis[b], lipodystrophy, myopathy[b] |
| Nonnucleoside RTIs | Efavirenz | Neuropsychiatric symptoms (dizziness, somnolence, sleep disturbance, vivid dreams, mood changes), rash, dyslipidemia |
| | Etravirine | Nausea, rash |
| | Nevirapine | Hypersensitivity[b], rash, hepatitis[b] |
| | Rilpivirine | Rash, headache, insomnia; requires food and gastric acid (no concomitant PPI use) for absorption |
| Protease inhibitors | Atazanavir | Nausea, hyperbilirubinemia, nephrolithiasis, rash; requires food and gastric acid (no concomitant PPI use) for absorption |
| | Darunavir | Nausea, diarrhea, rash |
| | Fosamprenavir | Nausea, diarrhea, rash |
| | Lopinavir | Nausea, diarrhea, hyperlipidemia, insulin resistance |
| | Saquinavir | Nausea, diarrhea, hyperlipidemia, QT prolongation |
| | Tipranavir | Nausea, diarrhea, hyperlipidemia, rash, hepatitis[b], intracranial hemorrhage[b] |
| CCR5 antagonist | Maraviroc | Hypersensitivity, hepatitis[b] |
| Integrase inhibitors | Dolutegravir | Elevated creatinine level (decrease in tubular secretion, not GFR), insomnia, headache (generally well tolerated) |
| | Elvitegravir | Nausea, diarrhea (generally well tolerated) |
| | Raltegravir | Rash, myopathy (generally well tolerated) |
| | Bictegravir | Elevated creatinine level (decrease in tubular secretion, not GFR), nausea, diarrhea, headache (generally well tolerated) |
| Pharmacokinetic boosters | Cobicistat | Elevated creatinine level (decrease in tubular creatinine secretion, not GFR), not recommended if CrCl <70 mL/min |
| | Ritonavir | Nausea, diarrhea, hyperlipidemia, insulin resistance, lipodystrophy, drug interactions[b] |

CrCl = creatinine clearance; GFR = glomerular filtration rate; HBV = hepatitis B virus; PPI = proton pump inhibitor; RTIs = reverse transcriptase inhibitors; TAF = tenofovir alafenamide; TDF = tenofovir disoproxil fumarate.

[a]Many agents are also available as components of combination medications.

[b]Black box warning. Note all nucleoside analogues have a black box warning about possible lactic acidosis, although it is far more likely with stavudine, didanosine, and zidovudine than the other agents.

**TABLE 67.** Preferred Regimens for Initial Treatment of HIV Infection[a]

| |
|---|
| Abacavir/lamivudine/dolutegravir |
| Tenofovir alafenamide/emtricitabine/dolutegravir |
| Tenofovir alafenamide/emtricitabine/cobicistat/elvitegravir |
| Tenofovir alafenamide/emtricitabine/raltegravir |
| Tenofovir alafenamide/emtricitabine/bictegravir |

[a]Endorsed by the 2016 International Antiviral Society–USA Panel guidelines and the 2018 Department of Health and Human Services guidelines.

**KEY POINTS**

- All persons with HIV infection should begin antiretroviral therapy as soon as they are ready, regardless of CD4 cell count.

- Standards for effective antiretroviral regimens include use of three drugs from two different classes; preferred regimens combine two nucleoside reverse transcriptase inhibitors with an integrase strand transfer inhibitor.

- HIV resistance testing may not be reliable if performed while the patient is not taking an antiretroviral regimen because resistance may not be detectable without the selective pressure of the antiretrovirals.

## Management of Pregnant Patients with HIV Infection

The management of pregnant women with HIV does not significantly differ from the management of nonpregnant women. Initiating antiretroviral therapy is recommended as soon as possible in pregnant women with HIV who are not already being treated, and it is especially important that women already receiving HIV treatment who become pregnant continue treatment without interruption. Antiretroviral therapy in pregnancy benefits the woman and significantly reduces the risk of perinatal transmission of HIV to her baby. Previous concerns about teratogenicity of some antiretrovirals, including concerns about neural tube defects with efavirenz, have been allayed by data showing no difference in birth defect rates compared with the general population regardless of when therapy was started. Initial treatment regimen selection in pregnant women does not typically differ from nonpregnant women; however, elvitegravir-cobicistat is not recommended because levels are inadequate in the second and third trimesters, and bictegravir and TAF are not recommended until safety and pharmacokinetic data in pregnancy are available. Dolutegravir is not recommended in the first 8 weeks of pregnancy until more data are available regarding possible increased risk of neural tube defects.

### KEY POINTS

- Pregnant women should promptly initiate or continue receiving HIV treatment without interruption; previous concerns about teratogenicity of efavirenz and tenofovir disoproxil fumarate have been allayed by data showing no difference in birth defect rates compared with the general population.

- In pregnant women with HIV, bictegravir and tenofovir alafenamide are not recommended until safety and pharmacokinetic data in pregnancy are available; dolutegravir should be avoided in the first 8 weeks of pregnancy until more safety data are available.

# Viral Infections

## Influenza Viruses

### Overview

Three types of influenza viruses primarily infect humans: A, B, and C. Influenza A viruses are divided into subtypes based on two surface proteins, hemagglutinin (H) and neuraminidase (N). Influenza A viruses can infect animals and humans and produce epidemics and pandemics. Influenza B viruses only affect humans and cause yearly epidemics but not pandemics. Influenza C causes mild illness and does not cause epidemics.

Minor changes in the H and N surface envelope glycoproteins (*antigenic drift*) of influenza A and B viruses cause yearly epidemics, and major changes (*antigenic shift*) in influenza A after genetic recombination from animals cause global pandemics. The last influenza pandemic occurred in 2009 and

was caused by H1N1. Emerging subtypes of importance include H7N9, which circulates among poultry in China and can cause severe illness in humans; H5N1, which infects humans through close contact with infected poultry and can spread from person to person; and variants circulating in pigs that can sporadically infect humans.

### Clinical Features and Evaluation

During the winter, influenza A causes a self-limiting illness with fever, cough, rhinorrhea, myalgia, and headache in most patients; influenza B causes a milder illness. Older adults (>65 years), young children, pregnant women, and patients with chronic medical conditions (especially chronic lung disease) are at higher risk for severe primary influenza, complications such as superimposed bacterial pneumonia caused by *Streptococcus pneumoniae* or *Staphylococcus aureus*, and death (see Community-Acquired Pneumonia). Less common but severe complications include asthma or chronic obstructive pulmonary disease exacerbations, myocarditis, encephalitis, rhabdomyolysis, myositis, sepsis, and multiorgan failure. Parotitis caused by influenza was reported during the 2015-2016 influenza season.

During the endemic season, patients can be diagnosed within 20 minutes using either rapid antigen tests or polymerase chain reaction (PCR) testing of nasopharyngeal swabs. Both tests are highly specific, but PCR has a sensitivity of nearly 100%; the rapid antigen tests have a sensitivity between 59% and 93%. Starting antiviral therapy following a negative antigen test result is reasonable if clinical suspicion is high. Serologic assays are not used clinically. Testing should be performed in patients at risk for complications (for example, those older than 65 years, patients with chronic medical conditions, immunocompromised patients, pregnant and postpartum women, those with a BMI of 40 or more, and persons with neuromuscular disease) and in health care workers, if the result will influence clinical management (decisions on initiation of antiviral treatment, impact on other diagnostic testing, antibiotic treatment decisions, and infection control practices).

### KEY POINTS

- Older adults (>65 years), young children, pregnant women, and patients with chronic medical conditions (especially chronic lung disease) are at higher risk for severe primary influenza, superimposed bacterial pneumonia caused by *Streptococcus pneumoniae* or *Staphylococcus aureus*, and death.

- Rapid antigen and polymerase chain reaction (PCR) tests of nasopharyngeal swabs are highly specific for influenza, but PCR has a higher sensitivity and can identify the virus subtype.

### Management

Antiviral therapy should be started within 48 hours of symptom onset in patients with a positive PCR or rapid antigen test result to speed up recovery and decrease hospitalization rates and complications. Antiviral therapy should also be initiated

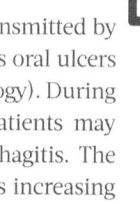
CONT.
as soon as possible in hospitalized patients because some observational studies have shown decreased adverse outcomes. Treatment initiation should not be delayed while waiting for the results of confirmatory testing.

Neuraminidase inhibitors are active against influenza A and B and can be given orally (oseltamivir), intranasally (zanamivir), or, more recently, intravenously (peramivir). Antiviral therapy is recommended for patients with severe disease, including all hospitalized patients, and those at high risk for complications with confirmed or suspected influenza infection. Antiviral therapy should be given for at least 5 days, but in severely ill or immunosuppressed patients, a longer duration should be considered with repeat follow-up testing to document clearance. Immunosuppressed patients are at risk for neuraminidase inhibitor resistance during or after therapy.

Widespread influenza vaccination is the most important preventive intervention; all persons aged 6 months or older without contraindications and all health care personnel should be vaccinated (see MKSAP 18 General Internal Medicine). Oral oseltamivir and inhaled zanamivir are FDA approved for chemoprophylaxis (zanamivir is not approved in patients with chronic lung diseases) to contain outbreaks in institutional settings (such as long-term care facilities) and hospitals in conjunction with droplet precautions and vaccination. Chemoprophylaxis is given for at least 2 weeks, continuing at least 1 week after the last identified infection. Good hand hygiene and face masks can prevent secondary infections in households.

### KEY POINTS

- Widespread influenza vaccination is the most important preventive intervention; all persons aged 6 months or older without contraindications and all health care personnel should be vaccinated.

- Antiviral therapy should be started within 48 hours of symptom onset but can be initiated up to 5 days after symptom onset in hospitalized patients; treatment should not be delayed while awaiting testing.

## Novel Coronaviruses

Coronaviruses are RNA viruses that cause respiratory and gastrointestinal diseases. Six known types infect humans, with some infecting animals as well. Two novel coronaviruses, severe acute respiratory syndrome–coronavirus (SARS-CoV) and Middle East respiratory syndrome–coronavirus (MERS-CoV), can infect animals and also cause severe disease and epidemics in humans. In 2002, SARS-CoV emerged in China, causing an acute pneumonia epidemic with a mortality rate of approximately 10%. No infections have been reported since 2004. Treatment is supportive. MERS-CoV emerged in 2012 in Saudi Arabia in humans and camels, with most infections occurring in the Arabian Peninsula. MERS-CoV causes pneumonia,

diarrhea, and kidney failure with a mortality rate of approximately 40%. Because all types of coronaviruses may spread from human to human, contact and airborne precautions should be implemented for hospitalized patients with suspected infection.

### KEY POINT

- Middle East respiratory syndrome–coronavirus infection occurs primarily in the Arabian Peninsula and can cause severe pneumonia with diarrhea, kidney failure, and death.

## Human Herpesvirus Infections

Human herpesviruses (HHVs) are a group of eight DNA viruses (Table 68). In humans, infection with HHV results in lifelong viral latency with the possibility of reactivation and oncogenesis. HHV can be transmitted by physical or sexual contact during active infection or through asymptomatic shedding of the virus (in saliva, semen, or cervical secretions); other routes include blood transfusion, organ transplantation, or maternofetal transmission. Varicella-zoster virus (VZV) is the only HHV that can be transmitted by the airborne route; it is also the only HHV with a vaccine that produces protective humoral immunity. Antivirals are available for some HHVs, and immunoglobulin therapy is available for cytomegalovirus and VZV.

### Herpes Simplex Virus Types 1 and 2

Herpes simplex virus (HSV) type 1 infection is transmitted by oral-oral or oral-genital contact. It typically causes oral ulcers and affects 90% of adults (see MKSAP 18 Dermatology). During stress, severe illness, or immunosuppression, patients may experience recurrence of oral stomatitis or esophagitis. The incidence of primary genital infection by HSV-1 is increasing (see Sexually Transmitted Infections). HSV-1 is the most common cause of viral encephalitis (see Central Nervous System Infections).

HSV-2 is sexually transmitted and typically causes genital and rectal ulcers with or without proctitis. HSV-2 affects approximately one sixth of adults in the United States and can also cause recurrent benign lymphocytic meningitis (Mollaret meningitis), myelitis, sacral radiculopathy, and neonatal infection or death (maternofetal transmission in primary genital infection). HSV-1 and HSV-2 can cause herpetic whitlow (on fingers), herpes gladiatorum (a skin infection typically associated with contact sports), keratoconjunctivitis, retinitis, and erythema multiforme.

HSV-1 and HSV-2 infections can be treated and suppressed with oral nucleoside analogues (acyclovir, valacyclovir, and famciclovir). Topical antiviral agents (trifluridine and vidarabine) are used for herpetic keratitis. Intravenous acyclovir is used for severe mucocutaneous disease, disseminated infections in immunosuppressed persons, esophagitis, and suspected HSV encephalitis.

**TABLE 68.** Human Herpesviruses and Associated Manifestations

| Type | Synonym | Subfamily | Manifestations | Latency Site |
|------|---------|-----------|----------------|--------------|
| HHV-1 | Herpes simplex virus 1 | α | Primary infection: oral and/or genital herpes (predominantly orofacial: gingivostomatitis, pharyngitis, herpes labialis)<br><br>Reactivation: Bell palsy, viral encephalitis; other sites, including skin and eye (recurrent herpes labialis) | Nerve ganglion |
| HHV-2 | Herpes simplex virus 2 | α | Primary infection: oral and/or genital herpes (predominantly genital); meningitis, sacral radiculopathy, and transverse myelitis | Nerve ganglion |
| HHV-3 | Varicella-zoster virus | α | Varicella (chickenpox), herpes zoster (shingles) | Nerve ganglion |
| HHV-4 | Epstein-Barr virus | γ | Infectious mononucleosis, nasopharyngeal carcinoma; in immunocompromised patients: Burkitt lymphoma, central nervous system lymphoma (in patients with AIDS), posttransplant lymphoproliferative disease, hairy leukoplakia | B cell |
| HHV-5 | CMV | β | CMV mononucleosis; in immunocompromised patients: CMV retinitis, leukopenia and thrombocytopenia, pneumonitis, colitis, esophagitis, or hepatitis | Monocyte, lymphocyte, endothelial cell, epithelial cell |
| HHV-6 (6A and 6B) | Roseolovirus, herpes lymphotropic virus | β | Mononucleosis-like syndrome, roseola (sixth disease, exanthema subitum) in children; may affect various organ systems in transplant patients | T cell |
| HHV-7 | Roseolovirus | β | Usually asymptomatic; may be associated with pityriasis rosea; roseola (sixth disease, exanthema subitum) in children | T cell |
| HHV-8 | Kaposi sarcoma-associated virus | γ | Kaposi sarcoma, PEL, multicentric Castleman disease | B cell, endothelial cell |

CMV = cytomegalovirus; HHV = human herpesvirus; PEL = primary effusion lymphoma.

**KEY POINTS**

- Herpes simplex virus (HSV) type 1 is the most common cause of viral encephalitis, and the incidence of primary genital infection caused by HSV-1 is increasing.

- Intravenous acyclovir is used for severe mucocutaneous herpes, disseminated infections in immunosuppressed persons, esophagitis, and suspected HSV encephalitis.

## Varicella-Zoster Virus

### Overview

VZV (HHV-3) is transmitted by inhalation and colonization of the respiratory tract, with subsequent viremic dissemination to skin, liver, spleen, and sensory ganglia (varicella, or chickenpox). VZV establishes latency in the ganglia and can later reactivate, causing herpes zoster (shingles), especially in adults older than 60 years or in immunosuppressed patients. Contact and airborne precautions should be used for all hospitalized patients with varicella, for patients with disseminated herpes zoster, and for those with dermatomal zoster who are immunosuppressed.

## Clinical Features and Diagnosis

Primary varicella infection (chickenpox) presents with a febrile pruritic vesicular rash affecting the skin and mucocutaneous surfaces (oropharynx, conjunctiva, genitals); the rash commonly begins on the face and trunk, then spreads to the extremities (centrifugal distribution). Lesions may comprise macules, papules, vesicles, and scabs in different stages of development. Skin lesions may become superinfected with *Streptococcus pyogenes* or *Staphylococcus aureus* (impetigo). Most children recover without sequelae, but adults may develop pneumonia, encephalitis, hepatitis, and cerebellar ataxia.

Herpes zoster typically causes a painful vesicular rash that follows a dermatomal distribution that does not cross the midline (see MKSAP 18 Dermatology). Young patients presenting with herpes zoster should be tested for HIV. Immunosuppressed patients can present with multiple dermatomes affected or with disseminated disease. Postherpetic neuralgia, defined as neuropathic pain lasting more than 1 month after resolution of the vesicular rash, is the most significant complication of herpes zoster. Other complications

CONT.

include herpes zoster ophthalmicus with visual loss, Ramsay-Hunt syndrome (vesicular rash in external ear associated with ipsilateral peripheral facial palsy and altered taste), pneumonia, hepatitis, and central nervous system complications such as meningitis, encephalitis, myelitis, and stroke caused by vasculitis (see Central Nervous System Infections).

Varicella or herpes zoster can be diagnosed clinically by the typical vesicular rash and confirmed with VZV PCR testing of the base of a vesicular lesion. VZV is underdiagnosed in the absence of a rash (zoster sine herpete); in such cases, cerebrospinal fluid serologic (VZV IgM and IgG) and PCR testing can be used to diagnose the infections.

## Management

 Antiviral therapy (acyclovir, valacyclovir, and famciclovir) speeds recovery and decreases the severity and duration of neuropathic pain if begun within 72 hours of VZV rash onset. Intravenous acyclovir should be used for immunosuppressed or hospitalized patients and those with neurologic involvement.

Vaccination is the most important preventive strategy (see MKSAP 18 General Internal Medicine). Postexposure prophylaxis should be provided to susceptible persons (VZV IgG negative): postexposure varicella vaccination is appropriate in immunocompetent persons, and varicella-zoster immune globulin should be used in immunocompromised adults and in pregnant women.

## Epstein-Barr Virus

Epstein-Barr virus (EBV) (HHV-4) is highly prevalent; serologic studies show evidence of previous EBV infection in almost all adults. It is most commonly transmitted by saliva and is the main cause of infectious mononucleosis in children and adolescents. Patients present with fever, severe fatigue, exudative pharyngitis, cervical and axillary lymphadenopathy, and splenomegaly. Atypical lymphocytosis and aminotransferase level

elevations are clues to the diagnosis, which is established by the presence of heterophile antibodies (Monospot test) or IgM to the EBV viral capsid antigen. The Monospot test result may be negative in the first week of illness. Treatment is supportive, with no role for acyclovir; glucocorticoids may be given to patients with autoimmune hemolytic anemia, central nervous system involvement, or tonsillar enlargement with a compromised airway. EBV is associated with the development of T-cell and B-cell lymphomas, Hodgkin and Burkitt lymphoma, nasopharyngeal carcinoma, and posttransplant lymphoproliferative disease in solid organ transplantation.

## Human Cytomegalovirus

Cytomegalovirus (HHV-5) infections are most commonly asymptomatic but may present with a mononucleosis-like syndrome without pharyngitis and with negative heterophile antibody results. Cytomegalovirus may be transmitted through the placenta (congenital cytomegalovirus), breastfeeding, saliva, blood transfusion, or organ transplantation (cytomegalovirus-positive donor to cytomegalovirus-seronegative recipient). Approximately 60% to 90% of adults have latent cytomegalovirus infection with reactivation of disease more common in immunosuppressed persons (those with AIDS, transplant recipients, those receiving glucocorticoid therapy). Cytomegalovirus can cause retinitis, pneumonitis, hepatitis, bone marrow suppression, colitis, esophagitis, and adrenalitis in immunocompromised persons. Immunocompetent patients occasionally also present with colitis.

Because cytomegalovirus can cause a myriad of clinical manifestations, a high index of clinical suspicion is important. Diagnosis is commonly confirmed with molecular tests, such as PCR testing of serum, bronchoalveolar lavage fluid, or cerebrospinal fluid, or by demonstrating typical cytopathic "owl's-eye" intracellular inclusions on biopsy specimens (Figure 25). Pathologic diagnosis is confirmed by cytomegalovirus immunostains. Serologic assays have limited diagnostic utility because most adults are seropositive; however, they are performed routinely in pretransplant evaluations to assess the risk of cytomegalovirus reactivation after transplantation and to determine appropriate prophylaxis.

Antiviral therapy with intravenous ganciclovir or oral valganciclovir is used in immunocompromised patients or in immunocompetent patients with severe disease. Oral valganciclovir is also used as prophylaxis or pre-emptive therapy (treat if the PCR serum testing result is positive) in transplant

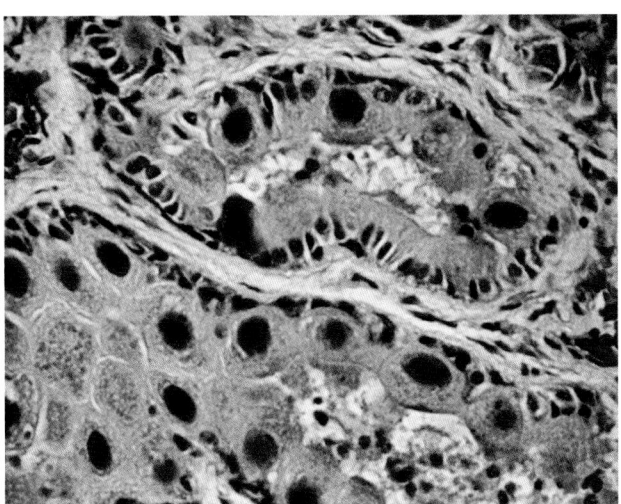

**FIGURE 25.** Under a magnification of 500X, a photomicrograph of a sample of kidney tissue reveals the presence of what are referred to as cytomegalic inclusion cells. With enlarged, darkly stained nuclei, such cells are also known as owl's-eye inclusion cells and are caused by cytomegalic inclusion disease resulting from cytomegalovirus.

CONT. recipients. Foscarnet and cidofovir can be used in instances of ganciclovir resistance or intolerance. **H**

**KEY POINTS**

- Serologic assays for cytomegalovirus have limited diagnostic utility because most adults are seropositive; however, they are performed routinely in pretransplant evaluations to assess the risk of cytomegalovirus reactivation following transplantation and to determine appropriate prophylaxis.

- Diagnosis of cytomegalovirus is confirmed with molecular tests of infected fluids, by demonstrating typical cytopathic "owl's-eye" intracellular inclusions on biopsy specimens, or by cytomegalovirus immunostaining of pathologic samples.

# Stewardship and Emerging Resistance

## Introduction

Emergence of antibiotic resistance is potentiated by all antibiotic use. Careful antibiotic use is essential to preserving the armamentarium. Among outpatient visits, 12.6% are associated with antibiotic prescriptions, and 30% of those prescriptions are considered inappropriate. Most prescriptions are for acute respiratory infections (usually caused by viruses) and asymptomatic bacteriuria not requiring antibiotic treatment. One fifth of emergency department visits for adverse drug events are related to antibiotics. Inpatient antibiotic use accounts for 38.5% of all antibiotic use; half of hospitalized patients receive antibiotics, and half of these medications are considered unnecessary or inappropriate. The World Health Organization has named carbapenem-resistant *Acinetobacter baumannii* and *Pseudomonas aeruginosa* and carbapenem-resistant and extended-spectrum β-lactamase (ESBL)–producing Enterobacteriaceae as priority-one pathogens, for which new antibiotics are critically needed.

## Antimicrobial Stewardship and the Value of Infectious Disease Consultation

Antibiotic stewardship refers to coordinated interventions to improve antibiotic use and clinical outcomes by promoting optimal antibiotic regimens. Goals include minimizing adverse events (5% risk per antibiotic per patient), risk of *Clostridium difficile* infection, and emergence of resistance. A key aspect of stewardship is avoiding antibiotic administration when not indicated. Antibiotic selection, dosing, therapy duration, and route of administration are also considered. Furthermore, antimicrobial stewardship programs include simplifying unnecessary combination therapy, avoiding redundant double anaerobic coverage, converting intravenous to oral agents, streamlining de-escalation, and minimizing duration of therapy.

Combination therapy does not prevent the emergence of resistance. However, it may be considered in specific circumstances, such as empiric therapy regimens, to broaden the spectrum of activity or provide coverage for potential antimicrobial-resistant organisms pending culture and susceptibility results. Antibiotic combination therapy may also provide synergistic activity in limited situations, such as enterococcal endocarditis and bacteremia caused by carbapenem-resistant Enterobacteriaceae (CRE).

Conversion from an intravenous to an oral antimicrobial **H** agent should be considered for ease of administration and to limit intravenous catheter access and use, thereby decreasing the risk of catheter-related bloodstream infection. Factors supporting readiness for conversion include a temperature of 38 °C (100.4 °F) or less, an improving leukocyte count, clinical stability and improvement of signs and symptoms related to infection, a functioning gastrointestinal tract and ability to swallow medications or having a nasogastric tube in place, no diagnostic indication for intravenous therapy (endocarditis, *Staphylococcus aureus* bacteremia), and availability of a suitable oral alternative with good oral bioavailability (fluoroquinolones, oxazolidinones, metronidazole, clindamycin, trimethoprim-sulfamethoxazole, fluconazole, doxycycline, voriconazole). **H**

Antimicrobial stewardship programs use various interventions to optimize antimicrobial use. Interventions that have been shown to be effective in improving outcomes, decreasing resistance, and decreasing costs include preauthorization and prospective audit with feedback to the

**TABLE 69.** Newer Antimicrobial Agents

| Agent | Class | Mechanism of Action | Route | Adverse Effects | Issues/Limitations | FDA Indications | Relative Cost |
|---|---|---|---|---|---|---|---|
| Ceftolozane-tazobactam | Antipseudomonal cephalosporin with β-lactamase inhibitor | Inhibits cell wall synthesis by binding to PBP; tazobactam irreversibly inhibits activity of many penicillinases and cephalosporinases | IV, every 8 hours | Similar to other cephalosporins | Reduced efficacy in patients with creatinine clearance ≤50 mL/min | Complicated intra-abdominal infections (combined with metronidazole); complicated urinary tract infections, including pyelonephritis. Active against many gram-negative organisms, including some ESBL-producing Enterobacteriaceae and multidrug-resistant *Pseudomonas aeruginosa*, including carbapenem-resistant strains | $$$ |
| Ceftaroline | Cephalosporin | Inhibits cell wall synthesis by high affinity binding to PBPs; high affinity for PBP2a that leads to activity against MRSA | IV, every 12 hours | Similar to other cephalosporins | Limited clinical experience for MRSA outside of skin infections | Community-acquired pneumonia (not caused by MRSA, clinical trial data lacking), ABSSSI caused by susceptible organisms (including MRSA) | $$ |
| Ceftazidime-avibactam | Third-generation cephalosporin with novel β-lactamase inhibitor | Inhibits cell wall synthesis by binding to PBP; avibactam inhibits broader range of β-lactamases than other available β-lactamase inhibitors | IV, every 8 hours | Similar to other cephalosporins | Approved on limited clinical safety and efficacy data. Reserve use for patients with limited or no alternative treatment options. Decreased efficacy in patients with baseline creatinine clearance between 30-50 mL/min. Monitor kidney function daily; adjust dose as needed | Complicated intra-abdominal infections (combined with metronidazole); complicated urinary tract infections, including pyelonephritis. Active against many multidrug-resistant gram-negative organisms, ESBL, and carbapenemases. Not active against metallo-β-lactamases or gram-negative organisms that overexpress efflux pumps or have porin mutations | $$$$$ |
| Dalbavancin | Lipoglycopeptide | Disrupts cell wall membrane synthesis | IV, once weekly | Nausea, headache, diarrhea, elevation of liver enzyme levels | Rapid IV infusion may cause flushing of the upper body, urticaria, pruritus, rash | ABSSSI caused by susceptible strains of gram-positive organisms (*Staphylococcus aureus* including MRSA, *Streptococcus pyogenes*, *Streptococcus agalactiae*, *Streptococcus anginosus* group) | $$$$ |

| | | | | | | |
|---|---|---|---|---|---|---|
| Delafloxacin | Fluoroquinolone | Acts on DNA gyrase and topoisomerase IV inhibiting DNA replication | IV, oral twice daily | Nausea, headache, diarrhea, aminotransferase elevation | Tendinitis, tendon rupture, peripheral neuropathy, central nervous system effects<br><br>Avoid coadministration of oral formulation with chelating agents, such as antacids | ABSSSI caused by susceptible gram-positive organisms, including MRSA<br><br>Has activity against gram-negative organisms, including *P. aeruginosa*<br><br>Studies ongoing for community-acquired pneumonia and complicated urinary tract infection | $$$ |
| Oritavancin | Lipoglycopeptide | Disrupts cell wall membrane synthesis, disrupts cell membrane integrity | IV, one dose | Headache, nausea, elevation of liver enzyme levels | Interaction with anticoagulation tests to monitor heparin; increases warfarin level by 30%, monitor patients for bleeding | ABSSSI caused by susceptible gram-positive organisms: *S. aureus* (MRSA and MSSA), *S. pyogenes, S. agalactiae, Streptococcus dysgalactiae, S. anginosus* group, and vancomycin-susceptible *Enterococcus faecalis* | $$$ |
| Tedizolid | Oxazolidinone | Disrupts bacterial protein synthesis initiation | IV, oral, once daily for 6 days | Nausea, headache, diarrhea | Patients taking selective serotonin reuptake inhibitors were excluded from clinical trials | ABSSSI caused by susceptible gram-positive organisms (MRSA, MSSA, linezolid-resistant *S. aureus, S. pyogenes, S. agalactiae, S. anginosus* group, *Streptococcus intermedius, Streptococcus constellatus, E. faecalis*) | $$ |
| Telavancin | Glycopeptide | Disrupts cell wall synthesis and function | IV, once daily | Nephrotoxicity | Interaction with coagulation tests to monitor heparin; may prolong QTc interval; decreased efficacy in pre-existing chronic kidney disease (eGFR <90 mL/min/1.73 m$^2$) | Complicated skin and soft tissue infections caused by susceptible organisms and *S. aureus* (including MRSA) hospital-acquired pneumonia | $$$ |

ABSSSI = acute bacterial skin and skin-structure infection; eGFR = estimated glomerular filtration rate; ESBL = extended-spectrum β-lactamase; IV = intravenous; MRSA = methicillin-resistant *Staphylococcus aureus*; MSSA = methicillin-sensitive *Staphylococcus aureus*; PBP = penicillin-binding protein.

prescriber, targeting antibiotics associated with a high risk of *C. difficile* infection (such as clindamycin, broad-spectrum antibiotics, and fluoroquinolones), using dedicated pharmacokinetic monitoring and adjustment programs, increasing the use of oral antimicrobial agents, and reducing antimicrobial therapy to the shortest effective duration.

**KEY POINT**

- Important components of antimicrobial stewardship programs include avoiding unnecessary antibiotic use, simplifying unnecessary combination therapy, avoiding double anaerobic coverage, converting intravenous to oral agents, streamlining de-escalation, and minimizing duration of therapy.

## Newer Antibacterial Drugs

Two newer cephalosporin antibiotics, ceftazidime-avibactam and ceftolozane-tazobactam, have enhanced activity against β-lactamase–producing organisms, particularly ESBLs, and against some carbapenemase-producing CRE. Three agents are available in the lipoglycopeptide class of antibiotics with activity against aerobic gram-positive organisms, such as *S. aureus* (including methicillin-resistant *S. aureus*), streptococci, and vancomycin-susceptible *Enterococcus faecalis*. Ceftaroline is a fifth-generation cephalosporin with a unique spectrum of activity that covers methicillin-resistant *S. aureus*. Delafloxacin is a new anionic fluoroquinolone with gram-positive (including methicillin-resistant *S. aureus*) and gram-negative activity (**Table 69**).

## Antibiotics for Antibiotic-Resistant Organisms

*Enterococcus faecium*, *S. aureus*, *Klebsiella pneumoniae*, *Acinetobacter* species, *Pseudomonas aeruginosa*, and *Enterobacter* species are particularly problematic antibiotic-resistant organisms. This group includes ESBL and carbapenemase-producing CRE (*Klebsiella pneumoniae* carbapenemases and New Delhi metallo-β-lactamase) that destroy carbapenems. Few effective antibiotics are available to treat infections with these pathogens. However, several older, less commonly used antibiotics retain their activity. Infectious disease consultation should be considered for infections with organisms in this group.

### Minocycline

Resurgence in the use of minocycline, available in intravenous and oral forms, is partly because of its activity against multidrug-resistant *Acinetobacter*. In vitro susceptibility to minocycline can be inferred from susceptibility to tetracycline; however, some tetracycline-resistant strains are sensitive to minocycline. Minocycline has been used to treat ventilator-associated pneumonia with an 80% clinical response rate and

is also useful for treating infections caused by *Stenotrophomonas maltophilia*, a problematic ICU pathogen with intrinsic antibiotic resistance. The adverse effects of minocycline are similar to those of tetracycline, including photosensitivity, gastrointestinal disturbance, and skin pigmentation changes with prolonged use.

**KEY POINT**

- Minocycline has activity against multidrug-resistant *Acinetobacter* and *Stenotrophomonas maltophilia*.

### Fosfomycin

Fosfomycin (available in the United States) is a bactericidal oral antibiotic with gram-negative and gram-positive activity (including methicillin-resistant *S. aureus* and vancomycin-resistant Enterobacteriaceae). It achieves high concentrations in the urine and may be used to treat cystitis caused by vancomycin-resistant Enterobacteriaceae and other multidrug-resistant uropathogens such as carbapenemase-producing *K. pneumoniae*.

**KEY POINT**

- Fosfomycin has gram-negative and gram-positive activity (including methicillin-resistant *S. aureus* and vancomycin-resistant Enterobacteriaceae) and achieves high concentrations in the urine, making it useful for treating cystitis.

### Colistin

Colistin (polymyxin E) is a bactericidal agent used to treat multidrug- and pan-resistant aerobic gram-negative infections, including *P. aeruginosa*. *Proteus*, *Providencia*, *Burkholderia*, *Morganella*, and *Serratia* species are resistant to colistin. Colistin resistance has been described in some multidrug-resistant gram-negative infections (mostly carbapenemase-producing *K. pneumoniae*), leading to completely untreatable infections. Colistin can be administered by nebulized aerosol or intravenously. The most common adverse effect is nephrotoxicity (up to 50% of patients), which is usually reversible.

**KEY POINT**

- Nephrotoxicity occurs in up to 50% of patients treated with colistin, although it is usually reversible.

## Outpatient Parenteral Antibiotic Therapy

Outpatient parenteral antibiotic therapy (OPAT) is defined as administration of at least two doses of intravenous antibiotics on different days without intervening hospitalization. Approximately 250,000 patients per year in the United States are treated with OPAT. OPAT allows patients to complete parenteral antibiotic therapy at home or in other outpatient settings when an oral antibiotic is not appropriate or available. Bone and joint infections compose most of the infections treated with OPAT; other candidates include endocarditis, cardiac device infections, abdominal infections, skin and soft tissue infections, and antibiotic-resistant infections for which parenteral antibiotics are the only option (such as urinary tract infection).

Patients should be clinically stable and their infection improving before starting OPAT; OPAT is not appropriate if the patient's care needs would be better met in the hospital. When considering OPAT, it is important to assess the type of infection being treated, the prescribed antibiotic and dosing frequency, the planned therapy duration, the administration site, the intravenous catheter type, and the monitoring process for possible complications. Increasingly, OPAT is being started without initial hospitalization after careful medical assessment by a well-established and organized OPAT program. OPAT requires close monitoring, including antibiotic levels (vancomycin, aminoglycosides), complete blood count, creatinine level, liver chemistry tests, and coagulation tests if relevant for the antibiotic; patients receiving daptomycin therapy in particular should undergo baseline measurement of kidney function and creatine kinase level, followed by weekly monitoring. Antibiotic doses and timing should be adjusted based on monitoring results. Treatment failure may result from relapse or progression of primary infection (60% and 21%, respectively) and therapeutic complications (19%). Successful OPAT requires patient participation; supervised infectious disease OPAT programs have been shown to be safe, efficient, and clinically effective.

## KEY POINT

- Bone and joint infections are the primary infections treated with outpatient parenteral antibiotic therapy (OPAT); other candidates for OPAT include serious infections (endocarditis, cardiac device infections, abdominal infections, and skin and soft tissue infections) and antibiotic-resistant infections for which parenteral antibiotics are the only option (such as urinary tract infection).

## Bibliography

### Central Nervous System Infections

Castelblanco RL, Lee M, Hasbun R. Epidemiology of bacterial meningitis in the USA from 1997 to 2010: a population-based observational study. Lancet Infect Dis. 2014;14:813-9. [PMID: 25104307] doi:10.1016/S1473-3099(14)70805-9

Hasbun R. Central nervous system device infections. Curr Infect Dis Rep. 2016;18:34. [PMID: 27686676] doi:10.1007/s11908-016-0541-x

Hasbun R, Rosenthal N, Balada-Llasat JM, Chung J, Duff S, Bozzette S, et al. Epidemiology of meningitis and encephalitis in the United States, 2011-2014. Clin Infect Dis. 2017;65:359-363. [PMID: 28419350] doi:10.1093/cid/cix319

McGill F, Heyderman RS, Michael BD, Defres S, Beeching NJ, Borrow R, et al. The UK joint specialist societies guideline on the diagnosis and management of acute meningitis and meningococcal sepsis in immunocompetent adults. J Infect. 2016;72:405-38. [PMID: 26845731] doi:10.1016/j.jinf.2016.01.007

Srihawan C, Castelblanco RL, Salazar L, Wootton SH, Aguilera E, Ostrosky-Zeichner L, et al. Clinical characteristics and predictors of adverse outcome in adult and pediatric patients with healthcare-associated ventriculitis and meningitis. Open Forum Infect Dis. 2016;3:ofw077. [PMID: 27419154] doi:10.1093/ofid/ofw077

Tunkel AR, Hasbun R, Bhimraj A, Byers K, Kaplan SL, Michael Scheld W, et al. 2017 Infectious Diseases Society of America's clinical practice guidelines for healthcare-associated ventriculitis and meningitis. Clin Infect Dis. 2017. [PMID: 28203777] doi:10.1093/cid/ciw861

van de Beek D, Brouwer M, Hasbun R, Koedel U, Whitney CG, Wijdicks E. Community-acquired bacterial meningitis. Nat Rev Dis Primers. 2016;2:16074. [PMID: 27808261] doi:10.1038/nrdp.2016.74

van de Beek D, Cabellos C, Dzupova O, Esposito S, Klein M, Kloek AT, et al; ESCMID Study Group for Infections of the Brain (ESGIB). ESCMID guideline: diagnosis and treatment of acute bacterial meningitis. Clin Microbiol Infect. 2016;22 Suppl 3:S37-62. [PMID: 27062097] doi:10.1016/j.cmi.2016.01.007

Venkatesan A, Tunkel AR, Bloch KC, Lauring AS, Sejvar J, Bitnun A, et al; International Encephalitis Consortium. Case definitions, diagnostic algorithms, and priorities in encephalitis: consensus statement of the international encephalitis consortium. Clin Infect Dis. 2013;57:1114-28. [PMID: 23861361] doi:10.1093/cid/cit458

Wang AY, Machicado JD, Khoury NT, Wootton SH, Salazar L, Hasbun R. Community-acquired meningitis in older adults: clinical features, etiology, and prognostic factors. J Am Geriatr Soc. 2014;62:2064-70. [PMID: 25370434] doi:10.1111/jgs.13110

### Prion Diseases of the Central Nervous System

Das AS, Zou WQ. Prions: beyond a single protein. Clin Microbiol Rev. 2016;29:633-58. [PMID: 27226089] doi:10.1128/CMR.00046-15

Geschwind MD. Prion diseases. Continuum (Minneap Minn). 2015;21:1612-38. [PMID: 26633779] doi:10.1212/CON.0000000000000251

Haïk S, Brandel JP. Infectious prion diseases in humans: cannibalism, iatrogenicity and zoonoses. Infect Genet Evol. 2014;26:303-12. [PMID: 24956437] doi:10.1016/j.meegid.2014.06.010

Kim MO, Geschwind MD. Clinical update of Jakob-Creutzfeldt disease. Curr Opin Neurol. 2015;28:302-10. [PMID: 25923128] doi:10.1097/WCO.0000000000000197

Knight R. Creutzfeldt-Jakob disease: a rare cause of dementia in elderly persons. Clin Infect Dis. 2006;43:340-6. [PMID: 16804850]

### Skin and Soft Tissue Infections

Bystritsky R, Chambers H. Cellulitis and soft tissue infections. Ann Intern Med. 2018;168:ITC17-ITC32. [PMID: 29404597] doi:10.7326/AITC201802060

Case definitions for infectious conditions under public health surveillance. Centers for Disease Control and Prevention. MMWR Recomm Rep. 1997;46:1-55. [PMID: 9148133]

Lipsky BA, Berendt AR, Cornia PB, Pile JC, Peters EJ, Armstrong DG, et al; Infectious Diseases Society of America. 2012 Infectious Diseases Society of America clinical practice guideline for the diagnosis and treatment of diabetic foot infections. Clin Infect Dis. 2012;54:e132-73. [PMID: 22619242] doi:10.1093/cid/cis346

Liu C, Bayer A, Cosgrove SE, Daum RS, Fridkin SK, Gorwitz RJ, et al; Infectious Diseases Society of America. Clinical practice guidelines by the Infectious Diseases Society of America for the treatment of methicillin-resistant Staphylococcus aureus infections in adults and children. Clin Infect Dis. 2011;52:e18-55. [PMID: 21208910] doi:10.1093/cid/ciq146

Poulakou G, Giannitsioti E, Tsiodras S. What is new in the management of skin and soft tissue infections in 2016? Curr Opin Infect Dis. 2017;30:158-171. [PMID: 28134678] doi:10.1097/QCO.0000000000000360

Stevens DL, Bisno AL, Chambers HF, Dellinger EP, Goldstein EJ, Gorbach SL, et al; Infectious Diseases Society of America. Practice guidelines for the diagnosis and management of skin and soft tissue infections: 2014 update by the Infectious Diseases Society of America. Clin Infect Dis. 2014;59:e10-52. [PMID: 24973422] doi:10.1093/cid/ciu444

Thomas KS, Crook AM, Nunn AJ, Foster KA, Mason JM, Chalmers JR, et al; U.K. Dermatology Clinical Trials Network's PATCH I Trial Team. Penicillin to prevent recurrent leg cellulitis. N Engl J Med. 2013;368:1695-703. [PMID: 23635049] doi:10.1056/NEJMoa1206300

Weng QY, Raff AB, Cohen JM, Gunasekera N, Okhovat JP, Vedak P, et al. Costs and consequences associated with misdiagnosed lower extremity cellulitis. JAMA Dermatol. 2016. [PMID: 27806170] doi:10.1001/jamadermatol.2016.3816

Wong CH, Khin LW, Heng KS, Tan KC, Low CO. The LRINEC (Laboratory Risk Indicator for Necrotizing Fasciitis) score: a tool for distinguishing necrotizing fasciitis from other soft tissue infections. Crit Care Med. 2004;32:1535-41. [PMID: 15241098]

# Bibliography

## Community-Acquired Pneumonia

Eliakim-Raz N, Robenshtok E, Shefet D, Gafter-Gvili A, Vidal L, Paul M, et al. Empiric antibiotic coverage of atypical pathogens for community-acquired pneumonia in hospitalized adults. Cochrane Database Syst Rev. 2012:CD004418. [PMID: 22972070] doi:10.1002/14651858.CD004418.pub4

Jain S, Self WH, Wunderink RG; CDC EPIC Study Team. Community-acquired pneumonia requiring hospitalization [Letter]. N Engl J Med. 2015;373:2382. [PMID: 26650159] doi:10.1056/NEJMc1511751

Kolditz M, Tesch F, Mocke L, Höffken G, Ewig S, Schmitt J. Burden and risk factors of ambulatory or hospitalized CAP: a population based cohort study. Respir Med. 2016;121:32–38. [PMID: 27888989] doi:10.1016/j.rmed.2016.10.015

Lee JS, Giesler DL, Gellad WF, Fine MJ. Antibiotic therapy for adults hospitalized with community-acquired pneumonia: a systematic review. JAMA. 2016;315:593–602. [PMID: 26864413] doi:10.1001/jama.2016.0115

Mandell LA, Wunderink RG, Anzueto A, Bartlett JG, Campbell GD, Dean NC, et al; Infectious Diseases Society of America. Infectious Diseases Society of America/American Thoracic Society consensus guidelines on the management of community-acquired pneumonia in adults. Clin Infect Dis. 2007;44 Suppl 2:S27-72. [PMID: 17278083]

Musher DM, Thorner AR. Community-acquired pneumonia. N Engl J Med. 2014;371:1619–28. [PMID: 25337751] doi:10.1056/NEJMra1312885

Postma DF, van Werkhoven CH, van Elden LJ, Thijsen SF, Hoepelman AI, Kluytmans JA, et al; CAP-START Study Group. Antibiotic treatment strategies for community-acquired pneumonia in adults. N Engl J Med. 2015;372:1312–23. [PMID: 25830421] doi:10.1056/NEJMoa1406330

Restrepo MI, Reyes LF, Anzueto A. Complication of community-acquired pneumonia (including cardiac complications). Semin Respir Crit Care Med. 2016;37:897–904. [PMID: 27960213]

Siemieniuk RA, Meade MO, Alonso-Coello P, Briel M, Evaniew N, Prasad M, et al. Corticosteroid therapy for patients hospitalized with community-acquired pneumonia: a systematic review and meta-analysis. Ann Intern Med. 2015;163:519–28. [PMID: 26258555] doi:10.7326/M15-0715

Tang KL, Eurich DT, Minhas-Sandhu JK, Marrie TJ, Majumdar SR. Incidence, correlates, and chest radiographic yield of new lung cancer diagnosis in 3398 patients with pneumonia. Arch Intern Med. 2011;171:1193-8. [PMID: 21518934] doi:10.1001/archinternmed.2011.15

## Tick-Borne Diseases

Biggs HM, Behravesh CB, Bradley KK, Dahlgren FS, Drexler NA, Dumler JS, et al. Diagnosis and management of tickborne rickettsial diseases: Rocky Mountain spotted fever and other spotted fever group rickettsioses, ehrlichioses, and anaplasmosis - United States. MMWR Recomm Rep. 2016;65:1-44. [PMID: 27172113] doi:10.15585/mmwr.rr6502a1

Goddard J. Not all erythema migrans lesions are Lyme disease. Am J Med. 2017;130:231–233. [PMID: 27612442] doi:10.1016/j.amjmed.2016.08.020

Hu LT. Lyme disease. Ann Intern Med. 2016;164:ITC65-ITC80. [PMID: 27136224] doi:10.7326/AITC201605030

Lantos PM. Chronic Lyme disease. Infect Dis Clin North Am. 2015;29:325–40. [PMID: 25999227] doi:10.1016/j.idc.2015.02.006

Moore A, Nelson C, Molins C, Mead P, Schriefer M. Current guidelines, common clinical pitfalls, and future directions for laboratory diagnosis of Lyme disease, United States. Emerg Infect Dis. 2016;22. [PMID: 27314832] doi:10.3201/eid2207.151694

Sanchez E, Vannier E, Wormser GP, Hu LT. Diagnosis, treatment, and prevention of Lyme disease, human granulocytic anaplasmosis, and babesiosis: a review. JAMA. 2016;315:1767–77. [PMID: 27115378] doi:10.1001/jama.2016.2884

Weitzner E, McKenna D, Nowakowski J, Scavarda C, Dornbush R, Bittker S, et al. Long-term assessment of post-treatment symptoms in patients with culture-confirmed early Lyme disease. Clin Infect Dis. 2015;61:1800–6. [PMID: 26385994] doi:10.1093/cid/civ735

## Urinary Tract Infections

Geerlings SE, Beerepoot MA, Prins JM. Prevention of recurrent urinary tract infections in women: antimicrobial and nonantimicrobial strategies. Infect Dis Clin North Am. 2014;28:135–47. [PMID: 24484580] doi:10.1016/j.idc.2013.10.001

Hooton TM. Clinical practice. Uncomplicated urinary tract infection. N Engl J Med. 2012;366:1028-37. [PMID: 22417256] doi:10.1056/NEJMcp1104429

Johnson JR, Russo TA. Acute pyelonephritis in adults. N Engl J Med. 2018;378:48–59. [PMID: 29298155]

Nicolle LE. Asymptomatic bacteriuria. Curr Opin Infect Dis. 2014;27:90–6. [PMID: 24275697] doi:10.1097/QCO.0000000000000019

Schaeffer AJ, Nicolle LE. Clinical practice. Urinary tract infections in older men. N Engl J Med. 2016;374:562-71. [PMID: 26863357] doi:10.1056/NEJMcp1503950

## *Mycobacterium tuberculosis* Infection

Horsburgh CR Jr, Barry CE 3rd, Lange C. Treatment of tuberculosis. N Engl J Med. 2015;373:2149-60. [PMID: 26605929] doi:10.1056/NEJMra1413919

Jamil SM, Oren E, Garrison GW, Srikanth S, Lewinsohn DM, Wilson KC, et al. Diagnosis of tuberculosis in adults and children. Ann Am Thorac Soc. 2017;14:275–278. [PMID: 28146376] doi:10.1513/AnnalsATS.201608-636CME

Lewinsohn DM, Leonard MK, LoBue PA, Cohn DL, Daley CL, Desmond E, et al. Official American Thoracic Society/Infectious Diseases Society of America/Centers for Disease Control and Prevention clinical practice guidelines: diagnosis of tuberculosis in adults and children. Clin Infect Dis. 2017;64:111-115. [PMID: 28052967] doi:10.1093/cid/ciw778

Nahid P, Dorman SE, Alipanah N, Barry PM, Brozek JL, Cattamanchi A, et al. Executive summary: official American Thoracic Society/Centers for Disease Control and Prevention/Infectious Diseases Society of America clinical practice guidelines: treatment of drug-susceptible tuberculosis. Clin Infect Dis. 2016;63:853–67. [PMID: 27621353] doi:10.1093/cid/ciw566

Pai M, Schito M. Tuberculosis diagnostics in 2015: landscape, priorities, needs, and prospects. J Infect Dis. 2015;211 Suppl 2:S21-8. [PMID: 25765103] doi:10.1093/infdis/jiu803

Salinas JL, Mindra G, Haddad MB, Pratt R, Price SF, Langer AJ. Leveling of tuberculosis incidence - United States, 2013-2015. MMWR Morb Mortal Wkly Rep. 2016;65:273-8. [PMID: 27010173] doi:10.15585/mmwr.mm6511a2

## Nontuberculous Mycobacterial Infections

Chand M, Lamagni T, Kranzer K, Hedge J, Moore G, Parks S, et al. Insidious risk of severe Mycobacterium chimaera infection in cardiac surgery patients. Clin Infect Dis. 2017;64:335–342. [PMID: 27927870] doi:10.1093/cid/ciw754

Griffith DE, Aksamit T, Brown-Elliott BA, Catanzaro A, Daley C, Gordin F, et al; ATS Mycobacterial Diseases Subcommittee. An official ATS/IDSA statement: diagnosis, treatment, and prevention of nontuberculous mycobacterial diseases. Am J Respir Crit Care Med. 2007;175:367–416. [PMID: 17277290]

Guglielmetti L, Mougari F, Lopes A, Raskine L, Cambau E. Human infections due to nontuberculous mycobacteria: the infectious diseases and clinical microbiology specialists' point of view. Future Microbiol. 2015;10:1467–83. [PMID: 26344005] doi:10.2217/fmb.15.64

Koh WJ, Jeong BH, Kim SY, Jeon K, Park KU, Jhun BW, et al. Mycobacterial characteristics and treatment outcomes in Mycobacterium abscessus lung disease. Clin Infect Dis. 2017;64:309–316. [PMID: 28011608] doi:10.1093/cid/ciw724

## Fungal Infections

Azie N, Neofytos D, Pfaller M, Meier-Kriesche HU, Quan SP, Horn D. The PATH (Prospective Antifungal Therapy) Alliance® registry and invasive fungal infections: update 2012. Diagn Microbiol Infect Dis. 2012;73:293–300. [PMID: 22789847] doi:10.1016/j.diagmicrobio.2012.06.012

Castillo CG, Kauffman CA, Miceli MH. Blastomycosis. Infect Dis Clin North Am. 2016;30:247–64. [PMID: 26739607] doi:10.1016/j.idc.2015.10.002

Farmakiotis D, Kontoyiannis DP. Mucormycoses. Infect Dis Clin North Am. 2016;30:143–63. [PMID: 26897065] doi:10.1016/j.idc.2015.10.011

Mahajan VK. Sporotrichosis: an overview and therapeutic options. Dermatol Res Pract. 2014;2014:272376. [PMID: 25614735] doi:10.1155/2014/272376

Maziarz EK, Perfect JR. Cryptococcosis. Infect Dis Clin North Am. 2016;30:179–206. [PMID: 26897067] doi:10.1016/j.idc.2015.10.006

McCarty TP, Pappas PG. Invasive candidiasis. Infect Dis Clin North Am. 2016;30:103–24. [PMID: 26739610] doi:10.1016/j.idc.2015.10.013

Pappas PG, Kauffman CA, Andes DR, Clancy CJ, Marr KA, Ostrosky-Zeichner L, et al. Executive summary: clinical practice guideline for the management of candidiasis: 2016 update by the Infectious Diseases Society of America. Clin Infect Dis. 2016;62:409–17. [PMID: 26810419] doi:10.1093/cid/civ1194

Patterson TF, Thompson GR 3rd, Denning DW, Fishman JA, Hadley S, Herbrecht R, et al. Executive summary: practice guidelines for the diagnosis and management of aspergillosis: 2016 update by the Infectious Diseases Society of America. Clin Infect Dis. 2016;63:433–42. [PMID: 27481947] doi:10.1093/cid/ciw444

Stockamp NW, Thompson GR 3rd. Coccidioidomycosis. Infect Dis Clin North Am. 2016;30:229–46. [PMID: 26739609] doi:10.1016/j.idc.2015.10.008

Wheat LJ, Azar MM, Bahr NC, Spec A, Relich RF, Hage C. Histoplasmosis. Infect Dis Clin North Am. 2016;30:207–27. [PMID: 26897068] doi:10.1016/j.idc.2015.10.009

**Sexually Transmitted Infections**

Bibbins-Domingo K, Grossman DC, Curry SJ, Davidson KW, Epling JW Jr, García FA, et al; US Preventive Services Task Force (USPSTF). Screening for syphilis infection in nonpregnant adults and adolescents: US Preventive Services Task Force Recommendation Statement. JAMA. 2016;315:2321-7. [PMID: 27272583] doi:10.1001/jama.2016.5824

Brunham RC, Gottlieb SL, Paavonen J. Pelvic inflammatory disease. N Engl J Med. 2015;372:2039-48. [PMID: 25992748] doi:10.1056/NEJMra1411426

Gnann JW Jr, Whitley RJ. Clinical practice. Genital herpes. N Engl J Med. 2016;375:666-74. [PMID: 27532832] doi:10.1056/NEJMcp1603178

Moi H, Blee K, Horner PJ. Management of non-gonococcal urethritis. BMC Infect Dis. 2015;15:294. [PMID: 26220178] doi:10.1186/s12879-015-1043-4

Stoner BP, Cohen SE. Lymphogranuloma venereum 2015: clinical presentation, diagnosis, and treatment. Clin Infect Dis. 2015;61 Suppl 8:S865-73. [PMID: 26602624] doi:10.1093/cid/civ756

Workowski KA, Bolan GA; Centers for Disease Control and Prevention. Sexually transmitted diseases treatment guidelines, 2015. MMWR Recomm Rep. 2015;64:1-137. [PMID: 26042815]

**Osteomyelitis**

American College of Radiology Appropriateness Criteria. Expert Panel on Musculoskeletal Imaging: suspected osteomyelitis, septic arthritis or soft tissue infection (excluding spine and diabetic foot) https://acsearch.acr.org/list (accessed 2/2/2017)

Berbari EF, Kanj SS, Kowalski TJ, Darouiche RO, Widmer AF, Schmitt SK, et al. 2015 Infectious Diseases Society of America (IDSA) clinical practice guidelines for the diagnosis and treatment of native vertebral osteomyelitis in adults. Clin Infect Dis. 2015;61:e26-46. [PMID: 26229122] doi:10.1093/cid/civ482

Choi SH, Sung H, Kim SH, Lee SO, Lee SH, Kim YS, et al. Usefulness of a direct 16S rRNA gene PCR assay of percutaneous biopsies or aspirates for etiological diagnosis of vertebral osteomyelitis. Diagn Microbiol Infect Dis. 2014;78:75-8. [PMID: 24231384] doi:10.1016/j.diagmicrobio.2013.10.007

Conterno LO, Turchi MD. Antibiotics for treating chronic osteomyelitis in adults. Cochrane Database Syst Rev. 2013:CD004439. [PMID: 24014191] doi:10.1002/14651858.CD004439.pub3

Grigoropoulou P, Eleftheriadou I, Jude EB, Tentolouris N. Diabetic foot infections: an update in diagnosis and management. Curr Diab Rep. 2017;17:3. [PMID: 28101794] doi:10.1007/s11892-017-0831-1

Lipsky BA, Berendt AR, Cornia PB, Pile JC, Peters EJ, Armstrong DG, et al; Infectious Diseases Society of America. 2012 Infectious Diseases Society of America clinical practice guideline for the diagnosis and treatment of diabetic foot infections. Clin Infect Dis. 2012;54:e132-73. [PMID: 22619242] doi:10.1093/cid/cis346

Mears SC, Edwards PK. Bone and joint infections in older adults. Clin Geriatr Med. 2016;32:555-70. [PMID: 27394023] doi:10.1016/j.cger.2016.02.003

**Fever of Unknown Origin**

Cunha BA, Lortholary O, Cunha CB. Fever of unknown origin: a clinical approach. Am J Med. 2015;128:1138.e1-1138.e15. [PMID: 26093175] doi:10.1016/j.amjmed.2015.06.001

**Primary Immunodeficiencies**

Abbott JK, Gelfand EW. Common variable immunodeficiency: diagnosis, management, and treatment. Immunol Allergy Clin North Am. 2015;35:637-58. [PMID: 26454311] doi:10.1016/j.iac.2015.07.009

Abolhassani H, Sagvand BT, Shokuhfar T, Mirminachi B, Rezaei N, Aghamohammadi A. A review on guidelines for management and treatment of common variable immunodeficiency. Expert Rev Clin Immunol. 2013;9:561-74; quiz 575. [PMID: 23730886] doi:10.1586/eci.13.30

Audemard-Verger A, Descloux E, Ponard D, Deroux A, Fantin B, Fieschi C, et al. Infections revealing complement deficiency in adults: a French nationwide study enrolling 41 patients. Medicine (Baltimore). 2016;95:e3548. [PMID: 27175654] doi:10.1097/MD.0000000000003548

Azar AE, Ballas ZK. Evaluation of the adult with suspected immunodeficiency. Am J Med. 2007;120:764-8. [PMID: 17765042]

Frazer-Abel A, Sepiashvili L, Mbughuni MM, Willrich MA. Overview of laboratory testing and clinical presentations of complement deficiencies and dysregulation. Adv Clin Chem. 2016;77:1-75. [PMID: 27717414] doi:10.1016/bs.acc.2016.06.001

**Bioterrorism**

Adalja AA, Toner E, Inglesby TV. Clinical management of potential bioterrorism-related conditions. N Engl J Med. 2015;372:954-62. [PMID: 25738671] doi:10.1056/NEJMra1409755

Breman JG, Henderson DA. Diagnosis and management of smallpox. N Engl J Med. 2002;346:1300-8. [PMID: 11923491]

Hendricks KA, Wright ME, Shadomy SV, Bradley JS, Morrow MG, Pavia AT, et al; Workgroup on Anthrax Clinical Guidelines. Centers for Disease Control and Prevention expert panel meetings on prevention and treatment of anthrax in adults. Emerg Infect Dis. 2014;20. [PMID: 24447897] doi:10.3201/eid2002.130687

McFee RB. Viral hemorrhagic fever viruses. Dis Mon. 2013;59:410-25. [PMID: 24314803] doi:10.1016/j.disamonth.2013.10.003

Prentice MB, Rahalison L. Plague. Lancet. 2007;369:1196-207. [PMID: 17416264]

Thomas LD, Schaffner W. Tularemia pneumonia. Infect Dis Clin North Am. 2010;24:43-55. [PMID: 20171544] doi:10.1016/j.idc.2009.10.012

Zhang JC, Sun L, Nie QH. Botulism, where are we now? Clin Toxicol (Phila). 2010;48:867-79. [PMID: 21171845] doi:10.3109/15563650.2010.535003

**Travel Medicine**

Delord M, Socolovschi C, Parola P. Rickettsioses and Q fever in travelers (2004-2013). Travel Med Infect Dis. 2014;12:443-58. [PMID: 25262433] doi:10.1016/j.tmaid.2014.08.006

Franco MP, Mulder M, Gilman RH, Smits HL. Human brucellosis. Lancet Infect Dis. 2007;7:775-86. [PMID: 18045560]

Freedman DO, Chen LH, Kozarsky PE. Medical considerations before international travel. N Engl J Med. 2016;375:247-60. [PMID: 27468061] doi:10.1056/NEJMra1508815

Giddings SL, Stevens AM, Leung DT. Traveler's diarrhea. Med Clin North Am. 2016;100:317-30. [PMID: 26900116] doi:10.1016/j.mcna.2015.08.017

Hahn WO, Pottinger PS. Malaria in the traveler: how to manage before departure and evaluate upon return. Med Clin North Am. 2016;100:289-302. [PMID: 26900114] doi:10.1016/j.mcna.2015.09.008

Patterson J, Sammon M, Garg M. Dengue, Zika and chikungunya: emerging arboviruses in the New World. West J Emerg Med. 2016;17:671-679. [PMID: 27833670]

Petersen LR, Jamieson DJ, Powers AM, Honein MA. Zika virus. N Engl J Med. 2016;374:1552-63. [PMID: 27028561] doi:10.1056/NEJMra1602113

Sanford CA, Jong EC. Immunizations. Med Clin North Am. 2016;100:247-59. [PMID: 26900111] doi:10.1016/j.mcna.2015.08.018

Suwannanee S, Luplertlop N. Dengue and Zika viruses: lessons learned from the similarities between these Aedes mosquito-vectored arboviruses. J Microbiol. 2017;55:81-89. [PMID: 28120186] doi:10.1007/s12275-017-6494-4

Weaver SC, Lecuit M. Chikungunya virus and the global spread of a mosquito-borne disease. N Engl J Med. 2015;372:1231-9. [PMID: 25806915] doi:10.1056/NEJMra1406035

**Infectious Gastrointestinal Syndromes**

Debast SB, Bauer MP, Kuijper EJ; European Society of Clinical Microbiology and Infectious Diseases. European Society of Clinical Microbiology and Infectious Diseases: update of the treatment guidance document for Clostridium difficile infection. Clin Microbiol Infect. 2014;20 Suppl 2:1-26. [PMID: 24118601] doi:10.1111/1469-0691.12418

DuPont HL. Acute infectious diarrhea in immunocompetent adults. N Engl J Med. 2014;370:1532-40. [PMID: 24738670] doi:10.1056/NEJMra1301069

McDonald LC, Gerding DN, Johnson S, Bakken JS, Carroll KC, Coffin SE, et al. Clinical practice guidelines for Clostridium difficile infection in adults and children: 2017 update by the Infectious Diseases Society of America (IDSA) and Society for Healthcare Epidemiology of America (SHEA). Clin Infect Dis. 2018 Feb 15. [Epub ahead of print] [PMID: 29462280] doi:10.1093/cid/cix1085.

Riddle MS, DuPont HL, Connor BA. ACG clinical guideline: diagnosis, treatment, and prevention of acute diarrheal infections in adults. Am J Gastroenterol. 2016;111:602-22. [PMID: 27068718] doi:10.1038/ajg.2016.126

Shane AL, Mody RK, Crump JA, Tarr PI, Steiner TS, Kotloff K, et al. 2017 Infectious Diseases Society of America clinical practice guidelines for the diagnosis and management of infectious diarrhea. Clin Infect Dis. 2017;65:e45-e80. [PMID: 29053792] doi:10.1093/cid/cix669

Surawicz CM, Brandt LJ, Binion DG, Ananthakrishnan AN, Curry SR, Gilligan PH, et al. Guidelines for diagnosis, treatment, and prevention of Clostridium difficile infections. Am J Gastroenterol. 2013;108:478-98; quiz 499. [PMID: 23439232] doi:10.1038/ajg.2013.4

**Infections in Transplant Recipients**

Ariza-Heredia EJ, Nesher L, Chemaly RF. Cytomegalovirus diseases after hematopoietic stem cell transplantation: a mini-review. Cancer Lett. 2014;342:1-8. [PMID: 24041869] doi:10.1016/j.canlet.2013.09.004

Fishman JA. From the classic concepts to modern practice. Clin Microbiol Infect. 2014;20 Suppl 7:4-9. [PMID: 24528498] doi:10.1111/1469-0691.12593

Fleming S, Yannakou CK, Haeusler GM, Clark J, Grigg A, Heath CH, et al. Consensus guidelines for antifungal prophylaxis in haematological malignancy and haemopoietic stem cell transplantation, 2014. Intern Med J. 2014;44:1283-97. [PMID: 25482741] doi:10.1111/imj.12595

Lumbreras C, Manuel O, Len O, ten Berge IJ, Sgarabotto D, Hirsch HH. Cytomegalovirus infection in solid organ transplant recipients. Clin Microbiol Infect. 2014;20 Suppl 7:19-26. [PMID: 26451404]

Rubin LG, Levin MJ, Ljungman P, Davies EG, Avery R, Tomblyn M, et al; Infectious Diseases Society of America. 2013 IDSA clinical practice guideline for vaccination of the immunocompromised host. Clin Infect Dis. 2014;58:309-18. [PMID: 24421306] doi:10.1093/cid/cit816

Ullmann AJ, Schmidt-Hieber M, Bertz H, Heinz WJ, Kiehl M, Krüger W, et al; Infectious Diseases Working Party of the German Society for Hematology and Medical Oncology (AGIHO/DGHO) and the DAG-KBT (German Working Group for Blood and Marrow Transplantation). Infectious diseases in allogeneic haematopoietic stem cell transplantation: prevention and prophylaxis strategy guidelines 2016. Ann Hematol. 2016;95:1435-55. [PMID: 27339055] doi:10.1007/s00277-016-2711-1

## Health Care–Associated Infections

Allegranzi B, Bischoff P, de Jonge S, Kubilay NZ, Zayed B, Gomes SM, et al; WHO Guidelines Development Group. New WHO recommendations on preoperative measures for surgical site infection prevention: an evidence-based global perspective. Lancet Infect Dis. 2016;16:e276-e287. [PMID: 27816413] doi:10.1016/S1473-3099(16)30398-X

Chenoweth CE, Saint S. Urinary tract infections. Infect Dis Clin North Am. 2016;30:869-885. [PMID: 27816141] doi:10.1016/j.idc.2016.07.007

Holland TL, Arnold C, Fowler VG Jr. Clinical management of Staphylococcus aureus bacteremia: a review. JAMA. 2014;312:1330-41. [PMID: 25268440] doi:10.1001/jama.2014.9743

Kalil AC, Metersky ML, Klompas M, Muscedere J, Sweeney DA, Palmer LB, et al. Management of adults with hospital-acquired and ventilator-associated pneumonia: 2016 clinical practice guidelines by the Infectious Diseases Society of America and the American Thoracic Society. Clin Infect Dis. 2016;63:e61-e111. [PMID: 27418577] doi:10.1093/cid/ciw353

Magill SS, Edwards JR, Bamberg W, Beldavs ZG, Dumyati G, Kainer MA, et al; Emerging Infections Program Healthcare-Associated Infections and Antimicrobial Use Prevalence Survey Team. Multistate point-prevalence survey of health care-associated infections. N Engl J Med. 2014;370:1198-208. [PMID: 24670166] doi:10.1056/NEJMoa1306801

Marston HD, Dixon DM, Knisely JM, Palmore TN, Fauci AS. Antimicrobial resistance. JAMA. 2016;316:1193-1204. [PMID: 27654605] doi:10.1001/jama.2016.11764

Meddings J, Saint S, Fowler KE, Gaies E, Hickner A, Krein SL, et al. The Ann Arbor criteria for appropriate urinary catheter use in hospitalized medical patients: results obtained by using the RAND/UCLA appropriateness method. Ann Intern Med. 2015;162:S1-34. [PMID: 25938928] doi:10.7326/M14-1304

Nuckols TK, Keeler E, Morton SC, Anderson L, Doyle B, Booth M, et al. Economic evaluation of quality improvement interventions for bloodstream infections related to central catheters: a systematic review. JAMA Intern Med. 2016;176:1843-1854. [PMID: 27757764] doi:10.1001/jamainternmed.2016.6610

Weiner LM, Fridkin SK, Aponte-Torres Z, Avery L, Coffin N, Dudeck MA, et al. Vital signs: preventing antibiotic-resistant infections in hospitals - United States, 2014. MMWR Morb Mortal Wkly Rep. 2016;65:235-41. [PMID: 26963489] doi:10.15585/mmwr.mm6509e1

Yokoe DS, Anderson DJ, Berenholtz SM, Calfee DP, Dubberke ER, Ellingson KD, et al. A compendium of strategies to prevent healthcare-associated infections in acute care hospitals: 2014 updates. Infect Control Hosp Epidemiol. 2014;35 Suppl 2:S21-31. [PMID: 25376067]

## HIV/AIDS

Brown TT, Hoy J, Borderi M, Guaraldi G, Renjifo B, Vescini F, et al. Recommendations for evaluation and management of bone disease in HIV. Clin Infect Dis. 2015;60:1242-51. [PMID: 25609682] doi:10.1093/cid/civ010

Centers for Disease Control and Prevention. Preexposure prophylaxis for the prevention of HIV infection in the United States—2014. A clinical practice guideline. Available at https://stacks.cdc.gov/view/cdc/23109.

Centers for Disease Control and Prevention. Updated guidelines for antiretroviral postexposure prophylaxis after sexual, injection drug use, or other nonoccupational exposure to HIV—United States, 2016. Available at https://stacks.cdc.gov/view/cdc/38856.

Centers for Disease Control and Prevention and Association of Public Health Laboratories. Laboratory testing for the diagnosis of HIV infection: updated recommendations. Available at http://dx.doi.org/10.15620/cdc.23447. Published June 27, 2014. Available at http://www.cdc.gov/hiv/testing/laboratorytests.html.

Günthard HF, Saag MS, Benson CA, del Rio C, Eron JJ, Gallant JE, et al. Antiretroviral drugs for treatment and prevention of HIV infection in adults: 2016 recommendations of the International Antiviral Society-USA Panel. JAMA. 2016;316:191-210. [PMID: 27404187] doi:10.1001/jama.2016.8900

Kay ES, Batey DS, Mugavero MJ. The HIV treatment cascade and care continuum: updates, goals, and recommendations for the future. AIDS Res Ther. 2016;13:35. [PMID: 27826353]

Lucas GM, Ross MJ, Stock PG, Shlipak MG, Wyatt CM, Gupta SK, et al; HIV Medicine Association of the Infectious Diseases Society of America. Clinical practice guideline for the management of chronic kidney disease in patients infected with HIV: 2014 update by the HIV Medicine Association of the Infectious Diseases Society of America. Clin Infect Dis. 2014;59:e96-138. [PMID: 25234519] doi:10.1093/cid/ciu617

Panel on Antiretroviral Guidelines for Adults and Adolescents. Guidelines for the use of antiretroviral agents in HIV-1-infected adults and adolescents. Department of Health and Human Services. Updated March 27, 2018. Available at https://aidsinfo.nih.gov/guidelines/html/1/adult-and-adolescent-arv/0

Panel on Opportunistic Infections in HIV-Infected Adults and Adolescents. Guidelines for the prevention and treatment of opportunistic infections in HIV-infected adults and adolescents: recommendations from the Centers for Disease Control and Prevention, the National Institutes of Health, and the HIV Medicine Association of the Infectious Diseases Society of America. Updated March 7, 2018. Available at https://aidsinfo.nih.gov/guidelines/html/4/adult-and-adolescent-opportunistic-infection/0

Panel on Treatment of HIV-Infected Pregnant Women and Prevention of Perinatal Transmission. Recommendations for use of antiretroviral drugs in pregnant HIV-1 infected women for maternal health and interventions to reduce perinatal HIV transmission in the United States. Updated March 27, 2018. Available at https://aidsinfo.nih.gov/guidelines/html/3/perinatal/0

Yarchoan R, Uldrick TS. HIV-associated cancers and related diseases. N Engl J Med. 2018;378:1029-1041. [PMID: 29539283] doi:10.1056/NEJMra1615896

## Viral Infections

Cohen JI. Clinical practice: Herpes zoster. N Engl J Med. 2013;369:255-63. [PMID: 23863052] doi:10.1056/NEJMcp1302674

Gnann JW Jr, Whitley RJ. Clinical practice. Genital herpes. N Engl J Med. 2016;375:666-74. [PMID: 27532832] doi:10.1056/NEJMcp1603178

Haagmans BL, Al Dhahiry SH, Reusken CB, Raj VS, Galiano M, Myers R, et al. Middle East respiratory syndrome coronavirus in dromedary camels: an outbreak investigation. Lancet Infect Dis. 2014;14:140-5. [PMID: 24355866] doi:10.1016/S1473-3099(13)70690-X

Harper SA, Bradley JS, Englund JA, File TM, Gravenstein S, Hayden FG, et al; Expert Panel of the Infectious Diseases Society of America. Seasonal influenza in adults and children—diagnosis, treatment, chemoprophylaxis, and institutional outbreak management: clinical practice guidelines of the Infectious Diseases Society of America. Clin Infect Dis. 2009;48:1003-32. [PMID: 19281331] doi:10.1086/598513

Paules C, Subbarao K. Influenza. Lancet. 2017. [PMID: 28302313] doi:10.1016/S0140-6736(17)30129-0

Zaki AM, van Boheemen S, Bestebroer TM, Osterhaus AD, Fouchier RA. Isolation of a novel coronavirus from a man with pneumonia in Saudi Arabia. N Engl J Med. 2012;367:1814-20. [PMID: 23075143] doi:10.1056/NEJMoa1211721

## Stewardship and Emerging Resistance

Barlam TF, Cosgrove SE, Abbo LM, MacDougall C, Schuetz AN, Septimus EJ, et al. Implementing an antibiotic stewardship program: guidelines by the Infectious Diseases Society of America and the Society for Healthcare Epidemiology of America. Clin Infect Dis. 2016;62:e51-77. [PMID: 27080992] doi:10.1093/cid/ciw118

Deak D, Outterson K, Powers JH, Kesselheim AS. Progress in the fight against multidrug-resistant bacteria? A review of U.S. Food and Drug Administration-approved antibiotics, 2010-2015. Ann Intern Med. 2016;165:363-72. [PMID: 27239977] doi:10.7326/M16-0291

Doi Y, Paterson DL. Carbapenemase-producing Enterobacteriaceae. Semin Respir Crit Care Med. 2015;36:74-84. [PMID: 25643272] doi:10.1055/s-0035-1544208

Petrak RM, Skorodin NC, Fliegelman RM, Hines DW, Chundi VV, Harting BP. Value and clinical impact of an infectious disease-supervised outpatient parenteral antibiotic therapy program. Open Forum Infect Dis. 2016; 3:ofw193. [PMID: 27807591]

Ritchie DJ, Garavaglia-Wilson A. A review of intravenous minocycline for treatment of multidrug-resistant Acinetobacter infections. Clin Infect Dis. 2014;59 Suppl 6:S374-80. [PMID: 25371513] doi:10.1093/cid/ciu613

Schmitt S, McQuillen DP, Nahass R, Martinelli L, Rubin M, Schwebke K, et al. Infectious diseases specialty intervention is associated with decreased mortality and lower healthcare costs. Clin Infect Dis. 2014;58:22-8. [PMID: 24072931] doi:10.1093/cid/cit610

# Infectious Disease Self-Assessment Test

This self-assessment test contains one-best-answer multiple-choice questions. Please read these directions carefully before answering the questions. Answers, critiques, and bibliographies immediately follow these multiple-choice questions. The American College of Physicians (ACP) is accredited by the Accreditation Council for Continuing Medical Education (ACCME) to provide continuing medical education for physicians.

The American College of Physicians designates MKSAP 18 Infectious Disease for a maximum of 25 *AMA PRA Category 1 Credits*™. Physicians should claim only the credit commensurate with the extent of their participation in the activity.

Successful completion of the CME activity, which includes participation in the evaluation component, enables the participant to earn up to 25 medical knowledge MOC points in the American Board of Internal Medicine's Maintenance of Certification (MOC) program. It is the CME activity provider's responsibility to submit participant completion information to ACCME for the purpose of granting MOC credit.

## Earn Instantaneous CME Credits or MOC Points Online

Print subscribers can enter their answers online to earn instantaneous CME credits or MOC points. You can submit your answers using online answer sheets that are provided at mksap.acponline.org, where a record of your MKSAP 18 credits will be available. To earn CME credits or to apply for MOC points, you need to answer all of the questions in a test and earn a score of at least 50% correct (number of correct answers divided by the total number of questions). Please note that if you are applying for MOC points, you must also enter your birth date and ABIM candidate number.

Take either of the following approaches:

- Use the printed answer sheet at the back of this book to record your answers. Go to mksap.acponline.org, access the appropriate online answer sheet, transcribe your answers, and submit your test for instantaneous CME credits or MOC points. There is no additional fee for this service.

- Go to mksap.acponline.org, access the appropriate online answer sheet, directly enter your answers, and submit your test for instantaneous CME credits or MOC points. There is no additional fee for this service.

## Earn CME Credits or MOC Points by Mail or Fax

Pay a $20 processing fee per answer sheet and submit the printed answer sheet at the back of this book by mail or fax, as instructed on the answer sheet. Make sure you calculate your score and enter your birth date and ABIM candidate number, and fax the answer sheet to 215-351-2799 or mail the answer sheet to Member and Customer Service, American College of Physicians, 190 N. Independence Mall West, Philadelphia, PA 19106-1572, using the courtesy envelope provided in your MKSAP 18 slipcase. You will need your 10-digit order number and 8-digit ACP ID number, which are printed on your packing slip. Please allow 4 to 6 weeks for your score report to be emailed back to you. Be sure to include your email address for a response.

If you do not have a 10-digit order number and 8-digit ACP ID number, or if you need help creating a username and password to access the MKSAP 18 online answer sheets, go to mksap.acponline.org or email custserv@acponline.org.

CME credits and MOC points are available from the publication date of December 31, 2018, until December 31, 2021. You may submit your answer sheet or enter your answers online at any time during this period.

# Directions

*Each of the numbered items is followed by lettered answers. Select the **ONE** lettered answer that is **BEST** in each case.*

## Item 1

A 68-year-old man is being evaluated for measures to decrease his risk of acquiring a surgical site infection; he is scheduled for coronary artery bypass graft surgery in 5 weeks for limiting chronic angina despite maximal medical therapy. Medical history includes chronic stable angina, hyperlipidemia, hypertension, and diabetes. Medications are low-dose aspirin, propranolol, isosorbide dinitrate, ranolazine, chlorthalidone, lisinopril, and atorvastatin.

On physical examination, blood pressure is 126/72 mm Hg; all other vital signs are normal. On cardiac examination, an $S_4$ is present. The remainder of the examination is noncontributory.

**Which of the following is the most appropriate measure to prevent surgical site infection?**

(A) Evaluate for *Staphylococcus aureus* nasal carriage
(B) Provide postoperative vancomycin prophylaxis for 7 days
(C) Provide preoperative vancomycin prophylaxis
(D) Shave patient's chest hair the morning of surgery

## Item 2

A 25-year-old man is evaluated in the emergency department for fever, productive cough, dyspnea, and pleuritic chest pain that began several days ago. He reports no other symptoms. Intravenous ceftriaxone and oral azithromycin are initiated, and he is hospitalized. Medical history is significant for a recent diagnosis of HIV infection, for which he began antiretroviral therapy 1 month ago. Other medications are lamivudine, abacavir, and dolutegravir.

On physical examination, temperature is 39.2 °C (102.6 °F), blood pressure is 136/84 mm Hg, pulse rate is 110/min, and respiration rate is 20/min. Oxygen saturation is 90% breathing ambient air. Cardiac examination is normal, and the lungs are clear bilaterally.

Laboratory studies at the time of HIV diagnosis showed a viral load of 95,420 copies/mL and CD4 cell count of 256/µL. The interferon-γ release assay for tuberculosis was indeterminate because of inadequate response to the positive control. One week ago, HIV viral load was 1077 copies/mL and CD4 cell count was 313/µL.

A chest radiograph shows an infiltrate in the right middle lobe and bilateral hilar enlargement.

Sputum acid-fast bacilli smear shows acid-fast bacilli; culture results are pending.

**Which of the following is the most appropriate management?**

(A) Await culture results
(B) Pause antiretroviral therapy
(C) Start prednisone
(D) Start rifabutin, isoniazid, ethambutol, and pyrazinamide

## Item 3

A 27-year-old man is evaluated in the hospital for a 1-month history of fever, drenching night sweats, malaise, fatigue, chest pain, and a nonproductive cough. He recently completed a 7-day course of levofloxacin with no improvement in symptoms. The patient is in the military, works as a car mechanic on base, and is stationed in Bakersfield, California.

On physical examination, temperature is 37.8 °C (100.0 °F), blood pressure is 128/76 mm Hg, pulse rate is 99/min, respiration rate is 24/min, and oxygen saturation is 92% with the patient breathing room air. The remainder of the physical examination is unremarkable.

**Laboratory studies:**

| | |
|---|---|
| Hemoglobin | 12.4 g/dL (124 g/L) |
| Leukocyte count | 11,900/µL ($11.9 \times 10^9$/L), with 30% eosinophils, 60% neutrophils, and 10% lymphocytes |
| Interferon-γ release assay | Negative |

A chest radiograph shows a right lower lobe infiltrate and ipsilateral hilar lymphadenopathy.

**Which of the following is the most likely diagnosis?**

(A) Coccidioidomycosis
(B) Sarcoidosis
(C) *Streptococcus pneumoniae* pneumonia
(D) Tuberculosis

## Item 4

A 44-year-old man is evaluated in the emergency department in January for a 3-day history of dyspnea, cough, and fever. Medical history is otherwise unremarkable, and he takes no medications.

On physical examination, temperature is 38.5 °C (101.3 °F), blood pressure is 118/80 mm Hg, pulse rate is 113/min, and respiration rate is 33/min. Oxygen saturation is 89% breathing 6 L/min oxygen by nasal cannula. The patient appears uncomfortable and is oriented only to person. Breath sounds are decreased bilaterally with scattered crackles. No rash is noted.

**Laboratory studies:**

| | |
|---|---|
| Leukocyte count | 19,000/µL ($19 \times 10^9$/L) |
| Platelet count | 274,000/µL ($274 \times 10^9$/L) |
| Blood urea nitrogen | 36 mg/dL (12.9 mmol/L) |
| Creatinine | 1.45 mg/dL (128 µmol/L) |

Sputum Gram stain shows 2+ polymorphonuclear cells and 1+ epithelial cells; no organisms are seen. A respiratory viral panel from a nasopharyngeal swab is positive for rhinovirus.

A chest radiograph is shown on the next page.

The patient will be transferred to the ICU.

**Which of the following is the most appropriate treatment?**

(A) Azithromycin
(B) Ceftazidime plus azithromycin
(C) Ceftriaxone plus levofloxacin
(D) Piperacillin–tazobactam plus ciprofloxacin

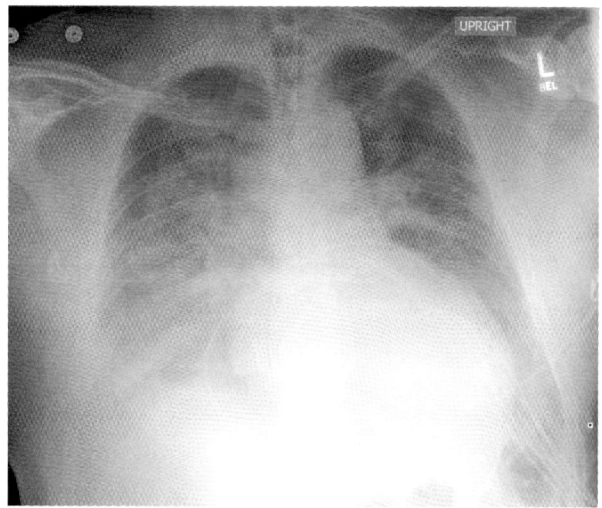

ITEM 4

## Item 5

A 43-year-old man is seen in follow-up for fever up to 38.3 °C (101 °F) occurring periodically over the past 3 months. He has no associated symptoms other than fatigue. He reports no recent travel, animal exposures, or tick or insect bites. He does not eat raw meats, raw seafood, or unpasteurized dairy products. He returns for further evaluation after initial testing. Family history is negative for undiagnosed fevers. He takes no medications.

On physical examination, temperature is 37.8 °C (100.1 °F), blood pressure is 114/72 mm Hg, pulse rate is 88/min, and respiration rate is 14/min. A complete physical examination is unremarkable.

**Laboratory studies:**

| | |
|---|---|
| Erythrocyte sedimentation rate | 10 mm/h |
| Hematocrit | 44% |
| Leukocyte count | 4200/µL ($4.2 \times 10^9$/L) with a normal differential |
| Platelet count | 320,000/µL ($320 \times 10^9$/L) |
| Alkaline phosphatase | Normal |
| Lactate dehydrogenase | Normal |
| Kidney and liver chemistry tests | Normal |
| Urinalysis | Normal |

HIV testing is negative. An interferon-γ release assay for tuberculosis is negative. Three sets of blood cultures are negative.

A chest radiograph is normal.

**Which of the following is the most appropriate diagnostic test to perform next?**

(A) Bone marrow biopsy
(B) CT of the abdomen and pelvis
(C) Liver biopsy
(D) Lumbar puncture

##  Item 6

A 34-year-old woman is evaluated in the emergency department for a 2-day history of fever, severe headache, malaise,

fatigue, dry cough, and shortness of breath. She underwent deceased-donor kidney transplantation 1 year ago; 2 weeks ago, she developed acute graft rejection and was treated with alemtuzumab. Other medications are tacrolimus, prednisone, and trimethoprim-sulfamethoxazole.

On physical examination, temperature is 37.5 °C (99.5 °F), blood pressure is 80/53 mm Hg, pulse rate is 90/min, and respiration rate is 22/min. Bibasilar crackles are heard on auscultation of the lungs.

Initial laboratory studies show a hemoglobin level of 6.9 mg/dL (69 g/L) and a leukocyte count of 4800/µL ($4.8 \times 10^9$/L).

A head CT scan shows multiple acute infarcts in the frontal lobe and cerebellum without superimposed hematomas. A lumbar puncture is performed.

**Cerebrospinal fluid studies:**

| | |
|---|---|
| Cell count | 2 erythrocytes/hpf; 77 leukocytes/hpf, with 90% neutrophils and 10% lymphocytes |
| Glucose | 80 mg/dL (4.4 mmol/L) |
| Pressure (opening) | 140 mm $H_2O$ |
| Protein | 100 mg/dL (1000 mg/L) |
| Cryptococcal antigen | Negative |
| Gram stain | No organisms |

A chest radiograph shows diffuse bilateral lung nodules.

**Which of the following is the most appropriate next diagnostic test?**

(A) Brain biopsy
(B) Bronchoscopy with biopsy and bronchoalveolar lavage
(C) Fungal blood culture
(D) Serum galactomannan assay

## Item 7

A 19-year-old woman is evaluated in the emergency department for a 2-day history of fever, headaches, and jaundice. She vacationed in Hawaii 1 month ago and reports swimming in lakes and rivers. She was diagnosed with a flu-like illness 2 weeks ago that resolved spontaneously. She reports no history of a rash. She is sexually active with one partner. She takes no medications other than an oral contraceptive.

On physical examination, she is alert and oriented. Temperature is 38.9 °C (102 °F), blood pressure is 92/60 mm Hg, pulse rate is 124/min, and respiration rate is 24/min. Generalized lymphadenopathy, conjunctival suffusion, and scleral icterus are noted. She has photophobia, and passive neck flexion elicits resistance and discomfort. The remainder of the examination is unremarkable.

**Laboratory studies:**

| | |
|---|---|
| Bilirubin, total | 5.6 mg/dL (95.8 µmol/L) |
| Creatinine | 2.3 mg/dL (203 µmol/L) |
| Cerebrospinal fluid | |
|    Leukocyte count | 152/µL ($152 \times 10^6$/L) |
|    Glucose | 72 mg/dL (4.0 mmol/L) |
|    Protein | 78 mg/dL (780 mg/L) |

Cerebrospinal fluid Gram stain is negative and culture results are pending.

**Which of the following is the most likely cause of the patient's findings?**

CONT.

(A) Acute retroviral syndrome

(B) Herpes simplex virus infection

(C) Leptospirosis

(D) Neurosyphilis

## Item 8

A 66-year-old woman is evaluated in the emergency department with a 2-day history of fever and nonbloody diarrhea occurring several times a day. She recently completed a 10-day course of cephalexin for cellulitis of the leg.

On physical examination, temperature is 39.0 °C (102.2 °F), blood pressure is 98/60 mm Hg, pulse rate is 110/min, and respiration rate is 23/min. She appears uncomfortable but is not confused. Her abdomen is distended and bowel sounds are decreased. She has tenderness and abdominal guarding to palpation. Cellulitis has resolved.

**Laboratory studies:**

| | |
|---|---|
| Leukocyte count | 30,000/µL (30 × 10⁹/L) (with 80% neutrophils, 15% band forms, and 5% lymphocytes) |
| Albumin | 2.5 mg/dL (25 g/L) |
| Creatinine | 2.5 mg/dL (221 µmol/L) (baseline 1.0 mg/dL [88.4 µmol/L]) |
| Lactate | 2.8 mEq/L (2.8 mmol/L) |

Stool polymerase chain reaction assay is positive for *Clostridium difficile* toxin gene. Abdominal imaging reveals evidence of toxic megacolon.

The patient is admitted to the ICU, and a surgical consultation is requested.

**Which of the following is the most appropriate medical treatment?**

(A) Fecal microbiota transplant

(B) Oral metronidazole

(C) Oral vancomycin

(D) Oral vancomycin and intravenous metronidazole

(E) Oral vancomycin and oral metronidazole

## Item 9

A 44-year-old woman is evaluated for persistent fatigue, headache, myalgia, and arthralgia. Early localized Lyme disease was diagnosed 2 months ago after the patient returned from a camping trip in western New Jersey with the symptoms described and a skin eruption of erythema migrans. She was treated with a 14-day course of doxycycline with resolution of the cutaneous lesions but continuation of the other symptoms, which now are adversely affecting her work and personal life. Her only medication is ibuprofen.

On physical examination, vital signs are normal. The patient has full range of motion of the joints. No skin lesions, synovitis, or effusions are noted.

Results of laboratory studies, including a complete blood count, comprehensive metabolic panel, and lactate dehydrogenase measurement, are all within normal limits.

**Which of the following is the most likely diagnosis?**

(A) Anaplasmosis

(B) Babesiosis

(C) Late-stage Lyme disease

(D) Post–Lyme disease syndrome

(E) Powassan virus infection

## Item 10

A 67-year-old man is evaluated for a chronic, nonhealing ulcer on his left foot of 3 months' duration. The patient states he was at a local sauna when he sustained an abrasion to the bottom of his foot after stepping on a sharp object. He subsequently developed an ulcer at the site of the injury and received several courses of antibiotics, including trimethoprim-sulfamethoxazole, doxycycline, and cephalexin, with no improvement. The ulcer continues to expand in size and deepen. Medical history is notable for hypertension and a 40-pack-year smoking history. His only medication is hydrochlorothiazide.

On physical examination, the vital signs are normal except for a temperature of 37.3 °C (99.2 °F). The legs and feet are without edema or discoloration. Pedal and popliteal pulses are symmetrical and intact. Lower extremity sensation is intact. He has a 2- × 2-cm ulcerated lesion on the plantar aspect of the metatarsal region of the great toe, with surrounding erythema, yellowish discharge, and firm edges.

**Which of the following is the most likely cause of his ulcer?**

(A) *Mycobacterium avium*

(B) *Mycobacterium fortuitum*

(C) *Mycobacterium kansasii*

(D) *Mycobacterium leprae*

## Item 11

A 26-year-old woman is evaluated in the emergency department for lower abdominal pain with vaginal discharge. She reports no nausea or vomiting but noted vaginal bleeding after intercourse the previous night. She is sexually active, with two partners in the past 3 months, but she does not use condoms consistently. She has an intrauterine device for contraception and takes no medications.

On physical examination, vital signs are normal. Pelvic examination is shown; uterine and cervical motion tenderness are noted, but she has no adnexal tenderness or masses.

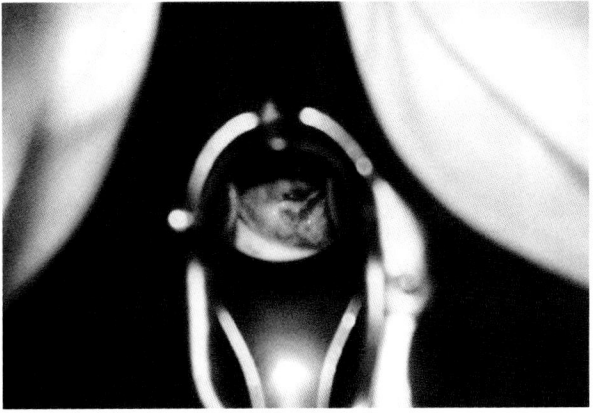

A urine pregnancy test is negative. Samples are obtained for nucleic acid amplification testing for *Neisseria gonorrhoeae* and *Chlamydia trachomatis*.

**Which of the following is the most appropriate empiric treatment?**

(A) Intramuscular ceftriaxone plus oral doxycycline
(B) Intravenous cefoxitin plus oral doxycycline
(C) Intravenous clindamycin plus intravenous gentamicin
(D) Oral amoxicillin-clavulanate plus oral doxycycline

## Item 12

A 72-year-old man undergoes preprocedural evaluation. He is scheduled to undergo cystoscopy and possible biopsy in follow-up for a previously diagnosed non–muscle invasive bladder cancer followed by an elective right total hip arthroplasty for chronic hip pain. He is otherwise asymptomatic. Medical history is significant for diabetes mellitus, hypertension, kidney transplantation, and osteoarthritis. Medications are metformin, amlodipine, pravastatin, prednisone, and tacrolimus.

On physical examination, vital signs are normal. External rotation of the right hip elicits pain. The examination is otherwise normal.

On microscopic urinalysis, leukocyte count is 20 to 40/hpf, erythrocyte count is 0 to 1/hpf, 2+ bacteria are present, and no squamous epithelial cells are seen. Urine culture grew 10,000 to 50,000 colony-forming units of *Proteus mirabilis*.

Kidney ultrasonography is unremarkable.

**Which of the following is the primary indication for antimicrobial therapy in this patient?**

(A) Cystoscopy and biopsy
(B) Diabetes mellitus
(C) Kidney transplant
(D) Total hip arthroplasty

## Item 13

A 33-year-old woman is evaluated after sustaining a needle-stick puncture in an infusion clinic, where she works as a nurse. The needle was being placed for intravenous therapy and had blood on it; it is from a patient at the clinic who is known to have HIV infection and is taking antiretrovirals, but the recent viral load is unknown. The nurse has already cleaned her wound. Medical history is unremarkable, and she takes no medications.

On physical examination, vital signs are normal, and other examination findings are noncontributory.

**Which of the following is the most appropriate immediate management?**

(A) Begin tenofovir and emtricitabine
(B) Begin tenofovir, emtricitabine, and dolutegravir
(C) Begin tenofovir, emtricitabine, and ritonavir-boosted darunavir
(D) Determine source patient's viral load

## Item 14

A 38-year-old woman undergoes follow-up evaluation in the office. She was evaluated in the emergency department 3 nights ago with fever and flank pain following 2 days of dysuria. A urine culture and two sets of blood cultures were collected. She was given intravenous ceftriaxone and discharged with a 7-day course of ciprofloxacin. She is now asymptomatic. Medications are ciprofloxacin and an oral contraceptive.

On physical examination, vital signs and other findings are normal.

*Escherichia coli* susceptible to ciprofloxacin was isolated from her urine culture and one blood culture.

**Which of the following is the most appropriate management?**

(A) Completion of oral ciprofloxacin course
(B) Completion of oral ciprofloxacin course with follow-up blood cultures
(C) Extended oral ciprofloxacin therapy for 2 weeks
(D) Intravenous ceftriaxone
(E) Kidney ultrasonography

## Item 15

A 25-year-old woman is evaluated for chronic intermittent nonbloody diarrhea with associated abdominal cramping, burping, and bloating. Symptoms began several months ago. She has a history of selective IgA deficiency with recurrent sinopulmonary infections. She has not taken antibiotics in the past 6 months.

On physical examination, temperature is 37.3 °C (99.1 °F); the vital signs are otherwise normal. On abdominal examination, bowel sounds are present with minimal diffuse tenderness to palpation.

Stool testing for occult blood is negative.

**Which of the following is the most likely cause of this patient's diarrheal illness?**

(A) *Clostridium difficile*
(B) Enterohemorrhagic *Escherichia coli*
(C) *Giardia lamblia*
(D) *Listeria monocytogenes*
(E) Nontyphoidal *Salmonella*

## Item 16

A 28-year-old woman arrives to discuss possible recent exposure to Zika virus. She is pregnant, at 8 weeks' gestation, and feels well. Her husband returned home from Brazil 4 weeks ago; while away, he experienced a 5-day febrile illness, which was accompanied by a faint rash, headache, and myalgias, all of which resolved before he arrived home. After his return, they engaged in unprotected sexual intercourse. Her only medication is a prenatal vitamin.

On physical examination, vital signs are normal, and other examination findings are unremarkable.

**Which of the following is the most appropriate test to perform next?**

(A) Dengue virus IgM and IgG antibodies test
(B) Uterine ultrasonography every 3 weeks

(C) Zika virus IgM antibody test

(D) Zika virus RNA nucleic acid amplification test

## Item 17

A 72-year-old woman is evaluated for a 2-day history of left facial droop and severe burning and stinging pain on the left ear helix and into the ear canal, with muffled hearing and tinnitus. She received the live-attenuated zoster vaccine at age 60 years. She takes no medications.

On physical examination, vital signs are normal. She has a left-sided peripheral facial droop. The tympanic membrane appears normal. No rash is present. Hearing is diminished to a whisper in the left ear. The remainder of the examination is unremarkable.

**Which of the following is the most likely cause of this patient's findings?**

(A) *Borrelia burgdorferi*

(B) Herpes simplex virus type 1

(C) Herpes simplex virus type 2

(D) Varicella-zoster virus

## Item 18

A 45-year-old man is evaluated for a 3-day history of fever, myalgia, headache, and nonproductive cough. He works as a large-animal veterinarian. Medical history is unremarkable, and he takes no medications.

On physical examination, vital signs are normal except for a temperature of 38.2 °C (100.8 °F). Oxygen saturation is 94% breathing ambient air. The examination is otherwise unremarkable.

A chest radiograph shows a patchy right lower lobe interstitial infiltrate.

**Which of the following is the most likely cause of his illness?**

(A) *Bacillus anthracis*

(B) *Coxiella burnetii*

(C) *Chlamydia psittaci*

(D) *Francisella tularensis*

(E) *Yersinia pestis*

## Item 19

A 46-year-old woman is evaluated for new-onset fever and discomfort at the site of a peripherally inserted central catheter (PICC). She was hospitalized for acute pancreatitis and required the PICC for intravenous access and hydration.

On physical examination, temperature is 37.8 °C (100.1 °F), and the remaining vital signs are normal. Right brachial PICC line site is tender, without erythema. Cardiac examination is without murmurs.

Two sets of peripheral blood cultures are obtained, showing gram-positive cocci and clusters. Both sets of blood cultures are growing coagulase-negative *Staphylococcus* resistant to methicillin. Vancomycin is initiated.

**Which of the following is the most appropriate additional management?**

(A) Maintain PICC line and continue vancomycin for 4 weeks

(B) Maintain PICC line and perform transesophageal echocardiography

(C) Remove PICC line

(D) Remove PICC line and repeat blood cultures

## Item 20

A 39-year-old man is evaluated in the hospital after a motorcycle accident that necessitated an open reduction and internal fixation of a femur fracture. During the emergency department evaluation, an indwelling urinary catheter was placed. Medical history is noncontributory, and he takes no medications.

On physical examination, he is alert and oriented. Vital signs are normal. The left leg is tender, with a sterile dressing over the incision.

**Which of the following is the most appropriate urinary catheter management?**

(A) Change catheter to an antimicrobial or antiseptic-coated catheter

(B) Initiate prophylactic antibiotics

(C) Maintain catheter placement until patient is ambulatory

(D) Remove catheter and observe for spontaneous voiding

## Item 21

A 50-year-old woman is evaluated in the emergency department for fever and tenderness at the site of a cat bite sustained on the dorsum of her right hand 2 days ago. She indicates that she works at an animal shelter. Medical history is significant for a methicillin-resistant *Staphylococcus aureus* skin infection 6 months ago; she is up to date on all vaccinations, including rabies and tetanus. She takes no medications.

On physical examination, temperature is 38.5 °C (101.3 °F), blood pressure is 98/66 mm Hg, pulse rate is 110/min, and respiration rate is 22/min. A tender puncture wound is noted on the dorsum of the right hand; it is warm and surrounded by significant erythema. Some purulent discharge is noted from the wound.

Blood cultures are obtained.

A plain radiograph of the right hand shows no evidence of gas, foreign body, or bony involvement.

**In addition to surgical consultation, which of the following antibiotic regimens is the most appropriate treatment at this time?**

(A) Ampicillin-sulbactam plus vancomycin

(B) Ceftriaxone plus metronidazole

(C) Ciprofloxacin plus aztreonam

(D) Imipenem

(E) Vancomycin and clindamycin

## Item 22

A 42-year-old man is evaluated for headache and progressive weakness. He was hospitalized yesterday with a 9-day history of fever, headache, and myalgia. He is a trail runner, and 10 days ago participated in a 10-kilometer race in North Carolina. He is not aware of any tick bite.

On physical examination, the patient appears ill. Temperature is 39.4 °C (102.9 °F), blood pressure is 102/78 mm Hg, pulse rate is 102/min, and respiration rate is 24/min. No tonsillar enlargement, cervical lymphadenopathy, hepatosplenomegaly, or skin lesion is noted.

### Laboratory studies:

| | |
|---|---|
| Leukocyte count | 1500/µL (1.5 × 10⁹/L), with 70% neutrophils and no atypical lymphocytes |
| Platelet count | 34,000/µL (34 × 10⁹/L) |
| Alanine aminotransferase | 667 U/L |
| Aspartate aminotransferase | 995 U/L |

Empiric doxycycline therapy is initiated for a possible tick-borne infection. Within 24 hours, he defervesces, and within 48 hours, the leukocyte and platelet counts normalize. Serologic tests for *Rickettsia rickettsii* and *Ehrlichia chaffeensis* obtained on admission have negative results.

**Which of the following is the most likely diagnosis?**

(A) Heartland virus infection
(B) Human monocytic ehrlichiosis
(C) Infectious mononucleosis
(D) Rocky Mountain spotted fever

## Item 23

A 32-year-old man is evaluated in the hospital for a 4-day history of fever and leukocytosis that began 1 week after cranial surgery and a 1-day history of worsening mental status. He experienced traumatic intracranial hemorrhage requiring a craniotomy for drainage and placement of an external ventricular drain. He remains intubated with mechanical ventilation. Medications are empiric vancomycin and cefepime, initiated 4 days ago.

On physical examination, temperature is 39.2 °C (102.5 °F), blood pressure is 108/62 mm Hg, pulse rate is 102/min, and respiration rate is 20/min. He was previously awake and able to follow simple commands, but now he is obtunded. Nuchal rigidity is noted. Other examination findings are unremarkable.

Cerebrospinal fluid (CSF) evaluation shows a leukocyte count of 134/µL (134 × 10⁶/L) with 50% neutrophils, erythrocyte count of 10,000/µL (10,000 × 10⁶/L), glucose level of 35 mg/dL (1.9 mmol/L), protein level of 112 mg/dL (1120 mg/L), and elevated lactate level of 5.4 mg/dL.

Blood cultures taken at onset of fever are negative, as are CSF cultures.

A chest radiograph shows no infiltrates.

**Which of the following is the most appropriate management?**

(A) Continue current care
(B) Discontinue vancomycin and cefepime and begin linezolid
(C) Remove the external ventricular drain
(D) Switch to intraventricular administration of antibiotics

## Item 24

A 19-year-old man is evaluated in the emergency department for fever, cough producing blood-tinged sputum, shortness of breath, and headache. He attended a political rally on his college campus 4 days ago. Six other people have been hospitalized with similar symptoms. Medical history is unremarkable, and he takes no medications.

On physical examination, the patient is alert and oriented. Temperature is 39.1 °C (102.4 °F), blood pressure is 98/58 mm Hg, pulse rate is 110/min, and respiration rate is 24/min. Oxygen saturation is 92% breathing oxygen 2 L/min by nasal cannula. Neurologic examination is nonfocal, and no meningeal signs are present. Dyspnea, bilateral pulmonary rhonchi, and tubular breath sounds are noted on pulmonary examination. No rash is present, and the abdomen is nontender.

Sputum Gram stain reveals many polymorphonuclear cells and abundant gram-negative coccobacilli demonstrating bipolar staining.

A chest radiograph shows bilateral patchy infiltrates.

**Which of the following is the most appropriate treatment?**

(A) Ceftriaxone and azithromycin
(B) Ciprofloxacin
(C) Gentamicin
(D) Piperacillin-tazobactam and levofloxacin

## Item 25

A 39-year-old man is hospitalized for tongue pain, abdominal pain, increased weakness, and a 2-week history of malaise and fever. He reports being in good health previously. He lives in the Ohio River Valley; approximately 1 month ago, he moved his antique business from a barn to an old store in the area, after which he developed "flu-like" symptoms lasting 2 to 3 days. He says that the barn was dusty and had pigeons and bats in the rafters. He also has rheumatoid arthritis. Medications are methotrexate and prednisone.

On physical examination, the patient is lethargic. Temperature is 39.7 °C (103.5 °F), blood pressure is 90/50 mm Hg, pulse rate is 128/min, and respiration rate is 24/min. A shallow ulceration is visible on the right buccal mucosa and left lateral tongue. His neck is supple. Lungs are clear to percussion and auscultation. There is moderate hepatosplenomegaly.

Results of laboratory studies show a hemoglobin level of 9 g/dL (90 g/L), a leukocyte count of 10,500/µL (10.5 × 10⁹/L), and a platelet count of 90,000/µL (90 × 10⁹/L).

Posteroanterior and lateral chest radiographs are unremarkable.

**Which of the following is the most appropriate treatment?**

(A) Ceftriaxone and azithromycin
(B) Colchicine
(C) Itraconazole
(D) Liposomal amphotericin B

## Item 26

A 45-year-old man is evaluated in the ICU for continued daily fevers. He was hospitalized 6 days ago after 4 days of left-sided pleuritic chest pain, fever, and cough productive of yellow sputum with occasional blood streaks. He has a history of injection drug use and last injected heroin 7 days ago. Chest radiograph obtained at admission revealed a left lower lobe infiltrate. A sputum Gram stain showed gram-positive cocci in clusters. Empiric antibiotic therapy including vancomycin was begun. Sputum and two sets of blood cultures taken at admission grew methicillin-resistant *Staphylococcus aureus*, and antibiotic therapy was de-escalated to vancomycin monotherapy on hospital day 3. His only medication is vancomycin.

On physical examination, temperature is 38.5 °C (101.3 °F), blood pressure is 94/68 mm Hg, pulse rate is 118/min, and respiration rate is 28/min. Oxygen saturation is 92% breathing 6 L/min oxygen by nasal cannula. Decreased breath sounds are heard at the left lung base.

A vancomycin trough measurement is therapeutic at 15 µg/mL. Repeat blood cultures from hospital day 3 were negative at 72 hours. Repeat sputum Gram stain shows 3+ leukocytes and 1+ gram-positive cocci.

A transthoracic echocardiogram was negative for valvular vegetations. A repeat chest radiograph is shown.

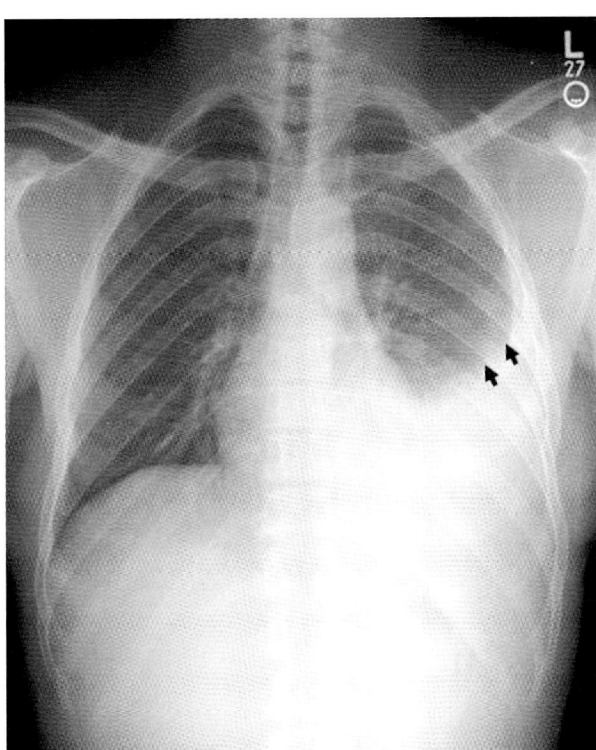

**Which of the following is the most appropriate management at this time?**

(A) Add methylprednisolone
(B) Add piperacillin-tazobactam
(C) Perform thoracentesis
(D) Procalcitonin measurement
(E) Switch to daptomycin

## Item 27

A 27-year-old woman is hospitalized with a 5-day history of intermittent fever, headache, muscle pains, and abdominal cramps. She returned 8 days ago from a 1-week trip to Kenya and Tanzania. She spent time outdoors in the evening and went hiking in a wooded park. She is pregnant at 20 weeks' gestation. She declined pretravel immunizations as well as antimalarial chemoprophylaxis. Her only medication is a prenatal vitamin.

On physical examination, temperature is 39.1 °C (102.3 °F), blood pressure is 98/64 mm Hg, pulse rate is 112/min, and respiration rate is 16/min. Her conjunctivae are icteric. Cardiopulmonary examination reveals regular tachycardia. The remainder of the examination is unremarkable.

A peripheral blood smear is shown.

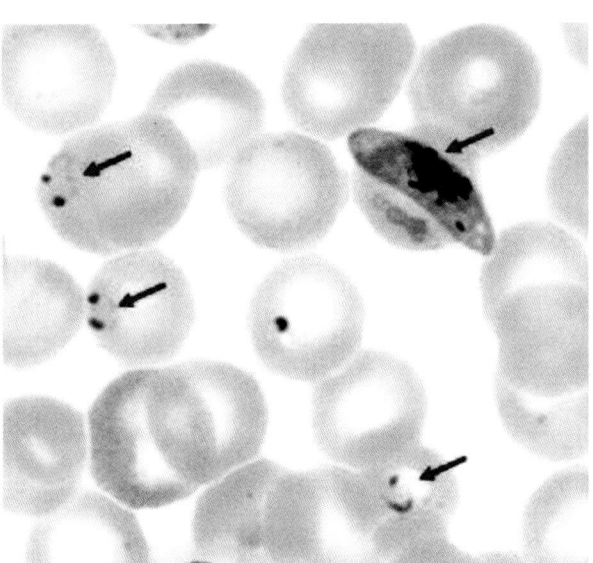

**Which of the following is the most likely causative agent?**

(A) *Plasmodium falciparum*
(B) *Plasmodium knowlesi*
(C) *Plasmodium malariae*
(D) *Plasmodium ovale*
(E) *Plasmodium vivax*

## Item 28

A 64-year-old man is evaluated in the emergency department for acute onset of severe lower back pain that radiates down his legs, with associated numbness and fever. Medical history is significant for end-stage kidney disease, for which he receives hemodialysis. Medications are erythropoietin, iron, lisinopril, nifedipine, and sevelamer.

On physical examination, temperature is 38.6 °C (101.5 °F), blood pressure is 110/62 mm Hg, pulse rate is 114/min, and respiration rate is 20/min. The lower extremities have decreased sensation to touch, diminished reflexes, and mild weakness.

Laboratory studies show a leukocyte count of 15,450/µL (15.5 × 10$^9$/L). Blood cultures are pending.

CONT.

MRI of the lumbar spine shows discitis in L2 to L3 with epidural abscess.

**Which of the following is the most appropriate management?**

(A) Await blood cultures before starting antimicrobial therapy
(B) Empiric antibiotic therapy alone
(C) Empiric antibiotic therapy and surgical drainage
(D) Surgical drainage alone

## Item 29

A 19-year-old man is hospitalized with a 6-day history of lightheadedness and nightly fevers. He also reports sore throat, headache, joint and muscle aches, and a dry cough. He recalls a blotchy rash on his trunk and arms, which has resolved. He returned home 12 days ago from a trip to Vietnam, for which he did not receive specific immunizations or other prophylaxis. During the second week of his trip, he experienced 2 days of diarrhea; he has had none since, but abdominal discomfort and anorexia persist.

On physical examination, the patient is lethargic. Temperature is 39.9 °C (103.9 °F), blood pressure is 98/58 mm Hg, pulse rate is 68/min, and respiration rate is 16/min. No skin rash or evidence of jaundice is present. The abdomen is distended, with diminished bowel sounds, but nontender. Neurologic examination is nonfocal.

**Which of the following is the most likely diagnosis?**

(A) Brucellosis
(B) Leptospirosis
(C) Melioidosis
(D) Typhoid (enteric) fever

## Item 30

A 31-year-old man arrives to establish care for newly diagnosed HIV infection. He is asymptomatic. Medical history is otherwise noncontributory, and he takes no medications.

On physical examination, vital signs are normal, and the remainder of the examination is unremarkable.

A review of his previous laboratory studies shows a normal complete blood count, and chemistries, including glucose, creatinine, and liver enzyme levels, are within normal limits. The HIV-1/2 antigen/antibody combination immunoassay is reactive. The HIV-1/2 antibody differentiation assay is positive for HIV-1 antibody, and HIV-1 RNA is quantified at 27,313 copies/mL. CD4 cell count is 455/µL.

**Which of the following is the most appropriate next step in management?**

(A) Genotypic viral resistance testing
(B) Glycohemoglobin level
(C) Phenotypic viral resistance testing
(D) Repeat HIV viral load and CD4 cell count in 1 month

 ## Item 31

A 33-year-old woman is evaluated in the emergency department in January with a 3-day history of fever, headache, stiff neck, and photophobia. She was previously well, and medical history is negative for recent travel; she takes no medications.

On physical examination, temperature is 38.5 °C (101.3 °F), blood pressure is 136/86 mm Hg, pulse rate is 100/min, and respiration rate is 18/min. The general medical examination is unremarkable. On neurologic examination, she shows photophobia, and a nondilated funduscopic examination shows no papilledema. The remainder of the examination is nonfocal.

Cerebrospinal fluid evaluation shows a leukocyte count of 324/µL (324 × 10⁶/L) with 60% neutrophils, glucose level of 58 mg/dL (3.2 mmol/L), and protein level of 125 mg/dL (1250 mg/L). Gram stain of the cerebrospinal fluid is negative, and culture is pending.

**Which of the following is the most likely cause of this patient's symptoms?**

(A) Enterovirus
(B) Herpes simplex virus type 2
(C) Mumps virus
(D) West Nile virus

## Item 32

A 22-year-old man returns for follow-up evaluation; he was recently diagnosed with HIV infection, and he began antiretroviral therapy 2 weeks ago. He also received influenza vaccination and the 13-valent pneumococcal conjugate vaccine at that time. He reports that he has sex with men. Medical history is notable for previous chlamydia infection and genital warts. Medications are tenofovir, emtricitabine, and dolutegravir.

On physical examination, vital signs are normal. A few small lesions consistent with warts are noted on the penis. The examination is otherwise unremarkable.

**Laboratory studies:**

| | |
|---|---|
| CD4 cell count | 527/µL |
| Hepatitis A IgG | Positive |
| Hepatitis A IgM | Negative |
| Hepatitis B surface antibody | Negative |
| Hepatitis B surface antigen | Positive |

**Which of the following is the most appropriate immunization to be given today?**

(A) 23-Valent pneumococcal polysaccharide vaccine
(B) Hepatitis A vaccine
(C) Hepatitis B vaccine
(D) Human papillomavirus vaccine

## Item 33

A 22-year-old man is evaluated in the emergency department 1 hour after awakening with right-sided facial weakness. He reports a 2-day history of headache but has had no fever. He lives in Minnesota and has removed two embedded ticks from himself and three from his dog over the past 3 weeks. The patient is otherwise healthy and takes no medication.

On physical examination, vital signs are normal. Nuchal rigidity and right facial nerve (cranial nerve VII) palsy are noted. Mental status is intact. Skin examination findings are shown on the next page.

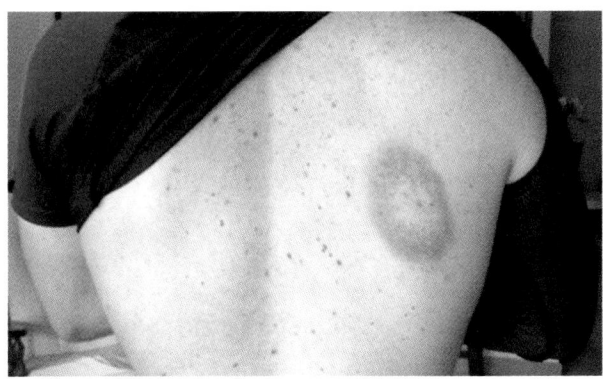

**Which of the following is the most appropriate preventive measure?**

(A) Reinforce consistent condom use and avoid antiretroviral therapy

(B) Tenofovir and emtricitabine single dose before each sexual encounter

(C) Tenofovir and emtricitabine single dose after each sexual encounter

(D) Tenofovir disoproxil fumarate and emtricitabine daily

CONT. All other physical examination findings are unremarkable. Results of laboratory studies show a leukocyte count of $11,500/\mu L$ $(11.5 \times 10^9/L)$.

**Which of the following is the most appropriate initial management?**

(A) *Borrelia burgdorferi* antibody testing

(B) Ceftriaxone administration

(C) Doxycycline administration

(D) Head CT

(E) Lumbar puncture

## Item 34

A 34-year-old woman is seeking medical advice. She is pregnant at 24 weeks' gestation. Her husband returned home 1 week ago from a medical mission in the Middle East. Spores of anthrax were discovered in the hospital where he was working. Her husband, who is asymptomatic, has begun taking ciprofloxacin and will receive a vaccination series. The patient questions if she is at risk for infection. Her only medication is a prenatal vitamin.

On physical examination, vital signs are normal. The examination is unremarkable.

**Which of the following is the most appropriate management?**

(A) Doxycycline and vaccination

(B) Nasopharyngeal swab and anthrax blood test

(C) Raxibacumab injection

(D) No treatment

## Item 35

A 27-year-old man is evaluated during a routine health maintenance visit with his internist. He asks about reducing his risk for HIV infection because he has sex with men, has multiple partners, and reports using condoms "sometimes." Medical history is unremarkable, and he takes no medications.

The physical examination is normal.

Laboratory studies show a normal serum creatinine level. A serum rapid plasma reagin test is negative. Nucleic acid amplification testing for gonorrhea and chlamydia from urine, pharynx, and rectum are all negative. An HIV test is negative.

## Item 36

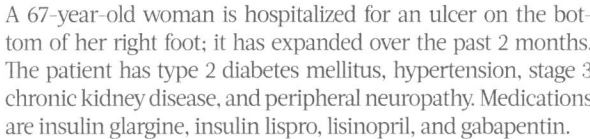

A 67-year-old woman is hospitalized for an ulcer on the bottom of her right foot; it has expanded over the past 2 months. The patient has type 2 diabetes mellitus, hypertension, stage 3 chronic kidney disease, and peripheral neuropathy. Medications are insulin glargine, insulin lispro, lisinopril, and gabapentin.

On physical examination, temperature is 37.3 °C (99.1 °F); the remaining vital signs are normal. A deep 3- × 4-cm ulcer is located on the distal medial compartment of the plantar surface of the right foot. The base of the ulcer is necrotic and malodorous; a probe-to-bone test is negative. No surrounding erythema or increased warmth is noted. Both feet are warm with palpable pulses.

Erythrocyte sedimentation rate and C-reactive protein level are elevated. Results of a complete blood count are normal.

A plain radiograph reveals soft tissue swelling and ulceration; an MRI reveals findings consistent with osteomyelitis of the distal head of the first metatarsal.

**Which of the following is the most appropriate management?**

(A) Bone biopsy and culture

(B) Forefoot amputation

(C) Swabbing and culture of wound base

(D) Vancomycin and piperacillin-tazobactam

## Item 37

A 32-year-old woman arrives to establish primary care. She is sexually active with a new male partner and reports consistent condom use. Medical history is significant for chlamydia cervicitis 5 years ago and treatment for syphilis 6 years ago. Her only medication is an oral contraceptive.

On physical examination, vital signs and the remainder of the examination are unremarkable.

A syphilis enzyme immunoassay is positive; rapid plasma reagin testing is negative. A fluorescent treponemal antibody test is positive. Nucleic acid amplification testing is negative for *Neisseria gonorrhoeae* and *Chlamydia trachomatis*. HIV antigen/antibody combination testing is negative.

**Which of the following is the most appropriate management?**

(A) Intramuscular benzathine penicillin, single dose

(B) Intramuscular benzathine penicillin, weekly for 3 weeks

(C) Repeat serology with *Treponema pallidum* particle agglutination assay

(D) No further testing or treatment

## Item 38

A 25-year-old woman returns for counseling regarding results of HIV testing completed during a recent routine health maintenance visit. She reports no known exposure or risk factors for HIV infection. Medical history is unremarkable, and she takes no medications.

Laboratory studies show a reactive HIV-1/2 antigen/antibody combination immunoassay, a negative HIV-1/2 antibody differentiation immunoassay, and no RNA detected on HIV-1 RNA nucleic acid amplification testing.

**Which of the following is the most appropriate management?**

(A) Initiate combination antiretroviral therapy after counseling

(B) Order T-cell subset testing to check CD4 cell count

(C) Perform HIV genotypic resistance testing

(D) Perform Western blot HIV antibody testing

(E) Tell the patient she does not have HIV infection

## Item 39

An 18-year-old man is evaluated for a 4-day history of frequent, large-volume diarrhea, with associated abdominal cramping, emesis, fever, and nausea. He is a lifeguard at a freshwater municipal pool, and several other swimmers who use the pool have recently developed similar symptoms.

On physical examination, temperature is 37.5 °C (99.5 °F); the vital signs are otherwise normal. On abdominal examination, bowel sounds are present, palpation elicits minimal tenderness, and no guarding or rebound is noted.

Modified acid-fast staining of the stool reveals oocysts that are about 5 microns in diameter.

**Which of the following is the most likely cause of this patient's diarrhea?**

(A) *Cryptosporidium*

(B) Enterohemorrhagic *Escherichia coli*

(C) Norovirus

(D) *Nocardia*

(E) *Vibrio parahaemolyticus*

## Item 40

A 31-year-old woman undergoes consultation regarding preventive strategies for travelers' diarrhea. She is planning a 7-day vacation to Mexico. Her itinerary includes 3 days in Mexico City followed by 4 days in the Yucatan Peninsula. Medical history is significant for Crohn colitis, which is currently in remission with maintenance therapy. Medications are adalimumab and as-needed loperamide; she is allergic to aspirin.

On physical examination, vital signs are normal, and other findings are unremarkable.

**Which of the following is the most appropriate preventive measure for this patient?**

(A) Azithromycin

(B) Bismuth subsalicylate

(C) Ciprofloxacin

(D) Probiotics

(E) No prophylaxis

## Item 41

An 82-year-old woman is hospitalized with hypotension and volume depletion resulting from gastroenteritis. Medical history is noncontributory, and she takes no medications.

On physical examination, temperature is 36.8 °C (98.3 °F), blood pressure is 92/66 mm Hg, pulse rate is 110/min, and respiration rate is 16/min. The remainder of the examination is unremarkable.

Because of difficulty in inserting a peripheral venous access line, an internal jugular central venous catheter will be placed for volume resuscitation.

**Which of the following is the most appropriate measure to prevent catheter-related bloodstream infection in this patient?**

(A) Assess catheter daily for necessity and potential removal

(B) Give one dose of vancomycin after catheter insertion

(C) Replace catheter every 7 days

(D) Use a small sterile drape when inserting the catheter

## Item 42

A 36-year-old man is evaluated for a 10-day history of abdominal cramping, diarrhea, malaise, and nausea. Diarrhea is watery without mucus or blood. He returned 2 weeks ago from a 7-day trip to Lima, Peru.

On physical examination, temperature is 37.7 °C (99.9 °F); the remaining vital signs are normal. On abdominal examination, bowel sounds are present with diffuse tenderness to palpation. The abdomen is not distended; no guarding or rebound is noted.

Stool polymerase chain reaction assay is positive for *Cyclospora*.

**Which of the following is the most appropriate treatment?**

(A) Atovaquone

(B) Metronidazole

(C) Pyrimethamine

(D) Quinacrine

(E) Trimethoprim-sulfamethoxazole

## Item 43

A 25-year-old woman is seen for counseling. She is newly pregnant at 7 weeks' gestation and has HIV infection diagnosed 6 years ago. HIV has been well controlled with an antiretroviral regimen, which she tolerates well. Medications are tenofovir disoproxil fumarate (TDF), emtricitabine, and efavirenz.

On physical examination, vital signs and other findings are normal.

Laboratory studies show HIV viral load is undetectable and the CD4 cell count is normal.

Which of the following is the most appropriate management?

(A) Continue TDF, emtricitabine, and efavirenz
(B) Pause antiretroviral therapy until after the first trimester
(C) Perform resistance testing
(D) Switch to zidovudine, lamivudine, and ritonavir-boosted lopinavir

## Item 44

A 31-year-old man undergoes pretravel consultation. He plans to leave in 8 days for a safari trip to Kenya. He received yellow fever and typhoid vaccinations 18 months ago, and he is undergoing a work-related three-dose hepatitis B vaccination series. He also has a prescription for prophylactic antimalarial medication. No serum IgG antibodies to hepatitis A were detected in a recent blood test. He smokes cigarettes and occasionally drinks an alcoholic beverage.

On physical examination, vital signs are normal, and other findings are unremarkable.

Which of the following is the most appropriate pretravel management for this patient?

(A) First dose of hepatitis A vaccine with a second dose in 7 days
(B) Immune globulin
(C) Single dose of hepatitis A vaccine
(D) Single dose of hepatitis A vaccine plus immune globulin
(E) No intervention

## Item 45

A 92-year-old man is hospitalized with a complicated urinary tract infection (UTI). He resides in a nursing home and has a chronic indwelling urinary catheter. In the nursing home, a urinalysis and urine culture were performed for possible UTI, and empiric ciprofloxacin therapy was initiated 1 day before transfer to the hospital. In the emergency department, ciprofloxacin was changed to piperacillin-tazobactam, and blood cultures were obtained. Medical history is notable for dementia, benign prostatic hyperplasia, chronic kidney disease, and recurrent UTIs. Medications are donepezil, memantine, and piperacillin-tazobactam.

On physical examination, temperature is 38.5 °C (101.3 °F), blood pressure is 108/70 mm Hg, pulse rate is 100/min, and respiration rate is 16/min. Suprapubic tenderness is noted, and the urinary catheter is draining cloudy urine. Other examination findings are noncontributory.

Laboratory studies show a leukocyte count of 15,200/µL (15.2 × 10⁹/L) and a serum creatinine level of 1.9 mg/dL (168 µmol/L). Urinalysis reveals leukocytes too numerous to count but no erythrocytes.

Urine culture obtained from the nursing home shows more than 10⁵ colony-forming units of *Escherichia coli* sensitive to piperacillin-tazobactam, gentamicin, cefepime, and meropenem (resistant to ceftriaxone, ceftazidime, cefotaxime, and ciprofloxacin); it is confirmed to be an extended-spectrum β-lactamase–producing organism. Blood cultures are pending.

No infiltrates are seen on the chest radiograph.

Which of the following is the most appropriate treatment?

(A) Add gentamicin
(B) Continue piperacillin-tazobactam
(C) Switch piperacillin-tazobactam to cefepime
(D) Switch piperacillin-tazobactam to meropenem

## Item 46

A 58-year-old man is assessed for discharge from the hospital. He was admitted 3 days ago with fever and chills. He has non-Hodgkin lymphoma and a tunneled subclavian venous catheter used for chemotherapy infusion. Blood cultures at admission grew vancomycin-resistant *Enterococcus faecium*. The patient's catheter was removed, a peripherally inserted central catheter (PICC) was placed for intravenous access, and daptomycin therapy was initiated. Blood cultures are now negative, and the patient is afebrile.

The patient is ready to be discharged to complete intravenous daptomycin therapy as an outpatient. At the time of discharge, his complete blood count and comprehensive chemistry profile are normal.

Which of the following is the most appropriate weekly monitoring of his daptomycin therapy?

(A) Electrocardiography and blood glucose
(B) Hemoglobin and platelet count
(C) Serum amylase and triglycerides
(D) Serum creatinine and creatine kinase

## Item 47

A 32-year-old man is evaluated for a 2-month history of painless, violaceous skin nodules with surrounding edema on the chest, back, and lower extremities. He reports that he has sex with men. Medical history is significant for AIDS, with a CD4 cell count of 54/µL. He is not following an antiretroviral therapy regimen.

On physical examination, temperature is 38.1 °C (100.5 °F), blood pressure is 135/62 mm Hg, pulse rate is 68/min, and respiration rate is 20/min. Several nodules are seen in the mouth during oral examination (shown).

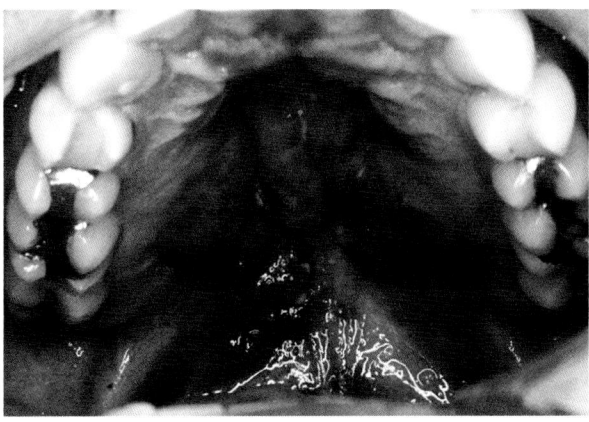

Which of the following is the most likely cause of these findings?

(A) Cytomegalovirus
(B) Epstein-Barr virus
(C) Human herpes virus type 6
(D) Human herpes virus type 8

## Item 48

A 42-year-old man is evaluated in the hospital for increased pain and drainage from a previously healed surgical wound over the left fibula. He underwent open reduction and internal fixation of a fracture 4 weeks ago. The patient has undergone incision and surgical debridement of the wound. A bone culture revealed methicillin-sensitive *Staphylococcus aureus*. Medical history is otherwise noncontributory, and his only medication is ibuprofen for pain.

On physical examination, vital signs are normal. A surgical wound over the left lateral leg is well approximated with no erythema or drainage.

A plain radiograph before debridement shows nonunion of the fracture with screws and K-wires in place.

Which of the following is the most appropriate treatment?

(A) Cefazolin
(B) Cefazolin and rifampin
(C) Ceftaroline
(D) Vancomycin and rifampin

## Item 49

A 34-year-old man is evaluated immediately after a dog bite to his thigh. Medical history is notable for splenectomy 5 years ago. The patient and dog are up to date on all immunizations. He takes no medications.

On physical examination, vital signs are normal. A tiny puncture wound is located on the right mid-thigh with minimal surrounding erythema.

Which of the following is the most appropriate management?

(A) Amoxicillin-clavulanate
(B) Ciprofloxacin
(C) Metronidazole
(D) Observation

## Item 50

A 76-year-old woman is evaluated in the hospital for recurrent diverticulitis. She has had multiple episodes of diverticulitis treated with ciprofloxacin and metronidazole over the past 18 months. During this hospitalization, an abscess was noted on a CT scan of the abdomen and pelvis, and a percutaneous drain was placed and the fluid sent for culture. Piperacillin-tazobactam is started empirically.

On physical examination, temperature is 39.2 °C (102.6 °F), blood pressure is 126/82 mm Hg, pulse rate is 100/min, and respiration rate is 15/min. She has diffuse abdominal tenderness to palpation.

Laboratory studies show a leukocyte count of 22,000/µL (22 × 10⁹/L) and a serum creatinine level of 1.3 mg/dL (115 µmol/L).

Gram stain of the abscess fluid reveals 4+ gram-negative rods; fluid culture grows *Pseudomonas aeruginosa* resistant to ceftazidime, piperacillin-tazobactam, ciprofloxacin, meropenem, and doripenem. Blood cultures are negative.

The *Pseudomonas* isolate should be tested for susceptibility to which of the following antibiotics?

(A) Ceftolozane-tazobactam and colistin
(B) Ertapenem and tobramycin
(C) Fosfomycin
(D) Minocycline

## Item 51

A 25-year-old woman is hospitalized with a 4-day history of fever and cough productive of brown sputum. She is at 14 weeks' gestation with her first pregnancy. Medical history is significant for mild persistent asthma. Medications are an albuterol inhaler, beclomethasone inhaler, and a prenatal vitamin.

On physical examination, temperature is 38.2 °C (100.8 °F), blood pressure is normal, pulse rate is 122/min, and respiration rate is 24/min. Oxygen saturation is 94% breathing ambient air. Crackles are heard at the left lung base on pulmonary auscultation.

Chest radiograph shows a left lower lobe infiltrate.

Which of the following is the most likely cause of pneumonia in this patient?

(A) *Escherichia coli*
(B) *Klebsiella pneumoniae*
(C) *Listeria monocytogenes*
(D) *Staphylococcus aureus*
(E) *Streptococcus pneumoniae*

## Item 52

A 67-year-old woman is evaluated in December for a 2-day history of runny nose, fever, headache, myalgia, cough, and sore throat. Medical history is notable for heart failure. She lives at home with her husband and is able to eat, drink, and take her oral medications. Her medications are carvedilol and enalapril. She received a standard-dose influenza immunization in October.

On physical examination, temperature is 38.6 °C (101.5 °F), blood pressure is 145/62 mm Hg, pulse rate is 98/min, and respiration rate is 20/min. The patient has rhinorrhea, and the pharynx is erythematous. Lungs are clear to auscultation.

A chest radiograph shows no infiltrates.

A nasopharyngeal swab is positive for influenza B.

Which of the following is the most appropriate treatment?

(A) Amantadine
(B) Oseltamivir
(C) Peramivir
(D) Rimantadine

**Item 53**

A 74-year-old man is evaluated in the emergency department for new onset of confusion and 2 days of fever and rigors. Medical history is significant for diabetes mellitus, hypertension, and benign prostatic hyperplasia. Medications are lisinopril, hydrochlorothiazide, metformin, tamsulosin, and aspirin.

On physical examination, the patient is confused. Temperature is 39.1 °C (102.4 °F), blood pressure is 102/56 mm Hg, pulse rate is 88/min, and respiration rate is 22/min. Oxygen saturation is 93% breathing ambient air. Neurologic examination is nonfocal and without meningeal signs. On abdominal examination, the abdomen is soft and the urinary bladder is distended. Other examination findings are noncontributory.

**Laboratory studies:**

| | |
|---|---|
| Hemoglobin | 15.2 g/dL (152 g/L) |
| Leukocyte count | 17,480/µL (17.5 × 10⁹/L) |
| Blood urea nitrogen | 72 mg/dL (25.7 mmol/L) |
| Creatinine | 2.1 mg/dL (186 µmol/L) |
| Urinalysis (catheterized sample) | Volume 780 mL (780 µL); cloudy; 1.244 specific gravity; >100 leukocytes/hpf; 0-5 erythrocytes/hpf; 4+ bacteria |

Urine culture and two sets of blood cultures are obtained.

A portable chest radiograph shows no signs of acute cardiopulmonary disease.

**In addition to supportive care, which of the following is the most appropriate management?**

(A) Intravenous cefepime and kidney ultrasonography

(B) Intravenous ciprofloxacin

(C) Intravenous levofloxacin and digital prostate massage

(D) Intravenous piperacillin-tazobactam and contrast-enhanced abdominal and pelvic CT

 **Item 54**

A 26-year-old woman is evaluated in the emergency department for fever and low back pain that has progressed for the past 3 weeks. She injects heroin daily. Medical history is unremarkable, and she takes no medications.

On physical examination, temperature is 38.1 °C (100.6 °F), blood pressure is 90/60 mm Hg, pulse rate is 110/min, and respiration rate is 28/min. The lower lumbar spine is tender to palpation. Neurologic examination and other physical examination findings are normal.

Aggressive fluid resuscitation is initiated. Complete blood count, metabolic profile, erythrocyte sedimentation rate, and blood culture and urinalysis are obtained.

MRI is shown (top of next column).

**Which of the following is the most appropriate antibiotic management?**

(A) Cefazolin and gentamicin

(B) Vancomycin

(C) Vancomycin and cefepime

(D) Withhold antibiotics while awaiting bone biopsy

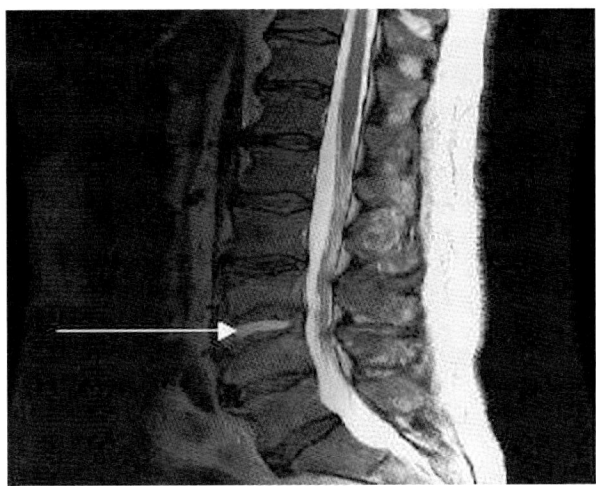

ITEM 54

**Item 55**

A 21-year-old man is evaluated for cold symptoms beginning last week, including malaise, fatigue, swollen lymph nodes in the neck, and sore throat, which resolved before his appointment today. He has no other symptoms. He reports occasionally having sex with men, usually using condoms, but has had no known HIV exposure. Medical history is unremarkable, and he takes no medications.

On physical examination, vital signs are normal. A few shotty cervical lymph nodes are palpable, but no other lymphadenopathy is noted. No rash is present. Other examination findings are normal.

Laboratory studies show a reactive HIV-1/2 antigen/antibody combination immunoassay. The HIV-1/HIV-2 antibody differentiation immunoassay is negative. HIV-1 RNA nucleic acid amplification testing is positive, with quantification of 11,540 copies/mL.

**Which of the following is the most likely diagnosis?**

(A) Acute HIV infection

(B) Chronic HIV infection

(C) False-positive HIV test

(D) HIV-2 infection

**Item 56**

A 19-year-old man is evaluated at an urgent care clinic for a 3-day history of dysuria, with purulent discharge at the urethral meatus this morning. He reports no urgency, frequency, or fever. He returned last week from a spring break trip, during which he had oral sex with a new female partner. Medical history is otherwise noncontributory, he takes no medications, and he has no medication allergies.

On physical examination, vital signs are normal. Purulent discharge is noted at the urethral meatus. The examination is otherwise unremarkable.

Nucleic acid amplification testing for *Neisseria gonorrhoeae* and *Chlamydia trachomatis* is performed on a first-catch urine sample.

CONT.

Which of the following is the most appropriate empiric treatment?

(A) Ceftriaxone plus azithromycin

(B) Doxycycline

(C) Trimethoprim-sulfamethoxazole

(D) Valacyclovir

## Item 57

A 30-year-old woman undergoes predischarge evaluation 1 month after allogeneic hematopoietic stem cell transplantation for acute myeloid leukemia. The posttransplant course was complicated by prolonged neutropenia and *Escherichia coli* bacteremia. The infection and neutropenia have resolved with broad-spectrum antibiotic therapy. She received all indicated pretransplant immunizations. Medications are trimethoprim-sulfamethoxazole for pneumocystis pneumonia prophylaxis and tacrolimus.

On physical examination, vital signs are normal. The indwelling central line site appears normal without erythema, swelling, or tenderness. Lungs are clear throughout. No skin lesions are present.

Laboratory studies show a leukocyte count of 2700/µL ($2.7 \times 10^9$/L) (differential of 57% polymorphonuclear cells, 30% lymphocytes, 10% monocytes, and 3% eosinophils) and a serum creatinine level of 0.7 mg/dL (61.9 µmol/L).

Pretransplant serologies were positive for cytomegalovirus, Epstein-Barr virus, varicella-zoster virus, and *Toxoplasma*.

**In addition to continuing the trimethoprim-sulfamethoxazole, which of the following is the most appropriate outpatient prophylaxis for this patient?**

(A) Acyclovir

(B) Ciprofloxacin

(C) Posaconazole

(D) Valganciclovir

 ## Item 58

A 34-year-old man is hospitalized with a 4-week history of fever, headaches, and stiff neck. He recently emigrated from Mexico, but his medical history is otherwise noncontributory, and he takes no medications.

On physical examination, the patient is alert. Temperature is 38.9 °C (102 °F), blood pressure is 92/60 mm Hg, pulse rate is 124/min, and respiration rate is 24/min. Neurologic examination is normal. Passive neck flexion elicits painful resistance.

Cerebrospinal fluid (CSF) analysis reveals a leukocyte count of 424/µL ($424 \times 10^6$/L) with 92% lymphocytes, glucose level of 22 mg/dL (1.2 mmol/L), and protein level of 278 mg/dL (2780 mg/L).

Rapid point-of-care antibody screening for HIV infection is negative. CSF Gram stain and cryptococcal antigen test results are negative. Results from cultures of the CSF and blood and from the interferon-γ release assay are pending.

The chest radiograph is normal.

Which of the following is the most appropriate management?

(A) Amphotericin B and 5-fluorocytosine

(B) Rifampin, isoniazid, pyrazinamide, and ethambutol

(C) Rifampin, isoniazid, pyrazinamide, ethambutol, and dexamethasone

(D) Vancomycin, ceftriaxone, and dexamethasone

## Item 59

A 25-year-old man undergoes follow-up consultation regarding a positive interferon-γ release assay. He reports working for the past year in Vietnam and having a negative tuberculin skin test before departing. He is asymptomatic. He has had no known exposure to anyone with a history of tuberculosis. He has otherwise been well and takes no medications.

On physical examination, vital signs and examination are normal.

HIV testing is negative.

Posteroanterior and lateral chest radiograph is normal.

**Which of the following is the most appropriate treatment?**

(A) Isoniazid and rifapentine once weekly for 24 weeks

(B) Isoniazid daily for 9 months

(C) Isoniazid, rifampin, pyrazinamide, and ethambutol for 8 weeks followed by isoniazid and rifampin for 4 months

(D) No treatment or testing

## Item 60

A 37-year-old man is hospitalized with abdominal pain, fever, and increasing diarrhea of 3 days' duration. He underwent kidney transplantation 3 weeks ago. The postoperative course has been complicated by pneumonia and wound infection, which resolved with antibiotic treatment. The patient was seronegative for cytomegalovirus before transplantation, but the transplant donor was seropositive. Medications are prednisone, tacrolimus, mycophenolate mofetil, valganciclovir, and trimethoprim-sulfamethoxazole.

On physical examination, temperature is 38.4 °C (101.2 °F), blood pressure is 122/85 mm Hg, pulse rate is 110/min, and respiration rate is 18/min. Abdominal palpation elicits tenderness, especially in the left lower quadrant, without rebound or guarding.

Which of the following is the most likely diagnosis?

(A) *Clostridium difficile* colitis

(B) Cytomegalovirus colitis

(C) Mycophenolate adverse effect

(D) Polyoma BK virus

## Item 61

A 22-year-old woman arrives for her annual gynecologic examination, including a Pap smear and refill of her oral contraceptive prescription. She indicates she recently became sexually active with a new partner. Medical history

CONT.

is otherwise unremarkable. Her only medication is her oral contraceptive.

On physical examination, vital signs are normal. Pelvic examination is normal. The remainder of the examination is noncontributory.

A urine pregnancy test is negative. The Pap smear is normal. Nucleic acid amplification testing is positive for *Neisseria gonorrhoeae* and negative for *Chlamydia trachomatis*. The HIV antigen/antibody combination immunoassay is negative.

**Which of the following is the most appropriate treatment?**

(A) Cefixime
(B) Ceftriaxone
(C) Ceftriaxone plus azithromycin
(D) Ciprofloxacin

## Item 62

A 51-year-old man is evaluated in the emergency department for a 12-hour history of fever, chills, headache, and weakness. He works on his farm in Maine and spends a considerable part of most days outside, but he is not aware of any tick or mosquito bites. He has had no diarrhea, cough, or rash. The patient had his spleen surgically removed 20 years ago after being involved in a motor vehicle collision. He has had no recent travel outside of the United States, and he is up to date on all immunizations.

On physical examination, temperature is 39.6 °C (103.3 °F), blood pressure is 88/42 mm Hg, pulse rate is 135/min, respiration rate is 28/min, and oxygen saturation is 90% with the patient receiving 4 L/min of oxygen via a nasal cannula. Lethargy, scleral icterus, jaundiced skin, hepatomegaly, and lower extremity petechiae are noted.

**Laboratory studies:**

| | |
|---|---|
| Haptoglobin | <8 mg/dL (80 mg/L) |
| Hematocrit | 25% |
| Leukocyte count | 4500/µL (4.5 × 10⁹/L) |
| Platelet count | 109,000/µL (109 × 10⁹/L) |
| Bilirubin, total | 3.9 mg/dL (66.7 µmol/L) |
| Creatinine | 1.0 mg/dL (88.4 µmol/L) |
| Lactate dehydrogenase | 909 U/L |

**A blood smear from this patient is most likely to show which of the following abnormalities?**

(A) Cytoplasmic morulae in leukocytes
(B) Intraerythrocytic banana-shaped gametocytes
(C) Intraerythrocytic tetrad forms
(D) Intraneutrophilic gram-positive diplococci
(E) Schistocytes

##  Item 63

A 55-year-old man is evaluated in the hospital for antibiotic management of a diabetic foot ulcer. He was hospitalized 3 days ago for debridement of a draining great toe ulcer. A radiograph of the left foot showed osteomyelitis of the great toe. Empiric piperacillin-tazobactam was started after debridement of the ulcer, and a bone biopsy was obtained

intraoperatively. Medical history is significant for diabetes mellitus with nephropathy. Medications are metformin, insulin glargine, and piperacillin-tazobactam. Today the patient is clinically improved.

On physical examination, vital signs are normal. A large, deep plantar ulcer penetrates to the bone of the left great toe with minimal surrounding erythema and no evidence of necrotic tissue.

The bone culture grows *Pseudomonas aeruginosa* (sensitive to piperacillin-tazobactam, ceftazidime, ciprofloxacin, aztreonam, and tobramycin) and *Bacteroides fragilis*.

**Which of the following is the most appropriate management?**

(A) Add tobramycin to piperacillin-tazobactam
(B) Switch piperacillin-tazobactam to aztreonam
(C) Switch piperacillin-tazobactam to ceftazidime
(D) Switch piperacillin-tazobactam to oral ciprofloxacin and metronidazole

## Item 64

A 55-year-old man is hospitalized for acute diverticulitis. Seventy-two hours after initiating treatment with piperacillin-tazobactam through a percutaneously inserted central venous catheter, he becomes hypotensive and tachycardic and is transferred to the ICU. He has a 5-year history of type 2 diabetes mellitus. His only medication is metformin.

On physical examination, temperature is 40 °C (104.0 °F), blood pressure is 89/46 mm Hg, pulse rate is 136/min, respiration rate is 32/min, and oxygen saturation is 92% with the patient breathing ambient air. The patient is somnolent. The funduscopic examination is unremarkable. Abdominal examination reveals a soft, slightly tender left lower quadrant. Other examination findings are unremarkable.

A blood culture is positive for yeast.

The intravenous catheter is removed, and a replacement catheter is inserted at a different site.

**Which of the following is the most appropriate management?**

(A) Begin empiric therapy with an echinocandin
(B) Begin empiric therapy with fluconazole
(C) Confirm candidemia with a second positive blood culture
(D) Perform antifungal susceptibility testing before initiating therapy
(E) No additional therapy is required

## Item 65

A 58-year-old man is evaluated in follow-up after being hospitalized with uncomplicated L3 vertebral osteomyelitis that presumably resulted from bacteremia during hemodialysis for end-stage kidney disease. In the hospital, a CT-guided bone biopsy identified a methicillin-susceptible *Staphylococcus aureus* infection. The patient completed 2 weeks of cefazolin antibiotic therapy and has responded with resolution of fever and improvement in pain. Other medications are sevelamer and amlodipine.

On physical examination, vital signs are normal. The lower lumbar spine is minimally tender to palpation. The remainder of the physical examination is noncontributory.

**Which of the following is the most appropriate treatment?**

(A) Continue cefazolin to complete 6 weeks of antibiotic therapy

(B) Continue cefazolin to complete 12 weeks of antibiotic therapy

(C) Discontinue cefazolin now

(D) Discontinue cefazolin when follow-up MRI demonstrates improvement

## Item 66

A 40-year-old man is hospitalized for a 2-day history of diarrhea. He has five liquid bowel movements per day. One week ago, he completed a course of levofloxacin for treatment of community-acquired pneumonia.

On physical examination, temperature is 38.1 °C (100.5 °F), blood pressure is 116/70 mm Hg, pulse rate is 98/min, and respiration rate is 19/min. The abdomen is nondistended with normal bowel sounds. Moderate abdominal tenderness is present, without guarding or rebound. Mental status is normal.

**Laboratory studies:**

Leukocyte count 18,000/µL (18.0 × 10 ⁹/L) (differential: 78% neutrophils, 3% band forms, 19% lymphocytes)
Albumin 2.8 g/dL (28 g/L)
Creatinine 1.6 mg/dL (141.4 µmol/L) (baseline, 1.0 mg/dL [88.4 µmol/L])
Lactate Normal

Stool polymerase chain reaction assay is positive for *Clostridium difficile* toxin gene.

**Which of the following is the most appropriate treatment?**

(A) Fecal microbiota transplant

(B) Intravenous vancomycin

(C) Oral metronidazole

(D) Oral vancomycin

(E) Oral vancomycin and intravenous metronidazole

## Item 67

An 18-year-old man is evaluated in the emergency department for new-onset seizures. The previous afternoon, he was evaluated in the university health service for acute onset of fever, severe myalgia, headache, and nausea; he was diagnosed with influenza and sent home with oseltamivir and ibuprofen. He received the quadrivalent meningococcal vaccine 7 months ago. Medical history is otherwise noncontributory. Other than oseltamivir and ibuprofen, he takes no medications.

On physical examination, temperature is 38.9 °C (102.0 °F), blood pressure is 90/55 mm Hg, pulse rate is 130/min, and respiration rate is 28/min. The patient is confused and lethargic. Photophobia, meningismus, and a diffuse petechial rash are present.

CT scan of the head is unremarkable.

Microscopic examination of the cerebrospinal fluid demonstrates gram-negative diplococci. Blood and cerebrospinal fluid cultures are pending.

**Which of the following is the most likely bacterial agent causing this patient's meningitis?**

(A) *Haemophilus influenzae*

(B) *Listeria monocytogenes*

(C) *Neisseria meningitides* group B

(D) *Streptococcus pneumoniae*

## Item 68

A 28-year-old man is evaluated for anal discharge accompanied by tenesmus of 3 days' duration. He reports no abdominal pain, diarrhea, or hematochezia. He is sexually active with men and women, practices anal receptive intercourse, and uses condoms inconsistently. Medical history is unremarkable, and he takes no medications.

On physical examination, vital signs are normal. Erythema and discharge are noted in the perianal region, but no ulcers are visible. Anoscopy is not available.

Nucleic acid amplification testing for *Neisseria gonorrhoeae* and *Chlamydia trachomatis* is performed on an anal swab sample. Testing for herpes, syphilis, and HIV infections is also initiated.

**Which of the following is the most appropriate treatment?**

(A) Azithromycin

(B) Budesonide foam

(C) Ceftriaxone and doxycycline

(D) Ciprofloxacin

## Item 69

A 42-year-old woman is hospitalized with dyspnea, dry cough, and fever that has been increasing over the past few days. She underwent allogeneic hematopoietic stem cell transplantation (HSCT) 7 months ago, with a recent occurrence of graft-versus-host disease of the skin and gastrointestinal tract. Donor and recipient were both cytomegalovirus seropositive before transplantation, the patient received monitoring for cytomegalovirus reactivation for 6 months after transplantation, and the cytomegalovirus nucleic acid amplification test was negative 1 month ago. Medications are prednisone, tacrolimus, trimethoprim-sulfamethoxazole, and acyclovir.

On physical examination, temperature is 38.1 °C (100.6 °F), blood pressure is 125/78 mm Hg, pulse rate is 104/min, and respiration rate is 24/min. Oxygen saturation is 88% breathing ambient air. Crackles are audible bilaterally on pulmonary examination. No lymphadenopathy is noted. The remainder of the examination is noncontributory.

Laboratory studies show a leukocyte count of 3500/µL (3.5 × 10⁹/L), with 85% polymorphonuclear cells, 8% lymphocytes, 5% monocytes, and 2% eosinophils.

A chest radiograph shows bilateral diffuse infiltrates. Chest CT scan shows bilateral diffuse ground-glass opacities without pleural effusions.

In addition to starting broad-spectrum antibacterial therapy, which of the following is the most appropriate initial treatment?

(A) Atovaquone
(B) Ganciclovir
(C) Liposomal amphotericin
(D) No additional therapy

## Item 70

A 47-year-old man is hospitalized with a 1-month history of increasingly severe low back pain and a 3-day history of fever and chills. He reports injection drug use (last injected 1 week ago). Medical history is otherwise unremarkable, and he takes no medications.

On physical examination, temperature is 38 °C (100.4 °F), blood pressure is 110/76 mm Hg, pulse rate is 88/min, and respiration rate is 16/min. Neurologic examination reveals no deficits, and no murmur is heard on cardiac auscultation. Palpation of the spine elicits point tenderness over L2-L4.

Laboratory studies show an erythrocyte sedimentation rate of 98 mm/h and a leukocyte count of 18,300/µL (18.3 × $10^9$/L).

MRI is positive for spondylodiskitis at L3-L4.

Blood samples were obtained, and empiric vancomycin was initiated.

Two sets of blood cultures are positive for methicillin-resistant *Staphylococcus aureus*, with a vancomycin minimum inhibitory concentration of 1.5 µg/mL; repeat blood cultures are pending. The vancomycin trough level is 19 µg/mL.

Transesophageal echocardiography shows no valvular vegetations.

**Which of the following is the most appropriate treatment?**

(A) Add gentamicin to vancomycin
(B) Add rifampin to vancomycin
(C) Change vancomycin to daptomycin
(D) Continue vancomycin

## Item 71

A 28-year-old woman undergoes follow-up evaluation after a recent hospitalization for meningococcal bacteremia. Lumbar puncture results during hospitalization were negative for meningitis. She completed a course of ceftriaxone 1 week ago and reports feeling well since stopping antibiotics. Medical history is notable for gonococcal arthritis of her knee 2 years ago. She has a sister with a history of meningococcal meningitis. She takes no medications.

On physical examination, vital signs are normal. The remainder of the examination is unremarkable.

**Which of the following is the most appropriate preventive measure?**

(A) Intravenous immune globulin
(B) Plasma infusion
(C) Prophylactic ciprofloxacin
(D) Quadrivalent meningococcal conjugate vaccine

## Item 72

A 33-year-old woman is evaluated for redness over her right calf at the site of a scratch that occurred 2 days ago. She has been well otherwise and takes no medications.

On physical examination, vital signs are normal. Tender erythema measuring 4 × 3 cm is noted over the right lower leg. No purulence, induration, or fluctuance is present.

**Which of the following is the most appropriate treatment?**

(A) Clindamycin
(B) Doxycycline
(C) Trimethoprim-sulfamethoxazole
(D) Vancomycin

## Item 73

An 82-year-old man is admitted to the ICU with a 7-day history of fever and cough productive of green sputum. He is unable to climb the stairs to his bedroom without becoming short of breath. Medical history is remarkable for bronchiectasis and polymyalgia rheumatica. His only medication is prednisone, 10 mg/d.

On physical examination, temperature is 38.8 °C (101.8 °F), blood pressure is normal, pulse rate is 115/min, and respiration rate is 25/min. Oxygen saturation is 88% breathing ambient air. Crackles are heard in the right lung base.

A sputum Gram stain shows 3+ polymorphonuclear cells and 2+ gram-negative organisms.

A chest radiograph is shown.

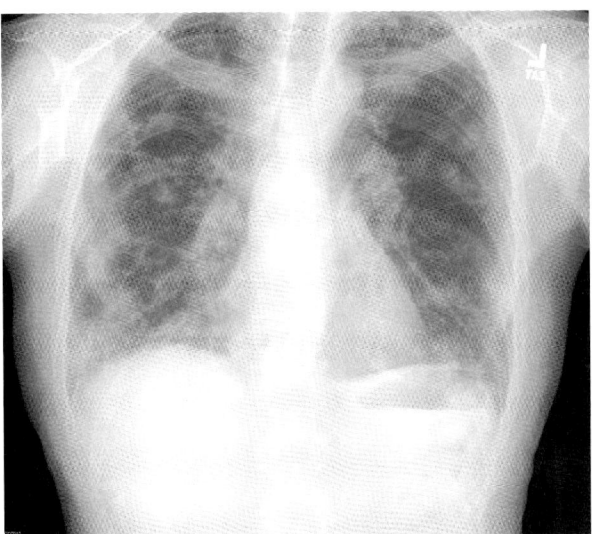

**Which of the following is the most appropriate treatment?**

(A) Ampicillin-sulbactam and levofloxacin
(B) Aztreonam and ciprofloxacin
(C) Cefepime and ciprofloxacin
(D) Ceftriaxone and azithromycin
(E) Ceftriaxone and levofloxacin

## Item 74

A 21-year-old man is hospitalized with a 3-day history of fever and cough productive of green sputum. He was in the hospital 2 months ago for giardiasis and a year ago for pneumonia. Medical history is also notable for frequent episodes of sinusitis, bronchitis, and otitis media dating back to childhood.

On physical examination, temperature is 38.2 °C (100.8 °F), blood pressure is 118/80 mm Hg, pulse rate is 108/min, and respiration rate is 24/min. Pulmonary examination reveals crackles at the right lung base.

Chest radiograph is significant for a right lower lobe consolidation, and empiric antibiotic therapy is initiated.

A sputum culture grows *Streptococcus pneumoniae*.

**Which of the following is the most likely underlying diagnosis?**

- (A) AIDS
- (B) Chronic granulomatous disease
- (C) Common variable immunodeficiency
- (D) Myeloperoxidase deficiency

## Item 75

A 28-year-old man undergoes follow-up evaluation of an injury to his right fourth finger sustained 10 weeks ago; he is a sport fisherman and obtained the injury from a tropical fish fin. He received separate 10-day courses of cephalexin and clindamycin without response. He takes no medications.

On physical examination, vital signs are normal. Swelling is present along the dorsum of the finger, with one 2- × 3-cm erythematous, papulonodular, fluctuant lesion located between the proximal and metacarpophalangeal joints. Pain is noted along the flexor tendon.

A plain radiograph of the finger shows no evidence of bony involvement or presence of a foreign body. Surgical exploration is performed, and intraoperative tissue specimens reveal noncaseating granulomas and inflammatory granulation tissue; Gram stain is negative.

**Which of the following is the most likely cause of this patient's infection?**

- (A) *Clostridium perfringens*
- (B) Herpes simplex virus type 1
- (C) *Mycobacterium marinum*
- (D) *Streptococcus pyogenes*

## Item 76

A 32-year-old woman is evaluated following a generalized erythematous rash that developed 1 week ago. The rash has now resolved, and she reports no additional symptoms. She was diagnosed with HIV infection and AIDS 6 months ago when she was treated for *Pneumocystis jirovecii* pneumonia. She began antiretroviral therapy and daily trimethoprim-sulfamethoxazole for secondary pneumonia prophylaxis. She stopped taking trimethoprim-sulfamethoxazole last week when the rash developed. Current therapy consists of lamivudine, abacavir, and dolutegravir.

On physical examination, vital signs are normal. No rash is noted. No lesions are present on the eyes or in the mouth. No lymphadenopathy is noted. The lungs are clear bilaterally, and the abdomen is soft and nontender.

Complete blood count with differential and liver enzyme levels are normal. CD4 cell count is 291/µL (130/µL 6 months ago). HIV quantitative RNA is undetectable (31,840 copies/mL 6 months ago); 3 months ago, the CD4 cell count was 209/µL, and viral load was undetectable.

**Which of the following is the most appropriate management?**

- (A) Begin atovaquone
- (B) Begin primaquine and clindamycin
- (C) Continue current therapy
- (D) Restart trimethoprim-sulfamethoxazole
- (E) Switch to tenofovir, emtricitabine, and dolutegravir

## Item 77

A 67-year-old woman is evaluated after a diagnosis of ventilator-associated pneumonia. She was transferred to the ICU 3 days ago for respiratory failure secondary to Guillain-Barré syndrome and was intubated. Yesterday, the ventilator-associated pneumonia diagnosis was made and empiric antibiotics were started. Today her antibiotic therapy was de-escalated to oxacillin after her sputum culture grew methicillin-sensitive *Staphylococcus aureus*. Blood cultures were negative. Her medications are oxacillin and low-molecular-weight heparin; she is also undergoing plasmapheresis.

On physical examination, temperature is 37.6 °C (99.6 °F), blood pressure and pulse rate are normal, and respiration rate is 15/min. Oxygen saturation is 97% breathing 40% $F_{IO_2}$. Pulmonary examination reveals scattered rhonchi.

A chest radiograph shows right middle and lower lobe infiltrates without effusions.

**Which of the following is the most appropriate antibiotic management?**

- (A) Continue antibiotic therapy for a total of 7 days
- (B) Continue antibiotic therapy for a total of 14 days
- (C) Continue antibiotics until extubation
- (D) Obtain sputum for Gram stain and culture before stopping antibiotics

## Item 78

A 29-year-old woman is evaluated in the emergency department in January for a 5-day history of fever, severe headaches, delusions, and paranoid behavior. Medical history is noncontributory, and she takes no medications.

On physical examination, she is confused and combative. Temperature is 37.9 °C (100.2 °F), blood pressure is 107/48 mm Hg, pulse rate is 102/min, and respiration rate is 20/min. The neck is supple. Occasionally, choreoathetoid movements of the bilateral upper extremities are observed. She has no paralysis. After the examination, she has a generalized seizure in the emergency department.

**CONT.** Lumbar puncture is performed, and results show a cerebrospinal fluid leukocyte count of 310/µL (310 × 10⁶/L) with 94% lymphocytes, glucose level of 60 mg/dL (3.3 mmol/L), and protein level of 55 mg/dL (550 mg/L).

Cerebrospinal fluid bacterial and fungal cultures are negative. Polymerase chain reaction for herpes simplex virus is negative.

An MRI scan of the brain is normal.

**Which of the following is the most likely diagnosis?**

(A) Anti-*N*-methyl-D-aspartate receptor encephalitis
(B) Lyme meningitis
(C) Tuberculous meningitis
(D) West Nile virus encephalitis

## Item 79

A 45-year-old man is evaluated for extreme fatigue accompanied by a 9.1-kg (20 lb) weight loss over the past 2 months. He also has had an occasional productive cough for 1 month. He is unemployed and has been sleeping in homeless shelters for approximately 6 months. He drinks alcohol daily, consuming a fifth of vodka approximately every 2 to 3 days; he does not smoke or use illicit drugs.

On physical examination, temperature is 38.3 °C (100.9 °F), blood pressure is 110/60 mm Hg, pulse rate is 90/min, and respiration rate is 18/min. Bilateral crackles are present throughout inspiration over the upper posterior thorax. The remainder of the examination is unremarkable.

Interferon-γ release assay is positive. HIV antibody testing is negative.

The chest radiograph is shown.

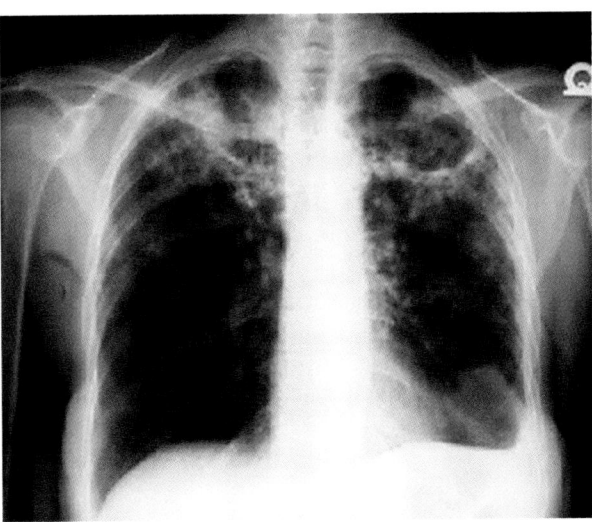

**Which of the following is the most appropriate management?**

(A) Initiate isoniazid plus pyridoxine
(B) Initiate isoniazid, rifampin, pyrazinamide, and ethambutol
(C) Initiate piperacillin–tazobactam
(D) Obtain sputum specimen for acid-fast bacilli stain and culture

## Item 80

A 19-year-old man is evaluated for multiple episodes of nonbloody diarrhea, fever, occasional vomiting, malaise, and crampy abdominal pain that began yesterday. He is a college student who adopted a pet corn snake 2 months ago; the snake is healthy.

On physical examination, temperature is 38.3 °C (100.9 °F), blood pressure is 110/60 mm Hg, pulse rate is 100/min, and respiration rate is 19/min. He appears to be in mild distress. On abdominal examination, bowel sounds are present, as is tenderness to palpation. No rebound or guarding is noted.

Stool testing for occult blood is positive.

**Which of the following is the most likely cause of this patient's diarrheal illness?**

(A) *Chlamydia psittaci*
(B) *Erysipelothrix rhusiopathiae*
(C) *Mycobacterium marinum*
(D) Nontyphoidal *Salmonella* species

## Item 81

A 72-year-old woman undergoes follow-up evaluation for persistent bacteremia. She was hospitalized 12 days ago with fever and chills, which started abruptly 1 week after a cardiac catheterization procedure. Blood cultures were positive for methicillin-sensitive *Staphylococcus aureus*, and cefazolin therapy was initiated. Medical history is otherwise noncontributory, and she takes no other medications.

On physical examination, temperature is 39.4 °C (100.8 °F), blood pressure is 116/76 mm Hg, pulse rate is 92/min, and respiration rate is 16/min. A systolic murmur is present and is unchanged from previous examinations. Abdominal examination reveals right upper quadrant tenderness. The remainder of the examination is noncontributory.

Laboratory studies show an alanine aminotransferase level of 53 U/L, aspartate aminotransferase level of 58 U/L, and alkaline phosphatase level of 104 U/L.

Repeated blood cultures are positive for *S. aureus*.

A transthoracic echocardiogram shows a small aortic valve vegetation. An electrocardiogram is normal.

**Which of the following is the most appropriate management?**

(A) Perform abdominal CT
(B) Perform head CT
(C) Switch cefazolin to daptomycin
(D) Switch cefazolin to vancomycin

## Item 82

A 48-year-old man is evaluated in the emergency department for skin trauma sustained in a freshwater lake 2 days ago, with abrasions and tiny lacerations over the right forearm; he developed a fever and pain at the site of trauma 1 day ago. Medical history is remarkable for cirrhosis secondary to alcohol use. He takes no medications.

On physical examination, temperature is 39.1 °C (102.4 °F), blood pressure is 100/70 mm Hg, pulse rate is 120/min, and

CONT.

respiration rate is 25/min. The right forearm is tender and warm, with several hemorrhagic bullae noted. The remainder of the examination is unremarkable.

A plain radiograph of the right forearm shows no evidence of gas or a foreign body. Surgical exploration and debridement is performed, confirming a diagnosis of necrotizing fasciitis. Gram stain of intraoperative tissue specimens reveals gram-negative bacilli. Empiric antibiotic treatment with vancomycin plus piperacillin-tazobactam is initiated. Twenty-four hours later, the tissue culture grows *Aeromonas hydrophila*.

**Which of the following is the most appropriate treatment?**

(A) Ciprofloxacin plus doxycycline
(B) Linezolid plus metronidazole
(C) Nafcillin plus rifampin
(D) Vancomycin plus clindamycin

## Item 83

A 33-year-old woman is evaluated 4 days after removing an embedded tick from her left arm. She reports that the tick was attached for less than 12 hours. She noticed itching at the site of tick attachment 2 days ago but otherwise has been asymptomatic. She preserved the tick in a bottle, and it is confirmed visually to be an adult black-legged deer tick (*Ixodes scapularis*).

On physical examination, vital signs are normal. A small area of induration is noted on the left arm, with no erythema, tenderness, or warmth. All other physical examination findings are unremarkable.

**Which of the following is the most appropriate initial management?**

(A) *Borrelia burgdorferi* polymerase chain reaction testing of the tick
(B) *Borrelia burgdorferi* serologies
(C) Doxycycline
(D) Reassurance that the risk of Lyme disease is low

## Item 84

A 34-year-old man is evaluated for smallpox (variola) exposure. He feels wells. He is an Air Force surgeon and returned 2 days ago from a mission to the Middle East. Two others who accompanied him on his mission are being evaluated for a febrile illness characterized by headache, sore throat, and a vesicular rash on their faces, arms, and legs. The other men have been placed in airborne precautions because their clinical presentation is consistent with probable active variola infection. Medical history is notable for Crohn disease; he is up to date on all recommended immunizations. His only medication is infliximab.

On physical examination, vital signs are normal, and other physical examination findings are unremarkable.

A complete blood count and comprehensive metabolic profile are normal.

**Which of the following is the most appropriate treatment?**

(A) Airborne precautions
(B) Tecovirimat
(C) Vaccinia immune globulin
(D) Vaccinia immunization

## Item 85

A 22-year-old man is evaluated in the emergency department for a 2-day history of painful rash on the left side of his posterior chest. Medical history is unremarkable, and he takes no medications.

On physical examination, temperature is 37.5 °C (99.5 °F), blood pressure is 115/62 mm Hg, pulse rate is 78/min, and respiration rate is 20/min. A vesicular rash is shown.

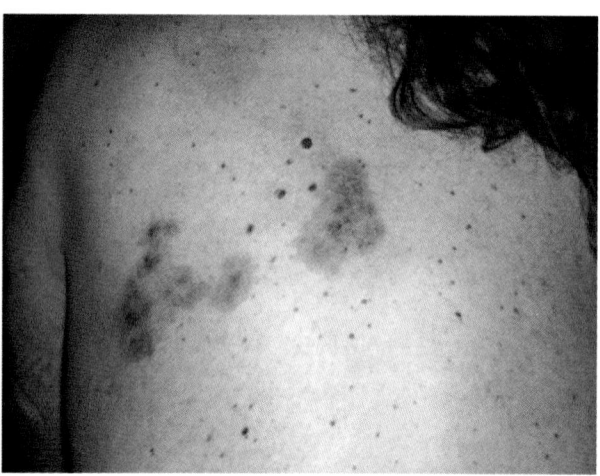

**Which of the following is the most appropriate test to perform next?**

(A) $CH_{50}$ activity
(B) Fourth generation HIV-1/2 antigen/antibody combination immunoassay
(C) IgA measurement
(D) Quantitative immunoglobulin measurement

## Item 86

A 57-year-old woman is hospitalized with a 1-month history of diminished concentration, memory, and judgment, with recent mental status fluctuations and gait disorder. Medical history is remarkable for hypertension. Medications are enalapril and hydrochlorothiazide.

On physical examination, vital signs are normal. She is somnolent but responds to verbal commands. The neck is supple. Deep-tendon reflexes are increased in the upper extremities and decreased in the lower extremities. Movement of the extremities is associated with myoclonus. The remainder of the examination is normal.

Complete blood count, comprehensive metabolic profile, thyroid studies, and vitamin $B_{12}$ measurements are normal.

**Lumbar puncture:**

| | |
|---|---|
| Opening pressure | 70 mm $H_2O$ |
| Leukocyte count | 4/µL ($4 \times 10^6$/L) |
| Erythrocyte count | 5/µL ($5 \times 10^6$/L) |
| Glucose | 108 mg/dL (6 mmol/L) |
| Protein | 57 mg/dL (570 mg/L) |

Gram stain of cerebrospinal fluid is negative. Polymerase chain reaction of cerebrospinal fluid for herpes simplex virus is negative.

Brain MRI shows abnormally increased T2 and FLAIR signal intensity in the putamen and head of the caudate.

**Which of the following is the most likely diagnosis?**

(A) Cryptococcal meningoencephalitis
(B) Sporadic Creutzfeldt-Jakob disease
(C) Tuberculous meningitis
(D) Vascular neurocognitive disorder

## Item 87

A 74-year-old homeless woman is evaluated for hospital discharge. She was admitted 6 days ago with a diagnosis of community-acquired pneumonia, and empiric ceftriaxone and azithromycin were begun. Her fever resolved within 48 hours of admission; however, hospital discharge was delayed because of difficulty arranging posthospitalization placement. Medical history is otherwise noncontributory. She takes no other medications.

On physical examination, vital signs are normal. Oxygen saturation is 96% breathing ambient air. The remainder of the examination is unremarkable.

Sputum culture obtained at admission is growing *Streptococcus pneumoniae* sensitive to penicillin, ceftriaxone, levofloxacin, and vancomycin and resistant to erythromycin. Blood cultures obtained at admission show no growth.

The patient has been accepted into a group home and is ready for hospital discharge.

**Which of the following is the most appropriate management at discharge?**

(A) Continue only azithromycin
(B) Continue only ceftriaxone
(C) Stop all antibiotics
(D) Stop ceftriaxone and azithromycin and switch to amoxicillin
(E) Stop ceftriaxone and azithromycin and switch to levofloxacin

## Item 88

A 46-year-old man is evaluated for pain and swelling of the left index finger that began 2 weeks ago. Ten weeks ago, the patient sustained a deep laceration to the finger while doing construction work. A plain radiograph at that time showed no evidence of fracture. The laceration was sutured, and the wound completely healed. History is significant for poorly controlled type 2 diabetes mellitus. Medications are metformin and glipizide.

On physical examination, vital signs are normal. A 4-cm wound along the medial aspect of the left index finger is completely healed. The finger is edematous and tender when palpated but without erythema.

Laboratory studies reveal an erythrocyte sedimentation rate of 120 mm/h, a leukocyte count of 7800/μL ($7.8 \times 10^9$/L), and a serum creatinine level of 0.6 mg/dL (53.0 μmol/L).

**Which of the following is the most appropriate diagnostic test to perform next?**

(A) CT with contrast
(B) MRI with gadolinium
(C) Plain radiography
(D) Three-phase nuclear bone scan
(E) Ultrasonography

## Item 89

A 42-year-old man is admitted to the ICU for nonresponsive pneumonia with a 7-day history of shortness of breath and cough. He was diagnosed with pneumonia and prescribed levofloxacin 3 days ago and has been adherent to his medication; however, his shortness of breath has worsened to the point he is unable to climb one flight of stairs. Medical history is remarkable for hospitalization 5 years ago for alcohol withdrawal and delirium tremens. He drinks a six-pack of beer every weekday and a case of beer on the weekends. His only medication is levofloxacin.

On physical examination, he is in mild respiratory distress but alert and oriented. Temperature is 38.7 °C (101.7 °F), blood pressure is normal, pulse rate is 122/min, and respiration rate is 24/min. Oxygen saturation is 89% breathing ambient air. Pulmonary auscultation reveals decreased breath sounds at the right lung base.

Laboratory studies show a leukocyte count of 18,700/μL ($18.7 \times 10^9$/L) and a serum creatinine level of 2.3 mg/dL (203 μmol/L).

A chest radiograph shows a right lower lobe infiltrate.

Levofloxacin is discontinued.

**In addition to initiating azithromycin, which of the following is the most appropriate antibiotic treatment?**

(A) Ceftriaxone
(B) Clindamycin
(C) Metronidazole
(D) Piperacillin-tazobactam

## Item 90

A 27-year-old man is evaluated in the emergency department for a 2-day history of bloody diarrhea with abdominal cramping. He reports attending a picnic 5 days before symptom onset where he ate a rare (undercooked) hamburger. Medical history is otherwise unremarkable, and he takes no medications.

On physical examination, temperature is 37.1 °C (98.8 °F), blood pressure is 120/76 mm Hg, pulse rate is 100/min, and respiration rate is 16/min. On abdominal examination, bowel sounds are present with diffuse tenderness to palpation but no guarding or rebound.

**Laboratory studies:**

| | |
|---|---|
| Hematocrit | 39% |
| Leukocyte count | 18,000/μL ($18.0 \times 10^9$/L) (differential: 80% neutrophils, 20% lymphocytes) |
| Platelet count | 190,000/μL ($190 \times 10^9$/L) |
| Creatinine | 1.3 mg/dL (114.9 μmol/L) |

Stool assay is positive for presence of Shiga-like toxin.

**Which of the following is the most appropriate management?**

(A) Ceftriaxone

(B) Ciprofloxacin

(C) Loperamide

(D) Trimethoprim-sulfamethoxazole

(E) Supportive care

 **Item 91**

A 45-year-old man is hospitalized with a 5-day history of fever, bloody diarrhea, and abdominal pain. Medical history is significant for end-stage kidney disease, for which he underwent kidney transplantation 1 year ago. Medications are prednisone, mycophenolate, and tacrolimus.

On physical examination, vital signs are normal. Conjunctival pallor is present. Abdominal palpation elicits diffuse abdominal pain. The remainder of the examination is unremarkable.

**Laboratory studies:**

| | |
|---|---|
| Hemoglobin | 9.5 mg/dL (95 g/L) |
| Leukocyte count | 3400/µL ($3.4 \times 10^9$/L) |
| Platelet count | 98,000/µL ($98 \times 10^9$/L) |
| Alanine aminotransferase | 99 U/L |
| Aspartate aminotransferase | 88 U/L |
| Creatinine | 1.5 mg/dL (133 µmol/L) |

**Which of the following is the most likely diagnosis?**

(A) Cytomegalovirus infection

(B) *Entamoeba histolytica* infection

(C) *Salmonella enteritidis* infection

(D) *Strongyloides stercoralis* infection

 **Item 92**

A 23-year-old man is evaluated for a 2-day history of erythema and drainage from a surgical incision site. He reports no fever or chills. He underwent a left inguinal hernia repair 10 days ago. Medical history is otherwise noncontributory, and he takes no medications.

On physical examination, vital signs are normal. The left inguinal incision is erythematous around the edges, is tender, and exudes a small amount of serosanguinous, cloudy drainage from a small area of incision breakdown. No induration is noted around the incision area.

Laboratory studies show a leukocyte count of 8700/µL ($8.7 \times 10^9$/L).

**Which of the following is the most appropriate diagnostic test to perform next?**

(A) Blood culture

(B) CT of upper thigh and pelvis

(C) Gram stain and culture of incision site drainage

(D) Gram stain and culture of incision site swabbing

**Item 93**

A 55-year-old man is evaluated in the emergency department for a 1-week history of chills and altered mental status

and a 2-week history of fever and severe headache. He has end-stage liver disease secondary to alcohol abuse. Medications are propranolol, furosemide, spironolactone, and lactulose.

On physical examination, temperature is 38.6 °C (101.5 °F), blood pressure is 110/85 mm Hg, pulse rate is 111/min, and respiration rate is 22/min. The patient is somnolent, cachectic, and jaundiced. Funduscopic examination shows no papilledema. Bibasilar crackles are heard on auscultation of the lungs. The abdomen is distended and tense. No focal neurologic findings are present.

A CT scan of the head with contrast shows cerebral atrophy. A lumbar puncture is performed.

**Cerebrospinal fluid studies:**

| | |
|---|---|
| Cell count | 2 erythrocytes/hpf; 98 leukocytes/hpf, with 70% neutrophils and 30% lymphocytes |
| Glucose | 20 mg/dL (1.1 mmol/L) |
| Pressure, opening | 180 mm $H_2O$ |
| Protein | 170 mg/dL (1700 mg/L) |
| Cryptococcal antigen titer | 1:2048 |
| Gram stain | Negative |

**Which of the following is the most appropriate treatment?**

(A) Fluconazole

(B) Itraconazole

(C) Liposomal amphotericin B and flucytosine

(D) Micafungin

**Item 94**

A 64-year-old woman is evaluated for a 6-week history of right knee swelling and pain. She has had no recent injury, fevers, or chills. She retired as a horticulturist and moved from Massachusetts to Florida 3 months ago. She takes NSAIDs, which provide partial pain relief, but the swelling persists.

On physical examination, vital signs are normal. The right knee has a moderately sized effusion but no erythema or warmth. Slight pain is present on passive movement of the knee.

Results of laboratory studies show an equivocal *Borrelia burgdorferi* enzyme immunoassay of 1.07; leukocyte count and rheumatoid factor titer are within normal limits.

**Which of the following is the most appropriate next diagnostic test?**

(A) *Borrelia burgdorferi* IgG Western blot

(B) C6 enzyme immunoassay antibody test

(C) Polymerase chain reaction of joint fluid

(D) No further testing

**Item 95**

A 63-year-old man undergoes discharge evaluation. He was hospitalized 24 hours ago after a diagnosis of acute bacterial prostatitis, for which ciprofloxacin was initiated. His fever has resolved. Medical history is otherwise unremarkable, and he takes no other medications.

He is being discharged home to complete 6 weeks of oral ciprofloxacin therapy.

**Which of the following is the most appropriate monitoring for this patient?**

CONT.

(A) Serum lipase level

(B) Serum sodium level

(C) Stool for *Clostridium difficile* toxin

(D) Symptoms of tendon or joint pain

## Item 96

A 30-year-old man is evaluated for a 1-week history of sore throat and odynophagia. He reports no fever, nausea, vomiting, diarrhea, or other symptoms. He was recently diagnosed with HIV infection and began antiretroviral therapy 2 weeks ago. Medications are tenofovir alafenamide, emtricitabine, dolutegravir, and trimethoprim-sulfamethoxazole.

On physical examination, vital signs are normal. Oral examination findings (shown) include whitish plaques on the posterior pharynx. Lymph nodes are palpable in the anterior and posterior cervical regions bilaterally. The remainder of the examination is normal.

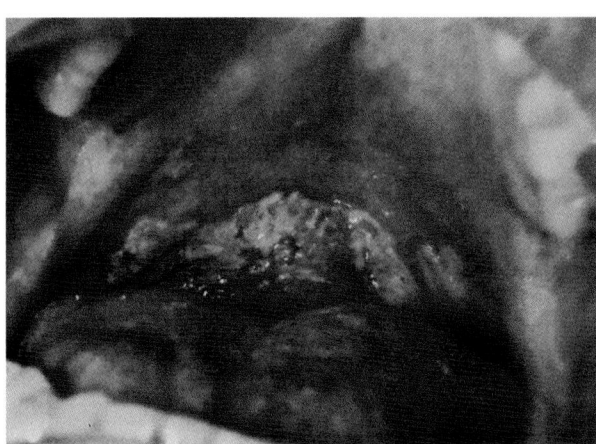

Laboratory studies at the time of HIV diagnosis showed a CD4 cell count of 55/µL and HIV viral load of 138,855 copies/mL.

**Which of the following is the most appropriate management?**

(A) Intravenous caspofungin

(B) Oral fluconazole

(C) Nystatin swish-and-swallow

(D) Upper endoscopy

(E) Valganciclovir

## Item 97

A 47-year-old woman is evaluated in the hospital for pyelonephritis not responding to antibiotic therapy. Five days ago she was evaluated in an urgent care center for abdominal and back pain, nausea, fever, and dysuria. She was started on oral ciprofloxacin for a urinary tract infection (UTI). Symptoms did not respond to this treatment, and two days ago, she was hospitalized. Acute pyelonephritis was diagnosed, and she was treated with intravenous fluids, vancomycin, and cefepime. Since hospitalization, her clinical condition has deteriorated, with continued fever and worsening flank pain. She also has stage 2 chronic kidney disease, recurrent UTIs, and a 6-year history of poorly controlled type 2 diabetes mellitus. Medications are amoxicillin, metformin, and insulin glargine.

On physical examination, temperature is 38.2 °C (100.8 °F), blood pressure is 130/60 mm Hg, pulse rate is 106/min, and respiration rate is 22/min. Abdominal examination reveals diminished bowel sounds, bilateral costovertebral angle tenderness, and suprapubic pain. Other examination findings are unremarkable.

**Laboratory studies:**

| | |
|---|---|
| Hemoglobin | 11 g/dL (110 g/L) |
| Leukocyte count | 21,000/µL (21 × 10⁹/L) with 91% neutrophils and 9% lymphocytes |
| Platelet count | 167,000/µL (167 × 10⁹/L) |
| Creatinine | 1.8 mg/mL (159 µmol/L) |
| Urinalysis | 10 erythrocytes/hpf, leukocytes too numerous to count, many yeast forms, trace protein, and 4+ glucose |

Urine culture results show 10,000 colony-forming units of *Candida glabrata*. Blood culture results are negative.

A CT scan of the abdomen with contrast shows bilateral perinephric stranding, no masses, and no renal abscesses.

**Which of the following is the most likely diagnosis?**

(A) Acute diverticulitis

(B) Antibiotic-resistant bacterial pyelonephritis

(C) *Candida* pyelonephritis

(D) Renal infarction

## Item 98

A 25-year-old man is evaluated for a 3-day history of painful lesions on his penis accompanied by generalized myalgia and malaise. He has been sexually active with one female partner for the past 6 months; he does not use condoms. Medical history is unremarkable for previous genital ulcers and is otherwise noncontributory. He takes no medications but indicates he develops a rash with penicillin use.

On physical examination, vital signs are normal except for a temperature of 38.2 °C (100.8 °F). Bilateral, tender inguinal lymphadenopathy is noted. Lesions on the penile shaft are shown on the next page.

**Which of the following is the most appropriate diagnostic test to perform next?**

(A) Darkfield examination

(B) Direct fluorescence assay

(C) Nucleic acid amplification testing

(D) Type-specific antibody testing

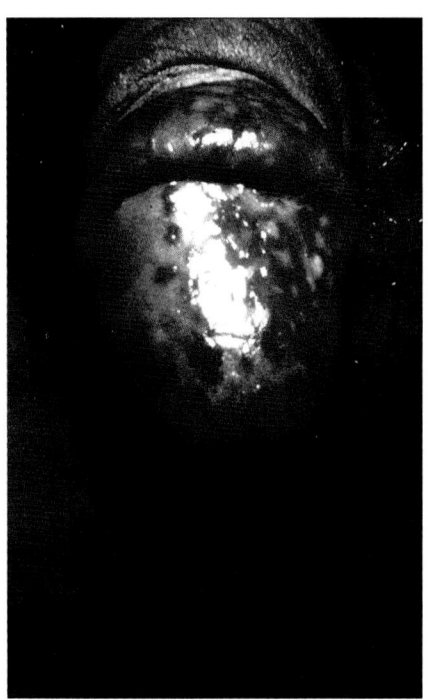

ITEM 98

## Item 99

A 25-year-old man is evaluated in the emergency department for left hand pain at the site of injection drug use. All of his immunizations are up to date. He takes no medications.

On physical examination, temperature is 39.3 °C (102.7 °F), blood pressure is 88/50 mm Hg, pulse rate is 110/min, and respiration rate is 26/min. A violaceous, swollen, indurated area is noted on the dorsum of the left hand at the site of recent injection drug use; it is warm to the touch and tender.

**Laboratory studies:**

| | |
|---|---|
| Hematocrit | 36% |
| Leukocyte count | 25,000/µL (25 × 10⁹/L) |
| Platelet count | 100,000/µL (100 × 10⁹/L) |
| Alanine aminotransferase | 65 U/L |
| Aspartate aminotransferase | 105 U/L |
| Creatinine | 2.5 mg/dL (221 µmol/L) |

Empiric treatment with vancomycin and piperacillin-tazobactam is initiated and he undergoes surgical debridement. Intraoperative findings confirm necrotizing fasciitis, and tissue and blood cultures grow group A *Streptococcus*.

**Which of the following is the most appropriate antibiotic treatment?**

(A) Continue vancomycin and piperacillin-tazobactam
(B) Change to doxycycline and ceftazidime
(C) Change to linezolid and imipenem
(D) Change to penicillin and clindamycin

## Item 100

A 78-year-old woman undergoes routine evaluation. She has been feeling relatively well but experiences occasional urinary incontinence when she coughs, sneezes, or laughs. Medical history is significant for hypertension. Medications are chlorthalidone and lisinopril.

On physical examination, vital signs and other physical examination findings are normal.

On dipstick urinalysis, urine is yellow and clear, specific gravity is 1.010, pH is 7.0, and moderate leukocyte esterase and nitrites are present; the urinalysis is negative for blood or glucose but 2+ for bacteria.

**Which of the following is the most appropriate management?**

(A) Ciprofloxacin
(B) Cystoscopy
(C) Microscopic urinalysis
(D) Urine culture and sensitivity
(E) No further investigation or treatment

## Item 101

A 52-year-old woman is evaluated in the emergency department for fever, headache, muscular pain, and a diffuse, nonpruritic rash that began on the arms. She returned 5 days ago from a 3-week trip in southern Spain. She recalls a dark, raised, scab-like lesion on her ankle that she attributed to an insect bite. Her medical history is otherwise unremarkable.

On physical examination, the patient is lethargic. Temperature is 38.7 °C (101.6 °F), blood pressure is 118/70 mm Hg, pulse rate is 82/min, and respiration rate is 16/min. Neurologic examination is nonfocal and without meningismus. A right inguinal lymph node is enlarged. A maculopapular pink rash is present on the trunk, arms, legs, palms, and soles. A black eschar is present on the right ankle that measures 1.5 × 1.5 cm. Other examination findings are normal.

**Which of the following is the most likely diagnosis?**

(A) Human granulocytic anaplasmosis
(B) Lyme disease
(C) Mediterranean spotted fever
(D) Rocky Mountain spotted fever

## Item 102

A 24-year-old man is evaluated in the emergency department in October for a 10-day history of headaches, fever, and stiff neck. He reports camping and hiking in the woods on Nantucket Island 2 months ago. Medical history is unremarkable, and he takes no medications.

On physical examination, he is alert and oriented. Temperature is 38.3 °C (101.0 °F), blood pressure is 134/85 mm Hg, pulse rate is 104/min, and respiration rate is 20/min. Right-sided facial palsy is noted, and neck flexion elicits resistance and discomfort, but the neurologic examination is otherwise normal. No rash is present.

A lumbar puncture is performed, and cerebrospinal fluid evaluation shows a leukocyte count of 235/µL (235 × 10⁶/L) with 84% lymphocytes. Gram stain is negative and cultures are pending.

**Which of the following is the most likely cause of the patient's findings?**

CONT.

(A) *Borrelia burgdorferi*

(B) Enterovirus

(C) Herpes simplex virus type 2

(D) Varicella-zoster virus

(E) West Nile virus

## Item 103

A 26-year-old man is hospitalized for a 3-month history of fever, night sweats, and weakness. Medical history is notable for kidney transplantation 5 years ago. Medications are prednisone and mycophenolate.

On physical examination, temperature is 38.1 °C (100.5 °F), blood pressure is 135/62 mm Hg, pulse rate is 68/min, and respiration rate is 20/min. The sclerae are pale. Cervical, supraclavicular, and axillary lymphadenopathy are noted. Abdominal examination reveals hepatosplenomegaly.

**Laboratory studies:**

| | |
|---|---|
| Hemoglobin | 8.4 mg/dL (84 g/L) |
| Leukocyte count | 2300/μL (2.3 × 10⁹/L) |
| Platelet count | 98,000/μL (98 × 10⁹/L) |
| Creatinine (stable) | 1.1 mg/dL (97.2 μmol/L) |

**Which of the following is the most likely cause of his symptoms?**

(A) Cytomegalovirus

(B) Epstein-Barr virus

(C) Herpes simplex virus type 1

(D) Polyoma BK virus

## Item 104

A 23-year-old man is evaluated for a furuncle on the left forearm that appeared 1 day ago. Medical history is notable only for anaphylaxis with administration of trimethoprim-sulfamethoxazole. He is otherwise well and takes no medications.

On physical examination, temperature is 38.3 °C (100.9 °F), blood pressure is 124/75 mm Hg, pulse rate is 95/min, and respiration rate is 15/min. A 2- × 2-cm fluctuant lesion is present on the right forearm with 1 cm of surrounding erythema. The remainder of the examination is unremarkable.

After incision and drainage of the abscess, a culture is obtained.

**Which of the following is the most appropriate additional treatment?**

(A) Oral cephalexin

(B) Oral clindamycin

(C) Oral doxycycline

(D) Oral penicillin

(E) Clinical follow-up

## Item 105

A 55-year-old woman undergoes annual tuberculin skin testing. An 8-mm induration is recorded after 48 hours. She reports no symptoms or exposures. She works as a clerk in an internal medicine outpatient clinic at a metropolitan hospital in New York City. Medical history is unremarkable, and she takes no medications.

On physical examination, vital signs and examination are normal.

**Which of the following is the most appropriate management?**

(A) Chest radiography

(B) Induce sputum for culture

(C) Initiate isoniazid for treatment of latent tuberculosis

(D) Move patient to nonpatient care areas

(E) No further testing or treatment

## Item 106

A 35-year-old man is evaluated during a follow-up consultation. He was diagnosed with HIV 6 months ago; at that time, his CD4 cell count was 30/μL. He immediately began antiretroviral therapy and has been adherent to his regimen. His initial screening tests included a nonreactive tuberculin skin test (TST). He states that he has been unemployed for more than 2 years and has lived in a variety of different homeless shelters. Medications are tenofovir-emtricitabine and raltegravir.

On physical examination, vital signs and other findings are unremarkable.

Today, a repeat CD4 cell count is 100/μL and a repeat TST results in 5 mm of induration.

A posteroanterior and lateral chest radiograph is unremarkable.

**Which of the following is the most appropriate management?**

(A) Initiate isoniazid plus pyridoxine

(B) Initiate isoniazid, rifampin, pyrazinamide, and ethambutol

(C) Obtain an interferon-γ release assay

(D) Repeat TST in 2 weeks

## Item 107

A 24-year-old woman is evaluated for cystitis symptoms of 4 days' duration. She reports no fever, chills, flank pain, or vaginal discharge. She has had similar symptoms three times within the past 10 months. She has been treated each time with trimethoprim-sulfamethoxazole at an urgent care center. The last episode was 5 weeks ago. She has sexual intercourse infrequently. Her only medication is an oral contraceptive.

On physical examination, vital signs and other findings are unremarkable.

On microscopic urinalysis, leukocytes are too numerous to count, erythrocyte count is 10/hpf, 4+ bacteria are present, and rare squamous epithelial cells are seen.

**Which of the following is the most appropriate management?**

(A) Nitrofurantoin

(B) Trimethoprim-sulfamethoxazole

(C) Urine culture plus ampicillin

(D) Urine culture plus cefpodoxime

(E) Urine culture plus ciprofloxacin

## Item 108

A 41-year-old woman is evaluated in the emergency depart-ment for total loss of vision in the left eye. She also reports a 3-day history of left-sided tunnel vision and a 2-week his-tory of sinus pain and rhinorrhea. The patient has a 20-year history of type 1 diabetes mellitus, which has been poorly controlled for the past 18 months. Medications are insulin glargine and insulin aspart.

On physical examination, temperature is 37.2 °C (99.0 °F), blood pressure is 140/66 mm Hg, pulse rate is 110/min, and respiration rate is 18/min. Left eye proptosis and chemosis are noted; the left pupil is nonreactive. The left nasal mucosa has gray-black exudate and an eschar. A 2- × 3-cm black eschar is seen on the hard palate. Neurologic examina-tion shows occulomotor, trochlear, trigeminal, and abducens nerve (cranial nerves III, IV, V, and VI) palsy on the left.

A CT scan of the head without contrast shows a mass in the maxillary sinus with extension into the left frontal lobe and surrounding edema.

**Which of the following is the most likely diagnosis?**

(A) Anthrax
(B) Aspergillosis
(C) Lemierre syndrome
(D) Mucormycosis

# Answers and Critiques

## Item 1     Answer:   A

**Educational Objective:** Prevent *Staphylococcus aureus* surgical site infection by evaluating for *S. aureus* nasal carriage.

The most appropriate measure to prevent surgical site infection is to evaluate for *Staphylococcus aureus* nasal carriage 2 weeks before surgery and decolonize if positive. *S. aureus* is the most common pathogen (23%) associated with surgical site infections (SSIs). SSIs after coronary artery bypass graft surgery can be serious and devastating, with mediastinitis related to *S. aureus* of particular concern. The 2016 World Health Organization guidelines recommend that patients known to be nasal carriers of *S. aureus* who are scheduled to undergo cardiothoracic or orthopedic surgery should have preoperative decolonization (mupirocin ointment for 5 days with or without chlorhexidine gluconate body wash) to decrease the risk of developing *S. aureus*–related SSI.

Data do not support extending antibiotic prophylaxis beyond 24 hours after cardiac surgery even while drains remain in place. For most other surgeries, no additional doses of antibiotic should be given postoperatively, even in cases of intraoperative spillage of gastrointestinal contents. Postoperative antibiotics are only indicated when treating an active infection.

Preoperative antibiotic prophylaxis reduces the risk of SSI by decreasing the concentration of pathogens at or around the incision site. The agent used and the timing of administration are key. For cardiac surgery, cefazolin is recommended unless a patient is known to have methicillin-resistant *S. aureus* colonization or has a severe (anaphylactic) β-lactam allergy, in which case vancomycin is used. For optimal benefit, the antibiotic should be administered 1 to 2 hours before incision. For procedures lasting more than several hours, the antibiotic should be redosed during surgery (for example, redose at 3-4 hours for cefazolin).

Preoperative shaving in the area of the planned incision increases the risk of SSI. Shaving causes microscopic abrasions of the skin, which promotes bacterial proliferation. Recommendations indicate only removing hair from the surgical site if it will interfere with the procedure, in which case clipping is preferred.

### KEY POINT

- Patients undergoing cardiothoracic or orthopedic surgery should be screened for nasal carriage of *Staphylococcus aureus* and, if positive, should have preoperative decolonization.

### Bibliography

Schweizer ML, Chiang HY, Septimus E, Moody J, Braun B, Hafner J, et al. Association of a bundled intervention with surgical site infections among patients undergoing cardiac, hip, or knee surgery. JAMA. 2015;313:2162-71. [PMID: 26034956] doi:10.1001/jama.2015.5387

## Item 2     Answer:   D

**Educational Objective:** Treat tuberculosis and immune reconstitution inflammatory syndrome in a patient with HIV.

The most appropriate management for this patient is to start rifabutin, isoniazid, ethambutol, and pyrazinamide therapy for tuberculosis. He began antiretroviral therapy 1 month ago and has responded well, with a significant decrease in viral load and increased CD4 cell count. The timing of his presentation is consistent with the immune reconstitution inflammatory syndrome (IRIS) (median 48 days), the return of a robust immune response resulting from treatment of the HIV that "unmasks" a pre-existing infection that appears like a new acute infection. This presentation is common with tuberculosis, which may present as a much more acute pulmonary illness resembling bacterial pneumonia. He had an indeterminate result on interferon-γ release assay (IGRA) because of an inadequate response to the positive control, which was the result of immunocompromise at the time of presentation; additionally, the results of IGRA testing are a poor indicator of active tuberculosis infection. He should begin four-drug antituberculous therapy while results of culture and susceptibility testing are pending. Nucleic acid amplification testing of the specimen may give information on the identification of the organisms and even the possibility of rifamycin resistance. Initial empiric treatment for tuberculosis should include a rifamycin as one of the four drugs, but rifabutin is often preferred over rifampin in patients with HIV because of fewer drug-drug interactions between rifabutin and antiretrovirals, including dolutegravir.

If this patient does have active tuberculosis, treatment is needed urgently; culture results may take weeks, so waiting would be inappropriate.

Antiretrovirals should not be stopped when IRIS occurs. Therapy should be continued while providing treatment for the newly diagnosed infection.

Prednisone can be added if IRIS is life threatening or involves the pericardium or central nervous system. None of these is the case in this patient; giving glucocorticoids without a known diagnosis increases the risk of worsening an infection that is not being directly treated.

### KEY POINT

- Immune reconstitution inflammatory syndrome is the return of a robust immune response resulting from treatment of HIV that may "unmask" a pre-existing infection; when this occurs, the underlying infection should be treated while antiretroviral therapy is continued.

### Bibliography

Panel on Opportunistic Infections in HIV-Infected Adults and Adolescents. Guidelines for the prevention and treatment of opportunistic infections in HIV-infected adults and adolescents: recommendations from the Centers for Disease Control and Prevention, the National Institutes of Health, and the HIV Medicine Association of the Infectious Diseases Society of America. Available at https://aidsinfo.nih.gov/guidelines/html/4/adult-and-adolescent-opportunistic-infection/0. Accessed April 12, 2018.

## Item 3    Answer:    A

**Educational Objective:**  Diagnose pulmonary coccidioidomycosis.

This patient has disseminated coccidioidomycosis manifesting as a pulmonary infection. The fungus *Coccidioides* is inhaled and causes an initial pulmonary infection. In endemic areas, as many as one third of cases of community-acquired pneumonia (CAP) are caused by *Coccidioides* species. Healthy persons generally contain the initial infection owing to intact cell-mediated immunity; however, immunocompromised persons are at risk for dissemination. This endemic dimorphic fungal infection is known to mimic other diseases, including tuberculosis, histoplasmosis, sarcoidosis, and cancer. The patient is stationed in Bakersfield, California, an epicenter for this infection. In addition, his assignment as a car mechanic, with much of his work likely conducted outside, increases the risk of infection. Another clue is his peripheral eosinophilia. A definitive diagnosis generally is made on the basis of serology and histopathologic analysis of tissue. When coccidioidomycosis is diagnosed, first-line therapy is fluconazole to prevent progressive or disseminated disease.

Sarcoidosis is a systemic disease of unknown cause. It is slightly more frequent in black persons in their 20s and 30s, especially women. It frequently presents in the respiratory tract as bilateral hilar lymphadenopathy, with or without diffuse parenchymal lung changes. Unilateral hilar lymphadenopathy is distinctly unusual, as is eosinophilia. In addition, sarcoidosis tends to be a much more indolent process, presenting over several months to years with progressive cough and dyspnea. This patient developed symptoms acutely, over a 1-month period.

The most commonly identified organism causing CAP is *Streptococcus pneumoniae*. Suggestive clinical symptoms include fever, cough, sputum production, and dyspnea. Radiographic findings can be characterized as interstitial infiltrates, lobar consolidation, or cavitary lesions; unilateral hilar lymphadenopathy would be distinctly unusual. Finally, symptoms lasting for a month and peripheral eosinophilia are not characteristic of a bacterial lung infection.

Primary pulmonary tuberculosis may present with mid- to lower-zone unilateral infiltrates, unilateral hilar lymphadenopathy, and pleural effusions. Early in the course of the disease, laboratory findings are often normal; eosinophilia is not present. Finally, pulmonary tuberculosis is excluded by the negative interferon-γ release assay.

### KEY POINT

• In endemic areas, as many as one third of cases of community-acquired pneumonia are caused by *Coccidioides* species.

**Bibliography**

Stockamp NW, Thompson GR 3rd. Coccidioidomycosis. Infect Dis Clin North Am. 2016;30:229-46. [PMID: 26739609] doi:10.1016/j.idc.2015.10.008

## Item 4    Answer:    C

**Educational Objective:**  Treat community-acquired pneumonia in a hospitalized patient requiring ICU support.

The most appropriate treatment is ceftriaxone plus levofloxacin. This otherwise healthy patient presents with severe community-acquired pneumonia (CAP). The initial evaluation reveals respiratory failure (tachypnea and hypoxia), uremia, altered mentation, and multilobar infiltrates, all of which are minor criteria for severe disease based on Infectious Diseases Society of America/American Thoracic Society (IDSA/ATS) criteria. Patients with at least three minor criteria for severe disease have increased risk of mortality and are best managed in the ICU. Guideline-based recommendations for empiric therapy of CAP requiring ICU care include a third-generation cephalosporin or ampicillin-sulbactam to treat *Streptococcus pneumoniae*, gram-negative bacilli, or *Haemophilus influenzae* plus an agent active against *Legionella*, such as a macrolide or quinolone. The initial evaluation of this patient was positive for rhinovirus on a respiratory viral panel (RVP). Respiratory viruses are increasingly recognized among hospitalized patients with CAP; however, the significance of this finding is uncertain. Respiratory viruses may predispose patients to a secondary bacterial pneumonia or be present as a copathogen. Considering the severity of this patient's illness, antibiotics should be initiated and continued despite the positive RVP until a bacterial cause is excluded.

Azithromycin monotherapy is an appropriate choice for treatment of CAP in a previously healthy outpatient. Patients with more severe CAP are at risk for infections with numerous organisms, as well as with drug-resistant pathogens. For this reason, patients with CAP admitted to the ICU should receive combination therapy with an antipneumococcal β-lactam and either a macrolide or a fluoroquinolone.

Ceftazidime is a third-generation cephalosporin that is effective against *Pseudomonas* but has minimal activity against gram-positive organisms, including *S. pneumoniae*, and therefore would not be an appropriate choice, even as combination therapy with a macrolide, to treat CAP.

Piperacillin-tazobactam plus ciprofloxacin would be indicated when concern for *Pseudomonas* pneumonia is present; however, in a previously healthy patient with minimal health care interactions or previous antibiotic use, *Pseudomonas* would be an unlikely pathogen.

### KEY POINT

• Guideline-based recommendations for empiric therapy of community-acquired pneumonia requiring ICU admission include a third-generation cephalosporin or ampicillin-sulbactam to treat *Streptococcus pneumoniae*, gram-negative bacilli, or *Haemophilus influenzae* plus an agent active against *Legionella*, such as a macrolide or quinolone.

## Bibliography

Mandell LA, Wunderink RG, Anzueto A, Bartlett JG, Campbell GD, Dean NC, et al; Infectious Diseases Society of America. Infectious Diseases Society of America/American Thoracic Society consensus guidelines on the management of community-acquired pneumonia in adults. Clin Infect Dis. 2007;44 Suppl 2:S27-72. [PMID: 17278083]

## Item 5        Answer:    B

**Educational Objective:**  Evaluate fever of unknown origin.

The most appropriate diagnostic test in this patient is CT of the abdomen and pelvis. He meets the criteria for classic fever of unknown origin, which is defined by fever of 38.3 °C (100.9 °F) or greater for 3 or more weeks that remains undiagnosed after two visits in the ambulatory setting. Taking a careful, detailed history is the starting point in evaluating a patient with fever of unknown cause. The history may need to be repeated on subsequent visits because subtle clues may be revealed only later. All symptoms should be considered relevant. A history of comorbid conditions and a surgical, obstetric or gynecologic (in women), medication, travel, and social history should be elicited followed by a careful physical examination that includes full neurologic, musculoskeletal, ear-nose-throat, eye or funduscopic, skin, lymphatic, and urogenital examinations. The results of basic laboratory and imaging studies along with the history and physical examination findings are used to guide further evaluation. In this patient, the initial evaluation for infectious causes (tuberculosis, endocarditis, urinary tract infection), neoplasms (lymphoma, leukemia), and connective tissue disease is unrevealing. Therefore, the patient should undergo CT of the abdomen and pelvis (with and without contrast) to evaluate for abscess, neoplasm (hepatoma, renal cell carcinoma), splenomegaly, and lymphadenopathy. The prognosis is good for adults who remain undiagnosed after extensive evaluation.

Bone marrow biopsy is generally considered when the complete blood count is abnormal and a process involving the bone marrow (such as tuberculosis, histoplasmosis, or malignancy) is evident.

Liver biopsy is considered in the setting of abnormal liver chemistry tests and a suggested abnormality on imaging. It would not be appropriate at this time.

If signs or symptoms referable to the central nervous system are evident, imaging of the head and lumbar puncture should be considered. However, this patient has no central nervous system findings.

### KEY POINT

- Initial studies for fever of unknown origin in most patients typically include a complete blood count with differential, complete metabolic profile with kidney and liver studies, at least three blood culture sets and cultures of other bodily fluids (such as urine or from other sources based on clinical suspicion), an erythrocyte sedimentation rate, tuberculosis testing, and serology for HIV; it is reasonable to perform chest imaging (radiography or CT) as initial diagnostic imaging.

## Bibliography

Mulders-Manders C, Simon A, Bleeker-Rovers C. Fever of unknown origin. Clin Med (Lond). 2015;15:280-4. [PMID: 26031980] doi:10.7861/clinmedicine.15-3-280

## Item 6        Answer:    B

**Educational Objective:**  Diagnose invasive aspergillosis.

This patient most likely has disseminated aspergillosis with lung and brain involvement. Aspergillus invades blood vessels and causes distal infarction of infected tissue. Patients with invasive pulmonary aspergillosis may have fever, cough, chest pain, and hemoptysis at presentation. Pulmonary infiltrates, nodules, or wedge-shaped densities resembling infarcts may also be seen on chest radiographs; CT scans may show a target lesion with a necrotic center surrounded by a ring of hemorrhage (halo sign). Central nervous system involvement may manifest as a brain abscess or infarction. Other sites of involvement include blood vessels in the heart, gastrointestinal tract, or skin. Risk factors for invasive or disseminated aspergillosis include profound and prolonged neutropenia and hematopoietic stem cell transplantation. The second most common risk group for invasive aspergillosis is solid organ (heart, lung, liver, kidney) transplant recipients. The infection has also increasingly been reported in patients who are critically ill and in ICUs, especially those with exposure to glucocorticoids. The most efficient way to establish a definitive diagnosis (and then initiate antifungal therapy) is with bronchoalveolar lavage (BAL) and biopsy. In patients with disseminated aspergillosis, the serum galactomannan assay has a sensitivity of less than 30% and is not very useful; in contrast, the BAL galactomannan assay has a much higher sensitivity and specificity. Therefore, BAL fluid samples should be collected for analysis, and tissue biopsy should be performed.

A brain biopsy is sometimes useful to establish a definitive diagnosis but carries a much greater risk of causing adverse effects than bronchoscopy and BAL. If the lung biopsy is negative, then a brain biopsy should be considered.

Fungal blood cultures have a low sensitivity in all invasive mold infections but especially in invasive aspergillosis, in which less than 1% of patients with infection have a positive culture.

### KEY POINT

- Risk factors for invasive or disseminated aspergillosis include profound and prolonged neutropenia and stem cell and solid organ transplantation; patients have fever, cough, chest pain, and hemoptysis at presentation, and pulmonary infiltrates, nodules, or wedge-shaped densities may be seen on chest radiographs.

## Bibliography

Cadena J, Thompson GR 3rd, Patterson TF. Invasive aspergillosis: current strategies for diagnosis and management. Infect Dis Clin North Am. 2016;30:125-42. [PMID: 26897064] doi:10.1016/j.idc.2015.10.015

**Item 7      Answer:   C**

**Educational Objective:**  Diagnose leptospiral meningitis.

The most likely diagnosis is leptospirosis. She presents with a biphasic illness after freshwater exposure in an area highly endemic for leptospirosis. Infection occurs by direct exposure to urine or tissues of infected animals or indirectly through contaminated water or soil. Rodents and other small mammals are the most significant sources of human disease. Leptospiral meningitis usually develops weeks after exposure, in the second phase of the illness, but may merge with the first phase in severe disease and can present with uveitis, rash, conjunctival suffusion (conjunctival redness without exudate), sepsis, lymphadenopathy, kidney injury, and hepatosplenomegaly. Subconjunctival suffusion may be subtle but is a finding that rarely occurs in other infections. The cerebrospinal fluid (CSF) findings resemble enteroviral meningitis, but empiric treatment with doxycycline should be started pending confirmation.

Most persons who develop HIV infection experience an acute symptomatic illness, referred to as acute retroviral syndrome, within a few weeks of acquiring the infection. Symptoms are most often consistent with an infectious mononucleosis with fever, malaise, lymphadenopathy, rash, and pharyngitis. Some of these patients will develop meningitis or meningoencephalitis. Meningitis caused by acute HIV infection is typically self-limited and may be clinically indistinguishable from other viral meningitis syndromes, but jaundice, kidney injury, and subconjunctival suffusion are not seen with acute HIV infection.

Patients with herpes simplex meningitis have typical meningitis symptoms, such as fever, nuchal rigidity, headache, and photophobia. Jaundice, kidney injury, and subconjunctival suffusion are not characteristic of herpes simplex meningitis.

*Treponema pallidum* meningitis can occur in the secondary or tertiary phase of syphilis. Headache and meningismus are common; decreased visual acuity secondary to uveitis, vitreitis, retinitis, or optic neuropathy can be seen, as well as other cranial neuropathies. The CSF usually shows a lymphocytic pleocytosis with an elevated protein level. This patient's clinical course is not compatible with syphilitic meningitis.

**KEY POINT**

- Leptospiral meningitis usually develops weeks after exposure, during the second phase of illness, and can present with uveitis, rash, conjunctival suffusion, sepsis, lymphadenopathy, kidney injury, and hepatosplenomegaly.

**Bibliography**

Londeree WA. Leptospirosis: the microscopic danger in paradise. Hawaii J Med Public Health. 2014;73:21-3. [PMID: 25478298]

 **Item 8      Answer:   D**

**Educational Objective:**  Treat fulminant *Clostridium difficile* infection.

The most appropriate treatment is oral vancomycin plus intravenous metronidazole. Treatment of *Clostridium dif-*ficile infection (CDI) should be stratified according to its severity. The Society for Healthcare Epidemiology of America and the Infectious Diseases Society of America define severe CDI by a leukocyte count $\geq$15,000/µL ($15 \times 10^9$/L) or a serum creatinine level >1.5 mg/dL (133 µmol/L). The American College of Gastroenterology defines severe CDI by the presence of hypoalbuminemia (<3 g/dL [30 g/L]) plus leukocytosis ($\geq$15,000/µL [$15 \times 10^9$/L]) or abdominal tenderness. Fulminant CDI is defined as severe infection complicated by ileus, hypotension, shock, or toxic megacolon.

Medical therapy for fulminant CDI includes oral vancomycin plus intravenous metronidazole; vancomycin enemas may also be added if ileus is present. Complications are treated on an individual basis, although the presence of toxic megacolon requires surgical consultation to determine if emergent colectomy is indicated.

Fecal microbiota transplant is effective for treatment of recurrent episodes of CDI, but it is not recommended for an initial episode of CDI, regardless of severity.

Oral metronidazole alone for 10 days can be used for patients who present with an initial episode of nonsevere CDI when oral vancomycin or fidaxomicin is not available.

Oral vancomycin alone for 10 days is recommended for treatment of an initial episode of nonsevere and severe CDI. Oral fidaxomicin can also be used.

Oral metronidazole does not add benefit when used in addition to oral vancomycin.

**KEY POINT**

- Fulminant *Clostridium difficile* infections require oral vancomycin plus intravenous metronidazole; vancomycin enemas may also be added if ileus is present.

**Bibliography**

McDonald LC, Gerding DN, Johnson S, Bakken JS, Carroll KC, Coffin SE, et al. Clinical practice guidelines for *Clostridium difficile* infection in adults and children: 2017 update by the Infectious Diseases Society of America (IDSA) and Society for Healthcare Epidemiology of America (SHEA). Clin Infect Dis. 2018;66:987-994. [PMID: 29562266] doi:10.1093/cid/ciy149

**Item 9      Answer:   D**

**Educational Objective:**  Diagnose post–Lyme disease syndrome.

This patient most likely now has post–Lyme disease syndrome (PLDS). In a patient who lives in or has visited an area endemic for Lyme disease, a skin lesion consistent with erythema migrans is sufficient to make a clinical diagnosis of early localized Lyme disease. Early localized Lyme disease is treated with doxycycline for 10 to 21 days. Despite appropriate therapy, this patient continues to experience nonspecific but debilitating symptoms that have persisted for several months. She most likely has PLDS, a poorly understood sequela of Lyme disease that sometimes is misclassified as "chronic Lyme disease" despite a lack of microbiologic evidence of a persistent viable organism. PLDS is thought to be due to a disordered immunologic response to the preceding infection. Most patients slowly improve over a period of

6 months, and treatment is directed toward symptom amelioration. Randomized controlled trials have shown that patients with PLDS do not respond to prolonged courses of antibiotic therapy, and such treatment is not warranted in this population.

*Anaplasma phagocytophilum, Babesia microti,* and Powassan virus are all transmitted by the same tick vector as *Borrelia burgdorferi,* the causative spirochete of Lyme disease, and coinfections may occur. Anaplasmosis is treated with doxycycline, and the patient's previous course of treatment should have eradicated any incubating disease.

In contrast, doxycycline is not effective therapy for babesiosis. Mild babesiosis may present as a nonspecific flu-like illness, although fever typically is present. The hallmark of babesiosis is hemolytic anemia, and normal laboratory studies in this patient essentially exclude this diagnosis.

In the United States, late-stage Lyme disease most commonly presents as an inflammatory arthritis involving larger joints. The patient has no physical findings consistent with this diagnosis and had appropriate treatment to prevent progression to late-stage Lyme disease.

Powassan virus causes meningoencephalitis rather than the nonspecific symptoms manifested by this patient.

### KEY POINT

- Post–Lyme disease syndrome is a poorly understood sequela of Lyme disease thought to be due to a disordered immunologic response to the preceding infection; most patients slowly improve over a 6-month course, and treatment is directed toward symptom amelioration.

### Bibliography

Aucott JN. Posttreatment Lyme disease syndrome. Infect Dis Clin North Am. 2015;29:309-23. [PMID: 25999226] doi:10.1016/j.idc.2015.02.012

## Item 10      Answer:      B

**Educational Objective:** Diagnose *Mycobacterium fortuitum* infection.

This patient most likely has an infection with *Mycobacterium fortuitum. M. fortuitum* is one of the rapidly growing, nontuberculous mycobacteria (NTM) capable of producing chronic, nonhealing wounds anywhere the bacteria has been introduced, including skin, soft tissue, surgical sites, and occasionally on prosthetic devices. Although *M. fortuitum* is not part of the differential diagnosis of acute wound infections, NTM should always be considered in chronic wounds, especially when conventional antimicrobial therapy has been ineffective. To diagnose an NTM infection, a deep biopsy of chronic wound tissue should be performed. The biopsy specimen should be sent for histopathology to stain for bacteria, mycobacteria, and fungi, and a portion should be sent to the microbiology laboratory for similar stains and cultures.

Pulmonary disease is the most common manifestation of NTM infection, and *Mycobacterium avium* complex (MAC) infection is the most common causative species. MAC is also responsible for most cases of NTM lymphadenitis. Disseminated MAC infection develops in patients with HIV who have CD4 cell counts less than 50/μL and are not receiving MAC prophylaxis. The clinical presentation often includes fever, night sweats, weight loss, and gastrointestinal symptoms. MAC would not be responsible for a solitary, nonhealing cutaneous ulcer.

*Mycobacterium kansasii* most commonly causes a lung infection that mimics tuberculosis, with cough, fever, weight loss, and cavitary lung disease. Risk factors for infection include COPD, cancer, HIV, alcohol abuse, and drug-associated immunosuppression. *M. kansasii* does not cause isolated chronic skin or soft tissue infections.

Leprosy is caused by the acid-fast bacillus *Mycobacterium leprae,* a slow-growing organism. Leprosy should be considered in the setting of chronic skin lesions that fail to respond to treatment of common skin conditions or when sensory loss is observed within lesions or in extremities. This patient's rapid development of a nonhealing ulcer after an initial injury 1 month ago is not compatible with infection caused by *M. leprae.*

### KEY POINT

- Rapidly growing, nontuberculous mycobacteria, such as *Mycobacterium fortuitum,* can produce chronic, nonhealing wounds that do not respond to conventional antimicrobial therapy.

### Bibliography

Guglielmetti L, Mougari F, Lopes A, Raskine L, Cambau E. Human infections due to nontuberculous mycobacteria: the infectious diseases and clinical microbiology specialists' point of view. Future Microbiol. 2015;10:1467-83. [PMID: 26344005] doi:10.2217/fmb.15.64

## Item 11      Answer:      A

**Educational Objective:** Treat pelvic inflammatory disease in an outpatient.

The most appropriate treatment for this patient is a single dose of intramuscular ceftriaxone (250 mg) plus oral doxycycline (100 mg twice daily) for 14 days. The patient has risk factors for sexually transmitted infections (multiple partners and inconsistent condom use) and presents with symptoms suggesting pelvic inflammatory disease (PID). Uterine and cervical motion tenderness are sensitive findings for the diagnosis of PID; the likelihood of PID is further increased by the presence of mucopurulent cervical discharge. Antibiotic therapy should begin before diagnostic testing results are received. Although PID is a polymicrobial infection, testing only for the common sexually transmitted pathogens, *Neisseria gonorrhoeae* and *Chlamydia trachomatis,* is recommended. Although a positive result for either pathogen significantly increases the probability of PID, even if the result is negative, a treatment course for PID should be completed based on clinical findings. Women with an intrauterine device can be treated successfully with the device in place in most cases. In addition to the diagnostic testing obtained from the cervical discharge, this patient should be screened for HIV and syphilis.

This patient has no signs of systemic toxicity or findings to suggest a potential surgical emergency, so hospitalization is not indicated. She is not pregnant and has no history suggesting she would be unable to tolerate oral therapy, so ambulatory treatment is appropriate. Intravenous cefoxitin plus doxycycline and intravenous clindamycin plus gentamicin are regimens for inpatient management of PID. Intravenous ampicillin-sulbactam plus doxycycline is an alternate regimen for hospitalized patients; however, oral amoxicillin-clavulanate is not recommended for the treatment of PID.

**KEY POINT**

- In patients with a high likelihood of pelvic inflammatory disease without indications for hospitalization, empiric therapy with intramuscular ceftriaxone and oral doxycycline is appropriate without waiting for microbiologic testing results.

**Bibliography**

Brunham RC, Gottlieb SL, Paavonen J. Pelvic inflammatory disease. N Engl J Med. 2015;372:2039-48. [PMID: 25992748] doi:10.1056/NEJMra1411426

## Item 12      Answer:   A

**Educational Objective:** Manage asymptomatic bacteriuria in a patient undergoing an invasive urologic procedure.

The indication for antimicrobial therapy in this patient is an invasive urologic procedure. Because urine is a sterile body fluid, the presence of significant bacteriuria is considered to be an infection. In men, either $10^5$ cfu/mL of bacteria from voided urine or at least $10^2$ cfu/mL of a single bacterial species from a clean intermittent catheterized sample is required to distinguish true bacteriuria from contamination. Asymptomatic bacteriuria (ASB) is diagnosed when no signs or symptoms of active infection referable to the urinary tract are present. Depending on variables such as age and genitourinary abnormalities, older adult men have an ASB prevalence of approximately 5% to 20% in the community, rising to 15% to 40% in long-term care facilities. It is important to recognize that screening for and possibly treating asymptomatic bacteriuria is supported by only two indications: pregnancy and risk mitigation before an invasive urologic procedure. The use of prophylactic antibiotics before minor noninvasive urologic interventions without mucosal bleeding does not provide any benefit and is not recommended.

Likewise, screening for and treating ASB in patients about to undergo orthopedic surgery, including total joint arthroplasty, is without proven merit because it is not a cause of postoperative surgical site infection.

Data are insufficient to advocate the routine treatment of ASB in kidney transplant recipients or patients with diabetes.

**KEY POINT**

- Screening for and possibly treating asymptomatic bacteriuria is supported by only two indications: pregnancy and medical clearance before an invasive urologic procedure.

**Bibliography**

Nicolle LE. Asymptomatic bacteriuria. Curr Opin Infect Dis. 2014;27:90-6. [PMID: 24275697] doi:10.1097/QCO.0000000000000019

## Item 13      Answer:   B

**Educational Objective:** Prevent HIV infection after exposure.

This patient has sustained a possible exposure to HIV and should begin postexposure prophylaxis as soon as possible with a three-drug regimen of tenofovir, emtricitabine, and dolutegravir. Significant risk factors for the exposure include that it was a hollow-bore needle with visible blood. If the source patient was known to have an undetectable viral load in blood, the risk would be reduced but not eliminated; however, the source patient's viral load is unknown at this time. Drug selection may be modified depending on the source patient's history of viral resistance, but the preferred empiric postexposure prophylaxis regimens include tenofovir disoproxil fumarate, emtricitabine, and either dolutegravir or raltegravir, and should be given for 4 weeks. The same recommendations are appropriate whether the exposure was occupational or nonoccupational. The exposed patient should be tested for HIV immediately, 4 to 6 weeks later, and 3 months after the exposure. Exposed persons should also be counseled on transmission, symptoms of acute infection, and toxicity of the medications being prescribed.

A two-drug regimen for postexposure prophylaxis (compared with pre-exposure prophylaxis) is no longer recommended.

Protease inhibitors such as darunavir, whether boosted or not, are not recommended for prophylaxis because of their higher rates of adverse effects.

Because postexposure prophylaxis must begin promptly to be most effective, it would not be appropriate to wait for results of the source patient's viral load before determining therapy. The source patient should also be tested for other blood-borne pathogens, such as hepatitis B and C.

**KEY POINT**

- Preferred HIV postexposure prophylaxis regimens include tenofovir disoproxil fumarate, emtricitabine, and either dolutegravir or raltegravir and are appropriate whether the exposure was occupational or nonoccupational.

**Bibliography**

Centers for Disease Control and Prevention. Updated guidelines for antiretroviral postexposure prophylaxis after sexual, injection drug use, or other nonoccupational exposure to HIV–United States, 2016. Available at https://stacks.cdc.gov/view/cdc/38856. Accessed November 2, 2017.

## Item 14    Answer:    A

**Educational Objective:** Manage acute pyelonephritis with bacteremia in a woman.

This patient should complete her prescribed 7-day course of oral ciprofloxacin. She has acute uncomplicated pyelonephritis, which can usually be managed with outpatient oral antimicrobial therapy. Ciprofloxacin for 1 week or levofloxacin for 5 days are the recommended first-line treatment regimens. An initial dose of a long-acting parenteral antibiotic (such as ceftriaxone or aminoglycoside) is suggested when local fluoroquinolone resistance (>10%) is a concern. When a fluoroquinolone antibiotic cannot be used or the bacterial isolate proves resistant, an alternative second-line oral antibiotic should be substituted. Available options include trimethoprim-sulfamethoxazole or the less well-studied oral β-lactam agents.

With the exception of pregnancy, follow-up microbiologic cultures and urinalysis are not required or indicated after resolution of infection.

Extending the duration of ciprofloxacin therapy beyond 7 days would be warranted for complicated pyelonephritis but should not be influenced by the discovery of the single bloodstream isolate in this otherwise healthy woman.

Transient bacteremia does not necessitate hospitalization for parenteral antimicrobial therapy except when the pathogen is found to be multidrug resistant or when complicating features are present (severe illness, obstruction, pregnancy).

In adult women with acute kidney infections, urinary tract imaging by ultrasonography or CT is not routinely performed. However, urologic imaging may be useful and is recommended in evaluating patients who do not clinically improve after 72 hours of adequate antimicrobial therapy or when complications such as obstruction or perinephric and renal abscesses are suspected. Such studies should also be considered when evaluating women who experience an excessive number of recurrent urinary tract infections.

### KEY POINT

- Acute, uncomplicated pyelonephritis can usually be managed with oral outpatient antimicrobial therapy, with the fluoroquinolones ciprofloxacin and levofloxacin being the preferred, first-line agents.

### Bibliography
Kumar S, Dave A, Wolf B, Lerma EV. Urinary tract infections. Dis Mon. 2015;61:45-59. [PMID: 25732782] doi:10.1016/j.disamonth.2014.12.002

## Item 15    Answer:    C

**Educational Objective:** Diagnose *Giardia lamblia* infection.

This patient with selective IgA deficiency most likely has chronic diarrhea due to a *Giardia lamblia* infection. Typical symptoms of *Giardia* include watery diarrhea that is fatty and foul smelling, bloating, crampy abdominal pain, flatulence, and nausea; fever is uncommon. In immunocompetent hosts, *Giardia* infection symptoms typically resolve within 2 to 4 weeks, but in patients with humoral immunodeficiency, such as hypogammaglobulinemia or selective IgA deficiency, *Giardia* infection may be prolonged because of impaired protection against *Giardia* adherence to the intestinal epithelium. Patients with selective IgA deficiency have impaired humoral immunity but no impairment in neutrophil, T-cell, or complement function. Infectious complications of selective IgA deficiency typically include recurrent respiratory tract infections and chronic diarrhea caused by *Giardia*.

Although *Clostridium difficile* can cause recurrent disease, this patient does not have a history of recent antibiotic use or any other risk factors for *C. difficile* infection such as advanced age, chemotherapy, gastrointestinal surgery, inflammatory bowel disease, or gastric acid suppression with proton pump inhibitors.

Enterohemorrhagic *Echerichia coli* (EHEC) infection is usually spread by ingestion of undercooked meat or fecally contaminated food. EHEC typically presents with bloody acute diarrhea, crampy abdominal pain, and no fever.

*Listeria monocytogenes* can cause an acute gastroenteritis syndrome associated with diarrhea, emesis, fever, headache, and nonbloody watery diarrhea associated with pain in muscles and joints. But such an infection typically lasts less than 2 days. Invasive complications of infection, including bacteremia and meningitis, are seen in conditions primarily associated with cell-mediated immune dysfunction such as pregnancy, use of glucocorticoids, and extremes of age (neonates or those older than 65 years).

Nontyphoidal *Salmonella* is the most common cause of foodborne illness. Infection usually results from ingesting fecally contaminated water or food of animal origin. Symptoms are typically self-limited and include crampy abdominal pain, fever, headache, nonbloody diarrhea, nausea, and vomiting. Severe invasive disease may occur in patients with cell-mediated immunodeficiency, but the clinical presentation is not significantly altered in selective IgA deficiency.

### KEY POINT

- Patients with selective IgA deficiency are susceptible to *Giardia lamblia* infection, manifesting as abdominal cramping, bloating, and chronic diarrhea.

### Bibliography
Einarsson E, Ma'ayeh S, Svärd SG. An up-date on Giardia and giardiasis. Curr Opin Microbiol. 2016;34:47-52. [PMID: 27501461] doi:10.1016/j.mib.2016.07.019

## Item 16    Answer:    C

**Educational Objective:** Evaluate a patient with recent Zika virus exposure.

Testing for Zika virus IgM antibodies is the most appropriate management for this pregnant patient, who has had possible exposure to Zika virus through unprotected sexual activity. Asymptomatic pregnant women not living in an area with active Zika virus transmission who may have been exposed more than 2 weeks previously require testing for Zika virus IgM antibodies; a positive result would indicate probable recent infection. Men who have had symptomatic or asymptomatic infection have been proven to have detectable Zika virus RNA in their semen for up to several weeks, with subsequent sexual transmission to their female partner. Under such circumstances, condoms should be used with each sexual encounter for at least 3 months. Her husband's recent viral-like illness occurring in an endemic geographic area, although unconfirmed, must be presumed to have been Zika virus infection. Evaluating her for evidence of asymptomatic infection is of paramount importance to provide counseling and investigate the possible risk of congenital Zika syndrome, of which microcephaly is the most frequent manifestation.

Patients with dengue may be asymptomatic or present with acute febrile illness associated with frontal headache, retro-orbital pain, myalgia, and arthralgia, with or without purpura, melena, or conjunctival injection. Gastrointestinal or respiratory symptoms may predominate. Severe lumbosacral pain is characteristic ("breakbone fever"). As the fever abates, a macular or scarlatiniform rash, which spares the palms and soles and evolves into areas of petechiae on extensor surfaces, may develop. The husband's symptoms are not compatible with dengue. Even if he did have dengue, he cannot transmit the infection to his wife, and testing her for dengue infection is not indicated.

Pregnant women with proven or presumptive recent Zika virus infection require serial ultrasonography every 3 to 4 weeks to assess fetal anatomy and growth. Frequent ultrasonographic monitoring may be appropriate if recent Zika infection is confirmed.

RNA nucleic acid amplification testing for the presence of Zika virus in serum and urine has a greatly diminished sensitivity if performed more than 2 weeks after symptomatic or asymptomatic exposure. In this case, Zika virus IgM antibody testing is preferred.

### KEY POINT

- In patients with potential Zika virus exposure more than 2 weeks previously, testing for Zika virus IgM antibodies is necessary.

### Bibliography

Petersen LR, Jamieson DJ, Powers AM, Honein MA. Zika virus. N Engl J Med. 2016;374:1552-63. [PMID: 27028561] doi:10.1056/NEJMra1602113

### Item 17    Answer:    D

**Educational Objective:** Diagnose Ramsay Hunt syndrome caused by varicella-zoster virus infection.

Varicella-zoster virus (VZV) is the most likely cause of this patient's findings. VZV reactivation presents with pain or paresthesias in a specific dermatome; the characteristic rash develops several days later. In order of frequency, the thoracic, trigeminal, lumbar, and cervical cutaneous dermatomes are most often involved. More than 50% of cases occur in persons older than 60 years; immunocompromised

patients are also at risk. Involvement of the geniculate ganglion may cause herpes zoster oticus, also known as the Ramsay Hunt syndrome, characterized by pain and vesicles in the external ear canal, ipsilateral peripheral facial palsy, and altered or absent taste. Patients may also experience hearing loss, tinnitus, and altered lacrimation. Most experts consider Ramsay Hunt syndrome to be a polycranial neuropathy, with frequent involvement of cranial nerves V, IX, and X. A vesicular rash may be absent in patients with VZV (zoster sine herpete) and should not deter physicians from ordering polymerase chain reaction testing for VZV. Acyclovir is typically prescribed for this syndrome. The live attenuated zoster vaccine has 64% efficacy that decreases to 36% after 6 years. A novel recombinant zoster vaccine, approved in 2017, has 97% efficacy and should be given to this patient.

The most common neurologic manifestation of early disseminated Lyme disease is facial nerve palsy, which may be unilateral or bilateral. Treatment of early localized disease prevents progression of infection. Untreated patients may progress to early disseminated infection. This stage typically presents as a febrile illness associated with erythema migrans at multiple sites distant from the initial tick attachment. Constitutional symptoms are common and include fever, myalgia, arthralgia, and headache. Neurologic Lyme disease without a history of tick bite, erythema migrans rash, or systemic symptoms is highly unlikely.

Bell palsy is defined as an isolated paralysis of the facial nerve that leads to complete unilateral facial paralysis. Herpes simplex virus (HSV) type 1 reactivation is the likely cause of Bell palsy in most cases. However, most cases of Bell palsy are diagnosed as "idiopathic" because it is difficult in clinical practice to prove that reactivation of HSV-1 is the cause of this peripheral neuropathy.

HSV type 2 is more commonly associated with genital ulcers, recurrent aseptic meningitis, or myelitis than with Bell palsy. Neither Lyme disease nor HSV reactivation can explain the burning and stinging ear pain, tinnitus, hearing loss, and facial palsy experienced by this patient as well as VZV reactivation can.

### KEY POINT

- Varicella-zoster virus is a cause of Ramsay Hunt syndrome, which usually presents with ear pain, a vesicular rash in the external ear (although the rash may be absent), and ipsilateral peripheral facial palsy.

### Bibliography

Cohen JI. Clinical practice: Herpes zoster. N Engl J Med. 2013;369:255-63. [PMID: 23863052] doi:10.1056/NEJMcp1302674

### Item 18    Answer:    B

**Educational Objective:** Diagnose Q fever pneumonia.

The most likely cause of this patient's illness is *Coxiella burnetii*. He presents with community-acquired pneumonia not requiring hospitalization, which is most frequently caused by atypical bacteria, *Streptococcus pneumoniae*, or a viral pathogen. His occupation puts him at risk for zoonotic causes of pneumonia as well. Many zoonotic organisms can potentially cause pulmonary infection, but they can usually be differentiated based on illness severity and animal reservoir. In this patient, the relatively mild infection coupled with exposure to livestock makes *C. burnetii* the most likely culprit. *C. burnetii*, which causes Q fever pneumonia, is most frequently associated with exposure to farm animals, parturient animals in particular. High rates of seropositivity have been reported in farmers, veterinarians, and abattoir workers. Infection can occur without direct animal exposure; increased rates of Q fever pneumonia have been found among persons residing in proximity to livestock farms. Infection occurs after inhalation of aerosolized bodily fluids from infected animals. Acute pulmonary infection ranges from subclinical to severe, but it is rarely fatal. Treatment with doxycycline is indicated to decrease symptom duration and to prevent progression to chronic Q fever.

*Bacillus anthracis* is the causative agent of anthrax. Cutaneous anthrax is the most common naturally occurring form of the disease. In the United States, inhalation anthrax is almost exclusively of concern as an agent of bioterrorism. In endemic areas, pulmonary infection may occur after inhalation of spores from the fur or hide of infected livestock, particularly goats and cattle. Inhalation anthrax is a fulminant, often fatal infection.

*Chlamydia psittaci* is the causative agent of psittacosis, which typically presents as pneumonia associated with abrupt onset of fever, severe headache, and dry cough. This organism is associated with inhalation of dried bird droppings, so bird owners or breeders and poultry farmers are at particularly high risk for this infection.

Pneumonic tularemia occurs either after direct inhalation or through secondary spread of *Francisella tularensis* into the lungs. Pneumonic tularemia is characterized by a nonproductive cough, dyspnea, and substernal or pleuritic chest pain. Chest radiographs show infiltrates, hilar lymphadenopathy, and pleural effusion. In the United States, most infections are transmitted through animal exposure. Hunters are at particularly high risk for primary tularemia pneumonia through skinning and dressing of infected rabbits or other wild game.

*Yersinia pestis* infection of the lung causes pneumonic plague. Rodents serve as the primary reservoir for plague. Pulmonary infection occurs through droplet transmission from an infected host or secondary spread from an extrapulmonary source. Patients present with sudden high fever, pleuritic chest pain, a productive cough, and hemoptysis. Pneumonic plague is almost uniformly fatal unless recognized and treated promptly.

**KEY POINT**

- Many zoonotic organisms have the potential to cause pulmonary infection, but they can be differentiated based on the severity of illness and animal reservoir; relatively mild infection coupled with exposure to livestock indicates likely *Coxiella burnetii* infection.

## Bibliography

Freidl GS, Spruijt IT, Borlée F, Smit LA, van Gageldonk-Lafeber AB, Heederik DJ, et al. Livestock-associated risk factors for pneumonia in an area of intensive animal farming in the Netherlands. PLoS One. 2017;12:e0174796. [PMID: 28362816] doi:10.1371/journal.pone.0174796

## Item 19          Answer:     D

**Educational Objective:** Treat coagulase-negative *Staphylococcus* central line–associated bloodstream infection.

The most appropriate management is to remove the peripherally inserted central catheter (PICC) and repeat blood cultures. Central line–associated bloodstream infections (CLABSIs) can occur with any type of catheter, including short-term peripheral intravenous catheters and PICCs. They are most commonly caused by coagulase-negative *Staphylococcus* followed by *S. aureus*. Coagulase-negative *Staphylococcus* is less virulent than *S. aureus* and is less likely to cause metastatic infection or endocarditis in patients without prosthetic devices or endovascular hardware (such as prosthetic heart valves) in place. Coagulase-negative *Staphylococcus* CLABSIs often resolve with removal of the catheter. Blood cultures should be repeated after catheter removal to document clearance of the organism. Alternatively, patients with coagulase-negative *Staphylococcus* CLABSIs can be treated with antibiotics for 5 to 7 days if the catheter is removed and for 10 to 14 days in combination with antibiotic lock therapy if the catheter is not removed.

Most uncomplicated CLABSIs are treated for 7 to 14 days; *S. aureus* CLABSIs may require treatment for 4 to 6 weeks after catheter removal. Shorter therapy durations (14 days) may be considered in select patients with *S. aureus* CLABSI whose catheters have been removed and who do not have diabetes mellitus, are not immunosuppressed, have no implanted prosthetic devices, have no evidence of endocarditis by echocardiography (preferably transesophageal), and have no evidence of infected thrombophlebitis; whose fever and bacteremia resolve within 72 hours of starting appropriate therapy; and whose physical examination and diagnostic tests do not suggest the presence of metastatic infection.

In patients with persistent bacteremia or endovascular hardware, transesophageal echocardiography may be pursued to evaluate for endocarditis. In patients with endovascular hardware, longer durations of antibiotics are generally required. Catheters should always be removed when endocarditis, metastatic infection, hemodynamic instability, suppurative thrombophlebitis, or persistent bacteremia is evident.

**KEY POINT**

- Coagulase-negative *Staphylococcus* is less virulent than *S. aureus* and is less likely to cause metastatic infection or endocarditis in patients without prosthetic devices or endovascular hardware in place (such as prosthetic heart valves) and may be treated with simple removal of the intravenous catheter.

## Bibliography

Mermel LA, Allon M, Bouza E, Craven DE, Flynn P, O'Grady NP, et al. Clinical practice guidelines for the diagnosis and management of intravascular catheter-related infection: 2009 update by the Infectious Diseases Society of America. Clin Infect Dis. 2009;49:1-45. [PMID: 19489710] doi:10.1086/599376

## Item 20    Answer:    D

**Educational Objective:** Prevent catheter-associated urinary tract infection by removing the catheter.

The proper management of the patient's urinary catheter is to remove it and observe the patient for spontaneous voiding. Catheters should be used for appropriate indications only, which include urinary retention and bladder outlet obstruction, measurement of urinary output in critically ill patients, perioperative use for selected surgical procedures, assistance with healing of perineal or sacral wounds in patients with incontinence, use in patients requiring prolonged immobilization, and contribution to comfort at the end of life. An indwelling urinary catheter is sometimes inserted in the emergency department during trauma evaluation; however, the need for continuing the catheter should be assessed when the initial evaluation has been completed. If this patient required prolonged immobilization (for example, multiple traumatic injuries such as pelvic fractures), continuing the indwelling urinary catheter may be appropriate. Patients should be monitored closely for their ability to void spontaneously when a catheter is removed. Bladder ultrasonography can be used to determine residual postvoid volume; if more than 200 mL remain, consider intermittent catheterization for a short amount of time rather than placing a new indwelling urinary catheter. Early removal of urinary catheters should be considered when possible and can be encouraged by reminder systems. Additionally, nurse-initiated removal protocols have been shown to be effective in limiting duration of catheterization. Catheter-associated urinary tract infection (CAUTI) prevention strategies are summarized by the acronym ABCDE: Adhere to general infection control principles, perform Bladder ultrasonography to potentially avoid catheterization, use Condom catheters or intermittent catheterization when appropriate, Do not use an indwelling catheter if criteria for use are not met, and remove catheters Early when they are no longer indicated using computerized reminders or nurse-driven removal protocols.

Antimicrobial-impregnated or antiseptic-coated catheters have not been shown to decrease CAUTIs with short-term (<14 days) catheterization. Information is scarce on their benefits with long-term urinary catheters. Early removal of the catheter is a better care strategy.

Administering antibiotics with the goal of preventing infection is not effective and promotes antibiotic-resistant bacteria and fungal CAUTIs and is not indicated in this case.

### KEY POINT

- Early removal of urinary catheters should be considered when possible, and patients should be monitored for their ability to void spontaneously after catheter removal.

## Bibliography

Chenoweth CE, Saint S. Urinary tract infections. Infect Dis Clin North Am. 2016;30:869-885. [PMID: 27816141] doi:10.1016/j.idc.2016.07.007

## Item 21    Answer:    A

**Educational Objective:** Treat an infected cat bite in a patient with risk factors for methicillin-resistant *Staphylococcus aureus.*

This patient should receive antibiotic treatment with ampicillin-sulbactam plus vancomycin in addition to undergoing surgical consultation. She has a cat bite–associated wound infection with accompanying low blood pressure and tachypnea and requires hospitalization. Cat bites are more likely than dog bites to cause infection because of cats' sharp, narrow teeth; infections are caused by organisms from the animal's mouth flora and the host's skin flora. This flora comprises a mix of anaerobic and aerobic organisms, including streptococci, staphylococci, and *Bacteroides, Fusobacterium, Porphyromonas,* and *Pasteurella* species. *Pasteurella* is a facultative anaerobic gram-negative rod that is the most common bacteria in a cat's mouth. Intravenous piperacillin-tazobactam, ampicillin-sulbactam, imipenem, or meropenem would address these organisms but not potential methicillin-resistant *Staphylococcus aureus* (MRSA). If pus is present, the patient has MRSA risk factors such as a previous MRSA infection or colonization within the last year, or local MRSA prevalence is high, then coverage should also include agents that target MRSA, such as vancomycin or daptomycin. Consequently, the combination of ampicillin-sulbactam and vancomycin would be the best choice for empiric antibiotic coverage because this regimen is effective against serious infections caused by MRSA and the microbiota of a cat's mouth.

Ceftriaxone and metronidazole would be effective against many of the organisms encountered in a cat bite–associated skin infection, but it would not cover the possibility of MRSA infection in this patient.

Ciprofloxacin and aztreonam also lack coverage for MRSA and some anaerobes likely to be associated with a bite wound.

Imipenem is a broad-spectrum antibiotic effective against many of the organisms associated with cat bite wounds, but it does not provide MRSA coverage.

Neither vancomycin nor clindamycin provides adequate coverage against *Pasteurella* species, so this regimen would not be effective for a cat bite–associated infection.

### KEY POINT

- Cat bite–associated wound infections comprise a mix of anaerobic and aerobic organisms, including *Pasteurella* species, which require treatment with antibiotic agents such as piperacillin-tazobactam, ampicillin-sulbactam, imipenem, and meropenem; coverage for methicillin-resistant *Staphylococcus aureus* must be included in select patients who have risk factors for this infection.

## Bibliography

Bystritsky R, Chambers H. Cellulitis and soft tissue infections. Ann Intern Med. 2018;168:ITC17-ITC32. [PMID: 29404597] doi:10.7326/AITC201802060

## Item 22     Answer:    B

**Educational Objective:** Diagnose human monocytic ehrlichiosis.

This patient most likely has human monocytic ehrlichiosis (HME), a tick-borne illness primarily caused by *Ehrlichia chaffeensis*. His symptoms include a nonfocal febrile illness associated with leukopenia, thrombocytopenia, and elevated hepatic enzyme levels, all of which are characteristic of HME. His participation in outdoor activities in wooded areas places him at risk for exposure to ticks. HME is endemic in the mid-Atlantic, southern, and southeastern United States; his clinical presentation is highly suggestive of this illness. The prompt response to doxycycline is classic for a tick-borne rickettsial illness, such as HME; a lack of response within 48 hours of therapy would suggest an alternative diagnosis or a coinfection. The negative serologic results for *E. chaffeensis* do not disprove the diagnosis and should not prompt early discontinuation of doxycycline. The sensitivity of antibody testing is low in the first week of illness; seroconversion typically occurs within 2 to 4 weeks of symptom onset, and acute and convalescent titers are useful for retrospective confirmation of infection. During the acute illness, buffy-coat staining (to reveal the presence of morulae, which are basophilic inclusion bodies in the cytoplasm of monocytes representing clusters of bacteria [shown]) or polymerase chain reaction of whole blood specimens may allow an early diagnosis.

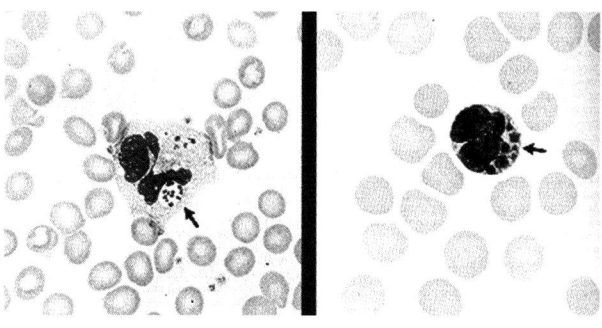

Although many infections present identically to HME, the salient feature in this patient was the rapid response to doxycycline therapy, which essentially excludes a viral process. Heartland virus, a newly described Bunyavirus transmitted by the same vector as *E. chaffeensis*, is clinically indistinguishable from HME and should be suspected when no improvement is seen within 48 hours of starting doxycycline therapy.

Infectious mononucleosis can present with fever, cytopenia, and elevated aminotransferase levels. However, other components of the infectious mononucleosis triad (fever,

pharyngitis, and cervical lymphadenopathy) were absent in this patient.

The rapid response to doxycycline treatment is consistent with Rocky Mountain spotted fever (RMSF) infection. However, the pronounced leukopenia and absence of a rash more than 1 week into the illness argue against this diagnosis.

> **KEY POINT**
>
> • Human monocytic ehrlichiosis infection is characterized by a nonfocal febrile illness associated with leukopenia, thrombocytopenia, elevated hepatic enzyme levels, and a rapid response to tetracycline.

## Bibliography

Biggs HM, Behravesh CB, Bradley KK, Dahlgren FS, Drexler NA, Dumler JS, et al. Diagnosis and management of tickborne rickettsial diseases: Rocky Mountain spotted fever and other spotted fever group rickettsioses, ehrlichioses, and anaplasmosis – United States. MMWR Recomm Rep. 2016;65:1-44. [PMID: 27172113] doi:10.15585/mmwr.rr6502a1

## Item 23     Answer:    C

**Educational Objective:** Treat health care–associated ventriculitis and meningitis.

The most appropriate management in this patient is removal of his ventricular drain. After drain removal, clinical monitoring for intracranial hypertension will be important. Health care–associated ventriculitis or meningitis (HCAVM) or nosocomial meningitis may present a diagnostic and treatment challenge to clinicians. It typically occurs after head trauma or a neurosurgical procedure (craniotomy, lumbar puncture) or secondary to device infection (for example, cerebrospinal fluid [CSF] shunts or drains, intrathecal pumps, deep brain stimulator). *Staphylococcus* species and enteric gram-negative bacteria are the most common causes, but up to 50% of patients can have negative cultures because more than 50% receive antibiotic therapy before CSF studies are performed, as occurred in this patient. Worsening mental status, new fever, or stiff neck in a patient who recently underwent surgery should raise the possibility of HCAVM. An elevated CSF lactate level greater than 4 mg/dL, an elevated CSF procalcitonin level, or a combination of both, may be useful in the diagnosis of health care–associated bacterial ventriculitis and meningitis in culture-negative cases. Empiric therapy should include vancomycin and a β-lactam with antipseudomonal activity (such as cefepime or meropenem) and device removal, if present.

For patients with health care–associated ventriculitis and meningitis caused by staphylococci in whom β-lactam agents or vancomycin cannot be used, treatment with linezolid, daptomycin, or trimethoprim-sulfamethoxazole is recommended with selection based on in vitro susceptibility testing. However, the priority in this patient is removing the ventricular drain, not changing the antibiotic regimen.

Intraventricular or intrathecal antimicrobial therapy should be considered for patients with health care–associated ventriculitis and meningitis in whom the infection responds poorly to systemic antimicrobial therapy alone. This strategy is not appropriate in a patient with a potentially infected ventricular drain.

### KEY POINT

- In patients with health care–associated ventriculitis or meningitis, device removal, if present, should accompany empiric antimicrobial therapy.

### Bibliography

Tunkel AR, Hasbun R, Bhimraj A. Byers K, Kaplan SL, Michael Scheld W, et al. 2017 Infectious Diseases Society of America's clinical practice guidelines for healthcare-associated ventriculitis and meningitis. Clin Infect Dis. 2017. [PMID: 28203777] doi:10.1093/cid/ciw861

## Item 24    Answer:    C

**Educational Objective:  Treat pneumonic plague.**

The most appropriate treatment is gentamicin. This patient most likely has pneumonic plague caused by the bacteria *Yersinia pestis*, one of the biologic agents classified as an A-list bioterrorism pathogen because of its high potential lethality and ease of dissemination. Sputum Gram stain (and possibly blood smear) may identify gram-negative coccobacilli demonstrating the classic bipolar staining or "safety pin" shape shown. Although most pulmonary involvement occurs through secondary hematogenous spread to the lungs from a bubo or other source, primary pneumonic plague can occur after close contact with another person with plague pneumonia, after animal exposure, or as a result of intentional aerosol release for the purpose of terrorism, as in this case. Recommended first-line treatment is either streptomycin or gentamicin.

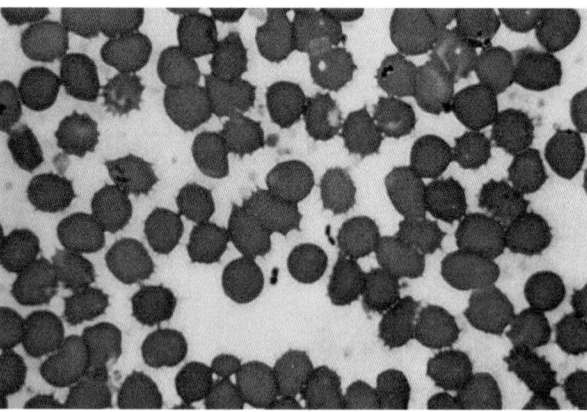

Anthrax is caused by *Bacillus anthracis*, a gram-positive, aerobic organism. It appears as a sporulating gram-positive rod on microscopic examination. Patients with inhalational anthrax present with low-grade fever, malaise, myalgia, and headache accompanied by cough, dyspnea, and chest pain. A chest radiograph showing mediastinal widening from hemorrhagic lymphadenitis is characteristic. Ciprofloxacin, levofloxacin, moxifloxacin, or doxycycline should be provided as

soon as possible after any actual or suspected case of anthrax that raises concern for a bioterrorism attack.

Ambulatory empiric therapy for community-acquired pneumonia (CAP) is directed against *Streptococcus pneumoniae*, *Haemophilus influenzae*, and atypical bacteria, even though a significant proportion of patients with CAP infected with viral pathogens do not benefit from antibiotic therapy. The combination of ceftriaxone and azithromycin would be an appropriate choice for the treatment of CAP but would be inadequate for treating plague, which requires either streptomycin or gentamicin.

When clinical concern for *Pseudomonas* is present, dual therapy with two active agents is indicated. Options include an antipseudomonal β-lactam (piperacillin-tazobactam, cefepime, or meropenem) in conjunction with either a quinolone (levofloxacin or ciprofloxacin) or an aminoglycoside. *Pseudomonas* infection should be considered in immunocompromised patients and patients with underlying structural lung disease (bronchiectasis or cystic fibrosis) or medical conditions requiring repeated courses of antibiotics. The combination of piperacillin-tazobactam and levofloxacin would be ideal for a seriously ill patient with CAP and concern for *Pseudomonas* infection but not for this patient most likely infected with *Yersinia pestis*.

### KEY POINT

- First-line treatment for primary pneumonic plague is either streptomycin or gentamicin.

### Bibliography

Adalja AA, Toner E, Inglesby TV. Clinical management of potential bioterrorism-related conditions. N Engl J Med. 2015;372:954-62. [PMID: 25738671] doi:10.1056/NEJMra1409755

## Item 25    Answer:    D

**Educational Objective:  Treat disseminated histoplasmosis.**

The most appropriate treatment for this patient is liposomal amphotericin B. He has disseminated histoplasmosis, for which he has numerous risk factors. He lives in an area endemic for histoplasmosis (Ohio River Valley), and because he takes prednisone and methotrexate for his rheumatoid arthritis, he is immunosuppressed. He has had significant exposure working in an old barn with bats. He also is hypotensive and diaphoretic and has oral ulcerations and hepatosplenomegaly, which are typical of disseminated infection, as is pancytopenia. Approximately 10% of patients with histoplasmosis develop disseminated infection; if not diagnosed early, the mortality rate is greater than 90%. The treatment of choice for disseminated histoplasmosis is liposomal amphotericin B initially, with de-escalation to itraconazole for several months. A definitive diagnosis can be established by detection of the urinary antigen for histoplasmosis (95% specificity), blood cultures, or a biopsy of the oral lesions.

Ceftriaxone and azithromycin are the recommended drugs of choice for community-acquired pneumonia. The

CONT.

patient's physical examination and chest radiograph are unremarkable, which effectively rules out pneumonia and the need for these antibiotics.

Behçet syndrome is a form of vasculitis associated with recurrent painful oral and genital ulcerations; patients also may demonstrate additional distinctive features, including hypopyon and pathergy. Central nervous system involvement can manifest as headaches, stroke, and behavioral changes. Gastrointestinal involvement may be hard to distinguish from inflammatory bowel disease. Low-dose prednisone or colchicine is used for oral or genital ulcers, and high-dose prednisone and immunomodulating agents are used for more severe disease. Behçet syndrome does not explain the patient's fever, hemodynamic instability, pancytopenia, or hepatomegaly, and colchicine therapy is not warranted.

Itraconazole is an azole triazole used to treat many endemic fungal infections, including histoplasmosis. However, it is not as effective as liposomal amphotericin B in disseminated infection. It may be used for subacute or chronic histoplasmosis, such as pulmonary histoplasmosis.

### KEY POINT

- Liposomal amphotericin B is the treatment of choice for disseminated histoplasmosis.

### Bibliography

Hage CA, Azar MM, Bahr N, Loyd J, Wheat LJ. Histoplasmosis: up-to-date evidence-based approach to diagnosis and management. Semin Respir Crit Care Med. 2015 Oct;36(5):729-45. doi: 10.1055/s-0035-1562899. Review. PMID: 26398539.

## Item 26　　Answer:　C

**Educational Objective:** Evaluate a patient for complications of pneumonia (empyema).

The most appropriate management at this time is to perform thoracentesis. This patient has nonresponsive pneumonia demonstrated by persistent fever of more than 72 hours despite directed therapy (vancomycin) against the causative organism (methicillin-resistant *Staphylococcus aureus* [MRSA]). Lack of response to therapy is a poor prognostic factor and is associated with excess mortality. Antibiotic therapy failure may indicate a noninfectious cause mimicking pneumonia, antibiotic-resistant bacterial infection, infection with a nonbacterial organism, or loculated infection such as an empyema. This patient's chest radiograph shows opacification of the left heart border and hemidiaphragm, raising concern for pleural fluid adjacent to a pulmonary infiltrate. Parapneumonic pleural effusions are present in up to 40% of patients hospitalized with CAP. Determining the need for chest tube drainage requires analysis of the pleural fluid. A finding of purulent or foul-smelling material or a positive Gram stain is diagnostic of an empyema, and a pleural fluid pH less than 7.2 or a pleural fluid glucose level less than 60 mg/dL (3.33 mmol/L) is highly suggestive. Chest tube placement in addition to antibiotics is necessary to treat infection localized to the pleural space. Delayed drainage

may result in ongoing fever, sepsis, or fibrosis ultimately requiring surgical intervention.

The role of glucocorticoids in CAP remains controversial. Evidence is accumulating that early administration of glucocorticoids may reduce the host inflammatory response, particularly in patients with acute respiratory distress syndrome; however, the routine use of glucocorticoids for CAP has not been established.

The addition of piperacillin-tazobactam would be indicated if a secondary hospital-acquired pulmonary infection were a concern, but the persistent fever and Gram stain showing only gram-positive cocci makes superinfection less likely.

Procalcitonin is produced by cells as a response to bacterial toxins, which result in elevated serum procalcitonin levels in bacterial infections. In viral infections, procalcitonin levels are reduced. Procalcitonin measurement is only one of several factors in determining a bacterial versus a viral cause and should be considered as adjunctive to other diagnostic tools. In this patient, there is little doubt concerning the microbiologic diagnosis, and determining the procalcitonin level will not be helpful.

Daptomycin is contraindicated for use in pulmonary infections because it binds to surfactant and does not achieve adequate levels in the alveoli.

### KEY POINT

- In patients with pneumonia unresponsive to appropriate antibiotic therapy, a noninfectious cause mimicking pneumonia, antibiotic-resistant bacterial infection, infection with a nonbacterial organism, or loculated infection such as an empyema may be the cause.

### Bibliography

McCauley L, Dean N. Pneumonia and empyema: causal, casual or unknown. J Thorac Dis. 2015;7:992-8. [PMID: 26150912] doi:10.3978/j.issn.2072-1439.2015.04.36

## Item 27　　Answer:　A

**Educational Objective:** Diagnose *Plasmodium falciparum* malaria.

This pregnant woman has contracted *Plasmodium falciparum* malaria after visiting a part of the world where malaria is endemic. Her clinical presentation and peripheral blood smear showing many parasitized erythrocytes demonstrating signet ring forms, together with the absence of trophozoites and schizonts, are typical for infection with *P. falciparum*. Of returning travelers with acute and potentially life-threatening febrile diseases, *P. falciparum* malaria accounts for most infections. Furthermore, pregnant women are at increased risk of severe disease and a heightened mortality rate, which is likely related to a reduced immune response. Additionally, effects on the microvasculature and sequestering of organisms in the placenta during pregnancy are known to significantly increase the risk of miscarriage,

CONT.

premature delivery, low-birth-weight neonates, congenital infection, and fetal demise.

Accurate identification of *P. falciparum* and *Plasmodium knowlesi* is critical because of the risk for severe and potentially lethal infection. *P. falciparum* should be suspected if the patient traveled to Africa, symptoms begin soon after return from an endemic area, and the peripheral blood smear shows a high level of parasitemia. *P. knowlesi* is a more recently recognized human pathogen; infection may be severe because of high levels of parasitemia. Examination of the peripheral blood smear reveals all stages of the parasite. The epidemiologic history is helpful because *P. knowlesi* is not encountered in Africa but rather South and Southeast Asia.

*Plasmodium malariae*, *Plasmodium ovale*, and *Plasmodium vivax* are all associated with a low or very low degree of parasitemia, typically less than 2%, and although the risk of recurrence is high, with the exception of *P. vivax*, the risk for severe disease is low.

### KEY POINT

- *Plasmodium falciparum* infection should be suspected if the patient traveled to Africa, symptoms begin soon after return from an endemic area, and the peripheral blood smear shows a high level of parasitemia.

### Bibliography

Hahn WO, Pottinger PS. Malaria in the traveler: how to manage before departure and evaluate upon return. Med Clin North Am. 2016;100:289-302. [PMID: 26900114] doi:10.1016/j.mcna.2015.09.008

 **Item 28      Answer:      C**

**Educational Objective:  Treat spinal epidural abscess.**

The most appropriate treatment of this patient is empiric antibiotic therapy and surgical drainage of the abscess. Spinal epidural abscesses (SEAs) usually result from contiguous spread from infected vertebrae or intervertebral body disc spaces or from hematogenous dissemination from a distant site. SEA can be challenging to diagnose because symptoms can be mild or nonspecific and fever may not always be present. A high index of suspicion, particularly in patients with atypical or persistent back pain, will facilitate more prompt diagnosis. Symptoms may progress from back pain to accompanying neurologic symptoms, such as bowel or bladder dysfunction, lower extremity weakness, paresthesias, and, in the last stages, paralysis. MRI of the spine with contrast is the preferred imaging modality for diagnosis. Blood cultures should be performed before starting antibiotic therapy to identify the cause, and, in certain cases, cultures may avoid the need for aspiration of the spinal abscess. Medical therapy alone is often successful if no neurologic deficits are present at the time of diagnosis or if substantial complications from surgery are likely because of comorbid conditions. However, surgical drainage is recommended in patients who present with neurologic symptoms or evidence

of progression or recurrence despite proper antimicrobial therapy. Serial clinical evaluations and follow-up MRI of the spine (at approximately 4-6 weeks into therapy or with any sign of clinical deterioration) are necessary adjuncts to management without surgery. Empiric parenteral antimicrobial therapy should include coverage for *Staphylococcus aureus* (accounts for approximately 50% of infections), *Streptococcus* species, and gram-negative bacilli and may be narrowed based on culture results, if available. Therapy typically lasts between 6 and 8 weeks (or until resolution of abscess on follow-up MRI) but may require modification depending on clinical and radiographic recovery.

Patients with sepsis or neurologic compromise, as in this patient, should start empiric broad-spectrum antimicrobial therapy pending blood and abscess cultures. Otherwise, empiric antimicrobial therapy may be withheld until a cause is confirmed. This patient has an indication for immediate empiric antibiotic therapy and surgical drainage.

### KEY POINT

- Patients with spinal epidural abscess who also have neurologic compromise should immediately begin broad-spectrum antimicrobial therapy and undergo surgical drainage.

### Bibliography

Berbari EF, Kanj SS, Kowalski TJ, Darouiche RO, Widmer AF, Schmitt SK, et al. 2015 Infectious Diseases Society of America (IDSA) clinical practice guidelines for the diagnosis and treatment of native vertebral osteomyelitis in adults. Clin Infect Dis. 2015;61:e26-46. [PMID: 26229122] doi:10.1093/cid/civ482

**Item 29      Answer:      D**

**Educational Objective:  Diagnose typhoid (enteric) fever.**

This patient most likely has typhoid fever, also known as enteric fever, caused by either of the typhoidal *Salmonella* strains, *S. typhi* or *S. paratyphi*. Infection is transmitted by ingestion of food or water contaminated by feces. In resource-poor areas, organisms may be spread in community food or, more frequently, by water. In developed countries, transmission is chiefly by food that has been contaminated during preparation by healthy carriers. Symptoms of enteric fever are generally nonspecific. Fever is the major manifestation, typically rising over 2 to 3 nights and persisting for several days. A pulse-temperature dissociation (relative bradycardia) is often present. A brief period of diarrhea followed by constipation, abdominal discomfort, nonproductive cough, mild confusion, and transient small blanching skin lesions (rose spots) are other clinical features. Ceftriaxone is the preferred empiric antibiotic agent, with ciprofloxacin and azithromycin as additional options if resistance is not encountered.

Human brucellosis can develop after exposure to one of four *Brucella* species through contact with viable organisms in secretions or excretions of infected animals, ingestion of undercooked meat or milk products, or, less often, inhalation. Patients experience numerous nonspecific symptoms as well as recurring or "undulating" waves of fever, but rash, gastrointestinal symptoms, and relative bradycardia are not typical.

Humans acquire leptospirosis after contact with infected urine spread by carrier animals. Classically, illness is biphasic, beginning with a septicemic phase followed by an immune phase, which correlates with the appearance of antibodies in serum. Clinically apparent leptospirosis presents with the abrupt onset of fever, rigors, myalgias, and headache. Conjunctival suffusion in a patient with a nonspecific febrile illness should raise suspicion for the diagnosis of leptospirosis. A more severe form, known as Weil syndrome (icteric leptospirosis), consisting of jaundice, azotemia, and anemia, may also occur. Gastrointestinal symptoms are infrequent.

The gram-negative bacillus *Burkholderia pseudomallei*, found in soil and water in endemic areas such as Southeast Asia, is the causative agent of melioidosis. After acquisition through direct skin contact, ingestion, or inhalation, an acute pulmonary, septicemic, or localized suppurative infection may occur. The patient's findings are not compatible with melioidosis.

**KEY POINT**

• Fever is the major manifestation of typhoid fever and is often associated with a relative bradycardia; additional symptoms may include a brief period of diarrhea followed by constipation, abdominal discomfort, nonproductive cough, mild confusion, and transient small blanching skin lesions (rose spots).

**Bibliography**
Thwaites GE, Day NP. Approach to fever in the returning traveler. N Engl J Med. 2017;376:548-560. [PMID: 28177860] doi:10.1056/NEJMra1508435

## Item 30   Answer:   A

**Educational Objective:**  Manage newly diagnosed HIV infection.

This patient needs baseline genotypic HIV resistance testing. Because of the possibility of transmitted virus having resistance mutations, it is recommended to obtain baseline resistance testing before starting an antiretroviral regimen. If the patient is ready, antiretrovirals can be started the same day, while waiting for resistance testing results, with regimen modification if necessary based on results. Virologic failure of a regimen (rebound of a suppressed viral load or failure to achieve undetectable viral load with therapy) is also an indication for resistance testing to guide the change in regimen. Genotypic testing looks for mutations in the viral genome associated with antiviral drug resistance. Phenotypic testing actually tests the virus's ability to grow in the presence of differing concentrations of the drug and is therefore more useful in the presence of multiple interacting mutations or unclear correlations of mutation and resistance, such as occurs with resistance to protease inhibitors. Genotypic testing is faster and less

expensive because all that is necessary is sequencing of the respective genes for the patient's viral isolate. When significant resistance is not expected and information is needed more quickly, genotypic testing would be preferred over phenotypic testing.

Some antiretroviral agents have been associated with increased insulin resistance and risk for hyperglycemia, and assessing for this at baseline and during therapy is recommended. This patient, however, already has a normal glucose level at baseline testing, so measuring the glycohemoglobin is not necessary at this time.

All patients with HIV should begin antiretroviral therapy as soon as they are ready. Prompt initiation of therapy benefits the patient and reduces the risk of transmission to others, so waiting for repeat viral load and CD4 cell count is inappropriate and unnecessary.

**KEY POINT**

• Genotypic viral resistance testing is recommended immediately after a diagnosis of HIV infection to guide the selection of active agents for the antiretroviral regimen or after virologic failure of a regimen to guide adjustment of antiretroviral therapy.

**Bibliography**
Panel on Antiretroviral Guidelines for Adults and Adolescents. Guidelines for the use of antiretroviral agents in adults and adolescents living with HIV. Department of Health and Human Services. Available at https://aidsinfo.nih.gov/guidelines/html/1/adult-and-adolescent-arv/0. Accessed April 12, 2018.

## Item 31   Answer:   B

**Educational Objective:**  Diagnose meningitis caused by herpes simplex virus type 2.

The most likely diagnosis in this patient is meningitis caused by herpes simplex virus (HSV) type 2. Viral meningitis is the most common cause of "aseptic" meningitis, in which cerebrospinal fluid (CSF) Gram stain and cultures are negative. Most patients have typical meningitis symptoms, such as fever, nuchal rigidity, headache, and photophobia. HSV meningitis syndromes can be related to primary infections, with central nervous system involvement as a secondary consequence, or reactivation of latent infection presenting as aseptic meningitis. HSV-2 is more commonly associated with meningitis and is the most common cause of recurrent meningitis (recurrent benign lymphocytic meningitis). HSV-1 is associated with encephalitis. HSV can cause meningitis year round. CSF findings resemble enteroviral meningitis, with lymphocytic pleocytosis, a normal glucose level, and a mildly elevated protein level as in this patient. CSF polymerase chain reaction studies may be used for diagnosing HSV and enterovirus meningitis.

Enteroviruses are the most common cause of viral meningitis, but they usually present between May and November in the Western Hemisphere, with symptoms including headache, fever, nuchal rigidity, photophobia, nausea, vomiting, myalgias, pharyngitis, maculopapular rash, and cough. This

CONT.

patient's presentation in the winter makes this an unlikely cause of her illness.

Mumps virus can cause meningitis, with typical symptoms of fever, headache, and neck stiffness. Since the advent of universal childhood vaccination for measles, mumps, and rubella, the incidence of mumps-related meningitis has dramatically decreased. Meningitis from mumps virus can occur at any point during the course of clinical mumps infection. Parotitis or orchitis may be present. The patient's clinical presentation is not consistent with mumps meningitis.

Focal motor weakness is a common finding in West Nile neuroinvasive disease (WNND), either combined with meningoencephalitis or as an isolated myelitis. In its most severe form, infection of the anterior horn cells can cause a symmetric or asymmetric flaccid paralysis, analogous to that seen with polio in the prevaccination era. The diagnosis of WNND can be confirmed through identification of the IgM antibody in CSF. West Nile virus is a mosquito-borne illness most commonly seen between June and October, making this an unlikely cause of this patient's illness.

**KEY POINT**

- Herpes simplex virus type 2 can cause acute aseptic meningitis year round and is the most common cause of recurrent viral meningitis.

**Bibliography**
Nigrovic LE. Aseptic meningitis. Handb Clin Neurol. 2013;112:1153-6. [PMID: 23622323] doi:10.1016/B978-0-444-52910-7.00035-0

## Item 32       Answer:    D

**Educational Objective:** Provide appropriate immunizations for a patient with HIV infection.

Human papillomavirus (HPV) is the most appropriate immunization for this patient at this time. He was recently diagnosed with HIV infection and has begun antiretroviral therapy. At baseline, his CD4 cell count is normal. He is in an age group for which HPV immunization is recommended, and that recommendation is the same regardless of HIV status. The presence of genital warts does not change the indication for HPV vaccination. He should begin the HPV vaccine series with the first injection today. Indications for influenza, tetanus-diphtheria-pertussis, and hepatitis A virus (HAV) vaccines are also the same for patients with HIV infection as for the general population.

Pneumococcal vaccination is important for all persons with HIV infection, regardless of CD4 cell count. As with other immunocompromised persons, patients with HIV should receive the 13-valent conjugate and 23-valent polysaccharide vaccines, in that order. This patient has already received the pneumococcal conjugate vaccine and needs the polysaccharide vaccine, but at least 8 weeks must elapse between these two vaccines to allow for better immune response in this prime-boost strategy. Therefore, giving him

the pneumococcal polysaccharide vaccine at this visit would be premature.

Serum IgM antibodies to HAV are detectable at the time of symptom onset and remain detectable for approximately 3 to 6 months. Serum IgG antibodies appear in convalescence and remain detectable for decades. The presence of anti-HAV IgG in the absence of anti-HAV IgM indicates past infection or vaccination. This patient does not need vaccination against HAV.

Hepatitis B virus (HBV) surface antibody testing is negative, indicating a lack of immunity to HBV; he also has risk factors for HBV that would warrant HBV vaccination. However, the patient tested positive for hepatitis B surface antigen, indicating he already has HBV infection and would not benefit from immunization with the HBV vaccine.

**KEY POINT**

- Indications for influenza, tetanus-diphtheria-pertussis, hepatitis A virus, and human papillomavirus vaccines are the same for patients with HIV infection as for the general population.

**Bibliography**
Panel on Opportunistic Infections in HIV-Infected Adults and Adolescents. Guidelines for the prevention and treatment of opportunistic infections in HIV-infected adults and adolescents: recommendations from the Centers for Disease Control and Prevention, the National Institutes of Health, and the HIV Medicine Association of the Infectious Diseases Society of America. Available at https://aidsinfo.nih.gov/guidelines/html/4/adult-and-adolescent-opportunistic-infection/0. Accessed April 12, 2018.

## Item 33       Answer:    E

**Educational Objective:** Diagnose neuroborreliosis.

This patient should undergo lumbar puncture. He has unilateral facial nerve palsy, headache, neck stiffness, and a circular rash with central clearing that is clinically consistent with erythema migrans. The presence of erythema migrans in a patient with risk factors for Lyme disease is diagnostic of infection. Neuroborreliosis occurs in 10% to 15% of patients with Lyme disease, and cranial nerve palsy, particularly of the facial nerve (cranial nerve VII), is the most common presentation. When unilateral or bilateral facial nerve palsy is present in isolation, oral doxycycline treatment for 14 to 28 days is sufficient for Lyme disease. However, when the central nervous system is involved, parenteral therapy with ceftriaxone, cefotaxime, or penicillin is recommended. In this patient, the presence of headache and nuchal rigidity raise concern for concomitant meningitis. Because confirmation of meningeal involvement would change therapy, a lumbar puncture is first necessary to determine appropriate therapy. Cerebrospinal fluid (CSF) findings in Lyme meningitis are indistinguishable from other forms of aseptic meningitis.

Testing for antibodies to *Borrelia burgdorferi* adds little to the diagnosis because the presence of erythema migrans with cranial neuropathy is sufficient for diagnosis of neuroborreliosis. Serum antibody testing for *B. burgdorferi*

CONT.

infection would be important in the absence of a compatible skin lesion or with inconsistent exposure history.

In neuroborreliosis, a delay in starting antimicrobial treatment is not associated with adverse outcomes as it is in bacterial meningitis, and empiric therapy can be deferred until CSF cell counts are available.

Performing a head CT is unnecessary because Lyme neuroborreliosis is rarely associated with intraparenchymal lesions, and thus the risk of lumbar puncture in this previously healthy, cognitively intact patient is low.

**KEY POINT**

- In a patient with Lyme disease and possible central nervous system involvement, positive findings on lumbar puncture can support the diagnosis of neuroborreliosis, which necessitates parenteral therapy with ceftriaxone, cefotaxime, or penicillin.

**Bibliography**

Halperin JJ. Neuroborreliosis. J Neurol. 2017;264:1292-1297. [PMID: 27885483] doi:10.1007/s00415-016-8346-2

## Item 34          Answer:    D

**Educational Objective:** Manage potential bioterrorism-related anthrax exposure.

Because this patient has no known direct exposure to anthrax, no treatment is necessary. In cases of proven or suspected anthrax in a family member, no specific treatment or isolation procedures are required for others in the household because spread in health care or household settings has never been demonstrated. In patients with confirmed or suspected bioterrorism-related anthrax exposure, postexposure prophylactic antibiotics, taken for 60 days, should be started as soon as possible. Ciprofloxacin, levofloxacin, and doxycycline are the approved drugs for postexposure prophylaxis in adult patients. In pregnant women, ciprofloxacin is the drug of choice, and although tetracyclines are not recommended during pregnancy, doxycycline can be used with caution when ciprofloxacin is contraindicated. Therapy can be completed with amoxicillin if the isolate is found to be penicillin susceptible. Because of the possibility that residual dormant spores may become active after antibiotics are completed, three subcutaneous injections of anthrax vaccine should be given at 2-week intervals as part of postexposure prophylaxis.

No test is available for the detection of anthrax infection in an asymptomatic person, so taking a swab or performing a blood test would provide no useful information.

The human monoclonal antibodies against anthrax toxin, raxibacumab (available only from the Centers for Disease Control and Prevention) and obiltoxaximab (FDA approved) can be combined with antibiotics for treatment of inhalation anthrax or for postexposure prophylaxis when alternative preventive therapies are not available or appropriate. In this scenario, they are not indicated for the patient or her husband who has received adequate prophylaxis for anthrax and does not have systemic disease.

**KEY POINT**

- Patients with no known direct exposure to anthrax do not require treatment or separation from those who may be infected.

**Bibliography**

Hendricks KA, Wright ME, Shadomy SV, Bradley JS, Morrow MG, Pavia AT, et al; Workgroup on Anthrax Clinical Guidelines. Centers for Disease Control and Prevention expert panel meetings on prevention and treatment of anthrax in adults. Emerg Infect Dis. 2014;20. [PMID: 24447897] doi:10.3201/eid2002.130687

## Item 35          Answer:    D

**Educational Objective:** Prevent HIV infection in persons at risk with pre-exposure prophylaxis.

The most appropriate preventive measure for this patient is daily tenofovir disoproxil fumarate and emtricitabine (TDF-FTC). He has multiple risk factors for acquiring HIV infection, including having sex with multiple partners without consistent condom use. Data support the use of pre-exposure prophylaxis (PrEP) in specific populations with ongoing high risk for infection, such as sexual partners of infected persons, men who have sex with men, and injection drug users. PrEP is recommended for persons in such groups who can adhere to the daily regimen. Efficacy has varied depending on adherence to the regimen; rates of reduction in new infections ranged from 42% to 75% and up to 92% in patients whose adherence was documented by monitoring drug blood levels. This patient is in a group shown in clinical trials to benefit from PrEP for HIV. Combination tenofovir alafenamide and emtricitabine is being studied for PrEP, but until results of these studies are known, only TDF should be used. Risk of kidney dysfunction from TDF is low, but kidney function should be checked every 6 months during PrEP. Patients taking PrEP should be counseled to continue using barrier precautions and should undergo testing for HIV, other sexually transmitted infections (STIs), and pregnancy in women, every 3 months.

TDF-FTC given as a single dose before or after each sexual exposure has not been proven effective, and because of concerns for lower effectiveness and possible selection for resistance, these methods should not be used for prevention.

Patients should be counseled regarding the need for continued barrier precautions during sex because the effectiveness of PrEP is less than 100% and to reduce transmission of other STIs. However, counseling the patient about consistent condom use without PrEP places the patient at unnecessary risk for HIV infection. PrEP and barrier protection is now the standard of prevention for men who have sex with men at risk for HIV infection.

**KEY POINT**

- The combination of tenofovir disoproxil fumarate plus emtricitabine taken once daily is more than 90% effective, if taken consistently, in preventing HIV acquisition.

## Bibliography

Riddell J 4th, Amico KR, Mayer KH. HIV preexposure prophylaxis: A review. JAMA. 2018;319:1261-1268. [PMID: 29584848] doi:10.1001/jama.2018.1917

## Item 36    Answer:    A

**Educational Objective:** Evaluate osteomyelitis in a diabetic foot infection.

A bone biopsy and culture is the next step in the management of osteomyelitis for this patient. Biopsies can be accomplished by open surgical procedure or percutaneously. Confirming a microbiologic diagnosis is needed before antibiotics can be administered.

Indications for amputation include persistent sepsis, inability to tolerate antibiotic therapy, progressive bone destruction despite therapy, and bone destruction that compromises the mechanical integrity of the foot. None of these indications are present in this patient. Surgical debridement of the ulcer may be needed to remove the necrotic tissue, but this can be done at the time of bone biopsy.

With the exception of *Staphylococcus aureus*, microorganisms isolated from culture samples obtained from superficial wounds or sinus tracts correlate poorly with deep cultures from bone; therefore, this practice is of limited value. Bone biopsy with histopathologic assessment and full microbiologic studies is important for diagnosing osteomyelitis, excluding other entities (such as neoplasm), and isolating the causative pathogen(s).

Because the patient has no signs of skin or soft tissue infection or of sepsis, antibiotics are not immediately needed; furthermore, the provision of empiric antibiotics would also decrease the yield of a subsequent bone biopsy. Vancomycin and piperacillin-tazobactam might be indicated in the future, pending the results of the bone biopsy. However, a histologic and microbiologic diagnosis confirmation is needed before antibiotics can be administered.

### KEY POINT

- Osteomyelitis in a patient with a diabetic foot infection and no evidence of skin or soft tissue infection or sepsis requires a bone biopsy before antibiotics are administered.

## Bibliography

Lipsky BA, Berendt AR, Cornia PB, Pile JC, Peters EJ, Armstrong DG, et al; Infectious Diseases Society of America. 2012 Infectious Diseases Society of America clinical practice guideline for the diagnosis and treatment of diabetic foot infections. Clin Infect Dis. 2012;54:e132-73. [PMID: 22619242] doi:10.1093/cid/cis346

## Item 37    Answer:    D

**Educational Objective:** Manage a patient based on syphilis serology results.

This woman's serologic results are consistent with successfully treated syphilis, and no additional testing or treatment is indicated. Many laboratories use a "reverse" screening strategy, whereby a treponemal test, such as an enzyme immunoassay (EIA), is performed first and, if positive, is followed by a nontreponemal test (rapid plasma regain [RPR] or Venereal Disease Research Laboratory [VDRL] test). If the EIA is positive and the RPR or VDRL is negative, the positive result should be confirmed by a second treponemal test (such as the fluorescent treponemal antibody test performed in this patient). A positive EIA (confirmed by a second test) with a negative RPR is the expected serologic result in a patient who has been treated for syphilis. The treponemal test (EIA) remains positive indefinitely, but the nontreponemal test (RPR or VDRL) should remain negative.

If the nontreponemal test became positive again, it would indicate a new infection, and treatment, based on disease stage, would be indicated. If this patient had reported no history of treatment for syphilis, she should be treated for syphilis of unknown duration, which consists of 3 weekly doses of intramuscular benzathine penicillin. Single-dose benzathine penicillin is indicated for the treatment of primary, secondary, and early latent syphilis.

Because the positive EIA result was already confirmed by a second treponemal test, the fluorescent treponemal antibody, additional testing with another treponemal test, such as the *Treponema pallidum* particle agglutination assay, is not necessary.

### KEY POINT

- In patients with previously treated syphilis, treponemal serology results will remain positive, but nontreponemal tests will be negative; these patients require no further testing or treatment.

## Bibliography

Workowski KA, Bolan GA; Centers for Disease Control and Prevention. Sexually transmitted diseases treatment guidelines, 2015. MMWR Recomm Rep. 2015;64:1-137. [PMID: 26042815]

## Item 38    Answer:    E

**Educational Objective:** Interpret the results of HIV testing.

This woman had a false-positive result for HIV and should be reassured she does not have HIV infection. She has no symptoms to suggest acute infection. The initial HIV combination immunoassay tests for HIV-1 or HIV-2 antibody and p24 antigen. If reactive, an HIV-1/2 antibody differentiation immunoassay is performed, which differentiates between HIV-1 and HIV-2 antibodies. If the antibody differentiation assay is reactive for HIV-1 antibody, then HIV-1 infection is confirmed. If the antibody differentiation assay is negative, then testing for HIV RNA by nucleic acid amplification is performed. A negative antibody differentiation assay with a positive HIV RNA test would indicate acute HIV infection (in the "window" period after infection but before antibody development). But if the HIV RNA assay is also negative (no HIV RNA detected), then no evidence for HIV infection exists, and the initial test was a false positive. Although false-positive findings are rare, in a population with low pre-test probability (such as in screening), false-positive results on the initial antigen/antibody combination immunoassay may be seen with higher frequency than true-positive results; waiting for the confirmatory testing results is crucial to avoid misdiagnosis and unnecessary additional testing and treatment.

Because the patient does not have HIV infection, it would be inappropriate to begin antiretroviral therapy. Likewise, baseline HIV resistance testing is not indicated, nor would it be possible because the patient has no detectable HIV RNA to be genotyped.

It is important to assess the CD4 cell count for all persons newly diagnosed with HIV infection so the level of immunocompromise and consequent risk for opportunistic infections can be determined and prophylaxis can be started, if indicated. But this patient does not have HIV infection. Testing CD4 cell count as a surrogate for HIV infection is inappropriate because the CD4 level is neither sensitive nor specific for HIV infection.

Western blot testing for HIV is no longer performed as part of the laboratory protocol for diagnosing HIV infection because of problems with sensitivity in acute infection and with interpretation of indeterminate results.

### KEY POINT

- A screening HIV test result that is positive on the initial antigen/antibody combination immunoassay but negative on the antibody differentiation immunoassay and nucleic acid amplification testing for HIV RNA represents a false-positive result.

### Bibliography

Centers for Disease Control and Prevention and Association of Public Health Laboratories. Laboratory testing for the diagnosis of HIV infection: updated recommendations. Available at http://dx.doi.org/10.15620/cdc.23447. Published June 27, 2014. Accessed November 2, 2017.

## Item 39    Answer:    A

**Educational Objective:** Diagnose *Cryptosporidium* infection.

This patient has watery diarrhea associated with swimming pool exposure, and the oocysts observed microscopically represent *Cryptosporidium*. This parasitic protozoan is tolerant to chlorine and can persist for days in a chlorinated pool. *Cryptosporidium* has become the leading cause of swimming pool–related outbreaks of diarrheal illness. Swallowing infected water can result in infection. The incubation period is about 1 week, and the clinical presentation typically includes watery diarrhea, crampy abdominal pain, dehydration, fever, malaise, nausea, vomiting, and weight loss. The infection typically resolves in immunocompetent persons, but infection can be more serious and prolonged in those with immunocompromise, particularly in persons with AIDS who are not receiving combination antiretroviral therapy. Diagnosis can be established microscopically

by visualization of oocysts with modified acid-fast staining. Because oocysts are shed intermittently, diagnosis may require stool antigen testing using polymerase chain reaction, enzyme immunoassay, or direct fluorescent antibody testing.

Although enterohemorrhagic *Escherichia coli* (EHEC) infection can be acquired by aspiration of contaminated swimming pool water, it typically produces bloody diarrhea. EHEC is a gram-negative rod that does not exhibit modified acid-fast staining.

Norovirus is the most common cause of gastroenteritis and is characterized by explosive vomiting and diarrhea. It is spread person to person through the fecal-oral route, leading to community outbreaks. But the virus is not visualized with modified acid-fast staining. A diagnostic assay for viral gastroenteritis with polymerase chain reaction testing is reserved for public health investigation.

Modified acid-fast staining can detect *Nocardia* species, but the organisms are filamentous branching rods. Infection usually involves the lungs, central nervous system, and skin, but not the gastrointestinal tract.

*Vibrio parahaemolyticus* lives in salt water and causes diarrhea, usually after consumption of undercooked shellfish, especially oysters. This gram-negative rod is not detected with a modified acid-fast stain and requires special culture media with high salt content for growth.

### KEY POINT

- The protozoan *Cryptosporidium* is the most common cause of swimming pool–related outbreaks of diarrhea; diagnosis is made by microscopic examination of the stool or by stool antigen testing.

### Bibliography

Wright SG. Protozoan infections of the gastrointestinal tract. Infect Dis Clin North Am. 2012;26:323–39. [PMID: 22632642] doi:10.1016/j.idc.2012.03.009

## Item 40    Answer:    C

**Educational Objective:** Prevent travelers' diarrhea in a patient with inflammatory bowel disease.

Ciprofloxacin is the most appropriate preventive measure for this patient. Travelers' diarrhea, defined as three or more loose or watery bowel movements per day associated with other signs or symptoms such as fever, abdominal pain, cramps, or blood in the stool, is the most common travel-associated infection; it has an incidence of 10% to 40% for trips lasting more than 1 week. Enterotoxigenic *Escherichia coli* is the causative agent in most cases. The risk of infection is related to certain geographic travel destinations (South and Southeast Asia, Central and South America, the Middle East and sub-Saharan Africa) as well as individual characteristics. Persons with chronic inflammatory bowel disease (Crohn and ulcerative colitis) or who are immunocompromised (HIV, organ transplantation, those taking immunosuppressant medications) are particularly susceptible. Although most diarrheal episodes are self-limited and resolve within a few days, they can sometimes be protracted and severe, causing significant volume depletion and electrolyte imbalance. In some persons, chronic diarrhea or irritable bowel syndrome may persist for many months after the initial travel diarrhea episode has subsided. Prevention strategies generally focus on advice for avoiding potentially contaminated water and food, but studies have not conclusively proven these measures to be significantly effective. Prophylactic administration of systemic antibiotics has been determined to be highly effective in preventing infection, but it should only be offered to those at greatest risk for complications should infection occur. Nevertheless, in these higher risk persons, the duration of antibiotic administration should not extend beyond 2 to 3 weeks in an effort to decrease the chances of medication-related adverse effects or the development of drug resistance. The fluoroquinolone antibiotics (ciprofloxacin or norfloxacin) are the preferred drugs.

The macrolide antibiotic azithromycin is a highly effective agent for the treatment of various bacterial pathogens causing enterocolitis, but it has not been adequately evaluated as a prophylactic medication.

More than two thirds of persons who took bismuth subsalicylate to prevent diarrhea while traveling found it effective. However, it requires multiple daily doses, has potential adverse effects, and would be contraindicated in this woman with an aspirin allergy.

Probiotics have been proposed for the prevention and treatment of numerous medical disorders, but proven benefit has been limited to only a handful of disorders; travelers' diarrhea is not one of them.

Even though the risk of infection is less than 50%, this woman has Crohn colitis, so not recommending chemoprophylaxis may place her at undue risk.

### KEY POINT

- Persons with chronic inflammatory bowel disease or who are immunocompromised are most susceptible to severe travelers' diarrhea or complications, and prophylaxis (fluoroquinolones preferred) should be provided to these patients.

### Bibliography
Steffen R, Hill DR, DuPont HL. Traveler's diarrhea: a clinical review. JAMA. 2015;313:71-80. [PMID: 25562268] doi:10.1001/jama.2014.17006

 **Item 41        Answer:    A**

**Educational Objective:** Prevent central line–associated bloodstream infection.

This patient's central venous catheter (CVC) should be assessed daily for continued necessity and potential removal. Approximately 250,000 central line–associated bloodstream infections (CLABSIs) occur in the United States every year, with 80,000 occurring in the ICU. CLABSIs increase length of hospital stay up to 24 days and have an attributable mortality rate of 35%. Approximately 55% of patients in the ICU

and 24% of those in other units have a central line. Antimicrobial resistance is a problem for most CLABSI pathogens. The risk of CLABSI can be reduced by routinely incorporating the CVC bundle as part of patient care. The CVC insertion bundle includes hand hygiene; use of full barrier precautions (including a large full-body sterile drape to cover the patient during catheter insertion) and personal protective equipment (mask, cap, sterile gown, and gloves); chlorhexidine skin antisepsis; selection of optimal catheter type (such as selecting the minimum number of ports or lumens needed) and site; sterile dressing; and daily review of line necessity with prompt removal of unnecessary catheters. The daily review of line necessity and documentation can be achieved with multidisciplinary rounds, daily reminders, and automated alerts. These practices are important for decreasing the risk of developing CLABSIs. Just as with the insertion bundle, a maintenance bundle helps decrease the risk of introducing organisms during use of the catheter. Components of the maintenance bundle include daily review of line necessity with prompt removal of unnecessary catheters, hand hygiene before manipulation of the intravenous system, care of injection ports, and proper monitoring of catheter site dressing and dressing changes.

Guidelines recommend against routinely replacing CVCs (or arterial catheters) and administering antimicrobial prophylaxis for short-term or tunneled catheter insertion. Neither practice has been shown to decrease central line–associated infections. In fact, routinely changing central catheters may increase the risk of infection by introducing bacteria from the skin at the time of insertion.

### KEY POINT

- Central venous catheters should be assessed daily for continued necessity and removed promptly when they are no longer needed.

### Bibliography
Marschall J, Mermel LA, Fakih M, Hadaway L, Kallen A, O'Grady NP, et al; Society for Healthcare Epidemiology of America. Strategies to prevent central line-associated bloodstream infections in acute care hospitals: 2014 update. Infect Control Hosp Epidemiol. 2014;35:753-71. [PMID: 24915204] doi:10.1086/676533

**Item 42        Answer:    E**

**Educational Objective:** Treat *Cyclospora* parasitic infection.

This patient has travel-associated *Cyclospora* infection and should be treated with trimethoprim-sulfamethoxazole. *Cyclospora* protozoan infections are typically acquired after consumption of fecal-contaminated food or water, particularly in countries where the parasite is endemic, such as Peru, Guatemala, Haiti, and Nepal. *Cyclospora* infections may also be acquired through consumption of fresh produce imported from tropical areas. The incubation period is approximately 1 week (range, 2 days to ≥2 weeks). The clinical presentation usually consists of crampy abdominal pain, anorexia, bloating, decreased appetite, fatigue, flatulence, low-grade fever, malaise, nausea, watery diarrhea, and weight loss. Persons with HIV infection may have more severe symptoms associated with wasting.

Diagnosis can be established microscopically by visualization of oocysts with modified acid-fast staining; fluorescence microscopy can be used as well. Several stool specimens may be required because *Cyclospora* oocysts may be shed intermittently and at low levels, even in persons with profuse diarrhea. Polymerase chain reaction assays appear to have the greatest sensitivity for the diagnosis of a *Cyclospora* infection.

The recommended treatment is one double-strength tablet of trimethoprim-sulfamethoxazole taken orally twice daily for 7 to 10 days. The Centers for Disease Control and Prevention states no effective alternative treatments have been identified for persons who are allergic to or cannot tolerate trimethoprim-sulfamethoxazole; observation and symptomatic care is recommended for those patients.

Atovaquone has activity against protozoans such as *Pneumocystis jirovecii*, *Toxoplasma*, *Plasmodium*, and *Babesia*, but not *Cyclospora*.

Metronidazole has activity against some protozoans, including *Giardia*, *Entamoeba*, and *Trichomonas*, but not *Cyclospora*.

Pyrimethamine has activity against protozoans such as *Toxoplasma*, *Pneumocystis jirovecii*, and *Isospora belli*, but not *Cyclospora*.

Quinacrine can be used to treat *Giardia* but is not effective against *Cyclospora*.

**KEY POINT**

- *Cyclospora* infection is treated with oral trimethoprim-sulfamethoxazole.

**Bibliography**
Wright SG. Protozoan infections of the gastrointestinal tract. Infect Dis Clin North Am. 2012;26:323-39. [PMID: 22632642] doi:10.1016/j.idc.2012.03.009

## Item 43    Answer:    A

**Educational Objective:** Prevent perinatal transmission of HIV.

This pregnant woman with well-controlled HIV infection should continue the same antiretroviral regimen. Antiretroviral therapy during pregnancy is crucial and significantly decreases the risk of perinatal transmission of HIV to the baby. Although most transmission in untreated women occurs at the time of delivery, in utero transmission also occurs, and maintaining therapy throughout pregnancy or starting therapy immediately is important to significantly reduce the risk. Although concerns have been raised regarding the safety of efavirenz and tenofovir disoproxil fumarate in pregnancy, more recent data demonstrate the safety of these agents, including in the first trimester. A woman whose HIV is well controlled and is found to be pregnant should continue the same regimen unless another reason exists to change it.

Pausing antiretroviral therapy would result in rebound of viral replication and viremia, which would significantly increase the risk of in utero transmission of HIV to the developing fetus.

Testing for HIV drug resistance can be genotypic (looking for specific mutations associated with resistance to specific drugs) or phenotypic (assessing whether HIV can replicate in the presence of achievable levels of specific drugs). Resistance testing should always be done before an initial drug regimen is chosen and when treatment failure occurs, as indicated by failure to suppress viral load or an increase in viral load that was previously suppressed. Resistance testing is unnecessary at this time because no virologic failure is evident that would necessitate changing therapy. Moreover, it would not be possible to perform resistance testing in a patient with an undetectable viral load because not enough virus is present to test. A viral load level greater than 500 copies/mL is usually necessary to successfully perform resistance testing.

Zidovudine, lamivudine, and ritonavir-boosted lopinavir is a valid alternative for treating HIV; it was previously a preferred regimen in pregnancy. However, changing this patient's therapy, which is well tolerated and controls her HIV infection well, is unnecessary and would only risk new adverse effects, poor adherence (because of more pills or more frequent dosing), or treatment failure.

**KEY POINT**

- Antiretroviral therapy during pregnancy is crucial and significantly decreases the risk of perinatal transmission of HIV to the baby.

**Bibliography**
Panel on Treatment of Pregnant Women with HIV Infection and Prevention of Perinatal Transmission. Recommendations for the use of antiretroviral drugs in pregnant women with HIV infection and interventions to reduce perinatal HIV transmission in the United States. Available at https://aidsinfo.nih.gov/guidelines/html/3/perinatal/0. Accessed April 12, 2018.

## Item 44    Answer:    C

**Educational Objective:** Prevent acute hepatitis A infection.

This patient should be given a single dose of hepatitis A vaccine. Worldwide, hepatitis A is the most common cause of acute viral hepatitis. Infection with this human-only RNA picornavirus is spread primarily through the fecal-oral route. Rates of endemicity are highest in developing nations, where hygiene and sanitary measures are less than optimal. Since the availability of effective hepatitis A vaccines in the mid-1990s, this enteric virus has been designated the leading cause of infection and death among vaccine-preventable diseases. Infected adolescents and adults usually present with fever, malaise, nausea, and anorexia, with more than 70% exhibiting jaundice. Most infection is benign and resolves uneventfully. Rarely, patients may experience fulminant hepatitis and acute liver failure. However, hepatitis A does not become a chronic disease. Either of the two inactivated cell culture–produced vaccines that have become part of the recommended routine childhood vaccine schedule can be used. In addition to avoiding potentially contaminated food and water, vaccination is also strongly advised for those planning to travel to areas that pose significant risk of infection. Ideally, vaccination should occur at least 2 to 4 weeks before departure. Nevertheless, a single dose of vaccine given any time before travel provides adequate protection in otherwise healthy persons. Depending on the particular vaccine product used, a second dose is administered between 6 to 18 months later.

Another dose of vaccine administered 7 days after the first would have no immunologic boosting effect.

Passive immunization with intramuscular immune globulin adds no benefit when administered alone or in combination with vaccination for most healthy patients when time before travel is short. However, to optimally guard against infection, immune globulin is recommended with vaccination in persons with chronic liver disease or other chronic medical conditions, immunocompromised states, and older adults if travel is scheduled in less than 2 weeks. Immune globulin alone would also be warranted in persons who are allergic to or decline vaccination and in children younger than 12 months for whom the vaccine is not approved.

Providing no intervention would place this traveler at undue risk of acquiring hepatitis A infection.

### KEY POINT

- Hepatitis A vaccination should ideally occur 2 to 4 weeks before travel to an endemic region; however, a single dose of the vaccine given any time before travel provides adequate protection to otherwise healthy persons.

### Bibliography

Fiore AE, Wasley A, Bell BP; Advisory Committee on Immunization Practices (ACIP). Prevention of hepatitis A through active or passive immunization: recommendations of the Advisory Committee on Immunization Practices (ACIP). MMWR Recomm Rep. 2006;55:1-23. [PMID: 16708058]

### Item 45       Answer:    D

**Educational Objective:** Treat multidrug-resistant urinary tract infection.

Antibiotic therapy should be switched from piperacillin-tazobactam to meropenem. This patient has a complicated urinary tract infection (UTI), defined by the presence of a chronic indwelling urinary catheter. The pattern of antibiotic susceptibility of *Escherichia coli* from the urine culture suggests an extended-spectrum β-lactamase (ESBL)–producing organism. ESBL-producing gram-negative organisms are capable of hydrolyzing higher generation cephalosporins that have an oxyimino side chain, including cefotaxime, ceftazidime, ceftriaxone, and cefepime. Laboratory identification of ESBLs is difficult because they are a heteroge-

neous group of enzymes. The carbapenem class of antibiotics (imipenem, meropenem, doripenem, ertapenem) is the preferred class of agents for treating infections with ESBL-producing organisms.

Adding gentamicin would provide no benefit. Additionally, this patient has kidney disease; thus, aminoglycosides should be avoided if at all possible.

On laboratory testing, ESBL-producing gram-negative organisms may appear susceptible to piperacillin-tazobactam; however, susceptibility breakpoints do not always reflect clinical success. Thus, piperacillin-tazobactam may be insufficient to treat infections with ESBL-producing organisms. An exception is uncomplicated UTI, in which piperacillin-tazobactam may be effective because high concentrations of the antibiotic are achievable in urine.

The oxyimino cephalosporins (such as cefepime) should not be used, even if an ESBL-producing organism appears to be susceptible on laboratory testing. Treatment failures are common, even with higher doses, so carbapenems are the preferred antibiotic.

### KEY POINT

- The carbapenem class of antibiotics (imipenem, meropenem, doripenem, ertapenem) is the preferred class of agents for treating infections with extended-spectrum β-lactamase–producing organisms.

### Bibliography

Kaye KS, Pogue JM. Infections caused by resistant gram-negative bacteria: epidemiology and management. Pharmacotherapy. 2015;35:949-62. [PMID: 26497481] doi:10.1002/phar.1636

### Item 46       Answer:    D

**Educational Objective:** Monitor for adverse effects of daptomycin therapy in an outpatient.

Patients receiving outpatient daptomycin therapy should undergo baseline measurement of kidney function and creatine kinase (CK) followed by weekly monitoring. Patients should also be screened for symptoms of myopathy. Daptomycin is commonly used for outpatient parenteral antibiotic therapy (OPAT) because of its safety profile, ease of administration (once daily), and good activity against gram-positive bacteria, including vancomycin-resistant enterococci and methicillin-resistant *Staphylococcus aureus*. However, daptomycin is known to cause elevated levels of CK and can contribute to the development of myopathy during therapy. Daptomycin should be discontinued in asymptomatic patients if CK levels increase to greater than 10 times the upper limit of normal or the CK level is greater than 5 times the upper limit of normal with symptoms of myopathy. Concomitant treatment with statins (particularly simvastatin and atorvastatin) may increase the chance of developing an elevated CK level; it is suggested that statins be discontinued if possible during daptomycin treatment. If statins cannot be discontinued, or if kidney dysfunction is evident, the CK level should be monitored more frequently than once weekly. Likewise, the creatinine level should also be monitored because daptomycin dosing may require adjustment (lower dose or dosing interval of every other day), and CK may require more frequent monitoring if the creatinine level increases.

Daptomycin use does not require electrocardiographic monitoring, and it has no effect on the bone marrow (for example, erythrocyte or platelet suppression), pancreas, lipid levels, or blood glucose level; so weekly amylase, triglyceride, glucose, and hemoglobin measurements and platelet count monitoring are unnecessary (although periodic leukocyte counts may be necessary in some patients for monitoring of the primary infection). It is important for patients undergoing OPAT to have close follow-up to monitor for any adverse effects from antibiotic therapy (including development of vascular access infections) as well as resolution of the infection being treated.

**KEY POINT**

- Patients receiving daptomycin therapy should undergo baseline measurement of kidney function and creatine kinase level followed by weekly monitoring.

**Bibliography**

Cervera C, Sanroma P, González-Ramallo V, García de la María C, Sanclemente G, Sopena N, et al; DAPTODOM Investigators. Safety and efficacy of daptomycin in outpatient parenteral antimicrobial therapy: a prospective and multicenter cohort study (DAPTODOM trial). Infect Dis (Lond). 2017;49:200-207. [PMID: 27820968] doi:10.1080/23744235.2016.1247292

## Item 47          Answer:    D

**Educational Objective:  Identify the cause of Kaposi sarcoma.**

This patient has Kaposi sarcoma caused by human herpes virus (HHV) type 8. It is found primarily in men who have sex with other men and who have AIDS. This patient's clinical presentation is typical for Kaposi sarcoma, with painless violaceous skin nodules with oral involvement. The treatment for Kaposi sarcoma includes antiretroviral therapy, local therapies (radiation therapy, intralesional chemotherapy, cryotherapy, or topical retinoids), and systemic therapies such as interferon or chemotherapy.

Cytomegalovirus (HHV-5) infections are most commonly asymptomatic, but they can also present with a mononucleosis-like syndrome and may reactivate in patients with cellular immunodeficiency such as AIDS or in those who have had a solid organ or bone marrow transplantation. Cytomegalovirus does not cause skin nodules but can present with retinitis (in AIDS), pneumonia, hepatitis, adrenalitis, pancytopenia, gastritis, or colitis.

Epstein–Barr virus (EBV) (HHV-4) is the main cause of infectious mononucleosis presenting with fever, exudative pharyngitis, cervical lymphadenopathy, and splenomegaly. EBV reactivation is associated with the development of T-cell and B-cell lymphomas, Hodgkin and Burkitt lymphoma, nasopharyngeal carcinoma, and posttransplant lymphoproliferative disease in solid organ transplantation.

Human herpes virus type 6 causes roseola infantum, febrile seizures in children, and cytomegalovirus-seronegative and EBV-seronegative mononucleosis. It does not cause skin nodules. Recipients of bone marrow transplantation may also develop encephalitis, hepatitis, pneumonia, rash, graft-versus-host disease, and delayed engraftment.

**KEY POINT**

- Kaposi sarcoma can develop in patients with AIDS infected with human herpes virus type 8, presenting with painless violaceous skin nodules with oral involvement.

**Bibliography**

De Paoli P, Carbone A. Kaposi's sarcoma herpesvirus: twenty years after its discovery. Eur Rev Med Pharmacol Sci. 2016;20:1288-94. [PMID: 27097948]

## Item 48          Answer:    B

**Educational Objective:  Treat osteomyelitis associated with orthopedic hardware.**

Cefazolin and rifampin are appropriate therapy for treatment of methicillin-sensitive *Staphylococcus aureus* (MSSA) osteomyelitis associated with orthopedic hardware. Identification of the causative pathogen, administration of adequate antimicrobials for a prolonged duration, surgical debridement (if warranted), and removal of orthopedic prosthetic devices (if feasible) influence the success of osteomyelitis treatment. Optimal management of this patient's infection includes hardware removal; however, this is not possible because the fracture has not yet healed. Hardware-associated infections caused by *S. aureus* are difficult to eradicate because of the biofilm that forms on the hardware. First-line treatment of MSSA osteomyelitis consists of a β-lactam agent such as cefazolin; a randomized controlled trial and systematic review of the literature have demonstrated that if infected hardware cannot be removed, the addition of rifampin increases the chances of therapeutic success compared with an antistaphylococcal agent alone.

Although cefazolin has activity against MSSA as well as good bone penetration, it would not be an appropriate therapeutic option for the treatment of hardware-associated osteomyelitis without the addition of rifampin.

Ceftaroline has coverage for MSSA, methicillin-resistant *S. aureus*, and Enterobacteriaceae, but it is unnecessarily broad coverage for the treatment of this patient's MSSA infection.

Vancomycin, a bacteriostatic agent, is less effective than β-lactam agents for the treatment of MSSA and is typically restricted to patients with drug intolerance or allergy.

**KEY POINT**

- Rifampin should be used in combination with another antistaphylococcal agent when managing *Staphylococcus aureus* osteomyelitis in the setting of orthopedic hardware if the hardware cannot be removed.

### Bibliography

Kim BN, Kim ES, Oh MD. Oral antibiotic treatment of staphylococcal bone and joint infections in adults. J Antimicrob Chemother. 2014;69:309-22. [PMID: 24072167] doi:10.1093/jac/dkt374

## Item 49        Answer:    A

**Educational Objective:**  Treat an immunocompromised patient after a dog bite.

The most appropriate management for this patient would be administration of amoxicillin-clavulanate. Because of asplenia, he is immunodeficient and should receive prophylactic antibiotic therapy after the dog bite, even without evidence of infection. Infections typically result from the host's skin flora and the animal's mouth flora. This flora is a mix of aerobic and anaerobic organisms, including staphylococci, streptococci, *Bacteroides* species, *Porphyromonas* species, *Fusobacterium* species, *Capnocytophaga canimorsus*, and *Pasteurella* species. *C. canimorsus* is a gram-negative bacillus that can cause overwhelming sepsis in patients with functional or anatomic asplenia who have experienced a dog bite or scratch. Because of its activity against pathogens associated with animal bite wounds, a 3- to 5-day course of amoxicillin-clavulanate is recommended for patients who are immunosuppressed (including patients with cirrhosis and asplenia); have wounds with associated edema, lymphatic or venous insufficiency, or crush injury; have wounds involving a joint or bone; have deep puncture wounds; or have moderate to severe injuries, especially when involving the face, genitalia, or hand. If a patient is allergic to penicillin, a combination of trimethoprim-sulfamethoxazole or a fluoroquinolone or doxycycline plus clindamycin or metronidazole can be used.

Because these infections are typically polymicrobial, consisting of aerobic and anaerobic bacteria, neither ciprofloxacin nor metronidazole alone would be adequate. Ciprofloxacin lacks anaerobic bacterial coverage, and metronidazole lacks aerobic activity.

Because of this the patient's immunodeficiency, observation alone would not be recommended by the Infectious Diseases Society of America guidelines.

### KEY POINT

- Amoxicillin-clavulanate is recommended for patients with animal bites who are immunosuppressed (including patients with cirrhosis and asplenia); have wounds with associated edema, lymphatic or venous insufficiency, or crush injury; have wounds involving a joint or bone; have deep puncture wounds; or have moderate to severe injuries, especially when involving the face, genitalia, or hand.

### Bibliography

Stevens DL, Bisno AL, Chambers HF, Dellinger EP, Goldstein EJ, Gorbach SL, et al. Practice guidelines for the diagnosis and management of skin and soft tissue infections: 2014 update by the infectious diseases society of America. Clin Infect Dis. 2014;59:147-59. [PMID: 24947530] doi:10.1093/cid/ciu296

## Item 50        Answer:    A

**Educational Objective:**  Treat multidrug-resistant intra-abdominal infection.

The *Pseudomonas* isolate should be tested for susceptibility to ceftolozane-tazobactam and colistin. This patient has an intra-abdominal infection caused by carbapenem-resistant (meropenem and doripenem) *Pseudomonas aeruginosa*. The antimicrobial options for treating carbapenem-resistant organisms are limited. Ceftolozane-tazobactam consists of a newer antipseudomonal cephalosporin combined with a β-lactamase inhibitor. It has activity against some extended-spectrum β-lactamase (ESBL)–producing gram-negative organisms as well as carbapenem-resistant strains of *Pseudomonas*. Its efficacy is reduced in patients whose creatinine clearance rate is 50 mL/min or less. Ceftolozane-tazobactam is approved to treat complicated urinary tract infections and complicated intra-abdominal infections. For complicated intra-abdominal infections, ceftolozane-tazobactam must be paired with metronidazole because it lacks antianaerobic activity. This patient's penicillin allergy is not an anaphylactic reaction, so it is reasonable to consider a cephalosporin in her treatment.

Colistin is an older antimicrobial agent that has made a resurgence because of its bactericidal activity against pan-resistant gram-negative organisms (including carbapenem-resistant, gram-negative organisms). Half of patients who are administered colistin develop nephrotoxicity, which limits the drug's usefulness in many cases. Kidney function should be closely monitored during administration, and colistin should be dose adjusted for patients with kidney disease. Paresthesias are a commonly reported neurotoxicity. Unfortunately, colistin resistance has been reported and appears to be increasing.

Ertapenem is a non-antipseudomonal carbapenem, so it would not be an option for this patient. Likewise, tobramycin is an aminoglycoside, which has poor activity and penetration into abscesses and would not be a consideration for this patient.

Fosfomycin is used to treat urinary tract infections caused by several multidrug-resistant organisms (such as vancomycin-resistant enterococci, methicillin-resistant *Staphylococcus aureus*, and resistant *Klebsiella pneumoniae*). Fosfomycin has poor tissue penetration and is not indicated for infections other than uncomplicated urinary tract infections.

Minocycline is another older antimicrobial agent that has been used recently to treat multidrug-resistant *Acinetobacter* as well as *Stenotrophomonas maltophilia* infections, but it does not have activity against *Pseudomonas*.

### KEY POINT

- Ceftolozane-tazobactam is a newer antipseudomonal cephalosporin combined with a β-lactamase inhibitor that can be used in the treatment of multidrug-resistant intra-abdominal infection.

## Bibliography

Morrill HJ, Pogue JM, Kaye KS, LaPlante KL. Treatment options for carbapenem-resistant Enterobacteriaceae infections. Open Forum Infect Dis. 2015;2:ofv050. [PMID: 26125030] doi:10.1093/ofid/ofv050

H **Item 51      Answer:    E**

**Educational Objective:** Evaluate community-acquired pneumonia in a pregnant patient.

*Streptococcus pneumoniae* is the most likely cause of this patient's community-acquired pneumonia (CAP). Pneumonia is the most common cause of fatal nonobstetric infection in pregnancy. The microbiology of CAP in pregnancy is similar to that seen in the general population. Among patients requiring hospitalization, the most common pathogens are *S. pneumoniae*, *Haemophilus influenzae*, and atypical organisms, including *Legionella* species, *Chlamydia pneumoniae*, and *Mycoplasma pneumoniae*. Empiric treatment of pregnant patients is similar to that in nonpregnant adults, although quinolones and tetracyclines are relatively contraindicated because of the potential for teratogenic effects. In addition to these common bacterial causes of CAP, pregnant women are at increased risk for serious viral pneumonia from influenza virus and varicella-zoster virus, so it is recommended that pregnant women receive seasonal influenza vaccination.

Gram-negative bacteria, including *Klebsiella pneumoniae*, *Pseudomonas aeruginosa*, *Acinetobacter* species, *Escherichia coli*, and *Enterobacter* species, are rarely implicated in CAP, including among pregnant women hospitalized for pneumonia. Most patients with CAP caused by gram-negative bacteria have a predisposing risk factor, such as bronchiectasis, cystic fibrosis, or COPD, and develop severe pneumonia necessitating admission and care in the ICU.

Pregnancy causes a decrease in T-cell function, and pregnant women are at increased risk for severe *Listeria* infections, including meningitis and sepsis. However, *Listeria* rarely causes pulmonary infection and would be an unlikely cause of infection in this patient.

*Staphylococcus aureus* is an increasingly recognized cause of CAP, with risk factors including antecedent viral infection or injection drug use. Maternal *S. aureus* infection can occur perinatally, related to delivery, surgery, or indwelling lines, but remains a rare cause of CAP in the prenatal period.

### KEY POINT

- The microbiology of community-acquired pneumonia in pregnancy is similar to that seen in the general population; among patients requiring hospitalization, the most common pathogens are *Streptococcus pneumoniae*, *Haemophilus influenzae*, and atypical organisms, including *Legionella* species, *Chlamydia pneumoniae*, and *Mycoplasma pneumoniae*.

## Bibliography

Mehta N, Chen K, Hardy E, Powrie R. Respiratory disease in pregnancy. Best Pract Res Clin Obstet Gynaecol. 2015;29:598-611. [PMID: 25997564] doi:10.1016/j.bpobgyn.2015.04.005

**Item 52      Answer:    B**

**Educational Objective:** Treat influenza virus infection with a neuraminidase inhibitor.

The most appropriate treatment for this patient is the neuraminidase inhibitor oseltamivir. During a confirmed local influenza outbreak, infection can be reliably diagnosed on the basis of clinical criteria alone. When confirmation is needed, rapid antigen tests of respiratory samples from nasopharyngeal swabs detect influenza A and B. Positive test results are highly specific. However, sensitivity ranges from 40% to 80%. Detection of viral nucleic acid by polymerase chain reaction (PCR) is rapid, has high sensitivity and specificity, and can determine the type and subtype of influenza virus. Annual influenza vaccination is the most effective intervention for preventing influenza and is recommended for all persons 6 months or older. Only a few randomized trials have assessed the efficacy of influenza vaccines in older individuals. These trials suggest that the vaccines are approximately 60% effective against influenza in adults 65 years and older. Nevertheless, immunization is likely to prevent hospitalization in older adults. Neuraminidase inhibitors have activity against influenza A and B. They can be given orally (oseltamivir), intranasally (zanamivir), or intravenously (peramivir). Antiviral therapy is recommended for severe disease, including all hospitalized patients or those with confirmed or suspected influenza infection at high risk for complications. Older adult patients (older than ≥65 years), young children, pregnant women, and patients with chronic medical conditions (especially chronic lung disease and heart disease) are at higher risk for severe primary influenza complications such as superimposed bacterial pneumonia caused by *Streptococcus pneumoniae* or *Staphylococcus aureus* and death.

M2 inhibitors, such as amantadine and rimantadine, were the first agents introduced for influenza treatment, but they are only active against influenza A. Therefore, these agents would be ineffective against this patient's infection with influenza B.

Antiviral therapy should be started within 48 hours of symptom onset in patients with a positive rapid influenza test because it decreases recovery time, hospitalization rates, and complications. Because this patient can be treated as an outpatient, either oseltamivir or zanamivir would be appropriate choices. Intravenous peramivir is typically reserved for patients who cannot tolerate or are otherwise incapable of taking inhaled or enteral agents.

### KEY POINT

- Neuraminidase inhibitors (oseltamivir, zanamivir, peramivir) are indicated for the treatment of influenza A and B and can be administered through various routes (oral, intranasal, intravenous).

## Bibliography

Uyeki TM. Influenza. Ann Intern Med. 2017;167:ITC33-ITC48. [PMID: 28869984] doi:10.7326/AITC201709050

**Item 53        Answer:    A**

**Educational Objective:** Manage urinary tract infections in men.

This patient should be given intravenous cefepime and fluids and should undergo kidney ultrasonography. According to the 2016 Critical Care Congress Third International Consensus Definition of Sepsis and Septic Shock (Sepsis-3), this man is septic. The probable source of his severe infection is the urinary tract (UTI), likely acute prostatitis, which is the most significant cause of bacteremia in older adult men. The prompt administration of adequate antimicrobial therapy is the most important factor in decreasing morbidity, mortality, and length of hospital stay in patients with sepsis. Cefepime is an appropriate choice because it possesses dependable bactericidal activity against common urinary pathogens as well as potentially drug-resistant organisms, including *Pseudomonas*. In addition to antimicrobial therapy and supportive medical care, men with febrile UTIs require anatomic assessment of the upper and lower urinary tract by either kidney ultrasonography or CT with contrast (more sensitive, but contraindicated with kidney disease) to determine the need for source control. When acute prostatitis is the presumed diagnosis, imaging generally is unnecessary, but assurance that this patient with sepsis does not have a prostatic abscess may prove beneficial if his fever persists beyond 72 hours.

The empiric use of ciprofloxacin or other fluoroquinolone antibiotics in a hospitalized patient with a complicated UTI is no longer recommended because several strains of *Escherichia coli* and other Enterobacteriaceae have become resistant to these agents.

Detection of a boggy and tender prostate gland on gentle digital rectal examination would suggest a prostate focus of infection, but vigorous prostate massage is not indicated in acute prostatitis because of a lack of diagnostic or therapeutic benefit and possibility of facilitating bacteremia.

The β-lactam and β-lactamase inhibitor, piperacillin-tazobactam, would be an adequate initial antibiotic selection but should be avoided in a patient with an undocumented penicillin allergy, even if he has tolerated cephalosporin medications.

**KEY POINT**

- Men with febrile urinary tract infections require prompt antimicrobial therapy and anatomic assessment of the upper and lower urinary tract.

**Bibliography**

Schaeffer AJ, Nicolle LE. Clinical practice. Urinary tract infections in older men. N Engl J Med. 2016;374:562-71. [PMID: 26863357] doi:10.1056/NEJMcp1503950

 **Item 54        Answer:    C**

**Educational Objective:** Treat vertebral osteomyelitis in a patient with signs of sepsis.

The patient has vertebral osteomyelitis and clinical findings suggestive of sepsis; empiric antibiotic therapy to cover the most likely pathogens should be initiated. A diagnosis of vertebral osteomyelitis should be considered in patients reporting worsening back or neck pain without an alternate explanation. Local tenderness over the site of spinal infection is frequently detected. Radicular pain, motor weakness, and sensory changes may be present. Common sources of hematogenous osteomyelitis are distant foci of infection (for example, skin and soft tissue, genitourinary, gastrointestinal), intravascular catheters, and infective endocarditis. Hematogenous osteomyelitis is typically monomicrobial, and *Staphylococcus aureus* is the most commonly isolated pathogen; however, aerobic, gram-negative bacilli cause disease in many patients. Certain patient-specific conditions are associated with less common bacterial organisms, including *Salmonella* osteomyelitis in persons with sickle cell disease and *Pseudomonas aeruginosa* bone infection in injection drug users. Lengthy parenteral antimicrobial therapy is the mainstay of treatment. An antistaphylococcal agent with methicillin-resistant *S. aureus* (MRSA) coverage (vancomycin) and a β-lactam with antipseudomonal coverage (cefepime) is an appropriate empiric regimen for suspected osteomyelitis in this patient who uses injection drugs.

Cefazolin does not provide coverage for MRSA, and aminoglycosides, such as gentamicin, have poor penetration into bone.

Vancomycin alone would not provide coverage for gram-negative organisms, which should be included in the empiric therapy for this patient.

Although microbiologic confirmation of the bacterial cause should always be sought, withholding antibiotics in a patient likely to have sepsis (fever, hypotension, tachycardia) is not appropriate. If the patient has positive blood cultures, a presumptive microbiologic diagnosis of vertebral osteomyelitis can usually be made. However, because injection drug users have frequent bacteremia and the patient's bloodstream infection may be unrelated to the vertebral osteomyelitis, some experts would recommend pursuing bone biopsy, even in patients with positive blood cultures.

**KEY POINT**

- When sepsis is suspected among patients with osteomyelitis, empiric antibiotic therapy should begin, even when the microbial cause of the infection has not yet been determined.

**Bibliography**

Berbari EF, Kanj SS, Kowalski TJ, Darouiche RO, Widmer AF, Schmitt SK, et al. 2015 Infectious Diseases Society of America (IDSA) clinical practice guidelines for the diagnosis and treatment of native vertebral osteomyelitis in adults. Clin Infect Dis. 2015;61:e26-46. [PMID: 26229122] doi:10.1093/cid/civ482

**Item 55        Answer:    A**

**Educational Objective:** Diagnose acute HIV infection.

This patient has acute HIV infection. His recent non-specific viral symptoms are consistent with the acute retroviral syndrome, although they are not diagnostic. Regardless of the presence or absence of symptoms, his HIV testing results support a diagnosis of acute HIV infection. His initial HIV-1/2 antigen/antibody combination immunoassay is reactive, indicating further testing is needed. The HIV-1/HIV-2 antibody differentiation assay is negative, indicating the absence of antibody to HIV; however, the RNA assay is positive for HIV-1 RNA. This finding indicates the patient does not have antibodies to HIV but does demonstrate the presence of virus by nucleic acid amplification testing. The initial combination immunoassay was reactive because of the presence of HIV p24 antigen rather than antibody, which indicates acute infection with HIV before antibody development. The ability to detect acute infection is a key advantage of and improvement in current HIV testing, allowing for earlier detection of infection, faster initiation of treatment, and, consequently, reduced risk of transmission.

In chronic HIV infection, the HIV antibody differentiation immunoassay would have demonstrated antibody to HIV, either HIV-1 (usually) or HIV-2 (rarely). Because no antibody was detected but HIV RNA is present, infection is still in the acute phase before antibody development.

Because the HIV-1 RNA assay was positive at a significant level, the initial HIV antigen/antibody immunoassay result was not a false positive. Although false-positive HIV RNA testing can occur, it is usually at a very low, barely detectable level. This patient's level is substantial, and he has known risk factors and consistent symptoms for acute HIV infection, increasing his pretest probability and making a positive result much more likely a true positive.

HIV-2 infection is rare in the United States. It is ruled out in this patient by the negative HIV-2 antibody result on the HIV-1/HIV-2 antibody differentiation assay.

**KEY POINT**

- On testing for HIV infection, a positive result on HIV-1/2 antigen/antibody combination immunoassay is followed by testing with the HIV-1/HIV-2 antibody differentiation immunoassay; a negative antibody differentiation immunoassay but a positive follow-up HIV-1 nucleic acid amplification test is diagnostic of acute HIV infection.

**Bibliography**

Centers for Disease Control and Prevention and Association of Public Health Laboratories. Laboratory testing for the diagnosis of HIV infection: updated recommendations. Available at http://dx.doi.org/10.15620/cdc.23447. Published June 27, 2014. Accessed November 2, 2017.

## Item 56          Answer:     A

**Educational Objective:** Treat urethritis with empiric therapy.

The most appropriate treatment is ceftriaxone plus azithromycin. The patient has dysuria and evidence of mucopurulent urethral discharge, which are consistent with urethritis.

Because he is being evaluated in an urgent care setting and may not return for follow-up, empiric therapy is appropriate. A single intramuscular dose of ceftriaxone (250 mg) plus a single oral dose of azithromycin (1 g) will treat *Neisseria gonorrhoeae* and *Chlamydia trachomatis*, the most common causes of urethritis. Diagnostic testing results are still important in case the patient does not respond to empiric therapy and for disease reporting and contact tracing. This man should also be offered HIV and syphilis testing and undergo counseling regarding the use of condoms for all sexual encounters, including oral sex. Some concern exists that sexually active persons, particularly young persons, may believe that oral sex is "safe" and does not pose a risk of sexually transmitted infection (STI) transmission. Most STIs can be acquired through oral sex; the risk of acquiring HIV infection may be lower, but precise data on the relative risk of STI acquisition from specific types of sexual activity are not available.

Doxycycline for 7 days is an alternate therapy for *C. trachomatis*; however, it should be used only when a macrolide allergy precludes the use of azithromycin. It also will not reliably treat *N. gonorrhoeae*.

Trimethoprim-sulfamethoxazole is not an effective treatment for urethritis. Trimethoprim-sulfamethoxazole can potentially be used for empiric therapy for cystitis; however, men with cystitis should not have purulent urethral discharge. Additionally, symptoms of bladder irritation, including increased frequency and urgency, are generally present.

Herpes simplex virus can present as urethritis, and penile ulcers may not be present on physical examination; however, this clinical presentation is less common and should only be considered if the infection fails to respond to treatment for the more common causes of urethritis. Therefore, valacyclovir is not the most appropriate initial empiric therapy for this patient.

**KEY POINT**

- In a patient with clinical signs and symptoms of urethritis, treatment with ceftriaxone and azithromycin provides appropriate empiric therapy without waiting for microbiologic testing results.

**Bibliography**

Workowski KA, Bolan GA; Centers for Disease Control and Prevention. Sexually transmitted diseases treatment guidelines, 2015. MMWR Recomm Rep. 2015;64:1-137. [PMID: 26042815]

## Item 57          Answer:     C

**Educational Objective:** Prevent opportunistic fungal infections after hematopoietic stem cell transplantation.

Posaconazole is the most appropriate prophylactic therapy for this patient after hospital discharge. Patients who undergo allogeneic hematopoietic stem cell transplantation (HSCT) usually experience a period of prolonged neutropenia after the pretransplant myeloablative conditioning regimen. This prolonged, severe neutropenia is a significant risk factor for invasive bacterial and fungal infections, and prophylaxis for both is indicated. The risk of invasive fungal infection remains elevated, however, even after recovery of neutrophils for the first few months after allogeneic HSCT and even later in the setting of graft-versus-host disease. Therefore, although this patient is doing well and her neutrophil count has recovered, antifungal prophylaxis should be provided in addition to continuing trimethoprim-sulfamethoxazole therapy. Posaconazole provides activity against *Candida* and *Aspergillus* and other moulds that are the cause of an increasing proportion of invasive fungal infections after HSCT.

Acyclovir is used to reduce reactivation of herpes simplex virus during periods of neutropenia, but its administration is no longer needed. Additionally, this patient is seropositive for varicella-zoster virus because of immunization, so varicella-zoster prophylaxis is unnecessary. Finally, acyclovir has no role in preventing reactivation of Epstein-Barr virus or cytomegalovirus, two other infections for which this patient is at risk.

Ciprofloxacin is a preferred agent for antibacterial prophylaxis during neutropenia because it has activity against most of the gram-negative bacteria of greatest concern. But with resolution of neutropenia and completion of therapy for known infection, continued antibacterial therapy should be avoided to lessen toxicities and complications such as *Clostridium difficile* colitis.

Valganciclovir is used to prevent or treat cytomegalovirus infection. This patient is at risk for reactivation cytomegalovirus because of her positive serology. However, because of the leukopenia that is a common toxicity of valganciclovir, a strategy of monitoring for cytomegalovirus and starting pre-emptive therapy only when indicated is preferred over prophylaxis after HSCT.

### KEY POINT

- In patients who have undergone hematopoietic stem cell transplantation, the risk of invasive fungal infection remains elevated for the first few months, even after recovery of neutrophil counts, so antifungal prophylaxis should be continued during this time.

### Bibliography
Ullmann AJ, Schmidt-Hieber M, Bertz H, Heinz WJ, Kiehl M, Krüger W, et al; Infectious Diseases Working Party of the German Society for Hematology and Medical Oncology (AGIHO/DGHO) and the DAG-KBT (German Working Group for Blood and Marrow Transplantation). Infectious diseases in allogeneic haematopoietic stem cell transplantation: prevention and prophylaxis strategy guidelines 2016. Ann Hematol. 2016;95:1435-55. [PMID: 27339055] doi:10.1007/s00277-016-2711-1

### Item 58    Answer:    C
**Educational Objective:** Treat suspected tuberculous meningitis.

The most appropriate management for this patient is four-drug antituberculous therapy (rifampin, isoniazid, pyrazinamide, and ethambutol) plus dexamethasone. Meningitis can be defined as either acute or chronic. The symptoms of acute meningitis typically progress over hours, sometimes days, whereas chronic meningitis generally progresses over 4 or more weeks. Tuberculosis and fungal infection are the most common causes of chronic meningitis. Tuberculous meningitis should be suspected in patients from highly endemic countries who have basilar lymphocytic meningitis associated with cranial neuropathies (particularly involving cranial nerve VI) and hypoglycorrhachia. A history of tuberculosis exposure, an abnormal chest radiograph, a positive tuberculin skin test, and a positive interferon-γ release assay may be clues to the diagnosis, but these can be absent. Cerebrospinal fluid (CSF) acid-fast bacilli stains and cultures are insensitive and may take up to 6 weeks to grow. Patients with a high suspicion for tuberculosis should be treated empirically with rifampin, isoniazid, pyrazinamide, and ethambutol pending culture results and clinical improvement. Adjunctive dexamethasone decreases mortality, especially in patients with normal mental status and no neurologic deficits; it should be started concomitantly with antituberculous therapy.

The most common fungal meningitis in the United States is cryptococcal meningitis. Cryptococcus is inhaled and causes an initial pulmonary infection. Risk factors for dissemination include AIDS, organ transplantation, glucocorticoid treatment, diabetes mellitus, liver dysfunction, and kidney injury. The central nervous system is the most common site of disseminated cryptococcosis. CSF analysis may resemble that of tuberculous meningitis, although monocytes may predominate and the opening pressure is often greater than 200 mm $H_2O$. An India ink preparation of the CSF will demonstrate cryptococcal organisms in up to 80% of patients with a high organism burden, such as patients with HIV infection, but is only 50% sensitive in patients without HIV. The CSF assay for cryptococcal antigen is highly sensitive and specific for the diagnosis of meningitis and can be obtained soon after lumbar puncture results are available. Recommended induction therapy for cryptococcal meningitis includes amphotericin B and 5-fluorocytosine but is not indicated in this patient who is at low risk for this infection.

Bacterial meningitis is an acute infection with progression of symptoms over hours to days. This patient has chronic lymphocytic meningitis with an extremely low CSF glucose level and a negative CSF Gram stain, making bacterial meningitis unlikely. Initiating vancomycin, ceftriaxone, and dexamethasone is not the most appropriate management.

### KEY POINT

- Tuberculosis and cryptococcus are the most common causes of chronic meningitis; empiric treatment for tuberculous meningitis includes four-drug antituberculous therapy (rifampin, isoniazid, pyrazinamide, and ethambutol) plus dexamethasone.

### Bibliography
Prasad K, Singh MB, Ryan H. Corticosteroids for managing tuberculous meningitis. Cochrane Database Syst Rev. 2016;4:CD002244. [PMID: 27121755] doi:10.1002/14651858.CD002244.pub4

## Item 59    Answer:    B

**Educational Objective:** Treat a patient with latent tuberculosis infection.

The most appropriate management for this patient is to initiate self-administered treatment with isoniazid. He has traveled to a high-risk area for *Mycobacterium tuberculosis*. Before departing for Vietnam, he had a negative tuberculin skin test; however, he returned with a positive screening result for tuberculosis. Because the chest radiograph is negative, he requires treatment for latent tuberculosis rather than treatment with the four-drug regimen for active tuberculosis. Several treatment options exist, and the regimen chosen should be based on comorbidities, knowledge of the drug-susceptibility data from the source patient, and possible drug interactions. Self-administered isoniazid for 9 months is approved for the treatment of latent tuberculosis by the Centers for Disease Control and Prevention for patients with and without HIV infection. In patients being treated for latent tuberculosis who have normal baseline aminotransferase levels and no risk factors for liver disease, routine testing of aminotransferase levels during treatment is unnecessary.

Once-weekly isoniazid and rifapentine only needs to be administered for 12 weeks, not 24 weeks. This regimen must be administered as directly observed therapy (that is, a health care worker directly observes the ingestion of a medication), as are all intermittent therapies. The 12-week regimen can be used instead of 9 months of isoniazid alone for healthy adult patients, including those with HIV coinfection who are not taking antiretroviral agents. It is not recommended for patients suspected of having rifampin- or isoniazid-resistant tuberculosis strains or for patients who are pregnant or plan to become pregnant while taking these agents.

Treatment of active tuberculosis usually consists of multiple drugs for 6 to 9 months administered in two phases: initial and continuation. The core first-line antituberculous agents are isoniazid, rifampin, pyrazinamide, and ethambutol. These agents are administered for 8 weeks as part of the initiation phase. Isoniazid and rifampin are then continued for 4 or 7 months as part of the continuation phase. This patient does not have active tuberculosis (absent symptoms and a normal chest radiograph) and does not require therapy with four antituberculosis drugs.

This patient has latent tuberculosis infection, as detected by the positive interferon-γ release assay. Providing no treatment would put him at risk of developing active disease or exposing close contacts who may then become ill.

### KEY POINT

- Prophylactic treatment with isoniazid is recommended for persons with latent tuberculosis infection, determined by a newly positive tuberculosis screening test but no signs or symptoms of active disease; 9 months of daily isoniazid can be self-administered.

**Bibliography**

Nahid P, Dorman SE, Alipanah N, Barry PM, Brozek JL, Cattamanchi A, et al. Executive summary: Official American Thoracic Society/Centers for Disease Control and Prevention/Infectious Diseases Society of America clinical practice guidelines: treatment of drug-susceptible tuberculosis. Clin Infect Dis. 2016;63:853-67. [PMID: 27621353] doi:10.1093/cid/ciw566

## Item 60    Answer:    A

**Educational Objective:** Diagnose *Clostridium difficile* colitis after transplantation.

The most likely diagnosis is colitis caused by *Clostridium difficile*. *C. difficile* infection is the most common cause of health care–associated colitis, and antibiotic use is the most significant risk factor. The patient presents within the first month after solid organ transplantation; this is a time when the most likely infections are nosocomial and similar to those in patients who have had other surgeries. This patient has recently completed antimicrobial treatment for pneumonia and wound infection, increasing his risk for *C. difficile* colitis, which is common in transplant recipients during this time frame. Testing for *C. difficile* colitis and providing treatment would be appropriate at this time. Polymerase chain reaction assays to detect the genes responsible for production of toxins A and B are very sensitive and are increasingly used in the diagnosis of *C. difficile* colitis.

The other concern of most significance in this patient would be cytomegalovirus infection, most likely manifesting as colitis in this scenario. Being a cytomegalovirus-seronegative recipient of an organ from a cytomegalovirus-seropositive donor puts the patient at significant risk for developing cytomegalovirus disease, most commonly in the gastrointestinal tract or as a nonspecific febrile illness. However, because of this risk, he is already receiving prophylaxis with valganciclovir, which significantly lowers the rate of occurrence. His presentation being so early after transplantation also makes cytomegalovirus less likely, because infection most often occurs in the "middle" period, 1 to 6 months after transplantation.

Mycophenolate toxicities include diarrhea, cytopenias, and infection. Although diarrhea is a common adverse effect of mycophenolate, the additional presence of fever and abdominal pain makes this an unlikely cause. *C. difficile* infection must be considered first and ruled out.

Polyoma BK virus causes a nephropathy after transplantation, not diarrhea, and usually occurs later than the first month after transplantation. Definitive diagnosis requires kidney biopsy. When polyoma BK nephropathy occurs, immunosuppression should be reduced to the minimum level necessary to avoid rejection.

### KEY POINT

- The first month after solid organ transplantation is when the most likely infections are nosocomial and similar to those in patients who have had other surgeries; patients who have recently completed antimicrobial treatment are particularly at increased risk for *Clostridium difficile* colitis.

## Bibliography

Fishman JA. From the classic concepts to modern practice. Clin Microbiol Infect. 2014;20 Suppl 7:4-9. [PMID: 24528498] doi:10.1111/1469-0691.12593

## Item 61     Answer:    C

**Educational Objective:** Treat *Neisseria gonorrhoeae* infection.

The most appropriate treatment is ceftriaxone plus azithromycin. This sexually active young woman presented for an annual Pap smear and renewal of oral contraceptives. She was appropriately screened for *Chlamydia trachomatis* and *Neisseria gonorrhoeae* infection using nucleic acid amplification testing. The U.S. Preventive Services Task Force recommends this screening for all sexually active women younger than 25 years. If the patient were older than 25 years, she should be tested because of her new sexual partner. Her screening results are positive for *N. gonorrhoeae*. Even without symptoms or findings on pelvic examination, she should be treated; a significant number of persons with *N. gonorrhoeae* infection are asymptomatic without evidence of cervicitis. Intramuscular ceftriaxone (250 mg) is the preferred therapy for treatment of *N. gonorrhoeae* infection, along with a single dose of oral azithromycin (1 g). Although this regimen is given empirically when *C. trachomatis* and *N. gonorrhoeae* coinfection is suspected (for example, empiric therapy for cervicitis), because of increasing minimum inhibitory concentrations (MIC) to ceftriaxone among *N. gonorrhoeae* isolates in the United States, azithromycin is used even when *C. trachomatis* infection is not present; this combination will increase the success of treatment of the *N. gonorrhoeae* infection.

Oral cefixime does not achieve adequate levels to exceed the MIC of many *N. gonorrhoeae* isolates, so this option should only be used if ceftriaxone is unavailable. In this circumstance, a single dose of oral azithromycin should be administered with the cefixime.

Ciprofloxacin was previously recommended for the treatment of *N. gonorrhoeae* infections; however, the prevalence of fluoroquinolone resistance among *N. gonorrhoeae* isolates has increased, and this antibiotic is no longer recommended.

### KEY POINT

- Because of increasing minimum inhibitory concentrations to ceftriaxone among *Neisseria gonorrhoeae* isolates in the United States, this agent should be combined with a single dose of azithromycin.

## Bibliography

Workowski KA, Bolan GA; Centers for Disease Control and Prevention. Sexually transmitted diseases treatment guidelines, 2015. MMWR Recomm Rep. 2015;64:1-137. [PMID: 26042815]

## Item 62     Answer:    C

**Educational Objective:** Diagnose babesiosis.

This patient's blood smear is most likely to show intraerythrocytic tetrad forms. He has a life-threatening illness characterized by fever and hemolysis and has no spleen. Given his residence in the northeastern United States and his outdoor vocation, severe babesiosis is likely. *Babesia* species are transmitted by the same tick that causes Lyme disease; infection also can be acquired through transfusion of infected erythrocytes outside of the endemic region. Asplenia is a major risk factor for fulminant *Babesia* infection, as is older age, HIV infection, or other immunocompromising conditions. Clinical manifestations are variable, with most relating to severe hemolytic anemia. Infection can be diagnosed by visualization of intraerythrocytic parasites, which appear as either ring forms or tetrads, with the latter often described as having the Maltese cross appearance shown. Complications, including acute respiratory distress syndrome, disseminated intravascular coagulation, heart failure, kidney failure, and coma, are associated with severe anemia (hematocrit level <30%) and parasitemia (exceeding 10%) and are indications for exchange transfusion.

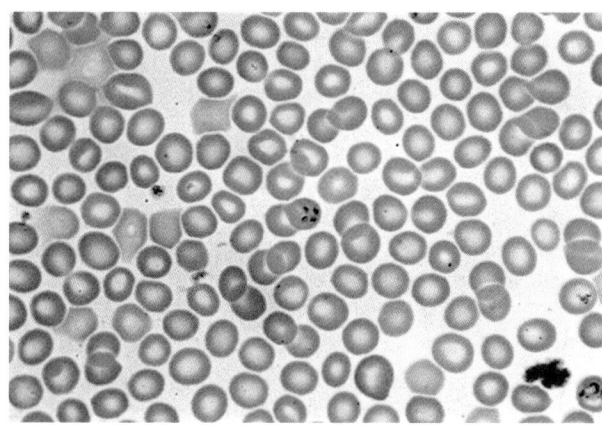

Morulae, basophilic inclusion bodies composed of clusters of bacteria, can be seen in the cytoplasm of monocytes and neutrophils of patients with ehrlichiosis and anaplasmacytosis, respectively. These tick-borne infections cause fever, leukopenia, and thrombocytopenia but are not associated with hemolytic anemia.

Both malaria and babesiosis cause a hemolytic anemia and may present with ring-shaped parasitic inclusions inside erythrocytes. However, banana-shaped gametocytes are seen only with *Plasmodium falciparum* malaria, and the absence of a compatible travel history excludes this diagnosis.

Asplenic patients are at risk for overwhelming pneumococcal sepsis with a high bacterial burden; gram-positive diplococci may be visualized inside neutrophils on buffy-coat stain. Although leukopenia and thrombocytopenia are common with fulminant infection, hemolytic anemia is not a feature of pneumococcal sepsis.

Schistocytes are a manifestation of microangiopathic hemolytic anemia caused by a thrombotic microangiopathy (TMA), such as hemolytic uremic syndrome or thrombotic thrombocytopenic purpura. Although both these syndromes can cause fever, hemolysis, and thrombocytopenia, the absence of acute kidney injury in this patient excludes a TMA.

**KEY POINT**

- Babesiosis can be diagnosed by visualization of intraerythrocytic parasites in a ring or tetrad form on a blood smear.

**Bibliography**

Akel T, Mobarakai N. Hematologic manifestations of babesiosis. Ann Clin Microbiol Antimicrob. 2017;16:6. [PMID: 28202022] doi:10.1186/s12941-017-0179-z

## Item 63    Answer:    D

**Educational Objective:** Manage conversion of intravenous antimicrobial therapy to oral antimicrobial therapy.

This patient's therapy should be switched from intravenous piperacillin-tazobactam to oral ciprofloxacin and metronidazole. He has a diabetic foot ulcer and osteomyelitis of the left great toe caused by *Pseudomonas aeruginosa* and *Bacteroides fragilis*. Ciprofloxacin and metronidazole have excellent bioavailability and will penetrate bone adequately with oral administration. Continuing intravenous therapy offers no advantage for this patient, and intravenous therapy has risks that include developing a venous catheter–associated bloodstream infection. Intravenous-to-oral antibiotic switching should be considered in patients who have an intact and functioning gastrointestinal tract, whose clinical status is improving, and who are not being treated for an infection for which parenteral therapy is preferred (for example, endocarditis or meningitis). Common infectious scenarios for which a switch from intravenous to oral therapy should be considered include community-acquired pneumonia, bacterial peritonitis, pyelonephritis, septic arthritis, and skin and soft tissue infections. When switching from a parenteral to an oral antibiotic agent, the bioavailability of the oral antibiotics must be considered.

A second antipseudomonal agent is not required for this patient's osteomyelitis. He also has kidney disease, which should discourage use of an aminoglycoside. Therefore, adding tobramycin while continuing intravenous antibiotic therapy would not be the best management for this patient who can de-escalate to oral therapy.

Although aztreonam and ceftazidime have good antipseudomonal activity, neither agent has any anaerobic activity to cover *B. fragilis*.

**KEY POINT**

- Intravenous-to-oral antibiotic switching should be considered in patients who have an intact and functioning gastrointestinal tract, whose clinical status is improving, and who are not being treated for an infection for which parenteral therapy is preferred.

**Bibliography**

Cyriac JM, James E. Switch over from intravenous to oral therapy: A concise overview. J Pharmacol Pharmacother. 2014;5:83-7. [PMID: 24799810] doi:10.4103/0976-500X.130042

## Item 64    Answer:    A

**Educational Objective:** Manage candidemia with empiric antifungal therapy.

This patient has candidemia. Candidemia occurs most frequently in the presence of an intravascular catheter and may lead to focal organ involvement or disseminated infection as a consequence of hematogenous spread. Risk factors for candidemia and other forms of systemic candidiasis include neutropenia, malignancies, organ transplantation, broad-spectrum antimicrobial agents, immunosuppressive agents, chemotherapeutic agents, intravascular catheters, hemodialysis, parenteral nutrition, and major abdominal surgery. Because systemic candidiasis has a high mortality rate, therapy should be initiated promptly when it is suspected or diagnosed. The finding of yeast in the blood culture is enough to initiate empiric antifungal therapy until the fungal identification is definitive. An echinocandin (anidulafungin, caspofungin, or micafungin) is recommended as empiric therapy for most patients with candidemia. If the *Candida* species is azole susceptible, the patient may be de-escalated to fluconazole to complete the 14-day course of therapy.

Fluconazole is not recommended as initial management for this patient. Several *Candida* species, such as *C. glabrata*, *C. auris*, and *C. krusei*, are known to be intrinsically resistant to azoles.

Systemic candidiasis is usually diagnosed by a positive culture from blood or a normally sterile body site. A positive blood culture should not be treated as a contaminant, and empiric therapy should be instituted immediately, particularly in seriously ill patients such as this one. *Candida* isolated from blood cultures should always prompt a search for the source.

Central venous catheters should be removed as soon as possible in patients with candidemia; however, removal of an implicated catheter is not sufficient treatment for candidemia. All patients must be treated with antifungal drugs.

**KEY POINT**

- A positive blood culture for *Candida* species should not be treated as a contaminant, and empiric therapy with an echinocandin should be instituted immediately.

**Bibliography**

Pappas PG, Kauffman CA, Andes DR, Clancy CJ, Marr KA, Ostrosky-Zeichner L, et al. Executive summary: clinical practice guideline for the management of candidiasis: 2016 update by the Infectious Diseases Society of America. Clin Infect Dis. 2016;62:409-17. [PMID: 26810419] doi:10.1093/cid/civ1194

## Item 65    Answer:    A

**Educational Objective:** Treat vertebral osteomyelitis.

This patient has a confirmed diagnosis of methicillin-susceptible *Staphylococcus aureus* osteomyelitis and should complete a 6-week course of antibiotics. Although there are no randomized controlled trials regarding the optimal duration of antibiotic therapy for osteomyelitis, a treatment course of 2 weeks is inadequate. For this patient, vertebral osteomyelitis at a single level, not associated with epidural abscess or hardware, has a favorable prognosis; older age, comorbidities, and infection with *S. aureus* are unfavorable factors. However, there is no evidence that antibiotics beyond 6 weeks will enhance therapeutic success. In a recently published clinical trial comparing 6 weeks to 12 weeks of antibiotics for vertebral osteomyelitis, cure rates were not significantly different between the treatment groups. Several retrospective studies have found similar results.

Prolonged courses of antibiotics place the patient at risk for adverse events, including drug-resistant pathogens and *Clostridium difficile*–associated diarrhea.

Cefazolin should not be discontinued now because the patient has only completed 2 weeks of treatment, and 6 weeks is considered the therapeutic minimum.

Monitoring of inflammatory markers during treatment can assist in assessing the success of therapy. Routine follow-up MRI is not recommended in patients who respond clinically. Follow-up MRI may suggest progressive infection and lead to unnecessary additional intervention. Follow-up MRI is indicated with clinical deterioration or if a concomitant epidural or paraspinal abscess was present that was managed medically.

**KEY POINT**

- The recommended duration of antibacterial therapy for acute vertebral osteomyelitis is 6 weeks.

**Bibliography**
Berbari EF, Kanj SS, Kowalski TJ, Darouiche RO, Widmer AF, Schmitt SK, et al. 2015 Infectious Diseases Society of America (IDSA) clinical practice guidelines for the diagnosis and treatment of native vertebral osteomyelitis in adults. Clin Infect Dis. 2015;61:e26-46. [PMID: 26229122] doi:10.1093/cid/civ482

## Item 66  Answer:  D

**Educational Objective:** Treat severe *Clostridium difficile* infection.

This patient has severe *Clostridium difficile* infection (CDI) and should receive oral vancomycin therapy. All patients with confirmed CDI require antimicrobial treatment, but optimal management depends on whether the episode represents the initial presentation or a recurrence, as well as the severity of the illness. The American College of Gastroenterology defines severe disease by the presence of hypoalbuminemia (<3 g/dL [30 g/L]) plus leukocytosis (leukocyte count ≥15,000/µL [15 × 10⁹/L]) or abdominal tenderness. The Society for Healthcare Epidemiology of America and the Infectious Diseases Society of America guidelines define severe disease by a serum creatinine level >1.5 mg/dL (133 µmol/L) or leukocyte count ≥15,000/µL (15 × 10⁹/L). Oral vancomycin for 10 days is recommended for the initial episode of a severe CDI infection. Oral fidaxomicin may also be used.

Fecal microbiota transplantation has been advocated as a treatment approach for patients with multiple relapses of CDI. The rationale is that exogenous feces will restore the normal colonic microbiota. Fecal microbiota transplantation is not recommended for an initial episode of CDI.

Intravenous vancomycin is not recommended for treatment of CDI because vancomycin delivered intravenously is not excreted into the large intestine and has no effect on CDI.

Oral metronidazole for 10 days can be used for patients who have an initial episode of nonsevere CDI when neither oral vancomycin nor fidaxomicin is available, but not in this patient with severe disease.

Oral vancomycin plus intravenous metronidazole is recommended for an initial episode of severe infection complicated (that is, fulminant disease) by ileus, hypotension, shock, or toxic megacolon. Fulminant CDI is often associated with ileus-limiting colonic transit of orally dosed medications; therefore, a vancomycin enema through a rectal tube should be considered to maximize colonic luminal concentrations.

**KEY POINT**

- Oral vancomycin (or fidaxomicin) therapy is recommended for the treatment of an initial episode of severe *Clostridium difficile* infection.

**Bibliography**
McDonald LC, Gerding DN, Johnson S, Bakken JS, Carroll KC, Coffin SE, et al. Clinical practice guidelines for *Clostridium difficile* infection in adults and children: 2017 update by the Infectious Diseases Society of America (IDSA) and Society for Healthcare Epidemiology of America (SHEA). Clin Infect Dis. 2018;66:987-994. [PMID: 29562266] doi:10.1093/cid/ciy149

## Item 67  Answer:  C

**Educational Objective:** Diagnose serogroup B *Neisseria meningitides* in a patient who received the quadrivalent meningococcal vaccine.

*Neisseria meningitides* serogroup B is the most likely cause of this patient's meningitis. Bacterial meningitis classically presents with fever, nuchal rigidity, and altered mental status. However, all three symptoms may not be present in many patients with confirmed disease. Other clinical manifestations that suggest bacterial meningitis include photophobia and headache. Serogroup B *N. meningitides* accounts for 40% of all bacterial meningitis infections in the United States because the quadrivalent conjugate vaccine (ACYW-135) does not include group B. College students are at higher risk for developing meningococcal meningitis because of risk factors such as living in dormitories, sharing drinks, and kissing multiple partners. Clinical findings that support the diagnosis of meningococcal meningitis include severe myalgia, rapid progression, hemodynamic instability, and early appearance of a petechial or hemorrhagic rash in a previously well person. Finally, the finding of gram-negative diplococci on cerebrospinal fluid (CSF) examination strongly supports the diagnosis.

CONT.

Prevalence of *Haemophilus influenzae* meningitis has decreased in the pediatric age group since the advent of the type B conjugate vaccine, and it is an uncommon cause of meningitis in adults. Adult patients with functional or anatomic asplenia are at greatest risk. Gram stain of the CSF would show small pleomorphic gram-negative coccobacilli, which is not consistent with this patient's findings.

*Listeria monocytogenes* is responsible for meningitis primarily in immunosuppressed patients with decreased cell-mediated immunity, owing to medications or medical conditions, as well as in the very old or very young. *L. monocytogenes* appears as gram-positive rods and coccobacilli, which are not consistent with this patient's findings. *Streptococcus pneumoniae* is the most common bacterial cause of meningitis in adults of all ages followed by *N. meningitidis*. Since the introduction of the pneumococcal conjugate vaccine in 2000, the rate of pneumococcal meningitis has decreased by about one third, and the greatest reduction is seen in children younger than 5 years. *S. pneumoniae* is a gram-positive diplococcus and is an unlikely cause of this patient's meningitis.

**KEY POINT**

- The quadrivalent meningococcal vaccine does not include coverage for serogroup B *Neisseria meningitides*, which now accounts for 40% of all meningitis infections in the United States.

**Bibliography**

van de Beek D, Brouwer M, Hasbun R, Koedel U, Whitney CG, Wijdicks E. Community-acquired bacterial meningitis. Nat Rev Dis Primers. 2016;2:16074. [PMID: 27808261] doi:10.1038/nrdp.2016.74

## Item 68    Answer:    C

**Educational Objective:** Treat proctitis in a patient at risk for sexually transmitted infection.

Ceftriaxone and doxycycline should be given empirically to patients with clinical evidence of proctitis who are at risk for sexually transmitted infections (STIs). The differential diagnosis of proctitis in this patient includes *Chlamydia trachomatis* (including the lymphogranuloma venereum serovars), *Neisseria gonorrhoeae*, syphilis, and herpes simplex virus (HSV) infection. In those who also have diarrhea (proctocolitis), *Campylobacter*, *Shigella*, and *Entamoeba histolytica* should be considered as well. In this patient with proctitis, diagnostic evaluation should include nucleic acid amplification testing (NAAT) of a rectal swab specimen for *N. gonorrhoeae*, *C. trachomatis*, and HSV-1 and HSV-2 (even if ulcers are not visible on external examination) as well as serologic testing for syphilis. If anoscopy is not available to further elucidate the most likely diagnosis, initial empiric therapy for *N. gonorrhoeae* and *C. trachomatis* should be prescribed pending diagnostic testing results. If the NAAT is positive for *C. trachomatis*, further testing for lymphogranuloma venereum should be performed, and consultation with an expert in STIs should be sought.

For initial empiric therapy of proctitis, azithromycin would not provide adequate coverage for the possibility of *N. gonorrhoeae* infection.

This patient could have inflammatory bowel disease; however, considering his high risk for STI and the acute nature of his symptoms, an STI is far more likely, and the use of a topical glucocorticoid preparation is not appropriate.

Although it may provide coverage for some of the enteric pathogens implicated in proctocolitis, ciprofloxacin cannot be used as part of empiric therapy for *N. gonorrhoeae* because of high rates of resistance.

**KEY POINT**

- Ceftriaxone and doxycycline should be given empirically to patients with clinical evidence of proctitis who are at risk for sexually transmitted infections.

**Bibliography**

Workowski KA, Bolan GA; Centers for Disease Control and Prevention. Sexually transmitted diseases treatment guidelines, 2015. MMWR Recomm Rep. 2015;64:1-137. [PMID: 26042815]

## Item 69    Answer:    B

**Educational Objective:** Treat pneumonia after hematopoietic stem cell transplantation.

Ganciclovir for cytomegalovirus is the most appropriate empiric treatment in this patient at this time. The risk of cytomegalovirus reactivation is related to serologic status of the donor and recipient and is unlikely when donor and recipient are both negative. Cytomegalovirus disease after transplantation may manifest as a nonspecific febrile illness; may cause leukopenia and thrombocytopenia; or may cause organ-specific disease, most often pneumonitis, colitis, esophagitis, or hepatitis. This patient is at significant risk for cytomegalovirus infection and has a clinical presentation consistent with cytomegalovirus pneumonia, specifically her presenting symptoms and radiographic findings of diffuse bilateral lung involvement. Although it has been more than 6 months from her hematopoietic stem cell transplantation (HSCT), her recent graft-versus-host disease increases infection risk. She is not receiving cytomegalovirus prophylaxis at this time; her acyclovir therapy is effective prophylaxis for herpes simplex virus and varicella-zoster virus but not for cytomegalovirus. Cytomegalovirus pneumonia after HSCT is associated with poor prognosis and significant mortality. Treatment with ganciclovir should be started while proceeding with the diagnostic evaluation, including nucleic acid amplification testing and bronchoscopy.

Atovaquone is an appropriate treatment for *Pneumocystis jirovecii* pneumonia. Although this patient is at risk for *P. jirovecii* and her presentation is consistent with it, she is taking trimethoprim-sulfamethoxazole, which is effective as prophylaxis, making this infection unlikely.

Liposomal amphotericin would provide broad-spectrum antifungal coverage in this patient who is at risk for fungal infection. However, her presentation and

CONT. radiographic findings are not consistent with invasive fungal infection, which is more likely to demonstrate nodules on CT. Moreover, the toxicity of amphotericin would preclude its use empirically in this setting.

**KEY POINT**

- Cytomegalovirus disease after transplantation may manifest as a nonspecific febrile illness; may cause leukopenia and thrombocytopenia; or may cause organ-specific disease, most often pneumonitis, colitis, esophagitis, or hepatitis; ganciclovir therapy should be initiated empirically in patients who present with signs and symptoms of cytomegalovirus infection.

**Bibliography**

Ariza-Heredia EJ, Nesher L, Chemaly RF. Cytomegalovirus diseases after hematopoietic stem cell transplantation: a mini-review. Cancer Lett. 2014;342:1-8. [PMID: 24041869] doi:10.1016/j.canlet.2013.09.004

## Item 70    Answer:    D

**Educational Objective:** Treat methicillin-resistant *Staphylococcus aureus* bacteremia.

The most appropriate management is to continue the vancomycin. Endocarditis and vertebral osteomyelitis are two important complications of *Staphylococcus aureus* bacteremia. Vancomycin is the preferred antimicrobial agent for treatment of bacteremia with methicillin-resistant *S. aureus* (MRSA). An alternative to vancomycin should be considered if the organism is not susceptible or if no clinical or microbiologic (such as persistent bacteremia) response occurs despite adequate source control. Daptomycin is an acceptable alternative if the isolate is susceptible. *S. aureus* with a vancomycin minimum inhibitory concentration (MIC) of 2 µg/mL or less is considered susceptible; intermediate susceptibility is defined as an MIC of 4 to 8 µg/mL. Vancomycin should not be used in the treatment of MRSA bacteremia when the vancomycin MIC is greater than 2 µg/mL because clinical failures have been reported. At MICs close to 2 µg/mL, clinical response (that is, clearance of bacteremia and resolution of fever and leukocytosis) should guide whether to continue vancomycin or change to daptomycin. Source control and appropriate antibiotic therapy are important for improving clinical outcomes. When using vancomycin to treat MRSA bacteremia, a trough level of 15 to 20 µg/mL should be targeted. At trough levels greater than 20 µg/mL, the risk for adverse effects increases without an increase in clinical benefit.

Adding rifampin or gentamicin to vancomycin has not been shown to improve outcomes of MRSA bacteremia and should be avoided. Combination therapy also increases the risk for adverse events (nephrotoxicity with gentamicin, hepatotoxicity and drug interactions with rifampin). Combination therapy is sometimes considered with prosthetic device infections, and an infectious diseases specialist should be consulted for guidance in such cases.

**KEY POINT**

- When treating methicillin-resistant *Staphylococcus aureus* bacteremia, vancomycin should be used only if the minimum inhibitory concentration is 2 µg/mL or less.

**Bibliography**

Choo EJ, Chambers HF. Treatment of methicillin-resistant Staphylococcus aureus bacteremia. Infect Chemother. 2016;48:267-273. [PMID: 28032484] doi:10.3947/ic.2016.48.4.267

## Item 71    Answer:    D

**Educational Objective:** Prevent infection in patients with terminal complement deficiency.

The most appropriate preventive measure for this patient is immunization with the quadrivalent meningococcal conjugate vaccine. A personal history of recurrent *Neisseria* infection or history of infection in multiple family members suggests a deficiency in one of the terminal complement components that make up the membrane attack complex (MAC). The MAC comprises C5 to C9, and a deficiency in any of these constituents leads to an impaired ability to combat *Neisseria* infections, particularly *N. meningitidis*. Patients are at risk for recurrent meningococcal infection, often caused by unusual serogroups. For unclear reasons, infection in this population is often uncharacteristically mild. Evaluation for terminal complement deficiency is performed by quantitation of total hemolytic complement ($CH_{50}$). If the $CH_{50}$ is low, more specific testing for individual components of the MAC may be performed. Immunization is the mainstay of infection prevention in patients with defects in terminal complement. The Advisory Committee on Immunization Practices recommends use of a conjugate quadrivalent meningococcal vaccine as well as a vaccine active against serogroup B meningococcal infection, with a booster of the conjugate quadrivalent meningococcal vaccine given every 5 years for adults with terminal complement deficiency. These patients should also receive both pneumococcal (polysaccharide and conjugate) and *Haemophilus influenzae* type B vaccines.

Intravenous immune globulin does not have appreciable levels of complement and would not be useful for infection prevention in a patient with terminal complement deficiency.

Although plasma is rich in complement, plasma infusion is not a feasible long-term approach to repletion of complement levels. Additionally, such treatment would be associated with an increased risk of bloodborne diseases and the potential development of antibody against the missing component.

Prophylactic ciprofloxacin has a role in reducing the risk of meningococcal disease after close exposure to an infected person, but no data support using chronic prophylactic antibiotics in patients with terminal complement deficiencies. Instead, patients should be counseled to be vigilant for development of fever, rash, headache, or other symptoms concerning for *Neisseria* infection.

**KEY POINT**

- Immunization with the quadrivalent meningococcal conjugate vaccine is the mainstay of infection prevention in patients with terminal complement deficiency.

**Bibliography**

Audemard-Verger A, Descloux E, Ponard D, Deroux A, Fantin B, Fieschi C, et al. Infections revealing complement deficiency in adults: a French nationwide study enrolling 41 patients. Medicine (Baltimore). 2016;95:e3548. [PMID: 27175654] doi:10.1097/MD.0000000000003548

**Item 72      Answer:   A**

**Educational Objective:  Treat a patient with mild nonpurulent cellulitis.**

The most appropriate treatment for this patient is clindamycin. Treatment of skin and soft tissue infections is guided by categorizing the infection as purulent or nonpurulent and by grading the severity of the infection as mild, moderate, or severe. This patient has a nonpurulent cellulitis without systemic signs of infection (mild infection). Nonpurulent infections are typically caused by streptococci, and outpatient treatment with an oral agent active against streptococci, including clindamycin, penicillin, cephalexin, or dicloxacillin, is recommended.

After incision and drainage, trimethoprim–sulfamethoxazole or doxycycline would be appropriate empiric therapy for moderate-severity (systemic signs of infection present) purulent skin infections (such as a furuncle or carbuncle) in which the usual cause is *Staphylococcus aureus* (including methicillin-resistant strains [MRSA]).

Because of the increased likelihood of MRSA contributing to infection, intravenous vancomycin would be appropriate to include for empiric treatment of severe purulent skin infections. Severe infections are those that do not improve with incision and drainage plus oral antibiotics or that have specific systemic signs of infection, including temperature greater than 38 °C (100.4 °F), heart rate greater than 90/min, respiration rate greater than 24/min, abnormal leukocyte count (>12,000/μL [12 × 10⁹/L] or <4000/μL [4 × 10⁹/L]), or infection in immunocompromised patients. Intravenous vancomycin is also appropriate for severe nonpurulent necrotizing skin infections (in addition to coverage of gram-negative bacilli and anaerobes). In select patients with cellulitis of moderate severity, vancomycin is recommended for coverage of streptococci and MRSA. These would include cellulitis in patients who are injection drug users, those with nasal MRSA colonization or extracutaneous MRSA infection, or those whose infection is associated with penetrating trauma.

**KEY POINT**

- Nonpurulent cellulitis without systemic signs of infection is usually caused by streptococci, which can be treated with an oral agent such as clindamycin, penicillin, cephalexin, or dicloxacillin.

**Bibliography**

Stevens DL, Bisno AL, Chambers HF, Dellinger EP, Goldstein EJ, Gorbach SL, et al; Infectious Diseases Society of America. Practice guidelines for the diagnosis and management of skin and soft tissue infections: 2014 update by the Infectious Diseases Society of America. Clin Infect Dis. 2014;59:e10-52. [PMID: 24973422] doi:10.1093/cid/ciu444

**Item 73      Answer:   C**

**Educational Objective:  Treat community-acquired pneumonia caused by *Pseudomonas aeruginosa*.**

The most appropriate empiric treatment regimen for this patient is cefepime and ciprofloxacin. *Pseudomonas aeruginosa* is an uncommon cause of community-acquired pneumonia (CAP), reported in 1% to 8% of patients in various case series. However, it is important to recognize risk factors predisposing patients to this organism because standard treatment regimens for CAP require modification when *Pseudomonas* is suspected. Risk factors for *Pseudomonas* infection include structural lung disease (such as bronchiectasis, COPD, and cystic fibrosis) and frequent COPD exacerbations requiring repeated courses of antibiotics or glucocorticoids. This patient has bronchiectasis, glucocorticoid use, and the presence of gram-negative bacilli on sputum Gram stain as risk factors for *Pseudomonas* infection. Initial treatment with an appropriate antibiotic regimen has been shown to decrease mortality in patients with CAP caused by *Pseudomonas*. For this reason, the use of two agents with antipseudomonal activity is advocated for empiric therapy, with de-escalation when culture and sensitivity results become available. Even in patients with risk factors for *Pseudomonas* infection, it is important to continue treatment with a combination that is also active against *Streptococcus pneumoniae* and *Legionella* species until culture results are available. Recommended regimens include dual therapy with an antipseudomonal, antipneumococcal β-lactam (such as cefepime or piperacillin–tazobactam) or an antipseudomonal carbapenem (such as imipenem or meropenem) and an antipseudomonal quinolone (ciprofloxacin or levofloxacin). The combination of cefepime and ciprofloxacin meets these requirements.

Neither ceftriaxone nor ampicillin-sulbactam is active against *Pseudomonas* and should not be used when this organism is a concern. Although levofloxacin is effective against quinolone-susceptible *Pseudomonas*, administration of a single antipseudomonal agent is not recommended because of the high rates of antibiotic resistance.

The combination of aztreonam and ciprofloxacin provides double coverage against *Pseudomonas*; however, it is inactive against *S. pneumoniae* and therefore is inappropriate for initial empiric therapy.

**KEY POINT**

- In patients with community-acquired pneumonia and risk factors for *Pseudomonas aeruginosa* infection, the use of dual therapy with antipseudomonal, antipneumococcal β-lactam, or an antipseudomonal carbapenem, and antipseudomonal quinolone agents is recommended for initial empiric therapy.

## Bibliography

Cillóniz C, Gabarrús A, Ferrer M, Puig de la Bellacasa J, Rinaudo M, Mensa J, et al. Community-acquired pneumonia due to multidrug- and non-multidrug-resistant Pseudomonas aeruginosa. Chest. 2016;150:415-25. [PMID: 27060725] doi:10.1016/j.chest.2016.03.042

## Item 74     Answer:    C

**Educational Objective:** Diagnose common variable immunodeficiency.

This patient has common variable immunodeficiency (CVID). The history of recurrent sinopulmonary and gastrointestinal infections in a young patient should trigger an investigation for an underlying immunodeficiency. CVID refers to a heterogeneous group of disorders that are linked by the presence of low levels of IgG and IgA and an impaired ability to produce antibody to antigenic stimuli. Clinically, patients with CVID are at increased risk for recurrent respiratory tract infections with encapsulated organisms such as *Streptococcus pneumoniae* and *Haemophilus influenzae* as well as *Mycoplasma pneumoniae*. These patients may also develop chronic diarrhea because of enteroviruses, norovirus, or *Giardia*. Based on this patient's history of previous infection with several of these pathogens, further evaluation with quantitative immunoglobulin levels is warranted. Diagnosis of CVID is important; patients with CVID benefit from replacement therapy with exogenous immune globulin. In addition to recurrent infection, patients with CVID are at increased risk for autoimmune diseases, bronchiectasis, enteropathy, and lymphoma.

Patients with advanced HIV infection or AIDS have low levels of CD4 cells and are at risk for opportunistic infections typically controlled through cellular immunity. Mucocutaneous candidiasis infection is one of the most common manifestations of HIV infection. *Cryptococcus* infection typically manifests as subacute or chronic meningitis. *Pneumocystis jirovecii* pneumonia is a common complication in patients with HIV infection who have not received prophylaxis. *Toxoplasma gondii* can cause encephalitis. Tuberculosis and *Mycobacterium avium* complex infection are the most common mycobacterial infections in patients with AIDS. Cytomegalovirus usually manifests as retinitis, esophagitis or colitis, and polyradiculitis or encephalitis. The nature of this patient's infections and history dating back to childhood make advanced AIDS an unlikely diagnosis.

Chronic granulomatous disease (CGD), which is usually diagnosed in childhood, is caused by a defect in neutrophil oxidation. A history of recurrent or unusually severe infections or infections with *Aspergillus* species, *Staphylococcus aureus*, *Burkholderia cepacia* complex, *Serratia marcescens*, or *Nocardia* species suggests the diagnosis. This patient's frequent episodes of sinusitis, bronchitis, otitis media, and giardiasis are not characteristic of CGD.

Myeloperoxidase is an intraleukocytic enzyme that plays a role in the destruction of fungal organisms. Complete deficiency of myeloperoxidase is rare, and most patients with this syndrome remain asymptomatic. This patient's recurrent episodes of infection since childhood are not compatible with myeloperoxidase deficiency.

**KEY POINT**

- Patients with common variable immunodeficiency are at increased risk of recurrent respiratory tract infections with encapsulated organisms (*Streptococcus pneumoniae*, *Haemophilus influenzae*), and they may develop chronic diarrhea because of enteroviruses, norovirus, or *Giardia*.

## Bibliography

Abbott JK, Gelfand EW. Common variable immunodeficiency: diagnosis, management, and treatment. Immunol Allergy Clin North Am. 2015;35:637-58. [PMID: 26454311] doi:10.1016/j.iac.2015.07.009

## Item 75     Answer:    C

**Educational Objective:** Diagnose *Mycobacterium marinum* skin infection.

The most likely cause of this patient's infection is *Mycobacterium marinum*. *M. marinum* is found worldwide in freshwater and saltwater aquatic environments, including swimming pools. Skin infections have typically been reported after skin trauma and contact with fish tanks ("fish tank granuloma"), fish, or shellfish. Hobbies and occupations predisposing to infection include aquatic sports enthusiasts, fishermen, seafood workers, and owners of fish tanks. The incubation period is usually less than 1 month, and the clinical course is often insidious. Infection usually manifests initially as a violaceous or erythematous papule or nodule that may ulcerate at the site of inoculation. Lesions may be solitary or multiple; occasionally, a sporotrichoid distribution along the lymphatic vessels may develop. The upper extremities, including the hands, fingers, or elbows, are commonly involved. Diagnosis is often delayed and is established by isolation of the organism from culture of a biopsy, aspirate, or drainage specimen. Granulomas may be present and provide evidence of potential mycobacterial infection.

This patient's course of infection is indolent and inconsistent with the more acute presentations of *Streptococcus pyogenes* and *Clostridium perfringens* skin and soft tissue infections. Additionally, Gram stain of the intraoperative specimen would have revealed bacterial organisms, and infections secondary to these organisms would have responded to the antibiotics already administered.

Herpes simplex virus type 1 can cause a painful infection of the finger (herpetic whitlow), manifesting as grouped vesicles on an erythematous base. Infection occurs when the virus is inoculated through breaks in the skin. Even without treatment, these infections usually resolve within several weeks and would not be expected to persist for months in an immunocompetent patient.

KEY POINT

- *Mycobacterium marinum* is found worldwide in freshwater and saltwater aquatic environments, typically causing indolent skin or soft tissue infection and usually appearing as papules on extremities after contact and trauma from fish tanks, fish, or shellfish.

## Bibliography

Aubry A, Chosidow O, Caumes E, Robert J, Cambau E. Sixty-three cases of Mycobacterium marinum infection: clinical features, treatment, and antibiotic susceptibility of causative isolates. Arch Intern Med. 2002;162:1746-52. [PMID: 12153378]

## Item 76    Answer:    C

**Educational Objective:** Discontinue *Pneumocystis* pneumonia prophylaxis in HIV infection.

This patient should discontinue taking trimethoprim-sulfamethoxazole regardless of whether it caused the reported rash the previous week, but she should continue her current antiretroviral regimen. The patient initially presented 6 months ago with *Pneumocystis jirovecii* pneumonia and was diagnosed with HIV and AIDS. Following successful treatment of the pneumonia and initiation of antiretroviral therapy, appropriate secondary prophylaxis was initiated with daily trimethoprim-sulfamethoxazole. She demonstrated an excellent response to antiretrovirals with achievement of undetectable viral load and rising CD4 cell count. Her CD4 cell count has now been higher than 200/µL for more than 3 months, meeting criteria for safe discontinuation of prophylaxis for *Pneumocystis*. Studies have shown that *Pneumocystis* prophylaxis, whether primary or secondary, can be safely discontinued in patients with this level of immune reconstitution.

Atovaquone would be an acceptable alternative to trimethoprim-sulfamethoxazole for prophylaxis of *Pneumocystis*, but this patient no longer requires *Pneumocystis* prophylaxis with any agent.

Primaquine and clindamycin is an appropriate alternative regimen to trimethoprim-sulfamethoxazole for treatment of *Pneumocystis* pneumonia but not for prophylaxis. However, this patient has no evidence of active pneumonia, so treatment is not indicated.

The patient has continued taking her previously prescribed antiretroviral regimen, and the rash resolved, so the rash was unlikely caused by these agents. With the excellent response to this regimen and no apparent adverse effects, the current regimen should be continued rather than switching regimens.

KEY POINT

- Patients with HIV who are taking antiretroviral therapy and achieve CD4 cell counts greater than 200/µL for more than 3 months may safely discontinue prophylaxis for *Pneumocystis jirovecii* infection.

## Bibliography

Panel on Opportunistic Infections in HIV-Infected Adults and Adolescents. Guidelines for the prevention and treatment of opportunistic infections in HIV-infected adults and adolescents: recommendations from the Centers for Disease Control and Prevention, the National Institutes of Health, and the HIV Medicine Association of the Infectious Diseases Society of America. Available at https://aidsinfo.nih.gov/guidelines/html/4/adult-and-adolescent-opportunistic-infection/0. Accessed April 12, 2018.

## Item 77    Answer:    A    H

**Educational Objective:** Treat ventilator-associated pneumonia for 7 days.

The recommended treatment duration for ventilator-associated pneumonia (VAP) is 7 days. VAP is defined as pneumonia developing 48 hours after endotracheal intubation. The most significant VAP risk factor is intubation and mechanical ventilation. Early onset (<5 days after hospitalization or intubation) generally results from antimicrobial-sensitive organisms (*Streptococcus pneumoniae*, *Haemophilus influenzae*, *Staphylococcus aureus*, and antibiotic-susceptible gram-negative bacteria); late onset (≥5 days after hospitalization or intubation) is more likely with multidrug-resistant organisms (MDROs), including *Pseudomonas aeruginosa*, *Klebsiella pneumoniae*, *Acinetobacter* species, *Stenotrophomonas maltophilia*, *Burkholderia cepacia*, and methicillin-resistant *S. aureus*. The recommended therapy duration for VAP is 7 days. A longer antibiotic duration does not improve outcomes, leads to the emergence of antibiotic-resistant organisms, and can increase the risk for adverse effects from antibiotic exposure.

Sputum Gram stain and culture are unnecessary for influencing the timing to stop antibiotics; the implicated organism may remain (colonizing) after treatment has been completed and the patient has improved clinically. Persistence of the infecting organism is not an indication to continue antibiotic therapy.

Antibiotics should not be continued until extubation. The antibiotic therapy duration is the same for patients who are successfully extubated during treatment and patients who remain intubated after 7 days of antibiotic therapy as long as clinical improvement occurs. If the patient does not improve clinically (resolution of fever, decrease in oxygenation and suction requirements) or initially improves and then worsens during treatment, the patient should be evaluated to identify development of infectious complications (pleural effusion, empyema, superinfection, antibiotic resistance) or noninfectious complications.

KEY POINT

- Ventilator-associated pneumonia should be treated with a 7-day course of antibiotics; longer courses contribute to the emergence of antibiotic resistance, increase the risk for antibiotic-related adverse effects, and do not improve outcomes.

## Bibliography

Kalil AC, Metersky ML, Klompas M, Muscedere J, Sweeney DA, Palmer LB, et al. Management of adults with hospital-acquired and ventilator-associated pneumonia: 2016 clinical practice guidelines by the Infectious Diseases Society of America and the American Thoracic Society. Clin Infect Dis. 2016;63:e61–e111. [PMID: 27418577] doi:10.1093/cid/ciw353

## Item 78     Answer:    A

**Educational Objective:** Diagnose anti-*N*-methyl-D-aspartate receptor encephalitis.

The most likely diagnosis is anti-*N*-methyl-D-aspartate receptor (anti-NMDAR) encephalitis. Anti-NMDAR encephalitis has emerged as an increasingly common cause of encephalitis. Anti-NMDAR encephalitis is associated with ovarian teratomas in more than 50% of patients with the disease because of antibody production to a tumor protein that cross-reacts with neuronal tissue. In patients without evidence of teratoma, an inciting antigenic stimulus is rarely identified. The diagnosis is suggested by the presence of choreoathetosis, psychiatric symptoms, seizures, and autonomic instability; detection of anti-NMDAR antibody in serum confirms it. Anti-NMDAR encephalitis should be suspected in young women presenting with encephalitis associated with changes in mood and behavior when initial evaluation for other causes, including herpes simplex virus infection, is negative. Anti-NMDAR encephalitis treatment can include tumor removal (if present), intravenous glucocorticoids, intravenous immune globulin, plasmapheresis, and rituximab.

The most common central nervous system manifestation of Lyme disease is lymphocytic meningitis that may be indistinguishable from viral meningitis with fever, headache, and meningismus. An inflammatory encephalomyelitis may very rarely be observed. Lyme meningitis usually occurs in the summer and fall; it is often associated with peripheral facial palsy and is not associated with altered mental status, psychiatric symptoms, choreoathetosis, or seizure as seen in this patient.

Tuberculous meningitis is a subacute febrile illness with a predilection for inflammatory changes at the base of the brain. After a 2- to 3-week prodromal period, patients often manifest meningismus and varying degrees of cranial nerve and long-tract signs. Tuberculosis is unlikely in this patient because of the lack of chronicity, normal glucose level in cerebrospinal fluid, absence of cranial nerve and long-track signs, and lack of evidence of basilar meningitis on MRI.

West Nile neuroinvasive disease may present with meningitis, encephalitis, or myelitis, either singly or as overlap syndromes in the endemic months between June and October. Limb weakness, which may be symmetric or involve a single extremity, is characteristic. A nonspecific viral exanthema may be found in less than 50% of patients. MRI may show focal lesions of the thalami, basal ganglia, and spinal cord in some patients.

### KEY POINT

- When other causes of encephalitis have been ruled out in a patient presenting with associated changes in mood and behavior, anti-*N*-methyl-D-aspartate receptor encephalitis should be suspected.

**Bibliography**

Dalmau J, Graus F. Antibody-mediated encephalitis. N Engl J Med. 2018;378:840–851. [PMID: 29490181] doi:10.1056/NEJMra1708712

## Item 79     Answer:    D

**Educational Objective:** Diagnose active tuberculosis infection.

The most appropriate management for this patient is to obtain a sputum specimen and perform acid-fast bacilli (AFB) staining and culture. The patient appears to have active pulmonary tuberculosis, based on an indolent course of cough, fever, fatigue, and weight loss and a posteroanterior chest radiograph showing bilateral upper lobe cavitary infiltrates and a left pleural effusion. Although it is essential to initiate antimicrobial therapy promptly, it is important to verify the microbiologic diagnosis of *Mycobacterium tuberculosis* infection first by submitting three sputum specimens for AFB staining and culture. If the AFB stain is positive, nucleic acid amplification testing (NAAT) can be used to differentiate *M. tuberculosis* from other types of mycobacteria, allowing for early initiation of treatment. It is also important to perform susceptibility testing because the frequency of antimicrobial resistance (for isoniazid and rifampin) is increasing.

The tuberculin skin test (TST) and interferon-γ release assay (IGRA) are the initial diagnostic studies used to evaluate for tuberculosis infection. However, neither test can distinguish between latent and active tuberculosis. Latent tuberculosis infection is diagnosed when an asymptomatic patient has a positive TST or IGRA result without clinical evidence of active tuberculosis infection by history, physical examination, or chest imaging. Because this patient has active tuberculosis, treatment for latent tuberculosis with isoniazid plus pyridoxine would not be appropriate. This regimen should only be used in patients with latent tuberculosis.

For active tuberculosis infection, the Centers for Disease Control and Prevention recommends initiating four-drug therapy with isoniazid, rifampin, pyrazinamide, and ethambutol for 8 weeks. In susceptible isolates, isoniazid and rifampin should then be continued for 18 weeks. This treatment regimen is appropriate only after *M. tuberculosis* infection has been confirmed with positive stain and NAAT.

Piperacillin-tazobactam would be an appropriate antibiotic choice if pneumococcus, *Klebsiella pneumoniae*, or *Pseudomonas aeruginosa* were the likely pathogens. However, the presentation of an indolent infection, a positive IGRA, and evidence of fibrocavitary disease in the upper lobes is highly suspicious for pulmonary tuberculosis, not acute bacterial pneumonia.

### KEY POINT

- The microbiologic diagnosis of tuberculosis should be verified by acid-fast bacilli staining of sputum samples and nucleic acid amplification testing before initiating antituberculous therapy.

**Bibliography**

Lewinsohn DM, Leonard MK, LoBue PA, Cohn DL, Daley CL, Desmond E, et al. Official American Thoracic Society/Infectious Diseases Society of America/Centers for Disease Control and Prevention clinical practice guidelines: diagnosis of tuberculosis in adults and children. Clin Infect Dis. 2017;64:111–115. [PMID: 28052967] doi:10.1093/cid/ciw778

## Item 80    Answer:    D

**Educational Objective:** Diagnose nontyphoidal *Salmonella* infection.

The most likely diagnosis is nontyphoidal *Salmonella* infection. This patient's fever and nonbloody diarrhea are most likely caused by nontyphoidal *Salmonella,* with infection resulting from contact with a colonized snake. Nontyphoidal *Salmonella* infection usually results from ingesting fecally contaminated water or food of animal origin, including poultry, beef, eggs, and milk. Intestinally colonized reptiles and amphibians are asymptomatic and intermittently shed the organism in their feces, creating the potential for fecal-oral route transmission. Handling infected snakes, turtles, iguanas, frogs, or toads or anything in the enclosures in which they live can result in infection. Surfaces contaminated by feces may also serve as a source of infection. The incubation period is usually less than 3 days, and symptoms typically include crampy abdominal pain, diarrhea (not usually visibly bloody), fever, headache, nausea, and vomiting.

Infection with *Chlamydia psittaci* is typically acquired by inhaling the organism in feces from a pet bird. The incubation period is about 1 week and the clinical presentation usually consists of chills, dry cough, fever, headache, and myalgia. Diarrhea may be present but is much less common. Chest radiograph abnormalities are common.

*Erysipelothrix rhusiopathiae* is a bacterium that infects animals such as fish, swine, and poultry. Human infection is usually occupationally acquired in butchers, fish handlers, and veterinarians. Localized cutaneous violaceous lesions of the fingers and hands are a classic finding, although more diffuse cutaneous infections, bacteremia, and even infective endocarditis can develop.

*Mycobacterium marinum* is a nontuberculous mycobacterium found worldwide in freshwater and saltwater aquatic environments. Skin infections result from skin trauma and contact with fish tanks ("fish tank granuloma"), fish, or shellfish. Persons predisposed to infection include aquatic sports enthusiasts, fish tank owners, fishermen, and seafood workers. The clinical course is often insidious, manifesting initially as a violaceous or erythematous papule or nodule at the site of inoculation, which may ulcerate. Lesions may be solitary or multiple; occasionally a sporotrichoid distribution along lymphatic vessels may develop. *M. marinum* does not cause diarrhea.

### KEY POINT

- Nontyphoidal *Salmonella* is commonly carried asymptomatically by reptiles and amphibians and transferred from the animals' feces to people; human symptoms include crampy abdominal pain, fever, nonbloody diarrhea, and vomiting.

**Bibliography**

Mermin J, Hutwagner L, Vugia D, Shallow S, Daily P, Bender J, et al; Emerging Infections Program FoodNet Working Group. Reptiles, amphibians, and human Salmonella infection: a population-based, case-control study. Clin Infect Dis. 2004;38 Suppl 3:S253-61. [PMID: 15095197]

## Item 81    Answer:    A    H

**Educational Objective:** Evaluate persistent *Staphylococcus aureus* bacteremia.

An abdominal CT is the most appropriate next step in the evaluation and management of this patient. Bacteremia persisting more than 72 hours after the start of appropriate antimicrobial therapy suggests a complicated infection, requiring additional evaluation with a longer treatment course. Endocarditis and vertebral osteomyelitis are two important complications of *Staphylococcus aureus* bacteremia. Patients with abdominal pain or flank pain should undergo abdominal CT to evaluate for the presence of metastatic infection of the liver, spleen, or kidney; psoas abscess; or other intra-abdominal source. This patient has aortic valve endocarditis, persistent *S. aureus* bacteremia and fever, new right upper quadrant pain, and abnormal liver chemistry tests, which are concerning for development of liver abscess. Metastatic infections are not uncommon with *S. aureus* bacteremia and require a careful history and physical examination to identify where to look and what tests to perform next. New right upper quadrant pain with liver chemistry test abnormalities should prompt investigation with imaging studies such as CT, which can also evaluate the spleen, kidney, and pararenal structures that may be seeded during bacteremia. Transesophageal echocardiography (TEE) will also need to be performed because of this patient's fever and persistent bacteremia. Development of a perivalvular abscess is a possibility, especially if conduction abnormalities are present on the electrocardiogram. Compared with transthoracic echocardiography, perivalvular abscesses are better visualized with TEE.

Several neurologic complications can arise from *S. aureus* endocarditis, including brain abscess, stroke, and meningitis. Neurologic symptoms can be the presenting signs in *S. aureus* endocarditis (for example, a patient presenting with stroke who has a heart murmur and unexplained fever should be evaluated for endocarditis). New neurologic symptoms that develop during the course of treatment for endocarditis should always be evaluated (such as with head CT). This patient has no neurologic symptoms, so a head CT is not indicated.

Daptomycin is rarely used to treat methicillin-sensitive *S. aureus* (MSSA) infections except in patients with multiple antibiotic allergies that preclude the use of β-lactams or glycopeptides. Persistent bacteremia is likely a failure of source control and requires careful investigation for possible sources of metastatic infection and drainage if amenable.

Cefazolin is more rapidly bactericidal than vancomycin and is preferred over vancomycin for treatment of MSSA. Therefore, switching would be inappropriate.

## KEY POINT

- *Staphylococcus aureus* bacteremia persisting more than 72 hours after the start of appropriate antimicrobial therapy suggests a complicated infection requiring additional evaluation; endocarditis, osteomyelitis, and intra-abdominal infections are important sites of metastatic infection.

### Bibliography

Tong SY, Davis JS, Eichenberger E, Holland TL, Fowler VG Jr. Staphylococcus aureus infections: epidemiology, pathophysiology, clinical manifestations, and management. Clin Microbiol Rev. 2015;28:603-61. [PMID: 26016486] doi:10.1128/CMR.00134-14

## Item 82          Answer:     A

**Educational Objective:** Treat necrotizing skin infection caused by *Aeromonas hydrophila.*

The most appropriate treatment for this patient is ciprofloxacin plus doxycycline. This patient has *Aeromonas hydrophila*-associated skin and soft tissue infection. *Aeromonas* species are found in aquatic environments, including fresh water and brackish water, and grow best during warmer months. Lacerations and puncture wounds sustained in these environments can result in wound infection. *Aeromonas* infections of the skin and soft tissue and of the bloodstream are more likely to occur in patients with underlying immunocompromising conditions, such as cirrhosis and cancer, and are more common in men. Necrotizing fasciitis caused by this gram-negative bacillus requires surgery, supportive care, and antibiotics. Pending culture data, empiric therapy for necrotizing skin infections typically consists of broad-spectrum antibiotics such as vancomycin plus piperacillin-tazobactam. When the diagnosis of *A. hydrophila* infection is established, doxycycline plus ciprofloxacin or ceftriaxone is recommended.

The combination of linezolid and metronidazole, although effective against aerobic gram-positive organisms, such as staphylococci and enterococci as well as many anaerobes, is not active against *Aeromonas.*

Nafcillin and rifampin would be active against methicillin-susceptible *S. aureus*, particularly prosthetic joint infections, but is not active against *A. hydrophila.*

Vancomycin plus clindamycin would be effective in necrotizing fasciitis with associated toxic shock caused by methicillin-resistant *S. aureus* but would not be active against *A. hydrophila.*

## KEY POINT

- Lacerations and puncture wounds sustained in fresh and brackish water environments can result in necrotizing infection with *Aeromonas hydrophila*; this infection should be treated with surgery, supportive care, and antibiotics with gram-negative coverage, such as doxycycline plus ciprofloxacin.

### Bibliography

Stevens DL, Bisno AL, Chambers HF, Dellinger EP, Goldstein EJ, Gorbach SL, et al. Practice guidelines for the diagnosis and management of skin and soft tissue infections: 2014 update by the infectious diseases society of America. Clin Infect Dis. 2014;59:147-59. [PMID: 24947530] doi:10.1093/cid/ciu296

## Item 83          Answer:     D

**Educational Objective:** Manage a tick bite.

The most appropriate initial management for this patient is reassurance that the risk of Lyme disease is low. In selected patients at high risk, doxycycline prophylaxis has been shown to decrease the risk of Lyme disease if given within 72 hours of tick removal, assuming that the tick has been attached for greater than 36 hours. Knowledge of the epidemiology of Lyme disease in the area of practice is important for making informed decisions about prophylaxis. Even in endemic regions, such as the northeastern and upper midwestern United States, few vector ticks are infected with *Borrelia burgdorferi.* Most patients in highly endemic areas do not develop symptomatic infection after a tick bite because bacterial transmission rarely occurs unless the vector tick has fed for at least 36 hours. In the subset of patients from highly endemic areas seen within 72 hours of tick removal in whom attachment with an *Ixodes* species tick for greater than 36 hours can be substantiated, a single dose of doxycycline (200 mg) has been shown to decrease the risk of developing infection. This patient was exposed to the tick that transmits Lyme disease. However, given the short duration of attachment, her risk for infection is negligible. Furthermore, she is beyond the 72-hour window during which prophylaxis has been shown to be beneficial. The most appropriate management is reassurance, with the caveat that she return for evaluation if she develops a rash, fever, or other suggestive symptoms within a month of the exposure.

Diagnostic testing with polymerase chain reaction to confirm tick infection is not routinely available and not informative because of the low risk of transmission, even if *B. burgdorferi* is identified in the vector.

Checking *B. burgdorferi* titers similarly has low yield because antibodies may not be present during the early stages of infection, and paired serologic testing with a subsequent convalescent specimen in the absence of symptoms is not cost effective.

## KEY POINT

- In patients at high risk, doxycycline prophylaxis has been shown to decrease the risk of Lyme disease if started within 72 hours of tick removal, assuming that the tick has been attached for at least 36 hours.

### Bibliography

Ogden NH, Lindsay LR, Schofield SW. Methods to prevent tick bites and Lyme disease. Clin Lab Med. 2015;35:883-99. [PMID: 26593263] doi:10.1016/j.cll.2015.07.003

## Item 84    Answer:    D

**Educational Objective:** Evaluate a patient with potential smallpox exposure.

This man has potentially been exposed to variola and requires active vaccinia immunization to prevent the development of smallpox. Ideally, vaccinia vaccination should be administered no more than 7 days (but preferably within 3) after the presumed exposure. In 1980, the World Health Organization declared that smallpox had been eradicated worldwide. However, because of its ease of deliberate airborne spread, highly contagious nature, and expected significant morbidity and mortality, smallpox has been identified as a member of the A list of potential agents of bioterrorism. Because routine childhood vaccinia immunization is no longer required or recommended in the United States, most of the population is not immune. Smallpox vaccines are available in the event of exposure. Although none of these vaccines contains the actual variola virus, when properly administered the vaccines elicit a significant protective immune response. Although serious adverse events are a greater risk after administration of any live virus vaccine, including those containing vaccinia, persons at high risk for complications from replication-component vaccines are also at higher risk for severe smallpox. Unless the patient is severely immunodeficient (within 4 months of bone marrow transplantation, HIV infection with CD4 cell counts <50/μL, or severe combined immunodeficiency), the vaccine should be given. This patient's use of infliximab would not exclude him from vaccination.

The core protein cysteine protease inhibitor tecovirimat, which has proven activity against members of the orthopox genus, has been approved for the treatment of smallpox in the event of a potential outbreak.

Airborne precautions after potential exposure would only be indicated if fever or other signs of active infection occurred.

Vaccinia immune globulin, available from the Centers for Disease Control and Prevention, consists of pooled human antibodies and is indicated for the treatment of severe vaccinia virus vaccine complications or when vaccination is contraindicated.

### KEY POINT

- Vaccinia immunization is appropriate in the event of possible exposure to smallpox (variola).

### Bibliography

Petersen BW, Damon IK, Pertowski CA, Meaney-Delman D, Guarnizo JT, Beigi RH, et al. Clinical guidance for smallpox vaccine use in a postevent vaccination program. MMWR Recomm Rep. 2015;64:1-26. [PMID: 25695372]

## Item 85    Answer:    B

**Educational Objective:** Evaluate a young patient with herpes zoster for HIV infection.

The most appropriate test to perform next is a fourth generation HIV-1/2 antigen/antibody combination immunoassay.

This test combines an immunoassay for HIV antibody with a test for HIV p24 antigen. This improves the ability of the test to detect early HIV infection because p24 antigen becomes detectable a week before antibody in acute infection. Detection of antigen may help diagnose patients as early as 2 weeks after infection. This patient's painful vesicular rash distributed over a thoracic dermatome is classic for infection with varicella-zoster virus. Older adults and immunocompromised patients, including patients with HIV infection, are at increased risk. Severe or recurrent varicella-zoster virus infections or infection at a young age should prompt an evaluation for HIV infection.

Patients with terminal complement component deficiencies usually present with recurrent, invasive infections with encapsulated bacteria such as *Neisseria meningitides*, *Haemophilus influenzae*, and *Streptococcus pneumoniae*. These patients should be screened for complement deficiency by assaying for $CH_{50}$ activity. If $CH_{50}$ activity is normal, alternate pathway function should be assessed with an alternative complement pathway ($AH_{50}$) assay. If results of either assay are abnormal, specific component concentrations should be determined.

Selective IgA deficiency is one of the most common B-cell immunodeficiencies. Inheritance may be autosomal dominant or recessive; most cases are sporadic. Patients with selective IgA deficiency may be asymptomatic or present with recurrent sinopulmonary infections (otitis media, sinusitis, pneumonia) or gastrointestinal infections (giardiasis). Other common manifestations include inflammatory bowel disease; celiac disease; an increased frequency of autoimmune disorders, including rheumatoid arthritis, systemic lupus erythematosus, and chronic active hepatitis; and allergic disorders, including asthma, allergic rhinitis, and food allergies.

Common variable immunodeficiency involves B- and T-cell abnormalities and results in clinically significant immune dysregulation. The primary manifestation is hypogammaglobulinemia, and recurrent respiratory infections are a common presentation in adults. The gastrointestinal tract is frequently involved and causes malabsorption or chronic diarrhea. Infection with *Giardia*, *Campylobacter*, or *Yersinia* species may occur, as may opportunistic infections. Concurrent autoimmune disorders occur in up to 25% of patients. The risk for malignancy is increased, including gastrointestinal cancers and non-Hodgkin lymphoma. Patients also have a poor or an absent response to protein and polysaccharide vaccines. Serum immunoglobulin levels are usually low, circulating B cells may be normal or low, and T-cell function varies. The diagnosis is made by confirming low levels of total IgG and IgA or IgM, as well as by a poor antibody response to vaccines.

### KEY POINT

- Infection with varicella-zoster virus in a young patient should prompt testing for HIV infection.

**Bibliography**

Cohen JI. Clinical practice: Herpes zoster. N Engl J Med. 2013;369:255-63. [PMID: 23863052] doi:10.1056/NEJMcp1302674

**Bibliography**

Kim MO, Geschwind MD. Clinical update of Jakob-Creutzfeldt disease. Curr Opin Neurol. 2015;28:302-10. [PMID: 25923128] doi:10.1097/WCO.0000000000000197

### Item 86        Answer:    B

**Educational Objective:** Diagnose sporadic Creutzfeldt-Jakob disease.

This patient most likely has sporadic Creutzfeldt-Jakob disease (sCJD). This is the most common form of prion disease and has no evidence of environmental risk factors. Involvement of several neurologic systems and a rapid onset of apparent dementia are classic manifestations of prion disease. On physical examination, ataxia, myoclonus, and a rapidly progressive dementia are present. MRI abnormalities are not specific for sCJD and vary with the clinical syndrome. Patients with increased T2 signal in the caudate and putamen are more likely to have early dementia and shorter survival. No simple, noninvasive assay is available to diagnose sCJD; however, the presence of T-tau or 14-3-3 protein in cerebrospinal fluid (CSF) can be suggestive. The definitive diagnostic test is a brain biopsy demonstrating widespread spongiform changes with gliosis. No definitive treatment exists for any prion disease, and most are rapidly fatal.

Cryptococcal meningitis may present initially with altered mentation. Cryptococcal meningitis can be seen in apparently immunocompetent persons; however, it is likely that most patients who develop this infection have some underlying immune deficiency. Lumbar puncture may show a high opening pressure, and the CSF typically shows a lymphocytic pleocytosis. The patient's findings are not compatible with this diagnosis.

Tuberculous meningitis may present with waxing and waning mental status changes. However, the CSF in tuberculous meningitis frequently shows high protein (>500 mg/dL [5000 mg/L]) and low glucose (<40 mg/dL [2.22 mmol/L]) levels. Additionally, MRI may reveal basilar pachymeningitis and occasional tuberculomas, which are not seen in this patient.

Vascular neurocognitive disorder (VND) is the term now used to describe cognitive impairment of any degree resulting from cerebrovascular disease. The diagnosis is made when neuroimaging or clinical history reveals evidence of a stroke or subclinical cerebrovascular disease that is responsible for impairment of at least one cognitive domain. The absence of infarcts on MRI and rapid progression of this patient's symptoms are not compatible with VND.

**KEY POINT**

- Sporadic Creutzfeldt-Jakob disease is the most common form of prion disease, involving several neurologic systems and rapid progression of apparent dementia.

### Item 87        Answer:    C

**Educational Objective:** Choose the appropriate treatment duration for uncomplicated community-acquired pneumonia.

The most appropriate management for this patient at discharge is to discontinue her antibiotics. She had pneumococcal pneumonia requiring hospitalization for treatment and stabilization. Her clinical status rapidly improved with appropriate empiric therapy. The Infectious Diseases Society of America/American Thoracic Society guidelines recommend an antibiotic treatment duration for uncomplicated community-acquired pneumonia of 5 to 7 days. A recent randomized trial found no difference in clinical response between patients treated for 5 days compared with control patients who received a median of 10 days of antibiotic therapy. This study was limited to immunocompetent patients who did not require admission to the ICU and who defervesced at least 48 hours before antibiotic discontinuation; short-course therapy has not been validated in patients with complicated infection, including those at risk for *Staphylococcus aureus* or *Pseudomonas* infection. Short-course therapy offers the advantages of minimizing the risk of adverse effects, lowering cost, and potentially decreasing length of hospital stay. Because this patient completed more than 5 days of therapy during hospitalization, no further antibiotics are indicated at discharge.

Under the same circumstances, azithromycin would be contraindicated because the isolate was resistant to erythromycin, indicating a class effect of macrolide resistance.

Continuing ceftriaxone would necessitate either continued inpatient intravenous treatment or placement of an indwelling intravenous line for outpatient therapy, both unnecessary interventions.

The management of patients who have clinically responded before completing 5 days of inpatient therapy can be challenging, especially if cultures are negative. Antibiotic de-escalation from parenteral to oral formulations is appropriate when patients have clinically improved. If this patient had been ready for discharge before completing 5 days of therapy, transition to oral amoxicillin would have been appropriate for completing the antibiotic course.

Although levofloxacin is active against this patient's infection, it is overly broad therapy for a penicillin-sensitive strain of *Streptococcus pneumoniae*.

**KEY POINT**

- In patients with uncomplicated community-acquired pneumonia not requiring ICU admission, a short course of antibiotic therapy (5-7 days) is sufficient.

## Bibliography

Uranga A, España PP, Bilbao A, Quintana JM, Arriaga I, Intxausti M, et al. Duration of antibiotic treatment in community-acquired pneumonia: a multicenter randomized clinical trial. JAMA Intern Med. 2016;176:1257-65. [PMID: 27455166] doi:10.1001/jamainternmed.2016.3633

## Item 88          Answer:   C

**Educational Objective:** Diagnose osteomyelitis using radiography.

Plain radiography is the appropriate initial diagnostic test for a patient with suspected osteomyelitis. This patient presents with pain and swelling in his finger after a traumatic injury that has healed. The clinical examination is not consistent with a skin and soft tissue infection (lack of erythema); however, inflammatory markers are elevated, so osteomyelitis due to a contiguous spread of organisms introduced by the injury should be considered. Cortical bone loss must be greater than 50% for a plain radiograph to show findings diagnostic of osteomyelitis, so plain radiography is not sufficiently sensitive to exclude this diagnosis. However, plain radiography is much less expensive than the other available imaging modalities and can be quite specific for bone infection if findings are positive, so this test should be done first. The utility of plain radiography in this patient may be higher because a film was taken at the time of the injury, and subtle changes may be apparent when compared.

If the plain radiograph is not diagnostic, a gadolinium-enhanced MRI would be the next imaging test to pursue. A contrast-enhanced CT can be performed if MRI is contraindicated (for example, because of the presence of hardware). A three-phase bone scan could be ordered with a labeled leukocyte scan, but it should only be done if an MRI or a CT with contrast cannot be obtained. Ultrasonography has limited utility in the diagnosis of osteomyelitis.

With the exception of ultrasonography, all these imaging modalities are expensive and, depending on the technique, unnecessarily expose the patient to contrast agents and excessive radiation; the clinician should always consult with the radiologist if the best imaging modality to confirm the suspected diagnosis is in question.

### KEY POINT

- Plain radiography is the most cost-effective diagnostic test that can confirm a suspected case of osteomyelitis, but it is not sufficiently sensitive to exclude the diagnosis.

## Bibliography

Beaman FD, von Herrmann PF, Kransdorf MJ, Adler RS, Amini B, Appel M, et al; Expert Panel on Musculoskeletal Imaging. ACR Appropriateness Criteria® suspected osteomyelitis, septic arthritis, or soft tissue infection (excluding spine and diabetic foot). J Am Coll Radiol. 2017;14:S326-S337. [PMID: 28473089] doi:10.1016/j.jacr.2017.02.008

## Item 89          Answer:   D

**Educational Objective:** Treat aspiration pneumonia.

In addition to starting azithromycin for empiric coverage of atypical organisms, piperacillin-tazobactam is the most appropriate antibiotic treatment for this patient. He requires ICU admission for severe, progressive community-acquired pneumonia (CAP) after outpatient therapy with levofloxacin has failed to improve his infection. Levofloxacin was an appropriate empiric treatment choice for CAP in this patient, considering his history of heavy alcohol use, which increases the risk of infection with Enterobacteriaceae, including *Klebsiella* species. Antibiotic treatment failure can result from poor adherence, a noninfectious cause of symptoms (such as pulmonary embolism), a nonbacterial infection (such as histoplasmosis), lack of source control (as with empyema), or infection with a resistant organism. The patient's history of heavy alcohol use suggests the possibility of aspiration pneumonia, whereby normal oropharyngeal organisms gain access to the lower airways and cause infection. Other risk factors for aspiration pneumonia include poor dentition, gastroesophageal reflux, dysphagia, vomiting, and reduced consciousness, as can be seen in patients with alcoholism, illicit drug use, or seizures. The localization to the right lower lobe is also consistent with aspiration because this area is dependent when patients are lying supine. In community-dwelling patients with aspiration pneumonia, the most common organisms are anaerobic bacteria, such as microaerophilic streptococci, *Fusobacterium*, *Peptostreptococcus*, and *Prevotella* species; however, Enterobacteriaceae may also be present. Therefore, an empiric agent active against anaerobic organisms and gram-negative bacteria is indicated; piperacillin-tazobactam meets these criteria.

Ceftriaxone has adequate coverage against Enterobacteriaceae (as well as other more common flora such as *Streptococcus pneumoniae*) but has limited activity against anaerobic organisms. Therefore, this agent would not be ideal when aspiration pneumonia is a concern.

Clindamycin is active against gram-positive anaerobic organisms but not against gram-negative agents, such as *Fusobacterium* or *Prevotella*. It also lacks activity against other aerobic gram-negative bacilli, such as *Haemophilus influenzae*.

Metronidazole has excellent activity against anaerobic gram-negative rods but limited utility against anaerobic gram-positive cocci and streptococcal species, so it would not be appropriate as empiric therapy for aspiration pneumonia.

### KEY POINT

- In community-dwelling patients with aspiration pneumonia, the most common organisms are anaerobic bacteria, such as microaerophilic streptococci, *Fusobacterium*, *Peptostreptococcus*, and *Prevotella* species as well as Enterobacteriaceae.

## Bibliography

DiBardino DM, Wunderink RG. Aspiration pneumonia: a review of modern trends. J Crit Care. 2015;30:40-8. [PMID: 25129577] doi:10.1016/j.jcrc.2014.07.011

## Item 90 Answer: E

**Educational Objective:** Treat enterohemorrhagic *Escherichia coli* infection with supportive care.

This patient has a diarrheal infection caused by enterohemorrhagic *Escherichia coli* (EHEC) and should receive supportive care and monitoring for the development of complications, such as hemolytic-uremic syndrome (HUS). EHEC strains such as *E. coli* O157:H7 and O104:H4 produce a Shiga-like toxin that can cause hemorrhagic colitis; consequently, EHEC is also referred to as Shiga toxin–producing *E. coli* (STEC). Supportive care typically consists of oral hydrations salts; salty liquids such as chicken soup are also effective. Bismuth subsalicylate compounds can help reduce the number of bowel movements.

*E. coli* infection is typically foodborne, with outbreaks often associated with consumption of a contaminated food source. Beef is commonly responsible when the intestinal contents from an infected animal contaminate the meat during processing. Consumption of fewer than 100 organisms can result in symptoms.

Although EHEC does not invade the mucosa, inflammation is caused by toxin release. The clinical presentation usually consists of abdominal pain, bloody diarrhea, and leukocytosis; fever is often absent or low grade. HUS complicates less than 10% of EHEC infections, manifesting as microangiopathic hemolytic anemia, thrombocytopenia, and kidney injury. It is more commonly seen in children than adults.

Diagnostic testing depends on laboratory protocol. Some laboratories routinely plate all stool samples on media capable of detecting *E. coli* O157:H7; other laboratories restrict testing to only grossly bloody stools or to clinician request. Considering this variability, the laboratory should be notified when STEC is a concern to ensure appropriate testing is performed.

Antibiotics (such as ceftriaxone, ciprofloxacin, and trimethoprim–sulfamethoxazole) and antimotility agents (such as loperamide) are usually not administered to patients with EHEC because they do not provide clinical benefit and their use is associated with an increased risk for HUS.

**KEY POINT**

- Primary enterohemorrhagic *Escherichia coli* infections should receive supportive care; administration of antibiotics or antimotility medications is associated with increased risk for hemolytic uremic syndrome.

### Bibliography

Freedman SB, Xie J, Neufeld MS, Hamilton WL, Hartling L, Tarr PI, et al; Alberta Provincial Pediatric Enteric Infection Team (APPETITE). Shiga toxin-producing Escherichia coli infection, antibiotics, and risk of developing hemolytic uremic syndrome: a meta-analysis. Clin Infect Dis. 2016;62:1251-1258. [PMID: 26917812] doi:10.1093/cid/ciw099

## Item 91 Answer: A

**Educational Objective:** Diagnose cytomegalovirus infection in a solid organ transplant recipient with colitis.

The most likely diagnosis in this patient is cytomegalovirus infection. Approximately 60% to 90% of adults have latent cytomegalovirus infection, with reactivation of disease common in persons who are immunosuppressed (patients with AIDS, transplant recipients, patients taking glucocorticoids). Cytomegalovirus is an important pathogen in kidney transplant recipients, and the risk of cytomegalovirus infection depends on the serologic status of the kidney donor and recipient at the time of transplantation. The highest risk occurs when a seronegative recipient (one who has never had a cytomegalovirus infection) receives a kidney from a seropositive donor. Cytomegalovirus can cause retinitis (especially in persons with AIDS), pneumonitis, hepatitis, bone marrow suppression, colitis with bloody diarrhea, esophagitis, and adrenalitis. This patient recently received a kidney transplant; he has bone marrow suppression (leukopenia and thrombocytopenia), hepatitis (elevated aminotransferase levels), and bloody diarrhea consistent with cytomegalovirus reactivation. Diagnosis relies on isolation of the virus from bodily fluids, such as urine; detection of cytomegalovirus pp65 antigen in leukocytes; cytopathic demonstration of "owl's eye" intracellular inclusions from tissue biopsy (colon in this case) (shown); polymerase chain reaction; and serologic assays. Antiviral treatment is typically indicated in cases of disease reactivation in immunocompromised patients and occasionally in immunocompetent hosts with severe disease. Valganciclovir is the first-line agent and is also used as prophylaxis or pre-emptive therapy in certain transplant patients.

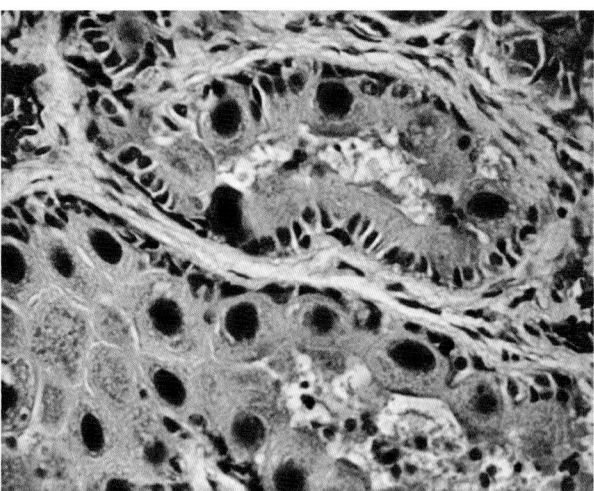

*Entamoeba histolytica* and *Salmonella enteritidis* can cause bloody diarrhea, but neither presents with pancytopenia. Therefore, they are unlikely possibilities in a solid organ transplant recipient. Furthermore, *E. histolytica* would not cause elevated aminotransferase levels in the absence of a liver abscess.

*Strongyloides stercoralis* is the only parasite that has an autoinfection route (ability to complete its life cycle entirely within the human host) resulting in an increasing burden of parasites that can survive for decades in patients. Disseminated strongyloidiasis after solid organ transplantation

CONT.

can present with abdominal pain and diarrhea, but it is usually nonbloody. Furthermore, disseminated *Strongyloides* infection may present with sepsis with colonic bacteria, serpiginous rash, meningitis, or eosinophilic pneumonia. All patients scheduled for solid organ transplantation are now screened with a *Strongyloides* antibody and treated with ivermectin to decrease the incidence of this infection.

**KEY POINT**

- Latent cytomegalovirus infection is present in 60% to 90% of adults, and patients who are immunosuppressed may experience disease reactivation with retinitis, pneumonitis, hepatitis, bone marrow suppression, colitis with bloody diarrhea, esophagitis, or adrenalitis.

**Bibliography**

Angarone M, Ison MG. Diarrhea in solid organ transplant recipients. Curr Opin Infect Dis. 2015;28:308-16. [PMID: 26098506] doi:10.1097/QCO.0000000000000172

## Item 92     Answer:   C

**Educational Objective:** Evaluate surgical site infection.

Gram stain and culture of the drainage from the incision site is the most appropriate test to perform next. Most surgical site infections (SSIs) occur within 30 days of surgery (90 days for surgery involving placement of an implant). The major sources of organisms causing SSIs are from the patient's skin and possibly the alimentary tract or female genital tract, depending on the type of surgery. The organism most often isolated is *Staphylococcus aureus*, followed by coagulase-negative staphylococci, *Escherichia coli*, *Enterococcus faecalis*, and *Pseudomonas aeruginosa*. SSIs are categorized as superficial incisional, deep incisional, and organ/deep organ space infections. A superficial incisional infection involves the underlying soft tissue and presents with inflammatory changes at the incision site (erythema, tenderness), with or without purulent drainage, and few if any systemic signs of infection, such as fever. Such incisions may require reopening to determine the extent of infection, allow complete drainage, and obtain proper specimens for Gram stain and culture to guide antibiotic therapy. Obtaining a culture is important to identify the pathogen involved and obtain antibiotic sensitivity information to determine if antibiotic-resistant organisms are present. Wound drainage fluid, purulent fluid, or infected tissue is the best culture source. Deep tissue or wound cultures are preferable to superficial wound swab cultures, which are more likely to reflect skin or wound colonization and do not necessarily yield the causative pathogen. The most narrow-spectrum oral antibiotic should be used whenever possible.

Deep incisional (involving fascia and/or muscle layers) SSIs usually present with some systemic signs of infection, such as fever and leukocytosis. These infections are managed with debridement and antibiotic therapy guided by results of deep-tissue cultures. Bacteremia may occur with deep or

organ space infections, and blood cultures should be considered in such circumstances but are unnecessary in patients with a superficial site infection such as this one.

CT is useful in cases of organ or deep space (tissue deep to the fascia) SSIs to identify abscesses and plan necessary drainage procedures. Imaging, such as ultrasonography or CT, does not provide additional information needed to manage this type of SSI.

A superficial swab of the incision site is likely to pick up skin flora and make interpreting the culture results difficult.

**KEY POINT**

- A superficial incisional infection involves the underlying soft tissue and presents with inflammatory changes at the incision site (erythema, tenderness), with or without purulent drainage, and few if any systemic signs of infection such as fever; therapy is guided by Gram stain and culture of the wound.

**Bibliography**

Garner BH, Anderson DJ. Surgical site infections: an update. Infect Dis Clin North Am. 2016;30:909-929. [PMID: 27816143] doi:10.1016/j.idc.2016.07.010

## Item 93     Answer:   C

**Educational Objective:** Treat cryptococcal meningitis.

This patient should be treated with liposomal amphotericin B and flucytosine. *Cryptococcus neoformans* is inhaled and causes an initial pulmonary infection. Healthy persons generally contain the initial infection because of intact cell-mediated immunity; however, immunocompromised persons are at risk for dissemination. Risk factors for dissemination include AIDS, organ transplantation, glucocorticoid treatment, diabetes mellitus, liver dysfunction, and kidney injury. The central nervous system is the most common site of disseminated cryptococcosis. The patient most likely has cryptococcal meningitis, as evidenced by the classic triad of headache, fever, and positive cryptococcal antigen titer in the cerebrospinal fluid (CSF). Because the mortality rate may approach 60% in patients without HIV with cryptococcal meningitis, it is imperative that the appropriate antifungal regimen of liposomal amphotericin B and flucytosine be initiated as soon as possible and continued for a minimum of 2 weeks. In addition, although no papilledema or focal neurologic findings are noted, the CSF opening pressure is elevated, and the patient may require serial lumbar punctures.

Fluconazole, an azole antifungal agent, has in vitro and in vivo activity against *C. neoformans*, but it is recommended as de-escalation therapy after the patient has received at least 2 weeks of amphotericin B and flucytosine and is clinically stable. Fluconazole should be continued for at least 2 months after diagnosis, assuming the patient improves and clinical disease manifestations respond to therapy.

Itraconazole, an azole antifungal agent, has some activity in vitro against *C. neoformans*. It is not recommended for primary therapy because of a lack of data. It may be used as an alternative agent and as suppressive therapy or prophylaxis if fluconazole is not available.

Micafungin, an echinocandin antifungal agent, is the drug of choice for candidemia and invasive candidiasis but has no activity against *C. neoformans*.

**KEY POINT**

- Combination therapy with liposomal amphotericin B and flucytosine is the treatment of choice for cryptococcal meningitis.

**Bibliography**

Maziarz EK, Perfect JR. Cryptococcosis. Infect Dis Clin North Am. 2016;30:179-206. [PMID: 26897067] doi:10.1016/j.idc.2015.10.006

## Item 94   Answer:   A

**Educational Objective:**  Diagnose late disseminated Lyme disease.

This patient should have IgG Western blotting to detect antigens to *Borrelia burgdorferi*. She has symptoms of monoarticular arthritis, which has a broad differential diagnosis. Her presentation is most compatible with late disseminated Lyme disease; her previous residence in a Lyme-endemic area and her occupation, with its increased likelihood of tick exposure, increase the probability of this diagnosis. Onset of symptoms of Lyme arthritis typically occurs months, and sometimes years, after the initial infection. Involvement of large joints, particularly the knees, is common. Confirmatory serologic testing using a two-tiered diagnostic approach is required for definitive diagnosis of late disseminated Lyme disease. The initial test is a Lyme enzyme immunoassay antibody titer. This test is very sensitive, and, in a patient suspected of having late disseminated Lyme disease, a negative result essentially excludes the diagnosis. In patients with a positive or equivocal result, as with this patient, a second-tier test is necessary to confirm the diagnosis. Early in the course of infection, both IgM and IgG Western blots are recommended because IgM antibody production predates IgG development. After 4 weeks or more of symptoms, IgG antibody is presumed to be positive, and thus a positive IgM Western blot with a negative IgG likely represents a false-positive result. For this reason, the testing algorithm from the Centers for Disease Control and Prevention specifies that when signs and symptoms are present for more than 30 days, only a confirmatory IgG Western blot should be performed.

The C6 antibody corresponds to a highly conserved protein common to all *Borrelia* strains. Testing using this assay may have a role in diagnosis of infections that occurred outside of the United States. For domestically acquired infections, this test is not currently recommended to replace either component of the conventional two-tier algorithm.

The sensitivity of synovial polymerase chain reaction is low, and this method is not recommended as an initial diagnostic test for Lyme arthritis.

**KEY POINT**

- Confirmatory serologic testing using a two-tiered diagnostic approach that includes enzyme immunoassay and IgG Western blotting (and, early in the course of disease, IgM Western blotting) is required for definitive diagnosis of late disseminated Lyme disease.

**Bibliography**

Arvikar SL, Steere AC. Diagnosis and treatment of Lyme arthritis. Infect Dis Clin North Am. 2015;29:269-80. [PMID: 25999223] doi:10.1016/j.idc.2015.02.004

## Item 95   Answer:   D

**Educational Objective:**  Monitor for ciprofloxacin adverse effects.

This patient should be monitored for tendon or joint pain. Fluoroquinolones (such as ciprofloxacin and delafloxacin) are associated with the development of tendinitis and tendon rupture. Most tendinitis occurrences (90%) involve the Achilles tendon and are more common in men and persons older than 60 years. Tendon rupture occurs in 40% of patients and is more common in women. Additional risk factors include concomitant glucocorticoid treatment and solid organ transplantation. Tendinitis can occur anytime during treatment and up to 6 months after discontinuation of the antibiotic. Patients should be counseled to immediately report tendon pain, swelling, or inflammation and stop taking the fluoroquinolone. Other adverse effects involve the nervous system and include headache, dizziness, insomnia, and alteration in mood. Peripheral neuropathy usually occurs early in therapy; symptoms can last years after fluoroquinolone discontinuation and may be irreversible. Another important adverse effect of fluoroquinolones is the potential for QT prolongation and the development of serious arrhythmias. Fluoroquinolones should be avoided in patients with known QT prolongation, risk factors for torsades de pointes, or concomitant administration of other medications that prolong the QT interval. The FDA advises restricting fluoroquinolone use in uncomplicated infections.

The gastrointestinal effects of fluoroquinolones (anorexia, nausea, vomiting, mild abdominal discomfort) do not include pancreatitis, so monitoring the serum lipase level is unnecessary; regardless, the serum lipase level would not be measured unless the patient had symptoms compatible with acute pancreatitis.

Fluoroquinolones are associated with hypoglycemia and hyperglycemia but not with disturbances in sodium level. Therefore, sodium levels do not require monitoring. Hypoglycemia occurs most often in older adult patients with diabetes mellitus but can occur in patients without diabetes. Hyperglycemia has also been associated with the use of fluoroquinolones. Patients should be monitored closely for signs and symptoms of disordered glucose regulation, but monitoring of glucose levels is not recommended in most patients without diabetes.

CONT.

Stool should be tested for *Clostridium difficile* toxin or with polymerase chain reaction assays to detect the genes responsible for production of toxins only if the patient develops diarrhea.

### KEY POINT

- Fluoroquinolone antibiotics such as ciprofloxacin are associated with the development of tendinitis and tendon rupture, so patients should be counseled to report tendon or joint pain and swelling.

### Bibliography

Lewis T, Cook J. Fluoroquinolones and tendinopathy: a guide for athletes and sports clinicians and a systematic review of the literature. J Athl Train. 2014;49:422-7. [PMID: 24762232] doi:10.4085/1062-6050-49.2.09

## Item 96      Answer:   B

### Educational Objective:  Treat *Candida* esophagitis.

Oral fluconazole is the most appropriate management for this patient's likely esophageal candidiasis; he should be treated presumptively and followed for response. The diagnosis of oropharyngeal candidiasis is usually made clinically; although whitish plaques are often prominent, oral candidiasis may also present as diffuse erythema without plaques. The presence of oral candidiasis and painful swallowing symptoms indicates likely esophageal involvement. The preferred treatment is oral fluconazole regardless if the disease is isolated to the oral cavity or extends into the esophagus; however, esophageal involvement warrants a more prolonged course (14-21 days rather than 7-14 days). Clinical response is usually apparent within a few days.

Because this patient is able to swallow pills, oral therapy is appropriate, and intravenous therapy is unnecessary. Additionally, fluconazole has higher rates for complete resolution without relapse of disease than the echinocandins and is preferred therapy unless resistance is documented, which would not be expected in a patient who has not been taking long-term azole therapy.

Topical agents such as nystatin are less effective than systemic fluconazole for oropharyngeal candidiasis and are especially ineffective for esophageal disease.

If presumptive treatment for candida esophagitis is ineffective in improving symptoms, then upper endoscopy is indicated to better define the cause.

Cytomegalovirus esophagitis is seen in immunocompromised patients and rarely occurs in patients with an intact immune system. Although herpes simplex virus (HSV) esophagitis can be seen in immunocompetent and immunocompromised patients, it is much more likely to be found in an immunocompromised person. These viral infections usually manifest as esophageal ulcerative lesions rather than plaques. Biopsies of the ulcer should be performed to confirm cytomegalovirus and HSV. Treatment of cytomegalovirus with valganciclovir (or HSV with acyclovir) would

not be appropriate without first seeing evidence for it on endoscopy.

### KEY POINT

- The preferred treatment for oropharyngeal candidiasis, including esophageal disease, is oral fluconazole, although esophageal involvement warrants a more prolonged treatment course.

### Bibliography

Panel on Opportunistic Infections in HIV-Infected Adults and Adolescents. Guidelines for the prevention and treatment of opportunistic infections in HIV-infected adults and adolescents: recommendations from the Centers for Disease Control and Prevention, the National Institutes of Health, and the HIV Medicine Association of the Infectious Diseases Society of America. Available at https://aidsinfo.nih.gov/guidelines/html/4/adult-and-adolescent-opportunistic-infection/0. Accessed April 12, 2018.

## Item 97      Answer:   C

### Educational Objective:  Diagnose invasive candidiasis.

This patient has *Candida* pyelonephritis, a form of invasive candidiasis. She has several risk factors for candidiasis, such as recently taking broad-spectrum antibiotics, uncontrolled diabetes mellitus, and a history of recurrent urinary tract infections. These risk factors, in combination with the findings of yeast, leukocytes, and erythrocytes in the urine, is classic for this infection. Although the urine culture only grew 10,000 colony-forming units of *Candida glabrata*, the colony count may not correlate with active infection in *Candida* infections of the urinary tract. Thus, antifungal therapy with an echinocandin should be initiated immediately. After identification of the species, the antifungal agent may be de-escalated to an oral azole if the *Candida* species is susceptible to azoles. The total duration should be 10 to 14 days of antifungal therapy.

Acute diverticulitis may present with the same manifestations this patient had. However, the bilateral flank pain and the lack of abdominal pain make diverticulitis less likely. In addition, the urinalysis results showing leukocytes too numerous to count and the classic CT scan finding of perinephric stranding point to a kidney infection.

Antibiotic-resistant bacterial pyelonephritis is a possibility and could explain her progressive symptoms despite appropriate antibiotic therapy for pyelonephritis. However, this diagnosis is excluded by the patient's urine culture, which showed only *Candida* species.

Patients with acute kidney infarction typically present with acute flank pain or generalized abdominal pain, often associated with nausea and vomiting and, less commonly, with fever; hematuria is present in one third of patients. Over half of kidney infarctions are cardioembolic, and atrial fibrillation is commonly found in patients with this diagnosis. A contrast-enhanced CT scan will show a wedge-shaped perfusion defect. This patient's normal abdominal

Answers and Critiques

CONT.

contrast-enhanced CT scan and urinalysis argue against kidney infarction.

**KEY POINT**

- In patients with invasive candidiasis, antifungal therapy with an echinocandin should be initiated immediately, followed by de-escalation to an oral azole if the identified *Candida* species is susceptible; the total duration of antifungal therapy should be 10 to 14 days.

**Bibliography**

Pappas PG, Kauffman CA, Andes DR, Clancy CJ, Marr KA, Ostrosky-Zeichner L, et al. Executive summary: clinical practice guideline for the management of candidiasis: 2016 update by the Infectious Diseases Society of America. Clin Infect Dis. 2016;62:409-17. [PMID: 26810419] doi:10.1093/cid/civ1194

## Item 98     Answer:    C

**Educational Objective:** Diagnose primary herpes simplex virus genital infection.

The patient's presentation is most consistent with primary genital infection with herpes simplex virus (HSV), and nucleic acid amplification testing (NAAT) for HSV-1 and HSV-2 is the preferred method to confirm the diagnosis. HSV is the most common cause of genital ulcer disease in the United States. The epidemiology of primary genital HSV infections has shifted, and up to half are now caused by HSV-1 rather than HSV-2. However, HSV-1 is less able to establish latency in the genital region, so most recurrent genital infections are caused by HSV-2. NAAT is highly sensitive and specific for HSV. Regardless of type, the initial treatment of primary genital HSV infection is the same (acyclovir, valacyclovir, or famciclovir), but patients with HSV-1 primary genital infection can be counseled that they are less likely to experience recurrent genital ulcers. This patient must also be counseled regarding the natural history of his infection, the need to inform sexual partners of his diagnosis, and the need to avoid sexual contact when ulcers are present. He should be screened for other sexually transmitted infections (STIs), including gonorrhea, chlamydia, syphilis, and HIV, and counseled on the use of condoms to reduce the risk of STI transmission.

Darkfield examination is the appropriate diagnostic test if genital ulcer disease caused by syphilis is suspected. Although syphilitic chancres may appear in multiples and are often accompanied by regional lymphadenopathy, single ulcers are far more common and appear as deeper ulcers with raised regular borders. Syphilitic chancres are generally painless.

Type-specific serologic testing for HSV-1 and HSV-2 should not be used to confirm the diagnosis of genital ulcer disease, especially when ulcers are present. Patients may have evidence of HSV infection on the basis of serologic testing with genital ulcers resulting from another cause.

Direct fluorescence assay testing of the ulcer is not as sensitive as NAAT. Viral culture is a better option if NAAT testing is unavailable.

For all diagnostic tests, sensitivity is improved by obtaining the sample by rotating the swab firmly on the ulcer base after a vesicle is unroofed or from a lesion that has been ulcerated for less than 24 hours.

**KEY POINT**

- Nucleic acid amplification testing is the most appropriate diagnostic choice for confirming genital ulcer disease caused by herpes simplex virus.

**Bibliography**

Gnann JW Jr, Whitley RJ. Clinical practice. Genital herpes. N Engl J Med. 2016;375:666-74. [PMID: 27532832] doi:10.1056/NEJMcp1603178

## Item 99     Answer:    D

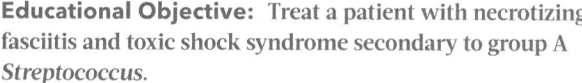

**Educational Objective:** Treat a patient with necrotizing fasciitis and toxic shock syndrome secondary to group A *Streptococcus*.

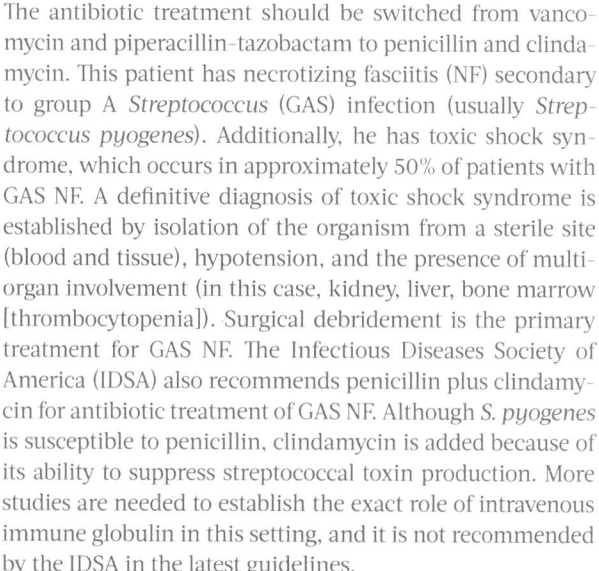

The antibiotic treatment should be switched from vancomycin and piperacillin-tazobactam to penicillin and clindamycin. This patient has necrotizing fasciitis (NF) secondary to group A *Streptococcus* (GAS) infection (usually *Streptococcus pyogenes*). Additionally, he has toxic shock syndrome, which occurs in approximately 50% of patients with GAS NF. A definitive diagnosis of toxic shock syndrome is established by isolation of the organism from a sterile site (blood and tissue), hypotension, and the presence of multiorgan involvement (in this case, kidney, liver, bone marrow [thrombocytopenia]). Surgical debridement is the primary treatment for GAS NF. The Infectious Diseases Society of America (IDSA) also recommends penicillin plus clindamycin for antibiotic treatment of GAS NF. Although *S. pyogenes* is susceptible to penicillin, clindamycin is added because of its ability to suppress streptococcal toxin production. More studies are needed to establish the exact role of intravenous immune globulin in this setting, and it is not recommended by the IDSA in the latest guidelines.

Doxycycline plus a third-generation cephalosporin, such as ceftazidime, ceftriaxone, or cefotaxime, is recommended by the IDSA for treatment of *Vibrio vulnificus*–associated necrotizing skin and soft tissue infections. This combination would not treat GAS NF adequately because it does not include a protein synthesis inhibitor to suppress toxin production.

Empiric therapy for necrotizing skin and soft tissue infections should address the possibility of mixed aerobic and anaerobic organisms, including methicillin-resistant *Staphylococcus aureus*. Vancomycin or linezolid plus imipenem or meropenem, or piperacillin-tazobactam, or metronidazole plus ceftriaxone, is recommended. When culture results are available, however, antibiotic stewardship principles would advocate discontinuing vancomycin and piperacillin-tazobactam and initiating targeted therapy consisting of penicillin and clindamycin against *S. pyogenes*. The combination of linezolid and imipenem would be too broad in its coverage after the culture results reveal GAS.

**KEY POINT**

- In patients with necrotizing fasciitis caused by group A *Streptococcus*, the combination of penicillin and clindamycin is indicated for antimicrobial therapy after surgical debridement.

**Bibliography**

Stevens DL, Bisno AL, Chambers HF, Dellinger EP, Goldstein EJ, Gorbach SL, et al. Practice guidelines for the diagnosis and management of skin and soft tissue infections: 2014 update by the infectious diseases society of America. Clin Infect Dis. 2014;59:147-59. [PMID: 24947530] doi:10.1093/cid/ciu296

## Item 100    Answer:    E

**Educational Objective:** Manage asymptomatic bacteriuria.

No treatment or further investigation is indicated in this asymptomatic older woman who has bacteriuria discovered on a routine dipstick urinalysis. Although commonly performed, analysis of the urine is not warranted, except when evaluating a patient who presents with clear signs or symptoms of a urinary tract infection (UTI), and may lead to unnecessary administration of antibiotics. Incontinence without urgency or dysuria is not unexpected in many older women. The prevalence of asymptomatic bacteriuria (ASB) is as low as 1% to 5% in healthy premenopausal women (2%-10% in pregnant women) and up to 100% in patients with long-term indwelling urinary catheters. However, most ASB occurs in older adult women and men, with a respective prevalence of 11% to 16% and 4% to 19% in the community, increasing to 25% to 50% and 15% to 40% in long-term care facilities. Except in specific patient groups, well-designed studies have proven that although persons with bacteriuria are at increased risk for symptomatic UTIs, ASB treatment does not decrease the frequency of symptomatic infections or improve other outcomes. ASB is associated with a higher prevalence of potentially dangerous antibiotic-resistant strains in women who progress to an active UTI. Except in pregnant women, who have a known increased prevalence of ASB, which has been demonstrated to lead to serious complications, routine screening for infection in women without symptoms is unwarranted. Screening and treatment are also indicated before invasive urologic procedures. The presence of pyuria accompanying ASB is not an indication for antimicrobial treatment.

This patient does not require treatment for her asymptomatic bacteriuria; additionally, fluoroquinolone antibiotics are no longer recommended for the treatment of symptomatic lower UTIs because of the significant rise in *Escherichia coli* isolates resistant to this class of agents.

Cystoscopy is recommended in the evaluation of microscopic hematuria for all patients older than 35 years or those with risk factors for urologic malignancy. Cystoscopy would possibly be warranted in patients with recurring symptomatic UTIs but is not indicated in this patient.

Culture and sensitivity testing as well as microscopic urinalysis are not necessary in women presenting with classic lower UTI symptoms, including frequency, urgency, and dysuria, without manifestations of systemic or upper tract disease. Urinalysis and urine culture are not indicated as part of routine health surveillance in asymptomatic patients and should not be performed. They are not necessary in this patient with asymptomatic bacteriuria.

**KEY POINT**

- No treatment is indicated for asymptomatic bacteriuria in otherwise healthy, nonpregnant patients.

**Bibliography**

Nicolle LE. Urinary tract infections in the older adult. Clin Geriatr Med. 2016;32:523-38. [PMID: 27394021] doi:10.1016/j.cger.2016.03.002

## Item 101    Answer:    C

**Educational Objective:** Diagnose Mediterranean spotted fever.

This patient most likely has Mediterranean spotted fever caused by *Rickettsia conorii*. Most rickettsial infections are transmitted by arthropod vectors. Outdoor activities, especially during the spring and summer months, present the greatest opportunity for infection. Mediterranean spotted fever is one of the most severe forms of the spotted fever group of rickettsial diseases likely to be contracted during international travel. Signs and symptoms of illness usually begin following an incubation period of 2 to 14 days after a tick bite, which frequently goes unnoticed. The risk of infection is greatest in northern and southern Europe but also occurs in Africa, India, and the Middle East. Characteristically, fever, myalgia, and headache mark the onset of infection followed shortly by the appearance of a maculopapular and oftentimes petechial rash, generally beginning on the ankles and wrists and typically involving the palms and soles. A distinct eschar (shown) is classically present

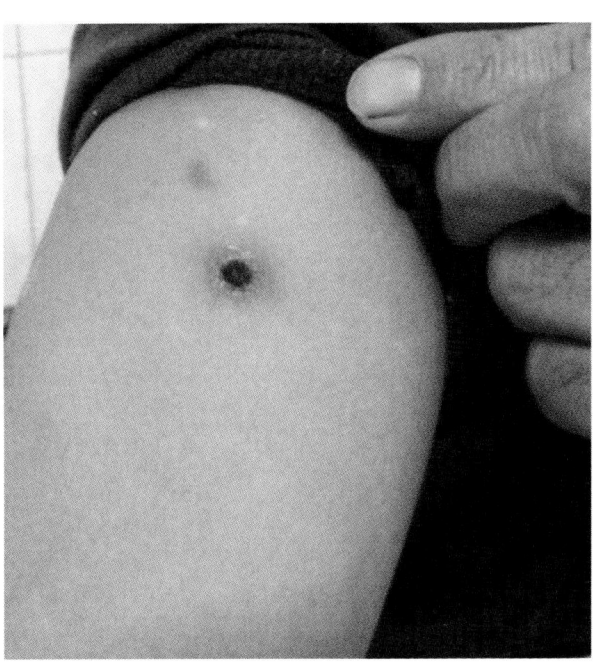

at the site of inoculation along with the development of localized regional lymphadenopathy. Disease is usually mild to moderate; however, vascular dissemination can lead to severe complications, of which neurologic manifestations are the most common. Laboratory findings are nonspecific, but diagnosis may be aided by polymerase chain reaction and serologic assays. A 7- to 10-day course of doxycycline is the treatment of choice.

*Anaplasma phagocytophilum*, the causative agent of human granulocytic anaplasmosis, can be found worldwide and is transmitted by various *Ixodes* tick species. However, rash is a very uncommon clinical manifestation (<10%).

Lyme disease in Europe mainly results from infection with *Borrelia garinii* or *Borrelia afzelii*, transmitted by *Ixodes ricinus* ticks. In nearly 75% of infected persons, it presents with an erythema migrans rash at the site of inoculation.

Rocky Mountain spotted fever, caused by *R. rickettsii*, is the most common rickettsial infection but is geographically restricted to certain areas of the United States, Central and South America, Mexico, and Canada. Eschar formation at the site of tick attachment is rare.

### KEY POINT

- Mediterranean spotted fever characteristically presents with fever, myalgia, and headache followed shortly by the appearance of a maculopapular and oftentimes petechial rash; a distinct black eschar is also classically present at the site of inoculation.

### Bibliography

Parola P, Paddock CD, Socolovschi C, Labruna MB, Mediannikov O, Kernif T, et al. Update on tick-borne rickettsioses around the world: a geographic approach. Clin Microbiol Rev. 2013;26:657-702. [PMID: 24092850] doi:10.1128/CMR.00032-13

## Item 102     Answer:   A

**Educational Objective:** Diagnose Lyme meningitis.

Lyme disease, caused by infection with *Borrelia burgdorferi*, is the most common vector-borne infection in the United States. The first stage involves localized symptoms occurring 1 to 4 weeks after infection. This early stage is usually characterized by erythema migrans present in 60% to 80% of localized infections. Untreated patients may progress to early disseminated infection, typically presenting as a febrile illness associated with erythema migrans at multiple sites distant from the initial tick attachment. Focal cardiac or neurologic symptoms may also occur in early disseminated disease, typically 2 to 10 weeks after the development of the erythema migrans rash. The most common neurologic manifestation of early disseminated Lyme disease is facial nerve palsy, which may be unilateral or bilateral. Because the cerebrospinal fluid (CSF) findings closely resemble those of other viral infections (enterovirus, herpes simplex virus, varicella-zoster virus, West Nile virus), the "rule of 7s" was derived and validated to accurately classify a patient at low

risk for having Lyme disease (headache duration <7 days, <70% mononuclear cells, and absence of a seventh facial nerve palsy). Nantucket Island is a highly endemic area for Lyme disease; the patient's history of camping 2 months before meningitis onset is consistent with the diagnosis of *Borrelia burgdorferi* infection. The treatment is intravenous ceftriaxone.

Aseptic meningitis caused by herpes simplex virus type 2, West Nile virus, or enterovirus would include a normal neurologic examination. The presence of right-sided facial palsy in this patient makes these unlikely causes.

Varicella-zoster virus can also present with a facial palsy, but this condition usually occurs as part of the Ramsay-Hunt syndrome (with vesicular rash of the external ear). Ramsay-Hunt syndrome is usually seen in young immunosuppressed persons (those with AIDS) or in older adults.

The normal mental status excludes West Nile virus encephalitis as does the presence of facial palsy.

### KEY POINT

- For patients presenting with aseptic meningitis and cerebrospinal fluid findings typical for viral infection, the "rule of 7s" can classify a patient at low risk for having Lyme disease (headache duration <7 days, <70% mononuclear cells, and absence of a seventh facial nerve palsy).

### Bibliography

Shapiro ED. Clinical practice. Lyme disease. N Engl J Med. 2014;370:1724-31. [PMID: 24785207] doi:10.1056/NEJMcp1314325

## Item 103     Answer:   B

**Educational Objective:** Diagnose Epstein-Barr virus infection in a kidney transplant recipient.

This patient's symptoms are most likely caused by infection with Epstein-Barr virus (EBV). He most likely has post-transplant lymphoproliferative disorder (PTLD). His clinical presentation of fever, pancytopenia, generalized lymphadenopathy, and hepatosplenomegaly is consistent with this diagnosis, considering his kidney transplantation and immunosuppressive therapy. PTLD risk is higher in patients with a history of pre-existing EBV infection treated with lymphocyte-depleting agents and in those receiving sirolimus and tacrolimus compared with those receiving mycophenolate and cyclosporine. PTLD can range from a benign monoclonal gammopathy to a malignant lymphoma. PTLD should be considered in any patient presenting with fever and lymphadenopathy or an extranodal mass; treatment includes reduction of immunosuppression and rituximab or other chemotherapy.

Although numerous viral infections can complicate transplantation, cytomegalovirus is the most significant. The risk for reactivation is related to serologic status of the donor and recipient and is most likely in seronegative recipients from a seropositive donor; it is unlikely when donor and recipient are both negative. Like EBV, cytomegalovirus can

CONT.

reactivate and cause pancytopenia, hepatitis, pneumonitis, esophagitis, colitis, or adrenalitis in solid-organ transplant recipients. Cytomegalovirus reactivation is also associated with organ rejection, secondary infection, and an increased risk for graft loss and death. However, cytomegalovirus does not cause generalized lymphadenopathy or hepatosplenomegaly. Cytomegalovirus-seropositive transplant recipients or cytomegalovirus-negative recipients with positive donors should receive prophylactic valganciclovir or undergo routine monitoring for cytomegalovirus viremia.

Herpes simplex virus can also reactivate in the setting of immunosuppressive therapy, but it would be more likely to present with oral or genital ulcers.

Polyoma BK virus reactivation occurs in approximately 5% of kidney transplant recipients and can cause kidney allograft dysfunction or loss. It can present with a gradual, asymptomatic increase in the serum creatinine level with tubulointerstitial nephritis or, less commonly, with ureteral stenosis. Patients may have polyoma BK virus on polymerase chain reaction of the urine or serum or may have polyoma BK virus inclusion-bearing epithelial cells called "decoy cells." The treatment is to reduce immunosuppression. This patient's stable serum creatinine level argues against this diagnosis.

**KEY POINT**

- Posttransplant lymphoproliferative disorder caused by Epstein-Barr virus can present several years after transplantation with fever, pancytopenia, generalized lymphadenopathy, and hepatosplenomegaly.

**Bibliography**

Petrara MR, Giunco S, Serraino D, Dolcetti R, De Rossi A. Post-transplant lymphoproliferative disorders: from epidemiology to pathogenesis-driven treatment. Cancer Lett. 2015;369:37-44. [PMID: 26279520] doi:10.1016/j.canlet.2015.08.007

## Item 104    Answer:    C

**Educational Objective:** Treat a patient with a moderate-severity purulent skin infection who is allergic to trimethoprim-sulfamethoxazole.

Empiric therapy with oral doxycycline is the most appropriate treatment for this patient after incision and drainage. Treatment of skin and soft tissue infections is guided by categorizing the infection as purulent or nonpurulent and by grading the severity of the infection as mild, moderate, or severe. The patient has a purulent skin infection (furuncle) of moderate severity (systemic signs of infection present, including fever and tachycardia). These infections are typically caused by methicillin-resistant *Staphylococcus aureus* (MRSA). Recommended treatment is incision and drainage and outpatient treatment with an oral agent active against MRSA. Oral trimethoprim-sulfamethoxazole or doxycycline is recommended by the Infectious Diseases Society of America (IDSA) for moderate-severity purulent skin infections; however, the patient has a known allergy to trimethoprim-sulfamethoxazole, eliminating it as an option.

Culture of the purulent material will allow for identification of the microbial agent and a reassessment of pathogen-directed therapy.

Mild (no evidence of systemic signs of infection), non-purulent skin infections are typically caused by streptococci, and empiric outpatient treatment with an oral agent such as clindamycin, penicillin, cephalexin, or dicloxacillin would be appropriate according to recommendations from the IDSA.

Incision and drainage alone with clinical follow-up is recommended by the IDSA for patients with mild purulent infections. However, in a 2017 randomized clinical trial of patients with skin abscess measuring 5 cm or less who underwent incision and drainage, higher cure rates were observed among those who received antibiotic therapy than those who received placebo. Because this patient has systemic signs of infection, he would be considered to have at least a moderate purulent skin and soft tissue infection and would, therefore, require antibiotics in addition to incision and drainage.

**KEY POINT**

- Purulent skin infections with systemic signs of infection should be managed with incision and drainage followed by empiric oral therapy with trimethoprim-sulfamethoxazole or doxycycline.

**Bibliography**

Stevens DL, Bisno AL, Chambers HF, Dellinger EP, Goldstein EJ, Gorbach SL, et al. Practice guidelines for the diagnosis and management of skin and soft tissue infections: 2014 update by the Infectious Diseases Society of America. Clin Infect Dis. 2014;59:147-59. [PMID: 24947530] doi:10.1093/cid/ciu296

## Item 105    Answer:    E

**Educational Objective:** Evaluate the results of a tuberculin skin test.

This patient has a negative tuberculin skin test (TST), so no treatment or further management is recommended. The criteria for a positive reaction have been established by the Centers for Disease Control and Prevention (CDC) based on the patient's risks for tuberculosis. A TST reaction of 5 mm or greater should be considered positive in persons at high risk, including patients with HIV, patients with recent known contact with a person with active tuberculosis, persons with chronic fibrotic changes on chest radiography consistent with old tuberculosis, patients who have undergone solid organ transplantation, and other persons who are immunosuppressed (patients taking prednisone >15 mg/d or a tumor necrosis factor-α antagonist). A TST reaction of 10 mm or greater should be considered positive in recent (<5 years) arrivals from high-prevalence countries, injection drug users, residents or employees of high-risk congregate settings (prisons and jails, nursing homes, and other long-term facilities for older adults), hospitals and other health care facilities (which would include this patient), homeless shelters, mycobacteriology laboratory personnel, persons with clinical conditions that put them at high risk for active disease, and children younger than 4 years or those exposed to adults in high-risk categories. In patients with no risk factors for tuberculosis, 15 mm or greater should be considered a positive result.

Because latent and active tuberculosis were ruled out in this patient, a chest radiograph is unnecessary.

Sputum induction for culture is not indicated in the absence of clinical signs or symptoms of active infection and without testing results indicating tuberculosis infection.

Because the patient did not have evidence of latent tuberculosis, isoniazid treatment is not indicated. Isoniazid should not be initiated empirically without evidence of infection.

Because the TST is considered negative and the chest radiograph is normal, latent and active tuberculosis have been ruled out in this patient, and she does not need to be removed from her work area.

### KEY POINT

- The criteria for a positive tuberculin skin test reaction have been established by the Centers for Disease Control and Prevention based on the patient's risks for tuberculosis; in patients with no risk factors for tuberculosis, 15 mm or greater should be considered a positive result.

### Bibliography

Lewinsohn DM, Leonard MK, LoBue PA, Cohn DL, Daley CL, Desmond E, et al. Official American Thoracic Society/Infectious Diseases Society of America/Centers for Disease Control and Prevention clinical practice guidelines: diagnosis of tuberculosis in adults and children. Clin Infect Dis. 2017;64:111-115. [PMID: 28052967] doi:10.1093/cid/ciw778

## Item 106      Answer:    A

**Educational Objective:** Treat latent tuberculosis infection in a patient who is HIV positive.

The most appropriate management for this patient is daily isoniazid plus pyridoxine. He has HIV, and a tuberculin skin test (TST) produces a 5-mm induration, which is considered positive in patients who are immunocompromised. Because the chest radiograph was negative, he should be treated as having latent tuberculosis infection (LTBI) with 9 months of isoniazid therapy. Pyridoxine is added to LTBI treatment in patients at risk for peripheral neuropathy (such as patients with HIV, diabetes, uremia, alcoholism, malnutrition, and pregnancy). It cannot be determined if the patient's tuberculosis infection is newly acquired or long standing because the previous negative TST was performed when his CD4 cell count was extremely low.

Because this patient has no evidence of active infection, four-drug antituberculous therapy is not necessary.

Routine use of a TST and interferon-γ release assay (IGRA) is not recommended. In certain circumstances, however, using a second test when the result of the initial test is negative might be helpful when the risk of infection or progression is increased or risk for poor outcome exists, such

as in children younger than 5 years who have been exposed to a patient with active tuberculosis or in patients with HIV infection. Use of a second test for diagnosing infection when the result of the first test is negative can also be considered when the suspicion of tuberculosis is strong based on clinical presentation or radiographic imaging. Conversely, using both tests when the result of the initial test is positive might be helpful when a suspected false-positive result is obtained in a person at low risk for infection and progression to active disease. This patient is at high risk for tuberculosis and has a positive TST; therefore, additional testing with IGRA is not necessary.

Repeating the TST would not provide additional information. The Centers for Disease Control and Prevention recommends initiating antituberculous prophylaxis in patients who are HIV positive who have a TST induration of 5 mm or greater.

### KEY POINT

- A 5-mm induration on tuberculin skin testing is considered positive in persons who are immunocompromised, including those with HIV; if no other signs of tuberculosis infection are present, treatment for latent tuberculosis infection should be initiated with isoniazid.

### Bibliography

Lewinsohn DM, Leonard MK, LoBue PA, Cohn DL, Daley CL, Desmond E, et al. Official American Thoracic Society/Infectious Diseases Society of America/Centers for Disease Control and Prevention clinical practice guidelines: diagnosis of tuberculosis in adults and children. Clin Infect Dis. 2017;64:111-115. [PMID: 28052967] doi:10.1093/cid/ciw778

## Item 107      Answer:    E

**Educational Objective:** Treat recurrent cystitis in women.

The most appropriate management of this patient is urine culture plus ciprofloxacin. This young woman has a classic presentation and typical dipstick urinalysis findings of a lower urinary tract infection (UTI). Urine cultures are not generally necessary to confirm the diagnosis; however, culture and susceptibility testing are indicated when infection is recurrent. Recurrent UTI is defined as three episodes of UTI in the preceding 12 months or two episodes in the preceding 6 months. Recurrent UTI is common in women. A recurrent UTI may be a relapse or reinfection. Relapse is defined as an infection caused by the same strain (by repeat culture) as the initial UTI and occurs within 2 weeks of completing initial therapy. Reinfection is diagnosed if the UTI is caused by a different strain than that causing the initial infection or if a sterile urine culture was documented between episodes. Most recurrences are reinfections. While awaiting results, she should begin empiric treatment with ciprofloxacin twice daily for 7 days. Although fluoroquinolone antibiotics are no longer recommended as first-line agents for the treatment of cystitis because of increasing concerns for potential adverse effects and uropathogen antimicro-

CONT.

bial resistance development, ciprofloxacin and levofloxacin are the preferred antimicrobial agents when trimethoprim-sulfamethoxazole local resistance rates are high (>20%) or the patient has been treated with an antibiotic for a UTI within the previous 3 months. Having recently received antibiotics defines this patient's UTI as complicated, warranting 7 to 10 days of treatment with a fluoroquinolone antibiotic.

Nitrofurantoin, trimethoprim-sulfamethoxazole, fosfomycin, and oral β-lactams are not recommended as first-line empiric oral therapy in complicated cystitis because of concerns regarding resistance to these agents. In the case of culture-proven sensitivity, these agents can be used in the treatment of complicated UTI.

Ampicillin and amoxicillin are no longer acceptable UTI treatment options because more than one third of community-acquired *Escherichia coli* harbor resistance to this agent.

**KEY POINT**

- Ciprofloxacin and levofloxacin are the preferred antimicrobial agents for the treatment of recurrent cystis when trimethoprim-sulfamethoxazole local resistance rates are high or the patient has been treated with an antibiotic for a urinary tract infection within the previous 3 months.

**Bibliography**
Gupta K, Hooton TM, Naber KG, Wullt B, Colgan R, Miller LG, et al; Infectious Diseases Society of America. International clinical practice guidelines for the treatment of acute uncomplicated cystitis and pyelonephritis in women: A 2010 update by the Infectious Diseases Society of America and the European Society for Microbiology and Infectious Diseases. Clin Infect Dis. 2011;52:e103-20. [PMID: 21292654] doi:10.1093/cid/ciq257

**Item 108      Answer:   D**

**Educational Objective:** Diagnose rhinocerebral mucormycosis.

This patient has mucormycosis (rhinocerebral form), which has a mortality rate of 60% to 80%. Various organisms are responsible for causing mucormycosis, with *Rhizopus* and *Mucor* species being the most common. Patients with uncontrolled diabetes or ketoacidosis have a unique susceptibility. Other risk factors include immunocompromise from hematologic malignancies, organ transplantation, and cancer chemotherapy. The most common presentation is rhinocerebral. This is a rapidly fatal infection that spreads from the sinuses retro-orbitally to the central nervous system. Symptoms and signs include headache, epistaxis, and ocular findings, including proptosis, periorbital edema, and

decreased vision. A pathognomonic finding on physical examination is the presence of a black eschar on the nose or palate. Mucormycosis is diagnosed by tissue biopsy and culture. The most important step in managing any form of mucormycosis is early, extensive, and repeated debridement of infected and necrotic tissue. The drug of choice is high-dose liposomal amphotericin B.

Cutaneous anthrax is the most common type of anthrax in the United States and results after causative microorganisms are introduced into a skin abrasion or open wound. Cutaneous lesions are initially pruritic and painless and subsequently progress to vesicular lesions surrounded by nonpitting edema. The lesions then become hemorrhagic or necrotic, and satellite lesions may form. Finally, a central black eschar can develop and usually resolves over 6 weeks. Anthrax does not cause rhinocerebral infection.

Rhinocerebral aspergillosis has a similar presentation to mucormycosis. A helpful clue to the correct diagnosis is the propensity of rhinocerebral aspergillosis to occur in patients with neutropenia, typically secondary to hematologic malignancy. In contrast, mucormycosis occurs most commonly in those with diabetes mellitus, especially with ketoacidosis, and typically is distinguished by the presence of the characteristic eschar. A biopsy is necessary to establish the correct diagnosis, which is important because treatment of the two conditions is different.

Lemierre syndrome (jugular vein suppurative thrombophlebitis) is a rare complication of acute pharyngitis that involves septic thrombosis of the internal jugular vein and bacteremia, typically involving *Fusobacterium necrophorum*. Lemierre syndrome should be considered in patients with antecedent pharyngitis and persistent fever despite antibiotic treatment. Soft-tissue CT of the neck with contrast typically shows a jugular vein thrombus with surrounding tissue enhancement. This disorder is not associated with necrotic involvement of the nose and sinuses.

**KEY POINT**

- Rhinocerebral mucormycosis is a rapidly fatal infection that spreads from the sinuses retro-orbitally to the central nervous system in immunocompromised patients, especially those with uncontrolled diabetes or ketoacidosis; a pathognomonic finding on physical examination of the nose or palate is the presence of a black eschar.

**Bibliography**
Farmakiotis D, Kontoyiannis DP. Mucormycoses. Infect Dis Clin North Am. 2016;30:143-63. [PMID: 26897065] doi:10.1016/j.idc.2015.10.011

# Index

Erythema multiforme, 94
Erythromycin, for STIs, 43t
*Escherichia coli*
bacterial prostatitis, 30
diarrhea related to, 67t, 69, 69t, Q90
epididymitis and, 45
traveler's diarrhea and, 59t, 61
UTIs and, 27
Ethambutol
for tuberculosis, 34, 35t, Q2
Ethionamide, for tuberculosis, 35t
Etravirine, for HIV infection, 92t

**F**
Facial palsy, Lyme disease and, 22
Famciclovir
for genital infections, 46t
for human herpesvirus infections, 94
Fatal familial insomnia, 8t
Fecal microbiota transplantation, 71
Fever of unknown origin (FUO), 52–53, 52t, Q5
Fidaxomicin, for *C. difficile* infection, 70, 71
Fluconazole
for *Candida* infections, 38
for coccidioidomycosis, 41
Flucytosine, for cryptococcosis, 40
Fluoroquinolones
adverse effects of, 99t, Q95
for anthrax exposure, 55
in bite wounds, 12
for diarrhea, 66
for osteomyelitis, 50
for *Salmonella* infection, 68
for travelers' diarrhea, 63
for typhoid fever, 60
for UTIs, 28
Fosamprenavir, for HIV infection, 92t
Foscarnet, for CMV, 97
Fosfomycin, 100
for UTIs, 28
Fungal infections, 37–42
Fungal meningitis, 4
Furuncles (boils), 10t, 11
*Fusobacterium*, in bite wound infections, 11–12

**G**
Ganciclovir, for CMV, 96, Q69
Gastroenteritis, viral, 71
Gastrointestinal infections
health care-associated, 76–77
syndromes, 66–73
Gemifloxacin, for *N. gonorrhoeae* infection, 44
Genital ulcers, 46–48, 46f, 47f, 48t
Genital warts, 48–49, 49f
Gentamicin
for brucellosis, 66
for *N. gonorrhoeae* infection, 44
for plague, 56t
for tularemia, 56t
*Giardia* spp.
diarrhea, clinical clues, 59t
*G. lamblia*, 71–72, Q15
infectious diarrhea and, 67t
Graft-versus-host disease (GVHD), 74

**H**
*Haemophilus* spp.
*H. ducreyi*, 48t
*H. influenzae*
community-acquired pneumonia and, 15t
detection of, 2
vaccines, 2
Health care-associated infections (HCAIs)
central line-associated bloodstream infections (CLABSIs), 81–82, 82t
epidemiology of, 76–77
prevention of, 77–78
*S. aureus* bacteremia, 82–83
surgical site infections, 80–81
transmission-based precautions, 78t
Health care-associated meningitis and ventriculitis, 4, Q23
Helminths, parasitic meningitis related to, 4

Hematopoietic stem cell transplantation (HSCT), 73
allogeneic, 75f
opportunistic infections after, 75f, Q57, Q69
Hemorrhagic fever viruses, 59t
Hepatitis viruses, 65
immunizations, 58t, 77t, Q44
infection in HIV, 89
in human bites, 12
Herpes lymphotropic virus (HHV-6), 95t
manifestations, 95t
Herpes simplex virus (HSV), 6, 94–95, 95t, Q31
anorectal infections and, 45
genital infections, 46–47, 46f, 46t, Q98
meningitis and, 1, Q31
Herpes zoster, 95–96, Q85
Herpesviruses, meningitis and, 1
Histoplasmosis, 41, Q25
clinical clues, 59t
diagnosis, 41
HIV/AIDS, 84–93
chronic infection and, 87, Q47
description of, 83
epidemiology, 85–86
opportunistic infections in, 88t, 90–91, Q76
prevention of, 85–86
HIV infection
acute infection, 86, 86t, Q55
brain abscesses in, 5t
complications of, 89–91, Q76
human bites and, 12
immunization recommendations in, 87, Q32
laboratory testing, 88f, 88t
management of, 87–89, 91–93, Q30
evaluation algorithm, 86f
in pregnancy, 93, Q43
postexposure prophylaxis antiretroviral therapy, 85
pre-exposure prophylaxis (PrEP), 85–86, 86f, Q13, Q35
screening and diagnosis, 87, Q38, Q85
transmission, 85, 85t
tuberculosis and, 34, Q2, Q106
Human bites, 12
Human granulocytic anaplasmosis (HGA), 25, 26f, 26t
Human herpesvirus 6 (HHV-6), 95t
encephalitis and, 6
meningitis and, 1
Human monocytic ehrlichiosis (HME), 25, 26t, Q22
Human papillomavirus (HPV)
genital warts and, 48, 49f
immunizations, 77t
Hydrochloroquine, for non-*falciparum* malaria, 62t

**I**
Imipenem
for acute pyelonephritis, 29
for animal bites, 12
Imiquimod, for genital warts, 49
Immune reconstitution inflammatory syndrome (IRIS), 34, 89–90, Q2
Immunizations
in HIV infection, 87
in transplant recipients, 77t
for travel, 58t
Immunocompromised patients
brain abscesses in, 5t
skin and soft tissue infections, 8–10, Q49
tuberculosis in, 31
Immunosuppression
surgical site infection risk and, 80t
in transplant recipients, 73–76, 73t
varicella-zoster virus in, 96
Incision dressings, SSI risk and, 80t
Infectious mononucleosis, EBV and, 96
Influenza virus infections, 93–94, Q52
community-acquired pneumonia and, 14
Interferon-γ release assay (IGRA), 31
Isavuconazole
for aspergillosis, 39
for mucormycosis, 42
Isoniazid, for tuberculosis, 34, 35t, Q2, Q59
Itraconazole
for histoplasmosis, 41
for sporotrichosis, 42

## A — NAME AND ADDRESS (Please complete.)

Last Name _____ First Name _____ Middle Initial

Address _____

Address cont. _____

City _____ State _____ ZIP Code

Country _____

Email address _____

**ACP®**
**American College of Physicians**
Leading Internal Medicine, Improving Lives

**Medical Knowledge Self-Assessment Program® 18**

---

### TO EARN *CME Credits and/or MOC Points* YOU MUST:

1. Answer all questions.
2. Score a minimum of 50% correct.

======================================

### TO EARN *FREE* INSTANTANEOUS *CME Credits and/or MOC Points* ONLINE:

1. Answer all of your questions.
2. Go to **mksap.acponline.org** and enter your ACP Online username and password to access an online answer sheet.
3. Enter your answers.
4. You can also enter your answers directly at **mksap.acponline.org** without first using this answer sheet.

### To Submit Your Answer Sheet by Mail or FAX for a $20 Administrative Fee per Answer Sheet:

1. Answer all of your questions and calculate your score.
2. Complete boxes A-H.
3. Complete payment information.
4. Send the answer sheet and payment information to ACP, using the FAX number/address listed below.

---

## B — Order Number

(Use the 10-digit Order Number on your MKSAP materials packing slip.)

## C — ACP ID Number

(Refer to packing slip in your MKSAP materials for your 8-digit ACP ID Number.)

---

## D — Required Submission Information if Applying for MOC

Birth Month and Day [ M M ] [ D D ]

ABIM Candidate Number [ ][ ][ ][ ][ ][ ]

---

### COMPLETE FORM BELOW ONLY IF YOU SUBMIT BY MAIL OR FAX

Last Name _____ First Name _____ MI

### Payment Information. Must remit in US funds, drawn on a US bank.
### The processing fee for each paper answer sheet is $20.

☐ Check, made payable to ACP, enclosed

Charge to  ☐ **VISA**  ☐ **MasterCard**  ☐ **AMERICAN EXPRESS**  ☐ **DISCOVER**

Card Number _____

Expiration Date _____ / _____
MM          YY

Security code (3 or 4 digit #s) _____

Signature _____

**Fax to:** 215-351-2799

**Mail to:**
Member and Customer Service
American College of Physicians
190 N. Independence Mall West
Philadelphia, PA 19106-1572

# E

## TEST TYPE

| | Maximum Number of CME Credits |
|---|---|
| ○ Cardiovascular Medicine | 30 |
| ○ Dermatology | 16 |
| ○ Gastroenterology and Hepatology | 22 |
| ○ Hematology and Oncology | 33 |
| ○ Neurology | 22 |
| ○ Rheumatology | 22 |
| ○ Endocrinology and Metabolism | 19 |
| ○ General Internal Medicine | 36 |
| ○ Infectious Disease | 25 |
| ○ Nephrology | 25 |
| ○ Pulmonary and Critical Care Medicine | 25 |

# F

## CREDITS OR POINTS CLAIMED ON SECTION
### 1 hour = 1 credit or 1 point

Enter the number of credits earned on the test to the nearest quarter hour. Physicians should claim only the credit commensurate with the extent of their participation in the activity.

# G

### Enter your score here.

Instructions for calculating your own score are found in front of the self-assessment test in each book. You must receive a minimum score of 50% correct.

_____ %

Credit Submission Date:_____

# H

☐ I want to submit for CME credits

☐ I want to submit for CME credits and MOC points.

1 Ⓐ Ⓑ Ⓒ Ⓓ Ⓔ
2 Ⓐ Ⓑ Ⓒ Ⓓ Ⓔ
3 Ⓐ Ⓑ Ⓒ Ⓓ Ⓔ
4 Ⓐ Ⓑ Ⓒ Ⓓ Ⓔ
5 Ⓐ Ⓑ Ⓒ Ⓓ Ⓔ

6 Ⓐ Ⓑ Ⓒ Ⓓ Ⓔ
7 Ⓐ Ⓑ Ⓒ Ⓓ Ⓔ
8 Ⓐ Ⓑ Ⓒ Ⓓ Ⓔ
9 Ⓐ Ⓑ Ⓒ Ⓓ Ⓔ
10 Ⓐ Ⓑ Ⓒ Ⓓ Ⓔ

11 Ⓐ Ⓑ Ⓒ Ⓓ Ⓔ
12 Ⓐ Ⓑ Ⓒ Ⓓ Ⓔ
13 Ⓐ Ⓑ Ⓒ Ⓓ Ⓔ
14 Ⓐ Ⓑ Ⓒ Ⓓ Ⓔ
15 Ⓐ Ⓑ Ⓒ Ⓓ Ⓔ

16 Ⓐ Ⓑ Ⓒ Ⓓ Ⓔ
17 Ⓐ Ⓑ Ⓒ Ⓓ Ⓔ
18 Ⓐ Ⓑ Ⓒ Ⓓ Ⓔ
19 Ⓐ Ⓑ Ⓒ Ⓓ Ⓔ
20 Ⓐ Ⓑ Ⓒ Ⓓ Ⓔ

21 Ⓐ Ⓑ Ⓒ Ⓓ Ⓔ
22 Ⓐ Ⓑ Ⓒ Ⓓ Ⓔ
23 Ⓐ Ⓑ Ⓒ Ⓓ Ⓔ
24 Ⓐ Ⓑ Ⓒ Ⓓ Ⓔ
25 Ⓐ Ⓑ Ⓒ Ⓓ Ⓔ

26 Ⓐ Ⓑ Ⓒ Ⓓ Ⓔ
27 Ⓐ Ⓑ Ⓒ Ⓓ Ⓔ
28 Ⓐ Ⓑ Ⓒ Ⓓ Ⓔ
29 Ⓐ Ⓑ Ⓒ Ⓓ Ⓔ
30 Ⓐ Ⓑ Ⓒ Ⓓ Ⓔ

31 Ⓐ Ⓑ Ⓒ Ⓓ Ⓔ
32 Ⓐ Ⓑ Ⓒ Ⓓ Ⓔ
33 Ⓐ Ⓑ Ⓒ Ⓓ Ⓔ
34 Ⓐ Ⓑ Ⓒ Ⓓ Ⓔ
35 Ⓐ Ⓑ Ⓒ Ⓓ Ⓔ

36 Ⓐ Ⓑ Ⓒ Ⓓ Ⓔ
37 Ⓐ Ⓑ Ⓒ Ⓓ Ⓔ
38 Ⓐ Ⓑ Ⓒ Ⓓ Ⓔ
39 Ⓐ Ⓑ Ⓒ Ⓓ Ⓔ
40 Ⓐ Ⓑ Ⓒ Ⓓ Ⓔ

41 Ⓐ Ⓑ Ⓒ Ⓓ Ⓔ
42 Ⓐ Ⓑ Ⓒ Ⓓ Ⓔ
43 Ⓐ Ⓑ Ⓒ Ⓓ Ⓔ
44 Ⓐ Ⓑ Ⓒ Ⓓ Ⓔ
45 Ⓐ Ⓑ Ⓒ Ⓓ Ⓔ

46 Ⓐ Ⓑ Ⓒ Ⓓ Ⓔ
47 Ⓐ Ⓑ Ⓒ Ⓓ Ⓔ
48 Ⓐ Ⓑ Ⓒ Ⓓ Ⓔ
49 Ⓐ Ⓑ Ⓒ Ⓓ Ⓔ
50 Ⓐ Ⓑ Ⓒ Ⓓ Ⓔ

51 Ⓐ Ⓑ Ⓒ Ⓓ Ⓔ
52 Ⓐ Ⓑ Ⓒ Ⓓ Ⓔ
53 Ⓐ Ⓑ Ⓒ Ⓓ Ⓔ
54 Ⓐ Ⓑ Ⓒ Ⓓ Ⓔ
55 Ⓐ Ⓑ Ⓒ Ⓓ Ⓔ

56 Ⓐ Ⓑ Ⓒ Ⓓ Ⓔ
57 Ⓐ Ⓑ Ⓒ Ⓓ Ⓔ
58 Ⓐ Ⓑ Ⓒ Ⓓ Ⓔ
59 Ⓐ Ⓑ Ⓒ Ⓓ Ⓔ
60 Ⓐ Ⓑ Ⓒ Ⓓ Ⓔ

61 Ⓐ Ⓑ Ⓒ Ⓓ Ⓔ
62 Ⓐ Ⓑ Ⓒ Ⓓ Ⓔ
63 Ⓐ Ⓑ Ⓒ Ⓓ Ⓔ
64 Ⓐ Ⓑ Ⓒ Ⓓ Ⓔ
65 Ⓐ Ⓑ Ⓒ Ⓓ Ⓔ

66 Ⓐ Ⓑ Ⓒ Ⓓ Ⓔ
67 Ⓐ Ⓑ Ⓒ Ⓓ Ⓔ
68 Ⓐ Ⓑ Ⓒ Ⓓ Ⓔ
69 Ⓐ Ⓑ Ⓒ Ⓓ Ⓔ
70 Ⓐ Ⓑ Ⓒ Ⓓ Ⓔ

71 Ⓐ Ⓑ Ⓒ Ⓓ Ⓔ
72 Ⓐ Ⓑ Ⓒ Ⓓ Ⓔ
73 Ⓐ Ⓑ Ⓒ Ⓓ Ⓔ
74 Ⓐ Ⓑ Ⓒ Ⓓ Ⓔ
75 Ⓐ Ⓑ Ⓒ Ⓓ Ⓔ

76 Ⓐ Ⓑ Ⓒ Ⓓ Ⓔ
77 Ⓐ Ⓑ Ⓒ Ⓓ Ⓔ
78 Ⓐ Ⓑ Ⓒ Ⓓ Ⓔ
79 Ⓐ Ⓑ Ⓒ Ⓓ Ⓔ
80 Ⓐ Ⓑ Ⓒ Ⓓ Ⓔ

81 Ⓐ Ⓑ Ⓒ Ⓓ Ⓔ
82 Ⓐ Ⓑ Ⓒ Ⓓ Ⓔ
83 Ⓐ Ⓑ Ⓒ Ⓓ Ⓔ
84 Ⓐ Ⓑ Ⓒ Ⓓ Ⓔ
85 Ⓐ Ⓑ Ⓒ Ⓓ Ⓔ

86 Ⓐ Ⓑ Ⓒ Ⓓ Ⓔ
87 Ⓐ Ⓑ Ⓒ Ⓓ Ⓔ
88 Ⓐ Ⓑ Ⓒ Ⓓ Ⓔ
89 Ⓐ Ⓑ Ⓒ Ⓓ Ⓔ
90 Ⓐ Ⓑ Ⓒ Ⓓ Ⓔ

91 Ⓐ Ⓑ Ⓒ Ⓓ Ⓔ
92 Ⓐ Ⓑ Ⓒ Ⓓ Ⓔ
93 Ⓐ Ⓑ Ⓒ Ⓓ Ⓔ
94 Ⓐ Ⓑ Ⓒ Ⓓ Ⓔ
95 Ⓐ Ⓑ Ⓒ Ⓓ Ⓔ

96 Ⓐ Ⓑ Ⓒ Ⓓ Ⓔ
97 Ⓐ Ⓑ Ⓒ Ⓓ Ⓔ
98 Ⓐ Ⓑ Ⓒ Ⓓ Ⓔ
99 Ⓐ Ⓑ Ⓒ Ⓓ Ⓔ
100 Ⓐ Ⓑ Ⓒ Ⓓ Ⓔ

101 Ⓐ Ⓑ Ⓒ Ⓓ Ⓔ
102 Ⓐ Ⓑ Ⓒ Ⓓ Ⓔ
103 Ⓐ Ⓑ Ⓒ Ⓓ Ⓔ
104 Ⓐ Ⓑ Ⓒ Ⓓ Ⓔ
105 Ⓐ Ⓑ Ⓒ Ⓓ Ⓔ

106 Ⓐ Ⓑ Ⓒ Ⓓ Ⓔ
107 Ⓐ Ⓑ Ⓒ Ⓓ Ⓔ
108 Ⓐ Ⓑ Ⓒ Ⓓ Ⓔ
109 Ⓐ Ⓑ Ⓒ Ⓓ Ⓔ
110 Ⓐ Ⓑ Ⓒ Ⓓ Ⓔ

111 Ⓐ Ⓑ Ⓒ Ⓓ Ⓔ
112 Ⓐ Ⓑ Ⓒ Ⓓ Ⓔ
113 Ⓐ Ⓑ Ⓒ Ⓓ Ⓔ
114 Ⓐ Ⓑ Ⓒ Ⓓ Ⓔ
115 Ⓐ Ⓑ Ⓒ Ⓓ Ⓔ

116 Ⓐ Ⓑ Ⓒ Ⓓ Ⓔ
117 Ⓐ Ⓑ Ⓒ Ⓓ Ⓔ
118 Ⓐ Ⓑ Ⓒ Ⓓ Ⓔ
119 Ⓐ Ⓑ Ⓒ Ⓓ Ⓔ
120 Ⓐ Ⓑ Ⓒ Ⓓ Ⓔ

121 Ⓐ Ⓑ Ⓒ Ⓓ Ⓔ
122 Ⓐ Ⓑ Ⓒ Ⓓ Ⓔ
123 Ⓐ Ⓑ Ⓒ Ⓓ Ⓔ
124 Ⓐ Ⓑ Ⓒ Ⓓ Ⓔ
125 Ⓐ Ⓑ Ⓒ Ⓓ Ⓔ

126 Ⓐ Ⓑ Ⓒ Ⓓ Ⓔ
127 Ⓐ Ⓑ Ⓒ Ⓓ Ⓔ
128 Ⓐ Ⓑ Ⓒ Ⓓ Ⓔ
129 Ⓐ Ⓑ Ⓒ Ⓓ Ⓔ
130 Ⓐ Ⓑ Ⓒ Ⓓ Ⓔ

131 Ⓐ Ⓑ Ⓒ Ⓓ Ⓔ
132 Ⓐ Ⓑ Ⓒ Ⓓ Ⓔ
133 Ⓐ Ⓑ Ⓒ Ⓓ Ⓔ
134 Ⓐ Ⓑ Ⓒ Ⓓ Ⓔ
135 Ⓐ Ⓑ Ⓒ Ⓓ Ⓔ

136 Ⓐ Ⓑ Ⓒ Ⓓ Ⓔ
137 Ⓐ Ⓑ Ⓒ Ⓓ Ⓔ
138 Ⓐ Ⓑ Ⓒ Ⓓ Ⓔ
139 Ⓐ Ⓑ Ⓒ Ⓓ Ⓔ
140 Ⓐ Ⓑ Ⓒ Ⓓ Ⓔ

141 Ⓐ Ⓑ Ⓒ Ⓓ Ⓔ
142 Ⓐ Ⓑ Ⓒ Ⓓ Ⓔ
143 Ⓐ Ⓑ Ⓒ Ⓓ Ⓔ
144 Ⓐ Ⓑ Ⓒ Ⓓ Ⓔ
145 Ⓐ Ⓑ Ⓒ Ⓓ Ⓔ

146 Ⓐ Ⓑ Ⓒ Ⓓ Ⓔ
147 Ⓐ Ⓑ Ⓒ Ⓓ Ⓔ
148 Ⓐ Ⓑ Ⓒ Ⓓ Ⓔ
149 Ⓐ Ⓑ Ⓒ Ⓓ Ⓔ
150 Ⓐ Ⓑ Ⓒ Ⓓ Ⓔ

151 Ⓐ Ⓑ Ⓒ Ⓓ Ⓔ
152 Ⓐ Ⓑ Ⓒ Ⓓ Ⓔ
153 Ⓐ Ⓑ Ⓒ Ⓓ Ⓔ
154 Ⓐ Ⓑ Ⓒ Ⓓ Ⓔ
155 Ⓐ Ⓑ Ⓒ Ⓓ Ⓔ

156 Ⓐ Ⓑ Ⓒ Ⓓ Ⓔ
157 Ⓐ Ⓑ Ⓒ Ⓓ Ⓔ
158 Ⓐ Ⓑ Ⓒ Ⓓ Ⓔ
159 Ⓐ Ⓑ Ⓒ Ⓓ Ⓔ
160 Ⓐ Ⓑ Ⓒ Ⓓ Ⓔ

161 Ⓐ Ⓑ Ⓒ Ⓓ Ⓔ
162 Ⓐ Ⓑ Ⓒ Ⓓ Ⓔ
163 Ⓐ Ⓑ Ⓒ Ⓓ Ⓔ
164 Ⓐ Ⓑ Ⓒ Ⓓ Ⓔ
165 Ⓐ Ⓑ Ⓒ Ⓓ Ⓔ

166 Ⓐ Ⓑ Ⓒ Ⓓ Ⓔ
167 Ⓐ Ⓑ Ⓒ Ⓓ Ⓔ
168 Ⓐ Ⓑ Ⓒ Ⓓ Ⓔ
169 Ⓐ Ⓑ Ⓒ Ⓓ Ⓔ
170 Ⓐ Ⓑ Ⓒ Ⓓ Ⓔ

171 Ⓐ Ⓑ Ⓒ Ⓓ Ⓔ
172 Ⓐ Ⓑ Ⓒ Ⓓ Ⓔ
173 Ⓐ Ⓑ Ⓒ Ⓓ Ⓔ
174 Ⓐ Ⓑ Ⓒ Ⓓ Ⓔ
175 Ⓐ Ⓑ Ⓒ Ⓓ Ⓔ

176 Ⓐ Ⓑ Ⓒ Ⓓ Ⓔ
177 Ⓐ Ⓑ Ⓒ Ⓓ Ⓔ
178 Ⓐ Ⓑ Ⓒ Ⓓ Ⓔ
179 Ⓐ Ⓑ Ⓒ Ⓓ Ⓔ
180 Ⓐ Ⓑ Ⓒ Ⓓ Ⓔ

MK7010

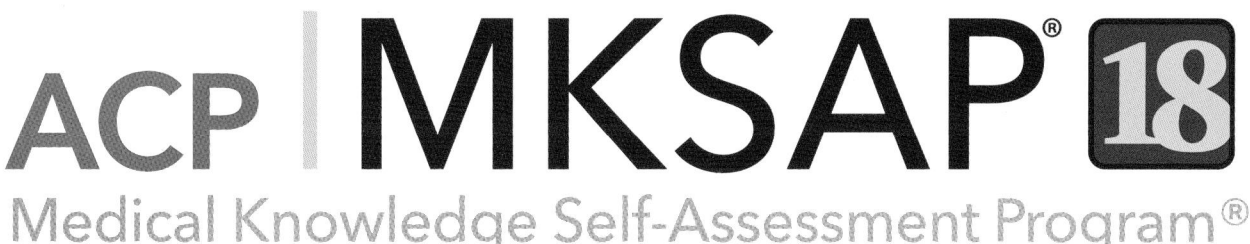

# Pulmonary and Critical Care Medicine

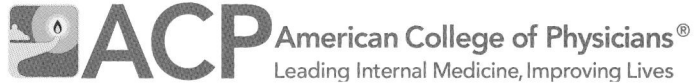
American College of Physicians®
Leading Internal Medicine, Improving Lives

# Welcome to the Pulmonary and Critical Care Medicine Section of MKSAP 18!

In these pages, you will find updated information on pulmonary diagnostic testing; airways disease; diffuse parenchymal lung disease; occupational lung disease; pleural disease; pulmonary vascular disease; lung tumors; sleep medicine; high-altitude–related illnesses; principles of ventilation in critical care; common ICU conditions such as upper airway emergencies, respiratory failure, sepsis, anaphylaxis, and toxicologic emergencies; and other clinical challenges. All of these topics are uniquely focused on the needs of generalists and subspecialists *outside* of pulmonary and critical care medicine.

The core content of MKSAP 18 has been developed as in previous editions—all essential information that is newly researched and written in 11 topic areas of internal medicine—created by dozens of leading generalists and subspecialists and guided by certification and recertification requirements, emerging knowledge in the field, and user feedback. MKSAP 18 also contains 1200 all-new peer-reviewed, psychometrically validated, multiple-choice questions (MCQs) for self-assessment and study, including 103 in Pulmonary and Critical Care Medicine. MKSAP 18 continues to include *High Value Care* (HVC) recommendations, based on the concept of balancing clinical benefit with costs and harms, with associated MCQs illustrating these principles and HVC Key Points called out in the text. Internists practicing in the hospital setting can easily find comprehensive *Hospitalist*-focused content and MCQs, specially designated in blue and with the █ symbol.

If you purchased MKSAP 18 Complete, you also have access to MKSAP 18 Digital, with additional tools allowing you to customize your learning experience. MKSAP Digital includes regular text updates with new, practice-changing information, 200 new self-assessment questions, and enhanced custom-quiz options. MKSAP Complete also includes more than 1200 electronic, adaptive learning–enhanced flashcards for quick review of important concepts, as well as an updated and enhanced version of Virtual Dx, MKSAP's image-based self-assessment tool. As before, MKSAP 18 Digital is optimized for use on your mobile devices, with iOS- and Android-based apps allowing you to sync between your apps and online account and submit for CME credits and MOC points online.

Please visit us at the MKSAP Resource Site (mksap.acponline.org) to find out how we can help you study, earn CME credit and MOC points, and stay up to date.

On behalf of the many internists who have offered their time and expertise to create the content for MKSAP 18 and the editorial staff who work to bring this material to you in the best possible way, we are honored that you have chosen to use MKSAP 18 and appreciate any feedback about the program you may have. Please feel free to send any comments to mksap_editors@acponline.org.

Sincerely,

*Patrick Alguire*

Patrick C. Alguire, MD, FACP
Editor-in-Chief
Senior Vice President Emeritus
Medical Education Division
American College of Physicians

# Pulmonary and Critical Care Medicine

## Committee

**Craig E. Daniels, MD, Section Editor[2]**
Associate Professor of Medicine
Division of Pulmonary and Critical Care Medicine
Mayo Clinic College of Medicine and Science
Rochester, Minnesota

**Rendell Ashton, MD, FACP[1]**
Program Director, Pulmonary and Critical Care Fellowship
Associate Director, Medical Intensive Care Unit
Cleveland Clinic Lerner College of Medicine of Case Western
    Reserve University
Cleveland, Ohio

**Sean M. Caples, DO, MS[2]**
Associate Professor of Medicine
Division of Pulmonary and Critical Care Medicine
Mayo Clinic College of Medicine and Science
Rochester, Minnesota

**Neal Chaisson, MD[2]**
Program Director, Critical Care Medicine Fellowship
Assistant Professor of Medicine
Cleveland Clinic Lerner College of Medicine of Case Western
    Reserve University
Cleveland, Ohio

**C. Jessica Dine, MD, MSHPR, FACP[2]**
Assistant Professor of Medicine
Perelman School of Medicine at the University
    of Pennsylvania
Perelman Center for Advanced Medicine
Philadelphia, Pennsylvania

**Melissa B. King-Biggs, MD[1]**
Assistant Professor of Medicine
Department Chair HealthPartners Medical Group
    Lung and Sleep Health
University of Minnesota Medical School
Minneapolis, Minnesota

**Eduardo Mireles-Cabodevila, MD[2]**
Director, Medical Intensive Care Unit
Assistant Professor of Medicine
Cleveland Clinic Lerner College of Medicine of Case
    Western Reserve University
Cleveland, Ohio

**Darlene R. Nelson, MD[1]**
Associate Program Director of PCCM fellowship
Assistant Professor of Medicine
Division of Pulmonary and Critical Care Medicine
Mayo Clinic College of Medicine and Science
Rochester, Minnesota

**Timothy Whelan, MD[2]**
Professor of Medicine
Medical Director of Lung Transplantation
Medical University of South Carolina
Charleston, South Carolina

## Consulting Editor

**Steven Weinberger, MD, MACP[2]**
Executive Vice President and CEO Emeritus
American College of Physicians
Adjunct Professor of Medicine
Perelman School of Medicine at the University
    of Pennsylvania
Philadelphia, Pennsylvania

## Editor-in-Chief

**Patrick C. Alguire, MD, FACP[2]**
Senior Vice President Emeritus, Medical Education
American College of Physicians
Philadelphia, Pennsylvania

## Deputy Editor

**Denise M. Dupras, MD, PhD, FACP[1]**
Associate Program Director
Department of Internal Medicine
Associate Professor of Medicine
Mayo Clinic College of Medicine
Rochester, Minnesota

## Pulmonary and Critical Care Medicine Reviewers

Mahmoud Amarna, MD, FACP[1]
Sameh G. Aziz, MD, FACP[1]
Thomas Bice, MD[1]
Martin M. Cearras, MD[1]

Sanjay Chawla, MD, FACP[2]
Jacob F. Collen, MD, FACP[1]
Oleg Epelbaum, MD, FACP[1]
Leila Hashemi, MD, FACP[1]
Ankur Kalra, MD, FACP[1]
Amay Parikh, MD, FACP[1]

## Hospital Medicine Pulmonary and Critical Care Medicine Reviewers

Shashi K Bellam, MD FACP[2]
Ehab G. Daoud, MD, FACP[1]

## Pulmonary and Critical Care Medicine ACP Editorial Staff

**Chuck Emig[1]**, Staff Editor
**Margaret Wells[1]**, Director, Self-Assessment and Educational Programs[1]
**Becky Krumm[1]**, Managing Editor, Self-Assessment and Educational Programs[1]

## ACP Principal Staff

**Davoren Chick, MD, FACP[2]**
*Senior Vice President, Medical Education*

**Patrick C. Alguire, MD, FACP[2]**
*Senior Vice President Emeritus, Medical Education*

**Sean McKinney[1]**
*Vice President, Medical Education*

**Margaret Wells[1]**
*Director, Self-Assessment and Educational Programs*

**Becky Krumm[1]**
*Managing Editor*

**Valerie Dangovetsky[1]**
*Administrator*

**Ellen McDonald, PhD[1]**
*Senior Staff Editor*

**Megan Zborowski[1]**
*Senior Staff Editor*

**Jackie Twomey[1]**
*Senior Staff Editor*

**Randy Hendrickson[1]**
*Production Administrator/Editor*

**Julia Nawrocki[1]**
*Digital Content Associate/Editor*

**Linnea Donnarumma[1]**
*Staff Editor*

**Chuck Emig[1]**
*Staff Editor*

**Joysa Winter[1]**
*Staff Editor*

**Kimberly Kerns[1]**
*Administrative Coordinator*

---

1. Has no relationships with any entity producing, marketing, reselling, or distributing health care goods or services consumed by, or used on, patients.

2. Has disclosed relationship(s) with any entity producing, marketing, reselling, or distributing health care goods or services consumed by, or used on, patients.

## Disclosure of Relationships with any entity producing, marketing, reselling, or distributing health care goods or services consumed by, or used on, patients.

**Patrick C. Alguire, MD, FACP**
*Royalties*
UpToDate

**Shashi K. Bellam, MD FACP**
*Speakers Bureau*
Genentech

**Sean M. Caples, DO, MS**
*Consultantship*
Zephyr Labs

**Neal Chaisson, MD**
*Consultantship*
Actelion Pharmaceuticals, Putnam Associates, Schlesinger Associates, Bayer
*Speakers Bureau*
Bayer, Gilead

**Sanjay Chawla, MD, FACP**
*Stock Options/Holdings*
Pfizer

**Davoren Chick, MD, FACP**
*Royalties*
Wolters Kluwer Publishing
*Consultantship*
EBSCO Health's DynaMed Plus
*Other:* Owner and sole proprietor of Coding 101, LLC; research consultant (spouse) for Vedanta Biosciences Inc.

**Craig E. Daniels, MD**
*Research Grants/Contracts*
Boehringer, Genentech/Roche
*Patent Holder*
Sanovas Inc.

**C. Jessica Dine, MD, MSHPR, FACP**
*Consultantship*
National Board of Medical Examiners

**Eduardo Mireles-Cabodevila, MD**
*Co-Patent Owner*
Co-owners Robert Chatburn and Cleveland Clinic:
    Ventilator Control System Utilizing a Mid-Frequency
    Ventilation Pattern

**Steven Weinberger, MD, MACP**
*Royalties*
Elsevier, Wolters Kluwer Publishing, UpToDate

**Timothy Whelan, MD**
*Consultantship*
Gilead Sciences, Boehringer Ingelheim, Sharing Hope SC,
    Genentech, France Foundation, RockPointe, Inc.
*Research Grants/Contracts*
Gilead Sciences, Boehringer Ingelheim, Genetech, Global
    Blood Therapeutics, Kadmon, National Institute of
    Health, Pulmonary Fibrosis Foundation, Celgene,
    Galapagos
*Board Member*
Sharing Hope SC

## Acknowledgments

The American College of Physicians (ACP) gratefully
acknowledges the special contributions to the development and production of the 18th edition of the Medical
Knowledge Self-Assessment Program® (MKSAP® 18) made
by the following people:

*Graphic Design:* Barry Moshinski (Director, Graphic
Services), Michael Ripca (Graphics Technical
Administrator), and Jennifer Gropper (Graphic
Designer).

*Production/Systems:* Dan Hoffmann (Director, Information
Technology), Scott Hurd (Manager, Content Systems),
Neil Kohl (Senior Architect), and Chris Patterson (Senior
Architect).

*MKSAP 18 Digital:* Under the direction of Steven Spadt
(Senior Vice President, Technology), the digital version
of MKSAP 18 was developed within the ACP's Digital
Products and Services Department, led by Brian
Sweigard (Director, Digital Products and Services). Other
members of the team included Dan Barron (Senior Web
Application Developer/Architect), Chris Forrest (Senior
Software Developer/Design Lead), Kathleen Hoover
(Senior Web Developer), Kara Regis (Manager, User
Interface Design and Development), Brad Lord (Senior
Web Application Developer), and John McKnight (Senior
Web Developer).

The College also wishes to acknowledge that many
other persons, too numerous to mention, have contributed to the production of this program. Without their
dedicated efforts, this program would not have been
possible.

## MKSAP Resource Site (mksap.acponline.org)

The MKSAP Resource Site (mksap.acponline.org) is a continually updated site that provides links to MKSAP 18 online answer
sheets for print subscribers; access to MKSAP 18 Digital; Board
Basics® e-book access instructions; information on Continuing
Medical Education (CME), Maintenance of Certification (MOC),
and international Continuing Professional Development (CPD)
and MOC; errata; and other new information.

## International MOC/CPD

For information and instructions on submission of international MOC/CPD, please go to the MKSAP Resource Site
(mksap.acponline.org).

## Continuing Medical Education

The American College of Physicians is accredited by the
Accreditation Council for Continuing Medical Education
(ACCME) to provide continuing medical education for
physicians.

The American College of Physicians designates this enduring material, MKSAP 18, for a maximum of 275 *AMA PRA
Category 1 Credits*™. Physicians should claim only the
credit commensurate with the extent of their participation
in the activity.

Up to 25 *AMA PRA Category 1 Credits*™ are available from
December 31, 2018, to December 31, 2021, for the MKSAP 18
Pulmonary and Critical Care Medicine section.

## Learning Objectives

The learning objectives of MKSAP 18 are to:

- Close gaps between actual care in your practice and pre-
  ferred standards of care, based on best evidence
- Diagnose disease states that are less common and some-
  times overlooked and confusing
- Improve management of comorbid conditions that can
  complicate patient care
- Determine when to refer patients for surgery or care by
  subspecialists
- Pass the ABIM Certification Examination
- Pass the ABIM Maintenance of Certification Examination

## Target Audience

- General internists and primary care physicians
- Subspecialists who need to remain up to date in internal
  medicine
- Residents preparing for the certifying examination in
  internal medicine
- Physicians preparing for maintenance of certification in
  internal medicine (recertification)

## ABIM Maintenance of Certification

Check the MKSAP Resource Site (mksap.acponline.org) for the latest information on how MKSAP tests can be used to apply to the American Board of Internal Medicine (ABIM) for Maintenance of Certification (MOC) points following completion of the CME activity.

Successful completion of the CME activity, which includes participation in the evaluation component, enables the participant to earn up to 275 medical knowledge MOC points in the ABIM's MOC program. It is the CME activity provider's responsibility to submit participant completion information to ACCME for the purpose of granting MOC credit.

## Earn Instantaneous CME Credits or MOC Points Online

Print subscribers can enter their answers online to earn instantaneous CME credits or MOC points. You can submit your answers using online answer sheets that are provided at mksap.acponline.org, where a record of your MKSAP 18 credits will be available. To earn CME credits or to apply for MOC points, you need to answer all of the questions in a test and earn a score of at least 50% correct (number of correct answers divided by the total number of questions). Please note that if you are applying for MOC points, you must also enter your birth date and ABIM candidate number.

Take either of the following approaches:

1. Use the printed answer sheet at the back of this book to record your answers. Go to mksap.acponline.org, access the appropriate online answer sheet, transcribe your answers, and submit your test for instantaneous CME credits or MOC points. There is no additional fee for this service.

2. Go to mksap.acponline.org, access the appropriate online answer sheet, directly enter your answers, and submit your test for instantaneous CME credits or MOC points. There is no additional fee for this service.

## Earn CME Credits or MOC Points by Mail or Fax

Pay a $20 processing fee per answer sheet and submit the printed answer sheet at the back of this book by mail or fax, as instructed on the answer sheet. Make sure you calculate your score and enter your birth date and ABIM candidate number, and fax the answer sheet to 215-351-2799 or mail the answer sheet to Member and Customer Service, American College of Physicians, 190 N. Independence Mall West, Philadelphia, PA 19106-1572, using the courtesy envelope provided in your MKSAP 18 slipcase. You will need your 10-digit order number and 8-digit ACP ID number, which are printed on your packing slip. Please allow 4 to 6 weeks for your score report to be emailed back to you. Be sure to include your email address for a response.

If you do not have a 10-digit order number and 8-digit ACP ID number, or if you need help creating a user-name and password to access the MKSAP 18 online answer sheets, go to mksap.acponline.org or email custserv@acponline.org.

## Disclosure Policy

It is the policy of the American College of Physicians (ACP) to ensure balance, independence, objectivity, and scientific rigor in all of its educational activities. To this end, and consistent with the policies of the ACP and the Accreditation Council for Continuing Medical Education (ACCME), contributors to all ACP continuing medical education activities are required to disclose all relevant financial relationships with any entity producing, marketing, re-selling, or distributing health care goods or services consumed by, or used on, patients. Contributors are required to use generic names in the discussion of therapeutic options and are required to identify any unapproved, off-label, or investigative use of commercial products or devices. Where a trade name is used, all available trade names for the same product type are also included. If trade-name products manufactured by companies with whom contributors have relationships are discussed, contributors are asked to provide evidence-based citations in support of the discussion. The information is reviewed by the committee responsible for producing this text. If necessary, adjustments to topics or contributors' roles in content development are made to balance the discussion. Further, all readers of this text are asked to evaluate the content for evidence of commercial bias and send any relevant comments to mksap_editors@acponline.org so that future decisions about content and contributors can be made in light of this information.

## Resolution of Conflicts

To resolve all conflicts of interest and influences of vested interests, ACP's content planners used best evidence and updated clinical care guidelines in developing content, when such evidence and guidelines were available. All content underwent review by peer reviewers not on the committee to ensure that the material was balanced and unbiased. Contributors' disclosure information can be found with the list of contributors' names and those of ACP principal staff listed in the beginning of this book.

## Hospital-Based Medicine

For the convenience of subscribers who provide care in hospital settings, content that is specific to the hospital setting has been highlighted in blue. Hospital icons (◨) highlight where the hospital-only content begins, continues over more than one page, and ends.

## High Value Care Key Points

Key Points in the text that relate to High Value Care concepts (that is, concepts that discuss balancing clinical benefit with costs and harms) are designated by the HVC icon [**HVC**].

## Educational Disclaimer

The editors and publisher of MKSAP 18 recognize that the development of new material offers many opportunities for error. Despite our best efforts, some errors may persist in print. Drug dosage schedules are, we believe, accurate and in accordance with current standards. Readers are advised, however, to ensure that the recommended dosages in MKSAP 18 concur with the information provided in the product information material. This is especially important in cases of new, infrequently used, or highly toxic drugs. Application of the information in MKSAP 18 remains the professional responsibility of the practitioner.

The primary purpose of MKSAP 18 is educational. Information presented, as well as publications, technologies, products, and/or services discussed, is intended to inform subscribers about the knowledge, techniques, and experiences of the contributors. A diversity of professional opinion exists, and the views of the contributors are their own and not those of the ACP. Inclusion of any material in the program does not constitute endorsement or recommendation by the ACP. The ACP does not warrant the safety, reliability, accuracy, completeness, or usefulness of and disclaims any and all liability for damages and claims that may result from the use of information, publications, technologies, products, and/or services discussed in this program.

## Publisher's Information

## Disclaimer Regarding Direct Purchases from Online Retailers

CME and/or MOC for MKSAP 18 is available only if you purchase the program directly from ACP. CME credits and MOC points cannot be awarded to those purchasers who have purchased the program from non-authorized sellers such as Amazon, eBay, or any other such online retailer.

## Unauthorized Use of This Book Is Against the Law

MKSAP 18 ISBN: 978-1-938245-47-3
(Pulmonary and Critical Care Medicine)
ISBN: 978-1-938245-58-9

Printed in the United States of America.

For order information in the U.S. or Canada call 800-ACP-1915. All other countries call 215-351-2600 (Monday to Friday, 9 AM – 5 PM ET). Fax inquiries to 215-351-2799 or email to custserv@acponline.org.

## Errata

Errata for MKSAP 18 will be available through the MKSAP Resource Site at mksap.acponline.org as new information becomes known to the editors.

# Table of Contents

# Pulmonary and Critical Care Medicine High Value Care Recommendations

The American College of Physicians, in collaboration with multiple other organizations, is engaged in a worldwide initiative to promote the practice of High Value Care (HVC). The goals of the HVC initiative are to improve health care outcomes by providing care of proven benefit and reducing costs by avoiding unnecessary and even harmful interventions. The initiative comprises several programs that integrate the important concept of health care value (balancing clinical benefit with costs and harms) for a given intervention into a broad range of educational materials to address the needs of trainees, practicing physicians, and patients.

HVC content has been integrated into MKSAP 18 in several important ways. MKSAP 18 includes HVC-identified key points in the text, HVC-focused multiple choice questions, and, for subscribers to MKSAP Digital, an HVC custom quiz. From the text and questions, we have generated the following list of HVC recommendations that meet the definition below of high value care and bring us closer to our goal of improving patient outcomes while conserving finite resources.

**High Value Care Recommendation:** A recommendation to choose diagnostic and management strategies for patients in specific clinical situations that balance clinical benefit with cost and harms with the goal of improving patient outcomes.

Below are the High Value Care Recommendations for the Pulmonary and Critical Care Medicine section of MKSAP 18.

- Spirometry before and after workplace exposures is a cost-effective way to confirm a suspected diagnosis of occupational asthma.
- A sputum culture is not routinely used to assess COPD exacerbations as it rarely affects management.

- The diagnosis of diffuse parenchymal lung disease can often be made based on high-resolution CT without a lung biopsy.
- Avoid mechanical ventilation for patients with idiopathic pulmonary fibrosis if lung transplantation is not an option.
- Uvulopalatopharyngoplasty and similar procedures are ineffective for treatment of obstructive sleep apnea.
- Do not routinely use haloperidol or atypical antipsychotics for the prevention of delirium.
- Do not routinely measure gastric residuals in critically ill malnourished patients because it delays achievement of feeding goals and may increase the risk of aspiration.
- Do not order diagnostic tests at regular intervals but rather in response to specific clinical questions.
- Do not use parenteral nutrition in adequately nourished critically ill patients within the first 7 days of an ICU stay.
- Adjunctive therapies for severe asthma exacerbation, including anesthetics with bronchodilator properties, inhalation of a helium-oxygen mixture, mucolytics, and leukotriene receptor antagonists lack evidence of clear efficacy.
- Pulmonary artery catheters have no benefit, and in some cases increase risk to patients when used to guide therapy for shock.
- Given the relative expense of colloids, crystalloid administration for distributive shock is generally preferred.
- There is no role for procalcitonin measurement in sepsis that is likely due to infection.
- There is no role for glucocorticoids in sepsis without shock.
- Home sleep testing is preferred in a patient with a high probability of obstructive sleep apnea without underlying cardiopulmonary or neuromuscular disease (see Item 4).

# Pulmonary and Critical Care Medicine

## Pulmonary Diagnostic Tests

### Pulmonary Function Testing

Pulmonary function testing is an essential tool to diagnose obstructive and restrictive pathophysiology and to quantify the severity of the abnormality. Pulmonary function testing can include spirometry, bronchial challenge testing, lung volume testing, and measurement of diffusion capacity of the lung for carbon monoxide ($D_{LCO}$). These findings are compared to age, sex, height, and race-adjusted population norms and expressed as a percent of the predicted value (**Table 1**). Values below 80% of the predicted value are considered reduced. Recent American Thoracic Society guidelines alternatively use the lower limit of normal (below the fifth percentile of healthy never-smokers) as a cutoff, but in most cases this is very similar to 80% of the predicted value.

> **KEY POINT**
>
> - Pulmonary function test results below 80% of predicted or below the lower limit of normal are indicative of pulmonary impairment.

### Spirometry

Measurement of expiratory airflow and volume is an essential diagnostic and management test for patients with lung diseases. Spirometry measures the maximal volume and flow of air during a best-effort, forced exhalation; reported values include the $FEV_1$, the FVC, and the $FEV_1$/FVC ratio. Measurement of maximal expiratory flow by peak flow meter is commonly used at home and in office settings to follow and manage patients with asthma, but is not considered a valid diagnostic tool for airways disease. Spirometry correlates with hand-held peak expiratory flow-meter measurements, but is more reliable, provides more data, and is used in both diagnosis and management of airways disease. Although spirometry is easily performed in the outpatient setting, technical test validation and patient factors—including poor effort, coughing, and failure to exhale for a minimum of 6 seconds—may result in suboptimal test performance and misinterpretation. ☐

### Bronchial Challenge Testing

Bronchial challenge testing is used to identify bronchial hyper-responsiveness, a diagnostic feature of asthma. This is particularly helpful in patients whose symptoms are suggestive of asthma but for whom other pulmonary function test results are normal. Patients inhale increasing doses of a substance known to induce bronchospasm, such as methacholine or histamine, in a stepwise fashion. This is followed by repeated measurements of $FEV_1$; if $FEV_1$ falls by 20% or more from the baseline value, the test is considered positive. Bronchial challenge testing has a high negative predictive value for diagnosing asthma; however, a positive test can be caused by other conditions including COPD, smoking, upper respiratory infections, allergic rhinitis, bronchiectasis, and cystic fibrosis.

> **KEY POINT**
>
> - Bronchial challenge testing is a helpful diagnostic tool in patients whose symptoms are suggestive of asthma but for whom other pulmonary function test results are normal.

### Lung Volumes and $D_{LCO}$

Measures of lung volume include total lung capacity (TLC), vital capacity (VC), and residual volume (RV). $D_{LCO}$ measurement estimates the amount of gas transfer through the alveolar/capillary unit and is proportional to the surface area of functional lung. $D_{LCO}$ is measured by inhalation of a gas mixture containing carbon monoxide and helium; the resulting value is corrected for hemoglobin level.

### Pulmonary Function Testing Interpretation

The purpose of pulmonary function testing interpretation is to classify abnormal results as an obstructive, a restrictive, or a mixed obstructive/restrictive pattern and to assess the severity of

| TABLE 1. Characterization of Impairment Severity in Pulmonary Function Tests | |
|---|---|
| **Severity of Impairment** | **% of Predicted** |
| $FEV_1$ | |
| Mild | 79-70 |
| Moderate | 60-69 |
| Moderately severe | 50-59 |
| Severe | 35-49 |
| Very severe | <35 |
| $D_{LCO}$ | |
| Mild | <LLN but >60 |
| Moderate | 40-60 |
| Severe | <40 |

LLN = lower limit of normal; below the fifth percentile of healthy never-smokers.

Reproduced with permission from ©ERS 2018. Pellegrino R, Viegi G, Brusasco V, Crapo RO, Burgos F, Casaburi R, et al. Interpretative strategies for lung function tests. Eur Respir J. 2005;26:948-68. [PMID: 16264058] doi: 10.1183/09031936.05.00035205

impairment (**Figure 1**). The initial step is to review the results of spirometry. An FEV$_1$/FVC ratio below 0.70 is consistent with obstruction, and the severity is determined based on the measured FEV$_1$ as a percent of the predicted value (see Table 1). Reversibility of obstruction is determined by the response to a short-acting inhaled bronchodilator. An increase from baseline in FEV$_1$, FVC, or both of at least 12% and at least 200 mL indicates a positive bronchodilator response (reversibility). The TLC is normal or even increased in pure obstructive disease. Elevation of TLC and residual volume (120% or greater of predicted) can be observed in obstruction and generally is indicative of hyperinflation and air trapping, a common pattern in severe COPD or asthma.

If FEV$_1$ or FVC is reduced and the FEV$_1$/FVC ratio is 0.70 or greater, then the pattern may be interpreted as restrictive, but measurement of TLC is needed to confirm this. If the TLC is below 80% of predicted (or the lower limit of normal) a restrictive pattern is present.

Some patients may present with coexisting obstructive and restrictive pulmonary disorders, such as a COPD patient who develops an interstitial lung disease. In these cases, a low FEV$_1$/FVC ratio (obstructive pattern) and a low TLC (restrictive pattern) are both present.

D$_{LCO}$ is reduced in conditions where functioning alveolar capillary units are destroyed (COPD), infiltrated (interstitial lung diseases), removed (lung resection), or their function is compromised (pulmonary parenchymal and vascular disorders). Conditions that increase pulmonary capillary blood volume, such as pulmonary alveolar hemorrhage, left-to-right shunt, or asthma, can cause an elevation in D$_{LCO}$.

The flow-volume loop is a graphic representation of maximally forced inspiratory and expiratory flow (on the Y-axis) against volume (on the X-axis). The shape of the spirometric flow-volume loop is also useful in differentiating obstructive from restrictive patterns (**Figure 2**).

**KEY POINTS**

- The purpose of pulmonary function testing interpretation is to classify abnormal results as either an obstructive or restrictive pattern and to assess the severity of impairment.
- The FEV$_1$/FVC ratio is the primary measurement that defines obstructive disease, and total lung capacity is the primary measurement to confirm restrictive disease.

## 6-Minute Walk Test

The 6-minute walk test provides a valid and reliable measurement of exercise capacity in patients with lung disease. Patients walk at their own pace along a course for 6 minutes,

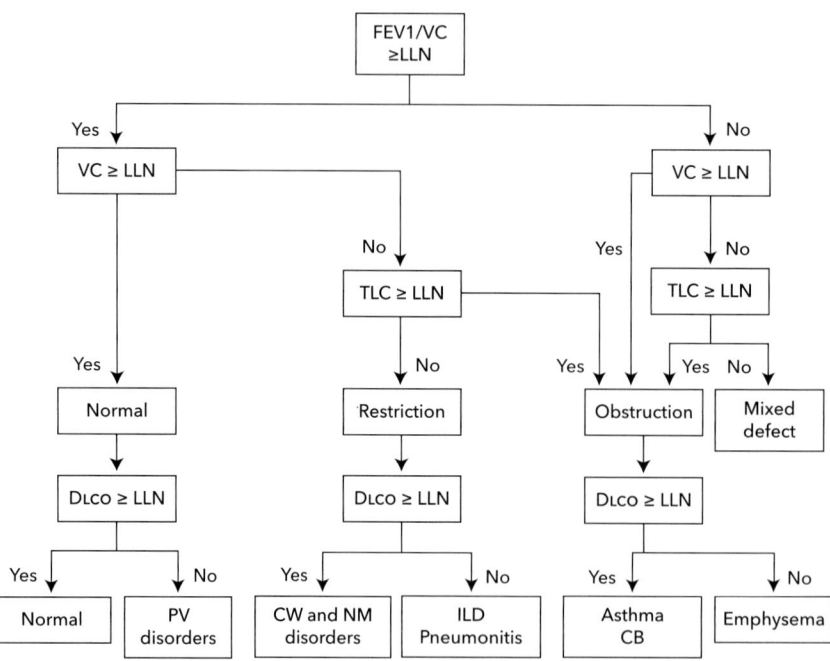

**FIGURE 1.** A simplified algorithm such as this may be used to assess lung function in clinical practice. It presents classic patterns for various pulmonary disorders. As in any such diagram, patients may or may not present with the classic patterns, depending on their illnesses, severity, and lung function prior to the disease onset (for example, did they start with a vital capacity [VC] close to the upper or lower limit of normal [LLN]?). The decisions about how far to follow this diagram are clinical, and will vary depending on the questions being asked and the clinical information available at the time of testing. The FEV$_1$/VC ratio and VC should be considered first. Total lung capacity (TLC) is necessary to confirm or exclude the presence of a restrictive defect when VC is below the LLN. The algorithm also includes D$_{LCO}$ measurement with the predicted value adjusted for hemoglobin. In the mixed defect group, the D$_{LCO}$ patterns are the same as those for restriction and obstruction. This flow chart is not suitable for assessing the severity of upper airway obstruction. CB = chronic bronchitis; CW = chest wall; ILD = interstitial lung diseases; NM = neuromuscular; PV = pulmonary vascular.

Reproduced with permission from ©ERS 2018. Pellegrino R, Viegi G, Brusasco V, Crapo RO, Burgos F, Casaburi R, et al. Interpretative strategies for lung function tests. Eur Respir J. 2005;26:948-68. [PMID: 16264058] doi: 10.1183/09031936.05.00035205

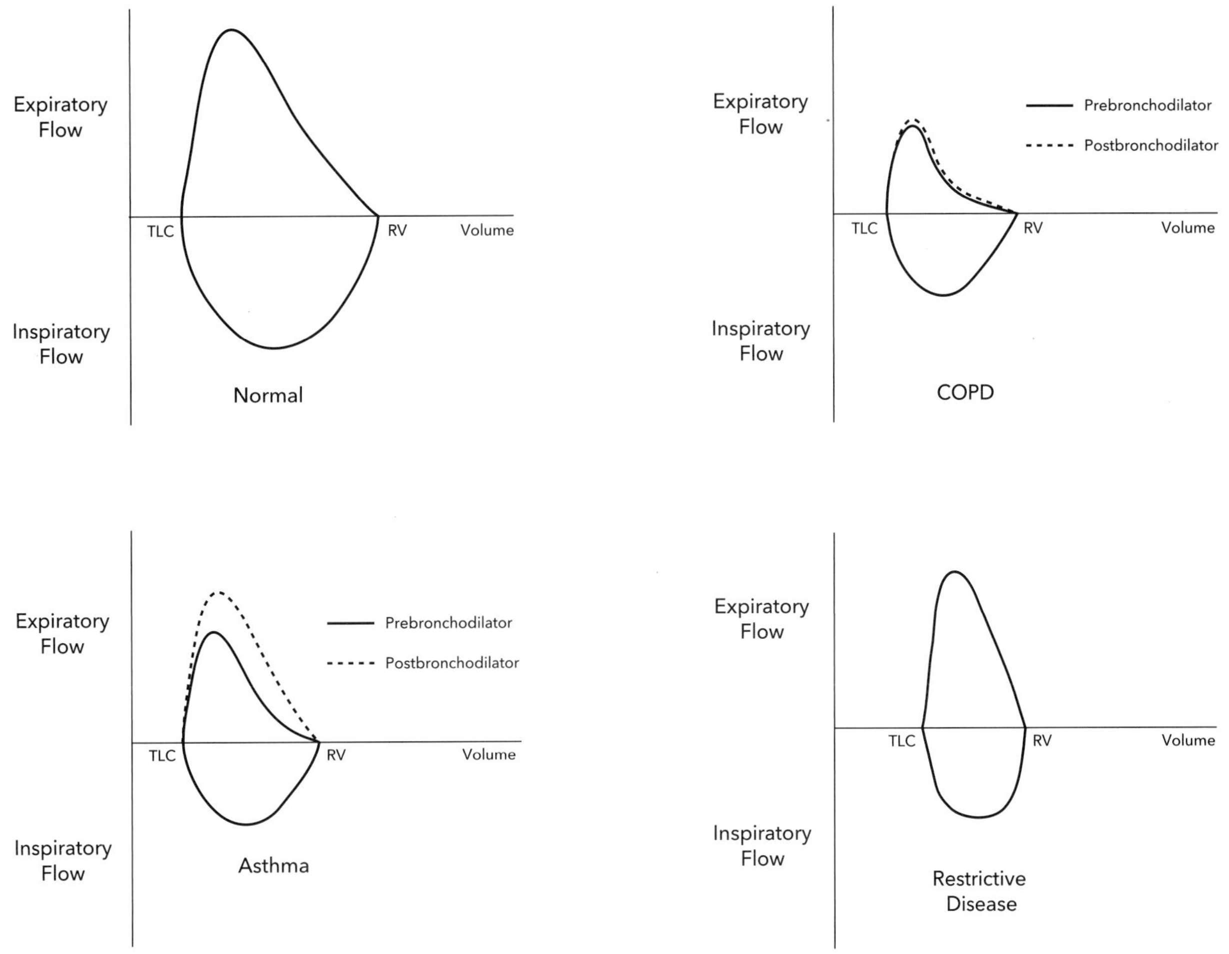

FIGURE 2. Pulmonary function test flow-volume patterns. RV = residual volume; TLC = total lung capacity.

and the total distance walked is recorded. Lower 6-minute walk test distances correlate with increased mortality in several lung diseases, including COPD, interstitial lung disease, and pulmonary arterial hypertension. Serial 6-minute walk testing may be used to assess response to therapy in patients with chronic respiratory disorders, especially pulmonary arterial hypertension.

## Pulse Oximetry

Pulse oximetry provides a readily available noninvasive measurement of oxygen-bound hemoglobin in the circulation. Oximeters work by calculating the differential between absorption of infrared light by oxygenated and deoxygenated blood. A normal hemoglobin saturation measured by pulse oximetry is 95% to 100% and values below 90% indicate hypoxemia. Substances in the blood that absorb infrared light may cause erroneous readings, including carboxyhemoglobin (present in carbon monoxide poisoning), methemoglobin (caused by nitrates), methylene blue, and some topical anesthetics. More commonly, patient factors such as cool extremities, poor circulation, and motion artifact result in erroneous

readings. In these cases, alternative methods of measuring oxygenation are needed.

# Imaging and Bronchoscopy

## Imaging

### Chest Radiography

Conventional chest radiographs are indicated as the initial imaging procedure for most patients with significant respiratory symptoms. Posteroanterior and lateral views should be obtained. Advantages are the availability of testing and low dose of radiation exposure for the patient. Limitations of chest radiographs include patient factors such as the need to take a deep inspiration, breath holding, image resolution, and the 2-dimensional nature of the images.

### Computed Tomography

CT of the thorax allows detailed, high-resolution imaging of the lungs and options for both static and dynamic imaging techniques. Helical scanners allow rapid scanning, but may require patients to hold their breath at full inspiration for 30 or

CONT.

more seconds. Reconstruction can include sagittal and coronal images, which result in 3-dimensional representation of the extent and distribution of disease. More specialized techniques reformat the data to highlight imaging of specific structures, such as maximum intensity projection (MIP), which focuses on the vasculature, and minimum intensity projection (MINIP), which focuses on the airways. Additional variables in CT imaging including slice thickness and interval; contrast enhancement may be used to augment the value of imaging based on the underlying disease.

The choice of examination will depend on the clinical context and information sought. For most patients, a routine (slice thickness of 2 or 2.5 mm) noncontrast CT is sufficient to provide the needed information. For patients suspected of having interstitial lung disease, a high-resolution (slice thickness of 1 mm) study should be ordered. Addition of expiratory views can evaluate for air trapping and further inform the diagnosis of small airways disease. However, because the slice interval (the distance between individual slices) with high-resolution CT is larger than with conventional CT, this technique "skips" interval sections of the lung and should not be used to evaluate lung nodules. Use of intravenous contrast dye helps delineate mediastinal structures and is particularly useful in patients with suspected lymphadenopathy or vascular pathology. CT angiography is used for detection of pulmonary embolism and utilizes a rapid, timed bolus of intravenous contrast.

CT scanning exposes the patient to a much higher dose of radiation than traditional chest radiographs, and CT is currently the primary source of imaging radiation exposure for patients. Efforts to reduce radiation doses are ongoing, and low-dose CT scanning of the chest is now the recommended choice for lung cancer screening in the United States (see Lung Tumors).

**KEY POINT**

- High-resolution CT techniques are preferred for evaluation of interstitial lung disease, conventional noncontrast CT is used to evaluate lung nodules, and CT angiography is used for detection of pulmonary embolism.

### Positron Emission Tomography Scanning
PET scans utilize the radionuclide 18-fluoro-2-deoxyglucose, which accumulates within highly metabolically active cells such as cancer cells, and can be visualized as discrete areas of uptake. Integrated PET/CT scanning allows improved localization of the metabolic activity. PET scans are widely used to evaluate risk of malignancy in lung nodules, to stage known thoracic tumors, and to evaluate for metastatic disease from other non-thoracic malignancies. False positive PET scans can occur in other hypermetabolic conditions where cells accumulate fluorodeoxyglucose, such as infection or inflammation. False negatives can occur when tumors have low rates of metabolic activity, such as carcinoid, adenocarcinoma in situ, and, rarely, metastatic kidney,

prostate, or testicular cancer. PET scanning is not useful for determination of malignant potential in lung nodules less than 8 mm in size.

### Bronchoscopy and Endobronchial Ultrasound
Bronchoscopy is a diagnostic and therapeutic tool for patients with lung disorders (**Table 2**). It is used for the diagnosis of localized and diffuse pulmonary diseases. It is important in the diagnostic evaluation for pulmonary infections, particularly in the immunocompromised host, and also has various therapeutic uses (**Table 3**). The addition of endobronchial ultrasound (EBUS) to visualize mediastinal and hilar lymph nodes for needle aspiration has made EBUS bronchoscopy the initial procedure of choice for obtaining tissue from mediastinal and hilar lymph nodes in the diagnosis and staging of patients with known or suspected thoracic malignancy.

**KEY POINT**

- Endobronchial ultrasound (EBUS) is the initial procedure of choice for obtaining tissue from mediastinal and hilar lymph nodes in the staging of patients with known or suspected thoracic malignancy.

# Airways Disease
## Asthma
### Epidemiology and Natural History
Asthma is an inflammatory disorder of the airways characterized by cough, wheezing, chest tightness, dyspnea, and variable airflow obstruction. Asthma is a major health burden throughout the world, and approximately 7.4% of the U.S. population has been diagnosed with asthma, accounting for more than 10 million office visits per year. Prevalence is increased among patients older than 65 years, women, blacks, and persons below the poverty level. Mortality in asthma is significant, causing 10.3 deaths per million Americans in 2015, with significantly higher mortality among patients who are black or are older than 65 years.

The onset of asthma can occur at any age, and the natural history varies with the duration and severity of symptoms, sex, and response to therapy. Children often have a family history of atopy, or exposure to sensitizing allergens such as dust mites or cockroaches. Childhood asthma may improve or resolve during teen and adult years, particularly in males. New-onset asthma in adults may have occupational exposures known to induce bronchial hyperreactivity. Those with severe symptoms generally have a more persistent course, lower pulmonary function, and increased risks of developing fixed airway obstruction. Diagnosis and treatment of asthma in older adults is often challenged by symptom overlap with other conditions (COPD, heart failure) and the normal effects of aging on pulmonary physiology.

| TABLE 2. | Bronchoscopic Diagnostic Procedures | |
|---|---|---|
| **Technique** | **Description** | **Examples of Indications** |
| Airway inspection | Visualization of the tracheobronchial tree to the level of segmental airways | Hemoptysis |
| | | Localized wheeze |
| | | Persistent atelectasis |
| | | Diagnosis of tracheobronchomalacia |
| | | Inhalational injury |
| Bronchial washings | Samples from large airways | Diagnosis of infections |
| Bronchoalveolar lavage | Samples from small bronchi and alveoli | Diagnosis of infections |
| | | Cell counts in diagnosis of parenchymal lung disease |
| | | Alveolar hemorrhage |
| | | Cytology for malignancy |
| Bronchial brushings | Brushings of the endobronchial mucosa for cells | Endobronchial lesions |
| Endobronchial biopsy | Biopsy within the airway lumen | Endobronchial mass or lesion |
| Transbronchial lung biopsy | Biopsy of the lung parenchyma or lung nodules/masses using small forceps; often aided by guidance technology including electromagnetic navigation and radial ultrasound | Diffuse lung disease |
| | | Persistent infiltrates |
| | | Lung nodules/masses |
| | | Posttransplant rejection |
| Transbronchial needle aspiration | Aspiration of a lymph node or mass adjacent to the airway | Lymphadenopathy |
| | | Pulmonary mass |
| | | Mediastinal mass |
| Endobronchial ultrasound | Use of an ultrasound probe at the distal end of the bronchoscope to guide transbronchial needle aspiration | Lymphadenopathy |
| | | Pulmonary mass |
| | | Mediastinal mass |
| Electromagnetic navigation | Images from a recent CT are "linked" with the bronchoscope. An electromagnetic guidance system at the bronchoscope creates a map of the airways and guides the physician to the area of interest. | Pulmonary mass or nodule |

| TABLE 3. | Bronchoscopic Therapeutic Procedures | |
|---|---|---|
| **Technique** | **Description** | **Examples of Indications** |
| Flexible bronchoscopy | Large airway suctioning | Lobar atelectasis from mucus plugs |
| | Basket and forceps | Foreign body |
| | Balloon tamponade of airway | Bleeding |
| Bronchial thermoplasty | Radiofrequency energy ablation of proximal airway smooth muscle | Severe asthma |
| Endobronchial stent placement | Bronchoscopic placement of silicon and metal prostheses to expand and support the airways | Malignant obstruction |
| | | Benign strictures |
| | | Tracheomalacia or bronchomalacia |
| | | Anastomotic dehiscence |
| Airway ablative therapies | Laser therapy | Malignant airway obstruction |
| | Electrocautery | Benign airway obstruction |
| | Argon plasma coagulation | Airway tumor ablation |
| | Cryotherapy | |
| | Brachytherapy | |
| Endobronchial valve placement | Airway placement of one-way valves | Bronchopleural fistula |
| | | Emphysema |
| Balloon dilation | Targeted endobronchial balloon inflation | Benign or malignant airway stricture |

- Approximately 7.4% of the U.S. population has been diagnosed with asthma, and prevalence is increased among patients older than 65 years, women, blacks, and persons below the poverty level.

## Pathogenesis

The pathophysiologic mechanisms of asthma include chronic airway inflammation, airway narrowing due to edema, subepithelial fibrosis, smooth muscle hypertrophy, and mucus hypersecretion, in addition to airway smooth muscle constriction causing bronchial hyperreactivity in response to various stimuli. The airway cellular inflammatory profile is variable; persists even during the absence of symptoms; and includes eosinophils, T lymphocytes, mast cells, and neutrophils. Eosinophilic inflammation is commonly recognized in allergic asthma, but patients may have other cellular profiles, with neutrophilic inflammation increasingly recognized in older patients. Bronchial hyperreactivity that causes airway obstruction is typically episodic and triggered by stimuli that would not induce symptoms in healthy people. Common triggers include allergens, dusts, fumes, exercise, extremes of temperature, and viral respiratory infections.

## Risk Factors

Risk factors for asthma include both host and environmental factors. Genes predisposing to atopy, bronchial hyperreactivity, and airway inflammation have been identified, but genetic predisposition is thought to interact with additional factors, including exposure to indoor allergens (mites, furred animals, cockroaches, molds) and outdoor allergens (pollens, molds), tobacco smoke, occupational sensitizers and allergens, viral respiratory infections, and air pollution. In addition, obesity is an important risk factor for asthma.

Asthma is heterogeneous, but distinct phenotypes are recognized and have implications for underlying mechanisms, treatment, and outcomes. Although specific phenotypes are not yet broadly accepted, many are commonly described. Clinically recognizable groups include allergic, nonallergic, late-onset, adult onset eosinophilic, and obesity-associated asthma. These subsets tend to have different cellular compositions of airway inflammation and may respond variably to anti-inflammatory therapies.

- Genetic predisposition to asthma is thought to interact with additional factors, including exposure to indoor allergens (mites, furred animals, cockroaches, molds) and outdoor allergens (pollens, molds), tobacco smoke, occupational sensitizers and allergens, viral respiratory infections, and air pollution.

## Symptoms and Clinical Evaluation

Common symptoms of asthma are cough, wheezing, chest tightness, and shortness of breath that are intermittent and occur in response to various potential stimuli, including allergens, infections, dusts, fumes, and exercise. Symptoms often have a diurnal variation, worsening in the evening and early morning. Viral respiratory infections are a particularly robust trigger for most patients. Variability of symptoms (both improvement and worsening of symptoms over time) is a key diagnostic feature of asthma.

History taking should establish whether the patient has ever smoked tobacco or other products, has pets, or has had environmental exposures (either recreationally or in the work place) to dust, fumes, or particulate matter known to cause bronchial hyperreactivity. A personal or family history of atopy or allergic sinus disease may be present. In particular, the presence of nasal polyps, sensitivity to aspirin, and wheezing is known as the "asthmatic triad." The physical examination may demonstrate wheezing, reduced airflow, or a prolonged expiratory phase. However, patients may also have a completely normal respiratory exam, particularly when they are symptom-free.

Confirmation of reversible airflow obstruction is a cornerstone of asthma diagnosis and can be assessed by spirometry, with measurement of forced expiratory volume in one second ($FEV_1$), forced vital capacity (FVC), and the $FEV_1$/FVC ratio, or by serial measurement of peak expiratory flow rates. Airway obstruction that improves with bronchodilators, on subsequent measurements, or after 4 weeks of anti-inflammatory treatment supports a diagnosis of asthma. For adults, a significant change in $FEV_1$ is an increase from baseline of at least 12% and at least 200 mL. For some patients, airflow obstruction is not present during the initial evaluation, and demonstration of bronchial hyperreactivity with bronchial challenge testing is indicated. This is usually performed with inhaled methacholine, although other stimuli (exercise, mannitol) have been validated. If a bronchial challenge test is negative, it is unlikely that a patient has asthma. A positive challenge test confirms bronchial hyperreactivity, but is not sufficient to confirm asthma because other disorders may demonstrate this finding. Therefore, clinical correlation of this finding with symptoms and other testing is needed.

A chest radiograph is helpful in many patients to rule out other diagnoses, such as COPD, heart failure, parenchymal lung disorders, central airway obstruction, and bronchiectasis. This is especially important in older adults, in whom asthma is often underrecognized and undertreated.

- Common symptoms of asthma are cough, wheezing, chest tightness, and shortness of breath that are intermittent and occur in response to various potential stimuli, including allergens, infections, dusts, fumes, and exercise.

- Confirmation of reversible airflow obstruction with bronchodilators is a cornerstone of asthma diagnosis and can be assessed by spirometry, with measurement of $FEV_1$, FVC, and the $FEV_1$/FVC ratio showing an increase from baseline of ≥12% and ≥200 mL.

*(Continued)*

- In patients with clinical symptoms suggestive of asthma but with normal spirometry, bronchial challenge testing (such as with methacholine) may be helpful to evaluate for asthma. A negative test excludes asthma, whereas a positive test requires clinical correlation and may require additional testing.

## Asthma Syndromes

### Allergic Asthma

Identifying the presence of atopy can identify an allergic asthma phenotype in a patient with respiratory symptoms. The most common tests are allergy skin prick tests, which may be administered in the outpatient setting by qualified personnel, or laboratory measurement of allergen-specific IgE in serum. Results of each method are generally concordant. Skin testing is more sensitive but subject to errors related to administration, whereas serum tests are more specific but have higher costs. Measurement of total serum IgE is not useful because a normal level does not preclude clinical allergies. However, IgE is a therapeutic target for advanced treatments such as omalizumab (monoclonal antibody targeting IgE in severe atopic asthma), so measurement of IgE can help guide the use of these agents.

Identifying eosinophilic airway inflammation through either elevated serum or sputum eosinophil counts, or measurement of exhaled nitric oxide levels, may help phenotype patients. A phenotype of severe adult-onset asthma with significant eosinophilia has been recognized, often without a significant component of allergies or atopy. These patients often require treatment with systemic glucocorticoids and may be appropriate for advanced anti-interleukin therapies such as mepolizumab.

### Cough-Variant Asthma

Patients with asthma whose primary symptom manifestation is chronic cough without other symptoms are considered to have cough-variant asthma. Diagnosis requires documentation of bronchial hyperreactivity, as most patients will have normal baseline spirometry. Recommended therapies are the same as those for other types of asthma. Other causes of chronic cough should be investigated, including gastroesophageal reflux and upper airway cough syndrome due to rhinitis. Frequently, these etiologies coexist and require concomitant therapy (see MKSAP 18 General Internal Medicine).

### Exercise-Induced Bronchospasm

Exercise-induced bronchospasm (EIB) refers to acute, measurable airway obstruction that occurs in response to exercise. EIB is one of the most common triggers of symptoms in patients with known asthma, and also occurs in patients without asthma, typically elite athletes, during periods of high-intensity exercise. Environmental factors play a key role in precipitating symptoms. Exercise in cold, dry air, such as during winter or in indoor ice rinks; exposure to high levels of trichloramines in swimming pools; and inhalation of airborne particulates and ozone have all been implicated.

Other disorders, such vocal cord dysfunction and cardiac disorders, can mimic EIB; therefore, establishing the presence of bronchial hyperreactivity is crucial to make an accurate diagnosis. For most patients this entails bronchial challenge testing with inhaled agents or, ideally, exercise. Initial pharmacologic therapy should consist of administration of an inhaled short-acting β2-agonist (SABA) 15 minutes before exercise. If patients require use of a SABA every day, or have inadequate symptom control, a second controller agent (inhaled glucocorticoid or a leukotriene receptor antagonist) should be added. Nonpharmacologic measures including preexercise warm-up and warming cold air before inhalation (such as a mask or scarf) are also recommended.

- Initial pharmacologic therapy for exercise-induced bronchospasm should consist of administration of a short-acting β2-agonist 15 minutes before exercise.

### Occupational Asthma

A careful occupational history is an essential part of asthma evaluation, as it is estimated that 15% of adult asthma is work-related. Occupational asthma includes asthma directly caused by exposure to sensitizing or irritant substances in the workplace, as well as preexisting asthma that is exacerbated by these same factors. Typical sensitizing agents are high molecular weight substances, such as proteins, that induce an IgE-mediated immunologic response. Examples include animal and plant allergens, latex, grains, and diisocyanates. Once sensitized, patients may subsequently react to very low levels of exposure. Those at risk include farmers and animal workers, health care workers, latex glove users, bakers, and manufacturers of polyurethane products. A key clinical indicator is the relationship of symptoms to work exposures; patients often improve during weekends and time away from work. Spirometry before and after workplace exposures is a cost-effective way to confirm a suspected diagnosis of occupational asthma. Alternatively, demonstration of bronchial hyperreactivity through bronchial challenge testing or serial peak flow measurements can be used. Treatment consists of reducing exposure to the offending agent through workplace modifications or removing patients from the workplace entirely, in addition to pharmacologic therapy. The overriding principle of treatment should be prevention, which includes workplace interventions to avoid exposures and monitoring for early identification of disease.

- A key clinical indicator of occupational asthma is symptom improvement during weekends and time away from work; spirometry before and after workplace exposures is a cost-effective way to confirm a suspected diagnosis.

**HVC**

7

## Reactive Airways Dysfunction Syndrome

Reactive airways dysfunction syndrome is a well-described subset of irritant-induced occupational asthma. This syndrome occurs in patients without preexisting asthma following a single, high-level exposure to fumes, gases, or vapors; usually the exposure is severe enough to prompt immediate medical evaluation. The diagnosis requires evidence of asthmatic symptoms for at least 3 months following the exposure and is confirmed by airway obstruction or bronchial hyperreactivity.

## Aspirin-Exacerbated Respiratory Disease

Aspirin-exacerbated respiratory disease describes asthma and rhinosinusitis that are precipitated by exposure to aspirin or other NSAIDs that inhibit cyclooxygenase-1. Clinical characteristics include an onset in adulthood; airway and peripheral eosinophilia; inflammatory sinusitis with polyposis; and persistent, often severe asthma. Ingestion of triggering substances can cause life-threatening bronchospasm within minutes to hours, sometimes accompanied by rhinorrhea, conjunctival injection, and flushing. Chronic management, in addition to the usual stepped asthma care includes discontinuing all NSAIDs and use of leukotriene-receptor antagonists that target the increased leukotriene production implicated in the mechanism of this particular asthma. Aspirin desensitization can improve control in a significant percentage of patients but requires specialized expertise.

## Allergic Bronchopulmonary Aspergillosis

Allergic bronchopulmonary aspergillosis is an ongoing immunologic response to inhaled *Aspergillus* species that leads to persistent eosinophilic airway inflammation, increased IgE levels (both total and *Aspergillus* specific), and eventually tissue damage with airway remodeling. Patients present with difficult-to-control asthma, productive cough, and expectoration of brownish mucus plugs. Radiographs may demonstrate pulmonary infiltrates and bronchiectasis. The diagnostic criteria are debated but include the presence of asthma, elevated IgE levels, positive skin tests to *Aspergillus* antigens, increased pulmonary *Aspergillus*-specific IgE and IgG levels, and either central bronchiectasis or infiltrates. Management is aimed at suppressing the enhanced immunologic response with systemic glucocorticoids and reducing the fungal antigenic burden with antifungal agents.

## Common Comorbidities

Comorbidities in asthma are common and should be considered and actively managed to reduce symptoms and potentially improve asthma control.

## Gastroesophageal Reflux Disease

Gastroesophageal reflux disease frequently coexists in asthma patients, and may be an independent cause of respiratory symptoms such as cough and chest pain. In patients with active gastroesophageal reflux disease symptoms, an empiric trial of a proton pump inhibitor for 2 months is indicated. Patients whose reflux symptoms do not improve should be considered for further testing such as endoscopy and 24-hour esophageal pH monitoring (see MKSAP 18 Gastroenterology and Hepatology).

## Sinus Disease

Disease of the upper airway, including rhinitis and sinusitis, is extremely common in patients with asthma and is associated with more severe asthma symptoms. Allergic rhinitis is an IgE-driven inflammatory response to sensitizing allergens, and is characterized by rhinorrhea, nasal obstruction, itching, and sneezing. Symptoms can be seasonal, intermittent, or perennial (usually caused by persistent exposure to indoor allergens such as dust mites). Patients with chronic rhinosinusitis have endogenous, ongoing inflammation of both the nose and paranasal sinuses, with additional symptoms of facial pain, sinus pressure, and sometimes anosmia. Those that develop nasal polyposis have more-difficult-to-control asthma. Guidelines suggest treating with intranasal glucocorticoids; more severe cases may require combined use of intranasal glucocorticoid and intranasal H1-antihistamines, oral antileukotrienes, oral glucocorticoids, biologics targeting IgE, and immunotherapy.

## Obstructive Sleep Apnea

Symptomatic obstructive sleep apnea (OSA) and polysomnographic evidence of OSA are more common in patients with asthma compared to those without asthma. The association becomes stronger with increasing severity of asthma. The presence of OSA also worsens asthma control, increases asthma-related health care utilization, and reduces quality of life. Although nocturnal worsening of asthma symptoms is common, patients should also be asked about snoring, excessive daytime sleepiness, and witnessed apneas, which are typical symptoms of OSA. If present, diagnostic testing to confirm the presence of OSA is indicated because treatment of OSA improves asthma outcomes, including symptoms, quality of life, bronchodilator use, and peak flow rates.

## Vocal Cord Dysfunction

Vocal cord dysfunction refers to paradoxical adduction of the vocal cords during inspiration, leading to functional upper airway obstruction. This entity is important as its symptoms mimic those of asthma. Vocal cord dysfunction should be considered in the differential diagnosis of asthma, particularly if patients complain of prominent inspiratory breathlessness, with throat tightness or voice dysfunction during attacks. Symptoms are often triggered by exercise, exposure to fumes or irritants, and stress. Patients with vocal cord dysfunction do not respond to standard asthma therapy. Vocal cord dysfunction also can coexist with asthma. The gold standard diagnosis is demonstration of the paradoxical vocal cord adduction using direct laryngoscopy during a symptomatic episode. However, patients are generally asymptomatic when evaluated or unable to tolerate the maneuver during an acute episode. Therefore, in patients with suggestive symptoms, a trial of treatment is often indicated. Management includes addressing factors known to worsen vocal cord dysfunction (gastro-esophageal reflux disease, postnasal drip), but the mainstay of treatment is speech therapy, which employs cognitive-behavioral techniques to self-identify triggers and symptoms and to reduce the functional obstruction.

**KEY POINT**

- Vocal cord dysfunction should be considered in the differential diagnosis of asthma, particularly if patients complain of prominent inspiratory breathlessness, with throat tightness or voice dysfunction during attacks.

## Obesity

Obese patients have a higher prevalence of asthma and poorer control of symptoms. Increased BMI appears to influence asthma through mechanisms related to both systemic inflammation and respiratory mechanics. Obese patients with asthma do not respond as well to standard controller therapies as nonobese patients, possibly because of an alternate inflammatory profile or the presence of comorbidities associated with obesity, such as gastroesophageal reflux disease and OSA. Asthma may be overdiagnosed and underdiagnosed in obese patients because of the overlap of symptoms of breathlessness and exertional wheezing. Therefore, it is important to measure BMI in all patients undergoing asthma evaluation and to objectively document reversible airway obstruction through pulmonary function testing. In patients with obesity-related asthma, weight loss has been demonstrated to improve asthma control and lung function and should be considered an essential part of the treatment plan. In some patients, bariatric surgery may be indicated because greater amounts of weight loss correlate with better outcomes, including reduction in asthma exacerbations, improved quality of life, improved lung function, and decreased systemic and bronchial inflammation (see MKSAP 18 General Internal Medicine).

## Management of Chronic Asthma

The goals of longitudinal asthma management are to control chronic asthma symptoms, prevent acute exacerbations, and minimize risks of developing fixed airway obstruction. This should be accomplished by assessing asthma severity, controlling symptoms on an ongoing basis, and then modifying therapies appropriately using a stepwise approach (**Figure 3**). There are three essential components to the management of asthma:

1. Assessment of symptom control and risk—Standardized, validated questionnaires that can discriminate between well-controlled and inadequately controlled asthma based on patient symptoms include the Asthma Control Test and the Asthma Control Questionnaire. Patients with daytime symptoms less than twice weekly and nocturnal symptoms less than twice monthly during the preceding 4 weeks are considered well controlled. Risk is based on measured lung function and the potential for future exacerbations, which is related to the presence of comorbidities and historical features known to predict future exacerbations.

2. Treatment—Once symptoms and risk are established, therapy should be initiated. All patients with asthma should be provided with rescue medication to use as needed for symptoms. Controller medications are used as a maintenance therapy to control symptoms and prevent exacerbations. A critical component of this therapy is teaching and assessing proper inhaler technique, as patients require skill and training to effectively use these devices. Use of a spacer can be helpful with compatible inhaler devices.

3. Review response and adjust therapy—After initiation of asthma therapies, patients should be reassessed after several months for their level of control and tolerance of medications. Controller medications can be stepped up or down with the goal to maintain symptom control and minimize medication exposure.

**KEY POINTS**

- Control of asthma should be assessed with the use of validated questionnaires.

- Inhaler skills training and adherence are essential for successful treatment.

### Quick Relief Medications

All patients with asthma should be provided with quick relief, or rescue, therapy. Short-acting $\beta_2$-agonists (SABAs) are the preferred medications to quickly reverse bronchospasm and relieve acute asthma symptoms (**Table 4**). These inhaled agents have a rapid onset of action and deliver medications directly through the airways, reducing systemic side effects; SABAs are generally well tolerated. Their main mechanism of action is induction of airway smooth muscle relaxation using stimulation of $\beta_2$-agonist receptors. SABAs should be used as needed for symptoms and are generally not administered on a scheduled basis. They may also be used before exercise to prevent EIB. Albuterol is the most commonly used SABA in the United States. Use of SABAs as single-agent asthma therapy is only indicated for patients with symptoms occurring not more than twice weekly, normal lung function between exacerbations, and nocturnal symptoms not more than twice monthly. For all others, rescue therapy is used in conjunction with controller therapy.

Short-acting inhaled anticholinergics are less effective than SABAs at relieving acute bronchospasm; however, they may be used as adjunctive therapy to SABA treatment in the management of acute exacerbations in the emergency department; this combination has been shown to reduce hospital admission rates. **H**

**KEY POINTS**

- All patients with asthma should be provided with quick relief, or rescue, therapy.

- Short-acting $\beta_2$-agonists are the preferred medications to quickly reverse bronchospasm and relieve acute asthma symptoms.

| Intermittent asthma | **Persistent asthma: Daily medication**<br>Consult with asthma specialist if step 4 care or higher is required<br>Consider consultation at step 3 |
|---|---|

**Step 1**

*Preferred:*
SABA PRN

**Step 2**

*Preferred:*
Low-dose IG

*Alternative:*
LTRA or
theophylline

**Step 3**

*Preferred:*
Low-dose IG
+ LABA

OR

Medium-dose IG

*Alternative:*
Low-dose
IG + LTRA,
theophylline,
or zileuton

**Step 4**

*Preferred:*
Medium-dose
IG + LABA

*Alternative:*
Medium-dose
IG + LTRA,
theophylline,
or zileuton

**Step 5**

*Preferred:*
High-dose
IG + LABA

AND

Consider
omalizumab for
patients who
have allergies

**Step 6**

*Preferred:*
High-dose IG
+ LABA + oral
glucocorticoid

AND

Consider
omalizumab for
patients who
have allergies

Step up if
needed

(first check
adherence,
environmental
control, and
comorbid
conditions)

Assess
control

Step down if
possible

(and asthma is
well controlled
at least
3 months)

**Each step: Patient education, environmental control, and management of comorbidities**

Steps 2-4: Consider subcutaneous allergen immunotherapy for patients who have allergic asthma

Quick-relief medication for all patients:

- SABA as needed for symptoms. Intensity of treatment depends on severity of symptoms: up to 3 treatments at 20-minute intervals as needed. Short course of oral systemic glucocorticoid may be needed.

- Use of SABA >2 days a week for symptom relief (not prevention of EIB) generally indicates inadequate control and the need to step up treatment.

**FIGURE 3.** Stepwise approach to asthma therapy. EIB = exercise-induced bronchospasm; IG = inhaled glucocorticoid; LABA = long-acting $\beta_2$-agonist; LTRA = leukotriene receptor antagonist; PRN = as needed; SABA = short-acting $\beta_2$-agonist.

Source: National Heart, Lung, and Blood Institute; National Institutes of Health; U.S. Department of Health and Human Services. National Asthma Education and Prevention Program. Expert Panel Report 3 (EPR-3): Guidelines for the Diagnosis and Management of Asthma. www.nhlbi.nih.gov/files/docs/guidelines/asthsumm.pdf. Published 2007. Accessed May 9, 2018.

## Controller Medications

Controller medications are used to provide ongoing symptom relief and to prevent asthma exacerbations. Several different classes of controllers exist that target different mechanisms of the asthmatic profile; therefore, medications can be effectively combined to achieve good control. The choice of therapy generally depends on the assessment of risk as described in **Management of Chronic Asthma**, and adjusted based on symptom response and patient tolerance (see Figure 3 and Table 4).

Inhaled glucocorticoids are the most effective class of asthma controller medications. These agents alleviate several pathologic processes that comprise the asthmatic response, including airway mucosal edema, mucus hypersecretion, and airway inflammation. Many strengths and formulations are available, and because individual patient response can vary, it is reasonable to try an alternate brand if the therapeutic response is not adequate. Side effects are dose-related and vary

with the steroid formulation. Side effects relate to local deposition (oral candidiasis, dysphonia) and can sometimes be generalized due to some degree of systemic absorption. Systemic adverse effects such as adrenocortical suppression, reduced bone mineral density, and cataracts do not generally occur at doses below 400 µg of inhaled budesonide daily or equivalent doses of other inhaled glucocorticoid formulations. An increased rate of pneumonia is found with high-dose and high-potency formulations. Despite these risks, use of inhaled glucocorticoids to prevent the need for oral glucocorticoids should outweigh these potential adverse effects. In active smokers, the effectiveness of these medications is diminished, and higher dosing may be required.

Inhaled long-acting $\beta_2$-agonists (LABAs) that provide sustained airway dilation with just once- or twice-daily dosing are an important tool for asthma treatment. When added to inhaled glucocorticoids, they provide improved control and

| TABLE 4. Asthma Medications | | |
|---|---|---|
| **Drug** | **Formulations** | **Side Effects** |
| **Short-Acting $\beta_2$-Agonists** | | |
| Albuterol | HFA-MDI, nebulizer solution | Tachycardia and hypokalemia |
| Levalbuterol | HFA-MDI, nebulizer solution | |
| **Short-Acting Anticholinergics (Muscarinic Antagonists)** | | |
| Ipratropium bromide | HFA-MDI, nebulizer solution | Dry mouth, tachycardia, acute narrow angle glaucoma (rare) |
| Albuterol/ipratropium bromide | HFA-MDI, nebulizer solution | Same and combined effects of both drug classes |
| **Long-Acting $\beta_2$-Agonists** | | |
| Formoterol | DPI | Tremor, tachycardia; black box warning for use in asthma |
| Salmeterol | DPI | |
| Arformoterol | Nebulizer solution | |
| Formoterol fumarate | Nebulizer solution | |
| Olodaterol | SMI | |
| Indacaterol maleate | DPI | |
| **Long-Acting Muscarinic Antagonists (Anticholinergics)** | | |
| Tiotropium | DPI, SMI | Dry mouth, tachycardia, urinary retention, acute narrow angle glaucoma (rare) |
| Aclidinium bromide | DPI | |
| Umeclidinium | DPI | |
| Glycopyrrolate | DPI | |
| **Inhaled Glucocorticoids** | | |
| Beclomethasone | HFA-MDI | Dysphonia, oral candidiasis, skin bruising, pneumonia, side effects of oral glucocorticoids (rare) |
| Budesonide | DPI, nebulizer solution | |
| Fluticasone propionate | HFA, DPI | |
| Fluticasone furoate | DPI | |
| Mometasone | DPI | |
| Ciclesonide | HFA-MDI | |
| Flunisolide | HFA-MDI | |
| **Inhaled Glucocorticoid and Long-Acting $\beta_2$-Agonist** | | |
| Budesonide and formoterol | HFA | Same as combined effects of both drug classes |
| Fluticasone and salmeterol | HFA, DPI | |
| Mometasone furoate and formoterol fumarate | HFA | |
| Fluticasone furoate and vilanterol | DPI | |
| **Oral Glucocorticoids** | | |
| Prednisone | Tablet, liquid | Bruising, adrenal suppression, osteoporosis, glaucoma, diabetes mellitus, opportunistic infection, insomnia, cataracts, hypertension |
| Prednisolone | IV infusion, tablet | |
| **Long-Acting Muscarinic Antagonist and Long-Acting $\beta_2$-Agonist** | | |
| Tiotropium and olodaterol | SMI | Same as combined effects of both drug classes |
| Umeclidinium and vilanterol | DPI | |
| Glycopyrrolate and formoterol | MDI | |
| Indacaterol and glycopyrrolate | DPI | |

*(Continued on the next page)*

**TABLE 4.** Asthma Medications (*Continued*)

| Drug | Formulations | Side Effects |
|------|--------------|--------------|
| **Leukotriene-Receptor Antagonists** | | |
| Montelukast | Tablet | Headache, liver disease (rare) |
| Zafirlukast | Tablet | |
| Zileuton (5-lipoxygenase inhibitor) | Tablet | |
| **Biologic Agents** | | |
| Omalizumab (Anti-IgE) | Subcutaneous injection | Anaphylaxis, increased risk of malignancy |
| Mepolizumab (Anti-IL5) | Subcutaneous injection | |
| Reslizumab (Anti-IL5) | IV infusion | |
| **Other** | | |
| Theophylline | Tablet, capsule, liquid | Tachycardia, nausea, overdose can be fatal |

DPI = dry powder inhaler; HFA = hydrofluoroalkane; IV = intravenous; MDI = metered dose inhaler; SMI = soft mist inhaler.

decrease risk of exacerbation. For patients whose asthma is not adequately controlled by moderate-strength inhaled glucocorticoids, addition of a LABA as combined therapy with inhaled glucocorticoids in a single inhaler device is the recommended next step. Administration in a single inhaler is preferred because of greater adherence and reduced cost compared with administration of each drug in a separate inhaler. Single-agent use of LABAs is not recommended because of the demonstrated increased risk of asthma-related death when used without a simultaneous controller medication, which led the FDA to place a black box warning on all medications containing these agents. However, the FDA recently removed the black box warning from combination inhaled glucocorticoids and LABA inhalers because five large clinical trials have shown that LABAs, when used with inhaled glucocorticoids, do not significantly increase the risk of asthma-related hospitalization, intubation, or death compared to inhaled glucocorticoids alone and result in significantly fewer asthma exacerbations.

Leukotriene-receptor antagonists have a modest bronchodilation effect and treat upper airway conditions such as allergic rhinitis. Patients with aspirin-exacerbated respiratory disease often respond well to these agents.

Oral glucocorticoids are a cornerstone of therapy for treatment of acute asthma exacerbations, but long-term use exposes patients to the well-known side effects of these agents (see Table 4).

Long-acting muscarinic antagonists (LAMAs) provide sustained airway dilation, and when added to therapy in patients not controlled with inhaled glucocorticoid/LABA combination therapy, tiotropium has been shown to improve lung function and reduce exacerbations. For patients with excessive side effects from LABAs, a LAMA can reasonably be substituted. However, there is not substantial evidence that LAMAs should be the first choice for long-acting airway dilation instead of LABAs.

Newer but expensive antibody therapies directed against specific mediators of the asthmatic response can be used in patients with severe asthma not adequately controlled on standard therapy. Currently, two types of biologic therapies are available: those targeting IgE and those targeting eosinophils through the interleukin-5 pathway. Anti-IgE therapy (such as omalizumab) is indicated for use in patients with elevated levels of IgE and sensitivity to allergens, as documented by skin testing or elevated serum allergen-specific IgE. Mepolizumab and reslizumab are anti-interleukin-5 monoclonal antibodies that act to reduce eosinophil levels in airway and sputum by blocking the action of interleukin-5, a cytokine that plays a significant role in eosinophil recruitment and maturation. These agents are effective in patients with eosinophil levels above 150 cells/μL ($0.15 \times 10^9$/L), regardless of IgE level. Both anti-IgE and anti-interleukin-5 therapies reduce symptoms, need for oral glucocorticoids, and exacerbations in eligible patients with moderate or severe persistent asthma.

Although expensive, omalizumab reduces emergency department visits and may be cost-effective in eligible patients with moderate to severe atopic asthma not well controlled with other therapies.

**KEY POINTS**

- Inhaled glucocorticoids are the most effective class of asthma controller medications.

- For patients whose asthma is not adequately controlled by moderate strength inhaled glucocorticoids, addition of a long-acting $\beta_2$-agonist as combined therapy with an inhaled glucocorticoid in a single inhaler device is the recommended next step.

- Single-agent use of long-acting $\beta_2$-agonists is not recommended because of the demonstrated increased risk of asthma-related death when used without another controller medication.

- Targeting elevated IgE or eosinophil levels with antibody therapies in eligible patients with severe persistent allergic asthma despite standard therapy reduces symptoms, need for oral glucocorticoids, and exacerbations.

## Nonpharmacologic Therapy

Comprehensive asthma-care strategies include avoidance of triggers with allergen management (mold abatement, pest control, air filters), reduced exposure to environmental tobacco smoke, and a healthy diet and exercise program to promote weight loss.

Bronchial thermoplasty is a radiofrequency airway treatment administered using bronchoscopy that can reduce exacerbations and improve quality of life. Candidates are patients with an $FEV_1$ above 60% and severe asthma that is poorly controlled despite high-dose inhaled glucocorticoid/LABA combination therapy.

## Management of Asthma Exacerbations

Asthma exacerbation refers to an acute worsening in symptoms or lung function from baseline that necessitates a step-up in therapy (see Figure 3). Prompt recognition and treatment of asthma exacerbations are needed to relieve symptoms and prevent hospitalizations. All asthma patients should have a written asthma management plan that helps them to recognize the symptoms of an exacerbation and begin self-treatment. Clinicians should screen for patient factors that contribute to an increased risk of death from asthma and counsel patients appropriately (Table 5). Self-treatment of an exacerbation consists of frequent use of reliever medications; increasing the dose, frequency, or both of controller medications; and adding a short course of oral glucocorticoids (typically 5 to 7 days of prednisone 40-50 mg/day). Patients who do not improve with self-care or who have signs that indicate a severe attack should be evaluated in an acute care facility. Management there should include close monitoring of

dyspnea, work of breathing, and vital signs; treatment should include frequent inhaled SABA administration, prompt glucocorticoid therapy, and administration of supplemental oxygen to maintain oxygen saturation above 93%. For further discussion of severe asthma exacerbations, see Common ICU Conditions. H

---

**KEY POINT**

- All asthma patients should have a written asthma management plan that helps them recognize the symptoms of an exacerbation and begin self-treatment.

---

## Severe Refractory Asthma

Severe refractory asthma is present in patients who require high doses of inhaled glucocorticoids plus a second controller and/or oral steroids to prevent worsening, or who experience 2 or more exacerbations within one year that require emergency department visits or hospitalization. This group of patients consumes most asthma-related health care resources. It is important to verify the diagnosis in these patients, document medication compliance, and correct inhaler technique before considering additional therapies. Additionally, comorbidities should be aggressively managed, and the possibility of coexisting vocal cord dysfunction should be considered. Treatment guided by specific phenotypes can be helpful in this group, such as biologic agents for patients with high IgE or high eosinophil levels, and leukotriene-receptor antagonists for patients with aspirin sensitivity. Referral to a team of subspecialists is often indicated.

## Asthma in Pregnancy

Pregnant patients should be advised that the advantages of treatment are significantly greater than the potential risk to the fetus from asthma therapies or exacerbations. Pregnancy can affect asthma control, leading to either worsening or improvement, and patients should be closely monitored for signs of exacerbation, which occurs most frequently during the second trimester. Inhaled glucocorticoids, oral glucocorticoids, SABAs, leukotriene-receptor antagonists (montelukast, zafirlukast), and LABAs have all been used extensively during pregnancy without data to suggest fetal harm.

# Chronic Obstructive Pulmonary Disease

## Definition

Chronic obstructive pulmonary disease (COPD) is a chronic lung disease defined by persistent respiratory symptoms and airflow limitation or obstruction that is not fully reversible.

## Epidemiology

COPD is a common disorder that currently affects 5% of the U.S. population. The worldwide prevalence continues to rise, and the World Health Organization predicts that by 2020 COPD will become the fifth most prevalent disorder and the third leading cause of death. COPD is associated with a high

---

**TABLE 5.** Severe Asthma Exacerbation Risk Factors and Signs

| Risk Factors |
| --- |
| History of near-fatal asthma attack or intubation |
| Emergency department or hospital visit in the last 12 months |
| Poor asthma medication adherence |
| Recent treatment with oral glucocorticoid |
| Psychosocial stressors or psychiatric disease |

| Signs |
| --- |
| Unable to speak in full sentences |
| Use of accessory muscles of respiration |
| Respiration rate >30/min, heart rate >120/min |
| $SpO_2$ <90% on ambient air |
| Agitation, confusion, or drowsiness |

$SpO_2$ = oxygen saturation as measured by pulse oximetry.

Data from Prasad Kerlin M. In the clinic. Asthma. Ann Intern Med. 2014;160: ITC3 2-15; quiz ITC3 16-9. [PMID: 24737276] doi:10.7326/0003-4819-160-5-201403040-01003 and Most Recent Asthma Data. Centers for Disease Control and Prevention Web site. www.cdc.gov/asthma/most_recent_data.htm. Updated February 27, 2017. Accessed May 9, 2018.

morbidity and mortality, and is the third leading cause of death in the United States.

## Pathophysiology

COPD is an inflammatory condition. Cigarette smoke and other irritants activate both macrophages and epithelial cells within the respiratory tract. The epithelial cells then release several neutrophil chemotactic factors. Macrophages and neutrophils release proteases that cause destruction of lung parenchyma. Proteases are typically inactivated by antiproteases, such as $\alpha_1$-antitrypsin, which may also be reduced in COPD. Oxidative stress from irritants and inflammatory cells may lead to additional inflammation and tissue destruction. Ultimately, patients develop fibrosis of the small airways and reduced elastic recoil of the lungs leading to static hyperinflation. As the degree of inflammation increases, airflow obstruction worsens and the ability to fully exhale decreases. Inhalation is initiated before exhalation is completed, resulting in dynamic hyperinflation, termed air trapping, which is seen as increased anteroposterior diameter of the chest and flattening of the diaphragm on chest radiographs. The diaphragmatic flattening limits the ability to increase breath volume during exertion. Compensatory use of accessory muscles, which increases tidal volume, and increased respiration rate augment minute ventilation. These changes increase the work of breathing and contribute to the sensation of dyspnea in patients with COPD.

## Risk Factors

Exposure to cigarette smoke (both first- and second-hand exposure) is the most important risk factor for COPD. Genetic predisposition seems to explain some of the variation in susceptibility to developing COPD when exposed to cigarette smoke. Long-term exposure to other irritants can also result in COPD. This includes exposure to air pollution (both indoor and outdoor) and occupational chemicals and dusts. An important example of indoor air pollution is the use of biomass fuel for cooking inside the home. Although it is uncommon in the United States, use of biomass fuel indoors is a common risk factor for COPD in the developing world. A family history of COPD is also considered a risk factor for the disease, as is a genetic condition that results in a deficiency of $\alpha_1$-antitrypsin.

### KEY POINT

- Exposure to cigarette smoke is the most important risk factor for COPD.

## Heterogeneity of COPD

COPD is a heterogeneous condition. Some patients present predominately with a chronic productive cough due to mucus hypersecretion, whereas others present predominately with progressive dyspnea secondary to hyperinflation. The heterogeneity extends beyond clinical symptoms. Phenotypic heterogeneity has been characterized on the basis of clinical, physiologic, molecular, and radiographic variables. For example, eosinophilia has been associated with increased responsiveness to glucocorticoids. There also appears to be a subgroup of patients who are more prone to developing acute exacerbations. Understanding such variables could potentially improve the accurate assessment of prognosis and individualize patient care. Because of the heterogeneity of the disease and its presentation, tools have been developed to aid in determining prognosis and best treatment strategies. Several staging assessments exist. For example, the Global Initiative for Chronic Obstructive Lung Disease (GOLD) system combines the degree of airflow obstruction obtained from spirometry with the number of previous exacerbations as well as symptoms to help determine treatment. The BODE index uses the variables of body mass index (B), airflow obstruction (O), dyspnea (D), and exercise capacity (E) to predict outcomes and response to therapy. Airflow obstruction is determined using the post-bronchodilator $FEV_1$ percent of predicted for age, gender, height, and race. The index uses the Modified British Medical Research Council (mMRC) questionnaire to grade perceived dyspnea ranging from dyspnea only with strenuous exercise to dyspnea even when getting dressed. The exercise capacity is determined by the walking distance on a 6-minute walk test. This index provides better prognostic information than the $FEV_1$ alone and has been used to approximate 4-year survival and risk of hospitalization for COPD.

## Comorbid Conditions

Patients with COPD often suffer from comorbid conditions that further increase morbidity and mortality. Some conditions, like cardiovascular disease, share common risk factors, but others seem to be independently associated with COPD or a consequence of treatment of COPD. These include muscle loss with associated weakness and weight loss, osteoporosis, and depression.

### KEY POINT

- COPD is a heterogeneous condition, and patients present with variable symptoms including cough, sputum production, and dyspnea.

### Diagnosis

The possibility of COPD should be considered and spirometry should be performed in patients 40 years of age or older with progressive dyspnea, chronic cough, or chronic sputum production, particularly in the presence of known risk factors for the disease, especially smoking. The role of screening spirometry in asymptomatic individuals with risk factors is controversial. The USPSTF guideline and the joint guideline developed by ACP/ATS/ACCP/ERS recommend against screening for COPD in asymptomatic adults, whereas GOLD advocates performing screening spirometry in individuals with risk factors for COPD. The diagnosis of COPD is made using spirometric measurement to document airflow obstruction. COPD is confirmed by a post-bronchodilator $FEV_1/FVC$ ratio of less than 0.70. This differs from the finding in asthmatic patients, whose airflow obstruction is fully reversible with bronchodilator therapy.

Some patients have bronchial inflammation with features of both asthma and COPD, referred to as asthma-COPD overlap syndrome. A GOLD and the Global Initiative for Asthma (GINA) consensus statement characterizes asthma-COPD overlap syndrome as persistent airflow limitation with several features usually associated with asthma and several features usually associated with COPD. Measuring lung volumes and diffusing capacity is not required to diagnose COPD but may help in determining the severity of disease. Clinicians should rule out other causes of chronic respiratory symptoms including heart failure, bronchiectasis, obliterative bronchiolitis, tuberculosis, and diffuse panbronchiolitis. H

### KEY POINTS

HVC
- There is no role for spirometric screening for COPD in asymptomatic individuals.
- COPD is defined as a post-bronchodilator $FEV_1/FVC$ ratio of less than 0.70.

## Disease Assessment

After a diagnosis of COPD has been established, the initial assessment focuses on disease severity, which is determined using a combination of symptoms, degree of airflow obstruction on spirometry, history of acute exacerbations, and presence of comorbid conditions. Several validated tools are available to assess patients' symptoms, including the COPD Assessment Test (CAT), the Clinical COPD Questionnaire (CCQ), and the mMRC scale (**Table 6**). The GOLD criteria use the CAT or mMRC scale to determine symptom severity, whereas the BODE index requires the use of the mMRC scale. The CCQ is often used to screen patients for symptoms of COPD. Symptoms are then combined with the results from spirometry (**Table 7**) to determine disease severity (**Table 8**).

Patients who have had two or more acute exacerbations within the last year, who have an $FEV_1$ of less than 50% of predicted, or who have ever been hospitalized for an acute exacerbation are considered to be at high risk for recurrent acute exacerbations. Clinicians should determine if the patient suffers from any of the common comorbid conditions associated with COPD that indicate a higher morbidity and mortality and treat appropriately.

Pulse oximetry at rest and at exertion should be used to determine the need of supplemental oxygen. Arterial blood gases should be measured to assess for underlying hypercapnia in patients with a low $FEV_1$, change in mental status, an acute exacerbation, an elevated level of serum bicarbonate, or oxygen saturation of less than 92% on pulse oximetry. H

An $\alpha_1$-antitrypsin level should be obtained in patients with COPD under the age of 45 who have a strong family history of COPD or who are without identifiable COPD risk factors. A pattern of basilar emphysema, associated liver disease

### TABLE 6. Modified Medical Research Council Dyspnea Scale

| Score | Description of Dyspnea | Severity |
|-------|------------------------|----------|
| 0 | I get breathless only with strenuous exercise. | None |
| 1 | I get short of breath when hurrying on level ground or walking up a slight hill. | Mild |
| 2 | On level ground, I walk slower than other people my age because of breathlessness, or I have to stop for breath when walking at my own pace. | Moderate |
| 3 | I stop for breath after walking approximately 100 yards or after a few minutes on level ground. | Severe |
| 4 | I am too breathless to leave the house or breathless when dressing. | Very severe |

Used with the permission of the Medical Research Council.

### TABLE 7. Classification of COPD Severity by Spirometry[a]

| Category | Severity | Spirometry |
|----------|----------|------------|
| GOLD 1 | Mild | $FEV_1 \geq 80\%$ of predicted |
| GOLD 2 | Moderate | $50\% \leq FEV_1 < 80\%$ of predicted |
| GOLD 3 | Severe | $30\% \leq FEV_1 < 50\%$ of predicted |
| GOLD 4 | Very severe | $FEV_1 < 30\%$ of predicted |

[a]In Patients with $FEV_1/FVC$ less than 70%.

Reprinted from Vogelmeier CF, Criner GJ, Martinez FJ, Anzueto A, Barnes PJ, Bourbeau J, et al. Global strategy for the diagnosis, management, and prevention of chronic obstructive lung disease 2017 report. GOLD executive summary. Am J Respir Crit Care Med. 2017;195:557-582. [PMID: 28128970] doi:10.1164/rccm.201701-0218PP

### TABLE 8. GOLD Model for Classifying Severity of Disease in COPD[a]

| Patient Category | Characteristics | Exacerbations Per Year | CAT Score | mMRC Score |
|------------------|-----------------|------------------------|-----------|------------|
| A | Low risk, fewer symptoms | ≤1 | <10 | 0-1 |
| B | Low risk, more symptoms | ≤1 | ≥10· | ≥2 |
| C | High risk, fewer symptoms | ≥2 | <10 | 0-1 |
| D | High risk, more symptoms | ≥2/≥1 with hospital admission | ≥10 | ≥2 |

CAT = COPD Assessment Test; mMRC = Modified Medical Research Council.

[a]See Table 7 for definitions of spirometric classifications.

Data from Vogelmeier CF, Criner GJ, Martinez FJ, Anzueto A, Barnes PJ, Bourbeau J, et al. Global strategy for the diagnosis, management, and prevention of chronic obstructive lung disease 2017 report. GOLD executive summary. Am J Respir Crit Care Med. 2017;195:557-582. [PMID: 28128970] doi:10.1164/rccm.201701-0218PP

or panniculitis, or a strong family history of emphysema in patients with COPD should also prompt consideration of α₁-antitrypsin deficiency in middle-aged and older patients. Some guidelines even recommend that all patients with COPD regardless of age be tested for α1-antitrypsin deficiency after weighing the risks and benefits of testing.

**KEY POINTS**

- After a diagnosis of COPD has been established, the initial assessment focuses on disease severity, which is determined using a combination of symptoms, degree of airflow obstruction on spirometry, history of acute exacerbations, and presence of comorbid conditions.

- Patients who have had two or more acute exacerbations within the last year, who have an $FEV_1$ of less than 50% of predicted, or who have ever been hospitalized for an acute exacerbation are considered to be at high risk for recurrent acute exacerbations.

## Management of COPD

A management plan for COPD should include the identification and reversal of risk factors, especially ongoing exposure to cigarette smoke. The severity of a patient's COPD should guide the choice of therapy (**Table 9**). No currently available treatments can prevent long-term decline in lung function, so patients should be monitored for evidence of disease progression that may guide additional therapy. The goals of therapy are to reduce symptoms, improve exercise tolerance and quality of life, as well as prevent and treat exacerbations, prevent disease progression, and decrease mortality.

### Smoking Cessation

Smoking cessation is essential in the management of COPD, as it can slow the decline of $FEV_1$. Providers should encourage patients to quit smoking and be aware that the success rates for smoking cessation increase when counseling is combined with medication therapy. Effective medications for cessation

**TABLE 9. Pharmacologic Management of COPD**

| Patient Group | Recommended Therapy | Alternative Therapy | Other Considerations |
|---|---|---|---|
| A | Short-acting bronchodilator *or* Long-acting bronchodilator | Evaluate effect of therapy and continue, stop, or try alternative bronchodilator as appropriate | All patients in Group A should receive bronchodilator therapy based on its effect on dyspnea; therapy should be continued if symptomatic benefit is documented. |
| B | Long-acting bronchodilator (LABA or LAMA) *or* Combination therapy with two bronchodilators may be considered for patients with severe dyspnea. | If symptoms persist after one long-acting bronchodilator, try combined therapy with LABA and LAMA | Long-acting inhaled bronchodilators are superior to short-acting bronchodilators taken as needed. There is no evidence to support use of one class of long-acting bronchodilators over another for initial relief of symptoms for patients in Group B. In the individual patient, the choice should depend on the patient's perception of symptom relief. Patients in Group B are likely to have comorbidities that affect symptoms and prognosis, and these should be investigated. |
| C | LAMA; if further exacerbations, LAMA and LABA | LABA and inhaled glucocorticoids | LABA and LAMA is preferred to LABA and inhaled glucocorticoids because inhaled glucocorticoids increase the risk of developing pneumonia in some patients. |
| D | LABA and LAMA; if further exacerbations, add inhaled glucocorticoids | If exacerbations continue, consider: roflumilast (patients with an $FEV_1$ <50% of predicted and chronic bronchitis, particularly if they have experienced at least one hospitalization for an exacerbation in the previous year); *or* macrolide therapy (the best available evidence exists for the use of azithromycin) | Initial therapy with LABA and inhaled glucocorticoids may be appropriate in some patients, including those with a history or findings suggestive of asthma-COPD overlap. |

LABA = long-acting β₂-agonist; LAMA = long-acting muscarinic agent.

Data from Vogelmeier CF, Criner GJ, Martinez FJ, Anzueto A, Barnes PJ, Bourbeau J, et al. Global strategy for the diagnosis, management, and prevention of chronic obstructive lung disease 2017 report. GOLD executive summary. Am J Respir Crit Care Med. 2017;195:557-582. [PMID: 28128970] doi:10.1164/rccm.201701-0218PP

include nicotine replacement, varenicline, and bupropion (see MKSAP 18 General Internal Medicine). **H**

**KEY POINT**

- Smoking cessation is essential in the management of COPD, as it can slow the decline of FEV$_1$.

## Pharmacologic Therapy

Pharmacologic therapies in COPD are used to reduce symptoms, improve quality of life, and reduce the frequency and severity of exacerbations (**Table 10**). Bronchodilators are mainstays of therapy in COPD irrespective of the severity of the disease. Any time bronchodilators or other inhalers are prescribed, the clinician should ensure that the patient receives education on proper inhaler technique. Initial management is outlined in Table 9.

### Bronchodilators

Inhaled bronchodilators include β$_2$-agonists and anticholinergics/antimuscarinic agents. Both are available as short-acting and long-acting inhalers and improve symptoms and expiratory airflow. Short-acting β$_2$-agonists and muscarinic antagonists result in similar bronchodilation, and either can be used as monotherapy. However, dual treatment results in a greater degree of bronchodilation and expiratory airflow, which may lead to symptom benefit in select patients.

If short-acting bronchodilators are insufficient to control symptoms in patients with more severe disease, a long-acting bronchodilator, either a LABA or a LAMA, can be added. Choosing the appropriate long-acting bronchodilator inhaler requires consideration of patient and physician preference, potential side effects, and cost. If symptoms persist on monotherapy, addition of a second long-acting bronchodilator from the alternate bronchodilator class may result in clinical improvement. Long-acting bronchodilators alone should not be used in patients with an asthma component to their COPD (asthma-COPD overlap syndrome) unless an inhaled glucocorticoid is also prescribed because of the potential for increased risk of mortality in this patient population when a LABA is used without an inhaled glucocorticoid.

### Inhaled Glucocorticoids

Inhaled glucocorticoids are typically used only in combination with a long-acting bronchodilator for treatment of COPD (see Table 9). Inhaled glucocorticoids are not used alone unless a patient is not able to use long-acting bronchodilators (see Table 10). Inhaled glucocorticoids, used alone and in combination with long-acting bronchodilators, improve lung function and reduce symptoms and exacerbations in patients with moderate to severe COPD, but are associated with an increased risk of pneumonia. In patients with severe COPD, triple inhaler therapy with a LABA, a LAMA, and an inhaled glucocorticoid may provide additional symptom benefit. **H**

**KEY POINT**

- Bronchodilators are mainstays of therapy in COPD irrespective of the severity of the COPD; any time bronchodilators or other inhalers are prescribed, the clinician should ensure that the patient receives education on proper inhaler technique.

### Systemic Glucocorticoids

Systemic glucocorticoids are recommended for short-duration treatment of acute exacerbations of COPD. (See Acute Exacerbations: Goals and Therapeutic Management section.) However, long-term use of systemic glucocorticoids should be avoided due to the risk of significant side effects, including diabetes and osteoporosis. **H**

### Methylxanthines

The methylxanthines (aminophylline and theophylline) are now rarely used to treat COPD. Theophylline has been shown to improve functional capacity and reduce the number of exacerbations. However, it has a narrow window between therapeutic and toxic dosages and is therefore only used for patients with advanced COPD who have refractory symptoms not controlled by standard therapy. Studies of the use of either aminophylline or theophylline during acute exacerbations have shown no benefit.

### Roflumilast

Roflumilast is a selective phosphodiesterase-4 inhibitor that is  used to reduce chronic symptoms and the frequency of exacerbations in patients with severe COPD who have either primarily symptoms of chronic bronchitis or frequent exacerbations. **H**

### α$_1$-Antitrypsin Augmentation Therapy

Antiproteases, including α$_1$-antitrypsin, typically inactivate proteases that may lead to permanent lung injury. In patients with α$_1$-antitrypsin deficiency, replacing this enzyme with augmentation therapy may slow the progression of related emphysema. However, it is costly, has not been shown to decrease exacerbations or the rate of FEV$_1$ decline, and is not effective for treatment of patients whose COPD is not caused by α$_1$-antitrypsin deficiency.

### Other Agents

Macrolide antibiotics have inflammatory and antimicrobial  effects. Long-term macrolide therapy may reduce the frequency of exacerbations when prescribed to patients with severe COPD and a history of frequent exacerbations. Mucolytics and antitussives are not routinely used in the management of COPD but may provide some symptomatic relief in patients with significant sputum production. **H**

### Immunization

Immunizations can prevent infections in patients with COPD. Because infections are the most common trigger of

| TABLE 10. Drug Treatment for COPD | | |
|---|---|---|
| **Agent** | **Side Effects** | **Notes** |
| **Bronchodilators** | | |
| Inhaled short-acting $\beta_2$-agonists (albuterol, fenoterol, levalbuterol, metaproterenol, pirbuterol, terbutaline) | Tachycardia and hypokalemia (usually dose dependent), but generally well tolerated by most patients | Generally used as needed for mild disease with few symptoms |
| Inhaled short-acting anticholinergic agents (ipratropium) | Dry mouth, mydriasis on contact with eye, tachycardia, tremors, rarely acute narrow angle glaucoma; this drug class has been shown to be safe in a wide range of doses and clinical settings | Generally used as needed for mild disease with few symptoms; avoid using both short- and long-acting anticholinergics |
| Inhaled long-acting anticholinergic agents (tiotropium, aclidinium, umeclidinium, glycopyrronium) | Dry mouth, mydriasis on contact with eye, tachycardia, tremors, rarely acute narrow angle glaucoma | Not to be used with ipratropium; use when short-acting bronchodilators provide insufficient control of symptoms for patients with an $FEV_1$ <60% of predicted |
| Inhaled long-acting $\beta_2$-agonists (salmeterol, formoterol, arformoterol, indacaterol, olodaterol) | Sympathomimetic symptoms such as tremor and tachycardia; overdose can be fatal | Use as maintenance therapy when short-acting bronchodilators provide insufficient control of symptoms for patients with an $FEV_1$ <60% of predicted; not intended to be used for treatment of exacerbations of COPD or acute bronchospasm |
| Methylxanthines (theophylline, aminophylline; sustained and short-acting) | Tachycardia, nausea, vomiting, and disturbed sleep; narrow therapeutic index; overdose can be fatal with seizures and arrhythmias | Used as maintenance therapy; generally use only after long-acting bronchodilator treatment to provide additional symptomatic relief of exacerbations; may also improve respiratory muscle function |
| Oral $\beta_2$-agonists (albuterol, metaproterenol, terbutaline) | Sympathomimetic symptoms such as tremor and tachycardia | Used as maintenance therapy; rarely used because of side effects but may be beneficial for patients who cannot use inhalers |
| **Oral Phosophodiesterase-4 Inhibitor** | | |
| Roflumilast | Diarrhea, nausea, backache, decreased appetite, dizziness | Used to reduce risk for exacerbations in patients with severe COPD (blood levels not required) with chronic bronchitis and history of exacerbations; roflumilast should not be used with methylxanthines owing to potential toxicity; very expensive and should be used only in select patients |
| **Anti-Inflammatory Agents** | | |
| Inhaled glucocorticoids (fluticasone, budesonide, mometasone, ciclesonide, beclomethasone) | Dysphonia, skin bruising, oral candidiasis, rarely side effects of oral glucocorticoids (see below) | Most effective in patients with a history of frequent exacerbations and when used in conjunction with long-acting bronchodilators |
| Oral glucocorticoids (prednisone, prednisolone) | Skin bruising, adrenal suppression, glaucoma, osteoporosis, diabetes mellitus, systemic hypertension, pneumonia, cataracts, opportunistic infection, insomnia, mood disturbance | Use for significant exacerbations of COPD; avoid, if possible, in stable COPD to limit glucocorticoid toxicity; consider inhaled glucocorticoids to facilitate weaning of systemic glucocorticoids |
| **Combination Agents** | | |
| Combined inhaled long-acting $\beta_2$-agonist and inhaled glucocorticoid in a single inhaler (fluticasone/salmeterol, budesonide/formoterol) | Same/combined effects of both drug classes | Fluticasone/salmeterol is approved by the FDA as maintenance therapy and for prevention of exacerbations; budesonide/formoterol metered-dose inhaler is approved by the FDA as maintenance therapy; combinations are not to be used for treatment of acute bronchospasm |
| Combined short-acting $\beta_2$-agonist plus short-acting anticholinergic in a single inhaler (fenoterol/ipratropium, salbutamol/ipratropium) | Same/combined effects of both drug classes | Generally used as needed for mild disease with few symptoms; avoid using both short- and long-acting anticholinergics; this combination therapy may be used for maintenance therapy only if patients have well-controlled disease on this combination treatment and do not require rescue therapy if/when expense is a determining factor |
| Combined inhaled glucocorticoid and ultra–long-acting $\beta_2$-agonist in a single inhaler (fluticasone/vilanterol) | Same/combined effects of both drug classes | Not to be used for treatment of acute bronchospasm |
| Combined long-acting anticholinergic plus ultra–long-acting $\beta_2$-agonist in a single inhaler (umeclidinium/vilanterol) | Same/combined effects of both drug classes | Not to be used for treatment of acute bronchospasm. Avoid using both short- and long-acting anticholinergics. |

acute exacerbations, routine immunizations are recommended for all patients with COPD. Patients should receive annual influenza immunization and the pneumococcal polysaccharide vaccine (PPSV23). Those above the age of 65 should also receive the pneumococcal conjugate vaccine (PCV13).

### KEY POINTS

- Systemic glucocorticoids are recommended for short-duration treatment of acute exacerbations of COPD; long-term use of systemic glucocorticoids should be avoided.
- All COPD patients should have annual influenza immunization and the pneumococcal polysaccharide vaccine; those above the age of 65 should also receive the pneumococcal conjugate vaccine.

### Nonpharmacologic Therapy
#### Pulmonary Rehabilitation
Pulmonary rehabilitation is a comprehensive program that combines exercise training, nutritional support, education, and social support for patients with chronic lung conditions. It has been shown to relieve symptoms, improve quality of life, and decrease frequency of hospitalizations in patients with COPD. Clinicians should consider adding this to appropriate medical therapy in symptomatic patients with an $FEV_1$ of less than 50% of predicted and to patients recovering from COPD exacerbation; particularly those recently hospitalized or treated with systemic steroids would benefit from pulmonary rehabilitation.

#### Oxygen Therapy
The use of supplemental oxygen has been shown to improve quality of life and decrease mortality in patients with COPD and resting hypoxemia with an arterial $Po_2$ of 55 mm Hg or less, or oxygen saturation as measured by pulse oximetry of 88% or less. Patients with cor pulmonale, heart failure, or erythrocytosis should be offered the use of supplemental oxygen if the $Po_2$ is 59 mm Hg or less or the oxygen saturation is 89% or less. Some patients may not qualify for oxygen at rest but may desaturate during sleep, exertion, or air travel. Supplemental oxygen is typically prescribed if the oxygen saturation as measured by pulse oximetry falls below 89% in these situations, but the benefits are less defined.

#### Noninvasive Mechanical Ventilation
Noninvasive mechanical ventilation (NIV), also termed noninvasive positive pressure ventilation (NIPPV), can be used for acute and chronic respiratory failure. For patients with a COPD exacerbation and acute hypercapnic respiratory failure with acidosis, NIV improves symptoms and reduces intubation rates, length of hospital stay, and mortality. It may also be beneficial in COPD patients with pneumonia, to help with discontinuing mechanical ventilation, and for palliative care. It does not replace intubation and mechanical ventilation in critically ill patients, comatose patients, or patients who have sustained a cardiac arrest. NIV is generally well tolerated, and improvement of the pH and $Pco_2$ within 1 to 2 hours predicts success. The benefit of using NIV in the treatment of chronic respiratory failure or in the outpatient setting is less clear. It may, especially if used at night, provide additional symptomatic relief when added to medical therapy in patients with severe COPD.

### Prognosis and Goals of Care
The current GOLD initiative recommends combining the degree of airflow limitation using the post-bronchodilator $FEV_1$ with the number of exacerbations and the patient's symptoms to classify the severity of disease. This will allow the clinician to guide escalation or de-escalation of medical therapies as appropriate.

The BODE index can be used as a prognostic indicator for patients with COPD. Using the BMI, the post-bronchodilator $FEV_1$ percent of predicted, dyspnea as defined using the mMRC scale (see Table 6), and the distance walked on a 6-minute walk test, it is possible to approximate the patient's 4-year survival. In patients with severe disease with an overall poor prognosis, referral for hospice and palliative care can provide significant improvements in symptom burden.

Palliative care can significantly aid in symptom management in patients with COPD at any stage of disease. Patients experience not only dyspnea, but also anxiety and depression, which may also be addressed. Opioids are commonly used to treat dyspnea that persists despite medical therapy. Current guidelines suggest a patient with severe COPD — defined by disabling symptoms despite medical therapy, progression of disease as evidenced by increasing emergency department evaluations or hospitalizations, and hypoxemia or hypercapnia — should be considered for hospice care.

### KEY POINT

- Current guidelines suggest a patient with severe COPD (defined by disabling symptoms despite medical therapy, progression of disease as evidenced by increasing emergency department evaluations or hospitalizations, and hypoxemia or hypercapnia), should be considered for hospice care.

#### Lung Volume Reduction Therapy
The National Emphysema Treatment Trial (NETT) demonstrated that patients with upper lobe–predominant and significant exercise limitations even after participation in a pulmonary rehabilitation program had improved quality of life, exercise tolerance, pulmonary function, and survival with lung volume reduction surgery. A key finding from NETT was that patient selection was critical to success and that patients with an $FEV_1$ of less than 20% of predicted, a diffusing capacity of less than 20% of predicted, or non–upper lobe predominant disease had a high operative mortality and should not be offered lung volume reduction surgery. The procedure should be considered in patients with upper lobe–predominant who have low exercise tolerance despite

maximal medical therapy and completion of a pulmonary rehabilitation program. Nonsurgical lung volume reduction procedures, including bronchoscopic placement of endobronchial one-way valves, plugs, or coils; administration of biologic sealants; and thermal ablation of the airway are being studied for treatment of emphysematous changes in patients with COPD. Early results suggest patients with severe air trapping and hyperinflation may get the most benefit from these new techniques.

### Lung Transplantation

Referral for lung transplantation can be considered in patients with severe COPD. The decision to refer should depend on the patient's life expectancy, quality of life, and patient preferences. In general, patients at high risk of dying in less than 2 years who have a high probability of 90-day postoperative survival are candidates. Patients with an elevated BODE index (5 or 6), resting hypoxemia, hypercapnia, an $FEV_1$ of less than 25% of predicted, or significant exercise limitation despite medical therapy, smoking cessation, and participation in a pulmonary rehabilitation program may be referred for evaluation for lung transplantation. Transplantation improves quality of life, and the median life expectancy is 5.7 years.

###  Acute Exacerbations

### Definition

An acute exacerbation of COPD is a change in a patient's typical symptoms that leads to a change in medical therapy or requires hospitalization. Most commonly, exacerbations are manifested by an increase in the severity or frequency of cough, worsening dyspnea, and an increase in the amount or change in the character of sputum produced. Most exacerbations are triggered by a respiratory infection (either viral or bacterial), smoking, and environmental exposures. An exacerbation can be triggered by other causes, but in some cases no trigger is ever identified. Studies suggest that exacerbations are underreported by patients and result in adverse outcomes. ▯

**KEY POINT**

- An acute exacerbation of COPD is a change in a patient's typical symptoms that leads to a change in medical therapy or hospitalization; the most common exacerbations are manifested by an increase in the severity or frequency of cough, worsening dyspnea, and an increase in the amount or change in the character of sputum produced.

### ▯ Prevention

Acute exacerbations of COPD can have substantial effects on quality of life and health care costs, and may accelerate the decline in lung function and increase mortality. It is therefore important to prevent exacerbations whenever possible. Strategies to prevent exacerbations include

smoking cessation, participating in pulmonary rehabilitation programs when appropriate, receiving recommended immunizations, and ensuring proper inhaler technique and use of medications. Long-term use of azithromycin or roflumilast has also been shown to prevent future exacerbations in patients who have a history of frequent exacerbations. ▯

**KEY POINT**

- Strategies to prevent COPD exacerbations include smoking cessation, participating in pulmonary rehabilitation programs when appropriate, receiving recommended immunizations, and ensuring proper inhaler technique and use of medications.

### Initial Assessment and Setting of Care

The first steps in managing a patient with a presumed COPD exacerbation are to confirm the diagnosis and determine the severity of the exacerbation for accurate triaging. A mild exacerbation is one that can be managed solely by increasing the dose of the regular medications the patient is already on. A moderate exacerbation requires treatment with antibiotics, steroids, or both; a severe exacerbation is defined by the need for an evaluation in the emergency department or hospitalization. Patients with respiratory distress or who are at risk of developing respiratory distress should be hospitalized; additional testing, including a chest radiograph, electrocardiogram, complete blood count, and basic metabolic panel, should be obtained to rule out other causes or comorbidities contributing to the acute presentation. Oxygen saturation should be measured by pulse oximetry. Arterial blood gas measurement is recommended for patients with a severe exacerbation to determine the presence of hypercapnia or hypoxemia. A sputum culture is not routinely used to assess COPD exacerbations as it rarely affects management. Patients with mild symptoms may not require any additional testing. ▯

**KEY POINTS**

- Patients who have COPD and respiratory distress or who are at risk of developing respiratory distress should be hospitalized and evaluated with a chest radiograph, electrocardiogram, complete blood count, basic metabolic panel, and oxygen saturation; arterial blood gas measurements can determine the presence of hypercapnia or hypoxemia.

- A sputum culture is not routinely used to assess COPD exacerbations as it rarely affects management. **HVC**

### Goals and Therapeutic Management

The management goals during an acute exacerbation are to relieve acute symptoms and to prevent future exacerbations. Supplemental oxygen should be used to maintain oxygen saturation between 89% and 92%. Noninvasive mechanical ventilation may be required if oxygenation or ventilation cannot be maintained. Patients may require mechanical intubation if they cannot tolerate noninvasive mechanical ventilation, have an altered mental status, or have worsening hypercapnic or hypoxemic respiratory failure despite the use of noninvasive mechanical ventilation. Short-acting $\beta_2$-agonists with or without anticholinergic agents should be used to relieve acute symptoms. The use of oral glucocorticoids during acute exacerbations has been shown to decrease the frequency of treatment failures, length of stay, and the time to subsequent exacerbations while improving $FEV_1$ and hypoxemia. Glucocorticoids have also been shown to decrease the need for hospitalization if used early. Recent randomized trials have demonstrated that short courses of lower-dose oral glucocorticoids, 40 mg for 5 days, are usually equivalent to longer courses, higher doses, and intravenous administration.

Antibiotics should be prescribed in cases of moderate or severe exacerbations or for patients with mild exacerbations who have noted an increase or change in sputum production. The most common infectious triggers are viruses, but bacterial causes include *Streptococcus pneumoniae, Haemophilus influenzae, Moraxella catarrhalis,* and *Mycoplasma pneumoniae.* If the patient is still smoking, treatment should also focus on smoking cessation because this can prevent future exacerbations. Because the prevalence of pulmonary embolism is higher in patients with COPD, a thromboembolic event should be considered as a potential trigger if patients do not improve with typical therapies for a COPD exacerbation, and appropriate testing should be performed. H

# Bronchiectasis

## Definition
Bronchiectasis is a chronic suppurative lung disease associated with irreversible enlargement of the airways due to destruction of airway architecture. An injury to the lung typically results in prolonged airway inflammation, which leads to localized injury with subsequent mucus stasis, which can lead to further airway obstruction, chronic infection, and inflammation with worsening bronchiectasis.

## Causes
In many cases of bronchiectasis, an underlying cause is not identified. The most common causes of bronchiectasis include cystic fibrosis, aspiration, immunodeficiencies, and connective tissue diseases (**Table 11**).

## Presentation
Bronchiectasis should be considered in the differential diagnosis of any patient with a chronic cough, especially if the patient has a history of frequent respiratory infections or if the cough is productive. Other possible symptoms include hemoptysis, wheezing, and chest pain. Features that should alert the clinician to consider bronchiectasis include previous

| TABLE 11. Common Causes of Bronchiectasis |
| --- |
| Airway obstruction |
|   Tumor |
|   Foreign body |
| Aspiration |
| COPD |
| Congenital |
|   Mounier-Kuhn syndrome |
|   Young syndrome |
| Connective tissue diseases |
|   Rheumatoid arthritis |
|   Sjögren's syndrome |
| Cystic fibrosis |
| Hypersensitivity |
|   Allergic bronchopulmonary aspergillosis |
| Immunodeficiency |
|   Common variable immunodeficiency |
|   HIV |
| Mucociliary dysfunction |
|   Primary ciliary dyskinesia |
| Postinfection |
|   Tuberculosis |
|   Pneumonia, especially recurrent |

sputum cultures growing uncommon pathogens such as *Pseudomonas aeruginosa, Aspergillus,* or nontuberculous mycobacteria; clubbing; and minimal or no smoking history.

Patients with bronchiectasis may also present with extrapulmonary symptoms, especially fatigue.

## Diagnosis
Initial evaluation should include a comprehensive medical history, including childhood diseases, family history, and careful evaluation to exclude known causes of bronchiectasis. Bronchiectasis is diagnosed by high-resolution chest CT. Diagnostic criteria include airway diameter that is greater than that of its accompanying vessel and lack of distal airway tapering (**Figure 4**). Bronchial wall thickening or cysts are often present. For every diagnosed patient, it should be determined whether there is an underlying cause that can be treated. This may involve testing for chronic bacterial or mycobacterial infections. These tests can identify causes of disease progression and help determine targeted antimicrobial therapy for exacerbations. Patients should also be evaluated for the presence of connective tissue disease and immune function. In selected patients, testing for cystic fibrosis, ciliary dysfunction, or $\alpha_1$-antitrypsin deficiency may be appropriate if suspected. However, even with rigorous evaluation, more than half of all cases are still considered idiopathic.

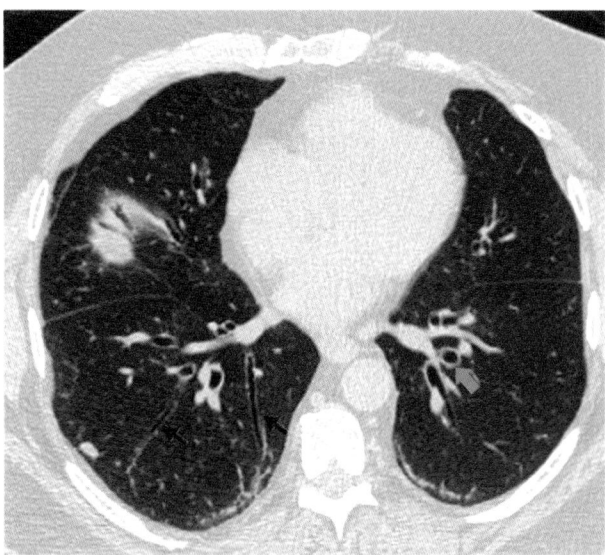

**FIGURE 4.** Bronchiectasis on chest CT. The airway is larger than its accompanying blood vessel (*thick arrow*), and the airway fails to taper distally (*thin arrows*).

## Treatment

The presence of chronic symptoms of cough and sputum production typically indicates irreversible airway dilation. Therefore, treatment of the underlying cause may not lead to improvement in current symptoms but could prevent further progression. Otherwise, treatment of bronchiectasis focuses on airway clearance, treating infections, and preventing exacerbations. The goal of airway clearance is to improve mucous clearance and thereby prevent chronic or recurrent infections. Bronchodilators, inhaled glucocorticoids, and combination inhalers have been shown to decrease symptoms but have no effect on the decline of lung function or frequency of exacerbations. Studies suggest that long-term use of macrolide antibiotics may prevent future exacerbations due to their anti-inflammatory effects. When deciding whether to use macrolide antibiotics, the risk of future exacerbations should be weighed against the possibility of developing macrolide resistance. Antibiotics may also be used in the management of chronic non–cystic fibrosis bronchiectasis to eradicate organisms such as *Pseudomonas aeruginosa* or methicillin-resistant *Staphylococcus aureus*. If eradication of bacterial colonization is not successful, there may be some symptomatic benefit from suppressive therapy with inhaled antibiotics. Patients should also be encouraged to exercise, which can improve airway clearance and symptoms. Surgical resection should be considered in patients who have localized disease with persistent symptoms despite therapy.

### Treatment of Exacerbations

Exacerbations of bronchiectasis may be difficult to differentiate from baseline symptoms. However, changes in sputum volume, viscosity, or purulence; increased cough; wheezing; shortness of breath; hemoptysis; or declines in lung function are considered evidence of an exacerbation. Therapy for an exacerbation is ideally guided by routine sputum and acid-fast bacilli culture results to identify a possible predominant organism for treatment. Empiric antibiotic therapy is recommended and may be based on previous culture data until the results of the current sputum culture become available. If previous data are not available, a fluoroquinolone can be started to ensure *Pseudomonas* coverage until sputum culture results are available.

# Cystic Fibrosis

Cystic fibrosis (CF) is an autosomal recessive disease affecting the CF transmembrane conductance regulator (*CFTR*) gene. It is diagnosed in approximately 1 of 2000-3000 live births with a predilection for disease in those of European descent. The most common genetic variant resulting in disease is ΔF508, but there are at least 1500 other genetic mutations. The pathogenesis for clinical manifestations of CF remains incompletely understood; however, the abnormal homozygous *CFTR* genotype results in abnormally thick secretions that are difficult to clear. There is an increased concentration of chloride in sweat gland secretions, and sweat chloride testing is a primary diagnostic tool for CF. The changes in respiratory secretions lead to bacterial colonization of airways and chronic bacterial infection, resulting in chronic inflammation and, ultimately, bronchiectasis. Further tissue destruction results from insufficient lung antiproteases to counteract the effect of elastase released from neutrophils. This ongoing inflammatory process also results in large amounts of free DNA and matrix protein deposition within areas of tissue destruction, which further drives increased viscosity of lung secretions.

Thickened secretions in the gastrointestinal tract impair flow of bile and pancreatic secretions, leading to pancreatic exocrine and endocrine deficiency, liver disease, and the development of malabsorption and maldigestion. The secretions increase the risk for bowel obstruction (distal ileal obstructive syndrome, intussusception, and rectal prolapse). Consequently, individuals with CF often present with malnutrition and weight loss.

## Diagnosis

Few patients with CF are diagnosed as adults. Adults diagnosed with CF most often present with pulmonary or gastrointestinal symptoms. Pulmonary manifestations often include chronic productive cough, recurrent sinusitis, and recurrent pulmonary infections requiring several courses of antibiotics. For those with gastrointestinal symptoms, loose and frequent stools with abdominal pain are the most common. Pancreatic insufficiency (either endocrine or exocrine) may occur but is less common. Chronic, persistent pulmonary or gastrointestinal symptoms requiring repetitive treatment should raise suspicion for CF. Radiographic findings of upper lobe–predominant with mucoid impaction may be present.

Often the greatest challenge to making the diagnosis is failing to include CF in the differential diagnosis. A family history of CF can be quite helpful in this regard. Sweat chloride testing is the initial test for CF, although it is less sensitive in adults. Abnormal results on repeat testing are diagnostic of CF. DNA testing confirms the diagnosis and helps with prognosis. A negative sweat chloride test in an adult patient does not rule out disease. Therefore, if the clinical suspicion remains high after negative repeat sweat chloride testing, consideration for referral to a center with expertise in CF or genetic testing is appropriate.

### KEY POINTS

- Adults diagnosed with cystic fibrosis most often present with pulmonary or gastrointestinal symptoms; pulmonary manifestations often include chronic productive cough, recurrent sinusitis, and recurrent pulmonary infections requiring several courses of antibiotics.

- A negative sweat chloride test in a patient who presents as an adult should not rule out cystic fibrosis.

## Treatment

The pillars of CF management are airway clearance, antibiotic therapy, nutritional support, and psychosocial support. The primary objectives of CF treatment are maintaining lung health and controlling/minimizing the impact of CF-affected organ disease. The Cystic Fibrosis Foundation practice guidelines recommend use of chronic medications to improve lung function and reduce exacerbations. These medications include mucolytics, hydrating agents, inhaled antibiotics, oral macrolide antibiotics, and *CFTR* potentiators. The treatment of CF lung disease is experiencing a period of rapid evolution, and management is suboptimal unless it involves a multidisciplinary approach best provided at a CF care center.

# Diffuse Parenchymal Lung Disease

Diffuse parenchymal lung diseases (DPLDs) are a group of disorders based on similar clinical, radiographic, physiologic, and pathologic changes that affect the alveolar walls and often the related small airways and distal pulmonary vasculature. Like other lung diseases, these disorders present primarily with shortness of breath. Imaging studies will typically demonstrate bilateral rather than unilateral lung disease. Although COPD and pulmonary hypertension affect the distal airways and vasculature, these are excluded from the category of DPLD.

## Classification and Epidemiology

Although there are hundreds of disorders that can present with diffuse parenchymal lung disease, they are typically divided into those with a known cause or those which are idiopathic (**Table 12**). The updated classification of idiopathic interstitial pneumonia will be discussed below. A thorough history that defines the time course is a critical first step in making the diagnosis.

DPLD is uncommon, compared to other pulmonary diseases such as asthma or COPD. The true prevalence of DPLDs is unknown; however, the literature estimates the prevalence at approximately 70 per 100,000 persons, with idiopathic cause accounting for 30% to 40% of disease in these patients.

## Diagnostic Approach and Evaluation

Nonproductive cough and dyspnea are the most common presenting symptoms of a DPLD. Dyspnea that comes on suddenly and is of short duration is more likely due to respiratory infection, asthma, pulmonary embolism, or heart failure than DPLD. In contrast, patients presenting with subacute or chronic dyspnea lasting weeks to months without response to treatment should be evaluated for DPLD. As opposed to the typical nonproductive cough of DPLD, a long history of cough with sputum production can suggest an underlying chronic infection, airways inflammation such as chronic bronchitis, or bronchiectasis.

When DPLD is suspected, questions should focus on determining the onset of symptoms, the disease course (improving or worsening), medications, and exposures. The most common identifiable etiologies of DPLDs are those associated with exposures, and the history should include a thorough review of occupations, home environment, hobbies, and other activities. Medication review should include current medications as well as those taken before the onset of symptoms.

Connective tissue diseases can lead to the development of DPLD; therefore, the review of systems should assess for symptoms of arthralgia, myalgia, arthritis, tenosynovitis, dry eyes, dry mouth, dysphagia, gastroesophageal reflux, and unexplained rash. A family history of DPLD due to connective tissue disease should substantially increase clinical suspicion.

Physical examination findings differ depending on the underlying cause of DPLD. In patients with connective tissue disorders, findings may include Raynaud phenomenon, skin

**TABLE 12. Classification and Distinguishing Features of Select Forms of Diffuse Parenchymal Lung Disease**

**Known Causes**

| | |
|---|---|
| Drug-induced | Examples: amiodarone, methotrexate, nitrofurantoin, chemotherapeutic agents (see www.pneumotox.com for a complete listing). |
| Smoking-related | "Smokers'" respiratory bronchiolitis characterized by gradual onset of persistent cough and dyspnea. Radiograph shows ground-glass opacities and thickened interstitium. Smoking cessation improves prognosis. |
| | Desquamative interstitial pneumonitis and pulmonary Langerhans cell histiocytosis are other histopathologic patterns associated with smoking and DPLD. |
| Radiation | May occur 6 weeks to months following radiation therapy. |
| Chronic aspiration | Aspiration is often subclinical and may exacerbate other forms of DPLD. |
| Pneumoconioses | Asbestosis, silicosis, berylliosis. |
| Connective tissue diseases | |
|    Rheumatoid arthritis | May affect the pleura (pleuritis and pleural effusion), parenchyma, airways (bronchitis, bronchiectasis), and vasculature. The parenchymal disease can range from nodules to organizing pneumonia to usual interstitial pneumonia. |
|    Systemic sclerosis | Nonspecific interstitial pneumonia pathology is most common; may be exacerbated by aspiration due to esophageal involvement; antibody to Scl-70 or pulmonary hypertension portends a poor prognosis. Monitoring of diffusing capacity for early detection is warranted. |
|    Polymyositis/dermatomyositis | Many different types of histology; poor prognosis. |
|    Other connective tissue diseases | Varying degrees of lung involvement and pathology can be seen in other forms of connective tissue disease. |
| Hypersensitivity pneumonitis | Immune reaction to an inhaled antigen; may be acute, subacute, or chronic. Noncaseating granulomas are seen. |

**Unknown Causes**

| | |
|---|---|
| Idiopathic interstitial pneumonias | |
|    Idiopathic pulmonary fibrosis | Chronic, insidious onset of cough and dyspnea, usually in a patient aged >50 years. Usual interstitial pneumonia pathology (honeycombing, bibasilar infiltrates with fibrosis). Diagnosis of exclusion. |
|    Acute interstitial pneumonia | Dense bilateral acute lung injury similar to acute respiratory distress syndrome; 50% mortality rate. |
|    Cryptogenic organizing pneumonia | May be preceded by flu-like illness. Radiograph shows focal areas of consolidation that may mimic infectious pneumonia or may migrate from one location to another. |
| Sarcoidosis | Variable clinical presentation, ranging from asymptomatic to multiorgan involvement. Stage 1: hilar lymphadenopathy. Stage 2: hilar lymphadenopathy plus interstitial lung disease. Stage 3: interstitial lung disease. Stage 4: fibrosis. Noncaseating granulomas are hallmark. |

**Rare DPLD with Well-Defined Features**

| | |
|---|---|
| Lymphangioleiomyomatosis | Affects women in their 30s and 40s. Associated with spontaneous pneumothorax and chylous effusions. Chest CT shows cystic disease. |
| Chronic eosinophilic pneumonia | Chest radiograph shows "radiographic negative" heart failure, with peripheral alveolar infiltrates predominating. Other findings may include peripheral blood eosinophilia and eosinophilia on bronchoalveolar lavage. |
| Pulmonary alveolar proteinosis | Median age of 39 years, and males predominate among smokers but not in nonsmokers. Diagnosed using bronchoalveolar lavage, which shows proteinaceous material in and around alveolar macrophages. Chest CT shows "crazy paving" pattern. |

DPLD = diffuse parenchymal lung disease.

thickening, sclerodactyly, malar rash, inflammatory arthritis, or tenosynovitis. Lung examination findings are variable and may be normal. This is more likely early in disease or in those with imaging findings of ground-glass opacity or micronodules. Decreased breath sounds and dullness to percussion may suggest a pleural effusion, which is atypical for many DPLDs. Wheezes may suggest small airways disease, while inspiratory dry "Velcro" crackles are more suggestive of fibrosis. In more severe disease there may be right heart strain on electrocardiography or evidence of right-sided heart failure with findings of jugular venous distention, peripheral edema, a pronounced pulmonic second sound, and an $S_3$. These findings are also suggestive of more long-standing disease.

The physical examination should include resting and exertional pulse oximetry. It is common for patients with DPLD to have normal resting pulse oximetry. However, because of reductions in the functional pulmonary capillary bed, individuals with DPLD will often demonstrate desaturation when ambulating. The desaturation may not require supplemental oxygen; however, desaturation of greater than 4% while ambulating is consistent with a diffusion limitation, which is a hallmark of interstitial lung disease.

Patients with a clinical suspicion of DPLD should undergo full pulmonary function testing, including lung volumes and $D_{LCO}$. The vast majority of DPLDs have restrictive physiology. However, there are a few diseases that have obstruction or exhibit a combined obstructive and restrictive deficit. Simple spirometry has a limited role because it can only identify obstruction and may be normal in the setting of restriction or reduced $D_{LCO}$.

Plain chest radiography is an appropriate initial test for the evaluation of dyspnea and cough in patients suspected of having DPLD. Chest radiography may show various findings in patients with DPLD, including diffuse reticular and reticulonodular patterns, increased septal line thickening, consolidation, pleural effusions with or without pleural calcification, bronchiectasis, and hilar or mediastinal lymphadenopathy. The

chest radiograph can be normal in patients with minimal disease, and a normal chest radiograph does not rule out DPLD.

**KEY POINTS**

- Patients presenting with subacute or chronic symptoms of dyspnea lasting weeks to months without response to treatments should be evaluated for diffuse parenchymal lung disease.
- Patients with a clinical suspicion of diffuse parenchymal lung disease should undergo full pulmonary function testing, including lung volumes and $D_{LCO}$.
- A normal chest radiograph does not rule out diffuse parenchymal lung disease.

## High-Resolution CT Scanning

High-resolution CT (HRCT) scan of the chest (slice thickness 1-2 mm) is the best imaging study to identify abnormalities that can help diagnose the underlying disease (**Table 13**). When disease of the small airways is suspected, HRCT imaging should be obtained both on inspiration and on expiration to accentuate air trapping. Prone images may be helpful if there is subtle septal thickening posteriorly that can be difficult to

**TABLE 13.** Patterns of Disease Associated with a Diagnosis of Diffuse Parenchymal Lung Disease

| Lung Disease | Imaging | Comments |
|---|---|---|
| Acute interstitial pneumonia | Diffuse ground glass with consolidation | Indistinguishable from ARDS but without a risk factor for ARDS |
| Organizing pneumonia | Patchy ground glass, alveolar consolidation, peripheral and basal predominance | Connective tissue diseases, infections, drug-related, or idiopathic |
| Idiopathic pulmonary fibrosis/usual interstitial pneumonia | Basal-predominant and peripheral-predominant septal line thickening with traction bronchiectasis and honeycomb changes | The usual interstitial pneumonia pattern can be seen in connective tissue disease, asbestosis, and chronic hypersensitivity pneumonitis; idiopathic pulmonary fibrosis is a diagnosis of exclusion |
| Nonspecific interstitial pneumonia | Ground glass, basal predominance | Idiopathic and common finding in connective tissue disease |
| Respiratory bronchiolitis | Centrilobular nodules and ground-glass opacity in an upper-lung predominant distribution | May be an asymptomatic finding in an active smoker |
| Desquamative interstitial pneumonia | Basal-predominant and peripheral-predominant ground-glass opacity with occasional cysts | |
| Hypersensitivity pneumonitis | Acute: ground-glass opacification; centrilobular micronodules that are upper- and mid-lung predominant<br><br>Chronic: mid- and upper-lung predominant septal lung thickening with traction bronchiectasis; usual interstitial pneumonia pattern may be seen | Acute: associated with flulike illness<br><br>Chronic: often cannot identify a causative antigen |
| Sarcoidosis | Upper lobe–predominant; mediastinal and hilar lymphadenopathy; cystic changes including development of aspergilloma; small nodules oriented along bronchovascular bundles | Findings for sarcoidosis are often not specific; DPLD with diffuse mediastinal and hilar lymphadenopathy greater than 2 cm in size should raise suspicion |

ARDS = acute respiratory distress syndrome; DPLD = diffuse parenchymal lung disease.

distinguish from dependent atelectasis. The findings on HRCT highly correlate with the histopathology identified on open lung biopsy. In fact, most of the time the diagnosis of idiopathic pulmonary fibrosis can be made without lung biopsy based on the results of HRCT.

## Serologic Testing

Although the American Thoracic Society guidelines recommend screening all patients with DPLD with an antinuclear antibody (ANA), rheumatoid factor, and anti-cyclic citrullinated peptide antibodies, it is most appropriate in younger patients, in particular those younger than 40 years of age, patients with symptoms of an underlying rheumatologic disorder, and patients with a family history of autoimmune or rheumatologic disease. Standard serological testing for individuals who have no clinical evidence of autoimmune disease remains controversial. Additional serologic tests for connective tissue and vascular diseases should be based on history and physical examination. See MKSAP 18 Rheumatology for further discussion of testing for connective tissue disease.

## Lung Biopsy

When pulmonary function tests and HRCT are insufficient for making the diagnosis, the physician must consider the risks and benefits of either a bronchoscopic or surgical lung biopsy, including the patient's general health and risk of intervention. Careful assessment of risk factors, alternate diagnostic strategies, and impact of the results of lung biopsy on treatment should be discussed within a multi-disciplinary team, including a thoracic radiologist, thoracic surgeon, and pulmonary specialist with expertise in DPLD. Although a bronchoscopic biopsy provides much less tissue than a surgical lung biopsy, it has a high yield for making a diagnosis of sarcoidosis and is typically performed as an outpatient procedure. Overall in-hospital mortality associated with a surgical lung biopsy (either thoracoscopic or open biopsy) for DPLD remains low for scheduled cases (1.7%), but is much higher for emergency cases (16%).

### KEY POINTS

HVC
- The diagnosis of diffuse parenchymal lung disease can often be made based on high-resolution CT without a lung biopsy.
- Serologic testing for diffuse parenchymal lung disease is most appropriate in young patients, those with symptoms of rheumatologic disease, or those with a family history of rheumatologic conditions.

# Diffuse Parenchymal Lung Diseases with a Known Cause

## Smoking-Related Diffuse Parenchymal Lung Disease

There are several DPLDs that occur almost exclusively in individuals who are current smokers. Examples include respiratory bronchiolitis-associated interstitial lung disease (RB-ILD), desquamative interstitial pneumonia (DIP), and pulmonary Langerhans cell histiocytosis (PLCH). A history of smoking is also believed to be a risk factor for the development of idiopathic pulmonary fibrosis.

RB-ILD is the histopathologic diagnosis associated with the HRCT finding of centrilobular micronodular disease in current smokers. This diagnosis may incidentally be made in asymptomatic smokers undergoing low-dose CT lung cancer screening. DIP is characterized by alveolar filling with macrophages and is associated with ground-glass opacities on CT imaging, although this imaging finding is not specific for DIP. Patients with DIP typically are symptomatic with a dry cough and dyspnea.

PLCH, on the other hand, has diffuse thin walled cysts and several pulmonary nodules that are mid- and upper-lung zone predominant on HRCT. PLCH can also be associated with the development of pulmonary hypertension. Demonstrating the presence of Langerhans cells with S100 or CD1a staining of tissue obtained by either transbronchial or open lung biopsy confirms the diagnosis.

On physiologic testing, RB-ILD may have combined restriction and obstruction, whereas DIP typically is associated with pure restrictive disease. PLCH often produces restrictive disease, but may have preserved total lung capacity and evidence of obstruction when significant cystic disease is present. D$_{LCO}$ is reduced in all of these conditions.

For all smoking-related DPLDs, the primary management is smoking cessation. The use of glucocorticoids for those with more severe smoking-related DPLD or who have quit smoking and have persistent symptoms is often attempted, but has uncertain treatment effect.

### KEY POINTS

- Respiratory bronchiolitis-associated interstitial lung disease may be diagnosed in asymptomatic smokers based on high-resolution CT findings and pulmonary function testing.
- The primary management of all smoking-related diffuse parenchymal lung diseases is smoking cessation.

## Connective Tissue Diseases

Individuals younger than 40 years of age who present with DPLD have a high prevalence of connective tissue disease (CTD). The review of systems should include a thorough review of rheumatologic symptoms. Signs and symptoms of CTD warrant serologic evaluation based on the most likely disorder. Ruling out this potential cause for DPLD is very important even in the older population, despite the lower prevalence of CTD, because of the implications for treatment with immunomodulating agents. Pulmonary abnormalities are extremely common in patients with rheumatoid arthritis and include bronchiolitis, organizing pneumonia, rheumatoid nodules, nonspecific interstitial pneumonia (NSIP), and usual interstitial pneumonia (the same pathology that is seen with idiopathic pulmonary fibrosis). Furthermore, patients with rheumatoid arthritis treated with methotrexate are also at risk for possible drug-induced DPLD.

Patients with systemic sclerosis are at high risk for the development of lung disease, which is the leading cause of death in these patients. NSIP is the most common histopathologic diagnosis on lung biopsy, and HRCT imaging typically demonstrates findings of bilateral lower lobe ground-glass opacities with or without septal line thickening and traction bronchiectasis. The pathologic pattern of NSIP can occasionally be diagnosed in a patient before the development of systemic disease. Although cyclophosphamide has been shown to be of modest benefit, it has high toxicity and has been replaced by mycophenolate mofetil, which has similar efficacy and is better tolerated with decreased side effects. As a result, mycophenolate mofetil is considered first-line therapy for those with progressive DPLD and systemic sclerosis. For patients thought to have idiopathic NSIP, rheumatology consultation and evaluation for immunosuppressive treatment is appropriate.

**KEY POINTS**

- Pulmonary abnormalities are extremely common in patients with rheumatoid arthritis and can include bronchiolitis, organizing pneumonia, rheumatoid nodules, nonspecific interstitial pneumonia, and usual interstitial pneumonia.

- Patients with systemic sclerosis are at high risk for the development of lung disease, which is the leading cause of death in these patients.

## Hypersensitivity Pneumonitis

Repetitive inhalation of antigens in a sensitized patient can result in hypersensitivity pneumonitis (HP), an immunologic response that results in noncaseating granulomas and peribronchial mononuclear cell infiltration with giant cells. The antigens are typically complex proteins, which can come from several sources including agricultural dusts, thermophilic fungi, and bacteria, but can also be some small-molecular-weight chemical compounds. There are three forms of HP, and they each present differently. The acute form, which is most easily identified, results after a large exposure to an inciting antigen. The patient will develop fevers, cough, and fatigue, typically within 12 hours of exposure. Chest radiography can demonstrate diffuse micronodular disease but may be normal. Physical examination will reveal inspiratory crackles. If a HRCT scan is performed, it will demonstrate diffuse centrilobular micronodules and ground-glass opacities (**Figure 5**). After removal from the offending antigen, symptoms will resolve within approximately 48 hours. The recurrence of symptoms if the patient is rechallenged is the hallmark of the disease.

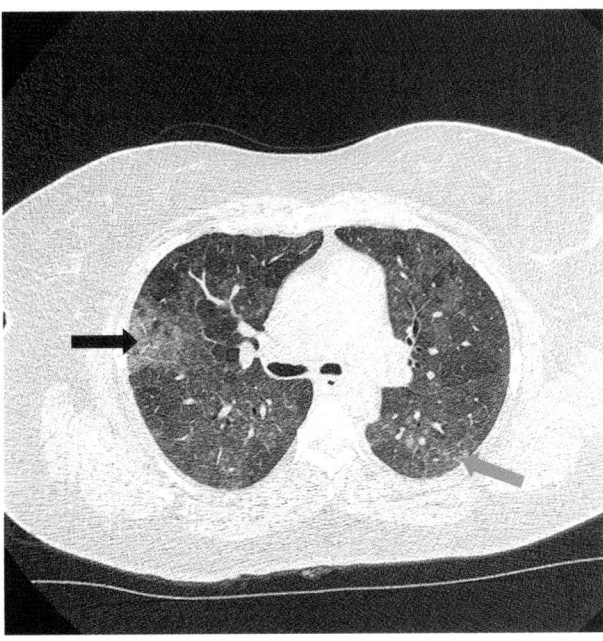

**FIGURE 5.** Chest CT scan demonstrating hypersensitivity pneumonitis with patchy, bilateral ground-glass opacities (*red arrow*) and centrilobular micronodules (*blue arrow*) in the mid-lung section.

Subacute and chronic forms of HP likely occur after more prolonged lower-level antigen exposure. Bird fanciers disease is an example of a chronic disorder. These patients have a chronic low-level exposure to avian antigens within the home and will ultimately experience cough, fatigue, weight loss, and shortness of breath. Similar to the acute form, the HRCT will show micronodules and ground-glass opacities, but there is also evidence of septal line thickening and fibrosis. In its most severe and chronic form, significant traction bronchiectasis and honeycomb changes will be evident. Evidence of severe fibrosis on CT imaging significantly increases the risk for progression of disease and death.

Removal of exposure to the offending antigen is essential in the treatment of HP. To identify potential antigens, careful history is vital, as serologic testing is often limited and may not include antibodies to the responsible antigen. Glucocorticoids are often used for those with more severe symptoms. Response to this therapy is variable. Prolonged glucocorticoid use is associated with significant side effects, and should be avoided without clear objective evidence of improved pulmonary function.

**KEY POINTS**

- The acute form of hypersensitivity pneumonitis is characterized by fever, cough, and fatigue within 12 hours of a major exposure to an inciting antigen; recurrence of symptoms with rechallenge is the hallmark of acute hypersensitivity pneumonitis.

- Removal of exposure to the offending antigen is essential in treatment of hypersensitivity pneumonitis.

## Drug-Induced Diffuse Parenchymal Lung Disease

Many medications have been implicated in the development of DPLD (**Table 14**). A review of medications should include those that are new and those taken for prolonged periods because the duration of exposure to the development of disease can vary, even for the same agent. For instance, amiodarone lung toxicity has an acute form consistent with acute lung injury/acute respiratory distress syndrome, and a chronic indolent form with reticular abnormalities and subpleural nodules. Prompt treatment by removal of the offending agent is important for resolution of symptoms. For those with more severe symptoms, glucocorticoids may have some benefit, although data are anecdotal.

## Radiation Pneumonitis

Radiation pneumonitis typically occurs 4 to 12 weeks after initial radiation exposure. Patients present with cough, shortness of breath, and a new radiographic infiltrate. Fever, pleuritic chest pain, fatigue, and weight loss are accompanying nonspecific symptoms. Differential diagnosis often includes infection and drug-induced lung injury. HRCT will demonstrate ground-glass opacities, usually within the field of

| TABLE 14. Select Drug-Induced Parenchymal Lung Diseases | | |
| --- | --- | --- |
| **Drug** | **Clinical Points** | **Radiographic Findings and Treatment** |
| Amiodarone | More common in:<br><br>Older patients<br><br>Increased dosage and higher cumulative dose<br><br>First year of therapy (but can occur late) | Multiple radiographic presentations possible, including ground-glass opacities, subpleural nodules, and reticular abnormalities<br><br>Very long half-life prevents clearance from the pulmonary parenchyma:<br><br>Rare improvement with discontinuation of the drug alone<br><br>High risk of recurrence with tapering of glucocorticoids |
| Methotrexate | Occurs in less than 5% of treated patients<br><br>Unpredictable time to presentation<br><br>No clear correlation between dose and disease severity | Diffuse reticular and ground-glass attenuation<br><br>Patients generally do well after stopping medication.<br><br>Glucocorticoids are often given and duration is based on response. |
| Nitrofurantoin | Acute (more common):<br><br>Fevers, chills, cough, shortness of breath, chest pain; rash can occur in 10%-20% of patients.<br><br>Peripheral eosinophilia common<br><br>Chronic:<br><br>Distinct from the acute form<br><br>Onset months to years after prolonged exposure | Acute: Faint bilateral lower lobe septal lines; moderate pleural effusions may be present. Treatment: Often will resolve with discontinuation but will recur with repeat exposure.<br><br>Chronic: Reticular opacities with subpleural lines and thickened peri-bronchovascular areas. Treatment: Possible benefit of glucocorticoids from anecdotal reports. |
| Busulfan | Occurs in less than 8% of treated patients.<br><br>Currently used solely as a conditioning regimen for HSCT; often combined with other agents associated with pulmonary toxicity.<br><br>Injury typically occurs 30 days to 1 year after exposure. | Multiple patterns including: ground glass opacities, reticulation, bibasilar septal lines, asymmetric peripheral and peribronchial consolidation, centrilobular nodules, and dependent consolidation<br><br>Optimal treatment unknown and is often supportive.<br><br>Glucocorticoids may be used for more progressive disease. |
| Bleomycin | Risk significantly increases with cumulative dose.<br><br>Increased age, renal insufficiency, concomitant chemotherapy and/or radiation also increases risk of toxicity.<br><br>Typically subacute presentation 1-6 months after exposure; may resemble hypersensitivity pneumonitis but with more rapid onset and progressive course. | Imaging patterns suggest the multiple possible pathologic findings seen:<br><br>Consolidation with ground glass (diffuse alveolar damage)<br><br>Septal line thickening, traction bronchiectasis, and honeycomb change (end-stage fibrosis)<br><br>Patchy ground glass with subpleural consolidation or peribronchial consolidation (organizing pneumonia)<br><br>Diffuse ground glass with centrilobular micronodules (hypersensitivity pneumonitis)<br><br>Glucocorticoids are used for more severe disease and disease may recur with tapering of steroids. |

HSCT = hematopoietic stem cell transplantation.

radiation exposure. A well-defined nonanatomic demarcation between normal and abnormal lung consistent with the radiation field is pathognomonic but not always present. Radiographic abnormalities, such as organizing pneumonia, may also be seen outside the field of exposure and can be nodular or alveolar. Treatment of radiation pneumonitis is typically glucocorticoids for severe disease with more extensive abnormalities on imaging, respiratory symptoms, or with hypoxemia. Observation may be appropriate for those with mild disease. From 6 to 12 months after radiation exposure, additional findings on HRCT may develop, including septal line thickening, traction bronchiectasis, and volume loss more consistent with chronic fibrosis. In addition, individuals exposed to radiation are at risk for the development of radiation-recall pneumonitis, which can occur when exposed to select chemotherapy agents including adriamycin, etoposide, gemcitabine, paclitaxel, and pemetrexed.

**KEY POINTS**

- Radiation pneumonitis typically presents 4 to 12 weeks after initial radiation exposure, with cough, shortness of breath, and a new radiographic infiltrate.

- Treatment of severe forms of radiation pneumonitis typically is glucocorticoids, whereas observation may be appropriate for those with mild disease.

# Diffuse Parenchymal Lung Diseases with an Unknown Cause

## Idiopathic Pulmonary Fibrosis

Idiopathic pulmonary fibrosis (IPF), which is associated with the histopathologic appearance of usual interstitial pneumonia (UIP), is the most common idiopathic form of DPLD. It typically presents in patients between 50 and 70 years of age who have a greater than 6-month duration of a dry cough and dyspnea on exertion. History will reveal no potential cause for the development of fibrosis, and lung examination is notable for Velcro inspiratory crackles that are predominant at the bases and may be subtle in early disease. Clubbing is present in up to 50% of patients and should raise suspicion for IPF. The diagnosis of IPF is challenging because it is uncommon and indolent. Because smoking is a risk factor, patients are often treated for COPD without significant improvement. Similarly, crackles on examination may lead to management for presumed heart failure. Chest radiographs may demonstrate bibasilar septal line thickening with reticular changes, and volume loss and bronchiectasis when the disease is more severe. The best diagnostic test is HRCT, which may show abnormalities, such as bilateral, peripheral, and basal predominant septal line thickening with honeycomb changes, when the chest radiograph is normal (**Figure 6**). When HRCT is consistent with UIP, lung biopsy may not be necessary for diagnosis.

IPF is progressive, with a median survival of 3 to 5 years after diagnosis. The progression of disease, however, is variable

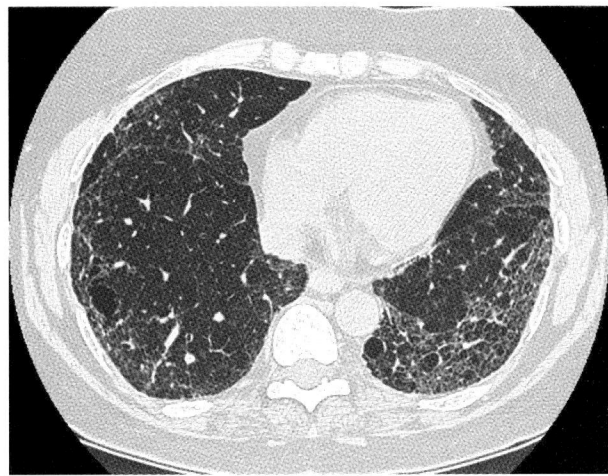

**FIGURE 6.** High-resolution chest CT demonstrating the typical findings in idiopathic pulmonary fibrosis, including increased reticular changes that are predominantly peripheral and basilar in distribution, honeycombing (at the left base), and absence of significant ground-glass opacification.

and may be associated with periods of stability with intermittent periods of acute decline. A subset of patients develop an acute exacerbation with a worsening of symptoms, typically of less than 1 month's duration, and associated new findings on chest CT of bilateral ground-glass opacities after having relatively stable disease over time. These events can be "triggered" by an inciting event such as an infection or may be "idiopathic." Heart failure and volume overload should be excluded as causes of the radiographic changes or clinical decompensation.

An important aspect of treatment of IPF includes optimum management of comorbidities such as obesity, heart failure, and deconditioning. Sleep-disordered breathing is common in this population due to nocturnal hypoxemia and increased prevalence of obstructive sleep apnea. Treatment of hypoxemia includes supplemental oxygen with exertion and at rest as needed based on pulse oximetry testing. For those with deconditioning, pulmonary rehabilitation has demonstrated benefits in exercise tolerance and quality of life in several small studies. In progressive and severe disease, pulmonary hypertension and right-sided heart failure are commonly observed. One preliminary study suggesting improvement in quality of life with sildenafil needs further study before recommending its use in this population.

In 2014, two FDA-approved therapies, nintedanib and pirfenidone, became available. Both therapies target the fibroblast, which is considered central in the progression of fibrosis. Although the mechanisms of these two medications differ, clinical response is quite similar, with both demonstrating a decline in the rate of progression of disease. Although these medications delay IPF progression, they are not curative. Referral to a pulmonologist or interstitial lung disease (ILD) center may be appropriate before initiating treatment with these medications.

CONT.

Lung transplantation is a life-prolonging therapy for those without comorbidities that may otherwise limit life expectancy. Typically, transplant centers exclude those with untreatable end-organ damage outside the lungs. Early referral of eligible patients to a transplant center is appropriate given the unpredictability of disease progression.

The most common cause of death in patients with IPF is respiratory failure. In patients with respiratory failure, the need for mechanical ventilation portends an extremely poor prognosis. As a result, consensus-based guidelines recommend against mechanical ventilation for IPF patients if lung transplantation is not an option. Palliative care consultation to establish advanced care plans should be considered for patients with IPF who are not candidates for lung transplantation and who have a severe exacerbation and poor performance status. Ideally, advance care planning, including end-of-life goals of care and palliative strategies, should be decided before urgently facing the decision of whether to begin mechanical ventilation in the setting of respiratory failure. **H**

- FDA-approved therapy with nintedanib and pirfenidone decreases the rate of progression of idiopathic pulmonary fibrosis but is not curative.

HVC
- Consensus-based guidelines recommend against mechanical ventilation for patients with idiopathic pulmonary fibrosis if lung transplantation is not an option.

## Nonspecific Interstitial Pneumonia

Nonspecific interstitial pneumonia (NSIP) is the most common DLPD associated with autoimmune disorders, but it can occasionally be idiopathic and not associated with an underlying connective tissue disease. There are two forms of NSIP: cellular and fibrotic. The fibrotic form has a worse prognosis and is poorly responsive to treatment. The cellular form has a better prognosis and will typically respond to immunosuppressive treatments. Although the overall prognosis is better than for IPF, the 5-year mortality of idiopathic NSIP remains approximately 15% to 25%. Individuals with progressive decline in pulmonary function are at increased risk of death regardless of the underlying pathology. Similar to IPF, select patients may benefit from lung transplantation. NSIP affects a younger population than IPF. HRCT will demonstrate bilateral lower-lobe reticular changes and an absence of honeycombing, but can also demonstrate areas of ground-glass opacification. These findings on HRCT have been associated with systemic sclerosis, systemic lupus erythematosus, Sjögren's syndrome, dermatomyositis, and polymyositis, as well as undifferentiated connective tissue disease. Because idiopathic NSIP is rare, a thorough investigation for an underlying autoimmune disorder is essential. NSIP was common in patients with AIDS in the pre-antiretroviral therapy era; however, it is much less common since the advent of antiretroviral therapy.

- Nonspecific interstitial pneumonia is the most common diffuse parenchymal lung disease associated with autoimmune disorders.

- Bilateral lower-lobe reticular changes and an absence of honeycombing on high-resolution CT scan, often accompanied by areas of ground-glass opacification, have been associated with systemic sclerosis, systemic lupus erythematosus, Sjögren's syndrome, dermatomyositis, and polymyositis, as well as undifferentiated connective tissue disease.

## Cryptogenic Organizing Pneumonia

Organizing pneumonia is defined by histopathologic findings of patchy proliferation of granulation tissue that affects the terminal bronchiole, and alveolar ducts and spaces, and is associated with surrounding inflammation. This pattern often follows or is associated with various types of injury to the lung, including acute infection, radiation exposure, drug-induced pneumonitis, and autoimmune diseases. In patients in whom no cause is identified, the diagnosis is termed cryptogenic organizing pneumonia (COP).

Patients with COP typically present with cough, fever, and malaise for 6 to 8 weeks. Initial chest radiographs will  demonstrate patchy opacities that mimic pneumonia and, as a result, patients are often initially misdiagnosed with community-acquired pneumonia and treated with standard antibiotics (**Figure 7**). However, nonresolving symptoms and failure to respond to antibiotics should raise suspicion for organizing pneumonia or COP. HRCT imaging will demonstrate ground-glass opacities or areas of alveolar consolidation resembling an infectious pneumonia, but findings can include peripheral nodules and nodules along the bronchovascular bundle. The diagnosis may not require lung biopsy if the clinical presentation and HRCT findings are consistent with COP. For cases with atypical presentation, lung biopsy may be necessary to make the diagnosis. **H**

Patients with COP typically respond to glucocorticoid therapy. In organizing pneumonia associated with an autoimmune disorder, treatment should focus on the autoimmune condition. Relapses of COP with tapering of glucocorticoids are common, and therefore a long taper of glucocorticoids or transition to alternate immunosuppressive therapy should be considered.

- Patients with cryptogenic organizing pneumonia typically present with complaints of cough, fever, and malaise for 6 to 8 weeks, which may mimic community-acquired pneumonia.

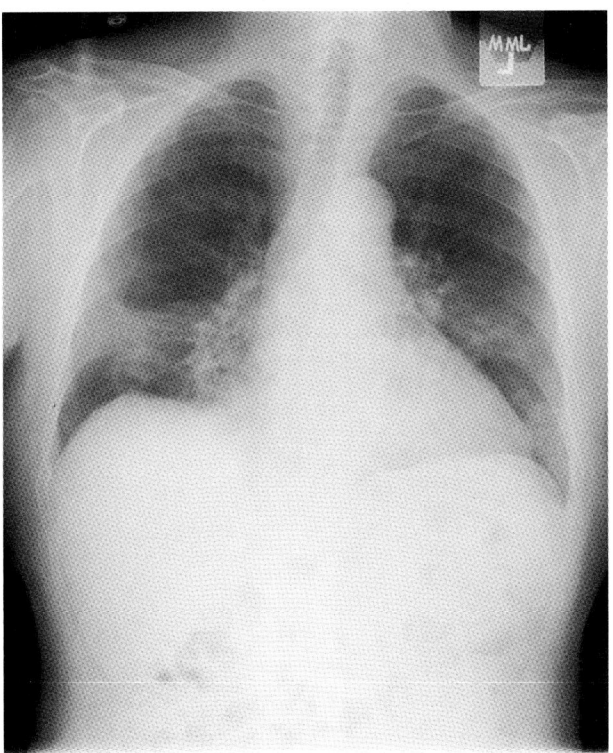

**FIGURE 7.** Chest radiograph showing cryptogenic organizing pneumonia, demonstrating multiple patchy bilateral alveolar opacities that are nonspecific and may be difficult to distinguish from more typical infectious pneumonia. Infiltrates may be migratory, with resolution of established opacities as new areas appear on serial imaging. Imaging may also be nonspecific, showing interstitial infiltrates and alveolar opacification or one or more rounded nodules that may be interpreted as malignancy.

## Acute Interstitial Pneumonia

Acute interstitial pneumonia develops rapidly during days to weeks, resulting in acute respiratory failure with bilateral alveolar opacities on HRCT of the chest consistent with pulmonary edema. The pathologic findings on open lung biopsy are those of diffuse alveolar damage. This process is clinically, radiographically, and pathologically indistinguishable from acute respiratory distress syndrome. The differentiating factor is the lack of risk factors for the development of acute respiratory distress syndrome. The history should carefully assess any history of aspiration, sepsis, or inhalational exposure that could result in acute lung injury.

Management includes supportive care, as for other patients with acute lung injury or acute respiratory distress syndrome. This includes low tidal volume ventilation if required and critical care management to avoid complications of illness. Although glucocorticoids are often used, there is little evidence other than case reports of improvement with their use. Mortality remains high (approximately 50%), and those who recover from the initial illness often have complications, are at risk for the development of chronic lung disease, and may have a relapse. Long-term management of these patients includes consideration of immunosuppression; however, there are limited data to guide therapy.

- Acute interstitial pneumonia is clinically, radiographically, and pathologically indistinguishable from acute respiratory distress syndrome; the differentiating point is the lack of risk factors for the development of acute respiratory distress syndrome.

## Sarcoidosis

Sarcoidosis is a granulomatous disease of unknown cause that can affect several organ systems. Greater than 90% of patients with sarcoidosis have lung involvement. The prevalence of sarcoidosis is approximately 10 to 20 per 100,000 individuals. Sarcoidosis affects blacks more frequently than whites and typically occurs in younger patients. Many patients are asymptomatic, and lung involvement is incidentally found on chest radiography done for other reasons (**Figure 8**). Findings from chest radiography can help predict the probability of spontaneous resolution (**Table 15**). CT scanning can show pulmonary parenchymal disease or intrathoracic lymphadenopathy, either alone or in combination. Although there are various appearances of sarcoidosis on chest CT scanning, a particularly characteristic finding is the presence of small nodules alongside bronchovascular bundles.

Pulmonary function testing is typically abnormal and findings can be obstructive, restrictive, or both. Sarcoidosis is a diagnosis of exclusion. Diagnosis, with a few exceptions (**Table 16**), typically requires bronchoscopic biopsy, with tissue obtained from a lymph node or from the pulmonary

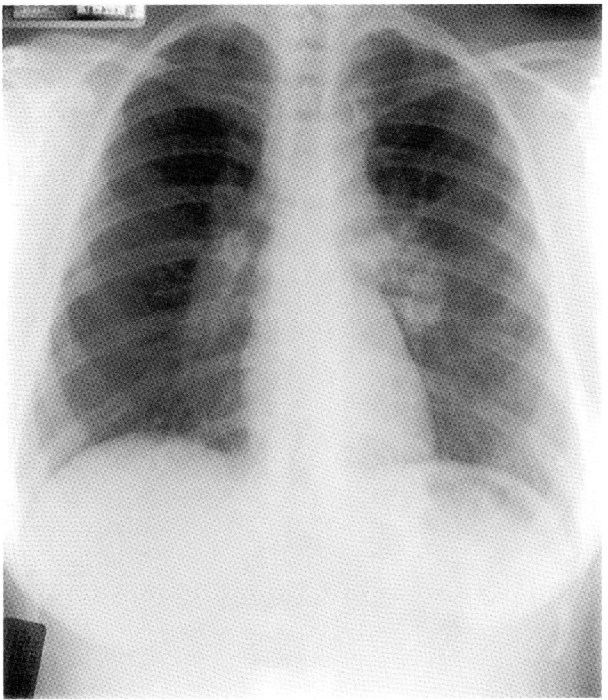

**FIGURE 8.** Chest radiograph showing stage I pulmonary sarcoidosis with hilar lymphadenopathy and normal lung parenchyma.

**TABLE 15.** Chest Radiograph Staging of Pulmonary Sarcoidosis

| Stage | Radiographic Pattern | Clinical Course and Comments |
|---|---|---|
| 0 | Normal | |
| I | Hilar lymphadenopathy with normal lung parenchyma | >90% will have spontaneous resolution without treatment |
| II | Hilar lymphadenopathy with abnormal lung parenchyma | Approximately 50% rate of spontaneous improvement without treatment |
| III | No lymphadenopathy with abnormal lung parenchyma | Approximately 20% rate of spontaneous improvement without treatment |
| IV | Parenchymal changes with fibrosis and architectural distortion | |

**TABLE 16.** Clinical Presentations of Sarcoidosis that Do Not Require a Biopsy

| Syndrome | Additional Findings/Symptoms |
|---|---|
| Asymptomatic bilateral hilar lymphadenopathy | No evidence of fevers, malaise, or night sweats to suggest a malignancy |
| Löfgren syndrome | Bilateral hilar lymphadenopathy, migratory polyarthralgia, erythema nodosum, and fever |
| Heerfordt syndrome | Anterior uveitis, parotiditis, fever (uveoparotid fever), and facial nerve palsy |

CONT.

parenchyma. The diagnosis is made by the finding of noncaseating granulomas with exclusion of potential mimicking infections (mycobacteria, fungi), exclusion of other systemic granulomatous diseases, and ideally with involvement of more than one organ system.

Pulmonary hypertension may develop through several different mechanisms, including chronic hypoxemia, destruction of the capillary bed resulting in severely reduced capillary surface area, granulomatous inflammation of the pulmonary arteries, compression of pulmonary arteries secondary to contiguous lymphadenopathy, pulmonary veno-occlusion from granulomatous inflammation, and left ventricular dysfunction from cardiac involvement. Development of pulmonary arterial hypertension is a poor prognostic indicator, with a median survival of approximately 3 years.

The primary treatment of sarcoidosis is glucocorticoids, although many patients do not need to be treated. In addition, spontaneous resolution without treatment is common and related to the radiographic stage of disease (see Table 15). The decision to treat and assessment of response should be based on symptoms and organ dysfunction, not radiographic findings. For those without symptoms or organ dysfunction, observation is appropriate. If treatment is required, low- to medium-dose glucocorticoid therapy, often on alternate days, is appropriate. Short-term symptomatic benefit is clear from retrospective study data; however, long-term benefits remain less clear. For patients with more severe or prolonged symptoms, side effects from chronic glucocorticoids should be

considered. In this setting, adjunctive glucocorticoid-sparing therapies are often used. Pulmonary consultation should be considered for management of persistent disease. For patients with pulmonary hypertension or severe disease with significant activity limitation due to lung disease, evaluation for lung transplantation is appropriate. ◨

**KEY POINTS**

- Greater than 90% of patients with sarcoidosis have lung involvement; radiographic staging can predict the probability of spontaneous resolution.
- The primary treatment of symptomatic sarcoidosis is glucocorticoids.

# Occupational Lung Disease
## When to Suspect an Occupational Lung Disease

Occupational lung disease can affect any part of the respiratory tract, including sinuses, airways, the lung parenchyma, and the surrounding pleura. As a result, signs and symptoms associated with occupational exposure include rhinitis, reactive airways disease, COPD, pleural disease, diffuse parenchymal lung disease, and malignancy. Occupational lung diseases can present acutely, subacutely, or slowly after many years of exposure. As a result, these diseases require that clinicians maintain suspicion for and obtain a careful history of occupational exposures. Clinical presentations related to silica and asbestos exposures are well characterized and recognized. However, new agents that may lead to respiratory diseases are frequently introduced in industry. Factors suggesting an underlying occupational lung disease include patient concerns about an exposure, a temporal association with an exposure, unexplained signs or symptoms, and evidence of coworkers with similar symptoms (**Table 17**). In addition, patients may experience relief of symptoms when away from the work environment and recurrence of symptoms upon their return. For the patient with occupational lung disease, similar to diffuse parenchymal lung disease, cough and dyspnea on exertion are common.

**TABLE 17.** Occupational Lung Disease Screening Questionnaire

**Occupation**

What do you do every day at your job?

Have you always done these tasks at work?

Have you had other duties?

How long have you been working in this job? Have you had a similar job elsewhere?

What other types of work have you done?*

**Type and Extent of Exposure**

Describe your work area. Is there adequate ventilation? Is there visible dust in the air? Is visibility across the work area limited due to the extent of dust in the air?

Are you exposed to vapors, gases, dust, or fumes in your work?

Does your employer require you to wear personal protective equipment? If so, do you wear it for the full extent of your exposure?

Do you know the amount and type of chemicals used?

Do you have Material Safety Data Sheets (MSDSs) from your workplace?

**Temporal Relationship of Symptoms to the Work Environment**

Before symptoms began, were there any changes in the processes at work or new exposures?

When you are off work, do your symptoms improve?

Are there others at work who have developed similar symptoms?

Has a process change at work resulted in improved symptoms?

**Other Relevant Exposures**

Do you perform activities at home that may expose you to organic or inorganic dust (for example, refurbishing old cars or wood working)?

Do you have any pet birds at home? Do you have any pets?

Have you always lived in the area?

Have you traveled recently?

*Obtain a full accounting of other jobs as well.

# Key Elements of the Exposure History

The time course from exposure to the development of signs and symptoms of occupational lung disease is highly variable. Therefore, it is essential to obtain a complete history, including employment history. Exposures within the same industry can vary based on use of best practices and on the type of workplace. For example, coal worker's pneumoconiosis in the United States has substantially decreased since the institution of federal safety standards. However, rates of coal worker's pneumoconiosis are higher for individuals who work for companies with fewer than 50 employees, and for those who work in thin-seam mines. Thin-seam mines appear to have higher crystalline silica exposure and pose greater risk. More than

95% of these mines are located in Kentucky, West Virginia, and Virginia. Adequate determination of exposure requires a clear description of job duties and determination of the extent of dust exposure. Clinicians should also obtain a history of additional exposures from hobbies or the home environment (see Table 17).

When an occupational lung disease is suspected, clinicians should request Material Safety Data Sheets (MSDSs) from the employer, which detail chemical properties and known health risks associated with substances within the workplace. The U.S. Occupational Safety and Health Administration (OSHA) requires that this information is available upon request for employees who work with potentially harmful materials.

For individuals who have undiagnosed disorders, persistent unexplained symptoms, or permanent impairment possibly due to an occupational lung disease, referral to an occupational and environmental lung disease specialist is appropriate.

**KEY POINTS**

- Presentations of occupational lung disease include rhinitis, reactive airways disease, COPD, pleural disease, diffuse parenchymal lung disease, or malignancy.

- When an occupational lung disease is suspected, it is essential to obtain a complete history, including occupation, type and extent of exposure, temporal relationship of exposure to symptoms and disease, and other exposures at home and from hobbies.

# Management

The key to management of occupational lung disease is removal of the offending agent from the workplace or the worker from the offending agent. Because workers typically have colleagues in a similar environment, further investigation of the workplace to ensure identification of all affected individuals is essential. Beyond one specific patient, prevention through mitigation of further exposures in the workplace is best practice.

Workers' compensation often becomes an issue during medical management. It may be difficult to define the degree of impairment resulting from the exposure, and the determination of disability related to the impairment may require referral to a specialist with expertise in occupational lung disease.

**KEY POINT**

- The key to management of occupational lung disease is removal of the offending agent from the workplace or the worker from the offending agent; further investigation of the workplace to ensure identification of all affected individuals is essential.

# Surveillance

For individuals at high risk for the development of pulmonary disease, the use of health questionnaires and pulmonary function screening is appropriate; such screening can also identify a new exposure and any associated risk of disease development. Surveillance systems that catalogue sentinel cases of disease can help identify clustering of cases. However, one major limitation of these databases is the failure of physicians to report events.

## Asbestos-Related Lung Disease

Asbestos includes a group of minerals that, when crushed, will break into fibers. These fibers are chemically heterogeneous hydrated silicates that are used in industry because of their high tensile strength, heat resistance, and acid resistance. In the past, asbestos fibers were widely used in insulation, brake linings, flooring, cement paint, and textiles. Because of the known toxicities associated with asbestos, these compounds are used far less frequently today.

Asbestos-associated diseases have a prolonged latency period (15 to 35 years), resulting in continued identification of new cases despite the decreased use of asbestos in the United States. Continued exposures within the United States and the developed world occur through updating, demolition, and abatement of older construction. Asbestos exposure remains an occupational hazard for workers in developing nations.

### Risk Factors

Duration and extent of exposure are key risk factors for the development of disease. Asbestos-related lung diseases are common in mine workers who procure the asbestos and in industries that make use of the products. In the United States, workers in construction, naval shipyards, and the automotive service industries are particularly at risk. Exposure is also possible in areas where manufacturing of asbestos leads to environmental contamination. Similarly, there are reports of people who develop asbestos-related lung diseases after exposure to asbestos dust from family members working in an asbestos-related industry.

### KEY POINT

- Asbestos-related lung diseases are common in mine workers who procure the asbestos and in industries that make use of products containing asbestos; in the United States, workers in construction, naval shipyards, and the automotive service industries are particularly at risk.

### Pathophysiology

Inhaled asbestos fibers deposit deep within the lung, reaching airway bifurcations; respiratory bronchioles; and the alveolus, where they promote alveolitis. Type I alveolar epithelial cells take up the fibers, which migrate to the interstitium. Lymphatic channels transport asbestos fibers to the pleural surface. Although activated macrophages phagocytose and remove fibers, remaining fibers stimulate the macrophage to produce inflammatory mediators. These and other cell mediators stimulate fibroblast proliferation and chemotaxis, resulting in collagen deposition and development of fibrosis.

Asbestos exposure increases the risk for development of lung cancer regardless of smoking status, but the risks are substantially higher in smokers. This risk of cancer is apparent when any form of asbestos-related lung disease is present; however, for those with a history of asbestosis (that is, diffuse parenchymal lung disease secondary to asbestos), the risk of lung cancer is 36 times higher than in those with no history of smoking. Smoking cessation is essential. Findings of parietal pleural calcifications or plaques on chest radiograph should alert the clinician to the possibility of asbestos exposure. Although most patients with pleural plaques are asymptomatic, the most common symptom is exertional dyspnea. Additional evaluation including evaluation for lung cancer or mesothelioma should be considered.

## Silicosis

Silicosis is a fibrotic lung disease caused by the inhalation of silica dust. Silica exposure typically occurs in industries that grind, cut, or drill silica-containing materials such as concrete, tile, and masonry. Pottery making, foundry work, and sand blasting can also result in exposure. Sandblasting of denim jeans (stone washing) recently resulted in an outbreak of disease in Turkey. Hydraulic fracturing for natural gas and oil may expose workers to hazards, as this process involves fine sand and a wide variety of chemicals.

There are four main types of silicosis (**Table 18**), and they are associated with altered cell immunity and macrophage function. Patients with silicosis are at increased risk for the development of mycobacterial infection and connective tissue disease. Chronic silicosis is associated with the development of infection, including tuberculosis, and clinicians should have a high index of suspicion for this complication. Once fibrosis develops in silicosis, there is little evidence that any therapies alter disease course. If individuals have continued exposure, removal from the environment will prevent further lung injury. Silica exposure is associated with increased risk of lung cancer, particularly for smokers. As a result, smoking cessation remains an essential intervention.

### KEY POINTS

- Silica exposure can occur in individuals who work with hydraulic fracturing, concrete, tile, masonry, pottery, sand blasting, or in those who do foundry work.
- Once fibrosis develops in patients with silicosis, no therapies alter the course of the disease.

## Pleural Disease

The two main abnormalities affecting the pleura result from the presence of fluid (pleural effusion) or air (pneumothorax) in the pleural space.

**TABLE 18. Key Features of Silica-Related Lung Diseases**

| Type | Latency | Exposure Level[a] | Imaging Findings | Clinical |
|---|---|---|---|---|
| Acute silicoproteinosis (acute silicosis) | A few weeks to 3 years | High level | Crazy-paving pattern (extensive ground-glass opacity and interlobular septal thickening) | Rapidly progressive dyspnea with constitutional symptoms. Typically fatal. BAL yields a thick, milky effluent |
| Chronic simple silicosis | 10-20 years | Low to moderate | Upper-zone predominant with centrilobular or peri-lymphatic nodules 1-9 mm in diameter<br><br>Hilar lymph nodes may have eggshell calcification. | Often asymptomatic<br><br>Rarely will progress to PMF |
| Chronic complicated silicosis (PMF)[b] | 10-20 years | Low to moderate for those who progress from simple silicosis | Coalescent fibrosis >1 cm in diameter, typically in the periphery, enlarging over time and progressing towards the hilum. May contain air bronchograms and calcifications | Debilitating disease marked by progressive dyspnea and functional impairment |
| Accelerated silicosis | 3-10 years | Accelerated disease may occur with very high exposure for a shorter period of time | Similar to chronic disease other than more rapid development | As for chronic disease |

BAL = bronchoalveolar lavage; PMF = progressive massive fibrosis.

[a]Exposure refers to both quantity of dust exposure and duration

[b]A form of chronic silicosis that may progress from simple silicosis

# Pleural Effusion

Each year more than 1.5 million new cases of pleural effusion are diagnosed in the United States. Most effusions are benign; however, approximately 16% of them are secondary to malignancy. Heart failure, pneumonia, and malignancy are the most common etiologies in the United States. The pleurae are thin membranes that cover the surface of the lung (visceral pleura) and the chest wall (parietal pleura). Normally the pleural space contains only a small amount of fluid (less than 15 mL). Pleural effusions result from conditions that affect the rate of fluid entry from pleural capillaries and the ability of lymphatics to absorb the fluid.

**KEY POINT**

- Heart failure, pneumonia, and malignancy are the most common causes of pleural effusion in the United States.

## Evaluation

### History and Physical Examination

The cause of a pleural effusion is often suggested by patient history and physical exam. Symptoms typically include dyspnea, cough, and pleuritic chest pain. Key questions include severity and duration of symptoms; constitutional symptoms such as fevers, night sweats, and weight loss; occupation; recent illness, injury, or travel; exposures (for example, asbestos); and medical history such as heart failure, previous surgeries, and medications. The chest examination may reveal dullness to percussion and diminished or absent fremitus and breath sounds if the effusion is larger than 300 mL. There are several other key physical examination findings that may suggest the cause of the effusion (Table 19).

### Diagnostic Imaging

A chest radiograph should be performed as the first test in an evaluation of a possible pleural effusion. The radiographic findings are variable, but abnormalities may be seen with as little as 200 mL on the posterior-anterior (PA) chest radiograph or 50 mL on the lateral view (Figure 9).

**TABLE 19. Key Physical Examination Findings in the Evaluation of a Pleural Effusion**

| Finding | Possible Cause of Pleural Effusion |
|---|---|
| Distended neck veins, $S_3$ gallop, pulmonary crackles | Heart failure |
| Bilateral peripheral edema | Heart failure, nephrotic syndrome, cirrhosis |
| Calf or thigh swelling, erythema, edema, tenderness, palpable cord | Pulmonary embolus |
| Accentuated cardiac pulmonic sound, right ventricular heave | Pulmonary embolus |
| Lymphadenopathy | Malignancy |
| Ascites | Cirrhosis |

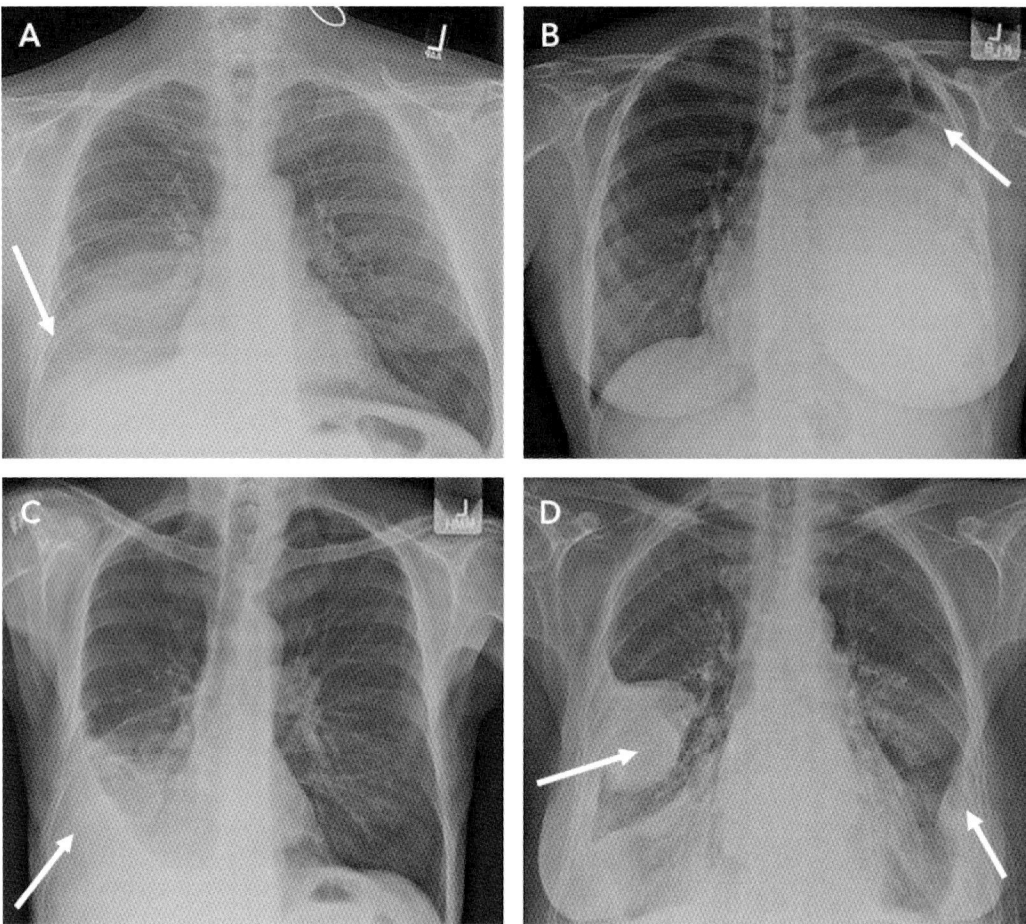

**FIGURE 9.** *A:* Moderate right pleural effusion which layers over the lower hemithorax; *B:* Large left pleural effusion with meniscus sign (a rim of fluid ascending the lateral chest wall); *C:* Loculated pleural effusion along the right lateral chest wall (presence of septations and separate compartments within the effusion); *D:* Bilateral multi-loculated pleural effusions.

CONT.

Thoracic ultrasound is a helpful addition to chest radiography for identification of small effusions, particularly in patients who are semirecumbent, such as those who are critically ill. This imaging allows estimation of the quantity of the fluid and determination of whether it is free-flowing or loculated (that is, with septations) (**Figure 10**). In addition, there is no radiation exposure with ultrasound.

Advantages of CT imaging include the ability to detect small amounts of pleural fluid; assessment of coexisting intrathoracic abnormalities, such as pulmonary masses and malignant pleural disease; and identification of an empyema, as enhancement of the pleura around the fluid creates a lenticular-shaped opacity (**Figure 11**).

### KEY POINTS

- A chest radiograph should be performed in the initial evaluation of possible pleural effusion.
- In supine patients and in those with small effusions, thoracic ultrasound is more sensitive than chest radiography for diagnosis of pleural effusion.

### Indications for Thoracentesis

Once a pleural effusion is identified, the next diagnostic test to consider is thoracentesis.

Indications include pleural effusion of unknown cause and greater than 1 cm of fluid thickness on ultrasound or lateral decubitus film. Fluid less than 1 cm thick is technically difficult to sample and less likely to be clinically meaningful, but still may be appropriate for thoracentesis based on clinical judgment. Thoracentesis should be done with ultrasound guidance, as it allows for both a greater success rate and a reduced risk of solid organ puncture and iatrogenic pneumothorax.

### Pleural Fluid Analysis

The first step in pleural fluid evaluation is assessing the appearance of the pleural fluid (**Table 20**). The next step is to determine whether it is a transudate or exudate. Transudates are due to an imbalance between hydrostatic and oncotic pressures, as occurs with heart failure and cirrhosis. Exudates are due to inflammation causing increased capillary permeability, impaired drainage by lymphatics, or both.

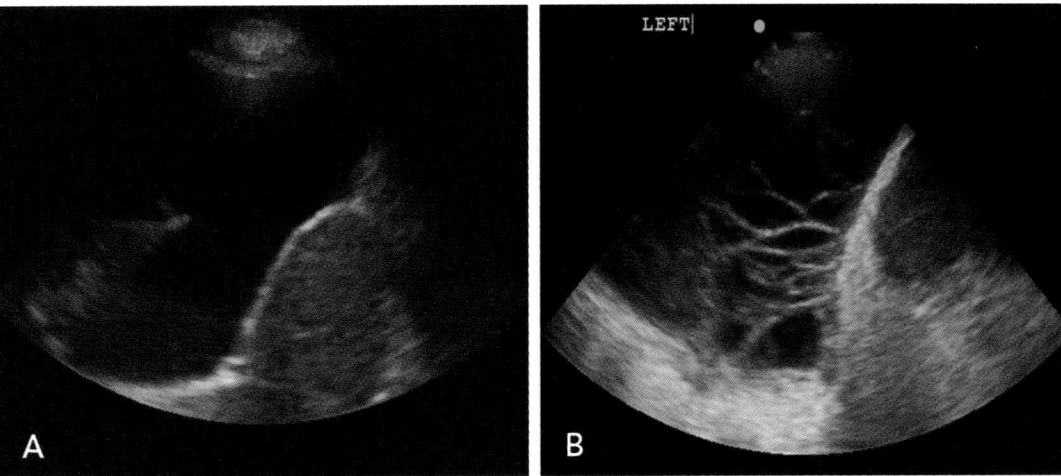

**FIGURE 10.** Comparison of a simple (*A*) and complicated (*B*) pleural effusion on thoracic ultrasound. A hypoechoic effusion (*A*) may be transudate or exudate. A multi-septated (loculated) effusion (*B*) is exudate.

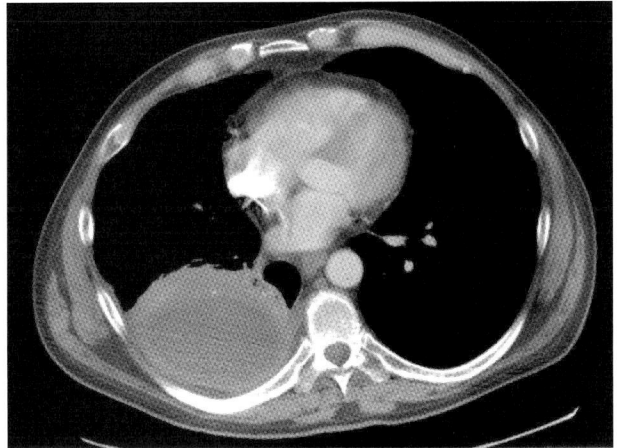

**FIGURE 11.** CT imaging reveals an empyema, as enhancement of the pleura around the fluid creates a lenticular-shaped opacity.

CONT.

There are many causes of exudative effusions but the most common are infection and malignancy. Differentiation is commonly made using Light's criteria, based on the levels of lactate dehydrogenase and total protein in both serum and pleural fluid (**Table 21**). However, a recent review also found that checking pleural fluid cholesterol was an accurate method for classifying the effusion as an exudate. Exudative and transudative effusions have a wide range of causes (**Table 22**).

In addition to characterizing a pleural effusion as a transudate or exudate, other tests are often performed depending on clinical suspicion. If infection is suspected then pH, glucose, cell count, Gram stain, and aerobic and anaerobic cultures should also be performed. If malignancy is suspected, then cytological analysis of fluid should be performed.

**TABLE 20. Pleural Fluid Characteristics and Diagnostic Considerations**

| Appearance | Possible Cause | Additional Tests to Perform |
|---|---|---|
| Bloody | Malignancy, pulmonary embolus, trauma, pneumonia, benign asbestos pleural effusion | Hematocrit. If >50% of the serum, it is a hemothorax; consider aortic rupture, myocardial rupture, and injuries to hilar structures, lung parenchyma, and intercostal vessels |
| Milky | Chylothorax or cholesterol effusion | Triglyceride level |
| Yellow-green | Rheumatoid pleurisy | Serum rheumatoid factor. Pleural fluid glucose <60 mg/dL (3.33 mmol/L) |
| Dark green | Bilothorax | Bilirubin |
| Dark brown/black | Long-standing hemothorax, fungal infection, malignancy | Hematocrit, cytology, fungal cultures |
| Purulent | Empyema | Aerobic and anaerobic cultures |

| TABLE 21. Criteria for Exudative Pleural Effusion | | |
|---|---|---|
| **Test** | **Sensitivity (%)** | **Specificity (%)** |
| Combined Light's criteria (1 or more of the following 3): | 97 | 85 |
|    Ratio of pleural-fluid protein to serum protein level >0.5 | 90 | 90 |
|    Ratio of pleural-fluid LDH level to serum LDH level >0.6 | 88 | 91 |
|    Pleural-fluid LDH level >2/3 the upper limit of normal for serum LDH | 88-89 | 93-100 |
| Pleural fluid cholesterol level >55 mg/dL | 85-94 | 95-99 |
| Ratio of pleural-fluid cholesterol to serum cholesterol >0.3 | 93 | 94 |

LDH = lactate dehydrogenase.

Data from Wilcox ME, Chong CA, Stanbrook MB, Tricco AC, Wong C, Straus SE. Does this patient have an exudative pleural effusion? The Rational Clinical Examination systematic review. JAMA. 2014;311:2422-31. [PMID: 24938565] doi:10.1001/jama.2014.5552

| TABLE 22. Causes of Transudates and Exudates | |
|---|---|
| **Transudates** | **Exudates** |
| **Very Common** | **Very Common** |
| Heart failure | Parapneumonic |
| Cirrhosis | Malignancy |
| **Less Common** | **Less Common** |
| Nephrotic syndrome | Pulmonary embolism |
| Hypoalbuminemia | Tuberculosis |
| Unexpandable (trapped) lung | Autoimmune diseases (RA, SLE) |
| Peritoneal dialysis | Benign asbestos effusion |
| Atelectasis | Post-coronary artery bypass |
| Urinothorax | Pancreatitis |
| Constrictive pericarditis | Post-myocardial infarction |
| Meigs syndrome (ovarian fibroma with ascites) | Yellow nail syndrome (lymphatic disorders) |
| | Drugs |

RA = rheumatoid arthritis; SLE = systemic lupus erythematosus.

*Cell Counts and Differential*

Cell counts are useful for determining the cause of a pleural effusion; however, they are not disease-specific. Neutrophil-predominant effusions are secondary to an acute process such as pneumonia (parapneumonic effusion) or pulmonary embolus. Lymphocyte predominance (more than 50%) is common in chronic effusions. The most common causes worldwide of lymphocyte-predominant effusions are tuberculosis and cancer. An eosinophilic effusion of greater than 10% is most commonly due to current or recent air or blood in the pleural space and is a nonspecific finding (**Table 23**).

*Chemical Analysis*

Pleural fluid acidosis (pH less than 7.3) is nonspecific and occurs in malignant effusions, complicated parapneumonic effusions, esophageal rupture, and inflammatory conditions such as rheumatoid and lupus pleuritis. Clinically, pH is most useful if an infection is suspected. A pH less than 7.2 in a parapneumonic effusion indicates a complicated pleural effusion is present and tube thoracostomy drainage is needed. Glucose normally diffuses freely across the pleural membrane. A pleural glucose concentration of less than 60 mg/dL (3.33 mmol/L) narrows the differential significantly and suggests that the effusion is secondary to malignancy, empyema or complicated parapneumonic effusion, tuberculosis, esophageal rupture, or rheumatoid or lupus pleuritis.

Pleural fluid amylase concentration should be checked if there is concern that the effusion may be due to pancreatitis or esophageal rupture. Pleural fluid amylase greater than the upper limit of normal for serum amylase, or a pleural fluid to serum amylase ratio greater than 1.0, is indicative of pancreatitis or esophageal rupture.

Pleural fluid triglycerides elevated above 110 mg/dL (1.24 mmol/L) support the diagnosis of chylothorax. If the triglyceride level is between 50 and 110 mg/dL (0.56 and 1.24 mmol/L), chylomicrons should be checked. A true chylothorax results from a disruption of the thoracic duct and is usually the result of thoracic surgery or trauma. Other causes include malignancy (lymphoma), tuberculosis, and lymphatic malformations.

*Tests for Tuberculous Effusions*

The diagnosis of tuberculosis should be considered in a patient with a lymphocyte-predominant exudative effusion of unclear cause; however, confirming the diagnosis may be challenging. An acid-fast smear of pleural fluid has a sensitivity of less than 5%, and mycobacterial culture has a sensitivity of only 10% to 20% due to the low mycobacterial load. Adenosine deaminase (ADA) is an enzyme present in lymphocytes that is elevated in most tuberculous pleural effusions (sensitivity 90%). In countries with a low incidence of tuberculosis, testing for ADA can be useful, as a negative test helps exclude tuberculosis. Pleural biopsy is useful for histology and is also the most likely source to yield a positive mycobacterial culture (greater than 70%).

| TABLE 23. | Pleural Cell Counts and Clinical Conditions | |
|---|---|---|
| Cell Type | Cell Count | Clinical Conditions |
| Erythrocyte | 5000-10,000/µL (5-10 × 10⁹/L) | Hemothorax if pleural fluid hematocrit >50% peripheral hematocrit |
| Nucleated cells | >50,000/µL (50 × 10⁹/L) | Complicated parapneumonic effusions and empyema |
| | >10,000/µL (10 × 10⁹/L) | Simple parapneumonic effusion, acute pancreatitis and lupus pleuritis |
| | <5000/µL (5 × 10⁹/L) | Chronic exudates (TB pleuritis and malignancy) |
| Lymphocytes | >80% | TB, lymphoma, malignancy, RA pleuritis, sarcoidosis, late post-CABG effusions |
| Eosinophils | >10% | Air or blood in the pleural space. Also parapneumonic effusions, drug-induced pleuritis, eosinophilic granulomatosis with polyangiitis, benign asbestos effusions, malignancy (lymphoma), pulmonary infarction, parasitic disease |

CABG = coronary artery bypass graft; RA = rheumatoid arthritis; TB = tuberculosis.

*Tests for Pleural Malignancy*

Cytologic examination of pleural fluid has an average sensitivity of 60%. This is slightly higher in adenocarcinoma and lower in mesothelioma, squamous cell carcinoma, and lymphoma. There is minimal benefit for obtaining and sending more than two fluid samples. If cytology is negative and malignancy is still suspected, thoracoscopy may be the next step in evaluation. This procedure allows for the direct visualization and biopsy of the pleural surface and has a diagnostic sensitivity for malignant disease of greater than 90%. Closed pleural biopsy provides only a random sample of pleural tissue without visualization of pleural abnormalities. It is less sensitive than fluid cytology and has been replaced by thoracoscopy in the diagnostic evaluation of pleural malignancy.

## Management
### Parapneumonic Effusions and Empyema

A pleural effusion associated with a bacterial pneumonia is called a parapneumonic effusion. It can be uncomplicated (sterile and free-flowing) or complicated (either infected or loculated). Uncomplicated effusions are typically small and resolve on their own with treatment of the pneumonia. Complicated parapneumonic effusions occur with significant inflammation or when bacteria invade the pleural space. An empyema is defined as a bacterial infection of the pleural space, which results in purulent fluid or a positive Gram stain. Pleural fluid cultures identify pathogens in only 60% of cases. If infection is suspected, culture bottles should be inoculated at the bedside to increase yield. Any pleural effusion greater than 10 mm in depth on lateral decubitus radiograph and associated with a pneumonic illness should be sampled with a diagnostic thoracentesis. Drainage is required if there is a positive Gram stain or culture, or when the pH is less than 7.2. The bacteriology of pleural space infection differs depending on if it is community-acquired or hospital-acquired. In the community, *Streptococcus pneumoniae*, *Streptococcus pyogenes*, *Staphylococcus aureus*, and *Streptococcus anginosus* group are the organisms typically associated with pleural infection. Methicillin-resistant *Staphylococcus aureus* and *Enterobacteriaceae* are more prevalent in nosocomial empyema. Anaerobic bacteria are cultured in greater than 20% of pleural-space infections and may be due to the common association with aspiration or the anaerobic environment of the pleural space. Polymicrobial infections are common, and empiric antibiotic regimens before obtaining culture results should include coverage for anaerobes.

Complicated parapneumonic effusions and empyema require drainage. The combined use of intrapleural fibrinolytics (streptokinase, urokinase, tissue plasminogen activator) and a mucolytic agent (deoxyribonuclease, or DNase) has demonstrated utility in decreasing the size of the effusion and lowering the rate of surgical referral for definitive treatment. The size of drainage tube needed to best manage pleural-space infection remains controversial, but several studies have demonstrated equal efficacy and improved patient comfort with the use of smaller (10 to 14 Fr) thoracostomy tubes. Effusions due to infection refractory to antibiotics and drainage require surgical debridement.

### Malignant Pleural Effusion

The diagnosis of a malignant pleural effusion signifies advanced disease and overall poor prognosis. As a result the goal of management is the relief of symptoms. Several therapeutic options exist, and treatment decisions should be based on symptoms, prognosis, degree of anticipated lung re-expansion, and patient performance status. Repeat therapeutic thoracentesis is appropriate for patients with poor prognosis (less than 3 months) and slow re-accumulation of fluid. Patients with rapid re-accumulation of fluid and dyspnea should be offered more definitive management. Indwelling pleural catheters with intermittent outpatient drainage provide significant symptom relief, and 50% to 70% of patients achieve spontaneous pleurodesis after 2 to 6 weeks. Chemical pleurodesis refers to obliteration of the pleural space with a sclerosing agent (typically talc). Talc can be introduced through a thoracostomy tube (talc slurry) or during a thoracoscopy (talc poudrage). Talc pleurodesis is very effective, with a success rate of 60% to 90% depending on the degree of lung re-expansion. Pleurectomy and pleuroperitoneal shunt are other management options but are rarely performed. ▣

# Pneumothorax

## Evaluation

Air in the pleural space is defined as a pneumothorax, which can occur spontaneously or as a result of trauma or a procedural complication. A primary spontaneous pneumothorax (PSP) occurs in someone without known underlying lung disease. A secondary spontaneous pneumothorax (SSP) occurs in someone with known underlying lung disease, such as COPD. Risk of recurrence for PSP is 23% to 50% over 1 to 5 years, and greater than 50% over 1 to 3 years in those with SSP. Risk factors for pneumothorax are listed in **Table 24**.

Symptoms include the sudden onset of dyspnea and sharp pleuritic chest pain. The symptoms are typically more severe with SSP, as patients have less respiratory reserve. Physical examination findings can be subtle but usually reveal reduced lung expansion, hyperresonance to percussion, and diminished breath sounds on the side of the pneumothorax. Tension pneumothorax should be suspected in patients presenting with significant cardiorespiratory distress (worsening dyspnea, hypotension, absent breath sounds on one side, tracheal deviation, and distended neck veins).

A chest radiograph is an appropriate initial test and can confirm the diagnosis and determine the size of the pneumothorax. If the lung margin is greater than 2 cm away from the chest wall at the level of the hilum, it is considered a large pneumothorax. A CT scan is the most sensitive imaging modality for small pneumothoraces and is particularly useful in patients with bullous emphysema.

## Management

Management of pneumothorax is driven by clinical symptoms. A tension pneumothorax (large and hemodynamically significant) should be managed by emergent needle thoracostomy followed by thoracostomy tube placement and hospitalization. Observation alone has been shown to be safe for small pneumothoraces in patients with minimal symptoms (**Table 25**).

Recurrence prevention is recommended after the second episode of pneumothorax on the ipsilateral side in PSP and after the first occurrence in SSP. Patients should be encouraged to stop smoking, as the lifetime incidence rates for PSP are much higher in men who are lifelong heavy smokers than men who have never smoked (12% vs 0.1%). Intervention to prevent recurrence includes both chemical and mechanical pleurodesis. Air travel should be avoided until complete resolution of the pneumothorax, and scuba diving is not recommended unless definitive therapy, such as surgical pleurectomy, has been applied. ◧

# Pulmonary Vascular Disease

## Pulmonary Hypertension

Pulmonary hypertension (PH) is defined as a resting mean pulmonary artery pressure of 25 mm Hg or greater measured during right heart catheterization. The normal mean pulmonary artery pressure is less than 20 mm Hg. Untreated PH eventually leads to right ventricular failure and may directly contribute to death; however, the rate of progression is highly variable and dependent upon the origin of disease and comorbidities.

The current classification system subdivides PH into five groups, which are based on similarities in mechanisms, hemodynamics, clinical presentation, and approach to treatment (**Table 26**).

| TABLE 24. Risk Factors for Pneumothorax |
| --- |
| **Risk Factors for PSP** |
| Smoking |
| Family history |
| Thoracic endometriosis |
| Tall stature |
| **Risk Factors for SSP** |
| COPD |
| Interstitial lung disease |
| Tuberculosis |
| Cystic fibrosis |
| Malignancy |
| Necrotizing pneumonia |
| Marfan syndrome |
| PSP = primary spontaneous pneumothorax; SSP = secondary spontaneous pneumothorax. |

| TABLE 25. Management of Pneumothorax | |
| --- | --- |
| **Size[a] and Clinical Symptoms** | **Management** |
| <2 cm on chest radiograph, minimal symptoms | Admit to hospital for observation and supplemental oxygen (PSP may be managed as an outpatient if good access to medical care) |
| >2 cm on chest radiograph, breathlessness, and chest pain | Insertion of a small-bore (<14 Fr) thoracostomy tube with connection to a high-volume low-pressure suction system |
| Cardiovascular compromise (hypotension, increasing breathlessness) regardless of size | Emergent needle decompression followed by thoracostomy tube insertion<br><br>Note: If persistent air leak (>48 hours) refer to a thoracic surgeon |
| [a]Measured between lung and chest wall | |
| PSP = primary spontaneous pneumothorax. | |

**TABLE 26.** Classification of Pulmonary Hypertension

| | |
|---|---|
| 1 | Pulmonary arterial hypertension (includes idiopathic and heritable, and disease related to drugs and toxins, connective tissue diseases, HIV infection, schistosomiasis, and portal hypertension) |
| 2 | Pulmonary hypertension due to left-sided heart disease |
| 3 | Pulmonary hypertension due to lung diseases and/or hypoxia |
| 4 | Chronic thromboembolic pulmonary hypertension and other pulmonary artery obstructions |
| 5 | Pulmonary hypertension with unclear or multifactorial causes |

Data from Simonneau G, Gatzoulis MA, Adatia I, Celermajer D, Denton C, Ghofrani A, et al. Updated clinical classification of pulmonary hypertension. J Am Coll Cardiol. 2013;62:D34-41. [PMID: 24355639] doi:10.1016/j.jacc.2013.10.029

**KEY POINT**

- Pulmonary hypertension is defined as a resting mean pulmonary artery pressure of 25 mm Hg or greater measured during right heart catheterization.

## Pathophysiology

Most cases of PH are caused by left-sided heart disease (group 2) and hypoxic respiratory disorders (group 3). Left-sided heart disease (heart failure with reduced or preserved ejection fraction, valvular disease) results in elevations in left atrial and pulmonary venous pressures. Chronic hypoxia is probably the primary contributor to PH in advanced respiratory disorders such as COPD, interstitial lung disease, and sleep hypoventilation syndromes; obliteration of the vascular bed in emphysema also contributes. Regardless of the underlying causes or disease associations, untreated PH is usually progressive, eventually leading to vascular remodeling and right ventricular hypertrophy and dilatation. PH is often a risk factor for death in patients with group 2 and 3 disease, and may be directly contributory in death due to right ventricular ischemia, arrhythmias, or heart failure.

**KEY POINT**

- Most cases of pulmonary hypertension are secondary and caused by left-sided heart disease and hypoxic respiratory disorders.

## Diagnosis

Because early symptoms of PH (exertional dyspnea and fatigue) are nonspecific and may be attributed to an underlying disorder such as heart failure or lung disease, a high index of suspicion can help identify PH in its earlier stages. Progressive disease, eventually resulting in right ventricular impairment, is associated with symptoms of exertional chest pain, syncope, and edema. Findings on physical examination depend on the severity of disease. An early sign is a prominent $S_2$; an audible split eventually widens. A prominent jugular venous a wave and a parasternal heave reflect right ventricular hypertrophy. As the right ventricle dilates, a holosystolic

tricuspid regurgitant murmur may be detected. Right ventricular failure leads to jugular venous distention, hepatomegaly, ascites, and peripheral edema. Pulmonary findings reflect underlying lung disease.

Enlarged central pulmonary arteries with peripheral pruning, along with a prominent right ventricle detectable on the lateral view on chest radiograph, are suggestive of PH (**Figure 12**). If PH is suspected, transthoracic echocardiography should be performed, as it allows an estimation of pulmonary arterial systolic pressure and assessment of both right and left heart size and function. However, echocardiography does not confirm the diagnosis because the estimation of true pulmonary artery pressure may be inaccurate. Right heart catheterization confirms the diagnosis of PH and is typically an essential component of the diagnostic evaluation, although it may be deferred in certain situations, such as in patients whose PH is attributable to advanced lung disease such as COPD.

Once PH is confirmed, further testing, guided by clinical history, helps determine underlying causes and important comorbid conditions. Left heart catheterization can assess the coronary arteries if ischemic cardiomyopathy is suspected. Additional diagnostics may include pulmonary function tests, high-resolution CT if interstitial lung disease is a consideration, and tests for nocturnal hypoxemia. Abnormal overnight pulse oximetry to detect nocturnal hypoxemia followed by polysomnography to characterize the cause can identify sleep-related breathing disorders as a cause of PH. Assessment of functional status with the 6-minute walk test should be performed to provide prognostic information and to determine a baseline for assessment of therapeutic response.

**KEY POINTS**

- If pulmonary hypertension is suspected, echocardiography should be performed, as it allows an estimation of pulmonary arterial systolic pressure and assessment of both right and left heart size and function.
- Right heart catheterization confirms the diagnosis of pulmonary hypertension and is an essential component of the diagnostic evaluation.

## Treatment of Pulmonary Hypertension

Therapy for patients with groups 2, 3, and 5 PH is directed at the underlying condition. Optimization of treatment of underlying left ventricular systolic and diastolic function and valvular disease is appropriate. COPD should be managed in a stepwise fashion. For a discussion of treatment of COPD, see Airways Disease. Supplemental oxygen for hypoxemia due to underlying lung disease causing PH may provide mortality benefit. Positive airway pressure therapy may be indicated for sleep-disordered breathing and hypoventilation syndromes. The use of advanced vasodilator therapy in groups 2 through 5 PH can be considered on a patient-by-patient basis. Treatment with such pulmonary vasodilators, however, may be harmful in patients with PH due to left ventricular dysfunction (group 2)

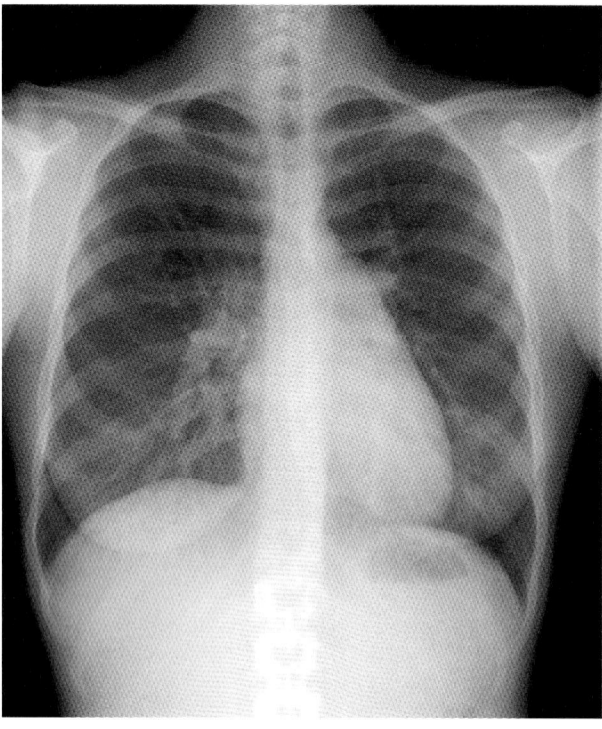 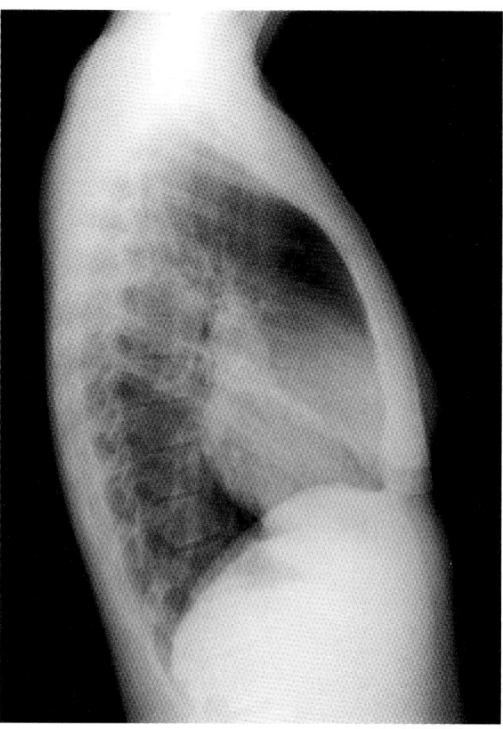

**FIGURE 12.** Posteroanterior chest radiograph (*left*) of a woman with pulmonary arterial hypertension showing right atrial dilatation (straightening of the right heart border), pulmonary artery enlargement, attenuation ("pruning") of the peripheral vessels, and oligemic lung fields. The lateral chest radiograph (*right*) demonstrates diminished retrosternal airspace, a sign of right ventricular hypertrophy.

or lung disease (group 3) because of the potential to overload a compromised left ventricle and to worsen ventilation-perfusion ($\dot{V}/\dot{Q}$) mismatching, respectively.

**KEY POINTS**

- Therapy for patients with pulmonary hypertension caused by left-sided heart disease, lung diseases, or hypoxia, is typically directed at the underlying condition.

- Treatment with pulmonary vasodilators may be harmful in patients with pulmonary hypertension due to left ventricular dysfunction or lung disease because of the potential to overload a compromised left ventricle and to worsen ventilation-perfusion mismatching, respectively.

# Chronic Thromboembolic Pulmonary Hypertension (Group 4)

Progressive exertional dyspnea is the most common symptom of chronic thromboembolic pulmonary hypertension (CTEPH). Less than 5% of patients who experience an acute pulmonary embolism (PE) develop CTEPH. Greater than 25% of patients diagnosed with CTEPH do not have a documented history of PE. For further discussion of pulmonary embolism, see MKSAP 18 Hematology and Oncology. In patients with CTEPH, the organized thrombus is incorporated into the pulmonary arterial endothelium, increasing pulmonary vascular resistance and pressures, eventually leading to right-sided

heart failure. Such patients are only occasionally diagnosed with an underlying hypercoagulable state.

## Diagnosis

Because PE (acute or previous) isn't always evident, CTEPH remains an underrecognized cause of PH and requires a high index of suspicion. The diagnosis is made in the setting of PH in the absence of left heart pressure overload accompanied by imaging evidence of chronic thromboembolism.

Ventilation/perfusion scanning is the most sensitive indicator of CTEPH and should be performed in all patients in whom the diagnosis is suspected. CT pulmonary angiography (CT-PA), which is often performed in the evaluation of a dyspneic patient, may demonstrate proximally located vascular abnormalities such as webs, intimal irregularities, and luminal narrowing, but may be less sensitive for more distal lesions. Conventional pulmonary angiography is used to best characterize the extent and distribution of organized thrombus to determine suitability for surgical intervention.

**KEY POINTS**

- The diagnosis of chronic thromboembolic pulmonary hypertension is made in the setting of pulmonary hypertension in the absence of left heart pressure overload accompanied by imaging evidence of chronic thromboembolism.

*(Continued)*

- Ventilation/perfusion scanning is the most sensitive indicator of chronic thromboembolic pulmonary hypertension and should be performed in all patients in whom the diagnosis is suspected.

## Management

Anticoagulation and consideration of thromboendarterectomy are indicated for CTEPH. Lifelong anticoagulant therapy is indicated in all patients to help prevent further thromboembolism. The only potentially curative therapy for CTEPH is pulmonary thromboendarterectomy. Because the disease usually irreversibly progresses, surgical evaluation at an experienced center is warranted in all patients with CTEPH regardless of disease severity. About half of patients with CTEPH will be eligible for surgery; a proportion will opt for the operation. Pulmonary thromboendarterectomy can result in normalization of pulmonary hemodynamics in about one-third of patients who undergo surgery. Riociguat, an advanced therapy vasodilator, may be used in those who are not candidates for surgery or have persistent PH following surgery. The role of inferior vena cava filters in patients with a coexisting clot in the lower extremities is controversial, and its effect on long-term outcomes is not known.

KEY POINT
- Lifelong anticoagulation and consideration of thromboendarterectomy are indicated for chronic thromboembolic pulmonary hypertension.

# Pulmonary Arterial Hypertension

Pulmonary arterial hypertension (PAH) is caused by changes in the small pulmonary arterioles resulting in high pulmonary vascular resistance. PAH is defined by a proliferative vasculopathy originating in the pulmonary arteriolar bed, with pathophysiologic contributions from endothelial cell proliferation, vasoconstriction, and in-situ thrombosis. Imbalances in nitric oxide, prostacyclin, and endothelin that affect vascular tone and endothelial and smooth muscle cellular growth drive the process and are targets for currently available therapy. PAH is classified as idiopathic (previously referred to as primary pulmonary hypertension), heritable, or associated with drugs, toxins, or other conditions.

Idiopathic PAH is typically seen in younger adults, particularly women. Heritable forms account for less than 10% of cases of PAH, with the majority due to mutations in bone morphogenetic protein receptor type 2 (*BMPR2*). Mutations in *BMPR2*, a gene related to the apoptotic process, might explain the propensity for cellular proliferation in PAH. Although otherwise clinically indistinguishable from sporadic disease, those with heritable PAH may have a worse prognosis.

PAH is most commonly associated with connective tissue diseases, portal hypertension, HIV infection, drug use, and toxin exposure.

In connective tissue disease, PAH is classically seen in systemic sclerosis, where it is a leading cause of death. Patients with limited cutaneous disease in association with CREST syndrome (calcinosis cutis, Raynaud phenomenon, esophageal dysmotility, sclerodactyly, and telangiectasia) may be at highest risk. PAH can also be seen in rheumatoid arthritis and systemic lupus erythematosus.

Portopulmonary hypertension affects some patients who have chronic liver disease (see MKSAP 18 Gastroenterology and Hepatology). The mechanism may relate to the diseased liver's inability to clear vasoactive substances.

PAH in patients with HIV infection is not common, but HIV-infected patients have an approximately 10-fold higher risk of PAH compared with patients without HIV infection. Both viral and host factors have been implicated, and disease can occur in the absence of AIDS-related complications.

The drugs most strongly associated with PAH are the anorectics, including fenfluramine, phentermine, and dexfenfluramine. The tyrosine kinase inhibitors dasatinib and imatinib have been implicated, as well as interferon alfa. There is an increasing association between PAH and illicit drugs such as methamphetamine and cocaine.

KEY POINT
- Pulmonary arterial hypertension is most commonly associated with connective tissue diseases, portal hypertension, HIV infection, drug use, and toxin exposure.

## Diagnosis

The diagnosis of PAH requires confirmation of high pulmonary vascular resistance as well as a normal pulmonary capillary wedge pressure to exclude left-sided heart disease. During right heart catheterization, vasoreactivity testing can help guide subsequent therapy (see below). Lung biopsy poses a significant risk in PAH and is not indicated in the diagnostic evaluation. The role of genetic testing is yet to be defined. Laboratory studies to investigate underlying cause of PAH depend on the clinical situation and may include HIV serologies, tests of liver function, and autoantibody titers.

KEY POINT
- The diagnosis of pulmonary arterial hypertension requires confirmation of high pulmonary vascular resistance as well as a normal pulmonary capillary wedge pressure to exclude left-sided heart disease.

## Treatment

Therapy for PAH is directed at PH itself, referred to as "advanced therapy." These vascular-targeted treatments are directed at reducing vasoconstriction and interrupting the pathways mediating cellular proliferation. Use of advanced agents may be guided by disease severity (Table 27). Before administering advanced therapy for patients with PAH, vasoreactivity testing with nitric oxide is performed to identify those who may respond to calcium channel blockers. Calcium channel

**TABLE 27. Pharmacologic Therapy for Pulmonary Arterial Hypertension**

| Class | Comments |
|---|---|
| Calcium channel blockers | Only for patients with acute vasodilator response at catheterization; acute response does not assure chronic response; side effects such as hypotension can occur. |
| Prostanoids (epoprostenol, treprostinil, iloprost) | Parenteral prostacyclin analogues such as epoprostenol, administered by a continuous central venous infusion, are first-line therapy for severe disease and for those in whom disease progresses despite oral therapy; inhaled iloprost requires frequent administration; prostanoids supplement endogenous levels of prostacyclin (PGI$_2$), a vasodilator with antismooth muscle proliferative properties. |
| Endothelin-1 receptor antagonists (bosentan, ambrisentan) | Reasonable initial oral therapies for mild to moderate disease. Blocks action of endogenous vasoconstrictor and smooth muscle mitogen endothelin; class-wide risk of liver injury and teratogenicity; liver chemistry testing and pregnancy testing for reproductive-aged women are required[a]. |
| Phosphodiesterase-5 inhibitors (sildenafil, tadalafil) | Reasonable initial oral therapies for mild to moderate disease. Prolongs effect of intrinsic vasodilator cyclic GMP by inhibiting hydrolysis by phosphodiesterase-5. |

GMP = guanosine monophosphate.

[a]Although not required for ambrisentan, some experts suggest that it is prudent to perform liver chemistry tests at the outset of treatment for pulmonary arterial hypertension and at periodic intervals thereafter at the discretion of the managing physician.

blockers are desirable therapy because they are less expensive and have fewer side effects than other forms of advanced therapy. Failure to achieve a favorable hemodynamic response with nitric oxide predicts unresponsiveness to calcium channel blockers and the need for other advanced therapy. Given the complexity of management, the increasing number of drugs available to treat PAH, and cost, these patients are best managed by specialists at a center experienced with PAH management.

Additional treatments include diuretic therapy to combat volume overload and supplemental oxygen for hypoxemia at rest or with exercise. Women of reproductive age who have PAH should be counseled on the risks of pregnancy; most specialists would advise against pregnancy. Because PAH predisposes patients to in-situ pulmonary vascular thrombosis and embolism, anticoagulation is often prescribed. Experience with direct oral anticoagulants in this setting is limited; therefore, warfarin remains the agent of choice. Digoxin might be used to improve right ventricular function or as a rate-control adjunct for supraventricular dysrhythmias or atrial fibrillation. Supervised exercise training has been shown to improve functional capacity.

Lung or heart-lung transplantation should be considered for patients in whom drug treatment is unsuccessful.

**KEY POINTS**

- Therapy for pulmonary arterial hypertension is directed at pulmonary hypertension itself, referred to as *advanced therapy*, and is best managed by specialists at a center experienced with pulmonary arterial hypertension management.
- Before administering advanced therapy for patients with pulmonary arterial hypertension, vasoreactivity testing with nitric oxide is performed to identify those who may respond to calcium channel blockers.

# Lung Tumors
## Pulmonary Nodule Evaluation

Pulmonary nodules are small rounded radiographic opacities that are less than 3 cm in size. A solitary pulmonary nodule is a nodule completely surrounded by aerated lung and not associated with atelectasis, hilar enlargement, or pleural effusion. These nodules are usually asymptomatic and found either incidentally or on screening. In contrast, a focal pulmonary opacity larger than 3 cm is considered a lung mass and is presumed malignant until proved otherwise.

The finding of a pulmonary nodule is increasingly common because of the frequency of CT scans done for other reasons, as well as lung cancer screening programs. Management of these lesions can be complicated and often requires subspecialty referral. Principles of pulmonary nodule evaluation include the review of imaging history, estimating the probability of malignancy, performing functional imaging tests (PET scan) to further characterize the nodule, and discussing management preferences with the patient. Guidelines recommend management based on nodule size and characteristics. When more than one nodule is present, follow-up is dictated by the size and characteristics of the largest lesion. Shared decision making is an integral part of the evaluation and management of pulmonary nodules.

**KEY POINTS**

- Principles of pulmonary nodule evaluation include the review of imaging history, estimating the probability of malignancy, performing functional imaging tests to further characterize the nodule, and discussing management preferences with the patient.
- A focal pulmonary opacity larger than 3 cm are presumed malignant until proved otherwise.

### Solid Indeterminate Nodule Larger Than 8 mm

The first step in evaluating a solid nodule that is larger than 8 mm in size is to estimate the probability of malignancy. Criteria included in the calculation include age, smoking history, nodule size, location within the lung, and presence of spiculated or lobular border (https://brocku.ca/lung-cancer-screening-and-risk-prediction/risk-calculators/). Solid nodules with low to moderate probability of malignancy should be characterized further with a PET scan. If the PET scan is negative for metabolic activity, continued surveillance is warranted (**Table 28**). A nodule with moderate or intense uptake is suggestive of malignancy and requires further evaluation, including complete staging followed by surgical resection or chemotherapy and radiation, for definitive management.

If the probability of malignancy is initially high, the next step is staging with a PET scan followed by definitive management with surgical resection or chemotherapy and radiation.

**TABLE 28.** Fleischner Society Recommendations for Single Pulmonary Nodule Follow-Up

| Risk Factors for Lung Cancer? | Size | Recommended Follow-Up |
|---|---|---|
| No (Low-risk patient) | <6 mm | No follow-up |
| | 6-8 mm | CT at 6-12 months then consider CT at 18-24 months |
| | >8 mm | Consider CT at 3 months, PET/CT, or tissue sampling |
| Yes (High-risk patient) | <6 mm | Optional CT at 12 months |
| | 6-8 mm | CT at 6-12 months then CT at 18-24 months |
| | >8 mm | Consider CT at 3 months, PET/CT, or tissue sampling |

Data from MacMahon H, Naidich DP, Goo JM, Lee KS, Leung ANC, Mayo JR, et al. Guidelines for management of incidental pulmonary nodules detected on CT images: From the Fleischner Society 2017. Radiology. 2017;284:228-243. [PMID: 28240562] doi:10.1148/radiol.2017161659

**KEY POINT**
- The first step in evaluating a solid pulmonary nodule larger than 8 mm in size is to estimate the probability of malignancy.

## Solid Indeterminate Nodule of 8 mm or Smaller

Solid indeterminate nodules of 8 mm or smaller are usually detected incidentally. The first step as with larger nodules is an estimation of the likelihood of malignancy (https://brocku.ca/lung-cancer-screening-and-risk-prediction/risk-calculators/). Nodules of 8 mm or smaller have a lower probability of being malignant, are difficult to biopsy, and are not reliably characterized by PET scan. As a result, these small nodules are usually followed by serial CT scans. The frequency and duration of follow-up is based on the recommendations of the Fleischner Society and endorsed by other professional societies (see Table 28).

## Subsolid Nodule

A subsolid nodule is a focal rounded opacity that is either pure ground glass in appearance (focal density with underlying lung architecture still preserved) or has a solid component (part solid) but is still more than 50% ground glass (**Figure 13**). These nodules often represent premalignant disease, such as adenocarcinoma in situ, and can be very slow growing. Observed growth rates for subsolid nodules can range between 400 to 800 days. This has implications for both the frequency and duration of follow-up. Subsolid nodules are not reliably characterized by PET scans and nonsurgical biopsies also have limited sensitivity. Development of a solid component in a pure ground-glass nodule or enlargement of the solid component suggests malignancy (see Figure 13). Recommendations for nonsolid and part-solid nodule follow-up are in **Table 29**.

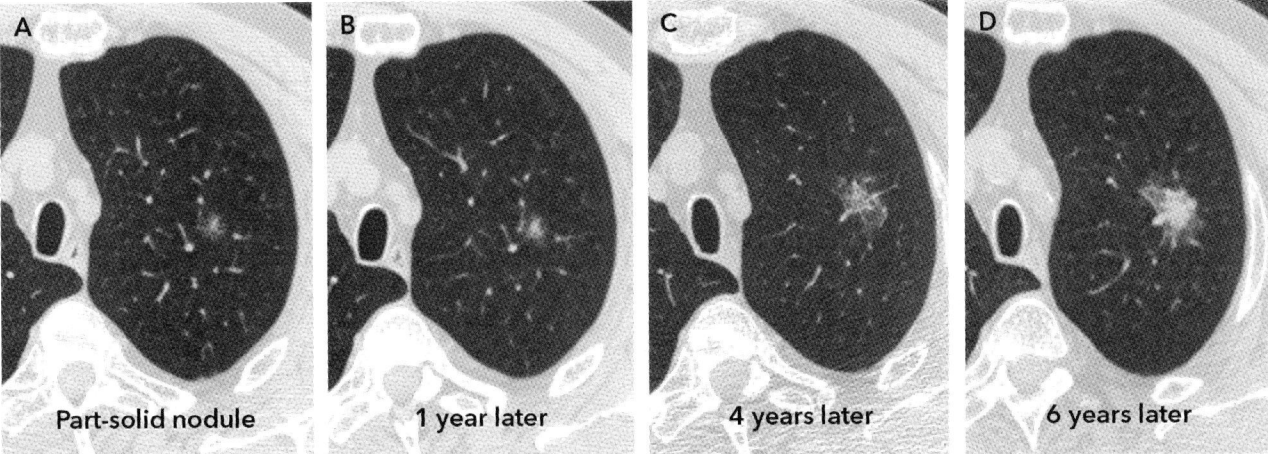

**FIGURE 13.** Radiographs show the evolution of a part-solid nodule from adenocarcinoma in situ to invasive adenocarcinoma: part-solid, part-ground-glass nodule in the left upper lobe (A); growth in the solid component of the nodule 1 year after initial imaging (B); an increase in size in the ground-glass component 4 years after initial imaging (C); and further increase in the solid component of the nodule 6 years after initial imaging (D). This growth rate is characteristic of a part-solid, part-ground-glass nodule and demonstrates why patients with this finding must be followed for at least 5 years.

**TABLE 29.** Fleischner Society Recommendations for Follow-Up of Solitary Subsolid Lung Nodule

| Imaging Findings | Size | Recommended Follow-Up |
|---|---|---|
| Pure ground glass | <6 mm | No follow-up |
| | ≥6 mm | CT at 6-12 months to confirm persistence, then CT every 2 years until 5 years |
| Part solid nodule | <6 mm | No follow-up |
| | ≥6 mm | CT at 3-6 months to confirm persistence. If unchanged and solid component remains <6 mm, annual CT should be performed for 5 years |

Data from MacMahon H, Naidich DP, Goo JM, Lee KS, Leung ANC, Mayo JR, et al. Guidelines for Management of Incidental Pulmonary Nodules Detected on CT Images: From the Fleischner Society 2017. Radiology. 2017;284:228-243. [PMID: 28240562] doi:10.1148/radiol.2017161659

# Lung Cancer

Lung cancer is the leading cause of cancer death worldwide. In the United States, it is estimated that 225,000 new cases will be diagnosed and more than 160,000 deaths occur each year. The overall 5-year survival rate remains low at 17.7%. However, much progress has been made recently regarding screening, diagnosis, and treatment.

### KEY POINT

- Lung cancer is the leading cause of cancer death worldwide, with an estimated 225,000 new cases and more than 160,000 deaths each year.

### Lung Cancer Types

There are two major classes of lung cancer: non–small cell lung cancer (NSCLC) and small cell lung cancer (SCLC). NSCLC accounts for most lung cancer cases (80%) and is divided into adenocarcinoma, squamous cell carcinoma, and large cell carcinoma. Adenocarcinoma is the most common NSCLC and accounts for almost all lung cancer diagnoses in nonsmokers. The most frequent location of adenocarcinoma is in the peripheral aspects of the lung parenchyma as a solitary nodule or mass.

Squamous cell carcinoma is the second most common subtype of NSCLC. It correlates highly with smoking history and usually originates in the central airways (trachea, main stem bronchi, lobar and segmental bronchi) (**Figure 14**). Individuals with squamous cell carcinoma often have symptoms of cough and hemoptysis due to central airway involvement. Radiographically, squamous cell carcinoma may present with postobstructive pneumonia or lobar collapse. Large cell carcinoma is an undifferentiated carcinoma and characteristically presents as a peripheral mass with prominent necrosis (**Figure 15**).

In the past decade the development of targeted therapy for specific gene mutations has revolutionized the treatment of lung cancer. The separation of adenocarcinoma and squamous cell carcinoma is important for determining the optimal therapy. Testing for epidermal growth factor receptor (*EGFR*) mutation, anaplastic lymphoma kinase receptor tyrosine kinase (*ALK*) translocation, and ROS proto-oncogene 1 receptor tyrosine kinase (*ROS1*) translocation is recommended in advanced-stage adenocarcinoma or mixed cancers. Targeted treatment has resulted in better responses than standard chemotherapy.

SCLC accounts for about 15% of all lung cancers. It is the most strongly associated with cigarette smoking and typically occurs adjacent to the central airways with extensive lymphadenopathy and distant metastasis at diagnosis. Imaging commonly shows a large mediastinal mass that encompasses lymph nodes with an uncertain primary site of origin (**Figure 16**). Paraneoplastic syndromes are most commonly associated with SCLC, including hyponatremia due to the syndrome of inappropriate antidiuretic hormone secretion (rare in other lung tumors), hypertrophic pulmonary osteoarthropathy, inflammatory myopathies, Cushing syndrome caused by ectopic adrenocorticotropic hormone secretion, and other hematologic and neurologic syndromes. 

### KEY POINTS

- There are two major classes of lung cancer: non–small cell lung cancer and small cell lung cancer; non–small cell lung cancer accounts for 80% of lung cancers and is divided into adenocarcinoma, squamous cell carcinoma, and large cell carcinoma.

*(Continued)*

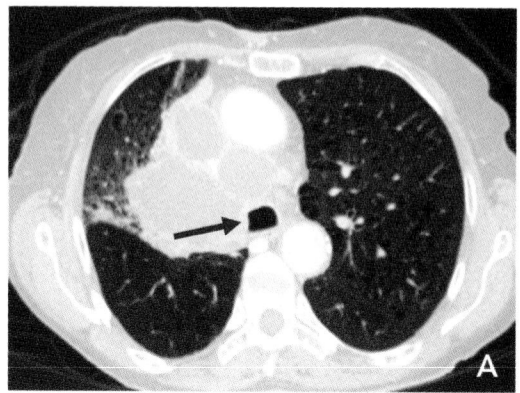
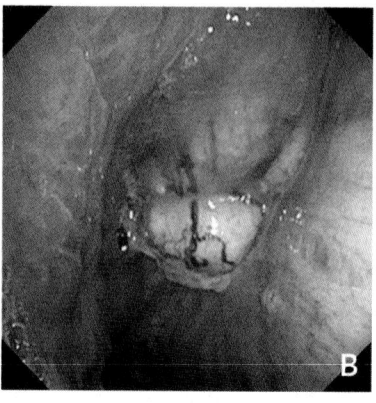

**FIGURE 14.** Metastatic squamous cell carcinoma can be seen as an 8-cm right hilar mass with invasion into the trachea on CT scan (*A*), and as tumor invasion into the distal trachea and occlusion of the right main stem on bronchoscopy (*B*).

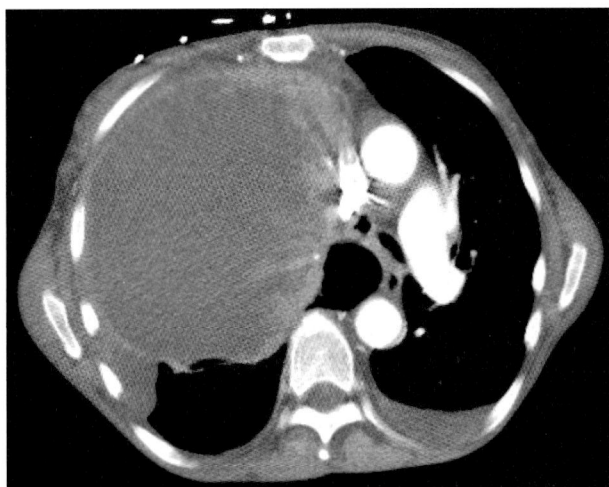

**FIGURE 15.** Large cell carcinoma with predominant necrosis can be seen on CT scan as a large necrotic tumor that has completely replaced the right upper and middle lobes, with deviation of the central airway structures to the left. Necrosis is noted by the mixed attenuation of the mass as noted on CT.

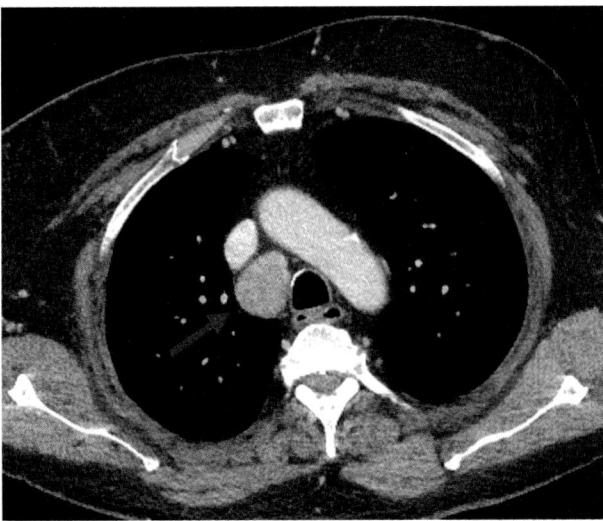

**FIGURE 16.** Small cell lung cancer can be seen on chest CT with a right paratracheal mass (*arrow*). This patient initially presented with encephalitis (paraneoplastic syndrome).

**KEY POINTS** *(continued)*

- Testing for epidermal growth factor receptor (*EGFR*) mutation, anaplastic lymphoma kinase receptor tyrosine kinase (*ALK*) translocation, and ROS proto-oncogene 1 receptor tyrosine kinase (*ROS1*) translocation is recommended in advanced-stage adenocarcinoma or mixed cancers.

## Risk Factors

The main risk factor for lung cancer is smoking tobacco (voluntary or secondhand). This risk increases based on the number of pack-years of smoking and other carcinogenic exposures. Any reduction in lung cancer mortality will be linked to an overall reduction of cigarette smoking. Other risk factors that have been associated with lung cancer include previous radiation therapy, exposure to environmental toxins (asbestos, radon, metals, and diesel fumes), pulmonary fibrosis, HIV infection, family history of lung cancer, and alcohol abuse.

## Screening

Until recently, screening for lung cancer was not widely done, as previous studies had not shown early detection resulted in any mortality benefit for lung cancer. The National Lung Screening Trial (NLST) was a randomized trial comparing CT screening to chest radiograph for detecting lung cancer in current or heavy smokers. The trial demonstrated a 20% reduction in lung cancer mortality in heavy smokers who were screened annually for 3 years. As a result, the U.S. Preventive Services Task Force has recommended annual lung cancer screening using low-dose CT scan for high-risk current and former smokers. The criteria for screening are based on the inclusion criteria for the NLST and include those who are age 55 to 80 years (other guidelines offer different ages to discontinue screening, ranging from 74 to 77 years), have at least a 30-pack-year smoking history, and are current smokers or have quit within the last 15 years. Cessation of screening should be considered in those with limited life expectancy or those who would not be candidates for or willing to undergo surgery.

### KEY POINT

- The U.S. Preventive Services Task Force recommends annual lung cancer screening using low-dose CT scan for those who are age 55 to 80 years, have at least a 30-pack-year smoking history, and are either current smokers or have quit smoking within the last 15 years.

## Diagnosis and Staging

When evaluating a patient who has a lung nodule or mass for possible lung cancer, two questions must be answered: first, what is the cell type?; and second, what is the stage? The radiographic abnormality should first be compared to any previous chest imaging studies the patient has undergone in order to determine the age and growth pattern of the lesion. A solid lung nodule that has been stable for 2 years or longer is unlikely to represent malignancy. However, ground-glass or part-solid lesions usually grow at a much slower rate (400 to 800 days) and need a longer period of time (5 years) to exclude cancer based on radiographic stability.

Initial evaluation should start with a full history, physical exam, complete blood count, serum chemistries, and CT scan of the chest. Most lung cancers present at a late stage. Symptoms result from the local effects of the tumor, metastatic spread involving other organs, or paraneoplastic syndromes. The most common symptoms at presentation include cough, dyspnea, chest pain, weight loss, and hemoptysis. NSCLC and SCLC present with similar symptoms. Similarly, the presence of findings on physical examination (consolidation, effusion, bone tenderness, neurological findings) will indicate advanced disease. CT

CONT.

scan findings that are suggestive of malignancy are listed in **Table 30**. A CT scan provides an accurate assessment of the location and size of the tumor within the chest and helps to direct tissue biopsy for diagnosis and staging. PET scans can be very helpful in the initial evaluation of potential lung cancer, as several studies have demonstrated that PET identifies unsuspected mediastinal involvement, distant disease, or both, which informs staging biopsies and reduces futile (noncurative) surgery. The sensitivity of a PET scan to detect lung cancer is affected by the mass of the nodule and its metabolic rate, with increased potential for false negative results for cancers smaller than 1 cm and slow-growing cancers, such as carcinoid tumors.

The definitive diagnosis of lung cancer requires tissue histopathology. If the nodule has a high probability for malignancy and the PET scan shows uptake only in the lesion, it is reasonable to offer surgical resection to diagnose and treat in a single procedure. In patients with radiographic evidence of advanced stage disease, diagnosis and staging are best accomplished with a single invasive test at a location that will establish both the diagnosis and the stage. Because there are many techniques available for tissue diagnosis, the strategy will depend on size and location of the tumor, patient characteristics, and surgical expertise. In general, mediastinal and central lesions are best approached with bronchoscopy, and smaller peripheral lesions are best approached with a transthoracic needle aspiration.

Definitive staging of lung cancer is essential, allows for accurate prognostication, and serves as a guide for treatment decision making. NSCLC is staged based on the TNM staging system, taking into account the characteristics of the primary tumor (T), regional lymph node involvement (N), and metastatic disease (M).

SCLC is generally staged as either "limited" or "extensive" disease. Limited disease is defined as disease limited to one hemithorax and ipsilateral supraclavicular lymph nodes. The presence of disease outside these locations defines extensive stage disease.

Treatment of lung cancer is discussed in MKSAP 18 Hematology and Oncology.

### KEY POINTS

- The definitive diagnosis of lung cancer requires tissue histopathology.
- In patients with radiographic evidence of advanced-stage lung cancer, diagnosis and staging are best accomplished with a single invasive test at a location that will establish both the diagnosis and the stage of disease.

| TABLE 30. CT Findings Suggestive of Lung Malignancy |
| --- |
| **Irregular or Spiculated Borders** |
| Upper-lobe location |
| Thick-walled cavitation |
| Solid component within a ground-glass lesion |
| Detection of growth on follow-up imaging |

## Other Pulmonary Neoplasms

Carcinoid tumors are low-grade neoplasms comprised of neuroendocrine cells and are uncommon, accounting for 1% to 2% of all lung cancers. Unlike the case for NSCLC and SCLC, smoking is not a risk factor. Most lung carcinoid tumors arise in the proximal airways, and the predominant symptoms or signs are those of an obstructing tumor mass (cough, dyspnea, monophonic wheezing) or bleeding. Bronchial obstruction may be responsible for lobar atelectasis and recurrent episodes of pneumonia in the same pulmonary segment, but may be asymptomatic (**Figure 17**). Misdiagnosing carcinoid tumors as asthma or pneumonia is responsible for delayed diagnosis. It is rare for lung carcinoid tumors to produce and release serotonin and other vasoactive substances into the systemic circulation and be associated with carcinoid syndrome. Surgical resection is often curative, and 10-year survival rates are higher than 90%.

Adenoid cystic carcinoma is a salivary gland tumor that occurs in the lower respiratory tract and accounts for less than 1% of all lung cancers. Surgical resection is the preferred treatment. Hamartomas are the most common benign lung neoplasm. These rare lesions are a combination of cartilage, connective tissue, smooth muscle, fat, and respiratory epithelium. On imaging they tend to be smooth-bordered nodules, which may contain fat. Additionally, they may be recognized by their classic appearance on CT of "popcorn" calcification; however, this only occurs 25% of the time.

The lung is a frequent site for metastatic disease from primary malignancies, which include head and neck, colon, kidney, breast, thyroid, and melanoma. Metastatic disease can present as solitary or multiple nodules; lymphangitic spread; and endobronchial, pleural, or embolic lesions. Surgical resection may be appropriate when a solitary pulmonary metastasis is identified without evidence of other metastatic disease.

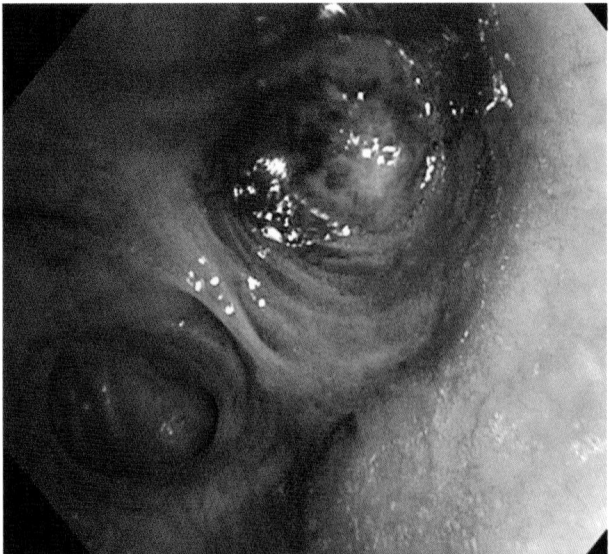

**FIGURE 17.** Endobronchial carcinoid can be seen on bronchoscopy as a smooth, polypoid, vascular-appearing mass that completely occludes a subsegmental airway of the right lower lobe.

- Surgical resection of carcinoid tumors is often curative, and 10-year survival rates are higher than 90%.

## Mesothelioma

Malignant pleural mesothelioma is a rare neoplasm that originates from the cells that line the pleural cavity (mesothelium). It can present as small nodules, plaque-like masses, or confluent sheets that can encase the lung. It is associated with inhalational exposure to asbestos fibers and has a latency of 20 to 40 years. Asbestos is a naturally occurring silicate mineral that is found in soil and rock as long fibers. It is valued for its resistance to heat and combustion and has been used in cement, ceiling tiles, pool tiles, automobile brake linings, and shipbuilding. In addition to malignant pleural mesothelioma and lung cancer, asbestos exposure has been linked to a spectrum of nonmalignant pleuropulmonary diseases (**Table 31**); for further discussion of asbestos-related disease, see Occupational Lung Disease. Because of environmental control of asbestos, the rate of mesothelioma in the United States has been declining since 2000.

Patients with malignant pleural mesothelioma usually present with advanced disease. Symptoms include chest pain, dyspnea, cough, hoarseness, night sweats, or dysphagia. Clinical suspicion for malignant pleural mesothelioma should arise in the setting of pleural thickening or exudative pleural effusion and a history of asbestos exposure. Pleural fluid cytology is typically negative in this scenario and the diagnosis requires a pleural biopsy. Medical or surgical thoracoscopy allows for direct visualization of the pleural surface and has a greater than 90% sensitivity for malignancy. Treatment options depend on the extent of disease and patient factors and preferences, and may include surgery, radiation therapy, and systemic chemotherapy. The overall prognosis of malignant pleural mesothelioma remains poor, with a median survival of 6 to 8 months.

- Mesothelioma is associated with inhalational exposure to asbestos fibers and has a latency of 20 to 40 years.

- Clinical suspicion for malignant pleural mesothelioma should arise in the setting of pleural thickening or exudative pleural effusion and a history of asbestos exposure.

**TABLE 31.** Nonmalignant Asbestos-Related Pleural and Pulmonary Diseases

| Disease | Characteristics |
|---|---|
| Asbestosis | Slowly progressive diffuse pulmonary fibrosis caused by inhalation of asbestos fibers |
| Benign asbestos pleural effusion | Small unilateral pleural effusion, may be associated with concomitant pleural plaques |
| Pleural plaques | Benign circumscribed areas of pleural thickening with linear or nodular appearance |

# Mediastinal Masses

The mediastinum is anatomically near the center of the thoracic cavity and is bound by the sternum anteriorly, the lungs and pleura laterally, and the vertebral column posteriorly. Tumors in the mediastinum can be either benign or malignant, and symptoms vary depending on size (mass effect) and systemic effects of the tumor. Dividing the mediastinum into compartments can be useful in developing a differential diagnosis when a mediastinal mass is discovered (**Figure 18**).

## Anterior Mediastinum

The anterior mediastinal compartment lies between the posterior sternum and the great vessels and heart. It is the most common mediastinal location where malignant tumors occur. Masses in this location are usually remembered as the "terrible T's": thymoma, teratoma/germ cell tumor, "terrible" lymphoma, and thyroid. Thymic lesions are the most common and are associated with various paraneoplastic syndromes, such as myasthenia gravis. Myasthenia gravis is an autoimmune disorder of the neuromuscular junction that commonly presents with muscular weakness, fatigability, ptosis, diplopia, and bulbar symptoms. Diagnosis can be confirmed with an acetylcholine receptor antibody test.

- Thymic lesions are the most common tumor in the anterior mediastinum and are associated with various paraneoplastic syndromes, such as myasthenia gravis.

## Middle Mediastinum

Masses in the middle mediastinum are common and are attributed to lymphadenopathy, cysts, esophageal disorders, or vascular lesions (aneurysm). Lymphadenopathy is most common and can be secondary to lymphoma, sarcoid, or metastatic disease.

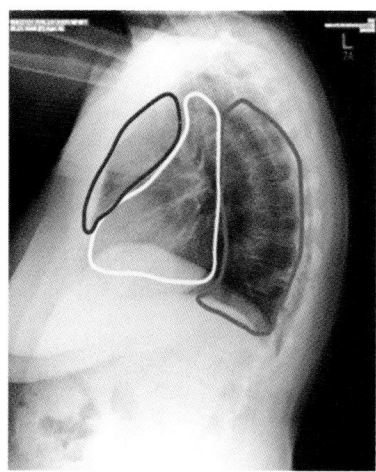

**FIGURE 18.** A lateral chest radiograph demonstrates the anterior (*red*), middle (*yellow*), and posterior (*blue*) mediastinal compartments.

- Lymphadenopathy is the most common mass in the middle mediastinum and can be secondary to lymphoma, sarcoid, or metastatic disease.

## Posterior Mediastinum

Masses in the posterior mediastinum include neurogenic tumors, meningoceles, and spine lesions. Neurogenic neoplasms are most common and are classified based on their neural origin.

- Neurogenic neoplasms are the most common tumors in the posterior mediastinum and are classified based on their neural origin.

# Sleep Medicine
## Classification of Sleep Disorders

Sleep disorders are broadly grouped into six classifications: insomnia, sleep-related breathing disorders, central disorders of hypersomnolence, circadian rhythm sleep-wake disorders, parasomnias, and sleep-related movement disorders (which includes restless leg syndrome).

## Excessive Daytime Sleepiness

Excessive daytime sleepiness refers to difficulty staying awake and alert during daytime hours. Sleepiness is most prominent during passive situations such as reading or watching television. Lack of self-recognition is common and can pose a safety hazard if sleepiness occurs while driving or operating machinery. When obtaining a history from the patient, it is important to distinguish sleepiness, a cardinal symptom of many sleep disorders, from fatigue, which refers to a lack of energy or sense of exhaustion that prevents mental or physical activity at the intensity or pace desired. Fatigue is unlikely to be explained solely by a sleep disorder, and is more likely to occur in the setting of certain medical conditions (malignancies, autoimmune disorders, anemia, endocrinopathies, infections), neurologic disorders (myasthenia gravis, multiple sclerosis, Parkinson disease), psychiatric conditions (mood disorders), and chronic fatigue syndrome.

Causes of excessive daytime sleepiness can be categorized as extrinsic (circumstantial) or intrinsic (disease-related) processes (**Table 32**).

Sleepiness can occur acutely when a person is deprived of the 7 to 8 hours of sleep most adults require. Functional impairment resulting from chronic sleep debt due to inadequate amount of sleep is termed insufficient sleep syndrome. It likely is the most common cause of excessive daytime sleepiness and has been associated with cardiovascular

**TABLE 32.** Extrinsic and Intrinsic Causes of Excessive Daytime Sleepiness

| **Extrinsic Causes** |
| --- |
| Insufficient sleep duration (or inadequate opportunity for sleep) |
| Circadian rhythm disturbance (shift work sleep disorder, jet lag) |
| Drug-, substance-, or medical condition–related hypersomnia |
| Environmental sleep disorder (ambient noise, pets) |
| **Intrinsic Causes** |
| Sleep-disordered breathing syndromes, such as obstructive sleep apnea and central sleep apnea |
| Narcolepsy |
| Idiopathic hypersomnia |
| Restless leg syndrome and periodic limb movement disorder |
| Circadian rhythm sleep disorders (misalignment of the intrinsic circadian timing with the desired sleep schedule; for example, dementia and blindness) |

disease and metabolic disorders such as glucose intolerance and obesity.

The initial evaluation of excessive daytime sleepiness should include a thorough history to assess the time available for and spent sleeping before pursuing additional testing. A 1- or 2-week diary of the sleep-wake schedule is a simple tool that promotes self-realization of suboptimal sleep habits. A more objective assessment of sleep and wakefulness can be obtained with a wrist actigraph, a device that measures movement and ambient light during a period of 1 or 2 weeks. Wrist-worn consumer fitness products using similar technology may provide useful feedback. Questionnaires such as the Epworth Sleepiness Scale can quantify sleepiness and help gauge the response to treatment.

Objective sleep testing, either in-lab or at-home multi-channel recordings, is often indicated when a primary sleep disorder (such as obstructive sleep apnea) is suggested by the history and physical examination. In certain cases a multiple sleep latency test, a sleep laboratory–based study that measures the time to sleep during a series of daytime nap opportunities following a normal night of sleep, provides an objective measure of sleepiness and is key to establishing the diagnoses of narcolepsy and idiopathic hypersomnia. A mean sleep latency of more than 15 minutes is considered normal and less than 5 minutes is indicative of pathologic sleepiness.

All patients with excessive daytime sleepiness should be counseled about the dangers of drowsy driving and the need to maintain a routine sleep-wake schedule that allows for 7 to 8 hours of sleep per night. Specific treatment depends on the underlying condition (positive airway pressure for obstructive sleep apnea or stimulant medications for narcolepsy). Short-term management of the occasional bout of acute sleepiness may include strategically timed naps or caffeinated beverages.

- The initial evaluation of excessive daytime sleepiness should include a thorough history to assess the time available for and spent sleeping before pursuing additional testing.

- All patients with excessive daytime sleepiness should be counseled about the dangers of drowsy driving and the need to maintain a routine sleep-wake schedule that allows for 7 to 8 hours of sleep per night.

- Functional impairment resulting from chronic sleep debt due to inadequate amount of sleep is termed insufficient sleep syndrome; it likely is the most common cause of excessive daytime sleepiness and has been associated with cardiovascular disease and metabolic disorders such as glucose intolerance and obesity.

- When obtaining a history from the patient, it is important to distinguish sleepiness, a cardinal symptom of many sleep disorders, from fatigue, which refers to a lack of energy or sense of exhaustion that prevents mental or physical activity at the intensity or pace desired.

# Conditions that Disrupt Circadian Rhythm

## Jet Lag

Jet lag results when the internal circadian clock is out of phase with the local time following air travel across multiple (typically more than five) time zones. Symptoms occur within one to two days following travel and may include insomnia, daytime sleepiness, and neuropsychiatric impairment. For short trips (one to two days), remaining on origin time might be preferable, if feasible. For longer trips, adjusting to the destination time may alleviate jet lag. Ways to promote adjustment include pretravel measures (avoidance of sleep deprivation and dehydration and, for the highly motivated, bright light therapy starting up to 3 days before travel with the intention to advance the circadian phase). In-flight hypnotic medications are popular, though they pose a risk of parasomnias, particularly if alcohol is consumed. Postarrival measures include timed bright light exposure and melatonin, depending upon the direction traveled, caffeine intake, and naps.

## Shift Work Sleep Disorder

As much as one fifth of the American work force maintains a job schedule outside the usual day shift hours. Although some people acclimate well to this schedule (and may even prefer it), many do not and suffer daytime symptoms such as excessive sleepiness, mood perturbations, and neurocognitive dysfunction. Such symptoms can render the next-morning drive home from work dangerous. Symptoms persisting at least 3 months meet criteria for shift work sleep disorder. Management should first include consideration of eliminating shift work by a change in work schedule. If this isn't feasible, interventions to improve daytime sleep may include bright light avoidance in the morning (wearing sunglasses if necessary), maintaining a structured sleep-wake pattern, and melatonin, which is of modest benefit in shifting the physiologic sleep cycle. Hypnotic medications have been used to promote daytime sleep but are of varying effectiveness and pose the risk of carryover effects into the nighttime work period. Interventions to promote nighttime wakefulness include bright light treatment in the evening before the night shift, caffeinated beverages or wake-promoting stimulants (such as modafinil) during work hours, and planned napping during work breaks.

# Obstructive Sleep Apnea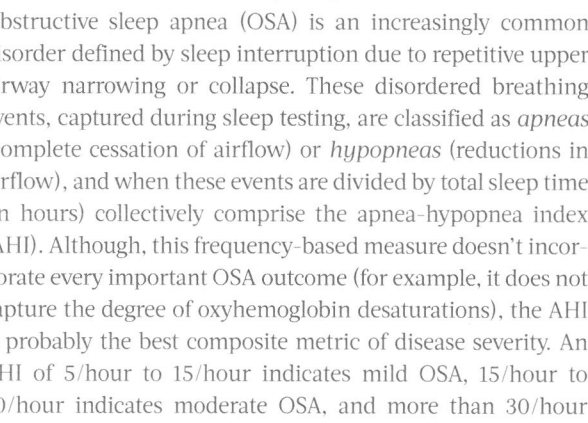

Obstructive sleep apnea (OSA) is an increasingly common disorder defined by sleep interruption due to repetitive upper airway narrowing or collapse. These disordered breathing events, captured during sleep testing, are classified as *apneas* (complete cessation of airflow) or *hypopneas* (reductions in airflow), and when these events are divided by total sleep time (in hours) collectively comprise the apnea-hypopnea index (AHI). Although, this frequency-based measure doesn't incorporate every important OSA outcome (for example, it does not capture the degree of oxyhemoglobin desaturations), the AHI is probably the best composite metric of disease severity. An AHI of 5/hour to 15/hour indicates mild OSA, 15/hour to 30/hour indicates moderate OSA, and more than 30/hour indicates severe OSA.

- Obstructive sleep apnea is an increasingly common disorder defined by sleep interruption due to repetitive upper airway narrowing or collapse.

- The apnea-hypopnea index (AHI) is the total number of apnea and hypopnea events divided by total sleep time (in hours) and can classify obstructive sleep apnea as mild (5/hour to 15/hour), moderate (15/hour to 30/hour), or severe (more than 30/hour).

## Pathophysiology

With sleep onset, pharyngeal muscles acting to maintain upper airway patency relax, resulting in redundancy of the soft tissues that line the airway. Snoring is often (though not universally) a result of this process, as inspired air collides with these tissues. In OSA, airflow is further compromised by forces (see Risk Factors) that overwhelm the neuromuscular mechanisms promoting upper airway patency. Posture and sleep stage are also important factors. The supine position promotes posterior displacement of the tongue, further narrowing the airway lumen. Disordered breathing events are most prominent during rapid eye movement (REM), a stage of sleep characterized by atonia of nearly all muscles, with the exception of the extraocular muscles and respiratory diaphragm. Efforts to breathe persist against the airway occlusion, resulting in intrathoracic pressure swings. The process is terminated with a brief awakening from sleep (called a microarousal), during which upper airway patency is restored and ventilation resumes, typically followed by resumption of sleep and continual repetition of the process.

Repetitive arousals and disruption of sleep architecture contribute to the development of excessive daytime sleepiness and neurocognitive symptoms of OSA. Oxyhemoglobin desaturations can be profound, particularly in those with underlying cardiopulmonary disease. This hypoxic stress, along with a host of other intermediary mechanisms including inflammation and high adrenergic tone, raise the question of whether OSA may directly contribute to commonly comorbid systemic disorders such as metabolic and cardiovascular disease. Current evidence, based in part on results of randomized controlled trials of positive airway pressure therapy, suggest a causal link between OSA and systemic hypertension. However, relationships with other disorders such as heart failure, cardiac arrhythmias, diabetes mellitus, and mortality are merely associative; causation remains unproven.

## Risk Factors

The most important risk factor for OSA is obesity, particularly in those with prominence of adipose tissue in the trunk and neck. Partially on account of gender-specific distribution of fat tissue, men are at higher risk than women, though rates equalize following menopause. The prevalence of OSA increases with age. Blacks and Asians are at higher risk. Alcohol and sedative drugs can exacerbate OSA. Tonsillar hypertrophy, macroglossia, retrognathia/micrognathia, and upper airway mass lesions can contribute to upper airway narrowing.

> **KEY POINT**
>
> - The most important risk factor for obstructive sleep apnea is obesity, particularly in those with prominence of adipose tissue in the trunk and neck.

## Clinical Features and Diagnosis

Patients are commonly brought to medical attention by the concerns of a bed partner who observes loud snoring, gasping, and breathing pauses. Nocturnal choking or gasping is probably the most sensitive pretest indicator of OSA. Other symptoms include overnight awakenings, nocturia, and feeling unrested after a night of sleep.

The most important established consequence of OSA is excessive daytime sleepiness. Although it is not a universal symptom, the lack of self-report may not reflect the true degree of impairment. Collateral history from a family member as well as questionnaires such as the Epworth Sleepiness Scale can help identify excessive daytime sleepiness. Neuropsychiatric symptoms are common, including mood alterations, difficulty in concentrating, and problems completing tasks at school or the workplace.

With increasing use of screening tools such as the STOP-BANG questionnaire and perioperative care pathways, unexpected patient events due to undiagnosed OSA following a surgical procedure involving general anesthesia or narcotic analgesics are less common than in the past.

Objective testing is required for a diagnosis of OSA. Physical examination findings (crowded oropharynx) and questionnaires might enhance pretest probability and guide decision-making about whether to pursue testing, but alone are insufficiently sensitive or specific. Overnight pulse oximetry is also poorly discriminative to diagnose OSA, but in those who are asymptomatic with a low pretest probability, normal overnight oximetry might be reassuring and support the decision to avoid further testing. The historic gold standard—in-laboratory polysomnography—which is costly and resource-intensive, is being replaced in many regions by home sleep testing. Home sleep testing doesn't measure electroencephalographic sleep like polysomnography. Yet, it is diagnostically similar in otherwise uncomplicated patients (without underlying cardiopulmonary or neuromuscular disease) who are felt to have at least moderate to severe OSA (to minimize false negatives that may occur in milder disease).

> **KEY POINTS**
>
> - Normal overnight pulse oximetry in those who are asymptomatic with a low pretest probability can be reassuring and supports the decision to avoid further testing for obstructive sleep apnea.
> - Home sleep testing may be most appropriate in patients without underlying cardiopulmonary or neuromuscular disease who are felt to have at least moderate to severe obstructive sleep apnea.

## Treatment

There are several treatment options for OSA, the efficacy of which are generally based upon the ability to reduce, if not abolish, apneas and hypopneas. Positive airway pressure therapy, which typically reduces the AHI toward zero, is the most reliable means to accomplish this, though because the AHI doesn't always correlate with important outcomes in OSA, other treatments may adequately manage OSA for a given patient, even in the face of residual sleep apnea.

Based upon clinical trial results, the strongest indication for treatment of OSA is excessive daytime sleepiness, which generally improves with effective therapy. Although they are not as easily measured as excessive daytime sleepiness, other associated symptoms such as choking or gasping would also be expected to respond to treatment. Neurocognitive and mood symptoms are probably indications for treatment. In patients who perform mission-critical work (truck drivers, pilots), the threshold for treatment may be lower than for others. The role of treatment in otherwise healthy or asymptomatic individuals is a matter of debate. Device therapy (positive airway pressure and oral appliances) has been shown to modestly reduce blood pressure in hypertensive patients with

OSA, but the effect of treatment to manage comorbid cardio-vascular disease or to prevent major cardiovascular events is unproven.

## Weight Loss, Behavioral Modifications

OSA severity improves with weight loss, so all overweight or obese patients with OSA should be counseled accordingly. In minimally symptomatic patients with mild OSA, weight loss might be preferred therapy. Weight loss associated with diet-ing programs or bariatric surgery generally improves but may not eradicate OSA, so close follow-up is required. Additional measures that may help manage mild OSA include reducing alcohol intake before bedtime and avoiding a supine posture if OSA is position-dependent. [H]

> **KEY POINT**
>
> - Obstructive sleep apnea severity improves with weight loss, so all overweight or obese patients with obstructive sleep apnea should be counseled accordingly.

## Positive Airway Pressure

Positive airway pressure remains the most effective therapy for preventing disordered breathing events and alleviating symp-toms in patients who have OSA. It acts by pressurizing the upper airway to maintain lumenal patency, thereby eliminat-ing snoring and airflow limitation.

As home sleep testing becomes more widespread in uncomplicated OSA, the traditional paradigm of in-lab poly-somnography titration performed by a sleep technologist to arrive at an optimal fixed and constant value referred to as continuous positive airway pressure will be less common. The diagnosis by home sleep testing is coupled to treatment with auto-adjusting positive airway pressure, which uses a com-puter algorithm to detect and overcome upper airway resist-ance in real time. Auto-adjusting positive airway pressure and continuous positive airway pressure are considered therapeu-tic equivalents in terms of reducing the AHI and adherence to treatment. Bilevel positive airway pressure, which delivers separate inspiratory and expiratory pressures (the gradient is referred to as pressure support) to augment alveolar ventila-tion, has no proved role in OSA without a hypoventilation syndrome (see below).

The effectiveness of positive airway pressure therapy hinges upon patient adherence. Symptom burden probably drives adherence but for those who lack motivation, educa-tional programs can help, as can direct-to-patient reports wirelessly transmitted from the device directly to smartphones or computers. Side effects such as xerostomia and nasal dry-ness and congestion can be ameliorated by in-line humidifica-tion. Intranasal glucocorticoids or anticholinergics may be useful for recalcitrant nasal congestion or rhinitis. Modified pressure profiles that slightly reduce pressure on exhalation may enhance comfort. Proper mask fit enhances comfort and mitigates air leak. Positive airway pressure interfaces, ranging from nasal pillows that sit at the nasal openings to nasal masks

that cover the nose to oronasal (full face) masks that cover the nose and mouth, are frequently updated and improved. [H]

> **KEY POINTS**
>
> - Positive airway pressure remains the most effective therapy for preventing disordered breathing events and alleviating symptoms in patients who have obstructive sleep apnea.
> - Auto-adjusting positive airway pressure and continuous positive airway pressure are considered therapeutic equivalents for reducing the apnea-hypopnea index and increasing adherence to treatment.

## Oral Appliances

Oral appliances increase upper airway caliber primarily by exerting traction to advance the mandible. They do not reduce the AHI or increase oxygen levels as reliably as positive airway pressure, and are, therefore, generally avoided in more severe cases of OSA. Oral appliances have some potential advantages over positive airway pressure, however, including a reduced incidence of side effects and a potentially higher rate of adher-ence. The most common side effects are morning occlusal changes, which are generally reversible, and sialorrhea.

## Upper Airway Surgery

Although surgical procedures are generally not first-line ther-apy for OSA, maxillomandibular advancement (MMA) signifi-cantly improves the AHI, even in severe disease, and can be considered for patients who do not benefit from or refuse posi-tive airway pressure therapy. Factors that predict surgical suc-cess are not fully known, though younger patients who are less obese probably fare better. Traditional soft palatal procedures such as uvulopalatopharyngoplasty (UPPP) are ineffective; tonsillectomy in adults may or may not be effective. Tracheotomy, which bypasses the entire upper airway, is an effective though uncommonly used treatment of OSA, limited by patient acceptance and aesthetics.

If surgery is performed, reassessment by objective testing should be performed within 3 to 6 months to assess effect.

> **KEY POINT**
>
> - Traditional soft palatal procedures such as uvulo-palatopharyngoplasty are ineffective for treatment of obstructive sleep apnea. **HVC**

## Other Devices

A hypoglossal nerve stimulator approved for use in OSA has been shown to improve the AHI in some patients. Implanted in the chest wall, it synchronizes with the respiratory cycle to contract the tongue muscles during inspiration. It is expensive, and those patients most likely to benefit from this treatment are yet to be determined.

A nasal end-expiratory positive airway pressure device applied to the nasal openings by way of an adhesive has also been shown to reduce the AHI in some but not all patients. No drug therapy is effective for OSA. Supplemental oxygen is not recommended as primary therapy for OSA. A direct comparison of supplemental oxygen versus positive airway pressure therapy found that blood pressure was reduced in the positive airway pressure group but not in the supplemental oxygen group.

# Central Sleep Apnea Syndromes
## Classification and Pathophysiology
Central sleep apnea (CSA) syndromes are defined by pauses in airflow due to loss of output from the central respiratory generators in the brainstem, resulting in lack of respiratory effort. Ventilation during sleep is primarily determined by the arterial $PCO_2$, particularly during non-REM sleep, which comprises about 75% of total sleep time. Under normal circumstances, a steady state exists where ventilation maintains the arterial $PCO_2$ in the normal range (approximately 40 mm Hg [5.3 kPa]). In CSA, the response to arterial $PCO_2$ is exaggerated, resulting in ventilatory overshoot, hyperventilation, and reduction of the arterial $PCO_2$ to a level near the apneic threshold, the level at which respiratory efforts cease. This central apnea further destabilizes ventilation and perpetuates the process. On polysomnography, a central apnea is identified by the absence of respiratory effort associated with loss of airflow for at least 10 seconds.

**KEY POINT**

- Central sleep apnea syndromes are defined by pauses in airflow due to loss of output from the central respiratory generators in the brainstem, resulting in lack of respiratory effort.

## Risk Factors
Comorbid illnesses that predispose to instability of the ventilatory control system are the most common risk factors for CSA. The most important and prevalent association is between CSA and heart failure, which classically manifests as Cheyne-Stokes breathing, characterized by a crescendo-decrescendo pattern of ventilation. Atrial fibrillation, both in the setting of heart failure and also in those with normal left ventricular systolic function, is a risk factor for CSA.

Known for their respiratory depressant effects in high doses, opioid analgesics are also associated with CSA. Opioids have destabilizing effects on ventilation, resulting in CSA and a chaotic breathing rhythm.

Approximately 10% percent of OSA patients treated with positive airway pressure exhibit "treatment–emergent CSA," the significance of which is a matter of debate. In many, the central apneas dissipate as patients acclimate to positive airway pressure therapy.

Other risk factors for CSA include stroke, brainstem lesions, and possibly kidney failure. Men may be at higher risk than woman. High-altitude periodic breathing is a form of CSA. Primary or idiopathic CSA, in which no risk factors are identified, is uncommon.

## Symptoms and Diagnosis
It can be difficult to determine which symptoms are specific to CSA and which are associated with the comorbid condition(s). Some symptoms may be indistinguishable from OSA, such as frequent awakenings from sleep and nocturnal dyspnea, although daytime sleepiness is uncommon in those with CSA and heart failure. In-lab polysomnography is required to accurately diagnose CSA, though the Cheyne-Stokes breathing pattern is sometimes recognizable on home sleep testing. It should also be noted that although the AHI is traditionally used to describe the severity of CSA, it hasn't been validated as a predictor of important clinical outcomes as it has been in OSA. Finally, abnormal oximetry does not reliably discriminate between OSA and CSA.

## Treatment
There are few clinical trials proving a role for specific treatment of CSA, so initial management should target modifiable risk factors. For example, reduction or elimination of opioids improves CSA. Medical optimization of heart failure (with drugs or devices, optimizing fluid balance in the setting of volume overload, or surgery such as valve repair or cardiac transplantation) has been shown to improve CSA and Cheyne-Stokes breathing, though it remains controversial as to whether CSA is an independent risk factor for worsened prognosis in those with heart failure.

Sleep-related symptoms probably represent an indication for treatment. Continuous positive airway pressure may occasionally be useful, especially in patients with overlapping OSA, though "treatment–emergent CSA" may persist. Adaptive servo-ventilation is a form of positive airway pressure therapy that effectively suppresses CSA. Its role in treatment, however, was called into question by the results of a recent large trial showing an unexpected increase in mortality in patients with CSA and heart failure with reduced ejection fraction.

**KEY POINT**

- Initial management of central sleep apnea should target modifiable risk factors such as heart failure and elimination of opioids.

# Sleep-Related Hypoventilation Syndromes
Sleep-related hypoventilation syndromes are associated with advanced COPD, obesity hypoventilation syndrome, and restrictive lung diseases related to kyphoscoliosis or neuromuscular disorders and others diseases (**Table 33**). These conditions are defined by impaired gas exchange during wakefulness that is further compromised with sleep, especially during the muscle atonia of REM. Capnometry (measurement of either transcutaneous or end-tidal carbon dioxide levels) are increasingly used to confirm hypoventilation during sleep, although oxygenation criteria are also used to diagnose

**TABLE 33. Causes of Sleep-Related Hypoventilation Syndromes**

| |
|---|
| COPD |
| Obesity hypoventilation syndrome |
| Myxedema |
| Neuromuscular disease |
|   Muscular dystrophy |
|   Amyotrophic lateral sclerosis |
|   Myasthenia gravis |
|   Guillain-Barré syndrome |
|   Phrenic nerve injury |
|   Poliomyelitis, post-polio syndrome |
|   Cervical spine injury |
| Kyphoscoliosis |

sleep-related hypoventilation syndromes. Sustained reductions in oxyhemoglobin saturation (less than 90% for at least 5 minutes or more than 30% total sleep time by oximetry or polysomnography) in the setting of a compatible medical condition signify a hypoventilation syndrome. Obstructive sleep apnea may or may not be an associated feature.

**KEY POINT**

- Sleep-related hypoventilation syndromes are defined by impaired gas exchange during wakefulness that is further compromised with sleep; common associated conditions include advanced COPD, obesity hypoventilation syndrome, and restrictive lung diseases related to kyphoscoliosis or neuromuscular disorders.

## Chronic Obstructive Pulmonary Disease

Patients with severe airflow obstruction due to COPD often exhibit sleep-related hypoventilation. In addition to optimization of COPD therapy, supplemental oxygen is often used. The noninvasive pressure support of bilevel positive airway pressure can be used if hypercapnia is confirmed. In the overlap syndrome where OSA is superimposed on COPD, continuous positive airway pressure therapy has been shown to decrease mortality rates.

## Obesity Hypoventilation Syndrome

The obesity hypoventilation syndrome (OHS) results from a combination of the mechanical load on the respiratory pump and blunting of the chemoreflex (ventilatory response to carbon dioxide) in those with marked obesity. The hallmark of OHS is daytime hypercapnia, defined as a $P_{CO_2}$ greater than 45 mm Hg (5.9 kPa). OSA is usually but not always superimposed. Biventricular heart failure, pulmonary hypertension, and volume overload are common.

Weight loss is essential and consideration can be given to bariatric surgery. Positive airway pressure therapy is indicated.

Although comparative trials are lacking, most would consider bilevel positive airway pressure the mode of choice to augment ventilation. Supplemental oxygen may need to be added and its continued need reassessed at a later date. See Principles of Critical Care for a discussion of acute respiratory failure associated with OHS.

**KEY POINT**

- The hallmark of obesity hypoventilation syndrome is daytime hypercapnia, defined as an arterial $P_{CO_2}$ greater than 45 mm Hg (5.9 kPa).

## Neuromuscular Diseases

Noninvasive positive pressure ventilation devices are often prescribed to alleviate sleep-related symptoms and support blood oxygen levels in patients with neuromuscular disorders (**Table 34**). Bilevel positive airway pressure or volume-assured devices (average volume-assured pressure support, or AVAPS), with or without supplemental oxygen, are indicated once there is evidence of daytime hypercapnia indicative of chronic respiratory failure. Polysomnography may aid in optimizing machine and oxygen settings and in assessing concomitant sleep disorders, but is not always needed. Tracheostomy and home mechanical ventilation are effective and may be appropriate for some patients. Supplemental oxygen may further depress ventilation in patients with respiratory muscle weakness and should generally not be prescribed without

**TABLE 34. Positive Airway Pressure Modes**

| Mode | Description | Indication |
|------|-------------|------------|
| CPAP | Fixed pressure derived from an in-lab titration attended by a technician | OSA<br>Occasionally CSA |
| APAP | Range of pressure delivered to maintain upper airway patency, determined by a proprietary computer algorithm | OSA |
| BPAP | Inspiratory pressure support delivered over and above a minimum expiratory pressure, derived from an in-lab titration | Hypoventilation syndromes<br>OSA when CPAP fails (including patient intolerance) |
| Auto-BPAP | Range of bilevel pressures determined by a proprietary computer algorithm | Same as BPAP |
| ASV | Breath-by-breath adjustment of inspiratory pressure support and back-up rate determined by a proprietary computer algorithm; expiratory pressure set by a technician | CSA (including mixed CSA and OSA) |
| Auto-ASV | Inspiratory and expiratory pressures determined by a proprietary algorithm | Same as ASV |

APAP = auto-adjusting positive airway pressure; ASV = adaptive servo ventilation; BPAP = bilevel positive airway pressure; CPAP = continuous positive airway pressure; CSA = central sleep apnea; OSA = obstructive sleep apnea.

adjunctive ventilatory support, either by noninvasive means or by tracheostomy.

**KEY POINT**

- Noninvasive positive pressure ventilation devices are often prescribed to alleviate sleep-related symptoms and support blood oxygen levels in patients with neuromuscular disorders.

# High-Altitude–Related Illnesses

## Sleep Disturbances and Periodic Breathing

Diminishing barometric pressure associated with an ascent to altitude reduces the amount of ambient oxygen available for gas exchange, a condition known as hypobaric hypoxia. Physiologic responses to hypobaric hypoxia mechanistically underlie many disorders collectively referred to as high-altitude illness. In general, high-altitude illnesses occur at elevations of 2500 meters (approximately 8200 feet) and higher but have been reported below this elevation. Susceptibility to high-altitude illness is individualized and difficult to predict. Although high-altitude illnesses can occur at all ages and in the fittest of sojourners, patients who have a history of high-altitude–related illness are at risk for recurrence. Higher altitudes and a rapid rate of ascent are two key risk factors. Prevention is the best method of management. Because high-altitude illnesses are likely to recur, prophylactic measures are indicated on subsequent trips to elevation.

With the onset of hypoxic stress associated with hypobaric hypoxia, there is stimulation of peripheral chemoreceptors that are sensitive to hypoxia, leading to an attendant increase in ventilation, which is a key pathophysiologic mechanism in the sleep disorder termed high-altitude periodic breathing. In high-altitude periodic breathing, arterial $P_{CO_2}$ is driven toward the apneic threshold, which, when crossed, results in a pause in breathing (central apnea). With this pause, arterial $P_{CO_2}$ eventually rises sufficiently to again stimulate breathing. The cycle of ventilatory overshoot, hypocapnia, and central apneas repeats, at night and at high altitude. Patients complain of interrupted sleep and insomnia and may experience paroxysms of dyspnea that awaken them. Alcohol ingestion, which promotes dehydration, can intensify the sequelae of high-altitude periodic breathing.

Gradual ascent of less than 1000 feet per day, especially at higher altitudes, is suggested to prevent high-altitude periodic breathing and other high-altitude illnesses. Spending one night at an intermediate altitude to allow acclimatization often suffices. Acetazolamide, a carbonic anhydrase inhibitor and weak diuretic, induces a slight metabolic acidosis, is used to stabilize ventilation and enhance gas exchange, and can be used prophylactically in patients who have previously suffered

high-altitude illness. Supplemental oxygen can relieve symptoms of disrupted sleep and paroxysmal nocturnal dyspnea, but because most cases of high-altitude periodic breathing are self-limited after a few nights, this is generally not indicated in otherwise healthy individuals.

**KEY POINTS**

- Gradual ascent of less than 1000 feet per day, especially at higher altitudes, is suggested to prevent high-altitude periodic breathing and other high-altitude illnesses.
- Acetazolamide is used to stabilize ventilation and enhance gas exchange at high altitude, and can be used prophylactically in patients who have previously suffered high-altitude illness.

## Acute Mountain Sickness

Cerebral blood flow and oxygen delivery to the brain are altered by the hypoxia and hypocapnia associated with the ascent to altitude. Cerebral autoregulatory mechanisms can dampen the stress on blood flow, and symptoms can be mild in acute mountain sickness (AMS), but when the compensatory pathways are overwhelmed, severe, life-threatening cerebral edema can ensue. In AMS, the most common high-altitude illness, symptoms are nonspecific and include headache, fatigue, nausea, and vomiting; disturbed sleep related to high-altitude periodic breathing is also common. AMS is probably more common than what comes to medical attention, with estimates of as many as 25% of visitors to an altitude of 2000 meters (approximately 6500 feet), the elevation at most major U.S. ski areas. Heavy exertion and dehydration tend to amplify symptoms, which, provided there is no further ascent, typically resolve within 24 to 48 hours. As in high-altitude periodic breathing, slow ascent helps prevent the syndrome. For mild symptoms, conservative treatment may include rest, fluid replacement, aspirin, NSAIDs, or antiemetics. Acetazolamide is best used as a prophylactic but has been used as a treatment as it is believed to accelerate acclimatization. Dexamethasone is equally effective to reduce symptoms of AMS and can be used as an alternative to acetazolamide, which is a sulfonamide, for either prophylaxis or treatment in patients with sulfonamide allergy. Supplemental oxygen or portable hyperbaric therapies to simulate descent, when available, are also used to treat more symptomatic cases of AMS. Descent should also be considered when feasible.

**KEY POINT**

- Symptoms of acute mountain sickness are nonspecific and include headache, fatigue, nausea, and vomiting; disturbed sleep related to high-altitude periodic breathing is common.

## High-Altitude Cerebral Edema

High-altitude cerebral edema is a feared manifestation of acute mountain sickness that tends to occur at higher elevations (above 3000 to 4000 meters, or approximately 9800 to 13,000 feet). Vascular leak leads to brain swelling, resulting in a range of manifestations from confusion and irritability, to ataxic gait, to coma and death. Prophylactic acetazolamide should be considered in individuals planning to ascend to these elevations. Recognition of cerebral edema mandates immediate intervention. Definitive treatment is immediate descent from altitude, particularly when the patient is still ambulatory, because incapacitation at high altitude exponentially complicates evacuation. Dexamethasone, supplemental oxygen, and hyperbaric therapy may be used in addition to descent in altitude.

**KEY POINT**

- Definitive treatment of high-altitude cerebral edema is immediate descent from altitude, particularly when the patient is still ambulatory, because incapacitation at high altitude exponentially complicates evacuation.

## High-Altitude Pulmonary Edema

Vascular leak resulting from hypoxia-induced high pulmonary vascular pressures is felt to be mechanistically important in the development of high-altitude pulmonary edema. Within 2 to 4 days of ascent (typically to at least 2500 meters, approximately 8200 feet), pulmonary artery pressures begin to rise in response to hypoxic stress. Cough, dyspnea, and exertional intolerance are usually insidious but may occur abruptly and awaken a patient from sleep. Other features of acute mountain sickness may or may not be present. A key feature of high-altitude pulmonary edema is dyspnea at rest. Patients are often tachypneic and tachycardic; crackles or wheezing can be heard on chest examination. Pink, frothy sputum or frank hemoptysis may occur, which heralds worsening gas exchange and respiratory failure. The treatment of choice is supplemental oxygen along with rest, both of which will acutely reduce pulmonary artery pressures. Descent from altitude should be considered. Salvage therapies in the absence of supplemental oxygen and descent include vasodilators such as nifedipine or phosphodiesterase-5 inhibitors (sildenafil or tadalafil). Conventional treatments for pulmonary edema in the setting of heart failure, such as diuretics and nitrates, are not recommended in this setting. Rarely, climbers may require assisted ventilation, including intubation.

## Air Travel in Pulmonary Disease

The principles of hypobaric hypoxia also apply to commercial airline travel. Cabins are pressurized to the equivalent of 1500 to 2500 meters (approximately 5000 to 8000 feet) in altitude, resulting in an inspired oxygen tension between 110 and 120 mm Hg (about 70% of the levels encountered at sea level). The resultant arterial $Po_2$ of approximately 60 mm Hg (8.0 kPa) is adequate for healthy individuals, but those with underlying pulmonary disease are at risk for significant hypoxemia during flight. Patients most at risk include those with advanced COPD

complicated by chronic hypercapnic respiratory failure, patients with pulmonary hypertension, and those with restrictive lung disease. Patients with a recent exacerbation of their chronic lung condition should be fully compensated back to baseline before air travel. Patients who have had previous in-flight symptoms are likely to have recurrent issues and warrant closer assessment. Pulse oximetry is a useful screening tool, where an oxyhemoglobin saturation less than 92% at sea level indicates a likely need for in-flight supplemental oxygen. In most cases, 2 to 3 liters per minute of supplemental oxygen by nasal cannula is adequate. In those with sea-level oxygen saturation between 92% and 95%, hypoxia altitude simulation testing, available at some centers, can be used to determine the need for oxygen supplementation. In patients who are already on long-term supplemental oxygen, doubling of the flow rate during flight is typically adequate.

Patients with advanced lung disease over time may develop air-filled bullae, blebs, or cysts. These noncommunicating cavities will expand under hypobaric conditions; however, because airline cabins are pressurized, the risk of in-flight rupture and subsequent pneumothorax is believed to be low. The risk of pneumothorax is probably higher in those who have had a recent exacerbation of obstructive airways disease (asthma or COPD), during which air trapping can be pronounced, and such patients should delay air travel until the acute phase resolves. Signs or symptoms indicative of a pneumothorax (acute chest pain, dyspnea) should prompt the in-flight administration of supplemental oxygen, which promotes resorption of pleural air.

Following cardiothoracic surgery, a delay of 3 to 4 weeks before air travel is reasonable. An existing pneumothorax has traditionally been considered a contraindication to flight owing to the potential risk of expansion and tension physiology. Air travel may be safe in the presence of a small postoperative pneumothorax that has been radiographically stable.

**KEY POINTS**

- Pulse oximetry is a useful screening tool for patients who have had previous in-flight symptoms of pulmonary disease, where an oxyhemoglobin saturation of less than 92% at sea level indicates a likely need for in-flight supplemental oxygen.

- In patients who are already on long-term supplemental oxygen, doubling of the flow rate during flight is typically adequate.

# Critical Care Medicine: ICU Ⓗ Utilization

## Recognizing the Critically Ill Patient

There are no commonly accepted criteria for admission to an ICU. Signs and symptoms of clinical instability including

CONT.

hypotension, hypoxemia, arrhythmias, and mental status changes may be useful to identify patients who require intense resources or may be at risk of deterioration. Several scoring systems (APACHE, SOFA, SAP) have been designed to help classify the severity of disease of patients admitted to the ICU. These scoring systems use vital signs and risk factors such as chronic disease, emergent surgery, and immunosuppression to calculate risk of mortality. Although they are rarely, if ever, used as ICU admission criteria, they are used to objectively compare severity and progression of disease and expected and observed mortality. Disease-specific scoring systems can also be used to triage patients based on risk of deterioration or death. Examples are the simplified Pulmonary Embolism Severity Index (sPESI), the Pneumonia Severity Index (PSI), or CURB 65 for predicting mortality in community-acquired pneumonia. Electronic early warning systems based on vital signs, age, and current or trending clinical information have also been developed to identify at-risk patients. These systems, which utilize telemedicine, have been available for some time, but data supporting their effectiveness are lacking.

## Organization of Critical Care

To improve early management and resuscitation of patients at risk or deteriorating, many health care systems have developed rapid response teams (RRT) or medical emergency response teams, with the aim of recognizing patients promptly, triggering early evaluation and management, and moving the patient to a higher level of care. A key element of this system is the ability for any member of the health care team to trigger the RRT. Systematic reviews and meta-analyses of the effectiveness of these teams have demonstrated a decrease in cardiac and respiratory arrests and unexpected deterioration but not decreased mortality in adults.

Determining the admission to a critical care bed is more complicated than simply assessing the level of patient illness. This is determined in a significant way by hospital and unit policies and resources unique to each institution. No standard admission model exists, although international societies have published guidelines. Hospitals have developed institution-specific protocols to better manage patients who require life support technology.

An ICU is equipped with technology that allows continuous monitoring and delivery of life-sustaining interventions, such as mechanical ventilation or extracorporeal circulation. Hospital units designated as ICUs typically have the sickest patients and require nurse-to-patient ratios of 1:1 or 1:2, whereas a progressive care unit (also called intermediate, transitional, or step-down unit) may have a nurse-to-patient ratio as high as 1:5, reflecting patients with less acuity.

Critical care is generally defined as open-unit versus closed-unit, and low-intensity versus high-intensity. In an open unit, patients are managed by their primary team, which may include, but does not require a critical care consultant. Patients in a closed unit are managed primarily by the critical care team. Low-intensity units are open units. Although high-intensity units can be open or closed units, the critical care team is present throughout the day providing consultation. High-intensity and closed models with continuous staffing of ICUs by intensivists have been controversial; recent systematic reviews and meta-analyses show no differences in mortality between the staffing models, and minimal differences in length of stay.

### KEY POINTS

- Rapid response teams have been shown to decrease the incidence of cardiac and respiratory arrests but not change hospital mortality in adults.

- Recent evidence shows no differences in mortality between open and closed ICUs, and minimal differences in length of stay.

- High-intensity and closed models of critical care with **HVC** continuous staffing of ICUs by intensivists have been controversial; recent systematic reviews and meta-analyses show no differences in mortality between the staffing models, and minimal differences in length of stay.

# Principles of Critical Care
## Comprehensive Management of Critically Ill Patients

The care of patients in an ICU must be multidisciplinary and team-based. Critical care teams often include pharmacists, respiratory therapists, physical therapists, occupational therapists, case managers, and social workers in addition to nurses and physicians. The goal of care is to restore health and allow the patient to return home while minimizing time in the hospital, medical complications, and long-term effects of critical illness.

Patients in the ICU are at risk for developing many hospital-acquired conditions. The most common are health care-associated infections (central line-associated bloodstream infection, ventilator-associated pneumonia, catheter-associated urinary tract infection, *Clostridium difficile* colitis), skin and soft tissue pressure injury (including ulceration), malnutrition, gastrointestinal bleeding, delirium, and neuromuscular weakness (see MKSAP 18 Infectious Disease). Protocolized care can improve safety and decrease the incidence of these conditions. Hospital-acquired infections are considered avoidable and unacceptable events. Infections have become quality metrics and the focus of protocols standardizing care, for example to reduce central line infections. Other interventions include the use of a checklist during rounding on patients to improve compliance with ICU prophylaxis measures.

Protocols used in the ICU should be evidence-based and periodically reviewed to ensure accuracy. For instance, although stress ulcer prophylaxis with acid suppression has been standard practice, recent recognition of its association with increased risk of ventilator-associated pneumonia, *C. difficile* colitis, respiratory failure, and coagulopathy has raised concerns about the risk versus benefit for acid suppression. Coupled with data suggesting that the incidence of stress ulcers is decreasing, which may be due to early low-volume enteral feeding in critically ill patients, this emphasizes the importance of critical review of protocols as new evidence becomes available.

Skin and soft tissue pressure injuries are a key quality metric in the performance of an ICU. Scoring systems such as the Braden scale use clinical criteria to define risk of pressure injury in an objective manner. This helps establish specific care to prevent development of such injuries. Essential nursing care includes skin integrity monitoring and avoidance of high-risk situations, such as ongoing contact on pressure points and excessive skin moisture (see MKSAP 18 General Internal Medicine).

The complexity of disease and interventions in a critically ill patient requires a methodical approach to daily care. Many ICUs use an organ system–based approach, which allows caregivers to review the main disease process, its effects on organs and systems, and prophylactic and maintenance interventions that are essential to patient well-being.

## Mechanical Ventilatory Support: General Ventilator Principles

Admission to the ICU for respiratory insufficiency is prompted by three basic conditions: (1) hypoxemic respiratory failure; (2) ventilatory (hypercapnic) respiratory failure; and (3) upper airway impairment. Acute hypoxemic respiratory failure is caused by ongoing perfusion of lung units that are no longer ventilating because of alveolar collapse or flooding with pus, edema fluid, or blood. Hypoxemia is reversed by application of positive end-expiratory pressure to the lung, which opens up flooded or collapsed alveoli. Adequate ventilation requires the generation of sufficient pressure by the respiratory muscles to create a pressure gradient that moves air from the mouth to the alveoli. The pressure generated has to overcome both elastic (chest wall and lung) and resistive (airway) forces. Ventilatory failure can result from elastic and resistive forces that are too high or respiratory muscles that are too weak to generate the necessary pressure gradient. Mechanical ventilator support for ventilatory failure can be accomplished by one of two methods: noninvasive, using a nasal or full face mask; or invasive, with an endotracheal tube or tracheostomy. Selection of noninvasive or invasive ventilation is dependent on the clinical situation and the goals of treatment. Initiation of any form of mechanical ventilatory support should be done in a monitored unit (for example, emergency department, ICU).

### Noninvasive Mechanical Ventilation
*Fundamental Concepts*

Noninvasive positive pressure ventilation is administered through a facial or nasal mask. Higher pressures usually require a full face mask to achieve the desired level of positive pressure.

There are two types of noninvasive mechanical ventilation (NIV): continuous positive airway pressure (CPAP) and bilevel positive airway pressure (BPAP). CPAP delivers a constant airway pressure during inspiration and expiration. BPAP delivers a higher level of positive airway pressure during inspiration than during expiration, thus providing additional inspiratory support. This additional inspiratory support with BPAP increases tidal volume and maintains an appropriate level of gas exchange while requiring less respiratory effort by the patient. **Table 35** highlights the physiological effects and indications for these different modes of ventilatory support.

| TABLE 35. | Modes of Noninvasive Ventilation | | |
|---|---|---|---|
| **Mode** | **Function** | **Physiologic Effects** | **Indications** |
| CPAP | Applies and maintains a constant airway pressure throughout the respiratory cycle | Maintains patent airway in setting of obstructive sleep apnea, increases functional residual capacity, increases mean airway pressure | Obstructive sleep apnea |
| | | | Pulmonary edema |
| | | | Excessive dynamic airway collapse |
| | | | Pre-intubation |
| | | | Post-extubation |
| BPAP | Applies two different levels of airway pressure: inspiratory (IPAP) and expiratory (EPAP) positive airway pressure | Same as CPAP, but also decreases work of breathing and augments tidal volume | COPD exacerbation |
| | | | Obesity hypoventilation syndrome |
| | | | Neuromuscular diseases |
| | | | Time-limited trial in selected "do not intubate" patients with clear goals of care |
| BPAP with S/T mode | BPAP with a minimum set respiration rate | In case of apnea it will continue to deliver breaths | Hypoventilation, central apneas |

BPAP = bilevel positive airway pressure; CPAP = continuous positive airway pressure; EPAP = expiratory positive airway pressure; IPAP = inspiratory positive airway pressure; S/T = spontaneous/timed.

CONT.

## Indications and Patient Selection

Evidence favors the use of NIV in the critical care setting in patients with COPD exacerbations, cardiogenic pulmonary edema, neuromuscular disease, obesity hypoventilation syndrome, and in patients who have been extubated, which places them at high risk of morbidity. However, NIV also increases the risk of mortality in some patients, such as those with COPD who require subsequent intubation. All patients placed on NIV need to be monitored and reevaluated within 2 hours to determine if the therapy is effective or if adjustments or more invasive therapy is needed.

The use of NIV has not been shown to benefit patients with asthma exacerbations, although the data are limited because of small numbers of patients and methodological design flaws. NIV is often used for patients who are not candidates for invasive mechanical ventilation, in part to decrease or palliate respiratory distress. NIV was thought to be beneficial for immunosuppressed patients, but recent trials have cast doubt about its effectiveness. Finally, the use of NIV in patients with hypoxemic respiratory failure remains controversial. Studies have not demonstrated benefit, and there is some evidence of harm.

Contraindications to the use of NIV include altered mental status, increased airway secretions, emesis, gastric distention, airway obstruction, recent esophageal surgery, cardiac arrest, inability to protect the airway, facial trauma/surgery (including oral, nasal, or sinus), and patient intolerance of the mask.

## Application

NIV can be delivered with a critical care ventilator, a portable ventilator, or a home device. Initiation of NIV for patients with acute respiratory failure should always be done in a monitored unit by trained providers. Proper mask sizing and patient adaptation to the device are essential; these require time and coaching of the patient. The timing of instituting NIV is essential, as late application (impending respiratory failure) is related to the need for subsequent intubation and to worse outcomes. After initiation, patients should be closely monitored for tolerance and adverse effects (patient comfort, skin integrity, gastric distention, and eye irritation), effectiveness of the ventilatory settings (measured using tidal volumes and respiration rate), and clinical improvement (blood pH, respiration rate, oxygen saturation as measured by pulse oximetry, and mental status). Failure to improve on NIV is associated with increased mortality.

## High-Flow Humidified Nasal Cannula Devices

High-flow humidified nasal cannula has surged as a new modality for oxygenation support in the critically ill. It consists of a device that mixes and humidifies high-flow air and oxygen (30 L/min or more) to deliver a reliable $FiO_2$ (0.21 to 1.0) through a nasal cannula. The high flow creates positive airway pressure; the amount of pressure depends on the flow rate and cannot be measured or monitored consistently. Delivery of inspired gas through high-flow humidified nasal cannula decreases the work of breathing, provides heated and humidified gas at a reliable $FiO_2$, and decreases dead space. High-flow humidified nasal cannula is effective for preoxygenating critically ill patients before intubation, as support for postoperative hypoxemic respiratory failure, and as support for acute hypoxemic respiratory failure. Its initial application should occur in the critical care setting with close monitoring for tolerance and effectiveness.

### Invasive Mechanical Ventilation

## Fundamental Concepts

Invasive mechanical ventilation involves the use of an endotracheal tube or tracheostomy to deliver positive pressure ventilation. Invasive mechanical ventilation allows the use of higher inspiratory pressures and addresses limitations of NIV, such as the ability to protect the airway. The indications for invasive mechanical ventilation are hypoxemic and ventilatory respiratory failure, contraindication to NIV, and inability to protect the airway. The timing, the ventilation mode, and the settings depend on the disease and the patient (**Table 36**).

The appropriate mode of invasive mechanical ventilation is chosen based on its ability to achieve safety, comfort, and ultimate liberation from the ventilator, as well as on the patient's disease and physiological status. Safe mechanical ventilation requires adequate minute ventilation and oxygenation while maintaining an appropriate tidal volume to prevent ventilator-induced lung injury (see Common ICU Conditions). Ventilator-induced lung injury can occur early or late in the course of inappropriate ventilation. Appropriate tidal volume is especially important for patients who cannot independently sustain minute ventilation because of paralysis or sedation, as well as for patients who require limited tidal volume, such as those with early acute respiratory distress syndrome.

When patients are awake and the risk of lung injury has decreased, patient-ventilator interaction should be optimized to provide comfort through adequate breath support. Important considerations include the patient's level of respiratory muscle weakness or fatigue, the presence of acidosis, and the patient's level of anesthesia.

## Weaning

Patients should be liberated from mechanical ventilation as soon as possible. The concurrent use of daily awakening or targeted light sedation protocols and spontaneous breathing trials reduces mechanical ventilation time and mortality (**Table 37**). Weaning strategies have shifted from gradual reduction of support to intermittent testing for readiness to breathe, with trials of minimal or no ventilator assistance. Spontaneous breathing trials of 30 minutes to 2 hours using low levels of pressure support (8 cm $H_2O$ or less) or T-piece can identify patients who will be successfully extubated. Recent guidelines suggest pressure support is the preferred method.

**TABLE 36.** Most Frequently Used Ventilator Modes

| Common Name | Mode Classification | Breath Control Variable | Breath Sequence | Targeting Scheme |
|---|---|---|---|---|
| Volume control and assist/control | VC-CMVs | VC: The ventilator controls the flow (volume) during the mandatory breath. If the patient's effort, lung compliance, or resistance changes, the ventilator will still deliver the set tidal volume (but the pressure will change). | CMV: All breaths are mandatory. The patient may or may not trigger the breath, but the ventilator always ends the breath when the tidal volume is delivered. The name "assist/control" is a misnomer from the past. | Set-point, s: The operator sets all the parameters of the breath (flow waveform, flow rate, and volume). The ventilator only delivers the breath and does not adjust to the patient's effort or change in lung characteristics. |
| Pressure control and assist/control | PC-CMVs | PC: The ventilator controls the pressure during the mandatory breath. If the patient's effort, lung compliance, or resistance changes, the ventilator will still deliver the set inspiratory pressure (but the tidal volume delivered will change). | CMV: All breaths are mandatory. The patient may or may not trigger the breath, but the ventilator always ends the breath when the preset inspiratory time elapses. | Set-point, s: The operator sets all the parameters of the breath (inspiratory pressure and inspiratory time). The ventilator only delivers the breath and does not adjust to the patient's effort or change in lung characteristics. |
| Pressure support, continuous positive airway pressure | PC-CSVs | PC: The ventilator controls the pressure during the breath. | CSV: All breaths are spontaneous. The patient triggers and cycles the breath. | Set-point, s: The operator sets all the parameters of the breath (inspiratory pressure). The ventilator delivers the breath and does not adjust to the patient's effort or change in lung characteristics. |
| Synchronized intermittent mandatory ventilation | PC-IMVs,s or VC-IMVs,s | PC or VC: The mandatory breaths can be set to be volume or pressure controlled, not both. | IMV: Preset mandatory breaths are delivered by the ventilator at a minimum set rate. Spontaneous breaths are permitted in between mandatory breaths. The triggering of the mandatory breath will be coordinated with the patient if the inspiratory effort occurs close to the scheduled time trigger (determined by the set frequency). | Set-point, s: One "s" refers to the mandatory breath and the other to the spontaneous breath. Generally, all spontaneous breaths in IMV are pressure supported (PC-CSVs). |

CMV = continuous mandatory ventilation; CSV = continuous spontaneous ventilation; IMV = intermittent mandatory ventilation; PC = pressure controlled; s = set-point; VC = volume controlled.

CONT.

Synchronized intermittent mechanical ventilation is a mode of ventilation that combines mandatory and spontaneous breaths. Some newer technologies are being marketed that use intermittent mandatory ventilation (IMV) sequences and different targeting algorithms, but evidence regarding their performance is scant, and synchronized IMV should not be used to wean patients from mechanical ventilation.

The use of NIV immediately (preemptive) after extubation prevents extubation failure in patients at high risk, such as those with heart failure, COPD, or hypercapnia. The delayed use of noninvasive ventilation after extubation, that is, when the patient develops features of respiratory failure, should be avoided as it is associated with increased mortality.

### Ventilator-Associated Pneumonia

Ventilator-associated pneumonia develops 48 hours or more after endotracheal intubation. Preventive strategies include minimizing sedation, early mobilization, minimizing pooling of supraglottic secretions, scheduled oral care with chlorhexidine, head of bed elevation, minimization of changes of the ventilator circuit, and proper hand hygiene. For further discussion of pneumonia see MKSAP 18 Infectious Disease.

**KEY POINTS**

- Spontaneous breathing trials of 30 minutes to 2 hours using low levels of pressure support (8 cm $H_2O$ or less) can identify patients who will be successfully extubated.

- The use of noninvasive mechanical ventilation immediately after extubation prevents extubation failure in patients at high risk, such as those with heart failure, COPD, or hypercapnia.

### Invasive Monitoring

Patients in the ICU often require intensive monitoring of vital signs or vascular pressures, which necessitates the use of invasive methods. Monitoring devices increase the risk of adverse

**TABLE 37.** Common Criteria for Spontaneous Breathing Trials (SBT) and Extubation[a]

| Criteria to Perform SBT |
| --- |
| Cause of respiratory failure improved |
| FIO$_2$ ≤40% and PEEP ≤5-8 cm H$_2$O |
| pH >7.25 |
| Hemodynamic stability |
| Able to spontaneously breathe |

| Criteria to Pass SBT: At Least 30 Minutes Without |
| --- |
| Clinical evidence of respiratory distress |
|    SpO$_2$ <90% |
|    Respiration rate >35/min |
| New arrhythmias |
| Tachycardia |
| Hypotension or hypertension |

| Additional Considerations Before Extubation |
| --- |
| Quantity of secretions |
| Adequacy of cough |
| Altered mental status |

[a]These criteria may differ between institutions.

PEEP = positive end-expiratory pressure; SpO$_2$ = peripheral arterial oxygen saturation.

CONT.

effects, so they should be used only when required to obtain information that cannot be obtained with noninvasive methods. For example, the routine use of pulmonary artery catheters does not lead to improved outcomes, is associated with increased side effects, and may increase mortality.

## Intravenous Access

There are different types of devices for central intravenous (IV) access. The determination of the type of access depends on many factors including urgency of access, expected duration, and reason for access (**Table 38**). Removal of intraosseus devices must be done as soon as IV access is obtained. Peripheral venous access with a short, wide-bore catheter is the route of choice for rapid volume resuscitation. In general, all IV access should be removed as soon as possible to decrease the risk of complications, mainly infection and thrombosis. Procedure-related complications, such as arterial injury, nerve injury, or pneumothorax can be minimized with the use of ultrasound-guided placement. Devices with lower risk of complications (for example, peripheral IV access) should be used whenever possible. **H**

### KEY POINTS

- All intravenous access should be removed as soon as possible to decrease the risk for complications.
- Peripheral intravenous access with a short, wide-bore catheter is the route of choice for volume resuscitation.

## Blood Pressure Support

Systemic arterial pressure is determined by cardiac output and systemic vascular resistance. Maintenance of arterial blood pressure requires compensatory adjustments when there is either a decrease in cardiac output or inappropriate reduction in systemic vascular resistance (vasodilation). A mean arterial pressure of 65 mm Hg is considered to be the threshold at which there is sufficient pressure for organ perfusion. A study comparing a lower (65-70 mm Hg) vs a higher (80-85 mm Hg) mean arterial pressures strategy in patients

**TABLE 38.** Types of Central Venous Access

| Type | Indications | Duration | Potential Complications | Contraindications |
| --- | --- | --- | --- | --- |
| Peripherally inserted central venous catheter | Delivery of potentially caustic medications such as vasoactive agents, sedatives or antibiotics; central venous access | Few days up to 1 year | Low risk overall, avoiding pneumothorax and reducing infectious risk; clot formation or occlusion due to smaller vessel diameter | Current or pending dialysis |
| Temporary non-tunneled | Same as peripherally inserted central venous catheter; short-term dialysis; central venous pressure monitoring | Usually not more than 6 weeks | Infection; site-specific complications such as pneumothorax for subclavian or low intrajugular approach | |
| Long-term tunneled (valved tip and nonvalved tip) | Long-term TPN; chemotherapy; long-term antibiotics; dialysis | More than 6 weeks | Infection; valves prevent back bleeding but have an increased risk of catheter malfunction | |
| Ports or totally implanted | Long-term intermittent access such as chemotherapy | More than 6 weeks | Lowest risk of infection but more difficult to implant with more costs; hidden extravasation beneath skin | |
| Intraosseous (tibia or humeral head [adults]) | When IV access otherwise not obtained but need emergency fluids and/or medications | About 24 hours | Low risk of infection; flow rates may be slower; if pain with infusion can use 2% preservative-free lidocaine injected slowly to control it | Do not place in a bone with a fracture, diagnosis of osteoporosis, or recent (24-48 h) intraosseous access attempt |

IV = intravenous; TPN = total parenteral nutrition.

with septic shock demonstrated no difference in mortality. Blood pressure is usually monitored noninvasively with a blood pressure cuff. An arterial line for continuous monitoring is useful when the systolic blood pressure is less than 90 mm Hg, when frequent measurements are needed (particularly for patients requiring IV medication for blood pressure management), or when the cuff readings are unreliable. Assessment of tissue perfusion includes physical examination (skin temperature, mottling, jugular venous distention), ultrasound assessment of inferior vena cava diameter and other dynamic indices, and cardiac examination (echocardiogram, invasive and noninvasive cardiac output monitors). However, in a patient with several physical examination findings suggestive of decreased intravascular volume, the physical examination, including basic vital signs, is sufficient. Management should focus on the underlying cause of blood pressure derangement. For instance, hypotension due to deceased preload should be initially treated with volume resuscitation. Support of blood pressure may require the use of vasopressors (**Table 39**). Norepinephrine is the most commonly used agent and has been shown to reduce mortality. However, other agents are available and may be used in specific situations. 

**KEY POINT**

- A study comparing a lower (65-70 mm Hg) vs a higher (80-85 mm Hg) mean arterial pressures strategy in patients with septic shock demonstrated no difference in mortality.

## Sedation and Analgesia

ICU patients often require sedation and analgesia. The need for analgesia should be monitored frequently, at least every 4 hours, and assessed using an objective scale such as the Behavioral Pain Scale or Critical Care Pain observation tool. Analgesics should be titrated to a goal and the patient should be monitored for side effects. Analgesia should include non-pharmacologic methods, such as relaxation techniques, non-narcotic and narcotic medication for general pain, and gabapentin or carbamazepine for neuropathic pain. Intravenous opioids are the drug of choice for treating non-neuropathic pain in critically ill patients, and all have similar efficacy and clinical outcomes when titrated to similar pain intensity endpoints. Additional analgesia should be given before painful procedures, such as thoracostomy tube placement. Most if not all patients requiring invasive mechanical ventilation will need some level of sedation. Sedation in the ICU requires monitoring and should be objectively assessed using a scale such as the Richmond Agitation Sedation Scale (RASS). Agents such as propofol or dexmedetomidine are preferred rather than benzodiazepines. If oversedation occurs, the drug should be stopped until the appropriate level of sedation is achieved, then restarted at half the previous dose.

### Interruption of Sedation and Analgesia

Daily interruption of sedation and analgesia is appropriate in critically ill patients and is associated with decreased length of mechanical ventilation, length of ICU stay, and incidence of

**TABLE 39.** Selection of Vasopressors

| Medication | Type of Shock | Receptor Target | Primary Impact | Comments |
|---|---|---|---|---|
| Dobutamine | Cardiogenic, Distributive | $\beta_1$, $\beta_2$ | ↑Inotropy | First choice for cardiogenic shock without hypotension; Add-on therapy for distributive shock with depressed cardiac function |
| Dopamine (high-dose) | Cardiogenic | D, $\alpha_1$, $\beta_1$ | ↑SVR, ↑inotropy | Alternative to norepinephrine in (distributive) shock associated with absolute or relative bradycardia |
| Dopamine (low-dose) | Cardiogenic, Distributive | D, $\beta_1$ | ↑Inotropy, ↑HR | Not recommended to augment renal blood flow |
| Epinephrine | Cardiogenic, Distributive, Hypovolemic | $\alpha_1$, $\alpha_2$, $\beta_1$, $\beta_2$ | ↑SVR, ↑inotropy | First choice anaphylactic (distributive) shock; May be added to norepinephrine in distributive shock |
| Norepinephrine | Cardiogenic, Distributive, Hypovolemic | $\alpha_1$, $\alpha_2$, $\beta_1$ | ↑SVR, ↑inotropy | First choice in cardiogenic, distributive, and hypovolemic shock |
| Phenylephrine | Distributive | $\alpha_1$ | ↑SVR | May be used when norepinephrine contraindicated (tachyarrhythmias) or failure of first-line drugs |
| Vasopressin | Distributive, Hypovolemic | V | ↑SVR | May be added to norepinephrine in septic shock |

HR = heart rate; SVR = systemic vascular resistance.

CONT.

delirium. Protocolized light sedation has shown similar patient outcomes to daily sedation interruption.

## Delirium

Delirium is characterized by an acute change in cognitive functioning occurring over hours to days, with fluctuations during the course of the day. Features of delirium include inattention, disorganized thinking, executive dysfunction, altered level of consciousness (lethargy or hypervigilance), perceptual disturbances (such as hallucinations or delusions), altered psychomotor activity (hyperactivity, hypoactivity, or alternating periods of hyperactivity and hypoactivity), sleep-wake disturbances, and labile mood. It is extremely common in ICU patients and is associated with increased length of ICU stay, morbidity, mortality, and post-intensive care cognitive impairment. Risk factors for delirium include preexisting dementia, hypertension, alcoholism, and high severity of illness on ICU admission. Patients should be monitored regularly and assessed using scales such as the Confusion Assessment Method-ICU (CAM-ICU) or Intensive Care Delirium Screening Checklist (ICDSC). Measures to decrease the risk of delirium include early mobilization, preservation of nocturnal sleep, adequate pain management, orientation of the patient, provision of visual and hearing aids, and minimization of nonessential medications. Early mobilization, consisting of interruption of sedation and physical and occupational therapy in the earliest days of critical illness, can be effective for treating and preventing delirium. In general, benzodiazepines should not be used for treating delirium in the ICU, unless needed in patients with alcohol withdrawal or seizures. Data do not support the routine use of haloperidol or atypical antipsychotics for the prevention of delirium. Treatment involves identification and correction of the underlying cause, maintaining adequate nutrition and hydration, and preventing complications. For further discussion of delirium see MKSAP 18 Neurology.

### KEY POINTS

- Sedation and analgesia should be monitored using objective standardized scales.
- **HVC** In general, benzodiazepines should not be used for treating delirium in the ICU, unless needed in patients with alcohol withdrawal or seizures; data do not support the routine use of haloperidol or atypical antipsychotics for the prevention of delirium.

## Nutrition

Malnutrition in critically ill patients leads to increased morbidity and mortality, and all patients admitted to the ICU should have a nutritional evaluation. Enteral nutrition is preferred unless a contraindication is present (perforation, hemorrhage, or surgery). Guidelines recommend that enteral nutrition should be started within 24 to 48 hours of admission in critically ill patients. There is evidence that early enteral nutrition is associated with decreases in mortality and

infections, yet the level of evidence remains low. Critically ill patients who cannot maintain volitional nutritional intake may be fed using a gastric tube, large-bore tube, small-bore tube, or post-pyloric tube; there is no evidence of increased incidence of ventilator-associated pneumonia or aspiration among these methods. Routine measurement of gastric residuals is discouraged because it delays achievement of feeding goals, increases the risk of clogging the enteral access, and may increase the risk of aspiration.

Guidelines recommend that in patients at either low or high risk of problems with nutrition, use of supplemental parenteral nutrition should be considered only after 7 to 10 days of not meeting more than 60% of energy and protein requirements by the enteral route alone. Administration of parenteral nutrition to supplement enteral nutrition may lead to harm and should be avoided. In contrast, parenteral nutrition should be started as soon as possible for severely malnourished patients, those at high risk of malnutrition, and those for whom enteral nutrition is not possible.

### KEY POINTS

- Enteral nutrition is preferred unless a contraindication is present and should be started within 24 to 48 hours of admission in patients anticipated to have prolonged critical illness.
- Parenteral nutrition should be started as soon as possible for severely malnourished patients, those at high risk of malnutrition, and those for whom enteral nutrition is not possible.
- **HVC** Routine measurement of gastric residuals is discouraged in malnourished patients who are critically ill because it delays achievement of feeding goals, increases the risk of clogging the enteral access, and may increase the risk of aspiration.
- **HVC** Administration of parenteral nutrition to supplement enteral nutrition may lead to harm and should be avoided.

## Early Mobilization

Many factors contribute to neuromuscular weakness in critically ill patients, including immobility, disease, medications, and medical interventions in the ICU. Immobility may result in muscular weakness, joint stiffness, ankylosis, pressure ulcers, osteoporosis, gastrointestinal dysmotility, and dysautonomia. Even a few days of immobility can have a prolonged effect on muscular strength; long-term follow-up of patients with critical illness demonstrates persistent muscular weakness at 1 and 5 years. The use of early mobilization strategies consisting of interruption of sedation and physical and occupational therapy in the earliest days of critical illness decreases length of time in the ICU and hospital stay, improves functional status, and decreases mortality. Despite the evidence favoring early mobilization and physical therapy, implementation remains low overall.

**KEY POINT**

- The use of early mobilization strategies decreases length of time in the ICU and hospital stay, improves functional status, and decreases mortality.

## ICU Care Bundles

An ICU care bundle is a series of evidenced-based interventions that have been shown to improve patient outcomes when used together. Bundles can help clinicians monitor patients and guide appropriate interventions. The Institute for Healthcare Improvement has defined three bundles that apply to critical care (**Table 40**).

## High Value Care in the ICU

The cost of health care in the United States is the highest per capita in the world. Critical care is responsible for a large proportion of health care costs. However, the survival and quality-of-life outcomes are not that different from those in other top-economy countries. Societal, organizational, and payment pressures have encouraged a focus on providing high value care, which is defined as care that maximizes benefit relative to harms and cost. The ICU is an environment in which high value care can have major effects, as the resources are expensive and the culture favors aggressive resource use. Internal medicine and critical care medical societies have joined the American Board of Internal Medicine (ABIM) Foundation's *Choosing Wisely*® campaign to promote cost-effective strategies that improve patient care (**Table 41**). The focus on resource utilization and cost will remain a central point of health care for the foreseeable future.

**KEY POINTS**

- Don't order diagnostic tests at regular intervals (such as every day), but rather in response to specific clinical questions. **HVC**
- Don't transfuse erythrocytes in hemodynamically stable, nonbleeding patients in the ICU who have a hemoglobin concentration greater than 7 g/dL (70 g/L). **HVC**
- Don't use parenteral nutrition in adequately nourished critically ill patients within the first 7 days of an ICU stay. **HVC**
- Don't deeply sedate mechanically ventilated patients without a specific indication and without daily attempts to lighten sedation. **HVC**
- Don't continue life support for patients at high risk for death or severely impaired functional recovery without offering patients and their families the alternative of care focused entirely on comfort. **HVC**

## ICU Complications

Critical care illness is no longer viewed as an acute event that ends at the time of discharge from the ICU. ICU complications may be classified as early, which occur during the hospitalization, or late, which persist after the critical care illness. During the last decade, there has been increased recognition of

**TABLE 40.  ICU Care Bundles**

**Prevention of Ventilator-Associated Pneumonia**

Head of bed elevation at least 30 degrees

Daily sedation interruption and assessment of readiness to extubate

Stress ulcer prophylaxis

Deep vein thrombosis prophylaxis

Daily oral care with chlorhexidine

**Central Line-Associated Bloodstream Infections**

Hand hygiene

Maximal barrier precautions

Chlorhexidine skin antisepsis

Avoid femoral access

Daily review of line necessity

**Sepsis**

3-hour bundle

  Measure lactate level

  Obtain blood cultures before antibiotics

  Administer broad-spectrum antibiotics

  Administer 30 mL/kg crystalloids for hypotension or lactate ≥4 mEq/L (4 mmol/L)

6-hour bundle

  Use vasopressors if no response to fluids; keep MAP above 65 mm Hg

  Repeat volume status and tissue perfusion assessment

MAP = mean arterial blood pressure, calculated as [(2 × diastolic) + systolic]/3.

**TABLE 41.  ICU *Choosing Wisely*® Top Five**

Don't order diagnostic tests at regular intervals (such as every day), but rather in response to specific clinical questions.

Don't transfuse erythrocytes in hemodynamically stable, nonbleeding patients in the ICU who have a hemoglobin concentration greater than 7 g/dL (70 g/L).

Don't use parenteral nutrition in adequately nourished critically ill patients within the first 7 days of an ICU stay.

Don't deeply sedate mechanically ventilated patients without a specific indication and without daily attempts to lighten sedation.

Don't continue life support for patients at high risk for death or severely impaired functional recovery without offering patients and their families the alternative of care focused entirely on comfort.

Reprinted with permission of the American Thoracic Society. Copyright © American Thoracic Society. Available at: http://www.choosingwisely.org/wp-content/uploads/2015/01/Choosing-Wisely-Recommendations.pdf. Accessed June 20, 2018.

persistent disability and a focus on treatment to prevent late consequences of critical illness.

## ICU-Acquired Weakness

Between 50% and 100% of critically ill patients develop muscle weakness. Muscle weakness may result from complications involving the nervous system (critical illness polyneuropathy), the muscles themselves (critical illness myopathy), or some combination thereof, or may be nonspecific (ICU-acquired weakness). It may also be related to prolonged neuromuscular blockade (**Table 42**). Identified risk factors include sepsis, multisystem organ failure, severe illness, prolonged immobility, and hyperglycemia. Evaluation for ICU-acquired weakness can initially be done at the bedside using the Medical Research Council muscle scale. ICU-acquired weakness generally improves over weeks to months, but may persist in a small percentage of patients for up to 2 years. Strategies to minimize ICU-acquired weakness include aggressive management of critical illness, early mobilization, and management of hyperglycemia. **H**

| TABLE 42. Definitions and Characteristics of ICU-Acquired Weakness |
|---|
| **ICU-Acquired Weakness** |
| Clinically detected weakness with no other explanation other than the critical illness |
| Proximal and distal symmetrical flaccid weakness with sparing of cranial nerves |
| Often failure to wean from mechanical ventilation is first indication of weakness |
| Diagnosis of exclusion |
| **Critical Illness Polyneuropathy** |
| ICU-acquired weakness with electrophysiological evidence of axonal polyneuropathy |
| Quadriparesis or quadriplegia, decreased muscle tone, sparing of facial muscles. Deep tendon reflexes decreased |
| **Critical Illness Myopathy** |
| ICU-acquired weakness with electrophysiological and/or histological evidence of myopathy |
| Examination is similar to critical illness polyneuropathy. New sensory loss is suggestive, CK may be elevated |
| **Critical Illness Neuromyopathy** |
| Coexistence of critical Illness polyneuropathy and critical Illness myopathy |
| Mixed features, perhaps most prevalent form |
| **Prolonged Neuromuscular Blockade** |
| Prolonged effects in patients with renal failure, liver failure, hypermagnesemia |
| Flaccid areflexic quadriplegia with cranial nerve involvement |
| Repetitive nerve stimulation shows decremental response |
| CK = creatine kinase. |

- Strategies to minimize ICU-acquired weakness include aggressive management of critical illness, early mobilization, and management of hyperglycemia.

## Long-Term Cognitive Impairment

As many as 30% to 80% of patients with critical care illness develop long-term impairment in cognition, which manifests clinically as cognitive impairment with similarities to acquired dementia. Observations have demonstrated that the level of impairment 1 year after critical illness is similar to mild Alzheimer disease. Although the specific risk factors and interventions related to developing cognitive impairment are not well defined, the development and duration of delirium during the ICU stay appear to be major predictors.

## Post-Intensive Care Syndrome

Post-intensive care syndrome describes a group of symptoms that present in patients after an episode of critical care. The symptoms have been grouped according to the area that they affect (physical impairment, mental health, and cognitive impairments). Patients with post-intensive care syndrome have increased health care use, increased morbidity and mortality, and impaired quality of life. Post-intensive care syndrome also affects the caregivers and family of the critically ill patient; it has been reported that family members experience anxiety, depression, and post-traumatic stress disorder. Current research and interventions are focusing on how to improve recognition, prevention, diagnosis, and management. **H**

# Common ICU Conditions **H**

## Acute Respiratory Failure

Acute respiratory failure occurs when a patient cannot adequately oxygenate blood (hypoxemia) or remove carbon dioxide (hypercarbia or hypercapnia) from the blood. It is essential to quickly stabilize the patient and identify the cause of respiratory failure. History and physical examination are essential, but tests such as chest radiograph (**Table 43**), CT scan, arterial blood gas, and pulse oximetry are also useful. A structured approach allows clinicians to both identify and treat factors leading to respiratory failure. This approach includes evaluation for airway compromise, inadequate oxygenation, and inadequate ventilation. (**Figure 19**)

## Acute Upper Airway Management

In patients who cannot maintain a patent airway or protect their airway against aspiration, a secure airway should be established by inserting a cuffed endotracheal or tracheostomy tube. High-flow oxygen; bag-valve mask ventilation; or oropharyngeal, nasopharyngeal, or laryngeal mask airway can aid oxygenation and ventilation when immediate intubation is not feasible and should be used until the airway can be secured. **H**

**TABLE 43.** Radiographic Findings and Differential Diagnosis in Acute Respiratory Failure

| Finding | Differential Diagnosis |
|---|---|
| No infiltrate | Asthma/COPD exacerbation |
| | Drug overdose |
| | Intracardiac shunt |
| | Neuromuscular weakness |
| | Pulmonary embolus |
| Diffuse infiltrates | Acute respiratory distress syndrome |
| | Cardiogenic pulmonary edema |
| | Acute exacerbation of idiopathic pulmonary fibrosis |
| | Pneumonia |
| | Other (for example, acute hypersensitivity pneumonitis, acute eosinophilic pneumonia) |
| Focal infiltrate | Airway obstruction |
| | Atelectasis |
| | Pneumonia |
| | Pulmonary infarction |

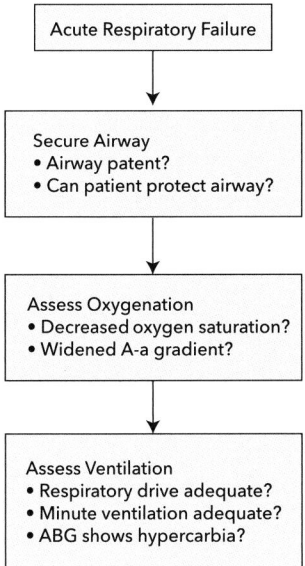

**FIGURE 19.** Key components to the assessment of acute respiratory failure. A-a = alveolar-arterial; ABG = arterial blood gas.

**KEY POINT**

- In patients who cannot maintain a patent airway or protect their airway against aspiration, a secure airway should be established by inserting a cuffed endotracheal or tracheostomy tube.

## Airway Obstruction

Respiratory failure can result from intraluminal obstruction or extraluminal compression of the upper airways. Patients with partial airway obstruction may have tachypnea, increased respiratory effort, or an upright (tripod) posture with use of accessory muscles. Absent air movement, inability to talk, or cyanosis suggests complete obstruction and signifies a medical emergency. Inspiratory stridor suggests an obstruction above the level of the vocal cords, whereas expiratory stridor and wheezing suggest an intrathoracic process. Pulse oximetry in the setting of partial upper airway obstruction and stridor is usually normal. Patients with potential upper airway obstruction should be cautiously examined to prevent exacerbation of the condition. In patients with respiratory distress or for whom the risk of respiratory deterioration is high, early intubation is indicated.

## Acute Inhalational Injuries
### Smoke Inhalation

Pulmonary complications are a leading cause of morbidity and mortality in patients who have been burned or experienced significant smoke exposure from fires. Direct thermal injury due to smoke inhalation is usually limited to the upper airways. However, steam inhalation causes direct thermal injury throughout the tracheobronchial tree due to its ability to carry heat more efficiently than dry, hot gas. Following smoke inhalation, one-third of patients develop airway edema or mucosal sloughing from epithelial necrosis. Chest physiotherapy and serial bronchoscopic suctioning are frequently necessary to facilitate continued airway clearance. Injury to the distal tracheobronchial tree and lung parenchyma is caused by chemicals in smoke that generate a complex cascade of bronchoconstriction, pulmonary edema, ventilation-perfusion ($\dot{V}/\dot{Q}$) mismatch, and bronchial cast formation. Treatment is largely supportive.

Secondary respiratory infections are common and are a major cause of morbidity and mortality. Pneumonia is the most common complication following smoke inhalation injury, especially from *Staphylococcus* and *Pseudomonas* specie. Systemic toxicity from substances like carbon monoxide (CO) and hydrogen cyanide (HCN) are common following smoke inhalation. Clinicians should suspect CO and HCN poisoning in all patients with smoke exposure. Both can cause a reduction in the oxygen-carrying capacity of hemoglobin. Unfortunately this may not be apparent, as CO and HCN are not detected by standard pulse oximetry, and oxygen saturation measurement may be falsely normal. Additional details of CO and HCN poisoning are reviewed in Toxicology.

### Other Forms of Inhalational Injury

Inhalational injuries related to chemical vapors are uncommon. War, industrial, or farming operations and exposure to home cleaning or pesticide agents constitute most chemical inhalational injuries. Water-soluble agents usually affect mucosal structures of the upper airway and have rapid onset of symptoms. Water insoluble agents affect deeper structures including lung parenchyma and distal airways, and symptoms are often delayed. Edema, bronchospasm, asphyxiation, and direct systemic toxicity are common. Key features of inhalational agents are listed in **Table 44**. Treatment is supportive, with a specific antidote, atropine, indicated only in cholinesterase inhibitor exposure.

## Hypoxemic Respiratory Failure

Hypoxemic respiratory failure is caused by inadequate oxygenation of hemoglobin. The most common causes of hypoxemic respiratory failure in the ICU are $\dot{V}/\dot{Q}$ mismatch and shunt ($\dot{V}/\dot{Q}$ = 0), which occur when perfused areas of the lung are not ventilated, whether because of alveolar collapse (atelectasis) or filling of alveoli with blood, pus, protein, or water. An increased alveolar-arterial oxygen difference (gradient) is the key feature of $\dot{V}/\dot{Q}$ mismatch and shunt. The gradient is derived by subtracting the measured arterial $P_{O_2}$ from the calculated alveolar $P_{O_2}$.

The alveolar $P_{O_2}$ is calculated using the alveolar gas equation:

$$\text{Alveolar } P_{O_2} = (F_{IO_2} \times [P_{atm} - 47]) - (1.25 \times P_{CO_2})$$

$F_{IO_2}$ is the fraction of inspired oxygen (0.21 in ambient air), $P_{atm}$ is the atmospheric pressure (760 mm Hg at sea level), and 47 represents the partial pressure of water in mm Hg at 37°C (98.6°F). The alveolar-arterial gradient increases with age, and normal gradients in individuals breathing ambient air (but not applicable in patients on supplemental oxygen) can be estimated with the equation:

$$\text{Expected alveolar-arterial oxygen gradient} = 2.5 + 0.21 \times \text{age in years}$$

| TABLE 44. | Key Features of Inhaled Agents | |
|---|---|---|
| **Agent** | **Characteristics** | **Clinical Features Following Exposure** |
| Ammonia | Colorless, ammonia odor | Cough, upper airway burns, pulmonary edema, asphyxiation in poorly vented areas |
| Chlorine | Yellow-green, chlorine odor | Upper airway irritation and burns, bronchospasm, pulmonary edema |
| Phosgene | Colorless, musty odor like fresh cut grass | Systemic toxicity including elevated methemoglobin level, cyanosis and metabolic acidosis. Pulmonary edema |
| Mustard gas | Yellow-brown vapor, odor like garlic or onions | Upper airways burns and obstruction can occur |
| Organophosphates and other cholinesterase inhibitors | Colorless, fruity odor | Systemic toxicity causing acetylcholine toxicity (rhinorrhea, bronchorrhea, diarrhea, bronchospasm, flaccid paralysis, apnea) |

Scenarios of acute and chronic hypoxemia are difficult to distinguish using arterial blood gases alone. A helpful distinguishing feature is the time course of development of symptoms; in addition, the presence of polycythemia suggests chronic hypoxemia. Findings on chest imaging studies may be helpful, as diffuse alveolar filling is more suggestive of acute hypoxemic respiratory failure, whereas interstitial lung disease is more suggestive of a chronic process.

Signs of acute hypoxemic respiratory failure include recent onset of increased work of breathing, tachypnea, and anxiety. Cyanosis of the lips or fingers may be present when oxygenation of hemoglobin is severely compromised, often below 80%. Findings on auscultation such as crackles, wheezing, egophony, or rhonchi may suggest an underlying cause.

Management of hypoxemic respiratory failure centers on administration of supplemental oxygen and measures to open alveoli that are fluid-filled or collapsed, such as mechanical ventilation with administration of both positive inspiratory and positive end-expiratory pressure (PEEP). In extreme cases where the technology and expertise are available, extracorporeal membrane oxygenation (ECMO) can be used to provide external oxygenation of, and removal of carbon dioxide from, the blood. Disease-specific management is discussed below.

**KEY POINTS**

- The most common causes of hypoxemic respiratory failure in the ICU are ventilation-perfusion mismatch and shunt, which occurs when perfused areas of the lung are not ventilated, whether because of alveolar collapse (atelectasis) or filling of alveoli with blood, pus, protein, or water.
- Management of hypoxemic respiratory failure centers on administration of supplemental oxygen and measures to open alveoli that are fluid-filled or collapsed.

## Acute Respiratory Distress Syndrome

Acute respiratory distress syndrome (ARDS) is characterized by a dysregulated inflammatory response within the lungs. The most common overall cause of ARDS is sepsis, but there are various other common causes of ARDS, including both direct and indirect pulmonary insults (**Table 45**).

In ARDS, disruption of surfactant production, vascular endothelial injury, and alveolar epithelial cell injury occur, leading to excess fluid and protein extravasation into interstitial and alveolar spaces. This results in interstitial and alveolar filling, microatelectasis, increased $\dot{V}/\dot{Q}$ mismatch, decreased lung compliance, and increases in both shunt and dead-space ventilation. Histology shows diffuse alveolar damage.

ARDS is a clinical diagnosis. The most recent guidelines defining ARDS were updated in the 2012 Berlin Definition of ARDS (**Table 46**). The Berlin definition emphasizes that ARDS occurs rapidly after an inciting event and is

**TABLE 45. Common Causes of Acute Respiratory Distress Syndrome**

| Direct Pulmonary Injury | Indirect Pulmonary Injury |
|---|---|
| Aspiration of gastric contents | Disseminated intravascular coagulation |
| Fat embolism | Non-thoracic trauma |
| Near drowning | Pancreatitis |
| Pneumonia | Pulmonary reperfusion injury (following lung transplantation) |
| Smoke or chemical inhalation | Sepsis/septic shock |
| Thoracic trauma/thoracic contusion | Transfusion of blood products |

**TABLE 46. 2012 Berlin Definition of Acute Respiratory Distress Syndrome**

The following criteria must be met:

Onset within 1 week of known ARDS insult (most cases occur within 72 hours)

Bilateral opacities on chest imaging consistent with pulmonary edema

Respiratory failure not related to cardiac failure or volume overload

Arterial $PO_2/FIO_2$ <300 on at least 5 cm $H_2O$ PEEP from noninvasive or invasive mechanical ventilator

Once criteria for diagnosis are met, severity of ARDS is based on the following criteria:

Mild = Arterial $PO_2/FIO_2$ >200 to <300

Moderate = Arterial $PO_2/FIO_2$ 100 to 200

Severe = Arterial $PO_2/FIO_2$ <100

ARDS = acute respiratory distress syndrome; PEEP = positive end-expiratory pressure.

Data from Ranieri VM, Rubenfeld GD, Thompson BT, Ferguson ND, Caldwell E, Fan E, et al; ARDS Definition Task Force. Acute respiratory distress syndrome: the Berlin definition. JAMA. 2012;307:2526-33. [PMID: 22797452] doi:10.1001/jama.2012.5669

characterized by diffuse, bilateral, noncardiogenic pulmonary edema. Patients with ARDS are at high risk of mortality, which increases with ARDS severity. However, mortality is usually the result of the underlying disease that triggered ARDS, secondary infection, or multi-organ dysfunction rather than refractory hypoxemia.

## Ventilatory Management

Most patients with ARDS are managed with invasive mechanical ventilation. PEEP and low tidal volume ventilation (LTVV) are the cornerstones of ARDS management, as they are associated with prevention of ventilator-associated lung injury. Because lungs affected by ARDS are frequently characterized by areas of noncompliant, diseased lung adjacent to lung with more normal compliance, high tidal volumes can lead to regional areas of lung overdistention and injury

(volutrauma). In 2000, the ARMA trial evaluated the benefits of LTVV (tidal volumes of 4 to 8 mL/kg) compared with higher tidal ventilation conventionally used at the time. The trial showed a significant, 11% absolute reduction in mortality with the use of LTVV. This trial also sought to prevent two other causes of ventilator-induced lung injury. Barotrauma, or lung injury due to high transpulmonary pressures, was prevented in the LTVV arm by avoiding plateau pressures greater than 30 cm $H_2O$. Current ARDS goals include both a tidal volume of ~6 mL/kg of predicted body weight and maintenance of the lowest possible plateau pressure. The ARMA trial also affirmed the utility of PEEP as having three benefits. First, it prevents lung injury associated with repeated opening and closing of distal airways and alveoli (atelectrauma). Second, it improves homogeneity of the lung parenchyma by reducing gross differences in regional lung compliance. Third, it improves $\dot{V}/\dot{Q}$ mismatch and shunt by maintaining alveolar recruitment. Although PEEP is now a standard part of lung protective ventilation, no definitive level of optimal PEEP has been designated for ventilation of patients with ARDS.

Despite the clear benefits of LTVV, adherence remains poor. Barriers to improved adherence include underrecognition of patients with ARDS, improper sedation of patients who do not initially tolerate LTVV, and a propensity for patients to develop respiratory acidosis from hypercapnia when using LTVV.

Ventilating patients in the prone position may reduce compression of portions of the lung behind the cardiac and mediastinal structures and improve $\dot{V}/\dot{Q}$ matching in ARDS patients. A recent large, randomized trial (PROSEVA) demonstrated improved mortality in patients with an arterial $PO_2/FIO_2$ ratio less than 150 who were treated with early prone positioning and LTVV. Early prone positioning for at least 12 hours a day should be considered in patients with severe ARDS.

The use of ECMO has been increasing, largely due to a single, prospective randomized controlled trial performed during the 2009 H1N1 influenza pandemic (CESAR trial). Although this trial suggested improved mortality in ARDS patients referred to a center capable of administering ECMO, many referred patients never received ECMO. This suggests that improved mortality may have simply been the result of referral to a center with improved expertise in ARDS management, not due to treatment with ECMO itself. In patients with severe, refractory hypoxemia, both prone positioning and ECMO may be considered; however, the effectiveness of prone positioning is better supported by data.

In patients with refractory hypoxemia, a recruitment maneuver—applying a high level of CPAP to open collapsed alveoli (for example, continuous pressure to 35 cm $H_2O$ for 40 seconds)—may be considered. Although controversial, the 2017 ATS/ESICM/SCCM Guideline on Mechanical Ventilation in Adults with Acute Respiratory Distress Syndrome provides

CONT.

a conditional recommendation for recruitment maneuvers. The guideline cautions that recruitment maneuvers should not be used in patients with preexisting hypovolemia or shock due to a high propensity for hemodynamic deterioration during the maneuver.

Other methods to optimize ventilator management in ARDS have been suggested, including inverse ratio ventilation, esophageal pressure and driving pressure-guided titration of PEEP, and high-frequency oscillator ventilation (HFOV). None of these have demonstrated mortality benefit in ARDS. [H]

**KEY POINT**

- Treating patients with severe acute respiratory distress syndrome using early prone positioning and low tidal volume ventilation has demonstrated clinically important mortality benefit.

### Nonventilatory Management

Although mortality in ARDS has decreased, most of this is attributed to improved mechanical ventilation strategies. Mechanically ventilated patients often require sedation to improve patient-ventilator interactions and achieve LTVV goals. Data support minimizing sedation to intermittent, bolus administration when possible and daily awakening of patients who require continuous sedation. Use of nursing-led sedation protocols can decrease the overall sedation required and improve patient outcomes. Excessive sedation increases risk of delirium and nosocomial infection, increases length of ICU stays, and is a likely contributor to many long-term psychological and physical effects now associated with ARDS.

ICU patients receive volume resuscitation for a host of reasons. In ARDS, the FACCT trial suggested excessive fluid resuscitation is harmful to ARDS patients. This trial compared conservative to liberal fluid strategies based on central venous pressure and pulmonary artery occlusion pressure (a surrogate for left atrial pressure) in patients with ARDS. Although mortality did not differ between groups, patients who were treated with conservative fluid management showed improved oxygenation and decreased time on the ventilator and in the ICU. In patients who are hemodynamically stable and do not have end-organ hypoperfusion, minimizing fluid administration is warranted.

The use of paralytic agents in ARDS to improve oxygenation and decrease ventilator-induced lung injury is controversial, as there have been concerns about the potential association of paralytics with critical illness myopathy. However, a recent study in patients with ARDS who were paralyzed within 48 hours of starting mechanical ventilation found no difference in critical illness myopathy and a lower mortality. Although further study is warranted, this practice has been recommended as an early intervention strategy in patients with severe ARDS.

Other therapies, including nutritional modifications, glucocorticoid administration, macrolide antibiotics, inhaled nitric oxide, prostacyclin analogues, and stem cells or granulocyte-macrophage colony-stimulating factor have conflicting or limited evidence and are not recommended in the management of ARDS.

### Heart Failure

Clinically, both acute cardiogenic pulmonary edema and ARDS present with pulmonary edema and hypoxemic respiratory failure. But unlike ARDS, cardiogenic pulmonary edema responds to aggressive diuresis and optimization of cardiac function. In patients who present with acute respiratory failure and features of ARDS, but no clear trigger, it is important to evaluate for cardiogenic causes, which include heart failure, mitral and aortic valve disease, myocardial ischemia, and arrhythmias (particularly atrial fibrillation with rapid ventricular rate). Evaluation for a cardiac cause of pulmonary edema should include an assessment for fluid overload (jugular venous distention, S₃, peripheral edema), an electrocardiogram, B-type natriuretic peptide, serial serum troponins, and an echocardiogram. [H]

**KEY POINT**

- Evaluation for a cardiac cause of pulmonary edema should include an assessment for fluid overload, an electrocardiogram, B-type natriuretic peptide, serial serum troponins, and an echocardiogram.

### Atelectasis

Atelectasis is a common postoperative complication. Inadequate postoperative analgesia or impaired respiratory mechanics following thoracic and abdominal surgeries can lead patients to adopt shallow breathing patterns or avoid airway clearance and cough. Presentation is often delayed following liberation from a ventilator and patients may be asymptomatic or present with diminished breath sounds at the lung bases, rhonchi, and labored breathing. Management of secretions with aggressive chest physiotherapy, suctioning, and incentive spirometry is recommended postoperatively. Bronchoscopy for airway mucous clearance offers no clear benefit compared to other methods of chest physiotherapy. If secretions are minimal, CPAP therapy to recruit collapsed alveoli may be considered. Use of mucolytics such as N-acetyl cysteine have not been adequately studied and are not indicated for treatment of atelectasis. [H]

**KEY POINT**

- Management of secretions with aggressive chest physiotherapy, suctioning, and incentive spirometry is recommended postoperatively to prevent atelectasis; bronchoscopy for airway mucous clearance offers no clear benefit compared to other methods of chest physiotherapy.

**HVC**

### Pneumonia

Pneumonia is a common cause of respiratory failure in the ICU and is the most common cause of ARDS that develops outside the hospital. In patients with an appropriate history, chest

CONT.

radiograph is the standard for diagnosis. However, a negative clinical examination or chest radiograph does not necessarily rule out community-acquired pneumonia in symptomatic patients, especially in elderly individuals. Therefore, absence of typical features or focal infiltrates on chest radiograph should not preclude early antibiotic administration to individuals with an otherwise high probability of pneumonia. For further discussion of pneumonia see MKSAP 18 Infectious Disease. In patients who do not respond appropriately to antibiotics, repeat sputum cultures should be obtained, and both nonbacterial causes of infection and noninfectious causes should be considered. In addition, further evaluation with chest CT scan, bronchoscopy, or both should be considered to evaluate for complicating factors such as pleural effusion, abscess, or airway obstruction stemming from malignancy or foreign body aspiration.

**KEY POINT**

- A negative clinical examination or chest radiograph does not necessarily rule out community-acquired pneumonia in symptomatic patients, especially in elderly individuals.

## Diffuse Parenchymal Lung Disease

Acute exacerbations of diffuse parenchymal lung disease (DPLD), particularly idiopathic pulmonary fibrosis (IPF) can occur either as a complication of an inciting event, or in many cases, for unknown reason. See the Diffuse Parenchymal Lung Disease section earlier for a detailed discussion of diagnosis and management. The mortality in patients with hypoxemic respiratory failure due to an exacerbation of IPF exceeds 50%. Most patients with hypoxemic respiratory failure due to IPF are treated empirically with high dose glucocorticoids, but the data are insufficient to support dose, duration, or certainty of benefit. Outcomes following intubation and mechanical ventilation are very poor, as mortality can approach 100%. Therefore, many clinicians recommend that goals of care discussion and palliative care be involved early and other therapies, such as ECMO, only be offered as a bridge for patients eligible for lung transplantation.

Patients in the ICU with an exacerbation of IPF are frequently given broad spectrum antibiotics if infection has not been ruled out. Although the cause of most IPF exacerbations is unclear, new data suggest that aspiration and infection may play a significant role.

**KEY POINT**

- Because outcomes following intubation and mechanical ventilation are very poor for patients with acute exacerbations of idiopathic pulmonary fibrosis, goals of care and palliative care should be discussed early, and other therapies, such as extracorporeal membrane oxygenation, should only be offered as a bridge for patients eligible for lung transplantation.

## Pulmonary Embolism

Pulmonary embolism (PE) causes respiratory failure primarily through $\dot{V}/\dot{Q}$ mismatch, and to a less common extent through shunting or low mixed venous oxygen saturation. Following an acute PE, resistance to pulmonary blood flow increases, due to both thrombosis and to vasospasm of adjacent pulmonary blood vessels from activated inflammatory mediators. Subsequently, blood flow is directed to unembolized areas of normal lung, which become overperfused. If ventilation of the normal lung is insufficient to fully oxygenate blood in the overperfused vessels, hypoxemia ensues. In addition, regional atelectasis is common following PE and lung infarction. Chest radiograph or chest CT scan may demonstrate peripheral, ground-glass, wedge-shaped opacities (Hampton hump sign) signifying the presence of infarcted lung and surrounding atelectasis. Blood flow through atelectatic lung can result in shunt and hypoxemia.

Pulmonary emboli can also cause strain on the right ventricle (RV) if the PE is sufficiently large. In these cases, cardiac output may be impaired. Low cardiac output leads to reduced mixed venous oxygen saturations, especially when metabolic demands exceed cardiac capacity. If this occurs in conjunction with $\dot{V}/\dot{Q}$ mismatch and shunt, blood cannot fully saturate with oxygen before leaving the alveolar capillaries. This adds to hypoxemia and subsequent respiratory failure.

Although most patients with hypoxemia following PE can be managed with supplemental oxygen alone, some patients require intubation and positive pressure ventilation.

Mechanical ventilation produces several physiologic effects that need to be considered in the patient with PE and RV dysfunction. Increased pleural pressure from mechanical ventilation can cause decreased venous return and result in low RV preload. Additionally, overdistention of alveoli increases RV afterload. These effects can lead to further RV dysfunction and hemodynamic instability. Although there is no absolute contraindication to mechanical ventilation in patients with underlying PE, the risks and benefits should be weighed carefully. In patients with hemodynamic collapse, treatment with thrombolytics is associated with decreased mortality, and the vast majority of patients demonstrate improvement in clinical and echocardiographic parameters following thrombolytic administration.

Thrombolytics carry a significant side effect profile, including an up to 2% risk of intracranial hemorrhage, but this should be considered relative to the life-threatening risk of massive PE leading to hemodynamic collapse. In patients with contraindications to thrombolysis, and in those in whom thrombolysis has failed to improve the hemodynamic status, surgical embolectomy is recommended if resources are available. For further discussion of PE, see MKSAP 18 Hematology and Oncology.

# Hypercapnic (Ventilatory) Respiratory Failure

Hypercapnic, or ventilatory, respiratory failure occurs when alveolar ventilation is inadequate to clear the $CO_2$ produced by cellular metabolism, and the level of $CO_2$ increases in the blood. Most commonly, hypercapnia reflects alveolar hypoventilation, but can also result from increased metabolic load (fever, increased work of breathing) that is not matched by an increase in alveolar ventilation. Alveolar hypoventilation occurs when the patient is unable to ventilate because of decreased respiratory drive, decreased tidal volume ($V_T$), or increased volume of dead space ($V_D$) relative to the overall tidal volume ($V_D/V_T$) (**Table 47**).

Clinical features of acute hypercapnic respiratory failure are variable and nonspecific. Symptoms may include somnolence and myoclonic jerks in the setting of $CO_2$ narcosis. In some cases, increased work of breathing may precede the development of acute hypercapnic respiratory failure. Underlying chest wall deformity, neurologic weakness, or polycythemia should also prompt evaluation for hypercapnia in the setting of respiratory failure.

Patients presenting with acute hypercapnic respiratory failure frequently have coexisting hypoxemia. Administration of supplemental oxygen may improve the hypoxemia, but will not necessarily improve hypercapnia. All patients who are suspected of acute hypercapnic respiratory failure should have

arterial blood gas analysis even if hypoxemia resolves with oxygen administration (**Table 48**). The pH helps to determine the acuity and severity of respiratory failure. In chronic hypercapnia, pH changes are less marked due to metabolic compensation resulting in increased serum bicarbonate levels. Management of an elevated arterial $P_{CO_2}$ depends on the clinical situation and the resultant pH. For instance, a moderately elevated arterial $P_{CO_2}$ may represent the baseline in patients with COPD; however, in an asthmatic, the development of elevated arterial $P_{CO_2}$ may indicate imminent respiratory failure requiring emergent intubation.

> **KEY POINT**
> - All patients who are suspected of acute hypercapnic respiratory failure should have arterial blood gas analysis even if hypoxemia resolves with oxygen administration.

## Management of Hypercapnic Respiratory Failure
### Decreased Respiratory Drive
Decreased respiratory drive leads to diminished alveolar $CO_2$ clearance and hypercapnia. Patients often present with somnolence and difficulty protecting their airway. Noninvasive positive pressure ventilation (NIPPV) should be considered if the patient can protect his or her airway. This improves minute ventilation and gas exchange. If airway protection is compromised, or if there is either significant respiratory acidosis (generally pH less than 7.25) or hemodynamic instability, intubation and mechanical ventilation are indicated. See MKSAP 18 Nephrology for further discussion of respiratory acidosis.

### Drug Overdose
Sedating drugs (illicit or prescribed), anesthetics, and severe alcohol intoxication can lead to depressed central respiratory drive. In cases of pharmacologic overdose, contact with a local poison control center is helpful to determine the most appropriate care of the patient. If opiate overdose is suspected, rapid reversal with naloxone is safe, effective, and may prevent the need for intubation. The benefits of flumazenil for patients with benzodiazepine overdose are less certain. Flumazenil carries the risk of precipitating withdrawal seizures in chronic users and is a short-acting agent, so several administrations

**TABLE 47.** Causes of Acute Hypercapnic Respiratory Failure

| Decreased Respiratory Drive | Decreased $V_T$ or Increased $V_D/V_T$ |
|---|---|
| Anesthesia | Amyotrophic lateral sclerosis |
| Central apnea | Ankylosing spondylitis |
| Obesity hypoventilation syndrome | Asthma exacerbation |
| | Botulism |
| Drugs (such as opioids, benzodiazepines, ethanol) | Bronchiectasis flare (including cystic fibrosis) |
| Encephalitis | COPD exacerbation |
| Hypothermia | Critical illness myopathy |
| Hypothyroidism | Electrolyte disorder (low magnesium, low phosphate) |
| Meningitis | Guillain-Barré syndrome |
| Stroke | Multiple rib fractures (flail chest) |
| | Myasthenia gravis |
| | Myositis (such as polymyositis, dermatomyositis) |
| | Polio |
| | Spinal or phrenic nerve injury |
| | Thoracic cage deformity (kyphoscoliosis) |

$V_T$ = tidal volume; $V_D$ = volume of dead space.

**TABLE 48.** Features of Acute and Chronic Hypercapnia

| | Acute Hypercapnia | Chronic Hypercapnia |
|---|---|---|
| pH | <7.35 | ~7.35-7.40 |
| Arterial $P_{CO_2}$ | >45 mm Hg (6.0 kPa) | >45 mm Hg (6.0 kPa) |
| Bicarbonate concentration [$HCO_3$] | 22-26 mEq/L (22-26 mmol/L) | >26 mEq/L (26 mmol/L) |
| Expected metabolic compensation | 1.0 mEq/L ↑ [$HCO_3$] for each 10 mm Hg (1.3 kPa) ↑ in arterial $P_{CO_2}$ | 3.5 mEq/L ↑ [$HCO_3$] for each 10 mm Hg (1.3 kPa) ↑ arterial $P_{CO_2}$ |

CONT.

may be required to keep respiratory failure from recurring, especially if long-acting benzodiazepines were ingested.

### Obesity Hypoventilation Syndrome

Obesity hypoventilation syndrome (OHS) is characterized by the presence of obesity, sleep-disordered breathing, and persistent daytime hypercapnia (arterial $Pco_2$ greater than 45 mm Hg [5.9 kPa]). Hypercapnia stems from low tidal volumes and from inappropriate central respiratory response to hypoxemia and elevated $Pco_2$ levels. Acute hypercapnic respiratory failure due to OHS should be a diagnosis of exclusion. Positive pressure ventilation is the key to improving hypercapnia in patients with OHS.

NIPPV is reasonable in patients who can protect their airway, but high levels of positive pressure are often needed because of poor chest wall compliance from obesity, diminished lung compliance from atelectasis, and cephalad displacement of the diaphragm from central adiposity. If NIPPV is used, arterial blood gases should be monitored to ensure clinical improvement. If patients are not improving, early intubation is warranted. Respiratory stimulants, such as acetazolamide, a progestin, and theophylline offer a compelling theoretical benefit to patients with chronic hypercapnia or depressed respiratory drive, but have limited data supporting their use in this setting.

### KEY POINT

- Acute hypercapnic respiratory failure due to obesity hyperventilation syndrome is a diagnosis of exclusion; if airway protection is compromised, or there is significant respiratory acidosis or hemodynamic instability, intubation and mechanical ventilation are indicated.

## Decreased Tidal Volume and Increased Dead Space

### Neuromuscular Weakness

The diaphragm is the main muscle responsible for inspiration and accounts for more than two-thirds of the ventilatory work in humans. The C3-C5 cervical nerve roots form the phrenic nerves, which directly innervate the diaphragm. Patients with diaphragmatic weakness develop orthopnea, shallow breathing, and often paradoxical movement of the chest wall and abdomen. Although exhalation is generally a passive process, intercostal and abdominal wall muscles are required for coughing. Lower cervical and upper thoracic nerve roots supply the intercostal and abdominal wall muscles. Weak cough, difficulty managing secretions, or a change in voice, which can become softer or more "breathy," may point to weakness in these areas.

Assessment of cranial nerves and respiratory muscle function is important in a patient with suspected neurologic disease. Specific components of pulmonary function testing can be helpful (**Table 49**) but are effort-dependent, and facial or postural weakness can complicate accurate measurement.

Guillain-Barré syndrome and myasthenic crisis are the most common causes of acute neurologic respiratory failure in

**TABLE 49.** Pulmonary Function Value Suggestive of Neuromuscular Weakness

| Function | Value |
|---|---|
| FVC | >20% decrement in supine position compared with upright position |
| Maximal inspiratory pressure (MIP) | Unable to achieve −30 cm $H_2O$ |
| Maximal expiratory pressure (MEP) | Unable to achieve +40 cm $H_2O$ |

the ICU. Infection can precipitate myasthenic crisis or Guillain-Barré syndrome. Myasthenic crisis can occur following medication changes or significant stressors.

Patients with Guillain-Barré syndrome generally present with rapid onset of ascending, symmetric paralysis and areflexia occurring over the course of 2 to 4 weeks. Dysautonomia is common and can cause hemodynamic instability or cardiac arrhythmias. In myasthenic crisis, the hallmark feature is muscle fatigability. Diplopia, ptosis, dysarthria, limb weakness, and weak cough are common. See MKSAP 18 Neurology for further discussion of Guillain-Barré syndrome and myasthenic crisis.

In the 25% of patients with Guillain-Barré syndrome who develop respiratory failure, intubation is necessary because respiratory function can take days to weeks to recover. In myasthenic crisis, early NIPPV may prevent the need for intubation. Therapy for both diseases includes plasma exchange or intravenous immune globulin. Glucocorticoids have no benefit in Guillain-Barré syndrome, but are indicated in addition to cholinesterase inhibitors in myasthenic crisis.

Acute spinal cord injuries at or above the C5 level invariably require mechanical ventilation. In some cases (complete spinal cord injury below C3 or incomplete injury above C3), recovery of independent respiratory function can occur. However, atelectasis, aspiration pneumonia, and pulmonary emboli are common and can lead to recurrent acute hypercapnic respiratory failure. Aggressive chest physiotherapy and use of mechanical cough assist devices are helpful and may lower the risk of these events.

### KEY POINTS

- Guillain-Barré syndrome and myasthenic crisis are the most common causes of acute neurologic respiratory failure in the ICU.

- Evaluation of maximum inspiratory and expiratory pressures and positional changes in vital capacity are helpful in assessing neuromuscular weakness as a cause of hypercapnic respiratory failure.

### Restrictive Chest Wall Disease

Restrictive disease from disorders affecting the pulmonary parenchyma (such as the various causes of diffuse parenchymal lung disease primarily leads to hypoxemia without

CONT.

hypercapnia. Acute hypercapnic respiratory failure is more common in patients with extrapulmonary chest wall restriction (pectus deformity, scoliosis, kyphosis), which causes compromised respiratory mechanics. Ascites and severe bowel distention can also compromise respiratory mechanics by exerting a significant cephalad force on the diaphragm. Commonly, extrapulmonary chest wall restriction causes poor ventilatory reserve without overt respiratory failure. However, acute insults such as infection or sedating medications can upset this delicate balance and precipitate hypercapnic respiratory failure. NIPPV and invasive positive pressure mechanical ventilation are both appropriate while the precipitating condition is managed. In patients with thoracic cage deformity, NIPPV in the outpatient setting is frequently beneficial. Improved $V_T$, especially during sleep when respiratory drive and minute ventilation decrease, can reduce the incidence of acute hypercapnic respiratory failure and improve patient function and quality of life.

### Obstructive Lung Diseases (Asthma and COPD)

Abnormal mechanical properties of the airways and the lung parenchyma cause both static and dynamic hyperinflation. A decrease in the lung's elastic recoil (as seen in emphysema) results in increased total lung capacity and is one of the factors leading to an increase in functional residual capacity (lung volume after a normal, not forced, exhalation). In addition, the ability to exhale is dependent on the elastic recoil of the lung, the degree of airflow obstruction (associated with structural changes, inflammation, increases in cholinergic tone, and mucous plugging), and the rate of breathing.

The degree of airflow obstruction and the respiration rate can each vary and cause greater air trapping during periods of exertion and exacerbation of disease, leading to increased lung volumes at the end of exhalation. This complication of airflow obstruction and insufficient time for exhalation is called dynamic hyperinflation and can result in intrathoracic pressure remaining positive at the end of exhalation, a phenomenon called auto-PEEP. Dynamic hyperinflation, auto-PEEP, and decreased elastic recoil of the lung all contribute to disordered lung mechanics, increased work of breathing, and respiratory muscle fatigue. Auto-PEEP may also decrease venous return and contribute to hemodynamic instability in patients receiving mechanical ventilation who are not given sufficient time for exhalation.

At the time of a COPD exacerbation, patients may present with signs of increased respiratory work. They may also have findings related to the presence of hypercapnia, such as altered sensorium or somnolence. See Airways Disease for more detailed information about management of COPD exacerbations.

In patients with COPD, excessive oxygen can increase $\dot{V}/\dot{Q}$ mismatch by disrupting compensatory vasoconstriction in poorly ventilated regions of lung, potentially leading to further elevation in $P_{CO_2}$. Therefore, in patients with COPD

exacerbation, oxygen therapy should be titrated to 88% to 92% oxyhemoglobin saturation. In patients with hypercapnic respiratory failure due to COPD exacerbation, NIPPV is preferred as the initial means to reduce $P_{CO_2}$. If patients cannot protect their airway, are hemodynamically unstable, or do not improve on NIPPV, intubation and mechanical ventilation are necessary. Strategies for mechanical ventilation in COPD include assuring sufficient expiratory time during the respiratory cycle to minimize auto-PEEP.

In patients with asthma, upright posture, inability to speak in full sentences, flaring of the nares, and contraction of the sternocleidomastoid muscles during inspiration, are signs of increased respiratory work and may herald respiratory failure. Blood gases usually demonstrate respiratory alkalosis due to rapid, shallow breathing patterns. Therefore, the presence of a normal or elevated arterial $P_{CO_2}$ may signal impending respiratory failure. Oxygen should be given to maintain a hemoglobin saturation of 90% to 95%. Hypoxemia can result from $\dot{V}/\dot{Q}$ mismatch, but should correct with oxygen. If oxygen saturation does not readily correct, other factors should be considered, including pneumonia, pneumothorax, or pulmonary embolism.

In cases of severe asthma exacerbation, magnesium sulfate may be used in addition to standard therapies to promote further bronchodilation. Adjunctive therapies, including anesthetics with bronchodilator properties (ketamine, isoflurane, sevoflurane), inhalation of a helium-oxygen mixture, mucolytics, and leukotriene receptor antagonists are not recommended because of lack of clear efficacy.

There is little objective evidence to support use of NIPPV in management of asthma exacerbations. Therefore, in asthmatic patients with respiratory failure, intubation is recommended. In these patients, efforts should be directed at maximizing expiratory time, as this improves dynamic hyperinflation and reduces auto-PEEP. The most effective way to do this is to minimize the patient's respiration rate. Doing so often requires sedation or paralytics and can lower a patient's overall minute ventilation. Because this may increase arterial $P_{CO_2}$, arterial blood gas analysis should be performed frequently in these patients.

### KEY POINTS

- Patients with hypercapnic respiratory failure and COPD exacerbation benefit from NIPPV provided they can protect their airway and are hemodynamically stable.

- In asthmatic patients with respiratory failure, intubation and mechanical evaluation are recommended rather than NIPPV.

- Adjunctive therapies for severe asthma exacerbation, including anesthetics with bronchodilator properties (ketamine, isoflurane, sevoflurane), inhalation of a helium-oxygen mixture, mucolytics, and leukotriene receptor antagonists are not recommended because of lack of clear efficacy.

**HVC**

# Shock

Shock occurs when systemic tissue perfusion is inadequate. In early states of tissue hypoperfusion, aerobic metabolism is supplanted by anaerobic metabolism and tissue injury is reversible. As compensatory mechanisms fail, sustained organ hypoperfusion can lead to cellular dysfunction and death. There are three primary mechanisms of shock: decreased circulating volume (hypovolemic), decreased cardiac output (cardiogenic), and inappropriate vasodilation (distributive).

Low blood pressure alone should not be considered diagnostic of end-organ hypoperfusion. Instead, blood pressure should be considered in the context of other physical examination findings that may suggest end-organ hypoperfusion (**Table 50**), as well as other general considerations for early shock assessment (**Figure 20**).

Treatment of a patient in shock is predicated on distinguishing the type of shock present and directing treatment toward correcting the root cause of the shock state (**Table 51**). Although many tools are available to aid in shock assessment and management, the use of bedside echocardiography has increased significantly during the last 10 years. Echocardiography can provide useful data regarding cardiac function and cardiac response to treatment. Other tools such as pulmonary artery catheters or those that predict response to volume replacement such as pulse pressure or stroke volume variation can also be considered; however, these technologies often carry higher risk due to their invasive nature, and the assessment of pulse pressure and stroke volume have procedural limitations (mechanical ventilation, receiving 8 mL/kg or greater of tidal volume, need for sinus rhythm, not triggering the ventilator) that may make them impractical. Pulmonary artery catheters have lost favorability in recent years because several large studies and meta-analyses that suggest no benefit, and in some cases increased risk to patients when used to guide therapy. Technologies that employ pulse contour, pulse pressure, or stroke volume variation assessment should be used with caution as well, given a broad array of clinical scenarios that can skew results and limited data to support their benefit in guiding therapy. ◪

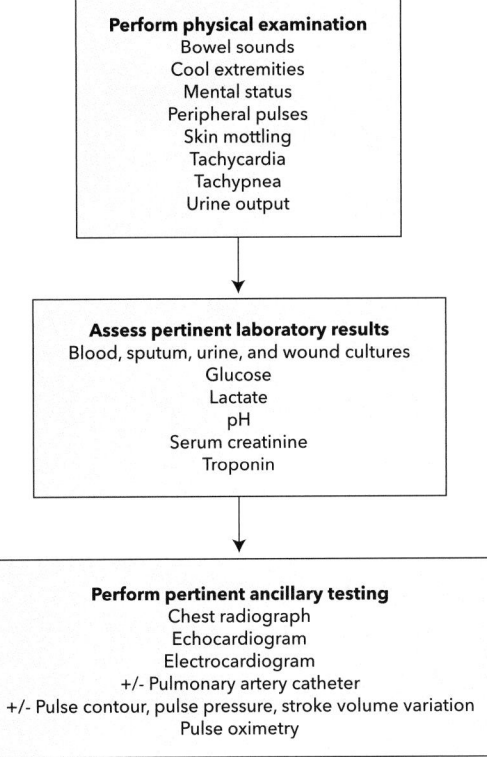

**FIGURE 20.** Early assessment of suspected shock.

- Treatment of a patient in shock is predicated on distinguishing the type of shock present and directed toward the root cause of the shock state.

- Pulmonary artery catheters have lost favorability in recent years because several large studies and meta-analyses that suggest no benefit, and in some cases increased risk to patients when used to guide therapy. **HVC**

## Distributive Shock

In distributive shock, the blood volume is generally normal, but a state of "relative" hypovolemia occurs from excessive vasodilation and microvascular dysfunction. This causes blood to bypass vital capillary beds, leading to tissue hypoxia. Cardiac output is often increased, but still cannot maintain a pressure sufficient for normal tissue perfusion. Initial treatment of distributive shock should focus on fluid resuscitation. Several studies have compared the effectiveness of crystalloid versus colloid administration, with no clear evidence that one is better than the other. Given the relative expense of colloids, crystalloid administration is generally preferred and recommended by guidelines. Vasopressor support is warranted if fluid administration alone is insufficient to support tissue perfusion. The selection of a vasopressor should be based on the patient's comorbidities and underlying cause of shock (see Table 39). ◪

**TABLE 50. Common Clinical Findings in Patients with Shock**

| |
|---|
| Altered mentation |
| Hypotension (SBP < 90 mm Hg) or 30 mm Hg drop in SBP from baseline |
| Mottled skin |
| Tachycardia (heart rate >100/min) |
| Tachypnea (respiration rate >25/min) |
| Urine output <0.5 mL/kg/h |
| Weak or absent peripheral pulses |
| Elevated serum lactate (>3 mEq/L [3 mmol/L]) |

SBP = systolic blood pressure.

| TABLE 51. | Selected Causes of Shock |
|---|---|
| **Distributive** | |
| Anaphylaxis | |
| Sepsis | |
| Spinal injury (usually above T4 level) | |
| Drugs (peripheral vasodilators, nitrates) | |
| **Hypovolemic** | |
| Acute blood loss (trauma, GI bleeding, surgery, uterine bleeding, obstetrical, retroperitoneal bleeding, aortic rupture) | |
| Crush injury, metabolic rhabdomyolysis | |
| Cutaneous losses (burns, toxic epidermal necrolysis, erythroderma, excessive sweating) | |
| Drugs (diuretics, laxatives) | |
| GI losses (vomiting/diarrhea) | |
| Kidney losses (diabetic ketoacidosis, hyperglycemic hyperosmolar syndrome, adrenal insufficiency, post-ATN osmotic diuresis) | |
| **Cardiogenic (Including Noncardiac Causes of Decreased Cardiac Output)** | |
| Abdominal compartment syndrome | |
| Arrhythmia (tachycardia, bradycardia) | |
| Atrial myxoma | |
| Heart failure | |
| Left ventricular infarction, right ventricular infarction | |
| Pericardial tamponade, constrictive pericarditis | |
| Pulmonary embolism | |
| Tension pneumothorax, severe dynamic hyperinflation (for example, excessive PEEP) | |
| Valvular heart disease (severe insufficiency, valve or chordae rupture, critical stenosis) | |
| Ventricular septal rupture, free ventricular wall rupture | |

ATN = acute tubular necrosis; GI = gastrointestinal; PEEP = positive end-expiratory pressure; T4 = fourth thoracic vertebra.

**KEY POINT**

HVC • Several studies have compared the effectiveness of crystalloid versus colloid administration for treatment of distributive shock, with no clear evidence that one is better than the other; given the relative expense of colloids, crystalloid administration is generally preferred and recommended by guidelines.

### Hypovolemic Shock

Hypovolemic shock occurs when decreased intravascular blood volume causes decreased preload, decreased ventricular filling, and diminished stroke volume. Initially, tachycardia and peripheral vasoconstriction help to preserve perfusion of vital organs but cannot compensate in the setting of severe hypovolemia. Treatment of hypovolemic shock includes aggressive volume or blood product replacement and, if possible, control of bleeding. Patients with hemorrhage may initially receive intravenous fluids to maintain hemodynamic stability, but ultimately need erythrocyte transfusion to prevent tissue ischemia. In stable ICU patients, hemoglobin levels should be maintained at about 7 g/dL (70 g/L); however, different thresholds and hemoglobin levels may trigger transfusion in actively bleeding patients who are in shock. Higher values may be necessary in patients with underlying cardiovascular disease. In patients with severe trauma, massive blood replacement requirements, and coagulopathy, evidence supports early resuscitation with a 1:1:1 ratio of erythrocytes, platelets, and fresh frozen plasma.

### Cardiogenic Shock

Cardiogenic shock occurs when a primary cardiac insult causes decreased cardiac output. This can result from any combination of obstructed filling or emptying of the ventricles, high or low heart rates, and decreased ejection fraction. It is essential to promptly identify the cause of cardiogenic shock to ensure appropriate medical therapy, surgical therapy, or both. In addition to a physical examination, evaluation should include laboratory testing for myocardial ischemia and heart failure, chest radiograph, electrocardiogram, and echocardiogram. In patients presenting with severe cardiogenic shock, additional supportive measures may include short-term mechanical support to allow a bridge toward definitive therapy. These include ECMO, intraaortic balloon pump, temporary pacemaker, and left or right ventricular assist device. However, recent technological advances have allowed many of these devices to be used for longer durations and even as destination therapy.

# Sepsis

### Definition, Pathophysiology, and Clinical Presentation of Sepsis

The Third International Definitions for Sepsis and Septic Shock (Sepsis-3) were published in 2016 and reflect evolving understanding of sepsis. Sepsis-3 defines sepsis as life-threatening organ dysfunction caused by a dysregulated host response to infection. Septic shock is defined as a subset of sepsis in which profound circulatory, cellular, and metabolic abnormalities are associated with a greater risk of mortality than with sepsis alone. The previous definition, combining known or suspected infection and systemic inflammatory response syndrome criteria, which can be appropriate (not necessarily dysregulated) responses to infection, is neither sensitive nor specific enough to diagnose sepsis. The terms *severe sepsis* and *septicemia* should no longer be used.

Infections giving rise to sepsis can include any agent and involve any organ, and need not be disseminated. The pathophysiology of sepsis is complex and involves dysfunction at many levels, from subcellular mitochondrial dysfunction to failure of entire organ systems. Loss of regulation of the body's finely balanced proinflammatory and antiinflammatory mediators and unregulated coagulation in the microvasculature are characteristic of the syndrome, although these features are difficult to assess clinically.

Operationally, sepsis can be identified whenever infection is known or suspected and clinical criteria defining organ dysfunction are met. The recommended criteria to assess organ dysfunction are included in the Sequential Organ Failure Assessment (SOFA) score, which assigns a value of 0-4 for each of six organ systems assessed: respiratory, coagulation, hepatic, cardiovascular, central nervous, and kidney, with increasing scores for more severe dysfunction (online SOFA score calculators are available: http://clincalc.com/IcuMortality/SOFA.aspx; https://www.mdcalc.com/sequential-organ-failure-assessment-sofa-score). An initial SOFA score of 2 or greater or an increase in SOFA score of 2 or more correlates with acute organ dysfunction and predicts hospital mortality of greater than 10%. The SOFA score should be used to assess patients in the ICU.

In the pre-ICU arena, Sepsis-3 guidelines recommend the use of the quick SOFA (qSOFA) score, a simplified clinical scoring system that includes only three criteria: respiration rate of 22/min or greater, altered mentation, and systolic blood pressure 100 mm Hg or less (**Table 52**). A qSOFA score of 2 or greater in the setting of known or suspected infection predicts increased mortality and should prompt evaluation for resuscitation and consideration of ICU admission. Failure to meet two or more qSOFA criteria should not be construed as ruling out sepsis, and investigation or treatment of infection should be pursued as deemed necessary by the responsible physicians. Although there is no definitive test for sepsis, the qSOFA score (specific but not sensitive) and the systemic inflammatory response syndrome (SIRS) criteria (sensitive but not specific) are complementary and can be used together to inform clinical judgment when diagnosing sepsis.

The criteria for diagnosing septic shock include hypotension requiring pressors to maintain a mean arterial pressure of greater than 65 mm Hg and serum lactate level of greater than 2 mEq/L (2 mmol/L) after adequate volume resuscitation. Patients who meet these criteria have a 40% or greater risk of in-hospital mortality. **H**

| TABLE 52. | qSOFA Score | |
|---|---|---|
| **Criterion** | **Value** | **qSOFA Points** |
| Respiration rate | >22/min | 1 |
| Systolic blood pressure | <100 mm Hg | 1 |
| Mental status | Altered from baseline | 1 |
| **qSOFA score** | **Predicted mortality** | |
| 0 | <1% | |
| 1 | 2-3% | |
| ≥2 | ≥10% | |

qSOFA = quick sequential organ failure assessment.

- Sepsis is defined as life-threatening organ dysfunction caused by a dysregulated host response to infection.
- Septic shock is defined as a subset of sepsis in which profound circulatory, cellular, and metabolic abnormalities are associated with a greater risk of mortality than with sepsis alone.

## Epidemiology of Sepsis

The epidemiology of sepsis is difficult to judge accurately because of its evolving definition, challenges with clinical recognition of the syndrome, and lack of standardized reporting. However, it is possible to estimate its incidence and clinical and economic effects. There are disparities in sepsis rates among different demographic groups. For example, sepsis is more common among black men than other racial groups or women. Sepsis is also more common among elderly patients, with incidence increasing with each year after the age of 65. Mortality from sepsis is high. A patient who is septic has a mortality rate 4 or more times greater for the same underlying condition and comorbidities without sepsis. Mortality increases by roughly 15% for each sepsis-related organ system failure.

## Management of Sepsis

Early diagnosis and timely treatment of sepsis are important to improve survival. In settings where sepsis is suspected, cultures and other investigations to identify infection, as well as the use of diagnostic instruments like the SOFA and qSOFA scoring tools to identify organ dysfunction, are helpful. Once sepsis is diagnosed, the two main pillars of management are: 1) supporting organ perfusion and function; and 2) controlling the infection. Various other adjunctive therapies may also affect survival. **H**

- The two main pillars of sepsis management are: 1) supporting organ perfusion and function; and 2) controlling the infection.

### Initial Resuscitation

Sepsis can have serious hemodynamics effects, with decreased preload (due to capillary leak), impaired cardiac contractility, and decreased vascular tone. Patients may present in shock, sometimes with profound hypotension requiring large volume resuscitation with intravenous fluids and often vasopressor therapy.

The fourth iteration of the Surviving Sepsis Guidelines, published in 2016, recommends early and aggressive fluid resuscitation for patients with hypoperfusion due to sepsis, with an initial bolus of 30 mL/kg of body weight. Additional fluids may be needed, and physiologic markers such as mean arterial pressure, pulse pressure variation, change in serum lactate level, bedside echocardiographic assessment of inferior vena cava filling, or other techniques are used as indicators of adequate fluid resuscitation. Although experts agree that aggressive fluid resuscitation is essential, the adequacy of fluid resuscitation requires clinical judgment in conjunction with the available data.

Fluid resuscitation should be with crystalloid, using normal saline or a balanced crystalloid solution. A balanced crystalloid solution has an electrolyte composition similar to plasma with the addition of a buffer, such as lactate (for example, Ringer's lactate solution). Data are emerging that suggest a balanced crystalloid solution may be associated with improved outcomes compared to normal saline, particularly in patients receiving a large volume of fluid, but current guidelines recommend either. There is weak evidence suggesting benefit from the use of albumin in patients requiring large volume resuscitation; however, sepsis guidelines offer this as a consideration rather than a recommendation.

**KEY POINT**

- Early and aggressive fluid resuscitation for patients with hypoperfusion due to sepsis begins with an initial bolus of 30 mL/kg body weight of normal saline or a balanced crystalloid solution.

## Antibiotic Therapy

Early administration of antibiotic therapy is crucial in treating sepsis. Broad spectrum antibiotics should be given within the first hour of suspected sepsis, and the regimen adjusted based on culture results. A delay in the first dose of antibiotic therapy increases sepsis mortality. The Surviving Sepsis Guidelines recommend empiric combination therapy for the initial management of septic shock, or when broad empiric coverage is needed for initial management of sepsis, bacteremia, or both. However, they recommend against combination therapy for the routine or ongoing treatment of sepsis and bacteremia without shock, even in the setting of neutropenia. The guidelines define combination therapy as the use of two different classes of antibiotics for a single putative pathogen expected to be sensitive to both, for purposes of accelerating pathogen clearance. The term is not used when the purpose of a multidrug strategy is to strictly broaden the range of antimicrobial activity. Antibiotic therapy should usually be continued for 7 to 10 days, depending on the clinical situation, and continually reassessed for efficacy and possible deescalation.

Procalcitonin, a serum marker for bacterial infection, should be measured when the probability of infection is estimated to be low. If the procalcitonin level is low, bacterial infection is unlikely and antibiotic therapy may not be warranted. There is no role for procalcitonin measurement in sepsis likely due to infection.

Prompt identification and control of any potential source of infection is essential in the management of sepsis. Examples include drainage of abscesses and removal of possibly infected intravenous catheters (once alternative intravenous access has been established). One exception is necrotizing pancreatitis, for which definitive resection should be delayed until the extent of necrosis is clear.

**KEY POINTS**

- Antibiotic therapy for patients with sepsis should usually be continued for 7 to 10 days, depending on the clinical situation, and continually reassessed for efficacy and for possible deescalation.

- Procalcitonin, a serum marker for infection, should be measured when the probability of infection is estimated to be low.

- There is no role for procalcitonin measurement in sepsis likely due to infection. **HVC**

- Prompt identification and control of any potential source of infection is essential in the management of sepsis.

## Adjunctive Therapies

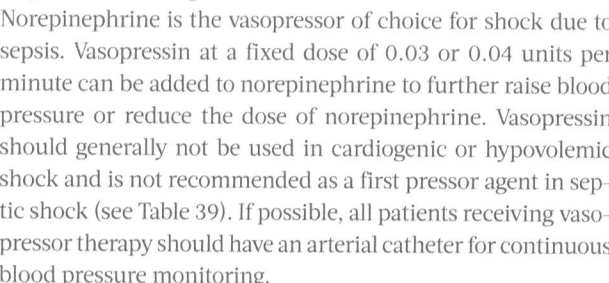

Norepinephrine is the vasopressor of choice for shock due to sepsis. Vasopressin at a fixed dose of 0.03 or 0.04 units per minute can be added to norepinephrine to further raise blood pressure or reduce the dose of norepinephrine. Vasopressin should generally not be used in cardiogenic or hypovolemic shock and is not recommended as a first pressor agent in septic shock (see Table 39). If possible, all patients receiving vasopressor therapy should have an arterial catheter for continuous blood pressure monitoring.

The use of glucocorticoids in the setting of sepsis is suggested to achieve hemodynamic stability when not achieved using intravenous fluids and vasopressor therapies. They have no role in sepsis without shock. If used, glucocorticoids can be added at a dose of not more than 200 mg daily of hydrocortisone (usually 50 mg intravenously every 6 hours). An adrenocorticotropic hormone stimulation test is not recommended.

**KEY POINTS**

- Norepinephrine is the vasopressor of choice in treatment of shock due to sepsis; vasopressin can be added to further raise the blood pressure or reduce the dose of norepinephrine.

- The use of glucocorticoids in the setting of sepsis is suggested if adequate fluid resuscitation and vasopressor therapy are unable to restore hemodynamic stability; there is no role for glucocorticoids in sepsis without shock. **HVC**

# Specific Critical Care Topics
## Anaphylaxis

Anaphylaxis is a severe reaction caused by acute mediator release into the circulation, usually triggered by IgE-linked immunological responses to specific foods, medications, insect venom, latex, or other antigens, but sometimes occurring without an allergic trigger. The mediator release results in various clinical manifestations including pruritus, hypotension, and tissue swelling (known as angioedema) caused by capillary leak from widespread inflammatory mediator release (**Table 53**). Onset of symptoms may be immediate after antigen exposure or delayed, sometimes for hours or even days, although more rapid onset usually signals a more severe reaction. This capillary leak can result in distributive shock with many of the same features as septic shock. Angioedema can be life-threatening when it compromises the airway.

Initial treatment is with epinephrine, which may be administered intramuscularly or intravenously. Adjunctive therapy with antihistamine medications may be used to relieve symptoms of pruritus and rash. Although commonly administered, evidence that glucocorticoids are useful in the treatment of anaphylaxis is sparse. Sometimes epinephrine must be given many times or continuously to achieve clinical stability. Patients should be given supplemental oxygen and watched closely for signs of airway compromise, which may require intubation to maintain airway patency. Patients often require fluid resuscitation, with or without vasopressor therapy. Removal of the precipitating antigen is also important if exposure is ongoing. Fortunately, anaphylaxis is rarely fatal but successful management requires early recognition and prompt attention to supportive and disease-reversing therapies, especially when shock or airway compromise is present.

Angioedema can occur without allergic stimulus (bradykinin-mediated), sometimes in response to medications (notably ACE inhibitors, even after long-term use), and sometimes for no identifiable reason. Nonallergic angioedema usually has slower onset and is not associated with urticaria, pruritus, or hypotension, but the tissue swelling can be clinically significant, especially in the airway, and may require intubation. Recurrent angioedema can be hereditary or acquired, as in C1 inhibitor deficiency. As in other forms of angioedema, treatment is supportive, sometimes with additional measures to control abnormal bradykinin, complement activation, or both. For more detail on angioedema see MKSAP 18 Dermatology.

**KEY POINT**

- Initial treatment of anaphylaxis is with epinephrine, which may be administered intramuscularly or intravenously.

## Hypertensive Emergencies

Hypertensive emergency refers to elevated blood pressure significantly above the normal range causing acute organ damage or dysfunction. The end-organ damage is the defining characteristic, particularly clinical dysfunction of the central nervous system (ischemic or hemorrhagic stroke, encephalopathy), the renal system (acute kidney injury), or the cardiovascular system (acute myocardial infarction, aortic dissection, acute heart failure). These effects often occur at blood pressures above 180/120 mm Hg, but there is no specific pressure threshold above which the syndrome is defined. When blood pressure is significantly elevated without evidence of end-organ damage, this is often labeled hypertensive urgency.

Hypertensive emergency should be treated by rapidly lowering the blood pressure, usually using intravenous short-acting agents in the ICU setting (**Table 54** and **Table 55**). The 2017 blood pressure guidelines from the American College of Cardiology/American Heart Association and nine other organizations recommend that for adults with a compelling condition (such as aortic dissection, severe preeclampsia or eclampsia, or pheochromocytoma crisis), systolic blood pressure (SBP) should be reduced to less than 140 mm Hg during the first hour and to less than 120 mm Hg in aortic dissection. For adults without a compelling condition, SBP should be reduced by no more than 25% within the first hour; then, if stable, to 160/100 mm Hg within the next 2 to 6 hours; and then cautiously to normal during the following 24 to 48 hours. See MKSAP 18 Neurology for further discussion of the treatment of hypertension associated with ischemic stroke and intracerebral hemorrhage.

| TABLE 53. | Organ System Involvement in Anaphylaxis | | |
|---|---|---|---|
| **Organ System** | **Symptoms** | **Signs** | **Patients with Organ Involved** |
| Skin and mucosa | Pruritus of skin, oropharynx, genitals, palms, soles | Flushing, urticaria, morbilliform rash, angioedema | 85% |
| Respiratory | Dyspnea, chest and throat tightness, stridor, cough, hoarseness, sneezing, rhinorrhea | Wheeze, stridor, respiratory distress | 70% |
| Cardiovascular | Lightheadedness, chest pain, palpitations | Hypotension, tachycardia > bradycardia | 45% |
| Gastrointestinal | Pain, nausea, vomiting, diarrhea | | 45% |
| Neurologic | Anxiety, headache | Encephalopathy | 15% |

**TABLE 54.** Intravenous Antihypertensive Drugs for Treatment of Hypertensive Emergencies without a Compelling Comorbidity

| Class | Examples | Comments |
|---|---|---|
| Dihydropyridine calcium channel blockers | Nicardipine | Nicardipine: Contraindicated in patients with severe aortic stenosis |
| | Clevidipine | Clevidipine: Contraindicated in patients with soy allergy, egg allergy, hyperlipidemia, lipoid nephrosis, and acute pancreatitis |
| Vasodilator-nitric oxide dependent | Sodium nitroprusside | Sodium nitroprusside: Intraarterial blood pressure monitoring recommended. Tachyphylaxis common with prolonged use. Irreversible cyanide toxicity possible with prolonged use |
| | Nitroglycerin | Nitroglycerin: Use only for patients with acute coronary syndrome or acute pulmonary edema; avoid in patients with right ventricular infarction and those taking PDE-5 inhibitors |
| Vasodilator-direct | Hydralazine | Not first-line drug due to unpredictable response and long duration of action |
| Adrenergic blocker-$\beta_1$ selective | Esmolol | Contraindicated with concurrent β-blocker therapy, bradycardia, pulmonary edema, severe HF |
| Adrenergic blocker-combined $\alpha_1$ and nonselective β blocker | Labetalol | Useful in hyperadrenergic syndromes. Contraindicated in patients with asthma, COPD, heart block. May worsen heart failure |
| Adrenergic blocker-nonselective α-blocker | Phentolamine | Useful in patients with pheochromocytoma, cocaine toxicity, amphetamine overdose, clonidine withdrawal |
| Dopamine$_1$-agonist | Fenoldopam | Contraindicated in patients with glaucoma or increased intracerebral pressure |
| ACE inhibitor | Enalaprilat | Useful in situations associated with high plasma renin activity (scleroderma renal crisis). Contraindicated in pregnancy, acute MI, bilateral renal artery stenosis |

HF = heart failure; MI = myocardial infarction; PDE = phosphodiesterase.

Data from Whelton PK, Carey RM, Aronow WS, Casey DE Jr, Collins KJ, Dennison Himmelfarb C, et al. 2017 ACC/AHA/AAPA/ABC/ACPM/AGS/APhA/ASH/ASPC/NMA/PCNA guideline for the prevention, detection, evaluation, and management of high blood pressure in adults: executive summary: A report of the American College of Cardiology/American Heart Association task force on clinical practice guidelines. Hypertension. 2018;71:1269-1324. [PMID: 29133354] doi:10.1161/HYP.0000000000000066

**TABLE 55.** Intravenous Antihypertensive Drugs for Treatment of Hypertensive Emergencies in Patients with a Compelling Comorbidity

| Comorbidity | Preferred Drugs[a] | Comments |
|---|---|---|
| Acute aortic dissection | Esmolol, labetalol | Rapid SBP lowering to ≤120 mm Hg. β-Blockade should precede vasodilator (such as with nicardipine or nitroprusside) administration. |
| Acute pulmonary edema | Nitroglycerin, nitroprusside, clevidipine | β-Blockers contraindicated |
| Acute coronary syndromes | Esmolol, labetalol, nicardipine, nitroglycerin | Esmolol and nitroglycerin are first-line drugs. |
| Acute kidney injury | Clevidipine, fenoldopam, nicardipine | |
| Eclampsia or preeclampsia | Hydralazine, labetalol, nicardipine | ACE inhibitors, ARBs, renin inhibitors, nitroprusside contraindicated |

[a]See Table 54 for specific drug contraindications.

ARB = angiotensin receptor blocker; SBP = systolic blood pressure.

Data from Whelton PK, Carey RM, Aronow WS, Casey DE Jr, Collins KJ, Dennison Himmelfarb C, et al. 2017 ACC/AHA/AAPA/ABC/ACPM/AGS/APhA/ASH/ASPC/NMA/PCNA guideline for the prevention, detection, evaluation, and management of high blood pressure in adults: executive summary: A report of the American College of Cardiology/American Heart Association task force on clinical practice guidelines. Hypertension. 2018;71:1269-1324. [PMID: 29133354] doi:10.1161/HYP.0000000000000066

**KEY POINTS**

- For adults with a hypertensive emergency and a compelling condition (such as aortic dissection, severe preeclampsia or eclampsia, or pheochromocytoma crisis), systolic blood pressure should be reduced to less than 140 mm Hg during the first hour and to less than 120 mm Hg in aortic dissection.

- For adults with a hypertensive emergency but without a compelling condition, systolic blood pressure should be reduced by no more than 25% within the first hour; then, if stable, to 160/100 mm Hg within the next 2 to 6 hours; and then cautiously to normal during the following 24 to 48 hours.

# Hyperthermic Emergencies

Hyperthermic emergency is defined as elevation of core body temperature, usually above 40°C (104°F), causing end-organ dysfunction or damage, which may include alteration in mental status, seizures, kidney injury, muscle rigidity, rhabdomyolysis, acute respiratory distress syndrome, and disseminated intravascular coagulation. Common causes of hyperthermia include heat stroke, malignant hyperthermia, and neuroleptic malignant syndrome, all of which can be fatal if not recognized and treated appropriately (**Table 56**).

## Heat Stroke

Heat stroke is a failure of the body's thermal regulatory system caused by dysfunction, as in elderly patients taking

**TABLE 56.** Causes of Severe Hyperthermia

| Diagnosis | Suggestive History | Key Examination Findings | Treatment | Notes |
|---|---|---|---|---|
| Heat stroke | Environmental exposure | Encephalopathy and fever | Evaporative cooling<br><br>Ice water immersion | Avoid ice water immersion if nonexertional |
| Malignant hyperthermia | Exposure to volatile anesthetic or succinylcholine | Masseter muscle rigidity; ↑ arterial $PCO_2$ | Stop inciting drug<br><br>Dantrolene | Monitor and treat ↑ $K^+$ and ↑ arterial $PCO_2$ |
| Neuroleptic malignant syndrome | Typical > atypical antipsychotic agent; onset over days to weeks | Altered mentation, severe rigidity, ↑ HR, ↑ BP, hyporeflexia, no clonus | Stop the inciting drug<br><br>Dantrolene<br><br>Bromocriptine | Resolves over days to weeks<br><br>Mentation change first |
| Severe serotonin syndrome[a] | Onset within 24 hours of initiation or increasing dose, gastrointestinal prodrome | Agitation, clonus, ↑ reflexes, rigidity | Stop inciting drug<br><br>Benzodiazepines<br><br>Cyproheptadine | Resolves in 24 hours |

[a]Not routinely considered a cause of severe hyperthermia but commonly confused with neuroleptic malignant syndrome.

BP = blood pressure; HR = heart rate; $K^+$ = potassium.

CONT.

anticholinergic medications; volume depletion (diuretics, insensible water loss); or because the system is overwhelmed, as in athletes or military recruits who train strenuously in hot, humid weather. When the core temperature rises above 40°C patients develop encephalopathy. They may also experience hypotension, nausea, and muscle weakness.

If untreated, mortality in heat stroke can be up to 60%. Centrally acting antipyretics such as NSAIDs or acetaminophen are not effective. For patients with nonexertional heat stroke, evaporative cooling with or without ice packs can be used to lower the core temperature to a safe target level, usually 38.5°C (101°F). For exertional heat stroke, evaporative cooling may be effective, but patients who remain severely symptomatic despite evaporative cooling efforts sometimes require immersion in ice water to bring the core temperature down rapidly. Because immersion therapy may be complicated by hypothermia, it is not recommended as first-line treatment. H

**KEY POINT**

- For patients with nonexertional heat stroke, evaporative cooling with or without ice packs can be used to lower the core temperature to a safe target level; for exertional heat stroke, immersion in ice water is sometimes required for severe cases.

## Malignant Hyperthermia

Malignant hyperthermia is a rare cause of severe hyperthermia in response to inhaled anesthetic agents (such as halothane and isoflurane) or depolarizing paralytic agents (such as succinylcholine). When a patient with inherited susceptibility is exposed to one of these agents, he or she may develop muscle rigidity, rhabdomyolysis, cardiac arrhythmias, and core body temperature elevation to 45°C

(113°F) or more. Mortality can reach 10%. Treatment consists of discontinuing the triggering agent, active cooling, and administration of the muscle relaxant dantrolene every 5 to 10 minutes until muscle rigidity and hyperthermia resolve.

## Neuroleptic Malignant Syndrome and Serotonin Syndrome

Neuroleptic malignant syndrome is an idiosyncratic response to neuroleptic agents such as haloperidol. It can occur with any neuroleptic medication, even after prolonged use, although it is more common at times of initiation or dose escalation. It can also occur with rapid withdrawal of dopaminergic medications for Parkinson disease. Dehydration may increase the risk of the syndrome, which includes fever, mental status changes, and rigidity. Mortality may exceed 10%. Treatment includes stopping the triggering agent (or reinstating the withdrawn dopaminergic agent), active cooling, and rehydration. Evidence for using dantrolene is weak. Neuroleptic medications can be reintroduced after a waiting period of at least 2 weeks, usually at lower dose, with care to avoid dehydration and concomitant administration with lithium.

Serotonin syndrome is a less severe hyperthermic reaction triggered by simultaneous use of two or more medications that affect release or reuptake of serotonin. Unlike neuroleptic malignant syndrome, serotonin syndrome usually includes hyperreflexia and myoclonus, and generally resolves after 24 hours. H

**KEY POINT**

- Treatment of neuroleptic malignant syndrome includes stopping the triggering agent, active cooling, and rehydration.

# Accidental Hypothermia

Accidental hypothermia results from heat loss significant enough to overwhelm the body's ability to maintain its core temperature. Shivering is the body's usual mechanism for raising a low core temperature and is quite effective. In the mild stage of hypothermia, shivering occurs, and patients may develop tachycardia, hyperventilation, poor judgment, loss of coordination, and diuresis. Clinical findings may progress to include hypotension, bradycardia, and further depression of mental status. As hypothermia worsens, victims stop shivering, lose consciousness, and can develop life-threatening complications, including pulmonary edema and ventricular arrhythmias (**Table 57**). In moderate to severe hypothermia Osborne waves may be present on electrocardiogram tracings (**Figure 21**).

If a severely hypothermic patient becomes pulseless and requires resuscitation, it is reasonable to continue cardiopulmonary resuscitation for a prolonged period of time until the patient can be rewarmed. There are reports of cardiopulmonary resuscitation lasting hours and resulting in full recovery when a severely hypothermic patient has a cardiac arrest.

Hypothermic patients who are shivering will passively rewarm themselves if they are removed from the cold environment and given adequate insulation to prevent heat loss, but as hypothermia progresses, shivering stops, usually when the core temperature drops below 32°C (89.6°F). At this point, a patient must be actively rewarmed to prevent complications. Active rewarming techniques include surface methods, such as heating pads and forced-air warming systems, as well as invasive methods such as rewarming by peritoneal or pleural space irrigation using peritoneal catheters or thoracostomy tubes. Extracorporeal support, including cardiopulmonary bypass, is recommended for patients in cardiac arrest because it maximizes the rewarming rate and can provide hemodynamic support. During active rewarming, core temperature should be monitored with an esophageal temperature probe, as rectal and bladder temperatures will lag behind the rising core temperature during the rewarming process.

# Toxicology

## Alcohol Poisoning

Ethanol and other ingested alcohols activate the γ-aminobutyric acid receptor, which is the primary central nervous system (CNS) inhibitor, thus leading to CNS depression, including loss of consciousness and suppression of respiratory drive at high doses. In addition to this acute toxicity, which can lead to life-threatening apnea or aspiration events, alcohol withdrawal can also be fatal, and patients should be monitored for signs of withdrawal, including seizures. Ethanol is the most commonly ingested alcohol and the most often encountered toxicity (**Table 58**). For further discussion of alcohol withdrawal see MKSAP 18 General Internal Medicine.

Other alcohols ingested include ethylene glycol (antifreeze), methanol (wood alcohol), and isopropyl alcohol (rubbing alcohol). These all have similar CNS depressant effects to those of ethanol. However, after ingestion, ethylene glycol is metabolized by alcohol dehydrogenase to oxalic acid, which crystalizes in the renal tubules and can lead to permanent kidney damage. Methanol is metabolized to formic acid, which is toxic to the retina and leads to blindness. When either of these alcohols has been ingested, there is an elevated anion gap metabolic acidosis as well as an osmolal gap (see MKSAP 18 Nephrology: Increased Anion Gap Metabolic Acidosis). Therapy includes elimination but also prevention of metabolism by alcohol dehydrogenase to toxic metabolites. The enzymatic process can be competitively inhibited by administering fomepizole.

Isopropyl alcohol has no toxic metabolites and does not elevate the anion gap, although it does increase the osmolal gap. Treatment is supportive. Dialysis removes all alcohols effectively, but is not necessary for patients who are inebriated but otherwise stable.

## Carbon Monoxide Poisoning

Carbon monoxide (CO) is a colorless, odorless product of hydrocarbon combustion that is readily absorbed into the circulation when inhaled, and binds avidly to hemoglobin to form carboxyhemoglobin, displacing oxygen and causing clinical tissue hypoxia and ischemia. CO toxicity occurs almost exclusively in enclosed areas where combustion is occurring and is often accidental, but may be intentional in suicide attempts. Exposed patients present with headache, nausea,

| TABLE 57. | Symptoms and Signs of Hypothermia | |
|-----------|-----------------------------------|---|
| **Severity** | **Temperature** | **Findings** |
| Mild | 32.0-35.0 °C (89.6-95.0 °F) | ↑ HR, ↑ BP, ↑ RR, shivering, alert, poor judgment |
| Moderate | 28.0-32.0 °C (82.4-89.6 °F) | ↓ HR, ↓ BP, ↓ RR, ↓ CO, ↓O$_2$ consumption, ↓ kidney function, somnolence, no shivering, supraventricular arrhythmia |
| Severe | <28.0 °C (82.4 °F) | Coma, absent reflexes, ventricular arrhythmia, asystole, apnea |

BP = blood pressure; CO = cardiac output; HR = heart rate; RR = respiration rate.

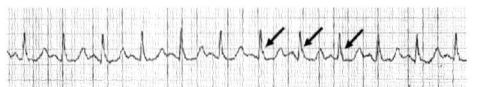

**FIGURE 21.** Electrocardiogram showing Osborne waves associated with hypothermia. They are best seen in the inferior and lateral chest leads. Osborne waves are defined by the shoulder or "hump" between QRS and ST segments.

| Alcohol | Common Sources | Major Findings | Anion Gap | Osmolar Gap | Antidote |
|---------|----------------|----------------|-----------|-------------|----------|
| Ethanol | Alcoholic beverages | CNS depression<br>Nausea, emesis | Possible | Yes | Supportive care |
| Isopropyl alcohol | Rubbing alcohol<br>Disinfectants<br>Antifreeze | CNS depression<br>Ketone elevation | No | Yes | Supportive care |
| Methanol | Windshield wiper fluid<br>De-icing solutions<br>Solvents<br>"Moonshine" | CNS depression<br>Vision loss<br>Hypotension | Yes | Yes | Fomepizole<br>HD for severe acidemia, very large ingestions, severe CNS depression, and any visual impairment |
| Ethylene glycol | Antifreeze<br>De-icing solutions<br>Solvents | CNS depression<br>AKI<br>Hypocalcemia<br>Hypotension | Yes | Yes | Fomepizole<br>HD for severe acidemia, very large ingestions, severe CNS depression, AKI, and systemic collapse |

**TABLE 58.** Presentation and Treatment of Alcohol Poisoning

AKI = acute kidney injury; CNS = central nervous system; HD = hemodialysis.

CONT.

malaise, confusion, syncope, seizures, or coma. Patients with coronary artery disease may develop signs and symptoms of cardiac ischemia.

Pulse oximetry is not helpful, as current transcutaneous oximetry technology does not differentiate between oxyhemoglobin and carboxyhemoglobin. Blood gas analysis, including cooximetry, will provide the carboxyhemoglobin level, which is less than 3% in normal individuals. Smokers may have up to 10% to 15% carboxyhemoglobin, and anything higher is consistent with CO poisoning.

The primary treatment is displacement of CO on the hemoglobin molecule with oxygen, which depends on the alveolar concentration of oxygen and the minute ventilation. Once the CO exposure has been stopped, the half-life of carboxyhemoglobin is 300 minutes if patients are breathing ambient air, 90 minutes if breathing 100% oxygen, and 30 minutes if given hyperbaric oxygen in a chamber where the pressure is gradually increased to 2 to 3 times the normal atmospheric pressure. Patients with high levels of carboxyhemoglobin (25% and greater) and evidence of organ ischemia should be treated with hyperbaric oxygen if possible.

Besides the immediate complications resulting from tissue hypoxia in the setting of CO toxicity, there are also delayed neurologic sequelae in approximately 40% of severe cases of CO poisoning. The mechanism is poorly understood, but probably relates to ischemic damage sustained in specific, oxygen-sensitive areas of the brain. These delayed neurocognitive and personality defects usually appear within 20 days of the exposure, but can appear later. They can last for a year or longer. There is weak evidence that hyperbaric oxygen therapy reduces the risk and severity of these delayed neurologic sequelae. ▪

**KEY POINTS**

- Pulse oximetry is not helpful in diagnosing carbon monoxide poisoning, as it does not differentiate between oxyhemoglobin and carboxyhemoglobin.
**HVC**
- Patients with high levels of carboxyhemoglobin (25% or higher) and evidence of organ dysfunction should be treated with hyperbaric oxygen if possible.

## Cyanide Poisoning

Cyanide is one of the most lethal poisons known. It inhibits cellular respiration by binding to cytochrome oxidase $a_3$ in the mitochondria, blocking the cells' ability to use oxygen for aerobic metabolism. This results in clinical signs of hypoxia, despite normal oxyhemoglobin saturation. Symptoms often include headache, anxiety, nausea, and either a metallic or bitter almond odor and taste. More severe or prolonged exposure can lead to coma, seizures, liver or kidney injury, vomiting, ischemic pain, rhabdomyolysis, and death. Serum lactate elevation is a sensitive but nonspecific marker for cyanide toxicity. A normal lactate concentration effectively rules out significant cyanide exposure.

Cyanide can be ingested or inhaled and is absorbed readily and acts quickly to inhibit cellular metabolism. Inhalation exposure is common in house fires where cyanide is produced and aerosolized when vinyl burns. Cyanide is a common co-exposure with carbon monoxide.

Successful treatment depends on early recognition of cyanide toxicity, elimination of ongoing exposure (for example, removal of contaminated clothing), and either neutralization or competitive binding of the cyanide to remove it from the mitochondrial respiration system. Hydroxocobalamin avidly binds to cyanide to produce

CONT.

cyanocobalamin, which is soluble, nontoxic, and readily excreted. The usual dose is 5 g for an adult. Other antidotes include nitrites (amyl nitrite and sodium nitrite) to induce methemoglobin, which in turn binds cyanide, as well as sodium thiosulfate, which donates sulfur to combine with cyanide, producing harmless thiocyanate. Inducing methemoglobinemia in inhalation-injury victims who may also have high levels of carboxyhemoglobin is not safe, so nitrite therapy should be avoided. Of these potential treatment strategies, hydroxocobalamin is the most commonly recommended due to ease and safety of administration. ▪

### KEY POINT

- Successful treatment of cyanide poisoning depends on early recognition of cyanide toxicity, elimination of ongoing exposure, and administration of hydroxocobalamin to remove the cyanide from the mitochondrial respiration system.

## Toxicity of Drugs of Abuse

Drugs of abuse may be taken singly or in combination, and an accurate history may be impossible to obtain due to alteration of mental status, reluctance on the part of the patient or others to admit what was taken, and insufficient or incorrect knowledge about the composition of illicit drugs. Clinical toxic syndromes, or constellations of symptoms and signs indicative of certain classes of drugs, can be recognized and provide clues as to what should be done for effective medical management of overdose (**Table 59** and **Table 60**).

In addition to seeking to identify the specific agent(s) or class(es) of drugs taken, care of overdose patients is primarily supportive; critically important is maintenance of airway patency and ventilation in patients with decreased mental status. Patients are often intubated to prevent aspiration and allow for mechanical ventilation in cases where respiratory drive is impaired by drugs.

An early empiric trial of the opioid antagonist naloxone is warranted when opioid overdose is suspected to reverse respiratory depression and depressed mental status. It is important to remember that naloxone has a very short half-life, and its antidote effects will usually wear off before the opioid effects are gone; patients should be observed for signs of opioid withdrawal (which is not fatal and requires only supportive care) and for continued or recurrent signs of respiratory distress, which may require repeated dosing of naloxone.

Administration of flumazenil for suspected benzodiazepine overdose is more problematic, as reversing the effect of benzodiazepines can lead to life-threatening CNS activation, including seizures, which are most likely in patients taking benzodiazepines chronically. It is usually best to manage patients with ventilator support and allow elimination of the agent over time.

In patients who have taken sympathomimetic agents, such as cocaine or amphetamines, benzodiazepines are the

| **TABLE 59.** | Toxic Syndromes and Their Manifestations | |
|---|---|---|
| **Syndrome** | **Manifestations** | **Representative Drugs** |
| Sympathomimetic | Tachycardia | Cocaine |
| | Hypertension | Amphetamines |
| | Diaphoresis | Ephedrine |
| | Agitation | Caffeine |
| | Seizures | |
| | Mydriasis | |
| Cholinergic | "SLUDGE" (Salivation, Lacrimation, increased Urination and Defecation, Gastrointestinal upset, and Emesis) | Organophosphates (insecticides, sarin) |
| | | Carbamates |
| | | Physostigmine |
| | | Edrophonium |
| | | Nicotine |
| | Confusion | |
| | Bronchorrhea | |
| | Bradycardia | |
| | Miosis | |
| Anticholinergic | Hyperthermia | Antihistamines |
| | Dry skin and mucous membranes | Tricyclic antidepressants |
| | Agitation, delirium | Anti-Parkinson agents |
| | Tachycardia, tachypnea | Atropine |
| | Hypertension | Scopolamine |
| | Mydriasis | |
| Opioids | Miosis | Morphine, fentanyl, oxycodone and related drugs |
| | Respiratory depression | |
| | Lethargy, confusion | Heroin |
| | Hypothermia | |
| | Bradycardia | |
| | Hypotension | |

cornerstone of therapy for agitation. Beta-blocker medications should be avoided, as they will block the beta-adrenergic receptors and theoretically leave the activated alpha receptors unopposed, thus leading to severe hypertension.

Hallucinogenic agents have no antidote, so care is supportive, including maintaining the airway, ventilation, and hemodynamic support. These patients may be extremely agitated and combative, requiring physical restraints or sedation to prevent them from harming themselves and others.

## Overdose of Therapeutic Drugs

Patients may overdose on prescribed medications either inadvertently or intentionally, and often many medications

**TABLE 60.** Presentation and Toxicity of Some Drugs of Abuse

| Drug Class | Examples | Examination Findings | Antidote |
|---|---|---|---|
| Opioids | Heroin, oxycodone, fentanyl analogs | ↓ HR, ↓ temp, ↓ BP, ↓ RR, miosis | Naloxone |
| Benzodiazepines | Lorazepam | CNS depression, usually normal vital signs and eye examination | Flumazenil (may be complicated by seizure) |
| Sympathomimetics | | Shared findings: ↑ HR, ↑ BP, ↑ temp, diaphoresis, mydriasis, agitation, seizure, ↑ CK, ↑ liver chemistry studies, ↑ Cr | Benzodiazepines are first line for agitation<br><br>Avoid β-blockers for hypertension<br><br>Haloperidol may worsen hyperthermia |
| | Cocaine | 30-minute duration, myocardial infarction prominent | |
| | Methamphetamine | Violent agitation prominent, ↓ Na, duration 20 hours | |
| | MDMA ("ecstasy") | ↓ Na, serotonin syndrome | |
| | Bath salts ("plant food") | Hallucinations, violent agitation common, duration up to 48 hours, negative urine drug screen | |
| Hallucinogens | Dextromethorphan | ↑ HR, ↑ BP, agitation, coma | Benzodiazepines are first line for agitation<br><br>Haloperidol is second line |
| | Lysergic acid diethylamide (LSD) | Mild ↑ HR, ↑ BP; rare ↑ temp and hemodynamic instability | |
| | Phencyclidine (PCP) | Variable mental status: ↑ agitation, CNS depression, nystagmus | |
| | Synthetic cannabinoids ("Spice," "K-2") | ↑ HR, agitation > marijuana, ↑Cr, negative urine drug screen | |

BP = blood pressure; CK = creatine kinase; CNS = central nervous system; Cr = creatinine; ECG = electrocardiogram; HR = heart rate; MDMA = 3-4 methylenedioxymethamphetamine; Na = sodium; RR = respiration rate; temp = temperature.

CONT.

are taken together, sometimes with alcohol. Information about suicidal ideation or intent, what medications a patient and family members have been prescribed, what prescriptions were filled, events reported by the patient or bystanders, and clinical signs and symptoms are all important in determining the nature of an overdose. If patients are alert and cooperative enough to protect their airway, administration of activated charcoal may be beneficial if it can be given within 1 to 2 hours of ingestion (**Table 61**). Acetaminophen overdose is discussed in MKSAP 18 Gastroenterology and Hepatology, and salicylate overdose in MKSAP 18 Nephrology.

## Acute Abdominal Surgical Emergencies

A large number of conditions can cause abdominal pain, distention, and rigidity. Although many of them can and should be managed medically, some require surgery, and timely diagnosis followed by surgical intervention is needed to improve survival. Imaging decisions should be based on history and examination findings, and should not delay intervention

(**Table 62**). For further discussion of abdominal compartment syndrome see MKSAP 18 Nephrology.

## Encephalopathy

Alterations in mental status are common in the ICU because of both critical illness and the ICU environment, which can provide sick patients few contextual clues to reorient themselves to time, place, and events. There are many situations that involve mental status change, but three are most important in the context of critical care medicine: delirium (addressed earlier in Principles of Critical Care), coma, and anoxic brain injury.

### Coma

Coma describes a condition of absent cortical function of the CNS, with intact brainstem function, whether due to illness, trauma, or medication. Patients in a coma do not respond to external stimuli. The Glasgow Coma Scale (GCS) is an instrument for assessing the severity of deficit based on three categories of stimulus response: eye response, verbal response, and motor response (**Table 63**). A GCS score of 15 means a normal,

| Medication | Key Clinical Findings | Treatment | Notes |
|---|---|---|---|
| **Nonopioid analgesics** | | | |
| Acetaminophen | ↑ liver chemistry studies, ↑Cr, ↑INR, encephalopathy, cerebral edema, vomiting | N-acetylcysteine | Transfer to liver transplant center if severe |
| Salicylates | Mixed respiratory alkalosis/anion gap metabolic acidosis, tinnitus, agitation, confusion, hyperthermia | Bicarbonate infusion, dextrose | Target urine pH 7.5 to 8.0; hemodialysis if acute kidney injury or severe toxicity |
| **Cardiovascular** | | | |
| β-Blocker, calcium channel blocker | ↓ HR, ↓ BP, heart block, altered mental status if β-blocker | Atropine 1 mg IV up to 3 doses, glucagon, calcium chloride, vasopressors, cardiac pacemaker (if indicated), high-dose insulin and glucose, IV lipid emulsion | Treatments may be added sequentially or initiated simultaneously depending on severity of case and response to treatment |
| Digoxin | ↓ HR, arrhythmia, nausea, emesis, abdominal pain, confusion, weakness | Digoxin-specific antibody | Use of antibody lowers $K^+$; hemodialysis not effective |
| **Anticholinergics** | | | |
| Tricyclic antidepressants | ↓ BP, sedation, seizure, anticholinergic signs, arrhythmia | Bicarbonate infusion titrated to QRS duration; benzodiazepines for seizure | Physostigmine contraindicated |
| Antihistamines | Anticholinergic signs including agitation and seizures | Benzodiazepines; physostigmine if isolated anticholinergic overdose | Physostigmine use requires continuous cardiac monitor and bedside atropine |
| **Hypoglycemic** | | | |
| Sulfonylurea | ↓ glucose, confusion, seizure, anxiety, diaphoresis, tremor | Dextrose + octreotide, glucagon IM = temporizing | Monitor for ↓ glucose for 48 hours if large ingestion |
| Metformin | ↑ lactate, abdominal pain | Hemodialysis for severe ↓ pH or acute kidney injury | Glucose usually normal if isolated metformin ingestion |
| **Others** | | | |
| Lithium | GI distress, confusion, ataxia, tremor, myoclonic jerks, diabetes insipidus | Hemodialysis if lithium level >4 mEq/L or severe symptoms | Serum level can guide need for hemodialysis, confirm diagnosis |
| SSRI/SNRI | Agitation, clonus, ↑ reflexes, rigidity, fever, ↑ HR | Benzodiazepines, cyproheptadine if severe | Venlafaxine has ↑ cardiac toxicity |

BP = blood pressure; Cr = creatinine; GI = gastrointestinal; HR = heart rate; IM = intramuscular; IV = intravenous; $K^+$ = potassium; SNRI = serotonin norepinephrine reuptake inhibitor; SSRI = selective serotonin reuptake inhibitor.

**CONT.**

alert (or fully arousable) patient, and a score of 3 means no response at all. Comatose patients are often hyperreflexic. In addition to a clinical examination, lumbar puncture and CNS imaging with MRI or CT scan are useful in diagnosing the cause of coma. Treatment is supportive with efforts to reverse the specific cause of the coma if possible.

## Anoxic Brain Injury

Anoxic brain injury refers to damage to the CNS caused by prolonged, profound tissue hypoxia. There are many possible causes of such hypoxia, including near drowning, seizures, obstructed airway, lung disease, cardiac arrest, asphyxiation, and other inhalational injury. Brain imaging shows edema and loss of grey-white matter demarcation. Electroencephalographic monitoring shows various patterns,

from diffuse slowing (typical of many types of encephalopathy) to burst suppression or seizure activity (indicative of more severe injury) to absence of brain electrical activity (which can indicate brain death). Prognosis is often not immediately apparent, and patients with anoxic brain injury require supportive care for 3 to 5 days or longer before the extent of injury can be understood well enough to be declared irreversible. **H**

### KEY POINT

- Prognosis for patients with anoxic brain injury is often not immediately apparent, and patients require supportive care for 3 to 5 days or longer before the extent of injury can be understood well enough to be declared irreversible.

**TABLE 62.** Acute Abdominal Emergencies

| Diagnosis | Presentation | Diagnostic Imaging | Notes |
|---|---|---|---|
| Acute cholecystitis and cholangitis | Persistent peritoneal RUQ or epigastric pain, fever, emesis, positive Murphy sign | Ultrasound<br><br>EUS and ERCP for diagnosis and treatment of cholangitis | ↑ alkaline phosphatase, ↑ bilirubin suggests cholangitis but typically not cholecystitis |
| Bowel obstruction | Cramping pain, emesis, distention, obstipation, dehydration | Radiograph: dilated loops of bowel with air-fluid levels<br><br>CT scan: identifies cause, complications | Top causes: incarcerated hernia, adhesions, volvulus, intussusception |
| Acute appendicitis | Classic: periumbilical then RLQ pain, emesis, ↑ leukocyte count | Often unnecessary<br><br>CT or ultrasound if unclear | Pain quality and location vary with appendix location |
| Peptic ulcer perforation | Abrupt peritoneal pain, later distention and hypovolemia | Radiograph: free air<br><br>CT scan if unclear | Surgery necessary in majority of cases |
| Acute mesenteric ischemia | Pain > examination findings, vomiting, hypotension, risk factors for clotting, embolism | CT angiography or conventional arteriography | ↑ amylase, ↑ phosphate common<br><br>Regular CT and lactate can be normal early in course |
| Toxic megacolon | Pain, diarrhea, fever, ↑ HR, ↓ BP, confusion | Radiograph: dilated colon, air-fluid levels in colon<br><br>CT scan if unclear | Causes: inflammatory bowel disease, *Clostridium difficile* infection |
| Ruptured abdominal aortic aneurysm | ↓ BP, abdominal and/or flank pain, pulsatile mass | Unnecessary if high suspicion and unstable<br><br>CT or ultrasound if unclear | Risk factors: older age, male, smoking, hypertension, family history of aneurysm |
| Ectopic pregnancy with tubal rupture | ↓ BP, ↓ Hb, ↑ hCG, abdominal pain, vaginal bleeding | Transvaginal ultrasound | High mortality without early surgery |

BP = blood pressure; ERCP = endoscopic retrograde cholangiopancreatography; EUS = endoscopic ultrasound; Hb = hemoglobin; hCG = human chorionic gonadotropin; HR = heart rate; RLQ = right lower quadrant; RUQ = right upper quadrant; temp = temperature.

**TABLE 63.** Glasgow Coma Scale

| | Score |
|---|---|
| Eyes | |
| Does not open eyes | 1 |
| Opens eyes in response to painful stimuli (when given pain) | 2 |
| Opens eyes in response to voice | 3 |
| Opens eyes spontaneously | 4 |
| Verbal | |
| Makes no sound | 1 |
| Incomprehensible sounds (mumbles) | 2 |
| Utters inappropriate words | 3 |
| Confused, disorientated | 4 |
| Oriented, chats normally | 5 |
| Motor (physical reflexes) | |
| Makes no movements | 1 |
| Extension (straightens limb when given painful stimulus) | 2 |
| Abnormal flexion (flexes limbs indiscriminately when given painful stimulus) | 3 |
| Flexion/withdrawal to painful stimuli (moves away when given painful stimulus) | 4 |
| Localizes painful stimuli (can pinpoint where pain is) | 5 |
| Obeys commands | 6 |
| **Brain Injury as Classified in the Glasgow Coma Scale (Eyes + Verbal + Motor)** | |
| Coma | 3 to 8 |
| Moderate brain injury | 9 to 12 |
| Mild brain injury | 13 to 15 |

## Bibliography

### Pulmonary Diagnostic Tests

Berrizbeitia LD. The lower limit of normal in the evaluation of pulmonary function [Editorial]. Heart Lung. 2014;43:267-8. [PMID: 24856225] doi:10.1016/j.hrtlng.2014.04.011

Johnson JD, Theurer WM. A stepwise approach to the interpretation of pulmonary function tests. Am Fam Physician. 2014;89:359-66. [PMID: 24695507]

Little BP. Approach to chest computed tomography. Clin Chest Med. 2015;36:127-45, vii. [PMID: 26024596] doi:10.1016/j.ccm.2015.02.001

Murgu SD. Diagnosing and staging lung cancer involving the mediastinum. Chest. 2015;147:1401-12. [PMID: 25940251] doi:10.1378/chest.14-1355

Parreira VF, Janaudis-Ferreira T, Evans RA, Mathur S, Goldstein RS, Brooks D. Measurement properties of the incremental shuttle walk test. a systematic review. Chest. 2014;145:1357-69. [PMID: 24384555]

Pellegrino R, Viegi G, Brusasco V, Crapo RO, Burgos F, Casaburi R, et al. Interpretative strategies for lung function tests. Eur Respir J. 2005;26:948-68. [PMID: 16264058]

Singh SJ, Puhan MA, Andrianopoulos V, Hernandes NA, Mitchell KE, Hill CJ, et al. An official systematic review of the European Respiratory Society/American Thoracic Society: measurement properties of field walking tests in chronic respiratory disease [Editorial]. Eur Respir J. 2014;44:1447-78. [PMID: 25359356] doi:10.1183/09031936.00150414

### Airways Disease

Altenburg J, de Graaff CS, Stienstra Y, Sloos JH, van Haren EH, Koppers RJ, et al. Effect of azithromycin maintenance treatment on infectious exacerbations among patients with non-cystic fibrosis bronchiectasis: the BAT randomized controlled trial. JAMA. 2013;309:1251-9. [PMID: 23532241] doi:10.1001/jama.2013.1937

Bel EH, Wenzel SE, Thompson PJ, Prazma CM, Keene ON, Yancey SW, et al; SIRIUS Investigators. Oral glucocorticoid-sparing effect of mepolizumab in eosinophilic asthma. N Engl J Med. 2014;371:1189-97. [PMID: 25199060] doi:10.1056/NEJMoa1403291

Boulet LP, O'Byrne PM. Asthma and exercise-induced bronchoconstriction in athletes. N Engl J Med. 2015;372:641-8. [PMID: 25671256] doi:10.1056/NEJMra1407552

Daniels JM, Snijders D, de Graaff CS, Vlaspolder F, Jansen HM, Boersma WG. Antibiotics in addition to systemic corticosteroids for acute exacerbations of chronic obstructive pulmonary disease. Am J Respir Crit Care Med. 2010;181:150-7. [PMID: 19875685] doi:10.1164/rccm.200906-0837OC

Evensen AE. Management of COPD exacerbations. Am Fam Physician. 2010;81:607-13. [PMID: 20187597]

Fishman A, Fessler H, Martinez F, McKenna RJ Jr, Naunheim K, Piantadosi S, et al; National Emphysema Treatment Trial Research Group. Patients at high risk of death after lung-volume-reduction surgery. N Engl J Med. 2001;345:1075-83. [PMID: 11596586]

Gilljam M, Ellis L, Corey M, Zielenski J, Durie P, Tullis DE. Clinical manifestations of CF among patients with diagnosis in adulthood. Chest. 2004;126:1215-24. [PMID: 15486385]

Global Strategy for Asthma. Global Strategy for Asthma Web site. www.ginasthma.org. Accessed May 9, 2018.

Herth FJ, Gompelmann D, Ernst A, Eberhardt R. Endoscopic lung volume reduction. Respiration. 2010;79:5-13. [PMID: 19923881] doi:10.1159/000256510

Leuppi JD, Schuetz P, Bingisser R, Bodmer M, Briel M, Drescher T, et al. Short-term vs conventional glucocorticoid therapy in acute exacerbations of chronic obstructive pulmonary disease: the REDUCE randomized clinical trial. JAMA. 2013;309:2223-31. [PMID: 23695200] doi:10.1001/jama.2013.5023

Maguire G. Bronchiectasis—a guide for primary care. Aust Fam Physician. 2012;41:842-50. [PMID: 23145413]

McShane PJ, Naureckas ET, Tino G, Strek ME. Non-cystic fibrosis bronchiectasis. Am J Respir Crit Care Med. 2013;188:647-56. [PMID: 23898922] doi:10.1164/rccm.201303-0411CI

Most Recent Asthma Data. Centers for Disease Control and Prevention Web site. https://www.cdc.gov/asthma/most_recent_data.htm. Updated February 13, 2018. Accessed May 9, 2018.

Mulhall P, Criner G. Non-pharmacological treatments for COPD. Respirology. 2016;21:791-809. [PMID: 27099216] doi:10.1111/resp.12782

Ong T, Ramsey BW. Update in cystic fibrosis 2014. Am J Respir Crit Care Med. 2015;192:669-75. [PMID: 26371812] doi:10.1164/rccm.201504-0656UP

Pakhale S, Baron J, Dent R, Vandemheen K, Aaron SD. Effects of weight loss on airway responsiveness in obese adults with asthma: does weight loss lead to reversibility of asthma? Chest. 2015;147:1582-90. [PMID: 25763936] doi:10.1378/chest.14-3105

Prasad Kerlin M. In the clinic. Asthma. Ann Intern Med. 2014;160:ITC3 2-15; quiz ITC3 16-9. [PMID: 24737276] doi:10.7326/0003-4819-160-5-201403040-01003

Qaseem A, Wilt TJ, Weinberger SE, Hanania NA, Criner G, van der Molen T, et al; American College of Physicians. Diagnosis and management of stable chronic obstructive pulmonary disease: a clinical practice guideline update from the American College of Physicians, American College of Chest Physicians, American Thoracic Society, and European Respiratory Society. Ann Intern Med. 2011;155:179-91. [PMID: 21810710] doi:10.7326/0003-4819-155-3-201108020-00008

Scheinberg P, Shore E. A pilot study of the safety and efficacy of tobramycin solution for inhalation in patients with severe bronchiectasis. Chest. 2005;127:1420-6. [PMID: 15821224]

Skloot GS, Busse PJ, Braman SS, Kovacs EJ, Dixon AE, Vaz Fragoso CA, et al; ATS ad hoc Committee on Asthma in the Elderly. An official American Thoracic Society Workshop report: evaluation and management of asthma in the elderly. Ann Am Thorac Soc. 2016;13:2064-2077. [PMID: 27831798]

Tarlo SM, Lemiere C. Occupational asthma. N Engl J Med. 2014;370:640-9. [PMID: 24521110] doi:10.1056/NEJMra1301758

Teodorescu M, Broytman O, Curran-Everett D, Sorkness RL, Crisafi G, Bleecker ER, et al; National Institutes of Health, National Heart, Lung and Blood Institute Severe Asthma Research Program (SARP) investigators. Obstructive sleep apnea risk, asthma burden, and lower airway inflammation in adults in the severe asthma research program (SARP) II. J Allergy Clin Immunol Pract. 2015;3:566-75.e1. [PMID: 26004304] doi:10.1016/j.jaip.2015.04.002

The Global Strategy for the Diagnosis, Management and Prevention of COPD, Global Initiative for Chronic Obstructive Lung Disease (GOLD) 2017. Available from: goldcopd.org. Accessed May 25, 2018.

Vogelmeier CF, Criner GJ, Martinez FJ, Anzueto A, Barnes PJ, Bourbeau J, et al. Global Strategy for the Diagnosis, Management, and Prevention of Chronic Obstructive Lung Disease 2017 Report. GOLD Executive Summary. Am J Respir Crit Care Med. 2017;195:557-582. [PMID: 28128970] doi:10.1164/rccm.201701-0218PP

Wechsler ME. Getting control of uncontrolled asthma. Am J Med. 2014;127:1049-59. [PMID: 24844737] doi:10.1016/j.amjmed.2014.05.006

### Diffuse Parenchymal Lung Disease

Collard HR, Ryerson CJ, Corte TJ, Jenkins G, Kondoh Y, Lederer DJ, et al. Acute exacerbation of idiopathic pulmonary fibrosis. An international working group report. Am J Respir Crit Care Med. 2016;194:265-75. [PMID: 27299520] doi:10.1164/rccm.201604-0801CI

Fischer A, Antoniou KM, Brown KK, Cadranel J, Corte TJ, du Bois RM, et al; ERS/ATS Task Force on Undifferentiated Forms of CTD-ILD. An official European Respiratory Society/American Thoracic Society research statement: interstitial pneumonia with autoimmune features. Eur Respir J. 2015;46:976-87. [PMID: 26160873] doi:10.1183/13993003.00150-2015

Hansell DM, Bankier AA, MacMahon H, McLoud TC, Müller NL, Remy J. Fleischner Society: glossary of terms for thoracic imaging. Radiology. 2008;246:697-722. [PMID: 18195376] doi:10.1148/radiol.2462070712

Hutchinson JP, Fogarty AW, McKeever TM, Hubbard RB. In-hospital mortality after surgical lung biopsy for interstitial lung disease in the United States. 2000 to 2011. Am J Respir Crit Care Med. 2016;193:1161-7. [PMID: 26646481] doi:10.1164/rccm.201508-1632OC

Raghu G, Chen SY, Hou Q, Yeh WS, Collard HR. Incidence and prevalence of idiopathic pulmonary fibrosis in US adults 18-64 years old. Eur Respir J. 2016;48:179-86. [PMID: 27126689] doi:10.1183/13993003.01653-2015

Raghu G, Rochwerg B, Zhang Y, Garcia CA, Azuma A, Behr J, et al; American Thoracic Society. An official ATS/ERS/JRS/ALAT Clinical Practice Guideline: treatment of idiopathic pulmonary fibrosis. An update of the 2011 Clinical Practice Guideline. Am J Respir Crit Care Med. 2015;192:e3-19. [PMID: 26177183] doi:10.1164/rccm.201506-1063ST

Schwaiblmair M, Behr W, Haeckel T, Märkl B, Foerg W, Berghaus T. Drug-induced interstitial lung disease. Open Respir Med J. 2012;6:63-74. [PMID: 22896776] doi:10.2174/1874306401206010063

Tashkin DP, Elashoff R, Clements PJ, Goldin J, Roth MD, Furst DE, et al; Scleroderma Lung Study Research Group. Cyclophosphamide versus placebo in scleroderma lung disease. N Engl J Med. 2006;354:2655-66. [PMID: 16790698]

Tashkin DP, Roth MD, Clements PJ, Furst DE, Khanna D, Kleerup EC, et al; Sclerodema Lung Study II Investigators. Mycophenolate mofetil versus oral cyclophosphamide in scleroderma-related interstitial lung disease (SLS II): a randomised controlled, double-blind, parallel group trial. Lancet Respir Med. 2016;4:708-19. [PMID: 27469583] doi:10.1016/S2213-2600(16)30152-7

Travis WD, Costabel U, Hansell DM, King TE Jr, Lynch DA, Nicholson AG, et al; ATS/ERS Committee on Idiopathic Interstitial Pneumonias. An official

American Thoracic Society/European Respiratory Society statement: update of the international multidisciplinary classification of the idiopathic interstitial pneumonias. Am J Respir Crit Care Med. 2013;188:733-48. [PMID: 24032382] doi:10.1164/rccm.201308-1483ST

Weill D, Benden C, Corris PA, Dark JH, Davis RD, Keshavjee S, et al. A consensus document for the selection of lung transplant candidates: 2014–an update from the Pulmonary Transplantation Council of the International Society for Heart and Lung Transplantation. J Heart Lung Transplant. 2015;34:1-15. [PMID: 25085497] doi:10.1016/j.healun.2014.06.014

**Occupational Lung Disease**

Bacchus L, Shah RD, Chung JH, Crabtree TP, Heitkamp DE, Iannettoni MD, et al; Expert Panel on Thoracic Imaging. ACR appropriateness criteria review ACR appropriateness criteria® occupational lung diseases. J Thorac Imaging. 2016;31:W1-3. [PMID: 26656194] doi:10.1097/RTI.0000000000000194

Curti S, Sauni R, Spreeuwers D, De Schryver A, Valenty M, Rivière S, et al. Interventions to increase the reporting of occupational diseases by physicians. Cochrane Database Syst Rev. 2015:CD010305. [PMID: 25805310] doi:10.1002/14651858.CD010305.pub2

Laney AS, Weissman DN. The classic pneumoconioses: new epidemiological and laboratory observations. Clin Chest Med. 2012;33:745-58. [PMID: 23153613] doi:10.1016/j.ccm.2012.08.005

Sauler M, Gulati M. Newly recognized occupational and environmental causes of chronic terminal airways and parenchymal lung disease. Clin Chest Med. 2012;33:667-80. [PMID: 23153608] doi:10.1016/j.ccm.2012.09.002

Seaman DM, Meyer CA, Kanne JP. Occupational and environmental lung disease. Clin Chest Med. 2015;36:249-68, viii-ix. [PMID: 26024603] doi:10.1016/j.ccm.2015.02.008

**Pleural Disease**

Baumann MH, Strange C, Heffner JE, Light R, Kirby TJ, Klein J, et al; AACP Pneumothorax Consensus Group. Management of spontaneous pneumothorax: an American College of Chest Physicians Delphi consensus statement. Chest. 2001;119:590-602. [PMID: 11171742]

Bhatnagar R, Corcoran JP, Maldonado F, Feller-Kopman D, Janssen J, Astoul P, et al. Advanced medical interventions in pleural disease. Eur Respir Rev. 2016;25:199-213. [PMID: 27246597] doi:10.1183/16000617.0020-2016

Davies HE, Davies RJ, Davies CW; BTS Pleural Disease Guideline Group. Management of pleural infection in adults: British Thoracic Society Pleural Disease Guideline 2010. Thorax. 2010;65 Suppl 2:ii41-53. [PMID: 20696693] doi:10.1136/thx.2010.137000

Davies HE, Mishra EK, Kahan BC, Wrightson JM, Stanton AE, Guhan A, et al. Effect of an indwelling pleural catheter vs chest tube and talc pleurodesis for relieving dyspnea in patients with malignant pleural effusion: the TIME2 randomized controlled trial. JAMA. 2012;307:2383-9. [PMID: 22610520] doi:10.1001/jama.2012.5535

Feller-Kopman D, Light R. Pleural disease. N Engl J Med. 2018;378:740-751.

MacDuff A, Arnold A, Harvey J; BTS Pleural Disease Guideline Group. Management of spontaneous pneumothorax: British Thoracic Society Pleural Disease Guideline 2010. Thorax. 2010;65 Suppl 2:ii18-31. [PMID: 20696690] doi:10.1136/thx.2010.136986

Rahman NM, Maskell NA, West A, Teoh R, Arnold A, Mackinlay C, et al. Intrapleural use of tissue plasminogen activator and DNase in pleural infection. N Engl J Med. 2011;365:518-26. [PMID: 21830966] doi:10.1056/NEJMoa1012740

Rahman NM, Mishra EK, Davies HE, Davies RJ, Lee YC. Clinically important factors influencing the diagnostic measurement of pleural fluid pH and glucose. Am J Respir Crit Care Med. 2008;178:483-90. [PMID: 18556632] doi:10.1164/rccm.200801-062OC

Roberts ME, Neville E, Berrisford RG, Antunes G, Ali NJ; BTS Pleural Disease Guideline Group. Management of a malignant pleural effusion: British Thoracic Society Pleural Disease Guideline 2010. Thorax. 2010;65 Suppl 2:ii32-40. [PMID: 20696691] doi:10.1136/thx.2010.136994

Wilcox ME, Chong CA, Stanbrook MB, Tricco AC, Wong C, Straus SE. Does this patient have an exudative pleural effusion? The Rational Clinical Examination systematic review. JAMA. 2014;311:2422-31. [PMID: 24938565] doi:10.1001/jama.2014.5552

**Pulmonary Vascular Disease**

Galiè N, Humbert M, Vachiery JL, Gibbs S, Lang I, Torbicki A, et al; ESC Scientific Document Group. 2015 ESC/ERS Guidelines for the diagnosis and treatment of pulmonary hypertension: The Joint Task Force for the Diagnosis and Treatment of Pulmonary Hypertension of the European Society of Cardiology (ESC) and the European Respiratory Society (ERS): Endorsed by: Association for European Paediatric and Congenital Cardiology (AEPC), International Society for Heart and Lung

Transplantation (ISHLT). Eur Heart J. 2016;37:67-119. [PMID: 26320113] doi:10.1093/eurheartj/ehv317

**Lung Tumors**

Aberle DR, Adams AM, Berg CD, Black WC, Clapp JD, Fagerstrom RM, et al; National Lung Screening Trial Research Team. Reduced lung-cancer mortality with low-dose computed tomographic screening. N Engl J Med. 2011;365:395-409. [PMID: 21714641] doi:10.1056/NEJMoa1102873

Gould MK, Donington J, Lynch WR, Mazzone PJ, Midthun DE, Naidich DP, et al. Evaluation of individuals with pulmonary nodules: when is it lung cancer? Diagnosis and management of lung cancer, 3rd ed: American College of Chest Physicians evidence-based clinical practice guidelines. Chest. 2013;143:e93S-e120S. [PMID: 23649456] doi:10.1378/chest.12-2351

Husain AN, Colby T, Ordonez N, Krausz T, Attanoos R, Beasley MB, et al; International Mesothelioma Interest Group. Guidelines for pathologic diagnosis of malignant mesothelioma: 2012 update of the consensus statement from the International Mesothelioma Interest Group. Arch Pathol Lab Med. 2013;137:647-67. [PMID: 22929121] doi:10.5858/arpa.2012-0214-OA

MacMahon H, Naidich DP, Goo JM, Lee KS, Leung ANC, Mayo JR, et al. Guidelines for management of incidental pulmonary nodules detected on CT images: from the Fleischner Society 2017. Radiology. 2017;284:228-243. [PMID: 28240562] doi:10.1148/radiol.2017161659

McWilliams A, Tammemagi MC, Mayo JR, Roberts H, Liu G, Soghrati K, et al. Probability of cancer in pulmonary nodules detected on first screening CT. N Engl J Med. 2013;369:910-9. [PMID: 24004118] doi:10.1056/NEJMoa1214726

Naidich DP, Bankier AA, MacMahon H, Schaefer-Prokop CM, Pistolesi M, Goo JM, et al. Recommendations for the management of subsolid pulmonary nodules detected at CT: a statement from the Fleischner Society. Radiology. 2013;266:304-17. [PMID: 23070270] doi:10.1148/radiol.12120628

Sholl LM. Biomarkers in lung adenocarcinoma: a decade of progress. Arch Pathol Lab Med. 2015;139:469-80. [PMID: 25255293] doi:10.5858/arpa.2014-0128-RA

Silvestri GA, Gonzalez AV, Jantz MA, Margolis ML, Gould MK, Tanoue LT, et al. Methods for staging non-small cell lung cancer: Diagnosis and management of lung cancer, 3rd ed: American College of Chest Physicians evidence-based clinical practice guidelines. Chest. 2013;143:e211S-e250S. [PMID: 23649440] doi:10.1378/chest.12-2355

Strollo DC, Rosado de Christenson ML, Jett JR. Primary mediastinal tumors. Part 1: tumors of the anterior mediastinum. Chest. 1997;112:511-22. [PMID: 9266892]

Strollo DC, Rosado-de-Christenson ML, Jett JR. Primary mediastinal tumors: part II. Tumors of the middle and posterior mediastinum. Chest. 1997;112:1344-57. [PMID: 9367479]

**Sleep Medicine**

Aurora RN, Chowdhuri S, Ramar K, Bista SR, Casey KR, Lamm CI, et al. The treatment of central sleep apnea syndromes in adults: practice parameters with an evidence-based literature review and meta-analyses. Sleep. 2012;35:17-40. [PMID: 22215916] doi:10.5665/sleep.1580

Caples SM, Rowley JA, Prinsell JR, Pallanch JF, Elamin MB, Katz SG, et al. Surgical modifications of the upper airway for obstructive sleep apnea in adults: a systematic review and meta-analysis. Sleep. 2010;33:1396-407. [PMID: 21061863]

Cowie MR, Woehrle H, Wegscheider K, Angermann C, d'Ortho MP, Erdmann E, et al. Adaptive servo-ventilation for central sleep apnea in systolic heart failure. N Engl J Med. 2015;373:1095-105. [PMID: 26323938] doi:10.1056/NEJMoa1506459

Kapur VK, Auckley DH, Chowdhuri S, Kuhlmann DC, Mehra R, Ramar K, et al. Clinical practice guideline for diagnostic testing for adult obstructive sleep apnea: an American Academy of Sleep Medicine clinical practice guideline. J Clin Sleep Med. 2017;13:479-504. [PMID: 28162150] doi:10.5664/jcsm.6506

Ramar K, Dort LC, Katz SG, Lettieri CJ, Harrod CG, Thomas SM, et al. Clinical practice guideline for the treatment of obstructive sleep apnea and snoring with oral appliance therapy: an update for 2015. J Clin Sleep Med. 2015;11:773-827. [PMID: 26094920] doi:10.5664/jcsm.4858

Sack RL. Clinical practice. Jet lag. N Engl J Med. 2010;362:440-7. [PMID: 20130253] doi:10.1056/NEJMcp0909838

Xie W, Zheng F, Song X. Obstructive sleep apnea and serious adverse outcomes in patients with cardiovascular or cerebrovascular disease: a PRISMA-compliant systematic review and meta-analysis. Medicine (Baltimore). 2014;93:e336. [PMID: 25546682] doi:10.1097/MD.0000000000000336

**High-Altitude–Related Illnesses**

Ahmedzai S, Balfour-Lynn IM, Bewick T, Buchdahl R, Coker RK, Cummin AR, et al; British Thoracic Society Standards of Care Committee. Managing passengers with stable respiratory disease planning air travel: British Thoracic

Society recommendations. Thorax. 2011;66 Suppl 1:i1-30. [PMID: 21856702] doi:10.1136/thoraxjnl-2011-200295

Bärtsch P, Swenson ER. Clinical practice: acute high-altitude illnesses. N Engl J Med. 2013;368:2294-302. [PMID: 23758234] doi:10.1056/NEJMcp1214870

Hu X, Cowl CT, Baqir M, Ryu JH. Air travel and pneumothorax. Chest. 2014;145:688-694. [PMID: 24687705] doi:10.1378/chest.13-2363

Silverman D, Gendreau M. Medical issues associated with commercial flights. Lancet. 2009;373:2067-77. [PMID: 19232708] doi:10.1016/S0140-6736(09)60209-9

West JB; American College of Physicians. The physiologic basis of high-altitude diseases. Ann Intern Med. 2004;141:789-800. [PMID: 15545679]

**Principles of Critical Care**

Barr J, Fraser GL, Puntillo K, Ely EW, Gélinas C, Dasta JF, et al; American College of Critical Care Medicine. Clinical practice guidelines for the management of pain, agitation, and delirium in adult patients in the intensive care unit. Crit Care Med. 2013;41:263-306. [PMID: 23269131] doi:10.1097/CCM.0b013e3182783b72

Connolly B, O'Neill B, Salisbury L, Blackwood B; Enhanced Recovery After Critical Illness Programme Group. Physical rehabilitation interventions for adult patients during critical illness: an overview of systematic reviews. Thorax. 2016;71:881-90. [PMID: 27220357] doi:10.1136/thoraxjnl-2015-208273

Girard TD, Alhazzani W, Kress JP, Ouellette DR, Schmidt GA, Truwit JD, et al; ATS/CHEST Ad Hoc Committee on Liberation from Mechanical Ventilation in Adults. An Official American Thoracic Society/American College of Chest Physicians Clinical Practice Guideline: Liberation from Mechanical Ventilation in Critically Ill Adults. Rehabilitation Protocols, Ventilator Liberation Protocols, and Cuff Leak Tests. Am J Respir Crit Care Med. 2017;195:120-133. [PMID: 27762595] doi:10.1164/rccm.201610-2075ST

Hermans G, Van den Berghe G. Clinical review: intensive care unit acquired weakness. Crit Care. 2015;19:274. [PMID: 26242743] doi:10.1186/s13054-015-0993-7

Schweickert WD, Pohlman MC, Pohlman AS, et al: Early physical and occupational therapy in mechanically ventilated, critically ill patients: A randomised controlled trial. Lancet 2009; 373:1874–1882. PMID 19446324

Taylor BE, McClave SA, Martindale RG, Warren MM, Johnson DR, Braunschweig C, et al; Society of Critical Care Medicine. Guidelines for the Provision and Assessment of Nutrition Support Therapy in the Adult Critically Ill Patient: Society of Critical Care Medicine (SCCM) and American Society for Parenteral and Enteral Nutrition (A.S.P.E.N.). Crit Care Med. 2016;44:390-438. [PMID: 26771786] doi:10.1097/CCM.0000000000001525

**Common ICU Conditions**

Briel M, Meade M, Mercat A, Brower RG, Talmor D, Walter SD, et al. Higher vs lower positive end-expiratory pressure in patients with acute lung injury and acute respiratory distress syndrome: systematic review and meta-analysis. JAMA. 2010;303:865-73. [PMID: 20197533] doi:10.1001/jama.2010.218

Brower RG, Matthay MA, Morris A, Schoenfeld D, Thompson BT, Wheeler A; Acute Respiratory Distress Syndrome Network. Ventilation with lower tidal volumes as compared with traditional tidal volumes for acute lung injury and the acute respiratory distress syndrome. N Engl J Med. 2000;342:1301-8. [PMID: 10793162]

Fan E, Del Sorbo L, Goligher EC, Hodgson CL, Munshi L, Walkey AJ, et al; American Thoracic Society, European Society of Intensive Care Medicine, and Society of Critical Care Medicine. An official American Thoracic Society/European Society of Intensive Care Medicine/Society of Critical Care Medicine clinical practice guideline: mechanical ventilation in adult patients with acute respiratory distress syndrome. Am J Respir Crit Care Med. 2017;195:1253-1263. [PMID: 28459336] doi:10.1164/rccm.201703-0548ST

Global Strategy for the Diagnosis, Management and Prevention of COPD, Global Initiative for Chronic Obstructive Lung Disease (GOLD) 2017. http://goldcopd.org. Accessed May 25, 2018.

Guérin C, Reignier J, Richard JC, Beuret P, Gacouin A, Boulain T, et al; PROSEVA Study Group. Prone positioning in severe acute respiratory distress syndrome. N Engl J Med. 2013;368:2159-68. [PMID: 23688302] doi:10.1056/NEJMoa1214103

National Heart, Lung and Blood Institute. National Asthma Education and Prevention Program. Expert Panel Report 3: Guidelines for the Diagnosis and Management of Asthma. August 28, 2007: www.nhlbi.nih.gov/guidelines/asthma/asthgdln.pdf. Accessed May 25, 2018.

Papazian L, Forel JM, Gacouin A, Penot-Ragon C, Perrin G, Loundou A, et al; ACURASYS Study Investigators. Neuromuscular blockers in early acute respiratory distress syndrome. N Engl J Med. 2010;363:1107-16. [PMID: 20843245] doi:10.1056/NEJMoa1005372

Ranieri VM, Rubenfeld GD, Thompson BT, Ferguson ND, Caldwell E, Fan E, et al; ARDS Definition Task Force. Acute respiratory distress syndrome: the berlin definition. JAMA. 2012;307:2526-33. [PMID: 22797452] doi:10.1001/jama.2012.5669

Rhodes A, Evans LE, Alhazzani W, Levy MM, Antonelli M, Ferrer R, et al. Surviving sepsis campaign: international guidelines for management of sepsis and septic shock: 2016. Crit Care Med. 2017;45:486-552. [PMID: 28098591] doi:10.1097/CCM.0000000000002255

Singer M, Deutschman CS, Seymour CW, Shankar-Hari M, Annane D, Bauer M, et al. The third international consensus definitions for sepsis and septic shock (Sepsis-3). JAMA. 2016;315:801-10. [PMID: 26903338] doi:10.1001/jama.2016.0287

Wiedemann HP, Wheeler AP, Bernard GR, Thompson BT, Hayden D, deBoisblanc B, et al; National Heart, Lung, and Blood Institute Acute Respiratory Distress Syndrome (ARDS) Clinical Trials Network. Comparison of two fluid-management strategies in acute lung injury. N Engl J Med. 2006; 354:2564-75. [PMID: 16714767]

**Specific Critical Care Topics**

Brooks DE, Levine M, O'Connor AD, French RNE, Curry SC. Toxicology in the ICU: part 2: specific toxins. Chest. 2011;140:1072-1085. [PMID: 21972388] doi:10.1378/chest.10-2726

Elmer J, Callaway CW. The brain after cardiac arrest. Semin Neurol. 2017;37:19-24. [PMID: 28147414] doi:10.1055/s-0036-1597833

Leon LR, Bouchama A. Heat stroke. Compr Physiol. 2015;5:611-47. [PMID: 25880507] doi:10.1002/cphy.c140017

Levine M, Brooks DE, Truitt CA, Wolk BJ, Boyer EW, Ruha AM. Toxicology in the ICU: Part 1: general overview and approach to treatment. Chest. 2011;140:795-806. [PMID: 21896525] doi:10.1378/chest.10-2548

Lieberman PL. Recognition and first-line treatment of anaphylaxis. Am J Med. 2014;127:S6-11. [PMID: 24384138] doi:10.1016/j.amjmed.2013.09.008

Rainer C, Scheinost NA, Lefeber EJ. Neuroleptic malignant syndrome. When levodopa withdrawal is the cause. Postgrad Med. 1991;89:175-8, 180. [PMID: 2008397]

Whelton PK, Carey RM, Aronow WS, Casey DE Jr, Collins KJ, Dennison Himmelfarb C, et al. 2017 ACC/AHA/AAPA/ABC/ACPM/AGS/APhA/ASH/ASPC/NMA/PCNA guideline for the prevention, detection, evaluation, and management of high blood pressure in adults: executive summary: A report of the American College of Cardiology/American Heart Association task force on clinical practice guidelines. Hypertension. 2018;71:1269-1324. [PMID: 29133354] doi:10.1161/HYP.0000000000000066

# Pulmonary and Critical Care Medicine Self-Assessment Test

This self-assessment test contains one-best-answer multiple-choice questions. Please read these directions carefully before answering the questions. Answers, critiques, and bibliographies immediately follow these multiple-choice questions. The American College of Physicians (ACP) is accredited by the Accreditation Council for Continuing Medical Education (ACCME) to provide continuing medical education for physicians.

The American College of Physicians designates MKSAP 18 Pulmonary and Critical Care Medicine for a maximum of 25 *AMA PRA Category 1 Credits*™. Physicians should claim only the credit commensurate with the extent of their participation in the activity.

Successful completion of the CME activity, which includes participation in the evaluation component, enables the participant to earn up to 25 medical knowledge MOC points in the American Board of Internal Medicine's Maintenance of Certification (MOC) program. It is the CME activity provider's responsibility to submit participant completion information to ACCME for the purpose of granting MOC credit.

## *Earn Instantaneous CME Credits or MOC Points Online*

Print subscribers can enter their answers online to earn instantaneous CME credits or MOC points. You can submit your answers using online answer sheets that are provided at mksap.acponline.org, where a record of your MKSAP 18 credits will be available. To earn CME credits or to apply for MOC points, you need to answer all of the questions in a test and earn a score of at least 50% correct (number of correct answers divided by the total number of questions). Please note that if you are applying for MOC points, you must also enter your birth date and ABIM candidate number. Take either of the following approaches:

- Use the printed answer sheet at the back of this book to record your answers. Go to mksap.acponline.org, access the appropriate online answer sheet, transcribe your answers, and submit your test for instantaneous CME credits or MOC points. There is no additional fee for this service.

- Go to mksap.acponline.org, access the appropriate online answer sheet, directly enter your answers, and submit your test for instantaneous CME credits or MOC points. There is no additional fee for this service.

## *Earn CME Credits or MOC Points by Mail or Fax*

Pay a $20 processing fee per answer sheet and submit the printed answer sheet at the back of this book by mail or fax, as instructed on the answer sheet. Make sure you calculate your score and enter your birth date and ABIM candidate number, and fax the answer sheet to 215-351-2799 or mail the answer sheet to Member and Customer Service, American College of Physicians, 190 N. Independence Mall West, Philadelphia, PA 19106-1572, using the courtesy envelope provided in your MKSAP 18 slipcase. You will need your 10-digit order number and 8-digit ACP ID number, which are printed on your packing slip. Please allow 4 to 6 weeks for your score report to be emailed back to you. Be sure to include your email address for a response.

If you do not have a 10-digit order number and 8-digit ACP ID number, or if you need help creating a username and password to access the MKSAP 18 online answer sheets, go to mksap.acponline.org or email custserv@acponline.org.

CME credits and MOC points are available from the publication date of December 31, 2018, until December 31, 2021. You may submit your answer sheet or enter your answers online at any time during this period.

## Directions

*Each of the numbered items is followed by lettered answers. Select the ONE lettered answer that is BEST in each case.*

## Item 1

A 52-year-old woman is evaluated in the emergency department for wheezing, dyspnea, and cough productive of clear sputum, which have worsened during the past 3 days despite use of her albuterol inhaler up to four times daily. She has no environmental triggers or recent respiratory infection. She smokes two packs of cigarettes per day and is unable to quit. History is notable for anxiety and a 20-year history of asthma. She has had two exacerbations in the past year and was hospitalized and briefly intubated for one of them. Her prescription for budesonide/formoterol controller inhaler ran out 2 weeks ago, and she has been unable to refill it. Other medications are albuterol, montelukast, and alprazolam.

On physical examination, temperature is 37.0 °C (98.6 °F), blood pressure is 140/82 mm Hg, pulse rate is 140/min, and respiration rate is 32/min with increased work of breathing. Oxygen saturation is 89% breathing ambient air. Chest examination demonstrates poor air movement with faint expiratory wheezing. The remainder of the examination is normal.

Chest radiograph demonstrates hyperinflation without infiltrates.

Albuterol improves her symptoms.

**Which of the following is the most appropriate management?**

(A) Admit patient to the hospital for inpatient management
(B) Begin prednisone and schedule outpatient follow-up
(C) Refill patient's prescription for budesonide/formoterol and schedule outpatient follow-up
(D) Refill patient's prescription for budesonide/formoterol, begin prednisone, and schedule outpatient follow-up

## Item 2

A 37-year-old man is evaluated for a 1-month history of worsening cough and wheezing requiring use of rescue therapy several times per week, as well as increasing nasal congestion and rhinorrhea. He has a history of moderate persistent asthma and rhinitis since his early twenties. One month ago the patient underwent repair of a traumatic anterior cruciate ligament tear and has some residual daily knee pain. His medical history is notable for sinusitis. He has no symptoms of gastroesophageal reflux disease. Medications are albuterol, budesonide/formoterol, and ibuprofen.

On physical examination, vital signs are normal. Oxygen saturation is 97% breathing ambient air. Examination demonstrates conjunctival injection and nasal polyps in both nostrils. Chest examination reveals wheezing on expiration. The remainder of the examination is noncontributory.

Laboratory studies reveal IgE is 265 U/mL (265 kU/L). Complete blood count reveals a leukocyte count of 4000/μL ($4 \times 10^9$/L) with 10% eosinophils.

Office spirometry demonstrates moderate airflow obstruction.

**Which of the following is the most appropriate initial management?**

(A) 24-Hour esophageal pH monitoring
(B) Add montelukast
(C) Discontinue ibuprofen, begin prednisone
(D) Nasal polypectomy

## Item 3

A 69-year-old man is evaluated for a 3-year history of dyspnea and chronic productive cough. He was diagnosed with COPD 2 years ago after spirometry confirmed severe airflow obstruction. He discontinued smoking at that time but in the past year he was treated for three COPD exacerbations, one requiring hospitalization. Medications are tiotropium, fluticasone/salmeterol, and albuterol inhalers.

On physical examination, vital signs are normal; oxygen saturation is 92% on ambient air. He intermittently coughs during the examination. He has a prolonged expiratory phase. The remainder of the examination is unremarkable.

Chest radiograph shows the lungs to be clear.

Spirometry demonstrates a postbronchodilator $FEV_1$ of 45% of predicted.

**Which of the following long-term treatments is most likely to reduce this patient's exacerbations of COPD?**

(A) Prednisone
(B) Roflumilast
(C) Theophylline
(D) Trimethoprim-sulfamethoxazole

## Item 4

A 57-year-old man is evaluated for a 6-month history of daytime sleepiness. His wife complains of his loud snoring and has observed breathing pauses; he sometimes awakens with a gasp. He has nocturia twice per night. He takes no medications.

On physical examination, vital signs are normal. Oxygen saturation is 96% breathing ambient air. BMI is 33. He has a crowded oropharynx with a low-lying soft palate; his neck is 46 cm (18 in) in circumference; he has trace edema at the ankles. Cardiovascular and neurologic examinations are normal.

**Which of the following is the most appropriate management?**

(A) Auto-adjusting positive airway pressure
(B) Home sleep testing
(C) Multiple sleep latency testing
(D) Overnight pulse oximetry

## Item 5

A 72-year-old man is evaluated during a follow-up visit. He was evaluated in the emergency department 2 weeks ago for the sudden onset of chest pain. A CT scan was negative for pulmonary embolism but demonstrated an 8-mm ground-glass nodule in the right upper lobe. He has had no recurrence of chest pain. His history is significant for hypertension treated with lisinopril.

Upon physical examination, vital signs are normal. The remainder of the physical examination is normal. The patient undergoes follow-up CT scans of his lung at 12 months and also at 2 years. The nodule is unchanged.

**Which of the following is the most appropriate management of the lung nodule?**

(A) Chest CT scans every 2 years for 5 years
(B) PET/CT scan
(C) Tissue sampling
(D) No further follow-up is needed

## Item 6

A 72-year-old man is hospitalized for progressive dyspnea and cough following a sore throat 3 weeks ago. Medical history is significant for idiopathic pulmonary fibrosis diagnosed 4 years ago that required 2 L/min of oxygen at rest. He is disabled because of his lung disease and is homebound. His only medication is pirfenidone.

On physical examination, blood pressure is 150/95 mm Hg, pulse rate is 105/min, and respiration rate is 28/min. Oxygen saturation is 89% on 6 L/min of oxygen. Lung examination demonstrates diffuse inspiratory crackles in all zones that are worse at the bases. He has clubbing and trace edema but no jugular venous distention.

Bronchoalveolar lavage is positive only for rhinovirus. B-type natriuretic peptide is 20 pg/mL.

High-resolution CT scan with contrast demonstrates new bilateral ground-glass opacities on a background of basal-predominant septal line thickening with traction bronchiectasis and honeycomb changes. CT angiography demonstrates no evidence of pulmonary embolism.

**Which of the following is the most likely diagnosis?**

(A) Acute exacerbation of idiopathic pulmonary fibrosis
(B) Acute heart failure
(C) Acute hypersensitivity pneumonitis
(D) Nonspecific interstitial pneumonia

## Item 7

A 32-year-old man is evaluated in the hospital for symptoms of persistent asthma. He was evaluated in the emergency department 2 days ago for dyspnea accompanied by wheezing, dysphonia, and upper chest and throat tightness. Symptoms persisted despite use of albuterol inhaler every 3 to 4 hours and intravenous methylprednisolone, and he was hospitalized. He was diagnosed with asthma in high school and generally requires several courses of prednisone per year. Current medications are albuterol and fluticasone/salmeterol inhalers, prednisone, and montelukast.

On physical examination, blood pressure is 130/85 mm Hg, pulse rate is 110/min, and respiration rate is 18/min. Oxygen saturation is 100% on 2 L/min of oxygen through nasal cannula. BMI is 25. Chest examination demonstrates monophonic wheezing on inspiration.

Laboratory studies, including complete blood count, metabolic panel, and IgE, are normal.

Chest radiograph is clear and bedside spirometry is normal.

**Which of the following is the most appropriate management?**

(A) CT scan of the sinuses
(B) Increase prednisone dosage
(C) Laryngoscopy
(D) Polysomnography

## Item 8

A 56-year-old man hospitalized for respiratory failure is evaluated for new-onset confusion. He has acute respiratory distress syndrome secondary to community-acquired pneumonia. He has been in the critical care unit for 3 days. He is orally intubated and placed on mechanical ventilation. Current medications are ceftriaxone, azithromycin, and propofol for light sedation according to protocol.

On physical examination, temperature is 38.3 °C (100.9 °F), blood pressure is 100/45 mm Hg, pulse rate is 112/min, and respiration rate is 24/min. He cannot focus his attention, does not follow simple commands, and has demonstrated fluctuating mental status during the past 8 hours. The neurological examination is otherwise normal. He appears to be comfortable and shows no signs of pain.

Arterial blood gas studies show a pH of 7.41, a $P_{CO_2}$ of 38 mm Hg (5.1 kPa), and a $P_{O_2}$ of 62 mm Hg (8.2 kPa). Serum sodium, serum creatinine, and blood urea nitrogen are normal.

Chest radiograph shows multifocal opacities consistent with pneumonia and acute respiratory distress syndrome.

**In addition to orientation strategies and promoting a normal sleep-wake cycle, which of the following is the most appropriate management?**

(A) Add haloperidol
(B) Add lorazepam
(C) Early mobilization
(D) Increase propofol

## Item 9

A 62-year-old man is evaluated during a general medical exam. He is a current smoker with a 42-pack-year history. He has a chronic cough but no shortness of breath or chronic health conditions.

On physical examination, vital signs and the remainder of the physical examination are normal.

**Which of the following interventions is most likely to improve this patient's long-term survival?**

(A) Annual chest radiograph
(B) Annual low-dose CT scan
(C) Annual sputum cytology
(D) Smoking cessation

## Item 10

A 56-year-old man is hospitalized for hematemesis. He vomited 300 mL of bright red blood 15 minutes ago. He has a history of heavy alcohol use and cirrhosis. He takes no medications.

On physical examination, blood pressure is 99/50 mm Hg, pulse rate is 110/min, and respiration rate is 25/min. Oxygen saturation is 93% breathing ambient air. He is only responsive to painful stimuli. He is jaundiced. His breathing is shallow but without accessory muscle use. Lung examination reveals rhonchi. There are telangiectasias on his chest. Ascites is present. The remainder of the examination is unremarkable.

Laboratory studies reveal a hemoglobin level of 8 g/dL (80 g/L), total bilirubin of 6.8 mg/dL (116.3 µmol/L), aspartate aminotransferase of 154 U/L, and alanine aminotransferase of 54 U/L.

Two large-bore intravenous lines have been placed and crystalloid resuscitation has been initiated.

**Which of the following should be done next?**

(A) Administer a nonselective β-blocker
(B) Administer oxygen by nasal cannula
(C) Emergency upper endoscopy
(D) Initiate noninvasive bilevel positive airway pressure
(E) Insert an endotracheal tube

## Item 11

A 30-year-old man presents for a refill on his albuterol inhaler. In the past he only needed albuterol once or twice a month, generally related to exercise. Over the last 4 to 5 months, he has noted that he needs his albuterol inhaler at least 3 or 4 times weekly for symptoms not associated with exercise. There are no apparent environmental triggers, symptoms of reflux, sinus symptoms, or recent respiratory infections. His medical and family history is otherwise unremarkable.

On physical examination, vital signs are normal. Oxygen saturation is 97% breathing ambient air. He has expiratory wheezing. Cardiac examination is normal.

Laboratory studies, including complete blood count and IgE level, are normal.

On spirometry FEV$_1$ is 82% of predicted and improves significantly following inhaled albuterol. His inhaler technique is excellent.

**Which of the following is the most appropriate treatment?**

(A) Beclomethasone
(B) Fluticasone/salmeterol
(C) Ipratropium
(D) Montelukast

## Item 12

A 72-year-old man is evaluated for nonproductive cough and progressively worsening dyspnea on exertion during the past year. He has no history of dry eyes, dry mouth, Raynaud phenomenon, arthralgia, myalgia, or arthritis. He has a 30-pack-year smoking history and quit 15 years ago.

Currently retired, he worked as a car insurance adjustor and reports no environmental exposures.

On physical examination, vital signs are normal. Oxygen saturation is 95% breathing ambient air. Findings on lung examination include late velcro inspiratory crackles at the bases. Bilateral clubbing is present. The remainder of the physical examination is normal.

Spirometry shows an FVC of 82% of predicted, an FEV$_1$ of 90% of predicted, an FEV$_1$/FVC ratio of 0.85, and a D$_{LCO}$ of 65% of predicted.

Chest radiograph shows an increase in reticular markings at the lung bases. High-resolution CT scan shows bilateral peripheral and basal predominant septal line thickening with honeycombing at the bases.

**Which of the following is the most likely diagnosis?**

(A) Desquamative interstitial pneumonia
(B) Hypersensitivity pneumonitis
(C) Idiopathic pulmonary fibrosis
(D) Pulmonary Langerhans cell histiocytosis
(E) Respiratory bronchiolitis–associated interstitial lung disease

## Item 13

A 38-year-old woman is evaluated for 24 hours of fever, myalgia, and confusion. She returned from a camping trip in the woods 5 days ago.

On physical examination, temperature is 39.0 °C (102.2 °F), blood pressure is 80/34 mm Hg, pulse rate is 125/min, and respiration rate is 24/min. Oxygen saturation is 95% breathing ambient air. She has right axillary lymphadenopathy. She is confused. The skin is warm and dry. Her right hand is erythematous and has a wound with purulent drainage. Lung examination reveals scattered basilar crackles. Cardiac examination shows no gallops, murmurs, or jugular venous distention. The remainder of the physical examination is noncontributory.

**Which of the following is required to assess this patient's intravascular volume status before fluid administration?**

(A) Central venous catheter measure of venous pressure
(B) Inferior vena cava collapsibility on echocardiography
(C) Pulmonary artery catheter measurements
(D) Pulse pressure variation
(E) No additional testing

## Item 14

A 67-year-old man is evaluated in the emergency department with a 3-day history of weakness and nausea and a 2-week history of difficulty swallowing. He has lost 22.7 kg (50 lb) during the past year. He has no other symptoms. History is significant for a 30-pack-year history of smoking. He quit smoking 4 years ago. He takes no medications.

On physical examination, vital signs are normal. Lung examination reveals decreased tactile fremitus above the lower portion of the right lung as well as dullness to percussion and decreased breath sounds. His neurologic examination is normal.

Laboratory studies reveal a serum sodium concentration of 127 mEq/L (127 mmol/L).

A chest CT scan is shown.

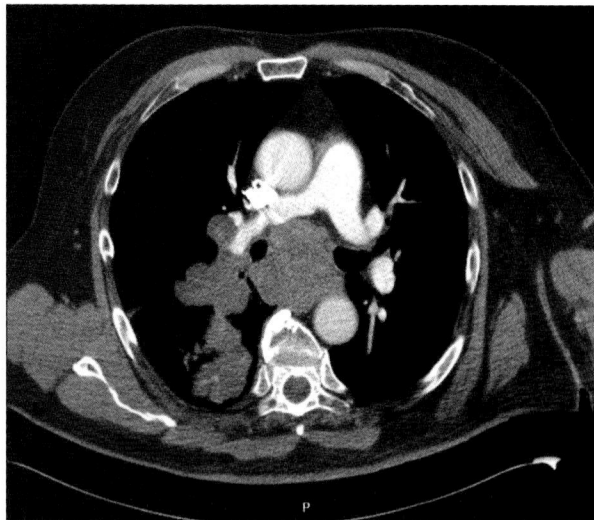

**Which of the following is the most likely diagnosis?**

(A) Adenocarcinoma of the lung

(B) Malignant pleural mesothelioma

(C) Small cell lung cancer

(D) Squamous cell carcinoma of the lung

## Item 15

A 62-year-old woman is evaluated in the emergency department for worsening dyspnea on exertion during the last 2 weeks. She has a history of severe COPD and an $FEV_1$ of 45% of predicted. She has a cough productive of yellow sputum and wheezing during the same time period. She has a 20-pack-year history of smoking but quit 10 years ago. Her albuterol inhaler and nebulizer have provided temporary relief at home. Current medications are umeclidinium/vilanterol, mometasone, and albuterol.

On physical examination, temperature is normal, blood pressure is 132/64 mm Hg, pulse rate is 110/min, and respiration rate is 30/min. Oxygen saturation is 90% on 6 L/min of oxygen by nasal cannula. Cardiopulmonary examination reveals tachycardia, tachypnea with accessory muscle use, and decreased breath sounds throughout with a prolonged expiratory phase and end expiratory wheezes. She has no jugular venous distention or edema.

Laboratory studies reveal an arterial $P_{CO_2}$ of 46 mm Hg (6.11 kPa). Complete blood count, serum electrolytes, and blood glucose are normal.

A chest radiograph shows hyperinflated lungs with flattening of the diaphragms but no infiltrate.

**Which of the following is the most appropriate next additional test?**

(A) CT pulmonary angiogram

(B) Electrocardiogram

(C) Sputum culture

(D) Sputum Gram stain

## Item 16

A 62-year-old man is evaluated for sleep apnea. He was recently hospitalized for atrial fibrillation with rapid ventricular rate. He sleeps 8 hours most nights but awakens feeling unrested. He is likely to doze off during the day while watching TV and reading the newspaper. He has hypertension and type 2 diabetes mellitus. Current medications are apixaban, lisinopril, metoprolol, and metformin.

On physical examination, blood pressure is 154/90 mm Hg and pulse rate is 82/min. Oxygen saturation is 98% breathing ambient air. BMI is 29. He has a low-lying soft palate, prominent tongue base, and an irregular heart rhythm. Cardiac examination reveals an irregular rhythm and variable intensity of $S_1$. There are no findings of heart failure.

Polysomnography demonstrates moderate obstructive sleep apnea (apnea–hypopnea index 18/hour).

Hemoglobin $A_{1c}$ measurement is 7.5%.

**Which of the patient's conditions is the strongest indication for positive airway pressure therapy?**

(A) Atrial fibrillation

(B) Diabetes

(C) Excessive daytime sleepiness

(D) Hypertension

## Item 17

A 39-year-old man with obesity hypoventilation syndrome is hospitalized for hypoxemia and altered mental status. Three hours ago he was placed on bilevel positive airway pressure (BPAP) with 50% oxygen. History is significant for obesity, diabetes, and obesity hypoventilation syndrome for which he is receiving home nocturnal BPAP ventilation and metformin. He has been unsuccessful in losing weight with diet and medications; he is being evaluated for bariatric surgery.

On physical examination, blood pressure is 150/78 mm Hg, pulse rate is 90/min, and respiration rate is 16/min. BMI is 42. Oxygen saturation is 96% on 50% oxygen. His respirations are shallow without wheezing. He is somnolent but awakens to light touch. He has an intact cough and gag reflex.

Chest radiograph shows small lung volumes, normal heart, and normal vascularization of the lung parenchyma.

**Arterial blood gas studies on BPAP and 50% oxygen:**

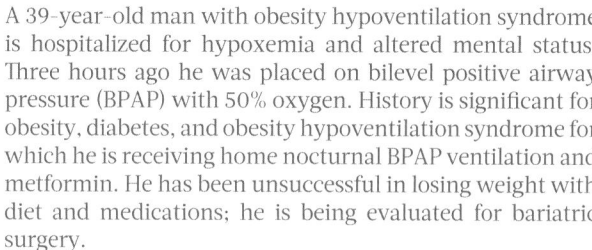

|  | 3 Hours Ago | Now |
|---|---|---|
| Bicarbonate | 29 mEq/L (29 mmol/L) | 28 mEq/L (28 mmol/L) |
| pH | 7.21 | 7.17 |
| $P_{O_2}$ | 114 mm Hg (15.1 kPa) | 108 mm Hg (14.4 kPa) |
| $P_{CO_2}$ | 74 mm Hg (9.8 kPa) | 80 mm Hg (10.6 kPa) |

**Which of the following is the most appropriate treatment?**

(A) Acetazolamide

(B) Endotracheal intubation

(C) Prednisone

(D) Theophylline

## Item 18

A 42-year-old man is evaluated in the office for follow-up of progressive dyspnea of 2 years' duration. He first noted dyspnea with exercise but now has symptoms when walking up a flight of stairs. He has intermittent wheezing but no coughing or nocturnal respiratory symptoms. At the time of his initial evaluation 2 years ago, pulmonary function tests demonstrated moderate airflow obstruction. He has a 1-pack-year smoking history but has not smoked in 20 years. He has no environmental exposures. His father and uncle both have emphysema without a history of smoking. He takes no medications.

On physical examination, vital signs are normal. Oxygen saturation is 94% breathing ambient air. Examination reveals no clubbing or jugular venous distention, extra cardiac sounds, edema, pulmonary crackles, or wheezing.

A chest radiograph shows hyperinflation and diaphragmatic flattening.

**Which of the following is the most appropriate test to perform next?**

(A) $\alpha_1$-Antitrypsin level
(B) Exhaled nitric oxide test
(C) High-resolution CT scan of the chest
(D) Vascular endothelial growth factor-D

## Item 19

A 46-year-old man is evaluated for problems with auto-adjusting positive airway pressure therapy that was prescribed 3 weeks ago for severe obstructive sleep apnea. He awakens with a sore throat, nasal congestion, and an occasional headache. Download from the device shows a residual apnea-hypopnea index of 3, which correlates with a decrease in his daytime sleepiness.

On physical examination, vital signs are normal. BMI is 33. He has a crowded oropharynx; low-hanging soft palate; 1+ tonsils; and boggy, erythematous nasal mucosa.

**Which of the following is the most appropriate treatment?**

(A) Bilevel positive airway pressure
(B) Eszopiclone
(C) Heated humidification
(D) Nasal fluticasone spray

## Item 20

A 49-year-old woman is evaluated in the office following a recent hospitalization for an asthma exacerbation. Her symptoms have improved but she continues to have dyspnea and intermittent wheezing. She has had two other hospitalizations within the past year for asthma exacerbations despite the chronic use of oral glucocorticoids. Other than a 3-year history of asthma, her medical history is unremarkable. Medications are mometasone/formoterol, montelukast, albuterol, tiotropium, and prednisone.

On physical examination, vital signs are normal. Oxygen saturation is 95% on ambient air. Pulmonary examination reveals expiratory wheezes with good air movement. The remainder of the physical examination is unremarkable.

Laboratory studies reveal leukocyte count of 10,000/µL (10 × 10⁹/L) with 650 eosinophils/µL (0.65 × 10⁹/L). Serum IgE level is 12 U/mL (12 kU/L) (normal range, 0-90 U/mL [0-90 kU/L]).

$FEV_1$ is 56% of predicted.
Chest radiograph is normal.

**Which of the following is the most appropriate treatment?**

(A) Begin doxycycline
(B) Change mometasone/formoterol to fluticasone/salmeterol
(C) Initiate a trial of mepolizumab therapy
(D) Initiate a trial of omalizumab therapy

## Item 21

A 79-year-old woman is brought into the emergency department after she was found unconscious in her apartment by a neighbor. She had been using a propane-fueled heater to heat her small apartment. No other medical history is available.

On physical examination, blood pressure is 100/64 mm Hg, pulse rate is 70/min, and respiration rate is 16/min. Pulse oximetry shows 100% oxygen saturation on mechanical ventilation using 50% oxygen. She is unresponsive to pain or voice but has intact normal deep tendon and brainstem reflexes.

Co-oximetry shows a carboxyhemoglobin level of 50%. CT scan of the head shows no acute changes.

**Which of the following is the most appropriate treatment?**

(A) Continue current management
(B) Decrease oxygen to 30%
(C) Hydroxocobalamin administration
(D) Hyperbaric oxygen therapy

## Item 22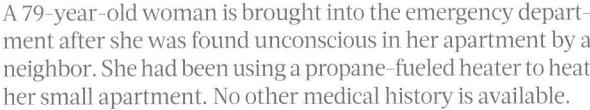

A 55-year-old man with COPD is evaluated in the emergency department for worsening dyspnea. He was doing well until 3 days ago when he developed fever, myalgia, increased cough productive of yellow sputum, and progressive dyspnea. He has no headaches, hypersomnolence, tremors, or extremity edema. Pulmonary function tests obtained 4 months ago demonstrated severe obstruction with air trapping. Current medications are albuterol and umeclidinium/vilanterol.

On physical examination, temperature is 38.2 °C (100.9 °F), blood pressure is 142/82 mm Hg, pulse rate is 94/min, and respiration rate is 18/min. Oxygen saturation is 90% breathing ambient air. He has end-expiratory wheezing throughout. There is no jugular venous distention or extra cardiac sounds.

A complete blood count and comprehensive metabolic profile are normal.

Other than tachycardia, an electrocardiogram is normal. Chest radiograph shows the lungs to be clear.

Therapy for a COPD exacerbation is initiated.

**Which of the following is the most appropriate next diagnostic test?**

(A) Arterial blood gas analysis
(B) B-type natriuretic peptide measurement
(C) CT pulmonary angiography
(D) Echocardiogram

## Item 23

A 35-year-old woman is evaluated for a 4-month history of exertional dyspnea and a 1-week history of chest pressure. She has no sputum production, cough, or wheezes. She has never smoked.

On physical examination, vital signs are normal. Oxygen saturation is 91% breathing ambient air. Cardiopulmonary examination reveals a widened split $S_2$ with a prominent pulmonic component and neck vein distention. Lungs are clear to auscultation.

Laboratory studies, including complete blood count and comprehensive metabolic profile, are normal.

Electrocardiogram is normal.

Chest radiograph shows clear lung fields and prominent hilae.

**Which of the following is the most appropriate initial test?**

(A) High resolution CT of the chest
(B) Pulmonary function testing
(C) Transthoracic echocardiogram
(D) Ventilation-perfusion ($\dot{V}/\dot{Q}$) scan

## Item 24

A 58-year-old man is evaluated for follow-up of an asthma exacerbation with no clear trigger, which improved with oral glucocorticoids and a short-acting $\beta_2$-agonist in addition to his outpatient medications. The patient has a 30-year history of asthma and has had two previous exacerbations during the preceding 12 months. He has no environmental triggers, allergies, atopy, symptoms of reflux, sinus symptoms, snoring, or recent respiratory infections. A recent sleep study was negative for obstructive sleep apnea. Medications are albuterol, budesonide/formoterol, montelukast, tiotropium, and prednisone.

On physical examination, vital signs are normal. Oxygen saturation is 97% breathing ambient air. BMI is 36. Pulmonary examination reveals scattered expiratory wheezing. Cardiac examination is normal.

Bedside spirometry demonstrates moderate airflow obstruction; $FEV_1$ improves by 15% following inhaled albuterol.

Laboratory studies, including IgE level and complete blood count, are normal.

CT scan of the sinuses is normal.

**Which of the following is the most appropriate management?**

(A) Add beclomethasone
(B) Perform methacholine challenge testing
(C) Start mepolizumab
(D) Start omalizumab
(E) Supervised weight loss program

## Item 25

A 71-year-old man is evaluated during a follow-up visit for sleep-related breathing pauses observed by the hospital staff when he was admitted for implantation of a cardioverter-defibrillator for ischemic cardiomyopathy (left ventricular ejection fraction of 30%). He has recently experienced dyspnea, a few episodes of which have awakened him from sleep. He has no insomnia or daytime sleepiness. He has dyslipidemia, stable coronary artery disease, and hypertension. Current medications are aspirin, atorvastatin, valsartan, metoprolol, and nitroglycerin as needed.

On physical examination, vital signs are normal. Oxygen saturation is 93% breathing ambient air. BMI is 23. Lung examination reveals bibasilar crackles, faint end-expiratory wheezing, neck vein distention, and 1+ ankle edema.

Polysomnography demonstrates central sleep apnea with a Cheyne-Stokes breathing pattern.

**Which of the following is the most appropriate treatment of the patient's central sleep apnea?**

(A) Adaptive servo-ventilation
(B) Auto-adjusting positive airway pressure
(C) Furosemide
(D) Supplemental oxygen

## Item 26

A 60-year-old woman is evaluated during a follow-up visit. She has a lifelong history of intermittent asthma previously provoked by exertion and exposure to cold air. During the past 2 years her symptoms have progressed, and she now has dyspnea after walking one block or going up any incline. COPD was diagnosed 4 days ago after spirometry revealed an $FEV_1$ of 65% of predicted that was only partially reversible with bronchodilator therapy. She has no history of acute exacerbations. She has recently discontinued cigarette smoking. She currently takes albuterol as needed.

On physical examination, vital signs are normal; oxygen saturation is 95% breathing ambient air. Lungs are clear to auscultation.

Laboratory studies reveal normal hemoglobin concentration and leukocyte count with 8% eosinophils.

Chest radiograph shows clear lungs.

**Which of the following is the most appropriate initial treatment?**

(A) Chronic macrolide therapy
(B) Inhaled glucocorticoid and long-acting $\beta_2$-agonist
(C) Long-acting $\beta_2$-agonists
(D) Long-acting muscarinic agent and long-acting $\beta_2$-agonists

## Item 27

A 68-year-old man develops abrupt, pleuritic, right-sided chest pain, and dyspnea 90 minutes into a flight from Nashville to Phoenix. He is on the second week of a prednisone taper for a recent COPD exacerbation in the setting of bullous emphysema. He is on supplemental oxygen at home at 2 L/min, which was augmented to 4 L/min for the flight. Current medications are a long-acting $\beta_2$-agonist, a long-acting muscarinic agent, and prednisone.

On physical examination, blood pressure is 138/78 mm Hg, pulse rate is 114/min, and respiration rate is 24/min. He appears moderately distressed. Lung examination reveals diminished breath sounds bilaterally, tympany to percussion bilaterally, and end-expiratory wheezing. He has strong symmetric peripheral pulses but no neck vein distention. Cardiac examination is unremarkable.

**Which of the following is the most likely diagnosis?**

(A) Descending aortic dissection
(B) *Pneumocystis jirovecii* pneumonia
(C) Pneumothorax
(D) Pulmonary embolism

## Item 28

A 58-year-old man with a history of severe COPD is evaluated for his chronic exertional dyspnea. He is taking his inhalers and medications as prescribed with excellent technique and has completed a pulmonary rehabilitation program within the last 6 months and is continuing his exercise program. He is using supplemental oxygen but despite adequate oxygenation still has significant exertional dyspnea. Current medications are umeclidinium/vilanterol, mometasone, and albuterol. He feels that his current quality of life is poor and would like other treatment options.

On physical examination, vital signs are normal. Oxygen saturation is 90% on 2 L/min of oxygen. BMI is normal. Pulmonary examination reveals decreased breath sounds throughout with a prolonged expiratory phase but no wheezing.

Spirometry demonstrates severe airflow obstruction. A recent chest CT shows heterogeneous emphysema without any nodules. A recent echocardiogram shows diastolic dysfunction but no evidence of pulmonary hypertension.

**Which of the following is the most appropriate management?**

(A) Add daily roflumilast
(B) Evaluation for lung volume reduction surgery
(C) Obtain a right heart catheterization
(D) Repeat pulmonary rehabilitation program

## Item 29

A 58-year-old man is evaluated for a 2-year history of slowly progressive exertional dyspnea with intermittent wheezing and a cough that is occasionally productive of clear sputum. He has no chest pain, palpitations, or lower extremity edema. He has a 40-pack-year history of smoking but quit 3 years ago. He has a history of coronary artery disease. He currently takes aspirin, metoprolol, rosuvastatin, and lisinopril.

On physical examination, vital signs are normal; oxygen saturation is 94% on ambient air. Pulmonary examination reveals a prolonged expiratory phase. The remainder of the physical examination is normal.

Chest radiograph shows the lungs to be clear. Electrocardiogram is normal.

**Which of the following is the most appropriate test to perform next?**

(A) Echocardiogram
(B) Exercise stress test
(C) High-resolution chest CT
(D) Spirometry

## Item 30

A 78-year-old woman is evaluated in the hospital for progressive dyspnea requiring increased oxygen. She was diagnosed with idiopathic pulmonary fibrosis 5 years ago. She was evaluated in the clinic 2 months ago; at that time she required 5 L/min of supplemental oxygen at rest and daily activities were limited to dressing and eating, both of which caused severe dyspnea. Currently, despite broad spectrum antibiotics and intravenous methylprednisolone, 1 g daily for 5 days, she is in severe respiratory distress requiring high-flow oxygen at 80%. She is alert and breathless, and understands her condition and treatment options.

On physical examination, blood pressure is 150/85 mm Hg, pulse rate is 110/min, and respiration rate is 36/min. Oxygen saturation is 88% on 80% high-flow oxygen. BMI is 24. Pulmonary examination reveals diffuse inspiratory crackles. She has clinical findings of pulmonary hypertension on cardiac examination, unchanged from 2 months ago. She has no edema or jugular venous distention.

Chest radiograph is unchanged.

**Which of the following is the most appropriate management?**

(A) Increase methylprednisolone
(B) Initiate albuterol
(C) Mechanical ventilation
(D) Palliative care

## Item 31

A 41-year-old woman is evaluated for nonproductive cough with dyspnea on exertion for the past 6 months. Her medical history is significant for diffuse cutaneous systemic sclerosis, gastroesophageal reflux disease, and Raynaud phenomenon. Her medications are omeprazole, nifedipine, and lisinopril.

On physical examination, vital signs are normal. Oxygen saturation is 98% breathing ambient air at rest but drops to 93% with exertion. She has sclerodactyly. The lung examination is normal.

Pulmonary function tests demonstrate restriction with a total lung capacity of 70% of predicted and D$_{LCO}$ of 65% of predicted.

Chest radiograph is normal.

**Which of the following is the most appropriate diagnostic test to perform next?**

(A) 6-Minute walk test
(B) Cardiopulmonary exercise testing
(C) High-resolution chest CT scan
(D) PET/CT scan

## Item 32

A 62-year-old woman is evaluated for a 1-year history of cough. She works in an office and has no environmental exposures, and cannot recall any specific initiating event. Her cough seems to be triggered by temperature changes, exercise, laughter, and strong scents and perfumes. She has no sputum production, rhinitis, postnasal drip, wheezing, or gastroesophageal reflux disease. She has recently been treated with intranasal fluticasone and oral antihistamines without significant improvement. She is not taking any medications currently.

On physical examination, oxygen saturation is 97% on ambient air. All vital signs and pulmonary and cardiac examinations are normal.

Laboratory studies, including complete blood count, are normal.

Chest radiograph is normal. Pulmonary function testing shows a normal FEV$_1$ and FEV$_1$/FVC ratio.

**Which of the following is the most appropriate management?**

(A) Begin daily inhaled budesonide and albuterol
(B) Obtain esophageal manometry and 24-hour pH monitoring study
(C) Obtain high-resolution CT scan of the chest
(D) Obtain methacholine challenge testing

### Item 33

A 45-year-old woman with hypovolemic shock is evaluated for rapid resuscitation in the ICU. She has sickle cell disease with recurrent pain and hemolytic crises, and osteoporosis.

On physical examination, temperature is 39 °C (102.3 °F), blood pressure is 70/40 mm Hg, pulse rate is 142/min and weak, and respiration rate is 22/min. Oxygen saturation is 99% breathing ambient air. There is a subcutaneous port in the right anterior chest wall.

**Which of the following is the most appropriate type of venous access for this patient?**

(A) Intraosseous port
(B) Peripheral wide-bore catheter
(C) Subcutaneous intravenous port
(D) Triple-lumen central catheter

### Item 34

A 66-year-old man is hospitalized in December for a 1-week history of increasing dyspnea on exertion, wheezing, and a nonproductive cough despite outpatient treatment with antibiotics and steroids. He now has awakenings with nocturnal dyspnea, which are only partially relieved by the use of his albuterol inhaler. He has started using his albuterol nebulizer four times a day, which provides only temporary relief. He does not have fever, headache, myalgia, runny nose, sputum production, chest pain, lower extremity edema, or palpitations. He has a history of COPD with an FEV$_1$ of 42% of predicted on spirometry obtained 3 months ago. In addition to albuterol, he takes umeclidinium and vilanterol and was started on azithromycin and prednisone 3 days ago.

On physical examination, temperature is 37.1 °C (98.8 °F), blood pressure is 135/80 mm Hg, pulse rate is 110/min, and respiration rate is 22/min. Oxygen saturation is 90% on ambient air. The patient is not using his accessory muscles. He has decreased breath sounds throughout, with diffuse end-expiratory wheezes. Other than tachycardia, the cardiovascular examination is normal without jugular venous distention or edema.

Laboratory studies, including complete blood count with differential, basic metabolic panel, B-type natriuretic peptide, and arterial blood gases, are unremarkable.

Electrocardiogram demonstrates sinus tachycardia, and a chest radiograph shows hyperinflation but no infiltrates.

**Which of the following is the most appropriate diagnostic test to perform next?**

(A) Bedside spirometry
(B) CT pulmonary angiography
(C) Polymerase chain reaction testing for influenza A and B
(D) Sputum culture

### Item 35

A 72-year-old woman is evaluated during a routine visit. She has a 30-pack-year smoking history and quit 5 years ago. She has a history of mild COPD and breast cancer diagnosed 15 years ago, currently in remission. A chest radiograph from 5 years ago showed no signs of disease recurrence. Medications are albuterol and tiotropium inhalers.

On physical examination, vital signs are normal. Lung examination reveals prolonged expiration and diminished breath sounds throughout. The breast examination is unremarkable.

A screening low-dose chest CT scan shows a peripheral 9-mm solid pulmonary nodule in the left upper lobe and emphysema but no mediastinal or hilar lymphadenopathy and no pleural effusion. A PET/CT scan using fluorodeoxyglucose (FDG) is performed and the nodule is intensely hypermetabolic. There is no evidence of distant uptake.

**Which of the following is the most appropriate management?**

(A) Bronchoscopy with biopsy
(B) Serial chest CT scans
(C) Surgical wedge resection
(D) Transthoracic needle aspiration

### Item 36

A 75-year-old man is evaluated for a 6-month history of dyspnea on exertion. He was a construction worker between 1972 and 1986. He notes that he was often in buildings with high levels of dust without respiratory protection. He finished his working career providing janitorial services for the public school system. He is an avid wood worker and has a shop in his garage. He has never smoked. He has no other medical problems and takes no medications.

On physical examination, vital signs are normal. Lung examination reveals inspiratory crackles at the lung bases bilaterally.

Spirometry shows an FVC of 80% of predicted, an FEV$_1$ of 85% of predicted, and a D$_{LCO}$ of 75% of predicted. CT scan shows pleural plaques, peripheral and basal predominant septal line thickening without ground-glass opacities, micronodules, or honeycombing.

**Which of the following is the most likely diagnosis?**

(A) Asbestosis

(B) Chronic hypersensitivity pneumonitis

(C) Idiopathic pulmonary fibrosis

(D) Respiratory bronchiolitis-associated interstitial lung disease

## Item 37

A 24-year-old woman is treated in the emergency department for an acute asthma exacerbation. She has received continuous albuterol and ipratropium nebulization and intravenous methylprednisolone. She has persistent wheezing and dyspnea. Her outpatient medications are inhaled albuterol and fluticasone/salmeterol.

On physical examination, blood pressure is 164/84 mm Hg, pulse rate is 121/min, and respiration rate is 28/min. Oxygen saturation is 95% on 4 L/min of oxygen through nasal cannula. Peak flow is less than 40% of her baseline. She is sitting upright and is using accessory muscles of respiration and can speak four words of a sentence. Lung examination demonstrates diffuse wheezing throughout both lungs.

**Which of the following is the most appropriate treatment?**

(A) Ketamine infusion

(B) Magnesium sulfate, intravenously

(C) Montelukast sodium

(D) Theophylline

## Item 38

A 65-year-old woman is admitted to the ICU with sepsis. She has become increasingly hypotensive despite intravenous fluid resuscitation of 30 mL/kg and the administration of increasing doses of norepinephrine and a standard dose of vasopressin. She has an arterial catheter in place. Appropriate antibiotics have been administered.

On physical examination, temperature is 37.7 °C (100 °F), blood pressure is 88/45 mm Hg, pulse rate is 116/min. Oxygen saturation is 98% on 2 L/min of oxygen through nasal cannula. She is alert and oriented. Her skin is cool. The remainder of the examination is normal.

Telemetry shows premature ventricular complexes.

**Which of the following is the most appropriate treatment?**

(A) Change norepinephrine to dopamine

(B) Hydrocortisone

(C) Increase the vasopressin infusion rate

(D) Intravenous immune globulin

## Item 39

A 73-year-old man is evaluated for a 6-month history of right-sided chest discomfort, fatigue, nonproductive cough, and progressive dyspnea. He has lost 9 kg (20 lb) during the last 6 months. His history is significant for COPD. He was a brake mechanic for 30 years. Medications are an albuterol inhaler as needed and tiotropium inhaler.

On physical examination, vital signs are normal. Lung examination reveals dullness to percussion and diminished breath sounds above the lower half of the right hemithorax. The physical examination is otherwise normal.

Laboratory studies, including complete blood count, are normal.

Chest radiograph shows a moderate right-sided loculated pleural effusion with pleural thickening.

A thoracentesis is performed that removes 600 mL of serosanguineous fluid.

**Pleural fluid analysis:**

| | |
|---|---|
| Cytology | Atypical mesothelial cells, negative for malignancy |
| Gram stain | Negative |
| Lactate dehydrogenase | 425 U/L |
| pH | 7.35 |
| Total protein | 4.6 g/dL (46 g/L) |

**Which of the following is the most likely diagnosis?**

(A) Empyema

(B) Heart failure

(C) Malignant pleural mesothelioma

(D) Rheumatoid pleuritis

## Item 40

A 60-year-old woman is evaluated for a 2-year history of dyspnea on exertion. She has dyspnea and wheezing when walking up an incline, especially if she is carrying something, but no other symptoms. She quit smoking 5 years ago and has a history of hypertension. Current medications are hydrochlorothiazide and ramipril.

On physical examination, vital signs are normal; oxygen saturation is 95% on ambient air. Lungs are clear on auscultation. Cardiovascular examination is unremarkable.

Laboratory studies reveal normal hemoglobin.

Spirometry shows a postbronchodilator $FEV_1$ of 75% of predicted and an $FEV_1/FVC$ ratio of 0.65. Electrocardiogram and chest radiograph are normal.

**Which of the following is the most appropriate initial treatment?**

(A) Roflumilast

(B) Short-acting and long-acting bronchodilator

(C) Short-acting bronchodilator

(D) Short-acting bronchodilator and inhaled glucocorticoid

(E) Short course of prednisone

## Item 41

A 54-year-old man is evaluated during a follow-up visit 1 month after an emergency appendectomy. He was diagnosed with amyotrophic lateral sclerosis 9 months ago. He was placed on supplemental oxygen for 2 nights after surgery because of nocturnal oxyhemoglobin desaturations.

Arterial blood gas studies revealed a pH of 7.42, $P_{CO_2}$ of 53 mm Hg (7.0 kPa), $P_{O_2}$ of 53 mm Hg (7.0 kPa), and bicarbonate of 33 mEq/L (33 mmol/L).

On physical examination, vital signs are normal. Oxygen saturation is 92% breathing ambient air. He has no difficulty managing his secretions. Examination reveals upper limb weakness, muscle fasciculations, hyperactive deep tendon reflexes, and dysarthria. Lung examination is unremarkable.

In-office measurement of FVC is 49% of predicted.

**Which of the following is the most appropriate management?**

(A) Bilevel positive airway pressure
(B) Continuous positive airway pressure
(C) Hypoglossal nerve stimulation
(D) Supplemental oxygen
(E) Tracheostomy

## Item 42

A 21-year-old man is hospitalized for sudden onset of dyspnea with chest pain that worsens with inspiration. He has a 3-pack-year history of smoking, but his medical history is otherwise unremarkable.

On physical examination, vital signs are normal. Oxygen saturation is 95% breathing ambient air. BMI is 18. Lung examination reveals reduced lung expansion, hyperresonance to percussion, and diminished breath sounds on the left side.

Chest radiograph demonstrates a large left-sided pneumothorax.

A thoracostomy tube is inserted that provides good lung reexpansion. Repeat chest radiograph is normal.

**Avoidance of which of the following is the most appropriate measure to prevent long-term recurrence of pneumothorax?**

(A) Air travel
(B) Mountain climbing
(C) Smoking
(D) Strenuous exercise

## Item 43

A 32-year-old woman is evaluated for a 10-day history of severe cough with increased sputum production, fever, wheezing, and dyspnea. She has a 12-year history of recurrent abdominal pain with watery stools and poor weight gain, recurrent sinusitis, and chronic cough that is productive of foul sputum. She takes no medications chronically.

On physical examination, temperature is 38.2 °C (100.8 °F), blood pressure is 92/64 mm Hg, pulse rate is 101/min, and respiration rate is 24/min. Oxygen saturation is 91% on ambient air. BMI is 18.2. Pulmonary examination reveals wheezes. Additional findings include a scaphoid abdomen and clubbing.

Laboratory studies reveal a leukocyte count of 16,000/μL $(16 \times 10^9/L)$, hemoglobin of 10 g/dL (100 g/L), and serum creatinine of 0.7 mg/dL (61.9 μmol/L). Serum immunoglobulin levels are normal.

Pulmonary function testing reveals an FVC of 80% of predicted, an $FEV_1$ of 50% of predicted, and an $FEV_1/FVC$ ratio of 0.55.

Chest radiograph is shown.

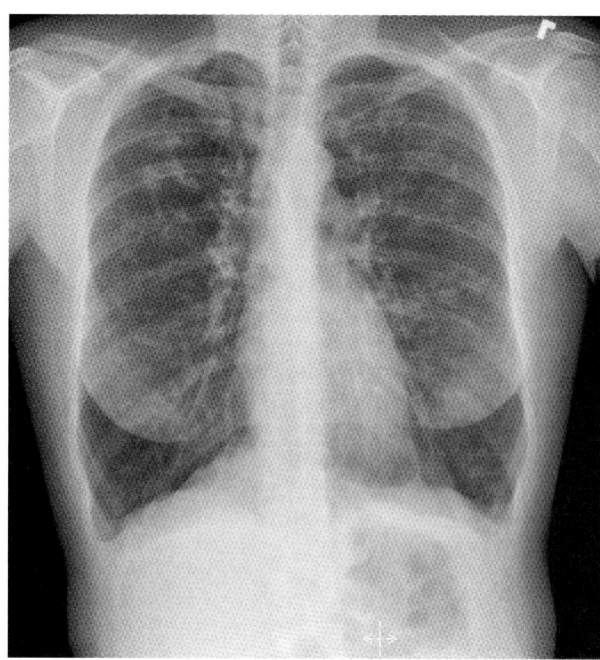

**Which of the following is the most likely underlying diagnosis?**

(A) Common variable immunodeficiency
(B) Complement component deficiency
(C) COPD
(D) Cystic fibrosis

## Item 44

A 62-year-old woman with a history of moderate COPD is evaluated in the emergency department for increasing dyspnea, cough, and sputum production. She had been doing well until 4 days ago when she developed rhinorrhea and a cough productive of purulent sputum. During the past two days she has noted increasing dyspnea on exertion that responds transiently to her albuterol inhaler. This is the patient's first episode of this nature. She stopped smoking 18 months ago. Current medications are albuterol and tiotropium inhalers.

On physical examination, temperature is 38.1 °C (100.6 °F), blood pressure is 130/80 mm Hg, pulse rate is 102/min, and respiration rate is 22/min. Oxygen saturation is 90% on ambient air. The patient is tachypneic and catches her breath between sentences but improves after a treatment of albuterol. She has diffuse end-expiratory wheezing.

A chest radiograph shows the lungs to be clear but hyperinflated.

Arterial blood gases on 2L/min of oxygen through nasal cannula show a pH 7.38, a $PCO_2$ of 42 mm Hg (5.58 kPa), and a $PO_2$ of 70 mm Hg (9.31 kPa).

**Which of the following is the most appropriate treatment?**

(A) Azithromycin and prednisone
(B) Mometasone inhaler
(C) Noninvasive positive pressure ventilation
(D) Roflumilast

## Item 45

A 62-year-old woman is evaluated for increasing exertional dyspnea during the past 6 months. She is a former smoker who was diagnosed with severe COPD 3 years ago ($FEV_1$ is 35% of predicted). For the past 18 months, she has used tiotropium and salmeterol; inhaled fluticasone was added 4 months ago, but without any perceived benefit. She takes no other medications.

On physical examination, blood pressure is 130/79 mm Hg, pulse rate is 88/min, and respiration rate is 18/min. Oxygen saturation is 89% breathing ambient air. Lung examination demonstrates diminished breath sounds. A prominent pulmonic sound is heard on cardiac examination.

Arterial blood gas studies breathing ambient air show a pH of 7.41, a $P_{CO_2}$ of 43 mm Hg (5.7 kPa), and a $P_{O_2}$ of 55 mm Hg (7.3 kPa).

Chest radiograph reveals hyperinflation. Echocardiography shows an estimated right ventricular systolic pressure of 58 mm Hg. Polysomnography showed an apnea–hypopnea index of 2 and a mean oxygen saturation of 87%.

**Which of the following is the most appropriate treatment?**

(A) Bilevel positive airway pressure
(B) Prednisone
(C) Sildenafil
(D) Supplemental oxygen

## Item 46

A 46-year-old man is evaluated for 6 months of exertional dyspnea, fatigue, and ankle edema. Recently he experienced near-syncope walking up two flights of stairs. He has no other medical problems and takes no medications.

On physical examination, blood pressure is 106/70 mm Hg, pulse rate is 94/min, and respiration rate is 18/min. Oxygen saturation is 90% breathing ambient air. On cardiac examination, a prominent jugular venous *a* wave is present along with widened splitting of $S_2$. Lung examination is unremarkable.

A transthoracic echocardiogram demonstrates a normal size left ventricle with ejection fraction of 65% and right ventricular enlargement. The estimated pulmonary artery systolic pressure is 58 mm Hg. Spirometry, lung volumes, and ventilation-perfusion scan are unremarkable; $D_{LCO}$ is 42% of predicted. CT angiogram of the chest is negative for pulmonary embolism and interstitial lung disease. Right heart catheterization demonstrates a mean pulmonary arterial pressure of 36 mm Hg, with no change with inhaled nitric oxide. Pulmonary capillary wedge pressure is normal.

**Which of the following is the most appropriate treatment?**

(A) Bosentan
(B) Diltiazem
(C) Metoprolol
(D) Pirfenidone

## Item 47

A 27-year-old woman is evaluated for concern about a 3-week history of a new chemical odor in her workplace. She has a history of mild asthma since childhood that is well-controlled with infrequent use of an albuterol inhaler. The plant safety manager at her job said there is no need for protective equipment, but she is experiencing increased cough and now uses her albuterol inhaler once daily.

On physical examination, vital signs are normal. Lungs are clear on auscultation with no wheeze.

Office spirometry shows an FVC of 98% of predicted, an $FEV_1$ of 93% of predicted, and an $FEV_1/FVC$ ratio of 0.78 of predicted.

**Which of the following is the most appropriate management?**

(A) Chest CT scan
(B) Obtain hair sample for toxic analysis
(C) Review employer Material Safety Data Sheet
(D) Transfer patient to other area of plant

## Item 48

A 49-year-old man is evaluated for a 4-month history of cough, chest pressure, and double vision. He has no fever, night sweats, or weight loss. He has never smoked.

On physical examination, vital signs are normal. There is ptosis bilaterally. The remainder of the physical examination is normal.

A CT scan of the chest is shown.

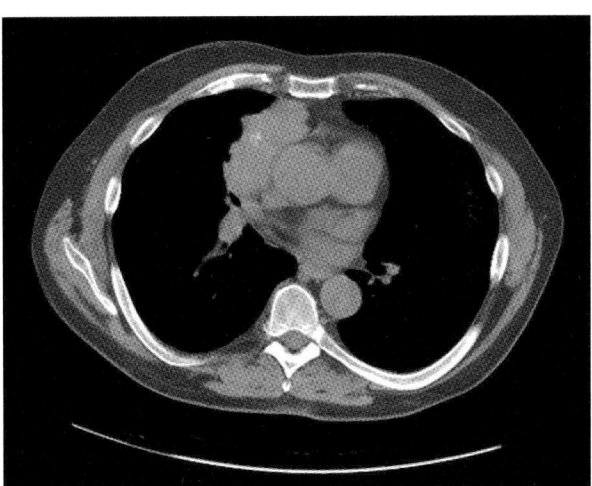

**Which of the following is the most appropriate test to perform next?**

(A) Acetylcholine receptor antibody
(B) α-Fetoprotein
(C) β-Human chorionic gonadotropin
(D) Lactate dehydrogenase

## Item 49

A 60-year-old woman is evaluated in the hospital for respiratory failure. She was hospitalized 3 weeks ago after a house fire. She suffered significant third-degree burns covering 40% of her body and mucosal burns to her nose. She was intubated, but was successfully liberated from the ventilator last week. A surveillance bronchoscopy performed before extubation was unremarkable. Last night she became progressively dyspneic and hypoxic, eventually requiring reintubation. Current medications are topical antibiotics and subcutaneous heparin.

On physical examination, temperature is 37.9 °C (100.2 °F), blood pressure is 104/60 mm Hg, pulse rate is 95/min, and respiration rate is 26/min. Oxygen saturation is 91% breathing from a ventilator ($F_{IO_2}$ of 0.6). Copious yellow sputum is present in the endotracheal tube when suctioned.

Laboratory studies reveal a leukocyte count of 16,000/μL ($16 \times 10^9$/L), increased from 12,000/μL ($12 \times 10^9$/L) yesterday.

A chest radiograph shows a focal consolidation in the lower left lobe.

**Which of the following is the most appropriate treatment?**

(A) Administer hydroxocobalamin
(B) Administer intravenous antibiotics
(C) Bronchoscopic airway stenting
(D) Insert a thoracostomy tube

## Item 50

A 30-year-old man with a history of alcohol and drug abuse is brought to the emergency department. He was found unresponsive and on arrival he was intubated and placed on mechanical ventilation for poor respiratory effort. Witnesses confirmed that he had been drinking alcohol and had also taken drugs at a party.

On physical examination, vital signs are normal. Respiration rate is 14/min on mechanical ventilation. He is not triggering the ventilator. Oxygen saturation is 100% on 35% oxygen. He responds to pain only. His pupils are dilated and reactive to light. He shows no signs of trauma.

Blood toxicology screening is positive for alcohol; urine toxicology screening is positive for benzodiazepines. Arterial pH and electrolyte anion gap are normal.

**Which of the following is the most appropriate management?**

(A) Administer flumazenil
(B) Administer fomepizole
(C) Administer hemodialysis
(D) Monitor for signs of agitation

## Item 51

A 22-year-old man is evaluated for acute onset of fever, chills, dyspnea, and nonproductive cough. He is a college student and spends summers using a combine to harvest wheat. He does not wear respiratory protective equipment. His symptoms start at the beginning of a work week, progress to the point that he must miss several days of work, and then the cycle begins again.

On physical examination, temperature is 37.8 °C (100.1 °F), blood pressure is 120/80 mm Hg, pulse rate is 98/min, and respiration rate is 22/min. Oxygen saturation is 94% breathing ambient air. Lung examination reveals diffuse crackles.

Chest radiograph demonstrates diffuse upper-lobe micronodular opacities.

**Which of the following is the most appropriate treatment?**

(A) Counsel the patient not to return to work
(B) Inhaled glucocorticoids
(C) Pirfenidone
(D) Sirolimus

## Item 52

A 64-year-old woman is evaluated during a posthospital visit for severe COPD with an $FEV_1$ of 30% of predicted. She has been admitted three times during the last year with acute exacerbations characterized by cough, increased purulent sputum production, and dyspnea. She is now at baseline of her exertional dyspnea and has no cough. She has already participated in a pulmonary rehabilitation program. She currently takes tiotropium, budesonide/formoterol, and albuterol.

On physical examination, vital signs are normal. Oxygen saturation is 90% on 3 L/min of supplemental oxygen at rest and with exertion. Pulmonary examination reveals decreased breath sounds throughout. The remainder of the examination is noncontributory.

**Which of the following is the most appropriate treatment to reduce this patient's COPD exacerbations?**

(A) Chronic low-dose oral glucocorticoid
(B) Chronic macrolide therapy
(C) Increase supplemental oxygen
(D) Nebulized hypertonic saline

## Item 53

A 52-year-old man is evaluated in the ICU for dyspnea that developed after aspiration of gastric contents during an upper endoscopy. The endoscopy was performed for evaluation of upper gastric bleeding due to peptic ulcer disease. His only medication is pantoprazole.

On physical examination, temperature is 37.3 °C (99.1 °F), blood pressure is 150/99 mm Hg, pulse rate is 110/min, and respiration rate is 28/min. Oxygen saturation is 90% on a 100% oxygen nonrebreather mask. He is awake, diaphoretic, and anxious. Lung examination reveals scant bilateral crackles and rhonchi as well as use of accessory muscles. The remainder of the physical examination is normal.

Arterial blood gas studies on a 100% oxygen nonrebreather mask show a pH of 7.35, a $P_{CO_2}$ of 46 mm Hg (6.1 kPa), and a $P_{O_2}$ of 55 mm Hg (7.3 kPa).

Chest radiograph reveals new bilateral opacities.

**Which of the following is the most appropriate treatment?**

(A) Continue current therapy
(B) High-flow humidified nasal cannula
(C) Intubation and mechanical ventilation
(D) Noninvasive mechanical ventilation

## Item 54

A 38-year-old man is evaluated for a 6-month history of dyspnea on exertion. He has gastroesophageal reflux disease and Raynaud phenomenon. He does not smoke and has no cough or wheezing. Current medications are lansoprazole and amlodipine.

On physical examination, vital signs are normal. Oxygen saturation is 91% breathing ambient air. He has scattered telangiectasias on the face and trunk and sclerodactyly. Lung fields are clear on auscultation.

The only abnormality on pulmonary function testing is a DLCO of 43% of predicted.

High-resolution CT of the chest shows no evidence of parenchymal lung disease.

**Which of the following is the most likely diagnosis?**

(A) Cryptogenic organizing pneumonia
(B) Lymphangioleiomyomatosis
(C) Lymphoid interstitial pneumonia
(D) Pulmonary arterial hypertension

## Item 55

A 58-year-old man is evaluated in the hospital for fever, hypotension, and altered mental status. He was hospitalized 2 days ago for an infected arm wound and was treated with intravenous piperacillin/tazobactam and vancomycin. This morning he developed new pain in the middle of his back and difficulty urinating. His medical history is significant for type 2 diabetes mellitus treated with metformin.

On physical examination, temperature is 39.1 °C (102.4 °F), blood pressure is 83/48 mm Hg, pulse rate is 109/min, and respiration rate is 21/min. Oxygen saturation is 98% breathing 2 L/min of oxygen through nasal cannula. He is somnolent but arousable and oriented when awake. There is erythema surrounding the wound on his right upper arm with no drainage or tenderness. There is tenderness to percussion in the middle of his back and a palpable bladder.

Laboratory studies reveal a blood serum leukocyte count of 22,000/μL (22 × 10⁹/L), and plasma glucose of 160 mg/dL (8.88 mmol/L).

Chest radiograph is unremarkable.

**Which of the following is the most appropriate next step in management?**

(A) Intravenous fluid bolus
(B) Intravenous insulin
(C) MRI of the spine
(D) Surgical exploration of the arm wound

## Item 56

A 72-year-old woman is evaluated in the hospital for a pneumothorax. The patient has severe, oxygen-dependent COPD complicated by several exacerbations. She was hospitalized 72 hours ago with abrupt onset of chest pain and dyspnea. Chest radiography confirmed the presence of a large left-sided pneumothorax and a thoracotomy tube was placed. She had 90% expansion of the lung following thoracostomy.

On physical examination, the patient is frail appearing but comfortable. Vital signs are normal. Oxygen saturation is 96% breathing 3 L/min of oxygen through nasal cannula. Pulmonary examination reveals diminished but present breath sounds bilaterally. A left thoracostomy tube is in place.

Chest radiograph demonstrates resolution of pneumothorax with a thoracostomy tube in place.

**Which of the following is the most appropriate management?**

(A) Clamp thoracostomy tube
(B) Place thoracostomy tube to high suction
(C) Pleurodesis
(D) Remove thoracostomy tube

## Item 57

A 66-year-old man with a history of COPD is evaluated during a routine visit. He is able to walk one flight of stairs and one block before he develops dyspnea. He was last treated for two acute exacerbations of COPD within the last year, one of which required hospitalization. He recently completed a pulmonary rehabilitation program. His medical history is significant for hypertension and a 60-pack-year smoking history. He quit smoking 5 years ago. Current medications are hydrochlorothiazide, glycopyrrolate/formoterol, and albuterol.

On physical examination, vital signs are normal; oxygen saturation is 94% on ambient air. Pulmonary examination reveals a prolonged expiratory phase. The cardiac and remainder of the physical examination are unremarkable.

Spirometry today shows a postbronchodilator FEV₁ of 35% of predicted. Chest radiograph at the time of his last exacerbation shows hyperinflation and no other findings. An electrocardiogram is normal.

**Which of the following patient characteristics places him at highest risk for a recurrent acute exacerbation?**

(A) Enrollment in a pulmonary rehabilitation program
(B) Hypertension
(C) Previous COPD exacerbations and FEV₁ level
(D) Smoking history and use of COPD medications

## Item 58

A 70-year-old man is hospitalized for a 4-week history of dyspnea, orthopnea, and daytime sleepiness. He was diagnosed with amyotrophic lateral sclerosis 6 months ago. His only medication is riluzole.

On physical examination, blood pressure is 128/73 mm Hg, pulse rate is 90/min, and respiration rate is 28/min. Oxygen saturation is 87% breathing ambient air. He has right-hand atrophy, decreased mobility, and fasciculations. Lung examination reveals abdominal paradox with breathing, use of accessory breathing muscles, and shallow tachypnea. He is awake, alert, and interactive, but dozes off easily. His speech is clear with no secretions. He is able to move all extremities and shows no cranial nerve abnormality.

On arterial blood gas testing, pH is 7.30, Pco₂ is 76 mm Hg (10.1 kPa), Po₂ is 50 mm Hg (6.65 kPa), and bicarbonate is 36 mEq/L (36 mmol/L) on room air. The calculated alveolar-arterial oxygen gradient is normal.

Chest radiograph reveals bilateral basal opacities consistent with atelectasis and shallow inspiration.

**CONT.** Which of the following is the most appropriate treatment?

(A) Invasive mechanical ventilation
(B) Noninvasive ventilation with bilevel positive airway pressure
(C) Noninvasive ventilation with continuous positive airway pressure
(D) Oxygen administration through nasal cannula

## Item 59

A 60-year-old man is evaluated in the emergency department for headache, nausea, vomiting, and confusion lasting 4 hours. He ran out of his hypertensive medications a few days ago. Current medications are lisinopril, metoprolol succinate, hydrochlorothiazide, and aspirin.

On physical examination, blood pressure is 230/140 mm Hg and pulse rate is 100/min. All other vital signs are normal. He is too uncooperative to perform a mental status examination or funduscopic examination. The cardiovascular examination is positive for an $S_4$ but otherwise normal.

Laboratory studies reveal normal electrolytes; serum creatinine is 1.6 mg/dL (141.4 µmol/L). It was 1.2 mg/dL (106 µmol/L) at his last outpatient appointment.

Electrocardiogram shows left ventricular hypertrophy and sinus tachycardia. Chest radiograph is normal. CT scan of the brain shows no acute findings.

Which of the following is the most appropriate treatment?

(A) Intravenous hypertensive therapy to lower systolic blood pressure (SBP) to 160 mm Hg within the first 6 hours
(B) Intravenous hypertensive therapy to lower SBP to 120 mm Hg within the first hour
(C) Intravenous hypertensive therapy to lower SBP to 160 mm Hg within the first 48 hours
(D) Resume usual oral antihypertensive regimen and observe

## Item 60

A 30-year-old woman is evaluated in the emergency department after she was rescued from her home where her vinyl sofa caught fire. She is intubated and unconscious.

On physical examination, blood pressure is 108/78 mm Hg, pulse rate is 100/min, and respiration rate is 24/min. Oxygen saturation by pulse oximetry is 100% on mechanical ventilation using 50% oxygen. She is unresponsive. She has no visible burns on her skin, and her airway secretions are clear. Brainstem reflexes are all intact.

**Laboratory studies:**

Serum electrolytes:
| | |
|---|---|
| Sodium | 140 mEq/L (140 mmol/L) |
| Potassium | 4.4 mEq/L (4.4 mmol/L) |
| Chloride | 99 mEq/L (99 mmol/L) |
| Bicarbonate | 13.1 mEq/L (13.1 mmol/L) |

Arterial blood gas studies:
| | |
|---|---|
| pH | 7.29 |
| $Pco_2$ | 28 mm Hg (3.7 kPa) |
| $Po_2$ | 233 mm Hg (31 kPa) |
| Carboxyhemoglobin | 5% |
| Methemoglobin | 2% |
| Lactate | 11 mEq/L (1.2 mmol/L) |

The oxygen is increased to 100%.

Which of the following is the most appropriate treatment?

(A) Hydroxocobalamin
(B) Hyperbaric oxygen therapy
(C) Methylene blue
(D) Sodium nitrite

## Item 61

A 35-year-old man is evaluated for chronic cough productive of foul-smelling sputum. He has been treated with four courses of antibiotics in the last 12 months; several infections have been associated with *Pseudomonas* species. His symptoms have been present for many years and are also associated with chronic sinusitis. He was recently diagnosed with infertility.

On physical examination, all vital signs are normal. Oxygen saturation is 98% on ambient air. Clubbing is present. Pulmonary examination reveals rhonchi and wheezes in the upper lobes bilaterally.

Chest radiograph reveals bilateral upper-lobe bronchiectasis.

Laboratory studies reveal a negative sweat chloride test of 39 mEq/L (39 mmol/L).

Which of the following is the most appropriate management?

(A) Begin chronic ciprofloxacin therapy
(B) Begin tiotropium
(C) Repeat sweat chloride testing
(D) Test for $\alpha_1$-antitrypsin deficiency

## Item 62

A 62-year-old man undergoes routine follow-up evaluation. His medical history is significant for tobacco use (35-pack–year) and hypertension controlled with lisinopril. He quit smoking 3 months ago and does not have any cough, wheezing, or shortness of breath.

On physical examination, vital signs are normal. BMI is 31. Cardiopulmonary examination is normal.

Which of the following is the most appropriate test?

(A) 6-Minute walk test
(B) Chest radiograph
(C) Low-dose CT scan of the chest
(D) Office spirometry
(E) Urinary cotinine test

## Item 63

A 22-year-old man is evaluated in the hospital for decreased responsiveness. He was hospitalized 4 days ago after a motor vehicle accident. He has multiple fractures and a chest contusion. He was intubated for respiratory distress in the emergency department and given morphine, propofol, and heparin. He is on volume-controlled continuous mandatory ventilation mode with an $FIO_2$ of 0.7.

On physical examination, temperature is 37.7 °C (99.9 °F), blood pressure is 124/65 mm Hg, pulse rate is 89/min, and

**CONT.** respiration rate is 27/min. Oxygen saturation is 93% on mechanical ventilation. He is unresponsive to voice or pain, and his pupils are 3 mm and reactive; the neurological examination is otherwise nonfocal. He has external fixators in both lower extremities. There are bruises on the anterior chest wall. The remainder of the physical examination is noncontributory.

**Which of the following is the most appropriate management?**

(A) Change propofol to dexmedetomidine
(B) CT of the head
(C) Continuous electroencephalography
(D) Stop sedation and analgesia

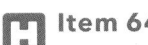 **Item 64**

A 61-year-old man is evaluated in the emergency department after he collapsed on a hot and humid day. He was playing in a marching band and had to stand in the sun for 2 hours while wearing a heavy uniform. No other medical information is available.

On physical examination, temperature is 40 °C (104 °F), blood pressure is 90/45 mm Hg, pulse rate is 110/min, and respiration rate is 20/min. His face is flushed, he is somnolent, and although he is arousable, he is not coherent. There are no signs of trauma.

His clothing is removed.

**Which of the following is the most appropriate treatment?**

(A) Acetaminophen and a cooling blanket
(B) Continuous alcohol sponge bath with cooling fans
(C) Ice water immersion
(D) Intravenous dantrolene
(E) Sprayed water and cooling fans

**Item 65**

A 53-year-old man is evaluated in the emergency department after 4 days of cough, fever, chills, myalgia, and poor appetite. He currently has increased dyspnea and lightheadedness. His child was diagnosed with influenza 2 weeks ago.

On physical examination, temperature is 38.8 °C (101.8 °F), blood pressure is 82/40 mm Hg, pulse rate is 128/min, and respiration rate is 17/min. Oxygen saturation is 92% on ambient air. The cardiac examination reveals regular rhythm and tachycardia without an $S_3$ or jugular venous distention. Lungs are clear on auscultation and extremities are warm. The remainder of the examination is normal.

**Laboratory studies:**

| | |
|---|---|
| Hemoglobin | 10 g/dL (100 g/L) |
| Lactate | 4.6 mEq/L (4.6 mmol/L) |
| Leukocyte count | 18,000/µL (18 × 10⁹/L) |
| Arterial blood gases: | |
|   pH | 7.32 |
|   $P_{CO_2}$ | 32 mm Hg (4.3 kPa) |
|   $P_{O_2}$ | 70 mm Hg (9.3 kPa) |
| Bicarbonate | 16 mEq/L (16 mmol/L) |

A chest radiograph shows basilar ground-glass opacities on the right. Electrocardiogram reveals sinus tachycardia but is otherwise normal.

**Which of the following is the most appropriate initial treatment?**

(A) 0.9% saline bolus
(B) Intravenous furosemide
(C) Norepinephrine
(D) Packed red blood cells

**Item 66**

A 19-year-old man is evaluated in the emergency department for cardiac arrest after he fell through the ice of a frozen lake. He was in the water for less than 10 minutes, but when he was pulled out onto the ice he was unresponsive and no pulse could be felt. Bystander cardiopulmonary resuscitation (CPR) was begun immediately and continued for 25 minutes until emergency medical services arrived. At the scene his rectal temperature was 27 °C (80.6 °F). He was intubated and bag ventilated and continued to receive CPR in the ambulance on the way to the emergency department.

On physical examination, temperature is 28 °C (82.4 °F). Oxygen saturation is 97% on mechanical ventilation with 65% oxygen. He is not responsive and shows no spontaneous movement or shivering. His heart rhythm on the monitor is ventricular fibrillation.

**Which of the following is the most appropriate management?**

(A) Continue CPR with active external rewarming
(B) Continue CPR with active internal (core) rewarming
(C) Continue CPR with passive external rewarming
(D) Discontinue CPR

**Item 67**

A 31-year-old man is evaluated near the end of a guided climb of a 3500-meter (11,482 feet) summit in the French Alps. He is confused and increasingly irritable. His only medication was prophylactic acetazolamide, which he discontinued due to bothersome nocturia.

On physical examination, pulse rate is 128/min and respiration rate is 22/min. In addition to confusion, his gait is ataxic. The neurological examination is otherwise nonfocal.

Supplemental oxygen is administered and arrangements are being made for descent.

**Which of the following is the most appropriate additional treatment?**

(A) Acetazolamide
(B) Dexamethasone
(C) Nifedipine
(D) Sildenafil

**Item 68**

A 42-year-old man was hospitalized 2 days ago with necrotizing fasciitis of the leg. He underwent extensive debridement and fasciotomy 2 hours earlier. He currently has severe pain in his leg wounds. He was well before this illness. Current medications are imipenem, clindamycin, vancomycin, and a morphine infusion.

On physical examination, blood pressure is 150/99 mm Hg, pulse rate is 110/min, and respiration rate is 24/min. He is awake, anxious, grimacing, and wriggling in bed. The remainder of the examination is noncontributory.

**Which of the following is the most appropriate treatment?**

(A) Add gabapentin
(B) Epidural for regional analgesia
(C) Intravenous bolus of morphine
(D) Replace morphine with intravenous fentanyl

## Item 69

A 24-year-old woman is evaluated during a follow-up visit. She was initially evaluated 6 weeks ago after a fall at work and had a chest radiograph performed for evaluation of pleuritic chest pain. This symptom has since resolved. She has no other symptoms and takes no medications.

Upon physical examination, vital signs are normal. The remainder of the physical examination is normal.

Chest radiograph is shown.

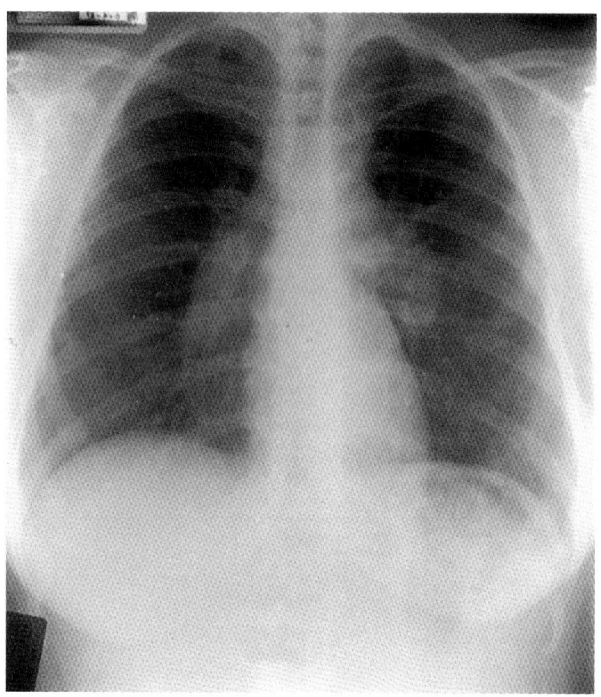

**Which of the following is the most appropriate management?**

(A) Endobronchial ultrasound and biopsy
(B) High-resolution CT scan of the chest
(C) Prednisone
(D) Observation

## Item 70

A 34-year-old male is hospitalized for acute respiratory failure following a heroin overdose and aspiration. Current

medications are piperacillin/tazobactam, propofol, heparin, and pantoprazole.

On physical examination, temperature is 37.7 °C (99.9 °F), blood pressure is 114/77 mm Hg, pulse rate is 74/min, and respiration rate is 16/min. His ideal body weight is 63 kg (138 lb). Ventilator settings are in the volume-controlled ventilation mode with tidal volume of 630 mL, a positive end-expiratory pressure (PEEP) of 8 cm $H_2O$, and $FIO_2$ of 0.5.

Arterial blood gas studies on an $FIO_2$ of 0.5 show a pH of 7.33, a $PCO_2$ of 46 mm Hg (6.1 kPa), and a $PO_2$ of 76 mm Hg (10.1 kPa).

Chest radiograph shows bilateral opacities.

**Which of the following is the most appropriate next step?**

(A) Decrease PEEP
(B) Increase PEEP
(C) Increase respiration rate
(D) Reduce tidal volume

## Item 71

A 51-year-old man is evaluated for fever, hypotension, and confusion. He was admitted to the ICU 8 days ago for observation after complications resulting from an outpatient surgical procedure. He had experienced unexpected bleeding in the recovery room and had a central venous catheter inserted emergently for blood transfusion. On the first postoperative day he was weaned from mechanical ventilation, vomited once but recovered, and has been receiving supplemental oxygen through nasal cannula. Today he developed a fever, hypotension, and confusion. His hemoglobin has remained stable.

On physical examination, temperature is 38.6 °C (101.5 °F), blood pressure is 89/50 mm Hg, pulse rate is 101/min, and respiration rate is 23/min. Oxygen saturation is 100% on 2L/min of oxygen through nasal cannula. Lung examination reveals clear breath sounds.

Laboratory studies reveal a leukocyte count of 15,000/μL (15 × 10⁹/L) and a serum creatinine of 1.2 mg/dL (106.1 μmol/L).

An intravenous fluid bolus of 30 mL/kg of body weight is now infusing. Blood and respiratory cultures have been obtained and broad spectrum antibiotics are administered.

**Which of the following is the most appropriate next step in management?**

(A) Administer glucocorticoids
(B) Administer norepinephrine
(C) Obtain procalcitonin level
(D) Remove the central venous catheter

## Item 72

A 31-year-old woman is evaluated for a 1-year history of daytime sleepiness. She falls asleep while watching TV, at the theater, and occasionally during a meal. She usually falls asleep between 10:00 PM and midnight and wakes during the workweek at 6:00 AM On weekends, she wakes at 9:00 AM. Her husband reports snoring but he hasn't observed breathing pauses. She has no cataplexy or symptoms of restless leg syndrome. She takes no medications.

On physical examination, vital signs are normal. BMI is 24.5. The physical examination, including inspection of nasal passages and oropharynx, is normal.

**Which of the following is the most appropriate management?**

(A) Actigraphy
(B) Modafinil
(C) Multiple sleep latency testing
(D) Polysomnography

## Item 73

A 43-year-old man is evaluated in the emergency department for a 1-week history of cough, shortness of breath, chest pain, and night sweats. He has a 25-pack-year smoking history.

On physical examination, temperature is 38.8 °C (102 °F), blood pressure is 134/82 mm Hg, pulse rate is 142/min, and respiration rate is 30/min. Oxygen saturation is 88% breathing ambient air. There are decreased breath sounds at the right base and dullness to percussion. The remainder of the examination is noncontributory.

Laboratory studies reveal a leukocyte count of 29,000/µL ($29.0 \times 10^9$/L).

Chest radiograph shows a large right pleural effusion with associated compressive atelectasis or consolidation, and consolidation in the right upper lobe.

The patient is prescribed broad-spectrum antibiotics and a diagnostic thoracentesis is performed that removes 100 mL of serous pleural fluid.

**Pleural fluid studies:**

| | |
|---|---|
| pH | 7.0 |
| Lactate dehydrogenase | 2310 U/L |
| Total protein | 5.2 g/dL (52 g/L) |
| Glucose | 42 mg/dL (2.3 mmol/L) |
| Gram stain | Negative |

**Which of the following is the most likely diagnosis?**

(A) Complicated parapneumonic effusion
(B) Empyema
(C) Malignant effusion
(D) Uncomplicated parapneumonic effusion

## Item 74

A 55-year-old woman is evaluated during a routine visit. She was previously diagnosed with spirometry-confirmed mild COPD for which she was prescribed a short-acting bronchodilator. She has a 20-pack-year history of cigarette smoking, but she quit 5 years ago. She is currently asymptomatic and has never received an influenza vaccination or pneumococcal vaccination. Her only medication is an albuterol inhaler.

On physical examination, vital signs are normal; oxygen saturation is 95% on ambient air. Lungs are clear to auscultation. The remainder of the physical examination is unremarkable.

**Which of the following vaccinations should the patient receive at this time?**

(A) High-dose influenza
(B) Pneumococcal polysaccharide (PPSV23) and standard influenza
(C) PPSV23 and pneumococcal conjugate (PCV13) and standard influenza
(D) PPSV23 and PCV13

## Item 75

A 48-year-old woman is evaluated for recurrent pulmonary embolism. Her first episode was 18 months ago; she was treated with warfarin for 3 months. She was hospitalized 9 months ago for pulmonary embolism and has been treated with warfarin since then. She reports progressive exertional dyspnea. She has no chest pain, cough, hemoptysis, or wheezing. Her only medication is warfarin.

On physical examination, blood pressure is 108/68 mm Hg, pulse rate is 90/min, and respiration rate is 16/min. Oxygen saturation is 90% breathing ambient air. BMI is 36. The cardiovascular examination shows jugular venous distention, a prominent jugular venous $a$ wave, and widened split $S_2$ with a prominent pulmonic component. Lung examination is unremarkable.

INR is 2.8.

Echocardiography reveals a normal left ventricle and dilated right ventricle with reduced function. Ventilation-perfusion scan shows multiple mismatched defects. Right heart catheterization reveals a mean pulmonary arterial pressure of 58 mm Hg and a normal pulmonary capillary wedge pressure. Pulmonary angiography is remarkable for pulmonary artery webs, intimal irregularities, and abrupt narrowing of the major pulmonary arteries.

**Which of the following is the definitive treatment?**

(A) Apixaban
(B) Inferior vena cava filter
(C) Nifedipine
(D) Pulmonary thromboendarterectomy

## Item 76

A 65-year-old woman is evaluated for discontinuation of mechanical ventilation. She was placed on mechanical ventilation 5 days ago for respiratory failure secondary to an exacerbation of COPD. Ventilator settings are in the volume-controlled continuous mandatory ventilation mode, with a set respiration rate of 10/min, a tidal volume of 370 mL, an $F_{IO_2}$ of 0.35, and a positive end-expiratory pressure of 5 cm $H_2O$. Current medications are albuterol/ipratropium, levofloxacin, prednisone, and fentanyl.

On physical examination, vital signs are normal. She is sleepy but arousable and can follow simple commands. Lung examination reveals distant breath sounds. The remainder of the examination is unremarkable.

Arterial blood gas studies show a pH of 7.46, $P_{CO_2}$ of 47 mm Hg (6.25 kPa), and a $P_{O_2}$ of 62 mm Hg (8.25 kPa). Other laboratory studies, including a leukocyte count, are normal.

Chest radiograph demonstrates hyperinflation but no infiltrates or evidence of heart failure.

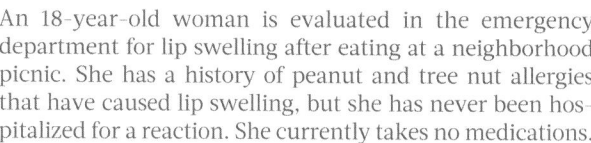

Which of the following is the most appropriate test or evaluation to perform next?

(A) 30-Minute spontaneous breathing trial
(B) Cuff leak test
(C) Glasgow Coma Scale
(D) Measure negative inspiratory force

## Item 77

A 48-year-old woman is hospitalized for a 2-week history of cough, sputum production, fever, and dyspnea.

On physical examination, temperature is 39.6 °C (103.3 °F), blood pressure is 110/63 mm Hg, pulse rate is 122/min, and respiration rate is 36/min. Oxygen saturation is 88% breathing ambient air. Lung examination reveals diminished breath sounds over the left base. Cardiac examination is notable only for tachycardia.

Chest radiograph reveals a small loculated effusion on the left.

A diagnostic thoracentesis is performed, which results in incomplete removal of the effusion.

**Pleural fluid analysis:**

| | |
|---|---|
| pH | 6.8 |
| Lactate dehydrogenase | 3289 U/L |
| Total protein | 3.7 g/dL (37 g/L) |
| Glucose | 9 mg/dL (0.5 mmol/L) |
| Gram stain | Gram-positive cocci in chains |

Appropriate intravenous antibiotics are initiated.

**Which of the following is the most appropriate intrapleural treatment of the effusion?**

(A) Antibiotics
(B) Streptokinase
(C) Tissue plasminogen activator-deoxyribonuclease
(D) No additional therapy required

## Item 78

A 67-year-old woman is evaluated for history of rhinorrhea, pharyngitis, nonproductive cough, and associated intermittent dyspnea. Her symptoms began 12 weeks ago associated with low-grade fevers, rhinorrhea, and pharyngitis. The fever, rhinorrhea, and pharyngitis resolved but her other symptoms persist. She has no chest pain, palpitations, edema, fever, chills, or orthopnea, and she has never smoked. Her medical history is significant for hypertension treated with an angiotensin receptor blocker.

On physical examination vital signs are normal. Cardiac examination, including jugular venous pressure, is normal. Lung examination is normal.

Laboratory studies, including complete blood count, are normal.

Chest radiograph and spirometry are normal.

**Which of the following is the most appropriate diagnostic test to perform next?**

(A) Echocardiography
(B) Exhaled nitric oxide testing
(C) High-resolution chest CT scan

(D) Methacholine challenge testing
(E) Nasal swab for influenza polymerase chain reaction

## Item 79

An 18-year-old woman is evaluated in the emergency department for lip swelling after eating at a neighborhood picnic. She has a history of peanut and tree nut allergies that have caused lip swelling, but she has never been hospitalized for a reaction. She currently takes no medications.

On physical examination, blood pressure is 100/64 mm Hg, pulse rate is 108/min, and respiration rate is 19/min. Oxygen saturation is 100% breathing ambient air. Bilateral lip swelling is evident that affects the upper lip more than the lower lip. She has no tongue swelling or stridor. Lungs are clear to auscultation. Urticaria is present on the hands and trunk.

**Which of the following is the most appropriate immediate treatment?**

(A) Diphenhydramine
(B) Epinephrine
(C) Intravenous fluid bolus
(D) Intravenous methylprednisolone

## Item 80

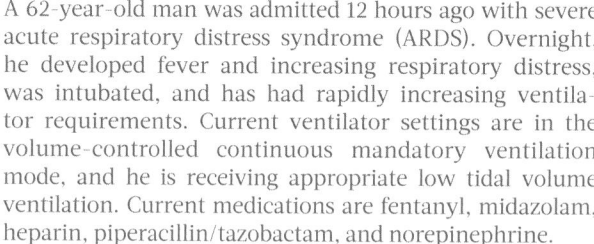

A 62-year-old man was admitted 12 hours ago with severe acute respiratory distress syndrome (ARDS). Overnight, he developed fever and increasing respiratory distress, was intubated, and has had rapidly increasing ventilator requirements. Current ventilator settings are in the volume-controlled continuous mandatory ventilation mode, and he is receiving appropriate low tidal volume ventilation. Current medications are fentanyl, midazolam, heparin, piperacillin/tazobactam, and norepinephrine.

On physical examination, temperature is 38.4 °C (101.2 °F), blood pressure is 89/45 mm Hg, pulse rate is 110/min, and his spontaneous respiration rate is 35/min with a positive end-expiratory pressure of 16 cm $H_2O$ and an $F_{IO_2}$ of 1.0.

**Arterial blood gases:**

| | |
|---|---|
| pH | 7.3 |
| $P_{CO_2}$ | 51 mm Hg (6.8 kPa) |
| $P_{O_2}$ | 55 mm Hg (7.3 kPa) |
| Bicarbonate | 24 mEq/L (24 mmol/L) |

Chest radiograph shows diffuse, bilateral infiltrates throughout the lung fields.

**Which of the following is the most appropriate management?**

(A) Perform a recruitment maneuver
(B) Start inhaled nitric oxide
(C) Transition the patient to high-frequency oscillator ventilation
(D) Ventilate the patient in the prone position

## Item 81

A 42-year-old man is evaluated in the office for chronic cough. He first developed a cough 3 years ago. It is productive of clear to yellow sputum that is occasionally blood-tinged. He has taken antibiotics when his sputum production increases, after which his cough improves but never completely resolves. He has no dyspnea. He does not smoke cigarettes. He currently is taking no medications.

On physical examination, vital signs are normal. Oxygen saturation is 96% breathing ambient air. BMI is normal. Pulmonary examination reveals scattered inspiratory squeaks.

A chest radiograph shows ill-defined linear atelectasis and irregular peripheral opacities in the right and left lower lobes. A CT scan of the chest with contrast is shown below.

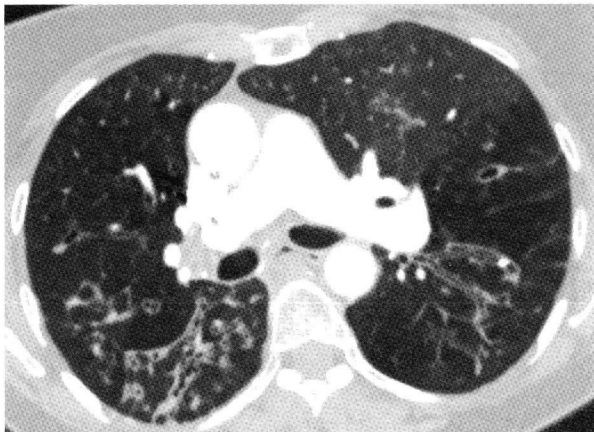

**Which of the following is the most likely diagnosis?**

(A) Bronchiectasis
(B) Centrilobular emphysema
(C) Chronic bronchitis
(D) Pulmonary Langerhans cell histiocytosis

## Item 82

A 35-year-old woman is evaluated in the emergency department for a 3-week history of worsening cough and dyspnea. She works as a sand mover operator at a hydraulic fracturing site and she notes that there is a large amount of dust that often clogs her respirator. She is otherwise healthy and has no history of fever, chills, sweats, or sick contacts. She has no current medications.

On physical examination, pulse rate is 110/min and respiration rate is 26/min. Other vital signs are normal. Oxygen saturation is 92% breathing ambient air. Lung examination reveals inspiratory crackles bilaterally. Cardiovascular examination is normal.

Chest radiograph shows patchy bilateral opacities with areas of consolidation in the lower lobes.

Bronchoalveolar lavage shows fluid with milky white return but no organisms; bacterial cultures are negative.

**Which of the following is the most likely diagnosis?**

(A) Acute interstitial pneumonia
(B) Acute silicosis
(C) Asbestosis
(D) Cryptogenic organizing pneumonia

## Item 83

A 66-year-old woman is evaluated for difficult weaning from mechanical ventilation. She was hospitalized 8 days ago with septic shock due to pneumococcal pneumonia and bacteremia. She required mechanical ventilation and was treated with glucocorticoids and neuromuscular blockers. Pneumonia and sepsis have resolved, but she is unable to be weaned from ventilation. Current medications are fentanyl and heparin.

On physical examination, temperature is 37.3 °C (99.1 °F), blood pressure is 133/88 mm Hg, pulse rate is 70/min, and respiration rate is 14/min. Oxygen saturation is 100% on an $F_{IO_2}$ of 0.35. She is awake and obeys commands but displays generalized weakness; she has decreased grip strength, distal lower extremity sensory loss, decreased tendon reflexes, and cannot raise her arms or legs.

Laboratory studies, including the complete blood count, metabolic profile, and electrolytes, are normal.

**Which of the following is the most appropriate next step in the evaluation?**

(A) Cervical spine MRI
(B) Electrodiagnostic testing
(C) Medical Research Council muscle scale
(D) Muscle biopsy

## Item 84

A 36-year-old woman is evaluated for dry cough and progressive dyspnea that limits her ability to exercise. She initially presented 8 weeks ago with cough, fever, sputum production, and dyspnea. A chest radiograph at that time revealed left-lower-lobe opacities; she was diagnosed with pneumonia and treated with azithromycin but had little improvement in her symptoms. Her fever and sputum production have resolved. She is a nonsmoker.

On physical examination, vital signs are normal. Lungs are clear to auscultation.

Repeat chest radiograph reveals patchy opacities bilaterally and several nodular densities that are peripherally predominant in different locations than previous radiographs. High-resolution CT scan of the chest shows extensive ground-glass changes bilaterally with several areas of nodular consolidation that are peripherally predominant and along bronchovascular bundles.

**Which of the following is the most likely diagnosis?**

(A) Acute HIV infection
(B) Community-acquired pneumonia
(C) Cryptogenic organizing pneumonia
(D) Idiopathic pulmonary fibrosis

## Item 85

A 56-year-old man is evaluated in the ICU for hypotension. He was admitted 3 hours ago for acute onset dyspnea. A CT angiogram performed upon admission showed a large, central pulmonary embolism. Treatment was started with subcutaneous low-molecular-weight heparin, and he was transferred to the ICU for monitoring. An hour later he became hypotensive.

CONT.

On physical examination, blood pressure is 78/54 mm Hg, pulse rate is 120/min, and respiration rate is 28/min. Oxygen saturation is 93% on 4 L/min of oxygen through nasal cannula. Lungs are clear on auscultation. Cardiac examination reveals a grade 2/6 systolic murmur above the left lower sternal border. The second heart sound is persistently split.

**Which of the following is the most appropriate treatment?**

(A)  Add recombinant tissue plasminogen activator (rtPA)
(B)  Change to apixaban
(C)  Change to intravenous unfractionated heparin infusion
(D)  Continue low-molecular-weight heparin

## Item 86

A 67-year-old woman is admitted to the ICU for abdominal distention, vomiting, and hypotension. She had a colectomy 3 weeks ago to treat recurrent diverticular bleeding, and postoperatively she had prolonged anorexia and nausea. She was discharged to an extended care facility on enteral nutrition through a small-bore nasogastric tube.

On physical examination, temperature is 36.8 °C (98.2 °F), blood pressure is 100/60 mm Hg, pulse rate is 109/min, and respiration rate is 19/min. BMI is 19. Preoperative BMI was 25. She has temporal wasting, colectomy wound with areas of dehiscence, lower extremity edema, decreased bowel sounds, and distended tympanitic abdomen.

Blood glucose is 65 mg/dL (3.6 mmol/L), albumin is 2.4 g/dL (24 g/L), creatinine is 0.6 mg/dL (53 μmol/L), and blood urea nitrogen is 6 mg/dL (2.14 mmol/L).

Radiograph and CT scan of the abdomen show dilated loops of small bowel. The nasogastric tube is in the proximal jejunum.

Intravenous fluid resuscitation is initiated and surgical consultation is obtained.

**Which of the following is the most appropriate nutritional management?**

(A)  Maintain current enteral nutrition
(B)  Measure gastric residual volume
(C)  Start metoclopramide
(D)  Switch to parenteral nutrition

## Item 87

A 56-year-old woman is evaluated following screening for lung cancer with low-dose chest CT scan. She has a 35-pack-year history of cigarette smoking and continues to smoke. She has no symptoms.

On physical examination, vital signs and the remainder of the physical examination are normal.

Low-dose chest CT scan demonstrates diffuse centrilobular micronodules that are predominant in the midlung and upper lung. There is no evidence of septal line thickening, traction bronchiectasis, honeycombing, ground-glass opacities, or mediastinal or hilar lymphadenopathy.

**Which of the following is the most likely diagnosis?**

(A)  Desquamative interstitial pneumonia
(B)  Idiopathic pulmonary fibrosis

(C)  Pulmonary Langerhans cell histiocytosis
(D)  Respiratory bronchiolitis-associated interstitial lung disease

## Item 88

A 73-year-old man is evaluated for a 3-month history of chronic productive cough, intermittent hemoptysis, night sweats, and 4.5 kg (10 lb) unintentional weight loss. He previously worked as a miner and has a history of chronic silicosis. He also has a 40-pack-year history of smoking, but quit 10 years ago.

On physical examination, vital signs are normal. He is thin and appears ill with temporal muscle wasting. Lung examination reveals bilateral upper-lobe crackles. Cardiac examination is unremarkable.

Chest radiograph reveals bilateral upper-lobe fibrosis with volume loss of the upper lobes and evidence of cavitation, traction of the hila upwards bilaterally, and bilateral calcified hilar lymphadenopathy.

**Which of the following is the most appropriate management?**

(A)  Aspergillus IgG antibody test
(B)  Bronchoscopy with transbronchial biopsy
(C)  High-resolution CT scan of the chest
(D)  Sputum sample for acid-fast bacillus

## Item 89

A 32-year-old woman is evaluated for a 2-month history of gradually worsening dyspnea on exertion. She has difficulty climbing one flight of stairs, but has no wheezing or cough. She was hospitalized 6 months ago for a cholecystectomy complicated by sepsis, with a 2-week ICU stay requiring mechanical ventilation, but she recovered without difficulty. She uses an albuterol inhaler as needed, but this does not provide significant relief.

On physical examination, vital signs are normal. Oxygen saturation is 97% breathing ambient air. Cardiopulmonary examination is normal.

Chest radiograph is normal; spirometry is performed, and a flow-volume loop is shown.

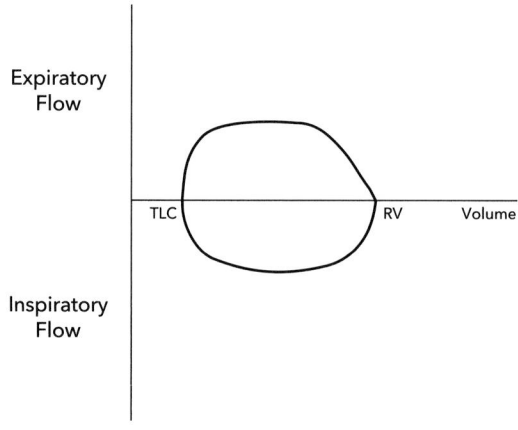

Which of the following is the most likely diagnosis?

(A) Asthma

(B) COPD

(C) Fixed upper airway obstruction

(D) Normal lung function

## Item 90

A 24-year-old woman is evaluated for recent onset of exertional dyspnea and chest tightness occurring three to four times weekly. She has a history of asthma since childhood that was previously well controlled with albuterol and budesonide. She is 14 weeks pregnant, and she stopped taking her medications 4 weeks ago out of concern for effects on the fetus. She has no other medical problems.

On physical examination, vital signs are normal. Oxygen saturation is 97% breathing ambient air. Chest examination shows good air movement with occasional expiratory wheezing. The remainder of the examination is normal.

Spirometry demonstrates mild airflow obstruction.

Which of the following is the most appropriate management?

(A) Begin fluticasone/salmeterol

(B) Begin low-dose prednisone

(C) Monitor serial peak flow measurements

(D) Restart previous medications

## Item 91

A 78-year-old man is evaluated for an 8-month history of nonproductive cough and dyspnea on exertion, particularly when going up an incline. He has a 40-pack-year smoking history but quit 15 years ago. His sister had pulmonary fibrosis.

On physical examination, vital signs are normal. Clubbing is present. Lung examination reveals inspiratory crackles at the bases. Cardiac examination is normal. Pulmonary function testing shows an FVC of 75% of predicted and an $FEV_1/FVC$ ratio of 0.85.

Chest radiograph demonstrates small lung volumes and interstitial opacities at the bases.

Which of the following is the most appropriate diagnostic test to perform next?

(A) Contrast-enhanced chest CT scan

(B) High-resolution chest CT scan

(C) Low-dose chest CT scan

(D) PET/CT imaging

## Item 92

A 62-year-old man is evaluated for a 2-month history of nonproductive cough, progressive dyspnea, and fatigue. He reports a 6.8-kg (15-lb) weight loss during this time. He has a 30-pack-year history of smoking. He worked in a navy ship yard 32 years ago. His history is otherwise unremarkable.

On physical examination, vital signs are normal. Oxygen saturation is 94% breathing ambient air. Lung examination findings are consistent with a right pleural effusion. The remainder of the examination is normal. A complete blood count and metabolic profile are normal.

Chest radiograph shows a large right pleural effusion.

Thoracentesis is performed and removes 1200 mL of serosanguineous fluid.

**Pleural fluid analysis:**

| | |
|---|---|
| Cytology | Negative |
| Glucose | 89 mg/dL (4.9 mmol/L) |
| Lactate dehydrogenase | 200 U/L |
| pH | 7.36 |
| Total protein | 3.8 g/dL (38 g/L) |

**Laboratory studies:**

| | |
|---|---|
| Serum lactate dehydrogenase | 235 U/L |
| Serum total protein | 6.2 g/dL (62 g/L) |

The patient returns 2 weeks later with a recurrent pleural effusion. CT scan of his chest demonstrates a moderate right pleural effusion with no parenchymal or pleural abnormalities noted. Thoracentesis is repeated; pleural fluid analysis is similar to the initial analysis, and cytology is again negative.

Which of the following is the most appropriate next step?

(A) Closed pleural biopsy

(B) Measure pleural fluid triglycerides

(C) Resend a pleural fluid specimen for cytology

(D) Thoracoscopy and pleural biopsy

## Item 93

A 63-year-old man is evaluated for symptoms of gradually increasing dyspnea on exertion. Symptoms began about 2 years ago with activities such as golfing, and recently he notes dyspnea and occasional nonproductive cough with stair climbing in his home. He has no palpitations, chest pressure, wheezing, orthopnea, or systemic symptoms. History is significant for hypertension, 30-pack-year tobacco use (quit smoking 1 year ago), and obesity. He currently takes chlorthalidone.

On physical examination, vital signs are normal. Oxygen saturation is 92% on ambient air. BMI is 31. Pulmonary examination demonstrates basilar inspiratory crackles; cardiac examination is normal. The remainder of the examination is unremarkable.

Laboratory studies, including a basic metabolic panel and complete blood count, are normal.

Pulmonary function testing reveals an $FEV_1$ of 70% of predicted, an FVC of 65% of predicted, an $FEV_1/FVC$ ratio of 0.78%, and a $D_{LCO}$ of 63% of predicted. Total lung capacity is 70% of predicted.

Chest radiograph demonstrates diffuse interstitial reticulonodular infiltrates.

Which of the following is the most appropriate test to perform next?

(A) Bronchoscopy with transbronchial lung biopsy

(B) Cardiopulmonary exercise test

(C) High-resolution CT scan of the chest

(D) Methacholine challenge testing

## Item 94

A 42-year-old man is evaluated for a 1-year history of disruptive snoring. His wife has not observed gasping, choking, or pauses in breathing. His normal sleep schedule is 10:30 PM to 6:30 AM. He awakens feeling refreshed and has no daytime sleepiness.

On physical examination, vital signs are normal. BMI is 34.6. He has a low-lying soft palate, his neck is 43 cm (17 in) in circumference, and he has patent nasal passages.

**Which of the following is the most appropriate management?**

(A) Home sleep testing
(B) Polysomnography
(C) Radiofrequency ablation of soft palate
(D) Weight loss program

## Item 95

A 58-year-old woman is evaluated for 6 months of progressive dyspnea and cough. She was treated for breast cancer 10 years ago with a radical mastectomy on the left side, lymph node dissection, chemotherapy, and radiation. Her functional status is limited only by the dyspnea.

On physical examination, vital signs are normal. Oxygen saturation is 94% breathing ambient air. Lung examination is consistent with a left-side pleural effusion. The remainder of the physical examination is normal.

Chest radiograph shows moderate left-sided pleural effusion.

Thoracentesis is performed removing 1100 mL of serosanguineous fluid, providing significant relief of her symptoms. Cytology is positive for adenocarcinoma. The patient initiates therapy for metastatic breast cancer. During the next 2 weeks the patient requires repeated thoracentesis to remove large quantities of pleural fluid. Each thoracentesis provides significant relief of dyspnea for about 2 to 3 days.

**Which of the following is the most appropriate management of the pleural effusions?**

(A) Indwelling pleural catheter placement
(B) Pleurectomy
(C) Serial thoracentesis
(D) Talc pleurodesis

## Item 96

A 19-year-old man is brought to the emergency department after he attended a party with friends. He is anxious and tremulous. He has a history of depression. His only medication is fluoxetine.

On physical examination, he is alert and oriented. Temperature is 38.9 °C (102 °F), blood pressure is 136/79 mm Hg, pulse rate is 112/min, and respiration rate is 20/min. Oxygen saturation is 98% breathing ambient air. Physical examination is notable for slow, continuous, horizontal eye movements, tremor of extremities, hyperreflexia, and sustained ankle clonus and spontaneous myoclonus. The physical examination is otherwise normal.

Urine toxicology screening is pending.

**Which of the following is the most likely diagnosis?**

(A) Anticholinergic toxicity
(B) Malignant hyperthermia
(C) Neuroleptic malignant syndrome
(D) Serotonin syndrome

## Item 97

A 62-year-old woman with alcoholic cirrhosis is evaluated for hypovolemic shock. She was hospitalized 24 hours ago with upper gastrointestinal bleeding. She underwent upper endoscopy, and a bleeding distal esophageal varix was controlled with epinephrine injection and banding. Gastric varices were also noted. Today she vomited 300 mL of bright red blood. Current medications are lactulose, rifaximin, pantoprazole, norfloxacin, and octreotide.

On physical examination, blood pressure is 79/54 mm Hg, pulse rate is 95/min, and respiration rate is 21/min. Oxygen saturation is 94% on 2 L/min of oxygen through nasal cannula. Ascites and splenomegaly are present.

Laboratory studies this morning reveal a hemoglobin level of 8 g/dL (80 g/L), platelet count of 74,000/µL (74 × 10⁹/L), and an INR of 1.4.

**Which of the following is the most appropriate immediate management?**

(A) Packed red blood cell transfusion
(B) Recombinant factor VII infusion
(C) Transjugular intrahepatic portosystemic shunting
(D) Upper endoscopy

## Item 98

A 45-year-old man is evaluated in the emergency department for alcohol intoxication, but the source and type of alcohol consumed are unknown. He has a history of heavy ethanol use and occasional isopropanol use.

On physical examination, vital signs are normal. Oxygen saturation is 97% on ambient air. He is somnolent but easily aroused.

**Laboratory studies**

| | |
|---|---|
| Bicarbonate | 24 mEq/L (24 mmol/L) |
| Blood urea nitrogen | 14 mg/dL (5 mmol/L) |
| Chloride | 106 mEq/L (106 mmol/L) |
| Creatinine | 1.6 mg/dL (141.4 µmol/L) |
| Ethanol | Negative |
| Glucose | 90 mg/dL (5 mmol/L) |
| Osmolality, plasma | 315 mOsm/kg H₂O |
| Potassium | 4.1 mEq/L (4.1 mmol/L) |
| Sodium | 139 mEq/L (139 mmol/L) |

**In addition to monitoring for signs of alcohol withdrawal, which of the following is the most appropriate treatment?**

(A) Fomepizole
(B) Hemodialysis
(C) Levetiracetam
(D) Supportive care

## Item 99

A 63-year-old man is evaluated in follow-up for a lung mass found during evaluation for a persistent cough. He is a current smoker with a 60-pack-year smoking history. His medical history is otherwise unremarkable, and he takes no medications.

Upon physical examination, vital signs are normal. The remainder of the physical examination is normal.

Laboratory studies, including liver chemistry tests, sodium, and calcium, are normal.

Chest radiograph shows a 2-cm nodule in the right upper lobe that was not seen on previous imaging. CT and PET scans demonstrate PET positivity of the lung lesion and in the mediastinal lymph nodes.

**Which of the following is the most appropriate diagnostic procedure to perform next?**

(A) CT-guided needle biopsy
(B) Endobronchial ultrasound and mediastinal lymph node biopsy
(C) Sputum cytology
(D) Thoracoscopic lung biopsy with lymph node dissection

## Item 100

A 38-year-old woman is evaluated in the emergency department for unresponsiveness. On arrival she was minimally responsive with miotic pupils and a respiration rate of 4/min, but 5 minutes after administration of two doses of intravenous naloxone, her respiration rate is 15/min, and she is awake, oriented, and able to converse. She does not remember what happened before her admission, but her history is significant for heroin use.

On physical examination, vital signs are normal. Oxygen saturation is 99% breathing ambient air. The physical examination is unremarkable save for miotic pupils and signs of "needle tracks" on the arms.

**Which of the following is the most appropriate management?**

(A) Administer regular doses of naloxone starting now
(B) Continue to observe for several hours
(C) Discharge now with outpatient follow-up
(D) Elective endotracheal tube placement now

## Item 101

A 74-year-old woman is evaluated in the hospital for loss of consciousness 1 day after total hip replacement. She suddenly became unresponsive and hypotensive while sitting in bed. Before this event she was doing well and discharge planning was under way. She has a remote history of penicillin allergy manifesting as hives. She received one dose of prophylactic cefazolin at the time of surgery. Her only medications are oxycodone and low-molecular-weight heparin.

On physical examination, blood pressure is 76/48 mm Hg, pulse rate is 116/min, and respiration rate is 26/min. Oxygen saturation is 80% on a 100% oxygen nonrebreather mask. The skin is cool and mottled but without rash. Cardiac sounds are soft, without murmur, but with persistent splitting of the second heart sound. Jugular venous distention is noted. The lungs are clear bilaterally.

**Which of the following is the most likely diagnosis?**

(A) Anaphylactic shock
(B) Opiate overdose
(C) Pulmonary embolism
(D) Tension pneumothorax

## Item 102

A 56-year-old woman is evaluated in follow-up after polysomnography documented an apnea-hypopnea index of 6, a mean oxyhemoglobin saturation of 86.4%, and 38% of sleep time with an oxygen saturation of less than 90% of predicted. She has type 2 diabetes mellitus and hypertension. Current medications are metformin and lisinopril.

On physical examination, vital signs are normal. Oxygen saturation is 91% breathing ambient air. BMI is 44. Other than +1 ankle edema, the remainder of the physical examination, including neurological examination, is unremarkable.

Laboratory studies reveal a hemoglobin level of 16.9 g/dL (169 g/L). Arterial blood gas studies show a pH of 7.36, a $P_{CO_2}$ of 58 mm Hg (7.7 kPa), and a $P_{O_2}$ of 59 mm Hg (7.8 kPa).

Chest radiograph demonstrates clear lung fields.

**Which of the following is the most likely diagnosis?**

(A) Amyotrophic lateral sclerosis
(B) Central sleep apnea
(C) Obesity hypoventilation syndrome
(D) Severe obstructive sleep apnea

## Item 103

A 54-year-old woman is evaluated in the office for an exacerbation of bronchiectasis characterized by low-grade fever, cough, and voluminous purulent sputum production progressing during the past 5 days. Her last exacerbation was 3 months ago and was treated with antibiotics. The results of the sputum culture from that episode are not available.

On physical examination, temperature is 38.0 °C (100.4 °F) and respiration rate is 18/min. All other vital signs are normal. Oxygen saturation is 96% breathing ambient air. Pulmonary examination reveals scattered inspiratory squeaks but no wheezes or crackles.

A chest radiograph does not show any infiltrates.

Sputum Gram stain shows gram-negative bacilli and a culture is pending.

**Which of the following is the most appropriate empiric treatment?**

(A) Amoxicillin
(B) Azithromycin
(C) Azithromycin and prednisone
(D) Inhaled tobramycin
(E) Levofloxacin

# Answers and Critiques

## Item 1     Answer:   A

**Educational Objective:** Treat an asthma exacerbation in the hospital.

This patient should be hospitalized for further management. She has an asthma exacerbation and factors that increase her risk of asthma-related death, including several recent exacerbations, history of intubation for asthma, history of anxiety, and poor compliance with her controller medications. She also has worrisome clinical signs, including tachycardia and diminished oxygen saturation, increased work of breathing and decreased air movement on chest examination. These physical findings suggest a severe degree of airflow obstruction and risk for impending respiratory failure; therefore, the most appropriate site of care is the hospital.

Management should include close monitoring of dyspnea, work of breathing, and vital signs; frequent bronchodilator treatment; and systemic glucocorticoids. Pulse oximetry may be falsely reassuring because patients maintain normal oxygen levels despite high work of breathing, and hypoxemia is a late sign of pending respiratory failure. In patients who are at high risk or have lack of symptom resolution with initial therapies, arterial blood gas assessment is vital and should initially reveal hyperventilation with a low arterial $P_{CO_2}$. Normalization of the arterial $P_{CO_2}$ could be an early indicator of respiratory muscle fatigue and impending respiratory arrest.

Outpatient treatment with prednisone and the patient's other medications would not be appropriate for this high-risk patient with severe asthma.

### KEY POINT

- Patients with asthma exacerbations who have signs that indicate a severe attack should be hospitalized.

### Bibliography

Prasad Kerlin M. In the clinic. Asthma. Ann Intern Med. 2014;160:ITC3 2-15; quiz ITC3 16-9. [PMID: 24737276]

## Item 2     Answer:   C

**Educational Objective:** Recognize the role of NSAIDs in poor control of asthma.

Treatment with ibuprofen should be discontinued for this patient, and therapy with prednisone should be started. This patient is presenting with signs of aspirin-exacerbated respiratory disease, triggered by his use of ibuprofen. This condition refers to upper and lower respiratory tract reactions to ingestion of substances inhibiting cyclooxygenase-1, which includes aspirin and many NSAIDs. Also known as aspirin-exacerbated respiratory disease or Samter's triad, aspirin-sensitive asthma includes severe persistent asthma, aspirin sensitivity, and hyperplastic eosinophilic sinusitis with nasal polyposis. Asthma is worsened by exposure to aspirin or other NSAIDs, likely because of the inhibition of cyclooxygenase and the resulting increase in leukotriene synthesis. Ingestion of cyclooxygenase-1–inhibiting substances can sometimes cause life-threatening bronchospasm, but patients can also have less severe symptoms, which often cause them to not recognize these substances as a trigger. In addition, the sensitivity to aspirin and other NSAIDs develops over time, generally after the onset of rhinosinusitis. Treatment consists of avoidance of aspirin or other NSAIDs along with typical asthma management. For patients who require aspirin use (such as those with coronary artery disease), an aspirin desensitization procedure can be performed. Successful desensitization down-regulates leukotriene receptors and modifies interleukin sensitivity, which may relieve asthma symptoms in some patients. For this reason, the addition of a leukotriene inhibitor such as montelukast or zafirlukast to an asthma maintenance regimen is helpful for most patients to modify the leukotriene dysregulation thought to contribute to the syndrome; however, addition of a leukotriene inhibitor alone would not be the appropriate next step for this patient.

24-Hour esophageal pH monitoring is helpful to diagnose gastroesophageal reflux disease, but the patient has no symptoms of this; moreover, a trial of empiric proton pump inhibitor therapy would be indicated before invasive testing.

A nasal polypectomy may be helpful in the long-term management of this syndrome, but it is not the initial step.

### KEY POINT

- Treatment of aspirin-exacerbated respiratory disease consists of symptom treatment with glucocorticoids and removal of the exposure; treatment can also include a leukotriene receptor antagonist.

### Bibliography

Ledford DK, Wenzel SE, Lockey RF. Aspirin or other nonsteroidal inflammatory agent exacerbated asthma. J Allergy Clin Immunol Pract. 2014;2:653-7. [PMID: 25439353] doi:10.1016/j.jaip.2014.09.009

## Item 3     Answer:   B

**Educational Objective:** Treat chronic bronchitis and prevent frequent COPD exacerbations with roflumilast.

Roflumilast is the most appropriate treatment. It is used primarily as add-on therapy in severe COPD associated with chronic bronchitis and a history of recurrent exacerbations despite other therapies; it has been shown to improve lung function and reduce risk and frequency of exacerbations in these individuals. However, it is not a bronchodilator, is expensive, and has not been shown to be effective in other groups of patients with COPD. Common side effects include diarrhea, nausea, weight loss, and headache. Recently the FDA has raised concerns regarding psychiatric adverse events with roflumilast (anxiety, depression, insomnia). Roflumilast is contraindicated in patients with liver impairment and has significant drug interactions.

Oral glucocorticoids, such as prednisone, are reserved for limited periodic use in treating exacerbations of COPD and may provide some benefit in decreasing hospital readmission rates after exacerbation. Long-term oral glucocorticoid therapy has limited, if any, benefit in COPD and carries a high risk for other significant side effects (such as muscle weakness and decreased functional status) and is generally not recommended.

Methylxanthines such as theophylline have shown modest treatment benefit in COPD, likely due to a bronchodilating effect mediated by nonselective inhibition of phosphodiesterase. However, the potential toxicity of this class of drugs coupled with their reduced efficacy has led to increasingly limited use. Although they may be helpful in any classification of COPD, they tend to be used in selected patients with late-stage disease or for patients in whom other preferred therapies have proved ineffective for symptomatic relief; they may also be used when other medications are not available or affordable.

Clinical trials have demonstrated that chronic macrolide therapy is associated with a reduction in the rate of exacerbation in patients with moderate to severe COPD despite optimal maintenance inhaler therapy. Macrolide antibiotic therapy and roflumilast have not been directly compared in patients with frequent exacerbations of COPD and the choice among the two is informed by benefits and risks on an individual patient basis. Trimethoprim–sulfamethoxazole has not been shown to prevent exacerbations of COPD.

**KEY POINT**

- Roflumilast, a selective phosphodiesterase-4 inhibitor, is used as add-on therapy in severe COPD associated with chronic bronchitis and a history of recurrent exacerbations to reduce risk and frequency of exacerbations.

**Bibliography**
Chong J, Leung B, Poole P. Phosphodiesterase 4 inhibitors for chronic obstructive pulmonary disease. Cochrane Database Syst Rev. 2017;9:CD002309. [PMID: 28922692] doi:10.1002/14651858.CD002309.pub5

**Item 4**  **Answer:**  **B**

**Educational Objective:** Evaluate a patient for obstructive sleep apnea.

The most appropriate next step is home sleep testing. This patient has signs (loud snoring, breathing pauses, gasping), symptoms (excessive daytime sleepiness, nocturia), and physical examination findings (BMI greater than 30, large neck size, crowded oropharynx, a low-lying soft palate) consistent with obstructive sleep apnea (OSA). Home sleep testing is

the preferred diagnostic test when there is a high likelihood of OSA and an absence of significant comorbidities such as cardiopulmonary or neuromuscular disease. If OSA is confirmed, daytime sleepiness represents a strong indication for treatment. Polysomnography performed in a sleep laboratory is the preferred diagnostic test for OSA in patients with underlying cardiopulmonary or neuromuscular disease who might require advanced positive airway pressure modes (such as bilevel positive airway pressure) or supplemental oxygen but would not be indicated for this patient who has no evidence of such comorbidities.

Objective testing should occur before treatment of OSA is prescribed. Auto-adjusting positive airway pressure generally follows home sleep testing that confirms OSA.

Occasionally, multiple sleep latency testing (MSLT) is used to provide an objective measure of sleepiness. MSLT requires a series of brief nap opportunities during the course of a full day in a sleep laboratory to determine the average time to fall asleep and is time and labor intensive; however, it is necessary to establish the diagnoses of narcolepsy and idiopathic hypersomnia. A mean sleep latency of less than 5 minutes is a clear indicator of pathologic sleepiness, whereas more than 15 minutes is considered normal. If these additional sleep disorders were suspected in a patient with obstructive sleep apnea, MSLT would occur only after positive airway pressure treatment has been optimized.

There is no established role for overnight pulse oximetry as a screening or diagnostic tool in OSA. With limited sensitivity and specificity in the symptomatic patient with a high pretest probability of OSA, overnight oximetry is not likely to add diagnostic information beyond home sleep testing, nor will it alter the decision to treat.

**KEY POINT**

- Home sleep testing is the first test indicated in a patient with a high probability of obstructive sleep apnea without underlying cardiopulmonary or neuromuscular disease.

**Bibliography**
Kapur VK, Auckley DH, Chowdhuri S, Kuhlmann DC, Mehra R, Ramar K, et al. Clinical practice guideline for diagnostic testing for adult obstructive sleep apnea: an American Academy of Sleep Medicine clinical practice guideline. J Clin Sleep Med. 2017;13:479-504. [PMID: 28162150] doi:10.5664/jcsm.6506

**Item 5**  **Answer:**  **A**

**Educational Objective:** Evaluate a subsolid solitary pulmonary nodule.

The most appropriate management of the pulmonary nodule is to perform follow-up chest CT scanning at 6-12 months and then every 2 years for 5 years, as recommended by the Fleischner Society Guidelines. Nodules are classified as solid or subsolid. Subsolid nodules are either pure ground-glass nodules (no solid component) or part-solid nodules (both ground-glass and solid components). A ground-glass nodule is defined as a focal area of increased attenuation in the lung through which normal parenchymal structures can still be seen. The classification of nodules helps in the assessment of malignant potential (for example, adenocarcinoma is more likely to present as a subsolid and part-solid nodule) and guides appropriate follow-up. This patient has a solitary pure ground-glass subsolid nodule that is larger than 6 mm. Earlier guidelines recommended initial follow-up at 3 months, but this was changed to 6-12 months because earlier follow-up is unlikely to affect the outcome of these characteristically indolent lesions. The average doubling time of subsolid, cancerous nodules typically is 3-5 years. Therefore, longer initial and total follow-up intervals are recommended for subsolid nodules than for solid nodules.

Evaluation with a PET/CT scan would be recommended for a solid nodule that is greater than 8 mm in size. This test most commonly uses fluorodeoxyglucose (FDG) as a metabolic marker to identify rapidly dividing cells such as tumor cells and, to a lesser degree, any inflammatory lesion. A nodule that demonstrates no FDG uptake is unlikely to be malignant. PET/CT imaging can also be used for staging a cancer by determining the presence or absence of metastatic disease.

Tissue sampling would not be appropriate at this stage because the vast majority of these lesions are not malignant.

**KEY POINT**

- Subsolid lung nodules 6-8 mm in size should be initially followed up at 6-12 months and then every 2 years for 5 years because of the slow rate of growth if such masses are malignant.

**Bibliography**

MacMahon H, Naidich DP, Goo JM, Lee KS, Leung ANC, Mayo JR, et al. Guidelines for management of incidental pulmonary nodules detected on CT images: from the Fleischner Society 2017. Radiology. 2017;284:228-243. [PMID: 28240562] doi:10.1148/radiol.2017161659

**Item 6    Answer:    A**

**Educational Objective:** Diagnose an acute exacerbation of idiopathic pulmonary fibrosis.

The most likely diagnosis is an acute exacerbation of idiopathic pulmonary fibrosis (IPF). The clinical course of an acute exacerbation is acute to subacute onset (typically shorter than 30 days) of worsening dyspnea, and the medical evaluation does not reveal another cause for dyspnea such as infection, heart failure, or pulmonary embolism. High-resolution CT scan shows new-onset diffuse bilateral ground-glass opacities. Patients may develop frank respiratory failure due to an exacerbation or stabilize at a new, worsened baseline. The proposed criteria for an acute IPF exacerbation have recently changed and now include the possibility of a "trigger" and, therefore, the history of a viral prodrome and presence of rhinovirus no longer exclude this diagnosis. Evidence-based treatment options are limited. The role for mechanical ventilation in this population is often futile if there is not a reversible cause and particularly if there is not a

path to lung transplantation. Glucocorticoids are often used in combination with broad spectrum antibiotics in the hopes of a clinical response. Many patients are now being treated for IPF with nintedanib or pirfenidone, although the value of continuing these antifibrotic therapies in the acute exacerbation phase of disease is currently unknown.

Heart failure does not fully explain the acute worsening of IPF because the B-type natriuretic peptide is low.

Hypersensitivity pneumonitis is the result of an immunologic response to repetitive inhalation of antigens and high-level exposure and will often be associated with fevers, flulike symptoms, cough, and shortness of breath, typically during a period of 48 hours. The most common sources of antigens are thermophilic actinomycetes, fungi, and bird droppings. High-resolution CT imaging of the chest shows findings of ground-glass opacities and centrilobular micronodules that are upper-lung and midlung predominant. The patient's history and radiological findings are not consistent with this diagnosis.

Nonspecific interstitial pneumonia (NSIP) is a disease that predominantly affects the lower lobes of the lung. Unlike IPF, NSIP tends to affect a younger patient population and is strongly associated with connective tissue disease. The ground glass opacities on this patient's CT scan indicate an acute exacerbation with a background of usual interstitial pneumonia and are not consistent with NSIP.

**KEY POINT**

- An acute exacerbation of idiopathic pulmonary fibrosis begins with an abrupt worsening during a few days to weeks in the absence of another cause for dyspnea such as infection, heart failure, or pulmonary embolism and is notable for new bilateral ground-glass opacities superimposed on findings consistent with usual interstitial pneumonia on CT scan.

**Bibliography**

Collard HR, Ryerson CJ, Corte TJ, Jenkins G, Kondoh Y, Lederer DJ, et al. Acute exacerbation of idiopathic pulmonary fibrosis. An international working group report. Am J Respir Crit Care Med. 2016;194:265-75. [PMID: 27299520] doi:10.1164/rccm.201604-0801CI

**Item 7    Answer:    C**

**Educational Objective:** Diagnose a patient with vocal cord dysfunction.

The most appropriate management is laryngoscopy. This patient has symptoms suggestive of vocal cord dysfunction, which is caused by paradoxical adduction of the vocal cords during inspiration, leading to functional upper airway obstruction. The diagnosis is suggested by dysphonia midchest or throat tightness with exposure to particular triggers such as strong irritants or emotions; difficulty breathing in; and symptoms that only partially respond to asthma medications. Patients may also experience midchest tightness, dyspnea, cough, and dysphonia, and stridor may be detected as inspiratory monophonic wheezing. Vocal cord dysfunction

CONT.

is commonly misdiagnosed as asthma, leading to excessive health care use. Diagnosis is ideally made by visualization of the abnormal vocal cord adduction during laryngoscopy. It may also be diagnosed if spirometry happens to capture a flat inspiratory limb on the flow-volume loop. However, if patients are unable to tolerate laryngoscopy while symptomatic, empiric therapy should be started if there is a high clinical suspicion of vocal cord dysfunction. Treatment consists of speech therapy utilizing cognitive behavioral techniques.

Because disorders affecting the upper respiratory tract may affect the lower tract, sinus disorders may be associated with worsening control of asthma. Patients with frequent asthma exacerbations should be evaluated for occult sinus disease, as untreated upper airway inflammation may contribute to poor asthma control. However, CT scan of the sinuses is not appropriate because sinus disease cannot explain the patient's upper chest and throat tightness, dysphonia, inspiratory monophonic wheezing, or unresponsiveness to intensive asthma treatment.

Increasing the prednisone dose is not likely to improve the patient's symptoms, which are not likely or entirely due to airway inflammation and will expose the patient to more potential side effects of glucocorticoids.

Asthma has been associated with obstructive sleep apnea (OSA). In difficult-to-control asthma, OSA is a significant risk factor for frequent exacerbations. Treatment of OSA improves asthma symptoms. However, this patient has no obvious risk factors for OSA and OSA cannot explain the patient's upper chest and throat tightness, dysphonia, or inspiratory monophonic wheezing. Therefore polysomnography is not indicated.

### KEY POINT

- The diagnosis of vocal cord dysfunction is suggested by midchest tightness with exposure to particular triggers such as strong irritants or emotions; difficulty breathing in; and symptoms that only partially respond to asthma medications.

### Bibliography

Idrees M, FitzGerald JM. Vocal cord dysfunction in bronchial asthma. A review article. J Asthma. 2015;52:327-35. [PMID: 25365113] doi:10.3109/02770903.2014.982288

### Item 8          Answer:     C

**Educational Objective:**  Treat a patient on mechanical ventilation for delirium using nonpharmacologic interventions.

Early mobilization with physical and occupational therapy and interruption of sedation should be used to decrease the duration of delirium. This patient has acute onset of cognitive dysfunction, impairment of attention, and fluctuating mental status, which are features of delirium. Increased or decreased psychomotor activity, disorganized thinking, disorientation, and perceptual disturbances are other supportive features. The use of a screening instrument (such as the Confusion Assessment Method) allows for improved recognition and diagnosis of delirium. Delirium contributes to length of ICU stay, morbidity, mortality, and post-intensive care cognitive impairment. A study of critically ill patients on mechanical ventilation demonstrated that an early physical and occupational therapy program reduced delirium by 2 days compared to controls.

Haloperidol is used to decrease hyperactive features of delirium. Currently, there is no strong evidence in favor of its use for treating delirium in critically ill patients.

Current guidelines for sedation in the ICU favor strategies that control pain, target lighter sedation, avoid benzodiazepines, and favor early mobility. The use of benzodiazepines is associated with an increased incidence of delirium, and would not be appropriate for this patient showing signs of delirium when compared with nonbenzodiazepine sedation strategies.

The practice of having all critically ill patients on mechanical ventilation receive continuous deep sedation is no longer followed, thus increasing the propofol dosage would not be appropriate. A practice-changing trial demonstrated that daily interruption of sedation decreased length of mechanical ventilation and stay in the ICU. Recent trials demonstrated that the use of a light sedation protocol had similar patient outcomes to daily interruption of sedation. Light levels of sedation using a protocol are associated with shorter length of mechanical ventilation and ICU stay.

### KEY POINT

- Early mobilization with physical and occupational therapy and interruption of sedation should be used to prevent and treat delirium in critically ill patients.

### Bibliography

Schweickert WD, Pohlman MC, Pohlman AS, et al: Early physical and occupational therapy in mechanically ventilated, critically ill patients: a randomised controlled trial. Lancet 2009; 373:1874– 1882 PMID 19446324

### Item 9          Answer:     D

**Educational Objective:**  Identify mortality benefits of smoking cessation.

Smoking cessation is the best way to prevent deaths and complications from lung cancer and other diseases. There is evidence of risk reduction within 5 years of quitting smoking. In addition, case-control studies have demonstrated an 80% to 90% relative risk reduction for lung cancer in former smokers who have been abstinent for 15 years.

Chest radiograph and sputum cytology are not recommended as screening tools for lung cancer. Several large-scale controlled clinical trials have been performed and none of them demonstrated a mortality benefit for screening with cytology or chest radiography.

Recently the national lung screening trial demonstrated that screening with low-dose CT (LDCT) reduced mortality in a high-risk population (based on age and smoking history) compared with screening by radiograph (relative risk reduction of 20%). However, smoking cessation is still more likely to save a life than LDCT. The U.S. Preventive Services Task Force does recommend annual screening for lung cancer with LDCT in adults age 55-80 years who have a 30-pack-year smoking history and currently smoke or have quit within the past 15 years. Candidates for screening should take part in shared decision making, which includes a discussion of benefits and risks. Ideally it should take place in the context of a multidisciplinary program to ensure that it is properly performed and downstream testing is managed appropriately. Active smokers engaged in lung cancer screening should be counseled and assessed for smoking cessation at every opportunity.

**KEY POINT**

- Smoking cessation is the best way to prevent deaths and complications from lung cancer and other diseases.

**Bibliography**

Aberle DR, Adams AM, Berg CD, Black WC, Clapp JD, Fagerstrom RM, et al; National Lung Screening Trial Research Team. Reduced lung-cancer mortality with low-dose computed tomographic screening. N Engl J Med. 2011;365:395-409. [PMID: 21714641] doi:10.1056/NEJMoa1102873

## Item 10    Answer:    E

**Educational Objective:** Prevent airway aspiration by establishing a secure airway in patients who are unable to protect their airway.

An endotracheal tube should be placed to establish a secure airway. This patient has upper gastrointestinal bleeding and several features of cirrhosis (telangiectasias, jaundice, ascites), and likely has an acute variceal bleed. Mortality in these patients is high and requires multidisciplinary management. Initial management of esophageal variceal bleeding includes placement of two large-bore intravenous lines, fluid resuscitation, and erythrocyte transfusion to a goal hemoglobin level of 7 g/dL (70 g/L) or greater. Up to 50% of patients with cirrhosis and gastrointestinal bleeding develop infections within 1 week, and prophylactic antimicrobial agents improve mortality rates. A splanchnic vasoconstrictor such as octreotide is recommended for 3 to 5 days. Upper endoscopy with band ligation should be performed urgently after the patient is stabilized, followed by addition of a nonselective β-blocker. For the 10% to 20% of patients with uncontrolled bleeding and those with early rebleeding, a transjugular intrahepatic portosystemic shunt (TIPS) should be placed. Early airway management to prevent aspiration is essential when a patient cannot protect the airway or is otherwise at risk for aspiration of blood or gastric contents. This patient has altered mental status and ongoing hemorrhage, both risk factors for airway aspiration.

A nonselective β-blocker is recommended as secondary prophylaxis against rebleeding after recovery from a variceal bleed, but it would not be warranted in the acute setting in this patient with hypotension.

Oxygen by nasal cannula is not indicated as the patient has adequate oxygenation; furthermore, additional oxygen though nasal cannula would not help establish a secure airway.

An upper endoscopy should be performed in this patient with presumed variceal hemorrhage, but only after his airway has been secured and he has been treated with standard pharmacotherapy (octreotide and antibiotics) and appropriately resuscitated to enable safe endoscopy.

Noninvasive bilevel positive airway pressure ventilation does not provide a secure airway and is contraindicated in patients with altered mental status or risk of vomiting because it can increase the risk of aspiration if the patient were to vomit into the mask.

**KEY POINT**

- In patients who cannot maintain a patent airway or protect the airway against aspiration, a secure airway should be established.

**Bibliography**

Long B, Koyfman A. The emergency medicine evaluation and management of the patient with cirrhosis. Am J Emerg Med. 2017 Dec 23. pii: S0735-6757(17)31049-5. doi: 10.1016/j.ajem.2017.12.047. [Epub ahead of print] [PMID:29290508]

## Item 11    Answer:    A

**Educational Objective:** Treat inadequately controlled mild persistent asthma by stepping up therapy.

This patient has mild persistent asthma (albuterol use more than twice weekly but no more than once per day, and $FEV_1$ greater than 80% predicted) and the most appropriate management is to begin low-dose inhaled glucocorticoids such as beclomethasone. An appropriate dosage would be 40 μg per puff with 1 inhalation twice daily. Patients with asthma who require a short-acting $β_2$-agonist more than twice per week for symptom control, rather than to prevent exercise-induced bronchospasm, are considered uncontrolled. The next step in treatment is the addition of low-dose inhaled glucocorticoids. An alternative would be to add montelukast but low-dose inhaled glucocorticoid therapy is preferred. Inhaler technique should be confirmed in all patients when beginning therapy and reviewed regularly.

When inhaled glucocorticoids alone do not achieve asthma control, the addition of a long-acting $β_2$-agonist (LABA) has proved to be effective as step-up therapy. Combination preparations that contain an inhaled glucocorticoid and a LABA are available, such as fluticasone/salmeterol. In addition to bronchodilation, LABAs appear to potentiate anti-inflammatory effects of inhaled glucocorticoids when taken together. However, beginning an inhaled glucocorticoid and a LABA combination is not appropriate, as this patient has mild persistent asthma and a combination inhaled glucocorticoid/LABA is indicated for moderate persistent asthma.

Anticholinergic agents dilate bronchial smooth muscle by decreasing the constrictive cholinergic tone in the

Answers and Critiques

# Answers and Critiques

airways. Although it is less effective than β₂-agonists, the short-acting agent ipratropium can be used as adjunctive quick-relief therapy during asthma exacerbations. However, this patient has poorly controlled asthma and it is appropriate to start controller therapy, such as an inhaled glucocorticoid, to reduce airway inflammation from asthma.

Leukotriene receptor antagonists (LTRAs), such as montelukast, are not considered preferred first-line controller therapy in any asthma population. LTRAs may have a particular role in aspirin-sensitive asthma and a protective role in exercise-induced asthma; however, low-dose inhaled glucocorticoids are preferred in this patient with uncontrolled mild persistent asthma.

### KEY POINT

- Patients with mild persistent asthma uncontrolled with a short-acting β₂-agonist should be stepped up to a controller medication; low-dose inhaled glucocorticoids are preferred.

### Bibliography

McCracken JL, Veeranki SP, Ameredes BT, Calhoun WJ. Diagnosis and management of asthma in adults: a review. JAMA. 2017;318:279-290. [PMID: 28719697] doi:10.1001/jama.2017.8372

## Item 12    Answer:    C

**Educational Objective:** Diagnose idiopathic pulmonary fibrosis.

The most likely diagnosis is idiopathic pulmonary fibrosis (IPF). Patients with IPF typically present with chronic shortness of breath on exertion and a dry cough. The prevalence of disease increases with increasing age and is rare in individuals younger than 50 years. Clubbing is common. A history of smoking is a risk factor for the development of IPF and is commonly seen in these patients. The finding of bilateral, peripheral, and basal predominant septal line thickening with honeycomb changes on CT scan is consistent with usual interstitial pneumonia pathologic pattern and can also be seen in connective tissue disease, asbestosis, and chronic hypersensitivity pneumonitis. However, the history is negative for symptoms suggestive of connective tissue disease and for significant environmental exposures. The exclusion of connective tissue diseases and environmental exposures combined with a definite usual interstitial pneumonia imaging pattern supports the diagnosis of IPF. Tobacco smoke is associated with the development of several diffuse parenchymal lung diseases (DPLDs), including IPF. There are also several disorders that generally develop only in individuals who are active smokers; these diseases are all subacute, evolving during weeks to months.

Desquamative interstitial pneumonia is due to extensive, diffuse macrophage filling of alveolar spaces and is accompanied by predominant cough and dyspnea symptoms and bilateral ground-glass opacities on chest imaging.

Hypersensitivity pneumonitis, in its chronic form, is the most common DPLD included in the differential diagnosis

for patients with IPF. When fibrosis occurs with chronic hypersensitivity pneumonitis, it is typically in the midlung and upper-lung zones and is associated with an environmental exposure, which was not elicited in this patient. Although many patients with chronic hypersensitivity pneumonitis may no longer have an exposure to a causative antigen, the typical age of onset, history, and basal predominant CT scan abnormalities favor a diagnosis of IPF rather than hypersensitivity pneumonitis.

Pulmonary Langerhans cell histiocytosis is characterized by thin-walled cysts with accompanying nodules and is often associated with pulmonary hypertension. All of these diseases are subacute, evolving during weeks to months and present in active smokers.

Respiratory bronchiolitis–associated interstitial lung disease is used to describe disease in active smokers who have imaging findings of centrilobular micronodules with a pathologic finding of respiratory bronchiolitis on biopsy.

### KEY POINT

- Idiopathic pulmonary fibrosis typically occurs in older individuals with nonproductive cough and progressive dyspnea on exertion; the diagnosis is supported by findings of usual interstitial pneumonitis on a high-resolution CT scan of the chest.

### Bibliography

Raghu G, Collard HR, Egan JJ, Martinez FJ, Behr J, Brown KK, et al; ATS/ERS/JRS/ALAT Committee on Idiopathic Pulmonary Fibrosis. An official ATS/ERS/JRS/ALAT statement: idiopathic pulmonary fibrosis: evidence-based guidelines for diagnosis and management. Am J Respir Crit Care Med. 2011;183:788-824. [PMID: 21471066] doi:10.1164/rccm.2009-040GL

## Item 13    Answer:    E

**Educational Objective:** Assess intravascular volume status.

No further testing is required. The physical examination has several features that suggest she has decreased intravascular volume and reduced systemic vascular resistance. The presence of warm and vasodilated skin, a very low diastolic pressure, absent jugular venous distention, and tachycardia all suggest severe vasodilation. There are several invasive and noninvasive devices available to aid the clinician to confirm the clinical diagnosis; however, none of them alone can provide a definite answer. Integrating the physical examination and basic vital signs remains the best clinical method to define intravascular volume status and the type of shock.

Central venous catheter measurement of venous pressure can provide information that helps confirm the diagnosis of low central venous pressure; however, it is invasive, subject to technical issues, and the presence of spontaneous breathing needs to be considered when obtaining readings. Studies have demonstrated that a single measurement does not help define intravascular volume status or volume responsiveness. Thus the value must be taken in the context of the history and physical exam.

CONT.

Fullness of the vena cava as detected by ultrasonography is thought to correlate with increased right atrial pressure, whereas a collapsing inferior vena cava at the end of expiration suggests volume responsiveness. Volume responsiveness refers to an increase in cardiac output upon the administration of fluid. A common inference is that intravascular volume is high when the patient is not volume responsive; however, this would be a limited assumption as the response to volume also involves cardiac function and infusion volume. In addition, the presence of increased respiratory effort will make the measurements unreliable.

A pulmonary artery catheter will provide a plethora of information on the intravascular pressures (by inference, the volume status) and cardiac output of the patient. However, placing a pulmonary artery catheter in a patient with sepsis is invasive, does not improve management, increases complications, and has not demonstrated improved outcome.

Pulse pressure is the difference between systolic and diastolic arterial blood pressure during respiration induced by positive pressure ventilation. A low variation in pulse pressure is believed to be an indicator of unresponsiveness to a fluid challenge whereas a pulse pressure variation of at least 13% to 15% is associated with volume responsiveness. However, this measurement is only reliable in patients who are mechanically ventilated (and not spontaneously triggering the ventilator), receiving 8 mL/kg or more of tidal volume, and in sinus rhythm.

**KEY POINT**

- The most appropriate method to evaluate volume status remains the physical examination; several technologies can help confirm the assessment.

**Bibliography**

Teboul JL, Saugel B, Cecconi M, De Backer D, Hofer CK, Monnet X, et al. Less invasive hemodynamic monitoring in critically ill patients. Intensive Care Med. 2016;42:1350-9. [PMID: 27155605] doi:10.1007/s00134-016-4375-7

**Item 14    Answer:    C**

**Educational Objective:** Diagnose small cell lung cancer.

The most likely diagnosis is small cell lung cancer (SCLC). SCLC is a neuroendocrine tumor that accounts for approximately 15% of all lung cancers and occurs predominantly in smokers.

This patient has signs and symptoms of hyponatremia and chest CT scan shows a large mediastinal right hilar mass and right-lower-lobe mass (arrows).

Imaging studies in SCLC commonly demonstrate a large hilar mass with bulky mediastinal lymphadenopathy; some patients may not have an obvious primary lesion. Signs and symptoms include cough, dyspnea, weight loss, and debility. Less commonly SCLC can present with endocrinologic or neurologic paraneoplastic syndromes. The

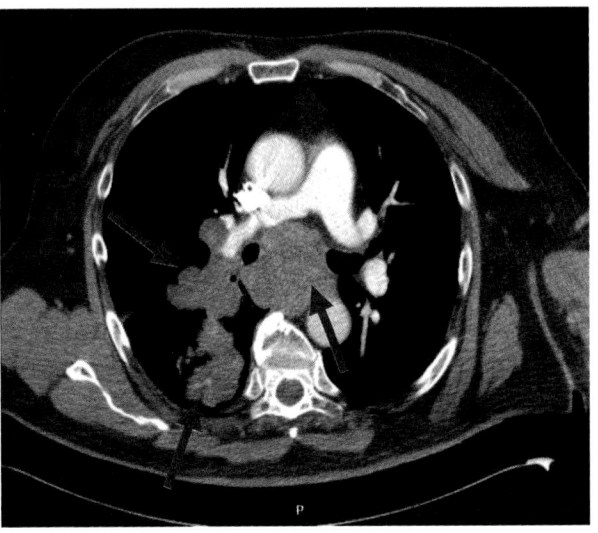

syndrome of inappropriate antidiuretic hormone secretion (SIADH) due to ectopic production of antidiuretic hormone (ADH) is most often due to a SCLC and is rarely seen with other lung tumors. It occurs in approximately 10% of patients and results in hyponatremia. The severity of symptoms is related to the degree of hyponatremia and rapidity of the decrease. They may include anorexia, nausea, and vomiting, but if the decrease is rapid, cerebral edema can occur and may result in irritability, restlessness, personality changes, confusion, coma, seizures, and respiratory arrest. SCLC is more aggressive than non-small cell lung cancer (NSCLC), is usually already disseminated at presentation, and requires prompt treatment; however, it is often initially more sensitive to chemotherapy and radiotherapy but typically relapses and becomes resistant to further treatment. Staging should not delay treatment.

NSCLC accounts for 80% of lung cancers, of which adenocarcinoma is the most common type, followed by squamous cell. Although NSCLC is in the differential diagnosis for this patient, hyponatremia and a large mediastinal mass are most consistent with SCLC.

Malignant pleural mesothelioma typically presents as a recurrent exudative pleural effusion with pleural thickening in a patient with exposure to asbestos. This patient did not present with a pleural effusion, which makes this diagnosis less likely.

**KEY POINT**

- Typical imaging findings in patients with small cell lung cancer (SCLC) include a large mediastinal mass; hyponatremia due to ectopic production of antidiuretic hormone is most often due to SCLC and is rarely seen with other lung tumors.

**Bibliography**

Jett JR, Schild SE, Kesler KA, Kalemkerian GP. Treatment of small cell lung cancer: diagnosis and management of lung cancer, 3rd ed: American College of Chest Physicians evidence-based clinical practice guidelines. Chest. 2013;143:e400S-e419S. [PMID: 23649448] doi:10.1378/chest.12-2363

## Item 15    Answer: B

**Educational Objective:** Evaluate an acute exacerbation of COPD.

An electrocardiogram should be obtained for this patient to evaluate other causes of her acute presentation, such as acute myocardial infarction, arrhythmia, and atrial fibrillation. The first steps in managing a patient with a presumed COPD exacerbation are to confirm the diagnosis. Studies helpful in the evaluation may include pulse oximetry to assess oxygenation or guide oxygen therapy; a chest radiograph to rule out an alternative diagnosis; a complete blood count to identify the presence of polycythemia, anemia, or leukocytosis; arterial blood gas studies; a biochemical panel to assess for electrolyte and glycemic abnormalities; and an electrocardiogram to evaluate tachycardia (as in this patient) and for other possible cardiac comorbidity. This patient has already had a chest radiograph and appropriate laboratory studies but an electrocardiogram is also indicated.

Patients with pulmonary embolism (PE) can present with symptoms similar to a COPD exacerbation. Because of this, pretest probability models such as the Wells criteria have been developed and validated to assist in clinical decision making. Patients who have a low pretest probability for PE using the Wells criteria, such as this patient, and who meet all Pulmonary Embolism Rule-Out Criteria do not need further testing to rule out PE. Physicians should obtain a D-dimer assay in patients with intermediate pretest probability for PE or for those with a low pretest probability for PE who do not meet all Pulmonary Embolism Rule-Out Criteria. In these patients, imaging studies should not be used for initial evaluation.

A sputum culture or Gram stain is not routinely used to assess COPD exacerbations as it rarely changes management. For patients with a confirmed COPD exacerbation with cough, increased sputum, and dyspnea, antibiotics are usually initiated regardless of the results of the sputum Gram stain or culture.

### KEY POINT

- The first steps in managing a patient with a presumed COPD exacerbation are to confirm the diagnosis and to evaluate other causes of the acute presentation.

**Bibliography**

Holden V, Slack III D, McCurdy MT, Shah NG. Diagnosis and management of acute exacerbations of chronic obstructive pulmonary disease. Emerg Med Pract. 2017;19:1-24. [PMID: 28926214]

## Item 16    Answer: C

**Educational Objective:** Identify the sequela of obstructive sleep apnea most responsive to therapy.

Excessive daytime sleepiness is the strongest indication for treatment of obstructive sleep apnea (OSA). Excessive daytime sleepiness is thought to result primarily from disruption of sleep architecture due to repetitive breathing events.

Randomized trials and meta-analyses of systematic reviews show that positive airway pressure therapy reduces the frequency of respiratory events during sleep and is associated with reduction in daytime sleepiness and improved sleep-related quality of life.

Observational studies that suggest benefit from positive airway pressure therapy on the natural history of atrial fibrillation is yet to be proved in randomized trials. There is a similar lack of proved benefit in other important conditions, such as cardiovascular death. In addition, a recent large multicenter trial failed to show mortality benefit afforded by positive airway pressure therapy in those with OSA and cardiovascular disease.

Trials assessing various measures of glucose homeostasis (fasting glucose, insulin resistance, hemoglobin $A_{1c}$) in patients with OSA treated with positive airway pressure have shown inconsistent results. This patient requires adjustment of his medication with the goal of reducing the hemoglobin $A_{1c}$ level.

Positive airway pressure therapy has been shown to modestly reduce blood pressure in those with OSA, but the effects are not always consistent. Those with excessive daytime sleepiness tend to be more responsive to these effects than those who are not sleepy. Also, comparative efficacy trials in those with OSA have shown greater reductions in blood pressure with antihypertensive drug therapy than positive airway pressure. This patient's antihypertensive medications should be adjusted with the goal of achieving the target blood pressure level recommended by the American College of Cardiology/American Heart Association of less than 130/80 mm Hg.

### KEY POINT

- Excessive daytime sleepiness is the strongest indication for treatment of obstructive sleep apnea.

**Bibliography**

McEvoy RD, Antic NA, Heeley E, Luo Y, Ou Q, Zhang X, et al; SAVE Investigators and Coordinators. CPAP for prevention of cardiovascular events in obstructive sleep apnea. N Engl J Med. 2016;375:919-31. [PMID: 27571048] doi:10.1056/NEJMoa1606599

## Item 17    Answer: B 

**Educational Objective:** Treat a patient with obesity hypoventilation syndrome and hypercarbic respiratory failure who does not improve quickly with noninvasive ventilation.

The most appropriate treatment is endotracheal intubation. This patient has developed acute on chronic hypercapnic respiratory failure in the setting of obesity hypoventilation syndrome. In a patient who is able to protect the airway, the initial management of acute hypercapnic respiratory failure due to obesity hypoventilation syndrome includes noninvasive positive pressure ventilation. Because he has an intact gag and cough reflex and is arousable, noninvasive positive pressure ventilation was an appropriate initial choice. However,

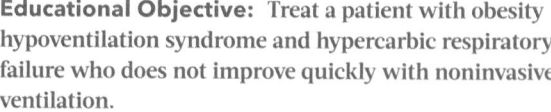

CONT.

when patients cannot protect their airway, do not tolerate bilevel positive airway pressure, or do not improve quickly, such as this patient, early intubation should be considered.

Respiratory stimulants such as acetazolamide have been considered adjunctive therapies of last resort for patients who chronically continue to have hypoventilation despite BPAP therapy and weight loss. Acetazolamide, by blocking carbon dioxide conversion to bicarbonate, can lower pH in the brain and theoretically increases central ventilatory drive. This patient already demonstrates significant acidemia with inadequate central respiratory drive. In addition, randomized trials demonstrating efficacy are lacking. Thus, acetazolamide is not recommended for either acute or chronic hypercapnic respiratory failure.

Although many patients with morbid obesity demonstrate features of obstruction or air trapping on pulmonary function testing, only a fraction have true reversible obstructive airways disease pathology. This patient has no clear evidence of obstruction on examination or chest radiograph and no history of asthma or other obstructive airways pathology. Therefore, prednisone use in this setting is not indicated.

Theophylline is a bronchodilator as well as a direct respiratory stimulant. Its use in obesity-hypoventilation syndrome has never been studied and thus is not recommended for treatment of this or other hypercapnic states.

**KEY POINT**

- Early intubation is indicated for patients with obesity hypoventilation syndrome and hypercapnic respiratory failure who do not improve with noninvasive positive pressure ventilation.

**Bibliography**

Manthous CA, Mokhlesi B. Avoiding management errors in patients with obesity hypoventilation syndrome. Ann Am Thorac Soc. 2016;13:109-14. [PMID: 26512908] doi:10.1513/AnnalsATS.201508-562OT

## Item 18          Answer:    A

**Educational Objective:** Diagnose a patient with $\alpha_1$-antitrypsin deficiency.

An $\alpha_1$-antitrypsin level should be obtained. This patient is younger than the usual age of presentation of COPD, and he does not have a significant smoking history. In this situation it is prudent to rule out other causes of dyspnea, especially in a patient where a diagnosis of COPD is unexpected. White patients experiencing symptoms of COPD and who are younger than 45 years of age or have a strong family history of COPD should be tested for $\alpha_1$-antitrypsin deficiency. Several guidelines even recommend that all patients with COPD regardless of age should be tested for $\alpha_1$-antitrypsin deficiency after weighing the risks and benefits of testing. Patients with this disorder are often misdiagnosed with asthma for many years. They may have a modest smoking history and basilar emphysema (although they may present with any pattern of emphysema), and they may have concurrent liver disease.

Patients with $\alpha_1$-antitrypsin deficiency who never smoke may develop symptoms later in life. If the diagnosis of $\alpha_1$-antitrypsin deficiency is confirmed, $\alpha_1$-antitrypsin augmentation therapy may slow disease progression, although data on its efficacy are limited.

Nitric oxide promotes dilation of bronchial blood vessels and airways. The fractional exhaled nitric oxide (FENO) is a noninvasive test most commonly used in patients with severe airflow obstruction when other techniques are difficult to perform (for example, assessing airflow in a child or mentally impaired adult). High levels of FENO are typically associated with asthma and other inflammatory airway conditions. Measurement of FENO is not indicated as the next diagnostic test in this patient with a history strongly suspicious for $\alpha_1$-antitrypsin deficiency.

High-resolution CT (HRCT) is indicated if diffuse parenchymal lung disease is suspected. HRCT can help narrow the differential diagnosis based on the distribution of the lung parenchymal abnormalities and the presence or absence of associated findings. Diffuse parenchymal lung disease should be suspected in the presence of restrictive or combined obstructive/restrictive diseases. HRCT is also diagnostically definitive for bronchiectasis, but this condition is typically characterized by cough and voluminous, often purulent, sputum production, which is not present in this patient.

A vascular endothelial growth factor-D level can help in the diagnosis of lymphangioleiomyomatosis (LAM). However, LAM is a cystic lung disease that mostly affects young women, so testing would not be indicated for this patient.

**KEY POINT**

- Measurement of $\alpha_1$-antitrypsin level is indicated for white patients experiencing symptoms of COPD and who are younger than 45 years of age or have a strong family history of COPD.

**Bibliography**

American Thoracic Society. American Thoracic Society/European Respiratory Society statement: standards for the diagnosis and management of individuals with alpha-1 antitrypsin deficiency. Am J Respir Crit Care Med. 2003;168:818-900. [PMID: 14522813]

## Item 19          Answer:    C

**Educational Objective:** Treat a patient for side effects of positive airway pressure therapy.

The most appropriate treatment is heated humidification. A common complication of positive airway pressure therapy is desiccation of the nasopharyngeal mucosa by the forced air, often resulting in throat irritation and nasal congestion. In-line heated humidification, available on all positive airway pressure machines, is a simple intervention to mitigate mucosal irritation. Patients can control the temperature and degree of humidity. Although there is conflicting evidence that in-line humidification improves adherence to positive airway pressure therapy, it does mitigate upper airway symptoms.

Bilevel positive airway pressure is indicated for hypoventilation syndromes caused by severe COPD or neuromuscular weakness. There is no evidence that bilevel positive airway pressure is superior to continuous positive airway pressure for the treatment of obstructive sleep apnea without hypoventilation. This patient does not suffer from a hypoventilation syndrome, and he is improving on current therapy; therefore, a change in therapy is not indicated. Finally, bilevel positive airway pressure without humidification will not relieve his upper airway symptoms.

The role of hypnotics in promoting positive airway pressure adherence is controversial and not generally recommended. One study showed nightly eszopiclone (a benzodiazepine receptor agonist) administered to unselected patients during the first 2 weeks of continuous positive airway pressure treatment improved adherence as long as 6 months later. Its continued use beyond initiation of positive airway pressure treatment has not been studied and the risk of side effects may outweigh its benefit. Finally, eszopiclone will not relieve this patient's throat irritation or nasal congestion.

Topical nasal steroids are often prescribed to reduce these side effects of nasal congestion and rhinorrhea, but evidence supporting their effectiveness in reducing upper airway symptoms is sparse. A recent randomized clinical study failed to show a reduction in nasal symptoms or improved adherence to therapy in patients treated with nasal fluticasone compared to placebo.

### KEY POINT

- In-line heated humidification is available on all positive airway pressure machines and is a simple intervention to mitigate mucosal irritation.

### Bibliography

Sommer JU, Kraus M, Birk R, Schultz JD, Hörmann K, Stuck BA. Functional short- and long-term effects of nasal CPAP with and without humidification on the ciliary function of the nasal respiratory epithelium. Sleep Breath. 2014;18:85-93. [PMID: 23657665] doi:10.1007/s11325-013-0853-0

### Item 20    Answer:    C

**Educational Objective:** Treat a patient with eosinophilic asthma with mepolizumab.

The most appropriate treatment is initiation of a trial of mepolizumab therapy. This patient has signs and symptoms of severe persistent asthma that is uncontrolled (more than two exacerbations per year), despite treatment with a high-dose inhaled glucocorticoid, long-acting $\beta_2$-agonist, long-acting anticholinergic agent, leukotriene-receptor antagonist, and oral glucocorticoids, so her therapy should be stepped up. Biologic therapies that target atopic pathways of asthma are indicated in appropriate patients. Currently available agents are directed against either eosinophils or their products (IgE). Interleukin (IL-5) is a pro-eosinophilic cytokine that promotes eosinophil production and contributes to eosinophilic inflammation in the airways. Mepolizumab and

reslizumab are monoclonal antibodies to IL-5 and both agents reduce exacerbations of severe asthma in patients who have blood eosinophil counts of 150/µL or 300/µL, respectively, or higher. Mepolizumab is administered subcutaneously every 4 weeks, whereas reslizumab is an infusion. Although these agents are expensive, patients with uncontrolled eosinophilic asthma treated with mepolizumab have reduced emergency department visits and hospitalizations, and both agents have reduced the requirement for inhaled and oral glucocorticoids. Use of these agents is contraindicated during acute asthma exacerbations.

Treatment with doxycycline is not indicated because there are no signs or symptoms of bacterial infection.

Changing from one inhaled glucocorticoid/long-acting $\beta_2$-agonist to another would not be expected to have a significant effect, as the inhaled glucocorticoid dose is similar and there is no apparent difference in the efficacy of the various combinations.

Omalizumab, a humanized monoclonal antibody directed at IgE, was the first biologic agent approved by the FDA for use in asthma. Administered subcutaneously every 2 to 4 weeks, omalizumab is indicated in patients with moderate to severe persistent asthma with the following characteristics: (1) symptoms inadequately controlled with inhaled glucocorticoids, (2) evidence of allergies to perennial aeroallergens, and (3) serum IgE levels between 30 and 700 U/mL (30-700 kU/L) (normal range, 0-90 U/mL [0-90 kU/L]). Omalizumab has been shown to reduce exacerbations and emergency department visits; it is not indicated for use in patients other than those meeting these treatment parameters.

### KEY POINT

- In patients with moderate to severe uncontrolled asthma with the eosinophilic phenotype, treatment with mepolizumab can reduce emergency department visits, hospitalizations, and requirements for inhaled and oral glucocorticoids.

### Bibliography

Israel E, Reddel HK. Severe and difficult-to-treat asthma in adults. N Engl J Med. 2017;377:965-976. [PMID: 28877019] doi:10.1056/NEJMra1608969

### Item 21    Answer:    D

**Educational Objective:** Treat severe carbon monoxide poisoning with hyperbaric oxygen therapy.

This patient should receive hyperbaric oxygen therapy. Inhaled carbon monoxide has a much higher affinity for hemoglobin binding sites than oxygen and readily forms carboxyhemoglobin, which is an ineffective oxygen transporter and results in reduced tissue oxygen content. Symptoms of carbon monoxide poisoning vary and include headache, confusion, nausea, vomiting, and, in severe cases, loss of consciousness. It is important to understand that carboxyhemoglobin does not lower oxygen saturation measured by standard pulse oximetry or reduce arterial $P_{O_2}$ determined by blood gas analysis.

CONT.

Co-oximetry, which measures carboxyhemoglobin levels, is used to make the diagnosis. She has severe carbon monoxide poisoning due to unvented combustion in a small, enclosed area. Cited indications for hyperbaric oxygen therapy include loss of consciousness, ischemic cardiac changes, neurological deficits, significant metabolic acidosis, or carboxyhemoglobin level greater than 25%. A carboxyhemoglobin level of 50% is critical and needs to be reduced as quickly as possible. Breathing 100% oxygen at normal atmospheric pressure, this patient will clear the carboxyhemoglobin with a half-life of 90 minutes, but hyperbaric oxygen therapy will lower the half-life to 30 minutes. Also, there is considerable risk of delayed neurocognitive impairment following a severe exposure such as this, and hyperbaric oxygen is believed to lower the risk of this long-term complication, although the strength of this evidence is disputed.

Maintaining the current ventilator settings of 50% oxygen or decreasing the oxygen to 30% will not clear the carboxyhemoglobin as rapidly as hyperbaric oxygen. If hyperbaric oxygen therapy is unavailable, or if the toxicity is less severe, administration of 100% oxygen is the most appropriate therapy. However, this patient has mental status changes and the carboxyhemoglobin level is 50%; hyperbaric treatment is clearly indicated.

Carbon monoxide poisoning resulting from smoke inhalation should prompt consideration of concomitant inhaled cyanide poisoning. Hydroxocobalamin effectively binds intracellular cyanide to form cyanocobalamin, which poses no harm. However, this patient's carbon monoxide poisoning is due to combustion of propane in an enclosed space, not a house fire; therefore, hydroxocobalamin is not indicated.

**KEY POINT**

- Cited indications for hyperbaric oxygen therapy include loss of consciousness, ischemic cardiac changes, neurological deficits, significant metabolic acidosis, or carboxyhemoglobin level greater than 25%.

**Bibliography**

Hampson NB, Piantadosi CA, Thom SR, Weaver LK. Practice recommendations in the diagnosis, management, and prevention of carbon monoxide poisoning. Am J Respir Crit Care Med. 2012;186:1095-101. [PMID: 23087025] doi:10.1164/rccm.201207-1284CI

 **Item 22       Answer:   A**

**Educational Objective:** Evaluate a patient who has an acute exacerbation of COPD with arterial blood gas analysis.

Arterial blood gas analysis is the most appropriate test for this patient with a COPD exacerbation. An exacerbation is considered mild when a change in the clinical condition is noted but no change in medication is necessary; moderate when medication changes are made; and severe if emergency department evaluation or hospitalization is required. A severe exacerbation can also be diagnosed if the patient has two of the three following symptoms: increased dyspnea, increased sputum volume, or increased sputum purulence. Studies helpful in the evaluation of a severe exacerbation may include pulse oximetry to assess oxygenation or guide oxygen therapy; a chest radiograph to rule out an alternative diagnosis; a complete blood count to identify the presence of polycythemia, anemia, or leukocytosis; a biochemical panel to assess for electrolyte and glycemic abnormalities; an electrocardiogram to evaluate for a possible cardiac comorbidity; and arterial blood gas analysis. Arterial blood gas analysis is recommended for patients with a severe exacerbation of COPD to assess for hypercapnia and hypoxemia. This information is helpful in determining site of care and the need for additional therapy such as noninvasive mechanical ventilation.

The patient has no signs or symptoms of heart failure or other cardiac disease to explain his presentation. Therefore, B-type natriuretic peptide measurement and echocardiogram are unlikely to change management at this time.

According to best practice advice from the Clinical Guidelines Committee of the American College of Physicians, patients who have a low pretest probability for pulmonary embolism (PE) using a validated clinical prediction rule (such as the Wells criteria for prediction of PE) and who meet all Pulmonary Embolism Rule-Out Criteria do not need further testing to rule out PE. Using the Wells criteria, this patient is a low risk for PE (0 points) and scores 2 points on the Pulmonary Embolism Rule-Out Criteria (fails to meet 2 criteria: age younger than 50 years and oxygen saturation greater than 94%). Additional evaluation for PE in this patient might include a D-dimer measurement as an initial test, but not an imaging study.

**KEY POINT**

- Arterial blood gas analysis is recommended for patients with a severe exacerbation of COPD to assess for hypercapnia and hypoxemia.

**Bibliography**

Qureshi H, Sharafkhaneh A, Hanania NA. Chronic obstructive pulmonary disease exacerbations: latest evidence and clinical implications. Ther Adv Chronic Dis. 2014;5:212-27. [PMID: 25177479] doi:10.1177/2040622314532862

**Item 23       Answer:   C**

**Educational Objective:** Evaluate suspected pulmonary arterial hypertension with transthoracic echocardiography.

The next most appropriate initial test is transthoracic echocardiography. Pulmonary hypertension is easily overlooked because early signs and symptoms, such as exertional dyspnea and fatigue, are nonspecific. As the disorder progresses, right ventricular impairment may be heralded by exertional chest pain, syncope, and peripheral edema. Findings on physical examination depend on the severity of disease. The cardiovascular examination may show jugular venous distention, a prominent jugular venous $a$ wave, parasternal heave, a widened split $S_2$ with a prominent pulmonic component,

Answers and Critiques

or murmurs of tricuspid regurgitation as the right ventricle dilates. Transthoracic echocardiography is a useful initial tool in the evaluation of suspected pulmonary hypertension as it allows an estimation of pulmonary artery pressures and right heart function as well as an assessment of the left heart. Because echocardiography may underestimate true pulmonary artery pressures, the evaluation should not end with an unrevealing echocardiogram if the index of suspicion for pulmonary hypertension is high. In such cases, right heart catheterization may be confirmatory. Once pulmonary hypertension is confirmed, further testing, guided by clinical history, helps determine identifiable causes. Left heart catheterization can assess coronary flow and left ventricular function. Diagnostic tests for respiratory diseases might include pulmonary function tests, chest imaging, ventilation-perfusion ($\dot{V}/\dot{Q}$) scanning, and overnight pulse oximetry.

High-resolution CT scanning of the chest allows a detailed assessment of the lung parenchyma and is useful in the evaluation of suspected interstitial lung diseases, but is unlikely to be helpful as an initial test in a patient with an unremarkable lung examination and clear lung fields on chest radiograph.

Pulmonary function testing is an important diagnostic test for suspected airways disease such as asthma, COPD, or interstitial lung disease. However, this patient has no symptoms or physical examination findings indicative of either obstructive or restrictive disease. In the patient with isolated pulmonary hypertension, pulmonary function tests demonstrate a reduction in diffusing capacity, which is a nonspecific finding.

$\dot{V}/\dot{Q}$ scanning is the diagnostic test of choice for suspected chronic thromboembolic pulmonary hypertension (CTEPH). Although CTEPH hasn't yet been excluded in this patient, $\dot{V}/\dot{Q}$ scanning would typically be performed after transthoracic echocardiography to first establish the presence of pulmonary hypertension.

**KEY POINT**

- Transthoracic echocardiography can estimate pulmonary artery pressures and is the preferred initial test if pulmonary hypertension is suspected.

### Bibliography
Vonk Noordegraaf A, Groeneveldt JA, Bogaard HJ. Pulmonary hypertension. Eur Respir Rev. 2016;25:4-11. [PMID: 26929415] doi:10.1183/16000617. 0096-2015

### Item 24        Answer:        E

**Educational Objective:** Manage obesity-related asthma with a supervised weight loss program.

This patient should be referred to a supervised weight loss program. He has poorly controlled asthma despite maximal medical therapy and in the absence of other factors known to exacerbate asthma (environmental triggers, uncontrolled gastroesophageal reflux disease, sinus disease, or obstructive sleep apnea). Obesity is associated with poor asthma control,

and the incidence of asthma is 1.47 times greater in obese patients than nonobese patients. Weight loss in patients with obesity-related asthma improves asthma control, lung function, and quality of life; reduces asthma medication use; and should be considered an essential part of the treatment plan.

Addition of beclomethasone is not appropriate because this patient is already on adequate inhaled therapy and glucocorticoids; increasing the inhaled steroid dose is unlikely to be beneficial.

Between attacks and exacerbations of asthma, spirometry can be normal in patients with suspected but undiagnosed asthma. Therefore, a bronchial challenge test, such as a methacholine challenge, may be helpful for diagnosis if positive or make the diagnosis less likely if negative. Methacholine challenge testing is not necessary in this patient because spirometry confirms reversible airflow obstruction (with a 12% or greater improvement in $FEV_1$ or FVC of 200 mL after administration of a bronchodilator), supporting a diagnosis of asthma.

Mepolizumab is a monoclonal antibody to IL-5 that has been shown to reduce asthma exacerbations in patients with difficult-to-control asthma and elevated blood eosinophil counts. This patient's eosinophil count was normal; therefore, add-on therapy with mepolizumab is not indicated.

Although omalizumab can reduce hospitalizations when added to standard therapy, it is a monoclonal antibody used for treatment of allergic asthma, and it targets elevated levels of IgE. Because this patient does not have a history of allergies and his IgE level is normal, treatment with omalizumab would not be appropriate.

**KEY POINT**

- Weight loss in patients with obesity-related asthma improves asthma control, lung function, and quality of life; reduces asthma medication use; and should be considered an essential part of the treatment plan.

### Bibliography
Pakhale S, Baron J, Dent R, Vandemheen K, Aaron SD. Effects of weight loss on airway responsiveness in obese adults with asthma: Does weight loss lead to reversibility of asthma? Chest. 2015;147:1582-1590. [PMID: 25763936] doi:10.1378/chest.14-3105

### Item 25        Answer:        C

**Educational Objective:** Treat heart failure in a patient with a Cheyne-Stokes breathing pattern.

Diuresis with furosemide is the most appropriate treatment option. This patient has central sleep apnea with Cheyne-Stokes breathing in the setting of decompensated heart failure, a state of ventilatory instability. Cheyne-Stokes breathing is an abnormal respiratory pattern characterized by cyclic crescendo-decrescendo respiratory effort during sleep (and sometimes during wakefulness), in the absence of upper airway obstruction. Apnea accompanying the decrescendo effort defines central sleep apnea. The degree of central sleep apnea tends to correlate with left ventricular dysfunction.

This patient has evidence on examination of volume overload (crackles and wheezing on lung exam, jugular venous distention, peripheral edema). Optimizing medical management of heart failure and improving fluid balance should precede other therapies for sleep apnea.

Adaptive servo-ventilation is a form of positive airway pressure therapy initially designed as a treatment of Cheyne-Stokes breathing. However, a large multicenter trial unexpectedly showed increased mortality in a subset of patients with systolic heart failure (left ventricular ejection fraction less than 45%) and central sleep apnea treated with adaptive servo-ventilation.

Auto-adjusting positive airway pressure is not an initial treatment for central sleep apnea. It is used to treat obstructive sleep apnea, where proprietary algorithms deliver varying pressure sufficient to prevent upper airway closure.

Supplemental oxygen is sometimes used in advanced heart failure where impaired gas exchange results in hypoxemia. This patient has preserved oxyhemoglobin saturation. Small trials have studied the use of nocturnal supplemental oxygen in the setting of central sleep apnea, with variable results. Such treatment would be premature before optimization of fluid status.

**KEY POINT**

- Initial treatment of central sleep apnea should target modifiable risk factors; medical optimization of heart failure has been shown to improve central sleep apnea and Cheyne-Stokes breathing and should precede other therapies for sleep apnea.

**Bibliography**
Hernandez AB, Patil SP. Pathophysiology of central sleep apneas. Sleep Breath. 2016;20:467-82. [PMID: 26782104] doi:10.1007/s11325-015-1290-z

## Item 26     Answer:     B

**Educational Objective:** Treat asthma-COPD overlap syndrome.

The most appropriate treatment is a combination inhaled glucocorticoid and a long-acting $\beta_2$-agonist. This patient has progressive symptoms, spirometry showing diminished $FEV_1$ that partially reversed with bronchodilation, and eosinophilia. Several diagnostic terms have been used to describe patients with both asthma and COPD, most including the word *overlap*, but there is no universally agreed upon term or defining diagnostic features for this condition. Given her progression of symptoms, her short-acting inhaler therapy should be augmented. Although a long-acting $\beta_2$-agonist is indicated in symptomatic patients with COPD and an $FEV_1$ of less than 60% of predicted, this may not be the best treatment for a patient with asthma. Patients with asthma are at increased risk of mortality when a long-acting bronchodilator is prescribed without a controller medication. Experts recommend that patients who have an asthma-COPD overlap syndrome who are receiving a long-acting bronchodilator should

ideally also be prescribed an inhaled glucocorticoid. Combination therapy seems to mitigate the excess risk of mortality observed in patients with asthma treated with long-acting $\beta_2$-agonist monotherapy. Therefore, the patient should be started on a combination therapy of an inhaled glucocorticoid and a long-acting $\beta_2$-agonist.

Chronic macrolide therapy can reduce the incidence of acute exacerbations but this patient has not had any exacerbations to warrant starting a macrolide.

Using a long-acting $\beta_2$-agonist or a long-acting muscarinic agent/long-acting $\beta_2$-agonist combination inhaler is likely not indicated for this patient with asthma-COPD overlap syndrome based on current guidelines. Long-acting bronchodilators should only be used in combination with inhaled glucocorticoids in patients with a history of asthma. Using long-acting bronchodilators alone has been linked to increased risk of asthma-related deaths.

**KEY POINT**

- Patients with a history of asthma-COPD overlap syndrome should not be prescribed a long-acting $\beta_2$-agonist without concurrent therapy with an inhaled glucocorticoid because of the increased risk of mortality in patients with asthma who are prescribed long-acting $\beta_2$-agonist monotherapy.

**Bibliography**
GINA/GOLD Joint Report. 2015 asthma, COPD and asthma-COPD overlap syndrome (ACOS) [Internet] Bethesda: Global Initiative for Asthma; 2016. Available from: http://ginasthma.org/asthma-copd-and-asthma-copdoverlap-syndrome-acos/. Accessed May 1, 2018.

## Item 27     Answer:     C

**Educational Objective:** Diagnose pneumothorax in a patient with lung disease in the setting of air travel.

The most likely diagnosis is pneumothorax. An estimated 12% of in-flight medical emergencies involve a respiratory complaint. Commercial airline cabins are partially pressurized, typically to the equivalent of approximately 1400 to 2500 meters (4000 to 8000 feet) above sea level, limiting exposure to extreme hypobaric conditions. The risk of pneumothorax is therefore mitigated but it is most likely to occur at cruising altitude in patients with bullous lung disease, particularly those with a recent exacerbation of airways disease who are, therefore, more prone to air trapping. Pain is typically pleuritic; dyspnea may be present, depending upon the volume of trapped air. If tension physiology develops (hypotension, shock, altered mental status), needle thoracostomy using the on-board equipment can be life-saving. Descending to a lower altitude may also be beneficial, because cabin pressure is inversely related to the altitude of the aircraft.

Descending aortic dissection typically presents with acute, severe back pain. Although chest pain can occur, it is less common. Radiation of pain to the abdomen can occur with disruption of blood flow to the abdominal viscera. Hypertension is the most important risk factor and is

Answers and Critiques

present in more than half of patients with descending aortic dissection. Pulse deficits are common. However, this patient does not have a history of hypertension and has normal peripheral pulses, making a diagnosis of descending aortic dissection unlikely.

*Pneumocystis jirovecii* pneumonia is unlikely to present in this manner. Although systemic glucocorticoids increase the risk for opportunistic lung infections such as *P. jirovecii* pneumonia, the risk is minimal during the course of a typical prednisone burst and taper used for a COPD exacerbation. In general, those taking prednisone dosage equivalents of at least 20 mg/day for more than 3 weeks should receive *P. jirovecii* pneumonia prophylaxis.

Air travel increases the risk of venous thromboembolism, though the risk is higher during relative immobilization on long flights and in those with other risk factors, such as cancer. The risk of pulmonary embolism does not really increase until the flight distance becomes greater than 5000 km (3000 miles). It is unlikely that a flight duration of only 90 minutes would heighten thrombotic risk in this patient.

### KEY POINT

- During air travel, pneumothorax is most likely to occur at cruising altitude in patients with bullous lung disease, particularly those with a recent exacerbation of airways disease who are, therefore, more prone to air trapping.

### Bibliography

Nable JV, Tupe CL, Gehle BD, Brady WJ. In-flight medical emergencies during commercial travel. N Engl J Med. 2015;373:939-45. [PMID: 26332548] doi:10.1056/NEJMra1409213

## Item 28    Answer:    B

**Educational Objective:** Evaluate a patient with upper-lobe emphysema and significant exercise limitations for lung volume reduction surgery.

Evaluation for lung volume reduction surgery is the most appropriate management for this patient with upper-lobe emphysema, significant exercise limitation, and poor quality of life. Lung volume reduction surgery excises areas of emphysematous lung, improves the mechanical efficiency of respiratory muscles, and increases the elastic recoil of the lungs to improve expiratory flow and reduce exacerbations. The National Emphysema Treatment Trial (NETT) demonstrated that carefully selected patients with upper-lobe predominant emphysema and significant exercise limitation despite participation in a pulmonary rehabilitation program had improved quality of life and survival with lung volume reduction surgery. Symptomatic improvement with the surgery appears to be durable.

Roflumilast is an oral selective phosphodiesterase-4 inhibitor. It is used primarily as add-on therapy in severe COPD associated with chronic bronchitis and a history of recurrent exacerbations despite other therapies; it has been shown to relieve symptoms and reduce risk and frequency

of exacerbations in these individuals. However, it is not a bronchodilator, is expensive, and has not been shown to be effective in other groups of patients with COPD. It is not indicated in the treatment of primary emphysema and has not been shown to decrease exertional dyspnea and would not benefit this patient.

Although patients with chronic lung conditions can develop pulmonary hypertension, this patient had an unremarkable echocardiogram and has no evidence of pulmonary hypertension on examination. Therefore, proceeding with a right heart catheterization is unnecessary and unlikely to change management at this time.

This patient has already participated in a pulmonary rehabilitation program. Although it is helpful for patients to continue exercise, restarting a formal pulmonary rehabilitation program is unlikely to provide him with any more significant symptomatic improvement.

### KEY POINT

- Lung volume reduction surgery improves quality of life and survival for patients with upper-lobe predominant emphysema and significant exercise limitations.

### Bibliography

Ginsburg ME, Thomashow BM, Bulman WA, Jellen PA, Whippo BA, Chiuzan C, et al. The safety, efficacy, and durability of lung-volume reduction surgery: a 10-year experience. J Thorac Cardiovasc Surg. 2016;151:717-724.e1. [PMID: 26670190] doi:10.1016/j.jtcvs.2015.10.095

## Item 29    Answer:    D

**Educational Objective:** Diagnose COPD with spirometry.

This patient's symptoms are consistent with a possible diagnosis of COPD and spirometry should be performed. Spirometric evaluation is required for the clinical diagnosis of COPD. Spirometry is warranted in any patient presenting with dyspnea, chronic cough, or sputum production. Screening for COPD with spirometry should not be performed in asymptomatic patients. For diagnosis of COPD, spirometry should be performed both before and after administration of an inhaled bronchodilator. A postbronchodilator $FEV_1/FVC$ of less than 0.70 is diagnostic of airflow obstruction that is not completely reversible with bronchodilator therapy and is consistent with a diagnosis of COPD.

Diagnostic testing for structural heart disease should be based on a thorough history and physical examination. New murmurs or a change in examination findings or symptoms in a patient with known structural heart disease should prompt further evaluation. The patient's examination is not consistent with pulmonary hypertension, heart failure, or valvular disease. Therefore, an echocardiogram is unlikely to be helpful.

In patients with a previous history of coronary artery disease and worsening cardiac symptoms, stress testing is helpful to assess for possible recurrent or progressive disease. Given this patient's cough, which would be an unusual presentation of heart disease in the absence of volume overload, a diagnosis of COPD is much more likely and should be investigated further. A cardiac stress test could be considered if his evaluation is otherwise unremarkable.

Although interstitial lung disease can present with similar symptoms, the absence of pulmonary crackles and normal chest radiograph do not support this diagnosis. Therefore, a high-resolution chest CT is currently not indicated.

**KEY POINT**

- A postbronchodilator $FEV_1$/FVC of less than 0.70 is diagnostic of airflow obstruction and is consistent with the diagnosis of COPD.

**Bibliography**

Qaseem A, Wilt TJ, Weinberger SE, Hanania NA, Criner G, van der Molen T, et al; American College of Physicians. Diagnosis and management of stable chronic obstructive pulmonary disease: a clinical practice guideline update from the American College of Physicians, American College of Chest Physicians, American Thoracic Society, and European Respiratory Society. Ann Intern Med. 2011;155:179-91. [PMID: 21810710] doi:10.7326/0003-4819-155-3-201108020-00008

## Item 30  Answer:  D

**Educational Objective:** Manage a patient with progressive idiopathic pulmonary fibrosis with palliative care.

This patient should receive palliative care including morphine for the symptom of dyspnea. Idiopathic pulmonary fibrosis (IPF) is the most common idiopathic interstitial pneumonia. It occurs predominantly in older individuals. Prognosis is poor, and individuals diagnosed with IPF have an estimated average survival of 3 to 5 years. The most common cause of death in IPF is respiratory failure. Patients with IPF may experience an acute exacerbation of IPF, diagnosed when the chest radiograph shows new alveolar infiltrates and medical evaluation does not reveal another cause for dyspnea such as infection, heart failure, or pulmonary embolism. Despite maximal supportive care during the past 5 days, this patient has progressed and is now on the brink of respiratory failure. Lung transplantation has been shown to provide a survival advantage in select patients with IPF. This patient gives a history consistent with severe and prolonged deconditioning associated with chronic respiratory failure. She now presents with frank respiratory failure and rapid progression of IPF with an unclear trigger. Consideration for transplant typically includes a full assessment of the patient for evidence of additional organ disease and education regarding the risks and benefits of the procedure. This is best accomplished long before the development of an acute exacerbation. Because of this patient's age, functional status, and lack of previous assessment by a transplant center, lung transplantation is not a viable option for her. At this time, she remains awake and alert and is able to participate in her end-of-life decision making. Patients with this presentation and functional status do not typically respond favorably to intubation and mechanical ventilation and, as such, recommending palliative medicines and comfort measures is most appropriate.

Although high-dose glucocorticoids are often used for acute exacerbation, their efficacy remains unknown. This patient has already been treated with glucocorticoids without apparent improvement; this indicates that administration of additional glucocorticoids is not likely to be of benefit.

Albuterol is a bronchial vasodilator. Unfortunately, the limitation in patients with IPF that results in hypoxemia and dyspnea is at the level of the interstitium, and bronchial dilators have little effect on these symptoms.

For individuals who develop severe respiratory distress that has no underlying reversible cause, supportive mechanical ventilation is of little long-term benefit. Therefore, the most recent evidence-based consensus statement recommends against mechanical ventilation for individuals with acute respiratory failure due to either progression or an acute exacerbation of IPF. In these circumstances, the focus should be on palliation of the patient's underlying dyspnea.

**KEY POINT**

- For individuals with idiopathic pulmonary fibrosis who develop severe respiratory distress that has no underlying reversible cause, supportive mechanical ventilation is of little long-term benefit; in these circumstances, the focus should be on palliation of the patient's underlying dyspnea.

**Bibliography**

Raghu G, Collard HR, Egan JJ, Martinez FJ, Behr J, Brown KK, et al; ATS/ERS/JRS/ALAT Committee on Idiopathic Pulmonary Fibrosis. An official ATS/ERS/JRS/ALAT statement: idiopathic pulmonary fibrosis: evidence-based guidelines for diagnosis and management. Am J Respir Crit Care Med. 2011;183:788-824. [PMID: 21471066] doi:10.1164/rccm.2009-040GL

## Item 31  Answer:  C

**Educational Objective:** Evaluate a patient with diffuse cutaneous systemic sclerosis for diffuse parenchymal lung disease.

This patient should receive a high-resolution CT (HRCT) scan of the chest. She has a history of diffuse cutaneous systemic sclerosis and has a chronic cough and dyspnea concerning for the possibility of scleroderma-associated interstitial lung disease. The most common cause of death from scleroderma is no longer kidney disease but progressive respiratory failure due to diffuse parenchymal lung disease. Among patients with the scleroderma spectrum disorders, patients with diffuse cutaneous systemic sclerosis and anti-Scl antibodies have the highest risk of interstitial lung disease. The most common pathologic finding in such patients is nonspecific interstitial pneumonia (NSIP). This patient has physiologic evidence of parenchymal lung disease with a mild restrictive defect and exercise-induced oxygen desaturation. Chest radiography can often miss mild disease and in these cases more advanced imaging is required. HRCT findings associated with NSIP include peripheral and basal predominant ground-glass opacities (cellular form) that spare the subpleural areas, basal predominant septal line thickening, and traction bronchiectasis in the fibrotic form.

Results of a 6-minute walk test (6MWT) are helpful to assess disability and prognosis in chronic lung conditions. During a 6MWT, oxygen saturation, heart rate, dyspnea and fatigue level, and distance walked in 6 minutes are recorded. The 6MWT is routinely used before, during, and after pulmonary rehabilitation programs. It would not be helpful in this patient with probable interstitial lung disease.

Cardiopulmonary exercise testing is routinely performed to assess prognosis in patients being evaluated for transplantation. Patients with low oxygen consumption or a high ratio of ventilation-to-carbon dioxide production have a poor 1-year prognosis. It may also be helpful in detecting deconditioning as a cause of dyspnea of unclear cause. It would not be appropriate in this patient with known restrictive lung disease.

Patients with a pulmonary nodule or other findings suggestive of malignancy may require PET/CT. This test most commonly uses fluorodeoxyglucose as a metabolic marker to identify rapidly dividing cells such as tumor cells and, to a lesser degree, any inflammatory lesion. It has no role in the evaluation on this patient with probable interstitial lung disease.

### KEY POINT

- Patients with diffuse cutaneous systemic sclerosis are at high risk for the development of diffuse parenchymal lung disease, which is the leading cause of death in these patients.

### Bibliography
Suliman S, Al Harash A, Roberts WN, Perez RL, Roman J. Scleroderma-related interstitial lung disease. Respir Med Case Rep. 2017;22:109-112. [PMID: 28761806] doi:10.1016/j.rmcr.2017.07.007

### Item 32          Answer:     D

**Educational Objective:  Diagnose cough-variant asthma.**

The most appropriate management is to perform methacholine challenge testing. This patient has a chronic cough with no cause identified by history or physical examination, and a normal chest radiograph. In such patients who are not taking ACE inhibitors and are not exposed to environmental irritants or tobacco smoke, the most common causes are asthma, gastroesophageal reflux disease (GERD), and rhinosinusitis. Cough-variant asthma refers to asthma in which the predominant manifestation is cough, without other typical asthma symptoms such as wheezing, breathlessness, and chest tightness. Although most patients with asthma have obstructive physiology on pulmonary function testing, in those patients with normal spirometry, methacholine challenge testing is indicated to evaluate for bronchial hyperreactivity, which supports a diagnosis of asthma. Bronchial challenge testing uses a controlled inhaled stimulus to induce bronchospasm in association with spirometry; a positive test is indicated by a drop in the measured $FEV_1$. Methacholine is a commonly used agent that induces cholinergic bronchospasm at low

concentrations in patients with asthma; levels of exhaled nitric oxide may also be elevated. Positive methacholine testing is not specific enough to diagnose asthma; therefore, patients with cough and a positive methacholine challenge must also respond clinically to treatment with asthma therapies to be considered to have cough-variant asthma.

Although an empiric trial of asthma treatment with budesonide and albuterol could be considered, expert consensus indicates that it is preferable to first establish a diagnosis to avoid making an incorrect diagnosis and prescribing unnecessary or incorrect treatment.

Esophageal manometry and 24-hour pH testing would not be appropriate because the patient has no symptoms of GERD. Current guidelines suggest an empiric trial of diet and lifestyle modification for cough due to GERD before invasive testing for the disease.

A high-resolution CT scan of the chest would be indicated in some patients with chronic cough to evaluate for interstitial lung disorders or bronchiectasis, but the chest radiograph and physical examination findings are normal and the more common condition of asthma should be excluded first.

### KEY POINT

- Cough-variant asthma refers to asthma in which the predominant manifestation is cough, and without other typical asthma symptoms; the diagnosis is supported by abnormal spirometry or methacholine challenge testing if spirometry is normal.

### Bibliography
Kahrilas PJ, Altman KW, Chang AB, Field SK, Harding SM, Lane AP, et al; CHEST Expert Cough Panel. Chronic cough due to gastroesophageal reflux in adults: CHEST Guideline and Expert Panel Report. Chest. 2016;150:1341-1360. [PMID: 27614002] doi:10.1016/j.chest.2016.08.1458

### Item 33          Answer:     B

**Educational Objective:  Treat a patient with shock using a peripheral wide-bore catheter.**

The most appropriate treatment is to insert a peripheral wide-bore central venous catheter. This patient is in shock with several possible causes. Flow of fluid through a catheter is inversely proportional to catheter length and proportional to the radius of the catheter to the fourth power. Therefore, the highest flow rates may be achieved through shorter, large-bore catheters. Peripheral intravenous (IV) catheters are shorter and larger than catheters used for central access or peripherally inserted central catheters and can deliver high volumes of fluid rapidly. For this reason, use of larger, shorter peripheral catheters is preferred for fluid resuscitation in patients requiring emergent treatment. However, peripheral IV catheters can sometimes be difficult to insert in patients in shock, and intraosseous ports and central venous catheters are the alternatives.

Intraosseous ports provide rapid access, but this patient has osteoporosis, which is a contraindication to this method.

When used, an initial dose of lidocaine is needed before infusing because pain levels are very high with initial flushes and infusion.

Subcutaneous intravenous ports are long and small bore, which makes them useful for blood draws and small-volume infusion administration but not for rapid, large-volume fluid resuscitation.

A triple-lumen central catheter is an acceptable alternative when no other intravenous access can be obtained; however, it takes longer to insert compared to a peripheral wide-bore central venous catheter. When used, care should be taken to choose wider-bore catheters to overcome the flow restriction from longer lengths.

**KEY POINT**

- Peripheral wide-bore venous catheters are the preferred method for rapid intravenous administration of large amounts of fluids.

**Bibliography**

Khoyratty SI, Gajendragadkar PR, Polisetty K, Ward S, Skinner T, Gajendragadkar PR. Flow rates through intravenous access devices: an in vitro study. J Clin Anesth. 2016;31:101-5. [PMID: 27185686] doi:10.1016/j.jclinane.2016.01.048

## Item 34    Answer:    B

**Educational Objective:** Diagnose pulmonary embolism as a potential trigger for acute COPD exacerbations.

This patient should undergo CT pulmonary angiography. Some COPD exacerbations thought to be of unknown cause may actually be due to other medical conditions, including a pulmonary embolism (PE). A meta-analysis suggests that the prevalence of PE in patients hospitalized for an acute COPD exacerbation is as high as 25%. Testing for PE is indicated for patients who are not responding to typical therapy for acute exacerbations unless the pretest probability for PE is unlikely. Other important entities in the differential diagnosis with high risk for mortality include heart failure and pneumonia. These entities are less likely in this patient because of the absence of fever, crackles, edema, normal chest radiograph, and normal B-type natriuretic peptide level.

Spirometry usually does not change management during an acute exacerbation. In addition, the patient may not be able to complete the testing given his symptoms and the increased work of breathing.

Evaluation for influenza may be useful in patients who present with compatible symptoms, including fever, headache, myalgia, pharyngeal irritation, and respiratory symptoms (nonproductive cough and nasal discharge), particularly during an influenza outbreak. During a confirmed local influenza outbreak, infection can be reliably diagnosed on the basis of clinical criteria alone. When confirmation is needed, polymerase chain reaction testing can be performed. Testing for influenza in this patient is not necessary in the absence of influenza symptoms.

Similarly, a sputum culture is usually not indicated as it infrequently changes management of COPD. An antibiotic is often added because infections are the most common triggers for an acute exacerbation.

**KEY POINT**

- Patients who are not responding to typical therapy for COPD exacerbations should be carefully evaluated for heart failure, pneumonia, and pulmonary embolism.

**Bibliography**

Aleva FE, Voets LWLM, Simons SO, de Mast Q, van der Ven AJAM, Heijdra YF. Prevalence and localization of pulmonary embolism in unexplained acute exacerbations of COPD: a systematic review and meta-analysis. Chest. 2017;151:544-554. [PMID: 27522956] doi:10.1016/j.chest.2016.07.034

## Item 35    Answer:    C

**Educational Objective:** Evaluate a solitary pulmonary nodule in a patient at high risk for malignancy.

Definitive treatment is recommended for this patient and, therefore, a surgical wedge resection is appropriate. She has several risk factors for malignancy, including age, size of the nodule, upper-lobe location of the nodule, smoking history, and history of malignancy. In addition, the PET/CT scan showed fludeoxyglucose avidity, confirming the high probability of malignancy but without evidence of distant metastasis. As with subcentimeter nodules, the availability of previous imaging of the chest to assess the stability or growth of these lesions is helpful. An enlarging or new pulmonary nodule warrants more aggressive evaluation with tissue diagnosis or excision depending on the nodule's pretest probability of malignancy. The first step when evaluating a solid pulmonary nodule that is larger than 8 mm is to estimate the probability of malignancy. This can be done either clinically or using quantitative models and should place the patient in one of three categories: low probability (less than 5%), intermediate probability (5% to 65%), or high probability (greater than 65%). This is most useful when nodules are 8-30 mm. If the lesion is larger than 30 mm, the likelihood of malignancy is so high that it typically is resected; in contrast, when the lesion is smaller than 8 mm, the likelihood of malignancy is low and the patient should undergo routine radiological surveillance with serial CT scans.

Biopsy of the nodule or a transthoracic approach is preferred when the probability of malignancy is intermediate (5% to 65%) and would not be appropriate for this patient with a hypermetabolic nodule on PET/CT scan suggesting a high probability of malignancy. Furthermore, the sampling procedure is chosen according to size and location of the nodule, availability, and local expertise. Typically, peripheral nodules are sampled using CT-guided transthoracic needle aspiration, and more central lesions are sampled using bronchoscopic techniques. This lesion is described as peripheral.

Radiologic surveillance with serial CT scans is preferred if the probability of malignancy is low (less than 5%).

This patient's lung nodule is highly suspicious for malignancy on CT/PET scan so sampling with CT-guided transthoracic needle aspiration is not indicated.

**KEY POINT**

- Patients with a solid indeterminate lung nodule larger than 8 mm and high probability of malignancy should be staged using a PET/CT scan followed by definitive management.

**Bibliography**

Gould MK, Donington J, Lynch WR, Mazzone PJ, Midthun DE, Naidich DP, et al. Evaluation of individuals with pulmonary nodules: When is it lung cancer? Diagnosis and management of lung cancer, 3rd ed: American College of Chest Physicians evidence-based clinical practice guidelines. Chest. 2013;143:e93S-e120S. [PMID: 23649456] doi:10.1378/chest.12-2351

**Item 36    Answer:    A**

**Educational Objective:** Diagnose a patient with asbestosis.

The most likely diagnosis is asbestosis. Asbestosis refers to the pneumoconiosis caused by inhalation of asbestos fibers. Asbestos is a silicate mineral fiber previously used as an insulating material that is a major cause of lung disease. Workers in construction, naval shipyards, and the automotive service industries are particularly at risk for asbestosis, with duration and extent of exposure being the key risk factors for the development of disease. Although asbestos use in the United States has been virtually eliminated since its peak in the 1980s, asbestos-related diseases will persist well into this century owing to the long latency period between exposure and disease development (15 to 35 years). Parietal pleural plaques are the most common finding and differentiate asbestos-induced parenchymal disease from other interstitial lung diseases. Diffuse parenchymal lung disease (DPLD) due to asbestos is related to the extent of the fiber burden. The most common symptom is exertional dyspnea; cough and sputum production are unusual unless the patient is a cigarette smoker. The CT scan imaging of pleural plaques and DPLD combined with the exposure history is adequate to make the diagnosis of asbestosis.

Chronic forms of hypersensitivity pneumonitis are believed to be associated with more chronic low-level exposures to inhaled antigen. This patient's hobby is wood working and wood dust is a potential source of antigen exposure. Patients with chronic hypersensitivity pneumonitis will ultimately present with cough, dyspnea, malaise, and weight loss. High-resolution CT findings include centrilobular micronodules in upper-lung and midlung distribution, as well as evidence of septal line thickening and fibrosis. Pleural plaques are not found. This patient's symptoms and CT findings are not compatible with this diagnosis.

Although this patient has some CT scan findings consistent with idiopathic pulmonary fibrosis, that diagnosis can only be made in a patient who does not have another plausible cause for fibrosis. In addition, the finding of pleural plaques makes idiopathic pulmonary fibrosis unlikely.

Respiratory bronchiolitis-associated DPLD is a disease in active smokers who have imaging findings of centrilobular micronodules. The patient's negative smoking history and presence of pleural plaques on imaging excludes this diagnosis.

**KEY POINT**

- Parietal plaques are the most common radiologic finding in patients with asbestos exposure and are the features that differentiate asbestosis from other interstitial lung diseases.

**Bibliography**

Fishwick D, Barber CM. Non-malignant asbestos-related diseases: a clinical view. Clin Med (Lond). 2014;14:68-71. [PMID: 24532750] doi:10.7861/clinmedicine.14-1-68

**Item 37    Answer:    B**

**Educational Objective:** Treat a patient for an acute asthma exacerbation with magnesium sulfate.

The most appropriate treatment is a single dose of magnesium sulfate. This patient is experiencing an acute asthma exacerbation. Treatment of acute asthma exacerbations can be difficult and requires prompt, aggressive management. The cornerstone of therapy in severe acute asthma exacerbation includes early administration of several doses of a short-acting β₂-agonist (SABA), a short-acting muscarinic antagonist (SAMA), and oral or intravenous glucocorticoids. In patients with a moderate to severe asthma exacerbation, combination therapy with a SAMA/SABA has been shown to reduce hospitalizations and improve lung function compared to SABA alone. Although use of a SAMA is not FDA-approved for treatment of an acute asthma exacerbation, several trials have demonstrated efficacy in both children and adults, and its use is supported by guidelines. Magnesium sulfate administration should also be considered early in the course of severe asthma exacerbation given its ability to relax bronchial smooth muscle tissue. A 2014 systematic review concluded that a single intravenous infusion of 1.2 g or 2 g of magnesium sulfate over 15 to 30 minutes reduces hospital admissions and improves lung function in adults with acute asthma who have not responded sufficiently to oxygen, nebulized SABAs and intravenous glucocorticoids.

Despite the theoretical bronchodilatory effect of intravenous ketamine, two randomized controlled trials have failed to demonstrate added bronchodilator effects when ketamine was compared to conventional management of asthma exacerbation.

Adjunct therapies such as a long-acting β₂-agonist, montelukast sodium, and theophylline have not demonstrated therapeutic benefit when used in the treatment of an acute asthma exacerbation and are not appropriate choices

CONT.

for this patient. However, their efficacy as long-term options in the outpatient setting should be considered in the overall treatment of asthma once the patient has been stabilized and is ready for hospital discharge.

> **KEY POINT**
>
> - Intravenous magnesium sulfate reduces hospital admissions and improves lung function in adults with acute asthma who have not responded sufficiently to oxygen, nebulized short-acting $\beta_2$-agonists, and intravenous glucocorticoids.

**Bibliography**

Albertson TE, Sutter ME, Chan AL. The acute management of asthma. Clin Rev Allergy Immunol. 2015;48:114-25. [PMID: 25213370] doi:10.1007/s12016-014-8448-5

## Item 38     Answer:    B

**Educational Objective:** Treat septic shock that persists after adequate fluid resuscitation using glucocorticoids.

Hydrocortisone is the most appropriate treatment. There is controversy about the role of glucocorticoids in the treatment of septic shock, but the Surviving Sepsis Guidelines published in 2016 recommend that if glucocorticoids are used, they should be used in refractory shock with persistent hypotension after adequate fluid resuscitation and after vasopressor medications have been titrated to high dose, and that the dose should be no more than 200 mg of hydrocortisone in 24 hours.

It is unlikely that substituting norepinephrine with another catecholamine vasopressor (dopamine) will lead to increased blood pressure. Dopamine also has a higher risk of inducing cardiac arrhythmias, and in this elderly patient who already has sinus tachycardia and frequent ectopic beats, dopamine would be an inappropriate substitution. Dopamine might best be reserved for selected patients with hypoperfusion and relative bradycardia.

Vasopressin levels in septic shock have been reported to be lower than anticipated for a shock state. Low doses of vasopressin may be effective in raising blood pressure in shock refractory to other vasopressors. Guidelines suggest adding vasopressin (up to 0.03 U/min) to norepinephrine with the intent of raising blood pressure to target or to decrease norepinephrine dosage. Vasopressin is not titrated like other pressors. Higher doses of vasopressin lead to ischemic complications, which more than offset any hemodynamic benefit.

Guidelines currently recommend against the use of intravenous (IV) immunoglobulins in patients with sepsis or septic shock. The most recent systematic review and meta-analysis differentiated between standard polyclonal IV immunoglobulins and M-enriched polyclonal immunoglobulin. Studies included in the review had low to moderate certainty of results based on risk of bias and heterogeneity. After excluding low-quality trials, no survival benefit was discernable with either immune globulin preparation.

> **KEY POINT**
>
> - Glucocorticoids are indicated in patients with sepsis who have not achieved hemodynamic stability from intravenous fluid administration and vasopressor therapies.

**Bibliography**

Rhodes A, Evans LE, Alhazzani W, Levy MM, Antonelli M, Ferrer R, et al. Surviving Sepsis Campaign: international guidelines for management of sepsis and septic shock: 2016. Intensive Care Med. 2017;43:304-377. [PMID: 28101605] doi:10.1007/s00134-017-4683-6

## Item 39     Answer:    C

**Educational Objective:** Diagnose malignant pleural mesothelioma.

The most likely diagnosis is malignant pleural mesothelioma. Asbestos exposure is the primary risk factor for mesothelioma, which has a latency period of 20 to 40 years, and this patient likely has a history of asbestos exposure from working as a brake mechanic. Occupational exposure to asbestos is most common in miners, electricians, plumbers, brake mechanics, shipyard workers, home remodelers, and selected military personnel. Patients most commonly present with symptoms of chest pain and a slowly enlarging pleural effusion. Chest imaging typically shows a unilateral pleural effusion, but patients can also present with pleural thickening, calcification, nodules, or masses. If malignant pleural mesothelioma is suspected, a thoracentesis should be performed, including pleural fluid cytology. Additional evaluation includes a chest CT scan to determine the extent of disease and evaluate for pleural lesions. Confirmation of the diagnosis requires pleural biopsy. Video-assisted thoracoscopic biopsy or open thoracotomy is required when the diagnosis remains uncertain, as diagnosis of mesothelioma cannot be made using cytology alone.

Empyema often presents with unilateral loculated exudative pleural effusion; however, the patient would not have a 6-month history of symptoms in the absence of fever and with a normal complete blood count. Finally, the pleural fluid characteristics are not consistent with empyema (typically pleural fluid pH less than 7.2, purulent effusion, or positive Gram stain).

Although cough, dyspnea, and pleural effusion could occur in patients with heart failure, the lack of physical examination findings consistent with volume overload and findings of a serosanguineous exudative effusion on thoracentesis would not be consistent with a diagnosis of heart failure (transudative effusion).

Rheumatoid pleuritis would also present with an exudative pleural effusion, but the patient has no other signs or symptoms of rheumatoid arthritis.

> **KEY POINT**
>
> - Asbestos exposure is the primary risk factor for malignant pleural mesothelioma, and patients most commonly present with symptoms of chest pain and a slowly enlarging pleural effusion.

## Bibliography

Scherpereel A, Astoul P, Baas P, Berghmans T, Clayson H, de Vuyst P, et al; European Respiratory Society/European Society of Thoracic Surgeons Task Force. Guidelines of the European Respiratory Society and the European Society of Thoracic Surgeons for the management of malignant pleural mesothelioma. Eur Respir J. 2010;35:479-95. [PMID: 19717482] doi:10.1183/09031936.00063109

## Item 40    Answer:    C

**Educational Objective:** Treat a patient with newly diagnosed mild COPD.

The most appropriate treatment is a short-acting bronchodilator. Two commonly used, evidence-based treatment schemes are available to guide therapy. The American College of Physicians, American College of Chest Physicians, American Thoracic Society, and European Respiratory Society classification and treatment scheme for stable COPD recommends an inhaled short-acting bronchodilator (anticholinergic or $\beta_2$-agonist) for patients with an $FEV_1$ between 60% and 80% of predicted. The Global Strategy for Diagnosis, Management and Prevention of COPD (GOLD) classification model allows for therapy for COPD based on spirometry, risk, and symptoms. According to the GOLD classification scheme, this patient is in group A (low risk, few symptoms, documented mild airflow obstruction with one or no exacerbations per year). Like the previous guideline, GOLD recommends a short-acting bronchodilator or a combination of short-acting bronchodilators.

Roflumilast is a phosphodiesterase-4 (PDE-4) inhibitor used as add-on therapy to reduce exacerbations in patients with severe COPD associated with chronic bronchitis and a history of recurrent exacerbations despite other therapies. Inhibition of PDE-4 decreases inflammation, which may be helpful in a limited number of patients with COPD in whom inflammation is a significant factor. Roflumilast has minimal bronchodilator activity and should always be used with at least one long-acting bronchodilator. This patient has no indication for roflumilast therapy and it should not be used as monotherapy.

If the patient's symptoms and airflow obstruction progress, both guidelines recommend the addition of a long-acting bronchodilator (either a long-acting $\beta_2$-agonist or long-acting muscarinic agent). If symptoms persist, either an inhaled glucocorticoid or long-acting muscarinic agent can be added to the regimen.

Because this patient has mild disease with minimal symptoms, it is not necessary to start an inhaled glucocorticoid at this time. Short prednisone bursts are used to treat patients with acute exacerbations but are not indicated for the management of mild chronic symptoms related to COPD.

### KEY POINT

- Patients whose symptoms and spirometry are consistent with mild COPD can begin treatment with a short-acting bronchodilator as needed.

## Bibliography

Qaseem A, Wilt TJ, Weinberger SE, Hanania NA, Criner G, van der Molen T, et al; American College of Physicians. Diagnosis and management of stable chronic obstructive pulmonary disease: a clinical practice guideline update from the American College of Physicians, American College of Chest Physicians, American Thoracic Society, and European Respiratory Society. Ann Intern Med. 2011;155:179-91. [PMID: 21810710] doi:10.7326/0003-4819-155-3-201108020-00008

## Item 41    Answer:    A

**Educational Objective:** Treat a patient with chronic hypoventilation due to neuromuscular disease with noninvasive ventilation.

Bilevel positive airway pressure is the most appropriate next step in management. This patient has chronic hypoventilation due to amyotrophic lateral sclerosis (ALS), as indicated by the elevated arterial $P_{CO_2}$ and a compensatory metabolic alkalosis, resulting in a normal pH on blood gas testing. ALS is marked by hypoventilation during sleep and may be exacerbated by acute illness and anesthesia. Bilevel positive airway pressure therapy augments ventilation by providing pressure support, improves quality of life, and may prolong survival in patients with ALS. Ventilatory support should be started in the presence of respiratory symptoms or hypercarbia. It also is essential to discuss prognosis and establish goals of care with patients and families, thereby avoiding unnecessary diagnostic and therapeutic measures.

Continuous positive airway pressure is designed to maintain upper airway patency in obstructive sleep apnea (OSA) and would not be appropriate ventilatory support in the setting of chronic respiratory failure due to hypoventilation.

Hypoglossal nerve stimulation is a treatment of OSA that activates the tongue muscles to increase upper airway caliber and prevent collapse. It has no effect on the respiratory pump muscles weakened by ALS.

Supplemental oxygen should generally not be prescribed for patients with hypoventilation due to neuromuscular disease without adjunctive ventilatory support because supplemental oxygen may further impair ventilation in patients with respiratory muscle weakness.

Tracheostomy may be appropriate for some patients with advanced respiratory failure due to neuromuscular disease, particularly those who experience difficulty in managing secretions or who require support during the waking hours. However, this patient is not yet affected by those issues, and noninvasive therapy should be the initial choice.

### KEY POINT

- Assisted breathing devices, such as bilevel positive airway pressure, can be prescribed to support gas exchange in patients with neuromuscular disorders and may prolong survival in amyotrophic lateral sclerosis.

## Bibliography

Radunovic A, Annane D, Rafiq MK, Brassington R, Mustfa N. Mechanical ventilation for amyotrophic lateral sclerosis/motor neuron disease. Cochrane Database Syst Rev. 2017;10:CD004427. [PMID: 28982219] doi:10.1002/14651858.CD004427.pub4

## Item 42    Answer:    C

**Educational Objective:** Prevent recurrent spontaneous pneumothorax with smoking cessation.

Smoking cessation is the most effective measure to prevent recurrent pneumothorax. This patient has a primary spontaneous pneumothorax (PSP) (air in the pleural space in someone without underlying lung disease). Cigarette smoking is a significant risk factor for PSP, likely because of airway inflammation. The lifetime risk of pneumothorax for men who are lifelong heavy smokers is 12%, compared to 0.1% for men who have never smoked. Because of the strong association between smoking and occurrence of PSP, smoking cessation may help prevent recurrence. Other risk factors for PSP are family history of PSP and thoracic endometriosis. PSP usually develops when the patient is at rest, and presenting patients are typically in their early 20s. Symptoms include the sudden onset of dyspnea and pleuritic chest pain. Recurrence is estimated at 23% to 50% during the first 5 years. Interventions to prevent recurrence includes chemical and mechanical pleurodesis, which are recommended after the second occurrence of PSP on the ipsilateral side, or first occurrence if the patient has a high-risk occupation such as deep sea diver or airplane pilot.

Air travel should be discouraged until resolution of the pneumothorax, but it is not in itself a risk factor for developing a pneumothorax.

There is no association between mountain climbing and development of a pneumothorax.

There is no association between the onset of pneumothorax and physical activity, with the occurrence being as likely when the patient is sedentary as when active.

### KEY POINT

- Patients with a primary spontaneous pneumothorax should be encouraged to stop smoking to prevent recurrence.

### Bibliography

MacDuff A, Arnold A, Harvey J; BTS Pleural Disease Guideline Group. Management of spontaneous pneumothorax: British Thoracic Society Pleural Disease Guideline 2010. Thorax. 2010;65 Suppl 2:ii18-31. [PMID: 20696690] doi:10.1136/thx.2010.136986

## Item 43    Answer:    D

**Educational Objective:** Diagnose an adult with cystic fibrosis.

The most likely underlying diagnosis is cystic fibrosis. This patient has acute symptoms of increased cough, sputum production, fever, chills, wheezing, dyspnea, clubbing, and a chest radiograph (shown) with bilateral upper-lobe predominant bronchiectasis with mucoid impaction (arrows), as well as a history of chronic pulmonary and gastrointestinal disease. This constellation of signs and symptoms is most consistent with an acute exacerbation of bronchiectasis in a patient with cystic fibrosis.

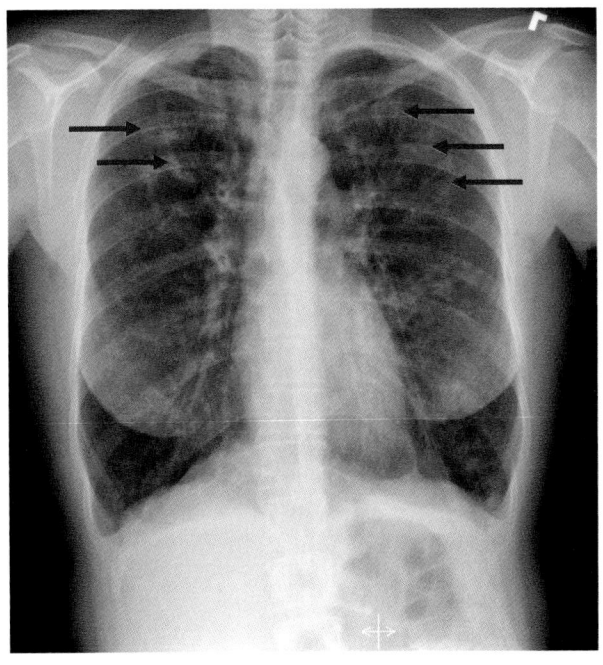

Common variable immunodeficiency involves B- and T-cell abnormalities and results in clinically significant immune dysregulation. The primary manifestation is hypogammaglobulinemia, and adults present with recurrent respiratory infections. The gastrointestinal tract is frequently involved with malabsorption or chronic diarrhea. The diagnosis is made by confirming low levels of total IgG and IgA or IgM, as well as by a poor antibody response to vaccines. The patient's normal serum immunoglobulin levels exclude this diagnosis.

The most common of the early complement disorders is C2 deficiency; C6 deficiency is the most common of the late complement disorders. Patients lacking one of the early components usually present with a rheumatologic disorder. Those with late complement component deficiencies usually present with recurrent, invasive meningococcal or gonococcal infections. The patient's history and findings are not consistent with either early or late complement component deficiency.

Although the patient has obstruction on pulmonary function testing, her age and history of chronic sinus and gastrointestinal disease make a diagnosis of COPD less likely than cystic fibrosis.

### KEY POINT

- Conditions suggesting the diagnosis of cystic fibrosis in adults include chronic asthma-like symptoms, chronic sinusitis, nasal polyposis, recurrent pancreatitis, infertility, and bronchiectasis.

### Bibliography

Nick JA, Nichols DP. Diagnosis of adult patients with cystic fibrosis. Clin Chest Med. 2016;37:47-57. [PMID: 26857767] doi:10.1016/j.ccm.2015.11.006

## Item 44     Answer:   A

**Educational Objective:** Treat a patient with an acute exacerbation of COPD.

The most appropriate treatment of the COPD exacerbation in this patient is azithromycin and prednisone. Exacerbations are marked by increased breathlessness and are usually accompanied by increased cough and sputum production. The degree of exacerbation is considered mild when a change in the clinical condition is noted but no change in medication is necessary. An exacerbation is considered moderate when medication changes are made. A severe exacerbation results in hospitalization. Short-acting bronchodilator therapy is a mainstay of therapy for treating COPD exacerbation. Glucocorticoids, such as prednisone, have been shown to reduce recovery time, improve lung function and arterial hypoxemia, decrease risk of early relapse, decrease treatment failure, and decrease length of hospital stay. Guidelines recommend 40 mg of prednisone or an oral equivalent for 5 to 7 days. The most recent Global Initiative for Chronic Obstructive Lung Disease report recommends that antibiotics should be considered in patients with moderate or severe COPD and symptoms of increased dyspnea, increased sputum, and sputum purulence. Recent studies in patients with moderate COPD have demonstrated improved patient outcomes. Commonly used regimens include an advanced macrolide (such as azithromycin), a cephalosporin, or doxycycline.

This patient's COPD appears to be well-controlled at baseline, so the addition of an inhaled glucocorticoid such as mometasone is not indicated for long-term COPD management. An inhaled glucocorticoid is not an effective treatment of an exacerbation of COPD.

Noninvasive positive pressure ventilation (NIPPV) has a significant role in the management of patients with very severe COPD during an acute exacerbation and may be helpful to avoid intubation. NIPPV is strongly recommended in patients with acute COPD exacerbations who have respiratory acidosis. This patient does not have an indication for NIPPV.

Although roflumilast has been shown to decrease the frequency of recurrent exacerbations, there is no role for this agent in the treatment of an acute exacerbation. As this is a first exacerbation of COPD, chronic roflumilast therapy is not indicated.

### KEY POINT

- An exacerbation of COPD is defined as a sustained worsening of symptoms, typically cough, dyspnea, and sputum production; standard treatment of moderate to severe exacerbations includes antibiotics and oral glucocorticoids.

### Bibliography

Holden V, Slack III D, McCurdy MT, Shah NG. Diagnosis and management of acute exacerbations of chronic obstructive pulmonary disease. Emerg Med Pract. 2017;19:1-24. [PMID: 28926214]

## Item 45     Answer:   D

**Educational Objective:** Treat pulmonary hypertension secondary to chronic hypoxemia.

The most appropriate treatment is supplemental oxygen. The clinical assessment and echocardiographic findings are consistent with pulmonary hypertension in the setting of advanced COPD (Group 3 pulmonary hypertension [PH]). The mainstay of treatment of Group 3 PH targets the underlying lung disease. This patient is on maximal inhaler therapy for COPD. Hypoxemia during daytime rest and, in the setting of cor pulmonale or secondary polycythemia, hypoxemia during sleep, is an indication for supplemental oxygen, which has proved benefit in pulmonary hemodynamics and survival in this population.

Bilevel positive airway pressure is indicated in patients with hypercapnia in the setting of COPD. Furthermore, in patients with overlap of COPD and sleep disordered breathing, continuous positive airway pressure has been shown to increase quality of life and prolong survival. The arterial blood gas study shows this patient to be normocapnic, and polysomnography demonstrates hypoxemia but no sleep apnea. Therefore, positive airway pressure therapy is not indicated.

A short course of prednisone is indicated in acute exacerbations of COPD, which typically present with acute dyspnea, cough, and sputum production. The more insidious course of this patient's symptoms is not consistent with an acute exacerbation of COPD, and there is no role for systemic glucocorticoids in patients with PH due to COPD.

Therapy with a vasodilator such as sildenafil is generally not indicated in patients with pulmonary hypertension related to lung disease or hypoxemia. Such drugs may cause harm by worsening ventilation-perfusion matching and further impairing gas exchange.

### KEY POINT

- Patients with pulmonary hypertension secondary to lung disease and associated hypoxemia should be treated with supplemental oxygen.

### Bibliography

Continuous or nocturnal oxygen therapy in hypoxemic chronic obstructive lung disease: a clinical trial. Nocturnal Oxygen Therapy Trial Group. Ann Intern Med. 1980;93:391-8. [PMID: 6776858]

## Item 46     Answer:   A

**Educational Objective:** Treat pulmonary arterial hypertension.

The most appropriate treatment is bosentan. This patient has pulmonary hypertension most consistent with Group 1 (pulmonary arterial hypertension [PAH]), based upon the right heart catheterization demonstrating high pulmonary arterial pressures in the absence of left-sided heart failure, lung disease, and venous thromboembolic disease. Before administering advanced therapy for patients with PAH, vasoreactivity testing with nitric oxide is performed to identify those who

Answers and Critiques

may respond to calcium channel blockers (CCBs). CCBs are desirable therapy because they are less expensive and have fewer side effects than other forms of advanced therapy. Failure to achieve a favorable hemodynamic response with nitric oxide predicts unresponsiveness to CCBs and the need for other advanced therapy. The endothelin receptor antagonist bosentan is one of many oral pulmonary vasoactive drugs that is indicated in PAH in patients with negative vasoreactivity testing, such as this patient, some of which have been shown to increase exercise capacity and improve echocardiographic parameters.

CCBs such as diltiazem may be used in the setting of PAH when a response to a vasodilator such as nitric oxide is demonstrated during right heart catheterization. When a response is not found, CCBs are not indicated.

β-Blockers such as metoprolol do not have a proved role specific to PAH, though they might be used as an adjunct agent for supraventricular tachyarrhythmias that are common in this population.

Pirfenidone is an antifibrotic agent indicated for the treatment of idiopathic pulmonary fibrosis. Pulmonary hypertension is frequently observed in patients with idiopathic pulmonary fibrosis, but pirfenidone would not be indicated for a patient with PAH without idiopathic pulmonary fibrosis.

## KEY POINT

- Before administering advance therapy for patients with pulmonary arterial hypertension (PAH), particularly idiopathic PAH, vasoreactivity testing directs agent selection by identifying those who may respond to calcium channel blockers.

### Bibliography

Galiè N, Humbert M, Vachiery JL, Gibbs S, Lang I, Torbicki A, et al. 2015 ESC/ERS Guidelines for the diagnosis and treatment of pulmonary hypertension: The Joint Task Force for the Diagnosis and Treatment of Pulmonary Hypertension of the European Society of Cardiology (ESC) and the European Respiratory Society (ERS): Endorsed by: Association for European Paediatric and Congenital Cardiology (AEPC), International Society for Heart and Lung Transplantation (ISHLT). Eur Respir J. 2015;46:903-75. [PMID: 26318161] doi:10.1183/13993003.01032-2015

## Item 47      Answer:      C

**Educational Objective:** Evaluate a patient for occupational exposure using a Material Safety Data Sheet.

The most appropriate management is to review the employer Material Safety Data Sheet (MSDS). This patient is concerned that an occupational exposure is causing new respiratory symptoms and potentially may worsen her asthma control. When an occupational lung disease is being considered, clinicians should request the MSDS, which details chemical properties and known health risks associated with substances within the workplace. The U.S. Occupational Safety and Health Administration (OSHA) requires that this information is available upon request for employees who work with potentially harmful materials. Establishing a clear causal link between this patient's symptoms of asthma and an occupa-

tional exposure is essential in diagnosis and management. Her history suggests a temporal relationship between the introduction of the new chemical and her cough. In addition, she feels the need to use her albuterol inhaler after exposure. Examples of known respiratory irritants include chlorine gas and sulfur dioxide, which are triggers of bronchospasm. Toluene diisocyanate is associated with allergic sensitization, cough, and bronchospasm that can develop weeks or months after initial exposure. Additional evaluation for occupational illness can include peak flow meter measurements before and after exposure, bronchoprovocation testing after prolonged time away from work and return to work, and, in select cases, specific inhalational challenges.

A chest CT scan is usually not needed for the evaluation of a patient with suspected occupational asthma. Exceptions to this rule include patients with abnormal chest radiography or suspected hypersensitivity pneumonitis. This patient has a normal lung examination, normal spirometry, and no symptoms compatible with acute hypersensitivity pneumonitis (fevers, flulike symptoms, cough, and shortness of breath). This patient has no indication for advanced imaging.

Although several commercial entities offer testing of hair samples for toxic chemicals, this testing is expensive, unlikely to be covered by insurance, and of questionable validity. It is, therefore, not recommended in the assessment of occupational exposure by primary care internists.

Supporting a patient's request to transfer work areas related to a health concern should be based on sound clinical assessment and judgment. A clinician's initial assessment should establish the presence of an occupational illness by assessing exposures, including known chemicals in the workplace, and establishing a temporal relationship between the introduction of the new chemical and symptoms.

## KEY POINT

- When an occupational lung disease is being considered, clinicians should request a Material Safety Data Sheet detailing chemical properties and known health risks associated with substances within the workplace.

### Bibliography

Friedman-Jimenez G, Harrison D, Luo H. Occupational asthma and work-exacerbated asthma. Semin Respir Crit Care Med. 2015;36:388-407. [PMID: 26024347] doi:10.1055/s-0035-1550157

## Item 48      Answer:      A

**Educational Objective:** Evaluate a patient with an anterior mediastinal mass and symptoms of myasthenia gravis.

An acetylcholine receptor (AChR) antibody test should be ordered. The mediastinum can be divided into three separate compartments (anterior, middle, and posterior), which can help narrow the differential diagnosis of a mediastinal mass. Each compartment normally contains separate and distinct anatomic structures that can lead to development of a mass. Patients may be asymptomatic and are often diagnosed after obtaining a chest radiograph for another reason, whereas others present with symptoms related to compression of adjacent structures. For example, they may present with dyspnea if the airway is compressed from a nearby mass or with upper extremity edema if vascular structures are compressed.

This patient has an anterior mediastinal mass (arrow) and neurologic symptoms. Masses in this location are usually remembered as the "terrible T's": thymoma, teratoma/germ cell tumor, "terrible" lymphoma, and thyroid. Additional considerations include thoracic aneurysm. Thymomas are the most common cause of an anterior mediastinal mass. Patients usually present as middle-age adults and may develop paraneoplastic syndromes. For example, myasthenia gravis can develop in 30% to 50% of patients with a thymoma. In comparison, only 10% to 15% of patients with myasthenia gravis have a thymoma. The second most common cause is lymphoma; these patients are typically younger at the time of presentation. Other less common paraneoplastic syndromes include pure red blood cell aplasia, nonthymic cancers, and acquired hypogammaglobulinemia.

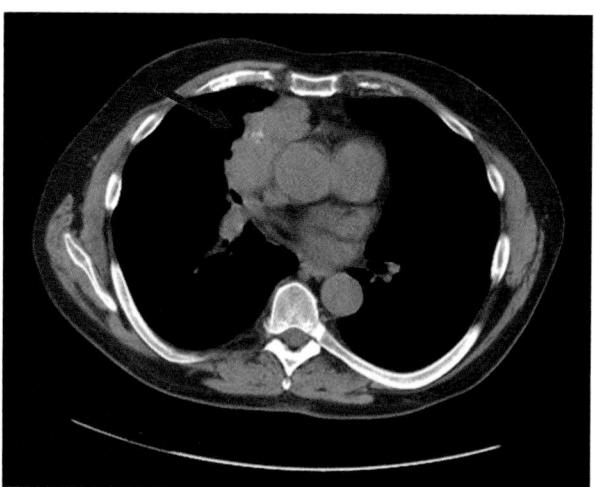

Myasthenia gravis is an autoimmune disorder of the neuromuscular junction that is characterized by fatigable (or fluctuating) muscular weakness. Common symptoms are ptosis and diplopia, which this patient has. Diagnosis of myasthenia gravis is based on clinical findings, detection of disease-specific antibodies (acetylcholine receptor antibodies in 90% of patients and anti–muscle-specific kinase [MuSK] antibodies in another 5% [with 5% of patients remaining antibody negative]), and electromyography findings (such as a characteristic decremental response to repetitive stimulation). Thymectomy should be performed in all patients with thymoma.

α-Fetoprotein and β-human chorionic gonadotropin are commonly elevated in germ cell tumors, which are also part of the differential diagnosis of an anterior mediastinal mass. However, this patient also has symptoms of myasthenia gravis, which is not associated with germ cell tumors.

Lactate dehydrogenase is commonly elevated in lymphoma and seminomas but is not as specific as other tumor markers and will not help determine the cause of this patient's symptoms.

**Bibliography**

Strollo DC, Rosado de Christenson ML, Jett JR. Primary mediastinal tumors. Part 1: tumors of the anterior mediastinum. Chest. 1997;112:511-22. [PMID: 9266892]

**Item 49      Answer:      B**

**Educational Objective:** Treat pneumonia in a patient with inhalational injury.

Administration of empiric intravenous antibiotics for presumed pneumonia is the most appropriate treatment. This patient suffered an inhalational injury as a result of her exposure to a house fire. Common acute complications of inhalational injury include systemic toxicity from carbon monoxide and hydrogen cyanide, upper airway obstruction from pharyngeal edema, mucosal sloughing, bronchial cast formation, bronchoconstriction, pneumonia, acute respiratory distress syndrome, and pulmonary edema. The most common complication following smoke inhalation injuries is pneumonia. Inhalational injury increases the risk for respiratory infections, especially from *Staphylococcus* and *Pseudomonas* species, because of several mechanisms, including impaired pulmonary macrophage activity, direct injury to the airway cilia and tracheobronchial mucosal epithelium, and impaired surfactant production. Although the patient is only borderline febrile, her increasing leukocyte count and the presence of a focal consolidation in her left lower lobe on chest radiograph increase the index of suspicion for pneumonia.

Acute cyanide poisoning primarily occurs through fire and occupational exposures. Although no reliable test for cyanide poisoning exists, patients suspected of cyanide poisoning should receive hydroxocobalamin. Because this patient's inhalational exposure occurred 3 weeks ago, it is unlikely that her acute respiratory failure is due to cyanide poisoning. Thus, hydroxocobalamin is not indicated.

Tracheobronchial stenosis is an infrequent but real complication of inhalational injury. However, it most commonly occurs several months postexposure. The patient's recent normal airway inspection also suggests stenosis is a less likely cause of her respiratory decline. Other long-term complications following smoke inhalation include vocal cord fixation, airway polyps, persistent dysphonia, bronchiolitis obliterans, and bronchiectasis.

Common indications for thoracostomy tube placement include empyema or pneumothorax. Although pneumothorax should be considered in a patient with acute respiratory failure, there is no pneumothorax on this patient's radiograph. A thoracentesis is indicated for any new unexplained pleural effusion. Observation and initiation of therapy without diagnostic thoracentesis is reasonable in the setting of a small parapneumonic effusion, as is seen in the left base of

CONT.

this patient's radiograph. If an empyema or other small fluid collection requires evaluation, the initial investigation with needle thoracentesis is generally indicated before consideration of thoracostomy tube placement.

**KEY POINT**

- Secondary respiratory infections are common in patients with inhalational injuries, especially from *Staphylococcus* and *Pseudomonas* species, and are a major cause of morbidity and mortality.

**Bibliography**
Walker PF, Buehner MF, Wood LA, Boyer NL, Driscoll IR, Lundy JB, et al. Diagnosis and management of inhalation injury: an updated review. Crit Care. 2015;19:351. [PMID: 26507130] doi:10.1186/s13054-015-1077-4

## Item 50    Answer:    D

**Educational Objective:** Treat a patient at risk for alcohol withdrawal who has overdosed on benzodiazepines.

This patient should be kept on mechanical ventilation and monitored for signs of agitation. He shows signs of benzodiazepine overdose, combined with alcohol abuse. His airway is secure, and he is easily supported with mechanical ventilation, which can continue until he has metabolized the drug and his mental status has improved. Because of his history of alcohol abuse, he is at risk for alcohol withdrawal. Alcohol withdrawal occurs with chronic heavy alcohol use within hours to days after alcohol cessation. Early withdrawal symptoms occur within a few hours of abstinence and include agitation, anxiety, tremulousness, headache, and symptoms of autonomic hyperactivity (fever, diaphoresis, tachycardia, hypertension). Generalized tonic-clonic seizures may occur usually within 6 to 24 hours and should be treated with benzodiazepines because if left untreated, up to one third of patients may progress to delirium tremens.

Flumazenil, a γ-aminobutyric acid (GABA)–receptor antagonist, is the antidote for benzodiazepine toxicity, but reversing the benzodiazepine he took could put him at risk for seizures, especially if he is a chronic user. The short half-life of flumazenil makes it challenging to use in patients requiring sustained reversal of long-acting benzodiazepines, and given the overall low risk of benzodiazepine overdose, it is safer to allow his body to metabolize the benzodiazepine and eliminate it along with the alcohol.

Fomepizole inhibits alcohol dehydrogenase. It is used to block the metabolism of ethylene glycol and methanol into toxic metabolites when either of these alcohols is ingested. There is no reason to suspect either agent, especially in a patient with normal blood pH and a normal anion gap. Administration would therefore not be appropriate.

Dialysis would not be appropriate because there is no acute indication for this invasive and costly intervention. In principle, hemodialysis is indicated for drug intoxications when the clearance of the drug by hemodialysis is significantly shorter than metabolic clearance and the patient is deteriorating or when measured drug concentrations are

predictive of a poor outcome without hemodialysis. Dialysis will remove alcohols effectively, but the patient is stable and does not require an invasive intervention.

**KEY POINT**

- Treatment for benzodiazepine overdose is supportive with assurance of adequate ventilation; flumazenil is generally not recommended for benzodiazepine overdose as it can precipitate seizures in chronic users and its short half-life makes it difficult to sustain reversal of long-acting benzodiazepines.

**Bibliography**
An H, Godwin J. Flumazenil in benzodiazepine overdose. CMAJ. 2016;188:E537. [PMID: 27920113]

## Item 51    Answer:    A

**Educational Objective:** Treat hypersensitivity pneumonitis.

This patient has acute hypersensitivity pneumonitis and should be counseled not to return to work. The acute form of hypersensitivity pneumonitis presents within 48 hours of a high-level exposure and will often be associated with fever, flu-like symptoms, cough, and shortness of breath. Radiographic imaging can demonstrate bilateral hazy opacities, whereas high-resolution CT imaging of the chest shows findings of ground-glass opacities and centrilobular micronodules that are upper- and midlung predominant. Symptoms typically wane within 24 to 48 hours after removal from the exposure. Recurrence of symptoms with exposure to the respiratory antigen is the hallmark of this disorder, and careful attention to the history will help identify the cause. Primary treatment of acute hypersensitivity pneumonitis is removal from the offending antigen. Studies indicate that pulmonary function can continue to gradually recover, with initial improvements in oxygen exchange followed by increased FVC and improved chest radiograph findings.

Although treatment of acute hypersensitivity pneumonitis with systemic glucocorticoids is appropriate for those with more severe disease, patient response is variable, and prolonged use is associated with significant side effects. There are no data to support the use of inhaled glucocorticoids for acute hypersensitivity pneumonitis and, again, the primary treatment is to remove the offending agent.

Idiopathic pulmonary fibrosis (IPF) is the most common idiopathic interstitial pneumonia. It occurs predominantly in older individuals; the diagnosis of IPF is rare in those younger than 50 years of age. Gradual onset of dyspnea and cough during months to years is typical. Pirfenidone is a novel therapeutic agent that regulates transforming growth factor β (TGF-β) and tumor necrosis factor α (TNF-α) activity through an unknown mechanism that is used in the treatment of idiopathic pulmonary fibrosis. Similarly, nintedanib is a tyrosine kinase inhibitor known to block pathways that lead to activation of the fibroblast. Although these therapies are an important step forward in the management of IPF, they are not curative. This patient does not have IPF and treatment with pirfenidone is not indicated.

Lymphangioleiomyomatosis is a rare disorder that occurs sporadically in women or in association with tuberous sclerosis. It manifests as a diffuse cystic lung disease due to infiltration of smooth muscle cells into the pulmonary parenchyma. Genetic mutations within the cells lead to activation of the mechanistic target of rapamycin (mTOR) pathway. Diagnosis is based on imaging studies with diffuse thin-walled cysts as well as spontaneous pneumothorax and angiomyolipomas. Treatment is inhibition of the mTOR with sirolimus. Such treatment is not indicated in this patient with hypersensitivity pneumonitis.

**KEY POINT**

• Removal of the offending antigen is the most appropriate treatment of acute hypersensitivity pneumonitis.

**Bibliography**

Vasakova M, Morell F, Walsh S, Leslie K, Raghu G. Hypersensitivity pneumonitis: perspectives in diagnosis and management. Am J Respir Crit Care Med. 2017;196:680-689. [PMID: 28598197] doi:10.1164/rccm.201611-2201PP

## Item 52    Answer:    B

**Educational Objective:** Treat a patient with a macrolide antibiotic to reduce frequent COPD exacerbations.

The most appropriate guideline-recommended (grade 2A) treatment of this patient with severe COPD and frequent exacerbations is chronic macrolide therapy. Macrolide antibiotics have inflammatory and antimicrobial effects and may reduce the frequency of exacerbations when used long-term by patients with severe COPD. Several clinical trials to assess prophylactic use and benefit have demonstrated a reduction in the rate of exacerbation in patients with moderate to severe COPD with one or more moderate or severe exacerbations in the previous year despite optimal maintenance inhaler therapy. The duration and exact dosage of macrolide therapy are unknown. The primary concerns with long-term macrolide therapy are development of antibiotic resistance, including macrolide-resistant strains of nontuberculous mycobacteria. In addition, hearing loss and potentially fatal arrhythmias due to prolongation of the QT interval have occurred in association with azithromycin.

The long-term use of systemic glucocorticoids is avoided in the chronic management of COPD due to lack of demonstrated benefit and recognized increased risk of significant side effects such as diabetes, hypertension, muscle weakness, and decreased functional status.

The use of supplemental oxygen in patients with COPD and hypoxemia has been shown to improve quality of life and mortality in patients who have resting hypoxemia with an arterial $P_{O_2}$ of 55 mm Hg (7.31 kPa) or lower, or oxygen saturation on pulse oximetry ($Sp_{O_2}$) of 88% or lower. This patient's $Sp_{O_2}$ is above 88% at rest and on exertion on her current level of supplemental oxygen. Increasing this further has not been shown to decrease the rate of acute exacerbations.

Mucolytics such as nebulized hypertonic saline and airway clearance maneuvers may provide some symptomatic relief in patients with significant sputum production, but this patient does not have cough or sputum production. Moreover, these interventions have not been shown to decrease the rate of acute exacerbations in patients with COPD.

**KEY POINT**

• In patients with severe COPD and frequent exacerbations, chronic macrolide therapy has been shown to decrease COPD exacerbations.

**Bibliography**

Criner GJ, Bourbeau J, Diekemper RL, Ouellette DR, Goodridge D, Hernandez P, et al. Prevention of acute exacerbations of COPD: American College of Chest Physicians and Canadian Thoracic Society Guideline. Chest. 2015;147:894-942. [PMID: 25321320] doi:10.1378/chest.14-1676

## Item 53    Answer:    C

**Educational Objective:** Treat a patient with acute hypoxemic respiratory failure with invasive mechanical ventilation.

The most appropriate treatment is intubation and mechanical ventilation. This patient has dyspnea, severe hypoxemia, bilateral opacities on chest radiograph, and acute hypoxemic respiratory failure after aspiration, all of which are diagnostic for acute respiratory distress syndrome (ARDS). ARDS is associated with heterogeneous but often widespread damage to the alveolar epithelium and vascular endothelium, as well as surfactant dysfunction leading to alveolar instability and collapse. The changes can severely reduce lung compliance, making adequate ventilation difficult and further worsening hypoxia. Most patients with ARDS require intubation and mechanical ventilation to ensure adequate delivery of high levels of inspired oxygen and positive end-expiratory pressure to stabilize alveoli.

Continuing oxygen through a face mask would not be appropriate. Although the patient is maintaining appropriate oxygen saturation, the presence of anxiety, diaphoresis, tachycardia, tachypnea, hypercapnia, and hypoxemia signal impending respiratory failure that should be treated with intubation and mechanical ventilation.

High-flow humidified nasal cannula devices decrease the work of breathing, provide heated and humidified air, provide a reliable $F_{IO_2}$, and decrease dead space. Their initial application should occur in the critical care setting with close monitoring for tolerance and effectiveness. A recent trial demonstrated that in patients with acute hypoxemic respiratory failure, the use of high flow nasal cannula led to decreased mortality compared to continuing face mask oxygen or noninvasive face mask ventilation; however, the study excluded patients with hypercapnia, such as this

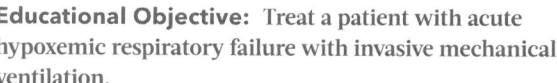

**CONT.**

patient. This patient shows features of respiratory muscle fatigue, including rapid breathing, diaphoresis, use of accessory muscles of respiration, and an elevated arterial $P_{CO_2}$, all indications for mechanical ventilation.

Noninvasive positive pressure ventilation (NIPPV) is the delivery of positive airway pressure using a cushioned face mask or helmet or without the use of an invasive connection directly in a patient's airway. In patients with hypoxemic respiratory failure, the use of NIPPV is controversial. Select patients may benefit from short-duration NIPPV to avoid intubation and associated complications but some studies have demonstrated increased mortality, likely due to delay in the implementation of appropriate invasive mechanical ventilation. This patient with deteriorating ventilation should be intubated and mechanically ventilated.

**KEY POINT**

- Most patients with acute respiratory distress syndrome require intubation and mechanical ventilation to ensure adequate delivery of high levels of inspired oxygen and positive end-expiratory pressure to stabilize alveoli.

**Bibliography**

Wilson JG, Matthay MA. Mechanical ventilation in acute hypoxemic respiratory failure: a review of new strategies for the practicing hospitalist. J Hosp Med. 2014;9:469-75. [PMID: 24733692] doi:10.1002/jhm.2192

## Item 54    Answer:    D

**Educational Objective:** Diagnose pulmonary arterial hypertension in a patient with limited cutaneous systemic sclerosis and CREST syndrome.

The most likely diagnosis is pulmonary arterial hypertension. Pulmonary involvement is frequent (greater than 70%) in patients with systemic sclerosis and can be symptomatic and disabling. The two principal clinical manifestations are interstitial lung disease and pulmonary vascular disease. Pulmonary vascular disease leading to pulmonary arterial hypertension may occur secondary to interstitial lung disease (typically in diffuse cutaneous systemic sclerosis) or as an isolated process (typically in limited cutaneous systemic sclerosis). This patient has several features of limited cutaneous systemic sclerosis with CREST syndrome (a condition defined by calcinosis cutis, Raynaud phenomenon, esophageal dysmotility, sclerodactyly, and telangiectasias). Patients are usually asymptomatic in early disease but later develop dyspnea on exertion and diminished exercise tolerance. Severe disease can lead to right-sided heart failure. Chest imaging is often normal and pulmonary function tests demonstrate a reduced $D_{LCO}$ with normal lung volumes.

Organizing pneumonia is a patchy process that involves proliferation of granulation tissue within alveolar ducts, alveolar spaces, and surrounding areas of chronic inflammation. There are many known causes of this pattern, including acute infections and autoimmune disorders such as rheumatoid arthritis. The term *cryptogenic organizing pneumonia*

(COP) is reserved for individuals who have this pattern but do not have a clear associated cause. Patients with COP will typically present with symptoms during 6 to 8 weeks that mimic community-acquired pneumonia. Evaluation typically demonstrates bilateral diffuse alveolar opacities on chest radiograph with normal lung volumes. This patient's presentation is not consistent with cryptogenic organizing pneumonia.

Lymphangioleiomyomatosis is a multisystem disease that almost exclusively affects young women. Pulmonary complications are prominent and include diffuse pulmonary cysts, pneumothorax, chylous pleural effusions, and obstructive airways disease. Lymphangioleiomyomatosis would be very unlikely in a patient with an unremarkable chest radiograph.

Lymphoid interstitial pneumonia is an interstitial lung disease characterized by lymphocytic infiltration of the pulmonary interstitium. It is observed in patients with Sjögren's syndrome and viral infections, especially HIV. Patients with lymphoid interstitial pneumonia often have crackles on the pulmonary examination, interstitial infiltrates on chest radiography, and decreased lung volumes and diffusing capacity on pulmonary function testing.

**KEY POINT**

- Pulmonary arterial hypertension is commonly associated with connective tissue diseases, such as limited cutaneous systemic sclerosis.

**Bibliography**

Kato M, Atsumi T. Pulmonary arterial hypertension associated with connective tissue diseases: A review focusing on distinctive clinical aspects. Eur J Clin Invest. 2018;48. [PMID: 29285766] doi:10.1111/eci.12876

## Item 55    Answer:    A

**Educational Objective:** Treat sepsis with immediate fluid resuscitation.

The most appropriate management is an intravenous fluid bolus of 30 mL/kg of body weight. Successful treatment of severe sepsis and septic shock depends on the rapid institution of hemodynamic support, empiric treatment of infection, and infection control. Crystalloid infusion (normal [0.9%] saline or lactated Ringer solution) to support circulating intravascular volume should be administered to all patients with severe sepsis and septic shock. The 2016 update to the Surviving Sepsis Guidelines recommends using an initial bolus of 30 mL/kg of body weight.

The 2018 American Diabetes Association Standards for Care recommend that insulin therapy be initiated for treatment of persistent hyperglycemia starting at a threshold of 180 mg/dL (10.0 mmol/L). Once insulin therapy is started, a target glucose range of 140 to 180 mg/dL (7.8–10.0 mmol/L) is recommended for most critically ill and noncritically ill patients. This patient's plasma glucose is not so high that it is an emergency; therefore, administration of insulin is a lower priority than treatment of shock.

CONT.

This patient may have also have developed a paraspinous abscess (fever, new-onset back pain, difficulty urinating). This patient may need spine imaging but the more urgent priority is his hemodynamic instability, which requires fluid resuscitation before he can undergo any diagnostic imaging study.

Before this patient can be evaluated for surgical source control, he needs to be resuscitated. He is not showing signs of necrotizing fasciitis, which would be a surgical emergency, but even if he were suspected of this diagnosis, he would need aggressive fluid resuscitation while arrangements were made for urgent surgical debridement.

**KEY POINT**

- Patients with hypoperfusion due to sepsis should be managed with aggressive crystalloid fluid resuscitation using an initial bolus of 30 mL/kg of body weight.

**Bibliography**

Rhodes A, Evans LE, Alhazzani W, Levy MM, Antonelli M, Ferrer R, et al. Surviving Sepsis Campaign: international guidelines for management of sepsis and septic shock: 2016. Intensive Care Med. 2017;43:304-377. [PMID: 28101605] doi:10.1007/s00134-017-4683-6

## Item 56    Answer:    C

**Educational Objective:** Treat secondary spontaneous pneumothorax with chemical pleurodesis.

The most appropriate management of this patient with severe COPD and secondary pneumothorax is pleurodesis. Pneumothorax (air in the pleural space) can occur spontaneously, as a result of trauma, or iatrogenically. Spontaneous pneumothorax is further characterized as a primary spontaneous pneumothorax (PSP) in a person without underlying lung disease or a secondary spontaneous pneumothorax (SSP) in a person with underlying lung disease. Patients presenting with SSP are at higher risk for persistent air leak, further expansion of the pneumothorax, or pneumothorax recurrence due to their underlying lung disease. Intervention to prevent recurrence includes both chemical and mechanical pleurodesis, which is recommended in all patients with SSP and after the second occurrence of a PSP. In patients with SSP the cause of persistent air leak following pneumothorax is usually subpleural bullae or cysts. Additional interventions are required to close the leak. For patients who are surgical candidates, video-assisted thoracoscopic surgery (VATS) is recommended to locate and staple or resect blebs followed by mechanical pleurodesis. Patients who cannot tolerate surgery are treated with blood patch or chemical pleurodesis. These procedures are designed to seal the leak and prevent recurrence of pneumothorax. A blood patch is performed by injecting a quantity of the patient's blood into the thoracostomy tube. Chemical pleurodesis is performed by instilling tetracycline or one of its derivatives or specialized talc powder through the thoracostomy tube. Success rate for chemical pleurodesis ranges from 60% to 90% but it is not as effective as mechanical pleurodesis using VATS.

Clamping or removing the thoracostomy tube would not be appropriate because the patient has a secondary spontaneous pneumothorax and the likelihood of recurrence is high.

Placing the thoracostomy tube to high suction would not be appropriate because high levels of suction can increase the risk for reexpansion and pulmonary edema; in addition, the pneumothorax has resolved so no additional suction is needed.

**KEY POINT**

- Recurrence prevention with pleurodesis is recommended after the first occurrence of secondary spontaneous pneumothorax.

**Bibliography**

MacDuff A, Arnold A, Harvey J; BTS Pleural Disease Guideline Group. Management of spontaneous pneumothorax: British Thoracic Society Pleural Disease Guideline 2010. Thorax. 2010;65 Suppl 2:ii18-31. [PMID: 20696690] doi:10.1136/thx.2010.136986

## Item 57    Answer:    C

**Educational Objective:** Identify risk factors of acute exacerbations of COPD.

The patient's previous COPD exacerbations and $FEV_1$ of 35% of predicted are most associated with high risk for recurrent acute exacerbations of COPD. In the Evaluation of COPD Longitudinally to Identify Predictive Surrogate Endpoints (ECLIPSE) prospective study, the best predictor of exacerbations was a history of exacerbations, regardless of COPD severity. In this study the number of exacerbations in the previous 12 months, degree of airflow obstruction, and number of hospitalizations for an exacerbation refined the risk estimate. A history of 0 or 1 exacerbation, $FEV_1$ of 50% or better, and no hospitalizations predicts a low risk of future exacerbations, whereas more than 1 exacerbation, $FEV_1$ less than 50% predicted, and hospitalization predicts a high future risk of exacerbation. Exacerbations of COPD can be prevented by optimizing treatment with appropriate interventions based on risk classification and overall disease management; this includes immunizations and lifestyle changes such as maintaining physical activity and addressing anxiety and depression.

Pulmonary rehabilitation is recommended for all symptomatic patients with an $FEV_1$ of less than 50% of predicted and specifically for those hospitalized with an acute exacerbation of COPD. Use of such a program is not causally linked with an increased risk of COPD exacerbation.

Several comorbidities are associated with an increased risk of acute exacerbation, including heart failure, ischemic heart disease, diabetes, kidney failure, and hepatic failure. However, hypertension has not been associated with an increased risk of acute COPD exacerbations.

Current tobacco use is an independent risk factor for the development of COPD. However, past tobacco use and significant pack-year history are not associated with an

Answers and Critiques

increased risk for acute exacerbation. Discontinuing maintenance COPD mediations is associated with COPD exacerbations, whereas the use of such medications is not.

**KEY POINT**

- Patients with COPD who have had two or more acute exacerbations within the last year, who have an $FEV_1$ of less than 50% of predicted, or who have ever been hospitalized for an acute exacerbation are considered to be at high risk for recurrent acute exacerbations.

**Bibliography**

Hurst JR, Vestbo J, Anzueto A, Locantore N, Müllerova H, Tal-Singer R, et al; Evaluation of COPD Longitudinally to Identify Predictive Surrogate Endpoints (ECLIPSE) Investigators. Susceptibility to exacerbation in chronic obstructive pulmonary disease. N Engl J Med. 2010;363:1128-38. [PMID: 20843247] doi:10.1056/NEJMoa0909883

## Item 58     Answer:   B

**Educational Objective:** Treat a patient with neurologic disease and hypercapnic respiratory failure with bilevel positive airway pressure.

The use of bilevel positive airway pressure (BPAP) ventilation is the most appropriate treatment. This patient has features consistent with chronic hypercapnic respiratory failure secondary to neuromuscular disease. He has dyspnea and, more characteristically, orthopnea. The patient has chronic respiratory acidosis with a normal alveolar-arterial (A-a) oxygen gradient. BPAP delivers both inspiratory positive airway pressure and expiratory positive airway pressure and improves survival and quality of life of patients with neuromuscular disease. The settings generate a pressure difference that augments the patient's own respiratory muscle activity, leading to an increase in the size of each breath. The $P_{CO_2}$ level will decrease due to the increase in minute ventilation and efficiency of breathing.

Invasive mechanical ventilation (mechanical ventilation with airway intubation or tracheostomy) is a therapeutic option in the setting of acute hypercapnic respiratory failure due to neuromuscular disease. However, the patient is awake, has excellent bulbar control (swallows and gags), and has a chronic disease that responds well to noninvasive ventilation.

Continuous positive airway pressure (CPAP) delivers positive airway pressure at a level that remains constant throughout the respiratory cycle preventing upper airway collapse or narrowing during sleep. No additional pressure above the level of CPAP is provided and patients must initiate every breath. CPAP does not increase minute ventilation, and it is not helpful in patients with hypercapnic respiratory failure due to neuromuscular disorders.

The patient has a normal A-a oxygen gradient and hypercapnia, which confirm that the hypoxemia is secondary to hypoventilation rather than a ventilation-perfusion mismatch or shunt; therefore, oxygen administration should not be needed once his $P_{CO_2}$ improves. More importantly,

the administration of oxygen in the absence of supportive ventilation should be avoided in patients with neuromuscular disease and chronic hypercapnic respiratory failure; it has been associated with acute hypercapnia, in some cases leading to death.

**KEY POINT**

- Bilevel positive airway pressure ventilation improves survival and quality of life in patients with neuromuscular disease.

**Bibliography**

Gregoretti C, Pisani L, Cortegiani A, Ranieri VM. Noninvasive ventilation in critically ill patients. Crit Care Clin. 2015;31:435-57. [PMID: 26118914] doi:10.1016/j.ccc.2015.03.002

## Item 59     Answer:   A

**Educational Objective:** Treat a patient with hypertensive encephalopathy.

The appropriate treatment is intravenous hypertensive therapy to lower the systolic blood pressure (SBP) to 160 mm Hg within the first 6 hours. Appropriate intravenous agents could include fenoldopam, nicardipine, or nitroprusside. Hypertensive emergency refers to elevation of SBP greater than 180 mm Hg, diastolic blood pressure (DBP) greater than 120 mm Hg, or both, that is associated with end-organ damage. Patients with hypertensive emergency require rapid, tightly controlled reductions in blood pressure that avoid overcorrection. Management typically occurs in an ICU with continuous arterial blood pressure monitoring and continuous infusion of antihypertensive agents. According to the 2017 American College of Cardiology/American Heart Association hypertension guidelines, for adults with a compelling condition (aortic dissection, severe preeclampsia or eclampsia, or pheochromocytoma crisis), SBP should be reduced to less than 140 mm Hg during the first hour and to less than 120 mm Hg in aortic dissection. For adults without a compelling condition, such as this patient, SBP should be reduced by no more than 25% within the first hour; then, if stable, to 160 mm Hg within the next 2 to 6 hours; and then cautiously to normal during the following 24 to 48 hours.

Because autoregulation of tissue perfusion is disturbed in hypertensive emergencies, reducing blood pressure too rapidly can result in ischemic organ damage. Therefore, targeting a blood pressure of 120/80 mm Hg during the first hour of treatment is inappropriate because it could result in further worsening of kidney injury, encephalopathy, or both.

Conversely, lowering the SBP to 160 mm Hg during 48 hours is likely too slow and not in keeping with current guidelines.

This patient's normal medication combined with observation is not aggressive enough. Eventually he will need a stable outpatient hypertension regimen with education on the importance of adherence to that regimen, but not in this acute setting.

**KEY POINT**

- For adults with a hypertensive emergency and without a compelling condition (such as aortic dissection) systolic blood pressure should be reduced by no more than 25% within the first hour; then, if stable, to 160 mm Hg within the next 2 to 6 hours; and then cautiously to normal during the following 24 to 48 hours.

**Bibliography**

Whelton PK, Carey RM, Aronow WS, Casey DE Jr, Collins KJ, Dennison Himmelfarb C, et al. 2017 ACC/AHA/AAPA/ABC/ACPM/AGS/APhA/ASH/ASPC/NMA/PCNA guideline for the prevention, detection, evaluation, and management of high blood pressure in adults: a report of the American College of Cardiology/American Heart Association Task Force on Clinical Practice Guidelines. Hypertension. 2017. [PMID: 29133356] doi:10.1161/HYP.0000000000000065

## Item 60     Answer:    A

**Educational Objective:** Treat a patient for cyanide poisoning as a coexposure to carbon monoxide poisoning after a house fire.

This patient should be treated with intravenous hydroxocobalamin, which is the preferred antidote for cyanide poisoning. Cyanide toxicity is common in victims of house fires, with up to 90% of rescued victims having elevated cyanide levels and 35% having significantly elevated levels, which is higher than the rate of carbon monoxide poisoning among such victims. Cyanide disrupts oxidative phosphorylation, forcing cells to convert to anaerobic metabolism despite adequate oxygen supply. The result in severe cases is multiorgan failure with coma, seizures, and cardiovascular symptoms, including hypotension, bradycardia, heart block, and ventricular arrhythmias. Early manifestations are nonspecific. Diagnostic clues include lactic acidosis and inappropriately elevated central venous oxyhemoglobin saturation, which manifests as bright red venous blood. Cyanide levels are not readily available and because toxicity is rapidly fatal, prompt empiric treatment is imperative in suspected cases. Hydroxocobalamin avidly binds to cyanide to produce cyanocobalamin, which is soluble, nontoxic, and readily excreted. In addition, ongoing exposure, such as contaminated clothing, should also be eliminated. Hydroxocobalamin can affect accuracy of lab results for methemoglobin, lactate, and other tests, so it is important to obtain blood for these tests before administering the antidote, if possible.

Carbon monoxide is removed by competitive binding of oxygen to hemoglobin. The initial treatment is administration of 100% oxygen, which reduces the half-life of carboxyhemoglobin from 5 hours to 90 minutes. Hyperbaric oxygen therapy yields an even higher alveolar $P_{O_2}$, thereby reducing the half-life to 30 minutes while substantially increasing the amount of oxygen directly dissolved in blood. However, hyperbaric oxygen therapy would not be appropriate because this patient's carboxyhemoglobin level is not high enough to suggest severe carbon monoxide poisoning.

Hyperbaric oxygen is usually recommended for levels of 25% to 40% or higher, or for victims with lower levels who are pregnant.

Methylene blue would be recommended for toxic levels of methemoglobin, usually 20% to 30% or higher, but it is not indicated for this patient.

Although sodium nitrite is an antidote for cyanide poisoning, it is contraindicated in victims of smoke inhalation because it works by inducing methemoglobinemia, which would further impair oxygen delivery by additive or synergistic effects on oxygen binding and delivery in cases of carbon monoxide toxicity.

Sodium thiosulfate is also used as an antidote for cyanide toxicity and is safer than sodium nitrite, but has a slower onset of action. It is considered second-line therapy after hydroxocobalamin, but the two agents can be given to the same patient, possibly with synergistic effect. However, they should not be administered simultaneously or through the same intravenous catheter.

**KEY POINT**

- Hydroxocobalamin effectively removes cyanide from the mitochondrial respiration system and is the preferred antidote for cyanide poisoning.

**Bibliography**

Hamad E, Babu K, Bebarta VS. Case files of the University of Massachusetts Toxicology Fellowship: Does this smoke inhalation victim require treatment with cyanide antidote? J Med Toxicol. 2016;12:192-8. [PMID: 26831054] doi:10.1007/s13181-016-0533-0

## Item 61     Answer:    C

**Educational Objective:** Manage a patient with clinical signs of cystic fibrosis and a negative sweat chloride test.

The most appropriate next step is to repeat the sweat chloride testing. Diagnosis of cystic fibrosis (CF) is based on a combination of CF-compatible clinical findings in conjunction with either biochemical (sweat testing, nasal potential difference) or genetic (*CFTR* mutations) techniques. Genetic counseling should always occur before any genetic test is performed. The essential components of counseling include informing the patient of the test purpose, implications of diagnosis, and alternative testing options. Ultimately, the decision of whether or not to be tested rests with the patient. Use of the sweat test has been the mainstay of laboratory confirmation. Negative sweat chloride testing does not exclude the diagnosis of CF. This patient has many findings suggestive of CF upper-lobe predominant bronchiectasis, chronic sinus disease, colonization with *Pseudomonas*, clubbing, and infertility. Therefore, the index of suspicion for CF, as well as ciliary dyskinesia disorders, is extremely high for this patient. Because sweat chloride testing can give variable results, it is appropriate to repeat the testing and, if still negative, refer the patient to a center with expertise in CF or genetic testing.

Chronic oral macrolide antibiotics and inhaled antibiotic therapy are beneficial in patients with a confirmed diagnosis of CF. However, individuals with bronchiectasis are often exposed to several courses of antibiotics, and resistance to quinolones is common. Therefore, initiation of chronic ciprofloxacin therapy is not indicated.

In a recent phase 3 trial, tiotropium was well tolerated in patients with CF, but lung function improvements compared with placebo were not statistically significant and such treatment is not generally recommended.

Patients with $\alpha_1$-antitrypsin deficiency can present with lung disease and liver disease. A characteristic radiographic finding of the emphysema associated with $\alpha_1$-antitrypsin deficiency is bullous changes most prominent at the bases, which are not present in this patient. Additionally, $\alpha_1$-antitrypsin deficiency cannot account for the patient's sinus disease or infertility. Therefore, $\alpha_1$-antitrypsin deficiency testing would not be the most appropriate next diagnostic test in this patient with a clinical history suggestive of possible CF.

**KEY POINT**

- Negative sweat chloride testing does not exclude the diagnosis of cystic fibrosis in patients with high pretest probability of disease.

**Bibliography**

Farrell PM, White TB, Ren CL, Hempstead SE, Accurso F, Derichs N, et al. Diagnosis of cystic fibrosis: consensus guidelines from the Cystic Fibrosis Foundation. J Pediatr. 2017;181S:S4-S15.e1. [PMID: 28129811] doi:10.1016/j.jpeds.2016.09.064.

## Item 62      Answer:      C

**Educational Objective:** Screen for lung cancer in a patient at high risk.

The most appropriate test is a low-dose CT scan of the chest. Annual low-radiation-dose CT has been shown to reduce lung cancer mortality (20% relative decrease in lung cancer deaths) among high-risk individuals and is now recommended by the U.S. Preventive Services Task Force and other expert groups. Patients recommended for screening are those aged 55 to 74-80 years (range differs among expert groups) with a greater than 30-pack-year history of tobacco use within the prior 15 years, and without signs or symptoms suggestive of lung cancer. This patient fulfills these criteria and is, therefore, an appropriate candidate for a low-dose CT scan of the chest. Patients must also receive in-office counseling regarding the potential benefits and harms of screening, and documentation of shared decision making.

Monitoring respiratory parameters during exertion with the 6-minute walk test (6MWT) is helpful to assess disability and prognosis in chronic lung conditions. During a 6MWT, oxygen saturation, heart rate, dyspnea and fatigue level, and distance walked in 6 minutes are recorded. This relatively simple maneuver quantifies exercise tolerance, determines effective interventions, and helps predict morbidity and mortality. This patient has no indication for a 6MWT.

Chest radiography has been shown to be ineffective in screening for lung cancer and is not indicated in an asymptomatic patient such as this one.

Spirometry is warranted in any patient presenting with dyspnea, chronic cough, or sputum production. Screening for lung disease with spirometry should not be performed in asymptomatic patients, even those with a history of smoking.

Urinary cotinine is a metabolite of nicotine that is excreted in the urine and can be measured to assess if patients are using tobacco products. It is sometimes used while patients are actively attempting to quit smoking to assess adequacy of nicotine replacement therapy and monitor abstinence. This patient is high risk and a candidate for screening regardless of his current smoking status, and this test is not indicated.

**KEY POINT**

- Patients recommended for lung cancer screening are those aged 55 to 74-80 years with a greater than 30-pack-year history of tobacco use within the previous 15 years, and without signs or symptoms suggestive of lung cancer.

**Bibliography**

Mazzone PJ, Silvestri GA, Patel S, Kanne JP, Kinsinger LS, Wiener RS, et al. Screening for lung cancer: CHEST guideline and expert panel report. Chest. 2018;153:954-985. [PMID: 29374513] doi:10.1016/j.chest.2018.01.016

## Item 63      Answer:      D

**Educational Objective:** Manage oversedation in a patient in the ICU.

The most appropriate management is to stop sedation and analgesia. Clinicians at the bedside may resist stopping sedation and analgesia in a patient with a clear need for both, or because of concerns with ventilator synchrony or oxygenation. Protocolized care can help guide nursing and respiratory therapy if these problems arise. In addition, daily protocolized interruptions of sedation and analgesia have been shown to decrease the incidence of delirium, the need for diagnostic testing, and the amount of time spent on mechanical ventilation and in the ICU. Stopping sedation and analgesia, rather than gradually decreasing them, allows for a faster return to awareness and titration of infusions to achieve the sedation and analgesia goal. Analgesia and sedation can be restarted, at lower doses, if the patient requires them later.

Dexmedetomidine has pharmacological properties that may benefit this patient (analgesia, allows arousal). However, there is currently no evidence that it is superior to appropriately titrated propofol.

Ordering a CT scan is not the most appropriate first step in management of an unresponsive patient with nonfocal physical examination findings currently being treated with propofol and morphine. Moreover, a CT would expose the patient to the risks of being moved while critically ill and

CONT.

unnecessary radiation. The rate of serious events during transport is important enough to warrant careful determination of need.

Ordering an electroencephalogram to assess his unresponsiveness would be part of the diagnostic evaluation if interruption of sedation did not lead to improved mental status. Nonconvulsive status epilepticus has been reported in up to 20% of patients with unexplained unresponsiveness. Current recommendations suggest continuous electroencephalogram as the diagnostic test of choice.

**KEY POINT**

- Daily protocolized interruptions of sedation and analgesia have been shown to decrease the incidence of delirium, the need for diagnostic testing, and the amount of time spent on mechanical ventilation and in the ICU.

**Bibliography**

Barr J, Fraser GL, Puntillo K, Ely EW, Gélinas C, Dasta JF, et al; American College of Critical Care Medicine. Clinical practice guidelines for the management of pain, agitation, and delirium in adult patients in the intensive care unit. Crit Care Med. 2013;41:263-306. [PMID: 23269131] doi:10.1097/CCM.0b013e3182783b72

 **Item 64        Answer:    E**

**Educational Objective:**  Treat heat stroke with evaporative cooling techniques.

This patient should be sprayed with water, and fans should be used to lower his body temperature to a safe level (usually 38.5 °C (101 °F) through evaporative cooling. Heat stroke occurs with high ambient temperature and humidity and is defined by the presence of a temperature greater than 40.0 °C (104.0 °F) and encephalopathy. It is often associated with hypotension, gastrointestinal distress, and weakness. Patients with advanced heat stroke exhibit shock, multiorgan failure, rhabdomyolysis, and myocardial ischemia. Exertional heat stroke typically occurs in healthy individuals undergoing vigorous physical activity in warm conditions. In contrast, most patients with nonexertional heat stroke are older than 70 years of age or have chronic medical conditions that impair thermal regulation. Medications and recreational drugs with anticholinergic, sympathomimetic, and diuretic effects, including alcohol, pose added risk. The primary treatment of nonexertional heat stroke is evaporative, external cooling. This involves removing all clothing and spraying the patient with a mist of lukewarm water while continuously blowing fans on the patient. Evaporative and convective cooling techniques are generally the safest and most effective.

Acetaminophen and other centrally acting antipyretics are ineffective in the treatment of heat stroke. A cooling blanket could be used as an adjunct, but it is not as effective as evaporative cooling.

Alcohol would evaporate and provide cooling as effective as that from applying water, but it would also be absorbed through the vasodilated skin and could lead to

alcohol toxicity similar to that observed in patients who have ingested alcohol and is therefore contraindicated.

Although ice water immersion is sometimes used in younger patients with exertional heat stroke to lower the body temperature rapidly, there is evidence for increased mortality when this method is used in older patients. Also, this patient's core temperature of 40 °C (104 °F) is not so severe that more aggressive measures need to be considered.

The muscle relaxant dantrolene is ineffective in the treatment of heat stroke. It is used for malignant hyperthermia and sometimes for neuroleptic malignant syndrome, although this is an off-label application.

**KEY POINT**

- Patients with nonexertional heat stroke should be treated with evaporative cooling to lower their core temperature to a safe level.

**Bibliography**

O'Connor JP. Simple and effective method to lower body core temperatures of hyperthermic patients. Am J Emerg Med. 2017;35:881-884. [PMID: 28162872] doi:10.1016/j.ajem.2017.01.053

**Item 65        Answer:    A**

**Educational Objective:**  Treat septic shock with crystalloid infusion as the initial resuscitative therapy.

This patient should receive a 0.9% saline bolus. He has signs of septic shock from influenza (fever, tachycardia, hypotension, elevated leukocyte count, and exposure to influenza). In patients with septic or distributive shock, initial resuscitation efforts should be aimed at giving crystalloid fluids (0.9% saline, Ringer's lactate). The 2016 Surviving Sepsis guidelines recommend giving 30 mL/kg crystalloid solution within 3 hours of presentation in patients who demonstrate signs of tissue hypoperfusion. Judicious fluid administration is warranted thereafter, as intravascular volume overload can contribute to pulmonary edema and pleural effusions. This patient has several features of hypoperfusion, including hypotension, tachycardia, metabolic acidosis, and an elevated blood lactate.

Furosemide would be appropriate if the patient were in cardiogenic shock and presenting with signs of volume overload. The history, examination, and chest radiograph are not consistent with cardiogenic shock or volume overload. Therefore, furosemide is not recommended and would only promote further hypotension.

If hypotension does not rapidly correct with fluids, vasopressors should be titrated to maintain a mean arterial pressure of 65 mm Hg or greater. Norepinephrine is considered first-line therapy. This patient has not received crystalloid solution yet so initial therapy with norepinephrine is incorrect. However, in patients who are refractory to volume loading, vasopressor therapy is recommended to help improve hemodynamic stability.

In the absence of extenuating circumstances (myocardial ischemia, severe hypoxemia, or active hemorrhage), the

Surviving Sepsis guidelines recommend that red blood cell transfusion only be given if hemoglobin is less than 7 g/dL (70 g/L). Because this patient has a hemoglobin level above 7 g/dL, there is no direct role for packed red blood cell transfusion.

**KEY POINT**

- Initial treatment of septic or distributive shock should focus on aggressive fluid resuscitation with crystalloids within the first 3 hours of presentation.

**Bibliography**

Rochwerg B, Alhazzani W, Sindi A et al. Fluid resuscitation in sepsis: a systematic review and network meta-analysis. Ann Intern Med. 2014;161:347. [PMID 25047428]

## Item 66     Answer:   B

**Educational Objective:** Treat a patient in cardiac arrest due to accidental hypothermia with prolonged cardiopulmonary resuscitation and active internal rewarming.

Cardiopulmonary resuscitation (CPR) should be continued with active internal (core) rewarming. Conventional treatment of ventricular arrhythmias and asystole is often ineffective until the temperature is raised to greater than 30.0 °C (86.0 °F). Because severe hypothermia may appear clinically similar to death, aggressive rewarming is appropriate in all patients in the absence of obvious irreversible signs of death. A critical first step entails removing wet clothing and covering the patient with insulating material, especially the head and neck. For mildly hypothermic, healthy individuals capable of shivering, this strategy of passive external rewarming alone suffices. Active external rewarming using warm blankets or a forced heated air blanket is commonly used in hemodynamically stable patients with moderate hypothermia. Body cavity lavage with warm fluids is an option for patients with hypothermia that is severe or does not respond to external rewarming. The colon, bladder, and stomach are readily accessible for irrigation but have a small surface area for heat exchange. Rewarming by peritoneal or pleural space irrigation is supported by case reports. Extracorporeal support, including cardiopulmonary bypass, is recommended for patients in cardiac arrest because it maximizes the rewarming rate and can provide hemodynamic support.

Although this man has already received nearly an hour of CPR, there are reports of full recovery in patients with cardiac arrest in the setting of accidental hypothermia, sometimes even after CPR has been performed for many hours. Therefore, continued CPR is indicated until the patient can be rewarmed. Discontinuation of CPR is not appropriate because hypothermia prevents reaching a definite conclusion about the futility or possible effectiveness of continued resuscitation.

**KEY POINT**

- Cardiopulmonary resuscitation should be continued in patients with accidental hypothermia accompanied by cardiac arrest until the patient can be rewarmed.

**Bibliography**

Hilmo J, Naesheim T, Gilbert M. "Nobody is dead until warm and dead": prolonged resuscitation is warranted in arrested hypothermic victims also in remote areas—a retrospective study from northern Norway. Resuscitation. 2014;85:1204-11. [PMID: 24882104] doi:10.1016/j.resuscitation.2014.04.029

## Item 67     Answer:   B

**Educational Objective:** Treat high-altitude cerebral edema with dexamethasone.

The most appropriate treatment is dexamethasone. Hypoxia and hypocapnia associated with altitude alter cerebral blood flow and oxygen delivery to the brain. When autoregulatory mechanisms are overcome, symptoms may be mild, as with acute mountain sickness, or severe, as with life-threatening cerebral edema. Acute mountain sickness is characterized by nonspecific symptoms such as headache, fatigue, nausea, and vomiting, in addition to disturbed sleep. High-altitude cerebral edema is a more extreme manifestation of acute mountain sickness. Vascular leak leads to brain swelling, resulting in manifestations that range from confusion and irritability to ataxic gait to coma and death. Recognition of cerebral edema mandates immediate intervention. This patient is exhibiting signs and symptoms of encephalopathy indicative of high-altitude cerebral edema, the risk of which increases at more extreme elevations (higher than 3000 meters [9842 feet]). Although the most important intervention is descent to lower elevation, dexamethasone should be administered immediately upon recognition of high-altitude cerebral edema. Supplemental oxygen should also be administered.

High-altitude illness can be prevented by gradually ascending, which can generally be accomplished by spending one night at an intermediate altitude to allow acclimatization. Acetazolamide accelerates the acclimatization process to high altitude by inducing a slight metabolic acidosis to stimulate ventilation and enhance gas exchange; it can be used prophylactically in patients with a history of altitude illness. However, it isn't an effective treatment once symptoms develop; although it may be used as an adjunct to dexamethasone, it has no role in high-altitude cerebral edema as monotherapy.

Nifedipine is used as a preventive and therapeutic agent for high-altitude pulmonary edema.

Another vasodilator, sildenafil, may be used as an alternative to nifedipine in high-altitude pulmonary edema. However, neither is useful in the treatment of high-altitude cerebral edema.

**KEY POINT**

- Although the most important treatment of high-altitude cerebral edema is descent to lower elevation, dexamethasone should be administered immediately upon recognition of high-altitude cerebral edema.

**Bibliography**

Luks AM, Swenson ER, Bärtsch P. Acute high-altitude sickness. Eur Respir Rev. 2017;26. [PMID: 28143879] doi:10.1183/16000617.0096-2016

## Item 68          Answer:   C

**Educational Objective:**  Treat a critically ill patient who has acute pain.

This patient should receive an intravenous push of morphine. He has acute postoperative pain of the leg and is experiencing severe pain despite a morphine infusion. Analgesia should be titrated to a specific pain management goal while preventing and monitoring for side effects. A bolus dose of morphine will reach therapeutic levels faster than changing rates of infusion. The bolus dose should be repeated until the patient achieves the therapeutic goal, a protocol limit is reached, or side effects occur. He should be monitored closely while receiving acute pain treatment. Common side effects include somnolence, depression of respiratory drive, urinary retention, and nausea and vomiting.

Adding gabapentin is a good strategy for patients with neuropathic pain. Enteral gabapentin added to parenteral opioids can reduce the doses of opiates needed and improve pain control in mechanically ventilated patients. However, this patient is experiencing acute nonneuropathic pain and an intravenous opioid is the drug class of choice.

Epidural analgesia is an effective means to control pain in critically ill patients. This has been demonstrated in patients with cardiac or thoracic surgery or in the setting of rib fractures. It can lead to a reduction of opiate dosing and improved pain control during dressing changes in patients such as this one; however, it takes time to implement and the patient should receive acute pain control before consideration of alternatives to improve his baseline pain control.

Changing the medication to fentanyl is not appropriate as all intravenously administered opioids have equi-analgesic efficacy and are associated with similar clinical outcomes when titrated to similar pain intensity end points. The choice of opiate should be based on pharmacological properties. Fentanyl has a shorter half-life than morphine, and this patient was not having any adverse effect or contraindication to morphine.

### KEY POINT

- Intravenous opioids are the first-line drug class of choice to treat nonneuropathic pain in critically ill patients; all intravenously administered opioids have equi-analgesic efficacy and are associated with similar clinical outcomes when titrated to similar pain intensity end points.

### Bibliography

Barr J, Fraser GL, Puntillo K, Ely EW, Gélinas C, Dasta JF, et al; American College of Critical Care Medicine. Clinical practice guidelines for the management of pain, agitation, and delirium in adult patients in the intensive care unit. Crit Care Med. 2013;41:263-306. [PMID: 23269131] doi:10.1097/CCM.0b013e3182783b72

## Item 69          Answer:   D

**Educational Objective:**  Manage an asymptomatic patient with stage I pulmonary sarcoidosis.

This patient should be managed with observation and clinical follow-up. She is incidentally discovered to have bilateral hilar lymphadenopathy likely representing pulmonary sarcoidosis.

Pulmonary sarcoidosis is classified based on the radiographic pattern: stage I, hilar lymphadenopathy with normal lung parenchyma; stage II, hilar lymphadenopathy with abnormal lung parenchyma; stage III, no lymphadenopathy with abnormal lung parenchyma; and, stage IV, parenchymal changes with fibrosis and architectural distortion. For patients such as this, a careful history and physical examination to rule out the possibility of lymphoma and infection are essential. In a series of 100 consecutive patients with bilateral hilar lymphadenopathy, none with either lymphoma or infection were asymptomatic. Furthermore, approximately 75% of patients with stage I pulmonary sarcoidosis, such as this patient, have spontaneous resolution of the hilar lymphadenopathy. Patients can, however, have extrapulmonary disease, and screening electrocardiography, assessment of serum calcium, and eye examination are appropriate initial tests in this population.

Endobronchial ultrasound is a bronchoscopic technique that involves the use of an ultrasound probe at the distal end of the bronchoscope. The ultrasound-tipped bronchoscope can identify mediastinal lymph nodes and increase the yield of a transbronchial needle aspiration by allowing direct visualization of the needle entering the lymph node. This can be used to visualize and biopsy structures adjacent to an airway. This patient has no need for endobronchial ultrasound and biopsy.

Obtaining a high-resolution CT of the chest in this patient may result in further findings of parenchymal lung disease; however, she is asymptomatic and the finding of parenchymal lung disease would not necessitate a change in management at this early stage.

Glucocorticoids are the mainstay of therapy for sarcoidosis. Treatment is usually limited to those with evidence of clinical symptoms from organ dysfunction. Because there is a high rate of spontaneous remission and stability, most treatment protocols favor a period of observation without therapy. The decision to initiate glucocorticoid therapy for sarcoidosis should be based on symptoms or physiologic impairment that is attributable to sarcoid disease. Therefore, treatment with prednisone is not indicated for this patient.

### KEY POINT

- Treatment of pulmonary sarcoidosis should be based on symptoms rather than radiographic findings.

### Bibliography

Baughman RP, Culver DA, Judson MA. A concise review of pulmonary sarcoidosis. Am J Respir Crit Care Med. 2011;183:573-81. [PMID: 21037016] doi:10.1164/rccm.201006-0865CI

## Item 70          Answer:   D

**Educational Objective:**  Prevent ventilator-associated lung injury.

The most appropriate next step is to reduce the tidal volume. This patient fulfills the definition of acute respiratory

CONT.

distress syndrome (ARDS) with presentation within 1 week of known insult, arterial $P_{O_2}/F_{IO_2}$ ratio of 300 with positive end-expiratory pressure (PEEP) of 5 cm $H_2O$ or greater, and bilateral otherwise unexplained opacities seen on frontal chest imaging. Common pulmonary causes of ARDS include pneumonia (most common), aspiration, inhalational injury, near drowning, and drugs. Although ARDS mortality remains high, significant reductions in mortality have been attributed to the use of lung protective ventilation strategies. These strategies generally include limiting the tidal volume given in mechanical ventilation to 6 mL/kg of ideal body weight, limiting the plateau pressure in the respiratory cycle to no more than 30 cm $H_2O$, and use of adequate PEEP to prevent the collapse of unstable alveolar units in the expiratory phase of the cycle. In the 2000 ARMA trial, low tidal volume ventilation (LTVV) was associated with a 9% absolute reduction in mortality when patients were ventilated at a goal of 6-8 mL/kg of ideal body weight compared with more liberal tidal volumes of 10-12 mL/kg. However, implementation of LTVV remains challenging for several reasons. Among them, patients who receive LTVV often demonstrate signs of air hunger. This can lead to ventilator dyssynchrony and increased sedation requirements.

Current recommendations are to use a PEEP level that achieves adequate oxygenation with an $F_{IO_2}$ of less than 0.6 and does not cause hypotension. These parameters are being met with the current level of PEEP; therefore, adjustment of PEEP is not the most appropriate next step.

If the respiration rate remains constant, a lower tidal volume will reduce the total minute ventilation and thus reduce $CO_2$ removal. This results in higher arterial $P_{CO_2}$ and lower arterial pH. In the ARMA trial, LTVV-related hypercapnea was permitted, provided the arterial pH did not go below 7.3. In cases where the pH did drop below 7.3, respiration rate was increased to improve minute ventilation and decrease the $P_{CO_2}$. The patient's $P_{CO_2}$ and pH are acceptable and adjustment of the respiration rate is not the most appropriate next step.

**KEY POINT**

- The use of low tidal volume ventilation and positive end-expiratory pressure is associated with prevention of ventilator-associated lung injury and a reduction in mortality related to acute respiratory distress syndrome.

**Bibliography**
Thompson BT, Chambers RC, Liu KD. Acute respiratory distress syndrome. N Engl J Med. 2017;377:562-572. [PMID: 28792873] doi:10.1056/NEJMra1608077

 **Item 71      Answer:    D**

**Educational Objective:** Recognize an emergently placed central venous catheter as a potential source of sepsis.

The most appropriate management for this patient is removal of the central venous catheter. Morbidity and mortality in patients with sepsis are heavily influenced by the care delivered during the first several hours after sepsis onset. Once sepsis is recognized, interventions focus on adequate fluid resuscitation. Crystalloid is recommended at a volume of 30 mL/kg of body weight. In septic shock, mortality increases with each hour that appropriate antibiotic therapy is delayed. Two sets of blood cultures should be obtained before antibiotic infusion in addition to cultures from the suspected infection site. Empiric antimicrobial treatment should cover all suspected pathogens, with special attention to risk factors for resistant or opportunistic organisms, including methicillin-resistant *Staphylococcus aureus* and *Pseudomonas* species. Identification and control of the source of infection are critical steps in managing sepsis. This patient may have sepsis due to a central line-associated bloodstream infection. Removal of the emergently placed central venous catheter is the next critical management step.

Glucocorticoid administration is not recommended for patients without shock or who have responded to fluids and vasopressors because it offers no benefit. Some studies suggest that glucocorticoid therapy might benefit patients who remain hypotensive following adequate fluid resuscitation and vasopressor therapy. It is premature to consider administering glucocorticoids to this patient without first assessing the response to the initial resuscitation attempts.

If hypotension does not rapidly correct with fluids, vasopressors should be titrated to maintain a mean arterial pressure of 65 mm Hg or greater. Norepinephrine is considered first-line therapy. Because fluid resuscitation has just been initiated, it is premature to consider vasopressor therapy. If vasopressor therapy is needed, a new intravenous catheter should be placed rather than using the existing catheter, which is suspected as the source of infection.

The biologic marker procalcitonin may help differentiate between bacterial and nonbacterial pneumonia and help exclude a bacterial community-acquired pneumonia diagnosis in outpatients where there is already low suspicion. Procalcitonin level has no evidence-based role in the management of sepsis in the hospital.

**KEY POINT**

- Fluid resuscitation, administration of antibiotics, and infection source control are essential in the early sepsis management.

**Bibliography**
Rhodes A, Evans LE, Alhazzani W, Levy MM, Antonelli M, Ferrer R, et al. Surviving Sepsis Campaign: international guidelines for management of sepsis and septic shock: 2016. Crit Care Med. 2017;45:486-552. [PMID: 28098591] doi:10.1097/CCM.0000000000002255

**Item 72      Answer:    A**

**Educational Objective:** Evaluate a patient with excessive daytime sleepiness with actigraphy.

The most appropriate management is testing with actigraphy. The initial step in the evaluation of the patient with excessive daytime sleepiness is to ensure adequate quantities (7 to 8 hours) of sleep on a regular basis. This patient's self-report of a variable bedtime and restricted sleep schedule during the workweek raises the possibility of insufficient sleep syndrome. Wrist actigraphy measures movement and ambient light to estimate nightly sleep periods during a 1 to 2 week time frame. Actigraphy is more accurate than patient reports of sleep duration and is likely more accurate than sleep diaries. When actigraphy isn't available, a sleep diary can be a useful alternative. Insufficient sleep syndrome suggested by either actigraphy or sleep diary should prompt a trial of sleep extension.

Modafinil is a stimulant medication used in hypersomnia syndromes such as narcolepsy. It would not be appropriate therapy without first excluding insufficient sleep syndrome.

Multiple sleep latency testing can be useful in the evaluation of pathologic daytime sleepiness (for example, narcolepsy) and may help establish a diagnosis of narcolepsy, but it is resource intensive and expensive. It should be performed only after addressing insufficient sleep quantities and polysomnography has ruled out common sleep disorders such as sleep apnea.

Polysomnography or home sleep testing would be indicated if the clinical history strongly suggested a primary sleep disorder such as obstructive sleep apnea. However, obstructive sleep apnea is unlikely in a young woman who is not overweight and does not have obvious upper airway abnormalities. In addition, the patient is suspected of having a restricted sleep schedule that should be evaluated first with actigraphy.

**KEY POINT**

- The initial step in the evaluation of the patient with excessive daytime sleepiness is to ensure adequate quantities of sleep on a regular basis using either actigraphy or a sleep diary.

**Bibliography**

Watson NF, Badr MS, Belenky G, Bliwise DL, Buxton OM, Buysse D, et al; Consensus Conference Panel. Recommended amount of sleep for a healthy adult: a joint consensus statement of the American Academy of Sleep Medicine and Sleep Research Society. J Clin Sleep Med. 2015;11:591-2. [PMID: 25979105] doi:10.5664/jcsm.4758

## Item 73      Answer:    A

**Educational Objective:** Diagnose a complicated parapneumonic effusion.

This patient has community-acquired pneumonia and complicated parapneumonic effusion. A complicated parapneumonic effusion is defined as an effusion associated with a pneumonia that has a pH less than 7.2 and glucose less than 60 mg/dL (3.3 mmol/L). Complicated parapneumonic effusions occur when bacteria invade the pleural space. However, because bacteria may be cleared rapidly from the pleural space, the Gram stain is typically negative and cultures are usually sterile. Complicated parapneumonic effusions have a variable response to antibiotics alone. Pleural effusions greater than 10 mm in depth on

chest radiograph and associated with a pneumonic illness should be sampled. In general, these require thoracostomy tube drainage when the pH is less than 7.2 or the pleural fluid glucose level is less than 60 mg/dL (3.3 mmol/L). The American College of Chest Physicians consensus guidelines concur as thoracostomy drainage speeds clinical recovery and hospital discharge.

An empyema is defined as a bacterial infection of the pleural space that results in frank pus on visual inspection of the pleural fluid or a positive Gram stain. A positive pleural fluid culture is not required for diagnosis as cultures are less sensitive than Gram stain in the detection of bacteria. The management of empyema includes early thoracic surgical consultation because thoracoscopic or open debridement and drainage is often required to successfully manage this condition. However, this patient's pleural fluid was described as serous and the Gram stain was negative making empyema an unlikely diagnosis.

Pleural fluid acidosis (pH less than 7.3) is seen in complicated parapneumonic effusions, tuberculous pleuritis, rheumatoid and lupus pleuritis, esophageal rupture, and malignancy. A low pleural fluid glucose level results from either increased utilization within the pleural space (bacteria, malignant cells) or decreased transport into the pleural space (rheumatoid pleurisy), and a concentration less than 60 mg/dL (3.3 mmol/L) narrows the differential diagnosis significantly. Although a malignant effusion can have a low pH and glucose, this patient's presentation is more consistent with a parapneumonic effusion.

An uncomplicated parapneumonic effusion is characterized by a pH greater than 7.2 and glucose greater than 60 mg/dL (3.3 mmol/L). These effusions do not require drainage and typically resolve with antibiotic therapy alone.

**KEY POINT**

- In general, parapneumonic effusions associated with a pH less than 7.2 or pleural fluid glucose level less than 60 mg/dL (3.3 mmol/L) require thoracostomy drainage in addition to antibiotics.

**Bibliography**

Colice GL, Curtis A, Deslauriers J, Heffner J, Light R, Littenberg B, et al. Medical and surgical treatment of parapneumonic effusions: an evidence-based guideline. Chest. 2000;118:1158-71. [PMID: 11035692]

## Item 74      Answer:    B

**Educational Objective:** Provide recommended vaccinations for patients with COPD.

This patient should receive the pneumococcal polysaccharide vaccine and an annual influenza vaccine. Influenza vaccination has been shown to reduce serious illness (such as lower respiratory tract infections that require hospitalization) and death in patients with COPD. These vaccines should be administered annually in all patients with COPD. There are currently three different types of influenza vaccine available in the United States:

inactivated influenza vaccine, live attenuated influenza vaccine, and recombinant trivalent influenza vaccine. Inactivated influenza vaccine is approved for use in all adults, including immunosuppressed persons and pregnant women.

A high-dose inactivated influenza vaccine is approved for use in adults age 65 years and older; it has been shown to be modestly more effective than the standard-dose inactivated influenza vaccine in this patient population.

Pneumococcal vaccination is indicated for all adults aged 65 years and older and for high-risk persons younger than 65 years. Two vaccines are currently available: pneumococcal polysaccharide vaccine (PPSV23) is composed of polysaccharide capsular material from 23 pneumococcal subtypes, whereas pneumococcal conjugate vaccine (PCV13) contains capsular material from 13 subtypes conjugated to a nontoxic protein, which increases its immunogenicity. For pneumococcal vaccine–naïve adults between the ages of 19 and 65 years with certain immunocompromising conditions or who are otherwise at high risk, a single dose of PCV13 should be given. These conditions include functional or anatomic asplenia, cerebrospinal fluid leaks, cochlear implants, and conditions causing immunosuppression. All patients should also receive the 13-valent pneumococcal conjugate vaccine at age 65 years, although the polysaccharide and conjugate vaccines should be given sequentially at least a year apart for immunocompetent adults over age 65 rather than together for optimal effect. COPD alone is not an indication for PCV13 vaccination.

PPSV23 has the same indications as the PCV13 vaccine, plus it is indicated in immunocompetent people with certain chronic medical conditions such as heart, liver, and lung disease (COPD, emphysema, asthma) and diabetes, as well as in cigarette smokers. PPSV23 revaccination should be given at age 65 years if 5 years have elapsed since the previous pneumococcal immunization. When possible, the PCV13 vaccine should be administered first, followed by a dose of PPSV23 at least 1 year later for most immunocompetent patients. Some patients with immunocompromising conditions, cochlear implants, or cerebrospinal fluid leaks should receive the dose of PPSV23 at least 8 weeks after the first dose of PCV13. If a patient has already received the PPSV23 vaccine, a single dose of PCV13 should be given at least 1 year after the administration of PPSV23.

**KEY POINT**

- Annual influenza vaccination and the pneumococcal polysaccharide vaccine are recommended for all patients with chronic lung disease (COPD, emphysema, asthma).

**Bibliography**

Kim DK, Riley LE, Hunter P; Advisory Committee on Immunization Practices. Recommended immunization schedule for adults aged 19 years or older, United States, 2018. Ann Intern Med. 2018;168:210-220. [PMID: 29404596]

## Item 75    Answer:    D

**Educational Objective:** Treat a patient with chronic thromboembolic pulmonary hypertension.

This patient has chronic thromboembolic pulmonary hypertension (CTEPH) and the preferred treatment is pulmonary thromboendarterectomy. There are two diagnostic criteria for CTEPH: (1) mean pulmonary artery pressure of 25 mm Hg or higher by right heart catheterization in the absence of left heart pressure overload and (2) compatible imaging evidence of chronic thromboembolism. CT pulmonary angiography (CT-PA) may demonstrate proximally located abnormalities such as vascular webs, intimal irregularities, and luminal narrowing but has limited sensitivity in more distal lesions. Ventilation-perfusion scanning is a more sensitive indicator of CTEPH and is generally the preferred first imaging modality. Once CTEPH is suggested by noninvasive testing, conventional pulmonary angiography should be performed to characterize the extent and distribution of organized thrombus and to determine suitability for surgical intervention. Surgical intervention is the only definitive therapy for CTEPH and can prevent irreversible remodeling of the pulmonary arterial vasculature. Surgical evaluation at an experienced center is warranted in all patients with CTEPH; however, only about half of patients will be surgical candidates and fewer than that will opt for surgery.

Lifelong anticoagulant therapy, traditionally with warfarin, is indicated in all patients to help prevent further thromboembolism. Experience with direct oral anticoagulants such as apixaban is limited in this patient population. Because this patient's INR is in the therapeutic range, there's no proved advantage of switching from warfarin to apixaban.

Inferior vena cava interruption is typically indicated in patients with venous thrombus for whom anticoagulation is ineffective or not tolerated. In patients with CTEPH and coexisting clot in the lower extremities, inferior vena cava interruption can be considered to help prevent further thromboembolism; however, its role in long-term outcomes is not known and of unclear benefit.

Calcium channel blockers such as nifedipine are used in the setting of pulmonary arterial hypertension when right heart catheterization reveals acute vasoreactivity. Their role in the treatment of CTEPH is unproved.

**KEY POINT**

- Surgical intervention is the only definitive therapy for chronic thromboembolic pulmonary hypertension (CTEPH), and most patients with CTEPH should be referred for evaluation at a specialty surgical center.

**Bibliography**

Edward JA, Mandras S. An Update on the management of chronic thromboembolic pulmonary hypertension. Curr Probl Cardiol. 2017;42:7-38. [PMID: 27989311] doi:10.1016/j.cpcardiol.2016.11.001

## Item 76     Answer:   A

**Educational Objective:** Evaluate readiness to liberate from mechanical ventilation in a patient with COPD.

A 30-minute spontaneous breathing trial (SBT) should be performed using low levels of pressure support (8 cm H$_2$O or less). Weaning from mechanical ventilation can start when the precipitating event or underlying condition that caused respiratory failure has resolved or is resolving. Patients should be assessed daily for their readiness to be removed from mechanical ventilation by performing an SBT. There are several methods used to assess if an SBT is successful. One criterion is the ability to tolerate a weaning trial for 30 minutes (in most patients, SBT failure will occur within approximately 20 minutes). 2-hour SBTs and 30-minute SBTs have a similar ability to recognize patients who are unable to breathe spontaneously. However a 30-minute trial has the benefits of less time on mechanical ventilation and less risk of respiratory muscle fatigue. If the patient successfully completes an SBT, the ability to follow commands, clear secretions, and a patent upper airway are other criteria that should be met to increase extubation success.

A "cuff leak" refers to measurable airflow around the endotracheal tube after the cuff of the endotracheal tube is deflated. Absent or minimal cuff leak following deflation of the cuff indicates reduced space between the endotracheal tube and the larynx. Minimal or absent cuff leak may be due to laryngeal edema, laryngeal stenosis, and thick secretions. The test is not standardized and not performed routinely and is not an initial routine test in the process of liberating a patient from mechanical ventilation. It might be considered in a patient who has a successful SBT but is at high risk for edema and stridor following extubation.

The Glasgow Coma Scale is pertinent to the actual extubation process, in which lack of awareness and ability to clear secretions and follow simple commands may increase the risk of aspiration and cooperation in the postextubation period. However, this patient should be placed on an SBT before being evaluated for extubation.

Negative inspiratory force has been used as a marker of inspiratory muscle strength to identify patients who will be able to be liberated from mechanical ventilation. However, there are technical issues that lead to variable predictive performance. A low negative inspiratory force by itself is not useful; however, serial measurements (for example, in patients with Guillain-Barré or myasthenia gravis) along with other measures (FVC, maximum tidal volume) may give a better picture of muscle strength recovery.

**KEY POINT**

- Patients should be assessed daily for their readiness to be removed from mechanical ventilation by performing a spontaneous breathing trial; one criterion for success is the ability to tolerate a spontaneous breathing trial for 30 minutes.

**Bibliography**

Schmidt GA, Girard TD, Kress JP, Morris PE, Ouellette DR, Alhazzani W, et al. Liberation from mechanical ventilation in critically ill adults: executive summary of an official American College of Chest Physicians/American Thoracic Society Clinical Practice Guideline. Chest. 2017;151:160–165. [PMID: 27818329] doi:10.1016/j.chest.2016.10.037

## Item 77     Answer:   C

**Educational Objective:** Treat a patient with empyema.

Instillation of intrapleural tissue plasminogen activator-deoxyribonuclease (tPA-DNase) is the most appropriate treatment to promote drainage. This patient has a community-acquired pneumonia complicated by an empyema. The diagnostic criterion for empyema is either visualization of frankly purulent pleural fluid or a positive Gram stain. The Gram stain supports the diagnosis of *group A pneumoniae* pneumonia. An empyema requires drainage to resolve the infection. A small-bore (14-Fr) tube can be placed to facilitate drainage. An empyema can become loculated (divided into small cavities or compartments) and will not resolve with simple thoracostomy drainage; loculated empyemas often require thorascopic or open surgical debridement. This patient has an incompletely drained empyema due to loculation. When performed twice daily for 3 days, intrapleural administration of tPA-DNase has been shown to decrease the radiographic pleural opacity, lower the rate of surgical intervention, and decrease hospital stay of patients with empyema (MIST-2 trial). It should be noted that the tPA-DNase has not been shown to decrease mortality. In addition, video-assisted thorascopic surgery has also been shown to effectively manage empyema in greater than 90% of cases, and a delay in surgery increases the risk of open thoracotomy. Given the lack of prospective data, a multidisciplinary discussion should be undertaken for any patient presenting with an empyema who is a good surgical candidate.

Instillation of intrapleural antibiotic solution may be used for postsurgical empyema but has no demonstrated efficacy in the initial management of a loculated empyema.

The MIST-1 trial compared the use of intrapleural instillation of streptokinase compared to saline and found no difference in mortality, need for surgery, radiographic outcome, or length of hospitalization. Consequently, use of fibrinolytics alone in empyema is not recommended.

Continued systemic antibiotic therapy without adequate drainage of the pleural space is inadequate therapy. Failure to adequately drain the pleural space of a complicated pleural effusion or empyema will result in failure to resolve the infection, increased morbidity, and the possibility of death by overwhelming infection.

**KEY POINT**

- Instillation of intrapleural tissue plasminogen activator-deoxyribonuclease has been shown to decrease the radiographic pleural opacity, lower the rate of surgical referral, and decrease hospital stay of patients with empyema.

## Bibliography

Rahman NM, Maskell NA, West A, Teoh R, Arnold A, Mackinlay C, et al. Intrapleural use of tissue plasminogen activator and DNase in pleural infection. N Engl J Med. 2011;365:518-26. [PMID: 21830966] doi:10.1056/NEJMoa1012740

## Item 78    Answer:    D

**Educational Objective:** Diagnose asthma in a symptomatic patient with normal spirometry.

Methacholine challenge testing is the most appropriate test to perform next for this patient with persistent cough and wheezing following a presumed viral upper respiratory tract infection. These symptoms can be the initial presentation of asthma, which is common in patients older than 65 years, with a prevalence of 8.1%; this age group also has the highest mortality rate, particularly in low-income Hispanic and black women. However, asthma is currently underdiagnosed and undertreated in patients older than 65 years in the United States. In patients with clinical symptoms suggestive of bronchospastic disease (such as cough or unexplained dyspnea) but with normal spirometry, bronchial challenge testing may be diagnostically helpful. Bronchial challenge testing uses a controlled inhaled stimulus to induce bronchospasm in association with spirometry; a positive test is indicated by a drop in the measured $FEV_1$. This symptomatic patient's spirometry is normal; therefore, methacholine challenge testing to evaluate for bronchial hyperresponsiveness is indicated.

Echocardiography could help evaluate cardiac function but the patient does not have findings of heart murmur or heart failure so this test would not be indicated.

Exhaled nitric oxide testing is a noninvasive breath test. Nitric oxide is normally present in airways but is increased in certain types of airway inflammation (asthma, eosinophilic airway inflammation). When elevated, it supports the diagnosis of asthma in the appropriate clinical context. Other factors may affect nitric oxide values such as age, sex, atopy, and cigarette smoking so a normal level in an older adult would not rule out asthma. The sensitivity and specificity of exhaled nitric oxide in the diagnosis of asthma are not well defined, particularly in patients with confounding variables, and it is not the preferred next test for this patient.

High-resolution CT (HRCT) is indicated if diffuse parenchymal lung disease is suspected. HRCT can help narrow the differential diagnosis based on the distribution of the lung parenchymal abnormalities and the presence or absence of associated findings. HRCT scan of the chest would not help confirm a diagnosis of asthma.

Nasal swab for influenza polymerase chain reaction would not be indicated because the patient's symptoms of a viral infection have resolved; furthermore, influenza testing in immunocompetent adults should be performed within 5 days of symptom onset.

**KEY POINT**

- The diagnosis of asthma requires demonstrating reversible airflow obstruction; for a patient with symptoms of asthma and normal spirometry, methacholine challenge testing to evaluate for bronchial hyperresponsiveness is indicated.

## Bibliography

Al-Alawi M, Hassan T, Chotirmall SH. Advances in the diagnosis and management of asthma in older adults. Am J Med. 2014;127:370-8. [PMID: 24380710] doi:10.1016/j.amjmed.2013.12.013

## Item 79    Answer:    B

**Educational Objective:** Treat a patient who has anaphylaxis with epinephrine.

This patient should be treated with epinephrine. Anaphylaxis is defined as a severe, potentially life-threatening allergic or hypersensitivity reaction that occurs within seconds to a few hours of allergen exposure, most commonly food, medication, or an insect sting. Classically, anaphylaxis occurs when allergen-specific IgE coating the surface of mast cells and basophils comes in contact with the triggering allergen, thereby precipitating cellular degranulation. The resulting abrupt systemic release of a host of mediators has various effects, including vasoconstriction, vasodilation, increased vascular permeability, and bronchoconstriction. The presentation is variable and findings may include flushing, urticaria, and angioedema (85%); wheeze, stridor, and respiratory distress (70%); and hypotension and tachycardia (less commonly bradycardia) (45%). Initial symptoms and findings may be mild but predicting the ultimate severity of the episode is difficult. The first step in treatment is immediate intramuscular or intravenous administration of epinephrine. There are studies showing increased mortality from anaphylaxis if epinephrine is delayed. The dose may be repeated after 5-15 minutes, or administered continuously as an intravenous solution (although at a lower concentration), until the effects are apparent. Patients can also be given supplemental oxygen and monitored for signs of airway compromise, which may require intubation to maintain airway patency. Following recovery, patients should maintain home access to an epinephrine auto-injector and may benefit from evaluation for anaphylactic triggers.

Diphenhydramine, a histamine$_1$-blocker, is often given because of its effect on itching and urticaria, but it has never been shown to effectively treat distributive shock, airway edema, or outcome in anaphylaxis. It is not a substitute for epinephrine.

Although intravenous fluids are often needed to manage anaphylaxis, they are reserved for use in cases where hypotension persists despite treatment with epinephrine.

Glucocorticoids are often given to reduce the risk of recurrent or persistent symptoms. However, there are no randomized controlled trials that confirm the effectiveness of glucocorticoids in preventing symptom recurrence.

More clinically relevant, a study of emergency department patients with anaphylaxis treated with glucocorticoids did not demonstrate a reduction in return visits to the emergency department for recurrent symptoms.

### KEY POINT

- Epinephrine is the appropriate initial treatment of anaphylaxis.

### Bibliography

Commins SP. Outpatient emergencies: anaphylaxis. Med Clin North Am. 2017;101:521-536. [PMID: 28372711] doi:10.1016/j.mcna.2016.12.003

## Item 80       Answer:   D

**Educational Objective:**  Treat a patient with severe acute respiratory distress syndrome using early prone positioning.

This patient should be ventilated in the prone position. In patients with acute respiratory distress syndrome (ARDS) low tidal volume ventilation (6-8 mL/kg ideal body weight) is optimal and is associated with significantly better outcomes than conventional, higher tidal volume ventilation (10-12 mL/kg). In patients with severe ARDS, several adjunctive therapies have been studied, but few have demonstrated additional improved outcomes beyond low tidal volume ventilation. However, in 2013, the PROSEVA trial evaluated patients with ARDS who had an arterial $Po_2/Fio_2$ ratio of less than 150 (defining severe ARDS) despite significant ventilator support. Patients were randomized to conventional therapy or low tidal volume ventilation plus prone positioning within 36 hours of developing ARDS and respiratory failure. The results suggested a 16.2% reduction in 28-day all-cause mortality in the prone-position group. The 2017 American Thoracic Society, European Society of Intensive Care Medicine, and Society of Critical Care Medicine (ATS/ESICM/SCCM) guideline makes a strong recommendation that all patients with ARDS receive ventilation with lower tidal volumes (4-8 mL/kg of predicted body weight). Patients with severe ARDS should be also ventilated in the prone position for at least 12 hours per day. Proning should be considered standard management for patients with severe ARDS, not a form of "rescue" or "salvage" therapy.

Recruitment is the application of a high level of continuous positive airway pressure to open up collapsed alveoli (for example, continuous pressure to 35 cm $H_2O$ for 40 seconds). The ATS/ESICM/SCCM guideline provides a conditional recommendation for recruitment maneuvers based on low to moderate confidence in the small to moderate magnitude of its effect on mortality. The guideline cautions that recruitment should not be used in patients with preexisting hypovolemia or shock due to hemodynamic deterioration, which can occur during the maneuver. This patient is hypotensive and, therefore, not a candidate for recruitment maneuvers.

Nitric oxide (NO) selectively dilates the pulmonary vasculature when administered by inhalation. Its use in acute hypoxemic respiratory failure is based on the rationale that inhaled NO may improve ventilation-perfusion mismatch. Studies of inhaled NO in patients with severe ARDS have

demonstrated temporary improvement in oxygenation but no improvement in survival.

In 2013 two large, prospective randomized trials demonstrated that compared to low tidal volume ventilation, high-frequency oscillator ventilation was either no different or harmful to patients with ARDS. In light of this, the ATS/ESICM/SCCM guideline strongly recommends against routine use of high-frequency oscillatory ventilation.

### KEY POINT

- Patients with severe acute respiratory distress syndrome have a demonstrated mortality benefit from low tidal volume ventilation in the prone position.

### Bibliography

Fan E, Del Sorbo L, Goligher EC, Hodgson CL, Munshi L, Walkey AJ, et al; American Thoracic Society, European Society of Intensive Care Medicine, and Society of Critical Care Medicine. An official American Thoracic Society/European Society of Intensive Care Medicine/Society of Critical Care Medicine clinical practice guideline: mechanical ventilation in adult patients with acute respiratory distress syndrome. Am J Respir Crit Care Med. 2017;195:1253-1263. [PMID: 28459336] doi:10.1164/rccm.201703-0548ST

## Item 81       Answer:   A

**Educational Objective:**  Diagnose bronchiectasis using chest CT imaging.

The most likely diagnosis is bronchiectasis. Bronchiectasis is irreversible pathologic dilation of the bronchi or bronchioles resulting from an infectious process occurring in the context of airway obstruction, impaired drainage, or abnormality in antimicrobial defenses. The pattern of lung involvement varies greatly with the underlying cause and may be focal or diffuse. Bronchiectasis causes a chronic or recurrent cough typically characterized by voluminous sputum production with purulent exacerbations. The vast majority of chest radiographs are abnormal, typically showing linear atelectasis, dilated and thickened airways, and irregular peripheral opacities. High-resolution CT (HRCT) of the chest is the definitive diagnostic test for bronchiectasis.

Typical findings (airway dilatation with lack of tapering [green arrow], bronchial wall thickening [yellow arrow], and cysts [red arrow]) may be seen on HRCT.

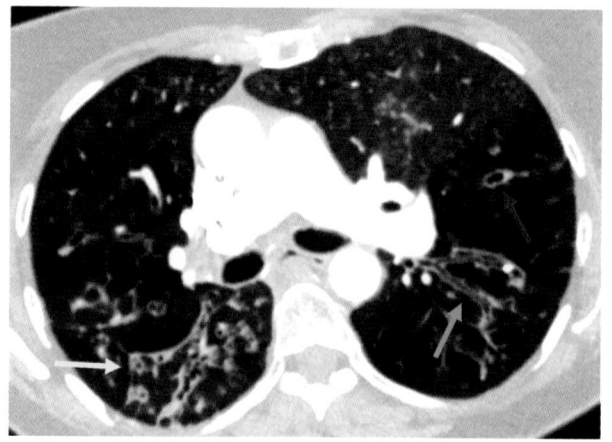

In addition to imaging, the cause of the bronchiectasis should be determined. This may involve testing for chronic bacterial or mycobacterial infections, assessing for the presence of connective tissue disease, and evaluating immune function. In selected patients, testing for cystic fibrosis or $\alpha_1$-antitrypsin deficiency may be appropriate if suspected.

There is no evidence of emphysema on his chest CT imaging, which would typically appear as dilated airspaces, classified based on the distribution of abnormalities as centrilobular, panlobular, or paraseptal. Bullous or cystic changes may be seen.

Although the duration of his symptoms are consistent with chronic bronchitis, the chest CT scan shows evidence of bronchiectasis. In chronic bronchitis, the walls of the airways are thickened without dilation of the airways themselves.

Pulmonary Langerhans cell histiocytosis is a rare subacute interstitial lung disease of young, actively smoking adults. Patients may present with cough, fever, weight loss, and abnormal chest radiography. The chest CT findings include pulmonary nodules and cysts with midlung to upper-lung zone predominance and are not associated with bronchiectasis.

**KEY POINT**

- Chest CT is the definitive diagnostic study for bronchiectasis; typical findings are airway dilatation with lack of tapering, bronchial wall thickening, and cysts.

**Bibliography**

Milliron B, Henry TS, Veeraraghavan S, Little BP. Bronchiectasis: mechanisms and imaging clues of associated common and uncommon diseases. Radiographics. 2015;35:1011-30. [PMID: 26024063] doi:10.1148/rg.2015140214

**Item 82      Answer:    B**

**Educational Objective:** Diagnose a patient with acute silicosis.

This patient most likely has acute silicosis, a fibrotic lung disease caused by the inhalation of silica dust. Silicosis is a spectrum of fibrotic lung diseases related to the inhalation of silica dust. Any occupation that disturbs the earth's crust involves potential risk. Workers in industries that process silica-containing rock or sand are also at risk. The typical disease course of simple silicosis can be accelerated (3 to 10 years after exposure) or latent (greater than 10 years after exposure). This patient has acute silicosis, a rare presentation characterized by onset of cough and dyspnea (but no fever) just a few weeks after intense exposure, patchy bilateral opacities on chest radiograph, and a milky effluent from bronchoalveolar lavage (BAL). Hydraulic fracturing, or fracking, is a process whereby large amounts of water and chemicals are injected into the ground; sand, which contains silica, is used to hold open the fissures created to enhance extraction of natural gas. Acute silicosis portends a

poor prognosis, as there is little evidence that any therapies can alter disease course. However, removal from the environment and smoking cessation will prevent further lung injury.

Acute interstitial pneumonia develops rapidly during days to weeks and results in progressive hypoxemic respiratory failure. Radiographic examination reveals bilateral alveolar opacities consistent with pulmonary edema. The findings on BAL are nonspecific. This patient's findings are not compatible with acute interstitial pneumonia.

Workers in the mining industry are at risk for asbestos exposure, but the typical latency period for asbestosis is decades rather than weeks, making this diagnosis unlikely. In addition, the most common radiographic finding of asbestosis is pleural plaques, which are not present on this patient's radiograph.

Patients with cryptogenic organizing pneumonia typically present with cough, dyspnea, fever, and malaise during 3 to 4 weeks that mimic community-acquired pneumonia. The chest radiograph reveals bilateral, patchy or diffuse, consolidative or ground-glass opacities and BAL effluent is not milky opaque.

**KEY POINT**

- Patients who work in industries that expose them to silica dust are at risk for silicosis.

**Bibliography**

Esswein EJ, Breitenstein M, Snawder J, Kiefer M, Sieber WK. Occupational exposures to respirable crystalline silica during hydraulic fracturing. J Occup Environ Hyg. 2013;10:347-56. [PMID: 23679563] doi:10.1080/15459624.2013.788352

**Item 83      Answer:    C**

**Educational Objective:** Diagnose ICU-acquired weakness in a critically ill patient using the Medical Research Council muscle scale.

Although rarely used in practice, the most appropriate initial test to perform is the Medical Research Council (MRC) muscle scale. This patient has symmetrical quadriparesis and distal sensory neuropathy after sepsis and should be evaluated for ICU-acquired weakness. ICU-acquired weakness is the presence of profound muscles weakness in the setting of a current or recent critical illness. The MRC scale is most appropriately used in awake and cooperative patients. In such a patient, muscle strength of each extremity can be tested and graded from 0 (no movement) to 5 (normal). Summing the maximum score for 3 movements of each upper extremity (shoulder abduction, elbow flexion, wrist extension) and each lower extremity (hip flexion, knee extension, ankle dorsiflexion) can result in a maximum score of 60. In the absence of other known causes of muscular weakness, a score less than 48 is considered diagnostic of ICU-acquired weakness. The MRC muscle scale has several limitations; however, it is universally available, easy to perform, and can guide management decisions.

CONT.

Cervical spine MRI is an excellent imaging modality to detect a cervical epidural abscess in a patient with a history of bacteremia and supportive physical examination findings. However, the patient does not have numbness of the arms or increased tone and hyperreflexia of the lower extremities to support the diagnosis of a cervical myelopathy.

Electrodiagnostic testing can help establish the diagnosis of critical care polyneuropathy, critical care myopathy, or their combination, and provide clues to other causes of prolonged weakness (for example, acute inflammatory demyelinating polyneuropathy). However, the test is not universally available in all ICU centers, is invasive, may not affect management of patients with ICU-acquired weakness, and should not precede careful evaluation of the patient with the MRC scale.

Similarly, a muscle biopsy can also aid diagnosis of critical illness myopathy, especially in the setting of elevated serum creatine kinase levels, but it would not be an appropriate initial test.

### KEY POINT

- Initial evaluation for ICU-acquired weakness can be done at the bedside using the Medical Research Council muscle scale.

### Bibliography

Fan E, Cheek F, Chlan L, Gosselink R, Hart N, Herridge MS, et al; ATS Committee on ICU-Acquired Weakness in Adults. An official American Thoracic Society Clinical Practice guideline: the diagnosis of intensive care unit-acquired weakness in adults. Am J Respir Crit Care Med. 2014;190:1437-46. [PMID: 25496103] doi:10.1164/rccm.201411-2011ST

## Item 84      Answer:      C

**Educational Objective:** Diagnose cryptogenic organizing pneumonia.

The most likely diagnosis is cryptogenic organizing pneumonia. This patient has a subacute history of progressive dyspnea and persistent cough after an initial history consistent with community-acquired pneumonia. Despite treatment with appropriate antibiotic therapy, she now has clear evidence of new opacities that are located in different areas, are peripherally predominant, and coalesce along bronchovascular bundles. These findings are consistent with a diagnosis of organizing pneumonia, which involves proliferation of granulation tissue within alveolar ducts, alveolar spaces, and surrounding areas of chronic inflammation. There are many known causes of this pattern, including acute infections and autoimmune disorders like rheumatoid arthritis. The term *cryptogenic organizing pneumonia* is reserved for individuals who have this pattern but do not have a clear associated cause. Patients with cryptogenic organizing pneumonia will typically present with a 6-to-8-week history of symptoms that mimic community-acquired pneumonia. Typically, an initial empiric treatment of infection is given but fails; subsequently, noninfectious causes are considered. This patient has a subacute illness that began with viral symptoms, persistent and progressive cough and dyspnea that are not responsive to past

antibiotics, and radiographic findings typical of cryptogenic organizing pneumonia. Patients with cryptogenic organizing pneumonia respond well to glucocorticoids. Glucocorticoids are slowly tapered during the subsequent 6 months.

Acute HIV is unlikely in this patient who initially presented with symptoms of community-acquired pneumonia and whose fever has resolved. Although acute HIV symptoms are not specific, the most common presentation includes persistence of symptoms including fever.

Recurrent community-acquired pneumonia is also unlikely in this patient who was appropriately treated with azithromycin and whose symptoms have partially improved with resolution of the fever and sputum production.

Idiopathic pulmonary fibrosis (IPF) is a disease that affects older patients (the mean age of presentation is in the mid- to late 60s) and presents with chronic (longer than 6 months) symptoms of dry cough and shortness of breath. This patient's presentation is not consistent with these criteria, making a diagnosis of IPF unlikely.

### KEY POINT

- A typical presentation of cryptogenic organizing pneumonia includes cough, fever, and malaise for 6 to 8 weeks that does not respond to antibiotics; patchy opacities on chest radiograph; and ground-glass opacities on CT scan that are peripherally distributed; glucocorticoids are first-line therapy.

### Bibliography

Lazor R, Vandevenne A, Pelletier A, Leclerc P, Court-Fortune I, Cordier JF. Cryptogenic organizing pneumonia. Characteristics of relapses in a series of 48 patients. The Groupe d'Etudes et de Recherche sur les Maladies "Orphelines" Pulmonaires (GERM"O"P). Am J Respir Crit Care Med. 2000;162:571-7. [PMID: 10934089]

## Item 85      Answer:      A

**Educational Objective:** Treat a patient with a hemodynamically unstable pulmonary embolism using thrombolytic therapy.

The most appropriate treatment is thrombolytic therapy with a recombinant tissue plasminogen activator (rtPA). This patient has a large pulmonary embolism and is most likely becoming hypotensive from acute right ventricular (RV) failure. RV failure is the leading cause of death among patients with acute pulmonary embolism. In patients with hemodynamic collapse, treatment with thrombolytics is associated with decreased mortality and improvement in clinical and echocardiographic parameters. Although this patient has no contraindications to rtPA, thrombolytics carry a significant side effect profile, including an up to 2% risk of intracranial hemorrhage, but this should be considered relative in patients with life-threatening, high-risk pulmonary embolism. In patients with contraindications to thrombolysis, and in those in whom thrombolysis has failed to improve the hemodynamic status, surgical or catheter-based embolectomy should be considered if surgical expertise and resources are available.

CONT.

According to the Apixaban for the Initial Management of Pulmonary Embolism and Deep-Vein Thrombosis as First-line Therapy (AMPLIFY) study, apixaban is an equivalent option to conventional heparin therapy for the initial treatment of pulmonary embolism. In this patient with hemodynamic collapse, it would not be more beneficial than low-molecular-weight heparin (LMWH) and is less beneficial than rtPA therapy.

In patients with acute pulmonary embolism, unfractionated heparin, LMWH, a new oral anticoagulant such as apixiban, or fondaparinux (a factor Xa inhibitor) should be started immediately unless otherwise contraindicated. Because this patient is experiencing hemodynamic collapse despite therapy with LMWH, continuing that treatment alone would not be appropriate.

Treatment of patients with acute pulmonary embolism with unfractionated heparin infusion appears to be associated with increased risk of adverse effect compared to LMWH administration. The 2014 European Society of Cardiology guidelines for diagnosis and management of pulmonary embolism recommends LMWH or fondaparinux rather than unfractionated heparin in hemodynamically stable patients because they are associated with a lower risk of heparin-induced thrombocytopenia and major bleeding events. However, the guidelines caution that LMWH and fondaparinux have not been tested in the setting of hypotension and shock and thus are not preferred modes of initial anticoagulation in that patient population.

**KEY POINT**

- In patients with pulmonary embolism and hemodynamic collapse, treatment with thrombolytics is associated with decreased mortality and improvement in clinical and echocardiographic parameters.

**Bibliography**

Konstantinides SV, Torbicki A, Agnelli G, Danchin N, Fitzmaurice D, Galiè N, et al; Task Force for the Diagnosis and Management of Acute Pulmonary Embolism of the European Society of Cardiology (ESC). 2014 ESC guidelines on the diagnosis and management of acute pulmonary embolism. Eur Heart J. 2014;35:3033-69, 3069a-3069k. [PMID: 25173341] doi:10.1093/eurheartj/ehu283

 **Item 86      Answer:   D**

**Educational Objective:** Treat a malnourished, critically ill patient using parenteral nutrition.

This patient should receive parenteral nutrition. Nutrition is an essential part of management for patients in the ICU and can be given enterally or parenterally, with the enteral route preferred. Initiation of enteral nutrition is recommended at 24 to 48 hours following admission if the patient is hemodynamically stable, with advancement to goal by 48 to 72 hours. Benefits include fewer infections and possibly reduced mortality. For patients with adequate nutritional status but who have contraindications to enteral nutrition or do not tolerate enteral nutrition, parenteral nutrition is delayed for 1 to 2 weeks based upon evidence that early parenteral

nutrition may increase the risk of infection. For patients with inadequate nutrition (or who are at high risk for malnutrition) who have contraindications or intolerance of enteral nutrition, parenteral nutrition should be initiated as soon as possible. This practice is based on two meta-analyses showing early parenteral nutrition in poorly nourished patients is associated with fewer complications and decreased mortality. This patient has several features consistent with severe malnutrition (temporal wasting, edema, hypoglycemia, poorly healing wounds), as well as ileus and evidence of enteral nutrition intolerance (nausea, vomiting).

The patient is obviously not tolerating enteral nutrition, as evidenced by her clinical nutritional status, nausea, vomiting, and distended abdomen. Continuing enteral nutrition would not be appropriate.

Measurement of gastric residual volume is no longer recommended for routine monitoring of enteral nutrition because it does not affect outcomes. In this patient, it is clinically apparent that she is not tolerating enteral nutrition, and measurement of gastric residual volume will not add clinically useful information.

Metoclopramide improves enteral nutrition tolerance but does not affect patient outcomes and is associated with adverse events (diarrhea, QT prolongation, tardive dyskinesia, cardiac toxicity). Because of this patient's recent surgery, she should first be started on parenteral nutrition and evaluated for a mechanical cause of bowel obstruction. Metoclopramide and other prokinetic agents are contraindicated in the presence of mechanical small bowel obstruction.

**KEY POINT**

- Parenteral nutrition should be started as soon as possible for severely malnourished patients or those at high risk of malnutrition for whom enteral nutrition is not possible.

**Bibliography**

Taylor BE, McClave SA, Martindale RG, Warren MM, Johnson DR, Braunschweig C, et al; Society of Critical Care Medicine. Guidelines for the provision and assessment of nutrition support therapy in the adult critically ill patient: Society of Critical Care Medicine (SCCM) and American Society for Parenteral and Enteral Nutrition (A.S.P.E.N.). Crit Care Med. 2016;44:390-438. [PMID: 26771786] doi:10.1097/CCM.0000000000001525

**Item 87      Answer:   D**

**Educational Objective:** Diagnose respiratory bronchiolitis-associated interstitial lung disease.

The most likely diagnosis is respiratory bronchiolitis-associated interstitial lung disease (RB-ILD). Evidence of RB-ILD is found on approximately 5% to 25% of cancer-screening CT scans. RB-ILD is used to describe disease in active smokers who have imaging findings of centrilobular micronodules with a pathologic finding of respiratory bronchiolitis and tan-pigmented macrophages (smokers' macrophages) on biopsy. Patients with RB-ILD are often asymptomatic. Symptomatic patients are typically smokers presenting in their fourth and fifth decades of smoking with cough and dyspnea and bibasilar inspiratory crackles. There are two other disorders that generally only develop in individuals who have an active smoking history. These are desquamative interstitial pneumonia and pulmonary Langerhans cell histiocytosis. Pulmonary function tests usually reveal an obstructive pattern with a decreased D$_{LCO}$ in individuals with more severe disease. For those with milder disease, pulmonary function tests can be normal, restrictive, or obstructive. Cessation of smoking is the primary management.

Desquamative interstitial pneumonia is due to extensive, diffuse macrophage filling of alveolar spaces with predominant cough and dyspnea symptoms and bilateral ground-glass opacities on chest imaging. This patient's symptoms and CT findings are not compatible with this disease.

CT scan findings of idiopathic pulmonary fibrosis include basal- and peripheral-predominant septal line thickening with traction bronchiectasis and honeycomb changes. This is the usual interstitial pneumonia pattern and can be seen in connective tissue disease, asbestosis, and chronic hypersensitivity pneumonitis; idiopathic pulmonary fibrosis is a diagnosis of exclusion. The CT scan findings are not consistent with this diagnosis.

Pulmonary Langerhans cell histiocytosis is characterized by middle and upper zone thin-walled cysts with accompanying nodules and is often associated with pulmonary hypertension. Patients tend to be young adults with cough and dyspnea. Thin-walled cysts are not present in this patient's CT scan, making this diagnosis unlikely.

**KEY POINT**

- Respiratory bronchiolitis–associated interstitial lung disease is found in active smokers who have chest CT scan findings of centrilobular micronodules.

**Bibliography**
Chung JH, Richards JC, Koelsch TL, MacMahon H, Lynch DA. Screening for lung cancer: incidental pulmonary parenchymal findings. AJR Am J Roentgenol. 2017:1-11. [PMID: 29231759] doi:10.2214/AJR.17.19003

## Item 88    Answer:    D

**Educational Objective:** Manage a patient with chronic silicosis and likely tuberculosis infection.

The most appropriate management is a sputum sample for acid-fast bacillus. This patient has constitutional symptoms that include night sweats, unintentional weight loss, hemoptysis, and upper-lobe cavitary disease on chest radiograph. Reactivation tuberculosis most commonly involves the apical-posterior segments of the upper lobe; cavitation is present in up to 40% of cases. Tuberculosis should be strongly considered when a patient with silicosis develops constitutional symptoms, worsening respiratory impairment, hemoptysis, or changes in the chest radiograph, particularly cavities. Chronic silicosis adversely affects macrophage function and is clearly associated with the development of infection with

tuberculosis. Concomitant silicosis and tuberculosis is associated with a substantially increased risk of mortality. Therefore, a high index of suspicion for this complication of chronic silicosis is essential to ensure early and appropriate medical therapy.

Aspergilloma is generally a consequence of colonization of a preexisting pulmonary cavity or cyst or in areas of devitalized lung. Symptoms include cough, hemoptysis, dyspnea, weight loss, fever, fatigue, and chest pain. Radiographic images show a round mass within a pulmonary cavity or cyst. Sputum cultures or IgG antibody are usually positive. This patient's chest radiograph is not consistent with an aspergilloma, and aspergillosis IgG antibody testing is not necessary.

Mine workers are often exposed to radon and several kinds of dust, and they have high rates of tobacco use; however, the development of silicosis is also an independent risk factor for the development of lung cancer. Nevertheless, bronchoscopy with transbronchial biopsy would not be appropriate for this patient. Although he has a substantially increased risk of lung cancer, the chest radiograph does not clearly demonstrate a target for biopsy. Furthermore, pursuing bronchoscopy without first ensuring there is not an active tuberculosis infection potentially places health care workers at risk for infection.

A high-resolution CT scan of the chest may identify additional findings not visible on the chest radiograph, but it will not change the need to rule out tuberculosis, which is a common comorbidity of chronic silicosis.

**KEY POINT**

- Tuberculosis should be strongly considered when a patient with silicosis develops constitutional symptoms, worsening respiratory impairment, hemoptysis, or changes in the chest radiograph, particularly cavities.

**Bibliography**
Nasrullah M, Mazurek JM, Wood JM, Bang KM, Kreiss K. Silicosis mortality with respiratory tuberculosis in the United States, 1968-2006. Am J Epidemiol. 2011;174:839-48. [PMID: 21828370] doi:10.1093/aje/kwr159

## Item 89    Answer:    C

**Educational Objective:** Diagnose upper airway obstruction using a flow-volume loop.

The most likely diagnosis is fixed upper airway obstruction. Flow-volume loops graphically plot pulmonary airflow during exhalation and inspiration, with characteristic patterns associated with specific clinical conditions. The normal expiratory portion of the flow-volume loop (above the x-axis) is characterized by a rapid rise to the peak flow rate, followed by a nearly linear fall in flow as the patient exhales. The inspiratory curve (below the x-axis) appears as a semicircle. Flattening of both the inspiratory and expiratory curve of the flow-volume loop suggests this patient has a fixed intrathoracic lesion, such as tracheal stenosis, which can be seen postintubation.

Spirometry is relatively insensitive to all but severe (greater than 71%) intrathoracic airway obstruction. Therefore, if intrathoracic airway obstruction is suspected, appearance of a normal flow-volume loop should not discourage further evaluation.

Patients with asthma would be expected to have this obstructive pattern, although patients without active symptoms can have a completely normal loop.

Patients with COPD demonstrate an obstructive pattern of the flow-volume loop. This is typically manifested by a fairly normal initial portion of the expiratory flow loop, with increased concavity of the terminal portion, indicating airway narrowing during exhalation.

The flow-volume loop demonstrates reduced inspiratory and expiratory volumes, and not the normal pattern described above.

### KEY POINT

- Flattening of both the inspiratory and expiratory curve of the flow-volume loop suggests a fixed intrathoracic lesion; direct examination of the airways is indicated to confirm the finding and identify the cause.

### Bibliography
Murgu SD, Egressy K, Laxmanan B, Doblare G, Ortiz-Comino R, Hogarth DK. Central airway obstruction: benign strictures, tracheobronchomalacia, and malignancy-related obstruction. Chest. 2016;150:426-41. [PMID: 26874192] doi:10.1016/j.chest.2016.02.001

## Item 90    Answer:    D

**Educational Objective:**  Treat asthma during pregnancy.

This patient's previous medications of albuterol and budesonide should be restarted. Asthma management during pregnancy should consist of optimization of anti-inflammatory therapy, management of gastroesophageal reflux, and smoking cessation. Inhaled glucocorticoids are considered safe in pregnancy, and abundant long-term safety evidence exists for budesonide. With the exception of zileuton, most leukotriene receptor antagonists are also considered safe in pregnancy. The treatment of asthma in pregnancy is very similar to treatment in nonpregnant patients. This patient has mild persistent asthma, with symptoms more than twice weekly, and use of low-dose inhaled glucocorticoids plus a short-acting $\beta_2$-agonist is the recommended therapy. The risks to the fetus of untreated asthma are significantly greater than the risks of asthma medications. Maternal asthma increases the risk of perinatal mortality, preterm birth, low-birth-weight infants, and preeclampsia. Budesonide is the preferred inhaled glucocorticoid to use in pregnant asthma patients because there are more data available concerning budesonide use in pregnancy than the other inhaled glucocorticoid formulations. However, there are no studies indicating that other inhaled glucocorticoid formulations are unsafe in pregnancy, so if a patient's asthma is well controlled on another inhaled glucocorticoid, it is not necessary to change to budesonide during pregnancy.

Combination fluticasone/salmeterol is not the recommended treatment regimen for mild persistent asthma and would be inappropriate for this patient.

Prednisone is used to treat asthma exacerbations, and all patients with asthma should have a written asthma action plan to manage an exacerbation and begin self-treatment. Therefore, although prednisone may be part of this patient's asthma management plan, it is not indicated for treatment of her current symptoms of mild persistent asthma.

This patient is experiencing frequent symptoms of asthma and would benefit from treatment. Therefore, peak flow monitoring alone is not appropriate without initiation of pharmacotherapy.

### KEY POINT

- Treatment of asthma during pregnancy is similar to treatment in nonpregnant patients.

### Bibliography
Bonham CA, Patterson KC, Strek ME. Asthma outcomes and management during pregnancy. Chest. 2018;153:515-527. [PMID: 28867295] doi:10.1016/j.chest.2017.08.029

## Item 91    Answer:    B

**Educational Objective:**  Evaluate a patient with diffuse parenchymal lung disease using high-resolution chest CT scan.

High-resolution CT (HRCT) scan of the chest is the most appropriate test. The choice of imaging modality in the evaluation of pulmonary disease is dependent on the information being sought based on the differential diagnosis. HRCT scan is indicated if diffuse parenchymal lung disease (DPLD) is suspected. The diagnostic approach to DPLD is grounded in the predominant pattern of abnormalities, distribution of disease, and associated findings (pleural plaques, calcifications, effusions, lymphadenopathy). HRCT scan provides more detail than either chest radiography or conventional CT scanning and can more accurately assess the pattern and distribution of DPLD. This patient's history, physical findings, pulmonary function tests, radiography results, and family history strongly suggest the diagnosis of idiopathic pulmonary fibrosis. An HRCT scan will allow for better characterization of pattern and distribution of the opacities on chest radiograph and will help diagnose the underlying disease.

Contrast-enhanced chest CT scan may be added to the study to better evaluate the mediastinal structures (for example, to assess for lymphadenopathy). However, there is no suggestion of mediastinal abnormality on the chest radiograph; rather, the patient's history, physical examination findings, and chest radiograph more strongly suggest DPLD, and HRCT is the preferred imaging modality in that situation.

Patients who meet criteria for lung-cancer screening should undergo imaging with low-dose chest CT scan to minimize radiation exposure. Low-dose chest CT images utilize a lower total radiation dose than standard CT chest protocols. The lower dose of radiation decreases the radiation to patients and is as effective as standard-dose CT in imaging lung nodules owing to the high inherent contrast between lung tissue and air. Low-dose CT scan is a good modality to screen for pulmonary nodules but not a good modality to assess DPLD.

Patients with a pulmonary nodule or other findings suggestive of malignancy may require PET/CT imaging. This test most commonly uses fluorodeoxyglucose (FDG) as a metabolic marker to identify rapidly dividing cells such as tumor cells. A nodule that demonstrates no FDG uptake is unlikely to be malignant. Any disease with metabolic activity, including infection, inflammation, and malignancy, can cause an FDG-avid nodule. PET/CT imaging would not be helpful in the evaluation of DPLD.

**KEY POINT**

- High-resolution chest CT scan is the preferred advanced imaging modality for suspected diffuse parenchymal lung disease; it can help narrow the differential diagnosis based on the character and distribution of the lung parenchymal abnormalities.

**Bibliography**

Walsh SL, Hansell DM. High-resolution CT of interstitial lung disease: a continuous evolution. Semin Respir Crit Care Med. 2014;35:129-44. [PMID: 24481766] doi:10.1055/s-0033-1363458

## Item 92    Answer:    D

**Educational Objective:** Evaluate recurrent unilateral exudative effusion for malignancy.

This patient should be referred for thoracoscopy and pleural biopsy. He has a recurrent exudative pleural effusion. The characterization of pleural fluid as a transudate or exudate helps narrow the differential diagnosis and direct subsequent investigations. An effusion is considered an exudate if any of the following criteria are met: pleural fluid total protein/serum total protein greater than 0.5; pleural fluid lactate dehydrogenase (LDH)/serum LDH greater than 0.6; pleural fluid LDH greater than 2/3 the upper limit of normal for serum LDH. This patient has an exudate. Despite the negative chest radiograph and CT scan, this exudate is concerning for malignancy considering his age, smoking history, and work in a shipyard with potential exposure to asbestos. The cytology of the pleural fluid was negative, but cytology is only 60% sensitive for malignancy.

Closed pleural biopsy is less sensitive than cytology and should not be performed.

A chylous effusion can be suspected by its milky appearance (seen in 50% of patients) and is associated with traumatic and nontraumatic etiologies. Nontraumatic chylous effusion is most commonly due to malignancy (lymphoma, chronic lymphocytic leukemia, metastatic cancer). Traumatic chylous effusions are most commonly associated with thoracic surgical procedures. A pleural fluid triglyceride level greater than 110 mg/dL (1.24 mmol/L) is characteristic of a

chylothorax. There is no reason to suspect a chylothorax at this point; thoracoscopic pleural biopsy will be of higher diagnostic yield.

The yield of sending more than two cytology specimens taken on different occasions is low. If cytology is negative and malignancy is still suspected, thoracoscopy with pleural biopsy allows for direct visualization of the pleural surface and has greater than 90% sensitivity for the diagnosis of malignancy.

**KEY POINT**

- For patients with negative cytology in whom malignancy is suspected, thoracoscopy with pleural biopsy allows for direct visualization of the pleural surface and has a diagnostic sensitivity for malignant disease of greater than 90%.

**Bibliography**

Hooper C, Lee YC, Maskell N; BTS Pleural Guideline Group. Investigation of a unilateral pleural effusion in adults: British Thoracic Society Pleural Disease Guideline 2010. Thorax. 2010;65 Suppl 2:ii4-17. [PMID: 20696692] doi:10.1136/thx.2010.136978

## Item 93    Answer:    C

**Educational Objective:** Diagnose interstitial lung disease with a high-resolution CT scan of the chest.

This patient should receive a high-resolution CT (HRCT) scan of the chest. He has symptoms of progressive dyspnea on exertion, inspiratory crackles, restrictive pulmonary function tests, and a chest radiograph demonstrating diffuse parenchymal lung disease. This constellation of findings suggests interstitial lung disease. Plain chest radiography findings may be highly variable in patients with diffuse parenchymal lung disease. Chest films may show increased interstitial reticular or nodular infiltrates in different patterns of distribution, but they may be normal in up to 10% of patients. Characteristics on HRCT of the chest have pulmonary pathology correlates that can help narrow the differential diagnosis. HRCT provides detailed resolution of the pulmonary parenchymal architecture. HRCT, clinical presentation (including time course of symptoms), physical findings, and, when necessary, lung biopsy and histopathology allow clinicians to reach selected diagnoses from an extensive list of diffuse parenchymal lung diseases.

In selected cases, bronchoscopic lung biopsy can provide enough tissue to demonstrate specific histopathologic features diagnostic of several specific disease processes, including carcinoma, sarcoidosis, and eosinophilic pneumonia. Bronchoalveolar lavage can provide additional diagnostic information, including culture, cytology, and cell differential. However, a lung biopsy and bronchoalveolar lavage would not be indicated until imaging studies confirmed the presence of diffuse parenchymal lung disease and have narrowed the differential diagnosis to entities that might be assessed with biopsy or bronchoalveolar lavage.

Cardiopulmonary exercise testing includes assessment of respiratory gas exchange during treadmill or bicycle exercise for a more detailed assessment of functional capacity and differentiation between potential causes of exercise limitation (cardiac, pulmonary, or deconditioning, versus volitional). It would not be the most appropriate next choice in a patient with increasing exercise limitation, pulmonary crackles, an abnormal chest radiograph, and restrictive findings on pulmonary function testing.

Methacholine challenge testing is used to evaluate bronchial hyperreactivity in patients with normal pulmonary function tests, and this patient's testing is abnormal, with a restrictive pattern, so such testing would not be indicated.

## KEY POINT

- High-resolution CT scan of the chest is standard care for evaluating parenchymal opacities seen on a plain radiograph.

### Bibliography
Meyer KC. Diagnosis and management of interstitial lung disease. Transl Respir Med. 2014;2:4. [PMID: 25505696] doi:10.1186/2213-0802-2-4

## Item 94    Answer:    D

**Educational Objective:** Treat disruptive snoring with weight loss.

The most appropriate next step in management is a trial of weight loss. In this obese but otherwise healthy patient without other sleep-related symptoms, weight loss is a reasonable first step that often relieves snoring. Obesity is the strongest risk factor for snoring and obstructive sleep apnea (OSA). Snoring occurs as the upper airway narrows during sleep, when inspired air collides with redundant soft tissue. Further airway collapse leads to OSA. Other treatments for snoring can include limiting time spent in the supine position (postural therapy) and curbing alcohol intake.

Home sleep testing should be reserved for patients with a high probability of moderate to severe apnea in whom positive airway pressure therapy is being considered. Although OSA hasn't been ruled out in this patient, his bed partner hasn't observed classic signs such as gasping or choking, nor does he exhibit strong indications for positive airway pressure therapy, such as excessive daytime sleepiness.

In-laboratory polysomnography allows more detailed analysis of the possible underlying sleep-related breathing disorder than out-of-center methods. Once the type of apnea is clarified during the diagnostic portion of the in-laboratory study, the technician may also then utilize the most appropriate mode of positive airway pressure therapy and assess the response to treatment. However, for this patient, testing of any kind should be preceded by a conservative approach that includes weight loss.

Upper airway surgical procedures, such as radiofrequency ablation of soft palate, are sometimes used to treat snoring and OSA but are variably effective and not considered first-line therapy.

## KEY POINT

- Obesity is the strongest risk factor for snoring and obstructive sleep apnea, and in obese but otherwise healthy patients without other sleep-related symptoms, weight loss is a reasonable first step that often relieves snoring and improves mild obstructive sleep apnea.

### Bibliography
Balachandran JS, Patel SR. In the clinic. Obstructive sleep apnea. Ann Intern Med. 2014;161:ITC1-15; quiz ITC16. [PMID: 25364899] doi:10.7326/0003-4819-161-9-201411040-01005

## Item 95    Answer:    A

**Educational Objective:** Manage a malignant pleural effusion.

This patient should be referred for an indwelling pleural catheter placement. Her diagnosis of a malignant pleural effusion signifies advanced disease and overall poor prognosis and the goal of management is the relief of symptoms. Several therapeutic options are available and should be made based on symptoms, prognosis, degree of lung reexpansion, and patient performance status. She has rapid reaccumulation of fluid and, therefore, should be offered more definitive management. Indwelling pleural catheters with intermittent drainage provide significant symptom relief, and 50% to 70% of patients achieve spontaneous pleurodesis after 2 to 6 weeks. In a recent randomized trial indwelling pleural catheters were found to be noninferior to talc pleurodesis, and patients who had an indwelling pleural catheter had a shorter hospital stay and less dyspnea at 6 months.

Pleurectomy is another management option but is rarely performed because it is invasive, associated with long recovery times, and appears to be no more effective than less invasive options.

Repeat therapeutic thoracentesis is appropriate for patients with poor prognosis (less than 3 months) and slow reaccumulation of fluid; given this patient's good performance status and rapid reaccumulation of pleural fluid, serial thoracentesis is not indicated.

Chemical pleurodesis refers to obliteration of the pleural space with a sclerosing agent (typically talc). Talc can be introduced through a thoracostomy tube (talc slurry) or during a thoracostomy or thoracotomy (talc poudrage). Talc pleurodesis is very effective, with a success rate of 60% to 90%, depending on the degree of lung reexpansion; however, it is associated with increased pain and longer initial hospital stay, so an indwelling pleural catheter would be preferable at this time.

## KEY POINT

- For patients with a malignant pleural effusion and rapid reaccumulation of fluid, indwelling pleural catheters provide significant symptom relief, and 50% to 70% of patients achieve spontaneous pleurodesis after 2 to 6 weeks.

## Bibliography

Feller-Kopman D, Light R. Pleural disease. N Engl J Med. 2018;378:740-751. doi: 10.1056/NEJMra1403503. [PMID: 29466146]

## Item 96    Answer:    D

**Educational Objective:** Diagnose serotonin syndrome.

The most likely diagnosis is serotonin syndrome. The features of hyperthermia, tremor, hyperreflexia, ocular clonus (slow, continuous, horizontal eye movements), other clonus (spontaneous or induced), and anxiety are classic features of this syndrome. Hyperreflexia and clonus help distinguish serotonin syndrome from other hyperthermic syndromes and toxic ingestions. This patient's history supports the diagnosis, which usually occurs after coingestion of several serotonergic medications—for example, fluoxetine and methylenedioxymethamphetamine ("ecstasy"). Treatment is mainly supportive, using benzodiazepines as needed to keep the patient calm and to control blood pressure and heart rate. Physical restraint can lead to agitated exertion and worsen hyperthermia. Autonomic instability is common, so close monitoring is recommended. Only in very severe cases of agitation or hyperthermia do patients need to be deeply sedated, intubated, paralyzed, and sometimes treated with cyproheptadine.

Anticholinergic toxicity is unlikely in this patient because he has no signs of mydriasis, dry mucus membranes, or urinary and bowel retention. He does exhibit hyperthermia and agitation, but has clonus and hyperreflexia, which are not associated with anticholinergic toxicity.

Malignant hyperthermia would be very unlikely without a history of inhaled anesthesia agents or neuromuscular blockade. Clinical features of malignant hyperthermia usually include higher fever, muscle rigidity, and, occasionally, hemorrhage but not hyperreflexia or clonus.

Neuroleptic malignant syndrome would be very unlikely without a history of neuroleptic medications, such as haloperidol. It usually develops subacutely during days or weeks, whereas serotonin syndrome typically develops within hours. Rigidity with hyporeflexia is more common, rather than hyperreflexia and myoclonus in serotonin syndrome. Hyperthermia, altered mental status, and rigidity are features of both syndromes. Neuroleptic malignant syndrome usually takes many days to resolve, whereas serotonin syndrome usually resolves within 24 hours.

### KEY POINT

- Classic features of serotonin syndrome include hyperthermia, tremor, hyperreflexia and clonus; treatment is mainly supportive, using benzodiazepines as needed to keep the patient calm and to control blood pressure and heart rate.

## Bibliography

Dobry Y, Rice T, Sher L. Ecstasy use and serotonin syndrome: a neglected danger to adolescents and young adults prescribed selective serotonin reuptake inhibitors. Int J Adolesc Med Health. 2013;25:193-9. [PMID: 24006318] doi:10.1515/ijamh-2013-0052

## Item 97    Answer:    A

**Educational Objective:** Treat a patient with acute hemorrhagic shock using volume resuscitation with blood products.

The most appropriate management for this patient is a transfusion of packed red blood cells. Clinicians should base decisions on blood transfusion on the full clinical picture, recognizing that overtransfusion may be as damaging as undertransfusion. A restrictive transfusion policy aiming for a hemoglobin level of 7 to 8 g/dL (70 to 80 g/L) is suggested in hemodynamically stable patients. More liberal blood transfusion thresholds lead to increased portal pressures and risk of further bleeding. This patient most likely is experiencing hemorrhagic shock from a recurrent variceal bleeding episode. Because the patient is hemodynamically unstable, initial guideline-based management includes volume resuscitation, and transfusion of blood products is the best method for achieving this. In patients who are bleeding and have a platelet count less than 50,000/µL ($50 \times 10^9$/L) or who have an INR greater than 1.5, transfusion of platelets or fresh frozen plasma, respectively, is indicated.

Historically, uncontrolled variceal bleeding offered a compelling rationale for use of recombinant factor VII, but a 2014 meta-analysis of almost 500 patients from two randomized clinical trials evaluated the role of factor VII following variceal bleed. In both trials, there was no indication that factor VII improved outcomes. Therefore, it would not be appropriate for this patient.

Emergent upper endoscopy and consideration of placing a transjugular intrahepatic portosystemic shunt are indicated in this patient, but are pursued after initial resuscitation efforts are completed. Because this patient is hemodynamically unstable and these procedures take time to coordinate, they would not supersede initial resuscitative efforts with blood products.

### KEY POINT

- In patients with hemorrhagic shock, initial management includes volume resuscitation with blood products to stabilize the patient.

## Bibliography

Tripathi D, Stanley AJ, Hayes PC, Patch D, Millson C, Mehrzad H, et al; Clinical Services and Standards Committee of the British Society of Gastroenterology. U.K. guidelines on the management of variceal haemorrhage in cirrhotic patients. Gut. 2015;64:1680-704. [PMID: 25887380] doi:10.1136/gutjnl-2015-309262

## Item 98    Answer:    D

**Educational Objective:** Treat a patient intoxicated with isopropyl alcohol.

The most appropriate management is supportive care. Calculation of the plasma osmolal gap is helpful in assessing the presence of unmeasured solutes, such as ingestion of certain toxins (for example, methanol or ethylene glycol). The plasma osmolal gap is the difference between the measured and calculated plasma osmolality. Plasma osmolality can be calculated using the following formula:

$$\text{Plasma Osmolality (mOsm/kg H}_2\text{O)} = 2 \times \text{Serum Sodium} \\ \text{(mEq/L) + Plasma Glucose (mg/dL)/} \\ 18 + \text{Blood Urea Nitrogen (mg/dL)/2.8.}$$

When the measured osmolality exceeds the calculated osmolality by greater than 10 mOsm/kg H₂O, the osmolal gap is considered elevated. This patient does not have an increased anion-gap metabolic acidosis, thus eliminating methanol and ethylene glycol poisoning. An elevated osmolal gap of 27 and absent blood ethanol support the diagnosis of isopropyl alcohol ingestion (rubbing alcohol), which does not cause a metabolic acidosis. It is metabolized by alcohol dehydrogenase (ADH) to acetone, which can cause a fruity odor on the patient's breath. There are no other toxic metabolites, and the main effect of isopropyl alcohol ingestion is central nervous system depression by both the isopropyl alcohol and the acetone.

There is no need to block the action of ADH with fomepizole. Administration of fomepizole would be advised for treatment of methanol or ethylene glycol ingestion, because these alcohols both have toxic metabolites that can lead to blindness, kidney failure, or death. Inhibiting ADH in patients who have ingested isopropyl alcohol only prolongs its elimination.

Hemodialysis is not normally needed to clear isopropyl alcohol from the blood, although it is a highly effective modality for eliminating all ingested alcohols. The risks of initiating hemodialysis in this patient who is inebriated but otherwise stable would not be justified.

Seizure prophylaxis with levetiracetam is not indicated for isopropyl alcohol ingestion, and this patient shows no clinical signs of withdrawal, a prelude to seizures. As long as he is closely monitored and treated appropriately with benzodiazepine medication for signs of withdrawal, antiepileptic medication should not be needed.

**KEY POINT**

- Patients with isopropyl alcohol poisoning can be treated effectively using supportive care.

**Bibliography**

Beauchamp GA, Valento M. Toxic alcohol ingestion: prompt recognition and management in the emergency department. Emerg Med Pract. 2016;18:1-20. [PMID: 27538060]

## Item 99    Answer:    B

**Educational Objective:** Evaluate potential lung cancer with the optimal diagnostic procedure.

The most appropriate diagnostic test for this patient with a lesion highly suspicious for lung cancer and PET-positive mediastinal lymphadenopathy is bronchoscopy with endobronchial ultrasound-guided transbronchial needle aspiration. The evaluation of a patient with suspected lung cancer aims to confirm whether the patient indeed has lung cancer, to determine the pathology (non-small cell lung cancer versus

small cell lung cancer), and to assess the stage at presentation. Most patients undergo chest CT scan as the first imaging modality, either after an abnormal chest radiograph or in evaluation of a symptom. The findings on the chest CT scan determine whether a PET/CT scan is necessary. A PET/CT scan can help in staging and therefore also help guide where to biopsy. For example, if a patient has a solitary pulmonary nodule, a PET/CT scan may help determine if any lymph node involvement is present that was not visible on the chest CT scan.

The next step is to obtain tissue diagnosis. The choice of initial diagnostic testing should be aimed first at identifying potential lymph node involvement or metastatic disease. Tissue diagnosis should then be targeted at the lesion that would result in the highest potential staging. In this patient, sampling the mediastinal lymph nodes is critical to both diagnose and stage the patient and will affect the clinical decision making for this patient. Endobronchial ultrasound-guided transbronchial needle aspiration is a minimally invasive way and preferred to more invasive surgical techniques. Endobronchial ultrasound-guided transbronchial needle aspiration can sample most mediastinal and some hilar lymph node stations, although some of the more posterior lymph nodes are not accessible with this technique.

CT-guided needle biopsy has a high accuracy for diagnosis of lung cancers, but has higher risks of procedural complications than endobronchial ultrasound-guided transbronchial needle aspiration (mainly pneumothorax), and the patient would require a second procedure to sample the mediastinum if the lung lesion is a non-small cell lung cancer.

Sputum cytology has a lower sensitivity than endobronchial ultrasound-guided transbronchial needle aspiration for diagnosis of lung cancer, does not produce sufficient sample material for molecular studies, and will not provide needed staging information.

Thoracoscopic lung biopsy with lymph node dissection is less preferable than a minimally invasive approach, due to cost and risks of complications.

**KEY POINT**

- Endobronchial ultrasound-guided transbronchial needle aspiration is the procedure of choice for diagnosing and staging mediastinal and hilar lymphadenopathy in patients with suspected thoracic malignancy.

**Bibliography**

Silvestri GA, Gonzalez AV, Jantz MA, Margolis ML, Gould MK, Tanoue LT, et al. Methods for staging non-small cell lung cancer: diagnosis and management of lung cancer, 3rd ed: American College of Chest Physicians evidence-based clinical practice guidelines. Chest. 2013;143:e211S-e250S. [PMID: 23649440] doi:10.1378/chest.12-2355

## Item 100    Answer:    B

**Educational Objective:** Treat acute opioid overdose with naloxone.

The most appropriate management is continued observation for signs of recurrent respiratory failure. Patients with opioid overdose have findings that suggest the diagnosis including:

CONT.

miosis, respiratory depression, lethargy, confusion, hypothermia, bradycardia, and hypotension. An early empiric trial of the opioid antagonist naloxone is warranted when opioid overdose is suspected. It is important to remember that naloxone has a very short half-life, and its antidote effects will usually wear off before the opioid effects are gone. Naloxone is given at higher doses to apneic patients, such as 2 mg intravenously (IV), which is larger than the typical starting dose of 0.4 mg IV usually given to overdose patients who are still breathing. The dose of naloxone is titrated to a respiration rate of at least 12/min, not to a normal mental status. Chronic opioid users require close monitoring for withdrawal.

Serial escalating doses of naloxone may be necessary in some patients, and patients who respond to serial dosing may require a continuous naloxone infusion. However, there is no immediate need for more naloxone because this patient has normal breathing and mentation. During the period of observation, more naloxone may be needed if her respiration rate slows or stops.

This patient cannot be discharged until it is known that her respiratory suppression will not return when the naloxone wears off. Patients should be observed for at least 60 minutes after the last dose of naloxone. Drug addiction resources should be accessed for this patient. It is also appropriate after overdose to rule out suicidal ideation or intent and refer the patient to a psychiatric clinician if needed.

Endotracheal intubation would not be appropriate because the patient is protecting her airway and is not in respiratory distress or failure. Intubation is required for patients whose respiratory suppression cannot be quickly reversed with naloxone.

### KEY POINT

- In the treatment of opioid overdose the antidote effects of naloxone will usually wear off before the opioid effects are gone; observation and repeated dosing are often necessary.

### Bibliography

Willman MW, Liss DB, Schwarz ES, Mullins ME. Do heroin overdose patients require observation after receiving naloxone? Clin Toxicol (Phila). 2017;55:81-87. [PMID: 27849133] doi:10.1080/15563650.2016.1253846

 **Item 101      Answer:      C**

**Educational Objective:** Diagnose pulmonary embolism as the cause of acute hypoxemic respiratory failure and shock.

This patient most likely has a pulmonary embolism. This patient has hypoxemic respiratory failure and shock. Severe hypoxemia is generally defined as an arterial $P_{O_2}$ of 60 mm Hg (8.0 kPa) or less or an oxygen saturation of 89% or less while breathing ambient air. The most common causes of hypoxemic respiratory failure are conditions that lead to mismatch between the ventilation of inspired air in the alveoli and perfusion of adjacent alveolar capillaries by blood (called ventilation-perfusion [$\dot{V}/\dot{Q}$] mismatch). Conditions such as pulmonary

embolism lead to $\dot{V}/\dot{Q}$ mismatch. Hypoxemia due to $\dot{V}/\dot{Q}$ mismatch should resolve with oxygen therapy. However, extremes of $\dot{V}/\dot{Q}$ mismatch (known as a shunt) do not fully resolve with supplemental oxygen because inspired gas does not interface with the shunted blood in the lungs. In addition, this patient has evidence of cardiogenic shock, including hypotension, elevated jugular venous pressure, fixed splitting of the second heart sound, and cool, mottled skin. Although cardiogenic shock can occur for many reasons, in this patient, it is the result of the pulmonary embolism causing a mechanical blockage in the pulmonary circulation, leading to impaired cardiac output from the right ventricle. Fat emboli following long-bone fractures can mimic pulmonary emboli.

Anaphylactic shock is a type of distributive shock, as might occur if a patient with an allergy to penicillin were given either penicillin or a related agent to which she reacted. Anaphylaxis is an IgE-mediated reaction and manifests within minutes to 1 hour after exposure to the implicated antigen. Anaphylactic shock would result in hypotension and warm extremities, typically with hives or rash. The patient is hypotensive, but does not have a rash. Respiratory failure could be present but would be associated with wheezing or stridor.

Opioid overdose can cause hypercapnic respiratory failure with hypoxemia occurring as the result of hypoventilation. Although the hypoxemia improves with oxygen, it does not improve the hypercapnea. Opioid overdose cannot account for the findings of obstructive shock.

Tension pneumothorax can cause respiratory failure and cardiogenic shock as a result of poor right ventricular filling. It should be suspected in patients with hypotension, diminished breath sounds on the affected side, distended neck veins, and tracheal deviation away from the affected side. Risk factors for tension pneumothorax include trauma, recent pulmonary procedure, mechanical ventilation, and underlying cystic lung disease. The patient has no risk factors for tension pneumothorax, and her lung findings do not support this diagnosis.

### KEY POINT

- The most common causes of hypoxemic respiratory failure are conditions that lead to ventilation-perfusion mismatch or shunt; hypoxemia due to ventilation-perfusion mismatch with shunting does not improve with supplemental oxygen.

### Bibliography

Wagner PD. The physiological basis of pulmonary gas exchange: implications for clinical interpretation of arterial blood gases. Eur Respir J. 2015;45:227-43. [PMID: 25323225] doi:10.1183/09031936.00039214

**Item 102      Answer:      C**

**Educational Objective:** Diagnose obesity hypoventilation syndrome.

The most likely diagnosis is obesity hypoventilation syndrome. Obesity hypoventilation syndrome is characterized by daytime hypercapnia (arterial $P_{CO_2}$ greater than 45 mm Hg [5.9 kPa]) that is thought to be a consequence of diminished ventilatory drive and capacity related to extreme obesity. Persons with a BMI of 35 or higher are considered at risk for obesity hypoventilation syndrome; it's estimated that more than half of patients with a BMI of 50 or higher have this condition. This patient's BMI of 44, compensated hypercapnic respiratory failure, hypoxemia during wakefulness but more pronounced during sleep, and polycythemia are all consistent with obesity hypoventilation syndrome. Positive airway pressure therapy (continuous positive airway pressure or bilevel positive airway pressure), sometimes with supplemental oxygen, is first-line therapy.

Neuromuscular diseases that can affect the respiratory system must be considered in the differential diagnosis of hypoventilation syndromes. Amyotrophic lateral sclerosis (ALS) often leads to hypercapnic respiratory failure. However, this patient has an unremarkable neurologic examination and none of the typical features of ALS, such as muscle weakness and fasciculations and hyperactive deep tendon reflexes.

Central sleep apnea (CSA) is defined by intermittent reduced central drive to breathe but is not a hypoventilation syndrome. In fact, the tendency to hyperventilate, as seen with the cyclic ventilatory pattern of Cheyne-Stokes breathing, is a key underlying mechanism of CSA. Patients with CSA are generally normocapnic or slightly hypocapnic on blood gas testing.

An apnea-hypopnea index (AHI) of 5 to 15 is indicative of mild obstructive sleep apnea (OSA). This patient has mild OSA based upon an AHI of 6. OSA is typically encountered on sleep testing in those with obesity hypoventilation syndrome, with upper airway collapse superimposed on obesity-related hypoventilation. Severe OSA is defined as an AHI of at least 30; OSA severity is not defined by degree or duration of hypoxemia.

**KEY POINT**

- Obesity hypoventilation syndrome is characterized by daytime hypercapnia, defined as an arterial $P_{CO_2}$ greater than 45 mm Hg that is thought to be a consequence of diminished ventilatory drive and capacity related to extreme obesity.

**Bibliography**

Randerath W, Verbraecken J, Andreas S, Arzt M, Bloch KE, Brack T, et al. Definition, discrimination, diagnosis and treatment of central breathing disturbances during sleep. Eur Respir J. 2017;49. [PMID: 27920092] doi:10.1183/13993003.00959-2016

## Item 103     Answer:    E

**Educational Objective:** Treat an acute exacerbation of bronchiectasis with antibiotics.

The most appropriate treatment of this patient is levofloxacin. Oral antibiotic treatment is appropriate for clinically stable patients with an acute exacerbation of bronchiectasis. The choice of antibiotic therapy can be based on previous sputum culture results, if available. If not available, a reasonable empiric antibiotic choice is a respiratory fluoroquinolone such as levofloxacin or moxifloxacin. Although duration of therapy is not well defined, most experts treat for 10 to 14 days.

Amoxicillin or a macrolide such as azithromycin is a reasonable choice for patients in the absence of β-lactamase-positive *Haemophilus influenzae* or *Pseudomonas*. Initial empiric therapy can also be deescalated to amoxicillin based on the results of sputum culture and sensitivity. However, in the absence of bacteriologic data from sputum culture, amoxicillin is an inadequate choice for empiric therapy in patients with recurrent acute exacerbations previously treated with antibiotics due to the high risk of β-lactamase producing organisms and *Pseudomonas*.

For similar reasons, azithromycin is not an appropriate empiric antibiotic for this patient. There is likely a role for long-term azithromycin therapy to prevent recurrent exacerbations of bronchiectasis. The salutary effect on chronic macrolide therapy in these situations may not be entirely due to its antimicrobial properties but rather its well-known antiinflammatory properties. However, the development of antibiotic resistance is a potential risk.

Oral or inhaled glucocorticoids would seem to be reasonable adjunctive therapy for patients with acute exacerbation of bronchiectasis, but supporting evidence for their use is sparse. Some experts may employ glucocorticoids in patients with coexistent asthma and wheezing or allergic bronchopulmonary aspergillosis, but the risk of routine use is related to immunosuppression and promotion of bacterial and fungal colonization and is not recommended.

Inhaled aerosols of antibiotics, including inhaled tobramycin solution, are not recommended for an acute exacerbation of bronchiectasis. This recommendation is based on a multicenter randomized trial that demonstrated the addition of inhaled tobramycin to ciprofloxacin was not superior to ciprofloxacin alone but was associated with more wheezing. There may be a role of inhaled antibiotics in the prophylaxis of acute exacerbations of bronchiectasis.

**KEY POINT**

- If previous data on bronchiectasis exacerbations are not available, a fluoroquinolone should be started to ensure *Pseudomonas* coverage until the sputum culture is completed.

**Bibliography**

Smith MP. Diagnosis and management of bronchiectasis. CMAJ. 2017;189: E828-E835. [PMID: 28630359] doi:10.1503/cmaj.160830

# Index

## A  NAME AND ADDRESS (Please complete.)

Last Name       First Name       Middle Initial

Address

Address cont.

City       State       ZIP Code

Country

Email address

**ACP®**
American College of Physicians
Leading Internal Medicine, Improving Lives

**Medical Knowledge Self-Assessment Program® 18**

### TO EARN *CME Credits and/or MOC Points* YOU MUST:

1. Answer all questions.
2. Score a minimum of 50% correct.

==========================================

### TO EARN *FREE* INSTANTANEOUS *CME Credits and/or MOC Points* ONLINE:

1. Answer all of your questions.
2. Go to **mksap.acponline.org** and enter your ACP Online username and password to access an online answer sheet.
3. Enter your answers.
4. You can also enter your answers directly at **mksap.acponline.org** without first using this answer sheet.

### To Submit Your Answer Sheet by Mail or FAX for a $20 Administrative Fee per Answer Sheet:

1. Answer all of your questions and calculate your score.
2. Complete boxes A-H.
3. Complete payment information.
4. Send the answer sheet and payment information to ACP, using the FAX number/address listed below.

## B  Order Number

(Use the 10-digit Order Number on your MKSAP materials packing slip.)

## C  ACP ID Number

(Refer to packing slip in your MKSAP materials for your 8-digit ACP ID Number.)

## D  Required Submission Information if Applying for MOC

Birth Month and Day    M M   D D       ABIM Candidate Number

### COMPLETE FORM BELOW ONLY IF YOU SUBMIT BY MAIL OR FAX

Last Name       First Name       MI

### Payment Information. Must remit in US funds, drawn on a US bank.
### The processing fee for each paper answer sheet is $20.

☐ Check, made payable to ACP, enclosed

Charge to   ☐ **VISA**   ☐ **MasterCard**   ☐ **AMERICAN EXPRESS**   ☐ **DISCOVER**

Card Number _____

Expiration Date _____ / _____
        MM      YY

Security code (3 or 4 digit #s) _____

Signature _____

**Fax to:** 215-351-2799

**Mail to:**
Member and Customer Service
American College of Physicians
190 N. Independence Mall West
Philadelphia, PA 19106-1572

1 Ⓐ Ⓑ Ⓒ Ⓓ Ⓔ
2 Ⓐ Ⓑ Ⓒ Ⓓ Ⓔ
3 Ⓐ Ⓑ Ⓒ Ⓓ Ⓔ
4 Ⓐ Ⓑ Ⓒ Ⓓ Ⓔ
5 Ⓐ Ⓑ Ⓒ Ⓓ Ⓔ

6 Ⓐ Ⓑ Ⓒ Ⓓ Ⓔ
7 Ⓐ Ⓑ Ⓒ Ⓓ Ⓔ
8 Ⓐ Ⓑ Ⓒ Ⓓ Ⓔ
9 Ⓐ Ⓑ Ⓒ Ⓓ Ⓔ
10 Ⓐ Ⓑ Ⓒ Ⓓ Ⓔ

11 Ⓐ Ⓑ Ⓒ Ⓓ Ⓔ
12 Ⓐ Ⓑ Ⓒ Ⓓ Ⓔ
13 Ⓐ Ⓑ Ⓒ Ⓓ Ⓔ
14 Ⓐ Ⓑ Ⓒ Ⓓ Ⓔ
15 Ⓐ Ⓑ Ⓒ Ⓓ Ⓔ

16 Ⓐ Ⓑ Ⓒ Ⓓ Ⓔ
17 Ⓐ Ⓑ Ⓒ Ⓓ Ⓔ
18 Ⓐ Ⓑ Ⓒ Ⓓ Ⓔ
19 Ⓐ Ⓑ Ⓒ Ⓓ Ⓔ
20 Ⓐ Ⓑ Ⓒ Ⓓ Ⓔ

21 Ⓐ Ⓑ Ⓒ Ⓓ Ⓔ
22 Ⓐ Ⓑ Ⓒ Ⓓ Ⓔ
23 Ⓐ Ⓑ Ⓒ Ⓓ Ⓔ
24 Ⓐ Ⓑ Ⓒ Ⓓ Ⓔ
25 Ⓐ Ⓑ Ⓒ Ⓓ Ⓔ

26 Ⓐ Ⓑ Ⓒ Ⓓ Ⓔ
27 Ⓐ Ⓑ Ⓒ Ⓓ Ⓔ
28 Ⓐ Ⓑ Ⓒ Ⓓ Ⓔ
29 Ⓐ Ⓑ Ⓒ Ⓓ Ⓔ
30 Ⓐ Ⓑ Ⓒ Ⓓ Ⓔ

31 Ⓐ Ⓑ Ⓒ Ⓓ Ⓔ
32 Ⓐ Ⓑ Ⓒ Ⓓ Ⓔ
33 Ⓐ Ⓑ Ⓒ Ⓓ Ⓔ
34 Ⓐ Ⓑ Ⓒ Ⓓ Ⓔ
35 Ⓐ Ⓑ Ⓒ Ⓓ Ⓔ

36 Ⓐ Ⓑ Ⓒ Ⓓ Ⓔ
37 Ⓐ Ⓑ Ⓒ Ⓓ Ⓔ
38 Ⓐ Ⓑ Ⓒ Ⓓ Ⓔ
39 Ⓐ Ⓑ Ⓒ Ⓓ Ⓔ
40 Ⓐ Ⓑ Ⓒ Ⓓ Ⓔ

41 Ⓐ Ⓑ Ⓒ Ⓓ Ⓔ
42 Ⓐ Ⓑ Ⓒ Ⓓ Ⓔ
43 Ⓐ Ⓑ Ⓒ Ⓓ Ⓔ
44 Ⓐ Ⓑ Ⓒ Ⓓ Ⓔ
45 Ⓐ Ⓑ Ⓒ Ⓓ Ⓔ

46 Ⓐ Ⓑ Ⓒ Ⓓ Ⓔ
47 Ⓐ Ⓑ Ⓒ Ⓓ Ⓔ
48 Ⓐ Ⓑ Ⓒ Ⓓ Ⓔ
49 Ⓐ Ⓑ Ⓒ Ⓓ Ⓔ
50 Ⓐ Ⓑ Ⓒ Ⓓ Ⓔ

51 Ⓐ Ⓑ Ⓒ Ⓓ Ⓔ
52 Ⓐ Ⓑ Ⓒ Ⓓ Ⓔ
53 Ⓐ Ⓑ Ⓒ Ⓓ Ⓔ
54 Ⓐ Ⓑ Ⓒ Ⓓ Ⓔ
55 Ⓐ Ⓑ Ⓒ Ⓓ Ⓔ

56 Ⓐ Ⓑ Ⓒ Ⓓ Ⓔ
57 Ⓐ Ⓑ Ⓒ Ⓓ Ⓔ
58 Ⓐ Ⓑ Ⓒ Ⓓ Ⓔ
59 Ⓐ Ⓑ Ⓒ Ⓓ Ⓔ
60 Ⓐ Ⓑ Ⓒ Ⓓ Ⓔ

61 Ⓐ Ⓑ Ⓒ Ⓓ Ⓔ
62 Ⓐ Ⓑ Ⓒ Ⓓ Ⓔ
63 Ⓐ Ⓑ Ⓒ Ⓓ Ⓔ
64 Ⓐ Ⓑ Ⓒ Ⓓ Ⓔ
65 Ⓐ Ⓑ Ⓒ Ⓓ Ⓔ

66 Ⓐ Ⓑ Ⓒ Ⓓ Ⓔ
67 Ⓐ Ⓑ Ⓒ Ⓓ Ⓔ
68 Ⓐ Ⓑ Ⓒ Ⓓ Ⓔ
69 Ⓐ Ⓑ Ⓒ Ⓓ Ⓔ
70 Ⓐ Ⓑ Ⓒ Ⓓ Ⓔ

71 Ⓐ Ⓑ Ⓒ Ⓓ Ⓔ
72 Ⓐ Ⓑ Ⓒ Ⓓ Ⓔ
73 Ⓐ Ⓑ Ⓒ Ⓓ Ⓔ
74 Ⓐ Ⓑ Ⓒ Ⓓ Ⓔ
75 Ⓐ Ⓑ Ⓒ Ⓓ Ⓔ

76 Ⓐ Ⓑ Ⓒ Ⓓ Ⓔ
77 Ⓐ Ⓑ Ⓒ Ⓓ Ⓔ
78 Ⓐ Ⓑ Ⓒ Ⓓ Ⓔ
79 Ⓐ Ⓑ Ⓒ Ⓓ Ⓔ
80 Ⓐ Ⓑ Ⓒ Ⓓ Ⓔ

81 Ⓐ Ⓑ Ⓒ Ⓓ Ⓔ
82 Ⓐ Ⓑ Ⓒ Ⓓ Ⓔ
83 Ⓐ Ⓑ Ⓒ Ⓓ Ⓔ
84 Ⓐ Ⓑ Ⓒ Ⓓ Ⓔ
85 Ⓐ Ⓑ Ⓒ Ⓓ Ⓔ

86 Ⓐ Ⓑ Ⓒ Ⓓ Ⓔ
87 Ⓐ Ⓑ Ⓒ Ⓓ Ⓔ
88 Ⓐ Ⓑ Ⓒ Ⓓ Ⓔ
89 Ⓐ Ⓑ Ⓒ Ⓓ Ⓔ
90 Ⓐ Ⓑ Ⓒ Ⓓ Ⓔ

91 Ⓐ Ⓑ Ⓒ Ⓓ Ⓔ
92 Ⓐ Ⓑ Ⓒ Ⓓ Ⓔ
93 Ⓐ Ⓑ Ⓒ Ⓓ Ⓔ
94 Ⓐ Ⓑ Ⓒ Ⓓ Ⓔ
95 Ⓐ Ⓑ Ⓒ Ⓓ Ⓔ

96 Ⓐ Ⓑ Ⓒ Ⓓ Ⓔ
97 Ⓐ Ⓑ Ⓒ Ⓓ Ⓔ
98 Ⓐ Ⓑ Ⓒ Ⓓ Ⓔ
99 Ⓐ Ⓑ Ⓒ Ⓓ Ⓔ
100 Ⓐ Ⓑ Ⓒ Ⓓ Ⓔ

101 Ⓐ Ⓑ Ⓒ Ⓓ Ⓔ
102 Ⓐ Ⓑ Ⓒ Ⓓ Ⓔ
103 Ⓐ Ⓑ Ⓒ Ⓓ Ⓔ
104 Ⓐ Ⓑ Ⓒ Ⓓ Ⓔ
105 Ⓐ Ⓑ Ⓒ Ⓓ Ⓔ

106 Ⓐ Ⓑ Ⓒ Ⓓ Ⓔ
107 Ⓐ Ⓑ Ⓒ Ⓓ Ⓔ
108 Ⓐ Ⓑ Ⓒ Ⓓ Ⓔ
109 Ⓐ Ⓑ Ⓒ Ⓓ Ⓔ
110 Ⓐ Ⓑ Ⓒ Ⓓ Ⓔ

111 Ⓐ Ⓑ Ⓒ Ⓓ Ⓔ
112 Ⓐ Ⓑ Ⓒ Ⓓ Ⓔ
113 Ⓐ Ⓑ Ⓒ Ⓓ Ⓔ
114 Ⓐ Ⓑ Ⓒ Ⓓ Ⓔ
115 Ⓐ Ⓑ Ⓒ Ⓓ Ⓔ

116 Ⓐ Ⓑ Ⓒ Ⓓ Ⓔ
117 Ⓐ Ⓑ Ⓒ Ⓓ Ⓔ
118 Ⓐ Ⓑ Ⓒ Ⓓ Ⓔ
119 Ⓐ Ⓑ Ⓒ Ⓓ Ⓔ
120 Ⓐ Ⓑ Ⓒ Ⓓ Ⓔ

121 Ⓐ Ⓑ Ⓒ Ⓓ Ⓔ
122 Ⓐ Ⓑ Ⓒ Ⓓ Ⓔ
123 Ⓐ Ⓑ Ⓒ Ⓓ Ⓔ
124 Ⓐ Ⓑ Ⓒ Ⓓ Ⓔ
125 Ⓐ Ⓑ Ⓒ Ⓓ Ⓔ

126 Ⓐ Ⓑ Ⓒ Ⓓ Ⓔ
127 Ⓐ Ⓑ Ⓒ Ⓓ Ⓔ
128 Ⓐ Ⓑ Ⓒ Ⓓ Ⓔ
129 Ⓐ Ⓑ Ⓒ Ⓓ Ⓔ
130 Ⓐ Ⓑ Ⓒ Ⓓ Ⓔ

131 Ⓐ Ⓑ Ⓒ Ⓓ Ⓔ
132 Ⓐ Ⓑ Ⓒ Ⓓ Ⓔ
133 Ⓐ Ⓑ Ⓒ Ⓓ Ⓔ
134 Ⓐ Ⓑ Ⓒ Ⓓ Ⓔ
135 Ⓐ Ⓑ Ⓒ Ⓓ Ⓔ

136 Ⓐ Ⓑ Ⓒ Ⓓ Ⓔ
137 Ⓐ Ⓑ Ⓒ Ⓓ Ⓔ
138 Ⓐ Ⓑ Ⓒ Ⓓ Ⓔ
139 Ⓐ Ⓑ Ⓒ Ⓓ Ⓔ
140 Ⓐ Ⓑ Ⓒ Ⓓ Ⓔ

141 Ⓐ Ⓑ Ⓒ Ⓓ Ⓔ
142 Ⓐ Ⓑ Ⓒ Ⓓ Ⓔ
143 Ⓐ Ⓑ Ⓒ Ⓓ Ⓔ
144 Ⓐ Ⓑ Ⓒ Ⓓ Ⓔ
145 Ⓐ Ⓑ Ⓒ Ⓓ Ⓔ

146 Ⓐ Ⓑ Ⓒ Ⓓ Ⓔ
147 Ⓐ Ⓑ Ⓒ Ⓓ Ⓔ
148 Ⓐ Ⓑ Ⓒ Ⓓ Ⓔ
149 Ⓐ Ⓑ Ⓒ Ⓓ Ⓔ
150 Ⓐ Ⓑ Ⓒ Ⓓ Ⓔ

151 Ⓐ Ⓑ Ⓒ Ⓓ Ⓔ
152 Ⓐ Ⓑ Ⓒ Ⓓ Ⓔ
153 Ⓐ Ⓑ Ⓒ Ⓓ Ⓔ
154 Ⓐ Ⓑ Ⓒ Ⓓ Ⓔ
155 Ⓐ Ⓑ Ⓒ Ⓓ Ⓔ

156 Ⓐ Ⓑ Ⓒ Ⓓ Ⓔ
157 Ⓐ Ⓑ Ⓒ Ⓓ Ⓔ
158 Ⓐ Ⓑ Ⓒ Ⓓ Ⓔ
159 Ⓐ Ⓑ Ⓒ Ⓓ Ⓔ
160 Ⓐ Ⓑ Ⓒ Ⓓ Ⓔ

161 Ⓐ Ⓑ Ⓒ Ⓓ Ⓔ
162 Ⓐ Ⓑ Ⓒ Ⓓ Ⓔ
163 Ⓐ Ⓑ Ⓒ Ⓓ Ⓔ
164 Ⓐ Ⓑ Ⓒ Ⓓ Ⓔ
165 Ⓐ Ⓑ Ⓒ Ⓓ Ⓔ

166 Ⓐ Ⓑ Ⓒ Ⓓ Ⓔ
167 Ⓐ Ⓑ Ⓒ Ⓓ Ⓔ
168 Ⓐ Ⓑ Ⓒ Ⓓ Ⓔ
169 Ⓐ Ⓑ Ⓒ Ⓓ Ⓔ
170 Ⓐ Ⓑ Ⓒ Ⓓ Ⓔ

171 Ⓐ Ⓑ Ⓒ Ⓓ Ⓔ
172 Ⓐ Ⓑ Ⓒ Ⓓ Ⓔ
173 Ⓐ Ⓑ Ⓒ Ⓓ Ⓔ
174 Ⓐ Ⓑ Ⓒ Ⓓ Ⓔ
175 Ⓐ Ⓑ Ⓒ Ⓓ Ⓔ

176 Ⓐ Ⓑ Ⓒ Ⓓ Ⓔ
177 Ⓐ Ⓑ Ⓒ Ⓓ Ⓔ
178 Ⓐ Ⓑ Ⓒ Ⓓ Ⓔ
179 Ⓐ Ⓑ Ⓒ Ⓓ Ⓔ
180 Ⓐ Ⓑ Ⓒ Ⓓ Ⓔ

MK7010

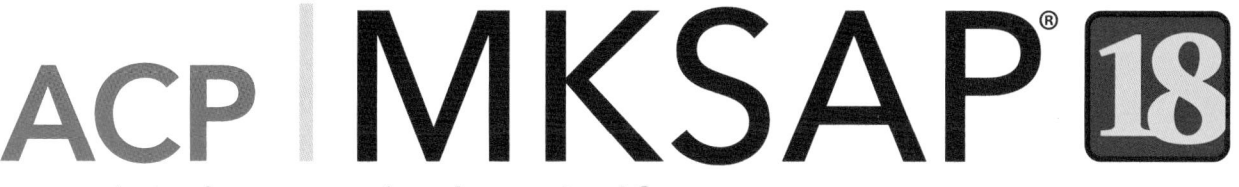

# ACP | MKSAP 18

## Medical Knowledge Self-Assessment Program®

# Nephrology

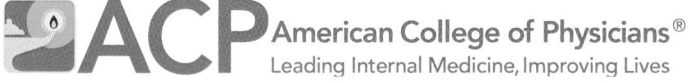

ACP American College of Physicians®
Leading Internal Medicine, Improving Lives

# Welcome to the Nephrology Section of MKSAP 18!

In these pages, you will find updated information on the clinical evaluation of kidney function, fluids and electrolytes, acid-base disorders, hypertension, chronic tubulointerstitial nephritis, glomerular diseases, kidney manifestations of deposition diseases, genetic disorders and kidney disease, acute kidney injury, kidney stones, the kidney in pregnancy, and chronic kidney disease. All of these topics are uniquely focused on the needs of generalists and subspecialists *outside* of nephrology.

The core content of MKSAP 18 has been developed as in previous editions—all essential information that is newly researched and written in 11 topic areas of internal medicine—created by dozens of leading generalists and subspecialists and guided by certification and recertification requirements, emerging knowledge in the field, and user feedback. MKSAP 18 also contains 1200 all-new peer-reviewed, psychometrically validated, multiple-choice questions (MCQs) for self-assessment and study, including 108 in Nephrology. MKSAP 18 continues to include *High Value Care* (HVC) recommendations, based on the concept of balancing clinical benefit with costs and harms, with associated MCQs illustrating these principles and HVC Key Points called out in the text. Internists practicing in the hospital setting can easily find comprehensive *Hospitalist*-focused content and MCQs, specially designated in blue and with the ■ symbol.

If you purchased MKSAP 18 Complete, you also have access to MKSAP 18 Digital, with additional tools allowing you to customize your learning experience. MKSAP Digital includes regular text updates with new, practice-changing information, 200 new self-assessment questions, and enhanced custom-quiz options. MKSAP Complete also includes more than 1200 electronic, adaptive learning-enhanced flashcards for quick review of important concepts, as well as an updated and enhanced version of Virtual Dx, MKSAP's image-based self-assessment tool. As before, MKSAP 18 Digital is optimized for use on your mobile devices, with iOS- and Android-based apps allowing you to sync between your apps and online account and submit for CME credits and MOC points online.

Please visit us at the MKSAP Resource Site (mksap.acponline.org) to find out how we can help you study, earn CME credit and MOC points, and stay up to date.

On behalf of the many internists who have offered their time and expertise to create the content for MKSAP 18 and the editorial staff who work to bring this material to you in the best possible way, we are honored that you have chosen to use MKSAP 18 and appreciate any feedback about the program you may have. Please feel free to send any comments to mksap_editors@acponline.org.

Sincerely,

*Patrick Alguire*

Patrick C. Alguire, MD, FACP
Editor-in-Chief
Senior Vice President Emeritus
Medical Education Division
American College of Physicians

# Nephrology

## Committee

**Michael J. Ross, MD, Section Editor[2]**
Chief, Division of Nephrology
Professor of Medicine
Professor of Developmental and Molecular Biology
Albert Einstein College of Medicine
Montefiore Medical Center
Bronx, New York

**Andrew S. Bomback, MD, MPH[2]**
Assistant Professor of Medicine
Division of Nephrology
Columbia University Medical Center
New York, New York

**Steven Coca, DO, MS[2]**
Associate Professor of Medicine
Division of Nephrology
Icahn School of Medicine at Mount Sinai
New York, New York

**Derek M. Fine, MD[2]**
Associate Professor of Medicine
Division of Nephrology
Johns Hopkins University School of Medicine
Baltimore, Maryland

**Susan Hedayati, MD, MSc[1]**
Professor of Medicine, Division of Nephrology
Yin Quan-Yuen Distinguished Professorship in Nephrology
Associate Vice Chair for Research, Department of Internal
  Medicine
Director of Nephrology Translational and Population Health
  Research
University of Texas Southwestern Medical Center
Dallas, Texas

**Harold M. Szerlip, MD, FACP[2]**
Director, Nephrology Division
Baylor University Medical Center at Dallas
Dallas, Texas

**Ashita Tolwani, MD, MSc[2]**
Professor of Medicine
Division of Nephrology
University of Alabama at Birmingham
Birmingham, Alabama

## Editor-in-Chief

**Patrick C. Alguire, MD, FACP[2]**
Senior Vice President Emeritus, Medical Education
American College of Physicians
Philadelphia, Pennsylvania

## Deputy Editor

**Davoren Chick, MD, FACP[2]**
Senior Vice President, Medical Education
American College of Physicians
Philadelphia, Pennsylvania

## Nephrology Reviewers

Faris A. Ahmed, MD, FACP[1]
Ayoola O. Akinbamowo, MBBS, FACP[1]
Fahad Aziz, MD[1]
Olurotimi J. Badero, MBchB, FACP[1]
Krishna M. Baradhi, MBBS, FACP[1]
Gautam Kantilal Bhanushali, MD, FACP[1]
Omar Hamze, MD, FACP[1]
Mira T. Keddis, MD, FACP[1]
Zeid J. Khitan, MD, FACP[1]
Wei Ling Lau, MD[2]

## Hospital Medicine Nephrology Reviewers

Corinne A. Ahmar, MD, FACP[1]
Rahul S. Koushik, MBBS, FACP[1]

## Nephrology ACP Editorial Staff

**Megan Zborowski[1]**, Senior Staff Editor, Self-Assessment and
  Educational Programs
**Margaret Wells[1]**, Director, Self-Assessment and Educational
  Programs
**Becky Krumm[1]**, Managing Editor, Self-Assessment and
  Educational Programs

## ACP Principal Staff

**Davoren Chick, MD, FACP[2]**
*Senior Vice President, Medical Education*

## Acknowledgments

The American College of Physicians (ACP) gratefully acknowledges the special contributions to the development and production of the 18th edition of the Medical Knowledge Self-Assessment Program® (MKSAP® 18) made by the following people:

*Graphic Design:* Barry Moshinski (Director, Graphic Services), Michael Ripca (Graphics Technical Administrator), and Jennifer Gropper (Graphic Designer).

*Production/Systems:* Dan Hoffmann (Director, Information Technology), Scott Hurd (Manager, Content Systems), Neil Kohl (Senior Architect), and Chris Patterson (Senior Architect).

*MKSAP 18 Digital:* Under the direction of Steven Spadt (Senior Vice President, Technology), the digital version of MKSAP 18 was developed within the ACP's Digital Products and Services Department, led by Brian Sweigard (Director, Digital Products and Services). Other members of the team included Dan Barron (Senior Web Application Developer/Architect), Chris Forrest (Senior Software Developer/Design Lead), Kathleen Hoover (Senior Web Developer), Kara Regis (Manager, User Interface Design and Development), Brad Lord (Senior Web Application Developer), and John McKnight (Senior Web Developer).

The College also wishes to acknowledge that many other persons, too numerous to mention, have contributed to the production of this program. Without their dedicated efforts, this program would not have been possible.

## MKSAP Resource Site (mksap.acponline.org)

The MKSAP Resource Site (mksap.acponline.org) is a continually updated site that provides links to MKSAP 18 online answer sheets for print subscribers; access to MKSAP 18 Digital; Board Basics® e-book access instructions; information on Continuing Medical Education (CME), Maintenance of Certification (MOC), and international Continuing Professional Development (CPD) and MOC; errata; and other new information.

## International MOC/CPD

For information and instructions on submission of international MOC/CPD, please go to the MKSAP Resource Site (mksap.acponline.org).

## Continuing Medical Education

The American College of Physicians is accredited by the Accreditation Council for Continuing Medical Education (ACCME) to provide continuing medical education for physicians.

The American College of Physicians designates this enduring material, MKSAP 18, for a maximum of 275 *AMA PRA Category 1 Credits*™. Physicians should claim only the credit commensurate with the extent of their participation in the activity.

Up to 25 *AMA PRA Category 1 Credits*™ are available from December 31, 2018, to December 31, 2021, for the MKSAP 18 Nephrology section.

## Learning Objectives

The learning objectives of MKSAP 18 are to:

- Close gaps between actual care in your practice and preferred standards of care, based on best evidence
- Diagnose disease states that are less common and sometimes overlooked and confusing
- Improve management of comorbid conditions that can complicate patient care
- Determine when to refer patients for surgery or care by subspecialists
- Pass the ABIM Certification Examination
- Pass the ABIM Maintenance of Certification Examination

## Target Audience

- General internists and primary care physicians
- Subspecialists who need to remain up to date in internal medicine
- Residents preparing for the certifying examination in internal medicine
- Physicians preparing for maintenance of certification in internal medicine (recertification)

## ABIM Maintenance of Certification

Check the MKSAP Resource Site (mksap.acponline.org) for the latest information on how MKSAP tests can be used to apply to the American Board of Internal Medicine (ABIM) for Maintenance of Certification (MOC) points following completion of the CME activity.

Successful completion of the CME activity, which includes participation in the evaluation component, enables the participant to earn up to 275 medical knowledge MOC points in the ABIM's MOC program. It is the CME activity provider's responsibility to submit participant completion information to ACCME for the purpose of granting MOC credit.

## Earn Instantaneous CME Credits or MOC Points Online

Print subscribers can enter their answers online to earn instantaneous CME credits or MOC points. You can submit your answers using online answer sheets that are provided at mksap.acponline.org, where a record of your MKSAP 18 credits will be available. To earn CME credits or to apply for MOC points, you need to answer all of the questions in a test and earn a score of at least 50% correct (number of correct answers divided by the total number of questions). Please note that if you are applying for MOC points, you must also enter your birth date and ABIM candidate number.

Take either of the following approaches:

1. Use the printed answer sheet at the back of this book to record your answers. Go to mksap.acponline.org, access the appropriate online answer sheet, transcribe your answers, and submit your test for instantaneous CME credits or MOC points. There is no additional fee for this service.

2. Go to mksap.acponline.org, access the appropriate online answer sheet, directly enter your answers, and submit your test for instantaneous CME credits or MOC points. There is no additional fee for this service.

## Earn CME Credits or MOC Points by Mail or Fax

Pay a $20 processing fee per answer sheet and submit the printed answer sheet at the back of this book by mail or fax, as instructed on the answer sheet. Make sure you calculate your score and enter your birth date and ABIM candidate number, and fax the answer sheet to 215-351-2799 or mail the answer sheet to Member and Customer Service, American College of Physicians, 190 N. Independence Mall West, Philadelphia, PA 19106-1572, using the courtesy envelope provided in your MKSAP 18 slipcase. You will need your 10-digit order number and 8-digit ACP ID number, which are printed on your packing slip. Please allow 4 to 6 weeks for your score report to be emailed back to you. Be sure to include your email address for a response.

If you do not have a 10-digit order number and 8-digit ACP ID number, or if you need help creating a user-name and password to access the MKSAP 18 online answer sheets, go to mksap.acponline.org or email custserv@acponline.org.

## Disclosure Policy

It is the policy of the American College of Physicians (ACP) to ensure balance, independence, objectivity, and scientific rigor in all of its educational activities. To this end, and consistent with the policies of the ACP and the Accreditation Council for Continuing Medical Education (ACCME), contributors to all ACP continuing medical education activities are required to disclose all relevant financial relationships with any entity producing, marketing, re-selling, or distributing health care goods or services consumed by, or used on, patients. Contributors are required to use generic names in the discussion of therapeutic options and are required to identify any unapproved, off-label, or investigative use of commercial products or devices. Where a trade name is used, all available trade names for the same product type are also included. If trade-name products manufactured by companies with whom contributors have relationships are discussed, contributors are asked to provide evidence-based citations in support of the discussion. The information is reviewed by the committee responsible for producing this text. If necessary, adjustments to topics or contributors' roles in content development are made to balance the discussion. Further, all readers of this text are asked to evaluate the content for evidence of commercial bias and send any relevant comments to mksap_editors@acponline.org so that future decisions about content and contributors can be made in light of this information.

## Resolution of Conflicts

To resolve all conflicts of interest and influences of vested interests, ACP's content planners used best evidence and updated clinical care guidelines in developing content, when such evidence and guidelines were available. All content underwent review by peer reviewers not on the committee to ensure that the material was balanced and unbiased. Contributors' disclosure information can be found with the list of contributors' names and those of ACP principal staff listed in the beginning of this book.

## Hospital-Based Medicine

For the convenience of subscribers who provide care in hospital settings, content that is specific to the hospital setting has been highlighted in blue. Hospital icons (🏥) highlight where the hospital-only content begins, continues over more than one page, and ends.

## High Value Care Key Points

Key Points in the text that relate to High Value Care concepts (that is, concepts that discuss balancing clinical benefit with costs and harms) are designated by the HVC icon [**HVC**].

## Educational Disclaimer

The editors and publisher of MKSAP 18 recognize that the development of new material offers many opportunities for error. Despite our best efforts, some errors may persist in print. Drug dosage schedules are, we believe, accurate and in accordance with current standards. Readers are advised, however, to ensure that the recommended dosages in MKSAP 18 concur with the information provided in the product information material. This is especially important in cases of new, infrequently used, or highly toxic drugs.

Application of the information in MKSAP 18 remains the professional responsibility of the practitioner.

The primary purpose of MKSAP 18 is educational. Information presented, as well as publications, technologies, products, and/or services discussed, is intended to inform subscribers about the knowledge, techniques, and experiences of the contributors. A diversity of professional opinion exists, and the views of the contributors are their own and not those of the ACP. Inclusion of any material in the program does not constitute endorsement or recommendation by the ACP. The ACP does not warrant the safety, reliability, accuracy, completeness, or usefulness of and disclaims any and all liability for damages and claims that may result from the use of information, publications, technologies, products, and/or services discussed in this program.

## Publisher's Information

## Disclaimer Regarding Direct Purchases from Online Retailers

## Unauthorized Use of This Book Is Against the Law

MKSAP 18 ISBN: 978-1-938245-47-3
Nephrology ISBN: 978-1-938245-57-2

Printed in the United States of America.

For order information in the U.S. or Canada call 800-ACP-1915. All other countries call 215-351-2600 (Monday to Friday, 9 AM – 5 PM ET). Fax inquiries to 215-351-2799 or email to custserv@acponline.org.

## Errata

Errata for MKSAP 18 will be available through the MKSAP Resource Site at mksap.acponline.org as new information becomes known to the editors.

# Table of Contents

# Nephrology High Value Care Recommendations

The American College of Physicians, in collaboration with multiple other organizations, is engaged in a worldwide initiative to promote the practice of High Value Care (HVC). The goals of the HVC initiative are to improve health care outcomes by providing care of proven benefit and reducing costs by avoiding unnecessary and even harmful interventions. The initiative comprises several programs that integrate the important concept of health care value (balancing clinical benefit with costs and harms) for a given intervention into a broad range of educational materials to address the needs of trainees, practicing physicians, and patients.

HVC content has been integrated into MKSAP 18 in several important ways. MKSAP 18 includes HVC-identified key points in the text, HVC-focused multiple choice questions, and, for subscribers to MKSAP Digital, an HVC custom quiz. From the text and questions, we have generated the following list of HVC recommendations that meet the definition below of high value care and bring us closer to our goal of improving patient outcomes while conserving finite resources.

**High Value Care Recommendation**: A recommendation to choose diagnostic and management strategies for patients in specific clinical situations that balance clinical benefit with cost and harms with the goal of improving patient outcomes.

Below are the High Value Care Recommendations for the Nephrology section of MKSAP 18.

- The random (spot) urine protein-creatinine ratio and albumin-creatinine ratio are sufficiently accurate for screening and monitoring proteinuria.
- Urinalysis should not be used for detection of bladder cancer in asymptomatic patients.
- Ultrasonography is the most commonly used imaging modality in the evaluation of the kidneys and upper urinary tract because of its safety, cost effectiveness, and availability.
- Obtaining blood pressure measurements outside of the clinical setting for diagnostic confirmation is recommended before starting treatment.

- Non-dialytic palliative therapy is a reasonable option for elderly patients with end-stage kidney disease and multiple comorbidities, with treatment focusing on symptom management and quality of life.
- Use of the potassium exchange resin, sodium polystyrene sulfonate, is controversial; its effectiveness is limited, and it produces adverse gastrointestinal effects.
- Initial antihypertensive treatment for black patients with or without diabetes mellitus includes a thiazide diuretic or calcium channel blocker.
- Kidney biopsy is required to diagnose and classify lupus nephritis, which guides therapy.
- Kidney ultrasonography, rather than other imaging modalities, should be obtained for suspected urinary tract obstruction or when the underlying cause of acute kidney injury is unclear.
- Normal pregnancy is associated with decreased blood pressure, increased glomerular filtration rate with decreased serum creatinine, and increased proteinuria.
- In properly selected individuals, peritoneal dialysis allows patients to preserve their independence and offers outcomes similar to those seen with hemodialysis (see Item 19).
- Patients with newly diagnosed primary membranous glomerulopathy are observed for 6 to 12 months while on conservative therapy to allow time for possible spontaneous remission before initiating immunosuppression (see Item 38).
- Nonpharmacologic therapy alone is especially useful for prevention of hypertension, including in adults with elevated blood pressure, and for management of high blood pressure in adults with milder forms of hypertension (see Item 105).
- There is no benefit in starting renal replacement therapy (RRT) in asymptomatic patients or at an arbitrary estimated glomerular filtration rate cutoff compared with careful clinical management and initiating RRT for symptoms or metabolic abnormalities that are refractory to medical treatment (see Item 108).

# Nephrology

## Clinical Evaluation of Kidney Function

### Assessment of Kidney Function

The kidney selectively removes waste while retaining needed substrate, maintains fluid and electrolyte homeostasis, and regulates blood pH. Glomerular filtration rate (GFR) measures total nephron filtration of blood and therefore correlates closely with toxin removal and overall kidney function. Early loss of kidney function is difficult to detect because nephron loss is not initially accompanied by GFR changes due to compensation through hypertrophy and hyperfiltration. Other markers of disordered glomerular filtration, such as proteinuria and hematuria, are also indicators of kidney disease that may precede any evidence of reduced filtration.

### Biochemical Markers of Kidney Function

Although numerous methods for estimating kidney function are available (**Table 1**), serum creatinine and serum cystatin C are the primary biomarkers used to estimate GFR.

### Serum Creatinine

Serum creatinine is the most extensively used measure of kidney function. Creatinine is freely filtered by the glomerulus, without metabolism or reabsorption. Therefore, changes in serum creatinine primarily reflect changes in GFR. However, the relationship of serum creatinine to GFR is nonlinear; significant losses in kidney function at higher GFR may be masked by only small changes in serum creatinine, and small filtration changes at lower GFR are associated with large changes in serum creatinine (**Figure 1**). Creatinine is also secreted into urine by the proximal tubule, and the contribution of secretion to total creatinine excretion increases as GFR declines. Therefore, when measured creatinine clearance is used to estimate GFR, secreted creatinine will contribute to overestimation of true GFR. With complete loss of kidney function (anuria), serum creatinine typically increases by about 1.0 mg/dL (88.4 µmol/L) per day in patients with average muscle mass.

Creatinine is a metabolite of creatine, which is mostly present in skeletal muscle. Persons with higher muscle mass (such as younger people, men, and black persons) have a higher serum creatinine compared with less muscular persons with the same GFR. Loss of muscle mass seen with aging, muscle wasting, malnutrition, or amputation will result in lower serum creatinine despite stable GFR. In persons with decreased muscle mass, serum creatinine therefore tends to overestimate the GFR.

Some medications reduce proximal tubule secretion of creatinine. Such drugs include cimetidine, trimethoprim, cobicistat, and dolutegravir. Resulting increases in serum creatinine occur despite stable GFR. Reassessment of the serum creatinine level 1 week after identification of the increase will confirm the drug's effect.

### Serum Cystatin C

Cystatin C is produced by all nucleated cells, freely filtered by glomeruli, and catabolized by tubules. Compared with serum creatinine, serum cystatin C levels are less affected by age, sex, or muscle mass but may be increased by acute disease (such as malignancy, inflammation, or HIV infection). Changes in serum cystatin C may identify small decreases in kidney function better than serum creatinine. Formulas using cystatin C to estimate GFR are helpful for patients in whom creatinine-based GFR may be inaccurate.

### Blood Urea Nitrogen

Blood urea nitrogen (BUN) is a product of protein metabolism. Levels increase with reduced GFR and with increased urea reabsorption caused by renal hypoperfusion. BUN is also affected by protein intake and by changes in catabolic rate as caused by glucocorticoids, starvation, or stress. Persons with liver disease have abnormally low levels. BUN may be useful in detecting renal hypoperfusion because elevation of BUN from increased reabsorption is disproportionate to the rise in serum creatinine level.

### Estimation of Glomerular Filtration Rate

Creatinine-based formulas are used to estimate GFR by adjusting for factors that affect serum creatinine and creatinine clearance. These formulas take into account the effects of age, race, sex, and muscle mass (estimated by weight) on serum creatinine levels (see Table 1).

The Chronic Kidney Disease Epidemiology (CKD-EPI) Collaboration creatinine equation is the most widely used method for estimating GFR and is the most accurate equation for most persons, particularly when GFR >60 mL/min/1.73 m². A newer CKD-EPI creatinine-cystatin C equation is the most accurate when serum cystatin creatinine-cystatin C is known. CKD-EPI equations presume standard body surface area and therefore require adjustment for very large or small persons.

The Modification of Diet in Renal Disease (MDRD) study equation does not accurately estimate high GFRs. It performs similarly to the CKD-EPI equation at GFRs

| TABLE 1. Methods for Estimating Kidney Function | | |
|---|---|---|
| **Method** | **Applications** | **Considerations** |
| **Serum Creatinine** | | |
| | Most frequently used assessment of kidney function | Nonlinear relationship with GFR<br><br>Nonkidney effects on blood levels (muscle mass, drugs affecting secretion) |
| **Serum Cystatin C** | | |
| | More accurate in elderly population and patients with cirrhosis due to their low muscle mass<br><br>More accurate in those with an increase in muscle mass<br><br>Sensitive to mild changes in GFR | Levels are affected by diabetes mellitus, thyroid disease, inflammation, glucocorticoid use, malignancy, HIV infection |
| **Chronic Kidney Disease Epidemiology (CKD-EPI) Collaboration Equation[a]** | | |
| ***CKD-EPI Creatinine*** | | |
| Variables include serum creatinine, age, race, and gender:<br><br>$eGFR = 141 \times min(S_{Cr}/\kappa, 1)^{\alpha}$<br><br>$\times max(S_{Cr}/\kappa, 1)^{-1.209}$<br><br>$\times 0.993^{Age}$<br><br>$\times 1.018$ [if female]<br><br>$\times 1.159$ [if black] | More accurate than MDRD and CGE equations in elderly population and in those with eGFR >60 mL/min/1.73 m$^2$ | Preferred formula for calculating creatinine-based eGFR |
| ***CKD-EPI Cystatin C*** | | |
| Variables include serum cystatin C, age, and gender:<br><br>$eGFR = 133 \times min(S_{Cr}/\kappa, 1)^{-0.499}$<br><br>$\times max(S_{Cr}/\kappa, 1)^{-1.328}$<br><br>$\times 0.996^{Age}$<br><br>$\times 0.932$ [if female] | Can be used as confirmatory test for CKD. May be more accurate than creatinine-based equation in those with muscle wasting, chronic illness, or high muscle mass. | Helpful in estimating GFR in those taking drugs that affect creatinine secretion (such as cobicistat, dolutegravir, bictegravir, trimethoprim, and cimetidine) |
| ***CKD-EPI Creatinine-Cystatin C*** | | |
| Equation uses same variables as CKD-EPI creatinine but different exponents and includes serum cystatin C:<br><br>$eGFR = 135 \times min(S_{Cr}/\kappa, 1)^{\alpha}$<br><br>$\times max(S_{Cr}/\kappa, 1)^{-0.601}$<br><br>$\times min(S_{Cys}/0.8, 1)^{-0.375}$<br><br>$\times max(S_{Cys}/0.8, 1)^{-0.711}$<br><br>$\times 0.995^{Age}$<br><br>$\times 0.969$ [if female]<br><br>$\times 1.08$ [if black] | Creatinine-cystatin C combination provides most accurate eGFR in most patient populations | — |
| **Modification of Diet in Renal Disease (MDRD) Study Equation[a]** | | |
| Variables include serum creatinine, age, race, and gender:<br><br>$eGFR = 175 \times (S_{Cr})^{-1.154}$<br><br>$\times (age)^{-0.203}$<br><br>$\times 0.742$ [if female]<br><br>$\times 1.212$ [if black] | Similar accuracy as CKD-EPI when eGFR is 15-60 mL/min/1.73 m$^2$ | Most accurate (but similar to CKD-EPI) when eGFR is 15-60 mL/min/1.73 m$^2$<br><br>Underestimates GFR when GFR >60 mL/min/1.73 m$^2$ |

*(Continued on the next page)*

| TABLE 1. | Methods for Estimating Kidney Function *(Continued)* | | |
|---|---|---|---|
| **Method** | **Applications** | **Considerations** | |
| **Creatinine Clearance (CrCl)** | | | |
| $U_{Cr}V/S_{Cr} = U_{Cr}$ (mg/dL) $\times$ 24-hour urine volume (mL/24 h)/$S_{Cr}$ (mg/dL) $\times$ 1440 (min/24 h) | Useful in pregnancy, extremes of age and weight, amputees, malnourished and cirrhotic patients (situations where creatinine is low so CKD-EPI and MDRD will overestimate GFR) | Overestimates GFR 10%-20% Overestimation worsens with lower GFR (due to increased ratio of creatinine secretion to filtration) Over- or undercollection limits accuracy | |
| **Cockcroft-Gault Equation (CGE)** | | | |
| Variables include serum creatinine, body weight, age, and gender: CrCl = (140 − age) × (weight in kg) × (0.85 if female)/(72 × $S_{Cr}$) | Improved accuracy when age is <65 years | Most accurate when eGFR is 15-60 mL/min/1.73 m² Underestimates GFR in obesity Overestimates GFR when BMI <25 | |
| **Radionuclide Kidney Clearance Scanning** | | | |
| Iothalamate GFR scan or diethylenetriamine pentaacetic acid (DTPA) GFR scan | Useful in kidney donor evaluation if eGFR is borderline for donation or other times when accurate prediction is essential | Most precise method; expensive | |

CKD = chronic kidney disease; eGFR = estimated glomerular filtration rate; GFR = glomerular filtration rate; $S_{Cr}$ = serum creatinine (mg/dL); $S_{Cys}$ = serum cystatin C (mg/L); $U_{Cr}$ = urine creatinine (mg/dL).

α = −0.329 for females, -0.411 for males; κ = 0.7 for females, 0.9 for males; min = minimum of $S_C/κ$ or 1; max = maximum of $S_C/κ$ or 1.

[a]Mathematical equations recommended by the National Kidney Foundation Kidney Disease Outcomes Quality Initiative for estimation of GFR.

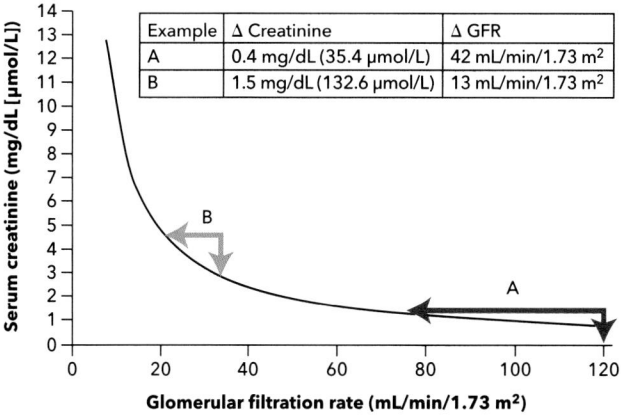

| Example | Δ Creatinine | Δ GFR |
|---|---|---|
| A | 0.4 mg/dL (35.4 µmol/L) | 42 mL/min/1.73 m² |
| B | 1.5 mg/dL (132.6 µmol/L) | 13 mL/min/1.73 m² |

**FIGURE 1.** The relationship between serum creatinine and glomerular filtration rate (GFR). Example A illustrates that a small increase in the serum creatinine level in the reference range (in this case, 0.8 to 1.2 mg/dL [70.7-106.1 µmol/L]) reflects a relatively large change in GFR (120 to 78 mL/min/1.73 m²). Example B illustrates that a relatively greater increase in the serum creatinine level (in the high range of 3.0 to 4.5 mg/dL [265.2-398 µmol/L]) reflects a proportionately smaller change in GFR (35 to 22 mL/min/1.73 m²).

<60 mL/min/1.73 m². Clinical laboratories that use the MDRD do not report GFRs >60 mL/min/1.73 m²; therefore, physicians may not be aware of the presence of kidney disease. However, an increasing serum creatinine level, proteinuria, or other urine abnormalities should alert the clinician to the presence of kidney disease despite high GFR. The MDRD study equation also requires adjustment for large or small body surface area.

The Cockcroft-Gault equation (CGE) is the least accurate method. It remains in use for drug dosing because it was used in pharmacokinetic studies for most medications.

Creatinine clearance obtained by using 24-hour urine collection is a better measure of GFR than serum creatinine, but it is not recommended for routine estimation of GFR because it is affected by the accuracy of collection and by creatinine secretion.

Radionuclide imaging provides the most accurate measurement of GFR and is the gold standard in research. It is useful for accurate determination of GFR during evaluation of kidney donors, evaluation of recipients for other organs, or assessment of the differential GFR of each kidney before nephrectomy.

**KEY POINTS**

- Serum creatinine changes nonlinearly with glomerular filtration rate (GFR), and significant losses in kidney function at higher GFR may cause only small changes in serum creatinine.

- The Chronic Kidney Disease Epidemiology (CKD-EPI) Collaboration equation is the most widely used equation to estimate glomerular filtration rate (GFR); it is the most accurate equation for most persons, particularly in the elderly and those with a GFR >60 mL/min/1.73 m².

## Interpretation of the Urinalysis

Urine dipstick and urine microscopy are indicated in the evaluation of both acute and chronic kidney disease (**Table 2**). Analysis is best performed on a fresh specimen within 30 to 60 minutes of voiding. Midstream collection is preferred with a clean catch in women and uncircumcised men.

### Urine Dipstick

See Table 2 for details on urine dipstick.

### Specific Gravity

Specific gravity measures hydration status and reflects the kidney's ability to concentrate urine.

### pH

Low urine pH may occur in persons eating high-protein diets. High alkaline pH ≥7.0 can occur in strict vegetarians and in persons with infections caused by urea-splitting organisms. Urine pH may be inappropriately high in some forms of renal tubular acidosis (type 1 distal) but may be appropriately low in others (type 4 distal).

| TABLE 2. Findings on Urinalysis | | |
|---|---|---|
| | **Normal Range** | **Comments** |
| **Dipstick** | | |
| Specific gravity | 1.005-1.030 | Low: dilute urine from excess hydration; impaired urine concentration (diabetes insipidus; sickle cell nephropathy; acute tubular injury) |
| | | High: volume depletion; renal hypoperfusion; excretion of hypertonic solute (glycosuria; contrast dye) |
| pH | 5.0-6.5 | Low/acidic: high protein diets; increases risk for uric acid and cystine calculi; type 4 distal RTA; some type 2 proximal RTA |
| | | High/alkaline: urease-splitting organisms (most commonly *Proteus* species; other potential organisms include *Escherichia coli* and *Pseudomonas*, *Klebsiella*, and some staphylococcal species); low acid ingestion; type 1 distal RTA; some type 2 RTA; increases risk for struvite and calcium phosphate calculi |
| Blood/heme pigments | None | Positive: hemoglobin or myoglobin; absence of erythrocytes suggests myoglobinuria or intravascular hemolysis |
| | | False positive: alkaline urine (pH >9) |
| Protein | None to trace | Dipsticks primarily detect albumin; concentration dependent (trace positive can be normal in a concentrated specimen); not sufficiently sensitive to detect moderately increased albuminuria |
| | | Graded as trace (10-30 mg/dL), 1+ (30 mg/dL), 2+ (100 mg/dL), 3+ (300 mg/dL), 4+ (>1000 mg/dL) |
| Glucose | None | Positive: plasma glucose exceeds ~180 mg/dL (10.0 mmol/L); proximal tubule defect (Fanconi syndrome); pregnancy (lower excretion threshold) |
| Ketones | None | Detects acetone and acetoacetic acid, not β-hydroxybutyrate |
| | | Positive: diabetic ketoacidosis; starvation; vomiting; pregnancy |
| Leukocyte esterase | None | Enzyme found in leukocytes; indicates pyuria (possibly from UTI); positive test requires ≥5 leukocytes/hpf |
| Nitrites | None | Produced by bacteria from nitrates |
| | | Positive: suggests UTI |
| | | Negative: does not rule out UTI (specific but not sensitive) |
| **Microscopic** | | |
| Erythrocytes | 0-2/hpf | Urine microscopy should be performed to evaluate erythrocyte morphology |
| Leukocytes | 0-4/hpf | The presence of any leukocytes may be abnormal depending on clinical circumstances |
| Squamous epithelial cells | <15/hpf | Increased epithelial cells indicates contamination |
| Casts | None or hyaline | Hyaline casts: indicative of poor kidney perfusion |
| | | Granular casts: acute tubular injury |
| | | Erythrocyte casts: glomerular bleeding/glomerulonephritis |
| | | Leukocyte casts: infection; acute interstitial nephritis |
| Crystals (see Table 3) | None | Most common are calcium oxalate, calcium phosphate, uric acid, and struvite |

RTA = renal tubular acidosis; UTI = urinary tract infection.

## Blood

Dipsticks detect peroxidase activity of blood and free heme pigments (hemoglobin and myoglobin). Three or more erythrocytes result in a positive test (1+ blood). A positive test in the absence of erythrocytes in the urine sediment may indicate myoglobinuria (due to rhabdomyolysis) or hemoglobinuria (due to intravascular hemolysis, transfusion, or shear stress related to mechanical heart valve and perivalvular leak). False-positive tests may occur with other substances with peroxidase activity, including peroxidase-expressing bacteria and drugs such as rifampin or chloroquine. Ascorbic acid can cause a false-negative result. Medications (rifampin, phenytoin) or food (beets) can cause red-colored urine that is heme negative.

## Protein

Although various proteins may be present in urine, the dipstick preferentially detects albumin. Because dipsticks are dependent on urine concentration, false negatives may result from dilute urine and false positives from highly concentrated urine. Because moderately increased albuminuria (microalbuminuria) may go undetected by dipstick, direct quantification of albuminuria and/or proteinuria using a random (spot) protein-creatinine ratio or albumin-creatinine ratio or a 24-hour urine collection is required in high-risk patients. False-positive tests can occur with highly alkaline urine specimens.

## Glucose

Glucosuria typically occurs when plasma glucose exceeds 180 mg/dL (10.0 mmol/L). Glucosuria in the absence of hyperglycemia suggests proximal tubular dysfunction, as seen with myeloma or exposure to drugs (including tenofovir disoproxil fumarate and sodium-glucose cotransporter-2 inhibitors such as empagliflozin and canagliflozin). Glucosuria may be present in normal pregnancy due to changes in tubular threshold for glucose reabsorption.

## Ketones

Ketonuria is most commonly seen in starvation, diabetic ketoacidosis, and alcoholic ketoacidosis. Urine ketones are also seen in salicylate toxicity and isopropyl alcohol poisoning. Urine dipstick detects acetone and acetoacetate but not β-hydroxybutyrate; therefore, in diabetic ketoacidosis and alcoholic ketoacidosis where β-hydroxybutyrate is the primary ketone, the dipstick underestimates ketone excretion. False-positive tests may occur with drugs containing sulfhydryl groups, such as captopril.

## Leukocyte Esterase and Nitrites

Leukocyte esterase is an enzyme present in leukocytes. A positive test suggests pyuria (≥5 leukocytes/hpf).

A positive nitrite test signifies the presence of gram-negative bacteria (*Escherichia coli*; *Klebsiella*, *Enterobacter*, *Citrobacter*, and *Proteus* species) capable of converting urine nitrates into nitrites. The test is falsely negative if there is inadequate contact time for urine nitrates with the bacteria. The nitrite test is negative in urinary tract infection (UTI) caused by nonconverting organisms (*Enterococcus*, *Staphylococcus*, *Streptococcus*, or *Haemophilus* species).

The presence of both leukocyte esterase and nitrites on urine dipstick is highly predictive of a UTI; conversely, the absence of both has a high negative predictive value for a UTI.

## Bilirubin

Bilirubin should be absent from the urine when serum levels are normal. Conjugated, water-soluble bilirubin is excreted in the urine in severe liver disease or obstructive hepatobiliary disease.

## Urobilinogen

Gut bacteria produce urobilinogen through metabolism of bilirubin. Urobilinogen is then absorbed via portal circulation and excreted in urine. Increased urobilinogen is associated with hemolytic anemia or parenchymal liver disease. Decreased levels are seen with severe cholestasis and obstructive disease.

### KEY POINTS

- Because moderately increased albuminuria (microalbuminuria) may go undetected by dipstick, direct quantification using a random (spot) protein-creatinine ratio or albumin-creatinine ratio or a 24-hour urine collection is required in high-risk patients.

- The urine nitrite test is negative in urinary tract infections caused by nonconverting organisms (*Enterococcus*, *Staphylococcus*, *Streptococcus*, or *Haemophilus* species).

- The presence of both leukocyte esterase and nitrites on **HVC** urine dipstick is highly predictive of a urinary tract infection (UTI); conversely, the absence of both has a high negative predictive value for a UTI.

## Urine Microscopy

Microscopic assessment of urine sediment (**Figure 2**) is indicated for patients with abnormalities on dipstick and in those with acute kidney injury, newly diagnosed chronic kidney disease, or suspected glomerulonephritis. See Table 2 for details on urine microscopy.

## Erythrocytes

Erythrocyte morphology may indicate their origin (see Figure 2). Isomorphic erythrocytes (round and of consistent size) suggest a nonglomerular origin as a result of infection, mass, cyst, or stone. Glomerular bleeding may be associated with erythrocyte fragmentation, leading to dysmorphic appearances with significant variability. Acanthocytes, a form of dysmorphic erythrocytes characterized by vesicle-shaped protrusions, are most suggestive of a glomerular source of bleeding and should result in prompt

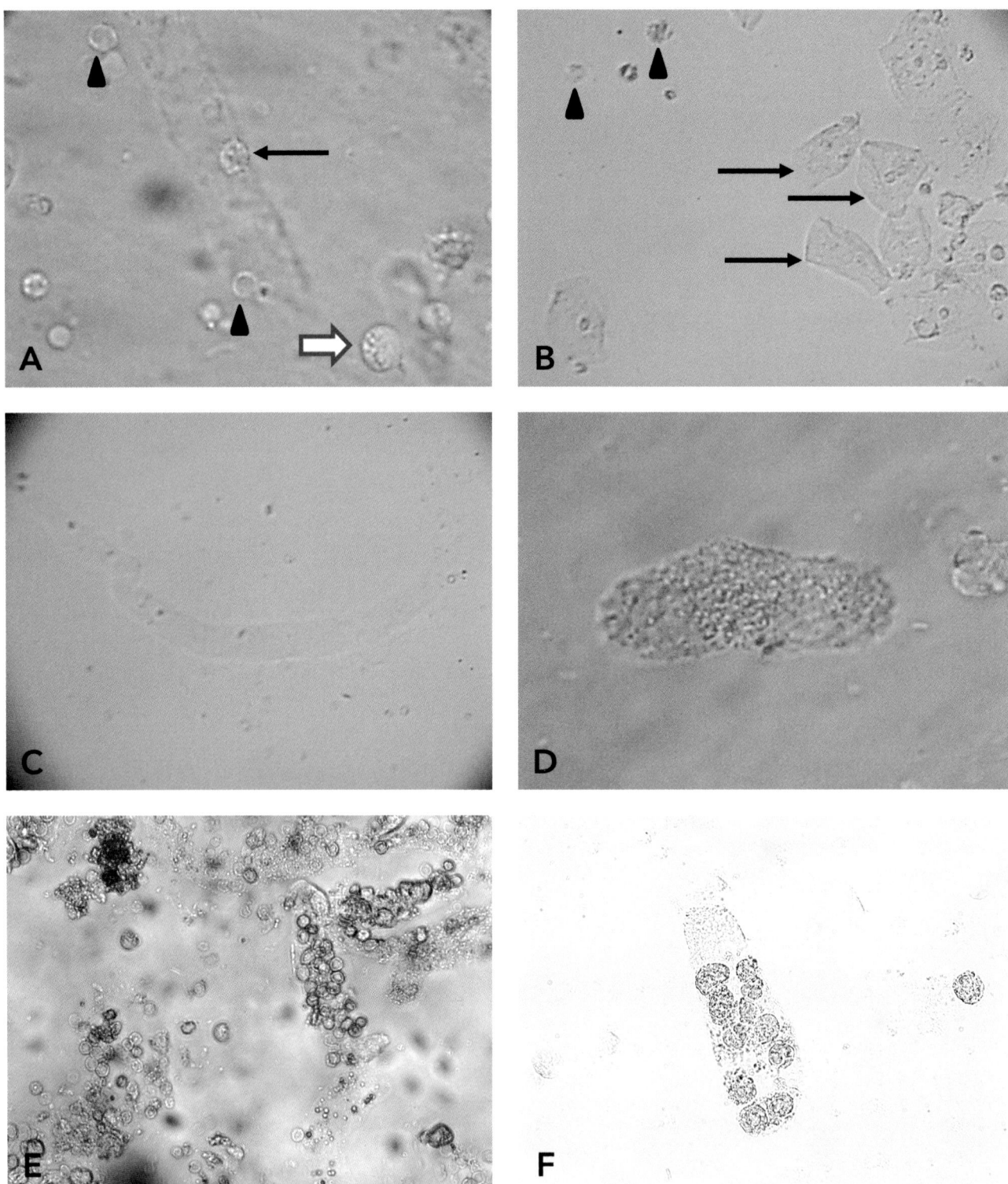

**FIGURE 2.** Findings on urine microscopy. **A**, Erythrocytes (*black arrowheads*). Also shown is a leukocyte (*black arrow*) embedded in a cast, as well as a tubular cell (*white arrow*). **B**, Leukocytes (*black arrowheads*): Note the large relative size of squamous epithelial cells (*black arrows*). **C**, Hyaline cast. **D**, Granular cast. **E**, Erythrocyte cast. **F**, Leukocyte cast.

evaluation for glomerulonephritis (**Figure 3**). See Clinical Evaluation of Hematuria for more information.

## Leukocytes

The presence of ≥5 leukocytes in the urine sediment indicates pyuria, which is most commonly caused by a UTI. Sterile pyuria is the presence of urine leukocytes in the setting of negative urine culture; common causes include vaginitis and cervicitis in women, prostatitis in men, acute interstitial nephritis (AIN), kidney stones, kidney transplant rejection, and, less commonly, UTIs due to organisms that do not grow by standard culture techniques (*Chlamydia* species, *Mycobacterium tuberculosis*, *Ureaplasma urealyticum*). The absence of leukocytes does not rule out AIN.

## Eosinophils

Urine eosinophils suggest interstitial nephritis, atheroembolic disease, glomerulonephritis, small-vessel vasculitis, UTI, prostatic disease, or parasitic infections. Poor sensitivity and specificity limit the utility of urine eosinophils in the diagnosis of interstitial nephritis.

## Epithelial Cells

Renal tubular, transitional, and squamous epithelial cells may be seen on urinalysis (see Figure 2). Renal tubular epithelial cells are round with central nuclei and are 1.5 to 3 times larger than leukocytes. Their presence in the context of granular casts suggests acute tubular necrosis. Transitional epithelial cells are slightly larger than renal tubular epithelial cells and may be binucleate; they originate anywhere from the renal pelvis to the proximal urethra. Squamous epithelial cells are the largest epithelial cells, and are flat and irregular with small central nuclei; they are derived from the distal urethra or external genitalia, and their presence in large numbers (>15/hpf) denotes contamination by genital secretions.

## Casts

The backbone of all urine casts is a matrix composed of Tamm-Horsfall protein (uromodulin). These cylindrical casts form in the distal tubular lumen. Any cells or debris in casts were present in the tubule at the time of cast formation, therefore originating from a more proximal part of the nephron. Erythrocyte casts are highly suggestive of glomerulonephritis. Leukocyte casts may be present in AIN and infections (pyelonephritis). Pigmented or granular (muddy brown) casts contain tubular cell debris (**Figure 4**) and are present in acute tubular necrosis. The severity of acute kidney injury correlates with the number of casts and presence of renal tubular epithelial cells.

## Crystals

Crystalluria results from the supersaturation of solutes in concentrated urine. These solutes are derived from metabolic disorders, inherited diseases, or drugs. **Table 3** describes features of common crystals. Certain drugs can crystallize in concentrated urine and when used in high doses, including sulfadiazine, sulfamethoxazole, intravenous acyclovir, methotrexate, and atazanavir.

### KEY POINTS

- Isomorphic erythrocytes suggest a nonglomerular origin of blood; dysmorphic erythrocytes, particularly acanthocytes, suggest a glomerular origin.

- Erythrocyte casts are highly suggestive of glomerulonephritis, leukocyte casts may be present in acute interstitial nephritis and infections, and granular (muddy brown) casts are present in acute tubular necrosis.

## Measurement of Albumin and Protein Excretion

Assessment for urine protein is indicated in patients with any suspected kidney disease. Concurrent increased serum creatinine or abnormal findings on urine sediment raise concern for active kidney disease in any patient with proteinuria.

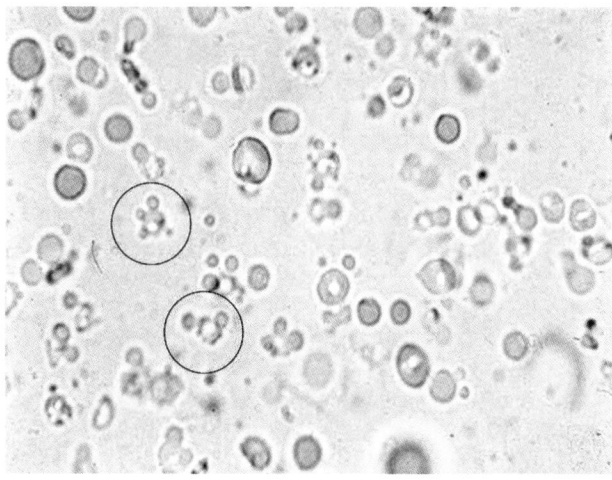

**FIGURE 3.** Urine microscopy demonstrating acanthocytes, indicated in the red circles. Acanthocytes, a form of dysmorphic erythrocytes characterized by vesicle-shaped protrusions, are most suggestive of glomerular bleeding.

Courtesy of J. Charles Jennette, MD.

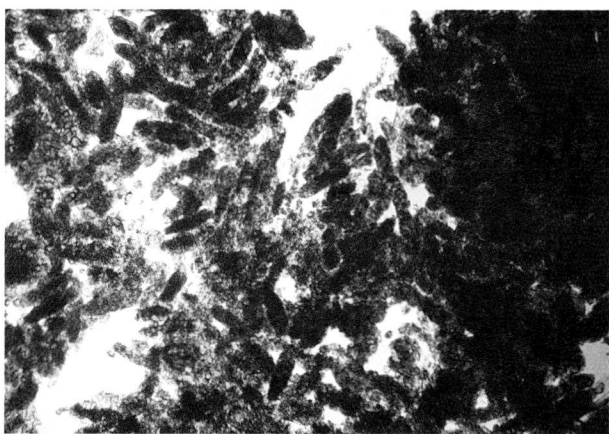

**FIGURE 4.** Tubular injury (for example, acute tubular necrosis) may lead to deposition of pigmented epithelial tubular debris in the proteinaceous matrix of the cast, with the formation of pigmented or granular (muddy brown) casts.

| Type | Morphology | Associated Conditions | Image |
|---|---|---|---|
| Calcium oxalate | Envelope; dumbbell; needle | Hypercalciuria; hyperoxaluria; ethylene glycol poisoning | |
| Calcium phosphate | Prism; needle; star-like clumps | Distal renal tubular acidosis; urine pH >6.5; tumor lysis syndrome; acute phosphate nephropathy | |
| Uric acid | Rhomboid; needle; rosette; barrels; hexagonal plates | Hyperuricemia; gout; diabetes mellitus; obesity; tumor lysis syndrome; urine pH <6.0 | |
| Struvite (magnesium ammonium phosphate) | Coffin-lid | Alkaline urine due to chronic urinary tract infection with urease-producing organisms | |
| Cystine | Hexagonal | Cystinuria | |

**TABLE 3. Urine Crystals**

Assays to detect protein in the urine include urine dipstick, random (spot) urine protein-creatinine ratio or albumin-creatinine ratio, and 24-hour urine collections. Due to the challenges of 24-hour urine collections, the random urine albumin-creatinine ratio and protein-creatinine ratio have been widely adopted. Both random tests adequately determine the presence of albuminuria, but the urine protein-creatinine ratio also detects nonalbumin proteins. Random collections correlate well with timed collections and are sufficiently accurate for screening and monitoring proteinuria despite inaccuracies due to diurnal fluctuations of urine protein and interindividual differences in urine creatinine excretion. **Table 4** outlines the definitions of proteinuria and albuminuria as well as normal values.

Urine albumin, when present at high levels, indicates glomerular injury; conversely, the absence of albuminuria essentially excludes most glomerular diseases. Smaller proteins are filtered at the level of the glomerulus but are reabsorbed by the proximal tubule; their presence in urine generally indicates

tubulointerstitial disease. Light chains present at high levels, such as in monoclonal gammopathy, are detected on urine protein electrophoresis or free light chain assay.

Transient, nonpathologic, usually small elevations in urine protein can occur with acute illness or fever, rigorous exercise, and pregnancy. Orthostatic proteinuria is a benign proteinuria that increases when the patient is upright but decreases when the patient is recumbent. This condition is more common in adolescents but should be considered in those up to age 30 years. Split urine collection (daytime versus nighttime collection that includes first morning void) can evaluate this diagnosis.

ACP recommends against screening for chronic kidney disease, including screening for proteinuria in asymptomatic adults without risk factors for chronic kidney disease, because there is no evidence of benefit from early treatment to outweigh the harms of screening, including false-positive results and unnecessary testing and treatment. However, screening

**TABLE 4.** Definitions of Proteinuria and Albuminuria

**Total Urine Protein**

| Urine Collection Method | Normal | Clinical Proteinuria | |
|---|---|---|---|
| 24-Hour Excretion | <150 mg/24 h | ≥150 mg/24 h | |
| Spot Urine Protein-Creatinine Ratio[a] | ≤150 mg/g ≈ ≤150 mg/24 h | >150 mg/g ≈ >150 mg/24 h | |

**Urine Albumin**

| Urine Collection Method | Normal[b] | Moderately Increased Albuminuria (Microalbuminuria)[b,c] | Severely Increased Albuminuria (Macroalbuminuria)[b,c] |
|---|---|---|---|
| 24-Hour Excretion | <30 mg/24 h | 30-300 mg/24 h | >300 mg/24 h |
| Conventional Spot Urine Dipstick[d] | Negative | Negative | Positive |
| Albumin-Specific Spot Urine Dipstick[e] | <3.0 mg/dL Negative | ≥3.0 mg/dL Positive | Positive |
| Spot Urine Albumin-Creatinine Ratio[a] | <30 mg/g ≈ <30 mg/24 h | 30-300 mg/g ≈ 30-300 mg/24 h | >300 mg/g ≈ >300 mg/24 h |

[a]Because of the difficulty of obtaining a 24-hour urine collection, urine protein-creatinine ratio or urine albumin-creatinine ratio on random (spot) urine samples is used to estimate 24-hour excretion. Measurement of either urine protein or albumin concentration in a sample is divided by the creatinine concentration of the same sample to derive a unitless value. These ratios correlate well with the 24-hour excretion of protein or albumin. Although these calculations are technically dimensionless, they may be expressed by different laboratories with their units of calculation, such as mg/g (mg protein or albumin/g creatinine) or with units to reflect the proportional 24-hour excretion amount (mg or g protein or albumin/g creatinine).

[b]Chronic kidney disease classification categories A1, A2, and A3 correspond to normal (or mildly increased), moderately increased, and severely increased albuminuria, respectively.

[c]The newer terminology of "moderately increased albuminuria" and "severely increased albuminuria" has been adopted due to the finding that even relatively low levels of urine protein have been associated with significant cardiovascular risk and risk of progression of underlying kidney disease.

[d]Conventional urine dipsticks are more sensitive for detection of albumin than non-albumin proteins; the detection limit is approximately 30 mg/dL, although they are not highly accurate for determining the degree of albuminuria if present.

[e]Urine dipsticks designed specifically to detect small amounts of albuminuria. Similar to conventional urine dipsticks, these dipsticks detect albumin above a concentration threshold but are sensitive to the presence of albumin at lower levels and can be used to indicate the presence of moderately increased albuminuria.

for proteinuria may be considered in high-risk patients, such as hypertensive, diabetic, and older patients.

In patients with diabetes mellitus, urine albumin screening is recommended due to its ability to detect early disease. The American Diabetes Association recommends yearly assessment in patients with type 2 diabetes, and assessment after 5 years of disease in patients with type 1 diabetes. Because there is no evidence that monitoring proteinuria levels in patients taking ACE inhibitors or angiotensin receptor blockers is beneficial or that reduced proteinuria levels translate into improved outcomes, ACP recommends against testing for proteinuria in adults with or without diabetes who are currently taking an ACE inhibitor or an angiotensin receptor blocker.

Urine protein electrophoresis can characterize proteins, allowing for classification of the proteinuria as glomerular or tubular. It also detects monoclonal gammopathy, although it is less sensitive than light chain assay.

**KEY POINTS**

HVC
- The random (spot) urine protein-creatinine ratio and albumin-creatinine ratio correlate with 24-hour urine collections and are sufficiently accurate for screening and monitoring proteinuria.

- High urine albumin levels indicate glomerular injury; the absence of albuminuria excludes most glomerular diseases.

## Clinical Evaluation of Hematuria

Hematuria is defined as the presence of ≥3 erythrocytes/hpf in the urine sediment and may be microscopic (detectable only on urine testing) or macroscopic (grossly visible). Hematuria is most often of nonglomerular origin. A glomerular origin is suggested by concurrent proteinuria, presence of dysmorphic erythrocytes, increased serum creatinine or decrease in estimated GFR (eGFR), or systemic signs and symptoms. Evaluation of hematuria is outlined in **Figure 5**.

Urinalysis should not be used for cancer screening in asymptomatic adults. However, a single incidental finding of hematuria is sufficient to warrant further investigation. Evaluation should be pursued even in patients with bleeding diatheses or those taking antiplatelet or anticoagulation therapy. If menstruation, viral illness, vigorous exercise, or some other benign cause is suspected, urinalysis should be repeated after the cause is resolved. If infection is confirmed, urinalysis should be repeated after treatment to document resolution of hematuria.

In a patient with asymptomatic microscopic hematuria, it is important to assess kidney function, erythrocyte morphology, and urine protein to evaluate for a nephrologic cause, particularly glomerulonephritis. The absence of proteinuria generally rules out a glomerular process; exceptions include very mild glomerular disease (most often IgA nephropathy) or thin glomerular basement membrane disease related to a type

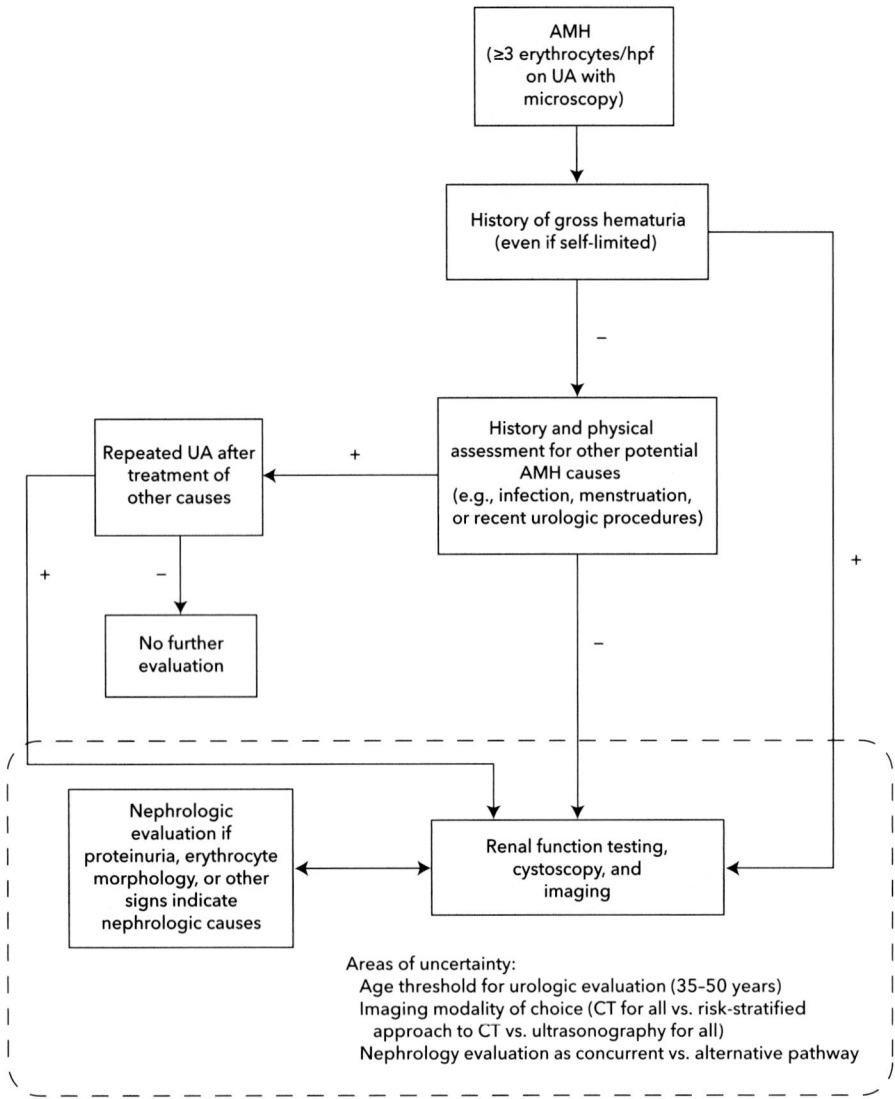

**FIGURE 5.** Summary of the American College of Physicians recommendations for the evaluation of patients with hematuria. AMH = asymptomatic microscopic hematuria; UA = urinalysis.

IV collagen defect that may present as isolated hematuria. Systemic signs and symptoms raise suspicion for nephrologic disease, particularly those associated with rheumatologic disorders and rapidly progressive glomerulonephritis.

Macroscopic hematuria should prompt urology referral even if self-limited, with further evaluation of nephrologic disease and malignancy as indicated.

If a nephrologic cause of hematuria is not suggested, hematuria may indicate a malignancy. The American Urological Association (AUA) guidelines recommend that patients older than 35 years or those with risk factors for malignancy undergo evaluation for malignancy. Although CT urography (contrast CT with kidney-specific imaging) has the highest sensitivity and specificity for renal malignancy, noncontrast helical CT is more appropriate if a kidney stone is suspected. Ultrasonography is a reasonable first imaging step because of availability, lower cost, and no ionizing radiation. MRI with contrast is useful when CT contrast studies cannot be performed. Cystoscopy is indicated when imaging is negative. ACP and the AUA recommend against obtaining urine cytology in the initial evaluation of hematuria. ☐

### KEY POINTS

- Urinalysis should not be used for detection of bladder cancer in asymptomatic patients.  **HVC**

- Hematuria requires thorough evaluation because of potentially life-threatening causes, such as rapidly progressive glomerulonephritis and urinary tract malignancy.

- Evaluation of nonglomerular hematuria in patients older than 35 years or those with risk factors for urologic malignancy includes CT urography unless contraindicated; if imaging is negative, cystoscopy should be performed.

## Imaging Studies

Ultrasonography is the most commonly used kidney imaging modality. It is easily available, safe, and relatively inexpensive. Ultrasonography can demonstrate hydronephrosis, kidney size and cortical thickness, echogenicity, and presence of cysts and tumors. Absence of hydronephrosis quickly rules out obstruction in most cases. Echogenicity is the ability of a tissue to "bounce back" or return the ultrasound signal and is recognized as brighter shades on the sonogram image. Echogenicity is nonspecific but implies acute or chronic parenchymal disease. Additionally, ultrasonography can measure pre- and postvoid bladder residual, for evaluation of bladder dysfunction or outlet obstruction. Ultrasonography is also useful for uncomplicated nephrolithiasis; a positive ultrasound may be adequate for initial diagnosis. Ultrasonography is less useful in evaluating diseases (including stones) of the mid or distal ureter. Doppler ultrasonography may detect renal artery stenosis or renal vein thrombosis, but is highly user dependent.

CT is appropriate for patients with a nondiagnostic ultrasound or a more complicated presentation. Noncontrast helical CT is the gold standard for diagnosis of nephrolithiasis, and is appropriate for evaluating renal colic. Most stones can be detected, including small stones and those in the distal ureter not detected on ultrasound. It may provide information regarding stone composition and, because the entire urinary tract and abdomen is visualized, alternative diagnoses may be suggested.

CT urography (contrast-enhanced kidney-specific CT) is the test of choice for patients with unexplained hematuria and allows characterization of renal tumors and cysts. CT with contrast is valuable for imaging the renal vasculature. The use of contrast confers risk for contrast-induced nephropathy, particularly in patients with an eGFR <50 mL/min/1.73 m².

MRI with contrast is an alternative for evaluation of renal masses and cysts when CT cannot be performed. MR angiography for detection of renal artery stenosis, and venography for detection of renal vein thrombosis, can be performed with or without gadolinium-based contrast, although contrast provides optimal imaging. MR angiography and CT angiography have mostly replaced standard angiography of renal arteries. Due to concerns for nephrogenic systemic fibrosis (NSF), gadolinium contrast must be avoided in patients with an eGFR <30 mL/min/1.73 m². In life-threatening situations in which benefit outweighs the risk for NSF, MRI is performed with low doses of stable gadolinium agents. See MKSAP 18 Dermatology for more information on NSF.

Radionuclide imaging provides the most accurate measurement of GFR and is the gold standard in research (see Estimation of Glomerular Filtration Rate).

**KEY POINTS**

HVC
- Ultrasonography is the most commonly used imaging modality in the evaluation of the kidneys and upper urinary tract because of its safety, cost effectiveness, and availability.
- CT urography is the test of choice for patients with unexplained hematuria and allows characterization of renal tumors and cysts; noncontrast helical CT is the gold standard for diagnosis of nephrolithiasis, and CT with contrast is valuable in imaging the renal vasculature.

## Kidney Biopsy

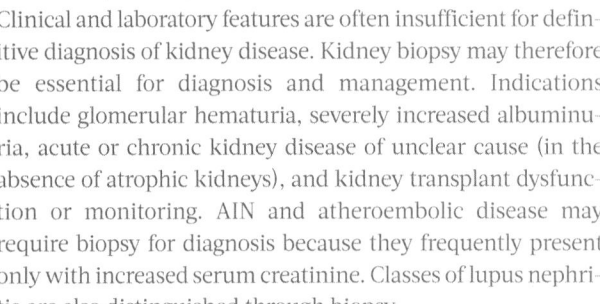

Clinical and laboratory features are often insufficient for definitive diagnosis of kidney disease. Kidney biopsy may therefore be essential for diagnosis and management. Indications include glomerular hematuria, severely increased albuminuria, acute or chronic kidney disease of unclear cause (in the absence of atrophic kidneys), and kidney transplant dysfunction or monitoring. AIN and atheroembolic disease may require biopsy for diagnosis because they frequently present only with increased serum creatinine. Classes of lupus nephritis are also distinguished through biopsy.

Percutaneous kidney biopsy with ultrasonography or CT guidance is most common. Open or laparoscopic surgical biopsy is performed when percutaneous biopsy is not possible. Contraindications to percutaneous biopsy include the uncooperative patient, bleeding diatheses (including antiplatelet use or anticoagulation), uncontrolled hypertension, poor kidney visualization, atrophic kidneys, and active UTI. Solitary kidney and pregnancy require weighing of risks and benefits.

The most common risks of biopsy are bleeding and injury to surrounding organs. The most common major complications (occurring in <3% of cases) are need for transfusion or angiography with or without embolization, as well as hemodynamic instability. Minor complications include pain and hematuria. Kidney loss and death are very rare complications.

**KEY POINT**

- Indications for kidney biopsy include glomerular hematuria, severely increased albuminuria, kidney disease of unclear cause, and kidney transplant dysfunction or monitoring.

# Fluids and Electrolytes
## Osmolality and Tonicity

The osmolality of a solution is determined by the number of solutes per kilogram. In serum or plasma, osmolality can be measured by freezing point depression or calculated using the following formula:

$$2 \times [Na^+] + Glucose\ (mg/dL)/18 + Blood\ Urea\ Nitrogen\ (mg/dL)/2.8 + Ethanol\ if\ present\ (mg/dL)/4.6$$

$$If\ using\ international\ units: 2 \times [Na^+] + Urea\ (mmol/L) + Glucose\ (mmol/L) + Ethanol\ (mmol/L)$$

Normal serum osmolality is between 275 and 295 mOsm/kg H₂O. The difference between measured osmolality and calculated osmolality (the osmolal gap) should be <10 mOsm/kg H₂O. A greater value suggests the presence of a low-molecular-weight alcohol. Because water moves freely between the intracellular and extracellular spaces based on the osmotic gradient, the osmolality of both compartments is virtually identical.

Tonicity is effective osmolality due to solutes that are not freely permeable across the cell membrane. Differences in tonicity determine the distribution of water between body compartments. The major solute determining plasma tonicity is sodium. Because urea and ethanol are freely permeable across the cell membrane, they do not contribute to tonicity or the movement of water.

Osmolality is tightly controlled within a narrow range by thirst and antidiuretic hormone (ADH; also known as vasopressin). ADH stimulates reabsorption of water in the collecting duct of the kidney. Increases in tonicity stimulate both thirst and ADH. As long as there is access to water, appropriate thirst, normal control of ADH, and a functioning nephron, serum osmolality should be maintained in the normal range. Disorders of osmolality reflect impaired water homeostasis. Because the body will defend volume status over tonicity, volume depletion (a decrease in total body sodium content) will stimulate ADH such that at any given osmolality, volume depletion will result in an exaggerated ADH response.

# Disorders of Serum Sodium

## Hyponatremia

Hyponatremia is defined as a serum sodium concentration <135 mEq/L (135 mmol/L). Evaluation begins with measurement of serum osmolality. Hyponatremia is then identified as hypertonic (osmolality >295 mOsm/kg $H_2O$), isotonic (osmolality 275-295 mOsm/kg $H_2O$), or hypotonic (osmolality <275 mOsm/kg $H_2O$) (**Figure 6**).

### Evaluation

Symptoms caused by hyponatremia depend on both the rapidity and degree of decline in serum sodium. Acute hyponatremia in <48 hours provides inadequate time for the brain to adapt. A sudden drop in serum sodium causes water to move into the brain, producing cerebral edema and possible headaches, seizures, or death. More chronic declines that allow cells to regulate their volume by decreasing intracellular electrolytes may be asymptomatic.

### Hypertonic Hyponatremia

Hypertonic hyponatremia (osmolality >295 mOsm/kg $H_2O$) results from an increased concentration of effective osmotic solute (typically glucose). The increase in osmolality pulls water out of cells, diluting the sodium. For every 100 mg/dL (5.6 mmol/L) increase in glucose, serum sodium decreases by 1.6 to 2.2 mEq/L (1.6-2.2 mmol/L).

### Isotonic (Pseudo) Hyponatremia

Isotonic (pseudo) hyponatremia (osmolality 275-295 mOsm/kg $H_2O$) is a laboratory artifact. Normally, plasma is 93% water (in which solutes are dissolved) and 7% solids (proteins and lipids). The normal sodium concentration in the water phase is 154 mEq/L (154 mmol/L) (hence, normal saline has a sodium concentration of 154 mEq/L [154 mmol/L]). The lower normal value (around 140 mEq/L [140 mmol/L]) is approximately 7% less because electrolytes are reported as a concentration per liter of plasma/serum. Conditions such as severe hypertriglyceridemia or multiple myeloma that increase the solid phase decrease the sodium concentration in plasma.

### Hypotonic Hyponatremia

Hypotonic hyponatremia (osmolality <275 mOsm/kg $H_2O$) reflects excess water for the sodium present and is further categorized by volume status into hypovolemic, hypervolemic, or isovolemic.

In hypovolemic hypotonic hyponatremia, renal sodium and water reabsorption are stimulated by sympathetic outflow, angiotensin, aldosterone, and ADH, leading to urine sodium concentration <20 mEq/L (20 mmol/L) and urine osmolality

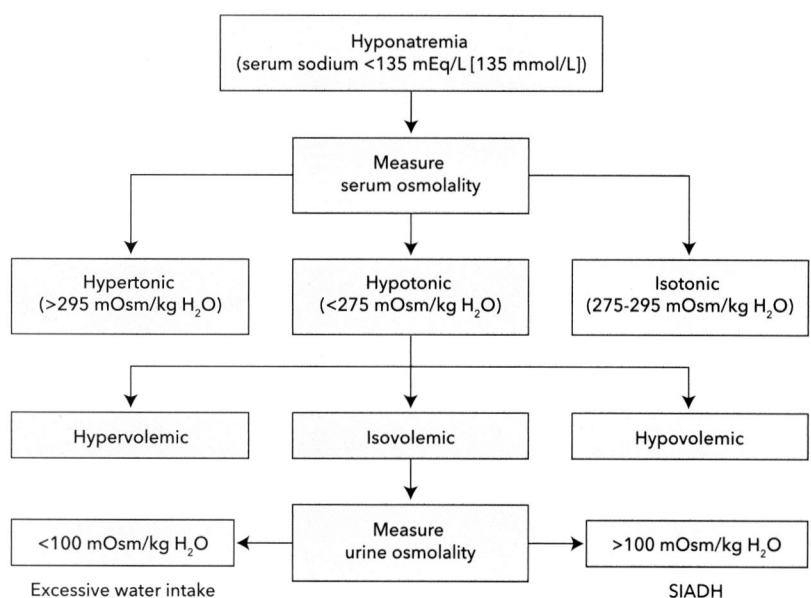

**FIGURE 6.** Evaluation of hyponatremia. SIADH = syndrome of inappropriate antidiuretic hormone secretion.

CONT.

>300 mOsm/kg $H_2O$ (except if taking diuretics). Common causes of volume depletion include gastrointestinal losses, excessive sweating, or renal salt wasting from diuretics.

In hypervolemic hypotonic hyponatremia resulting from heart failure or cirrhosis, effective circulating blood volume is inadequate despite total volume overload, resulting in similar urine chemistries.

Isovolemic hypotonic hyponatremia is secondary either to impaired dilution of urine or to water intake that exceeds the kidney's ability to excrete dilute urine. Urine osmolality distinguishes between these two entities. Urine osmolality <100 mOsm/kg $H_2O$ indicates excessive water intake, as seen with psychogenic polydipsia or poor solute intake. Because the kidney cannot excrete pure water, a minimal solute concentration of 50 mOsm/kg $H_2O$ is required. If solute intake is low while liquid intake remains high (as seen in beer potomania or chronic low food intake), water excretion is limited by available urinary solute.

Isovolemic hypotonic hyponatremia with urine osmolality >100 mOsm/kg $H_2O$ can occur in patients with late-stage chronic kidney disease because of impairment of urine dilution, causing hyponatremia after excessive dietary fluid intake. Urine osmolality >100 mOsm/kg $H_2O$ also occurs in isovolemic hypotonic hyponatremia due to the syndrome of inappropriate antidiuretic hormone secretion (SIADH) (**Table 5**). Medications are the most common cause of SIADH, with antidepressants and thiazide diuretics being the most common. 3,4-Methylenedioxymethamphetamine (ecstasy) is increasingly recognized as a cause of hyponatremia. This drug stimulates ADH and, because of the frequently associated fever and dry mouth, induces thirst. Hyponatremia has also been reported in inexperienced marathon runners who overhydrate. Of note, hyponatremia associated with thiazide diuretics, ecstasy, or extreme exertion occurs more frequently in women. A frequent finding in SIADH is a low serum urate level (<4.0 mg/dL [0.24 mmol/L]). Cortisol and thyroid hormone are required to suppress ADH; therefore, deficiencies of these hormones should be evaluated.

## Management

Treatment of hypotonic hyponatremia is determined by the underlying pathogenesis. In patients with volume overload, treatment is targeted to the underlying disease process along with water restriction. In hypovolemia, volume expansion with isotonic saline will suppress ADH, thereby increasing water excretion with correction of the hyponatremia.

Treatment of isovolemic hypotonic hyponatremia is determined by the severity of symptoms and the rapidity of the decline.

Symptomatic patients with isovolemic hypotonic hyponatremia and an acute decrease in serum sodium should be treated with a 100-mL bolus of 3% saline to increase the serum sodium by 2.0 to 3.0 mEq/L (2.0-3.0 mmol/L). This is usually adequate to decrease cerebral edema and relieve symptoms. If symptoms persist, the bolus can be repeated once or twice at

| TABLE 5. | Causes of the Syndrome of Inappropriate Antidiuretic Hormone Secretion |
|---|---|
| **Cause** | **Examples** |
| Drugs[a] | Thiazide diuretics |
| | Selective serotonin reuptake inhibitors |
| | Phenothiazines |
| | Haloperidol |
| | Clofibrate |
| | Carbamazepine |
| | Cyclophosphamide |
| | Tricyclic antidepressants |
| | Valproic acid |
| | Bromocriptine |
| | 3,4-Methylenedioxymethamphetamine (ecstasy) |
| Malignancy | Small cell carcinoma |
| | Squamous cell carcinoma of the head and neck |
| Central nervous system disease | — |
| Pulmonary disease | — |
| Endocrine disorders | Glucocorticoid deficiency |
| | Myxedema |
| Idiopathic | — |
| Endurance exercise (marathon running) | — |

[a]Drugs are the most common cause.

10-minute intervals as long as the serum sodium can be measured. If the acute decline in sodium is secondary to excess water intake, fluid restriction will rapidly correct the hyponatremia. Because it is often not possible to determine the acuity of the hyponatremia, some authorities recommend limiting the sodium increase in this population by using either hypotonic solutions or desmopressin.

In isovolemic hypotonic hyponatremia with a more chronic (>48 hours) decline in serum sodium, overly aggressive treatment can result in neuronal damage and osmotic demyelination. The serum sodium should not be increased >8.0 to 10 mEq/L (8.0-10 mmol/L) in 24 hours. If there is significant neurologic impairment (for example, seizures or coma), sodium can be acutely increased 2.0 to 4.0 mEq/L (2.0-4.0 mmol/L) using a bolus of 3% saline as long as the total increase remains ≤10 mEq/L (10 mmol/L) in 24 hours. Administration of potassium will also increase plasma sodium because it enters cells, increasing intracellular osmolality and causing water to move from the extracellular space into the intracellular space, thus raising the plasma sodium concentration.

In patients with asymptomatic isovolemic hypotonic hyponatremia or with only mild to moderate symptoms (headache, lethargy), water restriction is safe and effective.

CONT.

However, limiting fluid intake to <800 mL/24 h is often intolerable. If water restriction is not adequate, therapy is targeted at blocking ADH activity or increasing water excretion. Demeclocycline inhibits ADH action and can be used chronically but is frequently associated with photosensitivity and gastrointestinal symptoms. Tolvaptan, an ADH antagonist, is effective and usually well tolerated, but it is cost-prohibitive and its use is limited to 1 month because of potential liver toxicity. Loop diuretics can be used adjunctively to limit urine concentration, along with increased oral sodium intake. Oral urea, 15 to 30 g/d, is also effective in increasing water excretion, although its use is often limited by unpalatable taste. ▣

### KEY POINTS

- Hyponatremia is divided into three categories: hypertonic (osmolality >295 mOsm/kg $H_2O$), isotonic (osmolality 275-295 mOsm/kg $H_2O$), or hypotonic (osmolality <275 mOsm/kg $H_2O$); hypotonic hyponatremia is further categorized by volume status (hypovolemic, hypervolemic, or isovolemic).

- Treatment of acute symptomatic isovolemic hypotonic hyponatremia consists of a 100-mL bolus of 3% saline; if the acute decline in serum sodium is secondary to excess water intake, fluid restriction will rapidly correct the hyponatremia.

- Overly aggressive treatment of chronic isovolemic hypotonic hyponatremia can result in neuronal damage and osmotic demyelination; therefore, serum sodium should not be increased >8.0 to 10 mEq/L (8.0-10 mmol/L) in 24 hours.

## ▣ Hypernatremia

Hypernatremia is defined as a serum sodium concentration >145 mEq/L (145 mmol/L). Although less common than hyponatremia, hypernatremia is often seen in hospitalized patients and is associated with increased mortality in the critically ill.

Hypernatremia can be divided into three broad categories: inappropriate intake/administration of hypertonic solutions; loss of hypotonic fluids; and excessive water loss due to defects in ADH release or action. A detailed history and physical examination combined with measurement of urine electrolytes and osmolality help distinguish the pathogenesis of hypernatremia.

### Evaluation

The most common cause of hypernatremia is loss of hypotonic body fluids with inadequate water replacement because of lack of access or absence of thirst (adipsia). Hypotonic losses may result from diarrhea, the respiratory tract, excessive sweating, or renal losses from osmotic diuresis (such as with glucosuria). If the losses are nonrenal, urine osmolality will be elevated to >600 mOsm/kg $H_2O$. In osmotic diuresis, urine osmolality is usually between 300 and 600 mOsm/kg $H_2O$. Hypotonic losses

with inadequate replacement result in intravascular volume depletion with orthostasis or frank hypotension.

Hypertonic hypernatremia can also occur with administration of excessive quantities of hypertonic saline or sodium bicarbonate, or with salt ingestion. The acute increase in sodium causes water to move out of cells, causing shrinkage and neurologic findings. Symptoms can range from lethargy to seizures and coma. Physical examination frequently reveals intravascular volume overload with elevated jugular venous pressure and pulmonary crackles.

Less commonly, hypernatremia may be secondary to either an inadequate release (central diabetes insipidus) or action of ADH (nephrogenic diabetes insipidus). Common symptoms are polydipsia and polyuria. Urine osmolality <300 mOsm/kg $H_2O$ in a hypernatremic patient confirms the diagnosis. An increase in urine osmolality after a dose of desmopressin (ADH analogue) distinguishes between central and nephrogenic diabetes insipidus. Because solute loss is not excessive, hypernatremia from water loss is usually associated with minimal symptoms unless the sodium increases acutely.

### Management

Management of hypernatremia is determined by the underlying pathogenesis. When secondary to acute hypertonic gains, treatment of hypernatremia needs to rapidly restore normal sodium concentration. Water can be administered as 5% dextrose, along with intravenous loop diuretics, to abrogate the volume overload. If available, hemodialysis can be considered.

If hypernatremia has occurred over >24 hours, the brain adapts by uptake of electrolytes and other osmotically active solutes. Therefore, to prevent cerebral edema during water infusion, the correction should be <10 mEq/L/24 h (10 mmol/L/d). The change in the serum sodium for each liter of infusate can be calculated using the formula:

(Infusate Sodium) – (Serum Sodium) ÷ (Total Body Water + 1)

If possible, water should be administered orally or by means of a nasogastric tube. Because dextrose-containing solutions may cause glycosuria and increased free water losses, it is important to monitor serum glucose and maintain it below 180 mg/dL (10 mmol/L). In the presence of hemodynamic compromise due to intravascular volume depletion, replacement fluid should be isotonic saline; otherwise, a hypotonic solution (half [0.45%] or quarter [0.22%] normal saline) can be used.

In patients with diabetes insipidus, the first step is determining whether the defect is secondary to a defect in ADH secretion or an ADH action. Central diabetes insipidus can be treated with intranasal or oral desmopressin, a synthetic analogue of vasopressin. Nephrogenic diabetes insipidus is more difficult to treat. Therapy is aimed at limited solute intake to decrease the amount of free water that the kidney can excrete and induction of mild volume depletion using a thiazide diuretic to increase salt and water reabsorption proximal to the collecting duct. ▣

- The most common cause of hypernatremia is loss of hypotonic body fluids with inadequate water replacement because of lack of access or adipsia.

- Treatment of hypernatremia secondary to acute hypertonic gains is aggressive, with rapid restoration of normal sodium concentration

- If hypernatremia has occurred over >24 hours, correction should be <10 mEq/L/24 h (10 mmol/L/d) to prevent cerebral edema.

# Disorders of Serum Potassium

## Hypokalemia

Hypokalemia is defined as a serum potassium level <3.5 mEq/L (3.5 mmol/L). It can be divided into disorders of internal balance (movement of potassium between the intracellular and extracellular compartments) and disorders of external balance (potassium intake and output) (**Figure 7**). Serum potassium >3.0 mEq/L (3.0 mmol/L) is usually asymptomatic. Because the ratio of intracellular to extracellular potassium is the major determinant of the membrane potential of electrically active tissue, symptoms of hypokalemia include weakness or paralysis, decreased gastrointestinal motility or ileus with nausea, and cardiac arrhythmias. Electrocardiographic (ECG) manifestations include ST-segment depression, decreased T-wave amplitude, and increased U-wave amplitude. Severe hypokalemia can cause rhabdomyolysis.

## Evaluation

The cause of hypokalemia can usually be determined from the history and simple laboratory evaluation. Rarely, hypokalemia is spurious, as can occur in leukemia when delayed sample processing allows large numbers of metabolically active leukocytes to take up potassium. In addition to leukocytosis, a clue to pseudohypokalemia is the lack of signs and symptoms associated with hypokalemia.

Hypokalemia can occur secondary to disordered internal balance. Insulin or $\beta_2$-agonists shift potassium into cells, causing an acute, transient, and modest hypokalemia that is usually asymptomatic. Ingestion of soluble barium or cesium salts, which block potassium exit from cells, can produce severely symptomatic hypokalemia with levels below 2.0 mEq/L (2.0 mmol/L). Increased cell production after repletion of vitamin $B_{12}$ or folate in deficient individuals can also cause hypokalemia. Hypokalemic periodic paralysis, either an inherited autosomal dominant disorder or an acquired disorder seen in hyperthyroid patients usually of Japanese descent, may present with severe muscle weakness and paralysis.

Most cases of hypokalemia are due to disordered external balance with total body potassium depletion, secondary either to lack of potassium intake or to increased potassium excretion. Because the kidney can almost cease potassium excretion, only a severely compromised diet can cause hypokalemia. The major determinants of renal potassium secretion are distal tubular flow rate and aldosterone, both of which increase sodium reabsorption, increasing the electronegativity of the tubule lumen and promoting potassium secretion.

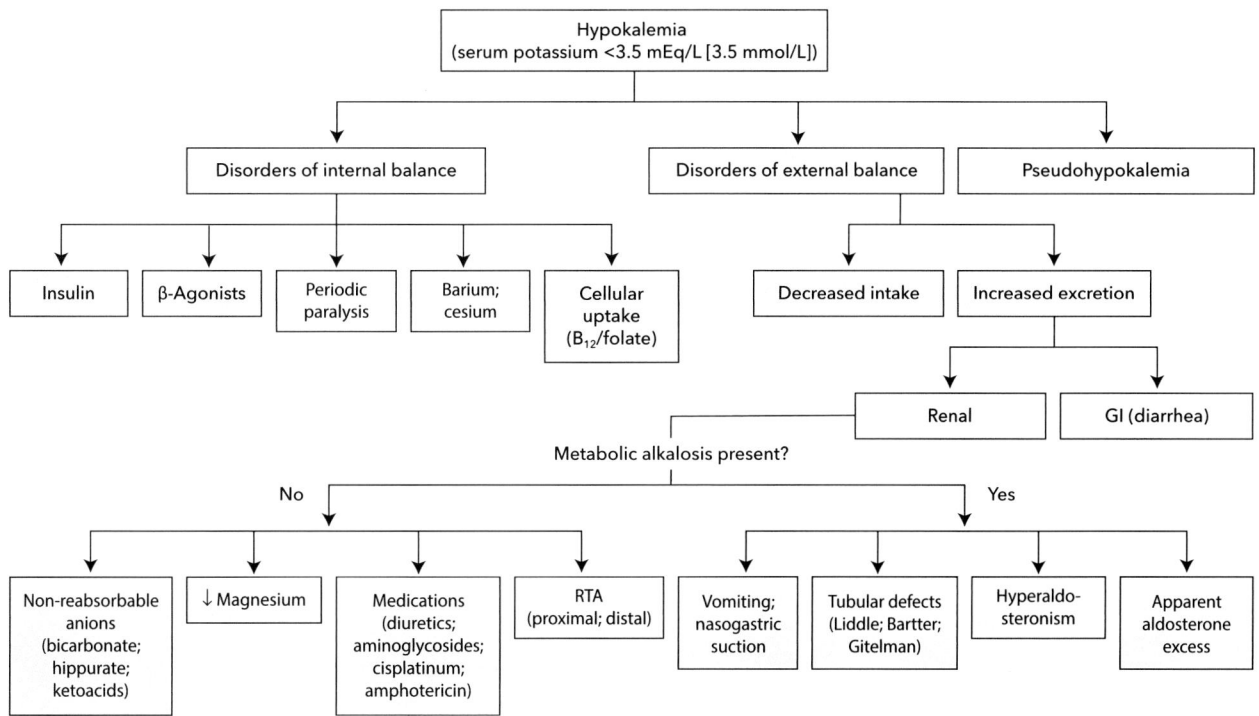

**FIGURE 7.** Causes of hypokalemia. GI = gastrointestinal; RTA = renal tubular acidosis.

CONT.

Under normal conditions, distal flow and aldosterone levels are inversely related, thus preventing disruptions in potassium homeostasis by changes in intravascular volume.

The gold standard to distinguish between renal and extra-renal causes of total body potassium depletion is a 24-hour urine potassium <30 mEq/24 h (30 mmol/d); however, this test is often impractical. The preferred alternative is a spot urine potassium-creatinine ratio. A value <13 mEq/g identifies hypokalemia secondary to lack of intake, transcellular shifts, or gastrointestinal losses.

Gastrointestinal losses are usually caused by diarrhea or laxative abuse. Frequently, a concomitant metabolic acidosis is present. Renal potassium wasting may be caused by numerous disorders, including medications (most commonly diuretics), delivery of non-reabsorbable anions to the distal tubule (such as bicarbonate), aldosterone excess, hypomagnesemia, and tubular defects (see Figure 7).

Hyperaldosteronism is associated with hypertension and a metabolic alkalosis. Hypomagnesemia can cause potassium wasting, and renal potassium wasting also occurs in inherited tubular defects, including Liddle, Bartter, and Gitelman syndromes. In Liddle syndrome, increased sodium reabsorption in the distal nephron causes hypertension, metabolic alkalosis, and potassium wasting. Bartter and Gitelman syndromes are caused by mutations in transporters that mimic the effects of diuretics on the tubule. Finally, proximal and distal renal tubular acidosis is associated with potassium wasting.

### Management

The total body potassium deficit is difficult to predict and can be up to 200 mEq (200 mmol) for each mEq/L decrease in plasma potassium. In patients with neuromuscular or cardiac symptoms, it is important to increase the potassium promptly. Intravenous potassium can be safely infused at 20 mEq/h (20 mmol/h). Infusion through a central vein can be increased to 40 mEq/h (40 mmol/h) with close monitoring. For mild hypokalemia (2.5-3.5 mEq/L [2.5-3.5 mmol/L]), oral supplementation using potassium chloride or potassium bicarbonate is usually adequate. Concurrent hypomagnesemia must be corrected to prevent ongoing potassium losses. In patients with potassium wasting, potassium-sparing diuretics can be helpful. When significant hypokalemia is secondary to acute transcellular shifts, total body potassium is normal and excessive potassium replacement may cause rebound hyperkalemia.

### KEY POINTS

- Symptoms of hypokalemia include weakness or paralysis, decreased gastrointestinal motility or ileus with nausea, and cardiac arrhythmias; electrocardiographic manifestations include ST-segment depression, decreased T-wave amplitude, and increased U-wave amplitude.

- In patients with hypokalemia and neuromuscular or cardiac symptoms, intravenous potassium (20 mEq/h [20 mmol/h]) can be used to increase the potassium promptly; oral supplementation is usually adequate for mild cases.

## Hyperkalemia

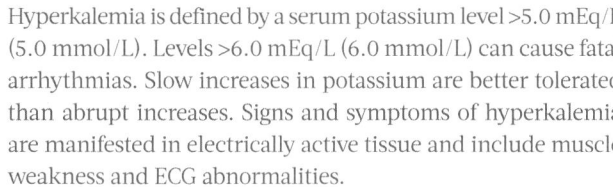

Hyperkalemia is defined by a serum potassium level >5.0 mEq/L (5.0 mmol/L). Levels >6.0 mEq/L (6.0 mmol/L) can cause fatal arrhythmias. Slow increases in potassium are better tolerated than abrupt increases. Signs and symptoms of hyperkalemia are manifested in electrically active tissue and include muscle weakness and ECG abnormalities.

### Evaluation

Initial evaluation of hyperkalemia requires a history and physical examination, review of all medications, assessment of kidney function, and an ECG. Initial ECG manifestations include peaked precordial T waves and a shortened QT interval. With progression of hyperkalemia, lengthening of the PR interval, loss of the P wave, widening of the QRS complex, a sine wave pattern, and asystole may occur (**Figure 8**). However, ECG findings do not always correlate with the serum potassium level and do not necessarily progress in an orderly fashion.

During the clotting process, cells are disrupted with the release of intracellular potassium, and pseudohyperkalemia may occur in serum specimens when there are extreme elevations of leukocytes or platelets. In these cases, repeating a plasma specimen will be normal. A tight tourniquet or excessively clenched fist during blood draw can also cause local potassium release.

Hyperkalemia may be caused by transcellular shifts, as occur in states of insulin deficiency or hypertonicity or with the use of β$_2$-adrenergic blockers. Rapid breakdown of cells such as that seen in rhabdomyolysis or in tumor lysis from treatment of leukemias and lymphomas can acutely raise serum potassium levels.

Hyperkalemia usually results from increased intake with decreased renal excretion. Hyperkalemia frequently occurs with

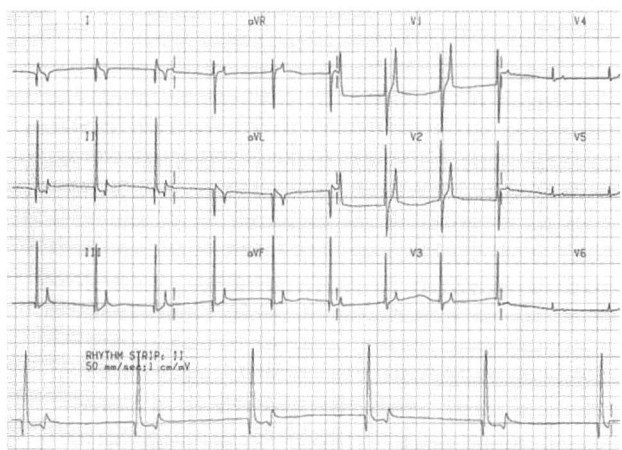

**FIGURE 8.** This electrocardiogram demonstrates tall, peaked T waves and decreased P waves, which are characteristic of hyperkalemia. T-wave peaking begins with mild to moderate elevations of serum potassium (5.5-7.0 mEq/L [5.5-7.0 mmol/L]) and tends to persist with more severe hyperkalemia. As serum potassium levels increase to above 7.0 to 8.0 mEq/L (7.0-8.0 mmol/L), decreases in P-wave amplitude and widening of the QRS complex are seen. With serum potassium levels above 9.0 to 10.0 mEq/L (9.0-10.0 mmol/L), the waveform will become sinusoidal, and cardiac arrest may follow.

CONT.

oliguric acute or chronic kidney disease with a glomerular filtration rate (GFR) <20 mL/min/1.73 m². Potassium-sparing diuretics (amiloride, triamterene, spironolactone) also commonly cause hyperkalemia through decreased excretion. Other medications that decrease potassium excretion include trimethoprim and pentamidine (by blocking the epithelial sodium channel) and NSAIDs (by decreasing renin). Hypoaldosteronism caused by inhibitors of the renin-angiotensin system, heparin, type 4 renal tubular acidosis (often seen in early diabetic nephropathy), or primary adrenal insufficiency also cause hyperkalemia, especially in the presence of excess potassium intake.

## Management

Elevation in the serum potassium level >6.5 mEq/L (6.5 mmol/L), or >6.0 mEq/L (6.0 mmol/L) with ECG changes, should be promptly treated. Treatment is directed at stabilizing the cardiac membrane, shifting potassium into cells, and removing potassium from the body. Intravenous administration of calcium gluconate (100 mg) quickly antagonizes the effects of hyperkalemia on the cardiac membrane. Its duration of action is relatively short and therefore is never definitive therapy. Intravenous administration of insulin alone if serum glucose is >250 mg/dL (13.9 mmol/L) or with 10% dextrose will drive potassium into cells, and is effective for up to 6 hours. Potassium can also be shifted into cells using high-dose nebulized albuterol. Sodium bicarbonate therapy has fallen out of favor because it does not promote redistribution of potassium.

Definitive treatment of severe hyperkalemia must include removal of potassium from the body. In patients without severe kidney disease, loop diuretics can be effective. Use of the potassium exchange resin sodium polystyrene sulfonate is controversial; its effectiveness is limited, and it produces adverse gastrointestinal effects. Hemodialysis is the treatment of choice in patients with severe hyperkalemia and oliguric kidney disease.

In chronic hyperkalemia, limiting potassium intake may be beneficial. Increased sodium intake along with a thiazide or loop diuretic will increase potassium excretion. In hypoaldosteronism, fludrocortisone will normalize the potassium; however, it may cause elevated blood pressure and edema, and long-term effects of fludrocortisone are unknown. All potentially causative medications should be discontinued if possible. If necessary, newer potassium binders (such as patiromer) may allow continuation of essential medications. H

### KEY POINTS

- Intravenous administration of calcium gluconate quickly antagonizes the effects of hyperkalemia on the cardiac membrane, but its duration of action is relatively short.

- Definitive treatment of severe hyperkalemia must include removal of potassium from the body; loop diuretics can be effective in patients without severe kidney disease, and hemodialysis is the treatment of choice in patients with severe hyperkalemia and oliguric kidney disease.

# Disorders of Serum Phosphate

## Hypophosphatemia

Hypophosphatemia is defined as a serum phosphate level <2.7 mg/dL (0.87 mmol/L). Phosphate ($PO_4$) is found primarily within bone and the intracellular space. Phosphate is required for metabolic pathways involved in energy production, cellular repair, and enzymatic activity. Mild hypophosphatemia is rarely symptomatic. Levels <2.0 mg/dL (0.65 mmol/L) are associated with muscle weakness. Severe hypophosphatemia (<1.0 mg/dL [0.32 mmol/L]) is associated with life-threatening symptoms, including delirium, seizures, coma, heart failure, respiratory failure, rhabdomyolysis, and hemolysis.

### Evaluation

Hypophosphatemia results from transcellular shifts, decreased intake, or increased excretion. Movement of phosphorous into cells occurs with respiratory alkalosis, insulin treatment, or refeeding of starved individuals. Medications that bind phosphate in the gut (calcium, antacids) can decrease effective intake. Because the kidney can decrease phosphate excretion to very low levels, low dietary phosphate rarely causes hypophosphatemia without coexisting malnutrition. Increased excretion may be caused by diarrhea or renal wasting. Excretion of >100 mg of phosphate in a 24-hour urine collection or a fractional excretion of phosphate ($FE_{PO_4}$) >5% suggests renal wasting. $FE_{PO_4}$ is calculated as follows:

$$FE_{PO_4} = (U_{PO_4} \times P_{Cr})/(P_{PO_4} \times U_{Cr}) \times 100$$

(where Cr = creatinine, P = plasma, $PO_4$ = phosphate, U = urine)

Renal losses of phosphate are seen in hyperparathyroidism and in proximal tubular dysfunction.

### Management

Mild decreases in serum phosphate can be treated with oral sodium or potassium phosphate. Levels <2.0 mg/dL (0.65 mmol/L) should be treated with intravenous sodium phosphate. Calcitriol is sometimes required to increase intestinal absorption of phosphate.

### KEY POINTS

- Severe hypophosphatemia (<1.0 mg/dL [0.32 mmol/L]) is associated with life-threatening symptoms, including delirium, seizures, coma, heart failure, respiratory failure, rhabdomyolysis, and hemolysis.

- Mild hypophosphatemia can be treated with oral sodium or potassium phosphate; levels <2.0 mg/dL (0.65 mmol/L) should be treated with intravenous sodium phosphate.

## Hyperphosphatemia

Hyperphosphatemia is defined by a serum phosphate level >4.5 mg/dL (1.45 mmol/L). Causes include cellular lysis with release of phosphate, excessive intake, and/or decreased renal

CONT.

excretion. Symptoms are usually related to co-occurring hypocalcemia. Acute elevations in phosphate can cause precipitation of calcium phosphate in the kidney, resulting in phosphate nephropathy.

### Evaluation

Hyperphosphatemia from reduced renal excretion does not occur due to reduced GFR unless patients have severe chronic kidney disease. Hypoparathyroidism decreases excretion through increased phosphate tubular reabsorption; hypocalcemia is often present. Rare defects in the action of fibroblast growth factor-23 (such as in tumoral calcinosis) also increase tubular reabsorption of phosphate.

Because phosphate is primarily an intracellular anion, widespread cellular damage as occurs in rhabdomyolysis and tumor lysis syndrome increases serum phosphate, especially if the GFR is decreased. Excessive phosphate intake rarely causes hyperphosphatemia because the kidney rapidly excretes phosphate. However, phosphate-containing cathartics can cause acute elevations in serum phosphate, especially in patients with reduced GFR.

### Management

If kidney function is adequate, serum phosphate levels should normalize in 12 to 24 hours. If necessary, phosphate excretion can be increased with intravenous saline. In patients with acute kidney injury, dialysis may be necessary. Because many foods contain phosphate, dietary phosphate restriction is difficult. Therefore, patients with chronic hyperphosphatemia must often use agents that bind phosphate in the gut. **H**

#### KEY POINTS

- Causes of hyperphosphatemia include cellular lysis with release of phosphate, excessive intake, and/or decreased renal excretion from decreased glomerular filtration rate or increased tubular reabsorption (hypoparathyroidism).
- If kidney function is adequate in patients with hyperphosphatemia, serum phosphate levels should normalize in 12 to 24 hours; if necessary, phosphate excretion can be increased with intravenous saline, and dialysis can be initiated for those with acute kidney injury.

## **H** Disorders of Serum Magnesium

There are approximately 24 grams of magnesium in the body, with 99% residing intracellularly and within bone. Magnesium is essential for protein and nucleic acid synthesis, cell adhesion, enzyme reactions, and modulating channel activity.

### Hypomagnesemia

Hypomagnesemia is defined by a serum magnesium level <1.7 mg/dL (0.7 mmol/L). Symptoms usually do not develop until serum magnesium is <1.2 mg/dL (0.5 mmol/L). Symptoms include tremors, fasciculations, muscle weakness,

carpopedal spasm, Chvostek (contraction of the ipsilateral facial muscles by tapping the facial nerve) and Trousseau (carpopedal spasm after inflation of blood pressure cuff above systolic blood pressure) signs, and seizures. Hypomagnesemia also appears to potentiate cardiac arrhythmogenicity due to hypokalemia, myocardial ischemia, and various drugs. In addition, hypomagnesemia causes hypokalemia due to renal potassium wasting, and it causes hypocalcemia by impeding parathyroid hormone release and action.

### Evaluation

Hypomagnesemia results from decreased gastrointestinal absorption or increased renal secretion. History and physical examination often delineate the cause. More than 10 mg of magnesium in a 24-hour urine collection or a fractional excretion of magnesium ($FE_{Mg}$) >2% suggests renal wasting in the setting of hypomagnesemia. $FE_{Mg}$ is calculated by using the following formula:

$$FE_{Mg} = ([U_{Mg} \times P_{Cr}]/[\{0.7 \times P_{Mg}\} \times U_{Cr}]) \times 100$$

(where Cr = creatinine, Mg = magnesium, P = plasma, U = urine. Magnesium is multiplied by 0.7 because only 70% of the magnesium is filtered.)

Causes of decreased magnesium absorption include severe malnutrition, diarrhea, and malabsorption. The use of proton pump inhibitors has become an important cause of hypomagnesemia, with most reported cases occurring after prolonged use; hypomagnesemia rapidly reverses upon discontinuation of the drug.

Hypomagnesemia from renal losses occurs with diuretics, cisplatin, aminoglycosides, or calcineurin inhibitors. Vascular endothelial growth factor inhibitors used in cancer treatment can cause significant magnesium wasting. Other causes of urine losses include volume expansion, alcohol ingestion, and diabetic ketoacidosis.

### Management

If significant symptoms are present, 4 grams of magnesium sulfate should be infused over 12 hours and repeated if necessary. Less severe symptoms can be treated with 1 to 2 grams of intravenous magnesium sulfate. Importantly, half of acutely infused intravenous magnesium is excreted by the kidney; therefore, slow-release oral magnesium or nasogastric tube delivery may be better to replete mild to moderate degrees of hypomagnesemia. **H**

#### KEY POINTS

- Significant symptoms of hypomagnesemia usually develop when the serum magnesium level is <1.2 mg/dL (0.50 mmol/L); these include tremors, fasciculations, muscle weakness, carpopedal spasm, Chvostek and Trousseau signs, seizures, and cardiac arrhythmogenicity.
- Treatment of significant symptoms of hypomagnesemia includes magnesium sulfate infusions; less severe symptoms can be treated with infusion or with slow-release oral magnesium.

### Hypermagnesemia

Hypermagnesemia is defined by a serum magnesium level of >2.4 mg/dL (0.99 mmol/L).

#### Evaluation

Hypermagnesemia occurs infrequently and most commonly results from excessive intake in the setting of decreased kidney function. Numerous medications such as antacids and laxatives contain magnesium, and magnesium sulfate can be used in the treatment of refractory asthma and remains the treatment of choice for prevention of preeclampsia.

Symptoms of hypermagnesemia do not occur until levels are >5.0 mg/dL (2.1 mmol/L). Early symptoms include loss of deep tendon reflexes, progressing to flaccid paralysis at higher levels. Hypermagnesemia also results in hypotension from vascular relaxation. Laboratory analysis often shows hypocalcemia.

#### Management

Prevention is the key to management of hypermagnesemia. Hypermagnesemia is usually self-limited; magnesium-containing agents should be limited or avoided in individuals with kidney disease. Magnesium-containing medications should be discontinued, and magnesium excretion can be enhanced with saline diuresis. For more severe symptoms, intravenous calcium will antagonize the effects of magnesium. H

**KEY POINTS**

- Early symptoms of hypermagnesemia include loss of deep tendon reflexes, progressing to flaccid paralysis at higher levels.

- For patients with hypermagnesemia, all magnesium-containing medications should be discontinued, and magnesium excretion can be enhanced with saline diuresis; for more severe symptoms, intravenous calcium will antagonize the effects of magnesium.

# Acid-Base Disorders

## Overview

Acid-base balance is essential to appropriate function of the human body. Hydrogen ions are maintained within narrow limits and determine pH (**Table 6**). Alterations of acid-base

**TABLE 6.** Physiologic Levels of Tests Used in the Assessment of Acid-Base Status

| | pH | $P_{CO_2}$ | Bicarbonate |
|---|---|---|---|
| Arterial blood | 7.37-7.44 | 36-44 mm Hg (4.8-5.9 kPa) | 22-26 mEq/L (22-26 mmol/L) |
| Venous blood | 7.32-7.38 | 42-50 mm Hg (5.6-6.7 kPa) | 23-27 mEq/L (23-27 mmol/L) |

balance can have dire consequences; therefore, any change in pH results in a predictable response to limit that change.

Causes of acid-base disorders can be determined by using blood gas results (pH, $P_{CO_2}$), serum bicarbonate measurements, and the serum anion gap. Arterial blood provides the most accurate measurement, although venous blood gases may be useful in following response to therapy. Venous gases are least useful in patients with shock, due to lower pH and higher $P_{CO_2}$ values than in arterial gases.

Primary acid-base disorders are classified according to the underlying mechanism (metabolic or respiratory) and their effect on acid-base balance (acidosis or alkalosis) (**Figure 9**). Expected compensatory response to the primary disorder is then assessed (**Table 7**). A mixed acid-base disorder is present when measured values fall outside the range of the predicted compensatory response. The primary disorder is usually reflected by the blood pH, although a normal pH may occur in the context of a mixed disorder. Appropriate compensation may result in near-normal pH.

**KEY POINTS**

- Primary metabolic acidosis is defined by low serum bicarbonate and primary metabolic alkalosis by elevated serum bicarbonate.

- In primary respiratory acidosis, arterial $P_{CO_2}$ is above the normal range; in primary respiratory alkalosis, $P_{CO_2}$ is below normal.

## Metabolic Acidosis
### General Approach

Metabolic acidosis is detected by low pH and low serum bicarbonate. A stepwise approach to assessment supports appropriate diagnosis of the underlying acid-base disorder. First, both pH and $P_{CO_2}$ are needed to confirm the primary disorder

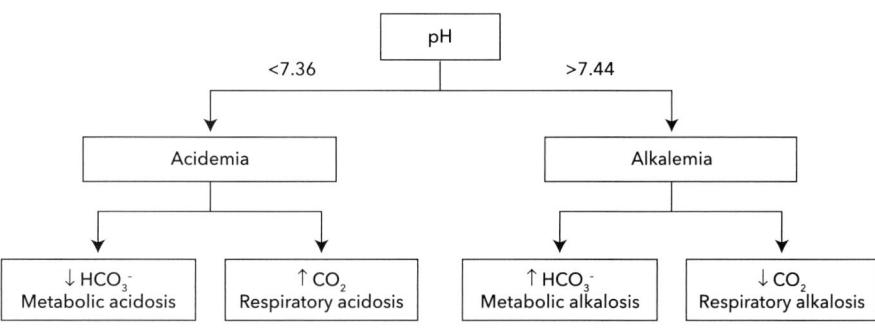

**FIGURE 9.** Classification of primary acid-base disorders.

| TABLE 7. | Compensation in Acid-Base Disorders |
|---|---|
| **Condition** | **Expected Compensation** |
| Metabolic acidosis | Maximally compensated: expected $P_{CO_2} = (1.5)[HCO_3] + 8 \pm 2$ (Winter's formula) |
| | Measured $P_{CO_2}$ > expected: complicating primary respiratory acidosis |
| | Measured $P_{CO_2}$ < expected: complicating primary respiratory alkalosis |
| Metabolic alkalosis | For each ↑ 1.0 mEq/L (1.0 mmol/L) in $[HCO_3]$, $P_{CO_2}$ ↑ 0.7 mm Hg (0.09 kPa) |
| Respiratory acidosis | Acute: 1.0 mEq/L (1.0 mmol/L) ↑ $[HCO_3]$ for each 10 mm Hg (1.3 kPa) ↑ in $P_{CO_2}$ |
| | Chronic: 3.5 mEq/L (3.5 mmol/L) ↑ $[HCO_3]$ for each 10 mm Hg (1.3 kPa) ↑ in $P_{CO_2}$ |
| | $[HCO_3]$ < expected value: complicating metabolic acidosis |
| | $[HCO_3]$ > expected value: complicating metabolic alkalosis |
| Respiratory alkalosis | Acute: 2.0 mEq/L (2.0 mmol/L) ↓ $[HCO_3]$ for each 10 mm Hg (1.3 kPa) ↓ in $P_{CO_2}$ |
| | Chronic: 4.0-5.0 mEq/L (4.0-5.0 mmol/L) ↓ $[HCO_3]$ for each 10 mm Hg (1.3 kPa) ↓ in $P_{CO_2}$ |
| | $[HCO_3]$ < expected value: complicating metabolic acidosis |
| | $[HCO_3]$ > expected value: complicating metabolic alkalosis |

because low serum bicarbonate may be a compensatory response to respiratory alkalosis.

Next, the serum anion gap is calculated to assess whether the low serum bicarbonate is due to loss of serum bicarbonate (no anion gap) or is a result of unmeasured anion (anion gap acidosis). The anion gap is calculated as follows:

$$\text{Anion Gap} = \text{Serum Sodium (mEq/L)} - (\text{Serum Chloride [mEq/L]} + \text{Serum Bicarbonate [mEq/L]})$$

The normal reference range for the anion gap is 8.0 to 10 mEq/L ± 2 mEq/L (8.0-10 mmol/L ± 2 mmol/L). In normal subjects, negatively charged albumin is a major contributor to the anion gap. Therefore, changes in albumin need to be taken into account. This is most important in the context of a low albumin wherein failure to correct the anion gap will result in underestimation of the true anion gap. The albumin-corrected anion gap (with normal albumin being 4.0 g/dL [40 g/L]) is calculated as follows:

$$\text{Albumin-Corrected Anion Gap} = \text{Anion Gap} + 2.5 \times (\text{Normal Albumin} - \text{Measured Albumin [g/dL]})$$

If the corrected anion gap is increased, patients should next be assessed for coexistent normal anion gap acidosis or metabolic alkalosis. One method for detection of a coexistent additional acid-base disorder is to assess the ratio of the amount of anion gap abnormality (Δ anion gap) to the amount of bicarbonate abnormality (Δ bicarbonate), or the "delta-delta (Δ-Δ) ratio."

$$\text{Δ-Δ Ratio} = \text{Δ Anion Gap}/\text{Δ Bicarbonate} = (\text{Anion Gap} - 12)/(25 - \text{Bicarbonate})$$

A ratio of <0.5 to 1 may reflect the presence of concurrent normal anion gap metabolic acidosis, whereas a ratio of >2 may indicate the presence of metabolic alkalosis.

Patients with metabolic acidosis due to acute or chronic kidney disease may have either a normal anion gap or an increased anion gap, depending on severity of loss of nephron mass. When the glomerular filtration rate (GFR) decreases to

<45 mL/min/1.73 m², decreased urine ammonium excretion leads to a normal anion gap metabolic acidosis, often associated with hyperkalemia. When the GFR decreases to <15 mL/min/1.73 m², retention of sulfates, phosphates, and organic acids results in an increased anion gap metabolic acidosis.

### KEY POINTS

- Metabolic acidosis is detected by low pH and low serum bicarbonate levels.

- When metabolic acidosis is present, the anion gap is useful in assessing whether the decreased serum bicarbonate is due to an unmeasured organic anion (increased anion gap metabolic acidosis) or to a loss of bicarbonate (normal anion gap metabolic acidosis).

- Metabolic acidosis due to acute or chronic kidney disease may have either a normal anion gap or an increased anion gap, depending on severity of nephron loss.

## Increased Anion Gap Metabolic Acidosis

Increased anion gap metabolic acidosis occurs when unmeasured anions accumulate. Lactic acidosis is the most common cause (**Table 8**). Less common causes include ketoacidosis (diabetic, alcoholic, or starvation), acute or chronic kidney injury, or poisoning (methanol, ethylene glycol, salicylate, or propylene glycol). The plasma osmolal gap may assist in identifying a cause. The plasma osmolal gap is the difference between the measured and calculated plasma osmolality. The calculated plasma osmolality is determined as follows:

$$\text{Plasma Osmolality (mOsm/kg } H_2O) = (2 \times \text{Serum Sodium [mEq/L]}) + \text{Plasma Glucose (mg/dL)}/18 + \text{Blood Urea Nitrogen (mg/dL)}/2.8$$

A high osmolal gap (>10 mOsm/kg $H_2O$) indicates the presence of unmeasured osmoles such as methanol or ethylene glycol, which are metabolized to organic acids, thereby increasing the anion gap. A high osmolal gap is also seen in

**TABLE 8.** Causes of Lactic Acidosis

| Condition | Cause | Clinical and Laboratory Manifestations | Treatment | Comments |
|---|---|---|---|---|
| Lactic Acidosis | See below. | Serum lactate level >4.0 mEq/L (4.0 mmol/L) | Treat underlying cause; sodium bicarbonate when arterial pH is <7.1 to raise pH to 7.2 | Most common cause of increased anion gap metabolic acidosis |
| Type A lactic acidosis | Tissue hypoperfusion | Multisystem organ dysfunction typically present | Correct cause of hypoperfusion | — |
| Type B lactic acidosis | | | | |
|   Propofol | Propofol >4 mg/kg/h for >24 h | Rhabdomyolysis; hyperlipidemia; cardiogenic shock | Discontinue propofol; hemodialysis | Seen with continuous infusion, not bolus dosing |
|   Metformin | Metformin use in patients with impaired kidney function | More likely to occur in those with acute kidney injury | Hemodialysis | Avoid in those with eGFR <30 mL/min/1.73 m$^2$ |
|   HIV nucleoside reverse transcriptase inhibitor | Mitochondrial toxicity | Type B lactic acidosis | Discontinue medication; supportive care | Risk factors: female sex, pregnancy, obesity, poor liver function, lower CD4 count; mostly: ddI, d4T > AZT; rare: TFV, ABC, FTC, 3TC |
|   Hematologic malignancy | Thought to be due to anaerobic metabolism in cancer cells | Type B lactic acidosis; hypoglycemia | Treat underlying malignancy | Portends very poor prognosis; seen in high-grade B-cell lymphomas |
| D-Lactic acidosis | Short-bowel syndrome[a]; undigested carbohydrates in the colon are metabolized to D-lactate by bacteria | Intermittent confusion; slurred speech; ataxia; increased anion gap metabolic acidosis with normal serum lactate level | Antibiotics (e.g., metronidazole or neomycin) directed toward bowel flora; restriction of dietary carbohydrates | Diagnosis requires measurement of D-lactate because D-isomer is not measured by conventional assays for serum lactate |

3TC = lamivudine; ABC = abacavir; AZT = zidovudine; d4T = stavudine; ddI = didanosine; eGFR = estimated glomerular filtration rate; FTC = emtricitabine; TFV = tenofovir.

[a]After jejunoileal bypass or small-bowel resection.

CONT.

pseudohyponatremia, in which plasma osmolality is normal while calculated osmolality is low. The patient's history should guide further testing for unmeasured anions.

Diabetic ketoacidosis usually presents with an increased anion gap metabolic acidosis due to accumulation of β-hydroxybutyrate and acetoacetate, although it may present with a normal anion gap due to excretion of ketoacids. Compensatory hyperventilation is characterized by increased tidal volume rather than increase in respiratory rate. Urine dipstick assays for ketones detect acetoacetate using the nitroprusside assay; however, β-hydroxybutyrate is the dominant ketoacid in diabetic ketoacidosis, so urine dipstick results can be falsely negative or underestimate the total ketone load (see MKSAP 18 Endocrinology and Metabolism).

Alcoholic ketoacidosis occurs in patients with chronic ethanol abuse who typically have a history of recent binge drinking, little food intake, and persistent vomiting. Liver chemistry test abnormalities may be present due to concomitant alcoholic hepatitis. Treatment with intravenous saline and intravenous glucose typically results in rapid resolution of ketones due to induction of insulin secretion and suppression of glucagon release. For patients with chronic malnutrition related to alcohol use, thiamine should be administered before glucose to decrease the risk of precipitating Wernicke encephalopathy.

Medication and toxin exposures that cause increased anion gap acidosis are described in **Table 9**.

**KEY POINTS**

- Lactic acidosis is defined as a serum lactate level >4.0 mEq/L (4.0 mmol/L); management includes treatment of the underlying cause and sodium bicarbonate when arterial pH is <7.1.

- Ethylene glycol or methanol ingestion should be suspected in patients with an increased anion gap acidosis associated with a serum bicarbonate level <10 mEq/L (10 mmol/L) and a plasma osmolal gap >10 mOsm/kg $H_2O$.

## Normal Anion Gap Metabolic Acidosis

Normal anion gap metabolic acidoses most often result from gastrointestinal bicarbonate losses (diarrhea), kidney bicarbonate losses (type 2 renal tubular acidosis), or inability of the kidney to adequately excrete acid (types 1 and 4 renal tubular acidosis; chronic kidney disease). Although a patient history

**TABLE 9. Medication and Toxin Exposures that Cause Increased Anion Gap Acidosis**

| Condition | Cause | Clinical and Laboratory Manifestations | Treatment | Comments |
|---|---|---|---|---|
| Ethylene glycol ingestion | Glycolic acid accumulation; calcium oxalate precipitation in renal tubules and crystals in the urine | Neurotoxicity/inebriation; AKI and flank pain due to precipitation of calcium oxalate in kidneys; hypocalcemic symptoms; cardiovascular collapse; pulmonary edema<br><br>Serum bicarbonate level <10 mEq/L (10 mmol/L); plasma osmolal gap >10 mOsm/kg $H_2O$ | Fomepizole<br><br>IV hydration<br><br>Hemodialysis: in severe acidemia, very large ingestions, severe CNS depression, AKI, systemic collapse<br><br>Pyridoxine and thiamine: in suspected ethylene glycol toxicity<br><br>Sodium bicarbonate | Found in antifreeze, solvents, cosmetics<br><br>May be difficult to differentiate from methanol ingestion |
| Methanol ingestion | Formic acid accumulation | CNS damage; optic nerve/eye damage with blindness; inebriation less prominent than with ethylene glycol; papilledema; mydriasis; afferent pupillary defect; abdominal pain; pancreatitis<br><br>Serum bicarbonate level <10 mEq/L (10 mmol/L); plasma osmolal gap >10 mOsm/kg $H_2O$ | Fomepizole<br><br>Hemodialysis: in severe acidemia, very large ingestions, severe CNS depression, any visual impairment<br><br>Folic acid: in suspected methanol toxicity<br><br>Sodium bicarbonate | Found in windshield-washing fluid, commercial solvents, paints, some antifreezes<br><br>May be difficult to differentiate from ethylene glycol ingestion<br><br>80%-90% mortality rate with methanol ingestion; permanent blindness may occur |
| Salicylate toxicity | Salicylate anion accumulation; ingestion of as little as 10 grams of aspirin in adults | Respiratory alkalosis; tinnitus; nausea/vomiting; impaired mental status; cerebral edema and fatal brainstem herniation; tachypnea; low-grade fever; noncardiogenic pulmonary edema; hepatic injury; with severe intoxication, lactic acidosis or ketoacidosis | Bicarbonate infusion: alkalinization mitigates CNS toxicity; aim for urine pH >7.5<br><br>Hemodialysis: in AKI, impaired mental status, cerebral edema, serum salicylate levels >100 mg/dL with acute ingestion and levels >60 mg/dL with chronic ingestion, refractory acidemia, pulmonary edema | Toxicity can develop from ingestion or mucocutaneous exposure to salicylate preparations such as methyl salicylate (oil of wintergreen) |
| Propylene glycol toxicity | Large doses of propylene glycol (a solvent used for IV medications), most commonly lorazepam diluted in propylene glycol (80%) | AKI; anion gap metabolic acidosis with increased plasma osmolal gap; toxicity when propylene glycol levels >25 mg/dL or plasma osmolal gap >10 mOsm/kg $H_2O$ | Discontinue the IV infusion<br><br>Hemodialysis | Monitor acid-base status and serum osmolality when lorazepam doses >1 mg/kg/d; unlikely to develop if 24-h lorazepam dose is limited to <166 mg/d |
| Pyroglutamic (5-oxoproline) acidosis | Resulting from chronic acetaminophen ingestion; most common in critically ill patients, those with poor nutrition, liver disease, or CKD, and in vegetarians | Impaired mental status; on urine testing for organic anions, high concentrations of urine pyroglutamate (5-oxoproline) | Discontinue acetaminophen<br><br>Consider N-acetylcysteine to regenerate depleted glutathione stores | Female preponderance (80%); genetic factors may play a role |

AKI = acute kidney injury; CKD = chronic kidney disease; CNS = central nervous system; IV = intravenous.

CONT.

may elucidate the cause, the urine anion gap may help to narrow down the cause.

The kidneys should increase acid excretion in response to acidemia. This is achieved primarily by increased tubular production of ammonia ($NH_3$) and secretion of protons, resulting in increased urine ammonium ($NH_4^+$). The amount of urine ammonium reflects the ability of the kidneys to respond appropriately to acidemia and indicates if the kidney is a cause of the acidosis. Because urine ammonium is difficult to obtain,

the urine anion gap is used as a surrogate to assess kidney acid excretion:

Urine Anion Gap = (Urine Sodium + Urine Potassium) – Urine Chloride

In patients with gastrointestinal losses of bicarbonate (diarrhea; laxative abuse) or those exposed to an acid load, urine $NH_4^+$ should increase. Ammonium cation excretion results in proportionately less excretion of sodium and

CONT.

potassium (the predominant urine cations). Chloride anion excretion continues with ammonium cation excretion to maintain electrical neutrality. In the context of increased urine $NH_4^+$ production, therefore, the urine anion gap will be negative (less than zero). A positive urine anion gap in a patient with acidemia suggests the presence of a distal renal tubular acidosis. Proton secretion in the distal nephron generates $NH_4^+$, and in distal renal tubular acidosis there is a defect in this proton secretion. Therefore, urine $NH_4^+$ will be low, with proportionately greater sodium and potassium excretion resulting in a positive urine anion gap.

The urine anion gap, together with serum potassium levels and urine pH, can help further distinguish the causes of normal anion gap metabolic acidosis (Table 10).

## Type 2 (Proximal) Renal Tubular Acidosis

The primary defect in type 2 (proximal) renal tubular acidosis (RTA) is failure of the proximal tubule to adequately absorb filtered bicarbonate, resulting in bicarbonate loss and acidosis. Type 2 RTA is usually accompanied by other evidence of proximal tubular dysfunction, including Fanconi syndrome (glycosuria, phosphaturia, aminoaciduria, hypouricemia). As blood bicarbonate levels decrease, less bicarbonate is filtered and eventually the resorptive threshold is reached, such that serum bicarbonate levels stabilize (around 12-14 mEq/L [12-14 mmol/L]). Because the distal nephron functions appropriately in type 2 RTA, urine can still be acidified to a pH <5.5 and $NH_4^+$ production will be normal, usually making the urine anion gap negative. Hypokalemia is also often present due to increased distal tubular potassium secretion. This occurs because sodium accompanies bicarbonate to the distal tubule, where sodium is reabsorbed in exchange for potassium.

Alkali replacement is the mainstay of treatment for type 2 RTA. Thiazide diuretics may help by causing mild volume depletion with subsequent aldosterone-driven proximal reabsorption of sodium and bicarbonate.

## Type 1 (Hypokalemic Distal) Renal Tubular Acidosis

In type 1 (hypokalemic distal) RTA, a distal tubular defect results in impaired excretion of hydrogen ions by the distal nephron (hence, low urine ammonium and positive urine anion gap) with inability to acidify urine below a pH of 6.0. Serum bicarbonate may fall below 10 mEq/L (10 mmol/L) as levels fail to stabilize as is seen with type 2 (proximal) RTA; despite lower filtered bicarbonate, continued impairment in acid excretion will worsen the acidosis.

The most common causes include Sjögren syndrome and other tubulointerstitial diseases, including reflux uropathy and obstructive uropathy. Type 1 RTA can also be caused by medications such as amphotericin B and lithium and has been described in dysproteinemias, sickle cell disease, and Wilson disease.

Urinary potassium wasting in the setting of diminished proton secretion underlies the development of hypokalemia. Hypercalciuria and hyperphosphatemia are frequent in untreated type 1 RTA due to increased calcium and phosphate release from bone due to buffering of acid. Reduced tubular calcium resorption in the context of acidosis exacerbates hypercalciuria. Increased proximal reabsorption of citrate in the context of acidosis and hypokalemia causes hypocitraturia. Citrate usually inhibits calcium crystallization; therefore, hypocitraturia, in addition to hypercalciuria, increases the risk of calcium phosphate stones and nephrocalcinosis.

Treatment consists of potassium citrate, 1 mEq/kg/d (which is subsequently metabolized to bicarbonate), with the dose titrated to response.

## Type 4 (Hyperkalemic Distal) Renal Tubular Acidosis

Type 4 (hyperkalemic distal) RTA is caused by aldosterone deficiency or resistance. Primary adrenal insufficiency (Addison disease) may cause aldosterone deficiency. Hyporeninemic hypoaldosteronism is a more common cause and may occur in the presence of various kidney diseases, most often diabetic nephropathy. Aldosterone resistance can occur in those with tubulointerstitial disease, including urinary obstruction, sickle cell disease, medullary cystic kidney disease, and kidney transplant rejection. Drug-induced type 4 RTA can be caused by numerous drugs that reduce aldosterone production, including ACE inhibitors, angiotensin receptor blockers, heparin, and cyclooxygenase-2 inhibitors.

Type 4 RTA is associated with a positive urine anion gap but a urine pH <5.5 (see Table 10). Hyperkalemia decreases $NH_3$ production (and therefore $NH_4^+$), resulting in a positive

| TABLE 10. Diagnostic Approach to Normal Anion Gap Metabolic Acidosis | | | |
|---|---|---|---|
| Diagnosis | Urine Anion Gap $(U_{Na} + U_K) - U_{Cl}$ | Serum Potassium | Urine pH |
| Ammonium chloride ingestion (acid load) | Negative | Normal | <5.5 |
| Diarrhea and acidosis | Negative | Normal | <5.5 |
| Type 2 (proximal) RTA[a] | Negative | Decreased | Variable[b] |
| Type 1 (hypokalemic distal) RTA | Positive | Decreased | >5.5 |
| Type 4 (hyperkalemic distal) RTA | Positive | Increased | <5.5 |

RTA = renal tubular acidosis; $U_{Cl}$ = urine chloride; $U_K$ = urine potassium; $U_{Na}$ = urine sodium.

[a]Type 2 (proximal) RTA is often associated with Fanconi syndrome (glycosuria, phosphaturia, aminoaciduria, hypouricemia).

[b]Patients with type 2 (proximal) RTA have normal distal renal tubular function and can acidify the urine once the serum bicarbonate drops to a point at which the filtered load of bicarbonate can be normally reabsorbed.

CONT.

urine anion gap. Even if the distal nephron is able to decrease urine pH appropriately, reduced $NH_4^+$ excretion will lead to insufficient acid excretion, generating a metabolic acidosis.

Treatment is focused on correcting the underlying cause if possible; offending medications should be discontinued when identified. Because many patients are also hypertensive and volume expanded, thiazide or loop diuretics may help increase bicarbonate and decrease serum potassium. Fludrocortisone can be used to replace mineralocorticoids in hyporeninemic hypoaldosteronism in those without hypertension or heart failure. Use of the potassium exchange resin sodium polystyrene sulfonate is controversial because its effectiveness is limited. The newer cation-exchanger patiromer is effective.

### Mixed Forms of Renal Tubular Acidosis
Topiramate inhibits carbonic anhydrase in both proximal and distal tubules, causing the acquired form of RTA. Due to consequent high urine pH (>6.0) and hypocitraturia, topiramate is associated with increased risk for calcium phosphate stones. Rare hereditary carbonic anhydrase deficiencies also result in combined proximal and distal RTAs. 🄷

### KEY POINTS

- In type 2 (proximal) renal tubular acidosis, failure of the proximal tubule to adequately absorb filtered bicarbonate causes bicarbonate loss; treatment consists of alkali replacement and a thiazide diuretic.

- In type 1 (hypokalemic distal) renal tubular acidosis, impaired distal hydrogen ion excretion causes citrate reabsorption and increases the risk for nephrocalcinosis; treatment consists of potassium citrate.

- In type 4 (hyperkalemic distal) renal tubular acidosis, aldosterone deficiency or resistance causes hyperkalemia and decreased $NH_4^+$ excretion; treatment includes correction of the underlying cause and treatment of hyperkalemia.

## 🄷 Metabolic Alkalosis

Metabolic alkalosis with high blood pH results either from a loss of acid or from administration or retention of bicarbonate (alkali). Metabolic alkalosis occurs in two phases: a generation phase in which the primary disorder (such as vomiting or the accumulation of alkali) occurs, and a maintenance phase in which typical renal compensatory excretion of excess bicarbonate is ineffective. The metabolic alkalosis generation phase usually involves the gastrointestinal (GI) tract (in vomiting-induced acid loss) or the kidney (typically a mineralocorticoid effect, either primary or in response to intravascular volume depletion, with resulting sodium and bicarbonate retention at the expense of acid and potassium secretion). Conditions that contribute to maintenance of metabolic alkalosis include volume contraction, ineffective arterial blood volume, hypokalemia, chloride depletion, and decreased glomerular filtration.

Symptoms of metabolic alkalosis are usually related to the underlying disorder. Coexisting hypokalemia markedly increases the risk for cardiac arrhythmias. Severe metabolic alkalosis (serum bicarbonate >50 mEq/L [50 mmol/L]) can cause hypocalcemia, hypoventilation, and hypoxemia, with potential neurologic consequences (seizures, delirium, stupor).

Thorough history and physical examination, including assessment of blood pressure and volume status, are essential to identifying the likely cause (**Figure 10**). Laboratory evaluation is based on urine chloride rather than urine sodium. Urine sodium can be high during appropriate compensatory urine bicarbonate excretion because sodium is the primary cation excreted with bicarbonate. Urine sodium measurement may also be misleading with diuretic use.

The most common causes of metabolic alkalosis are associated with chloride depletion: vomiting, nasogastric suction, and diuretic use. Although upper GI losses are far more common, lower GI chloride-secretory diarrheas (villous adenoma, congenital chloridorrhea) can rarely cause chloride depletion with bicarbonate retention. A "contraction alkalosis" results from loss of extracellular fluid containing low amounts of bicarbonate, leaving a contracted extracellular volume around a constant amount of existing circulating bicarbonate.

In patients with low urine chloride (<15 mEq/L [15 mmol/L]), normal/low intravascular volume, and normal/low extracellular volume, treatment consists of saline administration plus repletion of potassium (saline-responsive metabolic alkalosis) while addressing the primary cause of the alkalosis. In contrast, those with a low urine chloride (<15 mEq/L [15 mmol/L]) and normal/low intravascular volume but with an increased extravascular volume (heart failure, cirrhosis) have secondary hyperaldosteronism with sodium and bicarbonate retention manifested by edema; treatment is tailored to improving effective arterial blood volume and diuresis.

Mineralocorticoid excess presents with a high urine chloride (>15 mEq/L [15 mmol/L]) with elevated blood pressure and hypokalemia without volume overload (saline-resistant metabolic alkalosis). The lack of an overt increase in extravascular volume is often described as "aldosterone escape": after initial sodium retention, sodium balance is attained through spontaneous diuresis that returns vascular volume toward normal. Mineralocorticoid excess is treated with potassium repletion and treatment of the underlying condition.

Rarely, patients may have clinical features consistent with saline-responsive metabolic alkalosis but with a urine chloride of >15 mEq/L [15 mmol/L]; ongoing diuretic use can present this way. Two autosomal recessive genetic conditions, Bartter and Gitelman syndromes, result in disordered renal sodium and chloride transporters and clinically mimic loop diuretic

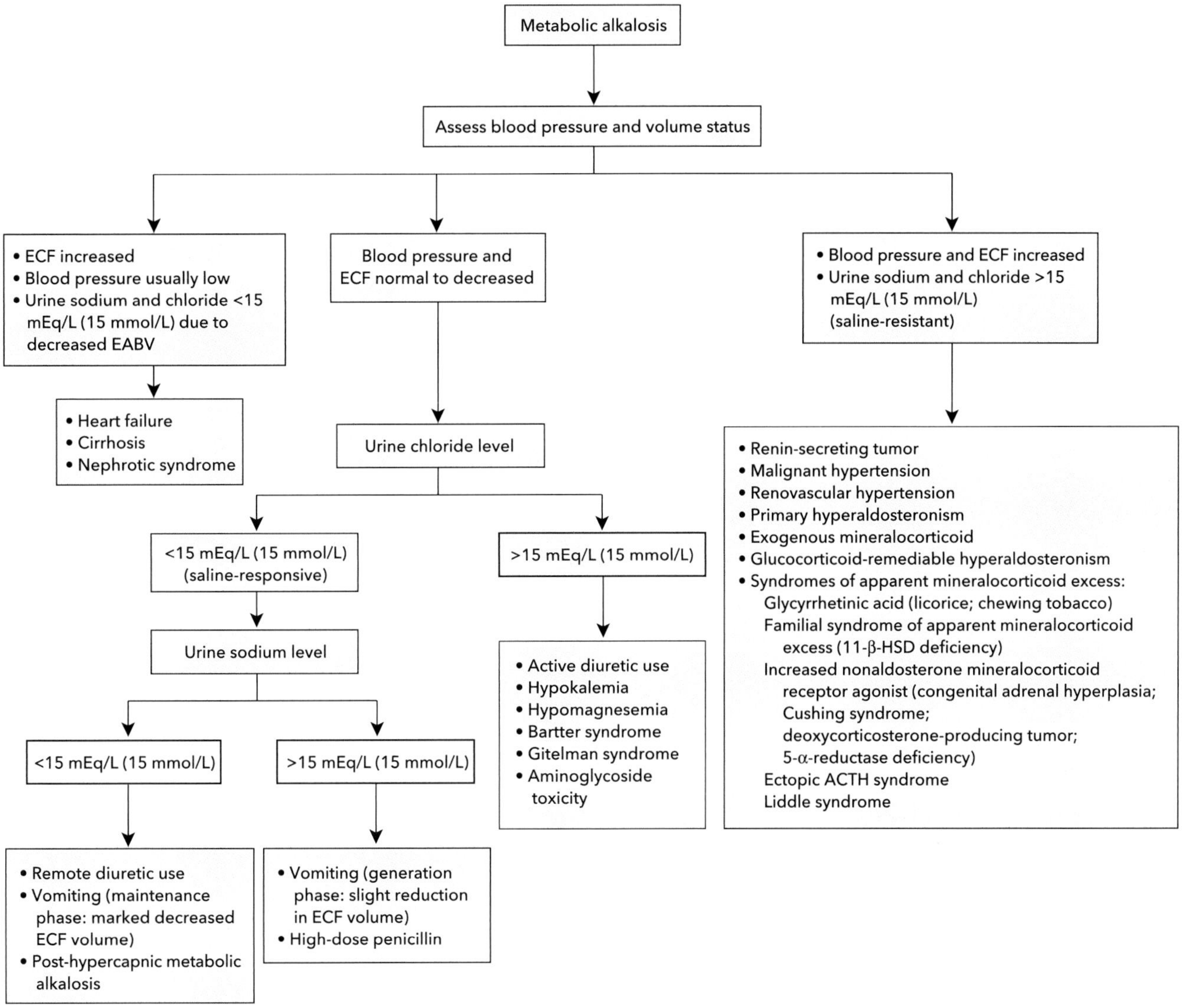

Metabolic alkalosis

↓

Assess blood pressure and volume status

**Branch 1:**
- ECF increased
- Blood pressure usually low
- Urine sodium and chloride <15 mEq/L (15 mmol/L) due to decreased EABV

↓

- Heart failure
- Cirrhosis
- Nephrotic syndrome

**Branch 2:**
Blood pressure and ECF normal to decreased

↓

Urine chloride level

- <15 mEq/L (15 mmol/L) (saline-responsive)

  ↓

  Urine sodium level

  - <15 mEq/L (15 mmol/L)

    ↓

    - Remote diuretic use
    - Vomiting (maintenance phase: marked decreased ECF volume)
    - Post-hypercapnic metabolic alkalosis

  - >15 mEq/L (15 mmol/L)

    ↓

    - Vomiting (generation phase: slight reduction in ECF volume)
    - High-dose penicillin

- >15 mEq/L (15 mmol/L)

  ↓

  - Active diuretic use
  - Hypokalemia
  - Hypomagnesemia
  - Bartter syndrome
  - Gitelman syndrome
  - Aminoglycoside toxicity

**Branch 3:**
- Blood pressure and ECF increased
- Urine sodium and chloride >15 mEq/L (15 mmol/L) (saline-resistant)

↓

- Renin-secreting tumor
- Malignant hypertension
- Renovascular hypertension
- Primary hyperaldosteronism
- Exogenous mineralocorticoid
- Glucocorticoid-remediable hyperaldosteronism
- Syndromes of apparent mineralocorticoid excess:
  Glycyrrhetinic acid (licorice; chewing tobacco)
  Familial syndrome of apparent mineralocorticoid excess (11-β-HSD deficiency)
  Increased nonaldosterone mineralocorticoid receptor agonist (congenital adrenal hyperplasia; Cushing syndrome; deoxycorticosterone-producing tumor; 5-α-reductase deficiency)
  Ectopic ACTH syndrome
  Liddle syndrome

**FIGURE 10.** Assessment of metabolic alkalosis. ACTH = adrenocorticotropic hormone; EABV = effective arterial blood volume; ECF = extracellular fluid; HSD = hydroxysteroid dehydrogenase.

and thiazide diuretic use, respectively. These diagnoses should be considered only after urine diuretic screening.

### KEY POINTS

- The most common causes of metabolic alkalosis are associated with chloride depletion: vomiting, nasogastric suction, and diuretic use.
- In metabolic alkalosis, blood pressure, volume status, and urine chloride are critical to identify the likely cause and to determine treatment.

## Respiratory Acidosis

Respiratory acidosis is characterized by retention of arterial $CO_2$ (hypercapnia). The most common causes are inadequate ventilation (decreased central respiratory drive, thoracic neuromuscular dysfunction, musculoskeletal disorders), impaired arterial-alveolar gas exchange (pneumonia, pulmonary edema, interstitial lung diseases), and airway obstruction (COPD, status asthmaticus, upper airway obstruction).

With acute respiratory acidosis, excess $CO_2$ is initially buffered by water, leading to formation of hydrogen ions and bicarbonate. Thus, the acute arterial blood gas reveals increased $P_{CO_2}$, decreased pH, and a slight increase in bicarbonate. Over 3 to 5 days, compensatory increases in renal acid excretion (with bicarbonate reabsorption) reach a new steady state (see Table 7).

Clinical manifestations of respiratory acidosis are complicated by frequently associated hypoxemia. Symptoms are predominantly neurologic, including headache, anxiety, blurred vision, and tremor. Severe acidosis can cause confusion, somnolence, or seizures. Chronic respiratory acidosis may have milder neurologic effects such as memory loss, inattentiveness, or irritability. Cardiovascular manifestations include vasodilation and tachycardia that may evolve to cardiac arrhythmias and decreased cardiac output. Renal vasoconstriction with enhanced sodium retention occurs in severe respiratory acidosis, typically in those with severe lung disease and right-sided heart failure.

Treatment involves correcting the underlying mechanism if possible, and may necessitate mechanical ventilation to reduce $CO_2$ and oxygen supplementation. **H**

### KEY POINTS

- In respiratory acidosis, arterial blood gases demonstrate elevated $P_{CO_2}$ (hypercapnia), decreased pH, and increased bicarbonate.
- Symptoms of acute respiratory acidosis are predominantly neurologic and can include confusion, somnolence, or seizures; chronic respiratory acidosis may result in memory loss, inattentiveness, or irritability.

## Respiratory Alkalosis

Respiratory alkalosis is defined by a reduction in arterial $P_{CO_2}$ (hypocapnia) due to increased ventilation. The most common causes of respiratory alkalosis are an enhanced respiratory drive (sepsis, hepatic failure, anxiety, iatrogenic hyperventilation, pregnancy, nicotine, salicylate intoxication, subarachnoid hemorrhage), hypoxemia, and pulmonary disease with stimulation of thoracic stretch receptors (pneumonia, acute respiratory distress syndrome, pulmonary embolism).

Acute hypocapnia leads to a rapid increase in arterial pH. However, immediate compensatory diffusion of hydrogen ions from intracellular stores, and subsequent reduction in serum bicarbonate through regeneration of $CO_2$, limits the magnitude of alkalosis. The typical arterial blood gas in this setting demonstrates a decrease in $P_{CO_2}$, an increase in pH, and a slight decrease in bicarbonate. Over 2 to 3 days, bicarbonate levels decrease further as compensatory kidney excretion of bicarbonate reaches a new steady state (see Table 7).

Respiratory alkalosis may cause increased cellular lactic acid production. Increases in negatively charged albumin may cause a mildly increased anion gap and decreased ionized calcium (from enhanced albumin binding). Finally, severe hypophosphatemia can occur due to a shift of phosphate from extracellular to intracellular fluid.

Clinical presentation includes underlying tachypnea and neurologic findings such as lightheadedness, numbness and paresthesias, cramps, confusion, and, rarely, seizures. An important consideration is the potential for salicylate intoxication, which in its early phases presents with mental status changes, respiratory alkalosis, and an increased anion gap metabolic acidosis.

Treatment of respiratory alkalosis is directed at correction of the primary disorder. Treatment of salicylate intoxication includes forced diuresis, urine alkalization, or hemodialysis. For anxiety-induced or psychogenic hyperventilation, increasing inspired $P_{CO_2}$ by closed bag rebreathing may be effective.

In rare circumstances of severe alkalemia (pH >7.55) with hemodynamic instability, arrhythmias, or altered mental status, strategies to reduce bicarbonate include acetazolamide or controlled mechanical hypoventilation. **H**

### KEY POINTS

- Respiratory alkalosis is associated with a decrease in $P_{CO_2}$, an increase in pH, and a slight decrease in bicarbonate.
- Salicylate intoxication presents in the early phase with mental status changes, respiratory alkalosis, and an increased anion gap metabolic acidosis; treatment includes forced diuresis, urine alkalization, or hemodialysis.

# Hypertension

## Epidemiology

In the United States, hypertension is second only to smoking as a risk factor for death and disability. In 2010, hypertension was the leading cause of death and disability-adjusted life-years worldwide. The prevalence of hypertension varies based on the cut-point used to define hypertension, with the prevalence increasing from 32% to 46% when the cutoff is changed from a blood pressure (BP) ≥140/90 mm Hg to ≥130/80 mm Hg. Prevalence increases as the population ages, such that in individuals without hypertension at age 45 years, the 40-year risk for developing hypertension is 93% for black adults, 92% for Hispanic adults, 86% for white adults, and 84% for Chinese adults. Overall, persons free of hypertension at 55 years have a 90% lifetime risk for developing hypertension. Although several clinical trials have revealed that treatment of hypertension with antihypertensive medications reduces cardiovascular events, hypertension control to a BP <140/90 mm Hg is achieved in only 50% of the U.S. population.

## Consequences of Sustained Hypertension

### End-Organ Injury

Exposure to chronic BP elevation and, in some cases, to hypertensive emergency (defined as severely elevated BP with symptoms or signs of acute target-organ damage) can significantly injure multiple organs.

### Eye

Chronically elevated BP can lead to elevated arteriolar pressure, resulting in hypertensive retinopathy, which manifests as vasoconstriction and arteriolar narrowing (visualized as "arteriovenous nicking" or "copper wiring" on funduscopic examination), endothelial damage and retinal hemorrhage (or "flame hemorrhages"), and choroidopathy. Optic neuropathy may result from ischemia to the nerve fiber secondary to fibrinoid necrosis of vessels, manifesting as "cotton wool spots" or optic disc pallor.

Hypertensive emergency can lead to papilledema, resulting from leakage, ischemia, and fibrinoid necrosis of arterioles supplying the optic disc, causing optic nerve hemorrhage and swelling. Loss of visual acuity and blindness can occur.

## Medium to Large Vessels

Long-standing hypertension can damage the vascular endothelium and, combined with elevated cholesterol and especially in the presence of diabetes mellitus, lead to peripheral vascular disease, including aortic aneurysms.

Hypertensive emergency may cause aortic aneurysmal rupture or aortic wall dissection.

## Brain

Arteriosclerosis related to long-standing hypertension can cause distal ischemia, including transient ischemic attacks, lacunar infarctions, cerebrovascular accidents, and vascular neurocognitive disorder.

Hypertensive emergency has serious manifestations such as hemorrhagic stroke or subarachnoid hemorrhage from cerebral aneurysmal rupture, resulting in paralysis or fatality.

## Heart

Left ventricular hypertrophy can occur as a compensatory mechanism, resulting in diastolic dysfunction, and can eventually lead to heart failure.

Hypertensive emergency can lead to acute myocardial infarction.

## Kidney

Injury to the renal vasculature results in arteriosclerosis and atherosclerosis and, ultimately, hypertensive nephrosclerosis and chronic kidney disease (CKD). Hypertension is a major cause of CKD and end-stage kidney disease (ESKD), especially in black persons. Additionally, uncontrolled hypertension can increase the rate of CKD progression in patients with other underlying CKD causes, such as diabetic nephropathy.

Hypertensive emergency can cause acute kidney injury (AKI), with arteriolar proliferation (onion skinning), fibrinoid necrosis, and features of thrombotic microangiopathy.

## Clinical Impact

Hypertension is one of the most significant but modifiable risk factors for cardiovascular disease, stroke, ESKD, and overall mortality. Systolic is more important than diastolic BP as an independent risk factor for coronary events, heart failure, stroke, and ESKD. Data suggest that BP-related cardiovascular disease, kidney disease, and vascular death risk is evident before development of hypertension per se; risk increases progressively throughout ranges of BP that were previously recognized as normal and are now referred to as "elevated blood pressure." Therefore, a large proportion of the U.S. population has BP below the traditional threshold for pharmacologic treatment but high enough to signify future risk. Worldwide, approximately 50% of strokes and of ischemic heart disease events are attributable to high BP, equivalent to 7.6 million premature deaths (13.5% of total) and 92 million disability-adjusted life-years (6% of total).

**KEY POINTS**

- Chronic elevation of blood pressure can lead to significant injury in multiple organs, including the eyes, blood vessels, brain, heart, and kidneys; hypertensive emergency is defined as severely elevated blood pressure and acute target-organ damage.
- Worldwide, approximately 50% of strokes and of ischemic heart disease events are attributable to high blood pressure.

# Blood Pressure Measurement

## Proper Technique

Repeat BP determinations with proper technique are necessary before making clinical decisions regarding management. Smoking, caffeinated beverages, or exercise within 30 minutes before BP measurements should be avoided. A properly calibrated and validated instrument using the oscillometric method (manual or calibrated automated device) should be employed. The patient should be quietly seated in a chair for ≥5 minutes, with the back supported, feet on the floor, legs uncrossed, and the arm bared and supported on a flat surface, with the upper arm at the heart level. The cuff size should be appropriately chosen to ensure that the bladder encircles at least 80% of the upper arm. Two common reasons for an elevated BP office reading include using a cuff that is too small or measuring the BP before the patient has rested in a seated position. At least two measurements should be taken and averaged, about 2 minutes apart; the process should be repeated if the initial measurements differ by more than 5 mm Hg. Office BP measurement(s) and the expected BP target should be communicated to the patient orally and in writing to increase awareness and adherence.

## Auscultatory Blood Pressure Monitoring

The sphygmomanometer is placed on the arm with the lower cuff edge about 2 to 3 cm above the antecubital fossa. A stethoscope is placed over the brachial artery in the antecubital fossa. The cuff is inflated at least 30 mm Hg above the point at which the palpated brachial pulse disappears (estimated systolic BP). Systolic BP is recorded at the point at which the first sound is heard (or onset of the first Korotkoff sound), and diastolic BP is recorded at the point the sound disappears (or disappearance of all Korotkoff sounds).

## Electronic Blood Pressure Monitoring

Electronic devices use the same oscillometric method as manual cuffs and may reduce the inter-individual variability of manual measurements. However, proper calibration is essential for accurate measurements, especially if used by the patient at home. In general, electronic devices underestimate systolic BP and overestimate diastolic BP compared with intra-arterial measurements, which is more of a problem than with nonautomated devices.

## Ambulatory Blood Pressure Monitoring

Ambulatory blood pressure monitoring (ABPM) is an electronic BP measuring device that can be worn continuously for periods of 24 hours or longer and programmed to measure and record BP every 15 to 60 minutes during daytime wakefulness and nighttime sleep. Average 24-hour, daytime, and nighttime systolic and diastolic BP are also generally reported. Normal BP by ABPM includes a 24-hour average BP <115/75 mm Hg; daytime average BP <120/80 mm Hg; and nighttime average BP <100/65 mm Hg. ABPM provides valuable information supplementary to office BP in the evaluation of scenarios such as the following:

- Suspected white coat hypertension (BP measures higher in the office)
- Suspected masked hypertension (BP measures lower in the office)
- Suspected episodic hypertension
- Apparent treatment-resistant hypertension
- Hypotensive symptoms with antihypertensive medication treatment
- Autonomic dysfunction
- Possible nondipping (<10% nocturnal decrease in BP, which is associated with increased risk for cardiovascular events). Presence of nondipping can be evaluated in patients at high risk for future cardiovascular events, such as in those with CKD, diabetes with microvascular complications, and history of previous myocardial infarction or stroke.

ABPM is clinically helpful in these scenarios and is a better prognosticator of both end-organ damage (such as left ventricular hypertrophy) and hard outcomes (such as cardiovascular death) compared with office or home BP measurements.

## Home Blood Pressure Monitoring

Home BP monitoring refers to the measurement of BP at home by the patient, often by using an electronic BP device. Observational data show that home systolic and diastolic BP readings are more predictive of cardiovascular death than office readings, but less predictive than ABPM average readings. The advantage of home BP monitoring over ABPM is that home monitoring is more readily available, less expensive, and less time consuming in that the patient does not have to come to the office to have the device put on and then return the device after the 24-hour period of monitoring. In addition, home BP monitoring encourages patients to play an active role in their own BP management and be more aware of the need for adherence to lifestyle modifications and antihypertensive medications. However, unlike ABPM, which provides information regarding continuous BP measurements during awake and asleep periods as well as during ambulatory and exertion periods, home BP measurements can only be taken during awake hours and when the patient is at rest. Home BP monitoring can provide additional information ancillary to office BP in the following ways:

- Assess response to lifestyle modifications or treatment with antihypertensive medications
- Improve patient adherence
- Evaluate for white coat and masked hypertension

Several issues should be considered to ensure accuracy of home BP measurements. First, upper arm cuffs are preferred over newer devices that measure BP more distally, such as at the wrist, given that systolic BP is higher and diastolic lower in distal arteries, and finger measurements are generally not accurate. Second, education should be given regarding the proper use of the device, frequency and timing of measurements, and avoidance of self-adjustment of antihypertensive medications based on home BP. The patient should be instructed to sit in a comfortable position with legs uncrossed and back supported, and to place the left arm raised and supported to the level of the heart. The cuff should be wrapped snugly around the upper part of the bare arm, and BP should be measured after at least 5 minutes of rest. BP readings and times of measurement should be recorded and a running list brought to office visits for evaluation and to assist with hypertension management. The device should be brought to the office initially and periodically to validate accuracy of readings. Those with home self-measured BP averaging ≥130/80 mm Hg are considered hypertensive.

### KEY POINTS

- Repeat blood pressure measurements using proper technique are necessary before making clinical decisions regarding management.
- Ambulatory blood pressure monitoring can be used to evaluate for white coat, masked, episodic, or treatment-resistant hypertension; hypotensive symptoms with antihypertensive medication treatment; autonomic dysfunction; and dipping status.
- Home blood pressure monitoring can be used to assess response to lifestyle modifications or treatment, improve patient adherence, and evaluate for white coat or masked hypertension.

## Definitions

The 2017 high BP guideline from the American College of Cardiology (ACC), the American Heart Association (AHA), and nine other organizations provides new BP definitions and recommendations (http://hyper.ahajournals.org/). This guideline is an update to the Seventh Report of the Joint National Committee on Prevention, Detection, Evaluation, and Treatment of High Blood Pressure (JNC 7). The new definitions of BP are listed in **Table 11**.

**KEY POINT**

- According to the 2017 high blood pressure guideline from the American College of Cardiology, the American Heart Association, and nine other organizations, hypertension is defined as blood pressure ≥130/80 mm Hg.

## Screening and Diagnosis

The U.S. Preventive Services Task Force (USPSTF) recommends screening for hypertension in adults ≥18 years of age to identify those at increased risk for cardiovascular disease from hypertension and to begin early interventions to decrease this risk. Adults aged 18 to 39 years with a BP <130/85 mm Hg and without cardiovascular risk factors should be rescreened every 3 to 5 years. Those aged ≥40 years and persons at increased risk for hypertension (for example, those who have BP that is 130-139/85-89 mm Hg, are overweight, or are black) should be screened annually.

A diagnosis of hypertension (BP ≥130/80 mm Hg) should be based on an average of two or more elevated systolic and/or diastolic BP measurements obtained on two or more occasions. Out-of-office automated monitoring or self-monitoring of BP measurements is recommended to confirm hypertension diagnosis. Compared with a single measurement, multiple measurements over time have better positive predictive values for hypertension diagnosis. More recent evidence regarding the prevalence of white coat and masked hypertension suggests that confirmation of elevated BP with 24-hour ABPM (≥125/75 mm Hg) or self-measured home BP monitoring (≥130/80 mm Hg) may be prudent for hypertension diagnosis.

**KEY POINTS**

- The U.S. Preventive Services Task Force recommends screening for hypertension in adults ≥18 years of age to identify those at increased risk for cardiovascular disease from hypertension and to begin early interventions to decrease this risk.

- A diagnosis of hypertension should be based on an average of two or more elevated systolic and/or diastolic blood pressure measurements obtained on two or more occasions; obtaining measurements outside of the clinical setting for diagnostic confirmation is recommended before starting treatment.

HVC

## Evaluation of the Patient with Newly Diagnosed Hypertension

Initial evaluation of a patient with newly diagnosed hypertension includes a complete history, physical examination, and screening laboratory studies to address the following:

- Establish whether a familial pattern of hypertension is present.
- Rule out secondary, potentially reversible, causes.
- Identify and eliminate modifiable factors that can elevate BP.
- Assess for the presence of other cardiovascular risk factors.
- Assess for end-organ damage.
- Identify potential barriers to lifestyle modification for lowering BP.

### History

A complete history should be elicited to identify a personal history of the following: stroke or myocardial infarction, thyroid disease, kidney disease, obstructive sleep apnea, and additional cardiovascular risk factors. Family history should be explored for a genetic pattern of hypertension and premature history of cardiovascular disease.

A complete review of the systems is warranted, especially to elicit the presence of episodic palpitations, headaches, or

| TABLE 11. | Definitions of Blood Pressure for Adults | | |
|---|---|---|---|
| Definitions[a] | Office-Based Readings (mm Hg)[a] | 24-Hour Ambulatory Readings (mm Hg)[b] | Self-Recorded Readings (mm Hg)[b] |
| Normal | <120/80 | <115/75 | <120/80 |
| Elevated Blood Pressure | 120-129/<80 | — | — |
| Hypertension, Stage 1 | 130-139/80-89 | ≥125/75 | ≥130/80 |
| Hypertension, Stage 2 | ≥140/90 | ≥130/80 | ≥135/85 |
| White Coat Hypertension | ≥130/80 | <125/75 | <130/80 |
| Masked Hypertension | <130/80 | ≥125/75 | ≥130/80 |

[a]Based on Whelton PK, Carey RM, Aronow WS, Casey DE Jr, Collins KJ, Dennison Himmelfarb C, et al. 2017 ACC/AHA/AAPA/ABC/ACPM/AGS/APhA/ASH/ASPC/NMA/PCNA guideline for the prevention, detection, evaluation, and management of high blood pressure in adults: a report of the American College of Cardiology/American Heart Association Task Force on Clinical Practice Guidelines. J Am Coll Cardiol. 2018;71:e127-e248. [PMID: 29146535]

[b]The corresponding thresholds of 24-hour ambulatory and self-recorded home blood pressure readings are provided as a guide and should be interpreted with caution, given that they are based on European, Australian, and Asian populations, with few available data in U.S. populations.

sweating (which may suggest pheochromocytoma); visual changes (to assess end-organ damage); or gross hematuria (which may suggest underlying kidney glomerular disease). Behavioral and psychosocial contributors to hypertension should also be explored, including a sedentary routine, illicit drug use, excessive alcohol, tobacco smoking, high dietary sodium intake, and emotional stress.

A complete list of prescription and nonprescription medications, including complementary and alternative medications (herbals) and illicit drugs, is of utmost importance because many medications can result in reversible BP elevations (**Table 12**). If the patient is taking any drugs that may result in BP elevation, the drug should be discontinued and BP remeasured in 1 month.

### Physical Examination
Physical examination should focus on the following:

- Measure BP accurately in both arms.
- Measure body weight and calculate BMI to ascertain cardiovascular risk.
- Recognize target organ damage: eye examination (retinopathy or papilledema); volume status (elevated jugular venous pressure or lower extremity edema suggesting heart failure or CKD); peripheral vascular examination (unequal pulses in all extremities, carotid or abdominal bruits suggesting vascular disease); cardiac examination (laterally displaced point of maximal impulse or $S_4$ gallop suggestive of left ventricular hypertrophy).
- Identify abnormalities that suggest potential secondary causes (tachycardia for pheochromocytoma; abdominal bruit for renovascular hypertension; enlarged thyroid gland suggestive of thyroid disease; violaceous abdominal striae or "buffalo hump" fat pad suggesting Cushing syndrome).

### Testing
Initial testing is performed to identify common secondary causes, assess for other cardiovascular risk factors, and detect end-organ damage.

- Baseline electrocardiography (ECG) to assess for left ventricular hypertrophy (end-organ damage) or previous silent myocardial infarction.
- Blood laboratory studies: complete blood count, serum creatinine, estimated glomerular filtration rate (GFR), serum sodium, potassium, calcium, bicarbonate, fasting glucose, lipid panel, thyroid-stimulating hormone.
- Urinalysis with microscopic examination; in addition, urine albumin-creatinine ratio in patients with diabetes mellitus and in those with a high clinical suspicion for underlying CKD, such as a positive family history or presence of other end-organ damage (left ventricular hypertrophy on ECG).

**TABLE 12. Drugs That Can Raise Blood Pressure**

| Drug/Drug Class | Potential Mechanisms |
|---|---|
| **Prescription Drugs** | |
| Antidepressants: monoamine oxidase inhibitors; selective serotonin reuptake inhibitors; serotonin-norepinephrine reuptake inhibitors | Adrenergic stimulation |
| Calcineurin inhibitors: cyclosporine A; tacrolimus | Vasoconstriction; sympathetic excitation; sodium retention |
| Contraceptives: estrogens; progesterones | Sodium retention; increased renin-angiotensin system activity |
| Glucocorticoids | Sodium retention; weight gain |
| Erythropoietin-stimulating agents | Vasoconstriction |
| NSAIDs | Sodium retention |
| Sympathomimetics (methylphenidate) | Adrenergic stimulation |
| Vascular endothelial growth factor antagonists | Endothelial dysfunction; vasoconstriction |
| **Nonprescription Drugs** | |
| Anabolic steroids | Sodium retention |
| Caffeine | Adrenergic stimulation |
| Ethanol | Adrenergic stimulation |
| Glycyrrhizic acid (in some licorice, cough drops, chewing tobacco) | Mineralocorticoid activity; sodium retention |
| Herbal supplements: ephedra; 1,3-dimethylamine; synephrine; N-methylamine; Citrus aurantium; Caulophyllum thalictroides | Sympathomimetic |
| Illicit drugs: amphetamines; cocaine; 3,4-methylenedioxymethamphetamine (ecstasy) | Sympathomimetic |
| NSAIDs | Sodium retention |
| Sympathomimetic nonprescription drugs: decongestants (phenylephrine, pseudoephedrine); appetite suppressants; vigilance enhancers | Sympathomimetic |

- Echocardiography is not routinely recommended but may be helpful in suspected white coat hypertension in which presence of left ventricular hypertrophy would necessitate treatment with antihypertensive medication, even in the absence of elevated home BP. Echocardiography may also be used to detect hypertrophy in the presence of left bundle branch block on ECG or to assess baseline wall function in persons with a known history of ischemic heart disease.

More extensive diagnostic testing can be pursued if the history, physical examination, or initial testing raises suspicion for secondary causes (**Table 13**).

**KEY POINTS**

- Initial evaluation of patients with newly diagnosed hypertension includes a complete history, physical examination, and screening laboratory studies to assess for a familial pattern, secondary causes, other cardiovascular risk factors, end-organ damage, and modifiable lifestyle factors.
- Baseline electrocardiography is appropriate for all patients with newly diagnosed hypertension.

# Primary Hypertension
## Pathogenesis

Ninety percent of patients with hypertension are identified as having primary (essential) hypertension, in which no secondary underlying etiology can be found. The pathogenesis is still not completely understood, but potential mechanisms include abnormal kidney sodium handling, increased activity of the renin-angiotensin system, and elevated sympathetic tone.

In general, hypertension is a complex polygenic disorder in which many genes or combinations may influence BP. Many genetic variants affect the distal tubular sodium transport and may result in excess sodium retention, leading to hypertension. Genetic polymorphisms involving oxidative stress, mediators of vascular smooth muscle tone, and vasoactive mechanisms have also been implicated. However, associated genetic variants have only small effects, such that the collective effect of all identified BP loci account for only about 3.5% of BP variability. Monogenic forms, in which single gene mutations explain the underlying pathophysiology of hypertension, are less common and include such diseases as glucocorticoid-remediable aldosteronism, Liddle disease, and Gordon syndrome.

**TABLE 13.** Secondary Causes of Hypertension

| Underlying Cause | Diagnostic Testing |
|---|---|
| Kidney disease | Serum creatinine; estimated glomerular filtration rate; urinalysis with microscopic examination; urine albumin-creatinine ratio; kidney ultrasonography |
| Renovascular disease | Renal duplex Doppler ultrasonography; CT or MR angiography; renal artery angiography |
| Obstructive sleep apnea | Polysomnography |
| Pheochromocytoma | Plasma fractionated metanephrines; 24-hour urine metanephrines and catecholamines |
| Hypo- or hyperthyroidism | Thyroid-stimulating hormone; free thyroxine |
| Primary hyperparathyroidism | Intact parathyroid hormone; serum calcium and phosphorus |
| Gordon syndrome (pseudohypoaldosteronism type II) | Clinical diagnosis; family history; aldosterone and renin levels; electrolytes |
| Aortic coarctation | Blood pressure measurements in arms and legs; CT or MR angiography; transthoracic echocardiography |

| Conditions Associated with Hypokalemia | Diagnostic Testing |
|---|---|
| High aldosterone conditions:<br><br>Primary hyperaldosteronism: adrenal adenoma (rarely carcinoma or ectopic); bilateral adrenal hyperplasia<br><br>Familial hyperaldosteronism type I (glucocorticoid-remediable aldosteronism; >50% normokalemic), type II, or type III<br><br>Secondary hyperaldosteronism: renal artery stenosis; renin-secreting tumor | Serum sodium and potassium concentrations; plasma aldosterone concentration/plasma renin activity ratio; saline suppression test; CT imaging; adrenal vein sampling; genetic testing |
| Cushing syndrome | Dexamethasone suppression test; 24-hour urine cortisol excretion; salivary cortisol |
| Congenital adrenal hyperplasia | Clinical diagnosis |
| Apparent mineralocorticoid excess | Clinical diagnosis; aldosterone and renin levels; electrolytes |
| Liddle syndrome | Clinical diagnosis; family history; aldosterone and renin levels; electrolytes |

Dietary factors have been implicated as contributors to hypertension development. Populations with low sodium intake have lower BP than those with high intake. Habitual high sodium intake along with low potassium intake seen in a modern diet is a critical factor contributing to the worldwide high prevalence of hypertension. This is especially true for those with salt sensitivity, common in black patients, older adults, and those with CKD or diabetes mellitus, in which an increase in sodium intake leads to a disproportionate increase in BP.

Positive correlations are also found between BP and physical inactivity, being overweight or obese, excess alcohol intake, hyperuricemia, and insulin resistance.

**KEY POINT**

- Habitual high sodium intake along with low potassium intake is a critical factor contributing to the worldwide high prevalence of hypertension.

## Management
### General Approach
Treatment recommendations for specific populations are elaborated upon in their respective sections. Importantly, consideration must be given to individual patient characteristics and circumstances to tailor management.

The 2017 ACC/AHA BP guideline provides treatment recommendations, including the following:

- Nonpharmacologic therapy is recommended for those with elevated BP (systolic BP between 120-129 mm Hg and diastolic BP <80 mm Hg) or stage 1 hypertension (systolic BP between 130-139 mm Hg or diastolic BP between 80-89 mm Hg) and a 10-year cardiovascular risk of <10%.

- Nonpharmacologic and drug treatment is recommended for those with BP ≥130/80 mm Hg and clinical cardiovascular disease or a 10-year cardiovascular risk ≥10% to a BP goal of <130/80 mm Hg.

- Nonpharmacologic and drug treatment is recommended for those with no cardiovascular disease and a 10-year cardiovascular risk of <10% for stage 2 hypertension (≥140/90 mm Hg).

- Adults with stage 2 hypertension and an average BP that is 20/10 mm Hg above their BP target should be treated with a combination of two first-line antihypertensive drugs of different classes.

- The target systolic BP goal for noninstitutionalized, ambulatory community-dwelling patients who are ≥65 years of age is <130 mm Hg.

- The target BP for patients with hypertension and diabetes mellitus is <130/80 mm Hg.

- The target BP for patients with hypertension and CKD is <130/80 mm Hg.

### Lifestyle Modifications
Lifestyle modifications and cardiovascular risk factors should be addressed in all patients with elevated BP or hypertension, even if pharmacologic treatment is necessary. Several nonpharmacologic interventions have been shown to have efficacy in reducing BP (**Table 14**). The best evidence for BP-lowering effects in individuals with elevated BP or hypertension exists for weight loss, the Dietary Approaches to Stop Hypertension (DASH) diet, and dietary sodium reduction. Of the lifestyle interventions tested in clinical trials, weight reduction was most efficacious, followed by sodium reduction. Although difficult to achieve, a combination of lifestyle modifications (such as DASH combined with a low sodium diet alone or in combination with weight loss) had BP-lowering effects greater than or equal to those of single-drug therapy in hypertensive patients. Other nonpharmacologic interventions supported by evidence include potassium supplementation (preferably in dietary modification), increased physical activity, and moderation in alcohol consumption. Controlled trials of an increase in magnesium or calcium intake revealed less robust BP-lowering effects. Regardless of BP effects, tobacco cessation should be encouraged given that smoking is a significant risk factor for cardiovascular disease.

Based on the level of evidence for behavioral therapies, transcendental meditation, yoga, and biofeedback had modest, mixed, or no consistent BP-lowering effects. More data

**TABLE 14.** Efficacy of Lifestyle Modifications for Reducing Blood Pressure

| Approach | Recommendation | Effect on Systolic Blood Pressure |
|---|---|---|
| Reduce weight | BMI <25 | 5 to 10 mm Hg reduction per 10-kg (22-lb) weight loss |
| Reduce dietary sodium | 1500 to 2400 mg/d | 2 to 8 mm Hg reduction |
| Consume DASH (Dietary Approaches to Stop Hypertension) diet | Fruits; vegetables; low-fat dairy; whole grains; legumes; low saturated fat and sodium; high potassium, magnesium, and calcium | 8 to 14 mm Hg reduction |
| Increase potassium intake | 4700 mg/d | Variable reductions |
| Moderate alcohol consumption | Men: ≤2 drinks per day; women: ≤1 drink per day | 2 to 4 mm Hg reduction |
| Exercise | 30 min/d, most days (not consistently independent of weight loss) | 4 to 9 mm Hg reduction |
| Alternative approaches | Device-guided breathing; yoga; meditation; biofeedback; acupuncture | Variable reductions |

support efficacy of device-guided breathing than acupuncture among the noninvasive procedures and devices that were evaluated.

It is imperative to tailor lifestyle modifications to the individual patient while considering patient needs, patient support systems and resources, and readiness for behavioral change.

- The 2017 high blood pressure guideline from the American College of Cardiology, the American Heart Association, and nine other organizations recommends a blood pressure goal of <130/80 mm Hg in most adult patient populations.

- Lifestyle modifications (weight loss, diet, dietary sodium reduction) and cardiovascular risk factors should be addressed in all patients with elevated blood pressure and hypertension.

## Pharmacologic Therapy

Clinical trials data suggest that antihypertensive medication therapy can be associated with up to a 40% reduction in stroke, 25% reduction in myocardial infarction, and 50% reduction in heart failure. In addition to lifestyle modification, treatment with antihypertensive medications should be initiated in patients with stage 1 hypertension and clinical cardiovascular disease or a 10-year cardiovascular risk ≥10% and in all patients with stage 2 hypertension.

Clinical trial evidence reveals that lowering BP is more important than the class of antihypertensive drug used to achieve control. Head-to-head trials of antihypertensive medications revealed comparable effects on cardiovascular outcomes, except that for preventing heart failure, initial therapy with a thiazide diuretic was more effective than a calcium channel blocker (CCB) or ACE inhibitor, and an ACE inhibitor was more effective than a CCB. The primary agents recommended are those that were shown to reduce clinical events and include a thiazide diuretic, CCB, ACE inhibitor, or angiotensin receptor blocker (ARB) for hypertension in the general nonblack population, including those with diabetes. In black patients, initial antihypertensive therapy should include a thiazide diuretic or a CCB (see Specific Populations, Black Patients).

There are not enough good quality head-to-head randomized trials comparing other antihypertensive classes (β-blockers, central- or peripheral-acting α-blockers, vasodilators, aldosterone receptor antagonists, or loop diuretics) to the four drug classes mentioned. Therefore, these drug classes are not recommended as first-line therapy but can be used in specific populations (β-blockers for post–myocardial infarction or heart failure; aldosterone receptor blockers for heart failure; loop diuretics for advanced CKD) or as add-on therapy for resistant hypertension.

See **Table 15** for more information on frequently used antihypertensive medications.

### Diuretics

Initial antihypertensive treatment may include thiazide diuretics, which act by inhibiting the sodium-chloride-cotransporter in the distal renal tubule. Although hydrochlorothiazide is the most commonly used thiazide diuretic, chlorthalidone is

**TABLE 15.** Frequently Used Antihypertensive Medications

| Class/Agent | Common Side Effects/Contraindications |
|---|---|
| Thiazide diuretics (e.g., hydrochlorothiazide; chlorthalidone) | Hypokalemia; hyponatremia; hyperlipidemia; hyperuricemia; hyperglycemia. Avoid in gout unless patient is on urate-lowering therapy. |
| ACE inhibitors (e.g., captopril; lisinopril; enalapril; benazepril) | Hyperkalemia; cough. Avoid use with angiotensin receptor blockers or direct renin inhibitors. Avoid in pregnancy. |
| Angiotensin receptor blockers (e.g., candesartan; losartan; valsartan; irbesartan) | Hyperkalemia. Avoid use with ACE inhibitors or direct renin inhibitors. Avoid in pregnancy. |
| Calcium channel blockers | |
| Dihydropyridines (e.g., amlodipine; felodipine; nifedipine) | Pedal edema; headache; flushing. |
| Non-dihydropyridines (e.g., diltiazem; verapamil) | Constipation. Avoid in HFrEF. Avoid routine use with β-blockers (heart block, bradycardia). Drug interactions (*CYP3A4* major substrate and moderate inhibitor). |
| β-Blockers (e.g., atenolol; metoprolol tartrate; metoprolol succinate; labetalol) | Fatigue; bronchospasm; sexual dysfunction; hyperglycemia. |
| Potassium channel openers (vasodilators) (e.g., hydralazine; minoxidil) | Edema. Hydralazine: lupus-like syndrome. Minoxidil: hypertrichosis. |
| α-Blockers (e.g., prazosin) | Orthostatic hypotension; dizziness. |
| Central α-agonists (e.g., clonidine, oral or patch) | Fatigue; depression; rebound hypertension. |
| Potassium-sparing diuretics (e.g., spironolactone; amiloride; eplerenone) | Hyperkalemia. Avoid if GFR <45 mL/min/1.73 m$^2$. Spironolactone: gynecomastia. |

GFR = glomerular filtration rate; HFrEF = heart failure with reduced ejection fraction.

preferred due to a prolonged half-life, which allows once-daily dosing, and evidence from trials demonstrating efficacy in reducing cardiovascular events. Loop diuretics are preferred in patients with symptomatic heart failure or CKD with an estimated GFR <30 mL/min/1.73 m$^2$ (see Kidney Disease, Management).

Suboptimal BP therapy in patients with difficult-to-control hypertension is frequently the result of not including a diuretic medication, which ensures that extracellular volume expansion is prevented or treated. This is particularly important in sodium-retentive, edematous conditions such as heart failure, liver cirrhosis, or CKD. Even in the absence of edematous conditions, persistent intravascular volume expansion without apparent edema can still contribute to hypertension that appears resistant to treatment. In addition, diuretic medication should be prescribed in adequate doses, with dosing frequency tailored appropriately to the diuretic half-life. For example, loop diuretics such as furosemide should be dosed at least twice to three times daily, and higher doses should be used in patients with low GFR.

Potassium-sparing diuretics, such as aldosterone receptor antagonists (spironolactone or eplerenone) or epithelial sodium channel blockers (amiloride), are weaker diuretics. These are often used in liver cirrhosis, heart failure, or resistant hypertension. Caution and close monitoring are advised when these medications are prescribed concomitantly with other drug classes that also raise the serum potassium, such as ACE inhibitors, ARBs, or direct renin inhibitors, and in patients with reduced GFR.

### Calcium Channel Blockers

There are two classes of CCBs: dihydropyridines (amlodipine, felodipine, nifedipine) and nondihydropyridines (diltiazem, verapamil). No data support the use of one class over the other for hypertension management, although long-acting dihydropyridines are usually chosen. Nondihydropyridines have more pronounced cardiac effects such as diminished cardiac contractility (negative inotropy) and atrioventricular nodal blockade, and caution should be taken in prescribing these medications concomitantly with β-blockers or in patients with heart failure with severely reduced ejection fraction, sick sinus syndrome, or second- or third-degree atrioventricular block. Additionally, short-acting nifedipine was associated with mortality if used immediately after acute myocardial infarction due to profound hypotension and sympathetic activation. Finally, there may be an increased risk for myopathy if a CCB (especially nondihydropyridines) is used concomitantly with a high-dose statin.

### Renin-Angiotensin System Agents

Renin-angiotensin system (RAS) agents are ACE inhibitors, ARBs, and direct renin inhibitors (such as aliskiren). Clinical trials reported similar efficacy of ACE inhibitors and ARBs on reducing BP, progression of albuminuria and CKD, and risk for cardiovascular events. Therefore, neither agent is preferred over the other.

Dry cough is a side effect of ACE inhibitors but is generally not reported with ARBs. Angioedema, a life-threatening condition, is a complication of both ACE inhibitors and renin inhibitors. Patients with a compelling indication for RAS inhibition who develop angioedema can be treated with an ARB with very careful monitoring, given a low but possible risk for occurrence. There are less outcomes data on the effects of aliskiren, although similar BP-lowering effect is expected. RAS agents should not be used in combination, and they are contraindicated in pregnancy.

### Combination Therapy

Combination therapy with more than one drug class (separately or as a single-dose pill) may be necessary to control BP. The 2017 ACC/AHA BP guideline recommends combination therapy with two first-line antihypertensive drugs of different classes for adults with stage 2 hypertension and an average BP of 20/10 mm Hg above their BP target (typically ≥150/90 mm Hg). There are no definitive recommendations for best drug combinations, but some data suggest an ACE inhibitor/CCB combination may be more efficacious than an ACE inhibitor/thiazide diuretic combination. Using a thiazide diuretic/CCB combination is also an option.

Combined use of any RAS drug classes (ACE inhibitors, ARBs, and direct renin inhibitors) is not recommended; several clinical trials (ONTARGET, NEPHRON-D, ALTITUDE) have revealed more adverse events with these combinations (hyperkalemia, hypotension, AKI), without additional cardiovascular or renal benefits.

## Assessment of Efficacy and Medication Titration

Adherence and response to treatment should be assessed 4 weeks after treatment initiation or sooner, based on the urgency for BP lowering. Further assessments are necessitated until target is achieved. Three strategies are possible for dose titration:

1. Maximize the first medication dose before adding a second.

2. Add a second medication before reaching the maximum dose of the first.

3. Start with two medication classes separately or as fixed-dose combinations.

There are no randomized controlled trials comparing these strategies; therefore, the strategy should be tailored to the individual patient, dose-related side effects, and adherence patterns. Generally, there is diminishing return in BP lowering if dose is titrated up from 50% to 100% of maximum. Also, it is unlikely that increasing the dose from 50% to 100% of maximum will result in an additional >5 mm Hg BP reduction; an additional agent may therefore need to be added. Finally, titration to maximum doses may more commonly result in side effects and reduce adherence.

- In addition to lifestyle modification, pharmacologic therapy should be initiated in patients with stage 1 hypertension and clinical cardiovascular disease or a 10-year cardiovascular risk ≥10% and in all patients with stage 2 hypertension.
- A thiazide diuretic, calcium channel blocker, ACE inhibitor, or angiotensin receptor blocker is recommended as initial therapy for hypertension in the general nonblack population, including those with diabetes mellitus.
- Combination therapy with two first-line antihypertensive drugs of different classes is recommended for adults with stage 2 hypertension and an average blood pressure (BP) that is 20/10 mm Hg above their BP target.

# White Coat Hypertension

White coat hypertension refers to elevated BP measured in the office, but out-of-office BP averages that are not elevated (see Table 11). In adults with untreated systolic BP >130 mm Hg but <160 mm Hg or diastolic BP >80 mm Hg but <100 mm Hg, it is reasonable to screen for white coat hypertension using either daytime ABPM or home BP monitoring. Before white coat hypertension is diagnosed, the reliability of out-of-office measurements must be confirmed; for example, the patient's home BP monitor should be calibrated against the office sphygmomanometer or, preferably, BP should be measured by ABPM.

The prevalence of white coat hypertension is approximately 13% and as high as 35% in some hypertensive populations. The risk for conversion of white coat hypertension to sustained hypertension is estimated to be about 1% to 5% per year by ABPM or home BP monitoring. Incidence of conversion is higher with older age, obesity, or black race. Additionally, such patients may have a slightly higher cardiovascular risk compared with normotensive patients, but a lower risk than in those with masked or sustained hypertension. Optimal management of such patients is uncertain. A 3-month trial of lifestyle modifications is suggested in those with suspected white coat hypertension. If this does not result in a decrease of daytime ABPM or home BP to <130/80 mm Hg, then initiation of an antihypertensive drug should be considered. Screening echocardiography may also be considered to evaluate for left ventricular hypertrophy, the presence of which necessitates treatment with antihypertensives.

- Lifestyle modifications and careful monitoring should be considered for patients with white coat hypertension due to increased risk for future development of hypertension and slightly higher cardiovascular risk compared with normotensive patients.

# Masked Hypertension

Masked hypertension is defined as BP that is normal in the office but elevated in the ambulatory setting (see Table 11). It is associated with an increased prevalence of target organ damage and risk of cardiovascular disease, stroke, and mortality compared with normotension. In adults with elevated office BP (120-129/<80 mm Hg) but not meeting the criteria for hypertension or with end-organ damage such as left ventricular hypertrophy, screening for masked hypertension with daytime ABPM or home BP is reasonable.

The prevalence of masked hypertension varies from 10% to 26% in population-based surveys and from 14% to 30% in normotensive clinic populations. A 3-month trial of lifestyle modifications should be considered in suspected cases of masked hypertension. Antihypertensive treatment should be initiated if daytime ABPM or home BP is still ≥130/80 mm Hg.

- Masked hypertension is associated with an increased risk for sustained hypertension and cardiovascular disease; after a 3-month trial of lifestyle modifications, antihypertensive medication should be initiated if daytime ambulatory or home blood pressure is still ≥130/80 mm Hg.

# Resistant Hypertension

Resistant hypertension is defined as BP that remains above goal despite concurrent use of three antihypertensive agents of different classes, or BP at goal but requiring four or more medications. One of these medications must be a diuretic to make the diagnosis. A prevalence of 2% to 10% is reported in the general population, but can be as high as 40% in patients with CKD. Risk factors include older age, male sex, black race, diabetes, and higher BMI.

Before the diagnosis is made, a systematic approach to BP control should include ensuring accuracy of BP readings, optimizing medication selection and dosing, and addressing potential secondary and reversible causes of hypertension. The importance of out-of-office BP measurements (home or ABPM) as a part of evaluation to rule out white coat hypertension and to confirm resistance is increasingly recognized. Behaviors that could lead to high BP, including excessive sodium consumption, should be reviewed, and use of recreational drugs and prescription or nonprescription medications (such as complementary and alternative medications) that may exacerbate hypertension should be excluded. Adherence to antihypertensive medications, including correct frequency and dosage, should be confirmed, and potential reasons for nonadherence, such as medication side effects, should be addressed.

The cornerstone of management includes a low sodium diet and treatment with an appropriate diuretic with attention to dosage and dosing frequency (see Diuretics). Patients should be treated with a combination of medications from different classes: a RAS blocker (either an ACE inhibitor, an ARB, or a direct renin inhibitor), a calcium antagonist, a diuretic, and possibly a β-blocker. Recent trials support the efficacy of adding a low-dose aldosterone receptor antagonist (spironolactone or eplerenone) for treatment of resistant hypertension. If additional agents are needed for BP control or the patient is intolerant of the aforementioned agents, then vasodilators (hydralazine or minoxidil), α-blockers (doxazosin, prazosin) or central sympathetic agonists (clonidine) can be added.

### KEY POINTS

- Resistant hypertension is defined as blood pressure (BP) that remains above goal despite the concurrent use of three antihypertensive agents of different classes, or BP at goal but requires four or more medications; one of the medications must be a diuretic to make the diagnosis.

- Management of resistant hypertension includes accurate out-of-office blood pressure (BP) measurement, addressing behaviors that contribute to high BP, avoiding drugs that exacerbate hypertension, reducing dietary sodium, and ensuring appropriate diuretic dose and frequency.

## Secondary Hypertension

In about 10% of adults with hypertension, a specific and remediable cause can be identified for hypertension. Diagnostic testing for secondary causes of hypertension can be pursued if a high clinical suspicion exists following history, physical examination, and initial laboratory testing (see Table 13). Factors that raise pretest probability for secondary hypertension include hypertension onset at <30 years of age, abrupt-onset or worsening BP if previously well controlled, drug resistance, clinical features indicating a secondary process, presence of target organ damage disproportionate to hypertension duration or severity, diastolic hypertension onset in those aged ≥65 years, and unprovoked or excessive hypokalemia.

### Kidney Disease
#### Pathophysiology and Epidemiology
Hypertension develops in the setting of both AKI and CKD. Underlying parenchymal kidney disease is an important cause of hypertension, and up to 85% of patients with CKD have high BP. Hypertension prevalence increases with GFR decline. Additionally, chronic uncontrolled hypertension is a leading cause of CKD and of CKD progression to ESKD. BP elevation in glomerular disease is primarily attributed to fluid overload, as evidenced by suppression of the RAS and increased release of atrial natriuretic peptide. In acute vascular diseases affecting the kidney (vasculitis or scleroderma renal crisis), elevated BP is thought to result from ischemia-induced activation of the RAS. Endothelial vascular injury, increased sympathetic tone, and impaired nitric oxide synthesis are also implicated.

### Clinical Manifestations
Underlying kidney disease is suggested by an elevated serum creatinine concentration and/or an abnormal urinalysis or albuminuria. Patients can present with other evidence of hypertension end-organ damage (such as left ventricular hypertrophy) and edema, but the absence of either does not exclude kidney disease as hypertension etiology.

### Diagnosis
Initial evaluation of hypertension in all patients includes assessment of serum creatinine and estimated GFR, urinalysis with microscopic examination to exclude hematuria and/or proteinuria, and urine albumin-creatinine ratio in those with diabetes mellitus or family history of kidney disease. Abnormalities in any of these tests can signify underlying kidney disease. In those with a normal serum creatinine but a high suspicion for certain kidney diseases, such as a positive family history of autosomal dominant polycystic disease, kidney ultrasonography can be undertaken.

### Management
The 2017 ACC/AHA BP guideline recommends a BP target of <130/80 mm Hg for patients with hypertension and CKD. An ACE inhibitor or an ARB is a preferred drug for treatment of hypertension for patients with stage G3 CKD or higher or for those with stage G1 or G2 CKD with albuminuria (albumin-creatinine ratio ≥300 mg/g).

Kidney function and serum potassium should be reassessed 2 to 3 weeks after medication initiation. An increase in serum creatinine of 25% to 30% is acceptable, but the dose may need to be lowered or medication discontinued if more severe decline in kidney function is observed; in such cases, bilateral renovascular disease should also be considered.

Given that sodium retention and volume overload are major contributory factors in the hypertension of CKD, dietary sodium restriction to <2000 mg/d and addition of a diuretic are both essential for control of BP, especially in advanced CKD. The following factors addressing appropriate dose and dosing interval for diuretics should be considered:

- Higher doses of diuretics are required in patients with CKD due to decreased GFR.

- Thiazide diuretics may be less effective if the estimated GFR is <30 mL/min/1.73 m$^2$; although there are no head-to-head trials, it seems preferable to use chlorthalidone instead of hydrochlorothiazide in patients with CKD due to a longer half-life.

- For an estimated GFR <20 to 30 mL/min/1.73 m$^2$, a loop diuretic can be used effectively, with more frequent dosing interval (for example, furosemide should be dosed at least two to three times daily).

- The combination of a thiazide and a loop diuretic can be used to augment diuresis, with careful monitoring.

- Volume overload refractory to medical management in those with stage G5 CKD (estimated GFR <15 mL/min/1.73 m$^2$) may necessitate dialysis.

## Renovascular Hypertension

### Pathophysiology and Epidemiology

Prevalence of renovascular hypertension is higher in white than black populations. Pathogenesis involves renal hypoperfusion as a result of renal artery stenosis, with subsequent release of renin and angiotensin resulting in systemic vasoconstriction, sodium retention, and hypertension. Disease can be unilateral or bilateral. Parenchymal kidney damage with loss of kidney function can occur.

There are two types of renovascular disease: (1) atherosclerotic renovascular disease, which usually occurs in patients >45 years of age, especially in those with diffuse atherosclerosis, but can also be isolated to the kidney; and (2) fibromuscular dysplasia, a nonatherosclerotic disorder that usually affects the mid and distal portions of the renal artery and usually occurs in young persons, particularly women.

### Clinical Manifestations

Patients with atherosclerotic renovascular disease often have other manifestations of atherosclerosis, including the presence of coronary artery, cerebrovascular, or peripheral vascular disease. Bruits may be auscultated, especially a systolic-diastolic abdominal bruit that lateralizes to one side. Clinical suspicion should be high in patients who present with onset of severe hypertension after age 55 years, recurrent flash pulmonary edema, refractory heart failure, AKI after initiation of an ACE inhibitor/ARB, or AKI after control of BP to target. Asymmetry in kidney sizes of >1.5 cm on imaging or the presence of a unilateral small kidney ≤9 cm also increases likelihood of renovascular disease.

Abrupt onset of hypertension at an age <35 years suggests fibromuscular dysplasia.

### Diagnosis

Routine testing for renovascular disease may not change management because recent data suggest that medical therapy may be as beneficial as invasive procedures, especially for those with atherosclerotic renovascular disease. However, in young patients with resistant hypertension and a high clinical suspicion for fibromuscular dysplasia, renal artery imaging may be considered. Plasma renin activity, captopril renal scintigraphy, and selective renal vein renin measurements are no longer recommended as diagnostic tests given the availability of more sensitive and specific imaging tests.

Renal duplex Doppler ultrasonography is a reasonable imaging modality if performed by experienced sonographers. MR or CT angiography have higher diagnostic utility but are potentially harmful in patients with severe CKD given the risk for contrast nephropathy and gadolinium-induced nephrogenic systemic fibrosis. A stenosis >75% in one or both renal arteries or >50% with post-stenotic dilatation suggests the diagnosis. Renal intra-arterial angiography is the gold standard and can be considered if other noninvasive tests are negative, clinical suspicion is high, and an invasive procedure is being considered. It is not recommended as a routine test due to adverse risks, such as contrast nephropathy and cholesterol emboli.

### Management

Three large randomized trials (STAR, ASTRAL, and CORAL) failed to show that renal artery angioplasty confers additional benefit above optimal medical therapy in patients with atherosclerotic renovascular disease and stable kidney function. Medical therapy in those suspected of having atherosclerotic renovascular disease includes treatment of underlying cardiovascular risk factors (such as hypercholesterolemia) and an ACE inhibitor or ARB. Patients who may benefit from percutaneous angioplasty and stenting or surgical intervention include those who present with a short hypertension duration; are refractory to medical therapy; have severe hypertension or recurrent acute flash pulmonary edema; have AKI following treatment with an ACE inhibitor or ARB; or have progressive impaired kidney function thought to result from bilateral renovascular disease or unilateral stenosis affecting a solitary functioning kidney. Patients with advanced CKD or with proteinuria >1000 mg/24 h are less likely to benefit from revascularization.

In young persons with fibromuscular dysplasia, studies have suggested that angioplasty alone may improve BP and even cure hypertension.

## Primary Hyperaldosteronism

A triad of resistant hypertension, metabolic alkalosis, and hypokalemia (including in patients treated with low-dose thiazide diuretics) should raise suspicion for primary aldosteronism (see Table 13). Primary hyperaldosteronism, in which aldosterone production cannot be suppressed with sodium loading, is the most common cause of secondary hypertension in middle-aged adults and an important cause of resistant hypertension. Screening for primary hyperaldosteronism is recommended if any of the following are present: resistant hypertension, hypokalemia (spontaneous or substantial, if diuretic induced), incidentally discovered adrenal mass, family history of early-onset hypertension, or stroke at age <40 years. Calculation of plasma aldosterone concentration (PAC)/plasma renin activity (PRA) ratio is used for screening, with a very high ratio of PAC/PRA suggestive of the diagnosis. Confirmatory diagnostic testing is needed with a saline suppression test.

PAC and PRA are usually suppressed in other disorders with hypokalemia and hypertension, including Cushing syndrome, syndrome of apparent mineralocorticoid excess, familial hyperaldosteronism type I (glucocorticoid-remediable aldosteronism), and Liddle syndrome (see Table 13). Renal artery stenosis and renin-secreting tumors generate high PRA and, therefore, lower PAC, with subsequent lowering of the PAC/PRA ratio, to usually <10. See MKSAP 18 Endocrinology and Metabolism for details.

## Pheochromocytomas

Pheochromocytomas are rare catecholamine-secreting neoplasms of the adrenal medulla or sympathetic ganglia that occur in <0.2% of patients with hypertension. Presence of the

CONT.

following characteristics raises clinical suspicion and may prompt testing: resistant hypertension; hypertension onset that is new or at a young age; paroxysmal hypertension; episodic tachycardia, headaches, and sweating; history of familial syndromes; adrenal adenoma found incidentally on imaging with or without hypertension; or pressor response during invasive procedures or anesthesia. Diagnostic tests include plasma fractionated metanephrines and 24-hour urine metanephrines and catecholamines. Positive test results should be followed by imaging to locate the tumor. Definitive treatment is surgical resection. See MKSAP 18 Endocrinology and Metabolism for details.

**KEY POINTS**

- The 2017 high blood pressure guideline from the American College of Cardiology, the American Heart Association, and nine other organizations recommends a target blood pressure of <130/80 mm Hg in patients with hypertension and chronic kidney disease.

- Treatment of hypertension in patients with chronic kidney disease includes an ACE inhibitor or angiotensin receptor blocker, dietary sodium restriction to <2000 mg/d, and addition of a diuretic as needed to control intravascular volume.

- Medical therapy for renovascular disease, including treatment of underlying cardiovascular risk factors and use of an ACE inhibitor or angiotensin receptor blocker, may be as beneficial as invasive procedures.

- Primary hyperaldosteronism is the most common cause of secondary hypertension in middle-aged adults and an important cause of resistant hypertension; the plasma aldosterone concentration/plasma renin activity ratio is used for screening.

## Hypertensive Urgency

Hypertensive urgency is defined as severely elevated BP—often a systolic BP ≥180 mm Hg and/or diastolic BP ≥110 mm Hg—in a patient without obvious signs or symptoms of acute or impending change in target organ damage or dysfunction. Patients are often asymptomatic or present with a mild headache in an ambulatory setting. The most important aspect of initial management is a focused history and physical examination to exclude the presence of acute end-organ damage in the setting of severely elevated BP, which would raise concern for hypertensive emergency. Referral to an emergency department may be required for further diagnostic testing to rule out target organ damage. See MKSAP 18 Pulmonary and Critical Care Medicine for information on hypertensive emergencies.

Management is very challenging and includes the assessment of imminent risk of cardiovascular events from severe hypertension versus risk of adverse sequelae from rapid BP reduction. These may include AKI, myocardial infarction, or

stroke resulting from decreased perfusion to organs and limited time for autoregulation to maintain perfusion. Therefore, recommendations regarding the rapidity of BP lowering in this setting are controversial and not based on strong evidence. Generally, systolic BP may be lowered in patients with imminent risk of target organ damage but without a compelling condition (aortic dissection, preeclampsia, or pheochromocytoma crisis) by no more than 25% within the first hour, then to <160/100 mm Hg within the next 2 to 6 hours, then cautiously to target during the following 24 to 48 hours. Choice of antihypertensive medication should be tailored to the specific patient. If there is concern for imminent end-organ damage, faster-acting antihypertensive agents, such as oral clonidine, can be given to lower BP. Several hours of observation in the ambulatory setting may be required to ensure that the patient remains asymptomatic and that BP is decreasing before discharge. In patients in whom hypertensive urgency developed because of medication nonadherence, antihypertensive medications can be resumed slowly and in a stepwise fashion, with care not to drop the BP precipitously. Close follow-up of such patients is necessary, and further management can include home monitoring of BP.

**KEY POINTS**

- Hypertensive urgency is defined as severely elevated blood pressure (BP)—often a systolic BP ≥180 mm Hg and/or diastolic BP ≥110 mm Hg—in a patient without obvious signs or symptoms of acute end-organ damage.

- Management of hypertensive urgency in patients with imminent risk of target organ damage but without a compelling condition includes lowering the systolic blood pressure by no more than 25% within the first hour, then to <160/100 mm Hg within the next 2 to 6 hours, then cautiously to target during the following 24 to 48 hours.

## Specific Populations
### Women

Hypertension prevalence is lower in women <50 years of age compared with men, but prevalence increases with older age and eventually becomes similar in both sexes. Women, particularly if premenopausal, are at a lower risk than men for hypertension complications, such as coronary artery disease, stroke, and left ventricular hypertrophy. Clinical trials suggest that women derive similar relative benefits from antihypertensive treatment as men, and recommendations for BP targets and agents are the same.

Women of childbearing age who anticipate pregnancy should not be prescribed RAS agents (ACE inhibitors, ARBs, or direct renin inhibitors) because of the risk for urogenital developmental abnormalities; these agents are contraindicated in pregnant women. Instead, transition to methyldopa, nifedipine, and/or labetalol during pregnancy is a reasonable choice. See The Kidney in Pregnancy for more information.

Oral contraceptives may be associated with modest increases in BP, which usually resolve with discontinuation; women prescribed these medications should be monitored. Hormone replacement therapy consists of much lower estrogen doses and is not associated with elevated BP.

## Patients with Diabetes Mellitus

The 2017 ACC/AHA BP guideline recommends a BP goal of <130/80 mm Hg for patients with diabetes. First-line therapy in nonblack patients with diabetes includes a thiazide diuretic, CCB, ACE inhibitor, or ARB; ACE inhibitors or ARBs are reasonable choices in the presence of albuminuria. In black patients with diabetes, a thiazide diuretic or CCB is recommended as initial therapy.

The American Diabetes Association (ADA) recommends that most patients with diabetes and hypertension should be treated to a BP goal of 140/90 mm Hg; lower systolic and diastolic BP targets, such as 130/80 mm Hg, may be appropriate for individuals at high risk of cardiovascular disease if they can be achieved without undue treatment burden. The ADA also recommends an ACE inhibitor or ARB, at the maximum tolerated dose indicated for BP treatment, as first-line treatment for hypertension in patients with diabetes and albuminuria.

## Black Patients

Although hypertension is more prevalent in black patients and correlates with a higher risk for cardiovascular and kidney outcomes, current recommendations for target BP are similar in black patients to those in other racial groups. The difference in management is with regard to the agent used. In general, ACE inhibitors are less efficacious in lowering BP in black patients than are CCBs. Additionally, a landmark trial (ALLHAT) revealed that in black patients, a thiazide diuretic was more effective in improving cardiovascular outcomes compared with an ACE inhibitor, and there was a higher risk of stroke with use of an ACE inhibitor as initial therapy compared with a CCB. Therefore, in the absence of CKD or heart failure, initial antihypertensive treatment should include a thiazide diuretic or CCB in black patients. If CKD is present, initial or add-on therapy should include an ACE inhibitor or ARB, especially in those with proteinuria, as illustrated by the AASK study. Choice of antihypertensive medication in patients with heart failure should be in accordance with appropriate guidelines.

## Older Patients

Prevalence of hypertension increases with age and is as high as 60% to 80% in patients >65 years of age. A wide pulse pressure and isolated systolic hypertension (>160 mm Hg with diastolic <90 mm Hg) are common.

According to the 2017 ACC/AHA BP guideline, the target systolic BP goal for noninstitutionalized, ambulatory community-dwelling patients who are ≥65 years of age is <130 mm Hg. In those with a high burden of comorbidity and limited life expectancy, clinical judgement, patient preference, and an assessment of risk-benefit ratio should be considered for decisions about the intensity of BP control and antihypertensive medication choice.

On the other hand, a 2017 guideline from the American College of Physicians and American Academy of Family Physicians (http://annals.org/aim/article/2598413/pharmacologic-treatment-hypertension-adultsaged-60-years-older-higher-versus) addressed the treatment of hypertension in patients ≥60 years of age, including three recommendations:

- Initiate treatment in patients ≥60 years of age with a systolic BP persistently ≥150 mm Hg to achieve a target systolic BP <150 mm Hg to reduce the risk for mortality, stroke, and cardiac events.
- Consider initiating or intensifying pharmacologic treatment in patients ≥60 years of age with a history of stroke or transient ischemic attack to achieve a target systolic BP <140 mm Hg to reduce the risk for recurrent stroke.
- Consider initiating or intensifying pharmacologic treatment in some patients ≥60 years of age at high cardiovascular risk, based on individualized assessment, to achieve a target systolic BP <140 mm Hg to reduce the risk for stroke or cardiac events.

Regarding antihypertensive class, nonblack older patients without CKD can be treated with a thiazide diuretic, CCB, or ACE inhibitor or ARB, similar to patients <65 years of age. Care must be taken in initiating antihypertensive medications at lower doses with close monitoring of BP and attention to adverse events, given that older patients are more prone to drug-drug interactions, hyponatremia from thiazide diuretics, and orthostatic hypotension when treated with diuretics, vasodilators, α-blockers, and central-acting drugs (such as clonidine).

### KEY POINTS

- Women of childbearing age who anticipate pregnancy should not be prescribed renin-angiotensin system agents because of the risk for urogenital developmental abnormalities; these agents are contraindicated in pregnant women.
- In the absence of chronic kidney disease, first-line therapy of hypertension in nonblack patients with diabetes is similar to treatment of patients without diabetes: a thiazide diuretic, calcium channel blocker, ACE inhibitor, or angiotensin receptor blocker.
- Initial antihypertensive treatment for black patients with or without diabetes mellitus includes a thiazide diuretic or calcium channel blocker.
- The 2017 ACC/AHA BP guideline recommends a target systolic BP goal of <130 mm Hg for noninstitutionalized, ambulatory community-dwelling patients who are ≥65 years, whereas the American College of Physicians and American Academy of Family Physicians recommend a target systolic BP goal of <150 mm Hg in patients ≥60 years of age.

# Chronic Tubulointerstitial Nephritis

## Epidemiology and Pathophysiology

Tubulointerstitial nephritis (TIN) is characterized by damage to the renal tubules and interstitium, resulting in tubulointerstitial edema and progressive fibrosis and tubular atrophy. TIN can be acute or chronic. Acute interstitial nephritis is commonly due to allergic drug reactions or infection and can cause acute kidney injury within days to weeks. It is characterized by inflammation of the renal interstitium and tubules, which is generally reversible after the offending drug is removed or the underlying disease is treated (see Acute Kidney Injury). Chronic TIN (CTIN) causes a slow decline in kidney function over months and years and is characterized by interstitial scarring, fibrosis, and tubular atrophy. Acute interstitial nephritis can progress to CTIN over time. CTIN can also develop in the setting of chronic primary glomerular disease, vascular diseases, and ischemia secondary to atherosclerosis and hypertension. Causes of CTIN are listed in **Table 16**.

## Diagnosis and Evaluation

CTIN is often asymptomatic until severe loss of kidney function occurs. Presenting symptoms include polyuria and nocturia due to renal concentrating defects.

A careful history with a review of medications should be performed to determine the cause of CTIN (see Table 16). A thorough physical examination may provide clues to the diagnosis and may reveal hypertension, but often no characteristic findings exist. Urinalysis may be normal or demonstrate pyuria and/or proteinuria <1500 mg/24 h. See **Table 17** for other laboratory manifestations of CTIN. Kidney ultrasound may show small kidneys. Kidney biopsy may be necessary to establish a definitive diagnosis.

### KEY POINTS

- Chronic tubulointerstitial nephritis is characterized by interstitial scarring, fibrosis, and tubular atrophy and results in a slow decline in kidney function over months and years.
- Features of chronic tubulointerstitial nephritis include polyuria and nocturia due to renal concentrating defects; hypertension; and a urinalysis that is normal or demonstrates pyuria and/or proteinuria <1500 mg/24 h.

## Causes

See Table 16 for a list of causes of CTIN.

## Immunologic Diseases

### Sjögren Syndrome

Kidney involvement in Sjögren syndrome may include interstitial nephritis, distal (type 1) renal tubular acidosis (RTA), and glomerulonephritis. Nephrolithiasis, nephrocalcinosis, and progressive kidney disease may also occur.

### Sarcoidosis

Kidney involvement in sarcoidosis is common and can manifest as nephrocalcinosis from hypercalcemia and hypercalciuria, obstructive uropathy, and TIN due to granulomatous interstitial nephritis. Urine findings of TIN include impaired urine concentration, mild proteinuria, and sterile pyuria. Kidney recovery is usually incomplete.

### Systemic Lupus Erythematosus

The TIN that may occur in systemic lupus erythematosus is often associated with concurrent glomerular disease but can also be the only manifestation of lupus nephritis. The severity of TIN is a useful predictor of hypertension, progressive kidney disease, and kidney failure.

### IgG4-Related Disease

IgG4-related disease can be associated with a TIN with an abundant IgG4-positive plasma cell interstitial infiltration. Other laboratory findings include decreased serum complement levels and peripheral eosinophilia.

## Infections

Infections associated with acute interstitial nephritis and CTIN include bacterial (such as brucellosis and tuberculosis), viral, fungal, and parasitic infections.

In immunosuppressed patients with transplanted organs, BK polyoma virus can cause interstitial nephritis. Diagnosis of BK virus nephropathy can be difficult to distinguish from acute cellular rejection. The most important treatment intervention is to decrease immunosuppressive therapy.

Chronic pyelonephritis resulting from chronic infections or vesicoureteral reflux is a common cause of CTIN. Patients can present with fever, chills, dysuria, flank or back pain, and hypertension. Kidney manifestations include distal tubular dysfunction, pyuria, and leukocyte casts. Persistent chronic pyelonephritis can progress to localized xanthogranulomatous pyelonephritis, which is characterized by a destructive mass that invades the renal parenchyma and is associated with urinary tract obstruction, infection, nephrolithiasis, diabetes mellitus, and/or immunosuppression.

## Malignancy

Lymphoproliferative disorders such as lymphoma and leukemia can infiltrate the kidney, causing TIN. Presenting features include proteinuria, sterile pyuria, and enlarged kidneys. Plasma cell dyscrasias such as multiple myeloma can cause TIN in the form of myeloma cast nephropathy, Fanconi syndrome, or interstitial light chain deposition.

| TABLE 16. | Causes of Chronic Tubulointerstitial Nephritis |
|---|---|
| **Immunologic Diseases** | |
| Anti–tubular basement membrane antibody-mediated tubulointerstitial nephritis | |
| Sarcoidosis | |
| Sjögren syndrome | |
| Systemic lupus erythematosus | |
| IgG4-related disease | |
| Tubulointerstitial nephritis with uveitis[a] | |
| **Toxic Causes** | |
| Balkan endemic nephropathy/aristolochic acid nephropathy (urologic evaluation is indicated due to increased risk of transitional cell carcinoma) | |
| Heavy metal nephropathy (e.g., lead, cadmium, mercury, arsenic, bismuth, chromium, copper, gold, iron, uranium) | |
| **Hereditary Tubulointerstitial Nephritis** | |
| Medullary cystic kidney disease | |
| Mitochondrial disorders | |
| Nephronophthisis | |
| **Infection-Related Causes** | |
| Polyoma BK virus (most commonly post–kidney transplantation) | |
| Brucellosis | |
| Cytomegalovirus | |
| Epstein-Barr virus | |
| Hantavirus | |
| HIV | |
| Hepatitis B virus | |
| Fungal infections | |
| *Legionella* species | |
| *Mycobacterium tuberculosis* | |
| Toxoplasmosis | |
| Chronic pyelonephritis | |
| **Malignancy-Related Causes** | |
| Leukemia | |
| Lymphoma | |
| Malignancy-associated monoclonal gammopathies (e.g., multiple myeloma, plasmacytoma) | |
| **Medication-Induced Causes** | |
| Analgesic nephropathy (e.g., acetaminophen, aspirin, caffeine, or NSAID combinations) | |
| Sodium phosphate (phosphate nephropathy) | |
| Orlistat; high doses of vitamin C (oxalate nephropathy) | |
| Calcineurin inhibitors (cyclosporine, tacrolimus) | |
| Lithium | |
| Cyclooxygenase-2 inhibitors (celecoxib) | |
| NSAIDs | |
| Proton pump inhibitors (esomeprazole, lansoprazole, omeprazole, pantoprazole, rabeprazole) | |
| $H_2$ blockers (famotidine, ranitidine, nizatidine, cimetidine) | |
| Allopurinol | |
| HIV medications (indinavir, abacavir, tenofovir) | |

*(Continued on the next page)*

**TABLE 16.** Causes of Chronic Tubulointerstitial Nephritis *(Continued)*

| Medication-Induced Causes |
|---|
| Diuretics (triamterene, furosemide, thiazides) |
| Anticonvulsants (e.g., phenytoin, carbamazepine, phenobarbital, valproate) |
| 5-Aminosalicylates (mesalamine) |
| Antibiotics (cephalosporins, fluoroquinolones, penicillins, rifampin, sulfonamides) |
| Antineoplastics (cisplatin, carboplatin, cyclophosphamide, ifosfamide, nitrosoureas) |
| Prolonged exposure to any medication that can cause acute interstitial nephritis |
| **Secondary Tubulointerstitial Injury Due to Glomerular and Vascular Disorders** |
| Hypertensive nephrosclerosis |
| **Urinary Tract Obstruction** |
| Obstructive uropathy |
| Nephrolithiasis |
| Reflux disease |

[a]Tubulointerstitial nephritis with uveitis is an uncommon immune-mediated syndrome with the combination of tubulointerstitial nephritis and uveitis associated with autoimmune disorders, including hypoparathyroidism, thyroid disease, IgG4-related disease, and rheumatoid arthritis.

**TABLE 17.** Laboratory Manifestations of Chronic Tubulointerstitial Nephritis

| Abnormality[a] | Causes |
|---|---|
| Decline in GFR | Obstruction of tubules; damage to microvasculature; interstitial fibrosis and sclerosis of glomeruli |
| Proximal tubular damage (Fanconi syndrome) | Incomplete absorption and kidney wasting of glucose, phosphate, uric acid, bicarbonate, and amino acids |
| Normal anion gap metabolic acidosis | Proximal and distal RTA; decreased ammonia production |
| Polyuria and isosthenuria | Decreased concentrating and diluting ability |
| Proteinuria | Decreased tubular protein reabsorption (usually <1500 mg/24 h) |
| Hyperkalemia | Defect in potassium secretion (type 4 [hyperkalemic] distal RTA) |
| Hypokalemia | Defect in potassium reabsorption (type 1 [hypokalemic] distal RTA) |
| Anemia | Injury to erythropoietin-producing cells in the kidney |

GFR = glomerular filtration rate; RTA = renal tubular acidosis.

[a]The degree of these abnormalities depends on the extent and location of injury.

## Medications
### Analgesics
Analgesic nephropathy is a chronic progressive TIN thought to be due to the long-term use of combinations of phenacetin (banned since 1983) with aspirin, caffeine, acetaminophen, or NSAIDs. It can also occur with the individual drugs. When severe, analgesic nephropathy is associated with renal papillary necrosis, which manifests as gross hematuria, flank pain, and, occasionally, obstruction and infection.

Patients with analgesic nephropathy are typically women over the age of 45 years with a history of heavy analgesic use, low back pain or chronic musculoskeletal pain, and kidney disease with low-grade proteinuria, sterile pyuria, and anemia. CT may demonstrate microcalcifications at the papillary tips.

### Calcineurin Inhibitors
The calcineurin inhibitors cyclosporine and tacrolimus can cause CTIN, in part via renal vasoconstriction. In kidney transplant recipients, cyclosporine- or tacrolimus-induced CTIN can be similar to chronic rejection. Clinical features of calcineurin inhibitor–induced TIN include hypertension and metabolic abnormalities from tubular dysfunction, including hyperkalemia, hyperuricemia, metabolic acidosis from type 4 (hyperkalemic distal) RTA, hypophosphatemia, hypomagnesemia, and hypercalciuria. Thrombotic microangiopathy might further contribute to both acute and chronic nephrotoxicity. Risk factors for CTIN are duration of exposure and cumulative dose.

### Lithium
Lithium causes several kidney disorders, including distal tubular dysfunction (type 1 hypokalemic distal RTA), nephrogenic diabetes insipidus, and CTIN. CTIN from long-term lithium use can occur in up to 15% to 20% of patients. Risk factors for CTIN include advanced age, duration of lithium exposure, the cumulative dose, and repeated episodes of lithium toxicity with high serum levels. Lithium nephropathy is characterized by cystic dilation of the distal tubules with formation of microcysts. Kidney dysfunction can progress to end-stage kidney disease even with discontinuation of lithium. Amiloride can attenuate lithium-induced nephrogenic diabetes insipidus by blocking distal tubular reabsorption of lithium.

### Antineoplastic Agents
Multiple chemotherapy agents can cause TIN, including cisplatin, carboplatin, cyclophosphamide, ifosfamide, and nitrosoureas (particularly streptozotocin and semustine). Newer

biologic agents such as immune checkpoint inhibitors have also been implicated.

## Lead

Lead can result in tubular dysfunction and CTIN. Occupational exposure to lead occurs from welding, smelting, the battery industry, and mining. Toxicity may also develop after months to years of exposure to lead in water, soil, paint, or food products. Lead nephropathy should be considered in any patient with a history of lead exposure, hypertension, gout, and progressive kidney disease. Gout is common because lead reduces urine excretion of uric acid. The clinical diagnosis of lead nephropathy is based on history of exposure, evidence of kidney dysfunction, and blood lead levels. Levels may be normal if high-level lead exposure has abated.

## Hyperuricemia

Both acute and chronic uric acid nephropathy can cause TIN from deposition of uric acid in renal tubules and interstitium. Clinical findings include elevated serum creatinine, bland urine sediment, mild proteinuria, and elevated serum urate levels. Kidney biopsy is necessary for definitive diagnosis.

## Obstruction

Obstructive uropathy from prostate disease, malignancy, nephrolithiasis, pelvic radiation, medications such as methysergide, and retroperitoneal fibrosis can cause CTIN and progressive kidney dysfunction. RTA, hyperkalemia, and mild proteinuria are common.

### KEY POINT

- Causes of chronic tubulointerstitial nephritis include various immunologic diseases, infections, malignancy, medications, lead, hyperuricemia, and obstruction.

## Management

Management of acute and chronic TIN involves treating the underlying cause: discontinuing offending agents, administering immunosuppressive therapy for immunologic or drug-related allergic causes, treating infection and malignancy, and relieving obstruction. Treatment of lead nephropathy consists of EDTA chelation therapy or oral succimer, which can slow the progression of chronic kidney disease. In patients with CTIN and progressive kidney disease, management includes control of blood pressure and treatment of proteinuria and metabolic abnormalities (see Chronic Kidney Disease).

### KEY POINT

- Management of chronic tubulointerstitial nephritis involves treating the underlying cause: discontinuing offending agents, administering immunosuppressive therapy for immunologic or drug-related allergic causes, treating infection and malignancy, and relieving obstruction.

# Glomerular Diseases
## Epidemiology and Pathophysiology

Glomerular diseases are the third leading cause of end-stage kidney disease (ESKD) in the United States, accounting for approximately 10,000 incident cases of ESKD per year and trailing only diabetes mellitus and hypertension. The term *glomerular disease* encompasses a wide array of conditions with etiologies that span autoimmune disease, malignancy-associated conditions, sequelae of infection, genetic mutations, and medication toxicities. These diseases are classified as either primary (idiopathic), in which the glomerular injury is an intrinsic process generally limited to the kidney, or secondary, in which the glomerular lesion is the result of a systemic disease with kidney involvement as one of many possible manifestations.

The normal, noninflamed glomerulus forms a tight barrier, largely due to the slit diaphragms that connect podocyte (visceral epithelial cell) foot processes on the outside surface of the glomerular basement membrane (**Figure 11**). When healthy, this filtration barrier prevents passage of blood and protein into the urinary filtrate. Glomerular diseases involve injury of the glomerular filter with subsequent passage of protein (proteinuria) and, in the setting of glomerulonephritis, blood (hematuria) into the urine. These urinary abnormalities are the earliest manifestation of a glomerular lesion. If the injury responsible for the hematuria and proteinuria goes unchecked, the result is scarring of the glomerular filters (glomerulosclerosis) with subsequent decline in kidney function that manifests as elevated serum creatinine.

Most etiologies of glomerular disease are diagnosed via kidney biopsy. No formal guidelines exist for the indications to perform a kidney biopsy in any age group. The decision to pursue a kidney biopsy should be individualized for each patient, but, in general, a kidney biopsy appears justified for

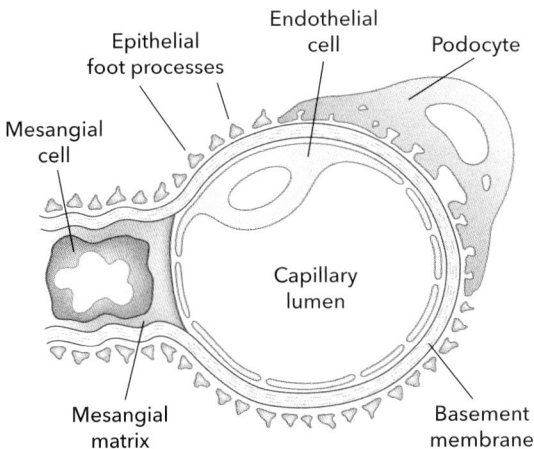

**FIGURE 11.** The podocyte, a visceral epithelial cell, sits on the outside surface of the glomerular basement membrane.

patients with two or more of the following four findings: hematuria, proteinuria >1000 mg/24 h, reduced kidney function (glomerular filtration rate <60 mL/min/1.73 m²), and/or positive serologies for systemic diseases with known potential for kidney involvement (for example, hepatitis B or C virus infection, systemic lupus erythematosus, and ANCA seropositivity).

# Clinical Manifestations of Glomerular Disease

The two main categories of glomerular disease are the nephrotic and nephritic syndromes, each of which has a distinct clinical presentation.

## The Nephrotic Syndrome

Clinical manifestations of the nephrotic syndrome stem from ongoing loss of protein, principally albumin, into the urine. This urinary loss of albumin causes hypoalbuminemia; in response, the liver increases its production of several proteins, including cholesterols, leading to hyperlipidemia. The resulting hallmark features of the nephrotic syndrome include the following:

- Urine protein excretion >3500 mg/24 h or a urine protein-creatinine ratio >3500 mg/g (nephrotic-range proteinuria)
- Hypoalbuminemia (usually <3.0 g/dL [30 g/L])
- Hypercholesterolemia
- Edema

Edema is typically most severe in the lower extremities. Many patients report periorbital edema upon awakening. Severe fluid retention can lead to pulmonary edema, pulmonary effusions, and anasarca. Despite avid salt and water retention, hypertension occurs only in a minority of patients.

Two explanations have been proposed for the edema seen in the nephrotic syndrome. The "underfill hypothesis" argues that low serum albumin concentrations lead to a reduction in intravascular oncotic pressure and a resultant shift of plasma from the capillary lumen to the interstitium. Further, the consequent intravascular depletion activates the renin-angiotensin system, which promotes salt and water retention throughout the nephron, exacerbating the edema. In contrast, the "overfill hypothesis" argues that sodium is primarily retained at the collecting duct, triggered by the abnormally filtered proteins themselves. Both hypotheses may be correct, and both provide a rationale for edema management in patients with the nephrotic syndrome. First, resolution of edema is only attainable long term by remission of proteinuria; lending support to the overfill hypothesis, edema will often subside when proteinuria has fallen but before albumin has returned to normal range. Second, diuretics are crucial to control the symptoms of edema, blocking the reabsorption of sodium (and water) at various points in the nephron.

The nephrotic syndrome is a hypercoagulable state due to urinary losses of protein. In addition to albuminuria, patients with the nephrotic syndrome lose in their urine a number of low-molecular-weight anticoagulants (for example, antithrombin III, protein S) and fibrinolytics (for example, plasminogen). Hepatic overproduction of proteins, as an intrinsic response to hypoalbuminemia, leads not only to hyperlipidemia but also to increased levels of procoagulants (for example, factor V, factor VIII, fibrinogen). As a result, patients with the nephrotic syndrome are at increased risk for lower extremity, pulmonary, and renal vein thrombosis. Clots are most often seen in patients with membranous glomerulopathy, but any patient with nephrotic-range proteinuria and significant hypoalbuminemia (usually <2.5 g/dL [25 g/L]) should be considered at risk.

Severe albuminuria should be treated with renin-angiotensin system blocking drugs to control blood pressure and reduce proteinuria. Hyperlipidemia should be treated with cholesterol-lowering medications. Edema should be managed with diuretics and dietary sodium restriction. This combination of renin-angiotensin system blocking drugs, cholesterol-lowering medications, and diuretics is generally considered conservative therapy for most forms of glomerular disease. A general strategy for edema management in a newly diagnosed patient with the nephrotic syndrome is to start with a loop diuretic, with a goal weight loss of 1 to 2 kg (2.2-4.4 lb) per week. In severe cases of edema when loop diuretics have been maximally uptitrated and weight loss/edema control is insufficient, it is often necessary to add a second diuretic (a thiazide diuretic and/or potassium-sparing diuretic) that works distal to the loop of Henle. In patients taking high doses of loop diuretics, increased delivery of salt and water to the distal portions of the nephron can lead to hypertrophy of these segments and overabsorption of sodium, undermining the effects of the loop diuretic.

## The Nephritic Syndrome

The nephritic syndrome, also termed glomerulonephritis, can present as a number of clinical variants. Common features are hematuria (microscopic or macroscopic) and proteinuria, with the more severe variants typically including hypertension, edema, and kidney dysfunction (elevated serum creatinine). The glomerular hematuria seen in the nephritic syndrome can be distinguished from other causes of urinary tract bleeding by the presence of either dysmorphic erythrocytes (resulting from passage through a damaged glomerular basement membrane) or erythrocyte casts on urine microscopy (see Clinical Evaluation of Kidney Function).

The mildest forms of the nephritic syndrome are asymptomatic, microscopic hematuria with or without proteinuria, often discovered on routine laboratory assessment. Recurrent gross hematuria, in which macroscopic hematuria occurs several days after an upper respiratory infection or physical exertion, is a classic presentation of IgA nephropathy, particularly in younger patients. This nephritic presentation also usually follows a benign clinical course without associated chronic kidney disease.

On the other hand, the term *acute glomerulonephritis* is used to denote the more classical nephritic syndrome presentation, with variable degrees of kidney dysfunction, hypertension, edema, proteinuria, and hematuria. The most severe form of the nephritic syndrome is termed *rapidly progressive glomerulonephritis*, in which patients experience a rapid decline of kidney function over days or weeks that will progress to ESKD if untreated.

**KEY POINTS**

- The hallmark features of the nephrotic syndrome include a urine protein excretion >3500 mg/24 h or a urine protein-creatinine ratio >3500 mg/g, hypoalbuminemia, hypercholesterolemia, and edema.

- Common features of the nephritic syndrome are hematuria (with dysmorphic erythrocytes or erythrocyte casts) and proteinuria; hypertension, edema, and kidney dysfunction may also occur.

# Conditions Associated With the Nephrotic Syndrome

## Focal Segmental Glomerulosclerosis

### Epidemiology and Pathophysiology

Focal segmental glomerulosclerosis (FSGS) is the most common form of the nephrotic syndrome in black patients and, in certain parts of the world, has replaced membranous glomerulopathy as the leading cause of the nephrotic syndrome in white patients. The prevalence of FSGS in the United States is more than 20,000 patients, with a yearly incidence of approximately 5000 newly diagnosed cases per year. In the United States, FSGS currently accounts for up to 40% of primary nephrotic syndromes in adults. Worldwide, the incidence of FSGS has been estimated at nearly 1 in 100,000 people per year.

FSGS stems from abnormalities in the podocyte. Podocyte detachment and death lead to the segmental sclerosis that is the hallmark histopathology of FSGS. The podocyte injury in FSGS, in turn, can stem from immunologic, genetic, and/or hyperfiltration causes. Immunologic injury is considered the main pathogenic mechanism behind primary forms of FSGS, with leukocytes producing a soluble circulating factor that directly targets podocytes. This mechanism is supported by cases of FSGS recurring almost immediately after kidney transplantation and responding briskly to plasmapheresis, although to date definitive identification of such a circulating factor has yet to occur. Identified genetic causes of FSGS are chiefly mutations in podocyte-specific proteins (for example, nephrin, podocin, formin). These mutations are more commonly found in infants, young (<25 years of age) patients who do not respond to glucocorticoid therapy, and patients with a family history of ESKD. Individuals of African ancestry carry approximately a five times higher risk of FSGS than those of

European descent, likely mediated in large part by variants in the *APOL1* gene (see Genetic Disorders and Kidney Disease). The third major cause of podocyte injury, hyperfiltration, causes a large proportion of secondary FSGS cases. This hyperfiltration form of FSGS is seen classically in obese patients but also can manifest in patients with a history of premature birth or solitary kidney. Finally, a drug-induced FSGS can occur as a rare complication of some commonly used treatments, including lithium, interferon, and pamidronate.

### Clinical Manifestations

All patients with FSGS have proteinuria. Primary forms of FSGS usually present with nephrotic-range proteinuria and can be accompanied by the full nephrotic syndrome, including severe edema, whereas secondary forms typically have asymptomatic subnephrotic proteinuria. Any form of FSGS can present with reduced glomerular filtration rate, particularly when diagnosed late in the disease course.

### Diagnosis

FSGS is diagnosed by kidney biopsy. On light microscopy, glomerulosclerosis (scarring of glomeruli) is seen in a focal (<50%) and segmental (affecting a portion but not the entirety of individual glomeruli) distribution (**Figure 12**). Histologic variants of FSGS include classic (or "not otherwise specified") FSGS, perihilar variant, glomerular tip lesion variant, cellular variant, and collapsing variant. The collapsing variant is often resistant to treatment and therefore carries the worst long-term prognosis, whereas the tip lesion usually responds to glucocorticoids and is unlikely to progress to ESKD.

### Treatment and Prognosis

For all patients with FSGS, conservative therapy includes renin-angiotensin system blocking drugs to control proteinuria,

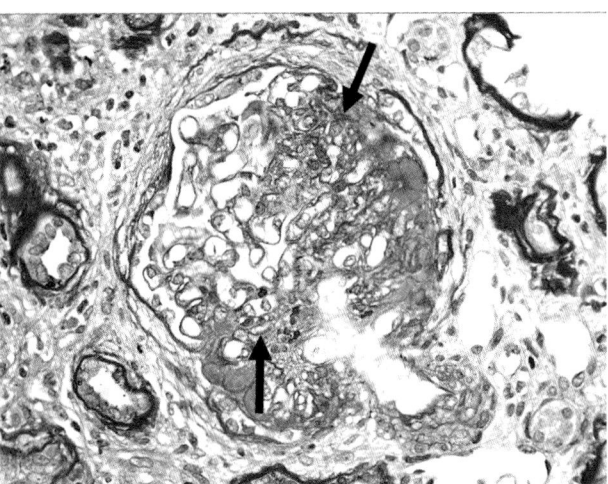

**FIGURE 12.** Light microscopy in focal segmental glomerulosclerosis shows scarring (*arrows*) in some, but not all, glomeruli in a segmental distribution, as demonstrated by this glomerulus.

Courtesy of Glen Markowitz, MD.

cholesterol-lowering medication, and edema management. Such conservative therapy measures suffice for FSGS patients with subnephrotic proteinuria.

When nephrotic-range proteinuria is present and if a primary form of FSGS is suspected, high-dose glucocorticoids remain the mainstay of initial therapy. Other immunosuppressants, including calcineurin inhibitors, mycophenolate mofetil, alkylating agents, and rituximab, have been reported to provide some benefit as second-line agents for patients who either do not respond to glucocorticoids or whose proteinuria relapses when glucocorticoids are tapered off.

Approximately 50% of patients with FSGS progress to ESKD within 10 years of diagnosis; this poor prognosis is rooted in low rates of treatment response.

## Membranous Glomerulopathy

### Epidemiology and Pathophysiology

Membranous glomerulopathy (membranous nephropathy) is a leading cause of the nephrotic syndrome in white adults. Epidemiology has remained constant over the past several decades. Disease occurs at an approximate rate of 1 case per 100,000 persons per year, with a peak incidence between 30 and 50 years of age. Approximately 75% of cases are considered primary; the remaining 25% are considered secondary to systemic diseases such as systemic lupus erythematosus, hepatitis B virus infection, and solid tumors.

In the past decade, target antigens and their associated autoantibodies responsible for the development of primary membranous glomerulopathy cases have been identified. The M-type phospholipase A2 receptor (PLA2R) is the specific podocyte antigen responsible for eliciting immune complex formation with circulating autoantibodies in most primary cases. Anti-PLA2R antibodies are detected in approximately 75% of primary cases and are rarely found in secondary forms. Additional alternative podocyte autoantigens have been reported in patients with primary membranous glomerulopathy, potentially filling in the missing gaps in PLA2R antibody–negative disease. Membranous glomerulopathy occurs when circulating antibodies permeate the glomerular basement membrane and, in the subepithelial space, form immune complexes with epitopes on podocyte membranes.

### Clinical Manifestations

Patients typically describe slowly progressive edema, and laboratory testing reveals proteinuria, hypoalbuminemia, and hyperlipidemia, most often with preserved kidney function. Patients with membranous glomerulopathy are particularly prone to thrombotic complications. These clots include lower extremity, pulmonary, and renal vein thromboses; they can occur in up to 25% of patients and are most likely to occur within the first 2 years of diagnosis. The risk of clotting increases when serum albumin is <2.8 g/dL (28 g/L) and is highest when serum albumin is <2.2 g/dL (22 g/L).

### Diagnosis

The diagnosis of membranous glomerulopathy is traditionally made by kidney biopsy, although FDA approval of serologic testing for anti-PLA2R antibodies in 2015 has introduced the possibility of diagnosing the disease noninvasively.

The hallmark biopsy finding is the presence of subepithelial immune deposits that alter the glomerular capillary wall, classically accompanied by intervening "spikes" of glomerular basement membrane extending between the immune deposits in more advanced cases. In addition to serologic testing for anti-PLA2R antibodies, the biopsy can be stained for the PLA2R antigen, which typically yields a higher sensitivity (>80%) than antibody testing in the serum. This testing is used not to make a diagnosis of membranous glomerulopathy but to help distinguish primary from secondary forms of the disease. Such a distinction is crucial because secondary forms are expected to remit if the underlying systemic disease responsible for the lesion is successfully treated. Notably, in patients with membranous glomerulopathy aged 65 years and older, malignancies have been detected in up to 25% within 1 year of their biopsy diagnosis. Therefore, age- and sex-appropriate cancer screening is recommended for all patients at the time of their diagnosis, even those with PLA2R positivity.

### Treatment and Prognosis

Patients with newly diagnosed primary forms of membranous glomerulopathy are usually observed for 6 to 12 months on conservative therapy (renin-angiotensin system blockade, cholesterol-lowering medication, and edema management) before initiating a course of immunosuppression for patients with persistent nephrotic-range proteinuria. The observation period allows patients a chance to achieve spontaneous remission, which occurs in approximately 30% within 1 to 2 years of diagnosis. Patients who remain nephrotic have the option of two first-line immunosuppressive regimens: (1) a combination of glucocorticoids and alkylating agents, which achieves remission in approximately 75% to 80% of patients within 12 months, or (2) calcineurin inhibitors (cyclosporine or tacrolimus), which have reported remission rates of 70% to 75% in the first year of therapy. Relapse rates are higher in patients treated with calcineurin inhibitors than alkylating agents. Recent reports also suggest that rituximab may have efficacy in membranous glomerulopathy. Treatment of secondary forms of membranous glomerulopathy should be aimed at the underlying systemic disease or etiology (for example, resection of a tumor in malignancy-associated membranous glomerulopathy, treatment of hepatitis B in viral-associated membranous glomerulopathy).

Progression to ESKD depends on remission of proteinuria: The 10-year incidence of ESKD in patients who undergo complete or partial remission of proteinuria ranges from 0 to 10%, compared with a >50% incidence of ESKD in patients who maintain nephrotic-range proteinuria.

## Minimal Change Glomerulopathy

### Epidemiology and Pathophysiology

Minimal change glomerulopathy (MCG; also known as minimal change disease) is the most common cause of the nephrotic syndrome in children (>90% of cases). For this reason, unless clinical and serologic evidence suggests the presence of a disease other than MCG, a kidney biopsy is not performed in children with the nephrotic syndrome unless they do not respond to glucocorticoid therapy. In adults, biopsy series have shown that MCG is the cause of up to 10% to 15% of cases of the nephrotic syndrome, with a greater representation in older patients (≥65 years of age) and elderly patients (≥80 years of age).

The pathophysiology of MCG is not well understood. Similar to FSGS, MCG is a podocytopathy; the presumed model of injury is immunologic, in which a circulating factor (produced by B or T cells) alters podocyte function, resulting in massive proteinuria. The rapid response of most cases (>90%) of MCG to nonspecific immunosuppression (usually glucocorticoids) fits this model of a circulating factor–inducing disease. Most cases of MCG are primary, but the disease is associated with various conditions, including malignancies (Hodgkin lymphoma, non-Hodgkin lymphoma, thymoma), medications (NSAIDs, lithium), infections (strongyloides, syphilis, mycoplasma, ehrlichiosis), and atopy (pollen, dairy products).

### Clinical Manifestations

The classic presentation of MCG is sudden-onset nephrotic syndrome. Microscopic hematuria is present in 10% to 30% of adult cases. Up to 25% of adults with MCG may also have acute kidney injury (AKI), more commonly occurring in older patients with hypertension, low serum albumin levels, and heavy proteinuria.

### Diagnosis

MCG is diagnosed with kidney biopsy demonstrating normal glomerular histology on light microscopy, negative immunofluorescence staining for immunoglobulin and complement proteins, and complete effacement of the podocyte foot processes on electron microscopy.

### Treatment and Prognosis

The 2012 Kidney Disease: Improving Global Outcomes (KDIGO) Clinical Practice Guideline for Glomerulonephritis recommends glucocorticoids as first-line therapy for children and adults with MCG, with remission achieved in more than 90% of children and 80% to 90% of adults. Time-to-response is prolonged in adults compared with children, and adults are not considered to have glucocorticoid-resistant disease until they have not responded to 16 weeks of glucocorticoid therapy. After an initial course of glucocorticoids, patients are subdivided into categories: glucocorticoid-sensitive MCG, glucocorticoid-dependent MCG, infrequently relapsing MCG, frequently relapsing MCG, and glucocorticoid-resistant MCG. Treatment of glucocorticoid-dependent, frequently relapsing, and glucocorticoid-resistant MCG has included calcineurin

inhibitors, mycophenolate mofetil, alkylating agents, and rituximab, with variable results.

## Diabetic Nephropathy

### Epidemiology and Pathophysiology

Diabetes mellitus is the leading cause of chronic kidney disease (CKD) and ESKD worldwide. In the United States, diabetes accounts for over 50,000 new cases of ESKD requiring dialysis each year. Diabetic nephropathy, defined as clinical evidence of kidney injury in response to chronic, long-standing hyperglycemia, has a 10% incidence over 25 years among patients with type 1 diabetes and a 12% incidence over 25 years among patients with type 2 diabetes.

Advanced glycation end products are felt to be the primary mediator of injury in diabetic nephropathy, activating signaling cascades that promote mesangial cell synthesis of profibrogenic cytokines, including platelet-derived growth factor and transforming growth factor β.

### Clinical Manifestations

Diabetic nephropathy manifests initially as moderately increased albuminuria (microalbuminuria). Over time, progressive proteinuria is followed by a decline in glomerular filtration rate, with progression to later stages of CKD and ESKD. When proteinuria is severe, it is typically accompanied by hypoalbuminemia, and many patients present with edema befitting a classic picture of the nephrotic syndrome.

Kidney disease due to diabetes is often accompanied by extrarenal microvascular complications of diabetes, including retinopathy and peripheral neuropathy, as well as macrovascular complications, such as peripheral vascular disease, coronary artery disease, and stroke.

### Diagnosis

The American Diabetes Association recommends yearly assessment of albuminuria in patients with type 2 diabetes, and assessment after 5 years of disease in patients with type 1 diabetes. The diagnosis of diabetic nephropathy is usually made clinically in the presence of hallmark features: proteinuric CKD in a patient with long-standing diabetes and evidence of other (microvascular and/or macrovascular) complications of disease. If the clinical presentation is not entirely consistent with diabetic nephropathy, a kidney biopsy is performed. The biopsy finding of nodular mesangial sclerosis with glomerular and tubular basement thickening, in the absence of immune deposits, is the classic description of diabetic nephropathy.

### Treatment and Prognosis

The cornerstone of treatment of diabetic nephropathy involves glycemic control and blood pressure control. Blockade of the renin-angiotensin system with an ACE inhibitor or angiotensin receptor blocker (ARB) is recommended, typically to the maximal tolerated dose, because these agents both reduce blood pressure and levels of proteinuria, which, along with glycemic control, are the most important modifiable risk factors for progression of diabetic nephropathy to ESKD. Combined use of any two of the three renin-angiotensin system drug classes (ACE inhibitor, ARB, and direct renin inhibitor) is not recommended given the results of several clinical trials that revealed more adverse events with these combinations (hyperkalemia, hypotension, AKI), without additional cardiovascular or renal benefits. Combining ACE inhibitors or ARBs with mineralocorticoid receptors (spironolactone or eplerenone) has been shown in small studies to be a safe and effective antiproteinuric strategy in diabetic nephropathy, but the risk for hyperkalemia should be considered.

The 2017 high blood pressure guideline from the American College of Cardiology (ACC), the American Heart Association (AHA), and nine other organizations recommends a blood pressure target of <130/80 mm Hg for patients with hypertension and diabetes mellitus and/or CKD. The American Diabetes Association recommends that most patients with diabetes and hypertension should be treated to a systolic blood pressure goal of <140 mm Hg and a diastolic blood pressure goal of <90 mm Hg; lower systolic and diastolic blood pressure targets, such as 130/80 mm Hg, may be appropriate for individuals at high risk of cardiovascular disease, if they can be achieved without undue treatment burden.

**KEY POINTS**

- Initial treatment of focal segmental glomerulosclerosis is high-dose glucocorticoids; other immunosuppressants (calcineurin inhibitors, mycophenolate mofetil, alkylating agents, rituximab) may provide some benefit for patients who do not respond to glucocorticoids or relapse when glucocorticoids are tapered off.

- Newly diagnosed primary membranous glomerulopathy is typically treated with conservative therapy for 6 to 12 months before initiating immunosuppression for patients with persistent nephrotic-range proteinuria.

- Minimal change glomerulopathy (MCG) is initially treated with glucocorticoids; treatment options for glucocorticoid-dependent, frequently relapsing, and glucocorticoid-resistant MCG include calcineurin inhibitors, mycophenolate mofetil, alkylating agents, or rituximab.

- The American Diabetes Association recommends yearly assessment of albuminuria in patients with type 2 diabetes mellitus, and assessment after 5 years of disease in patients with type 1 diabetes mellitus.

- The cornerstone of treatment of diabetic nephropathy involves glycemic control and renin-angiotensin system blockade using either an ACE inhibitor or an angiotensin receptor blocker.

## Conditions Associated With the Nephritic Syndrome

### Rapidly Progressive Glomerulonephritis

#### Epidemiology and Pathophysiology

Rapidly progressive glomerulonephritis (RPGN; also known as crescentic glomerulonephritis) is not a specific disease; rather, RPGN is a clinical entity that can be caused by multiple diseases and manifests as (1) at least a 50% decline in glomerular filtration rate over a short period (usually days to weeks) with (2) pathology findings of extensive glomerular crescents (**Figure 13**). Crescents signal focal rupture of the glomerular capillary walls, the most severe glomerular damage that can be seen on light microscopy. This rupture allows accumulation of fibrin and fibronectin in the urinary space, where they activate de-differentiated glomerular parietal epithelial cells to proliferate, surround, and compress the glomerular tuft.

#### Clinical Manifestations

RPGN typically presents with macroscopic or microscopic hematuria, erythrocyte casts, varying ranges of proteinuria, and AKI that can lead rapidly to dialysis dependence.

#### Diagnosis

The diagnosis of all forms of glomerulonephritis is traditionally made by kidney biopsy, which can distinguish among the three major categories of glomerulonephritis (**Table 18**) and their associated etiologies. Serologic testing (for example, ANCA, anti–glomerular basement membrane antibodies, antinuclear antibodies) aids in the diagnosis. An alternative classification scheme for glomerulonephritis is based on low versus normal complement levels (**Table 19**). Although any form of glomerulonephritis can display an aggressive disease course that would fit the definition of an RPGN, the most common etiologies seen in RPGN cases are ANCA-associated

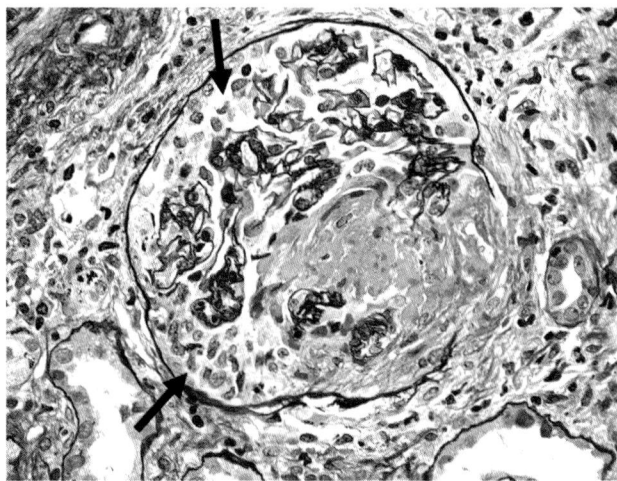

**FIGURE 13.** A glomerular crescent (*arrows*), named for its moon-shaped appearance, signals focal rupture of the glomerular capillary walls.

Courtesy of Glen Markowitz, MD.

**TABLE 18.** Categorization of Glomerulonephritis Based on Immunofluorescence Microscopy Findings

**Immunofluorescence Staining Pattern**

| Granular | Pauci-immune | Linear |
|---|---|---|
| Lupus nephritis | ANCA-associated GN | Anti-GBM antibody disease |
| Infection-related GN | | |
| IgA nephropathy | | |
| MPGN | | |
| Cryoglobulinemic GN | | |

GBM = glomerular basement membrane; GN = glomerulonephritis; MPGN = membranoproliferative glomerulonephritis.

**TABLE 19.** Categorization of Glomerulonephritis Based on Serum Complement Levels

| Low Serum C3 and/or C4 Levels | Normal Serum C3 and C4 Levels |
|---|---|
| Lupus nephritis | IgA nephropathy |
| Infection-related GN | ANCA-associated GN |
| MPGN | Anti-GBM antibody disease |
| Cryoglobulinemic GN | |

GBM = glomerular basement membrane; GN = glomerulonephritis; MPGN = membranoproliferative glomerulonephritis.

glomerulonephritis, lupus nephritis, and anti–glomerular basement membrane glomerulonephritis.

## Treatment and Prognosis

Treatment is based on the specific etiology of RPGN. If untreated, RPGN is expected to progress to dialysis dependence in a matter of days to weeks. If treated early, lesions can often be reversed, although CKD is often a lingering consequence.

## Anti–Glomerular Basement Membrane Antibody Disease

### Epidemiology and Pathophysiology

Anti–glomerular basement membrane (anti-GBM) antibody disease is a rare form of RPGN with an incidence of less than one case per million per year. Anti-GBM antibody disease accounts for about 20% of RPGN cases in adults. The lesion is more frequently seen in white patients and has a bimodal age and gender distribution, with peak incidences in young men in the second and third decades of life and in older women in the sixth and seventh decades of life. More than half of patients with anti-GBM antibody disease present with RPGN and pulmonary hemorrhage. About one third of patients present with isolated glomerulonephritis. Notably, up to one third of patients have concurrent circulating ANCA (usually antimyeloperoxidase [MPO]) antibodies.

Circulating anti-GBM antibodies target the alpha-3 chain of type IV collagen. When anti-GBM antibodies bind rapidly

and tightly to the GBM, they incite an intense inflammatory response that translates to the typically fulminant nature of this disease.

### Clinical Manifestations

The presentation of anti-GBM antibody disease is similar to that of other forms of RPGN previously described, with macroscopic or microscopic hematuria, erythrocyte casts, varying ranges of proteinuria, and usually moderate to severe AKI. Lung involvement (Goodpasture syndrome) occurs in >50% of patients; hemoptysis can be a presenting symptom, although shortness of breath or cough should also raise suspicion for a pulmonary-renal syndrome even in the absence of hemoptysis.

### Diagnosis

Kidney biopsy in anti-GBM disease shows a crescentic glomerulonephritis on light microscopy and pathognomonic linear staining for IgG along the glomerular capillaries, indicative of antibodies directed against the GBM. Serologic testing for anti-GBM antibodies is performed at the time of diagnosis. The serologic test is done by indirect immunofluorescence or direct enzyme-linked immunoassay (ELISA), with sensitivity ranging from 60% to 100%; therefore, a kidney biopsy to confirm diagnosis is recommended unless contraindicated. Even with a renal biopsy diagnosis, antibody levels should be measured because their titers can be followed to assess efficacy of therapy.

### Treatment and Prognosis

Outcomes in anti-GBM disease are based largely on the degree of AKI at the time of diagnosis and treatment. In an oft-cited series, patients with anti-GBM disease who presented with serum creatinine <5.65 mg/dL (500 µmol/L) had, at 10 years, a <5% overall mortality and a <20% risk for ESKD. In contrast, patients who presented with dialysis-dependent kidney failure had a 35% mortality rate within the first year of diagnosis, and only 8% were able to be taken off dialysis during this time. Treatment for anti-GBM disease consists of plasmapheresis, pulse glucocorticoids (high doses of intravenous glucocorticoids over a short period of time) followed by oral prednisone, and cyclophosphamide.

## ANCA-Associated Glomerulonephritis

See MKSAP 18 Rheumatology for more information on ANCA-associated vasculitis.

### Epidemiology and Pathophysiology

ANCA-associated glomerulonephritis (pauci-immune crescentic glomerulonephritis) accounts for more than half of all RPGN cases and has a particularly high prevalence in patients >65 years of age presenting with AKI and active urinary sediment. ANCA are autoantibodies that target proteins within neutrophil granules and monocyte lysosomes. There are two types of vasculitis-associated ANCA: p-ANCA (perinuclear) is directed against the neutrophil enzyme myeloperoxidase (MPO), and c-ANCA (cytoplasmic) is directed against the neutrophil proteinase 3 (PR3).

## Clinical Manifestations

Most patients with ANCA-associated glomerulonephritis report a vasculitic prodrome of malaise, arthralgia, myalgia, and flu-like symptoms that can include fever. Kidney involvement can produce dark brown (tea-colored) urine, and laboratory studies will confirm the presence of hematuria, proteinuria, and AKI. Lung and sinus involvement often occurs in ANCA-associated glomerulonephritis, with patients reporting hemoptysis and/or epistaxis.

## Diagnosis

Serologic testing for ANCA using enzyme-linked immunosorbent assay is usually performed at the time of presentation if RPGN is suspected. Light microscopy of the kidney biopsy shows a crescentic glomerulonephritis, but immunofluorescence shows a paucity or absence of immune-type deposits. Foci of necrosis or cellular crescents are highlighted by immunofluorescence staining for fibrinogen.

## Treatment and Prognosis

The initial treatment of organ-threatening disease is an area of ongoing controversy. Typical induction therapy consists of glucocorticoids combined with either cyclophosphamide or rituximab. Plasmapheresis is reserved for patients with evidence of alveolar hemorrhage or severe kidney failure. Other induction options include cyclophosphamide or rituximab-based therapies. After remission is induced, maintenance therapy is usually continued for at least 12 to 24 months using rituximab, azathioprine, or mycophenolate mofetil.

Patients with c-ANCA/anti-PR3 have a significantly higher rate of relapse than patients with p-ANCA/anti-MPO, particularly if there is a history of lung or sinus involvement. ANCA-associated glomerulonephritis is associated with an approximately 20% mortality rate within the first year of diagnosis and results in ESKD in up to 25% of surviving patients within the first 4 years after diagnosis.

**KEY POINTS**

- Rapidly progressive glomerulonephritis can be caused by multiple diseases; it is characterized by at least a 50% decline in glomerular filtration rate over a short period with pathology findings of extensive glomerular crescents.
- More than half of patients with anti–glomerular basement membrane antibody disease have lung involvement manifesting as hemoptysis, shortness of breath, or cough.
- Treatment of anti–glomerular basement membrane antibody disease consists of plasmapheresis, pulse glucocorticoids followed by oral prednisone, and cyclophosphamide.
- ANCA-associated glomerulonephritis is characterized by a prodrome of malaise, arthralgia, myalgia, and flu-like symptoms; dark brown (tea-colored) urine, hematuria, proteinuria, acute kidney injury, hemoptysis, and epistaxis may occur.

## Immune Complex–Mediated Glomerulonephritis

The glomerulonephritides with granular immunofluorescence microscopy staining patterns all fall under the umbrella category of immune complex–mediated glomerulonephritis, with antigen-antibody complexes depositing in the kidney at various locations and in various patterns (see Table 18). Immune complex deposition activates the classic complement pathway as a co-player in glomerular inflammation, injury, and, if unchecked, scarring. For this reason, most immune complex–mediated glomerulonephritides are associated with low levels of C3 and/or C4 (see Table 19). IgA nephropathy, which usually presents with normal C3 and C4 levels, is an exception due to the chronic, gradual nature of the disease; complement consumption is at a rate slow enough for hepatic production to replace complement proteins. In rare hyper-acute cases of IgA nephropathy that fulfill criteria for RPGN, however, complement levels are usually depressed.

### IgA Nephropathy
*Epidemiology and Pathophysiology*

IgA nephropathy (IgAN) is the most common primary glomerular disease worldwide, diagnosed in up to 10% of all kidney biopsies done in the United States and approximately one third of all kidney biopsies in Asian countries, where the disease is the leading cause of ESKD. In contrast, IgAN is very rare among patients of African ancestry. IgAN can be diagnosed at any age, particularly because a significant subgroup of patients is asymptomatic, but is most commonly diagnosed in youth or early adulthood, with a 2:1 male-to-female ratio. In the United States, the overall incidence of IgAN is estimated at 2.5 cases per 100,000 person-years, with a prevalence of approximately 80,000 individuals.

In IgAN, there is defect in IgA1-producing cells leading to hypogalactosylation of the hinge region of IgA1. Blood levels of galactose-deficient IgA1 (Gd-IgA1) are elevated in patients with IgAN. Patients then develop antibodies directed against Gd-IgA1 to form immune complexes that accumulate in the glomerular mesangium.

*Clinical Manifestations*

IgAN can present with any of the manifestations of the nephritic syndrome. The mildest presentation, seen in up to one third of patients, is asymptomatic microscopic hematuria with or without proteinuria, usually discovered incidentally as part of a routine examination. Recurrent gross hematuria, in which macroscopic hematuria occurs in the setting of an upper respiratory infection (synpharyngitic hematuria) is a common presentation in younger patients; it usually portends a benign clinical course with recurrent episodes of gross hematuria without progression to CKD. IgAN can also present as an acute glomerulonephritis or an even more aggressive RPGN, with variable degrees of AKI, hypertension, edema, proteinuria, and hematuria.

*Diagnosis*

The diagnosis of IgAN may be suspected clinically but can only be made by kidney biopsy showing dominant mesangial immune-deposits of IgA with C3, and occasionally IgG or IgM. In some centers, patients with microscopic hematuria, normal kidney function, and proteinuria <500 mg/24 h are given an empiric diagnosis of IgAN without a biopsy because the disease course is expected to be mild in these cases. In other centers, patients with microscopic hematuria that is deemed to be glomerular in origin (that is, presence of dysmorphic erythrocytes or erythrocyte casts in the urine sediment) elicits a biopsy regardless of kidney function or proteinuria.

*Treatment and Prognosis*

There are no current standard care therapies for IgAN other than conservative, nonimmunomodulatory therapies. Antiproteinuric therapy using an ACE inhibitor or ARB is a hallmark for treating IgAN; it is usually coupled with lipid-lowering therapy and fish oil, although the efficacy of the latter two as specific IgAN therapies is unproven. The use of immunosuppression in IgAN remains controversial. In the United States, it is common for most patients with IgAN who progress to ESKD to have done so despite long-term renin-angiotensin system blockade and at least one course of immunosuppressive therapy.

Approximately one third of patients with IgAN will have a benign long-term course, with continued microscopic hematuria but little to no proteinuria and no evidence of kidney dysfunction. The disease progresses to CKD or ESKD in the remainder of patients, with up to 40% reaching ESKD within 15 years of diagnosis. The recent Oxford histopathology classification of IgAN provides evidence that advanced disease chronicity, manifesting as >50% tubular atrophy and interstitial fibrosis on kidney biopsy, is the most reliable predictor of progression to ESKD. Among clinical parameters, proteinuria ≥1000 mg/24 h has been shown to be a risk factor for progression.

## IgA Vasculitis

IgA vasculitis (Henoch-Schönlein purpura) can present with the classic tetrad of rash, arthralgia, abdominal pain, and kidney disease. Considered a systemic version of IgAN, this vasculitis is often diagnosed empirically in the pediatric setting, because the differential diagnosis of vasculitis in children is extremely limited. In adults, the diagnosis should be confirmed with tissue biopsy (kidney or skin), because the presentation of IgA vasculitis can also fit with a non-IgA form of vasculitis. Skin biopsy is usually adequate to make the diagnosis when lesions less than 24 hours old in appearance are sampled. Kidney involvement in IgA vasculitis typically is more severe in adults than in children, with higher rates of AKI and the nephrotic syndrome. Treatment includes glucocorticoids and, in cases of associated RPGN, cyclophosphamide.

See MKSAP 18 Rheumatology for more information.

## Lupus Nephritis

See MKSAP 18 Rheumatology for more information on systemic lupus erythematosus.

*Epidemiology and Pathophysiology*

Kidney involvement in systemic lupus erythematosus (SLE), generally termed lupus nephritis (LN), is a major contributor to SLE-associated morbidity and mortality. Up to 50% of patients with SLE will have clinically evident kidney disease at presentation; during follow-up, kidney involvement occurs in up to 75% of patients. LN has been shown to affect clinical outcomes in SLE both directly via target organ damage and indirectly through complications of therapy.

The immune deposits that incite LN are primarily complexes of anti–double-stranded DNA antibodies directed against nucleosomal antigens. A smaller fraction of autoantibodies can also bind directly to chromatin in the glomerular basement membrane (GBM) and mesangium. These immune complexes, when deposited in the mesangium and subendothelial space, are proximal to the GBM and are in communication with the systemic circulation. Subsequent activation of the classical complement pathway, triggered by the DNA/anti-DNA antibody complex formation, generates the potent chemoattractants, C3a and C5a, which elicit an influx of neutrophils and mononuclear cells. The pattern on light microscopy is a proliferative glomerulonephritis that can be mesangial (class II), focal endocapillary (class III), or diffuse endocapillary (class IV) (**Table 20**). Endocapillary proliferation refers to an increased number of inflammatory cells within glomerular capillary lumina, causing luminal narrowing or obliteration. Immune complex deposits in the subepithelial space can also activate complement but only locally; C3a and C5a are separated from the circulation by the GBM, and hence no influx of inflammatory cells occurs into this space. The injury in this class V LN (membranous) is limited to the glomerular epithelial cells, the primary clinical manifestation is proteinuria, and the histologic pattern on light microscopy is similar to primary membranous nephropathy.

*Clinical Manifestations*

Typically, patients with SLE initially present with evidence of non–kidney organ involvement (malar rash, arthritis, oral ulcers). After a diagnosis of SLE is confirmed, evidence of kidney disease, if present, usually emerges within the first 3 years of diagnosis. Kidney involvement in SLE first manifests with proteinuria and/or microscopic hematuria on urinalysis; this eventually progresses to reduction in kidney function. Early in the course of disease, it is unusual for patients to present with decreased kidney function, except for very aggressive cases of LN that present as RPGN. The symptoms of kidney involvement tend to correlate with laboratory abnormalities. For example, patients with nephrotic-range proteinuria can present with edema. When kidney function is impaired, elevated blood pressure is a common clinical finding.

**TABLE 20.** Classification of Lupus Nephritis with Associated Presentation and Treatment Options

| ISN/RPS Class | Biopsy Findings | Clinical Features | Treatment | |
|---|---|---|---|---|
| | | | **Induction Phase** | **Maintenance Phase** |
| Class I: minimal mesangial LN | No LM abnormalities; isolated mesangial IC deposits on IF and/or EM | Normal urine or microscopic hematuria | Conservative, nonimmunomodulatory therapy (e.g., RAS blockade) | Not applicable |
| Class II: mesangial proliferative LN | Mesangial hypercellularity or matrix expansion with mesangial IC deposits on IF and/or EM | Microscopic hematuria and/or low-grade proteinuria | Conservative, nonimmunomodulatory therapy (e.g., RAS blockade) | Not applicable |
| Class III: focal LN | <50% of glomeruli on LM display segmental (<50% of glomerular tuft) or global (>50% of glomerular tuft) endocapillary and/or extracapillary proliferation or sclerosis; mesangial and focal subendothelial IC deposits on IF and EM | Nephritic urine sediment and subnephrotic proteinuria | Pulse IV glucocorticoids followed by tapering doses of oral glucocorticoids *and* IV cyclophosphamide for 6 doses (high-dose monthly vs. low-dose bimonthly) *or* Mycophenolate mofetil for 6 months | Lowest tolerable amount of oral glucocorticoids *and* Mycophenolate mofetil (tapered down every 3-6 months assuming stable disease) *or* Azathioprine (tapered down every 3-6 months assuming stable disease) |
| Class IV: diffuse LN | ≥50% of glomeruli on LM display endocapillary and/or extracapillary proliferation or sclerosis; class IV-S denotes that ≥50% of affected glomeruli have segmental lesions; class IV-G denotes that ≥50% of affected glomeruli have global lesions; mesangial and diffuse subendothelial IC deposits on IF and EM | Nephritic and nephrotic syndromes; hypertension; reduced kidney function | Pulse IV glucocorticoids followed by tapering doses of oral glucocorticoids *and* IV cyclophosphamide for 6 doses (high-dose monthly vs. low-dose bimonthly) *or* Mycophenolate mofetil for 6 months | Lowest tolerable amount of oral glucocorticoids *and* Mycophenolate mofetil (tapered down every 3-6 months assuming stable disease) *or* Azathioprine (tapered down every 3-6 months assuming stable disease) |
| Class V: membranous LN[a] | Diffuse thickening of the glomerular capillary walls on LM with subepithelial IC deposits on IF and EM, with or without mesangial IC deposits | Nephrotic syndrome | Pulse IV glucocorticoids followed by tapering doses of oral glucocorticoids *and* IV cyclophosphamide for 6 doses (high-dose monthly vs. low-dose bimonthly) *or* Cyclosporine *or* Tacrolimus *or* Mycophenolate mofetil for 6 months | Lowest tolerable amount of oral glucocorticoids *and* Mycophenolate mofetil (tapered down every 3-6 months assuming stable disease) *or* Azathioprine (tapered down every 3-6 months assuming stable disease) |
| Class VI: advanced sclerosing LN | >90% of glomeruli on LM are globally sclerosed with no residual activity | Advanced CKD or ESKD with varying degrees of hematuria and/or proteinuria | Conservative, nonimmunomodulatory therapy (e.g., RAS blockade) with preparation for renal replacement therapy | Not applicable |

CKD = chronic kidney disease; EM = electron microscopy; ESKD = end-stage kidney disease; IC = immune complex; IF = immunofluorescence; ISN/RPS = International Society of Nephrology/Renal Pathology Society; IV = intravenous; LM = light microscopy; LN = lupus nephritis; RAS = renin-angiotensin system.

[a]Class V may coexist with class III or class IV, in which case both classes are diagnosed.

*Diagnosis*

The diagnosis of LN is suspected by changes in laboratory parameters (elevated serum creatinine, hematuria and/or proteinuria, low serum complements) but can only be made definitively by kidney biopsy. The classic pattern of LN is an immune complex–mediated glomerulonephritis with a varied pathology that includes six distinct classes of disease (see Table 20). On immunofluorescence microscopy, the glomerular deposits in LN stain dominantly for IgG with co-deposits of IgA, IgM, C3, and C1q in a "full house" pattern. On electron microscopy, tubuloreticular inclusions, which represent "interferon footprints" in the glomerular endothelial cell cytoplasm, are essentially pathognomonic for LN.

*Treatment and Prognosis*

The current approach to treating LN is guided by histologic findings with appropriate consideration of presenting clinical parameters and the degree of kidney function impairment (see Table 20). Important recent changes in the management of LN include the preferential use of mycophenolate mofetil over cyclophosphamide as induction therapy for LN classes III, IV, and V based on similar efficacy rates and a more favorable side-effect profile with mycophenolate mofetil (in particular, the non-impact on fertility of mycophenolate mofetil compared with cyclophosphamide in a young patient population with childbearing potential). The landmark ALMS trial showed only a 56% response rate in the mycophenolate arm (compared with a 53% response rate in the cyclophosphamide arm).

Up to 30% of patients with LN will progress to ESKD within 10 years of diagnosis, depending in large part on the response to the initial course of immunosuppression. Severity of disease at the time of diagnosis as well as black race, Hispanic ethnicity, and socioeconomic status have also been reported to influence outcomes in LN.

## Infection-Related Glomerulonephritis

*Epidemiology and Pathophysiology*

Infection-related glomerulonephritis (IRGN) results from a recently resolved infection or an infection that is ongoing at the time of development of glomerulonephritis. IRGN is preferred to the formerly used term "postinfectious glomerulonephritis," which adequately described classic poststreptococcal glomerulonephritis but did not address the increasingly recognized forms of glomerulonephritis that are manifestations of ongoing infection and nonstreptococcal infectious agents. Diabetes is the most common comorbidity (malignancy, immunosuppression, AIDS, alcoholism, and injection drug use are other recognized comorbidities), and older age is a key risk factor. Patients over 65 years of age account for about one third of IRGN cases in the developed world.

The incidence of poststreptococcal glomerulonephritis has declined throughout most of the world due to improvements in infection control and sanitation. The entity, however, remains a health concern in developing countries: More than 450,000 cases of poststreptococcal glomerulonephritis occur worldwide annually, resulting in approximately 5000 deaths, with >95% of these cases in less developed countries. In industrialized countries, much of the burden of IRGN has shifted from children to adults, with a decrease in IRGN attributed to streptococcal infections and an increase in IRGN cases associated with *Staphylococcus aureus* and gram-negative bacteria.

In the classical view of the pathogenesis of IRGN, antibodies directed at bacterial antigens form immune complexes in the circulation that subsequently deposit in the glomerulus. Additionally, however, antibodies directed at bacterial antigens planted within glomeruli can result in *in situ* formation of glomerular immune complexes.

*Clinical Manifestations*

The variable presentation of IRGN ranges from asymptomatic microscopic hematuria to RPGN. Proteinuria is usually subnephrotic.

In classic poststreptococcal glomerulonephritis, symptomatic patients (typically children) present with an acute nephritic syndrome of hematuria, proteinuria, hypertension, edema, and, in some cases, kidney dysfunction. The urine sediment is active with dysmorphic erythrocytes, erythrocyte casts, and leukocyturia. Hypocomplementemia is very common, with decreased C3 in up to 90% of cases. There is usually a latent period (1 to 2 weeks after upper respiratory infections; 2 to 4 weeks after skin infections) between the resolution of the streptococcal infection and the onset of the nephritic syndrome. Serologic markers of a recent streptococcal infection, including elevated antistreptolysin O, antistreptokinase, antihyaluronidase, and antideoxyribonuclease B antibody levels, are often detected. In adults, most cases of IRGN are no longer poststreptococcal, and the glomerulonephritis often coexists with the triggering infection. Low complement levels may be absent in these peri-infectious cases.

*Diagnosis*

The diagnosis of IRGN can be made clinically in the appropriate setting (for example, classic nephritic presentation with low complements and clear evidence of a recent infection), although the only definitive way to make the diagnosis is by kidney biopsy. The most common finding on light microscopy is a proliferative glomerulonephritis with significant presence of infiltrating neutrophils. On electron microscopy, the classic finding in poststreptococcal glomerulonephritis is hump-shaped subepithelial electron dense deposits, although these are not required for the diagnosis of IRGN.

*Treatment and Prognosis*

Treatment is typically supportive and aimed at the infectious etiology, although in some cases with severe proliferative glomerulonephritis on biopsy, a trial of glucocorticoids is used.

In children, prognosis for complete recovery is excellent, and treatment usually is supportive and aimed at the infecting organism. The prognosis of the newly recognized forms of IRGN (for example, due to *S. aureus* and gram-negative organisms) in adults is different, with more patients developing severe kidney dysfunction and progressing to CKD and sometimes ESKD.

## Membranoproliferative Glomerulonephritis
### Epidemiology and Pathophysiology
Membranoproliferative glomerulonephritis (MPGN) is a rare form of chronic glomerulonephritis diagnosed primarily in children and young adults. The name stems from its pattern of glomerular injury. The entity is divided into immune-complex forms of MPGN (mediated by antigen-antibody interactions triggering the classical complement pathway) versus complement-mediated forms of MPGN (also termed C3 glomerulopathies, due to a hyperactive alternative complement pathway). An immune-complex MPGN, with or without cryoglobulinemia, is the classic form of kidney involvement seen in patients with hepatitis C virus infection. The alternative complement pathway abnormalities that drive the C3 glomerulopathies are either mutations in regulators (for example, complement factor H) or activators (for example, complement factor B) of the alternative pathway, or antibodies directed at regulator or activator complement proteins.

### Clinical Manifestations
Although MPGN can rarely present as an acute and severe form of glomerulonephritis, the more common presentation is a chronic glomerulonephritis that initially manifests with microscopic hematuria and subnephrotic proteinuria. As disease progresses, proteinuria can reach nephrotic range, and kidney dysfunction ensues.

### Diagnosis
The diagnosis of MPGN is made by kidney biopsy. The distinction between immune-complex and complement-mediated MPGN is based on immunofluorescence microscopy, in which the absence of immunoglobulin staining signals an antibody-independent manner of triggering complement and hence alternative pathway hyperactivity.

### Treatment and Prognosis
Currently, treatment of MPGN is nonspecific and includes immunosuppression (for example, glucocorticoids) when nephrotic-range proteinuria and/or kidney dysfunction is present. The advent of complement-targeting therapies such as the C5 monoclonal antibody, eculizumab, may bring disease-specific therapy for the complement-mediated forms of MPGN.

The overall prognosis of MPGN as a chronic form of glomerulonephritis is poor, with >50% of patients progressing to ESKD within 15 years of diagnosis.

## Cryoglobulinemia
Cryoglobulinemia can be associated with the nephritic syndrome. Of the three types of cryoglobulins, kidney involvement is typically due to type II cryoglobulins.

See MKSAP 18 Hematology and Oncology for details on cryoglobulinemia; MKSAP 18 Rheumatology for information on cryoglobulinemic vasculitis; and Kidney Manifestations of Deposition Diseases in MKSAP 18 Nephrology for information on kidney involvement in cryoglobulinemia.

## Collagen Type IV–Related Nephropathies
Type IV collagen is an integral component of the glomerular basement membrane. Structural defects in this protein due to genetic variations can result in a hereditary form of glomerulonephritis, discussed in more detail in Genetic Disorders and Kidney Disease.

**KEY POINTS**

- Treatment of IgA nephropathy consists of conservative therapy using an ACE inhibitor or angiotensin receptor blocker.
- Kidney biopsy is required to diagnose and classify lupus nephritis, which guides therapy.
- Treatment of classes I and II lupus nephritis (LN) includes conservative therapy with an ACE inhibitor or angiotensin receptor blocker; classes III, IV, and V LN may require aggressive immunosuppressive therapy; and class VI LN may be treated with conservative therapy.
- Infection-related glomerulonephritis results from a recently resolved infection or an infection that is ongoing at the time of development of glomerulonephritis; in industrialized countries, clinical disease is seen more often in adults and is associated with *Staphylococcus aureus* and gram-negative bacteria.
- Treatment of membranoproliferative glomerulonephritis is nonspecific and includes immunosuppression when nephrotic-range proteinuria and/or kidney dysfunction is present.

# Kidney Manifestations of Deposition Diseases
## Overview
Various kidney diseases are associated with deposition of immunoglobulin (Ig) and non-Ig proteins. On electron microscopy, these deposits can be unstructured or organized into fibrils or tubules (**Figure 14**). Monoclonal Ig deposits may be caused by myeloma, Waldenström macroglobulinemia, or chronic lymphocytic leukemia, or by the clonal expansion of Ig-secreting cells that do not meet the strict definition of these disorders, which has been termed *monoclonal gammopathy of renal significance* (MGRS). The pathological findings associated with monoclonal Ig deposition can include proliferative glomerulonephritis, AL amyloid, type 1 cryoglobulinemia, and, occasionally, immunotactoid and fibrillary glomerulopathy. Polyclonal Ig deposits include

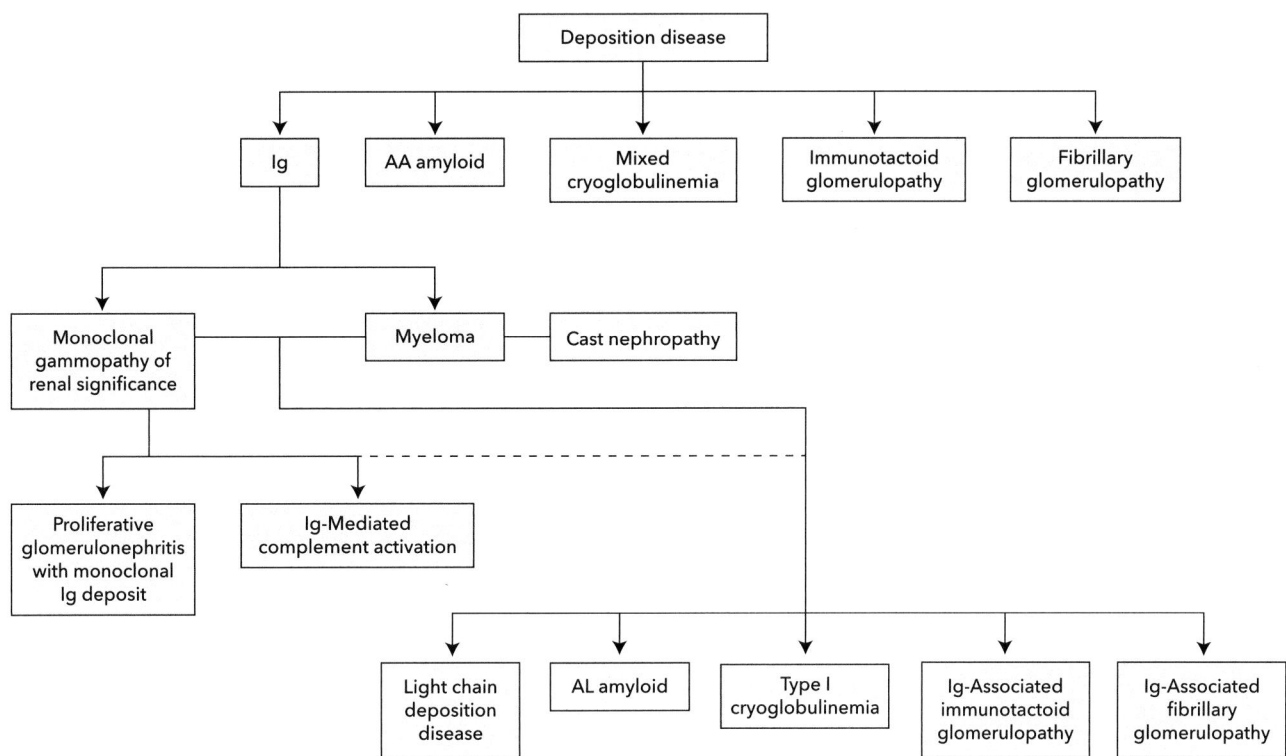

**FIGURE 14.** Deposition diseases can be divided into five major categories: immunoglobulin (Ig)-related disease, amyloid, cryoglobulinemia, immunotactoid glomerulopathy, and fibrillary glomerulopathy. Ig-related disease can be further divided into multiple myeloma and monoclonal gammopathy of renal significance (MGRS). Although some histopathological findings occur more commonly in either multiple myeloma (such as cast nephropathy) or MGRS, most have been reported in either disorder.

mixed cryoglobulinemia, whereas non-Ig proteins contribute to AA amyloid and to most cases of immunotactoid and fibrillary glomerulopathy.

## Monoclonal Immunoglobulin–Associated Kidney Disease

A wide array of renal lesions can be caused by clonal expansion of Ig-secreting cells. If there are greater than 10% plasma cells on bone marrow biopsy or the presence of an extramedullary plasmacytoma, a diagnosis of multiple myeloma can be made. However, as noted above, paraproteinemia caused by clonal expansion of Ig-secreting cells that do not meet the strict definition of myeloma, Waldenström macroglobulinemia, or chronic lymphocytic leukemia can be associated with nephrotoxicity. Although some of the findings noted pathologically occur more frequently with either MGRS or myeloma, except for myeloma cast nephropathy seen exclusively with myeloma, all the renal lesions can occur in each of these disorders. Because filtered light chains are endocytosed by proximal tubule cells and are nephrotoxic, patients may present with proximal tubular dysfunction with Fanconi syndrome; common features include glycosuria, phosphaturia, and normal anion gap metabolic acidosis. Kidney function may be normal or abnormal.

## Myeloma Cast Nephropathy

Myeloma cast nephropathy occurs in the presence of a markedly increased concentration of free light chains and is always associated with multiple myeloma. Light chains are freely filtered by the glomerulus and combine with secreted Tamm-Horsfall protein to form obstructing casts. These tubular casts have a characteristic fractured appearance on microscopic examination. Patients with cast nephropathy present with acute or slowly progressive kidney injury. Serum free light chains are extremely elevated. Treatment is aimed at reducing the concentration of free light chains using chemotherapy. Plasmapheresis may also be beneficial in selected patients.

## Monoclonal Gammopathy of Renal Significance

Monoclonal gammopathy of renal significance (MGRS) is characterized by kidney damage caused by monoclonal Ig that is secreted by a B cell or plasma cell clone not meeting diagnostic criteria for multiple myeloma or a lymphoproliferative disorder. All pathological findings associated with the clonal expansion of Ig-secreting cells can be seen in both myeloma and MGRS. The underlying pathology is likely determined by the characteristics of the secreted protein. Entities associated with MGRS include proliferative glomerulonephritis with monoclonal Ig deposits (PGNMID), C3 glomerulopathy with monoclonal gammopathy, AL amyloid, type 1 cryoglobulinemia, fibrillary glomerulonephritis, and immunotactoid glomerulopathy.

Kidney manifestations of MGRS are usually caused by deposition of monoclonal Ig light chains. Patients can present with both nephrotic and subnephrotic proteinuria, hematuria, and elevated serum creatinine.

Kidney biopsy is necessary to make the diagnosis. In addition to evaluating for underlying myeloma and chronic lymphocytic leukemia, further testing may include serum and urine protein electrophoresis, immunofixation, measurement of free light chains, and bone marrow biopsy. Because treatment is aimed at eradication of the expanded clonal line, it is important that the care of patients with MGRS be coordinated with a myeloma specialist.

# Amyloidosis

Amyloidosis is a disorder characterized by the fibrillary deposition of insoluble amyloid proteins that form β-pleated sheets, which exhibit green birefringence on polarizing microscopy when stained with Congo red. Amyloid fibrils are approximately 10 nm in diameter, as opposed to the larger microtubules seen in fibrillary glomerulonephritis and immunotactoid glomerulopathy. Although amyloid can be made up of numerous proteins, kidney disease is most commonly caused by AL amyloid or AA amyloid. AL amyloid is composed of monoclonal λ (most commonly) or κ light chains produced by either MGRS or myeloma; AA amyloid is formed by serum amyloid A protein, an acute phase reactant produced in various inflammatory diseases such as rheumatoid arthritis, inflammatory bowel disease, chronic osteomyelitis, and familial Mediterranean fever. Patients with renal amyloid frequently present with nephrotic-range proteinuria. Less commonly, amyloid can affect only the renal vasculature or tubular-interstitium and have minimal or no proteinuria. Treatment is aimed at the underlying disease.

# Monoclonal Immunoglobulin Deposition Disease

Monoclonal light chains (usually κ) or heavy chains can be deposited in the kidney and manifest as proteinuria and kidney failure. Unlike AL amyloid, these proteins do not form β-pleated sheets and do not stain with Congo red. These deposits can be limited to the basement membrane, giving a microscopic appearance similar to that of diabetic nodular sclerosis (light chain deposition disease), or can activate complement and induce a proliferative glomerulonephritis (PGNMID). In some cases, an underlying plasma cell dyscrasia or lymphoproliferative disorder can be identified, but

criteria for myeloma or chronic lymphocytic leukemia are often absent.

# Cryoglobulinemia

Of the three types of cryoglobulinemia, kidney involvement occurs most frequently with type II (mixed Ig) cryoglobulinemia and is usually associated with hepatitis C virus infection. Patients can present with a nephritic picture: elevated serum creatinine, hypertension, proteinuria, and hematuria. Membranoproliferative glomerulonephritis is usually noted on biopsy. Occasionally, a rapidly progressive glomerulonephritis with crescent formation can occur. A palpable purpuric rash is frequently present on the lower extremities. Because hepatitis C is the predominant cause, treatment is aimed at eradication of the virus.

# Fibrillary and Immunotactoid Glomerulopathy

Although rare, both fibrillary and immunotactoid glomerulopathy are becoming increasingly recognized causes of kidney disease. These diseases are caused by glomerular deposition of microtubular structures that are larger than amyloid (20 nm in fibrillary glomerulopathy and >30 nm in immunotactoid glomerulopathy) and do not stain with Congo red. Proteinuria, frequently in the nephrotic range, and hematuria are common. Although the pathogenesis of these entities is unknown, both have been associated with paraproteinemia. Treatment is usually unsuccessful, and kidney outcomes are poor.

**KEY POINTS**

- Patients with myeloma cast nephropathy present with acute or slowly progressive kidney injury and have extremely elevated serum free light chains; treatment is aimed at reducing the concentration of free light chains using chemotherapy.

- Diseases causing monoclonal gammopathy of renal significance can present with either nephrotic or subnephrotic proteinuria, hematuria, and elevated serum creatinine; kidney biopsy is necessary to make the diagnosis, and treatment is aimed at eradication of the expanded clonal line.

- Kidney disease in amyloidosis is most commonly caused by AL amyloid composed of monoclonal λ or κ light chains or AA amyloid formed by serum amyloid A protein; patients frequently present with nephrotic-range proteinuria, and treatment is aimed at the underlying disorder.

- Kidney involvement in cryoglobulinemia occurs most frequently with type II (mixed) cryoglobulins and is usually associated with hepatitis C virus infection; treatment is directed at eradication of hepatitis C virus.

# Genetic Disorders and Kidney Disease

## Genetic Cystic Kidney Disorders

Genetic cystic kidney disorders are categorized in **Table 21**.

### Autosomal Dominant Polycystic Kidney Disease

Autosomal dominant polycystic kidney disease (ADPKD) is the leading genetic cause of end-stage kidney disease (ESKD) and the fourth leading cause of ESKD. ADPKD manifests as large kidneys with multiple kidney cysts (**Figure 15**). Genetic mutations in *PKD1* and *PKD2*, which encode for proteins that regulate differentiation and proliferation of renal tubular epithelial cells, account for approximately 85% and 15% of cases, respectively. More than 90% of mutations are inherited as an autosomal dominant trait, with spontaneous germline mutations accounting for the remaining cases.

#### Screening and Diagnosis

Ultrasonography is the most common and least costly screening method for ADPKD. Ultrasonography criteria for diagnosing ADPKD are based on the number of visible cysts, the patient's age, and a family history of ADPKD. Direct DNA sequencing of the *PKD1* and *PKD2* genes is increasingly used to confirm diagnosis or, in some cases, is performed in lieu of imaging. Gene linkage testing, which identifies DNA markers in several members of a family, can also be used in patients with a family history of ADPKD.

#### Clinical Manifestations

Early in the disease, there are generally no symptoms. Diagnosis is therefore often delayed in patients without a known family history of ADPKD. The first sign of ADPKD is often hypertension; other early signs and symptoms include hematuria (macroscopic or microscopic), pain or bloating in the back or abdomen, urinary tract infection, or kidney

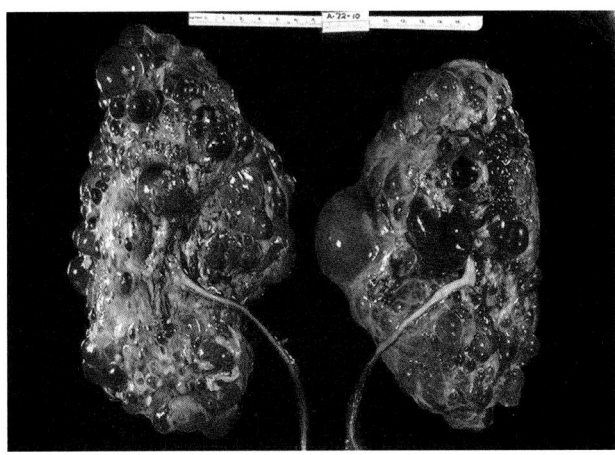

**FIGURE 15.** Autosomal dominant polycystic kidney disease with multiple bilateral cysts, which replace the normal smooth architecture of the kidneys and lead to markedly increased kidney size.

Image from the CDC Public Health Image Library.

stones. In patients without a family history, these presentations usually lead to imaging studies that reveal ADPKD. CT or MRI may be used to evaluate for complications in patients with known ADPKD, such as bleeding into a cyst or a suspected kidney stone.

Extrarenal manifestations include hepatic cysts (detected in >80% of patients over their lifetime), mitral valve prolapse, inguinal and umbilical hernias, and intracranial aneurysms (detected in 5%-10% of patients, with a strong familial pattern).

#### Management

Patients with ADPKD have a >50% chance of progressing to ESKD by age 70 years. No disease-specific therapies currently exist; therefore, management is focused on controlling blood pressure and addressing complications of disease. Vasopressin blockade with tolvaptan in patients with ADPKD has been shown in two randomized clinical trials to delay the need for

**TABLE 21.** Genetic Cystic Kidney Disorders

| Disorder | Inheritance | Gene(s) | Features/Comments |
|---|---|---|---|
| Autosomal dominant polycystic kidney disease | AD | *PKD1* <br> *PKD2* | Most common inherited kidney disorder (5% of ESKD cases); intracranial cerebral aneurysm; mitral valve prolapse; hepatic cysts; diverticulosis |
| Autosomal recessive polycystic kidney disease | AR | *PKHD1* | Causes ESKD in infancy or childhood; hepatic fibrosis; portal hypertension; homozygous mutations cause complete loss of function: severe cystic kidney disease, oligohydramnios, pulmonary hypoplasia, Potter syndrome (limb deformities, typical facial appearance, pulmonary hypoplasia) |
| Tuberous sclerosis complex | AD | *TSC1* <br> *TSC2* | Characterized by benign hamartomas; epilepsy, brain tumors, developmental delay, autism, and lung disease may also occur; renal angiomyolipomas are common; kidney cysts may develop |
| Nephronophthisis | AR | Multiple (13) | Most common genetic cause of ESKD detected in childhood/adolescence; interstitial fibrosis; renal medullary cysts; a renal concentrating defect and/or salt wasting; retinitis pigmentosa |

AD = autosomal dominant; AR = autosomal recessive; ESKD = end-stage kidney disease.

dialysis from 6 to 9 years. However, tolvaptan carries an FDA-mandated safety warning about the possibility of irreversible liver injury, and it has not been approved by the FDA for use in ADPKD.

The Guidelines for the Management of Patients with Unruptured Intracranial Aneurysms from the American Heart Association/American Stroke Association recommend that patients with a history of ADPKD, particularly those with a family history of intracranial aneurysm, should be offered screening by CT angiography or MR angiography. This is a class I recommendation (should be performed because benefit greatly exceeds risk) based on level B evidence (data derived from a single randomized trial or nonrandomized studies).

## Tuberous Sclerosis Complex

Tuberous sclerosis complex (TSC) is a genetic disorder with mutations in the tumor-suppressing genes *TSC1* or *TSC2* and resulting tumors in many organs, primarily in the brain, eyes, heart, kidney, skin, and lungs. Although TSC is most frequently diagnosed in the pediatric population, mild disease may escape detection until adulthood. Nearly 1 million people worldwide are estimated to have TSC, with approximately 50,000 in the United States.

Renal angiomyolipomas occur in 75% of patients with TSC and can be detected by CT, ultrasonography, or MRI. Renal cell carcinoma occurs in 1% to 2% of adults with TSC, and therefore screening with abdominal MRI is recommended every 1 to 3 years. Kidney cysts may also develop. The features of TSC that most strongly affect quality of life are generally associated with the brain: seizures, developmental delay, intellectual disability, and autism.

Therapy is rarely needed for the kidney manifestations of TSC. Surgery or related interventions (radiofrequency ablation, selective arterial embolization) may be required for large or hemorrhagic angiomyolipomas.

### KEY POINTS

- Autosomal dominant polycystic kidney disease is characterized by large kidneys with multiple kidney cysts, hypertension, hematuria, pain or bloating in the back or abdomen, urinary tract infection, or kidney stones.

- No disease-specific therapies currently exist for autosomal dominant polycystic kidney disease; therefore, management is focused on controlling blood pressure and addressing complications of disease.

- Kidney manifestations of tuberous sclerosis complex include renal angiomyolipomas, renal cell carcinoma, and cysts; surgery or related interventions may be required for large or hemorrhagic angiomyolipomas.

## Genetic Noncystic Kidney Disorders

Genetic noncystic kidney disorders are categorized in **Table 22**.

## Collagen Type IV-Related Nephropathies

Type IV collagen is an integral component of the glomerular basement membrane (GBM). Structural defects in this protein, due to genetic variations, can result in manifestations spanning from GBM thinning to progressive glomerular injury.

### Hereditary Nephritis

Hereditary nephritis (Alport syndrome) is a glomerular disease associated with sensorineural hearing loss and characteristic ocular findings that include corneal dystrophies, microcornea, arcus, iris atrophy, cataracts, spontaneous lens rupture, spherophakia, and anterior lenticonus. There are three genetic variants: X-linked (80%), autosomal recessive (15%), and autosomal dominant (5%). Females with the X-linked variant can be asymptomatic carriers or can develop kidney disease depending on activity of the X chromosome in somatic renal cells. The disease has a prevalence of 0.4% among U.S. adults.

Diagnosis has traditionally been made by kidney biopsy with electron microscopy; the hallmark finding is prominent thickening and lamellation of the GBM in a "basket-weave" appearance. In patients with a clearly documented family history and abnormal urinary findings, diagnosis is increasingly being made by genetic testing. Genetic testing is also the most reliable way to identify heterozygote carriers of type IV collagen mutations. Proteinuria, hypertension, and chronic kidney disease (CKD) usually progress to ESKD between the late teenage years and the fourth decade of life. Management is supportive, including blood pressure control via renin-angiotensin system blockade.

### Thin Glomerular Basement Membrane Disease

Thin glomerular basement membrane disease (benign familial hematuria) is associated with type IV collagen variants causing GBM thinning, which results in hematuria without significant proteinuria or ensuing glomerulosclerosis. Up to 5% of the population may be affected. Although diagnosis can be made using electron microscopy of kidney biopsy material, thin glomerular basement membrane disease is usually a clinical diagnosis based on benign presentation and course (normal kidney function with microscopic hematuria and little or no proteinuria) and positive family history of similarly benign phenotype (family history of isolated hematuria without kidney failure). The disease has excellent long-term prognosis with rare progression to CKD. Management is supportive.

### Fabry Disease

Fabry disease is an X-linked recessive inborn error of glycosphingolipid metabolism caused by deficiency of α-galactosidase A. The gene responsible for α-galactosidase is located on the long arm of the X chromosome, with almost 200 mutations identified. The enzyme deficiency leads to defective storage of sphingolipid and progressive endothelial

**TABLE 22.** Genetic Noncystic Kidney Disorders

| Disorder | Inheritance | Gene(s) | Features/Comments |
|---|---|---|---|
| Autosomal dominant tubulointerstitial kidney disease (also called medullary cystic kidney disease or uromodulin-associated kidney disease) | AD | *UMOD*; *REN*; *MUC1*; *HNF1B* | Rare; medullary cysts may or may not be present; slow progression to ESKD; bland urine sediment; may be associated with gout and anemia |
| Collagen type IV-related nephropathies | | | |
|    Hereditary nephritis (Alport syndrome) | X-linked | *COL4A5* | Sensorineural hearing loss; lenticonus (conical deformation of the lens) |
| | AD or AR | *COL4A3* | Similar phenotype as X-linked with some variability |
| | AD or AR | *COL4A4* | Similar to *COL4A3* |
|    Thin glomerular basement membrane disease (benign familial hematuria) | Primarily AD | *COL4A3*; *COL4A4* | Microscopic or macroscopic hematuria |
| Hereditary nephrotic syndromes | | | |
|    Congenital nephropathy (Finnish type) | AR | *NEPH1*; *NEPH2* | Severe perinatal nephrotic syndrome; ESKD; kidney transplantation is only treatment |
|    Familial FSGS | AR or AD | *NEPH2*; *ACTN4*; *TRPC6*; *INF2*; *APOL1* | The nephrotic syndrome; ESKD; should be considered in FSGS patients who are infants, are young (<25 years) and steroid-resistant, or have family history of ESKD |
|    Denys-Drash syndrome | AR | *WT1* | Cause of pediatric nephrotic syndrome; associated with urogenital abnormalities |
| Fabry disease | X-linked | *GLA* | Progressive kidney disease; premature coronary artery disease; severe neuropathic pain; telangiectasias; angiokeratomas |
| *APOL1* nephropathy | AR | *APOL1* | High-risk genotypes present in ~13% of black persons; account for a large fraction of nondiabetic kidney disease in black persons |

AD = autosomal dominant; *APOL1* = apolipoprotein 1; AR = autosomal recessive; ESKD = end-stage kidney disease; FSGS = focal segmental glomerulosclerosis.

accumulation, causing abnormalities in the skin, eye, kidney, heart, brain, and peripheral nervous system.

Fabry disease should be considered as a cause of CKD of unknown etiology in young adulthood. Diagnosis can be made by kidney biopsy but also can be made noninvasively with measurement of leukocyte enzymatic activity and subsequent genetic confirmation. Screening for the disease is recommended for family members of affected patients. Enzyme replacement therapy with recombinant human α-galactosidase A is available.

## Apolipoprotein L1 Nephropathy

Black persons develop kidney failure at rates four to five times higher than white persons. Recently, genetic variants in the apolipoprotein L1 (*APOL1*) gene were discovered that explain a large fraction of this health disparity. Two risk alleles for kidney disease (G1 and G2) have been identified in the *APOL1* gene. The transmission of disease risk is consistent with recessive inheritance: The high-risk *APOL1* genotype can be G1/G1, G1/G2, or G2/G2. Approximately 12% to 15% of black persons inherit a high-risk *APOL1* genotype; this accounts for a large fraction of nondiabetic kidney disease in black persons. High-risk *APOL1* alleles are unusually prevalent possibly because they conferred a survival advantage in sub-Saharan Africa by enhancing innate immunity against African trypanosomal disease (African sleeping sickness).

Persons with a high-risk *APOL1* genotype have an approximately 10-fold increased risk for focal segmental glomerulosclerosis, a 7-fold increased risk for hypertension-attributed ESKD, and, among those with HIV infection, a 29-fold increased risk for HIV-associated nephropathy. In addition, the *APOL1* risk genotype is associated with an increased risk for progression to CKD in other nondiabetic kidney diseases, including lupus nephritis and primary membranous nephropathy.

**KEY POINTS**

- Hereditary nephritis (Alport syndrome) is a glomerular disease associated with sensorineural hearing loss and characteristic ocular findings; proteinuria, hypertension, and chronic kidney disease usually progress to end-stage kidney disease between the late teenage years and the fourth decade of life.

- Thin glomerular basement membrane disease (benign familial hematuria) results in hematuria without significant proteinuria or ensuing glomerulosclerosis, with rare progression to chronic kidney disease.

*(Continued)*

- Fabry disease should be considered as a cause of chronic kidney disease of unknown etiology in young adulthood; treatment with recombinant human α-galactosidase A is available.

- High-risk *APOL1* genotype confers increased risk for chronic kidney disease in black persons, including an approximately 10-fold increased risk for focal segmental glomerulosclerosis, a 7-fold increased risk for hypertension-attributed end-stage kidney disease, and a 29-fold increased risk for HIV-associated nephropathy among those with HIV infection.

# Acute Kidney Injury

## Definition

Acute kidney injury (AKI) is characterized by a sudden decrease in kidney function resulting in an increase in serum creatinine concentration and the accumulation of nitrogenous excretory products over a course of hours to days. AKI is commonly accompanied by decreased urine output, fluid retention, metabolic acidosis, hyperkalemia, and hyperphosphatemia. The Kidney Disease: Improving Global Outcomes (KDIGO) Acute Kidney Injury Work Group definitions for AKI are described in **Table 23**. Multiple studies have shown a correlation between more severe stages of AKI and worse clinical outcomes.

AKI is associated with high morbidity, mortality, and health care costs. Patients with AKI have an increased risk for developing chronic kidney disease (CKD) and end-stage kidney disease (ESKD). Likewise, patients with preexisting CKD are at an increased risk for developing acute-on-chronic kidney failure. Given its substantial morbidity and mortality, AKI care should be focused on prevention, early recognition and diagnosis, and management of complications.

**TABLE 23.** KDIGO Definition of Acute Kidney Injury[a]

| Stage | Serum Creatinine Criteria | Urine Output Criteria |
|---|---|---|
| 1 | Increase in $S_{Cr}$ to 1.5 to 1.9 times baseline within 7 days or ≥0.3 mg/dL (26.5 μmol/L) within 48 h | <0.5 mL/kg/h for 6 to 12 h |
| 2 | Increase in $S_{Cr}$ to 2 to 2.9 times baseline | <0.5 mL/kg/h for ≥12 h |
| 3 | Increase in $S_{Cr}$ to 3 times baseline or ≥4.0 mg/dL (356.6 μmol/L) or initiation of RRT or, in patients <18 years, a decrease in eGFR <35 mL/min/1.73 m² | <0.3 mL/kg/h for ≥24 h or anuria for ≥12 h |

eGFR = estimated glomerular filtration rate; KDIGO = Kidney Disease: Improving Global Outcomes; RRT = renal replacement therapy; $S_{Cr}$ = serum creatinine.

[a]The KDIGO definition is based on the RIFLE (Risk, Injury, Failure, Loss, and ESKD) and AKIN (Acute Kidney Injury Network) criteria.

- The Kidney Disease: Improving Global Outcomes (KDIGO) Acute Kidney Injury Work Group defines acute kidney injury by any of the following: increase in serum creatinine by ≥0.3 mg/dL (26.5 μmol/L) within 48 hours; an increase in serum creatinine to ≥1.5 times baseline over 7 days; or a urine volume <0.5 mL/kg/h for 6 hours.

## Epidemiology and Pathophysiology

The reported incidence of AKI varies markedly depending on the definition of AKI applied and the patient population studied. The incidence of AKI based on the KDIGO definition is estimated to be 21% of all hospital admissions, with 11% requiring dialysis support. In the ICU, AKI affects >50% of patients. Mortality varies depending on the severity of AKI, underlying cause, and patient population. Critically ill patients with AKI in the context of multiorgan failure have been reported to have mortality rates >50%, especially when dialysis therapy is required.

AKI can be divided into prerenal, intrinsic, and postrenal causes (**Table 24**). Prerenal AKI (prerenal azotemia) is caused by decreased renal perfusion. The integrity of renal tissue is preserved, and tubular and glomerular function remains normal. Intrinsic AKI is caused by structural damage to the renal parenchyma. Postrenal AKI refers to AKI caused by urinary tract obstruction. Prerenal AKI and acute tubular necrosis (ATN) account for approximately 65% to 75% of AKI cases in hospitalized patients.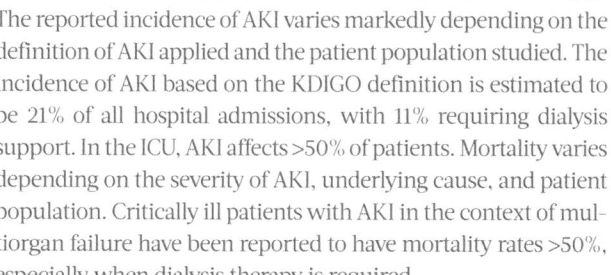

- Prerenal acute kidney injury and acute tubular necrosis account for approximately 65% to 75% of acute kidney injury cases in hospitalized patients.

## Clinical Manifestations

Patients with AKI can be asymptomatic until extreme loss of kidney function occurs, and patients with mild to moderate AKI are often diagnosed by laboratory studies only. Patients with AKI can also present with oliguria (urine output <500 mL/d or <0.3 mL/kg/h) or anuria (urine output <50 mL/d). Severe AKI can lead to symptoms from volume overload, electrolyte abnormalities, anemia, platelet dysfunction, and uremia. Uremic symptoms include nausea, vomiting, anorexia, weight loss, fatigue, muscle cramps, restless legs, mental status changes, pruritus, asterixis, seizures, and pericarditis.

- Patients with acute kidney injury (AKI) can be asymptomatic until extreme loss of kidney function occurs; severe AKI can lead to symptoms from volume overload, electrolyte abnormalities, anemia, platelet dysfunction, and uremia.

**TABLE 24.** Causes of Acute Kidney Injury

| Cause | Examples |
|---|---|
| **Prerenal** | |
| Volume depletion | Renal losses; GI fluid losses; hemorrhage; burns |
| Decreased cardiac output | Heart failure; massive pulmonary embolus; acute coronary syndrome |
| Systemic vasodilation | Sepsis; cirrhosis; anaphylaxis; anesthesia |
| Intrarenal vasoconstriction | Drugs (NSAIDs, COX-2 inhibitors, amphotericin B, calcineurin inhibitors, contrast agents); hypercalcemia; hepatorenal syndrome |
| Efferent arteriolar vasodilation | Renin inhibitors; ACE inhibitors; ARBs |
| **Intrinsic** | |
| Acute tubular necrosis | Ischemic: prolonged prerenal AKI; abdominal compartment syndrome |
| | Drug-induced: aminoglycosides; vancomycin; polymyxins; lithium; amphotericin B; pentamidine; cisplatin; foscarnet; tenofovir; cidofovir; carboplatin; ifosfamide; zoledronate; contrast agents; sucrose; immune globulins; mannitol; hydroxyethyl starch; dextran; NSAIDs; synthetic cannabinoids; amphetamines |
| | Pigment: rhabdomyolysis; intravascular hemolysis |
| Acute interstitial nephritis | Drug-induced: cephalosporins; penicillin; methicillin; fluoroquinolones; sulfonamides; rifampin; NSAIDs; COX-2 inhibitors; proton pump inhibitors; 5-aminosalicylates; indinavir; abacavir; allopurinol; phenytoin; triamterene; furosemide; thiazide diuretics; phenytoin; carbamazepine; Chinese herb nephropathy |
| | Infection: pyelonephritis; viral nephritides; leptospirosis; *Legionella*; *Mycobacterium tuberculosis* |
| | Autoimmune: Sjögren syndrome; sarcoidosis; SLE; TINU syndrome; IgG4-related disease |
| | Malignancy: lymphoma; leukemia; multiple myeloma |
| Acute glomerulonephritis | Infection-related glomerulonephritis; cryoglobulinemia; RPGN; IgA; lupus nephritis; renal vasculitis; anti-GBM antibody disease |
| Acute vascular syndromes | Macrovascular: renal artery occlusion; renal vein thrombosis; polyarteritis nodosa |
| | Microvascular:<br>  Disease-associated TMA: HUS; atypical HUS; TTP; HELLP; scleroderma renal crisis; hypertensive emergency |
| |   Drug-induced TMA: quinine; cancer therapies (gemcitabine, mitomycin, bevacizumab, bortezomib, sunitinib); calcineurin inhibitors (cyclosporine, tacrolimus); drugs of abuse (cocaine, ecstasy, intravenous extended-release oxymorphone) |
| |   Other drugs: clopidogrel; cyclosporine; tacrolimus; anti-angiogenesis drugs; interferon; mTOR inhibitors |
| | Atheroembolic disease |
| Intratubular obstruction | Paraprotein: myeloma |
| | Crystals: TLS; sulfonamides; triamterene; ciprofloxacin; ethylene glycol; acyclovir; indinavir; atazanavir; methotrexate; orlistat; large doses of vitamin C; sodium phosphate purgatives |
| **Postrenal** | |
| Upper tract obstruction | Nephrolithiasis; blood clots; external compression |
| Lower tract obstruction | BPH; neurogenic bladder; blood clots; cancer; urethral stricture |

AKI = acute kidney injury; ARB = angiotensin receptor blocker; BPH = benign prostatic hyperplasia; COX = cyclooxygenase; GBM = glomerular basement membrane; GI = gastrointestinal; HELLP = hemolysis, elevated liver enzymes, and low platelets; HUS = hemolytic uremic syndrome; mTOR = mammalian target of rapamycin; RPGN = rapidly progressive glomerulonephritis; SLE = systemic lupus erythematosus; TINU = tubulointerstitial nephritis and uveitis; TLS = tumor lysis syndrome; TMA = thrombotic microangiopathy; TTP = thrombotic thrombocytopenic purpura.

# Diagnosis

The diagnosis of AKI is based on increased levels of serum creatinine and blood urea nitrogen (BUN). The most reliable way to distinguish AKI from CKD is knowledge of previous serum creatinine levels; documentation of similarly elevated creatinine levels for ≥3 months suggests that the kidney failure is chronic. However, serum creatinine and BUN concentrations can be increased by multiple factors independent of kidney function, limiting their specificity for diagnosis of AKI (Table 25). Furthermore, serum creatinine is not a sensitive marker of kidney injury in patients with sepsis, liver disease, muscle wasting, or fluid overload and does not provide any information regarding the cause of AKI. BUN can also be normal in patients with AKI who are malnourished or have liver disease. Moreover, the rise in serum creatinine is delayed 24 to 36 hours after the onset of injury and decline in glomerular filtration rate (GFR).

A thorough patient history, physical examination, and analysis of laboratory and image findings are necessary to

**TABLE 25.** Selected Examples of Causes of Elevated Blood Urea Nitrogen and Serum Creatinine Without Acute Kidney Injury

| **Elevated Blood Urea Nitrogen** |
| --- |
| Gastrointestinal bleeding |
| Protein loading, including albumin infusions |
| Catabolic steroids |
| Tetracycline antibiotics |
| **Elevated Serum Creatinine** |
| Medications that block creatinine secretion: cimetidine; trimethoprim; cobicistat; dolutegravir |
| Creatine ethyl ester (an aid for athletic performance and for muscle development for body builders) |
| Substances that interfere with creatinine assay: acetoacetate; cefoxitin; flucytosine |

CONT.

identify the AKI as prerenal, intrinsic, or postrenal. The history focuses on identifying potential nephrotoxic medications (including over-the-counter medications, herbal products, and recreational drugs), recent exposure to iodinated contrast agents, predisposing conditions for AKI, and urinary obstructive symptoms (see Table 24). Physical examination focuses on volume status, signs of systemic illness that might impair kidney function, and evidence of urinary obstruction (such as a palpable bladder or flank pain). Laboratory evaluation includes BUN and creatinine concentrations, electrolytes, complete blood count, and assessment of the urine (urine indices, urinalysis, and microscopic evaluation of the urine sediment) (**Table 26**).

In patients with oliguria, the fractional excretion of sodium ($FE_{Na}$) can help distinguish between prerenal AKI and

ATN. $FE_{Na}$ measures the ratio of sodium excreted (urine sodium × volume) to sodium filtered (serum sodium × GFR) and is calculated as follows:

$$(U_{Sodium} \times P_{Creatinine})/(U_{Creatinine} \times P_{Sodium}) \times 100\%$$

In prerenal AKI, decreased renal perfusion increases sodium and water reabsorption, resulting in a decrease in urinary sodium excretion and $FE_{Na}$ <1%. However, $FE_{Na}$ <1% can occur with other causes of AKI that are not prerenal but have intact tubular function: contrast nephropathy, pigment nephropathy, glomerulonephritis, and early obstruction. $FE_{Na}$ >2% suggests impaired tubular ability to reabsorb sodium and is consistent with ATN. However, $FE_{Na}$ may be >2% in patients with prerenal AKI who have urinary sodium loss due to diuretics, adrenal insufficiency, or from bicarbonaturia in severe metabolic alkalosis. $FE_{Na}$ may also be >2% in prerenal patients with CKD as a result of impaired tubular function.

In the setting of diuretics, the fractional excretion of urea ($FE_{Urea}$) can be used to diagnose prerenal AKI, with $FE_{Urea}$ <35% suggesting the diagnosis. $FE_{Urea}$ is calculated as follows:

$$(U_{Urea} \times P_{Creatinine})/(U_{Creatinine} \times P_{Urea}) \times 100\%$$

Ultrasonography of the kidneys and bladder should be obtained for suspected urinary tract obstruction or when the underlying cause of AKI is unclear. Kidney size may help distinguish between AKI and CKD because diminished kidney size and cortical thinning suggest CKD. Kidney size can be normal in patients with CKD from infiltrative disorders such as diabetes mellitus, HIV-associated nephropathy, amyloidosis, or multiple myeloma. Kidney biopsy should be considered in patients with AKI from no apparent cause, suspected glomerulonephritis, or unexplained systemic disease.

**TABLE 26.** Diagnostic Findings in Acute Kidney Injury

| Condition | BUN-Creatinine Ratio | Urine Osmolality (mOsm/kg H₂O) | Urine Sodium (mEq/L [mmol/L]) | $FE_{Na}$ | Urinalysis and Microscopy |
| --- | --- | --- | --- | --- | --- |
| Prerenal | >20:1 | >500 | <20 | <1% | Specific gravity >1.020; normal or hyaline casts |
| Acute tubular necrosis | 10-15:1 | ~300 | >40 | >2%[a] | Specific gravity ~1.010; pigmented granular (muddy brown) casts and tubular epithelial cells |
| Acute interstitial nephritis | Variable | Variable, ~300 | Variable | Variable | Mild proteinuria; leukocytes; erythrocytes; leukocyte casts; eosinophiluria |
| Acute glomerulonephritis | Variable | Variable | Variable | Variable | Proteinuria; dysmorphic erythrocytes; erythrocyte casts |
| Intratubular obstruction | Variable | Variable | Variable | Variable | Crystalluria or Bence-Jones proteinuria |
| Acute vascular syndromes | Variable | Variable | Variable | Variable | Variable hematuria |
| Postrenal | Variable | Variable | Variable | Variable | Variable; bland |

BUN = blood urea nitrogen; $FE_{Na}$ = fractional excretion of sodium.

[a]$FE_{Na}$ can be low in contrast-induced nephropathy and pigment nephropathy.

- In patients with oliguria, the fractional excretion of sodium ($FE_{Na}$) can help distinguish between prerenal acute kidney injury (AKI) and acute tubular necrosis (ATN); $FE_{Na}$ <1% indicates prerenal AKI, and $FE_{Na}$ >2% is consistent with ATN.

- In the setting of diuretics, the fractional excretion of urea ($FE_{Urea}$) can be used to diagnose prerenal acute kidney injury, with $FE_{Urea}$ <35% suggesting the diagnosis.

- Ultrasonography of the kidneys and bladder should be obtained for suspected urinary tract obstruction or when the underlying cause of acute kidney injury is unclear.

# Causes

AKI can be divided into prerenal, intrinsic, and postrenal causes.

## Prerenal Acute Kidney Injury

See Table 24 for the causes of prerenal AKI.

Prerenal AKI (prerenal azotemia) is caused by underperfusion of the kidney with a subsequent decrease in GFR, which is reversible with appropriate therapy. Renal hypoperfusion can occur due to intravascular volume depletion, decreased effective arterial circulation, renal vasoconstriction, and/or medications. Patients may have a history of acute hemorrhage, loss of gastrointestinal fluids, heart failure, decompensated liver disease, sepsis, or recent diuretic or NSAID use. Physical signs of hypovolemia include hypotension, tachycardia, orthostasis, and decreased skin turgor. Patients with heart failure or cirrhosis have physical examination findings supporting these conditions.

In prerenal AKI, the kidney responds by reabsorbing urea, sodium, and water, often resulting in a BUN-creatinine ratio >20:1; however, a normal BUN-creatinine ratio does not exclude prerenal AKI. Other laboratory values that support a diagnosis of prerenal AKI are listed in Table 26. Prerenal AKI due to hypovolemia can be distinguished from ATN by the renal response to a fluid challenge. If serum creatinine recovers to baseline with fluid repletion, the cause of AKI is likely to be prerenal.

Drug-induced prerenal AKI typically results from decreased blood flow to the kidney or intraglomerular hemodynamic alterations. Diuretics can cause prerenal AKI from volume depletion. Drugs affecting vasodilatation of the afferent arterioles or vasoconstriction of the efferent arterioles can cause prerenal AKI, especially in the setting of volume depletion, decreased effective arterial circulation, or CKD. NSAIDs, including cyclooxygenase-2 inhibitors, cause AKI by diminishing the renal vasodilatory effect of prostaglandins. ACE inhibitors and angiotensin receptor blockers (ARBs) prevent efferent vasoconstriction by inhibiting angiotensin II. Calcineurin inhibitors such as cyclosporine and tacrolimus can cause prerenal AKI from afferent and efferent vasoconstriction.

Management of prerenal AKI includes discontinuing nephrotoxins and increasing renal perfusion by treating the underlying cause, such as correcting volume deficits. If prerenal AKI is not recognized and treated in a timely fashion, prolonged renal hypoperfusion will result in ATN and progressive intrinsic kidney failure.

- Prerenal acute kidney injury is caused by underperfusion of the kidney with a subsequent decrease in glomerular filtration rate, which is reversible with discontinuing nephrotoxins and treating the underlying cause.

## Intrinsic Kidney Diseases

Intrinsic AKI occurs from structural damage to the renal tubules, interstitium, glomerulus, or vascular structures, or intratubular obstruction (see Table 24).

### Acute Tubular Necrosis

ATN due to ischemia, nephrotoxins, and/or sepsis is the most common cause of AKI in hospitalized patients. A patient history of sepsis or nephrotoxin exposure along with assessment of hemodynamics and volume status can aid in the diagnosis. Laboratory values suggestive of ATN include a BUN-creatinine ratio <10 to 15:1, an $FE_{Na}$ >2%, and a urine osmolality of approximately 300 mOsm/kg $H_2O$ (see Table 26), reflecting the failure to maximally dilute or concentrate urine (isosthenuria). Urine sediment is characterized by many tubular epithelial cells and coarse granular (muddy brown) casts (**Figure 16**).

Unlike prerenal AKI, ATN does not rapidly improve with restoration of intravascular volume and blood flow to the kidneys. Treatment is supportive because no pharmacologic therapies exist. Complete or partial renal recovery can take days to weeks.

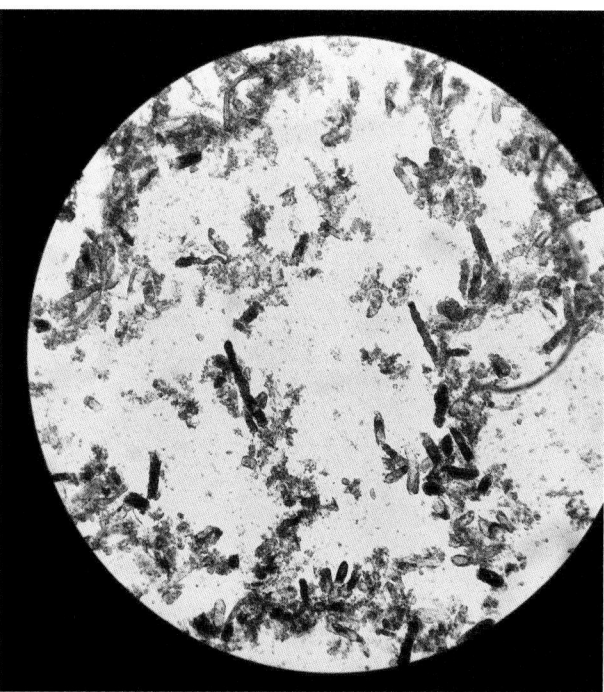

**FIGURE 16.** Urine sediment showing multiple coarse, granular (muddy brown) casts characteristic of acute tubular necrosis.

Compared with oliguric ATN, patients with nonoliguric ATN are thought to have less severe kidney injury and a better renal prognosis. Patients with baseline CKD are less likely to recover kidney function compared with patients with baseline normal kidney function. Patients with severe ATN who require acute dialysis may recover kidney function or progress to dialysis-dependent ESKD.

*Ischemic Acute Tubular Necrosis*

Severe ischemia due to prolonged hypotension or prolonged prerenal state can cause ATN (see Table 24). The ischemic injury leads to cytokine release, oxygen-free radical and enzyme production, endothelial activation and leukocyte adhesion, activation of coagulation, and apoptosis. GFR declines due to renal vasoconstriction, tubular back leak of filtrate into the bloodstream, and tubular obstruction from sloughed cellular debris. Ischemic ATN is mostly reversible but can result in permanent kidney failure.

Normotensive ischemic ATN can occur without overt hypotension in conditions with impaired renal autoregulation. These conditions include older age, hypertension, atherosclerotic or renovascular disease, and CKD. Patients with hypertension can develop normotensive ischemic ATN if their blood pressure is decreased to a value lower than what they are accustomed to but within normal range. Management involves treating any potential volume deficits and decreasing antihypertensive medications to allow the blood pressure to increase to baseline levels.

*Drug-Induced Acute Tubular Necrosis*

Drug-induced ATN can be a consequence of prolonged hemodynamic alterations or direct tubular injury (see Table 24). The drugs associated with prerenal AKI can cause ATN from prolonged hypoperfusion. Early recognition and prompt discontinuation of the drug are essential for renal recovery. The risk of drug-induced ATN increases in the elderly and in patients with decreased effective arterial circulation, CKD, or concomitant nephrotoxin exposure.

Osmotic nephrosis is a form of tubular injury due to hyperosmolar substances such as sucrose-containing intravenous immunoglobulin, mannitol, hydroxyethyl starch, dextran, and contrast media. It is characterized by vacuolization and swelling of the renal proximal tubular cells with resultant tubular obstruction and damage.

Contrast agents can cause nonoliguric ATN primarily through renal vasoconstriction. The serum creatinine increases within 24 to 48 hours after contrast administration. Aminoglycosides cause nonoliguric ATN through direct tubular toxicity with an increase in serum creatinine occurring 5 to 7 days after initiation of therapy. Hypomagnesemia, hypokalemia, hypocalcemia, and hypophosphatemia can be seen. Cisplatin causes ATN through direct tubular toxicity, renal vasoconstriction, and inflammation. Hypomagnesemia with urinary magnesium wasting is common. Amphotericin B causes dose-related AKI through both renal vasoconstriction and direct tubular toxicity. It can be associated with potassium

and magnesium wasting, metabolic acidosis due to type 1 (distal) renal tubular acidosis, and nephrogenic diabetes insipidus. Lipid-based preparations decrease the risk for nephrotoxicity. Vancomycin nephrotoxicity occurs in the setting of high trough levels (>15 mg/L), high vancomycin dose (≥4 g/d), prolonged duration of therapy, and/or concomitant nephrotoxic drugs (for example, an aminoglycoside or piperacillin-tazobactam). Certain types of synthetic cannabinoids used as recreational drugs have been associated with ATN.

*Pigment Nephropathy*

Heme pigment released from myoglobin or hemoglobin can cause AKI through intravascular volume depletion (seen in rhabdomyolysis), renal vasoconstriction, direct proximal tubular injury, and tubular obstruction. In rhabdomyolysis, myoglobin is released in the circulation from damaged skeletal muscle. Major causes of rhabdomyolysis include trauma, drugs and toxins, seizures, metabolic and electrolyte disorders, endocrinopathies (diabetic ketoacidosis, hyperglycemic hyperosmolar syndrome, hypothyroidism), and exercise. Rhabdomyolysis-induced AKI is more likely to occur with serum creatine kinase levels >5000 U/L. In addition to elevated serum creatine kinase and serum creatinine levels, hyperkalemia, hypocalcemia, hyperphosphatemia, hyperuricemia, metabolic acidosis, increased lactate dehydrogenase concentration, and increased aspartate and alanine aminotransferase levels can occur. Urinary findings include $FE_{Na}$ <1% (due to renal vasoconstriction), myoglobinuria, pigmented (red) granular casts, and a positive urine dipstick for blood with absence of erythrocytes.

In addition to correcting the underlying cause, prevention and management of AKI involve aggressive intravenous isotonic fluid resuscitation aimed at maintaining urine output >200 to 300 mL/h. Limited studies suggest that alkalinization of the urine with intravenous bicarbonate to increase the urine pH >6.5 may prevent tubular cast formation. If urine alkalinization is used, it should be discontinued if the patient develops symptomatic hypocalcemia or alkalosis, or if urine pH does not increase to >6.5 after several hours. Dialysis may be necessary for severe electrolyte and acid-base abnormalities. Most patients have partial or complete renal recovery.

Heme pigment nephropathy is less common and occurs when large amounts of heme pigment are released into circulation due to intravascular hemolysis. Causes include glucose-6-phosphate dehydrogenase (G6PD) deficiency, drug reactions, hemolysis related to cardiopulmonary bypass circuits, transfusion of stored red blood cells, paroxysmal nocturnal hemoglobinuria, malaria, certain poisonings, and snakebites. In addition to elevated serum creatinine concentration, other laboratory abnormalities include anemia, increased lactate dehydrogenase, and decreased haptoglobin. Urinary findings include $FE_{Na}$ <1%, hemoglobinuria, pigmented granular casts, and urine dipstick positive for blood with no erythrocytes. Both myoglobinuria and hemoglobinuria can cause tea-colored urine; however, only hemoglobin causes a reddish brown color of centrifuged serum

CONT.

because it is too large to be effectively filtered in kidneys. Treatment of hemoglobinuria involves treating the underlying cause as well as volume repletion with intravenous fluids.

## Acute Interstitial Nephritis

Acute interstitial nephritis (AIN) is a common cause of AKI characterized by inflammation and edema of the interstitium. The classic clinical presentation of fever, rash, and peripheral eosinophilia occurs in only 10% to 30% of patients with AIN. Urinary findings can include eosinophiluria by Hansel stain, leukocytes, erythrocytes, and leukocyte casts (see Table 26). Urine eosinophils are neither sensitive nor specific for AIN; AIN can still occur in their absence, and eosinophiluria can occur in other causes of AKI such as acute glomerulonephritis, atheroembolic disease, pyelonephritis, cystitis, and prostatitis.

Drug-induced AIN, especially due to antibiotics, is the most common cause of AIN and should be considered in any patient with AKI, a characteristic urinalysis, and history of any drug exposure. Other causes include infections, systemic diseases such as autoimmune disorders, and idiopathic cases (see Table 24). Typically, the serum creatinine gradually increases 7 to 10 days after drug exposure but can increase much sooner following repeat exposure of the drug.

Drug-induced AIN from NSAIDs, including selective cyclooxygenase-2 inhibitors, is usually not associated with fever, rash, or eosinophilia and develops 6 to 18 months after drug exposure. AIN from NSAIDs can be associated with the nephrotic syndrome due to minimal change glomerulopathy or membranous glomerulopathy. Proton pump inhibitors are also associated with AIN without fever, rash, and eosinophilia. The onset of AIN is variable but typically occurs 10 to 11 weeks after exposure. Proton pump inhibitors are thought to be a risk factor for the development of CKD.

Renal recovery from drug-induced AIN is usually complete if the drug is stopped immediately after the onset of kidney injury but may take weeks to several months. Irreversible interstitial fibrosis can develop after 2 weeks of continued exposure. Kidney biopsy should be considered if there is no improvement in kidney function after 5 to 7 days of drug discontinuation. Early glucocorticoid administration may limit damage associated with drug-induced AIN. ▣

## Acute Glomerulonephritis

Acute glomerulonephritis with AKI results from immune-mediated damage to glomeruli. Urinary findings include proteinuria, dysmorphic erythrocytes, and erythrocyte casts (see Table 26). Constitutional signs and symptoms are often present. Serologic assays and kidney biopsy identify most causes. Early recognition is extremely important because, without treatment, it can be fatal and result in irreversible kidney damage. See Glomerular Diseases for more information.

## Acute Vascular Syndromes

Macrovascular (large and medium vessel) or microvascular (small vessel) disease can cause AKI (see Table 24).

Examples of macrovascular disease include severe abdominal aortic disease, major renal artery occlusion, and renal vein thrombosis. Acute renal arterial occlusion and acute renal vein thrombosis cause acute renal infarction and present as abdominal or flank pain, elevated serum lactate dehydrogenase levels, and hematuria. Treatment usually consists of anticoagulation and supportive care.

AKI can also occur from polyarteritis nodosa, a systemic vasculitis that affects medium and occasionally small arteries at branching points. It causes microaneurysms that subsequently rupture, resulting in hemorrhage, thrombosis, and organ ischemia and infarction. AKI results from renovascular ischemic changes and renal artery vasculitis. See MKSAP 18 Rheumatology for more information.

Patients with atherosclerotic disease who undergo an invasive vascular procedure such as vascular surgery or angiography are at increased risk for atheroemboli-induced AKI (cholesterol emboli). Atheroembolic events can occur spontaneously or several days to weeks after manipulation of the aorta. Plaque rupture causes cholesterol embolization to distal small- and medium-sized arteries, resulting in ischemia with end-organ damage. In addition to the kidneys, atheroemboli can affect the arteries in the skin, muscle, gastrointestinal tract, liver, eyes, and central nervous system. Physical examination findings may include livedo reticularis (lacy network of bluish red vessels, usually seen on legs), Hollenhorst plaques on funduscopic examination (yellow refractile body within arteriole), ulcerations, and blue toes from ischemia (**Figure 17**). Laboratory findings can include low serum complements,

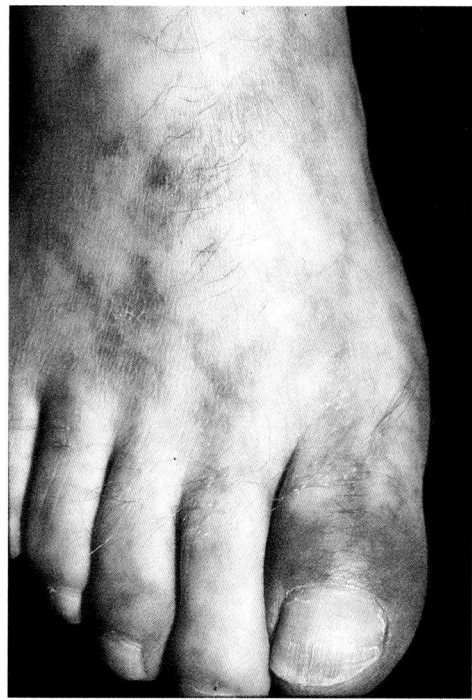

**FIGURE 17.** Blue toe syndrome presents as a cyanotic toe with necrosis of the skin caused by occlusion of the small vessels from cholesterol emboli, as seen in atheroembolic acute kidney injury.

peripheral eosinophilia, and eosinophiluria; urinalysis may be unremarkable or can have proteinuria, microscopic hematuria, or erythrocyte casts. Treatment of atheroemboli is supportive and consists of risk factor reduction: aspirin, statins, and hypertension management. The use of anticoagulants for treatment of cholesterol emboli is controversial because anticoagulants and thrombolytics can induce atheroemboli. Renal prognosis is poor.

AKI from microvascular disease can present as thrombotic microangiopathy (TMA) with microangiopathic hemolytic anemia, thrombocytopenia, and glomerular capillary thrombosis. Diseases that can lead to TMA include thrombotic thrombocytopenic purpura, hemolytic uremic syndrome, the HELLP (hemolysis, elevated liver enzymes, and low platelets) syndrome, hypertensive emergency, scleroderma renal crisis, complement-mediated TMA, and drug-induced TMA. Urine may show hematuria, erythrocyte casts, and/or proteinuria. Treatment of TMA is based on the underlying cause. Drug-induced TMA is treated by discontinuation of the drug.

### Intratubular Obstruction
Intratubular obstruction can cause AKI through precipitation of either protein or crystals within the tubular lumen. Examples include monoclonal light chain deposition in multiple myeloma, calcium oxalate deposition from ethylene glycol ingestion, crystals from drugs, and uric acid from tumor lysis syndrome (see Table 24).

In multiple myeloma, AKI from light chain cast nephropathy is the most common type of kidney disease. Cast nephropathy is due to direct tubular toxicity and obstruction from the precipitation of filtered free light chains. See Kidney Manifestations of Deposition Diseases for more information.

Ethylene glycol intoxication causes AKI from intratubular precipitation of calcium oxalate crystals, which can be seen on urine microscopy. Ethylene glycol should be suspected in a patient with a history of ingestion and whose laboratory studies demonstrate an increased anion gap metabolic acidosis and osmolal gap. Treatment consists of supportive care, the antidote fomepizole, and hemodialysis if needed. Orlistat, a gastrointestinal lipase inhibitor used to induce clinically significant weight loss by fat malabsorption, has also been associated with intratubular calcium oxalate deposition and AKI. High doses of vitamin C, which is metabolized to oxalate, can also lead to AKI from calcium oxalate precipitation in the tubules.

Drugs associated with crystal-induced AKI are listed in Table 24. Urinary findings include hematuria, pyuria, and crystals. AKI is usually reversed after discontinuation of the drug. Predisposing factors include volume depletion, CKD, and changes in urine pH. Correction of volume depletion with intravenous fluids is critical for both the prevention and treatment of crystal-induced AKI. Bolus intravenous acyclovir can cause acyclovir crystal deposition in the tubules, which can be prevented by prior intravenous fluid administration and slow rate of drug infusion. Because crystals from sulfonamide antibiotics and methotrexate are more likely to form in acidic

urine, urinary alkalinization can prevent crystal deposition. Crystals from protease inhibitors can cause AKI from both crystal deposition and nephrolithiasis.

Acute phosphate nephropathy is a potentially irreversible cause of AKI due to phosphate-containing bowel preparations. A transient severe increase in serum phosphate in the setting of volume depletion causes acute and chronic tubular injury from tubular and interstitial precipitation of calcium phosphate crystals. AKI can present days to months after exposure. Predisposing factors include volume depletion, CKD, older age, NSAIDs, and hypertension treated with ACE inhibitors, ARBs, or diuretics.

**KEY POINTS**

- Acute tubular necrosis due to ischemia, nephrotoxins, and/or sepsis is the most common cause of acute kidney injury in hospitalized patients; a history of sepsis or nephrotoxin exposure along with hemodynamic and volume status assessment can aid in the diagnosis.

- Drug-induced acute interstitial nephritis is associated with a gradual increase in serum creatinine 7 to 10 days after drug exposure; renal recovery is usually complete if the drug is stopped immediately after the onset of kidney injury.

- In atheroemboli-induced acute kidney injury, plaque rupture causes cholesterol embolization to distal small- and medium-sized arteries, resulting in ischemia with end-organ damage; treatment is supportive.

- Acute kidney injury from microvascular disease can present as thrombotic microangiopathy (TMA); conditions that can lead to TMA include thrombotic thrombocytopenic purpura, hemolytic uremic syndrome, the HELLP (hemolysis, elevated liver enzymes, and low platelets) syndrome, hypertensive emergency, scleroderma renal crisis, complement-mediated TMA, and drug-induced TMA.

- Intratubular obstruction causes of acute kidney injury include monoclonal light chain deposition in multiple myeloma; calcium oxalate deposition from ethylene glycol ingestion, orlistat, and high doses of vitamin C; crystals from drugs; and uric acid from tumor lysis syndrome.

### Postrenal Disease
Postrenal AKI can occur from obstruction anywhere from the renal pelvis to the external urethral meatus (see Table 24). Upper urinary tract obstruction (at the level of the ureters or renal pelvis) must be bilateral or affect a single functioning kidney to cause AKI. Obstruction of urinary flow leads to hydronephrosis and eventual renal parenchymal damage. If postrenal AKI is not treated promptly, the obstruction can predispose the patient to urinary tract infections and urosepsis, and it can also lead to CKD and ESKD.

Postrenal AKI should be suspected in patients with a history of benign prostatic hyperplasia, diabetes, nephrolithiasis, pelvic malignancies, abdominal or pelvic surgeries, or retroperitoneal adenopathy. Patients can present with anuria, oliguria, polyuria, or normal urine output. Symptoms of lower tract obstruction include abdominal fullness or pain, urinary frequency, urgency, hesitancy, nocturia, overflow incontinence, and incomplete voiding. Acute nephrolithiasis may present with flank pain and hematuria. Urine chemistries can be variable with obstruction (see Table 26).

Lower urinary tract obstruction can be diagnosed by placement of a urinary catheter with return of a large volume of urine or an elevated postvoid residual volume by ultrasound. Ultrasonography can yield false-negative results in the early stages of hydronephrosis or obstruction from encasement of the ureter or kidney, as seen in retroperitoneal disease. Noncontrast CT is indicated for suspected nephrolithiasis. Treatment focuses on removing the obstruction. Renal prognosis depends upon the severity and duration of the obstruction. Renal recovery is generally good if the obstruction is relieved within 1 to 2 weeks.

> **KEY POINT**
>
> - Postrenal acute kidney injury can occur from obstruction anywhere from the renal pelvis to the external urethral meatus; diagnosis can be made via ultrasonography or noncontrast CT, with generally good renal recovery if the obstruction is relieved within 1 to 2 weeks.

# Specific Clinical Settings

## Contrast-Induced Nephropathy

Contrast-induced nephropathy (CIN) is a common cause of reversible AKI in the hospital. CIN is defined as an increase in serum creatinine within 24 to 48 hours following contrast exposure. The pathogenesis is not completely understood, but CIN is thought to be due to ATN from contrast-induced vasoconstriction, decreased renal blood flow, medullary hypoxia, oxidative stress, and direct tubular cytotoxicity. AKI tends to be nonoliguric, with an $FE_{Na}$ <1%. The urinary sediment may be bland or show classic ATN findings. Risk factors include CKD, diabetic nephropathy, conditions of decreased renal perfusion (heart failure, hypovolemia, hypotension), multiple myeloma, concomitant nephrotoxins, high contrast dose, hyperosmolar contrast, and intra-arterial contrast administration.

Preventive strategies for patients at high risk for CIN include minimizing the amount of contrast, using low or iso-osmolar contrast, discontinuing nephrotoxins, and administering either intravenous isotonic saline or sodium bicarbonate. A randomized controlled trial demonstrated that oral acetylcysteine was no more effective than placebo for the prevention of CIN. Statins have been shown in observational studies and several randomized controlled trials to prevent CIN by acting as stabilizers of the endothelium and free radical scavengers in a model of ischemic nephropathy. Further studies are needed to establish their benefit. There is no role for prophylactic hemodialysis or hemofiltration following contrast exposure. Treatment of CIN is supportive.

## Cardiorenal Syndrome

Cardiorenal syndrome (CRS) is a disorder of the heart and kidneys whereby acute or long-term dysfunction in one organ induces acute or long-term dysfunction in the other. CRS is characterized by the triad of concomitant decreased kidney function, diuretic-resistant heart failure with congestion, and worsening kidney function during heart failure therapy. The decreased kidney function in CRS is thought to be due to neurohumoral activation, increased intra-abdominal pressure leading to venous congestion and increased renal venous pressure, reduced renal perfusion, and right ventricular dysfunction. CRS can be classified into five types (**Table 27**).

Management is challenging because treatment directed toward improving cardiac function (diuretics, ACE inhibitor/ARB, vasodilators, and inotropes) can worsen kidney function. Ultrafiltration has been used for volume overload refractory to diuretics. Current evidence does not support the use of ultrafiltration over intensive diuretic management. Decreased kidney function in patients with heart failure is an independent risk factor for all-cause mortality.

## Hepatorenal Syndrome

Hepatorenal syndrome (HRS) is a reversible functional kidney impairment that occurs in the setting of portal hypertension due to liver cirrhosis, severe alcoholic hepatitis, or acute liver failure. HRS is characterized by increased renal vasoconstriction and peripheral arterial vasodilation. Tubular function is preserved with the absence of significant hematuria and proteinuria, as well as lack of renal histological changes.

Type 1 HRS is a clinical diagnosis made after exclusion of other causes of kidney dysfunction. It is characterized by a rise in serum creatinine of at least 0.3 mg/dL (26.5 µmol/L) and/or ≥50% from baseline within 48 hours, bland urinalysis, and

**TABLE 27.** Classification of Cardiorenal Syndrome

| Type | Definition |
|------|-----------|
| Type 1 | Acute worsening of cardiac function (acute heart failure; acute coronary syndrome; cardiogenic shock) leading to acute kidney injury |
| Type 2 | Chronic abnormalities in cardiac function leading to progressive chronic kidney disease |
| Type 3 | Acute worsening of kidney function leading to acute cardiac dysfunction |
| Type 4 | Primary chronic kidney disease leading to cardiac injury (left ventricular remodeling and dysfunction; diastolic dysfunction; acute heart failure; acute coronary syndrome) |
| Type 5 | Systemic condition (such as diabetes mellitus, sepsis, amyloidosis) causing both cardiac and kidney dysfunction |

CONT.

normal findings on kidney ultrasound. It is also supported by a lack of improvement in kidney function after withdrawal of diuretics and 2 days of volume expansion with intravenous albumin. Often, patients also have low urine sodium, low $FE_{Na}$, and oliguria. Type 2 HRS is defined as a more gradual decline in kidney function associated with refractory ascites.

Patients with HRS have an overall poor prognosis without liver transplantation. General management includes discontinuing diuretics, restricting sodium, restricting water in hyponatremic patients, and searching for precipitating factors. Therapeutic interventions include treatment with vasoconstrictors and albumin, placement of a transjugular intrahepatic portosystemic shunt in select patients, renal replacement therapy, and liver transplant. Renal replacement therapy is usually reserved for patients with severe AKI who are liver transplant candidates.

### Tumor Lysis Syndrome

Tumor lysis syndrome (TLS) is characterized by the rapid lysis of malignant cells leading to hyperuricemia, hyperkalemia, hyperphosphatemia, hypocalcemia, and AKI. TLS typically occurs after initiation of chemotherapy in hematologic malignancies with high cell turnover rate, rapid growth rate, or high tumor bulk (acute lymphoblastic leukemia, Burkitt lymphoma, acute myeloid leukemia); however, it can also occur spontaneously. AKI occurs from deposition of uric acid and/or calcium phosphate crystals in the renal tubules.

Management of TLS requires the initiation of preventive measures in high-risk patients prior to cytotoxic therapy, as well as the timely initiation of supportive care for patients who develop TLS. Treatment of established TLS includes intravenous hydration, urate-lowering therapy, management of hyperkalemia and hyperphosphatemia, and renal replacement therapy in refractory cases. Patients at risk for or presenting with TLS require aggressive volume expansion to achieve a urine output of at least 80 to 100 mL/m²/h. Urinary alkalinization is no longer recommended because the high urine pH can cause an increase in calcium phosphate crystal deposition. Allopurinol, a competitive inhibitor of xanthine oxidase, prevents the formation of new uric acid and is recommended as prophylaxis for patients at intermediate risk for TLS (those with highly chemotherapy-sensitive solid tumors); it has no effect on existing serum urate levels. Rasburicase, a recombinant urate oxidase that makes uric acid more soluble in urine with rapid reduction in serum urate levels, is given to patients at high risk of TLS or those with TLS. Rasburicase is contraindicated in patients with G6PD deficiency.

### Abdominal Compartment Syndrome

Abdominal compartment syndrome is defined as a sustained intra-abdominal pressure (IAP) >20 mm Hg associated with at least one organ dysfunction. Abdominal compartment syndrome occurs in the setting of abdominal surgery, trauma, hemoperitoneum, retroperitoneal bleed, ascites, bowel obstruction, ileus,

and pancreatitis. It can also occur from capillary leak from massive fluid resuscitation or sepsis. Increasing IAP causes hypoperfusion and ischemia of the intestines and other peritoneal and retroperitoneal structures, leading to hemodynamic, respiratory, neurologic, and kidney impairment. Renal vein compression and renal artery vasoconstriction cause oliguric AKI.

Abdominal compartment syndrome is diagnosed by measuring IAP; measurement of bladder pressure with an indwelling catheter is the standard methodology. Management includes supportive therapy, abdominal compartment decompression, and correction of positive fluid balance.

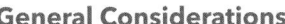

**KEY POINTS**

- Preventive strategies for patients at high risk for contrast-induced nephropathy include minimizing the amount of contrast, using low or iso-osmolar contrast, discontinuing nephrotoxins, and administering intravenous isotonic saline or sodium bicarbonate.

- Cardiorenal syndrome is characterized by the triad of concomitant decreased kidney function, diuretic-resistant heart failure with congestion, and worsening kidney function during heart failure therapy.

- Hepatorenal syndrome occurs in the setting of portal hypertension due to liver cirrhosis, severe alcoholic hepatitis, or acute liver failure and is characterized by increased renal vasoconstriction and peripheral arterial vasodilation.

- Acute kidney injury in the setting of tumor lysis syndrome (TLS) occurs from deposition of uric acid and/or calcium phosphate crystals in the renal tubules; management of TLS requires preventive measures in high-risk patients prior to cytotoxic therapy, and timely supportive care for established TLS.

- Abdominal compartment syndrome is defined as a sustained intra-abdominal pressure >20 mm Hg associated with at least one organ dysfunction; in this setting, renal vein compression and renal artery vasoconstriction cause oliguric acute kidney injury.

## Management

### General Considerations

In most cases of AKI, treatment of the underlying medical condition and discontinuation of nephrotoxic medications lead to improvement in kidney function. No specific pharmacologic therapy is effective in established ATN. Supportive measures include optimizing hemodynamics and renal perfusion, preventing further kidney injury, treating AKI complications, and providing appropriate nutrition. Diuretics can be used for volume overload. Bicarbonate can be administered to correct metabolic acidosis. Dietary potassium, magnesium, and phosphate should be restricted. Phosphate binders may be required to prevent severe hyperphosphatemia. In patients with severe AKI, initiation of renal replacement therapy may be the only option.

### Renal Replacement Therapy
Renal replacement therapy (RRT) is used to manage the urgent complications of severe AKI, including hyperkalemia, metabolic acidosis, volume overload refractory to diuretics, uremic manifestations, and dialyzable toxins. Options for RRT for AKI include intermittent hemodialysis (IHD), continuous renal replacement therapy (CRRT), "hybrid" therapies such as prolonged intermittent renal replacement therapy (PIRRT), and peritoneal dialysis (PD). IHD, CRRT, and PIRRT are extracorporeal therapies that require vascular access in the form of a large-bore, double-lumen central venous catheter; PD requires the placement of an intra-abdominal dialysis catheter.

IHD, typically delivered 3 to 6 times a week for 3 to 5 hours per session, allows for rapid correction of electrolyte disturbances and rapid removal of drugs or toxins. The main disadvantage of IHD is the risk for hypotension caused by the rapid solute and volume removal. Furthermore, rapid solute removal from the intravascular space can cause cerebral edema and increased intracranial pressure, limiting this therapy in patients with head trauma or hepatic encephalopathy. CRRT represents a variety of dialysis modalities developed specifically to manage critically ill patients with AKI who cannot tolerate IHD due to hemodynamic instability. CRRT is administered 24 hours a day and removes solutes and fluid much more slowly than IHD, resulting in better hemodynamic tolerance. PIRRT removes solutes and fluid more slowly than IHD but more quickly than CRRT and is administered 8 to 12 hours daily. PD is not as effective as the other forms of RRT but may be useful when the other types of RRT are unavailable or vascular access cannot be obtained.

Randomized clinical trials have not shown a survival benefit of CRRT over IHD or PIRRT for critically ill AKI patients. IHD is typically chosen for patients who are hemodynamically stable, whereas CRRT or PIRRT is chosen for patients who are unstable, are fluid overloaded, and/or have sepsis and multiorgan failure. IHD is favored in patients who need rapid solute removal, such as those with severe hyperkalemia or drug intoxications. CRRT is preferred in patients with cerebral edema because IHD may worsen neurologic status by compromising cerebral perfusion pressure. Transitions in therapy are common depending on the changing needs of the patient.

**KEY POINTS**

- In most cases of acute kidney injury, treatment of the underlying medical condition and discontinuation of nephrotoxic medications leads to improvement in kidney function.
- Renal replacement therapy is used to manage the urgent complications of severe acute kidney injury, including hyperkalemia, metabolic acidosis, volume overload refractory to diuretics, uremic manifestations, and dialyzable toxins.

# Kidney Stones

## Overview

Approximately 7% to 11% of the U.S. population will develop nephrolithiasis, and 50% will have recurrent disease. Risk factors for developing kidney stones include male gender, increased age, white race, obesity, diabetes mellitus, the metabolic syndrome, decreased fluid intake, chronic diarrheal states, and Roux-en-Y gastric bypass.

## Clinical Manifestations
Although kidney stones may be asymptomatic and diagnosed as an incidental finding on imaging, the typical presentation is waxing and waning "colicky" flank pain that radiates to the groin. Stone movement may result in pain migration to the lateralized genitalia. The patient frequently finds it difficult to achieve a comfortable position. Nausea, vomiting, and dysuria may also be present. Microscopic hematuria is usually noted, although its absence does not exclude a stone.

Similar symptoms may be present with pyelonephritis and acute abdominal processes, which need to be considered. In addition, the ureteral passage of blood clots can mimic renal colic pain.

**KEY POINT**

- Kidney stones typically present with waxing and waning "colicky" flank pain that radiates to the groin; nausea, vomiting, and dysuria may also be present.

## Diagnosis

Nephrolithiasis should be considered in all patients who present with flank pain. Costovertebral angle tenderness may be present. Microscopic examination of the urine for hematuria, leukocytes that may indicate infection, pH measurement, and crystals is mandatory but nonspecific. The presence of crystals may help to identify the type of stone. A complete blood count and complete metabolic panel should be obtained to exclude infection and acute kidney injury, and to screen for common metabolic causes of stone disease.

Definitive diagnosis is made with imaging. Noncontrast helical CT is the gold standard modality because of its high sensitivity and specificity. Although less sensitive than CT, kidney ultrasonography is less expensive, has no radiation exposure, and can be used in pregnant women or when CT is unavailable. Plain abdominal radiography has a low sensitivity and should not be ordered except to follow the stone burden in established disease.

**KEY POINT**

- Noncontrast helical CT is the gold standard modality to diagnose nephrolithiasis because of its high sensitivity and specificity; kidney ultrasonography, although less sensitive than CT, is less expensive and has no radiation exposure and can be used if CT is unavailable and in pregnant women.

# Types of Kidney Stones

See **Table 28** for details on kidney stones and Table 3 in Clinical Evaluation of Kidney Function for images of crystals.

## Calcium

Eighty percent of kidney stones contain calcium; most are composed of calcium oxalate, and the remainder are composed of calcium phosphate or a combination of the two.

Calcium oxalate stones are associated with hypercalciuria, hyperoxaluria, and hypocitraturia. Up to 50% of patients with recurrent stones have elevated 24-hour urine calcium levels. This increase may be secondary to elevated serum calcium as seen in hyperparathyroidism, sarcoidosis, or excessive vitamin D intake, but is more frequently idiopathic. Hyperoxaluria can be primary or can occur secondary to increased dietary oxalate intake; malabsorption syndrome due to the binding of gastrointestinal calcium to fatty acids, allowing for increased absorption of oxalate; decreased dietary calcium; and high vitamin C intake. Rous-en-Y gastric bypass surgery is associated with hyperoxaluria and an increase risk of stone formation. The weight loss drug orlistat, by inducing fat malabsorption, is also associated with hyperoxaluria and

the formation of calcium oxalate stones. Because citrate prevents calcium crystal formation, low urine levels are associated with increased stone formation. Citrate excretion is decreased in the presence of metabolic acidosis, as occurs with chronic diarrhea and distal renal tubular acidosis.

Calcium phosphate stones occur when there is persistently elevated urine pH and are therefore commonly associated with distal renal tubular acidosis and hyperparathyroidism. In addition, the use of carbonic anhydrase inhibitors such as acetazolamide or topiramate, by raising urine pH and decreasing citrate excretion, are associated with increased incidence of calcium phosphate stones. Imaging may reveal nephrocalcinosis.

## Struvite

Struvite stones occur in the presence of urea-splitting bacteria such as *Proteus*, *Klebsiella*, or, less frequently, *Pseudomonas* species. These bacteria split urea into ammonium, which markedly increases urine pH and results in the precipitation of magnesium ammonium phosphate (struvite). The pH of the urine will be >7.5. Struvite stones commonly produce staghorn calculi (stones that bridge two or more renal calyces) and occur most frequently in older women with chronic urinary tract infections. Because struvite stones are large and grow rapidly, they do not pass into the ureter to cause pain typical of smaller stones. Signs and symptoms typically are related to the underlying infection. Because of their association with infections, there is significant morbidity and mortality associated with these stones.

## Uric Acid

Uric acid stones (<10% of stones) develop in the presence of a persistently acidic urine, which decreases the solubility of uric acid. In addition, some individuals overproduce uric acid, resulting in increased urine uric acid; both gout and increased urine uric acid are associated with uric acid stones, but hyperuricosuria is not required for uric acid stone formation. Chronic diarrhea, resulting in metabolic acidosis and low urine volume, is a common cause of uric acid stones. The metabolic syndrome is also associated with uric acid stone formation. Uric stones are radiolucent but are visualized on ultrasound and CT.

## Cystine

Cystine stones (1%-2% of stones) result from cystinuria, an autosomal recessive disease that presents at a young age. These stones are recognized by characteristic hexagonal crystals in the urine. They may also form staghorn calculi, and are less radio-opaque then calcium-containing stones. H

| TABLE 28. | Kidney Stone Risk Factors and Therapy | |
|---|---|---|
| **Stone Type** | **Risk Factors** | **Therapy** |
| Calcium oxalate | Hypercalciuria; hyperoxaluria; hypocitraturia | Increase fluids |
| | | Decrease sodium intake |
| | | Thiazide diuretics |
| | | Low oxalate diet |
| | | Potassium citrate or bicarbonate |
| Calcium phosphate | Elevated urine pH; distal renal tubular acidosis; hyperparathyroidism | Increase fluids |
| | | Decrease sodium intake |
| | | Thiazide diuretics |
| | | Treat hyperparathyroidism |
| | | Potassium citrate or bicarbonate |
| Uric acid | Low urine pH; diarrhea; metabolic syndrome; gout; hyperuricosuria | Increase fluids |
| | | Potassium citrate or bicarbonate |
| | | Allopurinol |
| Struvite | Chronic urinary tract infections with urea-splitting organism | Treat infection |
| | | Urologic intervention |
| Cystine | Cystinuria; low urine pH | Increase fluids |
| | | Potassium citrate or bicarbonate |
| | | Acetazolamide |
| | | Penicillamine |
| | | Tiopronin |

**KEY POINTS**

- Eighty percent of kidney stones contain calcium; most are composed of calcium oxalate, which is associated with hypercalciuria, hyperoxaluria, and hypocitraturia.

*(Continued)*

**KEY POINTS** *(continued)*

- Struvite stones commonly produce staghorn calculi and occur most frequently in older women with chronic urinary infections; because of their association with infections, there is significant morbidity and mortality associated with these stones.

- Uric acid stones form in persistently acidic urine and are associated with chronic diarrhea, the metabolic syndrome, and gout.

- Cystine stones result from cystinuria, an autosomal recessive disease that presents at a young age; these stones produce characteristic hexagonal crystals in the urine.

## Management

Acute management of symptomatic nephrolithiasis is aimed at pain management and facilitation of stone passage. Pain can be relieved by NSAIDs and opioids as needed. Stone passage decreases with size. Only 50% of stones >6 mm will pass, and stones >10 mm are extremely unlikely to pass spontaneously. Medications, including tamsulosin, nifedipine, silodosin, and tadalafil, appear to increase the rate of spontaneous passage for most stones and can be considered for stones <10 mm.

Urologic intervention is required in all patients with evidence of infection, acute kidney injury, intractable nausea or pain, and stones that fail to pass. This may necessitate shock wave lithotripsy, ureteroscopy with laser ablation, or percutaneous nephrolithotomy.

Patients should strain their urine to collect stone fragments for chemical analysis if the type of stone is unknown. In addition to the initial evaluation previously described, a 24-hour urine for measurement of volume, calcium, oxalate, citrate, uric acid, and sodium should be collected on all recurrent stone formers.

Increased fluid intake is the most important intervention to prevent recurrent disease regardless of stone composition. Urine output should be >2500 mL/d to decrease urine solute concentration.

Other interventions should be based on findings in the metabolic workup and stone analysis (see Table 28). If hypercalciuria is present, calcium excretion can be decreased by the use of thiazide diuretics. Because calcium excretion parallels sodium excretion, limiting sodium intake will also lower urine calcium. Unless excessive, dietary calcium should not be restricted because this will increase oxalate absorption. Oxalate excretion can be decreased by limiting foods high in oxalate such as nuts, cocoa, spinach, rhubarb, and beets. Potassium citrate or potassium bicarbonate will increase urinary citrate excretion. An additional benefit of potassium citrate is a decrease in renal calcium excretion, possibly related to preventing calcium release from bone.

In patients with uric acid stones, management consists of increasing the solubility of uric acid by alkalinizing the urine with potassium citrate or bicarbonate; allopurinol can be beneficial if uric acid excretion is elevated.

Urinary cystine excretion can be reduced by limiting sodium intake and by alkalizing the urine to a pH >7.0. If unsuccessful, additional interventions may be required.

Struvite stones typically require urologic intervention. Before any surgical procedure, it is important that active infection be treated with antibiotics to avert sepsis. To prevent recurrent stone formation, all stone fragments must be removed from the kidney. In patients unable to undergo surgery, the urease inhibitor acetohydroxamic acid may reduce urine alkalinity and decrease stone growth; however, this is best used as an adjunct to urologic intervention.

**KEY POINTS**

- Acute management of symptomatic nephrolithiasis includes pain management and facilitation of stone passage.

- Urologic intervention is required in all patients with evidence of infection, acute kidney injury, intractable nausea or pain, and stones that fail to pass.

- Increased fluid intake to >2500 mL/d is the most important intervention to prevent recurrent kidney stones, regardless of stone composition.

# The Kidney in Pregnancy
## Normal Physiologic Changes in Pregnancy

Pregnancy is a state of volume expansion and vasodilation. Sodium and water retention increase plasma volume, augmenting renal blood flow and increasing glomerular filtration rate (GFR) by up to 50%. With the GFR increase, serum creatinine levels decrease. Therefore, high normal serum creatinine levels may indicate significant kidney impairment. Despite the volume expansion, blood pressure begins to decrease in the first trimester and reaches the nadir in the second trimester due to peripheral vasodilation.

Proteinuria increases, with the upper limit of normal increasing from 100 mg/24 h (in nonpregnant) to approximately 200 mg/24 h. Values >300 mg/24 h are considered abnormal. Prepartum proteinuria may also worsen during pregnancy, making pregnancy-related changes difficult to distinguish from a flare of an underlying kidney disease or development of preeclampsia.

Due to increased renal vascular and interstitial volume, kidney size may increase by 1 to 1.5 cm. Physiologic hydronephrosis and hydroureter, due in part to external compression of the ureters, are common in pregnancy, increase as pregnancy advances, and may take weeks to resolve postpartum. The dilated collecting system can lead to urinary stasis, which increases the risk for pyelonephritis. Therefore, screening for asymptomatic bacteriuria at least once in early pregnancy is recommended, and treatment is indicated.

Respiratory alkalosis due to progesterone-induced hyperventilation commonly decreases $P_{CO_2}$ to 27 to 32 mm Hg. Renal compensation results in serum bicarbonate levels between 18 and 20 mEq/L (18-20 mmol/L), with a serum pH of approximately 7.45.

Changes in antidiuretic hormone response to osmolality (reset osmostat) cause mild hyponatremia (decrease in serum sodium of 4-5 mEq/L [4-5 mmol/L]) with a decrease in serum osmolality by 8 to 10 mOsm/kg $H_2O$. No treatment is indicated. Rarely, transient gestational diabetes insipidus can develop due to excessive metabolism of antidiuretic hormone by placental vasopressinase.

**KEY POINTS**

- Pregnancy is associated with decreased blood pressure, increased glomerular filtration rate with decreased serum creatinine, and increased proteinuria.
- Dilatation of the urinary system during pregnancy increases the risk for pyelonephritis; therefore, screening for asymptomatic bacteriuria at least once in early pregnancy is recommended, and treatment is indicated.

# Hypertension in Pregnancy

## Chronic Hypertension

The American College of Obstetricians and Gynecologists (ACOG) defines chronic hypertension as a systolic blood pressure (BP) ≥140 mm Hg or diastolic BP ≥90 mm Hg starting before pregnancy or before 20 weeks of gestation or persists longer than 12 weeks postpartum. It is associated with worse maternal and fetal outcomes. Hypertension first recognized during pregnancy before 20 weeks' gestation usually indicates chronic hypertension. The lower BP measurements associated with physiologic changes of pregnancy can mask hypertension during the first trimester.

To avoid overtreatment of hypertension and associated fetal risk, the 2013 ACOG Taskforce on Hypertension in Pregnancy recommends treating persistent systolic BP ≥160 mm Hg or diastolic ≥105 mm Hg in women with chronic hypertension, and maintaining BP at 120-160/80-105 mm Hg. However, these goals remain controversial, with some suggesting lower targets. Antihypertensive treatment reduces the risk of progression to severe hypertension by 50% compared with placebo but has not been shown to prevent preeclampsia, preterm birth, being small for gestational age, or infant mortality. Any evidence of end-organ damage requires treatment, even with lower BPs. All antihypertensive medications cross the placenta; drug selection is based on safety profiles.

Renin-angiotensin system agents (ACE inhibitors, angiotensin receptor blockers, and direct renin inhibitors) are all contraindicated due to teratogenicity, even early in pregnancy, and should be stopped prior to conception. If conception has already occurred, they should be stopped immediately and the mother counseled regarding possible fetal effects.

First-line therapy includes methyldopa and labetalol, which have been used safely and extensively in pregnancy. Methyldopa monotherapy may be insufficient, in which case it can be replaced with labetalol. Calcium channel blockers can be added; nifedipine has been used most extensively. The β-blockers metoprolol and pindolol have also been used in pregnancy, but atenolol and propranolol may have adverse fetal effects. Diuretics must be used with caution because they may induce oligohydramnios if started during pregnancy.

## Gestational Hypertension

Gestational hypertension first manifests after 20 weeks of pregnancy without proteinuria or other end-organ damage (features of preeclampsia) and resolves within 12 weeks of delivery. Preeclampsia occurs in approximately one third of cases. Hypertension persisting beyond 12 weeks postpartum is considered chronic hypertension. Gestational hypertension can recur in subsequent pregnancies and is associated with an approximately fourfold risk for development of chronic hypertension.

**KEY POINTS**

- Chronic hypertension precedes pregnancy or is present before 20 weeks' gestation.
- The 2013 American College of Obstetricians and Gynecologists Taskforce on Hypertension in Pregnancy recommends treating persistent systolic blood pressure (BP) ≥160 mm Hg or diastolic BP ≥105 mm Hg in women with chronic hypertension.
- Renin-angiotensin system agents (ACE inhibitors, angiotensin receptor blockers, and direct renin inhibitors) are contraindicated in pregnancy due to teratogenicity; they must be stopped prior to conception or stopped immediately if conception has already occurred.
- First-line therapy of chronic hypertension in pregnancy includes methyldopa and labetalol.
- Gestational hypertension first manifests after 20 weeks of pregnancy without proteinuria or other end-organ damage and resolves within 12 weeks of delivery.

## Preeclampsia

Preeclampsia is defined by new-onset hypertension and proteinuria (≥300 mg/24 h from a timed collection or ≥300 mg/g by urine protein-creatinine ratio) that occurs after 20 weeks of pregnancy (**Table 29**). New-onset hypertension with new-onset end-organ damage (such as liver or kidney injury, pulmonary edema, cerebral or visual symptoms, or thrombocytopenia) is also diagnostic of preeclampsia. Severe preeclampsia is identified by persistent systolic BP >160 mm Hg or diastolic BP >110 mm Hg and end-organ damage. Eclampsia is the presence of seizures in context of preeclampsia without other cause. The HELLP (hemolysis, elevated liver enzymes, low platelets) syndrome is a life-threatening state complicating 10% to 20% of preeclampsia cases. Risk factors for preeclampsia include prior preeclampsia (with an approximate 20% recurrence rate), nulliparity, diabetes mellitus, advanced maternal age, multiple gestation, and family history.

The pathophysiology of preeclampsia is poorly understood. Abnormal placental vascular development and generalized endothelial dysfunction occur. Two angiogenic and antiangiogenic factors, soluble fms-like tyrosine kinase-1

**TABLE 29. Diagnostic Criteria for Preeclampsia**

| Blood pressure | ≥140 mm Hg systolic or ≥90 mm Hg diastolic on two occasions at least 4 hours apart after 20 weeks of gestation in a woman with a previously normal blood pressure |
| | ≥160 mm Hg systolic or ≥110 mm Hg diastolic; hypertension can be confirmed within a short interval (minutes) to facilitate timely antihypertensive therapy |
| and | |
| Proteinuria | ≥300 mg/24 h urine collection (or this amount extrapolated from a timed collection) |
| | or |
| | Urine protein-creatinine ratio ≥300 mg/g |
| | Dipstick reading of 1+ (used only if other quantitative methods are not available) |
| **Or, in the absence of proteinuria, new-onset hypertension with the new onset of any of the following:** | |
| Thrombocytopenia | Platelet count <100,000/μL (100 × 10⁹/L) |
| Kidney dysfunction | Serum creatinine concentrations >1.1 mg/dL (97.2 μmol/L) or a doubling of the serum creatinine concentration in the absence of other kidney disease |
| Impaired liver function | Elevated blood concentrations of liver aminotransaminases to twice the normal concentration |
| Pulmonary edema | — |
| Cerebral or visual symptoms | — |

With permission from American College of Obstetricians and Gynecologists; Task Force on Hypertension in Pregnancy. Hypertension in pregnancy. Report of the American College of Obstetricians and Gynecologists' Task Force on Hypertension in Pregnancy. Obstet Gynecol. 2013;122(5):1122-31. [PMID: 24150027]

(sFlt-1) and soluble endoglin (sEng), are elevated in women with preeclampsia; their role in treatment and diagnosis continues to be elucidated.

Symptoms of preeclampsia include rapid weight gain due to edema, nausea, vomiting, abdominal pain (particularly concerning if in the right upper quadrant, signifying possible HELLP syndrome), headaches, altered mental status, and blurred vision. If untreated, preeclampsia ultimately leads to maternal end-organ damage and fetal growth retardation, and it may cause maternal and/or fetal death.

Low-dose (81 mg/d) aspirin started after 12 weeks of pregnancy reduces the rate of preeclampsia in women at high risk. Antihypertensive medications do not prevent preeclampsia but reduce complications of stroke, heart failure, and kidney injury. Most experts initiate treatment at BP >150–160/100–110 mm Hg, although there is no consensus.

Definitive treatment of preeclampsia is delivery. Maternal risk for complications diminishes in the hours after delivery, although proteinuria may take months to resolve. Maternal benefits must be weighed against neonatal risks for a preterm delivery, but severe preeclampsia is an indication for immediate delivery regardless of gestational age. Mild preeclampsia may be managed conservatively, with maternal and fetal monitoring and treatment of hypertension. In all cases, close attention to hypertension is recommended in the postpartum period.

**KEY POINTS**

- Preeclampsia is defined by new-onset hypertension and proteinuria that occurs after 20 weeks of pregnancy.
- Low-dose (81 mg/d) aspirin started after 12 weeks of pregnancy reduces rates of preeclampsia in women at high risk.
- Definitive treatment of preeclampsia is delivery.

# Chronic Kidney Disease in Pregnancy

Chronic kidney disease (CKD) complicates management of pregnancy; the obstetric literature notes a serum creatinine cutoff of >1.4 mg/dL (124 μmol/L) as that at which complications are of most concern. Proteinuria may also increase risk, but reduced GFR has greater impact. Complications include preeclampsia, acute kidney injury, progression of CKD, end-stage kidney disease, preterm delivery, gestational hypertension, intrauterine growth retardation, and fetal loss. Preconception counseling regarding these risks is essential.

Pregnancy is uncommon in women receiving dialysis, which is frequently associated with infertility. Levels of β-human chorionic gonadotropin (β-hCG) may increase with dialysis in the absence of pregnancy; therefore, ultrasonography is usually necessary to confirm pregnancy. Pregnancy in the context of dialysis is associated with very high risk of preeclampsia and fetal loss, although live birth rates have improved to 60% to 80%. To optimize fetal outcomes, hemodialysis frequency and dose are increased to improve BP and volume status.

Pregnancy in women with kidney transplants is more common than in those receiving dialysis due to increased fertility after transplant. Outcomes are improved with better allograft function (serum creatinine <1.5 mg/dL [132.6 μmol/L]) and stable immunosuppression; transplant patients should await 1 to 2 years with a stable allograft before attempting conception. No immunosuppressive medication has been extensively studied in pregnancy, and all have some associated risk. Although calcineurin inhibitors (tacrolimus and cyclosporine) have been used safely, mycophenolate mofetil is teratogenic and needs to be replaced 3 to 6 months prior to conception with azathioprine, which has an extensive history of use in pregnancy. Sirolimus is contraindicated due to fetal toxicity. Glucocorticoids increase risk for pregnancy-induced hypertension and diabetes.

**KEY POINTS**

- Women with chronic kidney disease (CKD) have a greater risk for preeclampsia, acute kidney injury, progression of CKD, end-stage kidney disease, preterm delivery, gestational hypertension, intrauterine growth retardation, and fetal loss.
- Kidney transplant recipients should wait at least 1 to 2 years after transplantation with a stable allograft and stable immunosuppression before attempting conception.
- The immunosuppressive medications mycophenolate mofetil and sirolimus used in kidney transplant recipients are teratogenic and must be discontinued prior to attempting conception.

# Chronic Kidney Disease

## Definition and Staging

Chronic kidney disease (CKD) is defined as abnormal kidney structure or function present for >3 months. CKD is stratified into stages 1 to 5 based on the level of estimated glomerular filtration rate (eGFR). Stages G1 and G2 do not have reductions in eGFR and therefore are defined by the presence of anatomical defects or markers of kidney damage such as albuminuria, hematuria, or electrolyte abnormalities. Because albuminuria is associated with increased renal and cardiovascular morbidity and mortality, the Kidney Disease: Improving Global Outcomes (KDIGO) group further subdivides the eGFR-based kidney stages by degree of albuminuria (**Figure 18**). This dual eGFR and albuminuria staging algorithm provides a means for predicting which patients are at highest risk for developing progressive CKD into end-stage kidney disease (ESKD), defined as CKD stage G5 treated with chronic dialysis or kidney transplantation.

## Epidemiology and Pathophysiology

CKD, defined by either albuminuria or eGFR <60 mL/min/1.73 $m^2$, affects approximately 15% of the U.S. adult population. About 50% of patients with prevalent CKD have stage G3 disease or worse; the other 50% have CKD due to the presence of albuminuria. The prevalence of CKD is heavily influenced by age and has increased severalfold in elderly persons over the past 20 years. The largest increase over time, as assessed by the National Health and Nutrition Examination Survey (NHANES), is in stage G3 disease. In the United States, the prevalence of

| | | | | Persistent albuminuria categories Description and range | | |
|---|---|---|---|---|---|---|
| | | | | A1 | A2 | A3 |
| | | | | Normal to mildly increased | Moderately increased | Severely increased |
| | | | | <30 mg/g | 30-300 mg/g | >300 mg/g |
| GFR categories (mL/min/1.73 $m^2$) Description and range | G1 | Normal or high | ≥90 | | | |
| | G2 | Mildly decreased | 60-89 | | | |
| | G3a | Mildly to moderately decreased | 45-59 | | | |
| | G3b | Moderately to severely decreased | 30-44 | | | |
| | G4 | Severely decreased | 15-29 | | | |
| | G5 | Kidney failure | <15 | | | |

Green: low risk (if no other markers of kidney disease, no CKD); Yellow: moderately increased risk; Orange: high risk; Red: very high risk.

**FIGURE 18.** The Kidney Disease: Improving Global Outcomes (KDIGO) chronic kidney disease staging system. Prognosis of chronic kidney disease by glomerular filtration rate and albuminuria category. CKD = chronic kidney disease; GFR = glomerular filtration rate.

CKD stage G3 or worse is 0.3% in those aged 20 to 39 years, 3.3% in those aged 40 to 59 years, and 22.6% in those aged ≥60 years. In contrast, the prevalence of albuminuria is less age dependent. Approximately 6% of persons aged 40 to 59 years have a urine albumin-creatinine ratio ≥30 mg/g, compared with 8.5% of those aged ≥60 years. Advanced CKD, defined by stages G4 or G5, is present in <1% of the population. Compared with men, women have a slightly higher prevalence of both eGFR <60 mL/min/1.73 m² (7.9% versus 6.4%) and albuminuria (10.9% versus 8.8%).

CKD results from various etiologies that cause chronic damage to the glomeruli, tubulointerstitium, or both. Glomerular damage is reflected by proteinuria or albuminuria. Although a large degree of tubulointerstitial damage (both chronic inflammation and fibrosis) can exist subclinically and thus go unnoticed, eventually the underlying structural abnormalities affect kidney function, and GFR falls below normal levels.

Not all patients with CKD progress to ESKD. The most important predictors of progression are the baseline level of eGFR and the degree of albuminuria/proteinuria. eGFR trajectory over time also adds prognostic value for ESKD and cardiovascular outcomes. Patients with diabetic CKD usually progress faster than those without diabetes. The rate of eGFR decline ranges between -3 and -6 mL/min/1.73 m² per year in patients who have type 2 diabetes with high albuminuria. Renal risk variants in the apolipoprotein L1 (APOL1) gene are prevalent in black persons and are associated with higher rates of ESKD and progression of CKD, regardless of diabetes status (see Genetic Disorders and Kidney Disease).

# Screening

CKD is typically asymptomatic except in advanced stages (G4, G5). Controversy exists regarding screening patients for CKD. The U.S. Preventive Services Task Force (USPSTF) and the American College of Physicians recommend against screening for CKD in asymptomatic adults with or without risk factors for CKD. In contrast, the American Society of Nephrology advises screening all adults for CKD, including, but not limited to, those with a family history of kidney disease or adults with risk factors for CKD (diabetes, hypertension, or cardiovascular disease).

# Clinical Manifestations

CKD is typically asymptomatic except in advanced stages (G4, G5). When eGFR falls below 30 mL/min/1.73 m², numerous alterations in metabolic pathways, including 1,25-dihydroxyvitamin D production and erythrocyte production, become altered due to the lack of nephron mass and loss of 1α-hydroxylase and erythropoietin synthesis. Moderate to severe CKD can also result in impaired ability to excrete salt and water, and may manifest as edema. CKD in a patient with nephrotic-range proteinuria may also result in edema or anasarca.

When CKD progresses to ESKD, several nonspecific ("uremic") symptoms can occur such as fatigue, nausea, loss of appetite, insomnia, irritability, difficulty concentrating, confusion, or pruritus. Uremia can also induce serositis, including pleuritis and pericarditis. However, a large proportion of patients with CKD stage G5 manifest few or only intermittent uremic symptoms, for unexplained reasons. Although rarely seen today due to increased awareness and the widespread availability of dialysis, patients who have prolonged uremia that is untreated with renal replacement therapy may develop "uremic frost," which appears as chalky whitish skin and is due to crystallized urea deposits and other nitrogenous waste products that evaporated from sweat (**Figure 19**).

# Diagnosis

CKD may be clinically suspected, or it may be incidentally detected on a basic chemistry panel that includes serum creatinine. Initial assessment of GFR includes establishing eGFR based on serum creatinine using the Chronic Kidney Disease Epidemiology (CKD-EPI) Collaboration creatinine equation. If confirmation of GFR is required because of conditions that affect serum creatinine independent of GFR (such as extremes of muscle mass or diet), cystatin C should be measured to employ the CKD-EPI creatinine-cystatin equation, or GFR should be measured directly using a clearance procedure. Initial assessment of albuminuria includes a random urine albumin-creatinine ratio. If confirmation of albuminuria is required because of diurnal variation or conditions affecting creatinine excretion, the albumin excretion rate should be

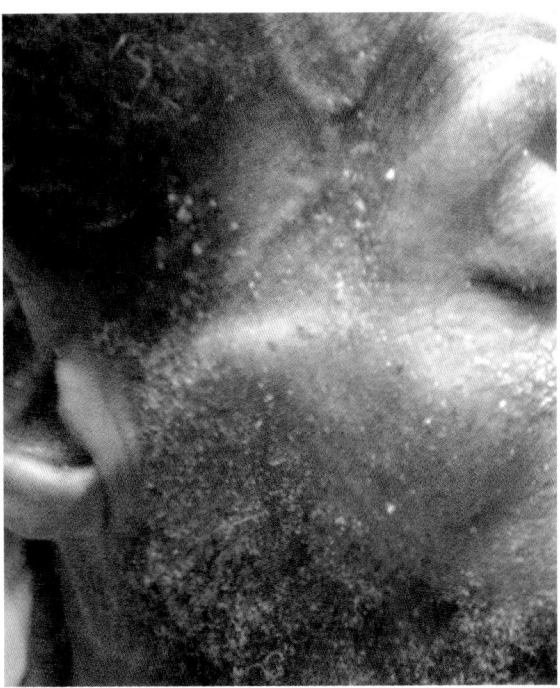

**FIGURE 19.** Uremic frost presenting as powdery deposits of urea and uric acid salts on the skin in a patient with untreated chronic kidney disease.

measured from a timed urine collection. See Clinical Evaluation of Kidney Function for more information.

Diagnosis of CKD requires a low eGFR confirmed at least 3 months after initial assessment, or persistent proteinuria or albuminuria. Kidney biopsy is used to determine the etiology of CKD when a glomerulonephritis, unexplained tubulointerstitial disease, or severe proteinuria is likely based upon clinical history, urine sediment, and laboratory results and/or antibody tests. Kidney biopsy is not indicated in the presence of shrunken kidneys (<9 cm), which generally indicate chronic irreversible disease. Occasionally, patients are noted to have "medical kidney disease" on imaging (such as ultrasound revealing hyperechoic kidneys). Urinalysis done for other nonspecific reasons may detect previously undiagnosed hematuria or proteinuria, which may suggest the presence of CKD and should prompt close observation or additional evaluation depending on the clinical scenario. There is currently a lack of evidence regarding the use of urinalysis as a routine screening test for CKD.

Patients who experience acute kidney injury (AKI) can have slow recovery; studies have demonstrated that kidney function can continue to recover for up to 1 year after an initial episode of AKI. Therefore, although diagnosis of CKD requires at least 3 months of persisting abnormalities in structure or function, a diagnosis of CKD after AKI may be premature in some patients between 3 and 12 months after the AKI episode.

### KEY POINTS

- Chronic kidney disease is defined as abnormal kidney structure or function present for >3 months.

- Staging of chronic kidney disease is based on estimated glomerular filtration rate and albuminuria.

- The U.S. Preventive Services Task Force and the American College of Physicians recommend against screening for chronic kidney disease (CKD) in asymptomatic adults with or without risk factors for CKD, whereas the American Society of Nephrology advises screening all adults for CKD, including, but not limited to, those with a family history of kidney disease or adults with risk factors for CKD (diabetes, hypertension, or cardiovascular disease).

## Complications and Management

According to KDIGO guidelines, referral to a nephrologist is indicated for evaluation and management of CKD in the presence of the following: AKI or an abrupt, sustained fall in GFR; GFR <30 mL/min/1.73 m$^2$; persistent albuminuria (>300 mg/g); progression of CKD; erythrocyte casts; >20 erythrocytes/hpf that is sustained and not readily explained; hypertension refractory to treatment with four or more antihypertensive agents; persistent abnormalities of serum potassium; recurrent or extensive nephrolithiasis; or hereditary kidney disease.

A kidney failure risk equation (KFRE) has been developed and validated. The KFRE uses four variables (age, sex, eGFR, and albuminuria) to predict 2-year and 5-year risk for ESKD in patients with CKD stages G3 to G5. The KFRE performs well across age, sex, race, and presence/absence of diabetes. The use of this equation is consistent with KDIGO guidelines, which recommend integration of risk prediction in the evaluation and management of CKD.

### Cardiovascular Disease

Cardiovascular disease is the leading cause of death among patients with CKD. The risk for cardiovascular-related death in patients with CKD stages G3 and G4 is 4 to 5 times higher than the risk for progression to ESKD. Mortality risk increases with decreasing eGFR and increasing albuminuria. Unfortunately, many landmark clinical trials that guide the prevention or treatment of cardiovascular disease did not include patients with advanced CKD, and the findings may not be generalizable to patients with CKD. However, most post-hoc analyses of randomized controlled trials that had participants with some degree of CKD demonstrated efficacy regardless of baseline CKD status, including for interventions such as percutaneous coronary interventions. Thus, experts recommend against withholding otherwise efficacious therapies from those with CKD due to unsubstantiated concerns of lack of efficacy or harm. These also include coronary angiography or thrombolysis and/or platelet antagonists for patients with acute coronary syndromes or acute strokes and contrast-based CT studies for patients with high pretest probability of pulmonary embolism or aortic dissection.

### Hypertension

Both KDIGO and the 2017 high blood pressure guideline from the American College of Cardiology (ACC), the American Heart Association (AHA), and nine other organizations recommend a blood pressure target of <130/80 mm Hg in patients with CKD.

An ACE inhibitor or an angiotensin receptor blocker is a preferred drug for treatment of hypertension for patients with stage G3 CKD or higher or for those with stage G1 or G2 CKD with albuminuria (albumin-creatinine ratio ≥300 mg/g). These medications may also slow the progression of CKD in some patients. Thiazide diuretics are a cornerstone of hypertension treatment but may lose efficacy with severe CKD. Loop diuretics therefore serve an important role in managing salt and water retention associated with proteinuria and CKD. Dietary sodium chloride restriction is essential for blood pressure control in most forms of CKD, and KDIGO recommends restricting sodium intake to <2000 mg/d.

See Hypertension for more information.

### Dyslipidemia

Elevated LDL cholesterol and triglyceride levels with low HDL cholesterol levels are common among patients with CKD. Conflicting data exist on the effect of treating dyslipidemia in reducing proteinuria and in slowing the progression of CKD. Statins have been shown to reduce cardiovascular and all-cause mortality in patients with CKD, although large trials have failed to demonstrate a mortality benefit for statins in patients with dialysis-dependent ESKD (unless initiated pre-dialysis). KDIGO guidelines recommend treatment with a statin in all patients aged ≥50 years with non-dialysis–dependent CKD and in adults aged 18 to 49 years with non-dialysis–dependent CKD and any one of the following: coronary disease, diabetes mellitus, prior ischemic stroke, or a >10% estimated risk of coronary death or nonfatal myocardial infarction. Statins are also recommended for adult kidney transplant recipients.

Dyslipidemia associated with the nephrotic syndrome helps maintain plasma oncotic pressure but, over time, may hasten the progression of glomerular injury. Dyslipidemia in the nephrotic syndrome requires aggressive treatment to prevent atherosclerotic disease, especially in patients with existing cardiovascular risk factors and in younger patients to prevent premature cardiovascular disease. See Glomerular Diseases for more information on the nephrotic syndrome.

### Coronary Artery Disease

There is a significantly increased prevalence of coronary artery disease (CAD) among patients with CKD compared with the general population. This is partly explained by the high prevalence of shared risk factors/comorbidities such as diabetes or hypertension. However, CKD is independently associated with CAD, and this association strengthens with declining eGFR and rising albuminuria. Despite high cardiovascular mortality among patients with CKD, these patients may be less likely to undergo coronary revascularization procedures, possibly because of the increased risk for contrast-induced nephropathy (see Special Considerations, Imaging Contrast Agents).

In patients with CKD, serum biomarkers for myocardial ischemia such as cardiac troponins may be chronically elevated due to decreased renal clearance. Serial troponin measurements and other markers such as creatine kinase-MB can help distinguish acute ischemia from stable elevations.

### KEY POINTS

- Both the Kidney Disease: Improving Global Outcomes group and the 2017 high blood pressure guideline from the American College of Cardiology (ACC), the American Heart Association (AHA), and nine other organizations recommend a target blood pressure of <130/80 mm Hg in patients with hypertension and chronic kidney disease.

- Treatment of hypertension in patients with chronic kidney disease includes an ACE inhibitor or angiotensin receptor blocker, dietary sodium restriction to <2000 mg/d, and addition of a diuretic as needed to control vascular volume.

*(Continued)*

**KEY POINTS** *(continued)*

- The Kidney Disease: Improving Global Outcomes guidelines recommend treatment with a statin in all patients with non-dialysis–dependent chronic kidney disease (CKD) who are over 50 years of age and in adults 18 to 49 years of age with non-dialysis–dependent CKD and any one of the following: coronary disease, diabetes mellitus, prior ischemic stroke, or a >10% estimated risk of coronary death or nonfatal myocardial infarction.

## Chronic Kidney Disease-Mineral and Bone Disorder

As kidney function declines, the normal homeostasis of calcium and phosphorus levels by the kidney becomes compromised, resulting in alterations in bone mineralization. The term *chronic kidney disease-mineral and bone disorder* (CKD-MBD) encompasses these changes. The KDIGO guidelines for CKD-MBD are available at kdigo.org.

### Calcium and Phosphorus Homeostasis

Three hormones are largely responsible for regulating calcium and phosphorus homeostasis: parathyroid hormone (PTH), vitamin D, and fibroblast growth factor 23 (FGF-23). PTH is the most important regulator of calcium and phosphorus concentrations. PTH has three separate mechanisms to increase serum calcium: It stimulates osteoclasts to resorb bone, stimulates hydroxylation of 25-hydroxyvitamin D in the kidneys, and stimulates tubular reabsorption of calcium (**Figure 20**). Concurrently, PTH induces renal phosphorus excretion.

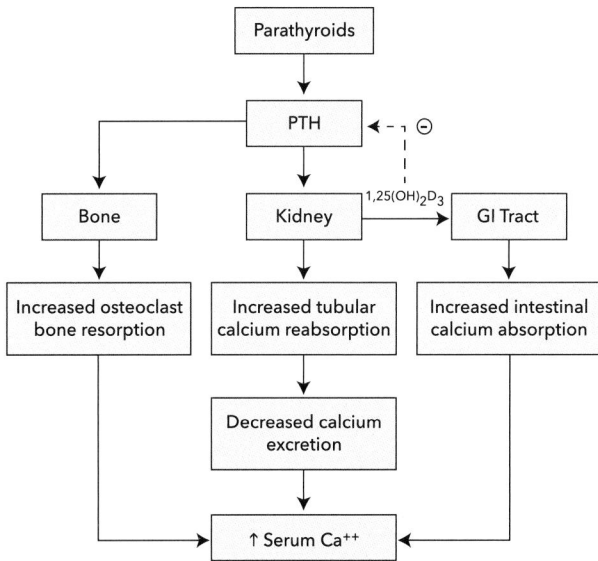

**FIGURE 20.** Overview of the metabolic systems that maintain calcium homeostasis. Parathyroid hormone (PTH) stimulates increased 1,25-dihydroxyvitamin $D_3$ [1,25(OH)$_2$D$_3$] synthesis by the kidneys, and 1,25(OH)$_2$D$_3$ causes feedback suppression of PTH production. Ca$^{++}$ = ionized calcium; GI = gastrointestinal; 1,25(OH)$_2$D$_3$ = 1,25-dihydroxyvitamin D$_3$; PTH = parathyroid hormone; ↑ = increased.

FGF-23 is a peptide secreted by osteocytes and osteoclasts. It acts on the kidney to induce phosphaturia and downregulates 1α-hydroxylase to inhibit synthesis of 1,25 dihydroxyvitamin D. FGF-23 rises in stage G3a CKD, preceding PTH elevation. As GFR falls and PTH rises, PTH directly stimulates further FGF-23 production by osteocytes, resulting in a massive increase of FGF-23 blood levels, upwards of 100-fold from normal. Initially, the high FGF-23 serves to increase renal phosphorus excretion and helps maintain normal phosphorus levels as GFR declines.

As CKD progresses, increased FGF-23 and decreased nephron mass reduce the conversion of 25-hydroxyvitamin D to 1,25-dihydroxyvitamin D by renal tubular cells. Reduction in 1,25-dihydroxyvitamin D levels results in lower intestinal absorption of calcium and phosphorus in the gut, mitigating phosphorus retention but also contributing to hypocalcemia, especially late in CKD. Reduced 1,25-dihydroxyvitamin D levels also increase PTH production by the parathyroid glands, and hypocalcemia is a potent stimulus for further increases in PTH levels.

Increased plasma PTH as a result of CKD is referred to as *secondary hyperparathyroidism*. Increased PTH levels result in reduced calcium excretion, increased calcium absorption from the gut, increased phosphorus excretion by the kidneys, and activation of osteoclast bone resorption. Early in CKD, the PTH-induced increase in renal phosphorus excretion enables normal phosphorus levels despite reduced renal excretory capacity. However, as CKD progresses, the kidney is unable to compensate for the increased release of phosphorus from bone, and phosphorus levels rise. This results in a vicious cycle as hyperphosphatemia stimulates PTH production.

If secondary hyperparathyroidism cannot be adequately controlled, tertiary hyperparathyroidism can ensue. Tertiary hyperparathyroidism is the result of the prolonged PTH stimulation needed to maintain eucalcemia. This prolonged stimulation results in increased calcium levels and severe hyperparathyroid hyperplasia with elevated PTH levels that are no longer responsive to the plasma calcium concentration.

## Laboratory Abnormalities

Serum calcium and phosphorus levels typically remain in the normal range until the eGFR drops below 20 to 30 mL/min/1.73 m$^2$ (stages G4-G5), at which point the ability of elevated FGF-23 and PTH levels to promote phosphorus excretion becomes overwhelmed, and hyperphosphatemia develops. Progressive decline in 1,25-dihydroxyvitamin D levels results in reduced intestinal calcium absorption, and hyperphosphatemia promotes precipitation of calcium and phosphorus in extraskeletal tissues, leading to hypocalcemia.

In addition to reduced conversion of 25-hydroxyvitamin D to 1,25-dihydroxyvitamin D, patients with CKD also have a higher prevalence of 25-hydroxyvitamin D deficiency. KDIGO guidelines recommend that patients with an eGFR <60 mL/min/1.73 m$^2$ (stage G3-G5) be evaluated for 25-hydroxyvitamin D deficiency and supplemented as per guidelines for the general population.

PTH levels are often elevated in patients with an eGFR <60 mL/min/1.73 m$^2$ (stage G3-G5) and progressively increase with worsening CKD. KDIGO guidelines recommend measuring intact PTH levels in these patients to aid in the detection and management of secondary hyperparathyroidism and its complications.

### Vascular Calcification

An increased prevalence of arterial calcification, including the coronary arteries, has been noted in patients with CKD; the burden of calcification is highest in patients with ESKD. Arterial calcification reduces vascular compliance and likely contributes to the increased prevalence of left ventricular hypertrophy observed in patients with CKD. Arterial calcification is also strongly associated with cardiovascular and all-cause mortality; KDIGO guidelines therefore suggest treating patients with CKD and arterial calcification as is appropriate for patients in the highest category of cardiovascular risk, although treatments specifically targeted at reducing vascular calcification have not been shown to improve clinical outcomes.

### Renal Osteodystrophy

*Renal osteodystrophy* refers to alteration of bone morphology in patients with CKD, which occurs as part of the systemic disorder of CKD-MBD. Four main types of histologic changes in bone can occur as part of renal osteodystrophy and are discussed in this section. KDIGO guidelines recommend a bone biopsy if knowledge of the type of renal osteodystrophy will affect treatment decisions in patients with CKD stages G3a to G5. This recommendation is based on the growing experience with osteoporosis medications in patients with CKD, low bone mineral density, and a high risk of fracture. The lack of ability to perform a bone biopsy may not justify withholding antiresorptive therapy from patients at high risk of fracture.

#### Osteitis Fibrosa Cystica

Osteitis fibrosa cystica is due to abnormally high bone turnover that can occur after prolonged exposure of bone to sustained high levels of PTH in secondary hyperparathyroidism. It is associated with an increased number and activity of osteoblasts and osteoclasts and expansion of osteoid surfaces, resulting in an increased risk for fracture. Patients can be asymptomatic or have bone pain. Classic skeletal changes on radiograph include subperiosteal resorption of bone, most prominently at the phalanges of the hands, and radiolucent bone cysts of the long bones.

#### Adynamic Bone Disease

Adynamic bone disease occurs when there is a lack of bone cell activity and a markedly reduced rate of bone turnover. Histopathologic abnormalities include decreased osteoclast activity with an increase in osteoid, resulting in an increased risk for fracture. Patients have suppressed PTH levels (due to chronic illness or aggressive treatment with vitamin D

**CONT.**

analogues) or skeletal resistance to PTH from down-regulation of the bone PTH receptor due to high circulating PTH levels. Patients may be asymptomatic or have bone pain. Adynamic bone disease should be excluded prior to bisphosphonate therapy because these drugs can cause and/or worsen the disease by inhibiting osteoclast activity.

*Osteomalacia*
Osteomalacia is characterized by decreased mineralization of osteoid at sites of bone turnover, with increased risk of fracture. The most common symptoms include bone pain and tenderness. Although patients with CKD are at increased risk for osteomalacia, CKD does not cause osteomalacia per se; vitamin D deficiency caused by coexisting factors such as intestinal malabsorption due to gastrointestinal disorders or restricted access to sunlight is often present.

*Osteoporosis*
Patients with CKD have many causes of reduced bone density. Current KDIGO guidelines indicate that in patients with CKD stages G3a to G5 with evidence of CKD-MBD and/or risk factors for osteoporosis, bone mineral density testing is suggested to assess fracture risk if results will affect treatment decisions. 

**Management**
In patients with CKD stages G3a to G5, treatment of CKD-MBD is based on serial assessments of phosphorus, calcium, and PTH levels. Current KDIGO guidelines recommend that in patients with CKD stages G3a to G5, elevated phosphorus levels should be lowered *toward* the normal range, not into the normal range, because there is an absence of data showing that efforts to maintain phosphorus in the normal range are of benefit and safety concerns. Thus, treatment should be aimed at overt hyperphosphatemia, and decisions to start phosphate-lowering treatment should be based solely on progressively or persistently elevated serum phosphorus levels.

KDIGO guidelines recommend avoiding hypercalcemia. Mild and asymptomatic hypocalcemia (for example, in the context of calcimimetic treatment) can be tolerated to avoid inappropriate calcium loading. KDIGO guidelines also now recommend restricting the dose of calcium-based phosphate binders (calcium carbonate and calcium acetate) in CKD stages G3a to G5, rather than restriction only in those with hypercalcemia. This change was based on published trials suggesting that exposure to exogenous calcium is harmful in terms of vascular calcification in all stages of CKD, along with data suggestive of lower mortality risk with non–calcium-containing phosphate binders (sevelamer and lanthanum) versus calcium-containing binders.

For patients with CKD stages G3a to G5 who are not on dialysis, optimal PTH levels are not known. Previously, patients with PTH levels above the upper normal limit were targeted for management. The 2016 KDIGO update suggests that patients with levels of intact PTH *"progressively rising or*

*persistently above the upper normal limit* for the assay be evaluated for modifiable factors, including hyperphosphatemia, hypocalcemia, high phosphate intake, and vitamin D deficiency." KDIGO guidelines recommend against routine use of calcitriol and vitamin D analogues to lower PTH levels in patients with CKD stages G3a to G5 not on dialysis, because trials of these agents failed to demonstrate improvements in clinically relevant outcomes. Instead, these agents should be reserved for patients with CKD stages G4 to G5 with severe and progressive hyperparathyroidism.

In patients on dialysis, KDIGO guidelines recommend use of calcimimetics, calcitriol, or vitamin D analogues, or a combination of calcimimetics and calcitriol or vitamin D analogues, to lower PTH levels. This recommendation was largely due to the EVOLVE (EValuation Of Cinacalcet Hydrochloride Therapy to Lower CardioVascular Events) trial and several secondary analyses of data from this trial. The EVOLVE trial evaluated the effect of cinacalcet versus placebo in hemodialysis patients by using a composite end point of all-cause mortality, nonfatal myocardial infarction, hospitalization for unstable angina, heart failure, and peripheral vascular events. Although the primary analysis demonstrated a nonsignificant reduction in the primary composite end point with cinacalcet, multiple sensitivity analyses demonstrated statistically significant reductions in the composite end point, including in those aged ≥65 years. Given these mostly positive but mixed findings, the KDIGO Work Group listed calcimimetic therapy among the acceptable treatment options while still recognizing the utility and efficacy of active vitamin D compounds.

Tertiary hyperparathyroidism does not respond to phosphate binders or calcitriol therapy, and patients often require parathyroidectomy for definitive treatment.

**KEY POINTS**
- Chronic kidney disease-mineral and bone disorder is defined by the changes to the normal homeostasis of calcium and phosphorus levels as kidney function declines, resulting in alterations in bone mineralization.
- According to current Kidney Disease: Improving Global Outcomes (KDIGO) guidelines, management of chronic kidney disease-mineral and bone disorder focuses upon normalizing serum phosphorus, avoiding hypercalcemia, and addressing modifiable factors.

**Anemia**
Anemia in the setting of CKD is common, and its prevalence increases as CKD progresses into stages G4 and G5. Most often normocytic, anemia in CKD largely results from lack of erythropoietin production due to the decline in functional renal mass. Other contributors include erythropoietin resistance, neocytolysis (decreased survival time of erythrocytes), and iron deficiency.

Although modest declines in hemoglobin are well tolerated, concern for inducing or contributing to the development

CONT.

of left ventricular hypertrophy has been the key driver in the belief that higher hemoglobin values are beneficial. Moreover, observational data suggest that higher hemoglobin values are associated with better outcomes in patients with CKD and ESKD. However, several large randomized controlled trials conducted in the past 15 to 20 years demonstrated no benefit or increased harm regarding some cardiovascular events in groups randomly assigned to higher hemoglobin targets via erythropoiesis-stimulating agents (ESAs). Moreover, these trials revealed only modest improvements in fatigue and no benefit in physical functioning with higher hemoglobin targets. The mechanisms underlying the lack of benefit or harm for the higher hemoglobin groups are not well understood but may include off-target effects of ESAs on extrarenal organs. Thus, current KDIGO recommendations are to consider ESAs for patients with CKD who have hemoglobin concentrations <10 g/dL (100 g/L). Black box warnings for use of ESAs include the risk for increased mortality and/or tumor progression in patients with active malignancy, increased risk for thromboembolic events in postsurgical patients not receiving anticoagulant therapy, and increased risk for serious cardiovascular events when ESAs are administered to patients with hemoglobin values >11 g/dL (110 g/L) or with a history of stroke.

All patients with CKD and anemia should have iron profiles assessed, including total iron-binding capacity and ferritin levels. KDIGO recommendations suggest maintaining transferrin saturation levels of >30% and serum ferritin levels of >500 ng/mL (500 µg/L) using either oral or intravenous iron supplementation. Inadequate iron stores will contribute to ESA hyporesponsiveness. Blood transfusions can be used in patients with severe anemia or modest anemia with symptoms; however, the goal is to minimize the number of erythrocyte transfusions in patients with CKD and ESKD due to concerns for iron overload and sensitization to HLA antigens, which may lead to allosensitization and increased waiting times for kidney transplantation.

KDIGO guidelines for the diagnosis and management of CKD-related anemia can be found at kdigo.org.

## Metabolic Acidosis

Metabolic acidosis frequently occurs in patients with CKD due to defective acid excretion (resulting in reduced bicarbonate generation), most commonly due to impaired ammoniagenesis. Untreated metabolic acidosis can lead to muscle loss (due to increased muscle proteolysis) and bone loss (due to increased bone resorption and impaired bone formation). In early CKD, metabolic acidosis is typically a normal anion gap hyperchloremic metabolic acidosis. As eGFR declines, organic and inorganic anions are retained, and an increased anion gap metabolic acidosis develops.

Large observational studies have shown a strong association between lower serum bicarbonate levels and both increased progression of CKD and mortality. Alkali therapy, most commonly sodium bicarbonate or sodium citrate, can

delay the progression of CKD. Therefore, KDIGO guidelines recommend starting alkali therapy when the serum bicarbonate is chronically <22 mEq/L (22 mmol/L). The alkali salt therapy dose should be titrated to achieve a serum bicarbonate level within the normal range; excessive alkali therapy in the setting of a reduced eGFR may induce a metabolic alkalosis, which is associated with increased mortality. Despite the administration of excess sodium, alkali salts are not associated with volume expansion, even among patients with chronic heart failure or overt edema, most likely because the accompanying anion is not chloride.

## Nephrotoxins

Two major issues exist regarding drug administration in patients with CKD: 1) Renally excreted drugs require dose adjustment to avoid accumulation and potential side effects; and 2) Reduced functional nephron mass increases the probability that a potentially nephrotoxic drug will cause nephrotoxicity.

Conceptually, it is useful to compartmentalize nephrotoxic medications by their main site of action. For example, several medications, including NSAIDs, calcineurin inhibitors, and ACE inhibitors/angiotensin receptor blockers, can have effects on glomerular blood flow. Patients with AKI who are on NSAIDs should have the medications immediately discontinued. For patients with CKD, the American Society of Nephrology recommends the avoidance of NSAIDs, including cyclooxygenase-2 inhibitors, due to the risk of worsening kidney function. ACE inhibitors or angiotensin receptor blockers are the cornerstone of treatment for patients with CKD; however, during episodes of acute illness and/or volume depletion, these drugs increase the risk for AKI due to their effects on intraglomerular pressure. Drugs that cause glomerular injury, tubular injury, or tubulointerstitial nephritis are reviewed in Acute Kidney Injury.

Emerging literature suggests that proton pump inhibitors, in addition to their classic association with acute interstitial nephritis/AKI, may contribute to the development and progression of CKD. The association is robust and has been confirmed in three independent cohorts. These studies used careful comparators, including the use of $H_2$ blockers, and adjusted for numerous potential confounding variables, including chronic NSAID use.

## Proteinuria

The severity of proteinuria is strongly associated with adverse clinical outcomes, including progression of CKD to ESKD, cardiovascular morbidity, and mortality. It is unclear whether proteinuria is simply a marker of the underlying severity of kidney damage and disease, or if proteinuria itself activates inflammatory pathways and contributes to tubulointerstitial fibrosis. Although dual renin-angiotensin system blockade via combinations of ACE inhibitors, angiotensin receptor blockers, or direct renin inhibitors have been shown to decrease proteinuria, several clinical trials have revealed that use of combination renin-angiotensin system antagonism results in more adverse events (hyperkalemia, hypotension, AKI) without additional cardiovascular or renal benefits.

## Protein Restriction

In animal models, protein-restricted diets have been shown to slow the progression of kidney disease by reducing glomerular filtration pressure, thereby preventing progressive injury and fibrosis. However, in the Modification of Diet in Renal Disease study, no definitive benefit was seen in renal outcomes in patients randomly assigned to the low protein (0.6 g/kg/d) group. Although there is insufficient evidence to recommend routine use of low protein diets to slow progression of CKD, high protein diets may precipitate or exacerbate symptoms of uremia in patients with stage G5 CKD. Small studies suggest that low protein diets might delay the onset of symptomatic uremia and the need for renal replacement therapy in patients with stage G5 CKD not yet on dialysis.

### KEY POINTS

- Erythropoiesis-stimulating agents are associated with an increased risk for serious cardiovascular events when administered to patients with hemoglobin values >11 g/dL (110 g/L) or a history of stroke.
- Kidney Disease: Improving Global Outcomes (KDIGO) guidelines recommend treatment of metabolic acidosis with alkali therapy in patients with chronic kidney disease when the serum bicarbonate is chronically <22 mEq/L (22 mmol/L).
- ACE inhibitors and angiotensin receptor blockers decrease proteinuria and slow progression of proteinuric kidney diseases, but use of both drug classes in combination results in more adverse events without additional cardiovascular or renal benefits.

# Special Considerations

## Imaging Contrast Agents

Intravenous iodinated contrast can cause contrast-induced nephropathy (CIN), and risk for CIN increases with increasing severity of CKD. Patients with CKD should receive intravenous hydration with isotonic saline or bicarbonate-containing solutions before and after receiving contrast unless there is evidence of frank pulmonary edema. See Acute Kidney Injury for more information on CIN.

Gadolinium contrast used in MRI is associated with risk for nephrogenic systemic fibrosis (NSF) and must be avoided in patients with an eGFR <30 mL/min/1.73 m². In life-threatening situations in which benefit outweighs the risk for NSF, MRI is performed with low doses of stable gadolinium agents. Prior nephrology consult should be obtained to assess risks of gadolinium administration and guide the use

of dialysis in advanced CKD and ESKD. In those with severe CKD who require gadolinium, daily dialysis for 3 days appears to be effective at clearing the gadolinium and reducing the risk for NSF. See MKSAP 18 Dermatology for more information on NSF.

## Vaccination

Patients with CKD are at increased risk for infections that can be prevented by vaccination; however, these patients also have impaired immune responses to vaccines. The Centers for Disease Control and Prevention guidelines state that vaccinations in patients with CKD may be more effective when performed before the need for chronic dialysis or kidney transplantation. Patients with CKD should otherwise receive vaccinations according to guidelines, with a few exceptions:

- Patients with advanced CKD near dialysis dependence or those with ESKD on hemodialysis should be vaccinated against hepatitis B virus.
- Patients with CKD (stage not specified) or the nephrotic syndrome should receive the 23- and 13-valent pneumococcal vaccines, with revaccination with the 23-valent vaccine after a minimum of 5 years.
- Influenza vaccine should be administered annually to patients with CKD, but patients with ESKD should only receive the inactivated influenza vaccine due to risks associated with the live vaccines in immunocompromised patients.

## Vascular Access

Patients with advanced CKD may ultimately require renal replacement therapy; for those who choose hemodialysis, timely vascular access creation is essential. Referral to an experienced surgeon many months before dialysis is critical because arteriovenous fistula placement can be technically challenging and may require several months for full maturation. Arteriovenous fistulas have superior clinical outcomes compared with arteriovenous grafts and tunneled catheters.

Protecting the nondominant arm veins is paramount and involves limiting phlebotomy and intravenous catheters in that arm. Peripherally inserted central venous catheters should be avoided in patients with an eGFR <60 mL/min/1.73 m². A recent study demonstrated that peripherally inserted central catheters placed before or after hemodialysis initiation were independently associated with approximately 15% to 20% lower likelihoods of transition to any working fistula or graft. Avoidance of subclavian venous catheters helps to limit subclavian stenosis, which could impair the proper functioning of an arteriovenous fistula or arteriovenous graft used for dialysis.

## Older Patients

CKD stages G1 through G3a in elderly patients without albuminuria is of minimal clinical importance; some may refer to this mild decrement in eGFR as normal aging. For elderly persons with progressing or severe CKD necessitating discussions about renal replacement therapy and/or referral for evaluation for kidney transplantation, a patient-centered approach is preferred. Comorbid medical conditions, functional status, expected outcomes, and patient preferences regarding goals of care should be considered. For patients aged ≥80 years at the start of hemodialysis treatment, data demonstrate better survival among those who received pre-hemodialysis nephrology care that followed a planned management pathway, those who had a good nutritional status, and those with an arteriovenous fistula as vascular access for hemodialysis at the time of hemodialysis initiation.

### KEY POINTS

- Gadolinium contrast used in MRI is associated with the risk for nephrogenic systemic fibrosis and must be avoided in patients with an estimated glomerular filtration rate <30 mL/min/1.73 m$^2$.

- In patients with chronic kidney disease, peripherally inserted central venous catheters and subclavian venous catheters should be avoided in the nondominant arm veins for possible future dialysis vascular access.

# End-Stage Kidney Disease

CKD stage G5 is defined as an eGFR <15 mL/min/1.73 m$^2$, and ESKD is defined as CKD stage G5 treated with chronic dialysis or kidney transplantation. About 10% of patients with CKD stage G3 progress to ESKD, but most die from cardiovascular disease or infection before they progress to advanced CKD.

Patients with an eGFR <30 mL/min/1.73 m$^2$ should be educated about renal replacement therapy (RRT) treatment options, including hemodialysis, peritoneal dialysis, and kidney transplantation. Patients with advanced age or multiple comorbidities may not want any of these life-sustaining options. There has been increasing support of "kidney supportive care," which involves services aimed at improving the quality of life for patients with advanced CKD. It includes aligning treatment with a patient's goals through culturally sensitive shared decision-making and advance care planning, along with treating symptoms resulting from uremia, hypervolemia, hyperkalemia, and/or acidosis. For patients amenable to RRT, studies demonstrate no benefit in starting RRT in asymptomatic patients or at a specific eGFR cutoff compared with watchful waiting and initiating RRT for symptoms or metabolic abnormalities that are refractory to medical treatment. For the elderly and frail patients, physicians need to balance the management of symptoms with optimal care, with less emphasis being placed on maximizing long-term health outcomes, such as survival. Care should align with patient preferences and maximize the patient's quality of life. **Table 30** compares goals of care for patients with ESKD treated with standard dialysis versus kidney supportive care.

## Dialysis

Patients who choose hemodialysis should be referred for arteriovenous fistula creation in a timely manner to allow for arteriovenous fistula maturation. Arteriovenous grafts for hemodialysis and peritoneal dialysis catheters for peritoneal dialysis can be placed weeks before starting RRT but ideally should be planned months in advance. Tunneled dialysis catheters can be placed within days or the same day prior to starting hemodialysis but are associated with increased risk for bloodstream infections and death. Therefore, arteriovenous fistula or arteriovenous graft is preferred.

## Hemodialysis

Hemodialysis achieves clearance of blood solutes by convection and diffusion against a concentration gradient provided

**TABLE 30.** Goals of Care for Patients with End-Stage Kidney Disease Treated with Dialysis Versus Kidney Supportive Care

| Issue | Current Disease-Focused Metrics for Conventional Delivery of Dialysis Care | Kidney Supportive Care |
|---|---|---|
| Vascular access | Creation and maintenance of an AVF; avoid central venous catheters as much as possible | Central venous catheter acceptable if patient chooses hemodialysis |
| Dialysis adequacy | Target small solute clearance based on current standards, intensifying the dialysis prescription as needed to achieve targets | Lower clearance acceptable if changes in dialysis prescription increase demands inconsistent with patient preference; may involve fewer hemodialysis sessions or more frequent but shorter sessions |
| Cardiovascular disease | Treat cardiovascular risk factors, potentially targeting BP and dyslipidemia | Tolerate hypertension to avoid symptoms; no indication for dyslipidemia treatment |
| Mineral and bone disorder | Dietary counseling; binders to control hyperphosphatemia; vitamin D analogues with or without calcimimetics for secondary hyperparathyroidism | Limited restrictions; more permissive hyperphosphatemia and hyperparathyroidism |
| Nutrition | Encourage dietary protein intake while limiting potassium, sodium, and phosphorus intake | Reduce dietary restrictions |
| Laboratory monitoring | Routine monthly laboratory tests | Minimal necessary |

AVF = arteriovenous fistula; BP = blood pressure.

CONT.

by dialysate flowing opposite to blood flow and separated by a semipermeable dialyzer membrane. Hemodialysis is commonly performed three times per week for 3- to 4-hour treatment sessions at an outpatient dialysis unit. Frequent and/or longer treatments provide better control of volume status and serum electrolytes. Some patients perform hemodialysis at home four to five times per week but with shorter treatment sessions.

## Peritoneal Dialysis

Peritoneal dialysis utilizes an indwelling catheter to perform exchanges of dialysate with a specified solute concentration and osmolality into the peritoneum, which serves as a semipermeable membrane and allows for diffusion of solutes and osmosis of water. Dialysate needs to be exchanged about three to five times per day to maintain a high concentration gradient and maintain adequate solute clearance. Patients can perform these exchanges during the day, or a cycler can be used to exchange the fluid overnight while the patient sleeps; these options provide greater autonomy because the patient can work or perform activities during the day, rather than the need to be present at a hemodialysis unit three times per week. Clinical outcomes are similar for patients on peritoneal dialysis compared with hemodialysis, although patients starting RRT who have residual renal function may have better outcomes with peritoneal dialysis. Furthermore, residual renal function is preserved longer in peritoneal dialysis compared with hemodialysis and, although small, helps maintain adequate solute clearance and euvolemia.

Peritonitis is an important complication because repeated infections can cause peritoneal fibrosis and reduce the efficacy of the dialysis treatments. Dialysis-associated peritoneal peritonitis is infrequent, with an average of one episode every 2 to 3 years. It is usually caused by gram-positive skin flora and less commonly by gram-negative intestinal flora. Proper skin hygiene and sterile technique when handling the peritoneal dialysis catheter are critical in preventing peritonitis.

## Non-dialytic Palliative Therapy

Some patients with CKD stage G5/ESKD may choose not to initiate RRT, or patients already on RRT may decide to discontinue treatment. Palliative care and hospice services play an important role in caring for these patients. Non-dialytic therapy is a reasonable treatment option for elderly patients with ESKD and multiple comorbidities. Treatment focuses on symptom management and results in less hospitalization with similar or better quality of life compared with patients on RRT. For patients who withdraw from RRT, death usually occurs within 2 weeks. Recent studies have shown that the withdrawal rate from dialysis is approximately 3 per 100 person-years of dialysis, and this rate is increasing over time. ◫

**KEY POINTS**

- Clinical outcomes are similar for patients on peritoneal dialysis compared with hemodialysis, although patients starting renal replacement therapy who have residual renal function may have better outcomes with peritoneal dialysis.
- Non-dialytic palliative therapy is a reasonable option for **HVC** elderly patients with end-stage kidney disease and multiple comorbidities, with treatment focusing on symptom management and quality of life.

## Kidney Transplantation

Kidney transplantation is the preferred treatment for ESKD. It improves life expectancy and quality of life, and provides a significant cost savings to the health care system compared with dialysis. However, demand far exceeds supply, and waiting lists for deceased-donor kidneys are several years long in most regions of the United States.

## Referral

Patients should be referred to a kidney transplant center for evaluation when the eGFR is <20 mL/min/1.73 m². Early referral is important because preemptive kidney transplants (transplants before needing dialysis) are associated with improved clinical outcomes compared with receiving a transplant after starting dialysis. Early referral also allows adequate time to identify suitable living donors; if no living donor is available, early listing is essential to begin the waiting process for a deceased-donor kidney.

Patients and donors undergo extensive health screening to identify issues that may affect the safety and/or outcome of the transplant. In the potential recipient, these include active malignancy, coronary ischemia, or active infections. An adequate social support system and financial resources are also important to ensure medication adherence and long-term survival of the transplanted allograft. Donors are screened for intrinsic kidney disease, hypertension, and diabetes to ensure there is minimal risk related to reduced renal mass resulting from donation nephrectomy.

Patients are generally managed by a transplant nephrologist for at least the first 6 months posttransplant and are then comanaged with a general nephrologist and/or internist, especially for comorbidities.

## Immunosuppressive Therapy

Immunosuppressive medications are required to prevent allograft rejection. Induction therapy is started perioperatively with polyclonal anti–T-cell antibodies (thymoglobulin) or monoclonal anti–interleukin-2 receptor antibody (basiliximab). Calcineurin inhibitors with pulse glucocorticoids are started at this time as well.

Long-term maintenance therapy for most patients includes a combination of calcineurin inhibitors (tacrolimus or cyclosporine), antimetabolites (mycophenolate mofetil or azathioprine), and glucocorticoids. However, some patients with well-matched allografts can discontinue glucocorticoids. Doses of these medications are highest immediately posttransplant and are gradually decreased over the next several months to minimize side effects (**Table 31**), including long-term nephrotoxicity, while maintaining adequate immunosuppression.

**Risks of Transplantation**

Immediately posttransplant, patients need to be monitored for acute rejection and postoperative complications. Thereafter, minimizing risk for infection and medication side effects becomes the focus while maintaining adequate immunosuppression to prevent acute and chronic rejection.

*Infection*

Immunosuppression significantly increases the risk for infection. Within the first month after surgery, the most common infectious complications are similar to other surgical patients and include urinary tract infections and wound infections. Afterward, opportunistic infections become more prevalent.

Cytomegalovirus (CMV) is an important pathogen, and the risk for infection depends on the serologic status of the donor and recipient at the time of transplant. The highest risk occurs when a seropositive donor kidney is transplanted into a seronegative recipient. Most patients receive prophylaxis against CMV with valganciclovir during the first 6 to 12 months; however, CMV infections can occur after the medication is discontinued. Signs and symptoms include fever, pneumonitis, hepatitis, and gastroenteritis/colitis.

**TABLE 31. Common Side Effects of Medications Used for Chronic Maintenance Immunosuppression After Kidney Transplantation**

| Class | Medication | Common Side Effects |
|---|---|---|
| Calcineurin inhibitor | Cyclosporine | Hypertension; decreased GFR; dyslipidemia; hirsutism; gingival hyperplasia |
| | Tacrolimus | New-onset diabetes mellitus; decreased GFR; hypertension; gastrointestinal symptoms |
| Antimetabolite | Mycophenolate mofetil | Diarrhea; nausea/vomiting; leukopenia; anemia |
| | Azathioprine | Leukopenia; hepatitis; pancreatitis |
| mTOR inhibitor | Sirolimus; everolimus | Proteinuria; dyslipidemia; new-onset diabetes mellitus; anemia; leukopenia |
| Glucocorticoid | Prednisone | Osteopenia, osteoporosis, osteonecrosis; hypertension; edema; new-onset diabetes mellitus; glaucoma; cataracts |

GFR = glomerular filtration rate; mTOR = mammalian target of rapamycin.

Prophylaxis against *Pneumocystis jirovecii* pneumonia with trimethoprim-sulfamethoxazole is most commonly used, but atovaquone can be used for sulfa-allergic or hyperkalemic patients.

Polyoma BK virus uniquely affects kidney transplant patients, only rarely occurring with other organ transplants or in other immunosuppressed states. The most common clinical manifestation is an acute or indolent rise in serum creatinine due to tubulointerstitial nephritis or ureteral stenosis. Treatment requires reduction in the immunosuppression dose, but this must be balanced against the risk of allograft rejection.

*Cancer*

Because kidney transplant recipients are at higher risk for developing cancer, it is important to screen recipients for the presence of active malignancy prior to transplant.

Immunosuppressive medications increase the risk for several forms of malignancy, with non-melanoma skin cancers being the most common. Transplant patients therefore should be screened regularly for skin cancer and other age- and sex-appropriate cancer.

Posttransplant lymphoproliferative disorders can occur with long-term immunosuppression. These malignancies are caused by uncontrolled B-lymphocyte proliferation associated with Epstein-Barr virus infection and impaired T-cell surveillance. Treatment involves reduction in immunosuppression and administration of the anti–B-cell monoclonal antibody rituximab. Additionally, calcineurin inhibitors may be switched to the mammalian target of rapamycin inhibitor sirolimus because of its antiproliferative effects.

Kaposi sarcoma is also common and is associated with human herpesvirus-8 infection. Treatment involves reduction in immunosuppression dosing and switching to a sirolimus-based regimen.

**Special Considerations in Transplant Recipients**

*Acute Kidney Injury*

AKI is a common posttransplant complication and can occur immediately posttransplant or any time in the future. Acute rejection should always be part of the differential diagnosis, because early recognition and treatment are associated with better long-term outcomes. Posttransplant AKI may also be due to renal vasoconstriction from calcineurin inhibitor toxicity, calcineurin inhibitor–induced thrombotic microangiopathy, BK nephropathy, acute tubular necrosis, acute interstitial nephritis, or volume depletion/prerenal causes.

*Disease Recurrence*

Glomerular diseases can recur in the transplant allograft. Focal segmental glomerulosclerosis is one of the most common forms of glomerular disease to recur posttransplant and can occur within a few days to weeks after transplantation. Focal segmental glomerulosclerosis and thrombotic microangiopathy should be treated aggressively if disease recurrence is seen in the transplanted kidney, because these conditions are associated with high rates of graft failure. Patients with lupus or ANCA vasculitis should have quiescent disease for several months preceding transplantation to reduce risk for disease recurrence posttransplant. Diabetic nephropathy and IgA nephropathy can affect allograft function after transplant but are unlikely to cause graft failure.

## Cardiovascular Disease

Cardiovascular disease is the leading cause of death in kidney transplant recipients (about 50% of deaths). Kidney transplantation, despite restoration of kidney function, should be treated as a cardiovascular disease equivalent for purposes of risk factor modification.

Calcineurin inhibitors induce hypertension by activating the sodium chloride cotransporter in the distal convoluted tubule of the kidney. Therefore, thiazide diuretics may be efficacious in these patients. Dyslipidemia is a common side effect of calcineurin inhibitors, sirolimus, and glucocorticoids. Treatment with a statin improves cardiac outcomes; however, statins have drug-drug interactions with calcineurin inhibitors and can increase toxicities of both drugs.

## Bone Disease

Secondary and tertiary hyperparathyroidism, common in patients with ESKD, can persist for several months posttransplant; continuation of vitamin D analogues or calcimimetics may be warranted if the patient is hypercalcemic. Additionally, hypophosphatemia secondary to hyperparathyroidism is common posttransplant due to renal phosphorus wasting. Long-term glucocorticoids can cause osteopenia, osteoporosis, and osteonecrosis. Calcineurin inhibitors induce magnesium wasting. See Chronic Kidney Disease-Mineral and Bone Disorder for more information.

## Vaccination

Most transplant centers do not recommend immunization within the first 3 to 6 months posttransplant due to increased immunosuppression and therefore decreased likelihood of developing long-term immunity from the vaccine. Influenza vaccine, however, may be administered within 1 month of transplant in the setting of an influenza outbreak. Live attenuated vaccines are generally contraindicated in transplant recipients.

**KEY POINTS**

- Patients should be referred to a kidney transplant center for evaluation when the estimated glomerular filtration rate is <20 mL/min/1.73 m².

- Preemptive kidney transplants are associated with improved clinical outcomes compared with transplantation after dialysis.

- Within the first month following kidney transplantation, the most common infectious complications are similar to other surgical patients and include urinary tract infections and wound infections; afterward, opportunistic infections (such as cytomegalovirus, *Pneumocystis jirovecii*, and polyoma BK virus) become more prevalent.

*(Continued)*

**KEY POINTS** *(continued)*

- Immunosuppression of kidney transplant recipients increases the risk for several malignancies, including non-melanoma skin cancers, Kaposi sarcoma, and posttransplant lymphoproliferative disorders; regular screening for skin cancer and other age- and sex-appropriate cancer is recommended.

## Complications of End-Stage Kidney Disease
### Cardiovascular Disease

Sudden cardiac death is the leading cause of death in ESKD. This population is at increased risk due to rapid shifts of serum electrolytes during dialysis and chronic volume overload that contribute to left ventricular hypertrophy and cardiac fibrosis. Uremic toxins also contribute to left ventricular hypertrophy and cardiac fibrosis and may play a role in arrhythmogenesis. Avoiding rapid changes in serum potassium during dialysis may help limit arrhythmias, and adherence to dietary salt and fluid restriction may help limit volume overload. However, intradialytic hypotension induced by rapid volume removal during dialysis may cause cardiovascular and central nervous system injury due to organ hypoperfusion. Vascular calcification is accelerated by uremic toxins, chronic inflammation, and calcium-based medications/vitamin D analogues. Limiting medications that raise serum calcium and achieving adequate clearance during dialysis may help delay the progression of atherosclerosis. KDGIO guidelines recommend continuing a statin if a patient with CKD progresses to ESKD, but statins should not be newly started if progression to ESKD has already occurred.

### Infection

Infection is the second leading cause of death in ESKD. Patients are at increased risk due to a relatively immunosuppressed state from chronic inflammation and frequent exposure to the health care environment. Tunneled dialysis catheters increase the risk for bacteremia, and empiric antibiotics should be administered while waiting for blood culture results in patients with suspected bacteremia. Tunneled catheters should be removed immediately for severe sepsis, evidence of metastatic infection, evidence of an exit-site or tunnel infection, persistent fever, or bacteremia despite antibiotics. Exchange of the catheter over a guidewire may be an option for clinically stable patients without a tunnel infection or for patients who clear the bacteremia within 48 hours of antibiotic administration. Antibiotic lock therapy consists of the instillation of a highly concentrated antibiotic solution into an intravascular catheter lumen to treat catheter-related bloodstream infections. Antibiotic lock therapy with vancomycin and/or ceftazidime is an alternative option for stable patients with less virulent organisms such as *Staphylococcus epidermitis*, but catheter salvage should not be attempted for *Staphylococcus aureus* infections and some gram-negative organisms.

## Acquired Cystic Kidney Disease

Acquired cystic kidney disease is common among patients with severe CKD and ESKD. Cysts are usually detected during routine kidney ultrasonography or incidentally found on abdominal CT or MRI. These cysts are at increased risk for transformation into renal cell carcinoma, but routine screening is not recommended for most patients. A high index of suspicion is warranted for patients with new gross hematuria or unexplained flank pain. For cysts that are highly suspicious for malignancy, partial nephrectomy and nephron-sparing approaches are indicated for less severe stages of CKD. For patients with advanced CKD or ESKD, radical nephrectomy is the most prudent option.

### KEY POINT

- Complications of end-stage kidney disease include cardiovascular disease, infection, and acquired cystic kidney disease.

## Bibliography

### Clinical Evaluation of Kidney Function

Corapi KM, Chen JL, Balk EM, Gordon CE. Bleeding complications of native kidney biopsy: a systematic review and meta-analysis. Am J Kidney Dis. 2012;60:62-73. [PMID: 22537423]

Davis R, Jones JS, Barocas DA, Castle EP, Lang EK, Leveillee RJ, et al; American Urological Association. Diagnosis, evaluation and follow-up of asymptomatic microhematuria (AMH) in adults: AUA guideline. J Urol. 2012;188:2473-81. [PMID: 23098784]

Fähling M, Seeliger E, Patzak A, Persson PB. Understanding and preventing contrast-induced acute kidney injury. Nat Rev Nephrol. 2017;13:169-180. [PMID: 28138128]

Inker LA, Schmid CH, Tighiouart H, Eckfeldt JH, Feldman HI, Greene T, et al; CKD-EPI Investigators. Estimating glomerular filtration rate from serum creatinine and cystatin C. N Engl J Med. 2012;367:20-9. [PMID: 22762315]

Ix JH, Wassel CL, Stevens LA, Beck GJ, Froissart M, Navis G, et al. Equations to estimate creatinine excretion rate: the CKD epidemiology collaboration. Clin J Am Soc Nephrol. 2011;6:184-91. [PMID: 20966119]

Levey AS, Fan L, Eckfeldt JH, Inker LA. Cystatin C for glomerular filtration rate estimation: coming of age [Editorial]. Clin Chem. 2014;60:916-9. [PMID: 24871681]

Margulis V, Sagalowsky AI. Assessment of hematuria. Med Clin North Am. 2011;95:153-9. [PMID: 21095418]

Moyer VA; U.S. Preventive Services Task Force. Screening for bladder cancer: U.S. Preventive Services Task Force recommendation statement. Ann Intern Med. 2011;155:246-51. [PMID: 21844550]

Nielsen M, Qaseem A; High Value Care Task Force of the American College of Physicians. Hematuria as a marker of occult urinary tract cancer: advice for high-value care from the American College of Physicians. Ann Intern Med. 2016;164:488-97. [PMID: 26810935]

Subramaniam RM, Suarez-Cuervo C, Wilson RF, Turban S, Zhang A, Sherrod C, et al. Effectiveness of prevention strategies for contrast-induced nephropathy: a systematic review and meta-analysis. Ann Intern Med. 2016;164:406-16. [PMID: 26830221]

### Fluids and Electrolytes

Adrogué HJ, Madias NE. Hypernatremia. N Engl J Med. 2000;342:1493-9. [PMID: 10816188]

Agus ZS. Hypomagnesemia. J Am Soc Nephrol. 1999;10:1616-22. [PMID: 10405219]

Ahamed S, Anpalahan M, Savvas S, Gibson S, Torres J, Janus E. Hyponatraemia in older medical patients: implications for falls and adverse outcomes of hospitalisation. Intern Med J. 2014;44:991-7. [PMID: 25039672]

Almond CS, Shin AY, Fortescue EB, Mannix RC, Wypij D, Binstadt BA, et al. Hyponatremia among runners in the Boston Marathon. N Engl J Med. 2005;352:1550-6. [PMID: 15829535]

Felsenfeld AJ, Levine BS. Approach to treatment of hypophosphatemia. Am J Kidney Dis. 2012;60:655-61. [PMID: 22863286]

Greenlee M, Wingo CS, McDonough AA, Youn JH, Kone BC. Narrative review: evolving concepts in potassium homeostasis and hypokalemia. Ann Intern Med. 2009;150:619-25. [PMID: 19414841]

Hoorn EJ, Betjes MG, Weigel J, Zietse R. Hypernatraemia in critically ill patients: too little water and too much salt. Nephrol Dial Transplant. 2008;23:1562-8. [PMID: 18065827]

Huang CL, Kuo E. Mechanism of hypokalemia in magnesium deficiency. J Am Soc Nephrol. 2007;18:2649-52. [PMID: 17804670]

Jain G, Ong S, Warnock DG. Genetic disorders of potassium homeostasis. Semin Nephrol. 2013;33:300-9. [PMID: 23953807]

Mohmand HK, Issa D, Ahmad Z, Cappuccio JD, Kouides RW, Sterns RH. Hypertonic saline for hyponatremia: risk of inadvertent overcorrection. Clin J Am Soc Nephrol. 2007;2:1110-7. [PMID: 17913972]

Moritz ML, Kalantar-Zadeh K, Ayus JC. Ecstasy-associated hyponatremia: why are women at risk? Nephrol Dial Transplant. 2013;28:2206-9. [PMID: 23804804]

Palmer BF. Regulation of potassium homeostasis. Clin J Am Soc Nephrol. 2015;10:1050-60. [PMID: 24721891]

Regolisti G, Cabassi A, Parenti E, Maggiore U, Fiaccadori E. Severe hypomagnesemia during long-term treatment with a proton pump inhibitor. Am J Kidney Dis. 2010;56:168-74. [PMID: 20493607]

Sterns RH, Silver SM. Complications and management of hyponatremia. Curr Opin Nephrol Hypertens. 2016;25:114-9. [PMID: 26735146]

### Acid-Base Disorders

Gennari FJ. Pathophysiology of metabolic alkalosis: a new classification based on the centrality of stimulated collecting duct ion transport. Am J Kidney Dis. 2011;58:626-36. [PMID: 21849227]

Kraut JA, Kurtz I. Toxic alcohol ingestions: clinical features, diagnosis, and management. Clin J Am Soc Nephrol. 2008;3:208-25. [PMID: 18045860]

Kraut JA, Madias NE. Metabolic acidosis of CKD: an update. Am J Kidney Dis. 2016;67:307-17. [PMID: 26477665] doi:10.1053/j.ajkd.2015.08.028

Kraut JA, Nagami GT. The serum anion gap in the evaluation of acid-base disorders: what are its limitations and can its effectiveness be improved? Clin J Am Soc Nephrol. 2013;8:2018-24. [PMID: 23833313]

Madias NE. Renal acidification responses to respiratory acid-base disorders. J Nephrol. 2010;23 Suppl 16:S85-91. [PMID: 21170892]

Melcescu E, Phillips J, Moll G, Subauste JS, Koch CA. 11Beta-hydroxylase deficiency and other syndromes of mineralocorticoid excess as a rare cause of endocrine hypertension. Horm Metab Res. 2012;44:867-78. [PMID: 22932914]

Raimondi GA, Gonzalez S, Zaltsman J, Menga G, Adrogué HJ. Acid-base patterns in acute severe asthma. J Asthma. 2013;50:1062-8. [PMID: 23947392]

Rastegar M, Nagami GT. Non-anion gap metabolic acidosis: a clinical approach to evaluation. Am J Kidney Dis. 2017;69:296-301. [PMID: 28029394]

Treger R, Pirouz S, Kamangar N, Corry D. Agreement between central venous and arterial blood gas measurements in the intensive care unit. Clin J Am Soc Nephrol. 2010;5:390-4. [PMID: 20019117]

Vichot AA, Rastegar A. Use of anion gap in the evaluation of a patient with metabolic acidosis. Am J Kidney Dis. 2014;64:653-7. [PMID: 25132207]

### Hypertension

ALLHAT Officers and Coordinators for the ALLHAT Collaborative Research Group. The Antihypertensive and Lipid-Lowering Treatment to Prevent Heart Attack Trial. Major outcomes in high-risk hypertensive patients randomized to angiotensin-converting enzyme inhibitor or calcium channel blocker vs diuretic: The Antihypertensive and Lipid-Lowering Treatment to Prevent Heart Attack Trial (ALLHAT). JAMA. 2002;288:2981-97. [PMID: 12479763]

Appel LJ, Wright JT Jr, Greene T, Agodoa LY, Astor BC, Bakris GL, et al; AASK Collaborative Research Group. Intensive blood-pressure control in hypertensive chronic kidney disease. N Engl J Med. 2010;363:918-29. [PMID: 20818902]

Braam B, Taler SJ, Rahman M, Fillaus JA, Greco BA, Forman JP, et al. Recognition and management of resistant hypertension. Clin J Am Soc Nephrol. 2017;12:524-535. [PMID: 27895136]

Brook RD, Appel LJ, Rubenfire M, Ogedegbe G, Bisognano JD, Elliott WJ, et al; American Heart Association Professional Education Committee of the Council for High Blood Pressure Research, Council on Cardiovascular and Stroke Nursing, Council on Epidemiology and Prevention, and Council on Nutrition, Physical Activity. Beyond medications and diet: alternative approaches to lowering blood pressure: a scientific statement from the american heart association. Hypertension. 2013;61:1360-83. [PMID: 23608661]

Eckel RH, Jakicic JM, Ard JD, de Jesus JM, Houston Miller N, Hubbard VS, et al; American College of Cardiology/American Heart Association Task Force on Practice Guidelines. 2013 AHA/ACC guideline on lifestyle management to reduce cardiovascular risk: a report of the American College of Cardiology/American Heart Association Task Force on Practice Guidelines. J Am Coll Cardiol. 2014;63:2960-84. [PMID: 24239922]

Fried LF, Emanuele N, Zhang JH, Brophy M, Conner TA, Duckworth W, et al; VA NEPHRON-D Investigators. Combined angiotensin inhibition for the treatment of diabetic nephropathy. N Engl J Med. 2013;369:1892-903. [PMID: 24206457]

Pierdomenico SD, Cuccurullo F. Prognostic value of white-coat and masked hypertension diagnosed by ambulatory monitoring in initially untreated subjects: an updated meta analysis. Am J Hypertens. 2011;24:52-8. [PMID: 20847724]

Qaseem A, Wilt TJ, Rich R, Humphrey LL, Frost J, Forciea MA; Clinical Guidelines Committee of the American College of Physicians and the Commission on Health of the Public and Science of the American Academy of Family Physicians. Pharmacologic treatment of hypertension in adults aged 60 years or older to higher versus lower blood pressure targets: a clinical practice guideline from the American College of Physicians and the American Academy of Family Physicians. Ann Intern Med. 2017;166:430-437. [PMID: 28135725]

Siu AL; U.S. Preventive Services Task Force. Screening for high blood pressure in adults: U.S. Preventive Services Task Force recommendation statement. Ann Intern Med. 2015;163:778-86. [PMID: 26458123]

Stergiou GS, Asayama K, Thijs L, Kollias A, Niiranen TJ, Hozawa A, et al; International Database on HOme blood pressure in relation to Cardiovascular Outcome (IDHOCO) Investigators. Prognosis of white-coat and masked hypertension: International Database of HOme blood pressure in relation to Cardiovascular Outcome. Hypertension. 2014;63:675-82. [PMID: 24420553]

Whelton PK, Carey RM, Aronow WS, Casey DE Jr, Collins KJ, Dennison Himmelfarb C, et al. 2017 ACC/AHA/AAPA/ABC/ACPM/AGS/APhA/ASH/ASPC/NMA/PCNA guideline for the prevention, detection, evaluation, and management of high blood pressure in adults: a report of the American College of Cardiology/American Heart Association Task Force on Clinical Practice Guidelines. J Am Coll Cardiol. 2017. [PMID: 29146535]

Yusuf S, Teo KK, Pogue J, Dyal L, Copland I, Schumacher H, et al; ONTARGET Investigators. Telmisartan, ramipril, or both in patients at high risk for vascular events. N Engl J Med. 2008;358:1547-59. [PMID: 18378520]

## Chronic Tubulointerstitial Nephritis

François H, Mariette X. Renal involvement in primary Sjögren syndrome. Nat Rev Nephrol. 2016;12:82-93. [PMID: 26568188]

Hutchison CA, Batuman V, Behrens J, Bridoux F, Sirac C, Dispenzieri A, et al; International Kidney and Monoclonal Gammopathy Research Group. The pathogenesis and diagnosis of acute kidney injury in multiple myeloma. Nat Rev Nephrol. 2011;8:43-51. [PMID: 22045243]

Lazarus B, Chen Y, Wilson FP, Sang Y, Chang AR, Coresh J, et al. Proton pump inhibitor use and the risk of chronic kidney disease. JAMA Intern Med. 2016;176:238-46. [PMID: 26752337]

Saeki T, Kawano M. IgG4-related kidney disease. Kidney Int. 2014;85:251-7. [PMID: 24107849]

Shah S, Carter-Monroe N, Atta MG. Granulomatous interstitial nephritis. Clin Kidney J. 2015;8:516-23. [PMID: 26413275]

Shirali AC, Perazella MA. Tubulointerstitial injury associated with chemotherapeutic agents. Adv Chronic Kidney Dis. 2014;21:56-63. [PMID: 24359987]

Stefanovic V, Toncheva D, Polenakovic M. Balkan nephropathy. Clin Nephrol. 2015;83:64-9. [PMID: 25725245]

## Glomerular Diseases

Almaani S, Meara A, Rovin BH. Update on lupus nephritis. Clin J Am Soc Nephrol. 2017;12:825-835. [PMID: 27821390]

Fogo AB, Lusco MA, Najafian B, Alpers CE. AJKD Atlas of Renal Pathology: membranoproliferative glomerulonephritis. Am J Kidney Dis. 2015;66:e19-20. [PMID: 26300204]

Geetha D, Specks U, Stone JH, Merkel PA, Seo P, Spiera R, et al; Rituximab for ANCA-Associated Vasculitis Immune Tolerance Network Research Group. Rituximab versus cyclophosphamide for ANCA-associated vasculitis with renal involvement. J Am Soc Nephrol. 2015;26:976-85. [PMID: 25381429]

Glassock RJ. Antiphospholipase A2 receptor autoantibody guided diagnosis and treatment of membranous nephropathy: a new personalized medical approach [Editorial]. Clin J Am Soc Nephrol. 2014;9:1341-3. [PMID: 25035274]

Glassock RJ, Alvarado A, Prosek J, Hebert C, Parikh S, Satoskar A, et al. Staphylococcus-related glomerulonephritis and poststreptococcal glomerulonephritis: why defining "post" is important in understanding and treating infection-related glomerulonephritis. Am J Kidney Dis. 2015;65:826-32. [PMID: 25890425]

Hogan JJ, Markowitz GS, Radhakrishnan J. Drug-induced glomerular disease: immune-mediated injury. Clin J Am Soc Nephrol. 2015;10:1300-10. [PMID: 26092827]

Maas RJ, Deegens JK, Smeets B, Moeller MJ, Wetzels JF. Minimal change disease and idiopathic FSGS: manifestations of the same disease. Nat Rev Nephrol. 2016;12:768-776. [PMID: 27748392]

Magistroni R, D'Agati VD, Appel GB, Kiryluk K. New developments in the genetics, pathogenesis, and therapy of IgA nephropathy. Kidney Int. 2015;88:974-89. [PMID: 26376134]

Markowitz GS, Bomback AS, Perazella MA. Drug-induced glomerular disease: direct cellular injury. Clin J Am Soc Nephrol. 2015;10:1291-9. [PMID: 25862776]

Sethi S, Haas M, Markowitz GS, D'Agati VD, Rennke HG, Jennette JC, et al. Mayo Clinic/Renal Pathology Society Consensus Report on pathologic classification, diagnosis, and reporting of GN. J Am Soc Nephrol. 2016;27:1278-87. [PMID: 26567243]

## Kidney Manifestations of Deposition Diseases

Alpers CE, Kowalewska J. Fibrillary glomerulonephritis and immunotactoid glomerulopathy. J Am Soc Nephrol. 2008;19:34-7. [PMID: 18045849]

Bridoux F, Leung N, Hutchison CA, Touchard G, Sethi S, Fermand JP, et al; International Kidney and Monoclonal Gammopathy Research Group. Diagnosis of monoclonal gammopathy of renal significance. Kidney Int. 2015;87:698-711. [PMID: 25607108]

Heher EC, Rennke HG, Laubach JP, Richardson PG. Kidney disease and multiple myeloma. Clin J Am Soc Nephrol. 2013;8:2007-17. [PMID: 23868898]

Rosner MH, Edeani A, Yanagita M, Glezerman IG, Leung N; American Society of Nephrology Onco-Nephrology Forum. Paraprotein-related kidney disease: diagnosing and treating monoclonal gammopathy of renal significance. Clin J Am Soc Nephrol. 2016;11:2280-2287. [PMID: 27526705]

## Genetic Disorders and Kidney Disease

Chapman AB, Devuyst O, Eckardt KU, Gansevoort RT, Harris T, Horie S, et al; Conference Participants. Autosomal-dominant polycystic kidney disease (ADPKD): executive summary from a Kidney Disease: Improving Global Outcomes (KDIGO) Controversies Conference. Kidney Int. 2015;88:17-27. [PMID: 25786098]

Eckardt KU, Alper SL, Antignac C, Bleyer AJ, Chauveau D, Dahan K, et al; Kidney Disease: Improving Global Outcomes. Autosomal dominant tubulointerstitial kidney disease: diagnosis, classification, and management–a KDIGO consensus report. Kidney Int. 2015;88:676-83. [PMID: 25738250]

El Dib R, Gomaa H, Carvalho RP, Camargo SE, Bazan R, Barretti P, et al. Enzyme replacement therapy for Anderson-Fabry disease. Cochrane Database Syst Rev. 2016;7:CD006663. [PMID: 27454104]

Friedman DJ, Pollak MR. Apolipoprotein L1 and kidney disease in African Americans. Trends Endocrinol Metab. 2016;27:204-215. [PMID: 26947522]

Hall G, Gbadegesin RA. Translating genetic findings in hereditary nephrotic syndrome: the missing loops. Am J Physiol Renal Physiol. 2015;309:F24-8. [PMID: 25810439]

Savige J, Storey H, Il Cheong H, Gyung Kang H, Park E, Hilbert P, et al. X-Linked and autosomal recessive alport syndrome: pathogenic variant features and further genotype-phenotype correlations. PLoS One. 2016;11:e0161802. [PMID: 27627812]

## Acute Kidney Injury

Durand F, Graupera I, Ginès P, Olson JC, Nadim MK. Pathogenesis of hepatorenal syndrome: implications for therapy. Am J Kidney Dis. 2016;67:318-28. [PMID: 26500178]

Grodin JL, Stevens SR, de Las Fuentes L, Kiernan M, Birati EY, Gupta D, et al. Intensification of medication therapy for cardiorenal syndrome in acute decompensated heart failure. J Card Fail. 2016;22:26-32. [PMID: 26209004]

Kidney Disease: Improving Global Outcomes (KDIGO) Acute Kidney Injury Work Group. KDIGO Clinical Practice Guideline for Acute Kidney Injury. Kidney inter., Suppl. 2012;2: 1-138.

Mehta RL, Cerdá J, Burdmann EA, Tonelli M, García-García G, Jha V, et al. International Society of Nephrology's 0by25 initiative for acute kidney injury (zero preventable deaths by 2025): a human rights case for nephrology. Lancet. 2015;385:2616-43. [PMID: 25777661]

Patel DM, Connor MJ Jr. Intra-abdominal hypertension and abdominal compartment syndrome: an underappreciated cause of acute kidney injury. Adv Chronic Kidney Dis. 2016;23:160-6. [PMID: 27113692]

Pendergraft WF 3rd, Herlitz LC, Thornley-Brown D, Rosner M, Niles JL. Nephrotoxic effects of common and emerging drugs of abuse. Clin J Am Soc Nephrol. 2014;9:1996-2005. [PMID: 25035273]

Raghavan R, Eknoyan G. Acute interstitial nephritis - a reappraisal and update. Clin Nephrol. 2014;82:149-62. [PMID: 25079860]

Wichmann JL, Katzberg RW, Litwin SE, Zwerner PL, De Cecco CN, Vogl TJ, et al. Contrast-induced nephropathy. Circulation. 2015;132:1931-6. [PMID: 26572669]

Wilson FP, Berns JS. Tumor lysis syndrome: new challenges and recent advances. Adv Chronic Kidney Dis. 2014;21:18-26. [PMID: 24359983]

**Kidney Stones**

Eisner BH, Goldfarb DS, Pareek G. Pharmacologic treatment of kidney stone disease. Urol Clin North Am. 2013;40:21-30. [PMID: 23177632]

Fink HA, Wilt TJ, Eidman KE, Garimella PS, MacDonald R, Rutks IR, et al. Medical management to prevent recurrent nephrolithiasis in adults: a systematic review for an American College of Physicians Clinical Guideline. Ann Intern Med. 2013;158:535-43. [PMID: 23546565]

Shoag J, Tasian GE, Goldfarb DS, Eisner BH. The new epidemiology of nephrolithiasis. Adv Chronic Kidney Dis. 2015;22:273-8. [PMID: 26088071]

Tan JA, Lerma EV. Nephrolithiasis for the primary care physician. Dis Mon. 2015;61:434-41. [PMID: 26362879]

**The Kidney in Pregnancy**

American College of Obstetricians and Gynecologists. Hypertension in Pregnancy. Report of the American College of Obstetricians and Gynecologists Task Force on Hypertension in Pregnancy. Obstet Gynecol. 2013;122:1122-31. [PMID: 24150027]

Cheung KL, Lafayette RA. Renal physiology of pregnancy. Adv Chronic Kidney Dis. 2013;20:209-14. [PMID: 23928384]

Coscia LA, Constantinescu S, Davison JM, Moritz MJ, Armenti VT. Immunosuppressive drugs and fetal outcome. Best Pract Res Clin Obstet Gynaecol. 2014;28:1174-87. [PMID: 25175414]

Hladunewich MA, Hou S, Odutayo A, Cornelis T, Pierratos A, Goldstein M, et al. Intensive hemodialysis associates with improved pregnancy outcomes: a Canadian and United States cohort comparison. J Am Soc Nephrol. 2014;25:1103-9. [PMID: 24525032]

Kattah AG, Garovic VD. The management of hypertension in pregnancy. Adv Chronic Kidney Dis. 2013;20:229-39. [PMID: 23928387]

Nadeau-Fredette AC, Hladunewich M, Hui D, Keunen J, Chan CT. End-stage renal disease and pregnancy. Adv Chronic Kidney Dis. 2013;20:246-52. [PMID: 23928389]

Vellanki K. Pregnancy in chronic kidney disease. Adv Chronic Kidney Dis. 2013;20:223-8. [PMID: 23928386]

Zhang JJ, Ma XX, Hao L, Liu LJ, Lv JC, Zhang H. A systematic review and meta-analysis of outcomes of pregnancy in CKD and CKD outcomes in pregnancy. Clin J Am Soc Nephrol. 2015;10:1964-78. [PMID: 26487769]

**Chronic Kidney Disease**

Coresh J, Turin TC, Matsushita K, Sang Y, Ballew SH, Appel LJ, et al. Decline in estimated glomerular filtration rate and subsequent risk of end-stage renal disease and mortality. JAMA. 2014;311:2518-2531. [PMID: 24892770]

Dierickx D, Habermann TM. Post-transplantation lymphoproliferative disorders in adults. N Engl J Med. 2018;378:549-562. [PMID: 29414277]

Grubbs V, Moss AH, Cohen LM, Fischer MJ, Germain MJ, Jassal SV, et al; Dialysis Advisory Group of the American Society of Nephrology. A palliative approach to dialysis care: a patient-centered transition to the end of life. Clin J Am Soc Nephrol. 2014;9:2203-9. [PMID: 25104274]

Kidney Disease: Improving Global Outcomes (KDIGO) Anemia Work Group. KDIGO Clinical Practice Guideline for Anemia in Chronic Kidney Disease. Kidney Int Suppl. 2012;2:279-335. Available at www.kdigo.org.

Kidney Disease: Improving Global Outcomes (KDIGO) CKD Work Group. KDIGO 2012 clinical practice guideline for the evaluation and management of chronic kidney disease. Kidney Int Suppl. 2013;3:1-150. Available at www.kdigo.org.

Kidney Disease: Improving Global Outcomes (KDIGO) CKD-MBD Update Work Group. KDIGO 2017 clinical practice guideline update for the diagnosis, evaluation, prevention, and treatment of chronic kidney disease–mineral and bone disorder (CKD-MBD). Kidney Int Suppl. 2017;7:1-59. Available at www.kdigo.org.

Kidney Disease: Improving Global Outcomes (KDIGO) Transplant Work Group. KDIGO clinical practice guideline for the care of kidney transplant recipients. Am J Transplant. 2009;9 Suppl 3:S1-155. [PMID: 19845597]

McMahon EJ, Campbell KL, Bauer JD, Mudge DW. Altered dietary salt intake for people with chronic kidney disease. Cochrane Database Syst Rev. 2015:CD010070. [PMID: 25691262]

Mills KT, Chen J, Yang W, Appel LJ, Kusek JW, Alper A, et al; Chronic Renal Insufficiency Cohort (CRIC) Study Investigators. Sodium excretion and the risk of cardiovascular disease in patients with chronic kidney disease. JAMA. 2016;315:2200-10. [PMID: 27218629]

Murphy D, McCulloch CE, Lin F, Banerjee T, Bragg-Gresham JL, Eberhardt MS, et al; Centers for Disease Control and Prevention Chronic Kidney Disease Surveillance Team. Trends in prevalence of chronic kidney disease in the United States. Ann Intern Med. 2016;165:473-481. [PMID: 27479614]

Saunders MR, Cifu A, Vela M. Screening for chronic kidney disease. JAMA. 2015;314:615-6. [PMID: 26262800]

Tangri N, Grams ME, Levey AS, Coresh J, Appel LJ, Astor BC, et al; CKD Prognosis Consortium. Multinational assessment of accuracy of equations for predicting risk of kidney failure: a meta-analysis. JAMA. 2016;315:164-74. [PMID: 26757465]

Whelton PK, Carey RM, Aronow WS, Casey DE Jr, Collins KJ, Dennison Himmelfarb C, et al. 2017 ACC/AHA/AAPA/ABC/ACPM/AGS/APhA/ASH/ASPC/NMA/PCNA guideline for the prevention, detection, evaluation, and management of high blood pressure in adults: a report of the American College of Cardiology/American Heart Association task force on clinical practice guidelines. J Am Coll Cardiol. 2017. [PMID: 29146535]

Xie Y, Bowe B, Li T, Xian H, Balasubramanian S, Al-Aly Z. Proton pump inhibitors and risk of incident CKD and progression to ESRD. J Am Soc Nephrol. 2016;27:3153-3163. [PMID: 27080976]

# Nephrology Self-Assessment Test

This self-assessment test contains one-best-answer multiple-choice questions. Please read these directions carefully before answering the questions. Answers, critiques, and bibliographies immediately follow these multiple-choice questions. The American College of Physicians (ACP) is accredited by the Accreditation Council for Continuing Medical Education (ACCME) to provide continuing medical education for physicians.

The American College of Physicians designates MKSAP 18 Nephrology for a maximum of 25 *AMA PRA Category 1 Credits*™. Physicians should claim only the credit commensurate with the extent of their participation in the activity.

Successful completion of the CME activity, which includes participation in the evaluation component, enables the participant to earn up to 25 medical knowledge MOC points in the American Board of Internal Medicine's Maintenance of Certification (MOC) program. It is the CME activity provider's responsibility to submit participant completion information to ACCME for the purpose of granting MOC credit.

## *Earn Instantaneous CME Credits or MOC Points Online*

Print subscribers can enter their answers online to earn instantaneous CME credits or MOC points. You can submit your answers using online answer sheets that are provided at mksap.acponline.org, where a record of your MKSAP 18 credits will be available. To earn CME credits or to apply for MOC points, you need to answer all of the questions in a test and earn a score of at least 50% correct (number of correct answers divided by the total number of questions). Please note that if you are applying for MOC points, you must also enter your birth date and ABIM candidate number. Take either of the following approaches:

- Use the printed answer sheet at the back of this book to record your answers. Go to mksap.acponline.org, access the appropriate online answer sheet, transcribe your answers, and submit your test for instantaneous CME credits or MOC points. There is no additional fee for this service.

- Go to mksap.acponline.org, access the appropriate online answer sheet, directly enter your answers, and submit your test for instantaneous CME credits or MOC points. There is no additional fee for this service.

## *Earn CME Credits or MOC Points by Mail or Fax*

Pay a $20 processing fee per answer sheet and submit the printed answer sheet at the back of this book by mail or fax, as instructed on the answer sheet. Make sure you calculate your score and enter your birth date and ABIM candidate number, and fax the answer sheet to 215-351-2799 or mail the answer sheet to Member and Customer Service, American College of Physicians, 190 N. Independence Mall West, Philadelphia, PA 19106-1572, using the courtesy envelope provided in your MKSAP 18 slipcase. You will need your 10-digit order number and 8-digit ACP ID number, which are printed on your packing slip. Please allow 4 to 6 weeks for your score report to be emailed back to you. Be sure to include your email address for a response.

If you do not have a 10-digit order number and 8-digit ACP ID number, or if you need help creating a username and password to access the MKSAP 18 online answer sheets, go to mksap.acponline.org or email custserv@acponline.org.

CME credits and MOC points are available from the publication date of December 31, 2018, until December 31, 2021. You may submit your answer sheet or enter your answers online at any time during this period.

# Directions

*Each of the numbered items is followed by lettered answers. Select the **ONE** lettered answer that is **BEST** in each case.*

## Item 1

A 72-year-old man is evaluated for near-syncope and a recent fall. History is significant for hypertension, hyperlipidemia, and coronary artery disease. Medications are hydrochlorothiazide, amlodipine, carvedilol, pravastatin, and aspirin. The hydrochlorothiazide dose was increased from 25 mg to 50 mg 1 month ago.

On physical examination, blood pressure is 164/88 mm Hg sitting and 140/76 mm Hg standing after 3 minutes, and pulse rate is 64/min sitting and 66/min standing; other vital signs are normal. Ecchymosis is noted over the left elbow. The remainder of the examination, including the neurologic examination, is unremarkable.

**Laboratory studies:**

| | |
|---|---|
| Creatinine | 1.4 mg/dL (123.8 µmol/L); 1 month ago: 1.0 mg/dL (88.4 µmol/L) |
| Bicarbonate | 30 mEq/L (30 mmol/L); 1 month ago: 26 mEq/L (26 mmol/L) |
| Potassium | 3.0 mEq/L (3.0 mmol/L); 1 month ago: 3.8 mEq/L (3.8 mmol/L) |
| Sodium | 132 mEq/L (132 mmol/L); 1 month ago: 136 mEq/L (136 mmol/L) |

A 12-lead electrocardiogram shows no changes from previous tracings.

**Which of the following is the most appropriate management?**

(A) Decrease hydrochlorothiazide dose and obtain ambulatory blood pressure monitoring
(B) Order telemetry and cardiac enzyme testing
(C) Schedule bilateral carotid ultrasonography
(D) Schedule head CT

## Item 2

An 81-year-old man is hospitalized for an acute onset of edema in his legs and abdomen. History is significant for chronic back pain, for which he takes daily ibuprofen. He has no other symptoms.

On physical examination, vital signs are normal. There is no rash. Cardiac examination is without extra sounds or murmurs, and the estimated central venous pressure is normal. The lungs are clear on examination. Ascites is noted. There is 3-mm pitting edema of the extremities to the mid thigh.

**Laboratory studies:**

| | |
|---|---|
| Albumin | 2.1 g/dL (21 g/L) |
| Creatinine | 2.9 mg/dL (256.4 µmol/L) |
| Electrolytes | Normal |
| Urinalysis | No blood; 4+ protein |
| Urine protein-creatinine ratio | 7200 mg/g |
| 24-Hour urine output | 1.5 L |

Doppler ultrasound of the kidneys is unremarkable.

**Which of the following is the most appropriate next step in management?**

(A) Initiate dialysis
(B) Schedule a kidney biopsy
(C) Start heparin
(D) Start intravenous glucocorticoids

## Item 3

A 56-year-old man is seen during a routine evaluation for stage G4 chronic kidney disease (CKD). History is also significant for hypertension. Medications are losartan, labetalol, furosemide, and amlodipine. He has no symptoms and remains physically active.

On physical examination, blood pressure is 129/76 mm Hg, and pulse rate is 68/min; other vital signs are normal. The physical examination is otherwise unremarkable.

**Laboratory studies:**

| | |
|---|---|
| Hemoglobin | 11 g/dL (110 g/L) |
| Bicarbonate | 19 mEq/L (19 mmol/L) |
| Creatinine | 3.1 mg/dL (274 µmol/L) |
| Phosphorus | 5.7 mg/dL (1.8 mmol/L) |
| Potassium | 5.1 mEq/L (5.1 mmol/L) |

**The addition of which of the following will most likely slow progression of this patient's CKD?**

(A) ACE inhibitor
(B) Erythropoiesis-stimulating agent
(C) Phosphate binder
(D) Sodium bicarbonate

## Item 4

A 69-year-old woman is evaluated in the emergency department for new-onset dependent edema that began 3 weeks ago. She says it is difficult to walk, and she has gained 4.5 kg (10 lb) of fluid weight. History is significant for obesity and hypertension. Her only medication is lisinopril.

On physical examination, vital signs are normal. BMI is 32. There is no rash. There is 3-mm bilateral dependent edema stopping just below the abdomen; it is equal on both sides. The remainder of the examination is unremarkable.

**Laboratory studies:**

| | |
|---|---|
| Albumin | 2.1 g/dL (21 g/L) |
| Creatinine | 1.3 mg/dL (114.9 µmol/L) |
| Urine protein-creatinine ratio | 8700 mg/g |

Kidney biopsy findings are consistent with a diagnosis of minimal change glomerulopathy with superimposed acute tubular necrosis.

**In addition to initiating diuretic therapy, which of the following is the most appropriate treatment?**

(A) Cyclosporine
(B) High-dose oral prednisone
(C) Rituximab
(D) No additional treatment

## Item 5

A 67-year-old man is seen for an increase in serum creatinine level and an abnormal urinalysis found during the evaluation of monoclonal gammopathy of undetermined significance. His evaluation revealed an M-protein spike of 1.5 g/dL, <10% clonal plasma cells on bone marrow biopsy, and no evidence of anemia, hypercalcemia, or lytic bone lesions on skeletal survey. Immunofixation revealed IgG as the monoclonal type. He has no constitutional symptoms, no other medical problems, and takes no medications.

On physical examination, vital signs are normal. Trace lower extremity edema is noted. The remainder of the examination is unremarkable.

**Laboratory studies:**

| | |
|---|---|
| Albumin | 3.6 g/dL (36 g/L) |
| Creatinine | 1.6 mg/dL (141.4 µmol/L) |
| Urinalysis | pH 5.5; 2+ blood; 3+ protein; 5-8 erythrocytes/hpf |
| Urine albumin-creatinine ratio | 400 mg/g |

**Which of the following is the most appropriate next diagnostic test?**

(A) ANCA testing
(B) $\beta_2$-Microglobulin levels
(C) Kidney biopsy
(D) Serum free light chains

## Item 6

A 31-year-old man is evaluated during a follow-up visit for IgA nephropathy found on kidney biopsy 3 months ago, at which time lisinopril was initiated. He is asymptomatic.

Physical examination and vital signs are unremarkable.

**Laboratory studies:**

| | Current | 3 Months Ago |
|---|---|---|
| Creatinine | 1.1 mg/dL (97. 2 µmol/L) | 1.0 mg/dL (88.4 µmol/L) |
| Potassium | 4.8 mEq/L (4.8 mmol/L) | 4.4 mEq/L (4.4 mmol/L) |
| Urinalysis | 3+ blood; 2+ protein | 3+ blood; 3+ protein |
| Urine protein-creatinine ratio | 700 mg/g | 1200 mg/g |

**Which of the following is the most appropriate next step in management?**

(A) Add losartan
(B) Add oral glucocorticoid therapy
(C) Start alternating courses of intravenous and oral glucocorticoid therapy
(D) Make no changes to the current medication regimen

## Item 7

A 48-year-old woman is evaluated in the emergency department for a 1-day history of hearing voices. History is significant for bipolar disorder. Medications are lithium carbonate and quetiapine.

On physical examination, the patient is disheveled and looks chronically ill. She is alert and oriented but appears anxious. Blood pressure is 138/78 mm Hg, and pulse rate is 80/min without orthostatic changes. There is no edema. The remainder of the examination is normal.

**Laboratory studies:**

| | |
|---|---|
| Blood urea nitrogen | 6 mg/dL (2.1 mmol/L) |
| Creatinine | 0.9 mg/dL (79.6 µmol/L) |
| Electrolytes: | |
| Sodium | 126 mEq/L (126 mmol/L) |
| Potassium | 3.5 mEq/L (3.5 mmol/L) |
| Chloride | 94 mEq/L (94 mmol/L) |
| Bicarbonate | 26 mEq/L (26 mmol/L) |
| Glucose | 156 mg/dL (8.7 mmol/L) |
| Urine sodium | 12 mEq/L (12 mmol/L) |
| Urine osmolality | 96 mOsm/kg $H_2O$ |

**Which of the following is the most likely cause of this patient's hyponatremia?**

(A) Hyperglycemia
(B) Nephrogenic diabetes insipidus
(C) Polydipsia
(D) Syndrome of inappropriate antidiuretic hormone secretion
(E) Volume depletion

## Item 8

A 38-year-old man is evaluated after passing his second kidney stone. History is significant for chronic pancreatitis secondary to a past history of alcohol abuse. He has three to four loose bowel movements each day. He reports no fever, flank pain, or dysuria. There is no family history of kidney disease, hyperparathyroidism, or nephrolithiasis. Current medications are pancreatic enzymes and multivitamins.

Physical examination reveals a thin man. Vital signs and the remainder of the examination are unremarkable.

**Laboratory studies:**

| | |
|---|---|
| Calcium | 8.5 mg/dL (2.1 mmol/L) |
| Creatinine | 0.7 mg/dL (61.9 µmol/L) |
| Electrolytes: | |
| Sodium | 137 mEq/L (137 mmol/L) |
| Potassium | 3.5 mEq/L (3.5 mmol/L) |
| Chloride | 104 mEq/L (104 mmol/L) |
| Bicarbonate | 21 mEq/L (21 mmol/L) |
| Urinalysis | Specific gravity; pH 5.0; negative dipstick; positive for calcium oxalate crystals |

**In addition to increasing fluid intake, which of the following is the most appropriate management?**

(A) Add allopurinol
(B) Add potassium citrate
(C) Add vitamin C
(D) Decrease calcium intake
(E) Increase protein intake

## Item 9

A 33-year-old man is hospitalized for headache, hypertension, and an elevated serum creatinine level. He has a 10-year history of poorly controlled type 2 diabetes mellitus and hypertension. Medications are insulin glargine, insulin lispro, atorvastatin, amlodipine, and low-dose aspirin.

On physical examination, blood pressure is 145/94 mm Hg; other vital signs are normal. Funduscopic examination reveals nonproliferative diabetic retinopathy. There is 1-mm pitting edema of the lower extremities to the ankles, equal on both sides. Dorsalis pedis and posterior tibial pulses are decreased bilaterally, and the feet are insensate.

**Laboratory studies:**

| | |
|---|---|
| Complete blood count | Normal |
| Albumin | 3.3 g/dL (33 g/L) |
| Creatinine | 1.8 mg/dL (159.1 µmol/L) |
| Hemoglobin A$_{1c}$ | 8.1% |
| Antinuclear antibodies | Negative |
| Hepatitis B virus antibodies | Negative |
| Hepatitis C virus antibodies | Negative |
| HIV antibodies | Negative |
| Urinalysis | No blood; 3+ protein |
| Urine protein-creatinine ratio | 6700 mg/g |

Kidney ultrasound reveals mildly increased echogenicity bilaterally, and both kidneys are enlarged at 12 cm.

**In addition to improved glycemic control, which of the following is the most appropriate management?**

(A) Add an ACE inhibitor
(B) Obtain ANCA titers
(C) Obtain serum and urine protein electrophoresis
(D) Schedule a kidney biopsy

## Item 10

A 32-year-old woman is brought to the emergency department by her boyfriend after she was found unresponsive and lying on the ground. She was last seen more than 24 hours ago. History is significant for substance use disorder. She has no other medical problems and takes no prescription drugs.

On physical examination, the patient is intubated and on mechanical ventilation. She is minimally responsive. Blood pressure is 120/75 mm Hg, and pulse rate is 110/min. The remainder of the vital signs and the cardiac, pulmonary, and abdominal examinations are unremarkable. The neurologic examination is nonfocal. Urine output has been <20 mL/h for the past 2 hours.

**Laboratory studies:**

| | |
|---|---|
| Calcium | 6.9 mg/dL (1.7 mmol/L) |
| Creatine kinase | 40,000 U/L |
| Creatinine | 2.8 mg/dL (247.5 µmol/L) |
| Electrolytes: | |
| Sodium | 150 mEq/L (150 mmol/L) |
| Potassium | 5.5 mEq/L (5.5 mmol/L) |
| Chloride | 110 mEq/L (110 mmol/L) |
| Bicarbonate | 16 mEq/L (16 mmol/L) |
| Phosphorous | 5.9 mg/dL (1.9 mmol/L) |
| Fractional excretion of sodium | <1% |
| Urine myoglobin | 300 mg/mL |
| Urinalysis | Reddish brown urine; pH 5.2; 4+ blood; 2+ protein; granular casts |
| Toxicology screen | Positive for cocaine and opiates |

**Which of the following is the most appropriate treatment?**

(A) Hemodialysis
(B) Intravenous 0.9% saline
(C) Intravenous 5% dextrose
(D) Intravenous calcium gluconate infusion
(E) Intravenous isotonic sodium bicarbonate in 5% dextrose

## Item 11

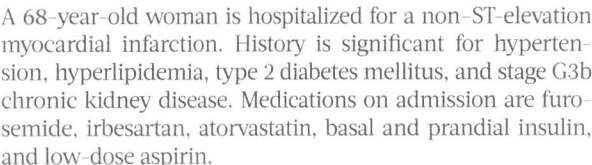

A 68-year-old woman is hospitalized for a non–ST-elevation myocardial infarction. History is significant for hypertension, hyperlipidemia, type 2 diabetes mellitus, and stage G3b chronic kidney disease. Medications on admission are furosemide, irbesartan, atorvastatin, basal and prandial insulin, and low-dose aspirin.

Vital signs and the physical examination are normal.

Transthoracic echocardiogram shows anterolateral hypokinesis with an estimated left ventricular ejection fraction of 35% to 40%.

Coronary angiography is scheduled.

**In addition to stopping furosemide, which of the following is the most appropriate measure to prevent acute kidney injury?**

(A) Begin intravenous 0.9% saline
(B) Begin oral N-acetylcysteine
(C) Discontinue atorvastatin
(D) Discontinue irbesartan

## Item 12

A 75-year-old woman is hospitalized for a 1-week history of dizziness, nausea, vomiting, increased urination, and decreased appetite. History is significant for hypertension treated with hydrochlorothiazide. She also takes calcium carbonate for bone health.

On physical examination, blood pressure is 150/85 mm Hg supine and 122/70 mm Hg standing, pulse rate is 78/min supine and 100/min standing, and respiration rate is 18/min. There is no neck vein distention. Cardiac, pulmonary, and abdominal examinations are unremarkable. There is no lower extremity edema.

**Laboratory studies:**

| | |
|---|---|
| Hematocrit | 30% |
| Leukocyte count | 3000/µL (3.0 × 10⁹/L) |
| Platelet count | 82,000/µL (82 × 10⁹/L) |
| Calcium | 12.8 mg/dL (3.2 mmol/L) |
| Creatinine | 3.7 mg/dL (327.1 µmol/L) |
| Electrolytes: | |
| Sodium | 132 mEq/L (132 mmol/L) |
| Potassium | 4.9 mEq/L (4.9 mmol/L) |
| Chloride | 115 mEq/L (115 mmol/L) |
| Bicarbonate | 17 mEq/L (17 mmol/L) |
| Phosphorus | 6.2 mg/dL (2.0 mmol/L) |
| Urine sodium | 15 mEq/L (15 mmol/L) |
| Urinalysis | Specific gravity 1.018; trace protein; few erythrocytes/hpf; occasional leukocytes/hpf; few granular casts; numerous hyaline casts |

CONT.

Which of the following is the most likely cause of this patient's hypercalcemia and acute kidney injury?

(A) Hydrochlorothiazide therapy

(B) Milk alkali syndrome

(C) Multiple myeloma

(D) Primary hyperparathyroidism

## Item 13

A 57-year-old man is evaluated during a routine visit. History is significant for hypertension. Medications are hydrochlorothiazide, 25 mg/d, and amlodipine, 5 mg/d.

On physical examination, blood pressure is 135/86 mm Hg, and pulse rate is 70/min; other vital signs are normal. There is 1+ bilateral ankle edema. The remainder of the examination is normal.

Laboratory studies show a serum creatinine level of 1.0 mg/dL (88.4 µmol/L), a serum potassium level of 3.6 mEq/L (3.6 mmol/L), and an estimated glomerular filtration rate >60 mL/min/1.73 m².

**Which of the following is the most appropriate treatment?**

(A) Add hydralazine

(B) Add losartan

(C) Double the amlodipine dose

(D) Double the hydrochlorothiazide dose

 ## Item 14

A 25-year-old woman is evaluated in the emergency department after a suicide attempt. History is significant for major depression. She takes no medication.

On physical examination, temperature is normal, blood pressure is 142/92 mm Hg, pulse rate is 110/min, and respiration rate is 22/min. The patient is obtunded. The remainder of the examination is normal.

**Laboratory studies:**

| | |
|---|---|
| Blood urea nitrogen | 28 mg/dL (10 mmol/L) |
| Creatinine | 2.2 mg/dL (194.5 µmol/L) |
| Electrolytes: | |
|   Sodium | 136 mEq/L (136 mmol/L) |
|   Potassium | 4.0 mEq/L (4.0 mmol/L) |
|   Chloride | 100 mEq/L (100 mmol/L) |
|   Bicarbonate | 12 mEq/L (12 mmol/L) |
| Ethanol | Undetected |
| Glucose | 90 mg/dL (5.0 mmol/L) |
| Osmolality | 314 mOsm/kg H₂O |
| Arterial blood gases: | |
|   pH | 7.25 |
|   P$_{CO_2}$ | 28 mm Hg (3.7 kPa) |

**Which of the following is the most appropriate management?**

(A) Activated charcoal gastric decontamination

(B) Intravenous ethanol

(C) Intravenous hydration, fomepizole, and hemodialysis

(D) Intravenous sodium bicarbonate

## Item 15

A 68-year-old woman is evaluated during a follow-up visit for a 3-week history of the nephrotic syndrome. She otherwise has been well and reports no additional symptoms. She has a 50-pack-year history of cigarette smoking with ongoing tobacco use.

On physical examination, vital signs are normal. Pitting edema to the ankles is present. The remainder of the examination is unremarkable.

**Laboratory studies:**

| | |
|---|---|
| Albumin | 2.9 g/dL (29 g/L) |
| C3 | Normal |
| C4 | Normal |
| Creatinine | Normal |
| Rapid plasma reagin | Normal |
| Antinuclear antibodies | Negative |
| Hepatitis B antibodies | Negative |
| Hepatitis C antibodies | Negative |
| 24-Hour urine protein excretion | 10,000 mg/24 h |

Kidney ultrasound shows normal-appearing kidneys with no evidence of thrombus in the renal veins. Lower extremity Doppler ultrasound shows no evidence of deep venous thrombosis.

Kidney biopsy shows membranous glomerulopathy with negative staining for the phospholipase A2 receptor (PLA2R) on immunofluorescence.

**Which of the following is the most appropriate management?**

(A) Age- and sex-appropriate cancer screening

(B) Immunosuppression therapy

(C) Prophylactic anticoagulation

(D) Serologic testing for anti-PLA2R antibodies

## Item 16

A 42-year-old man is evaluated for a 2-month history of painless gross hematuria. He was diagnosed with chronic kidney disease 4 years ago. His only medication is occasional ibuprofen. He is a recent immigrant from Bosnia.

On physical examination, blood pressure is 150/86 mm Hg. The remainder of the examination is unremarkable.

**Laboratory studies:**

| | |
|---|---|
| Hemoglobin | 10.5 g/dL (105 g/L) |
| Creatinine | 4.0 mg/dL (353.6 µmol/L) |
| Urinalysis | 1+ protein; numerous nondysmorphic erythrocytes; 5-8 leukocytes/hpf; occasional granular casts |
| Urine protein-creatinine ratio | 900 mg/g |

Kidney ultrasound shows echogenic kidneys measuring 8.0 cm and 8.5 cm in length; an irregular bladder wall is noted.

**Which of the following is the most appropriate diagnostic test to perform next?**

(A) CT urography

(B) Endoscopic urologic evaluation

(C) Kidney biopsy

(D) Urine cultures

## Item 17

A 46-year-old man is evaluated for increased urination and thirst of 3 days' duration. History is significant for pulmonary sarcoidosis diagnosed 4 months ago; prednisone, 40 mg/d, was initiated and subsequently tapered to 10 mg/d. Initial symptoms were cough and dyspnea on exertion, which had improved with treatment. He is taking no other medications.

Physical examination and vital signs are normal.

**Laboratory studies:**

| | |
|---|---|
| Blood urea nitrogen | 16 mg/dL (5.7 mmol/L) |
| Calcium | 9.9 mg/dL (2.5 mmol/L) |
| Creatinine | 1.1 mg/dL (97.2 µmol/L) |
| Electrolytes: | |
| Sodium | 146 mEq/L (146 mmol/L) |
| Chloride | 110 mEq/L (110 mmol/L) |
| Potassium | 3.8 mEq/L (3.8 mmol/L) |
| Bicarbonate | 26 mEq/L (26 mmol/L) |
| Urine sodium | 20 mEq/L (20 mmol/L) |
| Urine osmolality | 115 mOsm/kg H$_2$O |

In addition to increasing the prednisone, which of the following is the most appropriate treatment?

(A) Desmopressin acetate

(B) Hydrochlorothiazide

(C) Intravenous 5% dextrose

(D) Tolvaptan

## Item 18

A 52-year-old woman was hospitalized 3 days ago for laparoscopic resection of the sigmoid colon secondary to recurrent diverticulitis. Diet has been advanced to a full diet. She has a 20-year history of hypertension, stage G3 chronic kidney disease, and migraine headaches. Medications are amlodipine, heparin, topiramate, and as-needed intravenous morphine.

On physical examination, vital signs are normal. Mild incisional tenderness is present. The remainder of the physical examination is unremarkable.

**Laboratory studies:**

| | On Admission | Today |
|---|---|---|
| Creatinine | 1.6 mg/dL (141.4 µmol/L) | 1.9 mg/dL (168 µmol/L) |
| Electrolytes: | | |
| Sodium | 140 mEq/L (140 mmol/L) | 138 mEq/L (138 mmol/L) |
| Potassium | 4.9 mEq/L (4.9 mmol/L) | 5.6 mEq/L (5.6 mmol/L) |
| Chloride | 102 mEq/L (102 mmol/L) | 110 mEq/L (110 mmol/L) |
| Bicarbonate | 25 mEq/L (25 mmol/L) | 20 mEq/L (20 mmol/L) |
| Glucose | 116 mg/dL (6.4 mmol/L) | 128 mg/dL (7.1 mmol/L) |

Urine output during the past 24 hours is 1400 mL.

Which of the following is the most likely cause of this patient's elevated serum potassium?

(A) Acute kidney injury

(B) Heparin

(C) Hyperglycemia

(D) Metabolic acidosis

(E) Topiramate

## Item 19

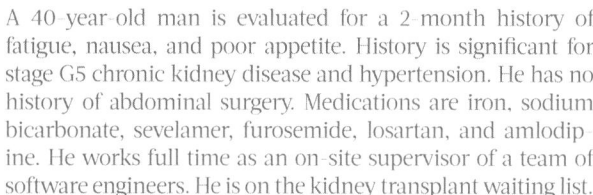

A 40-year-old man is evaluated for a 2-month history of fatigue, nausea, and poor appetite. History is significant for stage G5 chronic kidney disease and hypertension. He has no history of abdominal surgery. Medications are iron, sodium bicarbonate, sevelamer, furosemide, losartan, and amlodipine. He works full time as an on-site supervisor of a team of software engineers. He is on the kidney transplant waiting list.

On physical examination, vital signs are normal. BMI is 25. Conjunctival pallor is noted. There is no pericardial friction rub, jugular venous distention, lung crackles, or asterixis.

Laboratory studies are notable for a hemoglobin level of 8.7 g/dL (87 g/L) and an estimated glomerular filtration rate of 8 mL/min/1.73 m².

Which of the following considerations might favor the choice of peritoneal dialysis as the preferred pretransplant renal replacement therapy for this patient?

(A) Greater autonomy

(B) Improvement in anemia

(C) Improvement in mortality

(D) Lack of infectious complications

## Item 20

A 44-year-old man is evaluated during a follow-up visit for treatment of persistently elevated blood pressure. He takes no medications.

Physical examination reveals a well-developed muscular man in no apparent distress. Blood pressure is 165/98 mm Hg, and pulse rate is 70/min; other vital signs are normal. BMI is 26. Jugular venous pressure is normal. Cardiac examination is unremarkable.

**Laboratory studies:**

| | |
|---|---|
| Bicarbonate | 27 mEq/L (27 mmol/L) |
| Creatinine | 1.3 mg/dL (114.9 µmol/L) |
| Potassium | 4.5 mEq/L (4.5 mmol/L) |
| Estimated glomerular filtration rate | >60 mL/min/1.73 m² |
| Urine toxicology screen | Negative |

Electrocardiogram reveals normal sinus rhythm; voltage criteria for left ventricular hypertrophy are present.

Which of the following is the most appropriate treatment?

(A) Amlodipine/benazepril combination once daily

(B) Doxazosin and metoprolol, each once daily

(C) Hydralazine three times daily

(D) Telmisartan and ramipril, each once daily

## Item 21

An 83-year-old man is evaluated for a 1-week history of poor appetite, myalgia, fatigue, arthralgia, and low-grade fever. He was previously healthy and active. His only medication is acetaminophen as needed.

On physical examination, the patient is afebrile. Blood pressure is 155/95 mm Hg, and pulse rate is 80/min; there are no orthostatic changes. There is trace lower extremity edema. A faint red-blue reticular rash is present over the lower extremities.

**Laboratory studies:**

| | |
|---|---|
| Hemoglobin | 12 g/dL (120 g/L) |
| Calcium | 9.8 mg/dL (2.5 mmol/L) |
| Creatinine | Current: 3.1 mg/dL (274 µmol/L) |
| | Baseline 2 months ago: 0.9 mg/dL |
| | (79.6 µmol/L) |
| Urinalysis | 3+ blood; 2+ protein; 20-30 dysmorphic |
| | erythrocytes/hpf; 5-10 leukocytes/hpf |

Chest radiograph shows no acute infiltrates. Kidney ultrasound shows no masses or obstruction.

**Which of the following is the most likely diagnosis?**

(A) ANCA-associated glomerulonephritis

(B) Anti–glomerular basement membrane antibody disease

(C) Minimal change glomerulopathy

(D) Myeloma cast nephropathy

(E) Proliferative lupus nephritis

## Item 22

A 79-year-old woman is evaluated in the emergency department for worsening confusion over the past 5 days. She also reports lower back pain for the past 3 months. History is significant for hypertension and coronary artery disease with stenting of the left anterior descending artery 2 years ago. Daily medications are metoprolol, hydrochlorothiazide, atorvastatin, low-dose aspirin, and acetaminophen. Her husband confirms that the patient takes all medications as directed.

On physical examination, temperature is normal, blood pressure is 128/76 mm Hg, pulse rate is 72/min, respiration rate is 20/min, and oxygen saturation is 95% on ambient air. BMI is 19. There is no abdominal pain. The patient is weak, confused to time and place, and sleepy but easily arousable. The remainder of the neurologic examination is normal.

**Laboratory studies:**

| | |
|---|---|
| Blood urea nitrogen | 35 mg/dL (12.5 mmol/L) |
| Creatinine | 1.4 mg/dL (123.8 µmol/L) |
| Electrolytes: | |
|   Sodium | 138 mEq/L (138 mmol/L) |
|   Potassium | 4.8 mEq/L (4.8 mmol/L) |
|   Chloride | 102 mEq/L (102 mmol/L) |
|   Bicarbonate | 14 mEq/L (14 mmol/L) |
| Lactate | 0.7 mEq/L (0.7 mmol/L) |
| Arterial blood gases: | |
|   pH | 7.31 |
|   $P_{CO_2}$ | 29 mm Hg (3.9 kPa) |
| Urinalysis | Specific gravity 1.025; no protein, |
| | ketones, cells, or crystals |

**Which of the following is the most likely diagnosis?**

(A) D-Lactic acidosis

(B) Propylene glycol toxicity

(C) Pyroglutamic acidosis

(D) Salicylate toxicity

## Item 23

An 18-year-old man is evaluated in the ICU for oliguric acute kidney injury. Eighteen hours ago he underwent hepatectomy for a giant fibrolamellar hepatic carcinoma. During the procedure he developed coagulopathy and hepatic bleeding and required resuscitation with eight units of packed red blood cells, multiple units of fresh frozen plasma, and several liters of crystalloid fluids. He is receiving cefepime, gentamicin, propofol, and fentanyl. Urine output has decreased to 10 mL/h since ICU admission 14 hours ago.

On physical examination, the patient is mechanically ventilated. Blood pressure is 120/70 mm Hg, pulse rate is 115/min, and respiration rate is 12/min. Breath sounds are decreased bilaterally. The abdomen is distended and tense with intact midline incision and wall edema. The remainder of the examination is noncontributory.

**Laboratory studies:**

| | |
|---|---|
| Hemoglobin | 10 g/dL (100 g/L) |
| Creatine kinase | 1250 U/L |
| Creatinine | 1.7 mg/dL (150.3 µmol/L); on admission: |
| | 0.9 mg/dL (79.6 µmol/L) |
| Potassium | 5.2 mEq/L (5.2 mmol/L) |
| Urine sodium | <20 mEq/L (20 mmol/L) |
| Urinalysis | Specific gravity 1.030; pH 5.5; 4+ blood; |
| | trace protein; too numerous to count |
| | erythrocytes; few hyaline casts |

Kidney ultrasound reveals normal-sized kidneys and no hydronephrosis; a large volume of ascites is noted.

**Which of the following is the most appropriate diagnostic test to perform next?**

(A) Fractional excretion of sodium

(B) Intra-abdominal pressure measurement

(C) Urine myoglobin levels

(D) Urine stain for eosinophils

## Item 24

A 45-year-old man is evaluated for one episode of macroscopic hematuria. He currently does not see blood in his urine. He reports no flank pain and no associated trauma or exertion. He is a nonsmoker and takes no medications.

Physical examination and vital signs are normal.

Laboratory studies show a normal serum creatinine level; urinalysis shows 1+ blood, no protein, 10-15 isomorphic erythrocytes/hpf, 0-2 leukocytes/hpf, no nitrites, and no leukocyte esterase.

Contrast-enhanced CT urogram shows no kidney stones, masses, or cysts.

Which of the following is the most appropriate diagnostic test to perform next?

(A) Cystoscopy
(B) Kidney biopsy
(C) Kidney and renal vein Doppler ultrasonography
(D) Urine cytology

## Item 25

A 27-year-old woman is evaluated for a 6-month history of fatigue, arthralgia, and myalgia. She has a history of urinary tract infections. Medications are an oral contraceptive pill and as-needed naproxen for pain.

On physical examination, temperature is 38.2 °C (100.8 °F), blood pressure is 142/90 mm Hg, and pulse rate is 90/min. Cardiac, lung, and abdominal examinations are normal.

Laboratory studies show a serum creatinine level of 1.4 mg/dL (123.8 µmol/L); urinalysis shows 2+ blood, 3+ protein, positive leukocyte esterase, no nitrites, 10-15 erythrocytes/hpf, 5-10 leukocytes/hpf, and no crystals.

Urine microscopy is shown.

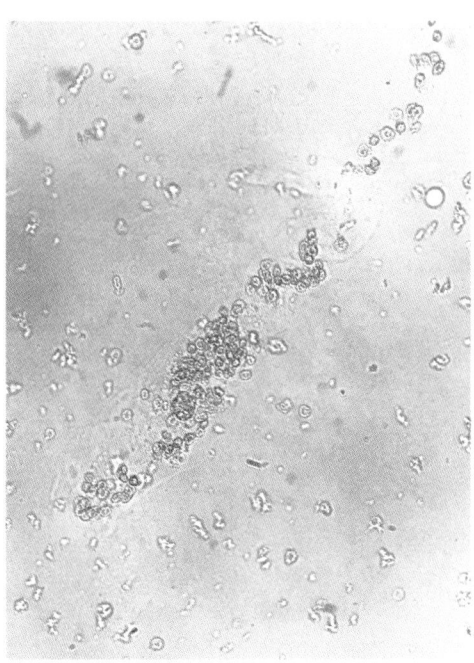

Which of the following is the most likely diagnosis?

(A) Bladder cancer
(B) Glomerulonephritis
(C) Tubulointerstitial nephritis
(D) Urinary tract infection

## Item 26

A 61-year-old woman is evaluated in the ICU for acute kidney injury. She was discharged from the hospital 10 days ago following elective cholecystectomy. Seven days ago she was readmitted to the hospital with sepsis. A CT scan of the abdomen with intravenous contrast did not show any abdominal pathology but confirmed pneumonia.

She was treated with intravenous fluids, norepinephrine infusion, vancomycin, and cefepime. The norepinephrine was stopped yesterday. History is significant for hypertension and stage G3a chronic kidney disease. Her baseline serum creatinine is 1.4 mg/dL (123.8 µmol/L). On admission the serum creatinine was 1.9 mg/dL (168 µmol/L) and returned to baseline by hospital day 2; it is 3.1 mg/dL (274 µmol/L) today. Outpatient medications are lisinopril and chlorthalidone.

On physical examination, temperature is 37.6 °C (99.7 °F), blood pressure is 140/82 mm Hg, pulse rate is 103/min, and respiration rate is 20/min. Examination of the lungs reveals bilateral crackles. There is 1+ pedal edema of the extremities. The remainder of the physical examination is noncontributory.

**Current laboratory studies:**

| | |
|---|---|
| Serum creatinine | 3.1 mg/dL (274 µmol/L) |
| Vancomycin trough | 25 mg/L |
| Fractional excretion of sodium | 2.5% |
| Urinalysis | Specific gravity 1.012; pH 5.5; no blood; 1+ protein; trace leukocyte esterase; no nitrites; no glucose; 2-4 leukocytes/hpf; 5-10 renal tubular epithelial cells/hpf; 5-10 coarse granular casts/hpf |

Kidney ultrasound reveals normal-sized kidneys and no hydronephrosis.

Which of the following is the most likely cause of this patient's acute kidney injury?

(A) Cefepime
(B) Intravenous contrast
(C) Omeprazole
(D) Vancomycin

## Item 27

An 18-year-old woman is brought to the emergency department by friends. She is confused and febrile. Her friends state that she took 3,4-methylenedioxymethamphetamine (ecstasy) at a party and was previously well. There is no other medical history.

On physical examination, the patient is confused and oriented to her name only. Temperature is 38.9 °C (102.0 °F), blood pressure is 148/94 mm Hg, pulse rate is 108/min, respiration rate is 20/min, and oxygen saturation is 96% breathing 2 L/min oxygen by nasal cannula. The remainder of the examination is unremarkable.

**Laboratory studies:**

| | |
|---|---|
| Blood urea nitrogen | 11 mg/dL (3.9 mmol/L) |
| Creatinine | 0.8 mg/dL (70.7 µmol/L) |
| Electrolytes: | |
|   Sodium | 118 mEq/L (118 mmol/L) |
|   Potassium | 3.5 mEq/L (3.5 mmol/L) |
|   Chloride | 88 mEq/L (88 mmol/L) |
|   Bicarbonate | 21 mEq/L (21 mmol/L) |
| Glucose | 88 mg/dL (4.9 mmol/L) |
| Urine osmolality | 405 mOsm/kg H$_2$O |

Which of the following is the most appropriate initial treatment?

(A) 0.9% sodium chloride, 100 mL/h
(B) 100-mL bolus of 3% saline
(C) Fluid restriction
(D) Oral urea
(E) Tolvaptan

## Item 28

A 26-year-old woman is evaluated during a follow-up visit for hypertension diagnosed 1 month ago. She is a marathon runner with previously normal blood pressure. Family history is significant for her mother who died of a ruptured cerebral aneurysm at the age of 50 years. Medications are lisinopril and an oral contraceptive.

On physical examination, blood pressure is 146/92 mm Hg, and pulse rate is 59/min. A systolic-diastolic abdominal bruit that lateralizes to the left side is heard. There is no lower extremity edema. The remainder of the examination is unremarkable.

Laboratory studies show a serum creatinine level of 1.4 mg/dL (123.8 µmol/L) (1 month ago: 0.8 mg/dL [70.7 µmol/L]). Urinalysis is normal with no blood, protein, or leukocyte esterase. A pregnancy test is negative.

A 12-lead electrocardiogram is normal.

Which of the following is the most appropriate diagnostic test to perform next?

(A) Plasma aldosterone concentration/plasma renin activity ratio
(B) Plasma fractionated metanephrines
(C) Renal artery imaging
(D) Transthoracic echocardiography

## Item 29

A 75-year-old man is evaluated in the hospital for an acute anterior ST-elevation myocardial infarction. He was hospitalized for chest pain and shortness of breath 45 minutes ago. History is significant for stage G4 chronic kidney disease (estimated glomerular filtration rate, 24 mL/min/1.73 m²), hypertension, and peripheral vascular disease. Medications are lisinopril, metoprolol, furosemide, sevelamer, sodium bicarbonate, aspirin, clopidogrel, and unfractionated heparin.

On physical examination, blood pressure is 145/88 mm Hg, pulse rate is 94/min, and respiration rate is 18/min. Cardiopulmonary examination reveals jugular venous distension, a grade 2/6 mitral regurgitation murmur, an $S_4$ gallop, and end-expiratory bilateral basilar crackles.

Which of the following is the most appropriate immediate management?

(A) Cardiac catheterization
(B) Cardiac magnetic resonance imaging
(C) Emergent dialysis followed by coronary catheterization
(D) Medical management

## Item 30

A 36-year-old man is evaluated in the emergency department for renal colic. He is in otherwise good health and takes no medications.

Physical examination reveals left costovertebral angle tenderness. The remainder of the examination is normal.

Noncontrast helical CT scan shows an 11-mm stone at the left ureteral pelvic junction and mild left caliectasis.

Analgesics are initiated.

Which of the following is the most appropriate next step in management?

(A) Extracorporeal shock wave lithotripsy
(B) Forced diuresis with intravenous normal saline
(C) Nifedipine
(D) Tamsulosin

## Item 31

A 41-year-old woman is evaluated for a 3-month history of increasing nonproductive cough, fatigue, anorexia, and malaise. History is significant for hypertension. Medications are hydrochlorothiazide, lisinopril, and self-prescribed vitamin D and calcium for bone health.

On physical examination, vital signs are normal. Bilateral crackles are heard on pulmonary auscultation. Trace pedal edema is present. The remainder of the examination is unremarkable.

**Laboratory studies:**

| | |
|---|---|
| Calcium | 11.3 mg/dL (2.8 mmol/L) |
| Creatinine | 1.6 mg/dL (141.4 µmol/L); 1 year ago: 1.0 mg/dL (88.4 µmol/L) |
| Phosphorus | 3.4 mg/dL (1.1 mmol/L) |
| Parathyroid hormone | 12 pg/mL (12 ng/L) |
| 25-Hydroxyvitamin D | 43 ng/mL (107.3 nmol/L) |
| Urinalysis | Specific gravity 1.010; 1+ protein; 5-20 leukocytes/hpf; occasional granular casts |
| Urine protein-creatinine ratio | 400 mg/g |
| 24-Hour urine calcium | Elevated |

Chest radiograph shows diffuse reticular opacities. Kidney ultrasound demonstrates nephrocalcinosis.

**Which of the following is the most likely cause of this patient's findings?**

(A) Hydrochlorothiazide
(B) Primary hyperparathyroidism
(C) Sarcoidosis
(D) Vitamin D intoxication

## Item 32

A 25-year-old woman is evaluated in the emergency department for chest pain after a belted motor vehicle accident. She is pregnant at approximately 23 weeks' gestation. She reports no additional symptoms and is otherwise well. Her only medication is a prenatal vitamin.

On physical examination, the patient is afebrile, blood pressure is 102/62 mm Hg, and pulse rate is 80/min. Pain and bruising over the left chest wall are noted. Abdominal examination findings are consistent with changes of pregnancy.

Laboratory studies are significant for a serum sodium level of 132 mEq/L (132 mmol/L).

**Which of the following is the most likely cause of this patient's low serum sodium level?**

(A) Excessive water intake
(B) Hypotension-induced antidiuretic hormone release
(C) Normal physiologic change in pregnancy
(D) Syndrome of inappropriate antidiuretic hormone secretion

## Item 33

A 51-year-old man is evaluated during a routine follow-up visit for stage G4 chronic kidney disease and hypertension. He is asymptomatic. Medications are valsartan, amlodipine, and furosemide.

On physical examination, blood pressure is 140/70 mm Hg, and pulse rate is 70/min. BMI is 32. The remainder of the physical examination is noncontributory.

**Laboratory studies:**

| | |
|---|---|
| HDL cholesterol | 32 mg/dL (0.83 mmol/L) |
| LDL cholesterol | 119 mg/dL (3.08 mmol/L) |
| Total cholesterol | 208 mg/dL (5.39 mmol/L) |
| Triglycerides | 289 mg/dL (3.27 mmol/L) |

**Which of the following is the most appropriate management for this patient's dyslipidemia?**

(A) Gemfibrozil
(B) Niacin
(C) Omega-3 fish oil
(D) Rosuvastatin

## Item 34

A 28-year-old man is evaluated in the emergency department for acute right-sided flank pain and blood in the urine. He reports no prior episodes of hematuria or flank pain. He takes no medications.

On physical examination, vital signs are normal. Costovertebral angle tenderness is noted. The abdomen is soft and nontender.

Urinalysis shows 3+ blood, trace protein, and too numerous to count erythrocytes.

A kidney ultrasound shows normal-appearing kidneys, no hydronephrosis, and no nephrolithiasis.

**Which of the following is the most appropriate test to perform next?**

(A) Contrast MRI
(B) Contrast-enhanced helical abdominal CT
(C) Kidney, ureter, and bladder plain radiography
(D) Noncontrast helical abdominal CT

## Item 35

A 26-year-old man is evaluated during a follow-up visit after presenting to an urgent care clinic for back pain 1 week ago. Laboratory studies at that time were significant for a serum creatinine level of 1.4 mg/dL (123.8 µmol/L); other laboratory studies, including urinalysis, were normal. A urine albumin-creatinine ratio obtained in preparation for this visit is 10 mg/g. He is a personal trainer, and his daily exercise regimen includes weightlifting. He states that his back pain has resolved. He occasionally takes ibuprofen; the last use was 1 week ago. He takes no over-the-counter supplements.

On physical examination today, vital signs are normal. BMI is 29. The patient is muscular, without signs of obesity. There is no muscle tenderness.

**Which of the following is the most appropriate management?**

(A) Avoid all NSAID medications
(B) Measure the serum creatine kinase level
(C) Measure the serum cystatin C level
(D) Schedule a kidney biopsy

## Item 36

A 42-year-old man is evaluated during a follow-up visit for kidney stones. He had his first stone 4 years ago. Despite increasing his water intake, he has had two additional episodes. Stone analysis has revealed only calcium oxalate. He is in otherwise good health. He has no history of urinary tract infections. There is no family history of kidney disease, hyperparathyroidism, or nephrolithiasis.

The physical examination and vital signs are unremarkable. The patient weighs 80 kg (176 lb).

**Laboratory studies:**

| | |
|---|---|
| Calcium | 9.6 mg/dL (2.4 mmol/L) |
| Creatinine | 0.9 mg/dL (79.6 µmol/L) |
| Electrolytes: | |
|   Sodium | 138 mEq/L (138 mmol/L) |
|   Potassium | 4.1 mEq/L (4.1 mmol/L) |
|   Chloride | 105 mEq/L (105 mmol/L) |
|   Bicarbonate | 25 mEq/L (25 mmol/L) |
| Urinalysis | Specific gravity 1.008; pH 5.5; no blood, protein, leukocyte esterase, or nitrites |
| 24-Hour Urine Studies: | |
|   Volume | 2945 mL |
|   pH | 5.2 |
|   Calcium | 320 mg/24 h (normal range, <320 mg/24 h) |
|   Citrate | 790 mg/24 h (normal range, 300-1100 mg/24 h) |
|   Oxalate | 32 mg/24 h (normal range, <40 mg/24 h) |
|   Sodium | 140 mEq/24 h (normal range, 40-220 mEq/24 h) |
|   Uric acid | 640 mg/24 h (normal range, <800 mg/24 h) |

Noncontrast helical CT scan shows a 4-mm stone in the lower pole of the left kidney and a 3-mm stone in the mid pole of the right kidney.

CONT.

Which of the following is the most appropriate next step to decrease this patient's stone recurrence?

(A) Add allopurinol
(B) Add hydrochlorothiazide
(C) Add potassium citrate
(D) Increase urine volume
(E) Recommend a low calcium diet

## Item 37

A 25-year-old man is evaluated during a physical examination for a new job. He is adopted, with no knowledge of his biological parents' medical history. He takes no medications.

On physical examination, blood pressure is 100/60 mm Hg; other vital signs are normal. The remainder of the examination, including cardiac examination, is unremarkable.

Urinalysis shows 2+ blood and no protein.

Kidney ultrasound shows a 15-cm right kidney, a 16-cm left kidney, and multiple cysts bilaterally.

Screening for *PKD* mutations is performed, and the *PKD1* variant associated with autosomal dominant polycystic kidney disease is detected.

Which of the following is the most appropriate next step in management?

(A) Obtain echocardiography
(B) Obtain MR angiography of the brain
(C) Start amlodipine
(D) Start tolvaptan

## Item 38

A 44-year-old man is evaluated during a follow-up visit for membranous glomerulopathy, which was diagnosed last week on kidney biopsy. He has no other pertinent personal or family history. His only medication is furosemide.

On physical examination, vital signs are normal. There is trace bilateral lower extremity edema to the ankles. The remainder of the examination is unremarkable.

**Laboratory studies performed before kidney biopsy:**

| | |
|---|---|
| Albumin | 3.0 g/dL (30 g/L) |
| Total cholesterol | 310 mg/dL (8.0 mmol/L) |
| Creatinine | 0.8 mg/dL (70.7 µmol/L) |
| Antinuclear antibodies | Negative |
| Anti-phospholipase A2 receptor antibodies | Titer: 1:80 |
| Hepatitis B surface Ag and Ab antibodies | Negative |
| Hepatitis C Ab antibodies | Negative |
| HIV antibodies | Negative |
| 24-Hour urine protein excretion | 6500 mg/24 h |

Ultrasound of the kidneys shows normal appearance with no evidence of thrombus in the renal veins.

An ACE inhibitor and a statin are initiated.

Which of the following is the most appropriate additional management?

(A) Alternating course of glucocorticoids and alkylating agents
(B) Anti–double-stranded DNA antibody measurement
(C) Cyclosporine
(D) Hepatitis B and hepatitis C viral polymerase chain reaction testing
(E) No additional management at this time

## Item 39

A 65-year-old man is seen in the hospital for preoperative evaluation prior to an umbilical hernia repair. Medical history is significant for hypertension, hyperlipidemia, and chronic kidney disease. Medications are metoprolol, amlodipine, furosemide, hydralazine, simvastatin, and aspirin.

On physical examination, average blood pressure is 150/96 mm Hg, and pulse rate is 54/min; other vital signs are normal. BMI is 26. Cardiac examination reveals no murmurs, gallops, or rubs. The lungs are clear. The abdomen is nontender, with a bruit heard over the umbilical region. Lower extremity pulses are diminished. The remainder of the examination is unremarkable.

**Laboratory studies:**

| | |
|---|---|
| Creatinine | 1.7 mg/dL (150.3 µmol/L); 3 months ago: 1.8 mg/dL (159.1 µmol/L) |
| HDL cholesterol | 46 mg/dL (1.2 mmol/L) |
| LDL cholesterol | 100 mg/dL (2.6 mmol/L) |
| Total cholesterol | 180 mg/dL (4.7 mmol/L) |
| Urine albumin-creatinine ratio | 300 mg/g |

Abdominal ultrasound with Doppler reveals 75% ostial right renal artery stenosis; there is no aortic aneurysm.

Which of the following is the most appropriate next step in management?

(A) Begin lisinopril
(B) Obtain renal intra-arterial angiography
(C) Perform percutaneous transluminal renal artery angioplasty and stenting
(D) Perform renal artery surgical revascularization

## Item 40

A 68-year-old woman is hospitalized for chest pain. History is significant for stage G3 chronic kidney disease, hypertension, coronary artery disease, and type 2 diabetes mellitus. Medications are aspirin, losartan, basal and prandial insulin, metoprolol, nitroglycerin paste, and unfractionated heparin.

On physical examination, blood pressure is 130/80 mm Hg; other vital signs are normal. S₁ and S₂ are normal. There is no S₃, lung crackles, or leg edema.

Laboratory studies show a serum creatinine level of 1.8 mg/dL (159.1 µmol/L) and an elevated serum troponin level.

CONT.

Electrocardiogram shows a 2-mm ST-segment depression in leads I, aVL, and V$_4$ through V$_6$.

Cardiac catheterization is planned.

**Which of the following is the most appropriate peri-procedure management?**

(A) Administer furosemide before cardiac catheterization

(B) Administer intravenous isotonic fluids before and after cardiac catheterization

(C) Administer oral sodium bicarbonate before catheterization

(D) Initiate hemodialysis following cardiac catheterization

## Item 41

A 40-year-old woman is evaluated for arthralgia, dry eyes, and dry mouth of several weeks' duration. She has been taking naproxen and acetaminophen daily for about 1 week. She has no pertinent personal or family history.

On physical examination, vital signs are normal. Mucous membranes and conjunctivae are dry. Bilateral parotid gland enlargement is present.

**Laboratory studies:**

| | |
|---|---|
| Creatinine | 0.9 mg/dL (79.6 µmol/L) |
| Electrolytes: | |
| Sodium | 138 mEq/L (138 mmol/L) |
| Potassium | 3.1 mEq/L (3.1 mmol/L) |
| Chloride | 118 mEq/L (118 mmol/L) |
| Bicarbonate | 12 mEq/L (12 mmol/L) |
| Glucose | 74 mg/dL (4.1 mmol/L) |
| Urinalysis | pH 7.0; no blood, protein, glucose, erythrocytes, or leukocytes |

Kidney ultrasound shows echogenic normal-sized kidneys.

**Which of the following is the most likely cause of the patient's laboratory findings?**

(A) Naproxen

(B) Type 1 (hypokalemic distal) renal tubular acidosis

(C) Type 2 (proximal) renal tubular acidosis

(D) Type 4 (hyperkalemic distal) renal tubular acidosis

## Item 42

A 49-year-old man is evaluated in the emergency department for abdominal pain, vomiting, and nausea after binge drinking. History is significant for alcohol abuse, with numerous hospitalizations for intoxications and withdrawal.

On physical examination, temperature is normal, blood pressure is 122/72 mm Hg sitting and 100/62 mm Hg standing, pulse rate is 100/min sitting and 118/min standing, respiration rate is 22/min, and oxygen saturation is 97% breathing ambient air. BMI is 18. Abdominal examination reveals diffuse abdominal tenderness to palpation; there is no rebound tenderness, ascites, or evidence of trauma. Neurologic examination is normal. There is no edema.

**Laboratory studies:**

| | |
|---|---|
| Electrolytes: | |
| Sodium | 137 mEq/L (137 mmol/L) |
| Potassium | 3.7 mEq/L (3.7 mmol/L) |
| Chloride | 96 mEq/L (96 mmol/L) |
| Bicarbonate | 10 mEq/L (10 mmol/L) |
| Ethanol | 10 mg/dL (2.2 mmol/L) |
| Glucose | 94 mg/dL (5.2 mmol/L) |
| Lactate | 0.8 mEq/L (0.8 mmol/L) |
| Arterial blood gases: | |
| pH | 7.26 |
| P$co_2$ | 23 mm Hg (3.1 kPa) |
| Urinalysis | Specific gravity 1.020; pH 5.5; positive ketones; no blood or cells |

Thiamine and B-complex vitamin are administered.

**Which of the following is the most appropriate treatment?**

(A) 0.9% saline

(B) 5% dextrose in 0.9% saline

(C) 5% dextrose in water with 150 mEq (150 mmol) of sodium bicarbonate

(D) Insulin and 5% dextrose in 0.9% saline

## Item 43

A 45-year-old man is evaluated during a follow-up visit for membranous glomerulopathy diagnosed 3 weeks ago. He reports persistent lower extremity edema and no weight loss despite adhering to a low-salt diet and taking maximal-dose furosemide. He does not have shortness of breath or abdominal discomfort. Other medications are enalapril and simvastatin.

On physical examination, vital signs are normal. The patient weighs 80 kg (176.4 lb), with a baseline weight of 75 kg (165.3 lb). There is no rash. Cardiac examination is normal, and there is no evidence of jugular venous distention. The lungs are clear on examination. There is pitting edema in the legs bilaterally to just below the patellae.

**Laboratory studies:**

| | |
|---|---|
| Albumin | 2.9 g/dL (29 g/L) |
| Blood urea nitrogen | Normal |
| Creatinine | 1.0 mg/dL (88.4 µmol/L) |
| Electrolytes | Normal |
| Urinalysis | No blood; 4+ protein |
| Urine protein-creatinine ratio | 6100 mg/g |

Doppler ultrasound of the lower extremities performed 3 weeks ago showed no evidence of deep venous thrombosis.

**Which of the following is the most appropriate management?**

(A) Add metolazone

(B) Change furosemide to bumetanide

(C) Hospitalize for intravenous diuresis

(D) Repeat lower extremity Doppler ultrasonography

## Item 44

A 27-year-old woman is evaluated for proteinuria identified on urinalysis performed for a life insurance examination. She reports no symptoms. History is significant for premature birth, a 2-year history of hypertriglyceridemia and prediabetes, and a 5-year history of obesity. The remainder of her medical history is unremarkable. Her only medication is gemfibrozil.

On physical examination, vital signs are normal. BMI is 37. The remainder of the examination is unremarkable.

**Laboratory studies:**

| | |
|---|---|
| Albumin | 3.8 g/dL (38 g/L) |
| Creatinine | 1.0 mg/dL (88.4 µmol/L) |
| Hemoglobin A$_{1c}$ | 6.4% |
| Urinalysis | No blood; 3+ protein |
| Urine protein-creatinine ratio | 2100 mg/g |

Kidney ultrasound shows normal-appearing kidneys with no masses or hydronephrosis.

**Which of the following is the most likely diagnosis?**

(A) Diabetic nephropathy
(B) Lipoprotein glomerulopathy
(C) Minimal change glomerulopathy
(D) Secondary focal segmental glomerulosclerosis

## Item 45

A 38-year-old woman is evaluated during a follow-up visit for primary membranous glomerulopathy. Diagnosis was made by kidney biopsy 4 months ago, and she was found to be positive for anti–phospholipase A2 receptor (PLA2R) antibodies. Medications are furosemide, losartan, and simvastatin. Recent age- and sex-appropriate cancer screening tests were normal.

On physical examination, vital signs are normal. There is pitting lower extremity edema to the mid shins bilaterally.

**Laboratory studies:**

| | |
|---|---|
| Albumin | 2.1 g/dL (21 g/L) |
| Total cholesterol | 288 mg/dL (7.5 mmol/L) |
| Creatinine | 1.1 mg/dL (97.2 µmol/L) |
| Urine protein-creatinine ratio | 9135 mg/g |

**Which of the following complications is this patient at greatest risk for developing?**

(A) Gout
(B) Malignancy
(C) Renal cell carcinoma
(D) Venous thromboembolism

## Item 46

A 50-year-old man is evaluated for elevated blood pressure measurements despite an increase in his hydrochlorothiazide dose 1 month ago. History is significant for hypertension and hyperlipidemia. Medications are hydrochlorothiazide and atorvastatin.

On physical examination, blood pressure is 150/92 mm Hg, and pulse rate is 69/min. BMI is 30. The remainder of the examination is normal.

Laboratory studies show a serum creatinine level of 1.0 mg/dL (88.4 µmol/L), a serum potassium level of 3.4 mEq/L (3.4 mmol/L), and a urine albumin-creatinine ratio of 550 mg/g.

**In addition to weight loss, which of the following is the most appropriate management?**

(A) Add amlodipine
(B) Add losartan
(C) Add spironolactone
(D) Schedule a follow-up visit for 3 months

## Item 47

A 37-year-old woman is evaluated for a headache lasting 1 day. She is in the third trimester of her first pregnancy. Until now, the pregnancy has been unremarkable, including blood pressure and urine protein measurements. Her only medication is a prenatal vitamin.

On physical examination, blood pressure is 166/115 mm Hg; other vital signs are normal. There is no papilledema. Cardiac examination is normal. On abdominal examination, the patient has a gravid uterus consistent with her stage of pregnancy, and there is no abdominal tenderness.

**Laboratory studies:**

| | |
|---|---|
| Hemoglobin | 12.3 g/dL (123 g/L) |
| Platelet count | 70,000/µL (70 × 10⁹/L) |
| Alanine aminotransferase | 72 U/L |
| Aspartate aminotransferase | 80 U/L |
| Bilirubin | Normal |
| Creatinine | 1.4 mg/dL (123.8 µmol/L) |
| Electrolytes | Normal |
| Peripheral blood smear | Normal |
| Urinalysis | 2+ protein |

**Which of the following is the most likely diagnosis?**

(A) Chronic hypertension
(B) Eclampsia
(C) Gestational hypertension
(D) HELLP syndrome
(E) Preeclampsia

## Item 48

A 29-year-old man is evaluated in the emergency department for a 3-week history of headaches. He reports a painful burning sensation in his toes and feet for the past few years, particularly after he exercises at the gym, and states that he does not sweat as much after exercise compared with his peers. He takes no medications. Family history is notable for the following: His maternal grandfather and maternal granduncle had similar burning sensations in their feet for years and died from strokes in their early 40s; and his mother has occasional burning sensations in her feet as well as corneal dystrophy.

On physical examination, blood pressure is 160/95 mm Hg; other vital signs are normal. Numerous angiokeratomas over the sternal area are present. Reduced pain and temperature sensation in the lower extremities bilaterally is noted.

Laboratory studies show a blood urea nitrogen level of 60 mg/dL (21.4 mmol/L) and a serum creatinine level of 4.1 mg/dL (362.4 µmol/L); urinalysis shows 2+ blood and 3+ protein.

Kidney ultrasound shows increased echogenicity in bilateral kidneys.

Which of the following is the most likely diagnosis?

(A)  Fabry disease

(B)  Hereditary nephritis

(C)  Medullary cystic kidney disease

(D)  Tuberous sclerosis complex

## Item 49

A 58-year-old woman is evaluated in the emergency department for fever and dysuria of 24 hours' duration. History is significant for frequent urinary tract infections. The patient takes no medications.

On physical examination, the patient appears ill. Temperature is 38.3 °C (101.0 °F), blood pressure is 148/84 mm Hg, pulse rate is 98/min, and respiration rate is 18/min. Abdominal examination reveals right costovertebral angle tenderness. The remainder of the examination is unremarkable.

Laboratory studies:
Creatinine   1.1 mg/dL (97.2 µmol/L)
Urinalysis   Specific gravity 1.010; pH 8.0; trace blood; trace protein; 2+ leukocyte esterase; 2+ nitrites; 3-4 erythrocytes/hpf; 10-12 leukocytes/hpf; positive for bacteria

Abdominal radiograph shows a staghorn calculus in the right kidney.
Empiric antibiotic therapy is initiated.

Which of the following is the most appropriate next step in management?

(A)  Chronic antibiotic suppression

(B)  Potassium citrate administration

(C)  Stone removal

(D)  Urease inhibitor administration

(E)  Urinary acidification

## Item 50

A 78-year-old woman is evaluated in the emergency department for severe pain in the left hip after a fall. History is significant for end-stage kidney disease as of 18 months ago, hypertension, and peripheral vascular disease. Medications are lisinopril, amlodipine, sevelamer, and epoetin alfa. She is also receiving morphine for the hip pain.

On physical examination, blood pressure is 132/70 mm Hg, and pulse rate is 72/min; other vital signs are normal. The left lower extremity is externally rotated at the hip. Peripheral pulses are diminished. The remainder of the physical examination is noncontributory.

Laboratory studies:
Alkaline phosphatase      78 U/L
Calcium                   9.7 mg/dL (2.4 mmol/L)
Phosphorus                4.2 mg/dL (1.4 mmol/L)
Parathyroid hormone       62 pg/mL (62 ng/L)
25-Hydroxyvitamin D       32 ng/mL (80 nmol/L)

Radiographs of the hips show a left hip fracture and calcified arteries.

Which of the following is the most likely diagnosis for the underlying bone disease?

(A)  Adynamic bone disease

(B)  $\beta_2$-Microglobulin–associated amyloidosis

(C)  Osteitis fibrosis cystica

(D)  Osteomalacia

## Item 51

A 72-year-old man is hospitalized for a 1-week history of worsening shortness of breath; he also has worsening lower extremity edema despite an increase in his furosemide dose 2 days ago. History is significant for hypertension, stage G3a chronic kidney disease, and heart failure with a preserved ejection fraction. Outpatient medications are amlodipine, lisinopril, furosemide, and low-dose aspirin.

On physical examination, blood pressure is 112/60 mm Hg, and pulse rate is 97/min. BMI is 28. Cardiac examination reveals an elevated jugular venous pressure and an $S_4$. Breath sounds are diminished at the lung bases. There is 2+ pitting edema of the lower legs.

Laboratory studies:
Blood urea nitrogen   64 mg/dL (22.8 mmol/L); 2 weeks ago, 40 mg/dL (14.3 mmol/L)
Creatinine            2.3 mg/dL (203.3 µmol/L); 2 weeks ago, 1.9 mg/dL (168 µmol/L)
Sodium                130 mEq/L (130 mmol/L); 2 weeks ago, 133 mEq/L (133 mmol/L)
Urinalysis            Specific gravity 1.009; 1+ protein; few hyaline casts

Chest radiograph shows bibasilar effusions and vascular congestion.

Which of the following is the most appropriate treatment?

(A)  Add conivaptan

(B)  Add dobutamine infusion

(C)  Increase furosemide

(D)  Start ultrafiltration

## Item 52

A 62-year-old woman is evaluated for fatigue and weakness. History is significant for stage G4 chronic kidney disease and hypertension. Her only medication is amlodipine.

On physical examination, blood pressure is 135/85 mm Hg; other vital signs are normal. There is no jaundice. Conjunctival rim pallor is noted, and there is no scleral icterus.

Laboratory studies:
Hemoglobin                              8.5 g/dL (85 g/L)
Leukocyte count                         Normal
Mean corpuscular volume                 80 fL
Platelet count                          Normal
Reticulocyte count                      1% of erythrocytes
Ferritin                                30 ng/mL (30 µg/L)
Transferrin saturation                  10%
Estimated glomerular filtration rate    18 mL/min/1.73 m²
Stool testing for occult blood          Negative

Colonoscopy performed at age 60 years was normal.

Which of the following is the most appropriate treatment?

(A) Blood transfusion
(B) Bone marrow biopsy
(C) Erythropoietin-stimulating agent
(D) Iron supplementation

### Item 53

A 45-year-old woman is evaluated for the recent onset of resistant hypertension. During her last visit, chlorthalidone was added to her medication regimen. She reports no symptoms, and review of the systems is otherwise unremarkable. Current medications are metoprolol, amlodipine, hydralazine, and chlorthalidone.

On physical examination, blood pressure is 160/96 mm Hg, and pulse rate is 65/min; other vital signs are normal. BMI is 24. There is no proptosis. The thyroid gland is not enlarged. The remainder of the examination is unremarkable.

**Laboratory studies:**

| | |
|---|---|
| Bicarbonate | 34 mEq/L (34 mmol/L) |
| Creatinine | 0.8 mg/dL (70.7 µmol/L) |
| Potassium | 2.9 mEq/L (2.9 mmol/L) |
| Urine albumin-creatinine ratio | 10 mg/g |

**Which of the following is the most appropriate diagnostic test to perform next?**

(A) Kidney ultrasonography with Doppler
(B) Plasma aldosterone concentration/plasma renin activity ratio
(C) Plasma fractionated metanephrines
(D) Polysomnography

### Item 54

A 28-year-old woman is evaluated in the emergency department for muscle cramps and weakness. She notes a weight loss of 15 kg (33 lb) over the past 3 months; baseline weight was 115 kg (254 lb). She reports no abdominal pain or diarrhea. She has a 1-year history of type 2 diabetes mellitus, for which she takes metformin.

On physical examination, temperature is normal, blood pressure is 122/72 mm Hg, pulse rate is 100/min, and respiration rate is 18/min. BMI is 36. Muscle strength of the lower and upper extremities is 4/5. Other than weakness, neurologic examination is normal.

**Laboratory studies:**

| | |
|---|---|
| Electrolytes: | |
|    Sodium | 138 mEq/L (138 mmol/L) |
|    Potassium | 2.4 mEq/L (2.4 mmol/L) |
|    Chloride | 92 mEq/L (92 mmol/L) |
|    Bicarbonate | 34 mEq/L (34 mmol/L) |
| Arterial blood gases: | |
|    pH | 7.50 |
|    $P_{CO_2}$ | 45 mm Hg (6.0 kPa) |
| Urine sodium | 40 mEq/L (40 mmol/L) |
| Urine potassium | 60 mEq/L (60 mmol/L) |
| Urine chloride | 5 mEq/L (5 mmol/L) |

Which of the following is the most likely diagnosis?

(A) Cushing syndrome
(B) Gitelman syndrome
(C) Primary hyperaldosteronism
(D) Surreptitious vomiting

### Item 55

A 64-year-old man is evaluated for a 2-month history of increasing fatigue and bilateral swelling of the submandibular region. History is significant for autoimmune pancreatitis treated with prednisone 2 years ago, hypertension, and allergic rhinitis. Medications are losartan and fluticasone propionate.

On physical examination, blood pressure is 148/84 mm Hg, and pulse rate is 78/min. There is no rash. Head and neck examination reveals bilateral submandibular gland swelling. Trace edema of the ankles is present. The remainder of the examination is normal.

**Laboratory studies:**

| | |
|---|---|
| Hemoglobin | 12 g/dL (120 g/L) |
| Leukocyte count | 10,000/µL (10 × 10⁹/L); 33% eosinophils |
| Platelet count | 180,000/µL (180 × 10⁹/L) |
| C3 | 65 mg/dL (650 mg/L) |
| C4 | 7 mg/dL (70 mg/L) |
| Creatinine | 3.1 mg/dL (274 µmol/L); 6 months ago: 1.8 mg/dL (159.1 µmol/L) |
| IgG | 2600 mg/dL (26 g/L) |
| IgE | 500 U/mL (500 kU/L) |
| Antinuclear antibodies | 1:640 |
| Urinalysis | Specific gravity 1.010; trace protein; 6-10 leukocytes/hpf |

Kidney ultrasound demonstrates bilateral markedly enlarged kidneys measuring 15 cm in size with hyperechoic cortex and peripheral cortical nodules.

**Which of the following is the most likely diagnosis?**

(A) IgG4-related disease
(B) Lupus nephritis
(C) Sarcoidosis
(D) Sjögren syndrome

### Item 56

A 70-year-old man is evaluated for new-onset swelling and fatigue for several weeks' duration, as well as right knee pain occurring during the same time period. History is significant for stage G3a chronic kidney disease and knee osteoarthritis. Medications are lisinopril and over-the-counter naproxen.

On physical examination, blood pressure is 150/80 mm Hg, and pulse rate is 70/min; other vital signs are normal. BMI is 30. There are no lung crackles or jugular venous distension. The bladder is not palpable. There is no abdominal bruit. Examination of the right knee reveals crepitus and

**H** CONT. pain at extremes of flexion and extension. There is 1+ pedal edema.

**Laboratory studies:**

| | |
|---|---|
| Bicarbonate | 23 mEq/L (23 mmol/L) |
| Creatinine | 2.4 mg/dL (212.2 µmol/L); baseline, 1.8 mg/dL (159.1 µmol/L) |
| Potassium | 5.6 mEq/L (5.6 mmol/L) |
| Urinalysis | No blood; trace protein |

**Which of the following is the most appropriate management?**

(A) Discontinue naproxen
(B) Obtain CT angiography of the renal arteries
(C) Obtain kidney biopsy
(D) Start furosemide

## Item 57

A 40-year-old man is evaluated during a follow-up visit for a kidney transplant he received 2 years ago. History is also significant for hypertension. Medications are tacrolimus, mycophenolate mofetil, prednisone, and nifedipine.

On physical examination, blood pressure is 150/95 mm Hg; other vital signs are normal. BMI is 26. The cardiovascular and pulmonary examinations are normal. The abdomen and renal allograft are nontender to palpation. Trace pedal edema is noted.

**Laboratory studies:**

| | |
|---|---|
| Potassium | 5.6 mEq/L (5.6 mmol/L) |
| Sodium | Normal |
| Estimated glomerular filtration rate | 90 mL/min/1.73 m² |

Duplex ultrasound of the kidneys shows no evidence of transplant renal artery stenosis.

**Which of the following is the most appropriate treatment?**

(A) Chlorthalidone
(B) Fludrocortisone
(C) Sodium polystyrene sulfonate
(D) Spironolactone

## **H** Item 58

A 48-year-old woman is evaluated in the emergency department for lower extremity weakness, nausea, and increased somnolence occurring during the past 24 hours. She had constipation for 3 days, for which she drank one bottle of milk of magnesia each night. History is significant for hypertension as well as stage G4 chronic kidney disease secondary to autosomal dominant polycystic kidney disease. Her only medication is lisinopril.

On physical examination, temperature is 36.6 °C (97.9 °F), blood pressure is 94/54 mm Hg, pulse rate is 58/min, respiration rate is 16/min, and oxygen saturation is 92% breathing ambient air. Bilateral flank fullness is present. Deep tendon reflexes are diminished diffusely. Strength in the lower extremities is 3/5.

**Laboratory studies:**

| | |
|---|---|
| Calcium | 8.0 mg/dL (2 mmol/L) |
| Creatinine | 3.9 mg/dL (344.8 µmol/L) |
| Electrolytes: | |
|   Sodium | 138 mEq/L (138 mmol/L) |
|   Potassium | 3.7 mEq/L (3.7 mmol/L) |
|   Chloride | 104 mEq/L (104 mmol/L) |
|   Bicarbonate | 22 mEq/L (22 mmol/L) |
| Magnesium | 8.1 mg/dL (3.3 mmol/L) |
| Phosphorous | 4.4 mg/dL (1.4 mmol/L) |

**In addition to administration of 0.9% saline and furosemide, which of the following is the most appropriate treatment?**

(A) Hemodialysis
(B) Intravenous calcium
(C) Intravenous potassium
(D) Intravenous sodium bicarbonate
(E) Oral sodium polystyrene sulfonate

## Item 59 **H**

A 72-year-old man is evaluated in the hospital after developing acute kidney injury 2 days following coronary artery bypass grafting. He is currently on mechanical ventilation and requires vasopressors for hypotension. He underwent coronary angiography 12 hours prior to surgery. The serum creatinine has increased from 0.8 mg/dL (70.7 µmol/L) at baseline to 2.2 mg/dL (194.5 µmol/L), and urine output has decreased to 350 mL/24 h. History is significant for type 2 diabetes mellitus and coronary artery disease. Current medications are intravenous furosemide, insulin, propofol, fentanyl, and norepinephrine.

On physical examination, the patient is intubated and mechanically ventilated. A urinary catheter is in place. Temperature is 37.9 °C (100.2 °F), blood pressure is 98/60 mm Hg, pulse rate is 105/min, respiration rate is 28/min, and oxygen saturation is 96% on 30% FIO₂. There is no rash. Decreased breath sounds are heard in the lung bases. The remainder of the examination is noncontributory.

**Which of the following is the most appropriate test to perform next?**

(A) Examination of urine sediment
(B) Fractional excretion of sodium
(C) Kidney ultrasonography
(D) Measurement of central venous pressure

## Item 60

A 42-year-old woman is evaluated during a routine visit. She recently had her blood pressure measured at her workplace; two measurements were taken, and both were elevated. The patient feels well, and review of systems is unremarkable. Family history is significant for hypertension in her father, mother, and two siblings; stroke in her father; and heart failure in her mother. She takes no medications.

On physical examination, the average of three blood pressure measurements is 128/78 mm Hg. BMI is 30. The remainder of the examination is normal.

**Laboratory studies:**

| | |
|---|---|
| Bicarbonate | 24 mEq/L (24 mmol/L) |
| Creatinine | 0.9 mg/dL (79.6 µmol/L) |
| Potassium | 4.0 mEq/L (4.0 mmol/L) |
| Urine albumin-creatinine ratio | 10 mg/g |

Electrocardiogram reveals normal sinus rhythm and positive voltage criteria for left ventricular hypertrophy.

**Which of the following is the most appropriate test to perform next?**

(A) 24-Hour ambulatory blood pressure monitoring
(B) Plasma aldosterone concentration/plasma renin activity ratio
(C) Polysomnography
(D) Thyroid-stimulating hormone measurement

## Item 61

A 46-year-old man is evaluated during a follow-up visit for recently diagnosed hypertension. Hydrochlorothiazide, 25 mg/d, was initiated 1 month ago. He tries to adhere to a low sodium, low fat diet. The patient is black.

On physical examination, the average of three blood pressure measurements is 147/97 mm Hg, and pulse rate is 74/min. The remainder of the examination is normal.

Laboratory studies show a serum creatinine level of 1.2 mg/dL (106.1 µmol/L), a serum potassium level of 3.5 mEq/L (3.5 mmol/L), and a urine albumin-creatinine ratio of 15 mg/g.

**Which of the following is the most appropriate next step in management?**

(A) Add amlodipine
(B) Add lisinopril
(C) Increase hydrochlorothiazide
(D) Reassess blood pressure in 3 months

## Item 62

A 28-year-old woman is evaluated during a follow-up visit for elevated blood pressure measurements during pregnancy. She is at 12 weeks' gestation of her first pregnancy. She feels well, and the pregnancy has been otherwise uncomplicated. She did not have routine medical care before her pregnancy. Family history is significant for hypertension in her father and sister. Her only medication is a prenatal vitamin.

On physical examination, blood pressure is 155/95 mm Hg; other vital signs are normal. Funduscopic, neurologic, and cardiac examinations are normal.

Laboratory studies are normal.

**Which of the following is the most likely cause of this patient's elevated blood pressure?**

(A) Chronic hypertension
(B) Gestational hypertension
(C) Normal physiologic changes in pregnancy
(D) Preeclampsia

## Item 63

A 73-year-old woman is hospitalized for an elevated serum creatinine level that has been unresponsive to intravenous fluids. She was evaluated in the emergency department 2 days ago for weakness, myalgia, arthralgia, and cough and admitted to the hospital. She has no other medical history and takes no medications.

On physical examination, the patient is afebrile. Blood pressure is 155/95 mm Hg, pulse rate is 70/min, and oxygen saturation is 98% breathing 2 L of oxygen per minute by nasal cannula. Cardiac examination is normal, without evidence of jugular venous distention. Dullness to percussion and diminished breath sounds are present at the posterior lung bases bilaterally. There is pitting lower extremity edema.

**Laboratory studies:**

| | |
|---|---|
| Hemoglobin | 9.9 g/dL (99 g/L) |
| Creatinine | Baseline 6 months ago: 0.7 mg/dL (61.9 µmol/L) |
| | Emergency department: 4.1 mg/dL (362.4 µmol/L) |
| | Hospital day 1: 4.3 mg/dL (380.1 µmol/L) |
| Antinuclear antibodies | Negative |
| Antimyeloperoxidase antibodies | Positive |
| Antiproteinase 3 antibodies | Negative |
| Urinalysis | 3+ blood; 2+ protein |

Chest radiograph shows diffuse infiltrates at the lung bases bilaterally.

Kidney biopsy shows necrotizing and crescentic glomerulonephritis with linear staining for IgG on immunofluorescence.

**Which of the following is the most appropriate diagnostic test to perform in this patient?**

(A) Anti–double-stranded DNA antibodies
(B) Anti–glomerular basement membrane antibodies
(C) Anti–phospholipase A2 receptor antibodies
(D) Antihistone antibodies

## Item 64

A 24-year-old woman is evaluated during a follow-up visit for elevated blood pressure measurements found on two separate occasions. The measurements were 144/94 mm Hg and 142/92 mm Hg. She states that going to the doctor makes her nervous, so she had her blood pressure measured at the local pharmacy, which was <130/80 mm Hg. Review of systems is otherwise unremarkable. She has no other pertinent personal or family history. She takes no medications.

On physical examination, the average of three blood pressure measurements is 143/93 mm Hg, and pulse rate is 80/min; other vital signs are normal. BMI is 21. The remainder of the examination is normal.

Laboratory studies show a serum creatinine level of 0.8 mg/dL (70.7 µmol/L), and a urine albumin-creatinine ratio is undetectable; pregnancy test results are negative.

Electrocardiogram is normal.

**Which of the following is the most appropriate next step in management?**

(A) Begin hydrochlorothiazide

(B) Obtain echocardiography

(C) Perform 24-hour ambulatory blood pressure monitoring

(D) Recheck blood pressure in 3 months

## Item 65

A 79-year-old woman is evaluated for hyperkalemia. She was admitted to the surgical ICU after having an urgent partial colectomy for a ruptured diverticulum with peritonitis. She was treated with intravenous fluids, antibiotics, and vasopressor therapy. Today, postoperative day 1, she is oliguric with urine output <5 mL/h for the past 4 hours. She is now weaned off the vasopressor therapy. History is significant for hypertension and stage G4 chronic kidney disease. Outpatient medications are amlodipine, irbesartan, and furosemide. Current medications are morphine, propofol, cefotaxime, and metronidazole.

On physical examination, the patient is intubated and mechanically ventilated. A urinary catheter is in place. Temperature is 38.9 °C (102.0 °F), blood pressure is 108/70 mm Hg, and pulse rate is 101/min. There is generalized anasarca. The abdomen is distended and quiet.

**Laboratory studies:**

| | |
|---|---|
| Creatinine | 3.6 mg/dL (318.2 µmol/L); baseline, 2.0 mg/dL (176.8 µmol/L) |
| Electrolytes: | |
| Sodium | 142 mEq/L (142 mmol/L) |
| Potassium | 7.1 mEq/L (7.1 mmol/L) |
| Chloride | 102 mEq/L (102 mmol/L) |
| Total bicarbonate | 17 mEq/L (17 mmol/L) |
| Arterial pH | 7.25 |
| Urine sediment | Brown granular casts |

Electrocardiogram shows peaked T waves with a QRS of 140 ms.

**In addition to intravenous calcium, insulin, and dextrose, which of the following is the most appropriate treatment?**

(A) Continuous renal replacement therapy

(B) Hemodialysis

(C) Intravenous furosemide

(D) Sodium bicarbonate

(E) Sodium polystyrene sulfonate enema

## Item 66

A 55-year-old man is evaluated for a 4-month history of persistent hyperkalemia. He also has long-standing type 2 diabetes mellitus complicated by retinopathy and nephropathy. Medications are basal and prandial insulin, atorvastatin, and aspirin.

On physical examination, vital signs are normal. Nonproliferative retinopathy is noted on funduscopic examination. The remainder of the physical examination is noncontributory.

**Laboratory studies:**

| | |
|---|---|
| Creatinine | 1.9 mg/dL (168 µmol/L) |
| Electrolytes: | |
| Sodium | 138 mEq/L (138 mmol/L) |
| Potassium | 5.1 mEq/L (5.1 mmol/L) |
| Chloride | 112 mEq/L (112 mmol/L) |
| Bicarbonate | 18 mEq/L (18 mmol/L) |
| Estimated glomerular filtration rate | 49 mL/min/1.73 m² |
| Urinalysis | pH 5.0; no blood, protein, glucose, erythrocytes, or leukocytes |
| Calculated urine anion gap | Positive |

**Which of the following is the most likely cause of the patient's acid-base disorder?**

(A) Chronic kidney disease

(B) Type 1 (hypokalemic distal) renal tubular acidosis

(C) Type 2 (proximal) renal tubular acidosis

(D) Type 4 (hyperkalemic distal) renal tubular acidosis

## Item 67

A 21-year-old woman is evaluated during a follow-up visit for a 1-year history of systemic lupus erythematosus. At the time of diagnosis, she presented with a malar rash and arthritis, along with positive antinuclear and anti–double-stranded DNA antibodies. Medications are hydroxychloroquine, low-dose prednisone, calcium, and vitamin D. She currently feels well and is asymptomatic.

Vital signs are normal, and the physical examination is unremarkable.

**Laboratory studies:**

| | |
|---|---|
| C3 | 40 mg/dL (400 mg/L) |
| C4 | 8 mg/dL (80 mg/L) |
| Anti–double-stranded DNA antibodies | Positive (titer: 1:320) |
| Urinalysis | 2+ blood; 2+ protein; dysmorphic erythrocytes; no casts |
| Urine protein-creatinine ratio | 600 mg/g |

Kidney ultrasound shows kidneys of normal size and echogenicity.

**Which of the following is the most appropriate next step in management?**

(A) Begin pulse glucocorticoids followed by cyclophosphamide

(B) Begin pulse glucocorticoids followed by mycophenolate mofetil

(C) Increase oral prednisone dose and add mycophenolate mofetil

(D) Schedule a kidney biopsy

## Item 68

A 45-year-old man is seen for a routine evaluation of his blood pressure. He has gained 1.5 kg (3.3 lb) since his last visit

CONT.

3 weeks ago. History is significant for stage G4 chronic kidney disease, hypertension, type 2 diabetes mellitus, and coronary artery disease. Medications are amlodipine, lisinopril, carvedilol, chlorthalidone, basal and prandial insulin, atorvastatin, and low-dose aspirin.

On physical examination, blood pressure is 165/100 mm Hg, pulse rate is 58/min, and respiration rate is 16/min. There is 1+ bilateral leg edema. The remainder of the physical examination is noncontributory.

**Laboratory studies:**

| | |
|---|---|
| Blood urea nitrogen | 44 mg/dL (15.7 mmol/L) |
| Creatinine | 2.8 mg/dL (247.5 µmol/L) |
| Potassium | 5.4 mEq/L (5.4 mmol/L) |
| Estimated glomerular filtration rate | 26 mL/min/1.73 m² |
| Urinalysis | Normal |

In addition to maintaining a low sodium diet, which of the following is the most appropriate treatment of this patient's blood pressure?

(A) Add hydralazine
(B) Add losartan
(C) Stop amlodipine; begin spironolactone
(D) Stop chlorthalidone; begin furosemide

## Item 69

A 52-year-old woman is hospitalized for a toe ulcer and foot pain occurring for 1 month. History is significant for stage G4 chronic kidney disease (estimated glomerular filtration rate, 22 mL/min/1.73 m²) and type 2 diabetes mellitus. Medications are lisinopril, sevelamer, sodium bicarbonate, insulin glargine, and insulin aspart.

On physical examination, vital signs are normal. A foul-smelling toe ulcer is present. Probe-to-bone test is positive.

A plain radiograph shows changes compatible with osteomyelitis. The patient undergoes wound débridement and bone biopsy.

Bone cultures are pending, and empiric antibiotic therapy is to be administered.

Which of the following is the most appropriate venous access strategy?

(A) Arteriovenous graft creation followed by peripherally inserted central catheter placement in opposite arm
(B) Peripherally inserted central catheter in the dominant arm
(C) Peripherally inserted central catheter in the nondominant arm
(D) Tunneled internal jugular central venous catheter

## Item 70

A 45-year-old woman is evaluated for elevated blood pressure found for the first time at her previous visit 1 month ago. She has a 7-year history of type 2 diabetes mellitus without retinopathy, as well as hyperlipidemia. Medications are metformin and atorvastatin.

On physical examination, blood pressure is 148/94 mm Hg (confirmed by home ambulatory blood pressure monitoring), and pulse rate is 74/min; other vital signs are normal. BMI is 32. The remainder of the physical examination is unremarkable.

Laboratory studies show a serum creatinine level of 0.9 mg/dL (79.6 µmol/L), a serum potassium level of 3.8 mEq/L (3.8 mmol/L), and a urine albumin-creatinine ratio of 50 mg/g.

The patient is instructed in appropriate lifestyle modifications.

Which of the following is the most appropriate treatment?

(A) Begin amlodipine
(B) Begin chlorthalidone
(C) Begin losartan
(D) Remeasure blood pressure in 2 months

## Item 71

A 50-year-old man is evaluated during a routine follow-up visit. History is significant for chronic kidney disease, long-standing hypertension, and HIV infection. His antiretroviral regimen was recently adjusted to a once-a-day dosing, with the integrase inhibitor raltegravir discontinued and dolutegravir started 3 weeks ago. In addition to dolutegravir, current medications are abacavir, lamivudine, and lisinopril.

Physical examination and vital signs are normal.

**Laboratory studies:**

| | |
|---|---|
| Serum creatinine | 1.5 mg/dL (132.6 µmol/L); baseline, 1.3 mg/dL (114.9 µmol/L) |
| Urinalysis | No blood, protein, or erythrocytes |
| Urine albumin-creatinine ratio | 100 mg/g (unchanged from baseline) |

Which of the following is the most appropriate next step in management?

(A) Discontinue lisinopril
(B) Measure a 24-hour urine creatinine clearance
(C) Reassess the serum creatinine level in 1 week
(D) No further assessment

## Item 72

A 42-year-old woman is evaluated in the emergency department for right flank pain of 3 hours' duration. History is significant for migraines. There is no family history of kidney stones. Medications are as-needed sumatriptan and daily topiramate.

On physical examination, right costovertebral angle tenderness is present.

**Laboratory studies:**

| | |
|---|---|
| Creatinine | 0.8 mg/dL (70.7 µmol/L) |
| Electrolytes: | |
|   Sodium | 138 mEq/L (138 mmol/L) |
|   Potassium | 3.5 mEq/L (3.5 mmol/L) |
|   Chloride | 104 mEq/L (104 mmol/L) |
|   Bicarbonate | 21 mEq/L (21 mmol/L) |
| Urinalysis | Specific gravity 1.005; pH 6.5; 1+ blood; negative leukocyte esterase; negative nitrites; 20-30 erythrocytes/hpf; 1-3 leukocytes/hpf; amorphous crystals |

CONT.

Noncontrast helical CT scan shows a 5-mm stone in the right proximal ureter.

**Which of the following is the most likely composition of this patient's kidney stone?**

(A) Calcium oxalate
(B) Calcium phosphate
(C) Cystine
(D) Struvite
(E) Uric acid

 **Item 73**

A 77-year-old man is evaluated for a 2-month history of worsening fatigue, increasing frequency of urination, nocturia, and anorexia. History is significant for hypertension, hypertriglyceridemia, gastroesophageal reflux disease, and depression. He has been taking low-dose aspirin and valsartan for more than 10 years, omeprazole and St. John's wort for 8 months, and fenofibrate for 2 months.

On physical examination, blood pressure is 150/79 mm Hg, and pulse rate is 82/min. The remainder of the examination is unremarkable.

**Laboratory studies:**
Creatinine  2.8 mg/dL (247.5 µmol/L); 9 months ago: 1.2 mg/dL (106.1 µmol/L)
Urinalysis  Specific gravity 1.008; trace blood; 2+ protein; 3-5 erythrocytes/hpf; 5-7 leukocytes/hpf

Kidney ultrasound shows 9-cm kidneys without hydronephrosis or calculi bilaterally.

**Which of the following is the most likely cause of the patient's kidney findings?**

(A) Aspirin
(B) Fenofibrate
(C) Omeprazole
(D) St. John's wort

 **Item 74**

A 54-year-old man is evaluated in the emergency department for a 5-day history of fever, fatigue, and bleeding gums. He was previously feeling well. He takes no medications.

On physical examination, the patient is pale and thin and appears chronically ill. Temperature is 39.0 °C (102.2 °F), blood pressure is 104/62 mm Hg, pulse rate is 108/min, respiration rate is 22/min, and oxygen saturation is 96% breathing ambient air. BMI is 22. Petechiae are present on the conjunctiva, forearms, and distal legs. Cardiac examination reveals tachycardia. There is no hepatosplenomegaly. There is no edema.

**Laboratory studies:**
Hemoglobin  8.8 g/dL (88 g/L)
Leukocyte count  111,000/µL (111 × 10⁹/L), 98% blasts
Platelet count  28,000/µL (28 × 10⁹/L)
Creatinine  1.2 mg/dL (106.1 µmol/L)

Electrolytes:
Sodium  134 mEq/L (134 mmol/L)
Potassium  6.4 mEq/L (6.4 mmol/L)
Chloride  104 mEq/L (104 mmol/L)
Bicarbonate  21 mEq/L (21 mmol/L)

Electrocardiogram reveals sinus tachycardia but is otherwise normal.

**Which of the following is the most appropriate next step in management?**

(A) Administer intravenous 0.9% saline
(B) Administer intravenous calcium gluconate
(C) Order a plasma potassium measurement
(D) Start inhaled albuterol
(E) Start sodium bicarbonate

 **Item 75**

A 65-year-old woman is evaluated for a 3-month history of increasing fatigue. History is significant for stage G4 chronic kidney disease and hypertension. Medications are sodium bicarbonate, sevelamer, furosemide, losartan, and amlodipine.

On physical examination, blood pressure is 120/60 mm Hg, and pulse rate is 75/min; other vital signs are normal. Conjunctival rim pallor is noted.

**Laboratory studies:**
Hemoglobin  8.5 g/dL (85 g/L)
Mean corpuscular volume  90 fL
Ferritin  600 ng/mL (600 µg/L)
Transferrin saturation  40%
Estimated glomerular filtration rate  25 mL/min/1.73 m²

Stool guaiac testing is negative.
Colonoscopy performed within the past 5 years was normal.

**Which of the following is the most appropriate treatment?**

(A) Discontinue losartan
(B) Schedule packed red blood cell transfusion
(C) Start an erythropoiesis-stimulating agent
(D) Start intravenous iron

 **Item 76**

A 52-year-old woman is evaluated in the emergency department for a 2-day history of lower extremity weakness and nausea. She reports no diarrhea. History is significant for hypertension treated with amlodipine. She has a history of alcohol abuse.

On physical examination, vital signs are normal. On neurologic examination, lower extremity strength is 4/5. The remainder of the examination is unremarkable.

**Laboratory studies:**
Albumin  3.0 g/dL (30 g/L)
Calcium  8.4 mg/dL (2.1 mmol/L)
Creatinine  0.7 mg/dL (61.9 µmol/L)

CONT.

Electrolytes:
| | |
|---|---|
| Sodium | 136 mEq/L (136 mmol/L) |
| Potassium | 2.1 mEq/L (2.1 mmol/L) |
| Chloride | 104 mEq/L (104 mmol/L) |
| Bicarbonate | 26 mEq/L (26 mmol/L) |
| Magnesium | 1.4 mg/dL (0.58 mmol/L) |
| Urine potassium | 30 mEq/L (30 mmol/L) |

**Which of the following is the most likely cause of this patient's hypokalemia?**

(A) Hypoalbuminemia
(B) Hypocalcemia
(C) Hypomagnesemia
(D) Poor nutrition

## Item 77

A 71-year-old man is evaluated in the hospital for an elevated serum creatinine level. He was hospitalized 2 days ago for a 4-day history of progressive right lower leg cellulitis. History is also significant for type 2 diabetes mellitus with prior episodes of cellulitis. Medications are basal and prandial insulin.

On physical examination, temperature is 38.9 °C (102.0 °F), blood pressure is 150/100 mm Hg, pulse rate is 100/min, and respiration rate is 20/min. A well-defined area of tender erythema and edema is present over the right foot and leg to just below the knee. The remainder of the examination is unremarkable.

**Laboratory studies:**
| | |
|---|---|
| Leukocyte count | 13,500/µL ($13.5 \times 10^9$/L) |
| C3 | 50 mg/dL (500 mg/L) |
| C4 | 12 mg/dL (120 mg/L) |
| Creatinine | On admission: 2.4 mg/dL (212.2 µmol/L); baseline: 1.1 mg/dL (97.2 µmol/L) |
| Urinalysis | 3+ blood; 3+ protein |
| Urine protein–creatinine ratio | 4100 mg/g |

Kidney biopsy shows endocapillary proliferation on light microscopy, co-dominant granular staining for C3 and IgA on immunofluorescence microscopy, and subepithelial hump-like deposits on electron microscopy.

**Which of the following is the most likely cause of this patient's kidney disease?**

(A) *Staphylococcus aureus*
(B) *Streptococcus agalactiae*
(C) *Streptococcus pneumoniae*
(D) *Streptococcus pyogenes*

## Item 78

A 72-year-old woman is evaluated during a routine visit. History is significant for hypertension treated with amlodipine and losartan. She has no other medical problems. She remains physically active and routinely plays tennis and golf.

On physical examination, blood pressure is 142/84 mm Hg, and pulse rate is 72/min; other vital signs are normal. BMI is 24. The remainder of the examination is unremarkable.

Laboratory studies show a serum creatinine level of 0.8 mg/dL (70.7 µmol/L) and a serum potassium level of 4.0 mEq/L (4.0 mmol/L).

**According to the target blood pressure goals recommended by the American College of Physicians and the American Academy of Family Physicians, which of the following would be an appropriate management?**

(A) Add chlorthalidone
(B) Increase the amlodipine dose
(C) Increase the losartan dose
(D) Make no changes to antihypertensive medications

## Item 79

A 56-year-old man is evaluated during a follow-up visit for diabetic nephropathy. He has a 15-year history of type 2 diabetes mellitus. Medications are insulin detemir, insulin aspart, lisinopril, furosemide, and atorvastatin.

On physical examination, blood pressure is 129/76 mm Hg; other vital signs are normal. The remainder of the examination is unremarkable.

**Laboratory studies:**
| | |
|---|---|
| Calcium | 9.5 mg/dL (2.4 mmol/L) |
| Phosphorus | 7.2 mg/dL (2.3 mmol/L) |
| Intact parathyroid hormone | 385 pg/mL (385 ng/L) |
| 25-Hydroxyvitamin D | 32 ng/mL (80 nmol/L) |
| Estimated glomerular filtration rate | 25 mL/min/1.73 m² |

**Which of the following is the most appropriate treatment?**

(A) Aluminum hydroxide
(B) Calcitriol
(C) Cinacalcet
(D) Sevelamer

## Item 80

A 38-year-old man is evaluated during a follow-up visit for elevated blood pressure found for the first time during his last visit. He reports back pain of several weeks' duration after an episode of heavy lifting at work. History is also notable for seasonal allergies. He currently takes ibuprofen daily for the back pain and loratadine as needed for allergies.

On physical examination, the patient is well developed and muscular, and in no apparent distress. The average of three blood pressure measurements is 139/84 mm Hg, and pulse rate is 52/min; other vital signs are normal. BMI is 26. The remainder of the examination is normal.

Office electrocardiogram is normal.

**In addition to follow-up in 1 month, which of the following is the most appropriate management?**

(A) Begin amlodipine
(B) Begin hydrochlorothiazide
(C) Discontinue ibuprofen
(D) Discontinue loratadine

## Item 81

A 29-year-old man is hospitalized for lower extremity edema and fatigue that has progressed over the past 6 months. Laboratory studies document kidney failure. History is notable for obesity. He has a remote history of intravenous drug use and a 5-year history of multiple sex partners (men and women). He takes no medications.

On physical examination, the patient is afebrile, and blood pressure is 148/94 mm Hg; other vital signs are normal. BMI is 38. There is no rash. There is pitting edema in the lower extremities to the ankles bilaterally. The remainder of the physical examination is unremarkable.

**Laboratory studies:**

| | |
|---|---|
| C3 | 60 mg/dL (600 mg/L) |
| C4 | 7.0 mg/dL (70 mg/L) |
| Creatinine | 2.8 mg/dL (247.5 µmol/L) |
| Urinalysis | 3+ blood; 3+protein |
| Urine protein-creatinine ratio | 2900 mg/g |

Kidney biopsy shows membranoproliferative glomerulonephritis on light microscopy, with immunofluorescence microscopy showing 3+ staining for IgG, 1+ staining for IgM, 2+ staining for C1q, and 2+ staining for C3.

**Results of which of the following tests will most likely explain this patient's findings?**

(A) Genetic mutations in alternative complement pathway proteins
(B) Hepatitis B surface antigen and surface antibodies
(C) Hepatitis C antibodies
(D) HIV antibodies

## Item 82

A 50-year-old man is evaluated for worsening right toe pain of 3 days' duration. He went to an urgent clinic 6 months ago for similar pain and was diagnosed with gout and hypertension. He has consumed illegally distilled alcohol (moonshine) for years. He is a native of Illinois, and his occupation history includes farming, tractor mechanic, and the postal service. His only medications are losartan and a 7-day course of ibuprofen for his previous gout attack. He reinitiated ibuprofen 2 days ago.

On physical examination, blood pressure is 148/84 mm Hg. The right great toe is red, swollen, warm, and tender to touch. There are no tophi. The remainder of the examination is unremarkable.

Kidney ultrasound shows echogenic but normal-sized kidneys bilaterally and no calculi.

**Laboratory studies:**

| | |
|---|---|
| Creatinine | 2.0 mg/dL (176.8 µmol/L) |
| Urate | 9.0 mg/dL (0.53 mmol/L) |
| Urinalysis | Specific gravity 1.009; pH 5.0; 2+ protein; 3-5 leukocytes/hpf; occasional fine granular and waxy casts |
| Urine protein-creatinine ratio | 1200 mg/g |

**Which of the following is the most likely diagnosis?**

(A) Analgesic nephropathy
(B) Balkan nephropathy
(C) Cadmium nephropathy
(D) Lead nephropathy

## Item 83

A 24-year-old woman is evaluated for progressive muscle weakness of several months' duration. She provides no pertinent personal or family history and takes no medications.

On physical examination, temperature is normal, blood pressure is 94/58 mm Hg, pulse rate is 98/min, and respiration rate is 16/min. BMI is 19. The remainder of the examination is normal.

**Laboratory studies:**

| | |
|---|---|
| Serum electrolytes: | |
|   Sodium | 142 mEq/L (142 mmol/L) |
|   Potassium | 2.8 mEq/L (2.8 mmol/L) |
|   Chloride | 120 mEq/L (120 mmol/L) |
|   Bicarbonate | 15 mEq/L (15 mmol/L) |
| Urine electrolytes: | |
|   Sodium | 18 mEq/L (18 mmol/L) |
|   Potassium | 8.0 mEq/L (8.0 mmol/L) |
|   Chloride | 32 mEq/L (32 mmol/L) |
| Urinalysis | pH 5.0; no blood or protein |

**Which of the following is the most likely cause of this patient's metabolic acidosis?**

(A) Laxative abuse
(B) Surreptitious vomiting
(C) Type 1 (hypokalemic distal) renal tubular acidosis
(D) Type 4 (hyperkalemic distal) renal tubular acidosis

## Item 84

A 51-year-old man is evaluated in the hospital for acute kidney injury. He was admitted 14 days ago with sepsis and community-acquired pneumonia requiring mechanical ventilation. He was treated empirically with ceftriaxone and azithromycin; additional medications included omeprazole, insulin, and subcutaneous heparin. On hospital day 3, blood cultures were positive for *Streptococcus pneumoniae*, and ceftriaxone was continued. Hospital course was complicated by the ICU stay, with mechanical ventilation and pneumothorax requiring thoracostomy tube placement. On admission, his serum creatinine level was 1.0 mg/dL (88.4 µmol/L), increasing to 1.9 mg/dL (168 µmol/L) on hospital day 10; omeprazole and ceftriaxone were discontinued, and he was transferred to the floor. Today, hospital day 14, he is oliguric. History is significant for hypertension and diabetes mellitus. Outpatient medications are losartan and metformin.

On hospital day 14, the patient is on 4-L oxygen by nasal cannula. A right-sided thoracostomy tube is in place. Temperature is 36.1 °C (97.0 °F), blood pressure is 145/78 mm Hg, pulse rate is 92/min, and respiration rate is 12/min. There are coarse rhonchi in the left lower lung field. The remainder of the examination is normal.

**Current (hospital day 14) laboratory studies:**

| | |
|---|---|
| Creatinine | 2.7 mg/dL (238.7 µmol/L) |
| Fractional excretion of sodium | 3% |
| Urinalysis | 2+ blood; 2+ protein; 5–10 erythrocytes/hpf; 5–10 leukocytes/hpf; 3–5 granular casts/hpf |
| Urine protein-creatinine ratio | 1100 mg/g |

Kidney ultrasound is normal and without hydronephrosis.

**Which of the following is the most appropriate next step in management?**

(A) Empiric glucocorticoids

(B) Kidney biopsy

(C) Normal saline fluid bolus

(D) Urinary catheter placement

## Item 85

A 30-year-old woman is evaluated because of her family history of kidney disease. Family history is notable for the following: older brother with end-stage kidney disease due to hereditary nephritis diagnosed by biopsy at age 18 years and now with a transplant at age 32 years; 50-year-old maternal uncle with end-stage kidney disease due to hereditary nephritis at age 31 years; mother and maternal grandmother with microscopic hematuria but normal kidney function; and younger brother and older sister without hematuria or proteinuria. The patient is planning for a pregnancy within the next year.

Physical examination and vital signs are normal.

Laboratory studies show a serum creatinine level of 0.7 mg/dL (61.9 µmol/L), and urinalysis shows 2+ blood and trace protein.

Kidney ultrasound shows bilateral kidneys of normal size and echogenicity with no masses or stones.

**Which of the following is the most appropriate to perform next?**

(A) Audiometry

(B) Genetic counseling

(C) Kidney biopsy

(D) Skin biopsy

## Item 86

A 46-year-old man is evaluated in the emergency department for right flank pain that began 3 hours ago. He describes the pain as sharp and severe with radiation to the right testicle. History is significant for chronic diarrhea from Crohn disease; he has two to three loose bowel movements each day. He reports no nausea, vomiting, or abdominal pain. He has no dysuria.

On physical examination, the patient appears uncomfortable. There is right costovertebral angle tenderness.

**Laboratory studies:**

Electrolytes:

| | |
|---|---|
| Sodium | 138 mEq/L (138 mmol/L) |
| Potassium | 3.9 mEq/L (3.9 mmol/L) |
| Chloride | 106 mEq/L (106 mmol/L) |
| Bicarbonate | 21 mEq/L (21 mmol/L) |
| Urinalysis | Specific gravity 1.025; pH 5.5; moderate blood; no protein, leukocyte esterase, or nitrites |

Kidney ultrasound shows a 6-mm stone at the right ureteral pelvic junction.

**Which of the following is the most likely composition of this patient's kidney stone?**

(A) Calcium oxalate

(B) Calcium phosphate

(C) Cystine

(D) Struvite

(E) Uric acid

## Item 87

A 54-year-old woman is evaluated in the emergency department for ataxia, confusion, and slurred speech occurring for several days. History is significant for antiphospholipid antibody syndrome with superior mesenteric artery embolus 1 year ago that required resection of a large segment of the small bowel. Her only medication is warfarin. There is no history of over-the-counter medication use.

On physical examination, blood pressure is 106/65 mm Hg, pulse rate is 95/min, and respiration rate is 20/min. The patient is confused, and her speech is slurred. She also has an unsteady, wide-based gait.

**Laboratory studies:**

| | |
|---|---|
| Blood urea nitrogen | 14 mg/dL (5.0 mmol/L) |

Electrolytes:

| | |
|---|---|
| Sodium | 141 mEq/L (141 mmol/L) |
| Potassium | 3.8 mEq/L (3.8 mmol/L) |
| Chloride | 105 mEq/L (105 mmol/L) |
| Bicarbonate | 16 mEq/L (16 mmol/L) |
| Glucose | 99 mg/dL (5.5 mmol/L) |
| Lactate | 0.8 mEq/L (0.8 mmol/L) |
| Osmolality | 298 mOsm/kg $H_2O$ |

Arterial blood gases:

| | |
|---|---|
| pH | 7.31 |
| $P_{CO_2}$ | 33 mm Hg (4.4 kPa) |
| Urinalysis | No protein, ketones, cells, or crystals |

Noncontrast CT of the head is normal.

**Which of the following is the most likely diagnosis?**

(A) D-Lactic acidosis

(B) Ethylene glycol toxicity

(C) Methanol toxicity

(D) Pyroglutamic acidosis

## Item 88

A 27-year-old woman seeks preconception counseling. She anticipates pregnancy within 3 to 6 months. She has a 10-year history of type 1 diabetes mellitus and a 3-year history of hypertension. Medications are basal and prandial insulin, losartan, and hydrochlorothiazide.

Vital signs include a blood pressure of 110/70 mm Hg and a pulse rate of 70/min. Physical examination findings are normal.

Laboratory studies show a urine albumin-creatinine ratio of 25 mg/g.

**Which of the following is the most appropriate next step in management?**

(A) Discontinue hydrochlorothiazide
(B) Discontinue losartan
(C) Discontinue losartan; begin lisinopril
(D) No changes until patient is pregnant

## Item 89

A 50-year-old man is evaluated during a follow-up visit for hypertension. Losartan was started 3 months ago. He is asymptomatic. Family history is notable for his father who was on chronic hemodialysis and died of a ruptured brain aneurysm at the age of 62 years.

On physical examination, blood pressure is 152/96 mm Hg, and pulse rate is 75/min; other vital signs are normal. BMI is 20. The thyroid gland is not enlarged. Abdominal examination reveals bilateral flank fullness and tenderness on deep palpation; the abdomen is otherwise soft and without bruits. The remainder of the examination is unremarkable.

**Laboratory studies:**

| | |
|---|---|
| Bicarbonate | 26 mEq/L (26 mmol/L) |
| Creatinine | 1.0 mg/dL (88.4 µmol/L) |
| Potassium | 4.7 mEq/L (4.7 mmol/L) |
| Urinalysis | Trace protein; 10–20 erythrocytes; 0-5 leukocytes |

**Which of the following is the most appropriate diagnostic test to perform next?**

(A) Kidney ultrasonography
(B) Plasma aldosterone concentration/plasma renin activity ratio
(C) Plasma fractionated metanephrines
(D) Thyroid-stimulating hormone

## Item 90

A 31-year-old woman seeks preconception counseling. She has end-stage kidney disease secondary to focal segmental glomerulosclerosis. She received a haploidentical kidney transplant from her brother 2 years ago. She had an acute rejection episode 18 months ago that was successfully treated with glucocorticoids, and kidney function has been stable since that time. She currently feels well and reports no symptoms. Current medications are mycophenolate mofetil, tacrolimus, and prednisone.

On physical examination, vital signs are normal. The allograft is palpable in the right lower quadrant and is nontender.

Laboratory studies show a serum creatinine level of 1.3 mg/dL (114.9 µmol/L).

**Which of the following is the most appropriate management?**

(A) Advise against pregnancy
(B) Discontinue mycophenolate mofetil; begin azathioprine
(C) Discontinue tacrolimus; begin cyclosporine
(D) Proceed with pregnancy without further intervention

## Item 91

A 54-year-old woman is evaluated for a 4-week history of dyspnea on exertion, malaise, fatigue, and anorexia. History is significant for hypertension, gout, and osteoarthritis. Medications are losartan, hydrochlorothiazide, allopurinol, naproxen, and aspirin.

On physical examination, blood pressure is 148/84 mm Hg, and pulse rate is 98/min; other vital signs are normal. Conjunctivae are pale. There is 2+ edema of the ankles.

**Laboratory studies:**

| | |
|---|---|
| Hemoglobin | 8.0 g/dL (80 g/L) |
| Albumin | 3.0 g/dL (30 g/L) |
| Calcium | 9.8 mg/dL (2.5 mmol/L) |
| Creatinine | 2.2 mg/dL (194.5 µmol/L); 3 weeks ago: 1.2 mg/dL (106.1 µmol/L) |
| Total protein | 8.4 g/dL (84 g/L) |
| Urate | 7.0 g/dL (0.41 mmol/L) |
| Urinalysis | 1+ protein; 2-5 granular casts/hpf; 1–2 erythrocytes/hpf |
| Urine protein-creatinine ratio | 6100 mg/g |

Chest radiograph is normal.

**Which of the following is the most likely diagnosis?**

(A) Light chain cast nephropathy
(B) NSAID-induced acute tubular injury
(C) Renal sarcoidosis
(D) Uric acid nephropathy

## Item 92

A 28-year-old woman is evaluated in the emergency department for hematuria of 12 hours' duration. She also reports upper respiratory infection symptoms for the past 2 days. She does not have dysuria or flank pain and is not currently menstruating. She reports a similar incident during college when she had the flu, but the urine cleared up after a few hours; she also had an episode of red urine after completing a half-marathon last year. She takes no medications.

Physical examination and vital signs are unremarkable.

**Laboratory studies:**

| | |
|---|---|
| C3 | Normal |
| C4 | Normal |
| Creatinine | Normal |
| Urinalysis | 4+ blood; 1+ protein; no leukocyte esterase; no nitrites |
| Pregnancy test | Negative |

Noncontrast CT scan of the abdomen shows no renal masses, no evidence of nephrolithiasis, and no hydronephrosis.

**Which of the following is the most likely diagnosis?**

(A) Acute postinfectious glomerulonephritis
(B) IgA nephropathy
(C) IgA vasculitis
(D) Lupus nephritis

## Item 93

A 76-year-old man is evaluated in the emergency department for confusion, an unsteady gait, tinnitus, nausea, and vomiting. His family has noticed progressive functional decline over the past 2 weeks. History is significant for osteoarthritis. His only medication is aspirin.

On physical examination, the patient is tachypneic and obtunded. Temperature is normal, blood pressure is 140/68 mm Hg, pulse rate is 96/min, respiration rate is 24/min, and oxygen saturation is 99% breathing ambient air. The neurologic examination is nonfocal.

**Laboratory studies:**
Electrolytes:
    Sodium          142 mEq/L (142 mmol/L)
    Potassium     3.2 mEq/L (3.2 mmol/L)
    Chloride       100 mEq/L (100 mmol/L)
    Bicarbonate   20 mEq/L (20 mmol/L)
Arterial blood gases:
    pH              7.56
    $P_{CO_2}$         22 mm Hg (2.9 kPa)

**Which of the following is the most likely acid–base diagnosis?**

(A) Respiratory alkalosis with chronic compensation
(B) Respiratory alkalosis and increased anion gap metabolic acidosis
(C) Respiratory alkalosis and metabolic alkalosis
(D) Respiratory alkalosis, increased anion gap metabolic acidosis, and metabolic alkalosis

## Item 94

A 65-year-old man is evaluated for a 2-month history of low back pain. The pain is worse with movement, but it does not radiate. He reports associated fatigue and a 4.5-kg (10-lb) weight loss. He has osteoarthritis and gastroesophageal reflux disease. He has been taking ibuprofen without any pain relief. His only other medication is omeprazole.

The physical examination, including vital signs and neurologic examination, is normal.

**Laboratory studies:**
Hemoglobin      9.2 g/dL (92 g/L)
Creatinine       3.0 mg/dL (265.2 µmol/L)
Urinalysis       Trace protein; no blood, erythrocytes, leukocytes, leukocyte esterase, or nitrites
Urine protein-
creatinine ratio   2500 mg/g

Ultrasound reveals normal-sized kidneys with slightly increased echogenicity; no hydronephrosis or abnormalities of the collecting system are seen.

**In addition to discontinuing ibuprofen, which of the following is the most appropriate next step in management?**

(A) Discontinue omeprazole
(B) Obtain a 24-hour urine protein collection
(C) Obtain a noncontrast helical abdominal CT
(D) Obtain a urine protein electrophoresis

## Item 95

A 60-year-old woman is evaluated for fatigue and weakness. She reports no nausea or vomiting. History is significant for hypertension, stage G4 chronic kidney disease, and type 2 diabetes mellitus. Medications are labetalol, amlodipine, insulin glargine, insulin lispro, and sodium bicarbonate.

On physical examination, blood pressure is 140/90 mm Hg; other vital signs are normal. A mature radiocephalic arteriovenous fistula (AVF) with a strong thrill and bruit is noted. There are no lung crackles. Trace pedal edema is present.

Laboratory studies show normal serum bicarbonate and potassium levels, a blood urea nitrogen level of 50 mg/dL (17.8 mmol/L), and an estimated glomerular filtration rate of 18 mL/min/1.73 m².

**Which of the following is the most appropriate management?**

(A) Clinical follow-up in 6 months
(B) Fistulography to evaluate patency of AVF
(C) Hemodialysis
(D) Kidney transplant evaluation

## Item 96

A 55-year-old woman is evaluated for increasing serum creatinine and oliguria; she has cirrhosis. She was hospitalized 3 days ago for worsening ascites, confusion, and an elevated serum creatinine level of 1.5 mg/dL ([132.6 µmol/L]; baseline, 1.1 mg/dL [97.2 µmol/L]). Her diuretics were held, and lactulose was continued. An abdominal paracentesis was negative for spontaneous bacterial peritonitis. Intravenous albumin was administered at 1 g/kg/d for 2 days, and today her serum creatinine level is 3.0 mg/dL (265.2 µmol/L). Urine output for the previous 24 hours was 300 mL. History is significant for cirrhosis secondary to nonalcoholic steatohepatitis. Outpatient medications are lactulose, spironolactone, furosemide, and propranolol.

On physical examination, the patient is confused. She is afebrile, blood pressure is 100/70 mm Hg (stable since admission), pulse rate is 84/min, and respiration rate is 16/min. Asterixis is noted. The skin and sclera are icteric. The jugular venous pressure is normal. Ascites is present. There is 3+ lower extremity edema. The remainder of the examination is normal.

CONT.

Current laboratory studies:

| | |
|---|---|
| Bicarbonate | 18 mEq/L (18 mmol/L) |
| Creatinine | 3.0 mg/dL (265.2 µmol/L) |
| Potassium | 5 mEq/L (5 mmol/L) |
| Sodium | 129 mEq/L (129 mmol/L) |
| Urine sodium | <10 mEq/L (10 mmol/L) |
| Urinalysis | Specific gravity 1.025; pH 5.0; trace protein; 2-4 erythrocytes/hpf; 1-3 pigmented granular casts/hpf |

Abdominal ultrasound demonstrates ascites, and normal-sized kidneys with no hydronephrosis.

**Which of the following is the most appropriate treatment?**

(A) Hemodialysis

(B) Isotonic crystalloid

(C) Octreotide and oral midodrine

(D) Transjugular intrahepatic portosystemic shunt

## Item 97

A 56-year-old woman is evaluated for hypernatremia. She was admitted to the ICU 6 days ago for pyelonephritis and septic shock requiring intubation, administration of fluids, norepinephrine, and cefepime. She developed nonoliguric acute kidney injury. She has been weaned off the norepinephrine, and she has been extubated. Her serum sodium level has increased from 142 mEq/L (142 mmol/L) to 148 mEq/L (148 mmol/L) over the past 72 hours.

Physical examination and vital signs are normal.
Urine output is 2.5 L over the past 24 hours.

Laboratory studies:

| | |
|---|---|
| Blood urea nitrogen | 74 mg/dL (26.4 mmol/L) |
| Creatinine | 2.8 mg/dL (247.5 µmol/L) |
| Electrolytes: | |
|    Sodium | 148 mEq/L (148 mmol/L) |
|    Potassium | 3.7 mEq/L (3.7 mmol/L) |
|    Chloride | 112 mEq/L (112 mmol/L) |
|    Bicarbonate | 26 mEq/L (26 mmol/L) |
| Glucose | 136 mg/dL (7.5 mmol/L) |
| Urine osmolality | 420 mOsm/kg $H_2O$ |

**Which of the following is the most likely cause of this patient's hypernatremia?**

(A) Adrenal insufficiency

(B) Central diabetes insipidus

(C) Glycosuria

(D) Osmotic diuresis

## Item 98

A 55-year-old man is evaluated for an increase in his serum creatinine level. History is significant for hypertension treated with lisinopril for 3 years. He reports no changes or additions to his medication regimen during the past year.

On physical examination, the patient is afebrile, blood pressure is 145/92 mm Hg, and pulse rate is 84/min. There is no rash, alopecia, or joint abnormalities. The remainder of the examination is unremarkable.

Laboratory studies:

| | |
|---|---|
| Complete blood count | Normal |
| Creatinine | First specimen, 1.3 mg/dL (114.9 µmol/L); repeat specimen, 1.5 mg/dL (132.6 µmol/L); baseline 6 months ago, 0.9 mg/dL (79.6 µmol/L) |
| Estimated glomerular filtration rate (eGFR), using the Chronic Kidney Disease Epidemiology (CKD-EPI) Collaboration creatinine formula | >60 mL/min/1.73 m² |
| Urinalysis | Trace protein |

Ultrasound reveals normal-sized kidneys with increased echogenicity, and no hydronephrosis or abnormalities of the collecting system are seen.

**Which of the following is the most appropriate management?**

(A) Discontinue lisinopril

(B) Obtain a 24-hour creatinine clearance

(C) Recalculate the eGFR using the CKD-EPI cystatin C formula

(D) Schedule a kidney biopsy

## Item 99

An 82-year-old woman is evaluated during a follow-up visit for stage G5 chronic kidney disease. History is also significant for coronary artery bypass graft surgery 10 years ago, peripheral vascular disease, oxygen-dependent COPD, anemia, mild-moderate vascular dementia, and a transient ischemic attack 2 years ago. She has increasing difficulty with activities of daily living and mobility. She has an 80-pack-year history of smoking, having quit 10 years ago. Medications are albuterol, tiotropium, fluticasone-salmeterol inhalers, metoprolol, atorvastatin, iron, and low-dose aspirin. She currently lives in a nursing home.

On physical examination, the patient appears thin and frail. Vital signs include a blood pressure of 108/62 mm Hg, a respiration rate of 22/min, and an oxygen saturation of 92% on 2-L/min oxygen by nasal cannula. BMI is 19. Diminished breath sounds are present throughout the lungs. There is no edema or asterixis.

Laboratory studies:

| | |
|---|---|
| Blood urea nitrogen | 79 mg/dL (28.2 mmol/L) |
| Creatinine | 4.6 mg/dL (406.6 µmol/L) |
| Potassium | 4.6 mEq/L (4.6 mmol/L) |
| Estimated glomerular filtration rate | 9.7 mL/min/1.73 m² |

**Which of the following is the most appropriate care strategy for this patient?**

(A) Creation of an arteriovenous fistula for dialysis access

(B) Discussion of non-dialytic options

(C) Placement of a double-lumen catheter for long-term hemodialysis

(D) Placement of a peritoneal dialysis catheter

## Item 100

A 62-year-old man is evaluated during a follow-up visit for difficult-to-control hypertension. He also has chronic kidney disease and hyperlipidemia. Medications are atorvastatin and carvedilol, as well as maximum doses of lisinopril, amlodipine, and hydralazine.

On physical examination, the average of three blood pressure measurements is 152/98 mm Hg, and pulse rate is 65/min. There is 1+ pitting pretibial lower extremity edema. The remainder of the examination is normal.

**Laboratory studies:**

| | |
|---|---|
| Creatinine | 2.5 mg/dL (221 µmol/L) |
| Potassium | 4.8 mEq/L (4.8 mmol/L) |
| Estimated glomerular filtration rate | 28 mL/min/1.73 m$^2$ |
| Urine albumin-creatinine ratio | 350 mg/g |

**Which of the following is the most appropriate additional treatment?**

(A) Chlorthalidone
(B) Furosemide
(C) Hydrochlorothiazide
(D) Losartan

## Item 101

A 64-year-old man is evaluated for a 5-day history of increased urination and weakness. He was recently diagnosed with non–small cell lung cancer and started on chemotherapy 10 days ago. Medications are cisplatin, gemcitabine, paclitaxel, bevacizumab, and ondansetron.

Physical examination reveals a chronically ill–appearing man. Blood pressure is 105/72 mm Hg, and pulse rate is 100/min; other vital signs are normal. The remainder of the examination is unremarkable.

**Laboratory studies:**

| | |
|---|---|
| Complete blood count | Normal |
| Calcium | 8 mg/dL (2 mmol/L) |
| Creatinine | 2.1 mg/dL (185.6 µmol/L); baseline, 0.9 mg/dL (79.6 µmol/L) |
| Electrolytes: | |
|   Sodium | 132 mEq/L (132 mmol/L) |
|   Potassium | 2.8 mEq/L (2.8 mmol/L) |
|   Chloride | 105 mEq/L (105 mmol/L) |
|   Bicarbonate | 18 mEq/L (18 mmol/L) |
| Glucose | 90 g/dL (5 mmol/L) |
| Magnesium | 1.5 mg/dL (0.62 mmol/L) |
| Phosphorous | 1.9 mg/dL (0.61 mmol/L) |
| Fractional excretion of sodium | 2% |
| Urinalysis | Specific gravity 1.010; pH 6.0; 1+ protein; 1+ glucose; occasional granular casts |

**Which of the following is the most likely cause of this patient's acute kidney injury?**

(A) Bevacizumab
(B) Cisplatin
(C) Gemcitabine
(D) Paclitaxel

## Item 102

A 55-year-old man is evaluated during a routine visit. He was diagnosed with primary focal segmental glomerulosclerosis 2 months ago. History is also significant for hypertension. Medications are furosemide, amlodipine, losartan, and prednisone. He has been instructed on a low-sodium diet.

On physical examination, blood pressure is 136/86 mm Hg, and pulse rate is 70/min; other vital signs are normal. Jugular venous pressure is elevated to 14 cm $H_2O$. Cardiac examination reveals an $S_3$ gallop. The lungs are clear to auscultation. There is 1+ pitting pretibial edema bilaterally.

**Laboratory studies:**

| | |
|---|---|
| Creatinine | 1.6 mg/dL (141.4 µmol/L) |
| Potassium | 4.5 mEq/L (4.5 mmol/L) |
| Estimated glomerular filtration rate | 40 mL/min/1.73 m$^2$ |
| Urine albumin-creatinine ratio | 1000 mg/g |

**Which of the following is the most appropriate treatment?**

(A) Increase the amlodipine dose
(B) Increase the furosemide dose
(C) Initiate treatment with lisinopril
(D) No changes to medication regimen

## Item 103

A 55-year-old man is evaluated during a follow-up visit for newly diagnosed chronic kidney disease (CKD). He also has a 10-year history of hypertension treated with losartan.

On physical examination, blood pressure is 135/78 mm Hg. BMI is 32. The remainder of the vital signs and examination is unremarkable.

**Laboratory studies:**

| | |
|---|---|
| Bicarbonate | 22 mEq/L (22 mmol/L) |
| Blood urea nitrogen | 27 mg/dL (9.6 mmol/L) |
| Creatinine | 2.1 mg/dL (185.6 µmol/L) |
| Potassium | 4.9 mEq/L (4.9 mmol/L) |
| Estimated glomerular filtration rate | 34 mL/min/1.73 m$^2$ |
| Urinalysis | No blood; 2+ protein |

**Which of the following additional measurement could best predict this patient's CKD progression?**

(A) Serum albumin
(B) Serum calcium
(C) Serum phosphate
(D) Urine albumin-creatinine ratio

## Item 104

A 48-year-old woman is evaluated for edema, dyspnea, and proteinuria. She has a 10-year history of rheumatoid arthritis. She was initially treated with NSAIDs, methotrexate, and prednisone. She stopped taking the NSAIDs 6 months ago because of gastritis. Three months ago she began noticing swelling of her legs, and two weeks ago she began experiencing dyspnea when walking. She has never received penicillamine, gold, or a biologic agent. Current medications are methotrexate, prednisone, and omeprazole.

On physical examination, the patient appears chronically ill. Temperature is 37.2 °C (99.0 °F), blood pressure is 158/90 mm Hg, pulse rate is 96/min, and respiration rate is 20/min. Jugular venous pressure is elevated. Cardiac examination reveals a summation gallop. The lungs are clear. Swelling and tenderness at the metacarpophalangeal joints and wrists are noted. There is 3+ lower extremity edema to the knees.

**Laboratory studies:**

| | |
|---|---|
| Albumin | 2.8 g/dL (28 g/L) |
| Creatinine | 1.1 mg/dL (97.2 µmol/L) |
| Serum protein electrophoresis | Polyclonal gammopathy |
| Urinalysis | Specific gravity 1.0120; pH 5.5; no blood; 4+ protein |
| Urine protein-creatinine ratio | 6000 mg/g |

Electrocardiogram reveals low voltage, pronounced in the limb leads, but without acute changes.

**Which of the following is the most likely cause of this patient's proteinuria?**

(A) AA amyloidosis
(B) Focal segmental glomerulosclerosis
(C) Minimal change glomerulopathy
(D) NSAID-associated interstitial nephritis
(E) Proton pump–associated interstitial nephritis

## Item 105

A 46-year-old man is evaluated during a follow-up visit for elevated blood pressure. His average blood pressure with home blood pressure monitoring is 126/77 mm Hg. He has no other pertinent medical history and takes no medications.

On physical examination, blood pressure is 128/78 mm Hg; other vital signs are normal. BMI is 28. The remainder of the examination is unremarkable.

**Which of the following is the most appropriate next step in management?**

(A) Initiate therapy with an angiotensin receptor blocker
(B) Initiate therapy with a thiazide diuretic
(C) Initiate a trial of lifestyle modification
(D) Remeasure blood pressure in 1 year

## Item 106

A 70-year-old man is evaluated for a recent onset of macroscopic hematuria. History is significant for end-stage kidney disease and hypertension. He has been on hemodialysis for 3 years. Urine output is approximately 250 mL/d. Medications are sevelamer, sodium bicarbonate, lisinopril, and amlodipine.

On physical examination, blood pressure is 150/90 mm Hg, and pulse rate is 70/min. Bilateral flank tenderness is noted. There is no abdominal mass.

Laboratory studies show a hemoglobin level of 15 g/dL (150 g/L).

Kidney ultrasound shows several complex cysts and two bilateral solid masses.

**Which of the following is the most appropriate management?**

(A) Bilateral partial nephrectomy
(B) Bilateral radical nephrectomy
(C) Percutaneous kidney biopsy
(D) Surveillance ultrasonography

## Item 107

A 42-year-old man is evaluated for an elevated blood pressure measurement of 136/86 mm Hg found during a routine screening at his workplace. He exercises 5 days a week for 45 minutes and adheres to a low fat, low salt diet. Family history is significant for hypertension in his father and mother; his father died of a stroke at the age of 55 years. He takes no medications. The patient is black.

On physical examination, the patient is well developed and muscular. The average of three blood pressure measurements is 126/75 mm Hg, and pulse rate is 52/min. BMI is 24.5. The remainder of the examination is unremarkable.

**Which of the following is the most appropriate management?**

(A) Amlodipine
(B) Annual blood pressure screening
(C) Blood pressure screening in 3 months
(D) Hydrochlorothiazide

## Item 108

A 62-year-old woman is evaluated during a follow-up visit for stage G5 chronic kidney disease. She is not a transplant candidate. She has opted for hemodialysis for her eventual dialysis modality; an arteriovenous fistula was created 6 months ago. She is active, has a fair appetite, and is sleeping well. She reports no nausea or vomiting. History is also significant for hypertension and secondary hyperparathyroidism. Medications are furosemide, amlodipine, epoetin alfa, sevelamer, calcitriol, and sodium bicarbonate.

On physical examination, blood pressure is 144/85 mm Hg; other vital signs are normal. The left upper extremity arteriovenous fistula appears functioning. There is no asterixis. There is 2+ lower extremity edema.

**Laboratory studies:**

| | |
|---|---|
| Bicarbonate | 21 mEq/L (21 mmol/L) |
| Blood urea nitrogen | 89 mg/dL (31.7 mmol/L) |
| Creatinine | 4.8 mg/dL (424.3 µmol/L) |
| Potassium | 4.8 mEq/L (4.8 mmol/L) |
| Estimated glomerular filtration rate | 9.7 mL/min/1.73 m² |

**Which of the following is the most appropriate management for this patient?**

(A) Delay dialysis until uremic symptoms occur
(B) Discontinue diuretics
(C) Refer for palliative care
(D) Start dialysis now

# Answers and Critiques

## Item 1    Answer:    A

**Educational Objective:** Use ambulatory blood pressure monitoring to evaluate antihypertensive treatment.

The most appropriate management is to decrease the hydrochlorothiazide dose and obtain ambulatory blood pressure monitoring (ABPM). The patient presents with orthostatic hypotension that likely resulted in his near-syncope and fall due to a recent increase in the dose of a thiazide diuretic. The maximal daily recommended dose for hydrochlorothiazide is 25 mg for the treatment of hypertension; side effects increase beyond this dose with little further antihypertensive effect. Increasing the daily dose to 50 mg likely resulted in an orthostatic drop in his blood pressure, and his pulse rate did not change because he is on a β-blocker. Additional evidence of overtreatment includes an increase in his serum creatinine level, hyponatremia, hypokalemia, and the development of metabolic alkalosis. The appropriate next step is to lower his hydrochlorothiazide dose and obtain ABPM, which is valuable in providing information supplementary to office blood pressure measurements in clinical situations such as hypotensive symptoms from antihypertensive medication treatment. ABPM may reveal that the patient has an element of white coat hypertension and that his blood pressures at home are well controlled on his previous lower dose of hydrochlorothiazide.

Bilateral carotid ultrasonography is not the appropriate next step for this patient. Although he has evidence of atherosclerotic vascular disease and may have carotid stenosis, it is an unlikely cause of near-syncope and falling. The dizziness and fall were most likely the result of orthostasis.

In a study of 1920 hospitalized patients with syncope, the most commonly ordered tests, in addition to electrocardiography, were telemetry (95%), cardiac enzymes (95%), and CT of the head (63%). These tests, along with echocardiography, carotid ultrasonography, and electroencephalography, aided diagnosis in <2% of patients and altered management decisions in <5% of patients. The most valuable diagnostic and management test was postural blood pressure. The American College of Physicians does not recommend brain imaging, with either CT or MRI, in the evaluation of a patient with simple syncope and a normal neurologic examination.

### KEY POINT

- Ambulatory blood pressure monitoring provides valuable information supplementary to office blood pressure measurements in the evaluation of antihypertensive treatment.

### Bibliography

Di Stefano C, Milazzo V, Totaro S, Sobrero G, Ravera A, Milan A, et al. Orthostatic hypotension in a cohort of hypertensive patients referring to a hypertension clinic. J Hum Hypertens. 2015;29:599-603. [PMID: 25631221]

## Item 2    Answer:    B

**Educational Objective:** Diagnose glomerulopathy with a kidney biopsy.

A kidney biopsy is the most appropriate next step for this patient who has the nephrotic syndrome most likely caused by minimal change glomerulopathy (MCG). MCG is the cause of the nephrotic syndrome in 10% to 15% of adults, with a significantly higher incidence in elderly patients (≥65 years of age) and very elderly patients (≥80 years of age). Most cases are idiopathic, but secondary causes must be considered in adults, including medications such as NSAIDs. Adults with MCG present with acute kidney injury (AKI) in up to 25% of cases. Factors associated with AKI include older age, male sex, hypertension, low serum albumin levels, and heavier proteinuria. The differential diagnosis for the nephrotic syndrome with AKI is limited to only a few entities: MCG with acute tubular necrosis or allergic interstitial nephritis, membranous glomerulopathy with bilateral renal vein thrombosis, amyloidosis with cast nephropathy, and collapsing focal segmental glomerulosclerosis. A kidney biopsy is therefore required to make the correct diagnosis.

Dialysis is used to control complications of severe AKI. Absolute indications for dialysis include hyperkalemia, metabolic acidosis, and pulmonary edema refractory to medical therapy; uremic symptoms; uremic pericarditis; and certain drug intoxications. This patient has no indication for dialysis.

The pathophysiology of hypercoagulability in the nephrotic syndrome is not well understood, nor has the mechanism underlying the higher propensity for thromboembolism in membranous glomerulopathy been well defined. There are no randomized clinical trials of prophylactic anticoagulation in patients with the nephrotic syndrome to guide clinical decision-making; in the absence of known risk and benefits, many experts recommend against prophylactic anticoagulation. Anticoagulation is typically recommended for patients with documented renal vein thrombosis to prevent further propagation of the thrombus and systemic embolization. The patient's ultrasound does not show evidence of renal vein thrombosis, and anticoagulation should be withheld.

Although this presentation is most suggestive of MCG given the patient's age, empiric glucocorticoids would not be indicated without a biopsy-confirmed diagnosis because glucocorticoids would not be efficacious in the treatment of membranous glomerulopathy or amyloidosis.

### KEY POINT

- A kidney biopsy is required to make the diagnosis of glomerulopathy associated with the nephrotic syndrome in adult patients.

## Bibliography

Waldman M, Crew RJ, Valeri A, Busch J, Stokes B, Markowitz G, et al. Adult minimal-change disease: clinical characteristics, treatment, and outcomes. Clin J Am Soc Nephrol. 2007;2:445-53. [PMID: 17699450]

## Item 3    Answer:    D

**Educational Objective:** Treat chronic metabolic acidosis in a patient with chronic kidney disease.

Sodium bicarbonate therapy is the most likely treatment to slow progression of this patient's chronic kidney disease (CKD). Metabolic acidosis frequently occurs in patients with CKD due to defective acid excretion (resulting in reduced bicarbonate generation), most commonly due to impaired ammoniagenesis. Untreated metabolic acidosis can lead to muscle loss and bone loss. In early CKD, metabolic acidosis is typically a normal anion gap hyperchloremic metabolic acidosis. As glomerular filtration rate (GFR) declines, organic and inorganic anions are retained, and an anion gap metabolic acidosis develops. Large observational studies have shown a strong association between lower serum bicarbonate levels and both increased progression of CKD and mortality. Alkali therapy, most commonly sodium bicarbonate or sodium citrate, can delay the progression of CKD. Therefore, the Kidney Disease: Improving Global Outcomes (KDIGO) guidelines recommend starting alkali therapy when the serum bicarbonate is chronically <22 mEq/L (22 mmol/L). The alkali salt therapy dose should be titrated to achieve a serum bicarbonate level within the normal range; excessive alkali therapy in the setting of a reduced GFR may induce a metabolic alkalosis, which is associated with increased mortality. Patients with CKD who are treated with alkali should be monitored for symptoms of volume overload.

Blood pressure control, particularly with renin-angiotensin system agents, has been shown to slow progression of proteinuric renal diseases and especially diabetes mellitus. However, this patient is already taking an angiotensin receptor blocker (ARB), and dual therapy with an ACE inhibitor and an ARB may instead be detrimental because studies of dual blockade have shown increased risks of acute kidney disease and hyperkalemia.

As the estimated GFR declines below 30 mL/min/1.73 m$^2$ (stages G4-G5), anemia can become symptomatic. Erythropoiesis-stimulating agents (ESAs) are highly effective in raising hemoglobin concentrations and alleviating symptoms but have not been shown to slow progression of CKD. These agents are associated with risks and are expensive. Black box warnings for use of ESAs include the risk of increased mortality and/or tumor progression in patients with active malignancy, increased risk of thromboembolic events for postsurgical patients not on anticoagulant therapy, and increased risk of serious cardiovascular events when ESAs are administered to patients with hemoglobin values >11 g/dL (110 g/L).

Although poorly controlled hyperphosphatemia is associated with a greater risk of CKD progression, optimizing mineral metabolism parameters with a phosphate binder has not been shown to slow progression of CKD.

### KEY POINT

- The Kidney Disease: Improving Global Outcomes (KDIGO) guidelines recommend treatment of metabolic acidosis with alkali therapy in patients with chronic kidney disease when the serum bicarbonate is chronically <22 mEq/L (22 mmol/L).

## Bibliography

Kraut JA, Madias NE. Metabolic acidosis of CKD: an update. Am J Kidney Dis. 2016;67:307-17. [PMID: 26477665]

## Item 4    Answer:    B

**Educational Objective:** Treat minimal change glomerulopathy.

Diuretics plus high-dose prednisone is the most appropriate treatment for this patient with minimal change glomerulopathy (MCG; also known as minimal change disease). MCG is the most common cause of the nephrotic syndrome in children and accounts for approximately 10% to 15% of cases in adults. Immunosuppressive therapy is indicated for treatment of primary MCG, which invariably presents with the full nephrotic syndrome. The concomitant acute tubular necrosis makes treatment even more imperative in this case, because primary MCG with acute kidney injury has been shown to be a treatment-responsive lesion if treated in a timely manner. First-line therapy is prednisone at a dose of 1 mg/kg per day or 2 mg/kg every other day for 8 to 12 weeks, followed by a taper. Patients typically respond to glucocorticoids within 8 to 16 weeks. However, relapse is common, and in a substantial percentage of patients, the course of MCG is one of remission followed by relapse. For frequently relapsing or glucocorticoid-dependent disease, treatment options include cyclophosphamide, calcineurin inhibitors (tacrolimus or cyclosporine), mycophenolate mofetil, and rituximab. In addition to immunosuppression, patients should receive standard therapy for the nephrotic syndrome, including an ACE inhibitor or angiotensin receptor blocker (this patient is already taking lisinopril, with well-controlled blood pressure), diuretics for edema management, and cholesterol-lowering medication if total cholesterol >200 mg/dL (5.1 mmol/L). In rare cases of MCG secondary to malignancies (Hodgkin lymphoma, non-Hodgkin lymphoma, thymoma), medications (NSAIDs, lithium), infections (strongyloides, syphilis, mycoplasma, ehrlichiosis), and atopy (pollen, dairy products), treatment of the underlying condition without immunosuppression may be sufficient.

Cyclosporine and rituximab are generally reserved for glucocorticoid-resistant or glucocorticoid-dependent cases of MCG and, except for a clear contraindication to glucocorticoids, should not be used as first-line therapy.

Diuretics alone are not sufficient to manage this patient and prevent progressive kidney disease; immunosuppressive therapy is therefore indicated.

**KEY POINT**

- Glucocorticoids are first-line therapy for primary minimal change glomerulopathy; standard treatment of the nephrotic syndrome (ACE inhibitor or angiotensin receptor blocker, diuretics for edema, and cholesterol-lowering medication if total cholesterol >200 mg/dL [5.1 mmol/L]) is also indicated as needed.

**Bibliography**

Vivarelli M, Massella L, Ruggiero B, Emma F. Minimal change disease. Clin J Am Soc Nephrol. 2017;12:332-345. [PMID: 27940460]

## Item 5      Answer:    C

**Educational Objective:** Diagnose monoclonal gammopathy of renal significance with a kidney biopsy.

The most appropriate next diagnostic test is a kidney biopsy. This patient appears to have monoclonal gammopathy of renal significance (MGRS). This is a recently defined set of kidney disorders found in patients who would otherwise meet the criteria for monoclonal gammopathy of undetermined significance but have an abnormal urinalysis and kidney insufficiency. This patient who otherwise meets the diagnostic criteria for monoclonal gammopathy of undetermined significance has an active urine sediment and an increase in the serum creatinine level and thus has underlying kidney disease. MGRS is an increasingly recognized disorder, and a kidney biopsy is necessary to make the diagnosis by demonstrating the presence of monoclonal immunoglobulin deposition in the kidney. MGRS can affect the kidney in various ways, including amyloidosis, proliferative glomerulonephritis, immunoglobulin deposition disease, C3 glomerulopathy, and proximal tubulopathy. Kidney manifestations of MGRS are usually caused by deposition of monoclonal light chains. Patients can present with both nephrotic and subnephrotic proteinuria, hematuria, and elevated serum creatinine. Despite not meeting the definition of multiple myeloma, MGRS increases morbidity and, in most cases, should be treated with therapy designed to eliminate or suppress the immunoglobulin clone.

Pauci-immune glomerulonephritis is caused by microscopic vessel vasculitis affecting the kidney, resulting in necrotizing lesions in the glomeruli with few or no immune deposits. The renal lesion may occur with or without systemic vasculitis and is the most common cause of rapidly progressive glomerulonephritis. Most patients have circulating ANCA directed against neutrophils. Other than proteinuria, this patient has a bland urinalysis that is not consistent with a pauci-immune glomerulonephritis, and testing for ANCA in lieu of a kidney biopsy will not establish a diagnosis.

$\beta_2$-Microglobulin levels can be helpful as prognostic indicators in myeloma but cannot be used to make a diagnosis of a plasma cell disorder.

Serum free light chains can be used to diagnose myeloma and predict the risk of progression in patients with monoclonal gammopathy of undetermined significance; however, a kidney biopsy, not serum free light chain determination, will confirm the cause of this patient's kidney disease.

**KEY POINT**

- Monoclonal gammopathy of renal significance is diagnosed in patients who would otherwise meet the criteria for monoclonal gammopathy of undetermined significance but have an abnormal urinalysis and kidney insufficiency; kidney biopsy confirms the diagnosis.

**Bibliography**

Rosner MH, Edeani A, Yanagita M, Glezerman IG, Leung N; American Society of Nephrology Onco-Nephrology Forum. Paraprotein-related kidney disease: diagnosing and treating monoclonal gammopathy of renal significance. Clin J Am Soc Nephrol. 2016;11:2280-2287. [PMID: 27526705]

## Item 6      Answer:    D

**Educational Objective:** Treat IgA nephropathy with an ACE inhibitor or angiotensin receptor blocker.

No changes need to be made to this patient's current medication regimen. He was diagnosed with IgA nephropathy 3 months ago, at which time the ACE inhibitor lisinopril was initiated. Antiproteinuric therapy using an ACE inhibitor or angiotensin receptor blocker (ARB) is the hallmark for treating IgA nephropathy and remains the most proven therapy in slowing progression of the disease. This patient currently has preserved kidney function and proteinuria <1000 mg/24 h; therefore, continuing conservative therapy with the ACE inhibitor lisinopril is appropriate.

Combined use of any of the three renin-angiotensin system drug classes (ACE inhibitor, ARB, and direct renin inhibitors) is not recommended given the results of several clinical trials that revealed more adverse events with these combinations (hyperkalemia, hypotension, acute kidney injury), without additional cardiovascular or renal benefits. Therefore, adding the ARB losartan to this patient's medication regimen is not recommended.

The risk for disease progression appears to be significantly increased when patients have proteinuria >1000 mg/24 h, particularly in the setting of reduced kidney function. Studies on using immunosuppression (particularly glucocorticoids) have used this 1000 mg/24 h proteinuria threshold for enrollment and have demonstrated conflicting results. Although earlier small studies have shown a clear benefit in adding glucocorticoids (oral or a combination of intravenous and oral) to ACE inhibitors or ARBs when proteinuria is >1000 mg/24 h, more recent larger studies (STOP-IgAN and TESTING studies) have raised concerns about the toxicity of this treatment strategy outweighing any potential benefits. Therefore, the use of immunosuppression in IgA nephropathy remains controversial.

**KEY POINT**

- Antiproteinuric therapy with an ACE inhibitor or angiotensin receptor blocker is the hallmark and most validated treatment strategy for IgA nephropathy.

**Bibliography**

Feehally J. Immunosuppression in IgA nephropathy: guideline medicine versus personalized medicine. Semin Nephrol. 2017;37:464-477. [PMID: 28863793]

## Item 7    Answer:    C

**Educational Objective:** Identify polydipsia as the cause of isovolemic hypotonic hyponatremia.

This patient has isovolemic hypotonic hyponatremia secondary to polydipsia. Isovolemia is documented by the presence of normal vital signs and physical examination findings. Hypotonicity is documented by the low calculated serum osmolality of 156 mOsm/kg $H_2O$, using the following equation:

$$\text{Serum Osmolality (mOsm/kg } H_2O) = (2 \times \text{Serum Sodium [mEq/L])} + \text{Plasma Glucose (mg/dL)}/18 + \text{Blood Urea Nitrogen (mg/dL)}/2.8$$

Isovolemic hypotonic hyponatremia is secondary either to impaired dilution of urine or to water intake that exceeds the kidney's ability to excrete dilute urine. Urine osmolality distinguishes between these two entities. Urine osmolality <100 mOsm/kg $H_2O$ indicates excessive water intake, as seen with psychogenic polydipsia or poor solute intake. Because the kidney cannot excrete pure water, a minimal solute concentration of 50 mOsm/kg $H_2O$ is required. If solute intake is low while liquid intake remains high (as seen in beer potomania or chronic low food intake), water excretion is limited by available urinary solute.

Hyperglycemia causes the osmotic translocation of water from the intracellular to the extracellular fluid compartment, which results in a decrease in the serum sodium level by approximately 1.6 to 2.0 mEq/L (1.6-2.0 mmol/L) for every 100 mg/dL (5.6 mmol/L) increase in the plasma glucose above 100 mg/dL (5.6 mmol/L). Although the patient has mild hyperglycemia, her glucose is not elevated enough to lower her sodium to 126 mEq/L (126 mmol/L).

Diabetes insipidus, due to either a lack of antidiuretic hormone (ADH) secretion from the posterior pituitary gland or kidney resistance to ADH (nephrogenic diabetes insipidus), will result in low urine osmolality as seen in this patient. In the absence of ADH, excessive water is excreted by the kidneys. Serum sodium is typically normal but may be elevated in patients who do not have access to water. Although lithium can cause nephrogenic diabetes insipidus, the fact that she is hyponatremic rules out this diagnosis.

Hyponatremia most often results from an increase in circulating ADH in response to a true or sensed reduction in effective arterial blood volume with resulting fluid retention. Hyponatremia may also be caused by elevated ADH levels associated with the syndrome of inappropriate antidiuretic hormone secretion. Because she has dilute urine indicating a lack of ADH, neither the syndrome of inappropriate antidiuretic hormone secretion nor volume depletion is the cause of her hyponatremia. Volume depletion is also excluded by the normal blood pressure and pulse measurement and absence of orthostatic changes.

**KEY POINT**

- Isovolemic hypotonic hyponatremia associated with urine osmolality <100 mOsm/kg $H_2O$ indicates excessive water intake, as seen with psychogenic polydipsia or poor solute intake.

**Bibliography**

Hoorn EJ, Zietse R. Diagnosis and treatment of hyponatremia: compilation of the guidelines. J Am Soc Nephrol. 2017;28:1340-1349. [PMID: 28174217]

## Item 8    Answer:    B    H

**Educational Objective:** Prevent calcium oxalate stones using potassium citrate in a patient who has malabsorption.

In addition to increasing fluid intake, potassium citrate is appropriate to prevent future calcium oxalate stones in this patient. Patients with chronic diarrhea and malabsorption are at increased risk for forming calcium oxalate stones for three reasons. First, because of the diarrhea and concomitant metabolic acidosis, urine citrate, an inhibitor of crystallization, is often reduced. In addition, volume depletion from the diarrhea decreases urine volume and thus increases the concentration of calcium and oxalate in the urine. Finally, in malabsorption, especially fat malabsorption as occurs in chronic pancreatitis, enteric calcium binds to fat as opposed to oxalate, leaving oxalate free to be absorbed and excreted in the urine. Although treatment should be based on the metabolic evaluation in this patient, his low urine pH and low serum bicarbonate level suggest that he has metabolic acidosis. Decreased systemic pH lowers urine citrate excretion. Supplementation with citrate as a base equivalent will help correct the acidosis and increase urine citrate, bind urinary calcium, and decrease the formation of calcium oxalate stones.

If the 24-hour urine metabolic evaluation showed elevated urine uric acid or if stone analysis revealed a uric acid nidus, allopurinol could be considered; however, in the absence of this information, allopurinol should not be prescribed.

Vitamin C increases urine oxalate excretion and would not have the desired effect of decreasing calcium oxalate stone formation.

Restricting dietary calcium intake in patients with hypercalciuria may paradoxically increase the risk of kidney stone formation by causing decreased binding of calcium with oxalate in the gut with increased absorption and urinary excretion of oxalate; therefore, dietary calcium should not be limited.

Increased protein intake increases glomerular filtration, and therefore the excretion of calcium, and would not

CONT.

contribute to decreased kidney stone formation. In addition, high protein diets may exacerbate hypocitraturia.

**KEY POINT**

- Potassium citrate can be used to help prevent calcium oxalate stones in patients with chronic diarrhea and malabsorption.

**Bibliography**
Pfau A, Knauf F. Update on nephrolithiasis: core curriculum 2016. Am J Kidney Dis. 2016;68:973-985. [PMID: 27497526]

 **Item 9** **Answer:** **A**

**Educational Objective:** Treat diabetic nephropathy.

The addition of an ACE inhibitor or angiotensin receptor blocker (ARB) is the most appropriate management for this patient with diabetic nephropathy. The hallmark clinical features include a proteinuric form of chronic kidney disease in a patient with long-standing diabetes mellitus and evidence of other (microvascular and/or macrovascular) complications of disease. Diagnosis can be made clinically for this patient, and he can be treated with the cornerstone of treatment: improved glucose control, and blockade of the renin-angiotensin system (RAS) with an ACE inhibitor or ARB using the maximal tolerated dose. Combined use of any RAS drug class (ACE inhibitors, ARBs, and direct renin inhibitors) is not recommended; several clinical trials have revealed more adverse events with these combinations (hyperkalemia, hypotension, acute kidney injury), without additional cardiovascular or renal benefits.

ANCA-associated glomerulonephritis is associated with the nephritic syndrome. The nephritic syndrome is characterized by hematuria, proteinuria, and leukocytes in the urine sediment. The hallmark is the presence of dysmorphic erythrocytes, with or without erythrocyte casts. Systemic findings may include edema, hypertension, and kidney failure. This patient does not have hematuria, making ANCA testing unnecessary.

Serum and urine protein electrophoresis is used to evaluate for kidney failure secondary to dysproteinemia, which is more common in older patients (>65 years of age). Other potential clues to the presence of dysproteinemia-related kidney disease include anemia, hypercalcemia, and evidence of proximal tubular dysfunction such as hypokalemia, metabolic acidosis, hypophosphatemia, glycosuria (with normoglycemia), or hypouricemia.

The diagnosis of diabetic nephropathy usually does not require a kidney biopsy if the clinical presentation is consistent with its diagnosis. The best predictors of finding diabetic nephropathy are duration of diabetes for more than 8 years followed by presence of the nephrotic syndrome. Therefore, this patient with a 10-year history of poorly controlled diabetes, nephrotic-range proteinuria, and findings of microvascular and macrovascular complications does not require a kidney biopsy or other testing to confirm the diagnosis of diabetic nephropathy.

**KEY POINT**

- The best predictors for the presence of diabetic nephropathy are duration of diabetes mellitus for more than 8 years followed by the presence of the nephrotic syndrome.

**Bibliography**
Wylie EC, Satchell SC. Diabetic nephropathy. Clin Med (Lond). 2012;12:480-2; quiz 483-5. [PMID: 23101153]

**Item 10** **Answer:** **B**

**Educational Objective:** Treat rhabdomyolysis-induced acute kidney injury.

Intravenous 0.9% saline is the most appropriate treatment for this patient who has severe rhabdomyolysis from cocaine and opiates. Major causes of rhabdomyolysis include trauma, drugs and toxins, seizures, metabolic and electrolyte disorders, endocrinopathies, and exercise. Rhabdomyolysis-induced acute kidney injury (AKI) is associated with elevated serum creatine kinase (usually >5000 U/L) and creatinine levels, hyperkalemia, hypocalcemia, hyperphosphatemia, hyperuricemia, and increased anion gap metabolic acidosis. Patients with rhabdomyolysis tend to be significantly volume depleted due to the sequestration of water in injured muscles. Therefore, initial management is early with aggressive repletion of fluids aimed at maintaining a urine output of 200 to 300 mL/h. Normal saline is the recommended initial fluid of choice, and patients can require 10 liters of fluid per day.

Hemodialysis is reserved for patients with severe AKI who remain oliguric with persistent hyperkalemia, persistent metabolic acidosis, and/or volume overload. This patient does not have an indication for hemodialysis at this time.

Although the patient has hypernatremia, intravenous 5% dextrose is not adequate to expand the extracellular fluid compartment. Due to the osmotic gradient, hypotonic fluids will leave the extracellular fluid compartment for the intracellular compartment.

Hypocalcemia is due to sequestration of calcium in damaged cells. Rebound hypercalcemia occurs during the recovery phase due to release of calcium from damaged muscles and is worsened by exogenous calcium treatment. Calcium should only be given in patients who are symptomatic or in patients at risk for arrhythmia due to severe hyperkalemia with electrocardiogram changes.

Although alkalinization of the urine to a pH >6.5 may prevent intratubular pigment cast formation, decrease the release of free iron from myoglobin, and decrease the risk for tubular precipitation of uric acid, clear benefit is lacking. Intravenous bicarbonate should only be used after diuresis is established with volume repletion. It should not be used if pH is >7.5, serum bicarbonate is >30 mEq/L (30 mmol/L), and/or severe hypocalcemia is present. Intravenous bicarbonate can cause symptomatic hypocalcemia and can promote deposition of calcium phosphate in the renal tubules.

Answers and Critiques

### Bibliography

Cervellin G, Comelli I, Benatti M, Sanchis-Gomar F, Bassi A, Lippi G. Nontraumatic rhabdomyolysis: background, laboratory features, and acute clinical management. Clin Biochem. 2017;50:656-662. [PMID: 28235546]

## Item 11          Answer:   A

**Educational Objective:**  Prevent contrast-induced nephropathy.

The administration of 0.9% saline is an appropriate measure to prevent contrast-induced nephropathy (CIN). CIN is a common cause of reversible acute kidney injury in the hospital. CIN is defined as an increase in serum creatinine within 24 to 48 hours following contrast exposure. Adequate intravenous volume expansion with isotonic crystalloids before the procedure and continued for 6 to 24 hours afterward has been shown to decrease the incidence of CIN in patients at risk. Intravenous hydration induces an increase of urine flow rate, reduces the concentration of contrast in the tubule, and increases the excretion of contrast. Because administration of intravenous crystalloid remains the primary strategy for reducing the risk of CIN, patients with compensated heart failure should still be given intravenous volume. Patients with uncompensated heart failure should undergo hemodynamic monitoring with continuation of diuretics. This patient has compensated heart failure noted on examination and should be given fluids.

A recent large randomized trial among patients at high risk for kidney complications compared three different strategies to prevent CIN: intravenous 1.26% sodium bicarbonate or intravenous 0.9% sodium chloride and 5 days of oral acetylcysteine or oral placebo. For fluid administration, this study used a protocol of 1 to 3 mL/kg/h before angiography, 1 to 1.5 mL/kg/h during angiography, and 1 to 3 mL/kg/h 2 to 12 hours after angiography. There was no benefit of intravenous sodium bicarbonate over intravenous sodium chloride or of oral acetylcysteine over placebo for the prevention of death, need for dialysis, or persistent decline in kidney function at 90 days or for the prevention of CIN.

Some but not all studies suggest that statins may reduce the risk of CIN. A 2016 meta-analysis suggested that statins given with N-acetylcysteine plus intravenous saline reduced the risk of CIN compared with N-acetylcysteine plus intravenous saline alone in relatively low-risk patients. Based on these results, there is no need to discontinue atorvastatin in this patient.

Discontinuation of ACE inhibitors or angiotensin receptor blockers such as irbesartan has not been clearly shown to decrease the risk of CIN.

### Bibliography

Weisbord SD, Gallagher M, Jneid H, Garcia S, Cass A, Thwin SS, et al; PRESERVE Trial Group. Outcomes after angiography with sodium bicarbonate and acetylcysteine. N Engl J Med. 2018;378:603-614. [PMID: 29130810]

## Item 12          Answer:   C

**Educational Objective:**  Diagnose multiple myeloma–associated hypercalcemia as a cause of acute kidney injury.

This patient's acute kidney injury (AKI) is due to hypercalcemia from multiple myeloma. Classic symptoms of polyuria, polydipsia, and nocturia sometimes occur with elevated serum calcium levels of 11 mg/dL (2.8 mmol/L) or less. Other symptoms such as anorexia, nausea, abdominal pain, constipation, increased serum creatinine levels, and mild mental status changes are more likely to occur with levels >11 mg/dL (2.8 mmol/L). Kidney dysfunction is found in about 30% of patients diagnosed with multiple myeloma, often due to cast nephropathy (also termed myeloma kidney), a condition in which excess monoclonal free light chains precipitate in the distal tubules and incite tubulointerstitial damage. Hypercalcemia and exposure to nephrotoxic agents are other frequent causes of kidney dysfunction. Hypercalcemia can decrease glomerular filtration rate through renal vasoconstriction, the natriuretic effects of high serum calcium levels, and impaired renal concentrating ability. This patient has orthostatic hypotension, a bland urinalysis with hyaline casts, and a fractional excretion of sodium <1%, consistent with a prerenal AKI from hypovolemia. The constellation of hypercalcemia, normal anion gap metabolic acidosis, pancytopenia, and AKI suggests multiple myeloma as the etiology.

Hydrochlorothiazide can cause volume depletion, decreased excretion of calcium and mild hypercalcemia, prerenal AKI, and metabolic alkalosis (due to hypovolemic stimulation of aldosterone release). However, the effect on serum calcium is usually minimal, and the patient has a metabolic acidosis, not metabolic alkalosis as might be seen with thiazide therapy.

Milk alkali syndrome occurs with the ingestion of large amounts of calcium and absorbable alkali (for example, calcium carbonate). It presents as hypercalcemia, metabolic alkalosis, and AKI. This patient has a metabolic acidosis, not a metabolic alkalosis, making this diagnosis unlikely.

Primary hyperparathyroidism is the most common cause of hypercalcemia in otherwise healthy outpatients and is diagnosed with a simultaneously elevated serum calcium level and an inappropriately normal or elevated intact parathyroid hormone level. Serum phosphorus levels are typically low or low-normal in these patients. This patient's phosphorus level is elevated, making the diagnosis of primary hyperparathyroidism unlikely.

**KEY POINT**

- A diagnosis of multiple myeloma is suggested by the constellation of anemia, hypercalcemia, normal anion gap metabolic acidosis, and acute kidney injury.

**Bibliography**

Rosner MH, Perazella MA. Acute kidney injury in patients with cancer. N Engl J Med. 2017;376:1770-1781. [PMID: 28467867]

## Item 13    Answer:    B

**Educational Objective:** Adjust an antihypertensive medication regimen to achieve a target blood pressure goal.

The addition of losartan is the most appropriate treatment. As antihypertensive agents are titrated or added when there is inadequate blood pressure control, it is important to recognize that there is a nonlinear and diminishing blood pressure–lowering effect when titrating from 50% maximal dose to 100% maximal dose of any agent. A general rule of thumb is that 75% of an agent's blood pressure–lowering effect may be achieved with 50% of its maximal dose. If blood pressure control requires an additional >5-mm Hg reduction, it is unlikely to be achieved by increasing the single agent from 50% to 100% maximal dose. The better strategy is to add a second drug or a third drug to a two-drug regimen, as seen in this patient.

Hydralazine is not the best option because it is a thrice-daily medication and may pose problems with adherence, considering that once-daily medication options have not been exhausted in this patient. In addition, hydralazine is a direct vasodilator and is associated with sodium and water retention and reflex tachycardia; use with a diuretic and a β-blocker is recommended. Hydralazine is typically reserved for patients with resistant hypertension or hypertensive urgencies.

Increasing the amlodipine or hydrochlorothiazide dose is not appropriate because there is diminishing return in blood pressure lowering if the dose is titrated up from 50% to 100% of maximum. Also, it is unlikely that increasing the dose from 50% to 100% of maximum will result in an additional >5-mm Hg reduction to bring this patient's blood pressure to a target of <130/80 mm Hg. In addition, titration to maximum doses may result in manifestation of undesirable side effects and decreased adherence. In this case, the patient already has dependent edema, which may increase with uptitration of the amlodipine dose. His serum potassium is borderline at 3.6 mEq/L (3.6 mmol/L), and increasing the dose of hydrochlorothiazide may further decrease his serum potassium and necessitate a potassium supplement, adding yet another medication to his drug regimen.

**KEY POINT**

- Three strategies can be used for antihypertensive dose adjustment in the treatment of hypertension: (1) maximize the medication dose before adding another; (2) add another class of medication before reaching the maximum dose of the first; and (3) start with two medication classes separately or as fixed-dose combinations.

**Bibliography**

Whelton PK, Carey RM, Aronow WS, Casey DE Jr, Collins KJ, Dennison Himmelfarb C, et al. 2017 ACC/AHA/AAPA/ABC/ACPM/AGS/APhA/ASH/ASPC/NMA/PCNA guideline for the prevention, detection, evaluation, and management of high blood pressure in adults: a report of the American College of Cardiology/American Heart Association Task Force on Clinical Practice Guidelines. Hypertension. 2017. [PMID: 29133356]

## Item 14    Answer:    C

**Educational Objective:** Treat ethylene glycol toxicity.

The most appropriate management is intravenous hydration, fomepizole, and hemodialysis. This patient has typical findings of ethylene glycol toxicity, including central nervous system depression, an increased anion gap metabolic acidosis, and an increased osmolal gap. In patients with an increased anion gap acidosis, calculation of the serum osmolal gap is helpful in assessing the presence of unmeasured solutes, such as ingestion of certain toxins (for example, methanol or ethylene glycol). The serum osmolal gap is the difference between the measured and calculated serum osmolality. Serum osmolality can be calculated using the following formula:

$$\text{Serum Osmolality (mOsm/kg } H_2O) = (2 \times \text{Serum Sodium [mEq/L]}) + \text{Plasma Glucose (mg/dL)}/18 + \text{Blood Urea Nitrogen (mg/dL)}/2.8$$

When the measured osmolality exceeds the calculated osmolality by >10 mOsm/kg $H_2O$, the osmolal gap is considered elevated. This patient has an osmolal gap of 27 mOsm/kg $H_2O$. Finally, this patient has kidney failure likely resulting from deposition of calcium oxalate crystals in the renal tubules. Because laboratory confirmation of ethylene glycol intoxication may take days, empiric therapy with fomepizole and aggressive fluid resuscitation with crystalloids (250-500 mL/h intravenous initially) should be instituted in all cases to increase kidney clearance of the toxin and to limit deposition of oxalate in the renal cortex. Hemodialysis to clear the alcohol and toxic metabolites should be instituted in the context of any organ-specific toxicity (central nervous system depression, acute kidney injury, systemic collapse), severe acidemia, or very large ingestions.

Activated charcoal gastric decontamination and nasogastric lavage have no role in toxic alcohol poisoning; both ethylene glycol and methanol are typically absorbed too rapidly for either of these modalities to be useful.

Intravenous ethanol was traditionally used as a competitive inhibitor of alcohol dehydrogenase. However, fomepizole has been found to be superior to alcohol with few side effects. Therefore, fomepizole is the preferred agent, and there is no additional benefit to coadministration of the two.

Adjunct therapy with intravenous sodium bicarbonate therapy in the context of pH <7.30 may reduce penetration of toxic metabolites of ethylene glycol (glycolate, glyoxylate, and oxalate) and methanol (formate) into the tissues and enhance renal excretion of glycolate and formate. However, the initiation of dialysis in this patient is more efficacious.

- Management of ethylene glycol toxicity in the context of organ-specific toxicity, severe acidemia, or very large ingestions includes aggressive fluid resuscitation, fomepizole, and hemodialysis.

**Bibliography**

Kruse JA. Methanol and ethylene glycol intoxication. Crit Care Clin. 2012;28:661-711. [PMID: 22998995]

## Item 15    Answer:    A

**Educational Objective:** Evaluate for secondary causes of membranous glomerulopathy.

Age- and sex-appropriate cancer screening is the most appropriate management. The initial step in the management of newly diagnosed membranous glomerulopathy is to evaluate for secondary forms of the disease, which account for approximately 25% of cases. Some of this evaluation is often done in the prebiopsy screening laboratory tests (for example, screening for hepatitis B and C viruses, lupus, and syphilis). Secondary forms of membranous glomerulopathy correlate with age. Cancer screening is particularly important in evaluating for secondary forms of membranous glomerulopathy in patients over the age of 65 years. Up to 25% of such patients will have a malignancy discovered within 1 year of diagnosis, essentially accounting for all forms of secondary membranous glomerulopathy in this age group. This 68-year-old woman with newly diagnosed membranous glomerulopathy has a 50-pack-year history of smoking. She should be sent for age- and sex-appropriate cancer screening, which would include cervical cytology and human papillomavirus testing, mammography, colonoscopy, and low-dose chest CT.

Immunosuppression should not be offered in this case until a secondary form has definitively been ruled out and the patient has been carefully monitored for at least 3 to 6 months to allow for the possibility, if this is a primary form of membranous glomerulopathy, for spontaneous remission, which occurs in approximately one third of primary cases.

Membranous glomerulopathy is associated with a higher risk for clotting, particularly when serum albumin is <2.8 g/dL (28 g/L). However, there is no consensus on whether such patients should be offered prophylactic anticoagulation, and most experts in the United States opt for vigilant monitoring rather than prophylactic anticoagulation.

The M-type phospholipase A2 receptor (PLA2R) is the specific podocyte antigen responsible for eliciting immune complex formation with circulating autoantibodies in most cases of primary membranous glomerulopathy. Anti-PLA2R antibodies are detected in approximately 75% of primary cases and rarely found in secondary forms. A negative staining on biopsy for this antigen (which is a more specific test than serum antibody assays) raises suspicion for a secondary form of the disease and does not require serum testing for confirmation.

- The initial step in the management of newly diagnosed membranous glomerulopathy is to evaluate for secondary forms of the disease, which account for approximately 25% of cases.

**Bibliography**

Leeaphorn N, Kue-A-Pai P, Thamcharoen N, Ungprasert P, Stokes MB, Knight EL. Prevalence of cancer in membranous nephropathy: a systematic review and meta-analysis of observational studies. Am J Nephrol. 2014;40:29-35. [PMID: 24993974]

## Item 16    Answer:    B

**Educational Objective:** Diagnose transitional cell (urothelial) cancer in a patient with Balkan endemic nephropathy.

The most appropriate next step for this patient is an endoscopic urologic evaluation with cystoscopy and upper tract imaging. The patient has Balkan endemic nephropathy (BEN), a slowly progressive tubulointerstitial disease that has been linked to aristolochic acid. Aristolochic acid is a nephrotoxic alkaloid from the plant *Aristolochia clematis*. BEN has a high prevalence rate in southeastern Europe (Serbia, Bulgaria, Romania, Bosnia and Herzegovina, and Croatia) and is the cause of kidney disease in up to 70% of patients receiving dialysis in some of the most heavily affected regions. Aristolochic acid is also sometimes found as a component of herbal therapies used for weight loss. Characteristics of BEN include chronic kidney disease due to tubulointerstitial injury, tubular dysfunction (polyuria and decreased concentrating ability, glucosuria without hyperglycemia, and tubular proteinuria), and anemia. Ultrasound demonstrates small echogenic kidneys. BEN has a familial but not inherited pattern of distribution. It is thought to be caused by exposure to aristolochic acid, and, because it is mutagenic, it is strongly associated with the development of upper tract transitional cell (urothelial) cancers. Therefore, urologic evaluation is indicated.

CT urography is the preferred test for patients with unexplained urologic/nonglomerular hematuria. However, CT urography involves the use of intravenous contrast, which would place this patient at a high risk of developing contrast-induced nephropathy given the severity of his kidney disease. Cystoscopy and retrograde ureteropyelography would be the preferred imaging techniques for this patient.

Kidney biopsy would not explain the nondysmorphic hematuria. Furthermore, kidney biopsy is not indicated in the setting of small echogenic kidneys <9 cm in size, which signifies chronic irreversible disease.

Pyuria, granular casts, and low-grade proteinuria are commonly found in patients with tubulointerstitial nephritis and contrasts with the isolated pyuria associated with most urinary tract infections. In addition, the small, echogenic kidneys, chronic hematuria, and irregular bladder wall are not consistent with a urinary tract infection and more strongly suggest the possibility of a malignancy. Therefore, urine cultures are not indicated.

- Balkan endemic nephropathy is strongly associated with the development of upper tract transitional cell (urothelial) cancers, and urologic evaluation is necessary.

**Bibliography**
Stefanovic V, Toncheva D, Polenakovic M. Balkan nephropathy. Clin Nephrol. 2015;83:64–9. [PMID: 25725245]

## Item 17     Answer:   A

**Educational Objective:** Treat hypernatremia caused by central diabetes insipidus.

In addition to increasing the prednisone, the antidiuretic hormone (ADH) analogue desmopressin acetate is the most appropriate treatment. This patient most likely has central nervous system sarcoidosis and central diabetes insipidus (DI). Nearly half of hypothalamic-pituitary sarcoidosis cases occur in the course of previously treated sarcoidosis. Central DI results from inadequate production of ADH by the posterior pituitary gland. In the presence of ADH, aquaporin water channels are inserted in the collecting tubules and allow water to be reabsorbed. In the absence of ADH, excessive water is excreted by the kidneys. Frank hypernatremia is unusual because patients develop extreme thirst and polydipsia, and with free access to water, can maintain serum sodium in the high normal range. When patients do not drink enough to replace the water lost in the urine, due to poor or absent thirst drive or lack of free access to water, they develop hypernatremia. DI is diagnosed with simultaneous laboratory evidence of inability to concentrate urine (urine osmolality <300 mOsm/kg $H_2O$) in the face of elevated serum sodium and osmolality. If necessary, a water deprivation test can confirm the diagnosis. A response to exogenous ADH would support a diagnosis of central DI, whereas a lack of response is seen in nephrogenic DI.

Although volume depletion induced by hydrochlorothiazide will help decrease urine output and conserve water, this treatment is reserved for patients with nephrogenic DI and is not necessary in central DI.

The hypernatremia in this case is mild, without symptoms, and can be rapidly treated with the administration of desmopressin acetate; therefore, it is not necessary to administer intravenous 5% dextrose.

Tolvaptan is a vasopressin receptor antagonist sometimes used for the syndrome of inappropriate antidiuretic hormone secretion, which is characterized by normal volume status, hyponatremia, and inappropriately elevated urine osmolality (not present in this patient).

**KEY POINT**

- Diabetes insipidus (DI) is diagnosed with simultaneous laboratory evidence of inability to concentrate urine in the face of elevated serum sodium and osmolality; a water deprivation test can confirm the diagnosis, and response to exogenous antidiuretic hormone supports the diagnosis of central DI.

**Bibliography**
Langrand C, Bihan H, Raverot G, Varron L, Androdias G, Borson-Chazot F, et al. Hypothalamo-pituitary sarcoidosis: a multicenter study of 24 patients. QJM. 2012;105:981–95. [PMID: 22753675]

## Item 18     Answer:   B

**Educational Objective:** Identify heparin as a cause of hyperkalemia.

The most likely cause of this patient's elevated serum potassium level is heparin. Hypoaldosteronism caused by heparin, inhibitors of the renin-angiotensin system, type 4 renal tubular acidosis, or primary adrenal disease can cause hyperkalemia. Both unfractionated and low-molecular-weight heparin use is associated with a decrease in aldosterone synthesis. This occurs more frequently in patients with chronic kidney disease or diabetes mellitus, or in those taking an ACE inhibitor or angiotensin receptor blocker.

Major underlying causes of persistent hyperkalemia are disorders in which urine potassium excretion is impaired. This can be due to a marked decrease in glomerular filtration rate, decreased sodium delivery to the distal potassium secretory sites, and hypoaldosteronism. The most common cause is chronic kidney disease with a glomerular filtration rate <20 mL/min/1.73 $m^2$ or acute oliguric kidney injury. Except in these cases, the kidney is able to maintain potassium homeostasis. The patient is not oliguric, and the slight increase in serum creatinine postoperatively is not sufficient to cause hyperkalemia.

Extreme elevations in glucose by increasing serum osmolality can directly cause hyperkalemia by pulling water from the intracellular space into the extracellular space, dragging potassium with it. This patient's glucose is only mildly elevated and would have little effect on osmolality and hyperkalemia.

In patients with metabolic acidosis caused by mineral acids (such as hydrochloric acid), buffering of intracellular hydrogen ions leads to potassium movement into the extracellular fluid to maintain electroneutrality. This does not occur with organic acids such as lactate or ketoacids. In most cases of hyperchloremic metabolic acidosis, hyperkalemia typically does not develop because there is concomitant urinary and/or gastrointestinal potassium loss. This is the case in patients with hyperchloremic metabolic acidosis with losses of potassium in the stool as the result of diarrhea or in the urine in patients with renal tubular acidosis.

Topiramate is a carbonic anhydrase inhibitor. Carbonic anhydrase inhibition results in proximal bicarbonate, sodium, and chloride urinary loss. The increased sodium loss causes hypovolemia and triggers secondary hyperaldosteronism, promoting potassium loss and hypokalemia.

**KEY POINT**

- Hypoaldosteronism caused by heparin, inhibitors of the renin-angiotensin system, type 4 renal tubular acidosis, or primary adrenal disease can cause hyperkalemia, especially in patients with chronic kidney disease or diabetes mellitus, or in those taking an ACE inhibitor or angiotensin receptor blocker.

**Bibliography**

Kovesdy CP. Updates in hyperkalemia: outcomes and therapeutic strategies. Rev Endocr Metab Disord. 2017;18:41-47. [PMID: 27600582]

**Bibliography**

Hansson JH, Watnick S. Update on peritoneal dialysis: core curriculum 2016. Am J Kidney Dis. 2016;67:151-64. [PMID: 26376606]

## Item 19    Answer:    A

**Educational Objective:** Select the most appropriate pre-transplant renal replacement therapy.

Due to this patient's full-time occupation and requirement to be present on-site at the workplace, peritoneal dialysis might be the preferred management for his end-stage kidney disease (ESKD). Peritoneal dialysis is a renal replacement therapy (RRT) modality utilizing the peritoneal membrane for diffusion of solutes and osmosis of water against a concentration gradient provided by infused dialysate. Patients exchange the dialysate three to five times per day rather than go to a dialysis center for 4 hours three times per week for hemodialysis. Control over one's dialysis is conducive for patients with full-time obligations, such as school or employment. The peritoneal dialysis exchanges can be performed overnight while the individual is sleeping and allow for greater independence during the day. The patient is otherwise healthy and independent. He has never had abdominal surgery, and his BMI is normal. He is an ideal candidate for peritoneal dialysis, and this modality will also allow him to preserve his independence and more easily transition to a life with ESKD. Planning for the right dialysis modality that best fits the patient's daily routine and lifestyle is important for patient satisfaction and long-term success.

A recent meta-analysis analyzing the effect of peritoneal dialysis versus hemodialysis on renal anemia in patients with ESKD found no significant difference for levels of hemoglobin, ferritin, parathyroid hormone, and transferrin saturation index between the hemodialysis and peritoneal dialysis groups. Both of the two dialysis strategies have a similar effect on renal anemia in patients with ESKD.

Clinical outcomes are similar for patients receiving peritoneal dialysis compared with those receiving hemodialysis, although patients starting RRT with residual kidney function may have better outcomes with peritoneal dialysis. Furthermore, residual kidney function is preserved longer with peritoneal dialysis than with hemodialysis and, although small, helps maintain adequate solute clearance and euvolemia. Finally, patients treated with peritoneal dialysis are more satisfied with their treatment and indicate a more satisfying shared decision-making experience.

Peritonitis is one of the most important complications of peritoneal dialysis and can damage the peritoneum, reducing the efficacy of dialysis. Peritoneal dialysis-associated peritonitis is uncommon, with one episode of peritonitis every 2 to 3 years, usually caused by bacteria from skin introduced by poor sterile technique and often easily treated with antibiotics.

**KEY POINT**

- In properly selected individuals, peritoneal dialysis allows patients to preserve their independence and offers outcomes similar to those seen with hemodialysis.

## Item 20    Answer:    A

**Educational Objective:** Initiate combination antihypertensive therapy for treatment of stage 2 hypertension.

Combination therapy with amlodipine/benazepril is appropriate treatment for this patient with stage 2 hypertension. The 2017 American College of Cardiology/American Heart Association blood pressure (BP) guideline recommends combination therapy with two first-line antihypertensive drugs of different classes (separately or as a single-dose pill) for adults with stage 2 hypertension and an average BP that is 20/10 mm Hg above their BP target. Stage 2 hypertension is defined as BP ≥140/90 mm Hg. This patient's target BP is <130/80 mm Hg. There are no definitive recommendations for best drug combinations, but some data suggest an ACE inhibitor/calcium channel blocker (CCB) combination may be more efficacious than an ACE inhibitor/thiazide diuretic combination. Using a thiazide diuretic/CCB combination is also an option. It is important to note that in black patients, ACE inhibitors are not as efficacious at reducing BP compared with thiazide diuretics or CCBs.

Specific non-recommended initial agents for the treatment of hypertension include β-blockers (due to higher rate of cardiovascular-related events and mortality compared with angiotensin receptor blockers) and α-blockers (due to higher rate of cardiovascular-related events and mortality compared with thiazides), although compelling clinical indications such as atrial fibrillation or benign prostatic hyperplasia may supersede these recommended restrictions.

Initiation of once-daily dosing of a combination pill simplifies the medication regimen and is appropriate in this patient to ensure adherence. Therefore, initiation of hydralazine is not correct because two-drug therapy is recommended for this patient, and adherence to a thrice-daily medication will be problematic.

Combination therapy with an ACE inhibitor (ramipril) and an angiotensin receptor blocker (telmisartan) is not recommended. Several clinical trials (ONTARGET, NEPHRON-D, ALTITUDE) have revealed more adverse events with these combinations (hyperkalemia, hypotension, acute kidney injury), without additional cardiovascular or renal benefits.

**KEY POINT**

- The 2017 American College of Cardiology/American Heart Association blood pressure (BP) guideline recommends combination therapy with two first-line antihypertensive drugs of different classes (separately or as a single-dose pill) for adults with stage 2 hypertension and an average BP of 20/10 mm Hg above BP target.

**Bibliography**

Whelton PK, Carey RM, Aronow WS, Casey DE Jr, Collins KJ, Dennison Himmelfarb C, et al. 2017 ACC/AHA/AAPA/ABC/ACPM/AGS/APhA/ASH/ASPC/NMA/PCNA guideline for the prevention, detection, evaluation, and management of high blood pressure in adults: a report of the American College of Cardiology/American Heart Association Task Force on Clinical Practice Guidelines. Hypertension. 2017. [PMID: 29133356]

## Item 21          Answer:     A

**Educational Objective:** Diagnose ANCA-associated glomerulonephritis.

The most likely diagnosis is ANCA-associated glomerulonephritis (pauci-immune crescentic glomerulonephritis). This patient's clinical picture suggests a rapidly progressive glomerulonephritis (RPGN), with an acute and steep rise in serum creatinine accompanied by hematuria and proteinuria. The differential diagnosis for RPGN is classically accounted for by three immunofluorescence findings seen on diagnostic kidney biopsy: pauci-immune staining (for example, ANCA-associated glomerulonephritis), linear staining (for example, anti–glomerular basement membrane glomerulonephritis), and granular staining (for example, lupus nephritis). ANCA-associated glomerulonephritis accounts for more than half of all RPGN cases and has a particularly high prevalence in patients >65 years of age presenting with acute kidney injury and active urine sediment. The patient's clinical presentation of acute onset of flu-like symptoms is a classic presentation for vasculitis, and the lacy or reticular rash on examination is likely related to active ANCA-associated vasculitis. He should be tested for antiproteinase-3 and antimyeloperoxidase ANCA antibodies and undergo kidney biopsy to confirm the diagnosis.

Anti–glomerular basement membrane antibody disease is a far rarer form of RPGN, with peak incidences in young men and older women. More than half of patients present with concomitant alveolar hemorrhage that may progress to life-threatening respiratory failure. These findings are not present in this patient.

Minimal change glomerulopathy is characterized by sudden-onset nephrotic syndrome. It can be associated with acute kidney injury in elderly patients, and the presentation is one of severe nephrotic syndrome without significant hematuria. This is distinctly different from this patient's presentation of rash, hypertension, rapidly progressive kidney failure, and active urine sediment.

Kidney dysfunction is found in 29% of patients with multiple myeloma, often due to cast nephropathy (also termed myeloma kidney), a condition in which excess monoclonal free light chains precipitate in the distal tubules and incite tubulointerstitial damage. Patients will typically have concomitant anemia and hypercalcemia. These findings are absent in this patient.

Proliferative lupus nephritis is a cause of RPGN that is usually limited to the pediatric and young adult patient population.

**KEY POINT**

- ANCA-associated glomerulonephritis is typically characterized by a vasculitic prodrome of malaise, arthralgia, myalgia, and skin findings; hematuria, proteinuria, and acute kidney injury are present, and kidney biopsy will confirm diagnosis.

**Bibliography**

Bomback AS, Appel GB, Radhakrishnan J, Shirazian S, Herlitz LC, Stokes B, et al. ANCA-associated glomerulonephritis in the very elderly. Kidney Int. 2011;79:757-64. [PMID: 21160463]

## Item 22          Answer:     C

**Educational Objective:** Diagnose pyroglutamic acidosis.

The most likely diagnosis is pyroglutamic acidosis. Pyroglutamic acidosis, which presents with mental status changes and an increased anion gap, occurs in selected patients receiving therapeutic doses of acetaminophen on a chronic basis. Susceptible patients are those with critical illness, poor nutrition, liver disease, or chronic kidney disease, as well as those on a strict vegetarian diet. In this context, acetaminophen leads to depletion of glutathione, altering the γ-glutamyl cycle to overproduce pyroglutamic acid (also known as 5-oxoproline). Diagnosis can be confirmed by measuring urine levels of pyroglutamic acid.

D-Lactic acidosis presents with an increased anion gap metabolic acidosis and characteristic neurologic findings of intermittent confusion, slurred speech, and ataxia in patients with short-bowel syndrome. Accumulation of the D-isomer of lactate can occur in patients with short-bowel syndrome following jejunoileal bypass or small-bowel resection. In these patients, excess carbohydrates that reach the colon are metabolized to D-lactate. Laboratory studies show increased anion gap metabolic acidosis with normal plasma lactate levels, because the D-isomer is not measured by conventional laboratory assays for lactate. Diagnosis is confirmed by specifically measuring D-lactate. This patient's lack of short-bowel syndrome rules out this diagnosis.

Propylene glycol, a solvent used to enhance the solubility of various intravenously administered medications, causes an increased anion gap metabolic acidosis through its acid metabolites, L-lactate and D-lactate. An increased osmolal gap accompanies the increased anion gap metabolic acidosis seen with propylene glycol. This patient's clinical history and lack of lactic acidosis are not consistent with propylene glycol toxicity.

Salicylate toxicity most commonly presents in adults as respiratory alkalosis or with features of both respiratory alkalosis and increased anion gap metabolic acidosis. This patient has appropriate respiratory compensation for the metabolic acidosis, not respiratory alkalosis, making salicylate toxicity unlikely.

### KEY POINT

- Pyroglutamic acidosis occurs in patients receiving therapeutic doses of acetaminophen on a chronic basis in the setting of critical illness, poor nutrition, liver disease, chronic kidney disease, or a strict vegetarian diet; diagnosis can be confirmed by measuring urine levels of pyroglutamic acid.

### Bibliography

Fenves AZ, Kirkpatrick HM 3rd, Patel VV, Sweetman L, Emmett M. Increased anion gap metabolic acidosis as a result of 5-oxoproline (pyroglutamic acid): a role for acetaminophen. Clin J Am Soc Nephrol. 2006;1:441-7. [PMID: 17699243]

## Item 23     Answer:   B

**Educational Objective:** Diagnose abdominal compartment syndrome.

The most appropriate diagnostic test to perform next is intra-abdominal pressure (IAP) measurement. This patient's findings are consistent with abdominal compartment syndrome, which occurs in the setting of abdominal surgery, large volume fluid resuscitation, and multiple transfusions. It can manifest as a distended abdomen, ascites, and sodium-avid acute kidney injury (AKI). The increased IAP causes direct compression of renal parenchyma and vasculature, resulting in oliguria and decreased glomerular filtration rate. The diagnosis of abdominal compartment syndrome is made by an IAP measurement >20 mm Hg and new organ dysfunction. Indirect measurement of IAP can be with intragastric, intracolonic, intravesical (bladder), or inferior vena cava catheters. Management includes supportive therapy, abdominal compartment decompression, and correction of positive fluid balance.

The increased specific gravity, low urine sodium, and presence of hyaline casts are consistent with a prerenal AKI. The fractional excretion of sodium would not provide any additional information to aid in the diagnosis.

Myoglobin is a heme pigment–containing protein that can cause AKI. The urine is reddish brown, pigmented casts are present, and the urine dipstick is positive for blood in the absence of erythrocytes. Abdominal compartment syndrome is a much more likely cause of this patient's AKI, and urine myoglobin levels do not need to be measured.

The patient is on a cephalosporin, which can cause acute interstitial nephritis (AIN). AIN is characterized by hematuria, pyuria, and/or leukocyte casts. However, the timing is too soon for AIN (unless the patient had been previously exposed), and the urine findings do not support it. Moreover, the urine eosinophil stain is neither sensitive nor specific for the diagnosis of AIN and does not need to be performed.

### KEY POINT

- Abdominal compartment syndrome is defined as a sustained intra-abdominal pressure >20 mm Hg associated with at least one organ dysfunction; management includes supportive therapy, abdominal compartment decompression, and correction of positive fluid balance.

### Bibliography

Patel DM, Connor MJ Jr. Intra-abdominal hypertension and abdominal compartment syndrome: an underappreciated cause of acute kidney injury. Adv Chronic Kidney Dis. 2016;23:160-6. [PMID: 27113692]

## Item 24     Answer:   A

**Educational Objective:** Identify the cause of nonglomerular hematuria.

Cystoscopy is the most appropriate diagnostic test to perform next in this patient. Hematuria is frequently encountered among adults in ambulatory care. For hematuria incidentally discovered on dipstick evaluation, clinicians should confirm the presence of hematuria with microscopic urinalysis that demonstrates ≥3 erythrocytes/hpf before initiating further evaluation in asymptomatic adults. Clinicians should also pursue evaluation of hematuria even if the patient is receiving antiplatelet or anticoagulant therapy. Macroscopic hematuria should prompt urology referral even if self-limited. Hematuria is most often of nonglomerular origin. If a nephrologic cause of hematuria is not suggested, hematuria may indicate a malignancy. Guidelines from the American Urological Association recommend that patients older than 35 years or with risk factors for lower urinary tract malignancy (such as irritative voiding symptoms, smoking, aniline dye exposure, or cyclophosphamide exposure) undergo evaluation for malignancy with imaging. If imaging is negative, cystoscopy should be performed. This male patient is 45 years old without evidence of glomerular disease (no proteinuria or increased serum creatinine) and negative imaging of the upper genitourinary tract. Therefore, it is appropriate to assess for bladder pathology using cystoscopy.

Kidney biopsy in a patient with hematuria is not indicated in the absence of evidence of glomerular disease or change in kidney function. This patient's lack of proteinuria rules out a significant glomerular process, and his normal serum creatinine and lack of systemic symptoms make other kidney disease unlikely.

Kidney ultrasonography will provide no additional information in this patient. Doppler is not indicated because the risk of renal vein thrombosis as a cause of hematuria in this patient is not suspected (normal kidney function, no flank pain, and no risk of thrombosis).

Routine cytologic evaluation of urine is no longer recommended in the initial evaluation of asymptomatic microscopic hematuria, and urine markers approved by the FDA for bladder cancer detection are specifically not recommended for patients with hematuria.

### KEY POINT

- Patients with hematuria who are older than 35 years or with risk factors for lower urinary tract malignancy (such as irritative voiding symptoms, smoking, aniline dye exposure, or cyclophosphamide exposure) should undergo evaluation for malignancy with imaging; if imaging is negative, cystoscopy is appropriate to assess for bladder pathology.

**Bibliography**
Davis R, Jones JS, Barocas DA, Castle EP, Lang EK, Leveillee RJ, et al; American Urological Association. Diagnosis, evaluation and follow-up of asymptomatic microhematuria (AMH) in adults. Available at: http://www.auanet.org/guidelines/asymptomatic-microhematuria-(2012-reviewed-and-validity-confirmed-2016). Accessed December 15, 2017.

## Item 25    Answer:    B

**Educational Objective:** Diagnose glomerulonephritis.

This patient likely has glomerulonephritis. Glomerular hematuria typically features brown- or tea-colored urine with dysmorphic erythrocytes (or acanthocytes) and/or erythrocyte casts on urine sediment examination. Erythrocyte casts are recognized by their cylindrical or tubular structure and inclusion of small, agranular spherocytes and, when present, are specific for hematuria of glomerular origin.

Isomorphic erythrocytes are of the same size and shape and usually arise from an extraglomerular urologic process causing bleeding into the genitourinary tract, such as a tumor, stone, or infection. Dysmorphic erythrocytes have varying sizes and shapes. Acanthocytes, a specific form of dysmorphic erythrocytes, are characterized by vesicle-shaped protrusions and suggest a glomerular source of bleeding. Acanthocytes and erythrocyte casts are highly specific for glomerulonephritis and exclude an extraglomerular cause of bleeding such as bladder cancer.

Sterile pyuria and leukocyte casts are hallmarks of tubulointerstitial nephritis, which can present acutely or may progress indolently and present as chronic kidney disease of unclear duration. Mild subnephrotic proteinuria also can be seen with interstitial nephritis. The cells comprising a leukocyte cast are larger than erythrocytes and appear more granular. The presence of erythrocyte casts excludes the diagnosis of tubulointerstitial nephritis.

Although this febrile patient has leukocytes (granular cells larger than erythrocytes) on urinalysis and positive leukocyte esterase on dipstick analysis, the presence of erythrocyte casts is specific for glomerulonephritis. This patient has the nephritic syndrome, which is associated with glomerular inflammation resulting in hematuria, proteinuria, and leukocytes in the urine sediment.

**KEY POINT**

- Glomerular macroscopic hematuria typically features brown- or tea-colored urine with dysmorphic erythrocytes (or acanthocytes) and/or erythrocyte casts on urine sediment examination.

**Bibliography**
Simerville JA, Maxted WC, Pahira JJ. Urinalysis: a comprehensive review. Am Fam Physician. 2005;71:1153-62. [PMID: 15791892]

## Item 26    Answer:    D

**Educational Objective:** Diagnose vancomycin-induced acute tubular necrosis.

The most likely cause of this patient's acute kidney injury (AKI) is vancomycin. The most common cause of hospital-acquired AKI is acute tubular necrosis (ATN), which represents damage and destruction of the renal tubular epithelial cells and is most commonly caused by ischemia or toxins. A careful evaluation of hemodynamics, volume status, medications, and physical findings of associated illness can help determine the cause of ATN. Most reported cases of vancomycin toxicity are due to acute interstitial nephritis; however, ATN has been reported. ATN is supported by the rapid rise in serum creatinine, fractional excretion of sodium >2%, and urine microscopy with numerous renal tubular epithelial cells and granular casts. Risk factors associated with vancomycin nephrotoxicity include chronic kidney disease, prolonged therapy, vancomycin doses ≥4 g/d, vancomycin trough concentrations >15 mg/L, and concomitant use of loop diuretics. Early recognition and prompt discontinuation of the drug are essential for renal recovery.

Some antibiotics (such as cefepime) and proton pump inhibitors (such as omeprazole) can cause acute interstitial nephritis (AIN). AIN may be associated with drugs, infection, autoimmune diseases, and malignancy. Only 10% to 30% of patients with AIN have the classic triad of fever, rash, and eosinophilia. Urine chemistries will reveal a variable (and unhelpful) fractional excretion of sodium, and urinalysis is characterized by hematuria, pyuria, and/or leukocyte casts and possibly eosinophiluria. Drug-induced AIN is characterized by a slowly increasing serum creatinine 7 to 10 days after exposure; however, it can occur within 1 day of exposure if the patient has been exposed previously. Drug-induced AIN can also occur months after exposure, as seen with NSAIDs and proton pump inhibitors. The patient's urine findings do not support AIN.

Contrast-induced nephropathy (CIN) results in ATN with an increase in serum creatinine within 48 hours of exposure. This patient's serum creatinine was at baseline 48 hours after exposure, making CIN an unlikely diagnosis.

**KEY POINT**

- Risk factors associated with vancomycin nephrotoxicity include chronic kidney disease, prolonged therapy, doses ≥4 g/d, trough concentrations >15 mg/L, and concomitant use of loop diuretics.

**Bibliography**
Bamgbola O. Review of vancomycin-induced renal toxicity: an update. Ther Adv Endocrinol Metab. 2016;7:136-47. [PMID: 27293542]

## Item 27    Answer:    B

**Educational Objective:** Treat acute hyponatremia in a symptomatic patient with hypertonic saline.

The most appropriate initial treatment is a 100-mL bolus of 3% saline. The hyponatremia in this young woman who presents confused and febrile is most likely due to ingestion of 3,4-methylenedioxymethamphetamine (ecstasy). Ecstasy is associated with hyponatremia both because it stimulates the release of antidiuretic hormone and because users often drink large quantities of water. When treating hyponatremia,

CONT.

the rate of correction of serum sodium concentration must be carefully considered to avoid the osmotic demyelination syndrome. Brain cells adapt to chronic hyponatremia by reducing intracellular concentration of organic osmolytes, such as myoinositol, to cope with hypotonicity. Acute hyponatremia is associated with an increase in brain water and cerebral edema and should be treated rapidly. Because the brain has not adapted to the hypotonic environment by the release of organic osmolytes, the risk of rapid correction and development of osmotic demyelination is absent. Treatment is with a bolus of 3% saline, and a 100-mL bolus should raise the serum sodium level by 2 to 3 mEq/L (2-3 mmol/L). If symptoms persist, this can be repeated one to two times.

In patients with neurologic symptoms, fluid restriction by itself is not an appropriate treatment. The immediate goal is to reduce brain swelling rapidly by the acutely raising the serum sodium level. Even in cases of chronic hyponatremia, the serum sodium can be increased acutely by 2 to 3 mEq/L (2-3 mmol/L) as long as the total change in the serum sodium is <10 mEq/L (10 mmol/L) in a 24-hour period. Except in cases of hypovolemic hyponatremia, the use of 0.9% sodium chloride is not recommended. In patients who are not volume depleted and have syndrome of inappropriate antidiuretic hormone secretion with a fixed urine osmolality, the infused saline can be excreted in the urine in a smaller volume, and thus the serum sodium can actually fall.

Both oral urea and tolvaptan are appropriate treatments for chronic hyponatremia, but they do not raise the serum sodium rapidly enough to reverse neurologic abnormalities and are therefore inappropriate for treatment of acute hyponatremia in this symptomatic patient.

### KEY POINT

- Treatment of acute symptomatic hyponatremia includes a 100-mL bolus of 3% saline to increase the serum sodium level by 2 to 3 mEq/L (2-3 mmol/L).

### Bibliography
Sterns RH. Disorders of plasma sodium–causes, consequences, and correction. N Engl J Med. 2015;372:55-65. [PMID: 25551526]

 **Item 28      Answer:      C**

**Educational Objective:** Diagnose fibromuscular dysplasia as the cause of secondary hypertension.

Renal artery imaging is the most appropriate diagnostic test to perform next to evaluate for fibromuscular dysplasia in this young woman with new-onset hypertension. Fibromuscular dysplasia is a nonatherosclerotic form of renovascular disease that usually affects the mid and distal portions of the renal artery. This disorder usually occurs in young persons, particularly young women, and abrupt onset of hypertension in a patient under the age of 35 years is suggestive. The elevation of serum creatinine more than 30% from baseline after the initiation of an ACE inhibitor is a clue that renovascular hypertension may be present. Fibromuscular dysplasia is associated with aneurysm and/or dissection in a variety of

vascular territories (for example, renal artery, carotid artery, and intracranial arteries). This has resulted in a recommendation that patients with fibromuscular dysplasia undergo one-time, head-to-pelvic cross-sectional imaging.

The importance of primary aldosteronism as a cause of hypertension is being increasingly recognized. Testing for primary aldosteronism should be considered in all patients with difficult-to-control hypertension. It should also be performed in patients with hypertension and an incidentally noted adrenal mass, spontaneous hypokalemia, or diuretic-induced hypokalemia. In these cases, the plasma aldosterone concentration/plasma renin activity ratio is obtained. Primary aldosteronism cannot account for this patient's renal bruit or serum creatinine elevation after the initiation of an ACE inhibitor.

Plasma fractionated metanephrines are obtained to screen for a pheochromocytoma. The absence of episodic palpitations, headaches, and tachycardia as well as the presence of an abdominal bruit make pheochromocytoma a less likely diagnosis.

Transthoracic echocardiography can be used for patients with clinical suspicion for white coat hypertension and/or to evaluate for end-organ damage. There are no pertinent findings from the history, physical examination, or electrocardiogram results to raise clinical suspicion for end-organ damage. More importantly, echocardiography will not be helpful in diagnosing the cause of this patient's hypertension or directing its treatment.

### KEY POINT

- Renal artery imaging is the most appropriate diagnostic test to evaluate for fibromuscular dysplasia in a young woman with new-onset hypertension.

### Bibliography
Olin JW, Gornik HL, Bacharach JM, Biller J, Fine LJ, Gray BH, et al; American Heart Association Council on Peripheral Vascular Disease. Fibromuscular dysplasia: state of the science and critical unanswered questions: a scientific statement from the American Heart Association. Circulation. 2014;129:1048-78. [PMID: 24548843]

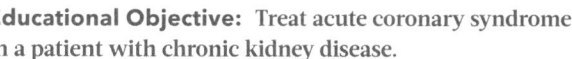 **Item 29      Answer:      A**

**Educational Objective:** Treat acute coronary syndrome in a patient with chronic kidney disease.

The most appropriate management for this patient with stage G4 chronic kidney disease (CKD) and ST-elevation myocardial infarction is immediate cardiac catheterization. Cardiovascular disease is the leading cause of death among patients with CKD. The risk of cardiovascular-related death in patients with CKD stages G3 and G4 is four to five times higher than the risk of progression to end-stage kidney disease. Mortality risk increases with decreasing estimated glomerular filtration rate and increasing albuminuria. Unfortunately, many clinical trials that guide the prevention or treatment of cardiovascular disease have not included patients with advanced CKD, and the findings may not be generalizable to patients with CKD. However, the recommendation from experts is to

CONT.

offer patients with CKD therapy for cardiovascular disease, including cardiac catheterization, percutaneous coronary intervention, and coronary bypass. The available data suggest that routine invasive management is associated with a statistically significant reduction in death, acute myocardial infarction, and rehospitalization, across most categories of CKD, at the predictable price of a significant increase in major and minor bleeding. Prognosis for patients following myocardial infarction, percutaneous intervention, and coronary artery bypass surgery is worse for patients with CKD than for those without CKD.

Suspected coronary anomalies, such as anomalous coronary origins, can be evaluated by cardiac magnetic resonance (CMR) imaging. CMR imaging is not a practical modality for patients with acute coronary syndrome because of the time necessary to generate the images and inability to provide revascularization therapy. In addition, CMR uses gadolinium contrast, which is associated with the development of nephrogenic systemic fibrosis in patients with CKD.

Studies have examined the potential efficacy of pre-catheterization dialysis to reduce the risk of contrast-induced nephropathy in patients with advanced CKD. The balance of the data suggests no benefit for this invasive maneuver, and it generally is not advocated.

This patient has acute coronary syndrome, and avoiding cardiac catheterization and potential intervention to treat this life-threatening condition in lieu of medical management will not be in the patient's best interest, regardless of the risk for contrast-induced nephropathy.

**KEY POINT**

- The available data suggest that routine invasive management of coronary artery disease is associated with a statistically significant reduction in death, acute myocardial infarction, and rehospitalization, across most categories of chronic kidney disease.

### Bibliography

Lingel JM, Srivastava MC, Gupta A. Management of coronary artery disease and acute coronary syndrome in the chronic kidney disease population–a review of the current literature. Hemodial Int. 2017;21:472–482. [PMID: 28093874]

 **Item 30        Answer:        A**

**Educational Objective:** Manage large kidney stones with extracorporeal shock wave lithotripsy.

The most appropriate next step in management is extracorporeal shock wave lithotripsy. Acute management of symptomatic nephrolithiasis is aimed at pain management and facilitation of stone passage. Pain can be relieved by NSAIDs and opioids as needed. Combination NSAID and opioid therapy seems more effective than treatment with either one alone. Stone passage decreases with increasing size of the stone. Only 50% of stones >6 mm will pass spontaneously, whereas stones >10 mm are extremely unlikely to pass spontaneously. Urologic intervention is required in all patients with evidence of infection, acute kidney injury, intractable nausea or pain,

and stones that fail to pass or are unlikely to pass. This patient has an 11-mm stone that is at the ureteral pelvic junction. There is associated dilation of the renal calyces suggesting obstruction to urine outflow. It is unlikely that a stone this size will pass. Appropriate management therefore is urology consultation. The patient will most likely require extracorporeal shock wave lithotripsy or percutaneous nephrolithotomy. Extracorporeal shock wave lithotripsy can be used for stones in the renal pelvis and proximal ureter, but it is less effective for stones located in the mid/distal ureter or the lower pole calyx, larger stones (>15 mm), and hard stones (calcium oxalate monohydrate or cystine). Potential complications of extracorporeal shock wave lithotripsy include incomplete stone fragmentation, kidney injury, and possibly increased blood pressure or new-onset hypertension.

Treatment of uncomplicated renal colic with analgesia and maintenance intravenous fluids is just as efficacious as with forced hydration with regard to patient pain perception and opioid use. Moreover, it appears the state of hydration has little impact on stone passage. This patient may require intravenous fluids to avoid dehydration if pain and nausea prevent adequate oral fluid intake, but not as a means to expel the kidney stone.

Stones up to 10 mm can be managed conservatively, although the likelihood of spontaneous passage decreases with increasing size. Medical expulsive therapy with α-blocker therapy (such as tamsulosin) or a calcium channel blocker (such as nifedipine) can aid the passage of small stones (≤10 mm in diameter). This large stone associated with probable obstruction is not a candidate for medical expulsive therapy with either tamsulosin or nifedipine.

**KEY POINT**

- Urologic intervention is required in all patients with evidence of infection, acute kidney injury, intractable nausea or pain, and stones that fail to pass or are unlikely to pass.

### Bibliography

Lawler AC, Ghiraldi EM, Tong C, Friedlander JI. Extracorporeal shock wave therapy: current perspectives and future directions. Curr Urol Rep. 2017;18:25. [PMID: 28247327]

### Item 31        Answer:        C

**Educational Objective:** Diagnose sarcoidosis with kidney involvement.

The most likely diagnosis is sarcoidosis, a systemic inflammatory disease that can affect multiple organs. The most common presentations of sarcoidosis are hilar lymphadenopathy and parenchymal lung disease; common extrapulmonary organ involvement includes the skin, joints, and eyes. More than 90% of patients with kidney involvement have thoracic sarcoid identified on chest radiograph. Kidney manifestations in sarcoidosis are common and include nephrocalcinosis from hypercalcemia and hypercalciuria, nephrolithiasis, and chronic interstitial nephritis with granuloma formation. Hypercalcemia occurs due to peripheral conversion of 25-hydroxyvitamin D to 1,25-dihydroxyvitamin D by activated macrophages. Parathyroid hormone is typically suppressed in response to the hypercalcemia. The urinalysis is typical of other chronic tubulointerstitial diseases and can be normal or show only sterile pyuria or mild proteinuria, as in this patient's case. Kidney manifestations of hypercalcemia and interstitial nephritis are treated with glucocorticoids.

Thiazide diuretics can be associated with a mild hypercalcemia but not nephrocalcinosis. Furthermore, they decrease urinary calcium excretion. This patient's urinary calcium excretion is increased.

Primary hyperparathyroidism is characterized by hypercalcemia, hypophosphatemia, and inappropriately normal or elevated parathyroid hormone. This patient's parathyroid hormone is suppressed, making this an unlikely diagnosis.

Increased levels of calcium absorption from the gut can be from markedly high vitamin D levels. Vitamin D intoxication is usually defined as a value >150 ng/mL (374.4 nmol/L). Vitamin D intoxication is not consistent with the laboratory findings because the phosphorus and 25-hydroxyvitamin D levels are normal.

Finally, thiazide diuretic use, primary hyperparathyroidism, or vitamin D intoxication cannot account for the patient's pulmonary findings.

### KEY POINT

- Kidney involvement in sarcoidosis can manifest as nephrocalcinosis from hypercalcemia and hypercalciuria, and as tubulointerstitial nephritis with granuloma formation.

### Bibliography

Löffler C, Löffler U, Tuleweit A, Waldherr R, Uppenkamp M, Bergner R. Renal sarcoidosis: epidemiological and follow-up data in a cohort of 27 patients. Sarcoidosis Vasc Diffuse Lung Dis. 2015;31:306-15. [PMID: 25591142]

## Item 32    Answer:    C

**Educational Objective:** Identify normal physiologic changes in pregnancy as a cause of low serum sodium.

Normal physiologic change in pregnancy is the most likely cause of this patient's low serum sodium level. Mild hyponatremia is common in normal pregnancy due to plasma volume increases with water retention (mediated by an increase in antidiuretic hormone levels) greater than sodium retention. An associated drop in serum osmolality of 8 to 10 mOsm/kg $H_2O$ and serum sodium concentration of 4 to 5 mEq/L (4-5 mmol/L) may occur. As the serum osmolality and sodium concentration decrease, a new set point is maintained, and thirst occurs in response to osmolality (reset osmostat). No treatment is necessary. Other conditions associated with reset osmostat include quadriplegia, tuberculosis, advanced age, psychiatric disorders, and chronic malnutrition.

Primary polydipsia should always be considered in the differential diagnosis of patients with mental illness and hyponatremia, particularly those with schizophrenia who are taking psychotropic drugs. Primary polydipsia presents with hyponatremia, decreased serum osmolality, and decreased urine osmolality, reflecting suppressed antidiuretic hormone (ADH) levels in response to water overload. Primary polydipsia is a rare cause of hyponatremia, and the volume of water intake would need to be very large to induce hyponatremia. This patient is not at risk for primary polydipsia.

Hypovolemia causes stimulation of the sympathetic nervous system, activation of the renin-angiotensin-aldosterone axis, and release of ADH. These adaptive responses allow volume maintenance at the expense of a low serum sodium with excessive water intake. Blood pressure in pregnant women begins to lower in the first trimester and reaches a nadir in the second. Furthermore, she is asymptomatic, and ADH release is therefore not likely to be induced by this level of blood pressure.

The syndrome of inappropriate antidiuretic hormone (SIADH) secretion may be associated with stress and pain; however, hyponatremia does not develop acutely. Although SIADH could have preceded the patient's car accident, she has no risk factors for SIADH (central nervous system disorders, pulmonary disorders, infection, drugs, postoperative status, tumors), and normal pregnancy is a more likely cause of her low serum sodium level.

### KEY POINT

- Mild hyponatremia is common in normal pregnancy due to plasma volume increases with water retention greater than sodium retention; no treatment is necessary.

### Bibliography

Cheung KL, Lafayette RA. Renal physiology of pregnancy. Adv Chronic Kidney Dis. 2013;20:209-14. [PMID: 23928384]

## Item 33    Answer:    D

**Educational Objective:** Treat dyslipidemia in a patient with stage G4 chronic kidney disease.

A statin is appropriate to treat dyslipidemia in this patient with stage G4 chronic kidney disease (CKD). Guidelines from the Kidney Disease: Improving Global Outcomes (KDIGO) group provide a grade 1A recommendation to treat adults aged ≥50 years with an estimated glomerular filtration rate (eGFR) <60 mL/min/1.73 m² , but not treated with chronic dialysis or kidney transplantation (GFR categories G3a-G5), with a statin or statin/ezetimibe combination. This recommendation largely emanates from results of the Study of Heart and Renal Protection (SHARP) trial, which included 9270 participants with CKD (mean eGFR, 27 mL/min/1.73 m²) who received simvastatin 20 mg plus ezetimibe 10 mg daily or placebo and were followed for 5 years. Statin plus ezetimibe therapy led to a significant 17% reduction in the relative hazard of the primary outcome of major atherosclerotic events (coronary death, myocardial infarction, nonhemorrhagic stroke, or any revascularization) compared with placebo (HR, 0.83; 95% CI, 0.74–0.94), driven by significant reductions in nonhemorrhagic stroke and coronary revascularization. It should be noted that simvastatin plus ezetimibe did not reduce the risk of progression to end-stage kidney disease.

Hypertriglyceridemia is the primary lipid abnormality in patients with CKD. However, the 2013 KDIGO update states that the evidence supporting the safety and efficacy of fibrates (such as gemfibrozil) is extremely weak, especially in patients with CKD. Therefore, KDIGO does not recommend fibrates for the treatment of hypertriglyceridemia. Finally, in patients taking a statin for dyslipidemia, the addition of a fibrate increases the risk of myalgia, muscle injury, and rhabdomyolysis.

Although niacin raises HDL cholesterol, several trials involving patients with and without CKD have demonstrated no evidence of improvement in cardiovascular events.

Although randomized controlled trials of omega-3 fatty acids have demonstrated a reduction in cardiovascular disease end points in persons with atherosclerotic cardiovascular disease (ASCVD), little to no data demonstrate the role for the benefits of omega-3 fatty acids for the primary prevention of ASCVD in patients at high cardiovascular disease risk.

**KEY POINT**

- The Kidney Disease: Improving Global Outcomes (KDIGO) guidelines recommend treatment of dyslipidemia with a statin in patients aged ≥50 years with an estimated glomerular filtration rate <60 mL/min/ 1.73 m², but not treated with chronic dialysis or kidney transplantation.

**Bibliography**

Kidney Disease: Improving Global Outcomes (KDIGO) Lipid Work Group. KDIGO clinical practice guideline for lipid management in chronic kidney disease. Kidney inter., Suppl. 2013;3:259–305. Available at www.kdigo.org.

## Item 34    Answer:    D

**Educational Objective:** Diagnose nephrolithiasis with noncontrast helical abdominal CT.

Noncontrast helical abdominal CT is the most appropriate next test for this patient with nephrolithiasis suggested by unilateral flank pain and hematuria. Ultrasonography is an appropriate initial diagnostic test for suspected nephrolithiasis; it is easily available, safe, and relatively inexpensive, and it is the study of choice in pregnant women. Ultrasonography can demonstrate hydronephrosis, kidney size and cortical thickness, echogenicity, and the presence of cysts and tumors. It is useful for uncomplicated nephrolithiasis; a positive ultrasound may be adequate for initial diagnosis. Ultrasonography is less useful in evaluating diseases of the mid or distal ureter, including stones. Furthermore, the

absence of hydronephrosis on ultrasound does not rule out kidney stones. Noncontrast helical CT is the gold standard for diagnosis of nephrolithiasis and is appropriate for evaluating renal colic. Most stones can be detected, including small stones and those in the distal ureter not detected on ultrasound. It may provide information regarding stone composition and, because the entire urinary tract and abdomen are visualized, alternative diagnoses may be suggested.

MRI with contrast is not as sensitive as CT in detecting suspected kidney stones. Due to lack of radiation, MRI may be useful in pregnant women with stone disease if ultrasound is nondiagnostic.

Contrast abdominal CT characterizes renal tumors and cysts, whereas CT urography is the preferred test for patients with unexplained urologic/nonglomerular hematuria. The decision to use contrast depends on the clinical scenario, the patient's risk factors for contrast-induced nephropathy, and the availability and utility of alternative imaging modalities. It is unnecessary in the evaluation of suspected nephrolithiasis and poses greater risk and cost in this situation compared with either ultrasonography or noncontrast helical abdominal CT.

Plain abdominal radiography has limited utility due to its inability to detect radiolucent uric acid stones and does not provide as much anatomic information as other modalities. However, it may be useful in assessing stone burden in patients with known radiopaque stones but is not the initial test of choice for acute nephrolithiasis.

**KEY POINT**

- Noncontrast helical CT is the gold standard for diagnosis of nephrolithiasis.

**Bibliography**

Brisbane W, Bailey MR, Sorensen MD. An overview of kidney stone imaging techniques. Nat Rev Urol. 2016;13:654–662. [PMID: 27578040]

## Item 35    Answer:    C

**Educational Objective:** Identify increased muscle mass as a cause of an increase in serum creatinine.

Measurement of the serum cystatin C level is appropriate for this patient. Cystatin C may be preferable to creatinine to assess kidney function in individuals with higher muscle mass. An increase in muscle mass would be expected to result in an increase in serum creatinine level in the absence of change in kidney function. This muscular man with a BMI of 29 has increase in muscle mass. Because serum creatinine is derived from the metabolism of creatinine produced by muscle, a significant increase in muscle mass would be expected to increase serum creatinine. An elevation in serum creatinine could also occur with creatine supplements, which he is not taking. This patient has a normal urinalysis and no proteinuria, all of which indicate no evidence of underlying kidney disease. Cystatin C, which is cleared by the kidney, is produced by all nucleated cells; therefore, levels are less dependent on muscle mass. Cystatin C can also be used for more accurate glomerular filtration rate estimation in these patients as a component of the Chronic Kidney Disease Epidemiology Collaboration equation.

Although NSAIDs can cause acute kidney injury, the remote and infrequent use by this patient is unlikely to have any effect on serum creatinine. The hemodynamic effects of NSAIDs will disappear within 24 hours of stopping the medication, and interstitial nephritis from NSAIDs is unlikely to present with occasional dosing and is usually associated with proteinuria. The adverse effects of renal fibrosis associated with NSAIDs are only seen with extensive and long-term use.

Creatine kinase levels can be measured to evaluate for the presence of rhabdomyolysis. Rhabdomyolysis significant enough to cause kidney injury would be expected to result in myoglobinuria reflected by heme-positive urine in the absence of red cells. No blood was seen on urinalysis.

In the absence of other changes suggesting glomerular or interstitial disease, a kidney biopsy is not necessary.

### KEY POINT

- Increased muscle mass can result in an increase in serum creatinine level in the absence of change in kidney function.

### Bibliography

Baxmann AC, Ahmed MS, Marques NC, Menon VB, Pereira AB, Kirsztajn GM, et al. Influence of muscle mass and physical activity on serum and urinary creatinine and serum cystatin C. Clin J Am Soc Nephrol. 2008;3:348-54. [PMID: 18235143]

## Item 36    Answer:    B

**Educational Objective:** Manage recurrent stone disease with hydrochlorothiazide.

The most appropriate next step to decrease this patient's stone recurrence is to add a thiazide diuretic such as hydrochlorothiazide. Hypercalciuria is the most common metabolic risk factor for calcium oxalate stones. In patients with hypercalcemia, increased filtered calcium results in hypercalciuria. However, hypercalciuria is often idiopathic and commonly familial, occurring without associated hypercalcemia. Hypercalciuria due to hypercalcemia is treated by addressing the cause of increased serum calcium. In patients with other forms of hypercalciuria, thiazide diuretics reduce calcium excretion in the urine by inducing mild hypovolemia, triggering increased proximal sodium reabsorption and passive calcium reabsorption. This effect can be enhanced by the addition of sodium restriction.

The patient's evaluation reveals a normal uric acid concentration. In calcium stones that form on a uric acid nidus, allopurinol has been associated with a decrease in stone formation. In this patient, however, stone analysis did not reveal a uric acid core and thus would not be the next step in management.

Urinary citrate inhibits stone formation by binding calcium in the tubular lumen, preventing it from precipitating with oxalate. Hypocitraturia is seen with diets high in animal protein and metabolic acidosis from chronic diarrhea, renal tubular acidosis, ureteral diversion, and carbonic anhydrase inhibitors (including seizure medications such as topiramate). The patient's urine citrate level is in the high-normal range, and the serum bicarbonate level is normal, thus increasing citrate in the urine would not be beneficial.

Although increasing urine volume will reduce the calcium saturation, the present urine volume is acceptable. Urine volume to prevent stone recurrence should be between 2500 and 3000 mL per day.

Recommending a low calcium diet is inappropriate for this patient because reducing calcium in the diet would provide less calcium in the gastrointestinal tract to bind oxalate and would increase oxalate absorption, and thus increase urine oxalate concentration and stone formation.

### KEY POINT

- In patients with hypercalciuria and kidney stones, calcium excretion and stone formation can be decreased by the use of thiazide diuretics.

### Bibliography

Qaseem A, Dallas P, Forciea MA, Starkey M, Denberg TD; Clinical Guidelines Committee of the American College of Physicians. Dietary and pharmacologic management to prevent recurrent nephrolithiasis in adults: a clinical practice guideline from the American College of Physicians. Ann Intern Med. 2014;161:659-67. [PMID: 25364887]

## Item 37    Answer:    B

**Educational Objective:** Screen for intracranial cerebral aneurysms in a patient with autosomal dominant polycystic kidney disease.

MR angiography of the brain is the most appropriate next step in management. This patient has autosomal dominant polycystic kidney disease (ADPKD), a genetic kidney disease characterized by enlarged kidneys with multiple cysts. Intracranial cerebral aneurysms are detected in 5% to 10% of patients with ADPKD and have a strong familial pattern. Guidelines for the Management of Patients with Unruptured Intracranial Aneurysms from the American Heart Association/American Stroke Association recommend that patients with a history of ADPKD, particularly those with a family history of intracranial aneurysm but even those without such history, should be offered screening by CT angiography or MR angiography. This is a class I recommendation (should be performed because benefit greatly exceeds risk) based on level B evidence (data derived from a single randomized trial or nonrandomized studies).

Mitral valve prolapse is an extrarenal manifestation seen in some patients with ADPKD, but screening with echocardiography should be limited to patients with findings of this valvular disorder, including chest pain, shortness of breath, edema, a systolic click(s) that is mobile (timing changes with squatting and standing), and a systolic murmur.

Blood pressure control is recommended to slow progression in ADPKD, but the utility of doing so in someone with low baseline blood pressures is unproven. The agent of choice when blood pressure medications are used in ADPKD is a blocker of the renin-angiotensin system and not a calcium channel blocker.

Vasopressin blockade with tolvaptan in patients with ADPKD has been shown in two randomized clinical trials to delay the need for dialysis from 6 to 9 years. Tolvaptan carries an FDA-mandated safety warning about the possibility of irreversible liver injury. Tolvaptan has not been approved for use in ADPKD in the United States.

**KEY POINT**

- Screening for intracranial cerebral aneurysms using CT or MR angiography is recommended for patients with autosomal dominant polycystic kidney disease.

**Bibliography**

Chapman AB, Devuyst O, Eckardt KU, Gansevoort RT, Harris T, Horie S, et al; Conference Participants. Autosomal-dominant polycystic kidney disease (ADPKD): executive summary from a Kidney Disease: Improving Global Outcomes (KDIGO) Controversies Conference. Kidney Int. 2015;88:17-27. [PMID: 25786098]

## Item 38    Answer:    E

**Educational Objective:** Manage primary membranous glomerulopathy.

An ACE inhibitor and statin are appropriate for this patient with recently diagnosed primary membranous glomerulopathy. His kidney biopsy findings are consistent with the diagnosis, and the presence of anti–phospholipase A2 receptor (PLA2R) antibodies has been shown to approach 100% specificity for the primary form of this disease. Approximately one third of patients with primary membranous glomerulopathy experience a spontaneous remission of disease over the first 6 to 24 months without immunosuppression. Therefore, within the first 6 months of diagnosis, barring signs of severe complications of the nephrotic syndrome (such as kidney failure, anasarca, or deep vein thrombosis), the recommended strategy is to treat patients with primary membranous glomerulopathy conservatively with renin-angiotensin system blockers, cholesterol-lowering medications (if cholesterol is above goal), and diuretics (for edema). The patient is then monitored with examinations and laboratory studies to gauge for spontaneous remission. If proteinuria increases in 6 to 12 months, a course of immunosuppression should be considered for those with persistent nephrotic-range proteinuria. With the advent of serologic testing for anti-PLA2R antibodies, these titers can now be followed during the observation period alongside traditional clinical parameters, such as proteinuria. Falling anti-PLA2R titers are associated with remission, whereas persistently high titers are associated with ongoing disease activity.

Alternating months of glucocorticoids and alkylating agents is first-line immunosuppressive therapy of choice for primary membranous glomerulopathy, and substituting with a calcineurin inhibitor such as cyclosporine is now considered a viable alternative for patients with contraindications to alkylating agents. However, utilization of such immunosuppressive therapies at this point is premature and runs the risk of treating a patient who may remit spontaneously.

Although hepatitis B and C virus infections, along with lupus, are well-known forms of secondary membranous glomerulopathy in adults, this patient's screening tests are negative and, with PLA2R antibody positivity, further testing is unnecessary.

**KEY POINT**

- Patients with newly diagnosed primary membranous glomerulopathy are usually observed for 6 to 12 months while on conservative therapy (renin-angiotensin blockade, cholesterol-lowering medication, and edema management) to allow time for possible spontaneous remission before initiating immunosuppression.

**Bibliography**

Couser WG. Primary membranous nephropathy. Clin J Am Soc Nephrol. 2017;12:983-997. [PMID: 28550082] doi:10.2215/CJN.11761116

## Item 39    Answer:    A

**Educational Objective:** Treat hypertension in a patient with atherosclerotic renovascular disease.

The most appropriate next step in management is to begin lisinopril. The patient most likely has atherosclerotic renovascular disease, given his age, diminished pulses, and resistant hypertension despite treatment with four antihypertensive medications, including a diuretic. Most patients with renovascular disease have atherosclerosis (>90%). In this patient, medical therapy should be optimized to include treatment of underlying cardiovascular risk factors such as hypercholesterolemia and addition of an ACE inhibitor or angiotensin receptor blocker (ARB) for blood pressure control. Kidney function should be checked 2 weeks after the addition of an ACE inhibitor or ARB to ensure that the serum creatinine does not increase, and the ACE inhibitor or ARB can be continued if there is not a >25% rise in the serum creatinine from baseline.

Although renal angiography is the gold standard for diagnosis of renovascular disease, it is not recommended as a routine test due to adverse risks such as contrast nephropathy and cholesterol emboli. It is undertaken only if an intervention to correct a discovered stenosis is planned. However, medical therapy is recommended for most adults with atherosclerotic renal artery stenosis.

Three randomized controlled trials (STAR, ASTRAL, and CORAL) failed to show that renal artery angioplasty confers additional benefit above optimal medical therapy for patients with atherosclerotic renovascular disease who have stable kidney function. Patients who may benefit from percutaneous angioplasty and stenting or surgical intervention include those who present with a short hypertension duration; fail medical therapy; or have severe hypertension or recurrent flash pulmonary edema, refractory heart failure, acute kidney injury following treatment with an ACE inhibitor or ARB, or progressive impaired kidney function. In patients who have an indication for renal artery revascularization, surgery is preferred only for those with complex anatomic lesions such as aneurysm or aortoiliac occlusive disease.

### KEY POINT

- In most patients with renal artery stenosis, the primary therapeutic intervention is medical management, including correction of modifiable cardiovascular risk factors.

### Bibliography

Cooper CJ, Murphy TP, Cutlip DE, Jamerson K, Henrich W, Reid DM, et al; CORAL Investigators. Stenting and medical therapy for atherosclerotic renal-artery stenosis. N Engl J Med. 2014;370:13-22. [PMID: 24245566]

### Item 40     Answer:    B

**Educational Objective:** Prevent contrast-induced nephropathy in a patient with chronic kidney disease.

Intravenous isotonic fluid (0.9% sodium chloride or 1.26% sodium bicarbonate) administered before and after cardiac catheterization is the most appropriate preventive measure for this patient with chronic kidney disease (CKD) who is at risk for contrast-induced nephropathy (CIN). CIN is a common cause of acute kidney injury in the hospital. Patients can be exposed to iodinated intravenous contrast during cardiac catheterization, angiography, and CT. Contrast agents are thought to cause acute tubular necrosis through renal vasoconstriction and direct cytotoxicity; however, the mechanisms are not completely understood. Risk factors for CIN include advanced age, diabetic nephropathy, multiple myeloma, concomitant use of nephrotoxins (for example, aminoglycoside antibiotics, NSAIDs), severity of CKD, reduced renal perfusion (due to poor cardiac function or volume depletion), higher dose of contrast, high osmolar contrast (rarely used in industrialized contrast), repeated doses of contrast, and intra-arterial administration. Intravenous isotonic fluids (1-1.5 mL/kg/h 3 to 4 hours before the procedure and continued for 6 to 12 hours) are the mainstay in preventing CIN and perform better than hypotonic fluids. However, among isotonic fluids, evidence does not support the superiority of any one particular fluid when comparing normal saline with sodium bicarbonate. Intravenous fluids should not be given to prevent CIN in patients who are hypervolemic.

Furosemide before catheterization is incorrect because diuresis would induce volume contraction, activate the renal angiotensin-aldosterone system, and increase the risk for CIN.

Oral bicarbonate does not have a role in the prevention of CIN, as studies using alkali therapy looked at intravenous forms only. However, intravenous infusion of 1.26% sodium

bicarbonate is as efficacious in preventing CIN as is 0.9% sodium chloride infusion.

This patient has no indications for renal replacement therapy. Hemodialysis does not improve CIN outcomes but rather may exacerbate kidney injury.

### KEY POINT

- Intravenous isotonic fluids are the mainstay in preventing contrast-induced nephropathy.

### Bibliography

Fähling M, Seeliger E, Patzak A, Persson PB. Understanding and preventing contrast-induced acute kidney injury. Nat Rev Nephrol. 2017;13:169-180. [PMID: 28138128]

### Item 41     Answer:    B

**Educational Objective:** Diagnose type 1 (hypokalemic distal) renal tubular acidosis.

The most likely cause of this patient's laboratory findings is type 1 (hypokalemic distal) renal tubular acidosis (RTA). It is due to a defect in urine acidification in the distal nephron and is most commonly caused by decreased activity of the proton pump in collecting duct intercalated-A cells. Because of the inability to excrete hydrogen ions, patients develop a metabolic acidosis with compensatory hyperchloremia, resulting in a normal anion gap, which is 8 mEq/L (8 mmol/L) in this patient, and the inability to acidify urine below a pH of 6.0, even in the context of an acidemia. The urine anion gap (using the equation: [Urine Sodium + Urine Potassium] – Urine Chloride) would be positive in this case, reflecting decreased acid excretion in the form of ammonium and chloride. The same defects also cause potassium wasting, and the increased proximal resorption of citrate that occurs with metabolic acidosis leads to hypocitraturia and increased risk of calcium phosphate kidney stones and nephrocalcinosis. This patient most likely has Sjögren syndrome (arthralgia, sicca, parotid gland enlargement) with concomitant interstitial nephritis (echogenicity seen on kidney ultrasound), one of the most common diseases associated with a distal RTA.

Naproxen, as well as other NSAIDs, can cause an interstitial nephritis usually accompanied by acute kidney injury and proteinuria, neither of which is seen in this case.

Type 2 (proximal) RTA involves a proximal tubular defect in reclaiming bicarbonate and is characterized by a normal anion gap metabolic acidosis, hypokalemia, glycosuria (without hyperglycemia), low-molecular-weight proteinuria, and renal phosphate wasting (known as Fanconi syndrome when all features are present). Because distal urine acidification remains intact, the urine pH is usually <5.5 without alkali therapy, and the urine anion gap should be negative, reflecting increased excretion of acid in the form of ammonium and chloride. This patient's high urine pH and absence of other characteristic features make type 2 (proximal) RTA unlikely.

Type 4 (hyperkalemic distal) RTA due to aldosterone deficiency or resistance is associated with hyperkalemia and a urine pH <5.5, neither of which is seen in this patient.

**KEY POINT**

- Type 1 (hypokalemic distal) renal tubular acidosis is due to a defect in urine acidification in the distal nephron and is characterized by a normal anion gap metabolic acidosis, positive urine anion gap, inability to acidify urine below a pH of 6.0, and potassium wasting.

**Bibliography**

Rastegar M, Nagami GT. Non-anion gap metabolic acidosis: a clinical approach to evaluation. Am J Kidney Dis. 2017;69:296-301. [PMID: 28029394]

## Item 42          Answer:    B

**Educational Objective:** Treat alcoholic ketoacidosis.

The most appropriate treatment is 5% dextrose in 0.9% saline for this patient who most likely has alcoholic ketoacidosis. Alcoholic ketoacidosis occurs in patients with chronic ethanol abuse, frequently with associated liver disease, and develops following an episode of acute intoxication. This patient has an increased anion gap metabolic acidosis (with an anion gap of 31), and ketoacidosis due to acute ethanol intoxication is the most likely cause. The ethanol level may be low or normal at the time of presentation because ingested ethanol may have already been extensively metabolized. Decreased insulin secretion (as a result of starvation) and increased counter-regulatory hormones cause lipolysis and generation of ketones, such as acetoacetate, which result in the anion gap. The urine in this case shows ketones, although ketone test results may be falsely negative in some cases because the nitroprusside reagent in the ketone assay detects only acetoacetate and the ketone β-hydroxybutyrate may predominate. Treatment with dextrose will increase insulin and decrease glucagon secretion, while saline will repair any volume deficit; the combination will correct ketoacidosis. In patients with alcoholism, thiamine should be administered before any glucose-containing solutions to decrease the risk of precipitating Wernicke encephalopathy.

Saline alone will correct the volume deficit, but glucose is needed to stimulate insulin secretion to correct the ketoacidosis.

Although dextrose with sodium bicarbonate may correct the underlying acidosis, there is no indication for additional bicarbonate in treating the ketoacidosis. In addition, alcoholic ketoacidosis may be associated with metabolic alkalosis due to concurrent vomiting. To determine if there is a concomitant metabolic alkalosis present, the corrected bicarbonate can be calculated. The corrected bicarbonate is the difference between the normal bicarbonate concentration and the delta anion gap. The delta anion gap is the difference between the measured anion gap and the normal anion gap. In this case the corrected bicarbonate concentration is 5 mEq/L (5 mmol/L) [24 - (31 - 12)]. Because the measured bicarbonate concentration (10 mEq/L [10 mmol/L]) is greater than the corrected, or expected, bicarbonate concentration, a concomitant metabolic alkalosis is present. Treatment with bicarbonate would be inappropriate.

Insulin treatment is not necessary because dextrose alone will increase insulin levels in patients who do not have diabetes mellitus.

**KEY POINT**

- For patients with alcoholic ketoacidosis, 5% dextrose in 0.9% saline is appropriate treatment.

**Bibliography**

Palmer BF, Clegg DJ. Electrolyte disturbances in patients with chronic alcohol-use disorder. N Engl J Med. 2017;377:1368-1377. [PMID: 28976856]

## Item 43          Answer:    A

**Educational Objective:** Treat edema associated with the nephrotic syndrome.

Addition of the thiazide diuretic metolazone is the most appropriate treatment. Edema management in a patient with newly diagnosed nephrotic syndrome generally starts with a salt-restricted diet and an oral loop diuretic, with a goal weight loss of 1 to 2 kg (2.2-4.4 lb) per week. Loop diuretics should be uptitrated toward this weight loss goal until a maximal dose is achieved, with close monitoring of electrolytes. It is appropriate for blood urea nitrogen, serum creatinine, and serum urate to rise slightly (≤10%) with effective diuresis. When oral loop diuretics have been maximally uptitrated, and weight loss and edema control are insufficient, it is often necessary to add a second oral diuretic (a thiazide diuretic and/or potassium-sparing diuretic) that works distal to the loop of Henle, which in this case can be accomplished via the addition of metolazone in this patient taking maximal-dose furosemide.

Loop diuretics are similarly effective when administered at equipotent doses. All loop diuretics have a similar dose-response curve characterized by an increased diuresis as more of the drug is renally excreted and flattening of the curve, at which further increases in dose are not associated with increased drug excretion and resultant diuresis.

Hospitalization for intravenous diuresis should be reserved for patients who have not responded to maximal doses of oral diuretics (that is, loop diuretic *and* thiazide diuretic) or for patients with severe symptoms of anasarca such as shortness of breath, swelling of genital regions, or gastrointestinal discomfort from ascites.

Repeating lower extremity Doppler ultrasonography is not indicated at this time given this patient's prior negative test results; serum albumin level >2.8 g/dL (28 g/L) (clotting risk in membranous glomerulopathy rises when albumin is ≤2.8 g/dL [28 g/L]); and the symmetric nature of his edema.

**KEY POINT**

- Edema management in a patient with newly diagnosed nephrotic syndrome starts with a salt-restricted diet and an oral loop diuretic; when loop diuretics have been maximally uptitrated and weight loss/edema control is insufficient, it is often necessary to add a thiazide and/or potassium-sparing diuretic.

## Bibliography

Kodner C. Diagnosis and management of nephrotic syndrome in adults. Am Fam Physician. 2016;93:479-85. [PMID: 26977832]

## Item 44          Answer:     D

**Educational Objective:** Diagnose secondary focal segmental glomerulosclerosis.

Secondary focal segmental glomerulosclerosis (FSGS) is the most likely diagnosis. FSGS is the most common form of the nephrotic syndrome in black persons. In the United States, FSGS currently accounts for up to 40% of idiopathic (primary) nephrotic syndromes in adults. The pathogenesis of FSGS stems from podocyte injury due to immunologic, genetic, and/or hyperfiltration causes. A large and growing proportion of FSGS cases are considered secondary forms of FSGS due to hyperfiltration injury in the setting of relatively reduced renal mass. The overworking of the glomerulus in this setting leads to adaptive podocyte injury and segmental sclerosis. This hyperfiltration form of FSGS is classically seen in obese patients but also can manifest in patients with a history of premature birth or solitary kidney. This patient has two risk factors for the secondary form of FSGS: obesity and a history of premature birth. In addition, her presentation is more typical of a secondary FSGS lesion, with subnephrotic proteinuria and no associated clinical findings. Electron microscopy of her kidney biopsy would be expected to show only mild to moderate effacement of the podocyte's foot processes. An immunologic route to injury is considered the main pathogenic mechanism behind primary forms of FSGS, with leukocytes producing a soluble circulating factor that directly targets podocytes. In such cases, proteinuria tends to be heavy (nephrotic range) with associated hypoalbuminemia, and edema is usually present on physical examination. Electron microscopy of a kidney biopsy with primary FSGS will typically show extensive effacement of the podocyte's foot process.

Diabetic nephropathy is the sequelae of chronic glycemic-induced damage to the glomerulus. On average, it occurs 8 years after the diagnosis of overt diabetes mellitus and is typically associated with other microvascular or macrovascular complications of diabetes. This patient's short history of prediabetes and lack of other microvascular/macrovascular findings makes diabetic nephropathy an unlikely diagnosis.

Lipoprotein glomerulopathy is a rare kidney disease characterized by moderate to severe proteinuria, progressive kidney failure, and distinct histopathologic findings of glomerular capillary dilatation by lipoprotein thrombi. To date, less than 100 cases have been reported in the medical literature, nearly all of which are from East Asian countries (predominantly Japan and China). This patient does not fit the profile for lipoprotein glomerulopathy.

Minimal change glomerulopathy typically presents with the full nephrotic syndrome (proteinuria >3500 mg/24 h, serum albumin usually <3.0 g/dL [30 g/L], hypercholesterolemia,

and edema on examination). These findings do not fit this patient's mild presentation.

**KEY POINT**

- Secondary focal segmental glomerulosclerosis is due to hyperfiltration injury in the setting of relatively reduced renal mass; it is classically seen in obese patients but also can manifest in those with a history of premature birth or solitary kidney.

## Bibliography

D'Agati VD, Kaskel FJ, Falk RJ. Focal segmental glomerulosclerosis. N Engl J Med. 2011;365:2398-411. [PMID: 22187987] doi:10.1056/NEJMra1106556

## Item 45          Answer:     D

**Educational Objective:** Identify the risk of venous thromboembolism in the nephrotic syndrome.

The nephrotic syndrome can be complicated by clotting manifestations due to a secondary hypercoagulable state. Of all the nephrotic syndromes, membranous glomerulopathy carries the greatest risk for clotting abnormalities, with some series reporting thrombotic complications in up to 35% of the most severe membranous glomerulopathy cases. The etiology for the hypercoagulable state in membranous glomerulopathy and other forms of heavy nephrosis is multifactorial. In response to the hypoalbuminemia induced by nephrotic-range proteinuria, the liver overproduces proteins. This is most classically seen in the form of hyperlipidemia. In addition, hepatic overproduction of proteins in response to hypoalbuminemia can also lead to increased levels of procoagulant proteins such as factor V, factor VIII, and fibrinogen. Urinary loss of albumin in high volume is also accompanied by similar urinary losses of low-molecular-weight anticoagulants (notably, antithrombin III and protein S) and fibrinolytics (such as plasminogen). In a large retrospective cohort of clotting complications in membranous glomerulopathy, >70% of the clots occurred within 2 years of diagnosis, and the risk of clotting markedly increased once albumin levels dropped below 2.8 g/dL (28 g/L) (OR, 2.53; $P = 0.02$, compared with albumin ≥2.8 g/dL [28 g/L]).

Chronic kidney disease is a risk factor for hyperuricemia and acute gout due to underexcretion of urate by the kidneys. In these patients, hyperuricemia may be due to impaired glomerular filtration and/or defects of urate handling in the renal proximal tubule. This patient's current kidney function does not place her at increased risk for gout.

Patients with membranous glomerulopathy have an increased risk of malignancy. Most cancers are diagnosed in men ≥65 years of age and are often solid tumors of the prostate, lung, or gastrointestinal tract. The risk for malignancy seems to be reduced in patients with anti-phospholipase A2 receptor (PLA2R) antibody. Taking into account her negative age- and sex-appropriate cancer screening, young age, and anti-PLA2R antibody status, this patient's risk of malignancy is low.

Patients with end-stage kidney disease have a markedly increased risk for renal cell carcinoma. Although current guidelines do not support routine screening for renal cell carcinoma in all patients with chronic kidney disease, a high level of suspicion is warranted in patients with symptoms such as new-onset gross hematuria or unexplained flank pain. In the absence of end-stage kidney disease, this patient is not at increased risk for renal cell carcinoma.

**KEY POINT**

- The nephrotic syndrome can be complicated by clotting manifestations due to a secondary hypercoagulable state, and risk is related to the degree of hypoalbuminemia.

**Bibliography**

Gyamlani G, Molnar MZ, Lu JL, Sumida K, Kalantar-Zadeh K, Kovesdy CP. Association of serum albumin level and venous thromboembolic events in a large cohort of patients with nephrotic syndrome. Nephrol Dial Transplant. 2017;32:157-164. [PMID: 28391310]

## Item 46    Answer:   B

**Educational Objective:** Treat hypertension in a patient with chronic kidney disease using an ACE inhibitor or angiotensin receptor blocker.

The addition of losartan is the most appropriate management. This patient has chronic kidney disease (CKD), given the presence of albuminuria, as well as uncontrolled hypertension. His antihypertensive medication regimen needs to be modified to control his blood pressure to target, given that uncontrolled hypertension will lead to CKD progression. The best option for this patient is to add an angiotensin receptor blocker (ARB) (such as losartan) or an ACE inhibitor, which are antihypertensive agents of choice in patients with CKD. Several studies have shown that use of an ARB or ACE inhibitor can result in decreased progression of albuminuria and CKD. Addition of losartan will also likely increase his serum potassium back to within normal range.

Adding amlodipine, a calcium channel blocker, is not the most appropriate next step in hypertension management for this patient and should be reserved if treatment with a maximum-tolerated dose of an ACE inhibitor or ARB does not result in blood pressure control.

Adding a low-dose aldosterone antagonist (such as spironolactone or eplerenone) may improve blood pressure control in patients with resistant hypertension. Treatment-resistant hypertension is defined as blood pressure that remains above goal despite concurrent use of three antihypertensive agents of different classes, one of which is a diuretic. Spironolactone is typically the fourth drug added to a three-drug regimen. This patient does not meet the definition of resistant hypertension.

Failure to act on this patient's blood pressure and albuminuria and reevaluating in 3 months misses the opportunity to slow the progression of CKD and albuminuria. In addition, guidelines recommend that adults initiating a new

or adjusted drug regimen for hypertension should have a follow-up evaluation of adherence and response to treatment at monthly intervals until control is achieved.

**KEY POINT**

- An ACE inhibitor or angiotensin receptor blocker is an agent of choice for treatment of hypertension in a patient with chronic kidney disease.

**Bibliography**

Whelton PK, Carey RM, Aronow WS, Casey DE Jr, Collins KJ, Dennison Himmelfarb C, et al. 2017 ACC/AHA/AAPA/ABC/ACPM/AGS/APhA/ASH/ASPC/NMA/PCNA guideline for the prevention, detection, evaluation, and management of high blood pressure in adults: a report of the American College of Cardiology/American Heart Association Task Force on Clinical Practice Guidelines. Hypertension. 2017. [PMID: 29133356]

## Item 47    Answer:   E

**Educational Objective:** Diagnose preeclampsia.

The most likely diagnosis is preeclampsia. Preeclampsia is defined by new-onset hypertension and proteinuria (≥300 mg/24 h from a timed collection or ≥300 mg/g by urine protein-creatinine ratio) that occurs after 20 weeks of pregnancy. New-onset hypertension with new-onset end-organ damage (such as liver or kidney injury, pulmonary edema, cerebral or visual symptoms, or thrombocytopenia) is also diagnostic of preeclampsia. Severe preeclampsia is identified by persistent systolic blood pressure >160 mm Hg or diastolic blood pressure >110 mm Hg and end-organ damage. Thrombocytopenia, liver enzyme elevation, and kidney involvement are all present in this pregnant patient with new-onset hypertension, making preeclampsia the most likely diagnosis.

Chronic hypertension is defined as a systolic blood pressure ≥140 mm Hg or diastolic pressure ≥90 mm Hg starting before pregnancy or before 20 weeks of gestation or persisting longer than 12 weeks' postpartum. In this case, the patient had normal blood pressures earlier in pregnancy.

Eclampsia is the presence of generalized tonic-clonic seizures in women with preeclampsia, which are not present in this patient.

Gestational hypertension first manifests after 20 weeks of pregnancy without proteinuria or other end-organ damage. Seen in 6% of pregnancies, gestational hypertension resolves within 12 weeks of delivery. Hypertension that persists beyond the 12 weeks is considered chronic hypertension. Of those who develop gestational hypertension, 15% to 25% progress to preeclampsia, and the rate increases to up to 50% in women who develop hypertension before 30 weeks. End-organ involvement in this case is inconsistent with gestational hypertension.

HELLP (hemolysis, elevated liver enzymes, and low platelets) syndrome is a life-threatening state that complicates 10% to 20% of cases of preeclampsia. The cause of HELLP syndrome is unknown, but it may be related to placental factors. However, it likely represents a separate disorder from preeclampsia. The diagnosis requires the presence of microangiopathic hemolytic anemia, which is excluded by the normal bilirubin level and peripheral blood smear.

### KEY POINT

- Preeclampsia is defined by new-onset hypertension and proteinuria that occurs after 20 weeks of pregnancy; new-onset hypertension with new-onset end-organ damage (such as liver or kidney injury, pulmonary edema, cerebral or visual symptoms, or thrombocytopenia) are also diagnostic.

### Bibliography

American College of Obstetricians and Gynecologists. Hypertension in pregnancy. Report of the American College of Obstetricians and Gynecologists' Task Force on Hypertension in Pregnancy. Obstet Gynecol. 2013;122:1122-31. [PMID: 24150027]

## Item 48      Answer:    A

**Educational Objective:** Diagnose Fabry disease.

The most likely disease is Fabry disease, an X-linked recessive inborn error of glycosphingolipid metabolism caused by deficiency of α-galactosidase A. The enzyme deficiency leads to defective storage of sphingolipid and progressive endothelial accumulation, causing abnormalities in the skin, eye, kidney, heart, brain, and peripheral nervous system. Typically, the disease begins in childhood with episodes of pain and burning sensations in the hands and feet. These painful episodes can be brought on by exercise, fever, fatigue, or other stressors. In addition, young patients often develop angiokeratomas (violaceous papules with overlying scale), decreased perspiration, and corneal and lens opacities of the eyes. The disease is progressive, and symptoms of kidney, heart, and/or neurologic involvement usually occur between the ages of 30 and 45 years. As an X-linked disorder, males who inherit a mutation in the gene responsible for α-galactosidase always display the disease phenotype. Females, on the other hand, who inherit only one copy of a disease-causing mutation, can show a wide range of clinical manifestations, ranging from asymptomatic carriers to severe heart and kidney failure no different from a hemizygous male's phenotype. This variability is likely due to varying degrees of random inactivation of one copy of the X chromosome in each cell (lyonization). The most common finding of Fabry disease seen in heterozygous females is corneal dystrophy, which occurs in more than half of females. Fabry disease should be considered as a cause of chronic kidney disease of unknown etiology in young adulthood, especially when there is a family history of early end-stage kidney disease or cardiovascular-related death (via myocardial infarction or cerebrovascular accident). Diagnosis can be made via kidney biopsy but also noninvasively with measurement of leukocyte enzymatic activity and subsequent genetic confirmation. Screening for the disease is recommended for family members of affected patients. Enzyme replacement therapy with recombinant human α-galactosidase A is available.

Hereditary nephritis (Alport syndrome), like Fabry disease, can present with kidney failure if diagnosed late but is not associated with abnormalities in the skin or peripheral nervous system.

Medullary cystic kidney disease is a familial form of kidney disease with no known extrarenal symptomatology and usually presents with bland urinary findings.

This degree of kidney failure in a patient with tuberous sclerosis complex would be associated with abnormal kidney imaging, such as angiomyolipomas and cysts, and the classic skin lesions in this condition are hamartoma formations, not angiokeratomas.

### KEY POINT

- Fabry disease should be considered as a cause of chronic kidney disease of unknown etiology in young adulthood.

### Bibliography

Pisani A, Visciano B, Imbriaco M, Di Nuzzi A, Mancini A, Marchetiello C, et al. The kidney in Fabry's disease. Clin Genet. 2014;86:301-9. [PMID: 24645664]

## Item 49      Answer:    C    H

**Educational Objective:** Manage a patient with a struvite stone.

In addition to starting antibiotics, stone removal should be considered to decrease future episodes of urinary tract infections in this patient who has a struvite stone. Struvite stones occur most frequently in older women with chronic urinary tract infections. These stones occur in the presence of urea-splitting bacteria such as *Proteus, Klebsiella*, or, less frequently, *Pseudomonas*. These bacteria split urea into ammonium, which markedly increases urine pH (>7.5) and results in the precipitation of magnesium ammonium phosphate (struvite). Struvite stones can form rapidly and commonly produce staghorn calculi (stones that bridge two or more renal calyces). Because bacteria can live within the interstices of the stone, limiting antibiotic access, the only intervention that will decrease recurrent infections is removal of the stone. Although this may be accomplished by means of shock wave lithotripsy, patients often require percutaneous nephrolithotomy and breakup of the stone. A percutaneous nephrostomy tube is often inserted to allow for irrigation and to ensure complete removal of all fragments.

Although antibiotics are needed to treat infection, chronic antibiotic suppression is rarely successful as a primary treatment. Continued use of antibiotics increases the risk of the development of antibiotic resistance.

Pure struvite stones often occur in women who have upper urinary tract infections, but oftentimes other components such as calcium oxalate serve as the initial nidus. Because this nidus may not be among the stone fragments submitted for analysis, it may be missed. It is therefore important that a metabolic evaluation be performed in all patients. If the evaluation reveals decreased levels of urine citrate, potassium citrate can be added. Potassium citrate should not, however, be used empirically.

CONT.

The urease inhibitor acetohydroxamic acid can decrease stone growth; however, it is associated with significant side effects (nausea, vomiting, diarrhea, headache, hallucinations, rash, abdominal discomfort, anemia) and is therefore not recommended as a primary treatment.

The use of acidifying agents such as ammonium chloride rarely is able to achieve acidic urine in patients with urea-splitting bacteria and therefore is not recommended.

### KEY POINT

• Patients with struvite stones require stone removal.

### Bibliography

Marien T, Miller NL. Treatment of the infected stone. Urol Clin North Am. 2015;42:459-72. [PMID: 26475943]

## Item 50    Answer:    A

**Educational Objective:** Diagnose adynamic bone disease in a patient with chronic kidney disease.

The most likely bone pathology is adynamic bone disease in this patient with end-stage kidney disease and normal serum calcium and phosphorus and relatively suppressed parathyroid hormone (PTH) and alkaline phosphatase levels. Adynamic bone disease can occur in patients with chronic kidney disease (CKD) or those on dialysis. It is typically associated with significant vascular calcifications. The gold standard for the diagnosis of adynamic bone disease is bone biopsy; however, this is rarely performed. Adynamic bone disease has no specific markers, but a constellation of findings may suggest this diagnosis. Patients with adynamic bone disease may present with fracture or bone pain. The latter has been attributed to the inability to repair microdamage because of low turnover. Serum calcium may be normal or elevated because the bone is unable to take up calcium. High PTH and alkaline phosphatase would exclude adynamic bone disease; in this disorder, both are typically normal. Treatment is targeted at factors that allow PTH secretion to rise. This includes avoiding calcium-based binders, conservative use of vitamin D, and decreasing the dialysate calcium concentration. It is important to note that, as with the general population, patients with CKD may also develop osteoporosis, particularly if they received glucocorticoid therapy for the primary kidney disorder or for immunosuppression in the setting of a kidney transplant.

β$_2$-Microglobulin–associated amyloidosis is usually seen in patients who have been on dialysis for at least 5 years. This disorder involves osteoarticular sites, and patients may present with carpal tunnel syndrome or shoulder pain. Bone cysts may be visible on radiograph.

Osteitis fibrosa cystica is the classic pathology associated with kidney disease. This disorder is associated with increased bone turnover and elevated PTH and alkaline phosphatase levels. Mixed uremic osteodystrophy has elements of both high and low bone turnover.

Osteomalacia refers to a defect with both low turnover and abnormal mineralization of bone. This disorder can be seen by vitamin D deficiency, but in the past, it was a common complication of aluminum toxicity. This patient's vitamin D level is in the "sufficient range," and there is no history of aluminum exposure.

### KEY POINT

• Adynamic bone disease can occur in patients with chronic kidney disease or those on dialysis and is associated with fracture or bone pain; parathyroid hormone and alkaline phosphatase levels are typically normal.

### Bibliography

Carvalho C, Alves CM, Frazão JM. The role of bone biopsy for the diagnosis of renal osteodystrophy: a short overview and future perspectives. J Nephrol. 2016;29:617-26. [PMID: 27473148]

## Item 51    Answer:    C

**Educational Objective:** Treat cardiorenal syndrome.

Increasing the furosemide dose is the most appropriate treatment in this patient with cardiorenal syndrome type 1 (CRS1). CRS is a disorder of the heart and kidneys in which acute or long-term dysfunction in one organ induces acute or long-term dysfunction in the other. CRS is characterized by the triad of concomitant decreased kidney function, diuretic-resistant heart failure with congestion, and worsening kidney function during heart failure therapy. CRS1 is defined as a worsening kidney function in patients with acute worsening of cardiac function (decompensated heart failure, acute coronary syndrome, cardiogenic shock). Management is challenging because treatment directed toward improving cardiac function can worsen kidney function. For this patient, an increase to his loop diuretic dose to a sufficient dose to induce a diuresis is appropriate. Among patients with decompensated heart failure, the best outcomes may occur with aggressive fluid removal even if associated with mild to moderate worsening of kidney function. An elevated blood urea nitrogen (BUN)-creatinine ratio should not discourage the use of diuretic therapy in patients with evidence of congestion. The decline in his kidney function with relative increase in BUN-creatinine ratio reflects the CRS1 physiology, rather than volume depletion due to diuresis.

Vasopressin receptor antagonists such as conivaptan can be used for the treatment of patients with hypervolemic or euvolemic hyponatremia. However, there is no evidence that treatment of hyponatremia improves clinical outcomes in patients with severe chronic heart failure.

Dobutamine, as well as milrinone, is used in the management of cardiogenic shock or decompensated acute heart failure with severe impaired left ventricular function and would not be indicated for a patient with preserved ejection fraction.

Ultrafiltration therapy is reserved for patients with severe volume overload refractory to medical management.

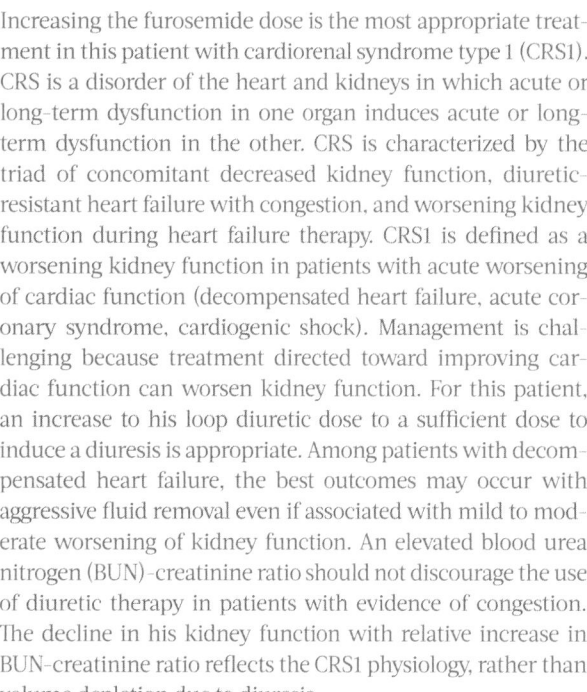

CONT.

In the Cardiorenal Rescue Study in Acute Decompensated Heart Failure (Caress-HF) study, the use of a stepwise pharmacologic therapy algorithm was superior to ultrafiltration for the preservation of kidney function at 96 hours, with a similar weight loss between the two strategies.

### KEY POINT

- In cardiorenal syndrome type 1, loop diuretics are first-line therapy for managing volume overload in patients with decompensated heart failure with evidence of peripheral and/or pulmonary edema.

### Bibliography

Verbrugge FH, Grieten L, Mullens W. Management of the cardiorenal syndrome in decompensated heart failure. Cardiorenal Med. 2014;4:176-88. [PMID: 25737682]

## Item 52        Answer:   D

**Educational Objective:** **Treat anemia associated with chronic kidney disease using iron supplementation.**

Iron supplementation is the most appropriate treatment for this patient with anemia associated with stage G4 chronic kidney disease (CKD). The prevalence of anemia increases as CKD progresses due to several factors, including impaired erythropoietin production, erythropoietin resistance, and reduced erythrocyte life span. Initial evaluation for the cause of anemia in patients with CKD includes laboratory studies as would be appropriate for patients without CKD. All patients with CKD and anemia should have iron profiles assessed, including total transferrin saturation (serum iron ÷ total iron-binding capacity × 100) and serum ferritin levels. The Kidney Disease: Improving Global Outcomes (KDIGO) recommendations suggest maintaining transferrin saturation levels of >30% and serum ferritin levels of >500 ng/mL (500 µg/L) using either oral or intravenous iron supplementation. Patients with stage G3 or G4 CKD can be treated with oral iron supplements but may need parenteral administration if oral iron is not effective. Patients with stage G5 CKD generally do not respond well to oral iron due to impaired gastrointestinal absorption and therefore often need intravenous administration. This patient with stage G4 CKD has iron deficiency and should have iron repletion.

Although blood transfusions are effective at acutely raising the hemoglobin, they are associated with adverse side effects. Specific to the advanced CKD population, blood transfusions should be avoided if possible to prevent HLA sensitization to foreign antigens, which may increase waiting time for kidney transplantation.

A bone marrow biopsy is not indicated because there is no evidence to suggest bone marrow dysfunction. Platelet count and leukocyte count are normal. The low hemoglobin and erythrocyte reticulocyte count reflect the inadequate iron stores. A brisk reticulocytosis should be observed within days of starting iron therapy.

Although many patients with advanced CKD and end-stage kidney disease require an erythropoietin-stimulating

agent (ESA), its use is indicated only when the patient has adequate iron stores. Iron deficiency is a common reason for ESA resistance. ESAs take several weeks to achieve full effect and are sometimes started at the same time as parenteral iron. Current KDIGO guidelines recommend consideration of ESAs for patients with CKD and hemoglobin concentrations <10 g/dL (100 g/L). However, it is premature to consider ESA in this patient for she may respond to supplemental iron administration alone with an increase in hemoglobin level.

### KEY POINT

- All patients with chronic kidney disease and anemia should have iron profiles assessed, including transferrin saturation and ferritin levels; treatment target levels are a transferrin saturation level >30% and a serum ferritin level >500 ng/mL (500 µg/L) using either oral or intravenous iron supplementation.

### Bibliography

Panwar B, Gutiérrez OM. Disorders of iron metabolism and anemia in chronic kidney disease. Semin Nephrol. 2016;36:252-61. [PMID: 27475656]

## Item 53        Answer:   B

**Educational Objective:** **Evaluate for primary hyperaldosteronism as the underlying cause of hypokalemia and resistant hypertension.**

The most appropriate diagnostic test to perform next is plasma aldosterone concentration (PAC)/plasma renin activity (PRA) ratio. The patient presents with a triad of resistant hypertension, metabolic alkalosis, and hypokalemia following the addition of a thiazide diuretic, which raises suspicion for primary hyperaldosteronism. Primary hyperaldosteronism, in which aldosterone production cannot be suppressed with sodium loading, is the most common cause of secondary hypertension in middle-aged adults and an important cause of resistant hypertension. Testing for primary hyperaldosteronism is recommended if any of the following are present: resistant hypertension, hypokalemia (spontaneous or substantial, if diuretic induced), incidentally discovered adrenal mass, family history of early-onset hypertension, or stroke at age <40 years. Diuretics should be discontinued prior to testing to assure euvolemia. Calculation of the PAC/PRA ratio is used for screening, with a very high ratio of PAC/PRA suggestive of diagnosis. A positive screening test would reveal a reduced or undetectable PRA or concentration and an inappropriately high (usually >15 ng/dL) PAC, which results in a high PAC/PRA ratio of >20. Confirmatory testing is performed except when initial testing is diagnostic, as in cases of spontaneous hypokalemia with undetectable PRA and PAC (>30 ng/dL [828 pmol/L]). Confirmatory tests include oral and intravenous salt loading and the fludrocortisone suppression and captopril challenge tests.

Kidney ultrasonography with Doppler is performed to diagnose renovascular disease, which can be a secondary cause of hypertension. However, no clinical trials have

CONT.

demonstrated that percutaneous intervention results in improvement of hypertension or lessens kidney deterioration; therefore, diagnostic testing is reserved for patients with otherwise strong indications for this study, such as a young woman with possible fibromuscular dysplasia, but not this patient.

Plasma fractionated metanephrines are obtained to screen for a pheochromocytoma, which could result in hypertension; however, this is a relatively rare diagnosis that cannot explain the patient's current findings, and there are no symptoms or signs (episodic headaches, palpitations) in this patient to indicate pheochromocytoma.

Polysomnography is used to diagnose obstructive sleep apnea, another secondary cause of hypertension. However, clinical suspicion for this diagnosis is low given that it cannot explain the patient's metabolic findings, and the patient is not obese and does not present with snoring and daytime sleepiness.

**KEY POINT**

- Calculation of the plasma aldosterone concentration/plasma renin activity ratio is used to diagnose primary hyperaldosteronism.

**Bibliography**
Braam B, Taler SJ, Rahman M, Fillaus JA, Greco BA, Forman JP, et al. Recognition and management of resistant hypertension. Clin J Am Soc Nephrol. 2017;12:524-535. [PMID: 27895136]

 **Item 54      Answer:    D**

**Educational Objective:  Diagnose surreptitious vomiting as a cause of metabolic alkalosis.**

The most likely cause of this patient's metabolic alkalosis is surreptitious vomiting. Metabolic alkalosis is diagnosed by an elevation in serum bicarbonate concentration. This disorder is caused either by a loss of acid or administration or retention of bicarbonate. Conditions that contribute to the maintenance of metabolic alkalosis include volume contraction, ineffective arterial blood volume, hypokalemia, chloride depletion, and decreased glomerular filtration. Laboratory evaluation of metabolic alkalosis is based on urine chloride concentration. Metabolic alkalosis is considered saline responsive when associated with true hypovolemia and responds to correction of the volume deficit with isotonic saline. Saline-responsive metabolic alkalosis presents with a low urine chloride of <15 mEq/L (15 mmol/L); the most common causes are vomiting, nasogastric suction, and diuretic use. Hypokalemia occurs secondarily due to aldosterone elevation and cation loss as the kidney attempts to lose bicarbonate. Although these patients are usually hypovolemic or normovolemic (with normal or low blood pressures), patients with preexisting chronic hypertension may present with high to normal blood pressures.

For those who have a high urine chloride (>15 mEq/L [15 mmol/L]) with elevated blood pressure and hypokalemia and do not appear to be overtly volume overloaded,

a mineralocorticoid excess disorder must be considered (saline-resistant metabolic alkalosis). Examples include Cushing syndrome and primary aldosteronism. Neither is a likely diagnosis based on the low urine chloride and absence of hypertension. Rarely, patients with metabolic alkalosis may appear to have clinical features consistent with saline-responsive metabolic alkalosis (normal/low extracellular fluid status, normal/low blood pressure) but have a urine chloride of >15 mEq/L (15 mmol/L). Diuretic use and inherited kidney disorders of sodium and chloride handling, such as Bartter and Gitelman syndromes, can mimic this presentation. These two autosomal recessive genetic disorders of renal sodium and chloride transporters clinically mimic loop diuretic and thiazide diuretic use, respectively. These diagnoses should be considered only after urine diuretic screening.

**KEY POINT**

- Saline-responsive metabolic alkalosis typically presents with hypovolemia and a low urine chloride of <15 mEq/L (15 mmol/L); the most common causes are vomiting, nasogastric suction, and diuretic use.

**Bibliography**
Soifer JT, Kim HT. Approach to metabolic alkalosis. Emerg Med Clin North Am. 2014;32:453-63. [PMID: 24766943]

**Item 55      Answer:    A**

**Educational Objective:  Diagnose IgG4-related disease.**

The patient's decline in kidney function is most likely due to IgG4-related disease, a syndrome that mostly affects middle-aged or older men. Plasma cell–rich tubulointerstitial nephritis (TIN) is the most common kidney manifestation. Other manifestations can include autoimmune pancreatitis, allergic rhinitis, submandibular gland swelling, an elevated antinuclear antibody (ANA) titer, low serum complement levels, elevated serum IgG, elevated serum IgE, and peripheral eosinophilia. Kidney imaging may show enlarged kidneys or renal masses that may present as small peripheral cortical nodules. This patient's urinalysis findings of trace protein and pyuria with progressive decline of kidney function are consistent with TIN. Definitive diagnosis of IgG4-related disease requires a tissue biopsy to demonstrate an infiltrate with IgG4-positive plasma cells. IgG4-related disease is readily treatable with glucocorticoids.

Although elevated ANA titers and hypocomplementemia are seen in lupus, lupus nephritis is usually characterized by proteinuria and a more active urine sediment (dysmorphic erythrocytes and cellular casts). Furthermore, lupus is more common in women and usually manifests at a much earlier age than in this patient.

Sarcoidosis can affect multiple organs and cause TIN. However, sarcoidosis is not associated with autoimmune pancreatitis, hypocomplementemia, elevated serum immunoglobulin levels, or cortical nodules on kidney ultrasound.

CONT.

Although Sjögren syndrome can affect lacrimal and salivary glands and cause TIN, this patient's constellation of symptoms is more consistent with IgG4-related disease. Dryness of the eyes and mouth is extremely common in Sjögren but not in IgG4-related disease. Allergy symptoms, such as asthma or allergic rhinitis, are rarely seen in Sjögren but are common in IgG4-related disease. Hypocomplementemia and the presence of cortical nodules on kidney ultrasound also favor the diagnosis of IgG4-related disease.

**KEY POINT**

- Tubulointerstitial nephritis is the most common kidney manifestation of IgG4-related disease and typically presents with pyuria, proteinuria, and elevated serum IgG and IgE levels; kidney imaging may show enlarged kidneys or renal masses.

**Bibliography**

Zhang P, Cornell LD. IgG4-related tubulointerstitial nephritis. Adv Chronic Kidney Dis. 2017;24:94-100. [PMID: 28284385]

**Item 56**       **Answer:    A**

**Educational Objective:** Identify NSAIDs as a cause of acute kidney injury in a patient with chronic kidney disease.

Discontinuation of naproxen is the most appropriate management for this patient with chronic kidney disease (CKD) who has developed acute kidney injury. NSAIDs are one of the most frequently used over-the-counter medications and a mainstay in many pain and inflammatory conditions. However, NSAIDs inhibit cyclooxygenase-1 and cyclooxygenase-2, which decrease vasodilatory prostaglandin production. In patients who are prostaglandin dependent (volume depleted, heart failure, CKD), this decreases renal blood flow and leads to decreased glomerular filtration rate. Patients with CKD are sensitive to the nephrotoxic effects of NSAIDs; therefore, these medications are a frequent cause of acute kidney injury in this patient population. The nephrotoxic effect of NSAIDs is augmented by concomitant use of renin-angiotensin system inhibitors due to concomitant effects on afferent and efferent vascular tone. Discontinuation of naproxen is the best treatment for this patient's acute kidney injury. The American Society of Nephrology recommends the avoidance of NSAIDs, including cyclooxygenase-2 inhibitors, in patients with CKD due to the risk of worsening kidney function. There are safer treatment alternatives for osteoarthritis (OA). Exercise is among the most important nonpharmacologic treatments for most patients with OA, and evidence for its efficacy is most convincing for knee OA. Because excessive weight contributes to both knee OA risk and symptomatology, measures to promote weight loss are appropriate for overweight patients with knee OA. Topical NSAIDs may be a safer, effective alternative to oral NSAIDs in this patient population.

CT angiography of the renal arteries with iodinated contrast is contraindicated in the setting of acute kidney injury.

There is no evidence to suggest that renal artery stenosis is contributing to this patient's acute kidney injury.

Kidney biopsy can be performed to diagnosis glomerulonephritis. Although NSAIDs can cause glomerulonephritis, there are no signs to suggest acute glomerulonephritis because the patient's urinalysis does not show blood or significant protein.

Starting furosemide would help with the new peripheral edema that has developed but would not reverse the acute kidney injury; in fact, it may worsen the acute kidney injury by decreasing intravascular volume and further decreasing renal blood flow.

**KEY POINT**

- In patients with chronic kidney disease, NSAIDs are potentially nephrotoxic and a frequent cause of acute kidney injury and should be avoided.

**Bibliography**

Zhang X, Donnan PT, Bell S, Guthrie B. Non-steroidal anti-inflammatory drug induced acute kidney injury in the community dwelling general population and people with chronic kidney disease: systematic review and meta-analysis. BMC Nephrol. 2017;18:256. [PMID: 28764659]

**Item 57**       **Answer:    A**

**Educational Objective:** Treat calcineurin inhibitor–induced hypertension and hyperkalemia in a kidney transplant recipient.

The most appropriate treatment for calcineurin inhibitor–induced hypertension and hyperkalemia in this kidney transplant recipient is a thiazide or thiazide-like diuretic such as chlorthalidone. Patients with kidney transplants must receive immunosuppressive medications to prevent their immune system from rejecting the kidney allograft. Doses are typically highest immediately after transplant and are tapered gradually over several months to minimize toxicities associated with these medications while maintaining adequate immunosuppression. The most commonly used immunosuppressants in the immediate posttransplant period for immunosuppression induction are anti–T-cell and interleukin-2 receptor–blocking antibodies. The most commonly prescribed medications for chronic maintenance immunosuppression include calcineurin inhibitors (tacrolimus or cyclosporine), antimetabolites (mycophenolate mofetil or azathioprine), and glucocorticoids. Although these medications are usually well tolerated, they can have significant side effects. Calcineurin inhibitors activate the sodium chloride cotransporter in the distal convoluted tubule, which reabsorbs sodium and chloride to cause hypertension. Decreased distal tubular flow impairs potassium secretion in the connecting tubule and collecting duct, leading to hyperkalemia. Calcineurin inhibitor–induced hypertension and hyperkalemia share the same phenotype as Gordon syndrome (familial hyperkalemic hypertension), which is due to a dysregulation of the WNK kinases in the distal convoluted tubule. Thiazide and thiazide-like diuretics such as chlorthalidone address the underlying mechanism of calcineurin inhibitor–induced hypertension and hyperkalemia by inhibiting the sodium chloride cotransporter.

Although fludrocortisone, a synthetic mineralocorticoid, would treat the hyperkalemia, this medication would exacerbate sodium retention and raise blood pressure in this patient with already uncontrolled hypertension. Sodium polystyrene sulfonate would also treat the hyperkalemia but provides a significant sodium load with each dose and may also raise the blood pressure. These medications do not address the underlying mechanism and are therefore not indicated.

Spironolactone may lower the blood pressure but would raise serum potassium and is therefore contraindicated in this patient who is already hyperkalemic.

**KEY POINT**

- Treatment using thiazide diuretics is appropriate for calcineurin inhibitor–induced hypertension and hyperkalemia in kidney transplant recipients.

**Bibliography**
Moes AD, Hesselink DA, Zietse R, van Schaik RH, van Gelder T, Hoorn EJ. Calcineurin inhibitors and hypertension: a role for pharmacogenetics? Pharmacogenomics. 2014;15:1243-51. [PMID: 25141899]

## Item 58    Answer:    B

**Educational Objective:** Treat hypermagnesemia using intravenous calcium.

In addition to administration of 0.9% saline and furosemide, intravenous calcium is appropriate treatment for this patient with hypermagnesemia. Because the kidney can efficiently eliminate magnesium, hypermagnesemia occurs infrequently and most commonly results from excessive intake in the setting of decreased kidney function. Numerous medications such as antacids and laxatives contain magnesium, and magnesium sulfate is the treatment of choice for prevention of eclampsia. Hypermagnesemia is usually not associated with significant symptoms until the level is >7.2 mg/dL (2.9 mmol/L). Symptoms include somnolence, headache, loss of deep tendon reflexes, bradycardia, hypotension, and hypocalcemia. At levels >12 mg/dL (4.9 mmol/L), flaccid paralysis, respiratory failure, and complete heart block can occur. Hypermagnesemia is usually self-limited. Magnesium-containing medications should be discontinued, and magnesium excretion can be enhanced with saline diuresis. In patients with hypotension and significant neuromuscular deficits, treatment is aimed at direct antagonism of the effects of hypermagnesemia, which is accomplished by intravenous administration of calcium. After this, efforts to lower the serum level should be instituted. If kidney function is adequate, a trial of 0.9% saline and furosemide will increase kidney excretion. Magnesium-containing agents should be limited or avoided in individuals with kidney disease.

If kidney failure is advanced, hemodialysis will effectively lower magnesium levels. However, this would require access to the central venous system and mobilization of the dialysis team, which can take several hours, and in the interim patients with symptomatic hypermagnesemia should be given intravenous calcium.

There is no role for either intravenous potassium or sodium bicarbonate other than correcting preexisting metabolic abnormalities.

Although sodium polystyrene sulfonate will bind a small amount of magnesium, this effect is minimal and not advocated as a treatment.

**KEY POINT**

- Management of hypermagnesemia includes discontinuation of magnesium-containing medications, administration of saline diuresis to enhance magnesium excretion, and administration of intravenous calcium to treat severe symptoms.

**Bibliography**
Van Hook JW. Endocrine crises. Hypermagnesemia. Crit Care Clin. 1991;7:215-23. [PMID: 2007216]

## Item 59    Answer:    A

**Educational Objective:** Diagnose the cause of acute kidney injury.

The most appropriate next step is examination of the urine sediment for cells and casts. This patient has developed oliguric acute kidney injury (AKI). He has multiple risk factors for AKI, including type 2 diabetes mellitus, recent coronary arteriography, hypotension, and cardiac surgery. The main consideration is whether the AKI is due to renal hypoperfusion (prerenal AKI) or whether the AKI is due to acute tubular necrosis (ATN). In the setting of diuretics, the fractional excretion of urea ($FE_{Urea}$) is more accurate than the fractional excretion of sodium because urea excretion is not promoted by diuretics and is still retained in volume-depleted states. $FE_{Urea}$ is calculated using the equation:

$$FE_{Urea} = (U_{Urea} \times P_{Creatinine})/(U_{Creatinine} \times P_{Urea}) \times 100\%$$

$FE_{Urea}$ <35% is suggestive of a prerenal state. The presence of granular casts and/or renal epithelial cells has strong predictive value for ATN. Urine microscopy can also help differentiate other causes of AKI, such as acute interstitial nephritis and glomerulonephritis.

The fractional excretion of sodium ($FE_{Na}$) is calculated as follows:

$$FE_{Na} = (U_{Sodium} \times P_{Creatinine})/(U_{Creatinine} \times P_{Sodium}) \times 100\%$$

$FE_{Na}$ <1% indicates prerenal AKI but can also be seen in contrast-induced nephropathy, acute interstitial nephritis, rhabdomyolysis, glomerulonephritis, and early obstruction because the tubular handling of sodium is intact in these conditions. $FE_{Na}$ >2% indicates ATN but is also seen in patients who are prerenal and are on diuretics or who have adrenal insufficiency, bicarbonaturia, or chronic kidney disease due to the increased distal tubular delivery of sodium in these conditions.

CONT.

Kidney ultrasonography should be performed to rule out obstructive uropathy as the cause of AKI. However, the patient already has a urinary catheter, so the likelihood of obstruction as the cause of AKI is low.

Central venous pressure is not a reliable indicator of organ perfusion and would not be able to differentiate prerenal AKI from ATN or other causes of AKI.

### KEY POINT

- The presence of granular casts and/or renal epithelial cells on urine microscopy has strong predictive value for acute tubular necrosis.

### Bibliography

Perazella MA, Coca SG, Kanbay M, Brewster UC, Parikh CR. Diagnostic value of urine microscopy for differential diagnosis of acute kidney injury in hospitalized patients. Clin J Am Soc Nephrol. 2008;3:1615-9. [PMID: 18784207]

### Item 60    Answer:    A

**Educational Objective:** Diagnose masked hypertension using ambulatory blood pressure monitoring.

The most appropriate test to perform next is 24-hour ambulatory blood pressure monitoring (ABPM) in this patient who has a strong family history of hypertension with cardiovascular complications. According to the American College of Cardiology/American Heart Association (ACC/AHA) blood pressure guideline, the patient has elevated blood pressure (BP), defined as systolic BP between 120-129 mm Hg and diastolic BP <80 mm Hg, and is at risk for development of hypertension (defined as systolic BP ≥130 mm Hg or diastolic BP ≥80 mm Hg). In addition, she has left ventricular hypertrophy on electrocardiogram, which raises concern for underlying long-standing hypertension. Therefore, masked hypertension, defined as BP that is normal in the office but elevated in the ambulatory setting, should be ruled out. Masked hypertension is associated with an increased risk of sustained hypertension and cardiovascular disease. The diagnostic test of choice is 24-hour ABPM; home blood pressure monitoring is an alternative strategy. Up to 10% to 40% of patients who are normotensive by clinic measurement may be hypertensive by ABPM or home blood pressure monitoring, which should be performed in patients referred for hypertension but with normal office BP and in those with end-organ damage such as left ventricular hypertrophy. Finally, the ACC/AHA notes that it is reasonable to evaluate for masked hypertension in patients with elevated BP, even in the absence of a strong family history of cardiovascular disease or evidence of sustained hypertension (for example, left ventricular hypertrophy on electrocardiogram).

A plasma aldosterone concentration/plasma renin activity ratio is often obtained in the evaluation of hyperaldosteronism. Such patients present with hypertension and often hypokalemia and metabolic alkalosis. It is premature to evaluate the patient for secondary causes of hypertension without first establishing the diagnosis of hypertension with ABPM or home blood pressure monitoring.

Disordered breathing events such as obstructive sleep apnea are associated with autonomic instability, increased vascular tone, hypertension, and alterations in heart rate. However, this patient has no symptoms to suggest obstructive sleep apnea (frequent awakenings, dry mouth, snoring, daytime sleepiness, nonrestorative sleep), and testing with polysomnography is not indicated at this time.

Measurement of thyroid-stimulating hormone levels is not the next best diagnostic test because the patient does not manifest any symptoms or signs concerning for hyperthyroidism, such as tachycardia, heat intolerance, palpitations, dyspnea, tremulousness, weight loss, fatigue, insomnia, and mood disturbances.

### KEY POINT

- Suspected masked hypertension (defined as blood pressure that is normal in the office but elevated in the ambulatory setting) should be confirmed with ambulatory blood pressure monitoring or home blood pressure monitoring.

### Bibliography

Whelton PK, Carey RM, Aronow WS, Casey DE Jr, Collins KJ, Dennison Himmelfarb C, et al. 2017 ACC/AHA/AAPA/ABC/ACPM/AGS/APhA/ASH/ASPC/NMA/PCNA guideline for the prevention, detection, evaluation, and management of high blood pressure in adults: a report of the American College of Cardiology/American Heart Association Task Force on Clinical Practice Guidelines. Hypertension. 2017. [PMID: 29133356]

### Item 61    Answer:    A

**Educational Objective:** Treat hypertension in a black patient using a thiazide diuretic and a calcium channel blocker.

Addition of the calcium channel blocker (CCB) amlodipine is the most appropriate next step in management. A landmark trial (ALLHAT) revealed that in black patients, a thiazide diuretic was more effective in improving cardiovascular outcomes compared with an ACE inhibitor, and there was a higher risk of stroke with use of an ACE inhibitor as initial therapy compared with a CCB. For these reasons, initial antihypertensive treatment in black patients, including those with diabetes mellitus, should include a thiazide diuretic or CCB, or combination of the two. However, if chronic kidney disease (CKD) is present, initial or add-on therapy should include an ACE inhibitor or angiotensin receptor blocker, especially in those with proteinuria, as illustrated by the AASK study. There is no evidence of CKD in this patient, given the normal serum creatinine and absence of an elevated urine albumin-creatinine ratio. Although hydrochlorothiazide was initiated 1 month ago, his blood pressure is still not at the target. Addition of the CCB amlodipine is therefore appropriate.

This patient is already on an adequate dose of hydrochlorothiazide, and his serum potassium level is borderline low at 3.5 mEq/L (3.5 mmol/L). Increasing the hydrochlorothiazide dose may further decrease his serum potassium and may be associated with adverse side effects, such as orthostasis and erectile dysfunction.

According to the American College of Cardiology/American Heart Association (ACC/AHA) blood pressure guideline, target blood pressure for most patients with hypertension, with or without coronary artery disease, diabetes, or CKD is <130/80 mm Hg. This patient is substantially above target, and reassessing in 3 months' time would not be adequate management. In addition, the ACC/AHA guideline recommends that adults initiating a new or adjusted drug regimen for hypertension should have a follow-up evaluation of adherence and response to treatment at monthly intervals until control is achieved. Waiting 3 months to reevaluate the patient is too long.

**KEY POINT**

- Initial antihypertensive treatment in black patients without chronic kidney disease should include a thiazide diuretic or calcium channel blocker, or combination of the two.

**Bibliography**

ALLHAT Officers and Coordinators for the ALLHAT Collaborative Research Group. The Antihypertensive and Lipid-Lowering Treatment to Prevent Heart Attack Trial. Major outcomes in high-risk hypertensive patients randomized to angiotensin-converting enzyme inhibitor or calcium channel blocker vs diuretic: the Antihypertensive and Lipid-Lowering Treatment to Prevent Heart Attack Trial (ALLHAT). JAMA. 2002;288:2981-97. [PMID: 12479763]

## Item 62     Answer:     A

**Educational Objective:** Diagnose chronic hypertension in a pregnant patient.

The most likely diagnosis in this pregnant patient is chronic hypertension. Hypertension first recognized during pregnancy at <20 weeks' gestation usually indicates chronic hypertension. The American College of Obstetricians and Gynecologists (ACOG) defines chronic hypertension as a systolic blood pressure ≥140 mm Hg or diastolic blood pressure ≥90 mm Hg starting before pregnancy or before 20 weeks of gestation or persists longer than 12 weeks' postpartum. In normal pregnancy, the blood pressure declines during the first trimester, reaches its lowest level in the second trimester, and rises slowly thereafter. A patient with hypertension in the first trimester suggests that the hypertension predates the pregnancy. To avoid overtreatment of hypertension and associated fetal risk, the 2013 ACOG guidelines recommend treating persistent systolic blood pressure ≥160 mm Hg or diastolic blood pressure ≥105 mm Hg in women with chronic hypertension. Blood pressure goals with medications are 120 to 160/80 to 105 mm Hg. Antihypertensive treatment reduces the risk of progression to severe hypertension by 50% compared with placebo but has not been shown to prevent preeclampsia, preterm birth, small size for gestational age, or infant mortality.

Gestational hypertension first manifests after 20 weeks of pregnancy without proteinuria or other end-organ damage and resolves within 12 weeks of delivery. This patient's early presentation is not consistent with gestational hypertension.

Normal physiologic changes in pregnancy are usually associated with decreased blood pressure in the first trimester with a nadir blood pressure in the second. In this patient, the high blood pressure is inconsistent with normal pregnancy changes.

Preeclampsia is defined clinically by new-onset hypertension and proteinuria that occur after 20 weeks of pregnancy. In addition to blood pressure criteria, there must be proteinuria or new-onset end-organ damage, including liver or kidney injury, pulmonary edema, cerebral or visual symptoms, or thrombocytopenia. This patient's early presentation in the first trimester and lack of end-organ involvement is not consistent with preeclampsia.

**KEY POINT**

- The American College of Obstetricians and Gynecologists defines chronic hypertension as a systolic blood pressure ≥140 mm Hg or diastolic blood pressure ≥90 mm Hg starting before pregnancy or before 20 weeks of gestation or persists longer than 12 weeks' postpartum.

**Bibliography**

American College of Obstetricians and Gynecologists. Hypertension in pregnancy. Report of the American College of Obstetricians and Gynecologists' Task Force on Hypertension in Pregnancy. Obstet Gynecol. 2013;122:1122-31. [PMID: 24150027]

## Item 63     Answer:     B

**Educational Objective:** Diagnose anti–glomerular basement membrane antibody disease.

The most appropriate diagnostic test to perform next is anti–glomerular basement membrane (GBM) antibodies. This patient presents with a rapidly progressive glomerulonephritis (RPGN), an acute and steep rise in serum creatinine accompanied by hematuria and proteinuria. The differential diagnosis for RPGN is divided histologically into three patterns on immunofluorescence microscopy of the kidney biopsy: pauci-immune staining (for example, ANCA-associated glomerulonephritis), linear staining (for example, anti-GBM antibody disease), and granular staining (for example, lupus nephritis). The patient's positive antimyeloperoxidase (MPO) antibodies predict that she will have pauci-immune staining on the biopsy, but the linear staining on her biopsy is more consistent with anti-GBM antibody disease. Therefore, testing for anti-GBM antibodies is required to confirm this diagnosis, although treatment for her condition should not be delayed while awaiting results. One in three patients with anti-GBM antibody disease will have positive ANCA serologies, usually MPO antibodies (or p-ANCA in older assays). This combined seropositivity is most commonly seen in the subset of anti-GBM patients who are older women, as in this case. Diagnosing anti-GBM antibody disease could affect treatment decisions in this case, particularly whether to pursue plasmapheresis, which is indicated for all cases of anti-GBM antibody disease. For ANCA-associated glomerulonephritis, plasmapheresis is reserved for those with alveolar hemorrhage and/or severe kidney failure (defined as requiring dialysis or a serum creatinine >5.8 mg/dL [512.7 µmol/L]).

This patient has negative antinuclear antibody testing and a biopsy not consistent with lupus nephritis, making testing for anti–double-stranded DNA antibodies unnecessary.

Anti–phospholipase A2 receptor (PLA2R) antibodies can be checked in patients suspected of having primary membranous glomerulopathy, which typically presents with the nephrotic syndrome and preserved kidney function, not RPGN.

Antihistone antibodies are measured if drug-induced vasculitis or drug-induced lupus erythematosus is suspected. This patient was not taking any medications, making this test unnecessary.

### KEY POINT

- Serologic testing for anti–glomerular basement membrane antibodies and kidney biopsy can confirm the diagnosis of anti–glomerular basement membrane antibody disease as the cause of rapidly progressive glomerulonephritis.

**Bibliography**

Sethi S, Haas M, Markowitz GS, D'Agati VD, Rennke HG, Jennette JC, et al. Mayo Clinic/Renal Pathology Society consensus report on pathologic classification, diagnosis, and reporting of GN. J Am Soc Nephrol. 2016;27:1278-87. [PMID: 26567243]

### Item 64    Answer:    C

**Educational Objective:** Diagnose white coat hypertension using ambulatory blood pressure monitoring.

The most appropriate next step is to evaluate for white coat hypertension using 24-hour ambulatory blood pressure monitoring (ABPM). ABPM uses a continuously worn device that can be programmed to measure blood pressure every 15 to 20 minutes during the day and every 30 to 60 minutes at night. White coat hypertension refers to elevated blood pressure measured in the office, but normal out-of-office blood pressure averages. According to the American College of Cardiology/American Heart Association blood pressure guideline, in adults with untreated systolic blood pressure >130 mm Hg but <160 mm Hg or diastolic blood pressure >80 mm Hg but <100 mm Hg, it is reasonable to screen for white coat hypertension using either ABPM (the gold standard) or home blood pressure monitoring. Before white coat hypertension is diagnosed, it needs to be confirmed that the out-of-office measurements are reliable; for example, the patient's home blood pressure monitor should be calibrated against the office sphygmomanometer or, preferably, blood pressure should be measured by ABPM. If white coat hypertension is con-

firmed, lifestyle modification and careful monitoring are indicated because there is risk for future development of hypertension.

Before initiating hydrochlorothiazide, 24-hour ABPM or home blood pressure monitoring should be performed to rule out white coat hypertension.

Screening echocardiography is not the correct next step in diagnosis, although it may be considered if the diagnosis of hypertension remains in doubt in order to evaluate for left ventricular hypertrophy. The presence of confirmed left ventricular hypertrophy will necessitate treatment with antihypertensive medication.

The patient's blood pressure has been elevated in the office on three different occasions, and it is unlikely that another measurement in 3 months' time will produce a different result. The issue at hand is the diagnosis of white coat hypertension, which will require out-of-office blood pressure measurements.

### KEY POINT

- White coat hypertension refers to elevated blood pressure measured in the office, but normal out-of-office blood pressure averages; diagnosis requires confirmation using 24-hour ambulatory blood pressure monitoring (gold standard) or home blood pressure monitoring.

**Bibliography**

Pierdomenico SD, Cuccurullo F. Prognostic value of white-coat and masked hypertension diagnosed by ambulatory monitoring in initially untreated subjects: an updated meta analysis. Am J Hypertens. 2011;24:52-8. [PMID: 20847724]

### Item 65    Answer:    B    H

**Educational Objective:** Treat hyperkalemia in a patient with acute kidney injury using hemodialysis.

Intermittent hemodialysis (IHD) is the most efficient way to correct this patient's hyperkalemia in the setting of anuric-oliguric acute kidney injury (AKI). IHD, typically delivered 3 to 6 times a week for 3 to 5 hours per session, allows for rapid correction of electrolyte disturbances and rapid removal of drugs or toxins. This patient has severe hyperkalemia with electrocardiographic changes, which should be corrected urgently to prevent lethal cardiac arrhythmias. Calcium, insulin, and dextrose are only temporizing measures and will not result in potassium removal from the body. Only dialysis will result in potassium removal from the body.

Continuous renal replacement therapy (CRRT) is a type of dialysis that is performed in critically ill patients who are hemodynamically unstable. CRRT provides hemodynamic stability by removing fluid and solutes at a much slower rate than IHD. As a result, CRRT would not be able to clear potassium rapidly but may be considered if the patient cannot tolerate IHD.

Furosemide can induce urinary potassium loss by increasing urine flow and delivery of sodium to the distal nephron for exchange with potassium. However, this patient

CONT.

is nearly anuric with acute tubular necrosis based on urine microscopy and unlikely to respond to furosemide.

Sodium bicarbonate causes a shift of hydrogen ion from the intracellular fluid compartment to the extracellular compartment, causing an opposing net intracellular potassium shift to maintain electroneutrality. The effect of bicarbonate is transient and ineffective in end-stage kidney disease or severe AKI.

Sodium polystyrene sulfonate is a cation exchange resin that removes potassium through the gastrointestinal tract. The onset of action is hours to days, and its effectiveness is disputed. It is contraindicated in patients with recent bowel surgery because of an increased risk for intestinal necrosis.

### KEY POINT

- In the setting of anuric-oliguric acute kidney injury, intermittent hemodialysis allows for rapid correction of electrolyte disturbances and rapid removal of drugs or toxins.

### Bibliography

Rossignol P, Legrand M, Kosiborod M, Hollenberg SM, Peacock WF, Emmett M, et al. Emergency management of severe hyperkalemia: guideline for best practice and opportunities for the future. Pharmacol Res. 2016;113:585-591. [PMID: 27693804]

 **Item 66          Answer:     D**

**Educational Objective:** Diagnose type 4 (hyperkalemic distal) renal tubular acidosis.

The most likely diagnosis is type 4 (hyperkalemic distal) renal tubular acidosis (RTA), which is caused by aldosterone deficiency or resistance. Primary adrenal insufficiency (Addison disease) may cause aldosterone deficiency, although hyporeninemic hypoaldosteronism is a more common cause and may occur in the presence of various kidney diseases, most often diabetes mellitus. Aldosterone resistance is seen in patients with tubulointerstitial disease, including urinary obstruction, sickle cell disease, medullary cystic kidney disease, and kidney transplant rejection. Drug-induced type 4 (hyperkalemic distal) RTA can be caused by numerous drugs that reduce aldosterone production, including ACE inhibitors, angiotensin receptor blockers, heparin, and NSAIDs. Patients with type 4 (hyperkalemic distal) RTA have a positive urine anion gap (using the equation: [Urine Sodium + Urine Potassium] – Urine Chloride), indicating a reduced excretion of acid in the form of ammonium and chloride, but a urine pH <5.5. Hyperkalemia decreases ammonia production with consequent lower ammonium excretion and therefore results in the positive urine anion gap. Due to the inadequate amount of ammonia available to buffer protons, the few protons that are secreted distally will result in the low urine pH (<5.5). Treatment is focused on correcting the underlying cause if possible. Fludrocortisone is used to replace mineralocorticoids in adrenal insufficiency and should be considered in hyporeninemic hypoaldosteronism in those without hypertension or heart failure.

Although chronic kidney disease may result in hyperkalemia and metabolic acidosis, the acidosis does not usually develop until later progression (glomerular filtration rate <40-45 mL/min/1.73 m$^2$), and hyperkalemia is usually not present until the glomerular filtration rate is at even lower levels (usually stage 4 or worse).

The normal anion gap of type 1 (hypokalemic distal) RTA results from a distal tubular defect and associated impaired excretion of hydrogen ions by the distal nephron. It is usually associated with hypokalemia and a negative urine anion gap, which are not present in this patient.

Type 2 (proximal) RTA results from failure of the proximal tubule to adequately reclaim filtered bicarbonate, driving the development of a normal anion gap metabolic acidosis and a positive urine anion gap. Type 2 (proximal) RTA is usually accompanied by other evidence of proximal tubular dysfunction (hypokalemia, glycosuria, and hypophosphatemia), none of which is present in this patient.

### KEY POINT

- Type 4 (hyperkalemic distal) renal tubular acidosis is characterized by hyperkalemia, a normal anion gap metabolic acidosis, impaired urine acidification (positive urine anion gap), and a urine pH <5.5.

### Bibliography

Yaxley J, Pirrone C. Review of the diagnostic evaluation of renal tubular acidosis. Ochsner J. 2016;16:525-530. [PMID: 27999512]

### Item 67          Answer:     D

**Educational Objective:** Diagnose lupus nephritis.

The most appropriate next step is a kidney biopsy. The presence of hematuria, dysmorphic erythrocytes, and proteinuria in a patient with known systemic lupus erythematosus (SLE) is highly suggestive of lupus nephritis; when serologies are positive and serum complement levels are low, this diagnosis is even more likely. Commonly cited indications for kidney biopsy include increasing serum creatinine without explanation, proteinuria >500 mg/24 h, or active urine sediment (dysmorphic erythrocytes, erythrocyte casts). Patients meeting these criteria are more likely to have focal or diffuse proliferative lupus nephritis or lupus membranous nephropathy requiring immunosuppressive therapy. Patients with proteinuria <500 mg/24 h and inactive urine sediment are more likely to have milder kidney involvement and may be followed with urinalysis, urine protein-creatinine ratio, and serum creatinine every 3 to 6 months.

Unless absolutely contraindicated (for example, bleeding diathesis or inability to stop anticoagulation), both rheumatology and nephrology guidelines support performing a kidney biopsy in patients with SLE who develop evidence of significant kidney involvement to establish the diagnosis and, of equal importance with regard to treatment decisions, to identify the International Society of Nephrology/Renal Pathology Society (ISN/RPS) class of lupus nephritis.

This patient's kidney biopsy could show a proliferative lupus nephritis (class III or IV), in which case treatment with glucocorticoids and mycophenolate mofetil or cyclophosphamide would be indicated (mycophenolate mofetil would likely be preferred given this patient's age). However, her biopsy could also conceivably show a milder, mesangial proliferative lupus nephritis (class II) or membranous lupus nephritis (class V), neither of which would require immunosuppression at this stage. Therefore, empiric therapy in this setting is substandard to biopsy-guided therapy according to ISN/RPS class of nephritis.

**KEY POINT**

- A kidney biopsy should be performed in patients with known systemic lupus erythematosus with suspected significant kidney involvement to establish the diagnosis and to identify the class, which will guide treatment decisions.

**Bibliography**

Hahn BH, McMahon MA, Wilkinson A, Wallace WD, Daikh DI, Fitzgerald JD, et al; American College of Rheumatology. American College of Rheumatology guidelines for screening, treatment, and management of lupus nephritis. Arthritis Care Res (Hoboken). 2012;64:797-808. [PMID: 22556106]

## Item 68    Answer:    D

**Educational Objective:** Treat hypertension associated with volume expansion in chronic kidney disease.

Stopping chlorthalidone and beginning furosemide is the most appropriate treatment for this patient's hypertension. Hypertension is a risk factor for cardiovascular morbidity and mortality. The most common cause of death in patients with chronic kidney disease (CKD) is cardiovascular disease. Therefore, blood pressure control is critical for preventing disease and death. Diuretics are central to the management of hypertension. Although thiazide diuretics (such as chlorthalidone) are recommended first-line agents for hypertension, efficacy decreases with advanced stages of CKD. Therefore, loop diuretics (furosemide, bumetanide, torsemide) are a cornerstone of blood pressure management in patients with advanced CKD. Sodium retention and impaired natriuresis lead to volume expansion and an increase in blood pressure. Loop diuretics are effective natriuretics and retain their activity even at low glomerular filtration rate (GFR); however, doses need to be increased as GFR declines to maintain appropriate urine output and negative fluid balance. Loop diuretics are equally effective if given in equipotent doses. The loop diuretic furosemide would effectively treat this patient's volume expansion and therefore reduce blood pressure. Additional benefit would include increased urine potassium and acid excretion to treat the mild hyperkalemia and metabolic acidosis associated with CKD. The most common side effects of loop diuretics are electrolyte and fluid abnormalities, hypersensitivity, and ototoxicity.

Hydralazine is not indicated for this patient who has volume expansion and needs diuresis; this drug is also relatively contraindicated in coronary artery disease.

Losartan is an angiotensin receptor blocker, which should not be combined with an ACE inhibitor due to the risk of hyperkalemia and acute kidney injury.

Although spironolactone can help reduce blood pressure and edema through its anti-aldosterone effects and blockade of sodium reabsorption in the cortical collecting duct, it would be contraindicated in this patient with advanced CKD and hyperkalemia.

**KEY POINT**

- Loop diuretics are a cornerstone of blood pressure management in patients with advanced chronic kidney disease.

**Bibliography**

Valika A, Peixoto AJ. Hypertension management in transition: from CKD to ESRD. Adv Chronic Kidney Dis. 2016;23:255-61. [PMID: 27324679]

## Item 69    Answer:    D

**Educational Objective:** Select the most appropriate venous access for a patient with advanced chronic kidney disease.

A tunneled internal jugular central venous catheter is the most appropriate venous access strategy for this patient. In patients with osteomyelitis, 6 weeks of antimicrobial therapy after surgical débridement is the preferred treatment course, and for most patients this requires long-term reliable venous access. However, this patient's advanced degree of kidney disease, relatively young age, and type 2 diabetes mellitus put her at high risk for progressing to end-stage kidney disease, and the upper extremity veins should be protected for future hemodialysis access creation. The American Society of Nephrology recommends nephrology consultation first before placing peripherally inserted central catheter (PICC) lines in patients with stage G3 to G5 CKD. PICCs are long catheters that are inserted peripherally and terminate in the central veins. PICCs are popular because of their ease of insertion and use. However, a national, population-based analysis revealed that PICCs placed before or after hemodialysis initiation were independently associated with lower likelihoods of transition to any working fistula or graft. PICC lines can lead to significant vein trauma and venous stenosis in the veins that may be used for arteriovenous fistula creation. This could impair blood flow through the fistula, impair maturation, and even lead to primary nonfunctioning of the hemodialysis access. Although central lines are associated with central venous stenosis, a central line is a better alternative than a PICC for long-term parenteral antibiotics because central lines are not inserted into a peripheral vein, which would be used for the creation of a hemodialysis site.

Arteriovenous fistula or graft creation is inappropriate due to the presence of active infection. Additionally, inserting a PICC line in the arm next to the fistula may also

CONT.

still cause damage to the access itself or damage one of the branching veins, which could impair the maturation of the access.

**KEY POINT**

- Peripherally inserted central catheter placement before or after hemodialysis initiation is associated with adverse vascular access outcomes in patients with chronic kidney disease.

**Bibliography**

McGill RL, Ruthazer R, Meyer KB, Miskulin DC, Weiner DE. Peripherally inserted central catheters and hemodialysis outcomes. Clin J Am Soc Nephrol. 2016;11:1434-40. [PMID: 27340280]

**Item 70      Answer:      C**

**Educational Objective: Treat hypertension in a patient with diabetes mellitus and albuminuria using an ACE inhibitor or angiotensin receptor blocker.**

In addition to lifestyle modifications, initiation of the angiotensin receptor blocker (ARB) losartan is the most appropriate treatment for this patient with newly diagnosed hypertension. She has a normal serum creatinine level but has moderately increased albuminuria. Her blood pressure has been elevated at two office visits and confirmed with home blood pressure monitoring, and she needs to be treated to target, given that uncontrolled hypertension will lead to progression of albuminuria and chronic kidney disease (CKD). A reasonable target blood pressure for this patient is <130/80 mm Hg. The 2017 high blood pressure guideline from the American College of Cardiology (ACC), American Heart Association (AHA), and nine other organizations recommends a treatment goal of <130/80 mm Hg. The ACC/AHA guideline notes that ACE inhibitors or ARBs may be considered as initial treatment choices in the presence of albuminuria. The American Diabetes Association (ADA) Standards of Medical Care in Diabetes 2018 recommends that most patients with diabetes mellitus and hypertension should be treated to a systolic blood pressure goal of <140 mm Hg and a diastolic blood pressure goal of <90 mm Hg. Lower systolic and diastolic blood pressure targets, such as 130/80 mm Hg, may be appropriate for individuals at high risk of cardiovascular disease if they can be achieved without undue treatment burden. In nonpregnant patients with diabetes and hypertension, the ADA recommends either an ACE inhibitor or an ARB for those with albuminuria. Several large randomized controlled trials and systematic reviews have shown that use of an ARB or ACE inhibitor can result in decreased progression of albuminuria and CKD in patients with diabetes.

The ACC/AHA blood pressure guideline recommends the following lifestyle modifications for individuals with elevated blood pressure or hypertension: weight loss in adults who are overweight or obese; a heart-healthy diet, such as DASH (Dietary Approaches to Stop Hypertension), that facilitates achieving a desirable weight; sodium reduction; potassium supplementation, preferably in dietary modification, unless

contraindicated by the presence of CKD or use of drugs that reduce potassium excretion; increased physical activity with a structured exercise program; and limiting alcohol consumption of standard drinks to two (men) and one (women) per day. Although these recommendations are appropriate for this patient, it is not the only recommended intervention to control hypertension in this patient with diabetes and albuminuria. Therefore, simply asking the patient to return in 2 months for a blood pressure measurement after initiating lifestyle changes is not sufficient.

Calcium channel blockers (such as amlodipine) and thiazide diuretics (such as chlorthalidone) are not initial choices for treating hypertension in patients with diabetes and albuminuria. If this patient's blood pressure is still not controlled to target after maximizing the dose of the ARB, then one of these agents can be added.

**KEY POINT**

- An ACE inhibitor or angiotensin receptor blocker is the initial treatment of choice for hypertension in patients with diabetes mellitus and albuminuria.

**Bibliography**

Palmer SC, Mavridis D, Navarese E, Craig JC, Tonelli M, Salanti G, et al. Comparative efficacy and safety of blood pressure-lowering agents in adults with diabetes and kidney disease: a network meta-analysis. Lancet. 2015;385:2047-56. [PMID: 26009228]

**Item 71      Answer:      C**

**Educational Objective: Identify medication as a cause of an increase in serum creatinine.**

Reassessing this patient's serum creatinine level in 1 week is the most appropriate next step in management. Some medications (such as cimetidine, trimethoprim, cobicistat, dolutegravir, bictegravir, and rilpivirine) reduce proximal tubule secretion of creatinine, resulting in increases in serum creatinine that are nonprogressive. This patient has chronic kidney disease (CKD), long-standing hypertension, and HIV infection. His antiretroviral medication regimen was recently adjusted to a once-a-day dosing, with the integrase inhibitor raltegravir discontinued and dolutegravir started 3 weeks ago. Dolutegravir is known to interfere with creatinine secretion without affecting glomerular filtration rate. Slight increases in serum creatinine of 0.2 to 0.3 mg/dL (17.7-26.5 µmol/L) may occur. This is more pronounced in those with preexisting CKD, in which creatinine secretion may contribute proportionately more to creatinine clearance. In patients with HIV taking the integrase inhibitors dolutegravir or bictegravir, the non-nucleoside reverse transcriptase inhibitor rilpivirine, or the pharmacokinetic enhancer (CYP3A inhibitor) cobicistat, serum creatinine elevations are nonprogressive and will remain unchanged within 1 to 2 weeks of initiation. Therefore, in the absence of other signs of kidney disease (hematuria, pyuria, or increasing proteinuria), reassessment of the serum creatinine level in 1 week will confirm the drug's effect in this patient.

Further increases in serum creatinine levels will require additional evaluation.

Discontinuation of the ACE inhibitor lisinopril is not necessary. This patient has long-standing hypertension and is likely benefiting from the lisinopril for his CKD and moderate albuminuria. It is unlikely to have caused this acute increase in serum creatinine because the hemodynamic effects of ACE inhibitors on glomerular filtration occur within days of initiating the medication and then stabilize.

A 24-hour urine creatinine clearance will be decreased in this case (due to drug-related lower creatinine secretion) and will not provide additional diagnostic information.

Should a repeat serum creatinine level be stable, no further evaluation will be necessary.

### KEY POINT

- Some medications (such as cimetidine, trimethoprim, cobicistat, dolutegravir, bictegravir, and rilpivirine) reduce proximal tubule secretion of creatinine, resulting in increases in serum creatinine that are nonprogressive; repeat serum creatinine measurement is required to confirm stable levels.

### Bibliography

Milburn J, Jones R, Levy JB. Renal effects of novel antiretroviral drugs. Nephrol Dial Transplant. 2017;32:434-439. [PMID: 27190354]

### Item 72      Answer:      B

**Educational Objective:** Identify calcium phosphate as the composition of a kidney stone in a patient taking topiramate.

The most likely composition of this patient's kidney stone is calcium phospate. Approximately 80% of kidney stones contain calcium oxalate, calcium phosphate, or both. Calcium stones are radiopaque on plain radiograph. Hypercalciuria, hyperoxaluria, and hypocitraturia are risk factors for calcium stones. Calcium phosphate stones occur when there is persistently elevated urine pH. These stones are therefore commonly associated with distal renal tubular acidosis and hyperparathyroidism. This patient is taking topiramate for migraine prophylaxis, a carbonic anhydrase inhibitor that is associated with calcium phosphate stones. Carbonic anhydrase promotes proximal tubule sodium, bicarbonate, and chloride reabsorption. Inhibitors of carbonic anhydrase produce both sodium chloride and bicarbonate urinary loss. The resultant mild metabolic acidosis causes decreased citrate excretion, and the persistent alkaline urine favors the precipitation of calcium phosphate.

Although calcium oxalate is the most common cause of kidney stones, there are no calcium oxalate crystals noted on this patient's urinalysis. The most common crystal formations of calcium oxalate in the urine are the dumbbell-shaped calcium oxalate monohydrate crystals and envelope-shaped calcium oxalate dihydrate crystals. She has amorphous crystals in alkaline urine, which are usually calcium phosphate crystals.

Cystine stones occur with cystinuria, which is a genetic disease. This patient has no family history of kidney stones, and the characteristic hexagonal-shaped crystals are not seen on urine microscopy.

Struvite stones occur in the presence of urea-splitting bacteria (*Proteus*, *Klebsiella*, or, less frequently, *Pseudomonas*). These bacteria split urea into ammonium, which markedly increases urine pH and results in the precipitation of magnesium ammonium phosphate (struvite). The pH of the urine will be >7.5. Struvite stones commonly produce staghorn calculi (stones that bridge two or more renal calyces) and occur most frequently in older women with chronic urinary infections. Coffin lid–shaped crystals may be seen in the urine. This patient does not demonstrate these findings.

Uric acid stones are uncommon (10% of stones), but the incidence increases in hotter, arid climates due to low urine volumes. The main risk factor is low urine pH, which decreases the solubility of uric acid. Hyperuricosuria is not a consistent finding. Comorbid risk factors for uric acid stones include gout, diabetes mellitus, the metabolic syndrome, and chronic diarrhea. Because uric acid stones occur in persistently acidic urine, this is an unlikely diagnosis for this patient.

### KEY POINT

- Topiramate, a carbonic anhydrase inhibitor, causes a decrease in urinary citrate excretion and formation of alkaline urine that favor the creation of calcium phosphate stones.

### Bibliography

Dell'Orto VG, Belotti EA, Goeggel-Simonetti B, Simonetti GD, Ramelli GP, Bianchetti MG, et al. Metabolic disturbances and renal stone promotion on treatment with topiramate: a systematic review. Br J Clin Pharmacol. 2014;77:958-64. [PMID: 24219102]

### Item 73      Answer:      C

**Educational Objective:** Diagnose proton pump inhibitor–induced tubulointerstitial nephritis.

The proton pump inhibitor omeprazole is the most likely cause of this patient's kidney findings. Nonspecific symptoms of tubulointerstitial disease include polyuria, malaise, and anorexia, as well as progressive kidney dysfunction. Urinary findings can range from minimal findings to the presence of sterile pyuria, proteinuria, and hematuria. Chronic tubulointerstitial diseases most commonly result from previous injury due to acute interstitial nephritis. Therefore, the history and physical examination should focus on conditions associated with acute tubulointerstitial disease and other potential treatable causes with a careful review of medications. Proton pump inhibitors are the most commonly prescribed drugs worldwide. The occurrence of interstitial nephritis is not dose related, and disease can recur with reexposure. The median time from drug initiation to interstitial nephritis diagnosis is variable but can exceed 6 months to 9 months, with 10 to 11 weeks the most common interval. There is also emerging

H CONT.

literature that proton pump inhibitors may contribute to the development and progression of chronic kidney disease.

Although large amounts of aspirin and NSAIDs can cause tubulointerstitial nephritis, a daily dose of low-dose aspirin (81 mg) is unlikely to cause interstitial nephritis. It is unlikely that therapeutic doses of aspirin alone cause chronic kidney disease in patients with normal underlying kidney function.

Fenofibrate nephrotoxicity is characterized by a rise in serum creatinine typically occurring ≥6 months after initiation of therapy. The sediment is bland, and there is usually no significant proteinuria. The mechanism of increase in creatinine is unknown. This patient has been taking fenofibrate for only 2 months, making this drug an unlikely cause of his interstitial nephritis.

St. John's wort (*Hypericum perforatum*) is most commonly used to treat depression. Adverse effects are uncommon but the following have been reported: gastrointestinal symptoms, dizziness, confusion, tiredness, sedation, photosensitivity, dry mouth, urinary frequency, anorgasmia, and swelling. St. John's wort has not been associated with tubulointerstitial nephritis.

KEY POINT

- Chronic tubulointerstitial nephritis can be caused by proton pump inhibitors, and the median time from drug initiation to diagnosis may exceed 6 to 9 months.

Bibliography

Moledina DG, Perazella MA. PPIs and kidney disease: from AIN to CKD. J Nephrol. 2016;29:611-6. [PMID: 27072818]

H

Item 74 Answer: C

Educational Objective: Diagnose pseudohyperkalemia.

The most appropriate next step in management is a repeat plasma potassium measurement. This patient has an elevated serum potassium level of 6.4 mEq/L (6.4 mmol/L) in the setting of leukocytosis likely due to acute leukemia. Hyperkalemia is defined as a serum potassium level >5.0 mEq/L (5.0 mmol/L). Any level >6.0 mEq/L (6.0 mmol/L) can be life-threatening. Because of the potential cardiac effects of hyperkalemia, immediate electrocardiography (ECG) is indicated. The earliest ECG changes of hyperkalemia are peaking of the T waves and shortening of the QT interval. As hyperkalemia progresses, there is prolongation of the PR interval, loss of P waves, and eventual widening of the QRS complexes with a "sine-wave" pattern that can precede asystole. This patient has no ECG evidence of hyperkalemia. Pseudohyperkalemia is therefore the most likely cause of his elevated serum potassium level. Pseudohyperkalemia occurs with a false rise in potassium values from cellular release of potassium during venipuncture due to hemolysis or prolonged tourniquet use. It also occurs with significant leukocytosis or thrombocytosis. During the clotting process, these cells are disrupted with the release of intracellular potassium, and pseudohyperkalemia may occur in serum specimens when there are extreme elevations of leukocytes or platelets. The next step is to obtain a plasma specimen and rapidly separate the plasma from the cells. Normally, the serum potassium is 0.3 to 0.4 mEq/L (0.3-0.4 mmol/L) greater than a plasma specimen obtained at the same time. In extreme cases of leukocytosis or thrombocytosis, the serum potassium can be more than 1.0 mEq/L (1.0 mmol/L) higher. In cases of pseudohyperkalemia, a rapidly processed plasma specimen will be normal.

In patients with normal kidney function, intravenous saline, usually with the concomitant administration of a loop diuretic, can increase potassium excretion. Intravenous calcium should be reserved for cases of hyperkalemia exhibiting ECG changes. The effect of calcium on stabilizing the cardiac membrane is a transient event that lasts only 30 minutes. Inhaled albuterol lowers potassium by shifting it into cells. However, this patient has no indication to rapidly reduce potassium levels or stabilize the cardiac membrane because his ECG is normal.

The use of sodium bicarbonate in hyperkalemia has fallen out of favor. It has minimal effects on potassium levels and is usually reserved for patients with metabolic acidosis.

KEY POINT

- Pseudohyperkalemia may occur in serum specimens when there are extreme elevations of leukocytes or platelets; repeat plasma potassium measurements can confirm a normal potassium level.

Bibliography

Meng QH, Wagar EA. Pseudohyperkalemia: a new twist on an old phenomenon. Crit Rev Clin Lab Sci. 2015;52:45-55. [PMID: 25319088]

Item 75 Answer: C

H

Educational Objective: Treat anemia associated with chronic kidney disease using an erythropoiesis-stimulating agent.

An erythropoiesis-stimulating agent (ESA) is appropriate to treat anemia in this patient with stage G4 chronic kidney disease (CKD). The prevalence of anemia increases as CKD progresses due to several factors, including impaired erythropoietin production, erythropoietin resistance, and reduced erythrocyte life span. Iron deficiency may contribute to erythropoietin resistance. The Kidney Disease: Improving Global Outcomes (KDIGO) recommendations suggest maintaining transferrin saturation levels of >30% and serum ferritin levels of >500 ng/mL (500 µg/L). The patient's iron stores are adequate based on the patient's transferrin saturation and ferritin levels, and the next step in treatment is to start an ESA. ESAs are highly effective in raising hemoglobin concentrations and alleviating symptoms, and can avoid the need for transfusion. ESAs should not be used in patients with active malignancy, history of malignancy, or history of stroke. ESAs should be started in symptomatic patients with CKD who have a hemoglobin concentration <10 g/dL (100 g/L), and the dose should be titrated to avoid hemoglobin concentrations increasing above 11.5 g/dL (115 g/L).

CONT.

ACE inhibitors and angiotensin receptor blockers (ARBs) inhibit erythropoiesis, and patients on maintenance dialysis taking either ACE inhibitors or ARBs may have increased erythropoietin requirements. However, the mechanisms by which this occurs are poorly defined. Discontinuing losartan is incorrect because renin–angiotensin system blockade in CKD is beneficial in delaying the progression of CKD to end-stage kidney disease, which outweighs any potential interaction with anemia. However, discontinuing the medication could be considered if the patient demonstrated signs of erythropoietin resistance or refractory anemia.

Packed red blood cell transfusion is not indicated at this time and would expose the patient to transfusion-related risks and side effects. Additionally, blood transfusions can cause allosensitization, which can lead to antibody formation, and may prolong transplant waiting times.

Starting iron is incorrect because the patient is iron replete. Iron repletion is recommended if the transferrin saturation is ≤30% and the ferritin is ≤500 ng/mL (500 µg/L).

**KEY POINT**

- The Kidney Disease: Improving Global Outcomes (KDIGO) guidelines recommend consideration of erythropoiesis-stimulating agents to treat anemia in patients with chronic kidney disease and adequate iron stores who have hemoglobin concentrations <10 g/dL (100 g/L); the dose should be titrated to avoid hemoglobin concentrations increasing above 11.5 g/dL (115 g/L).

**Bibliography**
Kidney Disease: Improving Global Outcomes (KDIGO) Anemia Work Group. KDIGO clinical practice guideline for anemia in chronic kidney disease. Kidney inter., Suppl. 2012;2:279–335. Available at www.kdigo.org.

 **Item 76      Answer:      C**

**Educational Objective:** Identify hypomagnesemia as a cause of hypokalemia.

The most likely cause of this patient's hypokalemia is hypomagnesemia. Symptoms of hypokalemia include weakness or paralysis; decreased gastrointestinal motility or ileus with nausea; and cardiac arrhythmias. This patient has symptomatic hypokalemia, presenting with lower extremity weakness and nausea. Hypokalemia can be caused by renal losses or nonrenal losses. In this case, the urine potassium is inappropriately high, pointing toward renal potassium wasting. Renal losses of potassium can occur with renal tubular acidosis; renal excretion of non-reabsorbable anions such as bicarbonate, hippurate, and ketones; drugs such as aminoglycosides or cisplatinum; Gitelman and Bartter syndromes; or hypomagnesemia. Hypomagnesemia is common, occurring in up to 12% of hospitalized patients. Chronic alcohol abuse results in excessive urinary excretion of magnesium and appears to reflect a reversible alcohol-induced tubular dysfunction. Intracellular magnesium is necessary to modulate the excretion of potassium through the potassium channel in the

cortical collecting tubule. Hypomagnesemia results in loss of potassium through this channel. Importantly, the hypokalemia will be refractory to therapy until magnesium is repleted. Target levels for magnesium replacement are at least 2 mg/dL (0.83 mmol/L).

Unlike calcium and magnesium, which have substantial binding to albumin, potassium levels are not affected by the concentration of albumin.

Low levels of magnesium (due to alcohol abuse or malnutrition) activate G-proteins that stimulate calcium-sensing receptors and decrease parathyroid hormone (PTH) secretion and are a cause of hypocalcemia. Low magnesium levels are also associated with resistance to PTH activity at the level of bone, further contributing to hypocalcemia. Hypocalcemia and hypokalemia in this patient are a direct result of chronic magnesium loss due to the patient's alcoholism. Hypocalcemia has no significant effect on potassium concentration.

Because the kidneys can reduce urine potassium excretion to <20 mEq/24 h (20 mmol/24 h), hypokalemia from inadequate intake is uncommon. Urinary or gastrointestinal losses of potassium are most common. Assessment of urine potassium excretion is critical to establish renal potassium wasting. Urine potassium loss >20 mEq/24 h (20 mmol/24 h), a spot urine potassium >20 mEq/L (20 mmol/L), or a spot urine potassium–creatinine ratio >13 mEq/g (1.5 mEq/mmol) suggests excessive urinary losses. Conversely, urine potassium loss <20 mEq/24 h (20 mmol/24 h) suggests cellular shift, decreased intake, or extrarenal losses of potassium. This patient's high urinary potassium suggests urinary loss rather than poor nutrition as the cause of hypokalemia.

**KEY POINT**

- Hypomagnesemia can cause symptomatic hypokalemia via renal losses of potassium; importantly, the hypokalemia will be refractory to therapy until magnesium is repleted.

**Bibliography**
Rodan AR, Cheng CJ, Huang CL. Recent advances in distal tubular potassium handling. Am J Physiol Renal Physiol. 2011;300:F821-7. [PMID: 21270092]

**Item 77      Answer:      A**

**Educational Objective:** Identify *Staphylococcus aureus* as a cause of infection-related glomerulonephritis.

*Staphylococcus aureus* is the most likely cause of this patient's infection-related glomerulonephritis (IRGN). This patient has acute kidney injury in the setting of cellulitis, with active urine sediment and low serum complement levels. The biopsy shows a proliferative glomerulonephritis on light microscopy with immunofluorescence of C3 and IgA and subepithelial hump-like deposits on electron microscopy, confirming a diagnosis of IRGN. In the developed world, the epidemiology of IRGN has drastically shifted over the past few decades, moving away from streptococcal-associated glomerulonephritides to infections caused primarily by *S. aureus* and, at a significantly lower rate, gram-negative bacteria. In this patient with cellulitis and IRGN occurring at the time of infection, *S. aureus* is the most likely culprit pathogen.

In patients with poststreptococcal glomerulonephritis (group A *Streptococcus*, or *Streptococcus pyogenes*), there is a latent period between the resolution of the streptococcal infection and the acute onset of the nephritic syndrome, usually 7 to 10 days after oropharyngeal infections and 2 to 4 weeks after skin infections. In adults with non–poststreptococcal IRGN, the glomerulonephritis often coexists with the triggering infection. Sites of infection can include the upper and lower respiratory tract, skin/soft tissue, bone, teeth/oral mucosa, heart, deep abscesses, shunts, and indwelling catheters. Notably, this patient's kidney failure has occurred at the same time as the cellulitis, consistent with a staphylococcal-mediated form of IRGN.

*Streptococcus pneumoniae* is an uncommon cause of cellulitis, and *Streptococcus agalactiae* (group B *Streptococcus*) is capable of causing cellulitis in nonpregnant adults in special circumstances (lymphedema, vascular insufficiency, chronic dermatitis, or radiation-induced cutaneous injury). *S. pyogenes* and *S. aureus* are much more common causes of cellulitis, and the co-occurrence of the infection and IRGN points to *S. aureus* as the most likely culprit.

### KEY POINT

- In adults, most cases of infection-related glomerulonephritis are no longer poststreptococcal, and the glomerulonephritis often coexists with the triggering infection.

### Bibliography
Glassock RJ, Alvarado A, Prosek J, Hebert C, Parikh S, Satoskar A, et al. Staphylococcus-related glomerulonephritis and poststreptococcal glomerulonephritis: why defining "post" is important in understanding and treating infection-related glomerulonephritis. Am J Kidney Dis. 2015;65:826-32. [PMID: 25890425]

### Item 78     Answer:    D

**Educational Objective:** Recognize differing guideline recommendations for blood pressure targets in older patients.

According to target blood pressure goals recommended by the American College of Physicians and the American Academy of Family Physicians, this 72-year-old woman's blood pressure is at target, and no changes are necessary. This guideline recommends that antihypertensive drugs be initiated in patients ≥60 years old if blood pressure is >150/90 mm Hg, with a goal of reducing systolic blood pressure to <150 mm Hg to reduce the risk for mortality, stroke, and cardiac events. The guideline further recommends that physicians consider initiating or intensifying pharmacologic treatment in patients ≥60 years of age with a history of stroke or transient ischemic attack to achieve a target systolic blood pressure <140 mm Hg to reduce the risk for recurrent stroke. The guideline also recommends

considering the initiation or intensification of pharmacologic treatment in some patients ≥60 years of age at high cardiovascular risk, based on individualized assessment, to achieve a target systolic blood pressure <140 mm Hg to reduce the risk for stroke or cardiac events. These recommendations are based on evidence that demonstrates the greatest absolute benefit of antihypertensive therapy is seen in patients with the highest blood pressure and cardiovascular risk.

On the other hand, the 2017 American College of Cardiology/American Heart Association blood pressure guideline recommends a target systolic blood pressure goal of <130 mm Hg for noninstitutionalized, ambulatory community-dwelling patients ≥65 years of age. In those with a high burden of comorbidity and limited life expectancy, clinical judgment, patient preference, and an assessment of risk-benefit ratio should be considered for decisions about the intensity of blood pressure control and antihypertensive medication choice. This recommendation is based upon randomized controlled trials of antihypertensive therapy that have included large numbers of older persons, which demonstrated that more intensive treatment safely reduced the risk of cardiovascular disease for those ≥65 years of age.

### KEY POINT

- Based on evidence that the greatest absolute benefit of antihypertensive therapy is seen in patients with the highest blood pressure and cardiovascular risk, the American College of Physicians and American Academy of Family Physicians recommend that antihypertensive drugs be initiated in patients ≥60 years old if blood pressure is >150/90 mm Hg, with a goal of reducing systolic blood pressure to <150 mm Hg; the American College of Cardiology/American Heart Association recommends a systolic blood pressure target of <130 mm Hg in patients ≥65 years old.

### Bibliography
Kansagara D, Wilt TJ, Frost J, Qaseem A. Pharmacologic treatment of hypertension in adults aged 60 years or older. Ann Intern Med. 2017;167:291-292. [PMID: 28806807]

### Item 79     Answer:    D   

**Educational Objective:** Treat hyperphosphatemia in a patient with stage G4 chronic kidney disease.

Sevelamer is the most appropriate treatment for this patient with secondary hyperparathyroidism and hyperphosphatemia associated with stage G4 chronic kidney disease (CKD). Increased plasma parathyroid hormone (PTH) occurring as a result of CKD is referred to as secondary hyperparathyroidism. Increased PTH levels result in reduced calcium excretion and increased phosphorus excretion by the kidneys. Early in CKD, the PTH-induced increase in renal phosphorus excretion enables normal serum phosphorus levels despite reduced renal excretory capacity. However, as CKD progresses, the kidney is unable to compensate for the increased phosphorus, and

CONT.

phosphorus levels rise. This results in a vicious cycle as phosphorus stimulates PTH production. Initial treatment of secondary hyperparathyroidism in CKD stages G3 through G5 is correction of serum calcium, phosphorus, and vitamin D levels. Current Kidney Disease: Improving Global Outcomes (KDIGO) guidelines recommend that elevated phosphorus levels should be lowered *toward* the normal range, not into the normal range, because there is an absence of data showing that efforts to maintain phosphorus in the normal range are of benefit to CKD stage G3a to G4. Thus, treatment should be aimed at overt hyperphosphatemia, and decisions to start phosphate-lowering treatment should be based solely on progressively or persistently elevated serum phosphorus levels. KDIGO guidelines also recommend avoiding hypercalcemia. In this patient, treatment of hyperphosphatemia with a phosphate binder and a low phosphorus diet is indicated. Sevelamer is a non–calcium-containing binder that might improve bone turnover, limit vascular calcification, and reduce all-cause mortality, compared with calcium-containing binders, although these potential benefits have not been consistently proven.

Aluminum hydroxide is an effective phosphate binder and is still used for very short-term treatment of severe secondary hyperparathyroidism. However, it would not be recommended in the chronic setting due to the toxic effects of aluminum (myalgia, weakness, osteomalacia, iron-resistant microcytic anemia, dementia), particularly because non–calcium-containing binders are now available.

This patient's 25-hydroxyvitamin D level is in the "sufficient" range. However, calcitriol may be warranted if hyperparathyroidism persists after normalization of serum calcium and phosphorus levels even in the setting of normal 25-hydroxyvitamin D levels, as impaired hydroxylation at the 1 position by the kidney can lead to functional deficiency.

Cinacalcet, a calcimimetic that decreases PTH levels, is currently FDA approved only for use in patients who are undergoing dialysis, although it has been used off-label for secondary hyperparathyroidism associated with hypercalcemia in cases in which use of vitamin D analogues has led to hypercalcemia.

**KEY POINT**

- Initial treatment of secondary hyperparathyroidism in chronic kidney disease stages G3 through G5 is correction of serum calcium, phosphorus, and vitamin D levels.

### Bibliography

Patel L, Bernard LM, Elder GJ. Sevelamer versus calcium-based binders for treatment of hyperphosphatemia in CKD: a meta-analysis of randomized controlled trials. Clin J Am Soc Nephrol. 2016;11:232-44. [PMID: 26668024]

## Item 80    Answer:    C

**Educational Objective:** Discontinue NSAIDs in a patient with elevated blood pressure.

The most appropriate management is to discontinue ibuprofen and measure the blood pressure (BP) in 1 month.

The American College of Cardiology/American Heart Association BP guideline defines stage 1 hypertension as a systolic BP of 130 to 139 mm Hg or diastolic BP of 80 to 89 mm Hg. This change is based on epidemiologic studies that indicate systolic BP >115 mm Hg and diastolic BP >75 mm Hg are associated in a linear fashion with cardiovascular events. In the initial assessment of a patient with elevated BP, before a diagnosis of hypertension is made, it is imperative that a complete history with a list of prescription, nonprescription (including complementary and alternative medications such as herbals), and illicit drugs is elicited. NSAIDs are one of the medication classes that can result in reversible elevations in BP, the mechanism for which is increased sodium retention. Therefore, ibuprofen, an NSAID, should be discontinued and BP remeasured. If the patient has ongoing pain, an alternative pain management strategy that does not result in BP elevation, such as nondrug interventions, topical analgesics (if appropriate), or acetaminophen, should be prescribed because pain can also result in BP elevation.

This patient's elevated BP would need to be confirmed 1 month after discontinuation of ibuprofen before antihypertensive medications such as amlodipine or hydrochlorothiazide are started in this otherwise healthy young individual.

Antihistamines such as loratadine generally do not result in BP elevation; therefore, loratadine does not need to be discontinued in this patient.

**KEY POINT**

- Many medications, such as NSAIDS, can result in reversible elevations in blood pressure; discontinuation of the drug and a reassessment of blood pressure 1 month later are necessary to confirm a return to normal blood pressure measurement.

### Bibliography

Weir MR. In the clinic: hypertension. Ann Intern Med. 2014;161:ITC1-15; quiz ITC16. [PMID: 25437425]

## Item 81    Answer:    C

**Educational Objective:** Identify hepatitis C virus infection as the cause of membranoproliferative glomerulonephritis.

The most appropriate test to perform next is measurement of hepatitis C antibodies. This patient presents with glomerulonephritis (elevated serum creatinine level, hematuria, and subnephrotic proteinuria), which shows a membranoproliferative (MPGN) pattern on kidney biopsy. The new approach to MPGN lesions is a bifurcation based on the pattern of staining on immunofluorescence microscopy. The more common pattern, as seen in this patient, is immune-complex deposition with the presence of both immunoglobulin (IgG, IgM, and/or IgA) and complement (C1q and/or C3) on immunofluorescence, which infers that the classical pathway has been activated by an inciting cause or event that generally falls into one of three major categories: infectious, autoimmune, or malignancy associated. The most common is infectious, specifically infection with hepatitis C virus (HCV).

When an MPGN lesion on immunofluorescence microscopy shows only C3 staining (that is, without immunoglobulin or C1q staining), this extremely rare finding is suggestive of an antibody-independent means of complement activation and points to hyperactivity of the alternative complement pathway. In these C3 glomerulopathies, named based on the isolated C3 staining pattern seen on immunofluorescence, screening for genetic abnormalities in alternative complement pathway proteins is an appropriate part of the diagnostic evaluation.

Hepatitis B virus infection and HIV infection have been linked to glomerular diseases, but these are classically associated with the nephrotic syndrome, specifically membranous glomerulopathy with hepatitis B virus infection and focal segmental glomerulosclerosis with HIV infection.

**KEY POINT**

• An immune-complex membranoproliferative glomerulonephritis is the classic form of kidney involvement seen in patients with hepatitis C virus infection.

**Bibliography**

Sethi S, Fervenza FC. Membranoproliferative glomerulonephritis–a new look at an old entity. N Engl J Med. 2012;366:1119-31. [PMID: 22435371]

## Item 82    Answer:    D

**Educational Objective:  Diagnose lead nephropathy.**

The most likely diagnosis is lead nephropathy, which causes a chronic tubulointerstitial disease after years of continuous or intermittent lead exposure. Lead nephropathy can occur in patients with occupational exposure to lead or exposure to lead in water, soil, paint, or food products. Chronic lead nephropathy is frequently associated with hyperuricemia, hypertension, and recurrent gouty attacks. This patient's lead exposure is likely due to lead-contaminated moonshine. Contamination occurs when lead-containing car radiators are used to condense the alcohol during the distilling process. The initial diagnostic test is measurement of blood lead levels, although lead levels may have normalized if exposure has been reduced or stopped.

Analgesic nephropathy occurs in patients with long-term excessive ingestion of analgesics such as aspirin, acetaminophen, and phenacetin, usually in combination. Patients frequently present with nocturia, sterile pyuria, hypertension, anemia, and chronic tubulointerstitial disease. This patient has no history of prolonged analgesic exposure.

Balkan nephropathy is a form of chronic tubulointerstitial disease that progresses to end-stage kidney disease in patients from southeastern Europe (Serbia, Bulgaria, Romania, Bosnia and Herzegovina, and Croatia). This patient is not from this region.

Cadmium nephropathy occurs in patients with prolonged exposure to plastic, metal, alloys, and electrical equipment manufacturing industries. Early manifestations are those of tubular dysfunction, including low-molecular-weight tubular proteinuria (for example, $\beta_2$-microglobulin), aminoaciduria, renal glucosuria, and hypercalciuria. Patients can develop osteomalacia and nephrolithiasis. Clinically, patients present with hypertension, bone pain, and chronic kidney disease. This patient does not give any history of an occupation that would result in cadmium exposure.

**KEY POINT**

• Lead nephropathy can occur in patients with occupational exposure to lead or exposure to lead in water, soil, paint, or food products; it is frequently associated with hyperuricemia, hypertension, and recurrent gouty attacks.

**Bibliography**

Lin JL, Lin-Tan DT, Li YJ, Chen KH, Huang YL. Low-level environmental exposure to lead and progressive chronic kidney diseases. Am J Med. 2006;119:707.e1-9. [PMID: 16887418]

## Item 83    Answer:    A

**Educational Objective:  Identify laxative abuse as a cause of a normal anion gap metabolic acidosis.**

Laxative abuse is the most likely cause of this patient's normal anion gap metabolic acidosis. Normal anion gap metabolic acidosis can be caused by gastrointestinal bicarbonate loss, renal loss of bicarbonate, or the inability of the kidney to excrete acid. The normal physiologic response to systemic acidosis is an increase in urine acid excretion. Therefore, an initial diagnostic step in normal anion gap metabolic acidosis is to determine whether the kidney is appropriately excreting acid or whether impaired kidney acid excretion is the cause of the metabolic acidosis. Increased acid excretion by the kidney is reflected as a marked increase in urine ammonium. However, urine ammonium is difficult to measure directly. Because ammonium carries a positive charge, chloride is excreted into the urine in equal amounts with ammonium to maintain electrical neutrality. Therefore, the amount of chloride in the urine reflects the amount of ammonium present, and the urine anion gap can be used as an indicator of the ability of the kidney to excrete acid. The urine anion gap is calculated as follows:

$$\text{Urine Anion Gap} = (\text{Urine Sodium} + \text{Urine Potassium}) - \text{Urine Chloride}$$

In the context of increased urinary ammonium excretion, therefore, the urine anion gap will be negative. The negative urine anion gap in this patient (-6 mEq/L [-6 mmol/L]) suggests a gastrointestinal cause of the normal anion gap metabolic acidosis, and laxative abuse is a possible, even likely explanation. In addition, the low urine potassium indicates appropriate renal compensation in context of laxative-induced hypokalemia.

Vomiting and gastric acid loss result in metabolic alkalosis, not metabolic acidosis.

CONT.

Renal causes of normal anion gap metabolic acidosis are due to specific defects in renal handling of bicarbonate reclamation (type 2/proximal RTA) or in hydrogen ion secretion (type 1/hypokalemic distal RTA). Type 1 (hypokalemic distal) RTA is caused by a defect in hydrogen secretion and a consequent decrease in ammonium excretion, and is therefore associated with a positive urine anion gap; it is also characterized by high urine potassium secretion and hypokalemia. Type 4 (hyperkalemic distal) RTA is usually caused by aldosterone deficiency or resistance and is characterized by a high serum potassium and positive urine anion gap.

### KEY POINT

- Normal anion gap metabolic acidosis can be caused by gastrointestinal bicarbonate loss, renal loss of bicarbonate, or the inability of the kidney to excrete acid.

### Bibliography

Rastegar M, Nagami GT. Non-anion gap metabolic acidosis: a clinical approach to evaluation. Am J Kidney Dis. 2017;69:296-301. [PMID: 28029394]

## Item 84    Answer:    B

**Educational Objective:** Diagnose the cause of acute kidney injury with a kidney biopsy.

The most appropriate next step in the evaluation of this patient's acute kidney injury (AKI) is a kidney biopsy. This patient with sepsis has developed AKI that has continued to worsen despite discontinuation of antibiotics 4 days ago. His urinalysis is notable for hematuria, pyuria, and proteinuria. The differential diagnosis includes ischemic or toxic acute tubular necrosis in the setting of hypotension, acute interstitial nephritis (AIN) from antibiotics or a proton pump inhibitor, and infection-associated glomerulonephritis. Given multiple potential contributing factors, a kidney biopsy is necessary to differentiate.

Glucocorticoids would be indicated if AIN is identified on biopsy, but empiric therapy is not justified because other causes may be contributing to his AKI. Moreover, glucocorticoids can cause significant adverse side effects, including worsening glycemic control in a patient with diabetes mellitus. If AIN is confirmed on kidney biopsy, a trial of glucocorticoids can be considered.

Prerenal AKI results from decreased renal perfusion and will typically respond to restoration of effective arterial circulation. However, the patient has no findings of hypoperfusion, and the elevated fractional excretion of sodium argues against this diagnosis (typically <1%) and the need for a fluid challenge. Such an intervention may be deleterious in a patient with oliguric AKI.

Postrenal AKI results from urinary tract obstruction. Bladder outlet obstruction should be suspected in patients with prostate enlargement or in the setting of diabetes mellitus (neurogenic bladder), pain medications, or anticholinergic medications. This patient's kidney ultrasound does not show obstruction; therefore, placement of a urinary catheter is not appropriate and would increase his risk of catheter-associated urinary tract infection.

### KEY POINT

- Kidney biopsy should be considered in patients with acute kidney injury from no apparent or unclear cause, suspected glomerulonephritis, or unexplained systemic disease.

### Bibliography

Levey AS, James MT. Acute kidney injury. Ann Intern Med. 2017;167:ITC66-ITC80. [PMID: 29114754]

## Item 85    Answer:    B

**Educational Objective:** Recognize the role of genetic counseling in the diagnosis and management of hereditary nephritis.

Genetic counseling potentially followed by genetic testing for hereditary nephritis (Alport syndrome) is appropriate for this patient. Hereditary nephritis is a familial form of glomerulonephritis that affects approximately 0.4% of U.S. adults. The earliest presentation is microscopic hematuria, with or without proteinuria. Heavier proteinuria, hypertension, and chronic kidney disease usually develop over time, with end-stage kidney disease occurring between the late teenage years and the fourth decade of life. There are three genetic variants: X-linked (80%), autosomal recessive (15%), and autosomal dominant (5%). This patient's family history fits the X-linked version of disease. Her mother and maternal grandmother are asymptomatic carriers; each has a 50% chance of passing the affected gene to male offspring (in this family, the maternal uncle and the patient's older brother), and their daughters likewise have a 50% chance of carrying the gene. Almost all female heterozygotes have some degree of hematuria. Females with the X-linked variant can develop kidney disease depending on activity of the X chromosome in somatic renal cells (lyonization), but that does not appear to be the case in this family. Given widespread access to genetic testing, in patients with a clearly documented family history and abnormal urinary findings, the diagnosis of hereditary nephritis is now increasingly being made by the noninvasive route using genetic testing. Genetic testing is the only way to diagnose a female with a family history of X-linked hereditary nephritis, such as this patient.

Hereditary nephritis is accompanied by sensorineural hearing loss that can be subtle and only picked up by audiometry, but this complication would not be expected in an asymptomatic carrier, such as this patient.

The diagnosis of hereditary nephritis for affected patients has traditionally been made by the more invasive route of kidney biopsy, with electron microscopy required for the hallmark finding of prominent thickening and lamellation of the glomerular basement membrane (a basket-weave appearance). Other than the expected microscopic hematuria, this patient has normal kidney function and does not require a kidney biopsy.

A diagnostic skin biopsy can be performed when X-linked hereditary nephritis is suspected. Type IV collagen alpha-5 chain (COL4A5) is normally present in the skin, and approximately 60% to 80% of patients with X-linked hereditary nephritis will show abnormal staining for COL4A5 in the skin biopsy, although these findings would not be expected in an asymptomatic carrier.

**KEY POINT**

- The diagnosis of hereditary nephritis is confirmed with kidney biopsy, skin biopsy, or molecular genetic analysis.

**Bibliography**

Gross O, Kashtan CE, Rheault MN, Flinter F, Savige J, Miner JH, et al. Advances and unmet needs in genetic, basic and clinical science in Alport syndrome: report from the 2015 International Workshop on Alport Syndrome. Nephrol Dial Transplant. 2017;32:916-924. [PMID: 27190345]

**Item 86      Answer:   A**

**Educational Objective:** Identify the composition of a kidney stone in a patient with Crohn disease.

The most likely composition of this patient's kidney stone is calcium oxalate. This patient has classic symptoms of renal colic, including flank pain that radiates to the groin. Stone movement may result in pain migration to the genitalia. Nausea, vomiting, and dysuria may also be present. Microscopic hematuria is usually noted, although its absence does not exclude a stone. Patients with diarrhea who are volume depleted and have a metabolic acidosis are at increased risk for developing a kidney stone, particularly stones composed of calcium oxalate and uric acid. In this patient with Crohn disease and chronic diarrhea, the most likely composition of the stone is calcium oxalate because the chronic metabolic acidosis (suggested by the low serum bicarbonate concentration and relatively low urine pH) increases calcium loss from bone and decreases citrate excretion. Citrate is the major inhibitor of calcium crystallization in the urine. In addition, if there is concomitant fat malabsorption, a common occurrence in inflammatory bowel disease, calcium will bind to fat in the gut, allowing increased absorption of oxalate.

Struvite stones are composed of magnesium ammonium phosphate (struvite) and calcium carbonate-apatite and occur in the presence of urea-splitting bacteria, such as *Proteus* or *Klebsiella*, in the upper urinary tract. These organisms convert urea to ammonium, which alkalinizes the urine, decreases the solubility of phosphate, and leads to struvite precipitation. Struvite stones can rapidly enlarge to fill the entire renal pelvis within weeks to months, taking on a characteristic "staghorn" shape. Calcium phosphate stones also form in alkaline urine. The low urine pH and absence of signs of infection on urinalysis make these diagnoses unlikely.

Cystine stones are caused by cystinuria, a rare autosomal recessive disorder of proximal tubular transport of dibasic amino acids such as cystine that presents at a young age.

The main risk factor for uric acid stones is low urine pH, usually ≤5.0, which decreases the solubility of uric acid. Hyperuricosuria is not a consistent finding. Comorbid risk factors for uric acid stones include gout, diabetes mellitus, the metabolic syndrome, and chronic diarrhea.

**KEY POINT**

- Patients with diarrhea who are volume depleted and have a metabolic acidosis are at increased risk for developing kidney stones, particularly calcium oxalate stones and, less commonly, uric acid stones.

**Bibliography**

Worcester EM, Coe FL. Clinical practice. Calcium kidney stones. N Engl J Med. 2010;363:954-63. [PMID: 20818905]

**Item 87      Answer:   A**

**Educational Objective:** Diagnose D-lactic acidosis.

The most likely diagnosis is D-lactic acidosis. D-lactic acidosis is an unusual cause of lactic acidosis that presents with an increased anion gap metabolic acidosis in patients with short-bowel syndrome, mostly in the context of small-bowel resection or jejunoileal bypass. D-lactate may accumulate when excess carbohydrates reach the colon and are metabolized to D-lactate by bacteria. Therefore, it is sometimes manifested after a large carbohydrate load. D-lactate is the stereoisomer of L-lactate, the isomer usually responsible for lactic acidosis. The conventional lactate assay measures the L-lactate isomer, and therefore lactic acid levels in this case are normal. Characteristic symptoms include intermittent confusion, slurred speech, and ataxia. The diagnosis should therefore be considered in a patient with characteristic neurologic findings who presents with an increased anion gap metabolic acidosis, normal lactate level, negative ketones, and short-bowel syndrome or other forms of malabsorption; it is confirmed by measuring a D-lactate level.

Ethylene glycol or methanol intoxication also presents with an increased anion gap metabolic acidosis and neurologic symptoms. However, they are usually accompanied by a serum osmolal gap >10 mOsm/kg $H_2O$ (6 mOsm/kg $H_2O$ in this case) and a serum bicarbonate level <10 mEq/L (10 mmol/L). The serum osmolal gap is calculated as the difference between the measured osmolality and calculated osmolality, which is determined as follows:

Serum Osmolality (mOsm/kg $H_2O$) = (2 × Serum Sodium [mEq/L]) + Plasma Glucose (mg/dL)/18 + Blood Urea Nitrogen (mg/dL)/2.8

Pyroglutamic acidosis also manifests as mental status changes in the context of an increased anion gap. This acidosis occurs in patients chronically receiving therapeutic doses of acetaminophen. Susceptible patients are those with critical illness, poor nutrition, liver disease, and chronic kidney

CONT.

disease, as well as those on a strict vegetarian diet. Diagnosis can be confirmed by measuring urine levels of pyroglutamic acid. This patient's history does not include acetaminophen ingestion and is more consistent with a D-lactic acidosis.

**KEY POINT**

- D-lactic acidosis is characterized by an increased anion gap metabolic acidosis in patients with short-bowel syndrome or other forms of malabsorption; diagnosis is confirmed by measuring the D-lactate level rather than the conventional L-lactate level.

**Bibliography**
Seheult J, Fitzpatrick G, Boran G. Lactic acidosis: an update. Clin Chem Lab Med. 2017;55:322-333. [PMID: 27522622]

## Item 88     Answer:   B

**Educational Objective:** Manage chronic hypertension prior to conception.

Discontinuation of the angiotensin receptor blocker (ARB) losartan is necessary for this patient who anticipates pregnancy. The renin-angiotensin system agents (ACE inhibitors, ARBs, and direct renin inhibitors) are contraindicated in pregnancy and should be stopped prior to conception. Exposure during the second and third trimesters of pregnancy has been associated with neonatal kidney failure and death. Although the level of risk for first trimester exposure is controversial, studies have suggested an association with cardiac abnormalities, and consensus is to stop these drugs prior to pregnancy. In patients with chronic hypertension, the 2013 American College of Obstetricians and Gynecologists guidelines recommend a goal blood pressure during pregnancy of 120-160/80-105 mm Hg. Antihypertensive treatment reduces the risk of progression to severe hypertension by 50% compared with placebo but has not been shown to prevent preeclampsia, preterm birth, small size for gestational age, or infant mortality. This patient's blood pressure is well below this goal of therapy, and her blood pressure would be expected to decline during pregnancy. Therefore, monitoring her blood pressure after discontinuation of losartan is a reasonable approach. If her blood pressure rises, initiation of a drug that is safe during pregnancy is recommended. Candidate drugs include methyldopa, nifedipine, and/or labetalol. No specific agent is first choice because no data support one over another. Therapeutic classes are not recommended because potential toxicity differs among agents within classes.

Diuretics may be continued in pregnancy, particularly if the woman is already taking them prior to pregnancy. If blood pressure remains low through the first trimester of pregnancy, the dose of the diuretic may be lowered. Although one could consider discontinuation of the diuretic if the patient's blood pressure remains within at or below target, there is no contraindication to its use.

Because ARBs and ACE inhibitors are contraindicated in pregnancy and carry similar risk, switching to the ACE inhibitor lisinopril is not recommended.

Although risks are less during the first trimester, recent data regarding first trimester risk of exposure suggest that the safest approach is to discontinue a renin-angiotensin system agent prior to conception. Waiting until the patient is pregnant is not recommended.

**KEY POINT**

- The renin-angiotensin system agents (ACE inhibitors, angiotensin receptor blockers, and direct renin inhibitors) are contraindicated in pregnancy and should be stopped prior to conception.

**Bibliography**
Whelton PK, Carey RM, Aronow WS, Casey DE Jr, Collins KJ, Dennison Himmelfarb C, et al. 2017 ACC/AHA/AAPA/ABC/ACPM/AGS/APhA/ASH/ASPC/NMA/PCNA guideline for the prevention, detection, evaluation, and management of high blood pressure in adults: a report of the American College of Cardiology/American Heart Association Task Force on Clinical Practice Guidelines. Hypertension. 2017. [PMID: 29133356]

## Item 89     Answer:   A

**Educational Objective:** Diagnose autosomal dominant polycystic kidney disease as a secondary cause of hypertension.

Kidney ultrasonography is the most appropriate diagnostic test to perform in this patient. The presence of hypertension, microhematuria, and a positive family history of chronic kidney disease requiring dialysis, as well as a brain aneurysm, raises clinical suspicion for autosomal dominant polycystic kidney disease (ADPKD). Clinical manifestations of ADPKD include gradual kidney enlargement, which may cause persistent abdominal pain and/or early satiety. Hypertension is common in patients with ADPKD, often preceding chronic kidney disease. Kidney cyst enlargement leads to stimulation of the intrarenal and circulating renin-angiotensin-aldosterone system. More than 50% of patients with ADPKD develop recurrent flank or back pain; causes include kidney stones, cyst rupture or hemorrhage, or infection. Nephrolithiasis occurs in approximately 20% of patients. A ruptured intracranial cerebral aneurysm resulting in a subarachnoid or intracerebral hemorrhage is the most serious extrarenal complication of ADPKD. Kidney ultrasonography is the most common and least costly screening and diagnostic method for ADPKD; it would reveal bilaterally enlarged kidneys with multiple cysts.

Calculation of the plasma aldosterone concentration/plasma renin activity ratio is used to screen for primary hyperaldosteronism, characterized by a triad of resistant hypertension, metabolic alkalosis, and hypokalemia. Although <50% of patients with primary hyperaldosteronism manifest hypokalemia, this diagnosis cannot account for the patient's flank fullness on palpation and hematuria or his family history of kidney failure.

Plasma fractionated metanephrines are obtained to screen for a pheochromocytoma, which could result in hypertension, but this patient has no symptoms or signs (for example, resistant hypertension, headaches, sweating) to indicate the presence of this tumor, and this diagnosis cannot account for the patient's flank fullness and hematuria.

CONT.

Although hyperthyroidism can be a secondary cause of hypertension, the patient does not manifest any symptoms or signs (heat intolerance, resting tachycardia, thyromegaly) to suggest this, making measurement of thyroid-stimulating hormone unnecessary.

**KEY POINT**

- Hypertension is common in patients with autosomal dominant polycystic kidney disease (ADPKD), often preceding chronic kidney disease; kidney ultrasonography is the most common and least costly screening and diagnostic method for ADPKD.

**Bibliography**

Krishnappa V, Vinod P, Deverakonda D, Raina R. Autosomal dominant polycystic kidney disease and the heart and brain. Cleve Clin J Med. 2017;84:471-481. [PMID: 28628430]

 **Item 90    Answer:    B**

**Educational Objective:** Discontinue mycophenolate mofetil in a woman who is planning pregnancy.

The most appropriate management for this kidney transplant recipient who is planning pregnancy is to discontinue mycophenolate mofetil and begin azathioprine. Fertility increases after kidney transplantation, although fertility rates remain lower and pregnancy complications are higher compared with the general population. Pregnancy planning for a kidney transplant recipient is essential to improve outcomes and includes adjusting medications and optimizing clinical status. Kidney transplant recipients should wait 1 to 2 years with a stable allograft before attempting conception. Other comorbid conditions (such as systemic lupus erythematosus) should also be stable prior to conception. Outcomes are improved with better allograft function (serum creatinine <1.5 mg/dL [132.6 µmol/L]) and stable immunosuppression. Mycophenolate mofetil (as well as sirolimus and everolimus) is teratogenic and needs to be replaced 3 to 6 months prior to conception with azathioprine, which is generally safer and well tolerated in pregnancy.

Calcineurin inhibitors (both tacrolimus and cyclosporine) have been used safely in pregnancy. Therefore, tacrolimus does not need to be discontinued and replaced with cyclosporine in this patient.

Although this would constitute a high-risk pregnancy, the success rate of pregnancies in patients with kidney transplants is high; with stable allograft function, a normotensive patient and her fetus have favorable prognoses, and therefore the patient could proceed with pregnancy following modification of her maintenance immunosuppression regimen.

**KEY POINT**

- In kidney transplant recipients who are planning pregnancy, mycophenolate mofetil, sirolimus, and everolimus must be discontinued 3 to 6 months prior to conception and replaced with azathioprine, which is generally safer and well tolerated in pregnancy.

**Bibliography**

Hou S. Pregnancy in renal transplant recipients. Adv Chronic Kidney Dis. 2013;20:253-9. [PMID: 23928390]

**Item 91    Answer:    A**

**Educational Objective:** Diagnose light chain cast nephropathy in a patient with multiple myeloma.

The most likely diagnosis is light chain cast nephropathy in this patient with multiple myeloma. In multiple myeloma, acute kidney injury from light chain cast nephropathy is the most common type of kidney disease. Cast nephropathy is characterized by intratubular obstruction with light chain casts that can result in acute tubular injury. A clinical clue to the diagnosis is the presence of an elevated urine protein-creatinine ratio, with minimal proteinuria detected by dipstick urinalysis (dipstick urinalysis detects albumin but not light chains). Other supporting findings are the presence of anemia and hypercalcemia (when calcium measurement is corrected for albumin).

Exposure to NSAIDs can cause tubular injury. However, NSAIDs do not cause a discrepancy in proteinuria between urinalysis and urine protein-creatinine ratio.

Renal sarcoidosis can result in tubulointerstitial dysfunction. Other kidney manifestations include direct ureteral involvement, retroperitoneal fibrosis, and, more commonly, hypercalcemia, hypercalciuria, nephrolithiasis, and nephrocalcinosis via excessive production of 1,25-dihydroxyvitamin D in granulomas. However, renal sarcoidosis is rare in patients without thoracic sarcoidosis and cannot account for the discrepancy in proteinuria between urinalysis and urine protein-creatinine ratio.

Uric acid nephropathy is unlikely given the modest elevation in the serum urate level. Furthermore, an elevated urine protein-creatinine ratio is not consistent with uric acid nephropathy.

**KEY POINT**

- Clinical clues to the diagnosis of light chain cast nephropathy from multiple myeloma include an elevated urine protein-creatinine ratio with minimal proteinuria by urine dipstick, anemia, and hypercalcemia.

**Bibliography**

Heher EC, Rennke HG, Laubach JP, Richardson PG. Kidney disease and multiple myeloma. Clin J Am Soc Nephrol. 2013;8:2007-17. [PMID: 23868898]

**Item 92    Answer:    B**

**Educational Objective:** Diagnose IgA nephropathy.

IgA nephropathy is the most likely diagnosis. Recurrent gross hematuria, in which macroscopic hematuria occurs concomitantly or within days after an upper respiratory infection (synpharyngitic nephritis) or physical exertion, is a classic presentation of IgA nephropathy, particularly in younger patients.

This nephritic presentation usually follows a benign clinical course without associated kidney insufficiency, although in a minority of cases intraluminal obstructive erythrocyte casts can be a cause of moderate to severe acute kidney injury that typically responds to supportive care measures. The diagnosis of IgA nephropathy can only be made by kidney biopsy, but some clinicians will make an empiric diagnosis for young patients with a classic history of recurrent gross hematuria, negative imaging for masses/stones, and normal kidney function with little to no proteinuria.

IgA vasculitis (Henoch-Schönlein purpura) is the most common childhood vasculitis and tends to appear after upper respiratory infections. IgA vasculitis is rarer among adults. Characteristic symptoms are abdominal pain and palpable purpura. Gastrointestinal ischemia may be severe enough to cause intestinal bleeding. Arthritis is common, other organ systems may be involved, and patients may present with glomerulonephritis. The patient's recurrent symptoms, lack of additional findings, benign clinical course, and urine findings are not compatible with a diagnosis of IgA vasculitis.

Lupus nephritis and postinfectious glomerulonephritis can present with macroscopic glomerular hematuria, but these disease states usually induce low complement levels (low C3 with or without low C4). Postinfectious glomerulonephritis, when associated with upper respiratory infections caused by streptococcal organisms, usually occurs 2 to 3 weeks after the resolution of the streptococcal infection. In the developed world, it is more common to see peri-infectious glomerulonephritis associated with staphylococcal infections (usually skin infections), with onset at the time of infection, but these are not usually associated with gross hematuria or a recurrent history of such episodes.

**KEY POINT**

- A classic presentation of IgA nephropathy is recurrent gross hematuria that occurs concomitantly or within days after an upper respiratory infection or physical exertion and usually follows a benign course.

**Bibliography**

Lai KN, Tang SC, Schena FP, Novak J, Tomino Y, Fogo AB, et al. IgA nephropathy. Nat Rev Dis Primers. 2016;2:16001. [PMID: 27189177]

**Item 93     Answer:   D**

**Educational Objective:** Diagnose a complex mixed acid-base disorder.

The most likely diagnosis is a complex mixed acid-base disorder consisting of respiratory alkalosis, increased anion gap metabolic acidosis, and metabolic alkalosis. Interpretation of acid-base disorders requires the identification of the likely dominant acid-base disorder, followed by an assessment of the compensatory response. When measured values fall outside the expected compensatory range, a mixed acid-base disorder is considered present. Multiple acid-base disturbances may coexist, as seen in this patient.

Because the blood pH is 7.56, the patient's dominant acid-base disorder is an alkalosis. The low $P_{CO_2}$ indicates a respiratory component to the alkalosis. The expected metabolic compensation for chronic respiratory alkalosis is a reduction in the serum bicarbonate of 4 to 5 mEq/L (4-5 mmol/L) for each 10 mm Hg (1.3 kPa) decrease in the $P_{CO_2}$ (in this case, the decrease in $P_{CO_2}$ is 20 mm Hg [2.7 kPa]). The expected serum bicarbonate concentration in this patient is calculated as follows:

Normal Bicarbonate - Expected Compensation
24 − (8-10) mEq/L (mmol/L) = 14-16 mEq/L (14-16 mmol/L)

Because the measured bicarbonate of 20 mEq/L (20 mmol/L) is higher than expected, this suggests coexistence of a metabolic alkalosis.

An elevated anion gap is also present, indicating the presence of an increased anion gap metabolic acidosis. Assessing the ratio of the change in the anion gap (Δ anion gap) to the change in bicarbonate level (Δ bicarbonate), or the "delta-delta (Δ-Δ) ratio," may indicate the presence of a coexistent acid-base disturbance. A ratio of <0.5 to 1 may reflect the presence of concurrent normal anion gap metabolic acidosis, whereas a ratio >2 may indicate the presence of metabolic alkalosis. This patient's Δ-Δ ratio is 2.5 [Δ anion gap/Δ bicarbonate = (22 - 12)/(24 - 20) = 2.5], confirming the coexistence of the metabolic alkalosis.

The clinical situation most likely to present with this acid-base disorder is salicylate toxicity. Central hyperventilation from salicylate will cause the respiratory alkalosis; salicylate itself will cause the anion gap metabolic acidosis; and vomiting will cause the metabolic alkalosis.

**KEY POINT**

- Interpretation of acid-base disorders requires the identification of the likely dominant acid-base disorder, followed by an assessment of the compensatory response; when measured values fall outside the range of the predicted compensatory response, a mixed acid-base disorder is considered present.

**Bibliography**

Seifter JL, Chang HY. Disorders of acid-base balance: new perspectives. Kidney Dis (Basel). 2017;2:170-186. [PMID: 28232934]

**Item 94     Answer:   D**

**Educational Objective:** Evaluate proteinuria in the absence of albuminuria.

The most appropriate next step in management is to obtain a urine protein electrophoresis. Albumin is the predominant protein detected on urine dipstick, which detects albumin excretion graded as trace (10-30 mg/dL), 1+ (30 mg/dL), 2+ (100 mg/dL), 3+ (300 mg/dL), and 4+ (>1000 mg/dL). Highly alkaline urine specimens can produce false-positive results on dipstick testing for protein. The sulfosalicylic acid (SSA) test can be used to detect the presence of not only albumin

CONT.

but also other proteins that are not detected with the urine dipstick, such as urine light chains or immunoglobulins. The possibility of cast nephropathy should be raised in patients with acute kidney injury and anemia when the urine dipstick reads negative or trace for protein, but the urine shows increased positivity for protein by the SSA test or by measuring the urine protein-creatinine ratio. Although these findings are most concerning for myeloma cast nephropathy, light chains are associated with other renal findings such as proximal tubulopathy. Proximal tubule involvement may be associated with hypophosphatemia and glucosuria (Fanconi syndrome).

Omeprazole and other proton pump inhibitors are well-described causes of acute interstitial nephritis. Although this is possible, this patient's proteinuria patterns are far more consistent with multiple myeloma.

Although a 24-hour urine collection is likely to provide a more accurate assessment of the total urine protein, the urine protein-creatinine ratio is sufficiently accurate to determine the presence of proteinuria.

Noncontrast helical abdominal CT may be helpful if the presence of a stone or mass in the kidney is suspected; however, in the absence of flank pain or hematuria, this imaging study is unlikely to provide additional diagnostic information.

**KEY POINT**

- The presence of significant measured proteinuria in the context of minimal proteinuria on urine dipstick suggests the presence of Bence-Jones (light chain) proteinuria, which can be confirmed by a urine protein electrophoresis.

**Bibliography**
Simerville JA, Maxted WC, Pahira JJ. Urinalysis: a comprehensive review. Am Fam Physician. 2005;71:1153-62. [PMID: 15791892]

## Item 95    Answer:   D

**Educational Objective:** Refer a patient with chronic kidney disease for kidney transplant evaluation.

Kidney transplant evaluation is the most appropriate management for this patient with stage G4 chronic kidney disease (CKD). Referral to a kidney transplant center is indicated when the estimated glomerular filtration rate (eGFR) is <20 mL/min/1.73 m². Kidney transplantation is the preferred treatment for patients with end-stage kidney disease, because it improves life expectancy and quality of life. It also provides a significant cost savings to the health care system compared with maintaining a patient on dialysis. Early referral allows adequate time to identify suitable living donors. If no living donor is available, early listing is essential to begin the waiting process for a deceased-donor kidney. Patients undergo an extensive health screening to identify potential issues that may affect the safety and/or outcome of the transplant. In the potential recipient, these include active malignancy, coronary ischemia, or active infections. An adequate social support system and financial resources also are important to ensure

medication adherence and long-term survival of the transplanted allograft.

Patients with stage G4 chronic kidney disease should be seen at least every 3 months, not 6 months. More importantly, clinical follow-up alone does not address the immediate problem of planning for renal replacement therapy, ideally with kidney transplantation.

Fistulography is not indicated because physical examination findings suggest that the fistula is mature and may be ready to use for hemodialysis. Invasive imaging is not required to confirm patency unless physical examination findings suggest a problem. Additionally, fistulography exposes the patient to nephrotoxic iodinated contrast and may reduce residual kidney function.

Although this patient has an arteriovenous fistula, hemodialysis is not indicated at this time because she has normal serum potassium and bicarbonate levels, does not have significant volume overload, and does not have uremic symptoms. Several recent studies have demonstrated no benefit in starting dialysis in asymptomatic patients early based upon an arbitrary eGFR cutoff compared with waiting until patients develop very low eGFR (<8-10 mL/min/1.73 m²) or clinical indications for dialysis are present.

**KEY POINT**

- Referral for kidney transplant evaluation is indicated when the estimated glomerular filtration rate is <20 mL/min/1.73 m² to allow for adequate time to identify suitable living donors or to be put on an early listing if no living donor is available.

**Bibliography**
Educational Guidance on Patient Referral to Kidney Transplantation-Organ Procurement and Transplantation Network, US Department of Health and Human Services. Available at: https://optn.transplant.hrsa.gov/resources/guidance/educational-guidance-on-patient-referral-to-kidney-transplantation/. Accessed October 30, 2017.

## Item 96    Answer:   C

**Educational Objective:** Treat type 1 hepatorenal syndrome.

Vasoconstrictor therapy with octreotide and oral midodrine is appropriate for this patient with type 1 hepatorenal syndrome (HRS). Type 1 HRS is a clinical diagnosis made after exclusion of other causes of kidney dysfunction. It is characterized by a rise in serum creatinine of at least 0.3 mg/dL (26.5 µmol/L) and/or ≥50% from baseline within 48 hours, bland urinalysis, and normal findings on kidney ultrasound. It is also supported by a lack of improvement in kidney function after withdrawal of diuretics and 2 days of volume expansion with intravenous albumin. Often, patients also have low urine sodium, low fractional excretion of sodium, and oliguria. Type 2 HRS is defined as a more gradual decline in kidney function associated with refractory ascites. General management of type 1 HRS includes discontinuing diuretics, restricting sodium, restricting water in hyponatremic patients, and searching for precipitating factors. Initial therapeutic interventions include

CONT.

treatment with vasoconstrictors in conjunction with intravenous albumin.

Dialysis should be initiated only if the patient does not respond to HRS medical therapy with midodrine and octreotide and/or if indications for dialysis develop. Absolute indications for dialysis include hyperkalemia, metabolic acidosis, and pulmonary edema refractory to medical therapy; uremic symptoms; uremic pericarditis; and certain drug intoxications. Currently, this patient has no acute indications for dialysis.

The patient was volume expanded with intravenous albumin, which should have corrected hypovolemia. Furthermore, she is not volume depleted on physical examination, has edema and ascites, and has stable blood pressure without tachycardia. Therefore, intravenous fluids are not indicated.

The transjugular intrahepatic portosystemic shunt is primarily used to treat variceal hemorrhage and ascites. It has been used as a last resort in the treatment of refractory ascites in highly selected patients with HRS who do not respond to medical therapy and who are awaiting liver transplantation. Complications include an increase in the rate of hepatic encephalopathy and risk of kidney injury associated with intravenous contrast. This procedure is not indicated at this time.

**KEY POINT**

- General management of type 1 hepatorenal syndrome includes discontinuing diuretics, volume replacement with albumin, and use of vasoconstrictors.

**Bibliography**
Colle I, Laterre PF. Hepatorenal syndrome: the clinical impact of vasoactive therapy. Expert Rev Gastroenterol Hepatol. 2018;12:173-188. [PMID: 29258378]

### Item 97     Answer:    D

**Educational Objective: Identify urea osmotic diuresis as a cause of hypernatremia.**

Urea osmotic diuresis is the most likely cause of this patient's hypernatremia. This patient is recovering from acute kidney injury and is having a urea diuresis, with an elevated urine osmolality of 420 mOsm/kg $H_2O$. In osmotic diuresis, urine osmolality is usually between 300 and 600 mOsm/kg $H_2O$. The majority of the osmolality of the urine is made up of nonelectrolytes. This loss of electrolyte-free water is causing her serum sodium level to increase. The two major nonelectrolytes found in urine are urea and glucose. Her glucose is only 136 mg/dL (7.5 mmol/L), below the threshold for glucose appearing in the urine; therefore, the likely cause is excretion of urea. This can be confirmed by measuring urea in the urine.

Hyponatremia is found in 70% to 80% of patients with adrenal insufficiency and is a consequence of sodium loss and volume depletion caused by mineralocorticoid deficiency and increased vasopressin secretion caused by cortisol deficiency. In addition, hyperkalemia and hyperchloremic

acidosis is found in approximately 50% of patients with adrenal insufficiency. Hypernatremia and hypokalemia would be unusual manifestations of adrenal insufficiency.

In the absence of antidiuretic hormone, excessive water is excreted by the kidneys, and the urine osmolality is low. The patient's urine osmolality is 420 mOsm/kg $H_2O$, making diabetes insipidus unlikely. In addition, there is no reason to suspect diabetes insipidus in this woman. Nevertheless, it would not be possible to rule out partial nephrogenic diabetes insipidus until her urea normalized.

Glycosuria is not the cause of this patient's hypernatremia because her glucose level is below the tubular threshold for reabsorption, approximately 180 mg/dL (10 mmol/L). A urine dipstick would verify the lack of glycosuria.

**KEY POINT**

- Hypernatremia may be caused by osmotic diuresis, in which the urine osmolality is usually between 300 and 600 mOsm/kg $H_2O$.

**Bibliography**
Lindner G, Schwarz C, Funk GC. Osmotic diuresis due to urea as the cause of hypernatraemia in critically ill patients. Nephrol Dial Transplant. 2012;27:962-7. [PMID: 21810766]

### Item 98     Answer:    D

**Educational Objective: Perform a kidney biopsy to evaluate a decline in kidney function.**

A kidney biopsy is appropriate for this patient with a decline in kidney function. Clinical and laboratory features are often insufficient for definitive diagnosis of kidney disease. Kidney biopsy may therefore be essential for diagnosis and management. Indications include glomerular hematuria, severely increased albuminuria, acute or chronic kidney disease of unclear cause, and kidney transplant dysfunction or monitoring. In this case, the patient has an elevated serum creatinine without clear cause. Although further serologic testing may be done to guide diagnosis, a kidney biopsy will provide definitive diagnosis.

Due to preferential dilation of the efferent arteriole, the ACE inhibitor lisinopril may reduce glomerular filtration rate (GFR) and hence increase serum creatinine; however, this change in serum creatinine will occur within days of drug initiation and then stabilize. In this case, the serum creatinine increased without a change in dose, suggesting an unrelated cause.

A 24-hour creatinine clearance may be helpful in estimating kidney function but will not change the evaluation at this time. Most studies show that the Chronic Kidney Disease Epidemiology (CKD-EPI) Collaboration equation or the Modification of Diet in Renal Disease (MDRD) study equation provides a more accurate estimated GFR (eGFR) compared with creatinine clearance.

Although this patient's CKD-EPI eGFR is reported as >60 mL/min/1.73 m², his increasing serum creatinine is consistent with a significantly declining eGFR. Although cystatin C will potentially add to the accuracy of the

CKD-EPI formula, it will not change the evaluation, as GFR is declining as documented by the serum creatinine elevation (and no baseline cystatin C is available to show otherwise).

**KEY POINT**

- Indications for kidney biopsy include glomerular hematuria, severely increased albuminuria, acute or chronic kidney disease of unclear cause, and kidney transplant dysfunction or monitoring.

**Bibliography**

Hogan JJ, Mocanu M, Berns JS. The native kidney biopsy: update and evidence for best practice. Clin J Am Soc Nephrol. 2016;11:354-62. [PMID: 26339068]

## Item 99      Answer:    B

**Educational Objective:** Manage end-stage kidney disease in an elderly patient with multiple comorbidities and poor prognosis.

Discussion of conservative management and non-dialytic options is appropriate for this 82-year-old patient with end-stage kidney disease (ESKD) who has multiple comorbidities and poor prognosis. The life expectancy of some patients with ESKD with advanced age and severe comorbidities can be extremely short and may not be improved by dialysis. In elderly persons with progressing or advanced chronic kidney disease, decisions need to be made about the desires and plans to initiate renal replacement therapy and/or referral for evaluation for kidney transplantation. Several factors, including comorbid medical conditions, functional status, expected outcomes, and patient preferences regarding goals of care, should be considered. There is growing recognition that clinicians need to ensure maximal involvement of patients and their families in treatment decisions. This shared decision-making is a process whereby patients and providers can discuss the benefits and burdens of potential treatment strategies in the context of each patient's priorities and needs.

Patients with low comorbidity levels and a predicted survival of >3 years should be considered for all kidney disease treatment modalities, including kidney transplantation. In contrast, patients with a high 3- and 6-month expected mortality may choose to delay initiation and may be candidates for non-dialytic conservative management. Patients who choose conservative therapy have relatively preserved functional status until the last months of life. Conservative management may be a reasonable choice for patients whose primary goal is to maintain their independence and to avoid the time, pain, and discomfort related to dialysis, as well as for patients with poor functional status and a predicted post-dialysis initiation projected survival of <3 months.

**KEY POINT**

- Non-dialytic therapy is a reasonable treatment option for elderly patients with end-stage kidney disease and multiple comorbidities; treatment focuses on symptom management.

**Bibliography**

Verberne WR, Geers AB, Jellema WT, Vincent HH, van Delden JJ, Bos WJ. Comparative survival among older adults with advanced kidney disease managed conservatively versus with dialysis. Clin J Am Soc Nephrol. 2016;11:633-40. [PMID: 26988748]

## Item 100      Answer:    B

**Educational Objective:** Manage difficult-to-control hypertension with the addition of a loop diuretic.

The addition of a loop diuretic such as furosemide is the most appropriate treatment. This patient has difficult-to-control hypertension in the setting of stage G4 chronic kidney disease (CKD), and his blood pressure is not at target. The American College of Cardiology/American Heart Association blood pressure guideline recommends a target blood pressure of <130/80 mm Hg for all patients, including those with CKD. The most appropriate treatment is the addition of a loop diuretic. Suboptimal blood pressure therapy in patients with difficult-to-control hypertension is frequently the result of not including a diuretic, which prevents or corrects extracellular volume expansion. Persistent volume expansion, even if not sufficient to produce clinically evident edema, contributes significantly to hypertension. This is particularly important in sodium-retentive, edematous conditions such as heart failure, liver cirrhosis, or CKD.

Although thiazide diuretics are frequently used as initial diuretic therapy, they are generally less effective in patients with lower glomerular filtration rates. At estimated glomerular filtration rates <30 mL/min/1.73 m$^2$, loop diuretics tend to be more effective at controlling extracellular volume expansion and should be used instead of (or added to) thiazide diuretics. The dosage of loop diuretics depends on the sodium intake and the severity of CKD. Generally, furosemide doses of 40 to 80 mg twice daily is initiated with a salt-restricted diet and adjusted according to the response. When it is appropriate to add a thiazide diuretic to a blood pressure regimen, chlorthalidone is often preferred because of its longer duration of action.

The patient is already on a maximum dose of the ACE inhibitor lisinopril, which is appropriate for the treatment of hypertension in patients with CKD. Although he still has albuminuria, addition of the angiotensin receptor blocker (ARB) losartan is inappropriate because several trials have shown that combination therapy with an ACE inhibitor and ARB may result in adverse events, such as acute kidney injury and hyperkalemia, and does not improve cardiovascular outcomes compared with treatment with an ACE inhibitor or ARB alone.

**KEY POINT**

- Patients with difficult-to-control hypertension typically require the addition of a diuretic, which prevents or corrects extracellular volume expansion in sodium-retentive, edematous conditions (heart failure, liver cirrhosis, chronic kidney disease).

**Bibliography**

Braam B, Taler SJ, Rahman M, Fillaus JA, Greco BA, Forman JP, et al. Recognition and management of resistant hypertension. Clin J Am Soc Nephrol. 2017;12:524-535. [PMID: 27895136]

## Item 101    Answer:    B

**Educational Objective:** Diagnose cisplatin-induced acute kidney injury.

The patient has cisplatin-induced acute kidney injury (AKI). AKI due to renal tubular dysfunction can occur following administration of cisplatin and ifosfamide. High-dose methotrexate can also cause renal tubular injury, which can be avoided with aggressive intravenous hydration, forced diuresis, urine alkalization, and administration of leucovorin. Cisplatin induces direct cellular toxicity as a result of their transport through tubular cells, induction of mitochondrial injury, oxidative stress, and activation of apoptotic signaling pathways. Cisplatin-induced AKI develops 7 to 10 days after administration and is characterized by polyuria, tubular injury, hypomagnesemia, and proximal renal tubular acidosis (RTA) with Fanconi syndrome. Cisplatin nephrotoxicity results in volume depletion from urinary excretion of sodium and hypomagnesemia from urinary magnesium loss with ensuing hypokalemia and hypocalcemia. Fanconi syndrome in this patient is supported by the normal anion gap metabolic acidosis, hypophosphatemia, and urinary findings of glycosuria (in the setting of normal blood glucose) and proteinuria. In patients receiving cisplatin, serum electrolyte levels and kidney function must be carefully monitored because early recognition and prompt discontinuation of the drug are essential for renal recovery.

Bevacizumab and gemcitabine can cause hypertension and AKI due to thrombotic microangiopathy, which manifests as thrombocytopenia with hemolytic anemia, elevated lactate dehydrogenase, decreased haptoglobin, and schistocytes on peripheral smear. Urinary findings usually demonstrate significant proteinuria and hematuria. No laboratory findings in this patient support this diagnosis, and these drugs do not cause renal tubular injury.

Paclitaxel has been associated with subacute diffuse interstitial lung disease and peripheral neuropathy. Paclitaxel does not cause AKI or the electrolyte abnormalities as seen in this patient.

### KEY POINT

- Cisplatin-induced acute kidney injury is characterized by polyuria, tubular injury, hypomagnesemia, and proximal renal tubular acidosis with Fanconi syndrome.

**Bibliography**

Rosner MH, Perazella MA. Acute kidney injury in patients with cancer. N Engl J Med. 2017;376:1770-1781. [PMID: 28467867]

## Item 102    Answer:    B

**Educational Objective:** Treat hypertension to a blood pressure target of <130/80 mm Hg in a patient with chronic kidney disease and hypervolemia.

The most appropriate management is to increase the furosemide dose. The patient has chronic kidney disease and proteinuria of 1000 mg/g, and he is taking prednisone for his primary focal segmental glomerulosclerosis. The pathophysiology of hypertension in kidney disease is complex, but sodium retention is the predominant mechanism and is related to a reduction in glomerular filtration rate (GFR), resistance to natriuretic peptides, and increased activity of the renin-angiotensin-aldosterone system. Control of sodium balance is an essential component of blood pressure management in patients with kidney disease. Dietary sodium restriction to <2000 mg/d combined with appropriate use of diuretics is advised. As the GFR declines, thiazide diuretics become less effective. Loop diuretics should be employed in such patients, with doses titrated to clinical response. Because this patient is hypervolemic (elevated jugular venous pressure, $S_3$, lower extremity edema), the dose of the loop diuretic needs to be increased.

Increasing the amlodipine dose is not the best option because it will not treat the underlying hypervolemia, and increasing the dose of amlodipine may worsen the lower extremity edema.

Adding an ACE inhibitor (such as lisinopril) is inappropriate because the patient is already on an angiotensin receptor blocker (losartan), and combination therapy with these agents and other renin-angiotensin system agents may result in adverse events such as hyperkalemia and acute kidney injury.

The 2017 American College of Cardiology/American Heart Association high blood pressure guideline recommends a target blood pressure of <130/80 mm Hg in patients with hypertension and chronic kidney disease. Therefore, maintaining this patient's current medication regimen would be inappropriate.

### KEY POINT

- Control of sodium balance is an essential component of blood pressure management in patients with kidney disease; dietary sodium restriction to <2000 mg/d combined with appropriate use of diuretics is recommended.

**Bibliography**

Gargiulo R, Suhail F, Lerma EV. Hypertension and chronic kidney disease. Dis Mon. 2015;61:387-95. [PMID: 26328515]

## Item 103    Answer:    D

**Educational Objective:** Predict chronic kidney disease progression using the four-variable kidney failure risk equation.

A urine albumin-creatinine ratio is needed to complete the four-variable kidney failure risk equation (KFRE) for this patient with newly diagnosed chronic kidney disease (CKD). Not all patients with CKD will progress to end-stage kidney disease. In 2011, Tangri and colleagues developed and validated a set of risk prediction models for progression to kidney failure among Canadian patients with moderate to severe CKD. They demonstrated that using laboratory data that are routinely obtained in patients with CKD provided excellent discrimination for prediction of progression of CKD to kidney failure over a 2- to 5-year period. Several models and variables were tested. Ultimately, the highest-performing models were the four-variable KFRE (age, sex, estimated glomerular filtration rate, and urine albumin-creatinine ratio) and the eight-variable KFRE (previous four variables, plus serum calcium, phosphate, bicarbonate, and albumin). The addition of diabetes mellitus, hypertension, blood pressure, and body weight did not improve the ability to discriminate risk for kidney failure.

In 2016, the KFRE was validated in 31 international cohorts comprised of 721,357 patients with stage G3 to G5 CKD. Calculation of the area under the receiver operating characteristic (ROC) curve quantifies the performance of a diagnostic test and allows comparison of different tests. A perfect test has an area under the curve (AUC) equal to 1; the closer the AUC is to 1, the better the test. The pooled AUC for the four-variable KFRE was 0.90 (95% CI, 0.89-0.92) to predict kidney failure at 2 years and 0.88 (95% CI, 0.86-0.90) at 5 years. Use of the eight-variable KFRE did not add to the predictive accuracy (AUC for 2 years, 0.89 [95% CI, 0.88-0.91]; AUC for 5 years, 0.86 [95% CI, 0.84-0.87]). Thus, the four-variable original risk equation appears generalizable and highly accurate in most cohorts and can be easily implemented across multiple health care systems. The KFRE performs well across age, sex, race, and the presence or absence of diabetes. The use of this equation is consistent with the Kidney Disease: Improving Global Outcomes (KDIGO) guidelines, which recommend integration of risk prediction in the evaluation and management of CKD.

### KEY POINT

- The kidney failure risk equation uses four variables (age, sex, estimated glomerular filtration rate, and albuminuria) to predict 2-year and 5-year risk of end-stage kidney disease in patients with stages G3 to G5 chronic kidney disease.

### Bibliography

Tangri N, Grams ME, Levey AS, Coresh J, Appel LJ, Astor BC, et al; CKD Prognosis Consortium. Multinational Assessment of Accuracy of Equations for Predicting Risk of Kidney Failure: A Meta-analysis. JAMA. 2016;315:164-74. [PMID: 26757465]

## Item 104      Answer:    A

**Educational Objective:  Diagnose AA amyloidosis in a patient with rheumatoid arthritis.**

AA amyloidosis is the most likely cause of this patient's proteinuria. Chronic inflammatory states, particularly rheumatoid arthritis, are associated with production of amyloid protein A. This acute phase reactant deposits in numerous tissues, most commonly the kidney (80%-90%) and heart, forming β-pleated sheets. In the kidney, amyloidosis presents with a bland urinary sediment and nephrotic-range proteinuria. Progression to end-stage kidney disease is frequent. Cardiac manifestations may include systolic or diastolic dysfunction

and heart failure; low voltage on electrocardiogram can be seen. Although serum amyloid P component scintigraphy can diagnose amyloid, it is not available in the United States. Confirmation would therefore require a kidney biopsy in this case. Current treatment strategies are aimed at the underlying disease. Tocilizumab, an anti–interleukin-6 antibody, has been used successfully in patients with AA amyloidosis from rheumatoid arthritis.

Both focal segmental glomerulosclerosis (FSGS) and minimal change glomerulopathy (MCG) are associated with the nephrotic syndrome. However, FSGS more frequently affects black persons, and MCG is the most common cause of the nephrotic syndrome in children. Finally, this patient's history of a chronic inflammatory disease and findings of heart failure and an abnormal electrocardiogram more strongly suggest the possibility of amyloidosis.

NSAIDs are associated with interstitial nephritis and the nephrotic syndrome due to MCG or membranous glomerulopathy; typical findings include hematuria, pyuria, leukocyte casts, proteinuria, and an acute rise in the plasma creatinine concentration. However, this patient has not been using NSAIDs for the past 6 months and her urinalysis is bland, making this diagnosis unlikely.

Proton pump inhibitors can cause acute interstitial nephritis but are not associated with nephrotic-range proteinuria.

### KEY POINT

- AA amyloid is formed by serum amyloid A protein, an acute phase reactant produced in various inflammatory diseases such as rheumatoid arthritis; confirmation of AA renal amyloidosis requires a kidney biopsy.

### Bibliography

Obici L, Raimondi S, Lavatelli F, Bellotti V, Merlini G. Susceptibility to AA amyloidosis in rheumatic diseases: a critical overview. Arthritis Rheum. 2009;61:1435-40. [PMID: 19790131]

## Item 105      Answer:    C

**Educational Objective:  Treat elevated blood pressure with lifestyle modification.**

The most appropriate next step in management is lifestyle modification. According to the American College of Cardiology/American Heart Association (ACC/AHA) blood pressure guideline, this patient has elevated blood pressure (BP), defined as systolic BP between 120-129 mm Hg and diastolic BP <80 mm Hg. Meta-analysis of observational studies has demonstrated that elevated BP and hypertension (systolic BP >130 mm Hg or diastolic BP >80 mm Hg) are associated with an increased risk of cardiovascular disease, end-stage kidney disease, subclinical atherosclerosis, and all-cause death. Nonpharmacologic therapy alone is especially useful for prevention of hypertension, including in adults with elevated BP, and for management of high BP in adults with milder forms of hypertension. Recommended lifestyle modifications include weight loss in adults who are overweight or obese; a heart-healthy diet that facilitates achieving a desirable weight; reduced sodium intake; high potassium intake (unless contra-indicated by the presence of chronic kidney disease or use of drugs that reduce potassium excretion); increase in physical activity; and limiting alcohol consumption of standard drinks to no more than two (men) or one (women) per day.

According to the ACC/AHA BP guideline, the use of antihypertensive medications is recommended for second-ary prevention of recurrent coronary events in patients with clinical coronary vascular disease and an average systolic BP of ≥130 mm Hg or an average diastolic BP of ≥80 mm Hg. Drug therapy is also recommended for primary prevention in adults with an estimated 10-year atherosclerotic cardio-vascular disease risk ≥10% and an average systolic BP ≥130 mm Hg or average diastolic BP ≥80 mm Hg. For initiation of antihypertensive drug therapy, first-line agents include thia-zide diuretics, calcium channel blockers, and ACE inhibitors or angiotensin receptor blockers. Because this patient has elevated BP (not hypertension), initiation of drug therapy is not indicated at this time.

The ACC/AHA recommends that adults with an elevated BP, such as this patient, should be managed with nonphar-macologic therapy and have a repeat BP evaluation within 3 to 6 months. Patients with normal BP (systolic BP <120 mm Hg and diastolic BP <80 mm Hg) can be reevaluated in 1 year.

### KEY POINT

- Nonpharmacologic therapy alone is especially useful for prevention of hypertension, including in adults with elevated blood pressure, and for management of high blood pressure in adults with milder forms of hypertension.

### Bibliography
Whelton PK, Carey RM, Aronow WS, Casey DE Jr, Collins KJ, Dennison Himmelfarb C, et al. 2017 ACC/AHA/AAPA/ABC/ACPM/AGS/APhA/ASH/ASPC/NMA/PCNA guideline for the prevention, detection, evaluation, and management of high blood pressure in adults: a report of the American College of Cardiology/American Heart Association Task Force on Clinical Practice Guidelines. Hypertension. 2017. [PMID: 29133356]

### Item 106      Answer:   B

**Educational Objective:** Manage acquired cystic kidney disease with suspected renal cell carcinoma in a patient with end-stage kidney disease.

Bilateral radical nephrectomy is the most appropriate man-agement for this patient with end-stage chronic kidney dis-ease (ESKD) and bilateral kidney solid masses. Acquired kid-ney cysts often develop in patients with severe chronic kidney disease (CKD) and are frequently detected during routine kidney ultrasound or incidentally noted on abdominal CT or MRI scan. Acquired cystic kidney disease becomes more com-mon and progresses during the course of ESKD, and some studies suggest that it may affect >50% of patients who have had ESKD for >3 years. The epithelial cells lining these cysts may undergo malignant transformation by poorly understood mechanisms. Patients with ESKD have a markedly increased

risk for renal cell carcinoma. Although current guidelines do not support routine screening for renal cell carcinoma in all patients with CKD, a high level of suspicion is warranted in patients with symptoms such as new-onset gross hematuria or unexplained flank pain.

Partial nephrectomy and nephron-sparing approaches would be indicated for less severe stages of CKD. However, this patient has ESKD, and maintaining residual kidney function is no longer a concern; therefore, radical nephrec-tomy would be the most appropriate option.

Kidney biopsy should be considered in patients with glomerular hematuria, severely increased albuminuria, acute or chronic kidney disease of unclear etiology, and kid-ney transplant dysfunction or monitoring. The role of kidney biopsy for a suspicious mass is more limited. It may be useful in the evaluation of a small mass if there is suspicion of a renal metastasis or lymphoma and is likely useful to confirm the diagnosis of renal cell carcinoma in patients who cannot tolerate surgery prior to initiating medical therapy. The best approach for this patient with a high likelihood of renal cell carcinoma is bilateral nephrectomy. The excised tissue will provide histological confirmation of the diagnosis and thus guide further therapy.

Surveillance ultrasonography would not be the best management of this patient with bilateral solid kidney masses. The new-onset hematuria and kidney masses in the context of advanced CKD are highly suspicious for renal cell carcinoma.

### KEY POINT

- Patients with end-stage kidney disease have a mark-edly increased risk for renal cell carcinoma, and a high level of suspicion is warranted in patients with symptoms such as new-onset gross hematuria or unexplained flank pain.

### Bibliography
Hu SL, Chang A, Perazella MA, Okusa MD, Jaimes EA, Weiss RH; American Society of Nephrology Onco-Nephrology Forum. The nephrologist's tumor: basic biology and management of renal cell carcinoma. J Am Soc Nephrol. 2016;27:2227-37. [PMID: 26961346]

### Item 107      Answer:   B

**Educational Objective:** Provide appropriate blood pres-sure screening for a patient at increased risk for cardiovas-cular disease.

Annual blood pressure screening is the most appropriate man-agement. This patient is healthy, physically active, not over-weight, and does not meet criteria for hypertension based on these office blood pressure (BP) readings measured during one visit. However, he is at risk for future hypertension given his age (>40 years), black race, and a positive family history of hypertension. In addition, according to the American College of Cardiology/American Heart Association (ACC/AHA) guide-line, the patient has elevated BP, defined as systolic BP between 120-129 mm Hg and diastolic BP <80 mm Hg. Although no interventions are needed during this visit, the patient does need to be screened for high BP at least annually or more frequently. The U.S. Preventive Services Task Force (USPSTF) recommendations have not been updated since the release of the ACC/AHA guideline, with borderline and normal BP defined by older guidelines; however, the USPSTF recommends screening for hypertension in adults ≥18 years of age to identify those at increased risk for cardiovascular disease from hypertension and to begin early interventions to decrease this risk. Adults aged 18 to 39 years with normal BP and without cardiovascular risk factors should be rescreened every 3 to 5 years. Those who are ≥40 years of age and persons at increased risk for hypertension should be screened annually.

Beginning antihypertensive therapy with medications such as amlodipine or hydrochlorothiazide is inappropriate for this patient who does not meet the criteria for hypertension (defined by the ACC/AHA as a systolic BP ≥130 mm Hg and/or a diastolic BP ≥80 mm Hg). According to this guideline, patients with clinical cardiovascular disease and an average systolic BP ≥130 mm Hg or an average diastolic BP ≥80 mm Hg should be treated with lifestyle changes and medications for secondary prevention of cardiovascular events. Adults without clinical cardiovascular disease but an estimated 10-year atherosclerotic cardiovascular disease risk ≥10% and an average systolic BP ≥130 mm Hg or an average diastolic BP ≥80 mm Hg should also be treated with lifestyle interventions and pharmacologic therapy for primary prevention of cardiovascular disease.

**KEY POINT**

- Annual blood pressure screening is appropriate for patients who are ≥40 years of age and persons at increased risk for hypertension.

**Bibliography**
Siu AL; U.S. Preventive Services Task Force. Screening for high blood pressure in adults: U.S. Preventive Services Task Force recommendation statement. Ann Intern Med. 2015;163:778-86. [PMID: 26458123]

## Item 108      Answer:     A

**Educational Objective: Manage stage G5 chronic kidney disease in a patient who will imminently require renal replacement therapy.**

The most appropriate management for this patient with stage G5 chronic kidney disease (CKD) is to delay dialysis until she has uremic symptoms. She is not a candidate for transplant and has opted for hemodialysis for her renal replacement therapy (RRT). The decision of when to start RRT for CKD is complicated and requires frank discussion between providers and the patient and their families. For many years, consensus guidelines suggested that dialysis be initiated on the basis of estimated glomerular filtration rate (eGFR) cutoffs, ranging between 10 and 15 mL/min/1.73 m². In 2010, results were published from the IDEAL (Initiating Dialysis Early and Late) trial, which demonstrated no significant difference between the early dialysis group (eGFR, 10-15 mL/min/1.73 m²) and late dialysis group (eGFR, 5-7 mL/min/1.73 m²) in the frequency of adverse events (cardiovascular events, infections, or complications of dialysis). Although 76% of the late-start group ultimately initiated dialysis with eGFR >7.0 mL/min/1.73 m², the median delay in onset of dialysis was 5.6 months compared with the early start group. Thus, this study demonstrated that with careful clinical management, dialysis may be delayed until either the GFR drops below 7.0 mL/min/1.73 m² or more traditional clinical indicators (such as uremic symptoms or metabolic abnormalities) for the initiation of dialysis are present.

Discontinuation of diuretics is inappropriate because the patient does have some evidence of total body sodium and water overload (2+ edema) and thus needs continued diuretic therapy to avoid frank volume overload.

Referral for palliative care is not indicated because the patient is functioning well and is without signs of terminal illness or symptoms that require palliation; moreover, she has already chosen hemodialysis for future RRT. However, if her condition worsens over time, it is strongly encouraged to practice "kidney supportive care" or "patient-centered dialysis," in which treatment goals are closely aligned with patient preferences in a shared decision-making process.

**KEY POINT**

- There is no benefit in starting renal replacement therapy (RRT) in asymptomatic patients or at an arbitrary estimated glomerular filtration rate cutoff compared with careful clinical management and initiating RRT for symptoms or metabolic abnormalities that are refractory to medical treatment.

**Bibliography**
Cooper BA, Branley P, Bulfone L, Collins JF, Craig JC, Fraenkel MB, et al; IDEAL Study. A randomized, controlled trial of early versus late initiation of dialysis. N Engl J Med. 2010;363:609-19. [PMID: 20581422]

# Index

**A**

## NAME AND ADDRESS (Please complete.)

_____
Last Name                First Name           Middle Initial

_____
Address

_____
Address cont.

_____
City                     State                ZIP Code

_____
Country

_____
Email address

**B**

### Order Number

(Use the 10-digit Order Number on your
MKSAP materials packing slip.)

| | | | | | | | | | |
|---|---|---|---|---|---|---|---|---|---|

**C**

### ACP ID Number

(Refer to packing slip in your MKSAP materials
for your 8-digit ACP ID Number.)

| | | | | | | | | | |
|---|---|---|---|---|---|---|---|---|---|

**ACP®**
American College of Physicians
Leading Internal Medicine, Improving Lives

**Medical Knowledge Self-Assessment Program® 18**

### TO EARN *CME Credits and/or MOC Points* YOU MUST:

1. Answer all questions.
2. Score a minimum of 50% correct.

========================================

### TO EARN *FREE* INSTANTANEOUS *CME Credits and/or MOC Points* ONLINE:

1. Answer all of your questions.
2. Go to **mksap.acponline.org** and enter your ACP Online username and password to access an online answer sheet.
3. Enter your answers.
4. You can also enter your answers directly at **mksap.acponline.org** without first using this answer sheet.

### To Submit Your Answer Sheet by Mail or FAX for a $20 Administrative Fee per Answer Sheet:

1. Answer all of your questions and calculate your score.
2. Complete boxes A-H.
3. Complete payment information.
4. Send the answer sheet and payment information to ACP, using the FAX number/address listed below.

**D**

### Required Submission Information if Applying for MOC

Birth Month and Day    [ ][ ] [ ][ ]
                        M M  D D

ABIM Candidate Number  [ ][ ][ ][ ][ ][ ]

---

### COMPLETE FORM BELOW ONLY IF YOU SUBMIT BY MAIL OR FAX

Last Name                                    First Name                              MI

| | | | | | | | | | | | | | | | | | | | | | | | | | | | | | | |
|---|---|---|---|---|---|---|---|---|---|---|---|---|---|---|---|---|---|---|---|---|---|---|---|---|---|---|---|---|---|---|---|

### Payment Information. Must remit in US funds, drawn on a US bank.
### The processing fee for each paper answer sheet is $20.

☐ Check, made payable to ACP, enclosed

Charge to    ☐ **VISA**    ☐ **MasterCard**    ☐ **AMERICAN EXPRESS**    ☐ **DISCOVER**

Card Number _____

Expiration Date _____ / _____     Security code (3 or 4 digit #s) _____
                 MM          YY

Signature _____

**Fax to:** 215-351-2799

**Mail to:**
Member and Customer Service
American College of Physicians
190 N. Independence Mall West
Philadelphia, PA 19106–1572

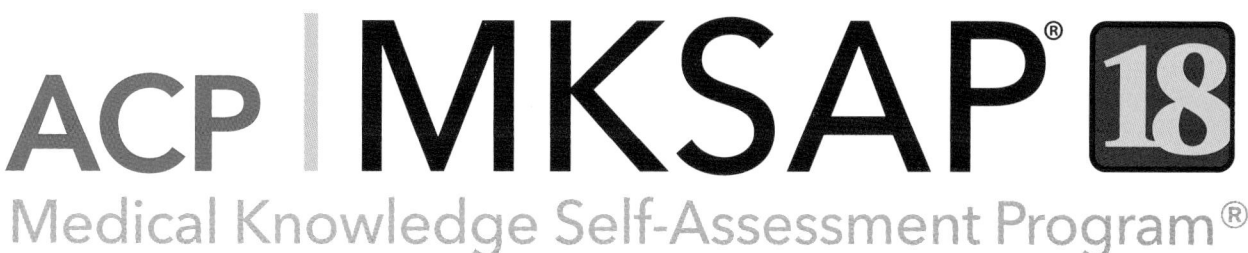

# General Internal Medicine

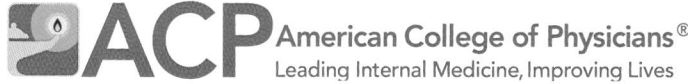
American College of Physicians®
Leading Internal Medicine, Improving Lives

# Welcome to the General Internal Medicine Section of MKSAP 18!

In these pages, you will find updated information on routine care of the healthy patient; patient safety and quality improvement; professionalism and ethics; palliative medicine; common symptoms, including chronic pain, medically unexplained symptoms, dyspnea, cough, fatigue, dizziness, syncope, insomnia, and lower extremity edema; musculoskeletal pain; dyslipidemia; obesity; men's and women's health; eye disorders; ear, nose, mouth, and throat disorders; mental and behavioral health; geriatric medicine; perioperative medicine; and other clinical challenges. All of these topics are uniquely focused on the needs of generalists and subspecialists in internal medicine.

The core content of MKSAP 18 has been developed as in previous editions—all essential information that is newly researched and written in 11 topic areas of internal medicine—created by dozens of leading generalists and subspecialists and guided by certification and recertification requirements, emerging knowledge in the field, and user feedback. MKSAP 18 also contains 1200 all-new peer-reviewed, psychometrically validated, multiple-choice questions (MCQs) for self-assessment and study, including 168 in General Internal Medicine. MKSAP 18 continues to include *High Value Care* (HVC) recommendations, based on the concept of balancing clinical benefit with costs and harms, with associated MCQs illustrating these principles and HVC Key Points called out in the text. Internists practicing in the hospital setting can easily find comprehensive *Hospitalist*-focused content and MCQs, specially designated in blue and with the 🄷 symbol.

If you purchased MKSAP 18 Complete, you also have access to MKSAP 18 Digital, with additional tools allowing you to customize your learning experience. MKSAP Digital includes regular text updates with new, practice-changing information, 200 new self-assessment questions, and enhanced custom-quiz options. MKSAP Complete also includes more than 1200 electronic, adaptive learning–enhanced flashcards for quick review of important concepts, as well as an updated and enhanced version of Virtual Dx, MKSAP's image-based self-assessment tool. As before, MKSAP 18 Digital is optimized for use on your mobile devices, with iOS- and Android-based apps allowing you to sync between your apps and online account and submit for CME credits and MOC points online.

Please visit us at the MKSAP Resource Site (mksap.acponline.org) to find out how we can help you study, earn CME credit and MOC points, and stay up to date.

On behalf of the many internists who have offered their time and expertise to create the content for MKSAP 18 and the editorial staff who work to bring this material to you in the best possible way, we are honored that you have chosen to use MKSAP 18 and appreciate any feedback about the program you may have. Please feel free to send any comments to mksap_editors@acponline.org.

Sincerely,

Patrick C. Alguire, MD, FACP
Editor-in-Chief
Senior Vice President Emeritus
Medical Education Division
American College of Physicians

# General Internal Medicine

## Committee

**Paul S. Mueller, MD, MPH, FACP, Section Editor[2]**
Consultant, Division of General Internal Medicine
Professor of Medicine and Professor of Biomedical Ethics
Mayo Clinic College of Medicine and Science
Rochester, Minnesota

**Karthik Ghosh, MD, MS, FACP[1]**
Director, Breast Clinic
Consultant, Division of General Internal Medicine
Professor of Medicine
Mayo Clinic College of Medicine and Science
Rochester, Minnesota

**Scott Herrle, MD, MS, FACP[1]**
Assistant Professor of Medicine
University of Pittsburgh School of Medicine
Pittsburgh, Pennsylvania

**Arya B. Mohabbat, MD, FACP[2]**
Consultant, Division of General Internal Medicine
Assistant Professor of Medicine
Mayo Clinic College of Medicine and Science
Rochester, Minnesota

**Kurt Pfeifer, MD, FACP[1]**
Professor of Medicine
Division of General Internal Medicine
Medical College of Wisconsin
Milwaukee, Wisconsin

**Mary Beth Poston, MD, FACP[1]**
Associate Professor
Internal Medicine Residency Program Director
Palmetto Health
University of South Carolina
Columbia, South Carolina

**Julie Rosenbaum, MD, FACP[2]**
Associate Professor of Medicine
Yale University School of Medicine
New Haven, Connecticut

**Jacob J. Strand, MD, FACP[1]**
Consultant, Division of General Internal Medicine
Chair, Center for Palliative Medicine
Assistant Professor of Medicine
Mayo Clinic College of Medicine and Science
Rochester, Minnesota

**Karna K. Sundsted, MD, FACP[1]**
Consultant, Division of General Internal Medicine
Assistant Professor of Medicine
Mayo Clinic College of Medicine and Science
Rochester, Minnesota

**Amy Tu Wang, MD, FACP[1]**
Assistant Professor of Medicine
David Geffen School of Medicine at UCLA
Director, Employee Health Services
Associate Director, Internal Medicine Residency Program
Harbor-UCLA Medical Center
Torrance, California

## Editor-in-Chief

**Patrick C. Alguire, MD, FACP[2]**
Senior Vice President Emeritus, Medical Education
American College of Physicians
Philadelphia, Pennsylvania

## Deputy Editor

**Robert L. Trowbridge, Jr., MD, FACP[2]**
Associate Professor of Medicine
Tufts University School of Medicine
Maine Medical Center
Portland, Maine

## General Internal Medicine Reviewers

Laura Greci Cooke, MD, FACP[1]
Preetivi Ellis, MD, FACP[1]
Major Frederick L. Flynt, MD, MC USAF, FACP[1]
Jason Higdon, MD, FACP[1]
Susan Hingle, MD, FACP[1]
Nadia Irshad, MD[2]
Michael LoCurcio, MD, FACP[1]
Ryan D. Mire, MD, FACP[1]
Anne Newland, MD, MPH, FACP[1]
Samuel C. Pan, MD[1]
Bonnie E. Gould Rothberg, MD, PhD, MPH[2]
Harlan L. South, MD, FACP[1]
Carola A. Tanna, MD[2]

## Hospital Medicine General Internal Medicine Reviewers

## General Internal Medicine ACP Editorial Staff

## ACP Principal Staff

---

## Acknowledgments

The American College of Physicians (ACP) gratefully acknowledges the special contributions to the development and production of the 18th edition of the Medical Knowledge Self-Assessment Program® (MKSAP® 18) made by the following people:

*Graphic Design:* Barry Moshinski (Director, Graphic Services), Michael Ripca (Graphics Technical Administrator), and Jennifer Gropper (Graphic Designer).

*Production/Systems:* Dan Hoffmann (Director, Information Technology), Scott Hurd (Manager, Content Systems), Neil Kohl (Senior Architect), and Chris Patterson (Senior Architect).

*MKSAP 18 Digital:* Under the direction of Steven Spadt (Senior Vice President, Technology), the digital version of MKSAP 18 was developed within the ACP's Digital Products and Services Department, led by Brian Sweigard (Director, Digital Products and Services). Other members of the team included Dan Barron (Senior Web Application Developer/ Architect), Chris Forrest (Senior Software Developer/Design Lead), Kathleen Hoover (Senior Web Developer), Kara Regis (Manager, User Interface Design and Development), Brad Lord (Senior Web Application Developer), and John McKnight (Senior Web Developer).

The College also wishes to acknowledge that many other persons, too numerous to mention, have contributed to the production of this program. Without their dedicated efforts, this program would not have been possible.

## MKSAP Resource Site (mksap.acponline.org)

The MKSAP Resource Site (mksap.acponline.org) is a continually updated site that provides links to MKSAP 18 online answer sheets for print subscribers; access to MKSAP 18 Digital; Board Basics® e-book access instructions; information on Continuing Medical Education (CME), Maintenance of Certification (MOC), and international Continuing Professional Development (CPD) and MOC; errata; and other new information.

## International MOC/CPD

For information and instructions on submission of international MOC/CPD, please go to the MKSAP Resource Site (mksap.acponline.org).

## Continuing Medical Education

The American College of Physicians is accredited by the Accreditation Council for Continuing Medical Education (ACCME) to provide continuing medical education for physicians.

The American College of Physicians designates this enduring material, MKSAP 18, for a maximum of 275 *AMA PRA Category 1 Credits*™. Physicians should claim only the credit commensurate with the extent of their participation in the activity.

Up to 36 *AMA PRA Category 1 Credits*™ are available from December 31, 2018, to December 31, 2021, for the MKSAP 18 General Internal Medicine section.

## Learning Objectives

The learning objectives of MKSAP 18 are to:

- Close gaps between actual care in your practice and preferred standards of care, based on best evidence
- Diagnose disease states that are less common and sometimes overlooked and confusing
- Improve management of comorbid conditions that can complicate patient care
- Determine when to refer patients for surgery or care by subspecialists
- Pass the ABIM Certification Examination
- Pass the ABIM Maintenance of Certification Examination

## Target Audience

- General internists and primary care physicians
- Subspecialists who need to remain up to date in internal medicine
- Residents preparing for the certifying examination in internal medicine
- Physicians preparing for maintenance of certification in internal medicine (recertification)

## ABIM Maintenance of Certification

Check the MKSAP Resource Site (mksap.acponline.org) for the latest information on how MKSAP tests can be used to apply to the American Board of Internal Medicine (ABIM) for Maintenance of Certification (MOC) points following completion of the CME activity.

Successful completion of the CME activity, which includes participation in the evaluation component, enables the participant to earn up to 275 medical knowledge MOC points and patient safety MOC credits in the ABIM's MOC program. It is the CME activity provider's responsibility to submit participant completion information to ACCME for the purpose of granting MOC credit.

## Earn Instantaneous CME Credits or MOC Points Online

Print subscribers can enter their answers online to earn instantaneous CME credits or MOC points. You can submit your answers using online answer sheets that are provided at mksap.acponline.org, where a record of your MKSAP 18 credits will be available. To earn CME credits or to apply for MOC points, you need to answer all of the questions in a test and earn a score of at least 50% correct (number of correct answers divided by the total number of questions). Please note that if you are applying for MOC points, you must also enter your birth date and ABIM candidate number.

Take either of the following approaches:

1. Use the printed answer sheet at the back of this book to record your answers. Go to mksap.acponline.org, access the appropriate online answer sheet, transcribe your answers, and submit your test for instantaneous CME credits or MOC points. There is no additional fee for this service.

2. Go to mksap.acponline.org, access the appropriate online answer sheet, directly enter your answers, and submit your test for instantaneous CME credits or MOC points. There is no additional fee for this service.

## Earn CME Credits or MOC Points by Mail or Fax

Pay a $20 processing fee per answer sheet and submit the printed answer sheet at the back of this book by mail or fax, as instructed on the answer sheet. Make sure you calculate your score and enter your birth date and ABIM candidate number, and fax the answer sheet to 215-351-2799 or mail the answer sheet to Member and Customer Service, American College of Physicians, 190 N. Independence Mall West, Philadelphia, PA 19106-1572, using the courtesy envelope provided in your MKSAP 18 slipcase. You will need your 10-digit order number and 8-digit ACP ID number, which are printed on your packing slip. Please allow 4 to 6 weeks for your score report to be emailed back to you. Be sure to include your email address for a response.

If you do not have a 10-digit order number and 8-digit ACP ID number, or if you need help creating a username and password to access the MKSAP 18 online answer sheets, go to mksap.acponline.org or email custserv@acponline.org.

## Disclosure Policy

It is the policy of the American College of Physicians (ACP) to ensure balance, independence, objectivity, and scientific rigor in all of its educational activities. To this end, and consistent with the policies of the ACP and the Accreditation Council for Continuing Medical Education (ACCME), contributors to all ACP continuing medical education activities are required to disclose all relevant financial relationships with any entity producing, marketing, reselling, or distributing health care goods or services consumed by, or used on, patients. Contributors are required to use generic names in the discussion of therapeutic options and are

required to identify any unapproved, off-label, or investigative use of commercial products or devices. Where a trade name is used, all available trade names for the same product type are also included. If trade-name products manufactured by companies with whom contributors have relationships are discussed, contributors are asked to provide evidence-based citations in support of the discussion. The information is reviewed by the committee responsible for producing this text. If necessary, adjustments to topics or contributors' roles in content development are made to balance the discussion. Further, all readers of this text are asked to evaluate the content for evidence of commercial bias and send any relevant comments to mksap_editors@acponline.org so that future decisions about content and contributors can be made in light of this information.

## Resolution of Conflicts

To resolve all conflicts of interest and influences of vested interests, ACP's content planners used best evidence and updated clinical care guidelines in developing content, when such evidence and guidelines were available. All content underwent review by peer reviewers not on the committee to ensure that the material was balanced and unbiased. Contributors' disclosure information can be found with the list of contributors' names and those of ACP principal staff listed in the beginning of this book.

## Hospital-Based Medicine

For the convenience of subscribers who provide care in hospital settings, content that is specific to the hospital setting has been highlighted in blue. Hospital icons (⊞) highlight where the hospital-only content begins, continues over more than one page, and ends.

## High Value Care Key Points

Key Points in the text that relate to High Value Care concepts (that is, concepts that discuss balancing clinical benefit with costs and harms) are designated by the HVC icon [HVC].

## Educational Disclaimer

The editors and publisher of MKSAP 18 recognize that the development of new material offers many opportunities for error. Despite our best efforts, some errors may persist in print. Drug dosage schedules are, we believe, accurate and in accordance with current standards. Readers are advised, however, to ensure that the recommended dosages in MKSAP 18 concur with the information provided in the product information material. This is especially important in cases of new, infrequently used, or highly toxic drugs. Application of the information in MKSAP 18 remains the professional responsibility of the practitioner.

The primary purpose of MKSAP 18 is educational. Information presented, as well as publications, technologies, products, and/or services discussed, is intended to inform subscribers about the knowledge, techniques, and experiences of the contributors. A diversity of professional opinion exists, and the views of the contributors are their own and not those of the ACP. Inclusion of any material in the program does not constitute endorsement or recommendation by the ACP. The ACP does not warrant the safety, reliability, accuracy, completeness, or usefulness of and disclaims any and all liability for damages and claims that may result from the use of information, publications, technologies, products, and/or services discussed in this program.

## Publisher's Information

## Disclaimer Regarding Direct Purchases from Online Retailers

CME and/or MOC for MKSAP 18 is available only if you purchase the program directly from ACP. CME credits and MOC points cannot be awarded to those purchasers who have purchased the program from non-authorized sellers such as Amazon, eBay, or any other such online retailer.

## Unauthorized Use of This Book Is Against the Law

MKSAP 18 ISBN: 978-1-938245-47-3
General Internal Medicine ISBN: 978-1-938245-55-8

Printed in the United States of America.

For order information in the U.S. or Canada call 800-ACP-1915. All other countries call 215-351-2600 (Monday to Friday, 9 AM – 5 PM ET). Fax inquiries to 215-351-2799 or email to custserv@acponline.org.

## Errata

Errata for MKSAP 18 will be available through the MKSAP Resource Site at mksap.acponline.org as new information becomes known to the editors.

# Table of Contents

# General Internal Medicine High Value Care Recommendations

The American College of Physicians, in collaboration with multiple other organizations, is engaged in a worldwide initiative to promote the practice of High Value Care (HVC). The goals of the HVC initiative are to improve health care outcomes by providing care of proven benefit and reducing costs by avoiding unnecessary and even harmful interventions. The initiative comprises several programs that integrate the important concept of health care value (balancing clinical benefit with costs and harms) for a given intervention into a broad range of educational materials to address the needs of trainees, practicing physicians, and patients.

HVC content has been integrated into MKSAP 18 in several important ways. MKSAP 18 includes HVC-identified key points in the text, HVC-focused multiple choice questions, and, for subscribers to MKSAP Digital, an HVC custom quiz. From the text and questions, we have generated the following list of HVC recommendations that meet the definition below of high value care and bring us closer to our goal of improving patient outcomes while conserving finite resources.

**High Value Care Recommendation**: A recommendation to choose diagnostic and management strategies for patients in specific clinical situations that balance clinical benefit with cost and harms with the goal of improving patient outcomes.

Below are the High Value Care Recommendations for the General Internal Medicine section of MKSAP 18.

- High breast density alone does not necessitate adjunctive breast imaging other than routine screening mammography (see Item 154).
- Direct-to-consumer genomic testing contributes very little to overall disease risk.
- The U.S. Preventive Services Task Force does not recommend multivitamins or herbal supplements for the prevention of cardiovascular disease or cancer.
- Enteral or parenteral artificial nutritional support at the end of life does not improve survival, is invasive, and can cause side effects.
- No evidence supports the use of long-term opioid therapy in patients with chronic noncancer pain; long-term opioid use is associated with poorer overall functional status, worse quality of life, and worse pain.
- In patients with medically unexplained symptoms, clinicians should limit diagnostic tests to those deemed medically necessary.

- In patients with acute cough, chest radiography is not indicated in the absence of abnormal vital signs or abnormal lung examination findings.
- Treatment of acute cough is primarily symptomatic; antibiotics are not recommended without a clear bacterial cause.
- Routine imaging is not recommended for benign paroxysmal positional vertigo.
- In patients with central vertigo, MRI is more sensitive than CT in detecting ischemic stroke, whereas CT provides an expedited, cost-effective assessment for hemorrhagic stroke.
- The American College of Physicians recommends against routinely performing brain imaging in cases of syncope that do not involve objective focal neurologic findings.
- Diagnostic testing, such as polysomnography, is usually unnecessary in the evaluation of insomnia.
- Pharmacologic therapies for insomnia are associated with adverse effects and should only be initiated in patients with insomnia refractory to nonpharmacologic interventions.
- Most patients with nonspecific low back pain do not require imaging or other diagnostic testing.
- Most patients with neck pain do not require imaging studies.
- Most patients with rotator cuff disease do not require imaging studies.
- In patients with asymptomatic popliteal (Baker) cysts, no treatment is necessary.
- In patients in whom statin therapy is being considered, an alanine aminotransferase level should be obtained at baseline to evaluate for liver dysfunction; further hepatic monitoring is unnecessary if the baseline level is normal (see Item 148).
- There is little evidence that over-the-counter weight loss supplements are effective.
- Treatment is not indicated in patients with low testosterone levels only; it should be reserved for patients with a low testosterone level associated with symptoms.
- Routine laboratory testing for the diagnosis of menopause is not recommended.
- Medications have not been shown to be of benefit in the management of tinnitus.
- Acute rhinosinusitis is usually caused by viruses, allergies, or irritants, and avoidance of unnecessary antibiotics represents high value care.
- Patients with pharyngitis who present with fewer than three of the four Centor criteria do not need to be tested or treated for group A *Streptococcus* infection.

- In tobacco cessation, combining behavioral counseling with pharmacotherapy is more effective than either modality alone, and combining more than one type of nicotine replacement therapy (short- and long-acting) is more effective than monotherapy.
- Cognitive impairment is best measured with assessment examinations, such as the Mini-Cog and the Mini–Mental State Examination, rather than laboratory testing or imaging (see Item 48).
- No pharmacologic therapies are recommended for the treatment of stress urinary incontinence or functional incontinence.
- Hydrocolloid or foam dressings are superior to standard gauze dressings in the treatment of pressure injuries (see Item 118).
- Preoperative laboratory testing should be performed based on the patient's medical conditions, physical examination findings, and preoperative symptoms; routine laboratory panels expose patients to unnecessary testing and are not recommended.
- Patients with low cardiovascular risk (<1% risk for a perioperative major adverse cardiac event) may proceed to surgery without preoperative cardiac stress testing.
- Preoperative cardiac stress testing should generally be reserved for patients at elevated risk for a major adverse cardiac event with a functional capacity less than 4 metabolic equivalents, but only if the results of the test will change perioperative management (see Item 34).
- Routine electrocardiography is not indicated in asymptomatic patients undergoing low-risk surgical procedures.
- In patients with coronary artery disease, routine coronary angiography or revascularization should not be performed exclusively to reduce perioperative cardiovascular events.
- Preoperative chest radiography is indicated only in patients with signs or symptoms of pulmonary disease and in patients with underlying cardiac or pulmonary disease and new or unstable symptoms.
- Spirometry should not be routinely performed preoperatively except in patients undergoing lung resection.
- Asymptomatic carotid bruit is not predictive of perioperative stroke and requires no preoperative evaluation.
- Pregnant patients should undergo the same preoperative medical evaluation as nonpregnant patients; additional diagnostic testing is unnecessary.

# General Internal Medicine

## High Value Care in Internal Medicine

Although the United States spends more on health care than all other developed nations, it has higher rates of medical care–related mortality and shorter life expectancy. Compared with other high-income countries, patients in the United States pay more for prescription drugs, undergo more diagnostic tests, and pay the highest hospital and physician prices for procedures. In response to this unsustainable spending, health policy organizations and other expert groups advocate implementing a high value approach to patient care.

High value care is individualized care that delivers proven benefits while minimizing risks and unnecessary costs. It requires a careful evaluation to determine whether the benefits of a diagnostic test or intervention justify the harms and costs. Importantly, when determining value, clinicians should consider the benefits of a test or intervention before the cost. Focusing primarily on cost increases the tendency to avoid an expensive test or intervention regardless of outcome or to continue a low-cost intervention that provides no benefit. Notably, some costly or risky tests and interventions, such as screening colonoscopy, are high value because their benefits may be substantial. Similarly, some inexpensive and low-risk tests and interventions, such as routine daily laboratory testing in hospitalized patients, represent low value care. Examples of high value and low value care are provided in **Table 1**.

Shared decision making is essential to high value care, particularly because perceived patient demand is one driver of inappropriate testing and interventions. Including patients in the decision-making process provides opportunities to educate patients on balancing benefits with potential harms and costs and to incorporate their values and preferences into the care process.

Resources to help clinicians determine the value of common tests and interventions are available from the American College of Physicians (https://www.acponline.org/clinical-information/high-value-care), Alliance for Academic Internal Medicine, and Society of Hospital Medicine. In addition, the Choosing Wisely campaign, an initiative of the American Board of Internal Medicine Foundation with medical specialty societies, has published specialty-specific lists of commonly used tests or procedures whose necessity should be questioned and discussed by clinicians and patients (www.choosingwisely.org). *Consumer Reports* works with many of the Choosing Wisely partners to develop patient-friendly materials from the lists of recommendations and to disseminate them to consumers through a network of Choosing Wisely consumer partners.

**TABLE 1.** Examples of High Value and Low Value Care Interventions

| Intervention | Cost | Benefit |
|---|---|---|
| **High Value Care** | | |
| High-sensitivity D-dimer testing to exclude venous thromboembolism in patients with low likelihood of disease | Low | High negative predictive value |
| Influenza vaccination | Low | High benefit for reducing disease burden and complications |
| **Low Value Care** | | |
| Antibiotic therapy in patients with upper respiratory tract infection | Low | No benefit for reducing duration or severity of illness |
| Carotid ultrasonography in patients with syncope | Intermediate | Low diagnostic value |
| Imaging studies in patients with low back pain in the absence of "red flag" findings (fever, involuntary weight loss, incontinence) | Intermediate | Low diagnostic value |

**KEY POINT**

- High value care is individualized care that delivers proven benefits while minimizing risks and unnecessary costs.

**HVC**

## Interpretation of the Medical Literature

### Introduction

The science of medicine is constantly evolving, and peer-reviewed literature is the primary means of disseminating new medical knowledge. The application of this information to patient-centered medical decision making requires an understanding of different study designs and how to interpret statistical tests for significance. Although research in the basic sciences (including pharmacology and physiology) provides the basis for many clinical advances, this chapter will review interpretation of the literature that may be immediately applicable to the clinical setting.

# Study Designs

Study designs can be divided into two broad categories: experimental studies and observational studies. The selection of a study design is guided by the suitability of the design to address the clinical question and the population being studied.

The validity, or trustworthiness, of a study's results may be limited by bias and/or confounders (see Validity of a Study).

## Experimental Study Designs

Experimental studies systematically expose some or all of the individuals in the study to a potential causative or protective factor (the exposure, often a treatment) (**Table 2**). Exposed and unexposed participants are compared with respect to developing the outcome of interest. As an example, an experimental study might compare patients with diabetes mellitus treated with a statin to those treated with a placebo to determine whether patients receiving active treatment are more or less likely than untreated patients to experience cardiovascular events.

The process for allocating the exposure or treatment to the study participants affects the study strength and the validity of the findings. The strongest experimental design is the randomized controlled trial. By randomly allocating the treatment, confounders (both known and unknown) are randomly distributed in the treatment and control groups. The least rigorous experimental design is the quasi-experimental design, in which participants are not randomly assigned. One example of a quasi-experimental design is a pre-post trial, in which

| TABLE 2. Experimental Study Designs | | | | |
|---|---|---|---|---|
| **Study Design** | **Description** | **Best Uses** | **Common Limitations to Use/Validity** | **Common Measure of Association** |
| Quasi-experimental study | All participants receive treatment of interest<br><br>Example: phase I drug trial | Establishing treatment effect, defining risks of adverse events | Difficult to clearly establish that treatment caused outcome<br><br>Risk for confounding, especially for factors not known | Before-and-after comparison of outcome of interest |
| Non-randomized controlled trial | Treatment is allocated in a prespecified manner but not using randomization; comparison is made between different treatment groups or between treatment and control groups<br><br>Example: study of surgical and nonsurgical treatment options in which enrolled participants are assigned to the treatment type they prefer to receive | When patients/participants may not be amenable to being randomly assigned to a treatment or when randomization is not ethically permitted | Risk for confounding, especially for factors not known<br><br>Risk for selection bias if patients are allowed choice in treatment allocated | Difference between treatment groups in outcome of interest<br><br>Measure reported varies depending on outcome of interest and statistical technique |
| Cluster randomized trial | Participants are randomly assigned as a unit instead of individually<br><br>Example: study of effect of diabetic education on average hemoglobin $A_{1c}$ value, in which participants are community primary care practices | Treatments for which randomization of individual patients is not feasible or ethical<br><br>When effect at a level larger than an individual level (i.e., institution or health system) is being studied | Complicated statistical analysis<br><br>May be difficult to ensure groups being compared are similar (risk for confounding) | Difference between treatment groups in outcome of interest<br><br>Measure reported varies depending on outcome of interest and statistical technique |
| Randomized controlled trial | Participants are randomly assigned to one of the treatment options (including control/placebo group) | Considered to be highest level of evidence for treatment studies<br><br>Confounding is minimized if study is large enough | Generalizability is limited to the population included in the trial<br><br>Expensive and resource intensive to conduct | Difference between treatment groups in outcome of interest<br><br>Measure reported varies depending on outcome of interest and statistical technique |

all participants receive the studied treatment and results are obtained by comparing measurements taken before and after the outcome; thus, participants serve as their own internal controls. Because there is no external control group, the ability of the quasi-experimental design to determine cause and effect is limited.

## Observational Study Designs

In observational studies, no treatment is imposed on the persons being studied. Instead, researchers observe naturally occurring events in individuals who have or have not been exposed to a risk factor or treatment. The relationships between risk factors and disease may be explored, but the ability to assess for causality is limited.

Common observational study designs include ecologic, cross-sectional, case-control, and cohort studies. Case reports or case series, which describe an individual case or a series of related cases, are not true studies but have the potential to identify new or unique relationships to be further studied.

Ecologic studies evaluate the prevalence or extent of an exposure across distinct populations. They are hypothesis generating and are used to identify compelling trends for an exposure of interest across different groups, which can be investigated subsequently in more focused studies. Ecologic studies cannot be used to determine causation. Incorrect assignment of causation based on ecologic study results is termed the ecologic fallacy.

Cross-sectional studies evaluate the relationship between exposures and health outcomes in a population of interest. These studies are characterized by the measurement of factors and outcomes at a single point in time. Because cross-sectional studies lack comparison groups and the temporal sequence is often unknown, these studies are best used to determine disease prevalence and generate hypotheses; they can also assess the relatedness between two exposures of interest. Surveys conducted by health services groups may serve as the basis for these studies. Examples include the National Health and Nutrition Examination Survey and the Behavioral Risk Factor Surveillance Survey, both conducted by the Centers for Disease Control and Prevention.

Case-control studies compare past exposures in patients with and without disease. The events being studied have already occurred; therefore, there is potential for recall bias, which arises when patients with the disease of interest are more likely to recall past exposures compared with controls. However, for the study of rare diseases, case-control studies may be the best way to collect enough data to determine meaningful relationships.

Cohort studies divide participants into groups based on the presence or absence of a critical exposure and evaluate for differences between the groups in the development of a disease or outcome. Cohort studies may enroll participants before the outcome develops and follow patients forward in time (prospective cohorts), or they may enroll participants after an event has occurred (retrospective cohorts). Cohort

studies are ideal for studying diseases or outcomes that develop over time, evaluating the effect of rare potential causative factors, and performing time-to-event (survival) analyses; however, these studies are subject to losses to follow-up. Similar to case-control studies, retrospective cohorts may also be subject to recall bias.

## Systematic Reviews and Meta-Analysis

Narrative review articles, a common source of information for clinicians, present an expert assessment of the known evidence on a certain topic. Although narrative reviews are valuable learning resources, the body of evidence they contain varies and is influenced by the experiences of the authors. In contrast, systematic reviews involve a systematic search of the literature using predefined criteria to collect all published and unpublished studies that address the topic. This systematic approach minimizes selection bias and increases the strength of the information presented. Systematic reviews that combine the results of the studies included in a statistical analysis are termed meta-analyses.

The value of meta-analysis often resides in the ability to pool data and increase sample size and statistical power, as the ability to detect a difference between two groups depends on the number of persons being studied. A larger sample size has a greater power to discriminate smaller differences between groups; however, larger studies carry a higher cost and are logistically more complicated to administer. Meta-analysis of high-quality randomized controlled trials is considered to be one of the highest levels of clinical evidence. Factors that limit the ability to combine study results meaningfully include differences in the study populations, research measures, and statistical techniques.

### KEY POINTS

- Experimental studies systematically expose some or all of the individuals in the study to a potential causative or protective factor; the strongest experimental design is the randomized controlled trial. **HVC**
- Cross-sectional studies lack comparison groups, and the temporal sequence is often unknown; therefore, these studies are best used in determining disease prevalence and generating hypotheses. **HVC**
- Case-control studies compare past exposures in patients with and without disease; these studies are advantageous for the study of rare diseases. **HVC**
- Cohort studies are ideal for studying diseases or outcomes that develop over time, evaluating the effect of rare potential causative factors, and performing time-to-event (survival) analyses. **HVC**

# Validity of a Study

Validity refers to the fidelity of the study results to what is correct or true. Validity can be further characterized as internal or external. Internal validity refers to how well study error is minimized and to what degree the results are true. External validity is the extent to which the study results can be applied to settings other than the study setting; it represents the generalizability of the study results. Threats to the validity of a study include systematic error and random error.

Systematic error is the influence of confounders and bias on the results of a study. Confounders, factors other than the variables being studied that are associated with the studied population and may affect the end point being assessed, are a common threat to validity. An observational study, for example, may show that patients receiving statin therapy have an increased risk for cardiovascular events compared with those not taking statin therapy. However, the presence of a powerful confounder, specifically that patients receiving statin therapy are at high risk for cardiovascular events, influences the outcome of the study. The impact of confounding can be reduced by design strategies, such as matching, and evaluation techniques, including stratification of the analysis and regression techniques (or regression adjustment).

Bias refers to the presence of factors that skew the study results in a specific direction. Bias can be introduced at any point in a study design, including patient recruitment and outcome measurement. Careful study design can decrease the likelihood of bias; however, once bias has been introduced into the study, it cannot be eliminated or minimized.

Random error is error that is introduced by random variability or purely by chance. The role of chance is expressed by the $P$ value or confidence interval and is determined by statistical analysis. The likelihood of random error can be decreased by increasing study size and using precise measurement strategies.

# Statistical Analysis

Statistical significance is reported using $P$ values or confidence intervals, which express the probability that chance alone accounts for the result. A $P$ value less than or equal to 0.05 ($\leq$5% probability that chance alone accounts for the result) is often considered as indicating a statistically significant finding. However, this determination is arbitrary, and some researchers may opt for a different level (typically more stringent).

Confidence intervals express the range of values within which the true result falls; the 95% confidence interval means that there is 95% confidence that the true value is within the confidence interval range. Narrower ranges imply greater confidence, or certainty, that the reported value is closer to the true value.

## Sensitivity, Specificity, and Predictive Values

Sensitivity and specificity reflect the accuracy of a diagnostic or screening test (**Table 3**). Sensitivity is the ability of the test to detect those who truly have a disease or condition, or the probability that the test result will be positive in a patient with the disease. Specificity is the ability of the test to correctly

identify those without the disease, or the probability that the test result will be negative in a patient without the disease. Therefore, sensitive tests are those with minimal rates of false-negative results, and specific tests are those with minimal rates of false-positive results.

Positive and negative predictive values reflect the validity of a positive or negative test result for predicting the presence or absence of disease in a specific population. The positive predictive value is the proportion of those with a positive test result who truly have the disease. The negative predictive value is the proportion of those with a negative test result who are truly free of the disease. Predictive values are determined not only by sensitivity and specificity but also by the prevalence of the disease in the population.

## Likelihood Ratios

Likelihood ratios (LRs) are used to translate the impact of sensitivity and specificity of a specific clinical finding on the probability of a disease or outcome in a given patient; they provide a measure of the strength of association between the clinical finding and the specific disease. Each clinical finding, inclusive of symptoms, physical findings, and laboratory and imaging results, has a positive and negative LR for a specific disease. The positive LR is used when the test result is positive, and the negative LR is used when the test result is negative.

LRs are used in conjunction with the pretest probability of disease (the probability of disease in the patient before the test result is considered). The interaction of the pretest probability and LR results in a posttest probability of disease. The posttest probability may then serve as the rationale for treating a patient for the disease in question (if the positive test resulted in a high posttest probability) or ruling out a diagnosis (if the negative test resulted in a very low posttest probability). Mathematically, the pretest probability (a percentage) is converted to pretest odds (a ratio), the odds are multiplied by the appropriate LR, and the posttest odds are converted to a posttest probability.

For ease of clinical use, several general LR rules apply. Positive LR values of 2, 5, and 10 correspond to an increase in disease probability by 15%, 30%, and 45%, respectively; negative LR values of 0.5, 0.2, and 0.1 correspond to a decrease in disease probability by 15%, 30%, and 45%, respectively. Larger positive LRs and smaller negative LRs are more apt to affect clinical decisions.

Clinical calculators that provide a quick means for calculating LRs and their effect on probability of disease, such as one from the Centre for Evidence-Based Medicine (https://www.cebm.net/2014/06/catmaker-ebm-calculators/), are widely available. Alternatively, nomograms may be used to extrapolate the posttest probability of disease from the pretest probability of disease based on the LR (**Figure 1**).

## Absolute and Relative Risk Reduction

Absolute risk reduction and relative risk reduction are measures commonly used to report the efficacy of an intervention

**TABLE 3.** Common Terms Used in Interpretation of the Medical Literature for Diagnostic Tests

| Term | Definition | Calculation | Notes |
|------|-----------|-------------|-------|
| Prevalence (Prev) | Proportion of patients with the disease in the population | Prev = (TP + FN) / (TP + FP + FN + TN) | |
| Sensitivity (Sn) | Proportion of patients with the disease who have a positive test result | Sn = TP / (TP + FN) | |
| Specificity (Sp) | Proportion of patients without the disease who have a negative test result | Sp = TN / (FP + TN) | |
| Positive predictive value (PPV) | Proportion of patients with a positive test result who have the disease | PPV = TP / (TP + FP) | Increases with *increasing* prevalence |
| Negative predictive value (NPV) | Proportion of patients with a negative test result who do not have the disease | NPV = TN / (TN + FN) | Increases with *decreasing* prevalence |
| Positive likelihood ratio (LR+) | The ratio of the probability of a positive test result among patients with the disease to the probability of a positive result among patients without the disease | LR+ = Sn / (1 − Sp) | |
| Negative likelihood ratio (LR−) | The ratio of the probability of a negative test result among patients with the disease to the probability of a negative result in patients without the disease | LR− = (1 − Sn) / Sp | |
| Pretest odds | The odds that a patient has the disease before the test is performed | Pretest odds = pretest probability / (1 − pretest probability) | |
| Posttest odds | The odds that a patient has the disease after a test is performed | Posttest odds = pretest odds × LR | LR+ is used if result of test is positive; LR− is used if result of test is negative. A nomogram is available to calculate posttest probability using pretest probability and LR without having to convert pretest probability to odds (see Figure 1) |
| Pretest probability | Proportion of patients with the disease before a test is performed | Pretest probability can be estimated from population prevalence, clinical risk calculators, or clinical experience if no evidence-based tools exist | |
| Posttest probability | Proportion of patients with the disease after a test is performed | Posttest probability = posttest odds / (1 + posttest odds) | |

FN = false negative; FP = false positive; TN = true negative; TP = true positive.

(**Table 4**). Absolute risk reduction is the difference in the response to treatment between experimental and control groups. Absolute risk reduction is particularly relevant when the measure reported is the rate of development of a clinically meaningful end point, such as the incidence of cardiovascular events or death in studies of lipid-lowering therapy. Because these differences may seem small, investigators will often also report the relative risk or risk ratio (the ratio of the risk for the event in the experimental group to the risk for the event in the control group) as well as relative risk reduction, or (1 − risk ratio) × 100%.

The difference in the magnitude of these measures can be illustrated with a study of lipid-lowering therapy in which the rate of acute coronary syndromes in 5 years is 3.6% in the treated group and 4.8% in the control group. The absolute risk reduction is 1.2%. The risk ratio, however, is 75%, and the relative risk reduction is 25%. Therefore, although the absolute difference in rates between the two groups is small (1.2%), the

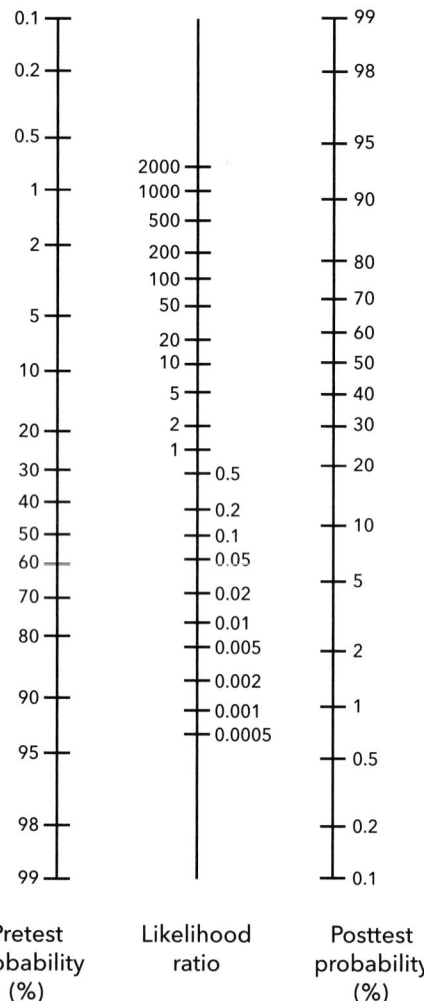

**FIGURE 1.** Nomogram for interpreting diagnostic test results. In this nomogram, a straight line drawn from a patient's pretest probability of disease (which is estimated from experience, local data, or published literature) through the likelihood ratio for the test result will indicate the posttest probability of disease.

Reproduced with permission from Fagan TJ. Letter: nomogram for Bayes theorem. N Engl J Med. 1975 Jul 31;293(5):257. [PMID: 1143310] Copyright 1975, Massachusetts Medical Society.

effect of a treatment may appear substantial when relative risk reduction (25%) is reported.

### Numbers Needed to Treat and Harm

The clinical impact of an intervention can be further assessed by using the number needed to treat (NNT) and the number needed to harm (NNH). The NNT is the inverse of the absolute risk reduction. It represents the number of patients who must receive a treatment to cause one additional patient to benefit, and it provides a quantifiable measure of the treatment effect that is easily understood by physicians and patients. The acceptability of the NNT depends on the risks associated with the condition, the cost and side effects of the treatment, and other treatments available.

The NNH can be similarly calculated for studies measuring adverse outcomes, but it also needs to be considered in the context of the benefits of the treatment and the severity of the harm incurred.

**KEY POINTS**

- Sensitivity is the ability of the test to detect those who truly have a disease or condition, whereas specificity is the ability of the test to correctly identify those without the disease.
- Likelihood ratios are used to translate the impact of sensitivity and specificity of a specific clinical finding on the probability of a disease or outcome in a given patient.
- Absolute risk reduction is the difference in the response to treatment between experimental and control groups.
- The number needed to treat is the inverse of the absolute risk reduction and represents the number of patients who must receive a treatment to cause one patient to benefit.

## Levels of Evidence

Levels of evidence describe the strength and quality of study results and can aid in clinical decision making. Systematic reviews, with or without meta-analysis, provide the highest level of evidence, followed by large, multicenter randomized, blinded, placebo-controlled trials. Large, meticulously controlled studies generally provide a higher level of evidence than smaller studies. Experimental studies provide a higher level of evidence than observational studies, and reports of expert opinion provide the lowest acceptable level of evidence. The U.S. Preventive Services Task Force and other organizations have developed grading systems to rank the relative rigor of clinical studies (**Table 5**). The grading system used by the U.S. Preventive Services Task Force for levels of benefit is provided in Routine Care of the Healthy Patient.

# Routine Care of the Healthy Patient

## History and Physical Examination

### Periodic Health Examination

The periodic health examination has played a central role in patient care for the past century, becoming an expectation for physicians and patients alike. Although evidence suggests periodic health examinations may improve surrogate outcomes, such as reduction in cardiovascular risk factors and increased receipt of preventive services, there is no evidence that they reduce mortality or other patient-important outcomes. A 2012 Cochrane systematic review confirmed that general health checks result in more diagnoses and medication prescriptions but do not reduce morbidity, hospitalizations, or mortality. The Danish Inter99 trial showed that screening for

**TABLE 4.** Common Terms Used in Interpretation of the Medical Literature for Therapeutics

| Term | Definition | Calculation | Notes |
|---|---|---|---|
| Absolute risk (AR) | The probability of an event occurring in a group during a specified time period | AR = patients with event in group / total patients in group | Also known as event rate; can be for benefits or harms. Often, an experimental event rate (EER) is compared with a control event rate (CER) |
| Relative risk (RR) | The ratio of the probability of developing a disease with a risk factor present to the probability of developing the disease without the risk factor present | RR = EER / CER | Used in cohort studies and randomized controlled trials |
| Absolute risk reduction (ARR) | The difference in rates of events between experimental group (EER) and control group (CER) | ARR = \| EER − CER \| | |
| Relative risk reduction (RRR) | The ratio of absolute risk reduction to the event rate among controls | RRR = \| EER − CER \| / CER | |
| Number needed to treat (NNT) | Number of patients needed to receive a treatment for one additional patient to benefit | NNT = 1 / ARR | A good estimate of the effect size |
| Number needed to harm (NNH) | Number of patients needed to receive a treatment for one additional patient to be harmed | NNH = 1 / ARI | ARI is the absolute risk increase and equals \| EER − CER \| when the event is an unfavorable outcome (e.g., drug side effect) |

**TABLE 5.** U.S. Preventive Services Task Force Hierarchy of Research Design

| Level | Description |
|---|---|
| I | Properly powered and conducted RCT; well-conducted systematic review or meta-analysis of homogeneous RCTs |
| II-1 | Well-designed controlled trial without randomization |
| II-2 | Well-designed cohort or case-control analytic study |
| II-3 | Multiple time series with or without the intervention; results from uncontrolled studies that yield results of large magnitude |
| III | Opinions of respected authorities, based on clinical experience; descriptive studies or case reports; reports of expert committees |

RCT = randomized controlled trial.

Reproduced from U.S. Preventive Services Task Force. Procedure Manual. https://www.uspreventiveservicestaskforce.org/Page/Name/procedure-manual. November 2017. Accessed June 27, 2018.

ischemic heart disease and repeated counseling over 5 years for those at high risk had no effect on risks for ischemic heart disease, stroke, or mortality after 10-year follow-up. Periodic health examinations also have a substantial financial impact, costing $5.2 billion annually without including costs of additional testing, visits, or missed work, according to a 2007 estimate. Overdiagnosis and overtreatment are other potential drawbacks to periodic health checks. Therefore, the Society of General Internal Medicine, through the Choosing Wisely campaign, specifically recommends against performing general health checks that include a comprehensive examination and laboratory testing for asymptomatic adults.

Despite this evidence, the periodic health examination may offer value that is difficult to measure in clinical trials. It provides dedicated time for screening and counseling and strengthens physician-patient relationships, which may improve adherence to physician recommendations. Notably, Medicare covers an initial preventive physical examination once in a lifetime within the first 12 months of a patient's enrollment in Medicare and an annual wellness visit thereafter. These visits are described as a focused physical and health review rather than a comprehensive head-to-toe physical examination.

## Routine History and Physical Examination

Obtaining a basic history is essential in establishing a clinician-patient relationship and understanding the patient's health history, concerns, and expectations (**Table 6**). Patients may be sensitive about sharing certain information, such as substance use and sexual practices, and open and nonjudgmental communication can encourage sharing. Clinicians should preface these inquiries by informing the patient that these questions are asked of everyone, the information is necessary to provide the best care, and responses are confidential.

A focused physical examination should always be performed to address the patient's concerns and relevant historical findings. Irrespective of gender presentation, physicians should provide care for the present anatomy in a

| TABLE 6. | Components of the History |
|---|---|

Past medical conditions and surgeries

   Hospitalizations

   Major childhood illnesses

   Allergies and corresponding reactions

Social history

   Alcohol use

   Tobacco use

   Illicit drug use

   Spirituality

Work and home situation

   Social support

   Safety

- Home safety: intimate partner violence and abuse, working smoke alarms, water heater set to ≤49 °C (120 °F), weapons safety
- Safety outside of the home: seatbelt use while driving, helmet use while motorcycling or bicycling, no electronic device use while driving

Diet

Physical activity

Family history

Medication history

   Prescription and over-the-counter medications

   Past and current hormone use for transgender patients

   Vitamins and supplements

   Herbal preparations and nontraditional therapies

Sexual history[a]

   Partners

- How many sex partners have you had in the past 2 months? 12 months?
- Have you had sex with men, women, or both?

   Practices

- What kind of sexual contact have you had? Vaginal (penis in vagina), anal (penis in rectum/anus), or oral sex (mouth on penis/vagina)?

   Protection/pregnancy

- Have you ever had a sexually transmitted infection?
- What do you do to protect yourself from sexually transmitted infections?
- Are you or your partner trying to get pregnant?
- What are you doing to prevent pregnancy?

Review of systems

[a]When taking a sexual history, do not assume heterosexuality, and use gender-neutral language when referring to partners ("partner" or "spouse" rather than "wife," "husband," "girlfriend," or "boyfriend").

sensitive, respectful, and affirming manner. In contrast to the focused physical examination, the value of the routine physical examination in asymptomatic patients has been debated.

Regularly obtaining height and weight (to calculate BMI) as well as blood pressure is universally recommended. Additionally, pulse palpation in individuals older than 65 years has been found effective for detection of atrial fibrillation. The U.S. Preventive Services Task Force (USPSTF) recommends against routine abdominal, testicular, and bimanual pelvic examinations for cancer screening. The USPSTF has also concluded that there is insufficient evidence to recommend routine cardiac and lung auscultation, thyroid palpation, skin examination, visual acuity assessment, and hearing assessment, although these evaluations may be appropriate as part of a comprehensive physical examination in persons at increased risk. Relatively no harms arise from these examinations save for the opportunity cost of providing another service that may be more valuable. Routine laboratory tests, such as screening complete blood count and urinalysis, are not recommended.

Preparticipation physical examination is required for adolescents before participation in organized sports. In conjunction with the American Academy of Family Physicians and several professional sports medicine organizations, the American Academy of Pediatrics (AAP) created the Preparticipation Physical Evaluation, now in its fourth edition. Additionally, free templates for history, physical examination, and clearance forms are available on the website of the AAP (https://www.aap.org/en-us/about-the-aap/Committees-Councils-Sections/Council-on-sports-medicine-and-fitness/Pages/PPE.aspx). Mandatory components include evaluating for exertional symptoms, family history of premature or sudden cardiac death, and presence of a heart murmur.

Digital stethoscopes, point-of-care ultrasonography, smart phone applications, and other technological advances are gradually becoming more commonplace in the physical examination. However, it is unclear whether these tools improve diagnosis or contribute to overdiagnosis.

**KEY POINT**

- The periodic health examination may improve surrogate outcomes, such as reduction in cardiovascular risk factors and increased receipt of preventive services; however, the periodic health examination has not been shown to reduce mortality or other patient-important outcomes.  **HVC**

## Screening
### Principles of Screening

Levels of prevention have traditionally been categorized as primary, secondary, and tertiary. Primary prevention is preventing disease or injury before it occurs (for example, through immunization). Secondary prevention is early detection and treatment of disease in asymptomatic patients to slow or stop disease progression. Most screening tests, such as those for colorectal and breast cancers, are secondary prevention measures. Tertiary prevention involves reducing morbidity and mortality due to established disease, such as cardiac rehabilitation after myocardial infarction.

Screening is appropriate for common conditions for which (1) early intervention can decrease morbidity and mortality and (2) safe, acceptable, widely available, and reasonably priced screening tests exist. Screening tests must also have adequate sensitivity and specificity to minimize false-positive and false-negative results.

The effectiveness of screening tests in reducing morbidity and mortality is evaluated through clinical trials; however, studies of screening tests are problematic and subject to three types of bias. Lead-time bias occurs when early detection artificially leads to an increase in measured survival. The time between early detection and clinical diagnosis is mistakenly counted as survival time; however, only the measured time with diagnosed disease, not survival time, has increased (**Figure 2**). Using disease-specific mortality rates rather than survival time as the primary outcome in studies of screening tests can help minimize lead-time bias. Length-time bias occurs when screening detects more cases of disease with a prolonged asymptomatic phase than cases of disease with a short asymptomatic phase. Slowly progressive disease is more likely than aggressive disease to be detected with screening, leading to an overestimation of survival benefit in those with screen-detected disease. Overdiagnosis, or finding and treating illness that otherwise would not have become clinically apparent or caused harm in the patient's lifetime, is an extreme example of length-time bias. Overdiagnosis is an increasingly recognized harm of breast and prostate cancer screening and may also occur with incidental detection of thyroid and kidney

cancers on imaging studies. Selection bias, also referred to as volunteer, referral, or compliance bias, occurs when patients who undergo screening tests are healthier and more interested in their health than nonadherent patients or the general population. Intention-to-treat analyses, in which patients are analyzed according to their original group assignment in randomized clinical trials regardless of intervention received, reduce selection bias.

## Screening Recommendations for Adults

The USPSTF and many specialty societies routinely aggregate and review available evidence to inform clinical practice guidelines for screening, counseling, and use of preventive medications. The American College of Physicians (ACP) has developed several different types of clinical recommendations, including clinical practice guidelines, clinical guidance statements, best practice advice, and recommendations regarding high value care, all of which are available at https://www.acponline.org/clinical-information/guidelines. Although there is much agreement among screening recommendations, guidelines often disagree when (1) sufficient evidence is lacking and expert opinion plays a larger role or (2) potential benefits and harms both exist and the balance depends on a person's risk, preferences, and values.

An additional resource to help clinicians identify appropriate screening tests and preventive services is the electronic Preventive Services Selector (ePSS) created by the Agency for Healthcare Research and Quality (available at epss.ahrq.gov in web-based or mobile application–based formats). With this tool, users can select USPSTF-recommended practices based

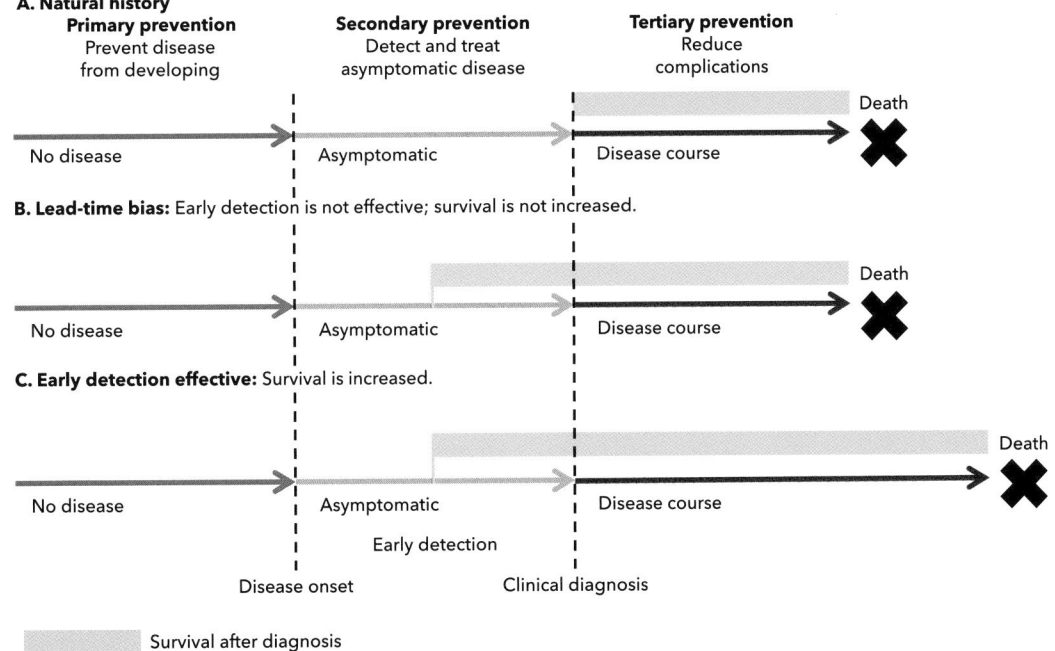

**FIGURE 2.** The effect of early detection (screening) on survival after diagnosis. (*A*) Screening is not implemented, and the disease takes its normal course. (*B*) Lead-time bias occurs when survival time appears to be lengthened because the screened patient is diagnosed earlier during the preclinical phase but does not live longer in actuality. (*C*) Screening effectively detects disease during the asymptomatic phase, and survival time is lengthened.

on patient age, sex, and other characteristics (such as tobacco use or pregnancy).

Screening recommendations frequently change as supportive evidence emerges. It is important to be aware of changes in recommendations as they occur, to reflect on the rationale and implications of the changes, to contemplate how to best help patients understand new recommendations, and to incorporate these changes appropriately into practice.

## Specific Screening Tests

The following section describes screening recommendations from the USPSTF and other organizations. The grading system of the USPSTF (A, B, C, D, and I) is explained in **Table 7**.

**TABLE 7.** U.S. Preventive Services Task Force Grading and Suggestions for Practice

| Grade | Definition | Suggestions for Practice |
|---|---|---|
| A | The USPSTF recommends the service. There is high certainty that the net benefit is substantial. | Offer or provide this service. |
| B | The USPSTF recommends the service. There is high certainty that the net benefit is moderate or there is moderate certainty that the net benefit is moderate to substantial. | Offer or provide this service. |
| C | The USPSTF recommends selectively offering or providing this service to individual patients based on professional judgment and patient preferences. There is at least moderate certainty that the net benefit is small. | Offer or provide this service for selected patients depending on individual circumstances. |
| D | The USPSTF recommends against the service. There is moderate or high certainty that the service has no net benefit or that the harms outweigh the benefits. | Discourage the use of this service. |
| I statement | The USPSTF concludes that the current evidence is insufficient to assess the balance of benefits and harms of the service. Evidence is lacking, of poor quality, or conflicting, and the balance of benefits and harms cannot be determined. | Read the Clinical Considerations section of USPSTF Recommendation Statement. If the service is offered, patients should understand the uncertainty about the balance of benefits and harms. |

USPSTF = U.S. Preventive Services Task Force.

Reproduced from U.S. Preventive Services Task Force. Procedure Manual. https://www.uspreventiveservicestaskforce.org/Page/Name/procedure-manual. November 2017. Accessed June 27, 2018.

## Screening for Chronic Diseases

### Abdominal Aortic Aneurysm

The USPSTF recommends one-time abdominal ultrasonography to screen for abdominal aortic aneurysm (AAA) in all men aged 65 to 75 years who have ever smoked (grade B). Ever-smokers are commonly defined as persons who have smoked more than 100 cigarettes in their lifetime. The number needed to screen (NNS) to prevent one death from AAA in this population is 667. The number needed to treat (NNT) with surgery to prevent one death is 1.5, owing to the high mortality rate associated with AAA rupture. In men aged 65 to 75 years who have never smoked, selective screening is recommended (grade C), especially in those with a first-degree relative with a history of treated or ruptured AAA. The USPSTF makes no recommendation regarding screening for AAA in women who have smoked and specifically recommends against routine screening in women who have never smoked (grade D).

### Cardiovascular and Cerebrovascular Disease

Cardiovascular risk assessment is performed in asymptomatic adults to evaluate a patient's risk for future cardiac events; it does not identify pre-existing disease and is therefore considered separate from screening (see MKSAP 18 Cardiovascular Medicine).

The USPSTF does not recommend screening for coronary artery disease with either resting or exercise electrocardiography (ECG) in asymptomatic patients at low risk, defined by the USPSTF as a 10-year cardiovascular event risk of less than 10% using the Pooled Cohort Equations (grade D). In patients at intermediate or high risk for such events, there was inadequate evidence to assess the relative benefits and harms of screening. Similarly, the ACP recommends against screening low-risk and asymptomatic adults with resting ECG or stress testing. No specialty organization recommends screening these populations with resting or exercise ECG, coronary calcium scoring, or coronary angiography.

The USPSTF also does not recommend screening for carotid artery stenosis in the general adult population (grade D).

### Depression

The USPSTF suggests that all adults, including pregnant and postpartum women, be screened for depression, with adequate systems in place for assessment, treatment, and follow-up (grade B). Most adults can be screened with the brief PHQ-2, which consists of two questions: "During the past 2 weeks, how often have you been bothered by feeling down, depressed, or hopeless?" and "During the past 2 weeks, have you often been bothered by having little interest or pleasure in doing things?" Answers are graded on a scale of 0 to 6, with a score of 3 indicating a positive screen. The PHQ-2 has a sensitivity of 83% and specificity of 90% for detecting depression; longer screening instruments, such as the PHQ-9, do not have a clear advantage over the PHQ-2. Patients with a positive screening result should complete the PHQ-9, which can be used for diagnosis and monitoring of depression.

Other screening instruments may be more accurate in specific patient populations, such as the Geriatric Depression Scale in older adults and the Edinburgh Postnatal Depression Scale in postpartum and pregnant women.

*Diabetes Mellitus*

The USPSTF recommends screening for diabetes mellitus in adults aged 40 to 70 years who are overweight or obese (grade B). Screening can be accomplished by measuring levels of fasting plasma glucose or hemoglobin $A_{1c}$. Those with a positive screening result should undergo intensive behavioral counseling to promote a healthful diet and physical activity. Earlier screening should be considered in persons at increased risk, including individuals who belong to certain racial or ethnic groups (blacks, American Indians, Asian Americans, Hispanics or Latinos, Native Hawaiians, Pacific Islanders), and those with a family history of diabetes or a personal history of gestational diabetes or polycystic ovary syndrome.

In contrast to the USPSTF, the American Diabetes Association (ADA) recommends that screening be performed in obese or overweight patients of any age with one or more risk factors for diabetes (**Table 8**). The ADA also recommends screening all adults beginning at age 45 years, regardless of risk factors, and repeating screening at 3-year intervals. Patients with prediabetes (hemoglobin $A_{1c} \geq 5.7\%$, impaired glucose tolerance, or impaired fasting glucose) should be screened annually.

*Dyslipidemia*

The USPSTF recommends lipid screening for adults aged 40 to 75 years for the purposes of calculating 10-year risk for atherosclerotic cardiovascular disease (ASCVD) and guiding initiation of statin therapy for primary prevention (see Dyslipidemia chapter on p. 79). Measuring lipid levels every 5 years is reasonable. If lipid levels are close to those that require therapy, testing may be performed at shorter intervals, whereas longer intervals can be considered for persons without cardiovascular risk factors who have repeatedly normal levels. For adults aged 21 to 39 years, the USPSTF recommends that clinicians use their clinical judgment regarding screening for and treating dyslipidemia due to a lack of supportive data.

The American Heart Association recommends assessing traditional cardiovascular risk factors, including total and HDL cholesterol levels, starting at age 20 years. Risk factor assessment should be performed every 4 to 6 years if the patient is at low 10-year risk (<7.5%). Patients with a family history of premature coronary artery disease or patients with a family history of or evidence on examination of familial hypercholesterolemia should also be screened at a younger age.

*Hypertension*

The USPSTF supports screening all adults for hypertension (grade A). Screening should occur annually in adults aged 40 years and older and in younger adults at increased risk (including patients with high-normal blood pressure [130 to 139/85 to 89 mm Hg], patients who are overweight or obese, and black patients). Screening should otherwise occur every 3 to 5 years. Before treatment is initiated, the diagnosis should be confirmed with blood pressure measurements outside of the clinical setting, such as ambulatory or home blood pressure monitoring.

The American Heart Association/American College of Cardiology recommend evaluating patients with a normal blood pressure (<120/<80 mm Hg) annually and patients with elevated blood pressure (120-129/<80 mm Hg) whose 10-year estimated ASCVD risk is less than 10% every 3 to 6 months.

*Obesity*

The USPSTF suggests that all adults should be screened for obesity by calculating BMI (grade B), without specifically delineating how frequently screening should be repeated. The American College of Cardiology, American Heart Association, and The Obesity Society recommend annual screening with BMI and waist circumference measurements. Adults with a BMI of 30 or higher should be offered or referred for intensive behavioral interventions, according to the USPSTF.

*Obstructive Sleep Apnea*

According to the USPSTF, there is insufficient evidence to assess the balance of benefits and harms of screening for obstructive sleep apnea in asymptomatic adults with the currently available tools. Because obstructive sleep apnea is widely underrecognized, clinicians should have a low threshold for investigating for sleep apnea in patients with symptoms consistent with the disease (see MKSAP 18 Pulmonary and Critical Care Medicine).

*Osteoporosis*

The USPSTF recommends screening for osteoporosis in women aged 65 years and older and in postmenopausal

| TABLE 8. | Risk Factors for Diabetes Mellitus |
|---|---|
| First-degree relative with diabetes ||
| High-risk race/ethnicity (e.g., African American, Latino, Native American, Asian American, Pacific Islander) ||
| History of cardiovascular disease ||
| Hypertension (≥140/90 mm Hg or on therapy for hypertension) ||
| HDL cholesterol level <35 mg/dL (0.90 mmol/L) and/or a triglyceride level >250 mg/dL (2.82 mmol/L) ||
| Women with polycystic ovary syndrome ||
| Physical inactivity ||
| Other clinical conditions associated with insulin resistance (e.g., severe obesity, acanthosis nigricans) ||
| History of gestational diabetes ||

Information from American Diabetes Association. 2. Classification and diagnosis of diabetes: Standards of Medical Care in Diabetes—2018. Diabetes Care. 2018;41:S13-S27. [PMID: 29222373] doi:10.2337/dc18-S002

women younger than 65 years at increased risk for osteoporosis, as determined by a formal clinical risk assessment tool. One commonly used clinical risk assessment tool is the Fracture Risk Assessment (FRAX), available at www.shef.ac.uk/FRAX. Women who have a 10-year FRAX risk for major osteoporotic fracture equal to or higher than that of a 65-year-old white woman without additional risk factors (10-year risk of 8.4%) should undergo screening for osteoporosis. Screening can be accomplished with bone mineral density measurement, most commonly with dual-energy x-ray absorptiometry (DEXA) of the hip and lumbar spine.

The USPSTF concludes that there is insufficient evidence to recommend routine screening for osteoporosis in men (I statement); however, the National Osteoporosis Foundation recommends osteoporosis screening in men aged 70 years or older. Screening may be considered in men at high risk for osteoporosis on the basis of risk factors, such as low body weight, recent weight loss, physical inactivity, use of oral glucocorticoids, previous fragility fracture, alcohol use, and androgen deprivation through pharmacologic agents or orchiectomy.

Risk assessment and screening for osteoporosis are further discussed in MKSAP 18 Endocrinology and Metabolism.

## Thyroid Disease

The USPSTF concludes that there is insufficient evidence to recommend for or against screening for thyroid disease (I statement). The American Thyroid Association and the American Association of Clinical Endocrinologists, however, recommend measuring thyroid-stimulating hormone in individuals at risk for hypothyroidism (for example, personal history of autoimmune disease, neck radiation, or thyroid surgery); they additionally recommend considering screening in adults aged 60 years and older.

## Screening for Infectious Diseases

Screening for infectious diseases is primarily recommended for individuals at increased risk (**Table 9** and **Table 10**), although there are several diseases for which average-risk patients should be screened.

According to the USPSTF, screening for chlamydia and gonorrhea should be performed in all sexually active women aged 24 years or younger because of increased prevalence in this population.

One-time hepatitis C screening is recommended for adults born between 1945 and 1965 and those who received

| TABLE 9. | U.S. Preventive Services Task Force Recommendations on Screening for Infectious Diseases | | |
|---|---|---|---|
| **Infectious Disease** | **Screening Recommendation** | **Screening Test** | **Populations at Risk** |
| Chlamydia and gonorrhea | Screen all sexually active women aged ≤24 y and women aged >24 y who are at increased risk for infection | Nucleic acid amplification test | Persons with a history of STIs, persons with new or multiple sexual partners, those who use condoms inconsistently, persons who exchange sex for money or drugs |
| HIV | Perform one-time screening for all adults aged 15-65 y; repeat screening for adults at high risk | Combination HIV antibody immunoassay/p24 antigen test | Men who have sex with men, active injection drug users, persons who engage in risky behaviors (unprotected vaginal or anal intercourse; sexual partners who are HIV infected, bisexual, or injection drug users; exchanging sex for drugs or money), persons with other STIs, persons who live and receive care in a high-prevalence setting (HIV seroprevalence of ≥1%) |
| HBV | Screen all adults at high risk | Hepatitis B surface antigen test; obtain antibodies (anti-HBs, anti-HBc) to differentiate between immunity and infection | Persons born in countries with ≥2% prevalence of HBV infection, persons receiving dialysis or cytotoxic or immunosuppressive treatments, persons with HIV infection, injection drug users, men who have sex with men, household contacts or sexual partners of persons with HBV infection |
| HCV | Screen all adults at high risk and perform one-time screening in adults born between 1945 and 1965 | Anti-HCV antibody test, followed by PCR viral load test if result is positive | Injection/intranasal drug users, persons who received a blood transfusion before 1992, persons receiving long-term hemodialysis, prisoners, and persons who received unregulated tattoos |
| Syphilis | Screen all adults at increased risk | VDRL or RPR test | Persons with HIV infection, prisoners, men who have sex with men, persons who exchange sex for money or drugs |
| Latent TB | Screen populations at increased risk | Tuberculin skin test or interferon-γ release assay | Persons born in or former residents of countries with high TB prevalence, close contacts of persons with known or suspected TB, persons who live or work in high-risk settings |

Anti-HBc = hepatitis B core antibody; Anti-HBs = hepatitis B surface antibody; HBV = hepatitis B virus; HCV = hepatitis C virus; PCR = polymerase chain reaction; RPR = rapid plasma reagin; STIs = sexually transmitted infections; TB = tuberculosis; VDRL = Venereal Disease Research Laboratory.

**TABLE 10.** Screening for Infectious Diseases in High-Risk Populations

| Specific Populations | Recommended Screening |
|---|---|
| Pregnant women | Chlamydia and gonorrhea, hepatitis B, HIV, syphilis |
| Persons engaging in high-risk sexual behavior | Hepatitis B and C, HIV, syphilis |
| Men who have sex with men | Chlamydia and gonorrhea[a], hepatitis B, HIV, syphilis |
| Injection drug users | Hepatitis B and C, HIV |
| Prisoners | Hepatitis C, syphilis, tuberculosis |
| Persons receiving hemodialysis | Hepatitis B and C, tuberculosis |
| Persons born in or living in certain countries[b] | Hepatitis B and tuberculosis depending on prevalence of disease |
| Health care workers | Tuberculosis (annually); pre-employment verification of immunity to hepatitis B virus, measles, mumps, rubella, and varicella |

[a]The Centers for Disease Control and Prevention recommends screening for chlamydia and gonorrhea in men who have sex with men; however, the U.S. Preventive Services Task Force has found insufficient evidence to recommend screening for these diseases in men.

[b]Countries with ≥2% hepatitis B virus prevalence, including most of sub-Saharan Africa, central and southeast Asia, and parts of South America. See https://wwwnc.cdc.gov/travel/yellowbook/2018/infectious-diseases-related-to-travel/hepatitis-b for further details.

a blood transfusion before 1992. Screening is accomplished by testing for antibodies to the disease, followed by polymerase chain reaction viral load testing if results of initial testing are positive (see MKSAP 18 Gastroenterology and Hepatology).

The USPSTF recommends that all persons aged 15 to 65 years receive one-time HIV screening regardless of risk, and the Centers for Disease Control and Prevention (CDC) recommends routine HIV screening for all persons aged 13 to 64 years. The USPSTF suggests screening persons at very high risk for HIV (men who have sex with men and active injection drug users) at least annually. The CDC recommends at least annual screening for men who have sex with men. Combination HIV antibody immunoassay/p24 antigen testing is recommended for screening. Diagnosis of HIV is discussed in MKSAP 18 Infectious Disease.

## Screening for Substance Use Disorders

The USPSTF recommends that clinicians ask all adults about tobacco use, advise them to stop using tobacco, and provide behavioral intervention and pharmacotherapy for tobacco cessation (grade A) (see Mental and Behavioral Health).

The USPSTF supports asking all adults about alcohol misuse and providing persons engaged in risky or hazardous drinking with brief behavioral counseling interventions to reduce alcohol misuse (grade B). Screening instruments to identify harmful drinking include the Alcohol Use Disorders Identification Test (AUDIT), the AUDIT-Consumption (AUDIT-C),

and single-item screening. The AUDIT (https://pubs.niaaa.nih.gov/publications/Audit.pdf) is a validated 10-item screening test that takes approximately 2 to 3 minutes to administer; the AUDIT-C is a briefer (three-item) version of the AUDIT. With single-item screening, the clinician asks, "How many times in the past year have you had five [four for women] or more drinks in 1 day?" A positive test result, defined as any answer other than zero, has a sensitivity and specificity of approximately 80% for unhealthy alcohol use.

The USPSTF concluded that there is insufficient evidence to assess the balance of benefits and harms of routine screening for illicit drug use. Screening tools include the Drug Abuse Screening Test (DAST-10) (https://www.integration.samhsa.gov/clinical-practice/DAST_-_10.pdf) and the CAGE questionnaire expanded to include drugs (CAGE-AID) (https://www.integration.samhsa.gov/images/res/CAGEAID.pdf). Prescription opioids are the most commonly abused opioids and are the leading cause of opioid overdoses in the United States. Clinicians must be aware of the potential for opioid abuse. The opioid risk tool can be useful to assess risk for abuse of opioid medications; however, this tool needs further validation in clinical practice.

## Screening for Abuse

The USPSTF recommends screening for intimate partner violence in all women of child-bearing age (grade B). Available screening tools include the Hurt, Insult, Threaten, Scream (HITS); Ongoing Abuse Screen/Ongoing Violence Assessment Tool (OAS/OVAT); Slapped, Threatened, and Throw (STaT); Humiliation, Afraid, Rape, Kick (HARK); Modified Childhood Trauma Questionnaire–Short Form (CTQ-SF); and Woman Abuse Screen Tool (WAST).

Screening for abuse in elderly and vulnerable adults may be considered, although there is currently insufficient evidence to recommend universal screening (I statement) (see Geriatric Medicine).

## Screening for Cancer

This section discusses cancer screening in asymptomatic, average-risk persons. Screening for cancer in patients at high risk is covered in the respective specialty books of MKSAP 18.

### Breast Cancer

The balance of benefits and harms of screening mammography has shifted with the advent of increasingly effective breast cancer treatments, which reduce the benefits of early detection, as well as emerging information about overdiagnosis. In women aged 50 to 74 years, there is a clear benefit to screening mammography, and all breast cancer guidelines recommend screening mammography in this age group. Biennial screening mammography imparts most of the benefits of annual screening mammography with fewer harms, although the recommended screening frequency differs between guidelines. In women younger than 50 years or aged 75 years and older, the balance of benefits and harms is less clear, and screening recommendations vary widely (**Table 11**).

**TABLE 11.** Recommendations for Breast Cancer Screening in Women at Average Risk

| Expert Group | Recommendation |
|---|---|
| American Cancer Society (2015) | Age 40-44 y: Provide women with the opportunity to begin annual screening mammography<br><br>Age 45-54 y: Perform annual screening mammography<br><br>Age ≥55 y: Perform biennial screening mammography with the opportunity to continue annual screening<br><br>Do not perform CBE for breast cancer screening |
| American College of Obstetricians and Gynecologists (2017) | Age 25-39 y: May offer CBE every 1-3 y<br><br>Age 40-49 y: Offer screening mammography and engage women in a shared decision-making process. May offer annual CBE<br><br>Age 50-75 y: Perform annual or biennial screening mammography based on a shared decision-making process<br><br>Age >75 y: Engage women in a shared decision-making process about discontinuing screening |
| American College of Physicians (2015) | Age <40 y: Do not perform screening<br><br>Age 40-49 y: Discuss the benefits and harms of screening mammography and order biennial mammography screening if an informed woman requests it<br><br>Age 50-74 y: Encourage biennial mammography screening<br><br>Age >75 y: Do not perform screening |
| American College of Radiology (2017) | Age 40 y: Begin annual screening mammography |
| National Comprehensive Cancer Network (2016) | Age 25-39 y: Perform CBE every 1-3 y<br><br>Age 40 y: Begin annual screening mammography and perform annual CBE |
| U.S. Preventive Services Task Force (2016) | Age 40-49 y: Decision to begin screening should be individualized (grade C)<br><br>Age 50-74 y: Perform biennial screening mammography (grade B)<br><br>Age ≥75 y: Insufficient evidence to assess the balance of benefits and harms of screening mammography (grade I) |

CBE = clinical breast examination.

**TABLE 12.** Breast Cancer Deaths Averted per 10,000 Women Screened Over 10 Years

| Variable | Patient Age | | | |
|---|---|---|---|---|
| | 40-49 Years | 50-59 Years | 60-69 Years | 70-74 Years |
| Breast cancer deaths averted (95% CI) | 3 (0-9) | 8 (2-17) | 21 (11-32) | 13 (0-32) |
| NNS | 3333 | 1250 | 476 | 769 |

NNS = number needed to screen for 10 years to avoid one breast cancer death.

Data from Nelson HD, Fu R, Cantor A, Pappas M, Daeges M, Humphrey L. Effectiveness of breast cancer screening: systematic review and meta-analysis to update the 2009 U.S. Preventive Services Task Force recommendation. Ann Intern Med. 2016;164:244-55. [PMID: 26756588] doi:10.7326/M15-0969

results may cause unnecessary biopsies and substantial patient anxiety. Overdiagnosis accounts for roughly 30% of all breast cancers diagnosed.

Approximately 50% of women have dense breasts on mammography. Increased breast density is associated with an increased breast cancer risk but decreased sensitivity of mammography (more so with film than digital mammography). As a result, legislation in many states requires that breast density be included on mammogram reports (**Table 13**). In women in whom increased breast density is the sole breast cancer risk factor, there is no evidence that adding MRI or ultrasonography to mammography affects breast cancer mortality, and most guidelines conclude that there is insufficient evidence to recommend adjunctive screening when dense breasts are present. The American College of Radiology, however, notes that ultrasonography may be considered in this circumstance. Women with dense breasts should undergo further risk stratification; for those at high risk, additional screening may be considered (see MKSAP 18 Hematology and Oncology).

### Prostate Cancer

Screening for prostate cancer in asymptomatic, average-risk men has been controversial, and recommendations among professional organizations continue to evolve (**Table 14**). For men aged 55 to 69 years, the USPSTF recommends that the decision to undergo periodic prostate-specific antigen (PSA)-based screening should be an individual one and should include discussion of the potential benefits and harms of screening with their clinician. The USPSTF recommends that clinicians should not screen men who do not express a preference for screening and recommends against PSA-based screening for prostate cancer in men aged 70 years and older.

Benefits of screening for men aged 55 to 69 years include prevention of one prostate cancer–related death for every 1000 men screened for 10 years (NNS, 1000). Risks include overdiagnosis, overtreatment, and false-positive results that trigger unnecessary biopsies and patient anxiety. Estimated rates of overdiagnosis and overtreatment vary widely.

If the decision is made to proceed with screening, the American Urological Association (AUA) recommends

When recommendations differ, shared decision making with consideration of the patient's level of risk, values, and preferences guides the screening decision. The benefit of screening is largest in those aged 60 to 69 years but is substantially lower for younger and older women (**Table 12**). Potential harms of screening include false-positive results and overdiagnosis. For patients starting mammography at age 40 or 50 years, the 10-year cumulative false-positive rates are 42% with biennial screening and 61% with annual screening. Such

| TABLE 13. | Breast Imaging Reporting and Data System (BI-RADS) Breast Composition Categories |
|---|---|
| a. | The breasts are almost entirely fatty |
| b. | There are scattered areas of fibroglandular density |
| c. | The breasts are heterogeneously dense, which may obscure small masses |
| d. | The breasts are extremely dense, which lowers the sensitivity of mammography |

Reproduced with permission of the American College of Radiology (ACR) from D'Orsi CJ, Sickles EA, Mendelson EB, et al. ACR BI-RADS® Atlas, Breast Imaging Reporting and Data System. Reston, VA, American College of Radiology; 2013. No other representation of this material is authorized without expressed, written permission from the ACR. Refer to the ACR website at https://www.acr.org/Clinical-Resources/Reporting-and-Data-Systems/Bi-Rads for the most current and complete version of the BI-RADS® Atlas.

| TABLE 14. | Recommendations for Prostate Cancer Screening |
|---|---|
| Expert Group | Recommendation |
| American Cancer Society (2010) | Age 40-44 y: Engage men at higher risk (≥2 first-degree relatives with prostate cancer before age 65 y) in shared decision making |
| | Age 45-49 y: Engage men at high risk (African American race or first-degree relative with prostate cancer before age 65 y) in shared decision making |
| | Age ≥50 y with life expectancy >10 y: Engage in shared decision making |
| American College of Physicians (2013) | Age 50-69 y: Inform men about the limited potential benefits and substantial harms of screening for prostate cancer; test only men who request screening after informed discussion |
| | Age <50 y, >69 y, or with a life expectancy <10 y: Recommend against screening |
| American Urological Association (2013, reviewed and confirmed 2015) | Men at higher risk (African American race or with positive family history): Individualize screening decisions |
| | Age <40 y: Recommend against screening |
| | Age 40-54 y: Do not recommend routine screening |
| | Age 55-69 y: Engage men considering PSA-based screening in shared decision making; proceed based on patient values and preferences. If proceeding with screening, consider PSA testing every 2 years or longer |
| | Age ≥70 y or with life expectancy <10-15 y: Do not recommend routine screening |
| U.S. Preventive Services Task Force (2018) | Age 55-69: Discuss potential benefits and harms of PSA-based screening for prostate cancer and individualize decision making by incorporating the patient's values and preferences |
| | Age ≥70 y: Recommend against PSA-based screening |

PSA = prostate-specific antigen.

choosing less frequent screening intervals (≥2 years), which may reduce overdiagnosis and the number of false-positive results while preserving most of the screening benefit. The AUA also recommends that the interval for rescreening may be based on the baseline PSA level. Screening is not recommended for men with less than a 10- to 15-year life expectancy.

Methods to better use PSA testing, including one-time PSA measurement at prespecified ages, adjusted-threshold testing, or PSA velocity and doubling time, are being investigated. However, there is currently insufficient evidence to support these methods.

### Colorectal Cancer

The USPSTF recommends screening for colorectal cancer in asymptomatic adults aged 50 to 75 years (grade A). In contrast, the American Cancer Society makes a qualified recommendation to initiate screening for colorectal cancer at age 45 years. According to the USPSTF, screening decisions in patients aged 76 to 85 years should be individualized according to life expectancy and ability to tolerate treatment of colorectal cancer if diagnosed. Screening history should also be considered because patients who have not undergone screening are the most likely to benefit (grade C). The USPSTF suggests that screening may be discontinued in patients older than 85 years; most other guidelines recommend stopping screening if life expectancy is less than 10 years.

There is little head-to-head comparative evidence that any one recommended screening modality provides a greater benefit than the others. In addition, despite unequivocal evidence that colon cancer screening reduces mortality, an estimated one in three U.S. adults who are eligible for colon cancer screening has not been screened. Therefore, the USPSTF supports using the test that is most likely to result in completion of screening. Understanding a patient's values and preferences and selecting a test to which the patient is most likely to adhere may improve screening rates. Clinicians should be familiar with the characteristics of each screening strategy to facilitate effective discussion with patients (**Table 15**).

The U.S. Multi-Society Task Force on Colorectal Cancer (MSTF), an initiative of U.S. gastroenterology societies, has ranked colorectal cancer screening tests in tiers based on the available evidence, cost-effectiveness, test availability, and several other factors. The MSTF recommends colonoscopy every 10 years or annual fecal immunochemical testing (FIT) as first-tier tests; CT colonography every 5 years, FIT-fecal DNA testing every 3 years, or flexible sigmoidoscopy every 5 to 10 years as second-tier tests; and capsule colonography every 5 years as a third-tier test. The serum circulating methylated *SEPT9* DNA test is an FDA-approved screening strategy that holds promise because blood tests may result in increased adherence. However, this test's sensitivity for detecting colorectal cancer is only 48%, and the MSTF does not recommend its use.

| TABLE 15. | Characteristics of Colorectal Cancer Screening Strategies | | |
|---|---|---|---|
| **Screening Strategy** | **Frequency** | **Reduction in Mortality Rate** | **Notes** |
| **Stool-based Tests (Cancer Detection)** | | | |
| gFOBT | Every year | 32% | High-sensitivity gFOBT has superior test performance characteristics than older tests |
| | | | Requires dietary restrictions; does not require bowel preparation, anesthesia, or transportation to and from the screening examination |
| FIT | Every year | Unknown | Improved accuracy compared with gFOBT |
| | | | Does not require bowel preparation, anesthesia, or transportation to and from the screening examination |
| FIT-DNA | Every 1 to 3 y | Unknown | Higher sensitivity but lower specificity than FIT, resulting in more false-positive results |
| **Direct Visualization Tests (Cancer Prevention)** | | | |
| Colonoscopy | Every 10 y | 68% | Requires full bowel preparation |
| | | | Usually requires sedation and a patient escort |
| | | | ACG/MSTF recommend split-dose preparation[a] |
| CT colonography | Every 5 y | Unknown | Requires bowel preparation |
| | | | Imaging only (cannot remove polyps or biopsy) |
| | | | Extracolonic findings are common |
| Flexible sigmoidoscopy | Every 5 y | 27% | Limited bowel preparation compared with colonoscopy |
| Flexible sigmoidoscopy with FIT | Flexible sigmoidoscopy every 10 y with FIT every year | 38% | |

ACG = American College of Gastroenterology; FIT = fecal immunochemical test; gFOBT = guaiac fecal occult blood test; MSTF = U.S. Multisociety Task Force on Colorectal Cancer.

[a]Split-dose preparation has been shown to increase detection rates for sessile polyps and possibly adenomas. It involves taking half of the preparation the evening before and half of the preparation on the day of colonoscopy, starting 4 to 5 hours before the procedure start and finishing 3 hours before the procedure start.

Adapted from U.S. Preventive Services Task Force. Final recommendation statement: colorectal cancer: screening. June 2017. https://www.uspreventiveservicestaskforce.org/Page/Document/RecommendationStatementFinal/colorectal-cancer-screening2. Accessed June 28, 2018. The Agency for Healthcare Research and Quality and the U.S. Department of Health and Human Services do not endorse derivative or excerpted materials and cannot be held liable for this content.

## Cervical Cancer

Cervical cancer incidence and mortality have steadily decreased over the last half-century, largely because of the implementation of widespread screening. The USPSTF, in a 2018 recommendation statement, recommends screening women aged 21 to 65 years every 3 years with cytology (Pap test). In women aged 30 to 65 years who want to lengthen the screening interval, high-risk human papillomavirus (HPV) testing (preferred) or cytology combined with high-risk HPV testing can be performed every 5 years. The USPSTF recommends against screening women younger than 21 years regardless of sexual history because screening has not been shown to reduce cervical cancer incidence or mortality compared with starting screening at age 21 years.

Screening can be discontinued at age 65 years in non–high-risk women with adequate prior screening, commonly defined as three consecutive negative cytology results or two consecutive negative cytology plus HPV test results within the last 10 years, with the most recent test occurring within 5 years. In women older than 65 years with life expectancy of at least 10 years and risk factors for cervical cancer (history of abnormal Pap smears, history of a high-grade precancerous lesion, in utero exposure to diethylstilbestrol, immunocompromise, previous HPV infection), continued screening should be considered.

Women who have never been screened have the highest incidence of and mortality from cervical cancer. The mortality reduction from screening in women who have not been previously screened may be as high as 74%. Women older than 65 years who have never been screened or in whom adequacy of prior screening cannot be confirmed should undergo screening with cytology every 3 years, high-risk HPV testing every 5 years, or combined high-risk HPV testing and cytology every 5 years.

Screening should not be performed in women who have had a hysterectomy with removal of the cervix unless a high-grade precancerous lesion (cervical intraepithelial neoplasia 2 or 3) was present, in which case screening should be continued for at least 20 years after hysterectomy.

### Additional Cancer Screening Tests

The USPSTF, Society of Gynecologic Oncology, and the American College of Obstetricians and Gynecologists all recommend against screening for ovarian cancer with serum CA-125 testing or ultrasonography in women at average risk. Women with a family history indicating a hereditary cancer syndrome should be referred to a genetic counselor for consideration of genetic testing (see MKSAP 18 Hematology and Oncology).

According to the USPSTF, evidence is insufficient to determine the balance of benefits and harms of screening for skin cancer with a visual skin examination. However, the USPSTF recommends that persons younger than 24 years who have fair skin receive counseling to minimize exposure to ultraviolet radiation to reduce risk for skin cancer (grade B) and recommends offering selective counseling to adults older than 24 years with fair skin types (grade C).

The USPSTF recommends against screening for pancreatic cancer in asymptomatic adults. Because up to 15% of pancreatic ductal adenocarcinomas are attributable to genetic factors, patients with a family history suggestive of a genetic syndrome associated with pancreatic cancer (*BRCA1/2* mutations, Peutz-Jeghers syndrome, Lynch syndrome) should be referred for genetic counseling and possible genetic testing.

There is insufficient evidence to recommend routine anal cancer screening in average-risk populations, but such screening may be considered in high-risk populations. The Infectious Diseases Society of America suggests screening patients with genital warts, men who have sex with men, and women who have a history of abnormal cervical cytology or participate in receptive anal intercourse.

Lung cancer screening with annual low-dose CT is recommended for persons aged 55 years to 74-80 years (guidelines vary) with a 30-pack-year smoking history, including former smokers who have quit in the last 15 years (see MKSAP 18 Pulmonary and Critical Care Medicine).

The USPSTF recommends against screening for testicular cancer and thyroid cancer in asymptomatic adults. Routine screening for bladder cancer is not recommended by any expert group, including the USPSTF.

### KEY POINTS

- The U.S. Preventive Services Task Force supports routine screening for depression, hypertension, obesity, tobacco use, and alcohol misuse in asymptomatic, average-risk adults.
- Lipid screening is indicated in adults aged 40 to 75 years for the purposes of calculating 10-year risk for atherosclerotic cardiovascular disease and guiding initiation of statin therapy for primary prevention.

*(Continued)*

### KEY POINTS *(continued)*

- Adults aged 40 to 70 years who are overweight or obese should be screened for diabetes mellitus, according to the U.S. Preventive Services Task Force.
- The U.S. Preventive Services Task Force recommends that all persons aged 15 to 65 years receive one-time HIV screening regardless of risk.
- All women aged 50 to 74 years should undergo screening mammography; the recommended screening interval varies by expert group.
- Evidence has not demonstrated that any one recommended screening test for colorectal cancer provides a greater benefit than the others; therefore, the U.S. Preventive Services Task Force supports using the test that is most likely to result in screening completion.

# Genetics and Genetic Testing

## Taking a Family History

Obtaining a family history is an inexpensive and important risk assessment tool that allows clinicians to identify persons at increased risk for certain conditions. Up to 40% of genetic risk factors that would have otherwise been missed can be detected with a family history. Features that suggest the presence of a genetically inherited condition include earlier age of onset than expected for a common disease; two or more relatives with the same disorder, especially if the disorder is uncommon or known to be caused by a single gene mutation; and the presence of a disease in the less-often-afflicted sex, such as breast cancer in a man.

Agreement on the essential components of a family history is lacking; however, obtaining a complete three-generation family history is a reasonable approach. Although time consuming, documenting the history in the form of a family pedigree provides a helpful pictorial representation of the relationship between family members and the presence of medical conditions (**Figure 3**). Several easy-to-use family history tools are also available. The My Family Health Portrait tool (https://familyhistory.hhs.gov) can be self-administered and updated over time by patients.

## Genetic Tests and Testing Strategies

Understanding different types of genetic tests and testing strategies is helpful in ensuring that genetic testing is used effectively (**Table 16**). Prenatal genetic testing is performed during pregnancy to identify conditions in utero, such as Down syndrome. In adults, genetic testing is most commonly performed in persons with a family history suggestive of a genetically inherited condition. Presymptomatic or predictive genetic testing is performed to detect the presence of a genetic mutation before the onset of symptoms. The presence of some genetic mutations, such as the *HD* gene for Huntington disease, will invariably lead to disease development. With other

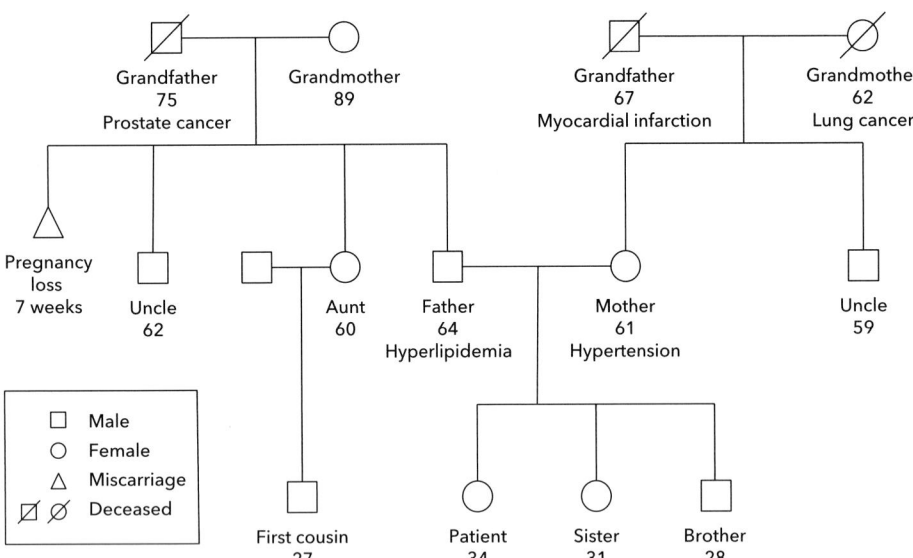

**FIGURE 3.** Example of a family history.

| TABLE 16. | Commonly Used Genetic Tests |
|---|---|
| **Type of Testing** | **Description** |
| Cytogenetic testing or karyotyping (Giemsa staining, in situ hybridization, microarray analysis) | Permits analysis of chromosomal structure<br><br>Giemsa staining produces banding pattern, allowing for gross structural analysis<br><br>In situ hybridization and microarray analysis allow for detection of more subtle abnormalities |
| Direct DNA testing (polymerase chain reaction analysis, Southern blot analysis) | Permits detection of specific genetic mutations |
| Indirect DNA testing (linkage analysis) | Useful when the genetic location for a condition is known but the genetic mutation is unknown |
| Biochemical testing | Involves measurement of metabolite levels to assess enzymatic activity |
| Whole exome sequencing | Useful when there is a clear family history of a genetic disorder based on pedigree but the affected gene is unknown |

genetic mutations, such as those involving the breast cancer susceptibility genes *BRCA1* and *BRCA2*, the risk for the disease is significantly increased, but not everyone with the mutation will develop disease. Diagnostic testing refers to genetic testing performed in those with a suspected genetic condition based on clinical features.

All patients for whom genetic testing is being considered should undergo genetic counseling. The basic components of genetic counseling are education on the condition being tested, including the natural history, possible treatments, and preventive measures; the risks and benefits of genetic testing;

alternatives to testing, including the option to forgo testing; and the implications for the patient and family members. Patients should be informed that the Genetic Information Nondiscrimination Act of 2008 protects against discrimination from obtaining employment and health insurance; however, this protection does not extend to discrimination involving other types of insurance, such as disability and life insurance. Clinicians can use a searchable database provided by the American College of Medical Genetics and Genomics (www.acmg.net/GIS) to locate a genetic counselor in their area.

## Pharmacogenetics

Pharmacogenetics is the study of how genetic differences lead to varying drug responses. Genetic testing for several common enzymes that affect drug metabolism, such as CYP2C19 and CYP2D6, are increasingly available. The CYP2C19 enzyme is involved in metabolizing the antiplatelet agent clopidogrel to its active form. Patients who have one or two copies of the reduced-function *CYP2C19* gene have an attenuated antiplatelet effect when taking clopidogrel, which may be associated with an increased risk for cardiovascular events. The CYP2D6 enzyme is responsible for converting codeine to its active metabolite, morphine. The presence of *CYP2D6* polymorphisms leads to variation in enzyme activity between individuals. Patients with high CYP2D6 activity may be subject to serious side effects of codeine, including respiratory depression and death, whereas patients with low CYP2D6 activity are unlikely to achieve adequate analgesia with codeine. The role of pharmacogenetic testing is unclear, and routine testing is not widespread at present.

## Direct-to-Consumer Genetic Testing

Direct-to-consumer (DTC) genomic testing is a commercial service that allows patients to obtain genetic information for a low cost. The FDA has approved DTC genetic testing for 10 disorders, including Parkinson disease and hemochromatosis, and physicians may be asked to provide guidance to persons who have undergone testing. DTC genomic testing typically estimates the risk for many common medical conditions by genotyping polymorphic nucleotides. Single-nucleotide polymorphisms (SNPs) that are disproportionately found in affected individuals are identified, and odds ratios for each SNP are determined. The SNPs are usually common but have low penetrance (that is, most people with an SNP do not develop disease). Individually, SNPs contribute very little to overall disease risk; most SNPs have an odds ratio of less than 1.5. As an example, if a condition has a general population prevalence of 8%, possessing an associated SNP with an odds ratio of 1.3 would increase one's risk for the condition to approximately 10%. Advocates of these services argue that they promote patient autonomy because patients can directly access information on genetic predispositions without physician referral. Critics counter that DTC testing is not usually accompanied by pre- or posttest genetic counseling, potentially leading to patient harms.

**KEY POINTS**

- Obtaining a three-generation family history is an inexpensive and important risk assessment tool that allows clinicians to identify persons at increased risk for certain conditions.

- Presymptomatic or predictive genetic testing is performed to detect the presence of a genetic mutation before the onset of symptoms, such as identification of the breast cancer susceptibility genes *BRCA1/2*; all patients for whom genetic testing is being considered should undergo genetic counseling.

HVC
- Direct-to-consumer genomic testing estimates the risk for many common medical conditions by genotyping polymorphic nucleotides; however, the identified single-nucleotide polymorphisms contribute very little to overall disease risk.

# Immunization

Immunization is a safe and cost-effective preventive health measure that is often underused in adult patients. In the United States, annual immunization recommendations are issued by the Advisory Committee on Immunization Practices (ACIP). ACIP recommendations can be accessed at https://www.cdc.gov/vaccines/acip.

It is important to adhere to recommended vaccine schedules as closely as possible. Administering doses at longer-than-recommended intervals does not appear to reduce immunologic response; however, doses should not be given at shorter-than-recommended intervals in order to allow for a complete immunologic response. If a vaccination series is interrupted, the series can be resumed at the point of interruption. Whenever possible, multiple vaccines should be given simultaneously to improve vaccination rates.

Vaccines can be safely administered to patients with mild acute febrile illness, during illness convalescence, and to patients who have previously developed low- or moderate-grade fever or local reactions with vaccination. Vaccines should be avoided if there is a history of anaphylaxis to the vaccine or the vaccine components. Contraindications to live vaccines are listed in **Table 17**.

## Vaccinations Recommended for All Adults
### Influenza
Influenza revaccination is necessary each year, owing to ongoing genetic changes in the influenza virus (antigenic drift). Annual vaccination is recommended for all individuals aged 6 months and older. The influenza vaccine should be administered as soon as it becomes available, preferably by October. The ACIP makes no preferential recommendation for one formulation over another, although use of the quadrivalent live attenuated influenza vaccine (LAIV4) was not recommended for the 2016 to 2018 influenza seasons as a result of poor efficacy against the H1N1 strain. A reformulated LAIV has received approval and a weak recommendation by the ACIP for the 2018 to 2019 influenza season. A high-dose, trivalent, inactivated formulation (IIV3-HD) is available for patients aged 65 years and older and is 24% more effective in preventing laboratory-confirmed influenza compared with its standard-dose counterpart.

Persons with a history of egg allergy of any severity can receive any influenza vaccine formulation; however, in persons who have had an egg-related reaction that caused symptoms other than hives, such as angioedema or respiratory distress, the vaccine should be administered by a provider trained in recognizing and managing severe allergic reactions.

### Tetanus, Diphtheria, and Pertussis
Primary vaccination against tetanus, diphtheria, and acellular pertussis consists of a five-dose vaccine series administered during childhood. Persons aged 11 to 18 years who have completed the primary series should receive a single dose of the tetanus toxoid, reduced diphtheria toxoid, and acellular pertussis (Tdap) vaccine. Adults aged 19 years and older should receive a tetanus and diphtheria toxoids (Td) booster every

| TABLE 17. | Contraindications to Administration of Live Vaccines |
|---|
| Pregnancy or probable pregnancy within 4 weeks |
| HIV with CD4 count ≤200/μL or CD4% ≤15% of total lymphocytes |
| Immunosuppressant therapy, including high-dose glucocorticoids (≥20 mg/d of prednisone or equivalent for ≥2 wk) |
| Leukemia, lymphoma, or other bone marrow and lymphatic system malignancies |
| Cellular immunodeficiency |
| Solid organ transplant recipient |
| Recent hematopoietic stem cell transplantation |

10 years. In adults who did not receive Tdap during adolescence, one of the 10-year Td booster doses should be replaced with a dose of the Tdap vaccine.

Unvaccinated adults should receive a three-dose series consisting of Td doses and at least one Tdap dose. Adults who have received fewer than three doses of the primary series should complete the series with the Td or Tdap (if not previously administered) vaccine.

Pregnant women should receive one dose of the Tdap vaccine between 27 weeks' and 36 weeks' gestation with every pregnancy, regardless of when the Td or Tdap vaccine was last administered.

## Vaccinations Recommended for Some Adults

### Varicella and Herpes Zoster

All immunocompetent adults without evidence of varicella immunity should receive two varicella vaccine doses. Evidence of varicella immunity includes laboratory-confirmed disease or immunity, diagnosis or verification of varicella or zoster by a provider, or documentation of age-appropriate varicella vaccination. U.S. birth before 1980 is also considered to be evidence of immunity, except in pregnant women and immunocompromised persons (who are at risk for severe disease) and health care workers (who are at risk for repeated varicella exposure and spreading the disease to those at high risk for severe disease). These patient groups must meet the other criteria for varicella immunity.

All adults aged 50 years and older, including those with a previous episode of zoster, should receive the recombinant (inactivated) herpes zoster vaccine to reduce the incidence of zoster and postherpetic neuralgia. The recombinant vaccine has demonstrated 97% efficacy in persons aged 50 to 69 years and 91% efficacy in those aged 70 years and older. It is recommended in preference to the live attenuated zoster vaccine, and adults who have been previously vaccinated with the live attenuated zoster vaccine should be revaccinated with the recombinant zoster vaccine after at least 8 weeks. The recombinant vaccine is administered intramuscularly in two doses, with an interval of 2 to 6 months between doses. The safety of the vaccine in pregnant women and patients with significant immunosuppression has not been determined. Healthy adults aged 60 years or older may receive either the recombinant vaccine (preferred) or the live attenuated vaccine. The live attenuated vaccine is administered subcutaneously in one dose.

### Pneumococcal Disease

Pneumococcal vaccination is recommended in all adults aged 65 years and older and adults aged 19 to 64 years with certain high-risk conditions (**Table 18**). Two pneumococcal vaccines are available: the 13-valent conjugate vaccine (PCV13) and the 23-valent polysaccharide vaccine (PPSV23). In a randomized controlled trial involving more than 80,000 persons aged 65 years and older, the efficacy of PCV13 was 75% against vaccine-type invasive disease and 46% against vaccine-type pneumonia. PPSV23 is 60% to 70% effective in preventing vaccine-type invasive disease, although its effect on noninvasive disease is unclear.

All adults aged 65 years and older who have not previously been vaccinated should receive PCV13, followed by a dose of PPSV23 1 year later. In immunocompetent adults aged 65 years and older who have already received a dose of PPSV23, PCV13 should be administered no sooner than 1 year later. In adults aged 19 to 64 years with high-risk conditions who require vaccination with both PCV13 and PPSV23 but who have not yet received either vaccine, a single dose of PCV13 should be given first, followed by a single dose of PPSV23 given at least 8 weeks later. Adults aged 19 to 64 years with high-risk conditions who require vaccination with both PCV13 and PPSV23 and who have already received PPSV23 should be administered a single dose of PCV13 no sooner than 1 year after receiving the most recent PPSV23. A second dose of PPSV23 should also be administered 5 years after the first PPSV23 dose in adults aged 19 to 64 years with certain immunocompromising conditions (see Table 18).

### Human Papillomavirus

HPV vaccination prevents persistent HPV infection, which can lead to cervical, anogenital, and nasopharyngeal cancers. Bivalent, quadrivalent, and nine-valent HPV vaccines are approved for use in females; quadrivalent and nine-valent vaccines are approved for use in males. Females should be administered the vaccine series at age 11 or 12 years or between the ages of 13 and 26 years if not given previously. In males, the series should be administered at age 11 or 12 years, between the ages of 13 and 21 years if not previously administered, or through age 26 years for immunocompromised men (including those with HIV infection) and men who have sex with men. If administered before the age of 15 years, a two-dose series is recommended, whereas a three-dose series is recommended in older individuals. Vaccination is not recommended during pregnancy, although no harmful effects have been noted when inadvertently given to pregnant women.

### Measles, Mumps, and Rubella

All U.S. adults born before 1957 are considered to be immune to measles and mumps. Adults born in 1957 or later without documented evidence of receiving one or more doses of the measles, mumps, and rubella (MMR) vaccine or laboratory-confirmed immunity against all three diseases should receive at least one MMR dose. A second MMR dose should be administered to postsecondary students, health care workers, and international travelers. For persons who have been previously vaccinated with two doses of a mumps virus–containing vaccine but are at increased risk because of an outbreak, the ACIP recommends administering a third dose of mumps virus–containing vaccine to improve protection.

In women of childbearing age, it is necessary to determine rubella immunity. Nonpregnant women who lack immunity should be vaccinated. Pregnant women who lack

**TABLE 18.** Pneumococcal Vaccination Recommendations for Adults Aged 19 Years and Older With Underlying Medical Conditions

| Risk Group | Underlying Medical Condition | PCV13 Recommended | PPSV23 Recommended | PPSV23 Revaccination at 5 Years After First Dose |
|---|---|---|---|---|
| Immunocompetent persons | Chronic heart disease[a] | | X | |
| | Chronic lung disease[b] | | X | |
| | Diabetes mellitus | | X | |
| | CSF leaks | X | X | |
| | Cochlear implants | X | X | |
| | Alcoholism | | X | |
| | Chronic liver disease | | X | |
| | Cigarette smoking | | X | |
| Persons with functional or anatomic asplenia | Sickle cell disease/other hemoglobinopathies | X | X | X |
| | Congenital or acquired asplenia | X | X | X |
| Immunocompromised persons | Congenital or acquired immunodeficiencies[c] | X | X | X |
| | HIV infection | X | X | X |
| | Chronic kidney failure | X | X | X |
| | Nephrotic syndrome | X | X | X |
| | Leukemia | X | X | X |
| | Lymphoma | X | X | X |
| | Hodgkin lymphoma | X | X | X |
| | Generalized malignancy | X | X | X |
| | Iatrogenic immunosuppression[d] | X | X | X |
| | Solid-organ transplant | X | X | X |
| | Multiple myeloma | X | X | X |

CSF = cerebrospinal fluid; PCV13 = 13-valent pneumococcal conjugate vaccine; PPSV23 = 23-valent pneumococcal polysaccharide vaccine.

[a]Including heart failure and cardiomyopathies.

[b]Including COPD, emphysema, and asthma.

[c]Including B- (humoral) or T-lymphocyte deficiency, complement deficiencies (particularly C1, C2, C3, and C4 deficiencies), and phagocytic disorders (excluding chronic granulomatous disease).

[d]Diseases requiring treatment with immunosuppressive drugs, including long-term systemic glucocorticoids and radiation therapy.

Adapted from Centers for Disease Control and Prevention (CDC). Use of 13-valent pneumococcal conjugate vaccine and 23-valent pneumococcal polysaccharide vaccine for adults with immunocompromising conditions: recommendations of the Advisory Committee on Immunization Practices (ACIP). MMWR Morb Mortal Wkly Rep. 2012 Oct 12;61(40):816-9. [PMID: 23051612]

immunity should be vaccinated at the time of delivery before leaving the hospital or at the time of pregnancy termination.

The MMR vaccine is a live virus vaccine and should not be administered to immunocompromised individuals.

## Meningococcal Disease
Meningococcal vaccines used in the adult population include the quadrivalent meningococcal conjugate vaccine (MenACWY), which protects against serogroups A, C, W135, and Y, and the MenB vaccine, which protects against serogroup B disease. The quadrivalent conjugate vaccine is used in most patients, whereas the MenB vaccine is reserved for specific high-risk situations.

Indications for meningococcal vaccination in adults are summarized in **Table 19**.

## Hepatitis A
Vaccination against hepatitis A is recommended for all persons who desire vaccination and for persons who are at increased risk for infection or complications of infection. Persons at increased risk include those who work in or travel to endemic areas, men who have sex with men, individuals with chronic liver disease, illicit drug users, persons with clotting disorders, persons who conduct hepatitis A–related research, and household or close contacts of children adopted from endemic areas.

| TABLE 19. | Indications for Meningococcal Vaccination in Adults |
|---|---|
| **Vaccine** | **Indicated Populations** |
| Quadrivalent meningococcal conjugate vaccine (MenACWY) | |
| Single dose[a] | First-year college students living in a dormitory |
| | Travelers to endemic areas |
| | Microbiologists exposed to *Neisseria meningitidis* |
| | Military recruits |
| | Adults at increased risk because of serogroup A, C, W, or Y meningococcal outbreak |
| Two-dose primary series[b] | Adults with anatomic or functional asplenia |
| | Adults with persistent complement component deficiencies (C5-C9, factor H, factor D, properdin, or patients taking eculizumab) |
| | Adults with HIV infection |
| Serogroup B meningococcal vaccine (MenB)[c,d] | Adults with persistent complement component deficiencies (C5-C9, factor H, factor D, properdin, or patients taking eculizumab) |
| | Adults with functional or anatomic asplenia |
| | Microbiologists exposed to *Neisseria meningitidis* |
| | Adults at increased risk because of serogroup B meningococcal outbreak |
| | May be administered to patients aged 16-23 years for short-term protection, preferably between age 16 and 18 years |

[a]A single dose should be administered unless the patient has been vaccinated with MenACWY within the past 5 years. If exposure is ongoing, revaccination is indicated every 5 years.

[b]Doses should be administered 8-12 weeks apart, followed by a booster dose every 5 years.

[c]MenB vaccine is approved for use in persons aged ≥10 years.

[d]Persons who are considered to be at increased risk for infection should be given three separate doses at 0, 1-2, and 6 months. If the second dose is administered at >6 months, a third dose is not necessary.

## Hepatitis B

Hepatitis B vaccination is recommended for any nonimmune adult who desires vaccination or who is considered to be at high risk for infection (**Table 20**). The typical hepatitis B vaccination series is a three-dose series, with doses administered at 0, 1, and 6 months. In adults aged 40 years and younger, 30% to 55% of patients will mount a protective antibody response after being administered one dose, 75% after the second dose, and more than 90% after the third dose. Older adults and patients undergoing hemodialysis have lower protective antibody response rates. A newer vaccine with a novel adjuvant, which was released in 2017 and endorsed by the ACIP in 2018, requires only two doses over a 1-month period and appears to be more immunogenic than previous vaccines.

Checking serum antibodies is not typically recommended after routine vaccination but is indicated in persons in whom subsequent clinical management is dependent upon knowledge of serologic response (chronic hemodialysis patients, persons with HIV, health care and public safety workers, and needle-sharing partners of persons with positive hepatitis B surface antigen).

## Vaccinations Recommended for Specific Populations

Health care workers (HCWs) are at increased risk for acquiring and transmitting hepatitis B, influenza, measles, mumps,

| TABLE 20. | Populations With an Indication for Hepatitis B Vaccination |
|---|
| Any nonimmune adult desiring vaccination |
| Sexually active persons who are not in a monogamous relationship (any person with more than one sexual partner within the past 6 months) |
| Sexual partners of persons who are HBsAg positive |
| Persons seeking evaluation or treatment for sexually transmitted infection |
| Men who have sex with men |
| Household contacts of persons who are HBsAg positive |
| Residents and staff members of institutions for persons who are developmentally disabled |
| Current or recent injection drug users |
| Health care and public safety workers with anticipated risk for exposure |
| Persons with end-stage kidney disease, including those receiving hemodialysis and peritoneal dialysis |
| International travelers to regions with intermediate or high levels of endemic hepatitis B infection |
| Persons with chronic liver disease |
| Persons with HIV infection |

HBsAg = hepatitis B surface antigen.

rubella, pertussis, and varicella viruses. All HCWs, regardless of patient contact, should receive the influenza vaccine annually. HCWs without immunity should be vaccinated against hepatitis B; measles, mumps, and rubella; and varicella. Additionally, all HCWs who have not previously received the Tdap vaccine should receive one dose, irrespective of when they last received the Td vaccine.

Patients with anatomic or functional asplenia are at increased risk for infection from encapsulated organisms, such as *Haemophilus influenzae* type B, meningococcus, and pneumococcus, and should be appropriately vaccinated.

Vaccination recommendations for international travelers vary depending on the destination. Trip-specific recommendations from the CDC can be accessed at https://wwwnc.cdc.gov/travel. For more information on vaccination in travelers, see MKSAP 18 Infectious Disease, Travel Medicine.

**KEY POINTS**

- Annual influenza vaccination is recommended for all individuals aged 6 months and older.

- Pregnant women should receive one dose of the tetanus toxoid, reduced diphtheria toxoid, and acellular pertussis (Tdap) vaccine during each pregnancy between 27 weeks' and 36 weeks' gestation.

HVC
- All adults aged 50 years and older should receive the recombinant (inactivated) herpes zoster vaccine, regardless of previous immunization or clinical infection, to reduce the incidence of zoster and postherpetic neuralgia.

- Pneumococcal vaccination is recommended in all adults aged 65 years and older and adults aged 19 to 64 years with certain high-risk conditions.

- Patients with anatomic or functional asplenia should be vaccinated against *Haemophilus influenzae* type B, meningococcal, and pneumococcal diseases.

# Aspirin as Primary Prevention

Aspirin therapy for primary prevention is a continually debated and constantly evolving topic. The decision to initiate low-dose aspirin for primary prevention of ASCVD and colorectal cancer is predominantly based on weighing the benefits of prevention with the harms of increased bleeding. Factors that increase bleeding risk include concurrent anticoagulant or NSAID use, history of gastrointestinal ulcer, upper gastrointestinal pain, uncontrolled hypertension, male sex, and increasing age. Other factors, such as patient preferences on taking aspirin, may also shift the balance.

Aspirin has been found to reduce nonfatal myocardial infarction (relative risk [RR], 0.78; 95% CI, 0.71-0.87) but not nonfatal stroke, cardiovascular mortality, or all-cause mortality. The benefits of ASCVD prevention are apparent within the first 5 years of therapy and continue for as long as aspirin is taken. The evidence for cancer prevention is stronger, with a 34% to 40% reduction in colorectal cancer mortality with at least 5 to 10 years of aspirin therapy. The benefit is not apparent until 10 to 20 years after initiation of aspirin; no mortality benefit was observed in the first 10 years of follow-up. Therefore, adults older than 60 years are less likely to experience these benefits.

The USPSTF recommends low-dose aspirin for the primary prevention of ASCVD and colorectal cancer in adults aged 50 to 59 years with a 10-year ASCVD risk of 10% or higher who do not have an increased risk for bleeding, have a life expectancy of at least 10 years, and are willing to take low-dose aspirin daily for at least 10 years (grade B). ASCVD risk can be calculated by using the American College of Cardiology/American Heart Association risk calculator based on the Pooled Cohort Equations, available at http://tools.acc.org/ASCVD-Risk-Estimator/. In those aged 60 to 69 years with a 10-year ASCVD risk of 10% or higher, the benefits of aspirin use for primary prevention are smaller but still outweigh the risk for bleeding; the decision to initiate low-dose aspirin in this population should be individualized (grade C). Owing to limited evidence, the USPSTF does not make a recommendation on aspirin use for primary prevention in persons younger than 50 years and older than 70 years (I statement).

In contrast to the USPSTF, the American Diabetes Association and American Heart Association suggest low-dose aspirin for primary prevention in adults with diabetes with a 10-year ASCVD risk greater than 10% who are not at increased risk for bleeding. Low-dose aspirin therapy may be considered in patients with diabetes and intermediate risk for ASCVD (10-year risk, 5%-10%). Notably, the European Society of Cardiology does not recommend any antiplatelet therapy for individuals without ASCVD because of the increased risk for bleeding and lack of convincing data on cardiovascular mortality benefit.

For patients in whom the balance of benefits and harms is unclear, the Aspirin Guide, a clinical decision making support tool available online (www.aspiringuide.com) and as a mobile application, may offer guidance. The Aspirin Guide uses internal algorithms to calculate the patient's ASCVD risk and bleeding risk as well as the NNT with aspirin to prevent one ASCVD event and the number needed to harm (NNH) to cause one excess bleeding event due to aspirin. The tool has not yet been validated in clinical trials and does not include NNT for cancer prevention. In general, the Aspirin Guide advises initiating low-dose aspirin if the NNT is less than the NNH; however, clinical judgment is warranted.

**KEY POINT**

- The U.S. Preventive Services Task Force recommends aspirin for primary prevention of atherosclerotic cardiovascular disease (ASCVD) and colorectal cancer in adults aged 50 to 59 years with a 10-year ASCVD risk of 10% or greater who do not have an increased risk for bleeding, have a life expectancy of at least 10 years, and are willing to take low-dose aspirin daily for at least 10 years.

# Healthy Lifestyle Counseling

Healthy lifestyle counseling is directed at the leading preventable causes of death. More than one third of preventable deaths are attributable to tobacco use and obesity and the resulting increased risks for cancer and cardiovascular disease. Other preventable causes of death include alcohol use, infectious diseases, toxins, accidents, deaths from firearms, and drug use.

Tobacco cessation is a high priority health intervention from a health and cost-effectiveness standpoint. Smokers should be offered pharmacologic therapy and behavioral interventions (see Mental and Behavioral Health).

All overweight and obese patients should undergo counseling on the benefits of a healthy weight, regular exercise, and a healthy diet (see Behavioral Counseling).

Injury prevention, including seat belt use, use of safety helmets for motorcycles and bicycles, and home safety measures (such as weapons safety), should be emphasized. Patients should be counseled to use smoke alarms in the home and to set water heaters to lower than 49 °C (120 °F). The "5 Ls" may be used for firearm safety counseling; they involve asking the following questions regarding a firearm in the home:

- Is it Locked?
- Is it Loaded?
- Are there Little children present?
- Anyone feeling Low in the house?
- Is the operator Learned about firearm safety?

Sleep and stress reduction are also components of a healthy lifestyle. The American Heart Association and the American Academy of Sleep Medicine recommend that adults obtain at least 7 hours of sleep per night for optimal health. Stress reduction, development of strong social ties, and community involvement are also associated with better health outcomes.

Even small changes at the population level, such as improving social determinants of health, can create large preventive benefits. Healthy People 2020 is a CDC initiative with the goal of creating social and physical environments that promote good health. Using strategies from behavioral economics, such as making healthy choices the default option or nudging (gently steering people in a certain direction), may help improve health outcomes. Pricing and taxation strategies and food stamp programs can help promote the purchase of fruits and vegetables and inhibit the purchase of unhealthy processed foods. Making neighborhoods and cities safer and improving bicycle lanes, walking paths, and stairs may encourage physical activity and reduce inequalities in health.

Climate change could cause numerous deleterious effects on human health, including higher rates of respiratory and heat-related illness, increased prevalence of vector-borne (malaria, chikungunya, dengue fever) and waterborne (cholera) diseases, food and water insecurity, and malnutrition. The ACP advises that physicians become educated about climate change, its effect on human health, and how to respond to future challenges.

## Behavioral Counseling

For adults who are overweight or obese and have additional risk factors for cardiovascular disease (hypertension, dyslipidemia, impaired fasting glucose/diabetes), the USPSTF recommends offering or referral to intensive behavioral counseling interventions to promote a healthful diet and physical activity (grade B). Because the benefit of behavioral counseling is small in adults who do not meet these criteria, the USPSTF recommends an individualized approach to offering or referring these patients to behavioral counseling to promote a healthy lifestyle (grade C). Strategies such as motivational interviewing and setting specific and attainable goals can help facilitate lifestyle changes. Using a multidisciplinary team of health care professionals (dieticians, nurses, and psychologists) can be helpful when available.

Behavioral counseling does not need to be complex or time consuming. An analysis of more than 5000 patients who participated in the National Health and Nutritional Examination Survey found that patients who were informed that they were overweight by their physicians were more likely to report significant weight loss, although it has been shown that overweight and obesity are commonly unmentioned and undiagnosed. Advising patients to maintain a healthy weight and adopt healthy practices, including eliminating sugar-containing beverages, implementing a reduced-calorie diet, avoiding processed foods, and practicing mindful eating can be beneficial. Providers may also help patients by modeling healthy behaviors; evidence shows that doctors who improve their health habits may be better able to counsel their patients regarding preventive and healthful behaviors.

## Diet and Physical Activity

Adults who adhere to a healthful diet and engage in regular physical activity have lower cardiovascular mortality and may have improved cognitive function and decreased disability. Dietary guidelines from the U.S. Department of Health and Human Services recommend following a healthy eating pattern that consists of vegetables, whole fruits, whole grains, low-fat dairy, protein (poultry, fish, legumes), and oils (including nuts), while limiting consumption of added sugars, saturated and *trans* fats, and sodium. Adults of legal drinking age should be advised to limit consumption of alcohol to no more than one drink per day for women and two drinks per day for men.

Adults should perform at least 150 minutes of moderate-intensity physical activity per week or 75 minutes of vigorous-intensity physical activity per week. For increased benefit, 300 minutes of moderate-intensity activity or 150 minutes of vigorous-intensity activity is recommended. Muscle-strengthening activities (resistance training and weight lifting) are also beneficial, and adults should perform moderate- or high-intensity muscle-strengthening activities that involve all major muscle groups 2 or more days per week. It is important to note that any physical activity is better than no activity. Physical activity need not be formal exercise; incorporating natural movement into the day offers some health benefits.

**KEY POINTS**

- For adults who are overweight or obese and have additional risk factors for cardiovascular disease, the U.S. Preventive Services Task Force recommends offering or referral to intensive behavioral counseling interventions to promote healthful diet and physical activity.
- Dietary guidelines from the U.S. Department of Health and Human Services recommend following a healthy eating pattern that consists of vegetables, whole fruits, whole grains, low-fat dairy, protein, and oils, while limiting consumption of added sugars, saturated and *trans* fats, and sodium.

## Supplements and Herbal Therapies

Dietary supplements, including vitamins, minerals, botanicals, herbals, metabolites, and amino acids, are categorized as foods by the FDA and are therefore not subject to the same regulations as over-the-counter and prescription drugs. Manufacturers are not required to demonstrate efficacy or safety unless the supplement includes ingredients that were introduced after 1994. Manufacturers are also not allowed to make specific medical claims; however, the product's purported effect on body structure or function may be described.

Patients take dietary supplements for various reasons, such as to prevent illness, enhance health, and correct perceived deficiencies. In the United States, approximately 50% of adults report using vitamins or dietary supplements, with total consumer spending of more than $20 billion each year.

Despite their prevalent use, the USPSTF does not recommend multivitamins or herbal supplements for the prevention of cardiovascular disease or cancer. The USPSTF also concludes that there is insufficient evidence for use of vitamin D and calcium to prevent fractures. Evidence has shown that supplementation with vitamin D and calcium together increases the incidence of kidney stones. Multivitamins should not be used in the absence of a specific indication and are not effective in compensating for a poor diet. Smokers should avoid β-carotene altogether, as evidence has linked β-carotene with increased risk for lung cancer.

There are several populations for which vitamin or supplement use is strongly recommended. Women of childbearing age are advised to take 0.4 to 0.8 mg (400 to 800 μg) of folic acid daily to prevent fetal neural tube defects. Vegans and older adults may consider vitamin B$_{12}$ supplementation to address dietary deficiency.

In addition to questionable efficacy, supplement use is associated with risk for both direct and indirect harms. Direct harms include side effects, interactions with other drugs, and harms related to inclusion of unadvertised additives, compounds, or

toxins. Many supplements, such as St. John's wort, affect the cytochrome P450 system, which may affect warfarin and antidepressant metabolism. *Ginkgo biloba*, ginseng, garlic, vitamin E, and fish oil may interact with anticoagulant or antiplatelet medications, potentially causing increased risk for bleeding or inadequate anticoagulation. Harms may also occur indirectly when herbal supplement use replaces or delays standard treatments.

Despite these risks, many patients strongly believe in supplement use, and the role of the physician is to inform these patients of harmful supplements and suggest safer alternatives (**Table 21**). The National Institute of Health's MedlinePlus directory of herbs and supplements (https://medlineplus.gov/druginfo/herb_All.html) and Nutrition.gov (https://www.nutrition.gov/dietary-supplements) are useful resources.

**KEY POINTS**

- Manufacturers of dietary supplements are not required to demonstrate efficacy or safety unless the supplement includes ingredients that were introduced after 1994.
- The U.S. Preventive Services Task Force does not recommend multivitamins or herbal supplements for the prevention of cardiovascular disease or cancer. **HVC**

# Patient Safety and Quality Improvement

## Introduction

Patient safety is defined by the World Health Organization as the prevention of errors and adverse events related to medical care. Although it is a necessary component of high-quality health care, integrating safety into medical practice is a complex process that requires involvement and action at both the clinician and systems levels. Importantly, health care systems must be built on a culture of safety and structured to prevent errors, empower individuals to promote safety, and recognize and respond to errors that occur.

Quality in health care refers to the extent to which the clinician or organization meets or exceeds the needs and expectations of patients. Quality improvement involves the systematic and continuous implementation of changes that measurably improve patient care. Because quality improvement is based on the understanding that it is easier to improve that which can be measured, quality improvement usually entails ongoing monitoring and assessment.

## Patient Safety and Quality Issues at the Clinician Level

Common patient safety and quality issues that occur at the clinician level include diagnostic errors, medication errors, and errors occurring during transitions of care.

| TABLE 21. | Common Herbal Supplements | | | |
|---|---|---|---|---|
| **Name** | **Common Uses** | **Effectiveness** | **Adverse Effects** | **Important Drug Interactions** |
| Black cohosh | Treatment of menopausal hot flashes | Likely effective, low-quality evidence | Possible estrogenic effect on breast<br><br>Avoid in women with estrogen receptor–positive breast cancer<br><br>Reports of hepatotoxicity | |
| Cranberry | Prevention of urinary tract infections | Likely ineffective, low-quality evidence | Increased glucose intake with juice, GI upset | |
| *Echinacea* | Prevention of common colds | Small effect | GI upset, nausea, allergic reactions | |
| | Treatment of common colds | Not effective | | |
| Evening primrose oil | Treatment of breast pain | Mixed data on effectiveness | GI upset, headache<br><br>May increase risk for pregnancy complications | May increase bleeding if used with warfarin |
| | Treatment of eczema | Not effective | | |
| | Treatment of diabetic neuropathy | Possibly effective | | |
| Garlic | Treatment of high cholesterol | Not effective | Increased bleeding risk, breath and body odor, heartburn | May decrease effectiveness of isoniazid and saquinavir<br><br>May increase bleeding if used with warfarin, likely due to antiplatelet effect |
| | Treatment of hypertension | Possibly effective, weak evidence | | |
| Ginger | Treatment of nausea | Likely effective for pregnancy-related and chemotherapy-related nausea | Increased bleeding | May increase risk for bleeding when used with anticoagulants |
| | Treatment of inflammation | Possibly effective | | |
| *Ginkgo biloba* | Treatment and prevention of cognitive decline | Not effective | Headache, GI upset, allergic skin reactions, increased risk for bleeding | May increase risk for bleeding when used with anticoagulants and NSAIDs; potentiates MAOIs |
| | Treatment of claudication | Not effective | | |
| Kava | Treatment of anxiety | Likely effective | Hepatotoxicity<br><br>Use with caution in patients with liver disease or at risk for liver disease | |
| Milk thistle | Reduction in liver inflammation | Not effective | Nausea, indigestion, diarrhea | May interact with medications metabolized by CYP2C9 |
| Red yeast rice (contains monacolin K, identical active ingredient to lovastatin) | Treatment of hyperlipidemia | Likely effective; risks likely outweigh benefits | Myalgia, liver function abnormalities<br><br>Some may contain citrinin (a harmful contaminant), which can cause kidney failure | May interact with medications metabolized by CYP3A4 enzymes |
| Saw palmetto | Treatment of benign prostatic hyperplasia | Likely not effective | Headache, nausea, dizziness<br><br>Contraindicated in pregnancy and lactation | |
| Soy (isoflavones) | Treatment of menopausal symptoms | Likely effective, low-quality evidence | GI upset, allergic reaction<br><br>Avoid high doses in patients with breast cancer | |

*(Continued on the next page)*

| TABLE 21. | Common Herbal Supplements *(Continued)* | | | |
|---|---|---|---|---|
| Name | Common Uses | Effectiveness | Adverse Effects | Important Drug Interactions |
| St. John's wort | Treatment of depression | Mixed data on effectiveness | GI upset, fatigue, headache, dizziness | Inducer of CYP3A4 and CYP2C9 enzymes<br><br>Many interactions<br><br>Do not use with antidepressants |
| Valerian | Treatment of anxiety | Not effective | Tremor, headache, sedation, hepatotoxicity | |
| | Treatment of sleep disorders, insomnia | Inconclusive | | |

CYP2C9 = cytochrome P-450 2C9; CYP3A4 = cytochrome P-450 3A4; GI = gastrointestinal; MAOIs = monoamine oxidase inhibitors.

## Diagnostic Errors

CONT.

A diagnostic error occurs when a patient is not provided with a timely and correct diagnosis or the diagnosis is not communicated to the patient. More specifically, a diagnostic error is present when there was a missed opportunity to make the correct diagnosis in a timely manner. The rate of diagnostic error is approximately 10%, and most patients will be subject to a diagnostic error at some point in their lifetime. Diagnostic errors are also the leading cause of malpractice claims against internists.

Diagnostic errors are usually multifactorial in etiology, with flawed cognitive processes on the part of the clinician and issues at the systems level contributing to most errors. Examples of cognitive errors include premature closure, diagnostic momentum, confirmation bias, and faulty knowledge or knowledge application. Premature closure involves accepting a diagnosis and discontinuing the diagnostic process before the data necessary to establish the diagnosis have been obtained. Diagnostic momentum is a similar phenomenon in which a diagnosis is suggested early in the diagnostic process, and the diagnostic evaluation continues to move toward this diagnosis even if the data do not support it. Confirmation bias, the predisposition to seek evidence to confirm a suspected diagnosis without looking for evidence that disproves it, is a common feature of premature closure and diagnostic momentum. Faulty application of knowledge occurs when the clinician does not possess the underlying knowledge necessary to make the diagnosis or does not apply the knowledge properly.

Systems factors common to diagnostic error include poor communication, lack of test availability, and productivity pressures. Poor communication of crucial laboratory and imaging results (for example, the incidental finding of a pulmonary nodule) may result in delayed diagnosis and patient harm. Similarly, lack of test availability (such as advanced imaging in resource-poor environments) may result in delayed diagnoses. Productivity pressures and their effect on clinician time with patients may also contribute to diagnostic errors. **Table 22** provides techniques for avoiding some common diagnostic errors.

## Medication Errors

Medication errors can occur from the time of prescription to the time of administration and may or may not result in patient harm. Medication errors are often caused by prescribing faults (inappropriate prescribing, underprescribing, or overprescribing) or prescription errors (errors in drug dose, route of administration, frequency of use, or duration of therapy; duplicative orders; prescription of drugs that interact; or prescription to the incorrect patient). In contrast, an adverse drug event is harm experienced by a patient as a result of exposure to a medication. Adverse drug events, which account for 100,000 hospitalizations in the United States each year, may be secondary to an accepted risk of a medication or may be the result of a medication error.

There are several known risk factors for medication errors. Polypharmacy, advanced patient age, and impaired kidney or liver function are patient-specific factors that increase the risk for medication errors. Clinician-specific risk factors include illegible handwriting and use of nonstandard abbreviations. Errors are also more likely to occur with the use of specific drugs, including those with look-alike or sound-alike names.

Measures to reduce medication errors include computerized physician order entry (CPOE) systems, medication reconciliation, improved labeling for medications with similar names, and barcode-assisted medication administration. The Institute for Healthcare Improvement (www.ihi.org) and the Institute for Safe Medication Practices (www.ismp.org/tools) have issued tools and resources to reduce harms related to medications. In addition, the Agency for Healthcare Research and Quality (AHRQ) has developed several strategies to prevent adverse drug events (**Table 23**).

## Transitions of Care

Patient transitions between inpatient and outpatient settings, institutions, or hospital units present unique challenges to patient safety. A medication error occurs in almost 50% of patients at the time of hospital admission and is the most common form of postdischarge adverse event. The risk for diagnostic error at the time of hospital discharge is similarly high, as almost 40% of patients have test results pending or require

| TABLE 22. | Twelve Tips for Avoiding Diagnostic Errors |
|---|---|
| **Technique** | **Comments** |
| 1. Understand heuristics[a] | Availability heuristic: Diagnosing based on what is most easily available in the physician's memory (e.g., because of a patient recently seen) rather than what is most probable |
| | Anchoring heuristic: Settling on a diagnosis early in the diagnostic process despite data that refute the diagnosis or support another diagnosis (premature closure) |
| | Representativeness heuristic: Application of pattern recognition (a patient's presentation fits a "typical" case; therefore, it must be that case) |
| 2. Use "diagnostic timeouts" | Taking time to periodically review a case based on data but without assuming that the diagnosis is that which was previously reached |
| 3. Practice "worst-case scenario medicine" | Consider the most life-threatening diagnoses first: <br> • Lessens chance of missing these diagnoses <br> • Does not mandate testing for them |
| 4. Use systematic approach to common problems | For example, anatomic approach to abdominal pain beginning from exterior to interior |
| 5. Ask why | For example, when a patient presents with diabetic ketoacidosis or a COPD exacerbation, ask what prompted this acute exacerbation of a chronic condition |
| 6. Use the clinical examination | Decreases reliance on a single test and decreases chance of premature closure |
| 7. Use Bayes theorem | Use pre- and posttest probabilities <br> • Helps avert premature closure based on a single test result |
| 8. Acknowledge the effect of the patient | How does the patient make the physician feel? <br> • Physicians may avoid making unfavorable diagnoses in patients with whom they identify <br> • Physicians may discount important data in patients with whom they have difficult encounters |
| 9. Look for clinical findings that do not fit the diagnosis | Encourages a comprehensive approach and incorporates healthy skepticism |
| 10. Consider "zebras" | Resist temptation to lock onto common diagnoses at risk of missing the uncommon |
| 11. Slow down and reflect | Difficult to do in most health care systems, which stress the economy of "getting it right the first time" |
| 12. Admit mistakes | Awareness of one's own fallibility may lead to fewer diagnostic errors later |

[a]Heuristics are shortcuts in reasoning used in discovery, learning, or problem solving.

Information from Trowbridge RL. Twelve tips for teaching avoidance of diagnostic errors. Med Teach. 2008;30:496-500. [PMID: 18576188] doi:10.1080/01421590801965137

CONT.

completion of a diagnostic evaluation as an outpatient. Furthermore, almost one fifth of discharged Medicare patients are rehospitalized within 30 days of discharge; at least 25% of these readmissions are potentially preventable.

Medication reconciliation, predischarge patient education, and timely scheduling of posthospitalization appointments can improve safety during care transitions. Medication reconciliation entails creating an accurate, comprehensive list of the patient's prescription and nonprescription medications (including the dosage, frequency, and route of administration) and comparing the list to medication orders (at admission, transfer, or discharge) to resolve inconsistencies. Completion of medication reconciliation has been shown to decrease adverse drug events, and although the effect on hospital readmissions is less clear, medication reconciliation should occur at all care transitions to prevent medication errors. The Institute for Healthcare Improvement has published a guide to implementing medication reconciliation and measuring improvement, available at www.ihi.org/Topics/ADEsMedicationReconciliation.

Detailed communication between the hospital discharge and receiving teams is also recommended to promote patient safety. A discharge summary that includes the evaluations performed, medication reconciliation, pending test results, required follow-up tests, and follow-up appointments is an important tool in the communication between the hospital and the follow-up physician. A meta-analysis, however, revealed that crucial information on pending test results and required follow-up testing is omitted from up to two thirds of discharge summaries, and only one third of summaries are received by the accepting outpatient clinician by the time of the initial posthospitalization visit. █

### KEY POINTS

- Diagnostic error is a common cause of patient harm and is usually the result of a combination of cognitive and systems errors.

- Measures to reduce medication errors include computerized physician order entry systems, medication reconciliation, improved labeling for medications with similar names, and barcode-assisted medication administration.

HVC

*(Continued)*

**TABLE 23.** Strategies to Prevent Adverse Drug Events

| Stage | Safety Strategy |
|---|---|
| Prescribing | Avoid unnecessary medications by adhering to conservative prescribing principles |
| | Use computerized provider order entry, especially when paired with clinical decision support systems |
| | Perform medication reconciliation at times of transitions in care |
| Transcribing | Use computerized provider order entry to eliminate handwriting errors |
| Dispensing | Have clinical pharmacists oversee the medication dispensing process |
| | Use "tall man" lettering and other strategies to minimize confusion between look-alike, sound-alike medications (for example, **DOP**amine and **DOBUT**amine) |
| Administration | Adhere to the "five rights" of medication safety (administering the right medication, in the right dose, at the right time, by the right route, to the right patient) |
| | Use barcode medication administration to ensure medications are given to the correct patient |
| | Minimize interruptions to allow nurses to administer medications safely |
| | Use smart infusion pumps for intravenous infusions |
| | Use patient education and revised medication labels to improve patient comprehension of administration instructions |

Adapted from Agency for Healthcare Research and Quality. Patient safety primer: medication errors. https://psnet.ahrq.gov/primers/primer/23/medication-errors. Updated June 2017. Accessed June 27, 2018.

**KEY POINTS** (continued)

**HVC**
- A discharge summary that includes the evaluations performed, medication reconciliation, pending test results, required follow-up tests, and follow-up appointments is an important tool in the communication between the hospital and the follow-up physician.

# Patient Safety and Quality Issues at the Systems Level

Diagnostic errors, medication errors, and communication errors (especially errors associated with care transitions) are among the many patient safety issues that require systems-level interventions to effect improvement. Similarly, improvement of many quality measures (such as readmission rates, health care–associated infections, and appropriate treatment) largely depends on systems-level changes. Individual clinicians play an important role in systems-level quality and safety programs by identifying areas in need of improvement and participating in improvement activities.

## Quality Improvement Models

Successful quality improvement programs include the following components: (1) a health care delivery system with resources (people, information, technology), processes (what is done and how it is done), and outcomes (change in health behavior, patient satisfaction); (2) the objective of meeting the needs and expectations of the patient; (3) a team-based interprofessional approach; and (4) outcome assessment using both qualitative and quantitative data. Several different quality improvement models are used in the health care setting; these models focus on identifying, measuring, and correcting areas that need improvement.

### Model for Improvement

The Model for Improvement focuses on achieving specific and measurable results in a specified population. This model relies on identifying a goal to be accomplished with a change, determining how the results of a change will be measured, and deciding on the changes that will bring about an improvement. These changes are tested and implemented by using a Plan-Do-Study-Act (PDSA) cycle. PDSA cycles are rapid tests of improvement, and additional PDSA cycles are completed until the desired results are achieved. A medical center, for example, may set the specific goal of decreasing central line–associated bloodstream infections and use a PDSA cycle to rapidly implement and assess the impact of changes, such as using a central line bundle.

### Lean

The Lean model aims to maximize value and minimize waste by closely examining a system's processes and eliminating non–value-added activities within the system. Value stream mapping can be used to graphically display the steps of a process and the time required for each step, thereby highlighting process inefficiencies or areas of waste and allowing for their improvement. Lean also uses a 5S strategy (Sort, Shine, Straighten, Systemize, and Sustain) to create an organized workplace. Lean, for example, may be used to improve the time used to obtain, submit, analyze, and report the results of a laboratory test.

### Six Sigma

Six Sigma is a quality improvement model that improves processes by identifying and removing causes of error and minimizing variability in patient care. The term Six Sigma is derived from statistical quality control measures in manufacturing processes and refers to a process that delivers nearly perfect production quality. The Six Sigma model achieves quality improvement by implementing several methods, including the stepwise DMAIC (Define, Measure, Analyze, Improve, and Control) process. The Define step of DMAIC involves developing the objectives of the project. In the Measure step, baseline data on the number and types of defects within the system are measured. The Analyze stage uses the data collected to determine the magnitude of the effects. The Improve step involves implementation of tools to improve the process. Finally, in the Control phase, future processes are controlled to sustain the gains. Six Sigma may be applied to complex, multistep health care processes, such as the ordering and administration of high-risk medications like chemotherapy, to decrease medication errors.

### Operational Excellence

As its name suggests, Operational Excellence is a management system that focuses on the consistent and reliable operation of an institutional strategy. It also involves building and sustaining a culture in which each person is empowered and engaged, often by using aspects of Lean, Six Sigma, and other improvement methods. Operational Excellence can be used to improve quality by focusing key performance indicators on quality and safety metrics, such as timely completion of medication reconciliation.

### KEY POINTS

HVC • Successful quality improvement programs include a health care delivery system, the objective of meeting the needs and expectations of the patient, a team-based approach, and outcome assessment using both qualitative and quantitative data.

HVC • The Model for Improvement, Lean, Six Sigma, and Operational Excellence are examples of quality improvement models that can be used in the health care setting.

## Measurement of Quality Improvement

Multiple organizations and payers now assess quality of care as a condition of accreditation or participation. For example, quality of care and patient safety are important elements in the Joint Commission accreditation process. The Joint Commission assesses a wide variety of quality metrics, such as timely provision of reperfusion therapy in acute myocardial infarction, the incidence of potentially preventable venous thromboembolic disease cases, and rates of immunization.

Medicare also has a significant impact on measurement of health care quality. The Medicare Access and CHIP Reauthorization Act of 2015 (MACRA) includes a new payment structure, the Merit-based Incentive Payment System (MIPS). MIPS consolidates previous quality-based programs and includes elements of the Physicians Quality Reporting System and Meaningful Use programs. More specifically, MIPS includes payment incentives and penalties related to quality and safety, value-based care, improvement activities, and meaningful use of the electronic health record (EHR). Clinicians will be required to report clinical quality metrics, participate in improvement activities (such as the patient-centered medical home), and continue to implement the EHR.

Medicare will adjust reimbursement, with bonuses and penalties based on overall performance, as determined by these measures. For American College of Physicians (ACP) resources on MACRA, see https://www.acponline.org/practice-resources/business-resources/payment/medicare/macra.

## Patient Safety and Quality Improvement Initiatives

### Patient-Centered Medical Home

The patient-centered medical home is a model of providing health care in which the patient's care is coordinated by a primary provider in a team-based practice. The functions of the patient-centered medical home include providing comprehensive care (including preventive, acute, and chronic care), supporting and partnering with patients to make care patient centered, coordinating care across settings with a specific focus on care transitions, delivering accessible services with extended clinician availability, and engaging in quality and safety improvement programs. Further information about the patient-centered medical home is available from AHRQ (www.pcmh.ahrq.gov/page/defining-pcmh).

The concept of the patient-centered medical home has been expanded in the patient-centered medical neighborhood, which includes other clinicians and institutions involved in an individual patient's care (such as specialists and hospitals).

### High Value Care

The ACP High Value Care initiative aims to improve health, avoid harms, and eliminate wasteful practices. This initiative addresses high value care broadly, offering learning resources for clinicians and medical educators, curricula, clinical guidelines, best practice advice, case studies, and patient resources on a wide variety of related topics (https://www.acponline.org/clinical-information/high-value-care). Some learning opportunities offer free Continuing Medical Education credits and Maintenance of Certification points. Components of the High Value Care initiative that are evident in MKSAP 18 include the identification of High Value Care key points in the text and a list of high value care recommendations assembled for each MKSAP section.

### Choosing Wisely

The Choosing Wisely initiative was developed by the American Board of Internal Medicine Foundation in collaboration with *Consumer Reports* to encourage discussions between clinicians and patients on selecting tests, treatments, and procedures that are evidence based and truly necessary, thereby avoiding unnecessary evaluations and treatments. More than 80 specialist organizations have participated to create lists of overused tests and treatments in their specialties (www.choosingwisely.org/clinician-lists), and *Consumer Reports* has generated patient education materials based on these lists to engage and empower patients to participate in care discussions.

## National Patient Safety Goals

The Joint Commission establishes annual National Patient Safety Goals to address important issues in health care safety (https://www.jointcommission.org/standards_information/npsgs.aspx). The National Patient Safety Goals are recommended by a panel of patient safety experts and apply to a variety of patient care settings. The Joint Commission focuses on goals that will have the highest impact on both quality and safety and provides specific metrics for each goal to facilitate implementation. The 2018 National Patient Safety Goals for the hospital setting emphasize improving the accuracy of patient identification, improving staff communication, using medications safely, reducing harms associated with alarm systems, preventing infection, identifying patient safety risks, and preventing surgical mistakes.

## Health Information Technology and Patient Safety

Health information technology (HIT) is the use of an electronic environment to share patient health information. The EHR, CPOE, and clinical decision support (CDS) are some common examples of HIT.

The EHR is a compilation of all health data for a specific patient, including medical notes and test results, in a digital format. The EHR enables the timely sharing of patient information by multiple users, including those spread across several geographic sites, resulting in improved communication and care efficiency.

CPOE is a system by which clinicians electronically enter medication, radiology, and laboratory orders, thereby eliminating errors related to illegible handwriting, improving efficiency by reducing delays between order entry and receipt, and ensuring that directions for use are shared exactly as ordered.

CDS refers to the use of information technology to facilitate clinical decision making. When integrated into a CPOE system, for example, CDS can highlight potential contraindications to diagnostic tests, specify dose recommendations, identify potential drug interactions, and suggest modifications to drug dosage in patients with kidney or liver dysfunction. When integrated into EHR systems, CDS can promote protocols to improve care and provide ready access to clinical guidelines.

Limitations of HIT include the expense associated with system implementation and maintenance as well as concerns related to protection of patient privacy. Although useful for preventing many types of errors, HIT does not provide a failsafe against errors and may facilitate errors itself, such as those resulting from charting templates and use of the copy-and-paste function in composing notes.

For more information on how to incorporate HIT in practice, useful resources are available from ACP (https://www.acponline.org/practice-resources/business-resources/health-information-technology) and AHRQ (https://www.ahrq.gov/professionals/prevention-chronic-care/improve/health-it).

## Health Literacy

As defined by AHRQ, health literacy is the degree to which individuals have the capacity to obtain, process, and understand the information required to make informed health decisions. Low health literacy is more common among older adults, minority populations, persons with lower socioeconomic status, and medically underserved groups. Low health literacy may hinder patients' ability to describe their health concerns, complete health forms accurately, understand medical information, and manage their health conditions. Furthermore, evidence shows that low health literacy is associated with poorer health outcomes as well as decreased utilization of care.

Clinicians need to be aware of the health literacy of their patients and identify those who may need assistance. Tools to assess health literacy in specific populations are available at the Health Literacy Tool Shed (http://healthliteracy.bu.edu). Steps the clinician can take to improve patient understanding include using simple sentences, repeating information, providing an opportunity for the patient to ask questions, and supplying the patient with educational materials written in plain language. ACP offers a collection of patient education materials developed to help patients and their families understand health conditions and facilitate communication between patients and the health care team at https://www.acponline.org/practice-resources/patient-education-resources-and-tools.

# Professionalism and Ethics

## Professionalism

Professionalism is the foundation of medicine's relationship with society and governs the conduct of the physician community. Professionalism in medicine is specifically characterized by the placement of the patient's interests above the physician's self-interests (the fiduciary relationship); acquisition, maintenance, and expansion of specialized medical knowledge; adherence to ethical principles; and self-regulation of members and responsibilities. The Charter on Medical Professionalism from the American Board of Internal Medicine Foundation, the American College of Physicians–American Society of Internal Medicine Foundation, and the European Federation of Internal Medicine sets forth three fundamental principles along with 10 professional commitments that form the ideals and values to be pursued by all physicians (Table 24).

## Primacy of Patient Welfare

The principle of primacy of patient welfare is rooted in the importance of placing the patient's interests at the heart of the clinical enterprise. The patient's welfare must supersede all economic, personal, societal, and administrative forces. Under this principle, the physician has a duty to act for the benefit of the patient (beneficence) and to minimize patient harm

**TABLE 24.** Principles and Commitments of Professionalism

| Principle or Commitment | Comment |
| --- | --- |
| **Fundamental Principle** | |
| Primacy of patient welfare | Altruism is a central trust factor in the physician-patient relationship. Market forces, societal pressures, and administrative exigencies must not compromise this principle. |
| Patient autonomy | Patients' decisions about their care must be paramount, as long as those decisions are in keeping with ethical practice and do not lead to demands for inappropriate care. |
| Social justice | Physicians should work actively to eliminate discrimination in health care, whether based on race, gender, socioeconomic status, ethnicity, religion, or any other social category. |
| **Professional Commitment** | |
| Competence | Physicians must be committed to lifelong learning and to maintaining the medical knowledge and clinical and team skills necessary for the provision of quality care. |
| Honesty with patients | Obtain informed consent for treatment or research. Report and analyze medical errors in order to maintain trust, improve care, and provide appropriate compensation to injured parties. |
| Patient confidentiality | Privacy of information is essential to patient trust and even more pressing with electronic health records. |
| Appropriate patient relations | Given the inherent vulnerability and dependency of patients, physicians should never exploit patients for any sexual advantage, personal financial gain, or other private purpose. |
| Improve quality of care | Work collaboratively with other professionals to reduce medical errors, increase patient safety, minimize overuse of health care resources, and optimize the outcomes of care. |
| Improve access to care | Work to eliminate barriers to access based on education, laws, finances, geography, and social discrimination. Equity requires the promotion of public health and preventive medicine, as well as public advocacy, without concern for the self-interest of the physician or the profession. |
| Just distribution of resources | Work with other physicians, hospitals, and payers to develop guidelines for cost-effective care. Providing unnecessary services not only exposes one's patients to avoidable harm and expense but also diminishes the resources available for others. |
| Scientific knowledge | Uphold scientific standards, promote research, create new knowledge, and ensure its appropriate use. |
| Manage conflicts of interest | Medical professionals and their organizations have many opportunities to compromise their professional responsibilities by pursuing private gain or personal advantage. Such compromises are especially threatening with for-profit industries, including medical equipment manufacturers, insurance companies, and pharmaceutical firms. Physicians have an obligation to recognize, disclose to the general public, and deal with conflicts of interest that arise. |
| Professional responsibilities | Undergo self-assessment and external scrutiny of all aspects of one's performance. Participate in the processes of self-regulation, including remediation and discipline of members who have failed to meet professional standards. |

Adapted with permission from ABIM Foundation; American Board of Internal Medicine; ACP-ASIM Foundation; American College of Physicians-American Society of Internal Medicine; European Federation of Internal Medicine. Medical professionalism in the new millennium: a physician charter. Ann Intern Med. 2002;136:243-6. [PMID: 11827500] Copyright 2002, American College of Physicians.

CONT.

(nonmaleficence). This is especially important in the context of the physician-patient relationship, given the inherent vulnerability of many patients. The altruism of serving the patient's interests before the physician's interests creates the trust that is essential to the physician-patient relationship.

Physicians must perform their duties irrespective of the health care setting or the patient's characteristics, including age, religion, gender, sexual orientation, decision-making capacity, insurance status, or immigration status. Care should be provided with respect, competence, compassion, and attention to the uniqueness of the patient and his or her circumstances.

## Appropriate Patient Relationships

The physician-patient relationship should be based on mutual agreement. Once this relationship has been established, the physician should strive to understand the patient's health concerns, values, goals, and expectations to guide the provision of care.

Appropriate boundaries between the physician and patient must always be maintained. It is unethical for a physician to become sexually involved with a current patient, and sexual relationships with former patients should be avoided owing to concerns of continued vulnerability and transference (unconscious redirection of the feelings a person has about a second person to feelings that person has about a third person). Physicians must also maintain boundaries during the history, physical examination, and treatment maneuvers by communicating the planned actions in advance and effectively conveying the purpose of these actions (for example, "I will now lift the gown to examine your abdomen more closely"). During the examination of intimate areas, a chaperone should be present.

CONT.

Physicians may be asked to care for persons with whom they have an existing nonprofessional relationship, including close friends and family members. Caring for these persons may be associated with impaired objectivity, insufficient history taking (for example, failure to obtain an adequate sexual history), incomplete examination, and incomplete or biased assessment. Physicians should weigh these considerations carefully and encourage alternative sources of care whenever feasible.

When communicating with patients online, physicians should conduct themselves according to the usual standards for professional interactions, including treating the patient with respect and maintaining privacy and confidentiality. Social media can lead to confusion over the boundaries between personal and professional interactions, and physicians should keep these spheres separate and behave professionally in both because their behavior reflects upon themselves and upon the profession as a whole. Importantly, all electronic physician-patient communications should be maintained in a secure electronic health record. Benefits, pitfalls, and recommended safeguards for online physician activities are described in **Table 25**.

Physician-patient relationships should generally be established based on an in-person professional encounter. Telemedicine, or the use of electronic communication and technologies to provide health care to patients at a distance, may improve physician-patient collaboration, access to care, and reduce costs. The American College of Physicians holds the position that a valid patient–physician relationship must be established for professionally responsible telemedicine services to occur; however, the patient–physician relationship may be formed during a telemedicine encounter through real-time audiovisual technology.

| TABLE 25. | Online Physician Activities: Benefits, Pitfalls, and Recommended Safeguards | | |
|---|---|---|---|
| **Activity** | **Potential Benefits** | **Potential Pitfalls** | **Recommended Safeguards** |
| Communications with patients using e-mail, text, and instant messaging | Greater accessibility<br><br>Immediate answers to nonurgent issues | Confidentiality concerns<br><br>Replacement of face-to-face or telephone interaction<br><br>Ambiguity or misinterpretation of digital interactions | Establish guidelines for types of issues appropriate for digital communication<br><br>Reserve digital communication only for patients who maintain face-to-face follow-up |
| Use of social media sites to gather information about patients | Observe and counsel patients on risk-taking or health-averse behaviors<br><br>Intervene in emergency | Sensitivity to source of information<br><br>Threaten trust in patient-physician relationship | Consider intent of search and application of findings<br><br>Consider implications for ongoing care |
| Use of online educational resources and related information with patients | Encourage patient empowerment through self-education<br><br>Supplement resource-poor environments | Non–peer-reviewed materials may provide inaccurate information<br><br>Scam "patient" sites that misrepresent therapies and outcomes | Vet information to ensure accuracy of content<br><br>Refer patients only to reputable sites and sources |
| Physician-produced blogs, microblogs, and physician posting of comments by others | Advocacy and public health enhancement<br><br>Introduction of physician "voice" into such conversations | Negative online content, such as "venting" or ranting, that disparages patients and colleagues | "Pause before posting"<br><br>Consider the content and the message it sends about a physician as an individual and the profession |
| Physician posting of physician personal information on public social media sites | Networking and communications | Blurring of professional and personal boundaries<br><br>Impact on representation of the individual and the profession | Maintain separate personas, personal and professional, for online social behavior<br><br>Scrutinize material available for public consumption |
| Physician use of digital venues (e.g., text and Web) for communicating with colleagues about patient care | Ease of communication with colleagues | Confidentiality concerns<br><br>Unsecured networks and accessibility of protected health information | Implement health information technology solutions for secure messaging and information sharing<br><br>Follow institutional practice and policy for remote and mobile access of protected health information |

CONT.

## Challenging Physician-Patient Relationships

Conflicts between the physician and patient can arise for many reasons. Common causes of conflict include patient requests for inappropriate or nonindicated tests or treatments and patient refusal of a recommended course of treatment. Patients may disagree with the physician's recommendation because of a lack of understanding of the appropriate diagnostic or therapeutic approach, which can be exacerbated by a lack of trust or low health literacy. Other factors include financial or socioeconomic status, which can hinder patient participation in the recommended plan, and cultural considerations, which may lead to a divergent understanding of the cause of the health problem or appropriate approaches to treatment. In response to these conflicts, the physician should offer the rationale for the proposed intervention and explore the patient's reasoning. Physicians also should work to understand the social determinants of health for local communities and how these forces may affect the intersection of health and health care delivery. Furthermore, physicians have a responsibility to develop cultural responsiveness and to sensitively inquire and learn about how a patient's belief system can affect his or her understanding of the health condition. Physicians should consider cultural traditions, the specific social context, and communication standards when discussing care with patients and their families. A deeper understanding of the patient's background and rationale for decision making may allow for conflict resolution or prompt a search for more appropriate alternatives.

There are circumstances in which the physician-patient relationship becomes irreparably compromised because of lack of trust, lack of mutual goals, or failure to maintain an effective working relationship despite efforts to resolve differences. In these cases, the patient and physician can mutually terminate the relationship so long as the patient's health is stable enough for such a transition. The physician should provide formal, written documentation of the termination and provide the patient with information on obtaining a new provider. Patient abandonment (withdrawing from an established relationship without giving reasonable notice or providing a competent replacement) is unethical and may be a cause for legal action.

## Requests for Interventions

Patients and their family members may request specific diagnostic or therapeutic interventions that challenge the physician's sense of what is best for the patient. Examples include requests for antibiotic therapy for a suspected viral infection and demands for aggressive chemotherapy in a debilitated patient with cancer. Although the physician needs to respect patient autonomy, this duty must be weighed against the physician's professional judgment and integrity, the potential harms of inappropriate interventions, possible secondary effects (for example, antimicrobial resistance caused by inappropriate antibiotic prescribing), and responsible stewardship of medical resources. When there is no evidence that the desired diagnostic or therapeutic intervention will provide clinical benefit, physicians are not obligated to provide these treatments.

Particularly difficult requests may occur in the setting of ambiguous or conflicting goals of care. For example, a physician may perceive that a patient with multiorgan failure will not achieve the goal of returning to his or her previous level of functioning and therefore conclude that continued intensive care is inappropriate. However, family members may have the goal of extending their loved one's life for as long as possible, regardless of the incurred risk and costs.

Effective communication regarding the preferences and goals of the patient and family members can often help adjudicate conflicts of values, clarify prognosis and uncertainties, and lead to conflict resolution. When resolution cannot be achieved, ethics consultation can be beneficial. Prompt transfer of care to a physician who concurs with the patient's or family's plan and is willing to provide the requested intervention may be necessary when resolution is not possible.

## Conflicts of Interest

Conflicts of interest are financial, professional, or other personal concerns that have the potential to compromise the physician's objectivity. Real or potential conflicts threaten the physician's ability to ensure that the patient's welfare is the primary motivating factor in patient care and may undermine trust in the profession. Conflicts of interest may also exist in research and medical education.

Physicians should recognize, disclose, and manage all conflicts of interest. Researchers should disclose sources of funding and minimize opportunities for bias, and medical educators should disclose pertinent conflicts to learners. Disclosure of conflicts, however, may not be an adequate safeguard against bias in decision making, and potential conflicts should be removed if at all possible.

Physician acceptance of gifts, hospitality, and other items and services of value is also strongly discouraged, as even small and seemingly inconsequential gestures may lead to bias. To help guide decision making, physicians can consider whether they think it would be appropriate for their own physician to accept such an inducement and what the public or patient perception of the inducement might be. Other strategies for controlling conflicts of interest are listed in **Table 26**. Physicians should also recognize that the Physician Payments Sunshine Act requires medical product and pharmaceutical manufacturers to disclose payments and gifts to physicians and teaching hospitals, a list of which is published annually in a searchable database. H

### KEY POINTS

- Patient abandonment, or withdrawing from an established relationship without giving reasonable notice or providing a competent replacement, is unethical and may be a cause for legal action.

*(Continued)*

**TABLE 26.** A Selection of Institute of Medicine Recommendations for Individual Physicians to Control Conflicts of Interest

Do not accept items of material value from pharmaceutical, medical device, and biotechnology companies, except when a transaction involves payment at fair market value for a legitimate service.

Do not make educational presentations or publish scientific articles that are controlled by industry or contain substantial portions written by someone who is not identified as an author or who is not properly acknowledged.

Do not enter into consulting arrangements unless they are based on written contracts for expert services to be paid for at fair market value.

Do not meet with pharmaceutical and medical device sales representatives except by documented appointment and at the physician's express invitation.

Do not accept drug samples except in certain situations for patients who lack financial access to medications.

Reproduced with permission from Institute of Medicine. Conflict of Interest in Medical Research, Education, and Practice. Washington, DC: National Academies Press, 2009. https://www.ncbi.nlm.nih.gov/books/NBK22942/. Accessed June 28, 2018. Copyright 2009, The National Academy of Sciences.

**KEY POINTS (continued)**

HVC
- If a patient requests diagnostic or therapeutic interventions for which there is no evidence of clinical benefit, physicians are not obligated to provide these interventions.

- Conflicts of interest threaten the physician's objectivity and the public's trust in the profession; physicians must avoid acceptance of financial, professional, or other personal inducements from health care companies and manufacturers.

# Respecting Patient Autonomy

## Confidentiality

Physicians are required to protect the privacy and confidentiality of a patient's medical information. The promise of confidentiality fosters trust and encourages honest disclosure of sensitive personal details, thereby improving patient care.

Physicians must recognize that disclosure of medical information outside of the physician-patient relationship requires patient consent and that there is real risk for inadvertent disclosure. Physicians should be vigilant about protecting patient confidentiality in the era of electronic health records, e-mail, patient portals, and social media. Communication with and regarding patients should involve secure communication systems and storage, and physicians should follow best practices. Discussing patients outside of a clinical or educational setting, such as in a hospital cafeteria, violates confidentiality and may compromise trust in the physician and profession. Physicians must also be knowledgeable in the relevant state and federal statutes regarding confidentiality, including the Health Insurance Portability and Accountability Act of 1996 (HIPAA).

There are circumstances in which competing interests may conflict with the need for confidentiality, and disclosure becomes necessary to minimize a greater harm. For example, physicians may be required to breach confidentiality in situations of child or elder abuse, on behalf of public health concerns (for example, sexually transmitted infections), or when patients may be a threat to themselves or others. In these situations, the duty to the public good and other patients overrides the duty to maintain patient confidentiality.

## Informed Consent and Refusal

Informed consent and refusal is the process of engaging the patient in meaningful dialogue about his or her health conditions, assessing the patient's understanding, and respecting the patient's autonomy to accept or refuse care. Informed consent requires that a patient be provided with all of the information necessary to determine the individual acceptability and appropriateness of the proposed treatment or intervention. Pertinent information includes the nature of the underlying condition; the goals of treatment; and the risks, benefits, and alternatives to treatment (including the option to forgo treatment). Information should be communicated in ways that are sensitive, appropriate for the patient's literacy level, and attentive to the cultural context. For informed consent to be considered valid, the patient must have decision-making capacity and be free from coercion. An exception to informed consent is a medical emergency in which a patient is unable to participate in the decision-making process; in these instances, consent for life-saving therapies should be presumed unless available information or directives suggest otherwise.

Therapeutic privilege, or the withholding of information due to concern that the disclosure will cause the patient harm, bypasses the process of informed consent and should rarely, if ever, be used. Therapeutic privilege may be used only after consultation with a colleague and a thorough weighing of the risks and benefits of the disclosure.

## Advance Care Planning

Advance care planning is the process by which a patient articulates preferences, goals, and values regarding his or her future medical care. Advance care planning should consist of ongoing conversations between the patient, the physician, and loved ones to inform decisions and direct medical care in the event that the patient loses decision-making capacity. These conversations should be a routine component of care and ideally occur before an acute event or medical crisis. Advance care planning should include written documentation of the patient's preferences (advance directives) and be documented in the medical record.

Advance directives may include a living will or durable power of attorney for health care. In a living will, a patient can outline specific preferences for treatment decisions (for example, use of dialysis or mechanical ventilation). A durable power of attorney allows the patient to designate a surrogate to be the primary medical decision maker when the patient cannot make his or her own decisions.

The legal requirements for and implementation of advance directives vary by state, and physicians should be familiar with

CONT.

the laws pertaining to advance directives in the state in which they practice. State laws regarding the withdrawal of artificial nutrition and hydration may be particularly variable, and patients who have preferences regarding these interventions should clearly document these preferences in a living will.

## Decision-Making Capacity

All adult patients should be presumed legally competent to make medical decisions unless found otherwise by judicial determination. However, in routine clinical care, physicians must frequently determine the patient's decision-making capacity, including the patient's ability to understand the relevant information, appreciate the medical consequences of the situation, consider various treatment options, and communicate a choice. Decision-making capacity should be evaluated for each decision to be made, and frequent reassessment is necessary to confirm previous determinations of capacity (**Table 27**). The presence of depression or early dementia may complicate the evaluation but

| TABLE 27. | Legally Relevant Criteria for Decision-Making Capacity and Approaches to Assessment of the Patient | | | |
|---|---|---|---|---|
| **Criterion** | **Patient's Task** | **Physician's Assessment Approach** | **Questions for Clinical Assessment**[a] | **Comments** |
| Communicate a choice | Clearly indicate preferred treatment option | Ask patient to indicate a treatment choice | Have you decided whether to follow your doctor's (or my) recommendation for treatment? Can you tell me what the decision is? (If no decision) What is making it hard for you to decide? | Frequent reversals of choice because psychiatric or neurologic conditions may indicate lack of capacity |
| Understand the relevant information | Grasp the fundamental meaning of information communicated by the physician | Encourage patient to paraphrase disclosed information regarding medical condition and treatment | Please tell me in your own words what your doctor (or I) told you about: • The problem with your health now • The recommended treatment • The possible benefits and risks (or discomforts) of the treatment • Any alternative treatments and their risks and benefits • The risks and benefits of no treatment | Information to be understood includes nature of patient's condition, nature and purpose of proposed treatment, possible benefits and risks of that treatment, and alternating approaches (including no treatment) and their benefits and risks |
| Appreciate the situation and its consequences | Acknowledge medical condition and likely consequences of treatment options | Ask patient to describe views of medical condition, proposed treatment, and likely outcomes | What do you believe is wrong with your health now? Do you believe that you need some kind of treatment? What is treatment likely to do for you? What makes you believe it will have that effect? What do you believe will happen if you are not treated? Why do you think your doctor has (or I have) recommended this treatment? | Courts have recognized that patients who do not acknowledge their illnesses (often referred to as "lack of insight") cannot make valid decisions about treatment Delusions or pathologic levels of distortion or denial are the most common cause of impairment |
| Reason about treatment options | Engage in a rational process of manipulating the relevant information | Ask patient to compare treatment options and consequences and to offer reasons for selection of option | How did you decide to accept or reject the recommended treatment? What makes (chosen option) better than (alternative option)? | This criterion focuses on the process by which a decision is reached, not the outcome of the patient's choice, because patients have the right to make "unreasonable" choices |

[a]Questions are adapted from Grisso T, Appelbaum PS. Assessing Competence to Consent to Treatment: A Guide for Physicians and Other Health Professionals. New York: Oxford University Press; 1998. Patients' responses to these questions need not be verbal.

Reproduced with permission from Appelbaum PS. Clinical practice. Assessment of patients' competence to consent to treatment. N Engl J Med. 2007;357:1836. [PMID: 17978292] Copyright 2007, Massachusetts Medical Society.

CONT.

does not necessarily preclude the presence of decision-making capacity, highlighting the importance of an appropriate assessment. When a decision may result in serious consequences, determination of capacity is of even greater importance. Decisions are likely more valid when consistent with previously stated values, beliefs, and choices. Decisions that run counter to previously expressed preferences may be equally valid; however, when such changes occur, it must be clear that the patient maintains capacity and understands the ramifications of the decisions.

## Surrogate Decision Making

In the absence of patient decision-making capacity, a surrogate is required to make health care decisions. The most appropriate surrogate is the person who has been legally appointed by the patient as a health care proxy. If the patient has not designated a surrogate, a person who is knowledgeable about the patient's preferences should serve as decision maker. Many states have laws that provide a hierarchy of preferred surrogates based upon relationship to the patient (typically in the sequence of spouse, adult child, parent, and adult sibling).

The surrogate should adhere to the instructions described in the living will, and physicians should assist surrogate decision makers in fulfilling these duties. If there is no living will, the surrogate should make decisions based on knowledge of the patient's preferences and values, also known as substituted judgment. If the surrogate does not have first-hand knowledge of the patient's preferences or values, he or she should make decisions based on what he or she perceives to be the patient's best interests.

## Withholding or Withdrawing Treatment

When a patient with decision-making capacity refuses further treatment, even life-saving care, patient autonomy must be respected, and treatment should be stopped. If the patient lacks decision-making capacity but has articulated future wishes through an advance directive or surrogate, those preferences should guide the treatment decision. Ethically and legally, there is no distinction between withholding (not initiating) or withdrawing (removing) treatment. The decision to withdraw care can be fraught with guilt or concerns about suffering for some family members, and the physician can play an important role in explaining the process and ameliorating these concerns. An ethics committee or ethics consultation can also be helpful in assisting family members. If the patient or surrogate decides to withhold or withdraw life-sustaining treatment, other care (including symptom management and palliative care) should be continued.

## Physician-Assisted Suicide

Physician-assisted suicide, or physician-assisted death, occurs when a physician provides a lethal prescription to a competent patient who has requested a means to end his or her life. The patient self-administers the drug with the intent to cause death. Physician-assisted suicide must be distinguished from euthanasia, in which a physician directly and intentionally administers an agent to cause death, and from interventions that are administered with the intent of relieving suffering but unintentionally hasten the patient's death.

Physician-assisted suicide raises profound legal, clinical, and social concerns. It may erode trust in the profession, cause harm to the most vulnerable, and hinder progress in improving end-of-life care. The American College of Physicians does not support legalization of physician-assisted suicide or euthanasia and instead emphasizes the need to provide palliative care, relief from suffering, and emotional support to the patient and family members during the end of life. Several states, however, have legalized physician-assisted suicide, and physicians may be asked to participate in discussions regarding the practice.

### KEY POINTS

- Physicians may be required to breach confidentiality in situations of child or elder abuse, on behalf of public health concerns, or when patients may be a threat to themselves or others.
- Informed consent requires that the patient be informed of the nature of the underlying condition; the goals of treatment; and the risks, benefits, and alternatives to treatment (including the option to forgo treatment).
- The presence of depression or early dementia does not necessarily preclude the presence of decision-making capacity, but these conditions increase the importance of an appropriate assessment.
- Surrogates and physicians are required to act in accordance with the patient's expressed preferences for medical care, and if these are not available, they should serve the patient's best interests.
- The American College of Physicians does not support legalization of physician-assisted suicide or euthanasia and instead emphasizes the need to provide palliative care, relief from suffering, and emotional support to the patient and family members during the end of life.

# Justice

The principle of justice is predicated on fairness. Physicians have an obligation to promote and respect patients' rights and to justly allocate health care resources. Physicians should work to reduce disparities in the allocation of such resources based on patient characteristics, including sex, race, ethnicity, socioeconomic status, sexual orientation, or gender identify. However, resource allocation or rationing decisions should not be made at the bedside. Rather, these decisions are best made on the societal and policy levels; physicians should work at these levels (for example, through professional societies) to reduce disparities.

Physicians also have the responsibility to provide effective and efficient health care that uses health care resources responsibly (that is, high value care). At times, attention to just distribution of societal resources may seem contradictory to

CONT.

the principles of primacy of patient welfare and patient autonomy; however, physicians must weigh each of these considerations in a particular context to determine the appropriate course of action. By practicing high value care, physicians can ensure excellent care while also using resources wisely and ensuring that resources are equitably available.

## Medical Error Disclosure

In the 1999 report *To Err Is Human: Building a Safer Health System*, the Institute of Medicine (now called the National Academy of Medicine) defined a medical error as "the failure of a planned action to be completed as intended or the use of a wrong plan to achieve an aim." Full disclosure of medical errors is recommended practice, and several states mandate such disclosures. Disclosure of errors is necessary to respect the patient's autonomy, promote trust through honesty, and promote justice through appropriate compensation. Disclosure may also benefit physicians by alleviating distress, improving physician-patient communication, and reducing litigation. Strategies that focus on early communication and response after an error have been associated with fewer malpractice lawsuits and lower litigation costs, although these outcomes are not the primary drivers of such initiatives.

The process of error disclosure should include an explanation of the course of events and how the error occurred, an apology by the physician, a description of how the effects of the error will be minimized or rectified, and steps the physician or system will take to reduce recurrences. Disclosure should be performed thoughtfully and sensitively, accounting for the emotional effect on both the patient and provider.

### KEY POINT

- Medical error disclosure should include an explanation of the course of events and how the error occurred, an apology by the physician, a description of how the effects of the error will be minimized or rectified, and steps the physician or system will take to reduce recurrences.

## Colleague Responsibility

Physicians have the responsibility to maintain professional competence, create and share new knowledge with colleagues and trainees, and work collaboratively to optimize patient care. These behaviors must be governed by self-regulation and mutual respect for the members of the health care team.

In accordance with these tenets of professionalism, physicians also have the responsibility to safeguard patients from impaired physicians and to assist impaired colleagues by identifying appropriate sources of help. Physicians have an individual obligation to report an impaired physician to the appropriate authorities and should also work collectively with institutions to develop methods for reporting, treating, and remediating impaired or disruptive colleagues.

## Approaching Ethical Dilemmas

Clinical ethical dilemmas can often be resolved by analyzing (1) the patient's medical indications, including the medical condition, problems, and treatment options; (2) patient preferences, including a consideration of decision-making capacity and need for a surrogate; (3) patient quality of life, including the likelihood of restoring the patient to his or her previous state, possible harms to the patient with treatment, and patient and physician impressions of these considerations; and (4) contextual factors, including family, social, legal, religious, and other issues that might affect the decision. When ethical dilemmas are difficult to resolve, physicians may obtain assistance through an ethics consultation.

## Providing Care as a Physician Bystander

Physicians' specialized knowledge creates a unique opportunity to intervene and benefit other citizens in emergency situations, and in this context, physicians may provide care outside of the clinical setting to persons who are not their patients. When physicians assist in emergency situations, patient consent to receive treatment is usually presumed or implied. If the treatment is provided in good faith, Good Samaritan laws usually protect the physician from liability, except in cases of gross negligence. Providing medical care as a bystander is typically voluntary; however, state laws vary on this point, and several states have "failure to act" laws that are not specific to physicians.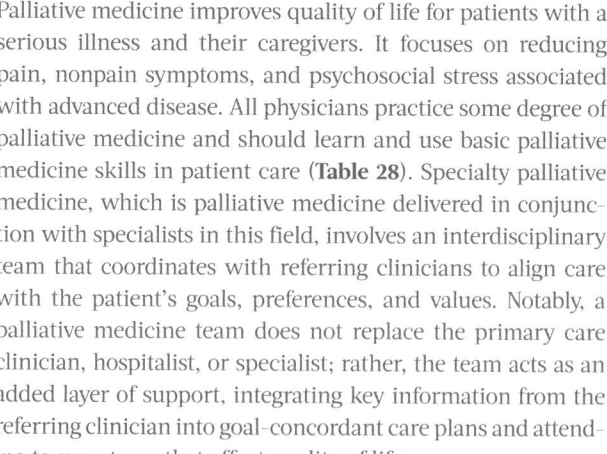

# Palliative Medicine
## Introduction

Palliative medicine improves quality of life for patients with a serious illness and their caregivers. It focuses on reducing pain, nonpain symptoms, and psychosocial stress associated with advanced disease. All physicians practice some degree of palliative medicine and should learn and use basic palliative medicine skills in patient care (**Table 28**). Specialty palliative medicine, which is palliative medicine delivered in conjunction with specialists in this field, involves an interdisciplinary team that coordinates with referring clinicians to align care with the patient's goals, preferences, and values. Notably, a palliative medicine team does not replace the primary care clinician, hospitalist, or specialist; rather, the team acts as an added layer of support, integrating key information from the referring clinician into goal-concordant care plans and attending to symptoms that affect quality of life.

Evidence has shown that specialty palliative medicine improves overall quality of life, physical symptom burden, mood, and caregiver satisfaction with patient care in the setting of serious or life-threatening illness. Although referral to palliative care historically occurred at the end of life, an

**TABLE 28.** Representative Skill Sets for Primary and Specialty Palliative Care

**Primary Palliative Care**

Basic management of pain and symptoms

Basic management of depression and anxiety

Basic discussions about:

    Prognosis

    Goals of treatment

    Suffering

    Code status

**Specialty Palliative Care**

Management of refractory pain or other symptoms

Management of more complex depression, anxiety, grief, and existential distress

Assistance with conflict resolution regarding goals or methods of treatment

    Within families

    Between staff and families

    Among treatment teams

Assistance in addressing cases of near futility

Reproduced with permission from Quill TE, Abernethy AP. Generalist plus specialist palliative care—creating a more sustainable model. N Engl J Med. 2013;368:1174. [PMID: 23465068] doi:10.1056/NEJMp1215620. Copyright 2013, Massachusetts Medical Society.

 CONT.

emerging consensus of research indicates that early initiation during a serious or life-threating illness is associated with substantial advantages. Much of the evidence on the benefits of subspecialty palliative care has involved patients with incurable cancer; however, numerous guidelines highlight the need for early palliative care in patients with advanced cardiac, pulmonary, or kidney disease; patients with advanced dementia; critically ill patients; and patients undergoing potentially curative interventions, such as hematopoietic stem cell transplantation. ◧

**KEY POINT**

HVC   • Specialty palliative medicine improves overall quality of life, physical symptom burden, mood, and caregiver satisfaction with patient care in the setting of serious or life-threatening illness.

## ◧ Communicating with Patients with Serious Illness

For patients with serious illness, there are considerable disparities between the care that patients report they want and the care that they receive. Patients report a strong desire to have serious illness and end-of-life conversations and wish to have them with the clinicians they view as their primary physician contacts. Timely and skillful communication with patients, family members, and caregivers is essential to align

care with patients' wishes. However, many clinicians report that they do not have the training for conversations about end-of-life care, and many conversations occur too late, with poor quality, and outside of the patient's primary clinician-patient relationship. Even among clinicians caring for populations for whom consistent advance care and end-of-life planning are considered to be standard care, it may be unclear who should facilitate end-of-life discussions, and such clinicians may feel ill-equipped. One study of clinicians caring for patients with advanced heart failure found that primary care clinicians, cardiologists, and heart failure clinicians all felt unprepared for conversations related to advance care planning, despite guideline recommendations that such conversations should occur yearly.

Structured conversations are associated with improved goal-concordant care and reduced patient anxiety. One model for skilled conversations with patients facing a serious illness is outlined in **Table 29**. The Serious Illness Conversation Guide provides sample phrases that are designed to elicit a patient's goals, preferences, and values after the patient's illness understanding is assessed. In contrast to discussion techniques in which information is shared and patients are subsequently asked to choose from a list of medical interventions, the Serious Illness Conversation Guide encourages shared decision making and enables the physician to help patients understand the illness and prognosis, elicit important patient goals, and make recommendations for care. The output of these conversations should be communicated to the patient's family and surrogate decision maker. Institutional advance directives, commercial advance directive forms or electronic applications, physician orders for life-sustaining treatment (POLST) paradigm forms, and medical orders for life-sustaining treatment (MOLST) forms should be viewed as mechanisms to record the outcomes of these discussions rather than as conversation guides. For further discussion of advance care planning and advance directives, see Professionalism and Ethics. ◧

**KEY POINTS**

• Patients report a strong desire to have serious illness   **HVC** and end-of-life conversations and wish to have them with the clinicians they view as their primary physician contact.

• Structured conversations about serious illness are asso-   **HVC** ciated with improved goal-concordant care and reduced patient anxiety.

## Symptom Management

Effective and proactive symptom management is critical to the  success of both basic and specialty palliative care interventions. Management of debilitating and distressing symptoms, such as pain or nausea, can markedly improve a patient's mood, sense of hope, and quality of life. ◧

| TABLE 29. Serious Illness Conversation Guide | |
|---|---|
| **Conversation Flow** | **Patient-Tested Language** |
| 1. Set up the conversation: | |
|     Introduce the idea and benefits. | "I'm hoping we can talk about where things are with your illness and where they might be going. Is this okay?" |
|     Ask permission. | |
| 2. Assess illness understanding and information preferences. | "What is your understanding now of where you are with your illness?" |
| | "How much information about what is likely to be ahead with your illness would you like from me?" |
| 3. Share prognosis: | |
|     Tailor information to patient preference. | Prognosis: "I'm worried that time may be short." |
| |     or "This may be as strong as you feel." |
|     Allow silence; explore emotion. | |
| 4. Explore key topics: | |
|     Goals | "What are your most important goals if your health situation worsens?" |
|     Fears and worries | "What are your biggest fears and worries about the future with your health?" |
|     Sources of strength | "What gives you strength as you think about the future with your illness?" |
|     Critical abilities | "What abilities are so critical to your life that you can't imagine living without them?" |
|     Tradeoffs | "If you become sicker, how much are you willing to go through for the possibility of gaining more time?" |
|     Family | "How much does your family know about your priorities and wishes?" |
| 5. Close the conversation: | |
|     Summarize what you've heard. | "It sounds like _____ is very important to you." |
|     Make a recommendation. | "Given your goals and priorities and what we know about your illness at this stage, I recommend…." |
|     Affirm your commitment to the patient. | "We're in this together." |
| 6. Document your conversation. | |

## Pain

 Although pain in advanced illness shares some features with chronic noncancer pain, pain management in palliative care has several unique attributes, which will be discussed in this section. For a discussion of pain mechanisms as well as the evaluation and initial treatment of patients with pain, refer to Common Symptoms.

Pain commonly occurs in patients with serious illness, and recognition and constant evaluation of pain are integral to effective management. Up to 90% of patients with advanced cancer have pain. Unfortunately, cancer pain remains undertreated, with about one third of patients with cancer receiving inadequate analgesia. The incidence of pain in patients with other serious illnesses is also underappreciated. Most patients with advanced COPD, severe heart failure, amyotrophic lateral sclerosis, or end-stage kidney disease undergoing hemodialysis have undertreated pain.

Many patients additionally face complex psychosocial and spiritual issues related to their illness and may experience total pain, defined as physical, social, psychological, and spiritual suffering. Engaging interdisciplinary team members, such as nurses, psychologists, chaplains, and social workers, is important in addressing the nonphysical components of pain.

The pharmacologic management of pain in patients with a serious illness requires a multimodal approach that uses both opioids and nonopioid analgesics, such as acetaminophen, NSAIDs, glucocorticoids, topical therapies, neuropathic agents, and antidepressants with analgesic properties. (See Common Symptoms for a discussion of common coanalgesic agents.) Current approaches eschew the use of opioid-acetaminophen combination medications because of the risk for acetaminophen overdose with titration of the opioid component, particularly when used concurrently with other acetaminophen-containing drugs. Additionally, the so-called "weak opioids" (codeine, tramadol) should be avoided in this population because of significant drug-drug interactions, marginal effectiveness, and wide variations in hepatic metabolism. For patients in whom nonopioid treatment is ineffective or not tolerated, opioids are appropriate, with careful attention paid to dosing, frequency, and side effect profile. **Table 30** outlines the most commonly used opioids in the treatment of pain resulting from a serious illness, as well as specific patient population concerns.

Short-acting opioids should be titrated to achieve symptom relief. In patients using short-acting opioids who require longer-lasting relief, long-acting agents are appropriate; however, long-acting opioids should not be initiated in opioid-naïve patients. Selection of a long-acting opioid should be based on underlying organ function and previous response to the equivalent short-acting formulation (for example, oxycodone immediate-release and controlled-release forms).

Fentanyl patches are commonly used for long-acting pain relief, although they have a more complex pharmacokinetic profile than oral agents and are less easily titrated. Fentanyl patches must be used with caution in patients with a serious illness, especially those who lack adipose tissue or are subject to recurrent infections. Absence of adipose tissue may result in irregular transdermal absorption, whereas fever may cause increased absorption with a greater potential for adverse events.

Orally administered transmucosal immediate-release fentanyl (TIRF) products are approved for the treatment of cancer-related pain. TIRF formulations are rapidly absorbed and offer immediate onset for patients who are not achieving adequate analgesia with high-dose morphine. Management of these medications is challenging because the dosing regimen, escalation, and frequency differ among brands. Additionally, clinicians require specialized education and certification (TIRF Risk Evaluation and Mitigation Strategy program) to initiate these medications. Methadone is another long-acting agent used to treat pain from a serious illness; however, its complex dosing and variable half-life restrict its general use. Owing to their complicated management, TIRF formulations and methadone should be prescribed in collaboration with an expert in pain management or a palliative medicine specialist with experience in their use.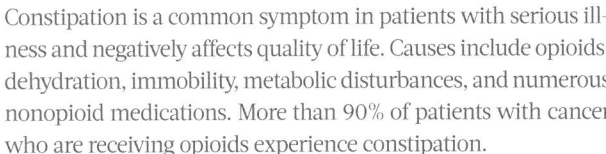

Medical cannabis has long been used in the management of symptoms associated with serious illness. It has been studied for numerous clinical indications and is approved in many states for the treatment of cancer symptoms or symptoms associated with other terminal illnesses. Cannabis extracts, predominantly those containing higher concentrations of cannabidiol, have shown a moderate degree of benefit in the treatment of patients with chronic pain and patients with pain symptoms from spasticity in the setting of neurodegenerative disorders. However, given the lack of data on medical cannabis in managing complex cancer pain and the need for multimodal analgesic therapy in seriously ill patients, the role of medical cannabis for this indication remains unclear.

## Constipation

Constipation is a common symptom in patients with serious illness and negatively affects quality of life. Causes include opioids, dehydration, immobility, metabolic disturbances, and numerous nonopioid medications. More than 90% of patients with cancer who are receiving opioids experience constipation.

Patients with constipation in the setting of serious illness should be educated on increasing their intake of fluids and dietary fiber. Patients taking opioids, however, should not receive supplemental fiber, owing to concerns for worsening constipation in the setting of opioid-reduced gastrointestinal motility. Pharmacologic therapy for constipation and for all patients taking scheduled opioids should include a stimulant laxative, such as senna or bisacodyl. Osmotic laxatives, such as

| TABLE 30. | Opioids Commonly Used in Palliative Care | | |
|---|---|---|---|
| **Opioid** | **Protein Binding** | **Metabolism** | **Comments** |
| Hydrocodone | Low | Liver enzyme CYP2D6 | Variable efficacy; combination with acetaminophen limits use |
| | | | Increased time to analgesic onset in liver failure |
| Hydromorphone | Low | Liver (glucuronidation) | Better choice if kidney disease is present |
| | | | Reduce dose and frequency in liver failure/cirrhosis |
| Tramadol | Low/moderate | Liver enzymes CYP2D6/CYP3A4 | Variable time to onset and analgesic efficacy in liver failure |
| | | | Interactions with other serotonergic medications, potentially leading to serotonin syndrome (agitation, clonus, muscle rigidity, hyperreflexia) |
| Oxycodone | Moderate/high | Liver enzymes CYP2D6/CYP3A4 | Increased half-life and variable onset in liver failure; if used, reduce dose and frequency |
| Morphine | Moderate/high | Liver (glucuronidation) | Avoid in liver failure/cirrhosis, kidney failure |
| | | | Increased bioavailability with liver failure |
| | | | Increased toxic metabolites with kidney failure |
| Fentanyl | High | Liver enzyme CYP3A4 | Safest long-acting drug in kidney and liver failure |
| | | | Increased bioavailability with liver failure; start lower-dose patch in liver failure |

CYP2D6 = cytochrome P-450 2D6; CYP3A4 = cytochrome P-450 3A4.

polyethylene glycol, are often added to achieve a regular bowel pattern. Docusate, alone or in combination, is no more effective than placebo for constipation in patients with a serious illness. Third-line therapy consists of rectal suppositories and/or enema preparations. Phosphate- or magnesium-containing enema preparations are contraindicated in seriously ill patients because of the potential for dangerous electrolyte shifts. If maximal medical therapy has failed to achieve laxation in patients taking opioids, peripheral opioid antagonists (such as methylnaltrexone) should be considered; these medications do not cross the blood-brain barrier and therefore do not affect analgesia.

## Nausea

Nausea and vomiting are common and debilitating symptoms in patients with a serious illness, with many patients rating nausea as more distressing than unrelieved pain. Management of nausea should be tailored to address the underlying mechanism and associated neurotransmitter pathway (**Table 31**). More than one agent is frequently required for symptom relief. In hospitalized patients, parenteral forms should be administered on a scheduled basis to achieve symptom control and not just reduce the number of emesis events.

## Other Symptoms

Anorexia and weight loss frequently occur in patients at the end of life. Clinicians should identify and treat any reversible conditions that may contribute to anorexia to ease patient and family distress. Although some medications are marketed for patients with anorexia and weight loss, they are marginally effective in a minority of terminally ill patients and often have unacceptable side effects. The use of enteral or parenteral artificial nutritional support at the end of life does not improve survival, is invasive, and can cause side effects, including increased terminal secretions and painful edema. Discussing the dying process, including the common presence of weight loss and anorexia and the lack of effective treatment for these

expected changes, can prepare patients and their family members and set realistic expectations.

Audible oropharyngeal secretions at the end of life ("death rattle") are often distressing for families and clinicians alike and may occur in up to 50% of dying patients. However, these secretions rarely affect respiratory status or cause patient distress, and educating family members on the normal process of dying can ease concerns. Treatment is often initiated in anticipation of family distress but is generally ineffective. Current literature does not support the routine use of antimuscarinic drugs in the treatment of death rattle. There is also no evidence that scopolamine, glycopyrronium, hyoscine butylbromide, atropine, or octreotide are superior to no treatment. The use of anticholinergic agents in patients who are awake can lead to undesirable symptoms, such as dry mouth and urinary retention. Suctioning by catheter should be avoided unless secretions are causing obvious respiratory distress.

Although symptoms of anticipatory grief are common at the end of life, clinical depression is not experienced by most patients and should not be expected. Clinical depression worsens quality of life and should be aggressively treated if present. In contrast to neurovegetative symptoms that accompany terminal illness (such as poor appetite and low energy), symptoms of unrelenting helplessness, hopelessness, and lack of pleasure should raise concerns for clinical depression. If depression is diagnosed, pharmacotherapy consists of antidepressant agents that are appropriate for the patient's estimated prognosis. Selective serotonin reuptake inhibitors are effective and safe in patients with end-organ dysfunction; however, their therapeutic effects may not be reached for several weeks. In patients with an estimated life expectancy of less than 6 weeks, psychostimulants, such as methylphenidate, are favored.

Delirium is a common symptom in patients at the end of life. It can result from many potentially reversible causes (medication side effects, inadequate analgesia, urinary retention, constipation), although a cause is often not identified.

| TABLE 31. Treatment of Nausea in the Palliative Care Patient | | |
|---|---|---|
| **Cause of Nausea** | **Mediating Receptor Pathway** | **Treatment** |
| Gut wall stretching or dilatation (constipation, bowel obstruction, ileus) | Dopamine type 2 ($D_2$) receptors in the gastrointestinal tract | Antidopaminergic antiemetics (metoclopramide, prochlorperazine, haloperidol) |
| Gut mucosal injury (radiation, chemotherapy, infection, inflammation, direct tumor invasion) | Serotonin (5-hydroxytryptamine-3 [5-$HT_3$]) receptors in the gastrointestinal tract | Serotonin antagonists (ondansetron, granisetron) |
| Drugs, metabolic by-products, bacterial toxins | $D_2$ receptors, 5-$HT_3$ receptors, and neurokinin type 1 receptors in the chemoreceptor trigger zone | Antidopaminergic antiemetics and serotonin antagonists |
| Motion sickness, labyrinthine disorders | Histamine type 1 ($H_1$) receptors and muscarinic acetylcholine receptors in the vestibular system | Anticholinergic antiemetics (scopolamine, diphenhydramine, promethazine) |
| Anticipatory nausea | Unknown, presumed cerebral cortex | Benzodiazepines |
| Increased intracranial pressure | Unknown | Glucocorticoids |

Nonpharmacologic interventions remain standard care; however, for some patients, medications may be required to maintain patient and caregiver safety and to ensure relief from suffering. First-generation antipsychotics, such as haloperidol or chlorpromazine, are effective and have not been shown to be inferior to newer-generation antipsychotics. The combination of benzodiazepines and antipsychotics may be more effective than antipsychotics alone in the treatment of delirium at the end of life.

Dyspnea can be a prominent and distressing symptom in patients with advanced illness and those at the end of life. The patient's subjective sensation of difficulty breathing should be measured on an iterative basis during evaluation and treatment. Although the initial goal of treatment is to address the underlying cause of dyspnea, many patients with advanced illness will have persistent dyspnea despite maximal medical management. In these patients, opioids are the treatment of choice. Opioids reduce the sensation of dyspnea and, when appropriately selected and dosed, do not cause respiratory depression. Refer to Common Symptoms for further discussion of the evaluation and management of dyspnea.

**KEY POINTS**

- The pharmacologic management of pain in patients with serious illness requires a multimodal approach that uses opioids and nonopioid analgesics such as acetaminophen, NSAIDs, glucocorticoids, topical therapies, neuropathic agents, and antidepressants with analgesic properties.
- For patients in whom nonopioid analgesic agents are ineffective or not tolerated, opioids are appropriate, with careful attention paid to dosing, frequency, and side effect profile.
- Pharmacologic therapy for patients with constipation and for all patients taking opioids should include a scheduled stimulant laxative, such as senna or bisacodyl.
- **HVC** Enteral or parenteral artificial nutritional support at the end of life does not improve survival, is invasive, and can cause side effects, such as increased terminal secretions and painful edema.
- Clinical depression should not be expected in patients at the end of life; if present, it should be aggressively treated.

## Hospice

Hospice is a form of palliative medicine that delivers specialized interdisciplinary care to patients with an expected prognosis of 6 months or less. Hospice care can be provided to patients in multiple settings, including the home, skilled nursing facilities, and residential hospice homes. Hospice teams are skilled in managing the symptoms of advanced and terminal illness and improve overall satisfaction with care.

# Common Symptoms

## Introduction

Specific symptom concerns account for nearly half of all outpatient visits. Although most symptoms resolve in several weeks, they sometimes present clinicians with the challenge of how to best determine their significance and the role of testing in the diagnostic approach. Unnecessary testing accounts for nearly 30% of health care costs. Hence, when evaluating symptoms, physicians have a responsibility to use testing strategies that offer the highest value. Fortunately, a thorough history alone generates the highest diagnostic yield, up to 75% in some studies, with the physical examination contributing an additional 10% to 15%. In contrast, testing results in less than 10% of diagnoses. Although diagnostic testing may provide crucial information and justify the costs incurred, physicians should consider the value of diagnostic testing and the effects of test results on patient management.

This chapter focuses on high-value approaches to the diagnosis and treatment of commonly encountered symptoms, including chronic noncancer pain, medically unexplained symptoms, dyspnea, cough, fatigue, dizziness, syncope, insomnia, and lower extremity edema. In addition, in-flight emergencies, a common event encountered by physicians, are reviewed.

## Chronic Noncancer Pain

The classification, assessment, and management of chronic noncancer pain are discussed in this section. For a discussion of cancer-related pain and pain in the setting of advanced illness, refer to Palliative Medicine.

Chronic pain is defined as a painful sensation lasting for more than 3 months or beyond the time frame expected for normal healing. Chronic pain has substantial negative effects on patient quality of life and physical, social, financial, and functional status. More than 10% of the U.S. population has symptoms consistent with chronic pain.

The approach to the patient with chronic pain is guided by the type of pain the patient experiences. Classification of chronic pain as nociceptive or neuropathic can be helpful in designing a tailored therapeutic approach; however, many patients with chronic noncancer pain syndromes will experience both nociceptive and neuropathic pain from multiple sources.

Nociceptive pain syndromes are caused by involvement of either visceral or somatic nociceptors. Visceral pain syndromes classically result from injury to or abnormal firing of visceral pain fibers; patients typically report poorly localized cramping or aching. In contrast, somatic pain syndromes are more commonly associated with injury to somatic pain fibers that convey signals from muscles, bones, and joints. Types of somatic pain include musculoskeletal pain (see Musculoskeletal Pain) and inflammatory pain. Often described by patients as sharp and stabbing pain, somatic nociception is easier to localize than visceral pain.

Neuropathic pain syndromes result from injury to peripheral nerve structures or central nervous system damage. Peripheral nerve syndromes, such as postherpetic neuralgia, are common and can be diagnosed by identifying sensory symptoms within the distribution of the affected peripheral nerve or nerves. Central neuropathic pain syndromes, such as those caused by cerebrovascular accidents or spinal cord injuries, often have widely varying presentations and symptom expression and can evade initial diagnostic approaches. A high index of suspicion is required because pain is often vaguely localized. Clinicians should look for key features, such as hyperalgesia (oversensitivity to a normally painful stimulus) or allodynia (pain from a normally nonpainful stimulus) occurring in the setting of underlying central nervous system injury.

In addition to nociceptive and neuropathic pain, pain induced by opioid therapy can occur paradoxically. Opioid-induced hyperalgesia is thought to result from repeated exposure to systemic opioids. Patients with this pain syndrome may experience a change in the character of their pain during the course of opioid therapy, a worsening of pain with increased opioid dosages, and a reduction in pain when opioid dosages are decreased.

## Assessment

The first step in the assessment of chronic pain is a thorough history and physical examination. Determination of pain location, duration, severity, temporal nature, and responsiveness to treatment is crucial in identifying the pain generator and tailoring the diagnostic and therapeutic approaches. In most cases of chronic pain, additional testing and imaging are unlikely to produce further diagnostic yield.

A key component of the assessment is a thorough review of the patient's functional status, including physical functioning, ability to perform basic activities of daily living, and psycho-social-spiritual functioning. Psychological comorbidities influence and are influenced by experiences of chronic pain, and they affect response and adherence to a multimodal treatment strategy. Patients should be screened for mental health disorders, and if present, these disorders should be treated in conjunction with the patient's chronic pain whenever possible. Depending on severity, treatment of concomitant mental health conditions may take precedence over interventions targeting chronic pain.

Patients with chronic pain are up to four times more likely to have concomitant depression. Depression increases as pain symptoms magnify, and depression may also manifest as pain. Aggressive treatment of depression, with both pharmacologic and nonpharmacologic behaviorally based therapies, can lead to substantial improvement in both chronic pain and depressive symptoms. Iterative evaluation of depressive symptoms during chronic pain treatment is critical to ensuring that patients are able to sustain improvements.

Substance abuse screening is another essential part of the assessment of patients with chronic pain (see Routine Care of the Healthy Patient). Substance use disorders are more common in patients with chronic pain syndromes and increase the risk for opioid misuse.

In the setting of chronic pain without a treatable underlying cause, clinicians should monitor for significant changes in pain experience, new acute pain syndromes superimposed on chronic pain, and development of "red flag" symptoms. Red flags include pain occurring with constitutional symptoms (such as fever and involuntary weight loss), change in bowel or bladder function, and weakness or sensory deficits. These signs and symptoms should trigger further investigation.

## Management

Management is determined by the cause of the patient's pain; the pain severity (as it relates to functional status); medical and psychosocial comorbid conditions; and barriers to treatment, such as health care access and concomitant mental health disorders. Developing a therapeutic relationship in which patients feel that their physician takes their pain seriously and in which patients, as well as family, friends, or other social supports, are active participants in the treatment strategy are important for success over time. Physical activity, engagement in work activities, and behavioral interventions should be encouraged regardless of pain score. Pharmacologic therapy should be viewed as adjunctive to nonpharmacologic therapy in the treatment of chronic pain. Patients receiving treatment should undergo periodic evaluation of pain, functional status, response to interventions, and quality of life.

### Nonpharmacologic Therapy

All patients with chronic pain should be referred to a structured physical therapy program for evaluation and treatment. Physical therapy teaches patients safe, self-guided exercises to improve functional status. High-quality evidence suggests that physical therapy programs improve both pain and function in patients with debilitation due to pain symptoms. Continuation of physical therapy beyond 12 weeks should be based on iterative clinical assessments and documented gains. Like physical therapy, exercise programs improve pain and function in patients with chronic pain, although no specific regimen has proved superior. Low- to moderate-quality evidence supports the use of complementary and integrative therapies, such as massage and acupuncture, to manage chronic pain.

Cognitive behavioral techniques, including cognitive behavioral therapy (CBT), mindfulness practices, and biofeedback, have been associated with reduced pain and improved overall function and mood. Referral to practices or specialized pain centers that provide these therapies should be explored when available.

Interventional approaches may be appropriate for patients with pain syndromes that can be anatomically targeted with injection-based therapy. In addition, advanced therapies, such as high-frequency neurostimulation, hold promise for appropriately selected patients. Patients may be referred to a pain specialist for consideration of these therapies.

**Pharmacologic Therapy**

Pharmacologic therapy should be used as adjunctive treatment for chronic pain when nonpharmacologic therapies have not achieved their desired effect. Clinicians should emphasize that pharmacologic therapies have limited efficacy in the long-term management of chronic pain and are intended to improve function and quality of life, not pain scores. Patients should be informed that adjuvant pharmacologic therapies may take weeks to be effective and that a combination of medications with differing mechanisms may be necessary to provide optimal benefit. When selecting pharmacologic therapies to add to a multimodal treatment regimen, attention to comorbid illness (particularly organ dysfunction) and concurrent medications is critical to limit side effects.

For chronic musculoskeletal or inflammatory nociceptive pain, trials of acetaminophen (≤3 g/d) or NSAIDs can be considered as initial pharmacologic therapy in patients without contraindications to their use. In cases of inflammatory nociceptive pain, NSAIDs can be given both orally and topically. NSAIDs are typically used for periodic pain flares or potentially while opioid therapy is being down-titrated but not for long-term therapy. Topical NSAIDs, such as topical diclofenac, have few systemic side effects, are generally well tolerated, and are effective for short-term treatment of musculoskeletal nociceptive conditions. Although short courses of muscle relaxants may be beneficial in some patients with acute pain, long-term use should be avoided because of the potential for side effects and drug-drug interactions.

In chronic neuropathic pain syndromes, gabapentinoids (such as gabapentin and pregabalin) and serotonin-norepinephrine reuptake inhibitors (such as duloxetine) are first-line therapy. When pain generators are topically located, capsaicin and topical lidocaine can be considered. Tricyclic antidepressants, such as nortriptyline and desipramine, are also effective for neuropathic pain syndromes, although titration to effective dosages is often limited by side effects and drug-drug interactions.

Medical cannabis is increasingly available for use in patients with chronic pain. Many states have passed laws legalizing the use of cannabis or allowing its use for medical conditions, although it is still classified by the U.S. Drug Enforcement Administration as a schedule I agent. Current data on the effectiveness of medical cannabis for chronic pain are characterized by significant heterogeneity in both patient populations and cannabis preparations, although recent systematic reviews have demonstrated that cannabis has some efficacy in the treatment of chronic noncancer pain. The most robust data originate from studies of compounds available outside the United States (such as nabiximols), which contain higher ratios of cannabidiol to tetrahydrocannabinol (THC) than the existing FDA-approved synthetic THC (dronabinol). Little is known about the comparative efficacy of cannabis preparations in states where medical cannabis is available.

*Opioids*

Patients who present to physicians' offices with chronic pain are frequently provided with prescriptions for opioids. Despite high prescribing rates, no evidence supports the use of long-term opioid therapy in patients with chronic noncancer pain. In fact, evidence demonstrates that long-term opioid use is associated with poorer overall functional status, worse quality of life, and worse pain (possibly mediated through opioid tolerance and hyperalgesic mechanisms). In addition, although often well intentioned, these prescribing patterns lead to substantial morbidity and mortality. From 1999 to 2015, more than 183,000 Americans died from overdose related to prescription opioids, and in 2011, an estimated 400,000 emergency department visits were attributable to opioid misuse or abuse. Importantly, most opioid-related overdoses occurred in patients taking opioids as prescribed. Opioids should not be considered first-line therapy in any patient with a chronic noncancer pain syndrome.

In patients in whom multimodal analgesic therapy has not improved function and quality of life or in patients already receiving opioids, the decision to initiate or continue opioids should include a thorough assessment of the benefits and burdens of therapy. In 2016, the Centers for Disease Control and Prevention (CDC) released a comprehensive guideline for prescribing opioids in patients with chronic pain syndromes, not including patients with active cancer, patients receiving palliative care, and patients at the end of life. Central to these guidelines are a robust discussion of risks and benefits, close monitoring, and use of risk-mitigation strategies (**Table 32**). The CDC provides a checklist to assist clinicians in the prescribing of opioids in the setting of chronic noncancer pain, available at https://stacks.cdc.gov/view/cdc/38025.

When discussing opioid therapy with patients, it is important to emphasize the lack of evidence for long-term opioid therapy in chronic pain syndromes and the substantial risks associated with long-term use of these medications. **Table 33** summarizes some of the important risks associated with long-term opioid therapy.

Clear treatment goals based on functional improvement and quality-of-life considerations should be established to manage patient expectations and provide a means for measuring the success or failure of treatment. These goals can be incorporated into a patient-physician prescribing agreement, which can also be used to communicate expectations for follow-up, monitoring, and risk mitigation.

The CDC guideline recommends that before starting and periodically during continuation of opioid therapy, clinicians should evaluate risk factors for opioid-related harms. A commonly used risk assessment instrument, the Opioid Risk Tool, is available at https://www.drugabuse.gov/sites/default/files/files/OpioidRiskTool.pdf. Urine drug screening and surveillance of state prescription monitoring databases are important

**TABLE 32.** Centers for Disease Control and Prevention Recommendations for Prescribing Opioids for Chronic Pain Outside of Active Cancer, Palliative, and End-of-Life Care[a]

**Determining When to Initiate or Continue Opioids for Chronic Pain**

1. Nonpharmacologic therapy and nonopioid pharmacologic therapy are preferred for chronic pain. Clinicians should consider opioid therapy only if expected benefits for both pain and function are anticipated to outweigh risks to the patient. If opioids are used, they should be combined with nonpharmacologic therapy and nonopioid pharmacologic therapy, as appropriate.

2. Before starting opioid therapy for chronic pain, clinicians should establish treatment goals with all patients, including realistic goals for pain and function, and should consider how therapy will be discontinued if benefits do not outweigh risks. Clinicians should continue opioid therapy only if there is clinically meaningful improvement in pain and function that outweighs risks to patient safety.

3. Before starting and periodically during opioid therapy, clinicians should discuss with patients known risks and realistic benefits of opioid therapy and patient and clinician responsibilities for managing therapy.

**Opioid Selection, Dosage, Duration, Follow-up, and Discontinuation**

4. When starting opioid therapy for chronic pain, clinicians should prescribe immediate-release opioids instead of extended-release/long-acting (ER/LA) opioids.

5. When opioids are started, clinicians should prescribe the lowest effective dosage. Clinicians should use caution when prescribing opioids at any dosage, should carefully reassess evidence of individual benefits and risks when increasing dosage to ≥50 morphine milligram equivalents (MME)/day, and should avoid increasing dosage to ≥90 MME/day or carefully justify a decision to titrate dosage to ≥90 MME/day.

6. Long-term opioid use often begins with treatment of acute pain. When opioids are used for acute pain, clinicians should prescribe the lowest effective dosage of immediate-release opioids and should prescribe no greater quantity than needed for the expected duration of pain severe enough to require opioids. Three days or less will often be sufficient; more than 7 days will rarely be needed.

7. Clinicians should evaluate benefits and harms with patients within 1 to 4 weeks of starting opioid therapy for chronic pain or of dose escalation. Clinicians should evaluate benefits and harms of continued therapy with patients every 3 months or more frequently. If benefits do not outweigh harms of continued opioid therapy, clinicians should optimize other therapies and work with patients to taper opioids to lower dosages or to taper and discontinue opioids.

**Assessing Risk and Addressing Harms of Opioid Use**

8. Before starting and periodically during continuation of opioid therapy, clinicians should evaluate risk factors for opioid-related harms. Clinicians should incorporate into the management plan strategies to mitigate risk, including considering offering naloxone when factors that increase risk for opioid overdose, such as history of overdose, history of substance use disorder, higher opioid dosages (≥50 MME/day), or concurrent benzodiazepine use, are present.

9. Clinicians should review the patient's history of controlled substance prescriptions using state prescription drug monitoring program (PDMP) data to determine whether the patient is receiving opioid dosages or dangerous combinations that put him or her at high risk for overdose. Clinicians should review PDMP data when starting opioid therapy for chronic pain and periodically during opioid therapy for chronic pain, ranging from every prescription to every 3 months.

10. When prescribing opioids for chronic pain, clinicians should use urine drug testing before starting opioid therapy and consider urine drug testing at least annually to assess for prescribed medications as well as other controlled prescription drugs and illicit drugs.

11. Clinicians should avoid prescribing opioid pain medication and benzodiazepines concurrently whenever possible.

12. Clinicians should offer or arrange evidence-based treatment (usually medication-assisted treatment with buprenorphine or methadone in combination with behavioral therapies) for patients with opioid use disorder.

[a]All recommendations are category A (apply to all patients outside of active cancer treatment, palliative care, and end-of-life care) except recommendation 10 (designated category B, with individual decision making required); see full guideline at https://www.cdc.gov/mmwr/volumes/65/rr/rr6501e1.htm for evidence ratings.

Reproduced from Dowell D, Haegerich TM, Chou R. CDC guideline for prescribing opioids for chronic pain—United States, 2016. MMWR Recomm Rep. 2016;65:16. [PMID: 26987082] doi:10.15585/mmwr.rr6501e1

**TABLE 33.** Risks of Long-Term Opioid Therapy

Endocrinopathies (e.g., osteoporosis, hypogonadism)

Increased risk for opioid addiction

Increased risk for overdose and death

Increasing pain through mechanisms of opioid-induced hyperalgesia

Opioid tolerance resulting from adaptive central nervous system mechanisms

risk–mitigation strategies for patients receiving opioids in the setting of chronic pain. Although the optimal frequency of urine drug screening is unclear, patients taking long-term opioid therapy should undergo urine screening at least yearly to assess for adherence to the prescribed agent and for the presence of substances that could increase the risk for opioid overdose. More frequent screening may be recommended based on individual patient characteristics. State prescription monitoring databases (where available) should also be reviewed on a regular basis for adherence to the terms of the prescribing agreement.

The CDC guideline also provides recommendations on safe dosing. The risk for opioid-related overdose is dose dependent, with significantly increased risk for overdose in patients receiving dosages higher than 90 morphine milligram equivalents per day. The lowest possible dosage should be used to achieve the functional and quality-of-life goals established by the patient and prescriber. Given the risks and limited efficacy of opioid therapy in treating chronic noncancer pain, these dosages should not typically exceed more than 50 morphine milligram equivalents per day. Follow-up evaluation should occur at frequent intervals after therapy initiation or dosage changes and at least every 3 months. Dosages exceeding 50 morphine milligram equivalents per day should prompt re-evaluation and closer follow-up intervals. Dosages higher than 90 morphine milligram equivalents per day are considered high risk and should be prescribed only in consultation with pain specialists. Co-prescription of opioids and benzodiazepines is associated with an increased risk for death from overdose and should be avoided.

Evidence shows that naloxone, an opioid antagonist that reverses life-threatening respiratory depression, is effective in preventing opioid-related overdose death at the community level through community-based distribution. Primary care clinicians should consider offering naloxone kits and associated overdose prevention education to patients at increased risk for overdose, such as those receiving daily doses of 50 morphine milligram equivalents per day or more, concurrently taking a benzodiazepine, or with a history of substance use disorder, as well as to the patient's family members or caregivers.

For patients who previously received prescriptions for opioids in the setting of chronic pain and present to a physician for referral or as a new patient, a discussion on opioid prescribing best practices should be framed by the CDC guideline recommendations. Discussions on tapering opioid therapy, incorporating a nonopioid multimodal pain strategy as the cornerstone of pain management, and setting appropriate goals are fundamental to these prescribing relationships.

For a discussion on the treatment of opioid use disorder, see Mental and Behavioral Health.

### KEY POINTS

- **HVC** In patients with chronic pain, determining the pain location, duration, severity, temporal nature, and responsiveness to treatment is crucial in identifying the pain generator and tailoring the diagnostic and therapeutic approaches; in most cases of chronic pain, additional testing and imaging is unlikely to produce further diagnostic yield.
- In the setting of chronic pain without a treatable underlying cause, clinicians should monitor for significant changes in pain experience, new acute pain syndromes superimposed on chronic pain, and the development of red flag symptoms.

*(Continued)*

### KEY POINTS *(continued)*

- Physical therapy improves both pain and function in patients with debilitation due to chronic pain. **HVC**
- Cognitive behavioral techniques, including cognitive behavioral therapy, mindfulness practices, and biofeedback, have been associated with reduced pain and improved overall function and mood in patients with chronic pain. **HVC**
- For chronic musculoskeletal or inflammatory nociceptive pain, trials of acetaminophen (≤3 g/d) or NSAIDs can be considered as initial pharmacologic therapy in patients without contraindications to their use. **HVC**
- In chronic neuropathic pain syndromes, gabapentinoids and serotonin-norepinephrine reuptake inhibitors are first-line therapy.
- No evidence supports long-term opioid therapy in patients with chronic noncancer pain, and evidence demonstrates that long-term opioid use is associated with poorer overall functional status, worse quality of life, and worse pain. **HVC**
- The decision to initiate opioid therapy in patients with chronic pain should involve a robust discussion of risks and benefits, close monitoring for benefits and harms, avoidance of long-acting opioid formulations, and use of risk-mitigation strategies.
- Primary care clinicians should consider offering naloxone kits and associated overdose prevention education to patients at increased risk for overdose, such as those receiving daily doses of 50 morphine milligram equivalents per day or more, concurrently taking a benzodiazepine, or with a history of substance use disorder.

## Medically Unexplained Symptoms

Medically unexplained symptoms (MUS) are symptoms that cannot be attributed to a specific medical cause after a thorough medical evaluation. The prevalence of MUS is high; a recent systematic review of 32 studies involving 70,085 patients determined that the prevalence of patients with at least one unexplained symptom ranges from 40% to 49%. Patients with MUS are frequently seen in both primary and subspecialty clinics, resulting in significantly increased health care utilization. The costs associated with MUS are estimated at more than $250 billion annually. Unsurprisingly, the high prevalence, increased resource utilization and frequency of visits, ongoing inexplicable symptoms, and looming fear of a missed diagnosis all contribute to patient and clinician dissatisfaction.

Many terms have been incorrectly and interchangeably used to describe and diagnose MUS, further complicating an already challenging scenario. Patients with MUS must be distinguished from those with somatic symptom and related disorders, which are psychiatric conditions with specific diagnostic criteria (see Mental and Behavioral Health). Although many somatic symptom and related disorders involve MUS, most patients with MUS do not meet the diagnostic criteria for these disorders.

## Clinical Presentation and Evaluation

Symptoms that are common in patients with MUS include fatigue, headache, abdominal pain, musculoskeletal pain (back pain, myalgia, and arthralgia), dizziness, paresthesia, generalized weakness, transient edema, insomnia, dyspnea, chest pain, chronic facial pain, chronic pelvic pain, and chemical sensitivities. MUS appear more frequently in women, persons with lower levels of education, and those with lower socioeconomic status.

There is no formal approach to the diagnostic evaluation of MUS; however, the initial evaluation should involve a thorough history and physical examination related to each symptom. Clinicians must approach each symptom in a focused manner and diligently review any previous diagnostic evaluations. Laboratory and radiographic studies should be guided by the findings on the history and physical examination, and subspecialty referrals should be used judiciously. Given the high comorbidity of mood disturbances in patients with MUS, patients with features concerning for an underlying mood disorder should be evaluated accordingly.

If an underlying medical cause cannot be identified after an appropriately thorough evaluation, it is imperative that clinicians have an open and honest discussion of the results with the patient, being mindful to acknowledge the patient's concerns and frustrations. Frequently, patients will request, or even demand, additional testing and consultations that may not be clinically indicated. Although doing so may be challenging, clinicians should limit additional evaluations to those deemed medically necessary, as unnecessary studies provide negligible reassurance, pose iatrogenic risks, and result in additional patient anxiety.

## Management

The foundation of management of patients with MUS is an open, honest, and effective therapeutic relationship. Patients should be treated respectfully and cared for in a nonjudgmental manner. It is important to not only expect but to accept the patient's feelings of frustration, acknowledging these feelings early in the patient's management course can help to build and strengthen the therapeutic alliance.

Management of MUS requires a patient-focused, holistic, and multimodal approach. The goals of management are functional restoration, decreased symptom focus, and acquisition of coping mechanisms rather than abatement of symptoms. Office visits should be scheduled at regular intervals, allowing for additional discussion, educational opportunities, and longitudinal reassessment. Frequency of appointments can gradually be decreased over time as tolerated by the patient. It should be made clear to patients that the treatment of MUS will not likely be curative and that symptoms may persist.

Patients should be encouraged to develop short-term and long-term goals with the recognition that many goals will change from a physical symptom focus to a psychosocial focus. If additional symptoms arise, clinicians should respond empathically and perform an appropriately thorough investigation.

Interventions that may benefit patients with MUS include CBT, physical therapy, occupational therapy, individual or group psychotherapy, social support, biofeedback therapy, graded exercise therapy, stress management activities, and training in coping mechanisms. Patients with comorbid mood conditions should be considered for a trial of antidepressant therapy and referral to a psychiatrist or psychologist. Given the wide-ranging effects of MUS, treatment should be focused on both physical and psychosocial aspects (**Table 34**).

Knowledge of barriers to the treatment of patients with MUS can help clinicians prevent unnecessary missteps and provide ongoing value-based care. Common barriers include a poor physician-patient relationship, the heterogeneity of symptoms, varying diagnostic labels, and ongoing changes in the health care system (insurance coverage, access to care, and value-based metrics).

**KEY POINTS**

- In patients with medically unexplained symptoms, clinicians should limit diagnostic tests to those deemed medically necessary because unrevealing studies provide negligible reassurance, pose iatrogenic risks, and result in additional patient anxiety.  **HVC**

- The goals of management in patients with medically unexplained symptoms are functional restoration, decreased symptom focus, and acquisition of coping mechanisms rather than abatement of symptoms.  **HVC**

## Dyspnea

Dyspnea is a common symptom with a diverse pathophysiologic basis and substantial variation in patient experience. The American Thoracic Society defines dyspnea as "a subjective experience of breathing discomfort that consists of qualitatively distinct sensations that vary in intensity." Patients may describe this symptom as breathlessness or tightness, an inability to catch their breath, or a feeling of drowning. The prevalence of dyspnea increases with age, with more than one third of those older than 70 years reporting sensations of dyspnea in an ambulatory setting. Dyspnea affects up to half of hospitalized patients and is a common reason for patients to seek care in urgent and emergent care settings.

Dyspnea results from multiple underlying neurophysiologic mechanisms, including greater work of breathing, air hunger, and airway irritation or damage. These mechanisms may be triggered by poor functional status, organ-specific pathology, medication effects, or physiologic stimuli (including hypoxia and hypercapnia).

**TABLE 34.** Follow-up Management of the Patient With Medically Unexplained Symptoms

| Category | Issue | How? | How Often? | Notes |
|---|---|---|---|---|
| Nonpharmacologic therapy | Maintaining an effective relationship with the patient | Elicit and address the patient's emotional concerns; use a negotiated rather than a prescriptive approach; tailor care to patient's personality; address your own negative reactions to the patient. | Each visit | Monitor the provider-patient relationship regularly as you would, for example, monitor blood pressure in a patient with hypertension. Ask, "So how is all this going; how are you and I working together?" Examples of indicators of an effective relationship are adherence to the treatment plan, friendliness, improved eye contact, positive statements about the provider and the treatment. |
| | Dissociating treatment regimen from symptoms | Schedule regular, consistent, time-contingent visits rather than ad hoc (as-needed) visits; give all medications on a scheduled rather than on an as-needed basis. | Each visit | Titrate number of scheduled visits and amount of treatment to patient's needs and progress. |
| Pharmacologic therapy | MUS symptoms | Consider lowest effective dose of antidepressant and nonopioid analgesics. | Each visit | Minimize or avoid use of opioids and tranquilizers. |
| | Comorbid depression and anxiety | Treat depression as indicated. | As needed | |
| Patient education | Overall management | Review patient's diary and facilitate understanding of how his or her thoughts, emotions, and behaviors are related to symptoms. | Ongoing | |
| | Education and treatment plan | Educate the patient so that the patient understands the plan of care and its purpose. | Each visit | |
| | Reinforcing patient commitment to treatment | Give appropriate praise for commitment behavior, such as completing homework; address noncommittal behavior, such as not keeping appointments or visiting an acute care facility without prior discussion. | Each visit | |
| | Reviewing and revising patient goals | Reinforce previous short-term goals or negotiate new ones to operationalize patient's long-term goals. | Each visit | Help patient to identify solutions to roadblocks. |
| | Negotiating new plans | Negotiate plans to adjust physical activity; recommend relaxation techniques; refer for physical therapy. | Each visit | Continuously encourage the patient to add new healthy behaviors and to progress in what he or she is already doing. |

MUS = medically unexplained symptoms.

Adapted with permission from Dwamena FC, Fortin AH, Smith RC. Medically unexplained symptoms. In ACP Smart Medicine (online database). Philadelphia: American College of Physicians, 2015. Accessed June 25, 2015.

## Evaluation

The history and physical examination are the most important components of the evaluation of dyspnea. A crucial aspect of the history is determining whether the patient's dyspnea is new in onset or an acute-on-chronic exacerbation of a known disease. Evaluation of the patient with acute-on-chronic symptoms should include an investigation for a potentially new generator of dyspnea (such as pleural effusion in the setting of existing lung malignancy) or progression of the underlying cause.

Dyspnea has many causes (**Table 35**). A cardiac or respiratory origin is most common, although some patients will have a mixed presentation. In the absence of an obvious cause, the initial evaluation in most patients will include measurement of oxygen saturation and hemoglobin, as well as electrocardiography and chest radiography. Depending on the results of these tests, further evaluation may entail measurement of B-type natriuretic peptide, D-dimer assay, pulmonary function testing, and advanced imaging of the cardiac or pulmonary systems. Such testing, however, should be pursued only when the

| TABLE 35. | Common Causes of Dyspnea |
|---|---|
| **Acute Dyspnea** | |
| Decreased cardiac output/function | |
| Ischemic heart disease | |
| Pulmonary infection | |
| Pneumothorax | |
| Pleural effusion | |
| Bronchospasm | |
| Pulmonary vascular disease (e.g., pulmonary embolism or hemorrhage) | |
| **Chronic Dyspnea** | |
| Airflow obstruction (e.g., COPD) | |
| Restrictive lung diseases | |
| Decreased cardiac output/function | |
| Deconditioning | |

CONT.

initial evaluation reveals a reasonable likelihood of disease; scattershot testing should be avoided. Referral to a cardiologist or pulmonologist may be appropriate when the diagnosis remains elusive or when conditions require subspecialty input.

Dyspnea should be assessed on an iterative basis during the patient's care. Many validated dyspnea scoring systems are available; however, these instruments are lengthy, take significant time to complete, and may not account for contributing factors in the patient's experience of dyspnea. Standard measurement with a numeric scale akin to a pain-rating scale is advantageous for its ease of use, but it must be paired with a functional assessment of quality of life and dyspnea-related impairment.

## Management

Initial treatment strategies are aimed at treating or modifying the patient's dyspnea generator and the underlying disease state responsible for causing the symptom. In patients with chronic conditions, the first step in reducing dyspnea is to maximize standard therapies, with regular assessment of symptomatic response.

In patients with persistent debilitating symptoms despite maximal medical therapy, there are nonpharmacologic and pharmacologic strategies to reduce dyspnea severity, with varying levels of evidence to support each one. Of these therapies, pursed-lip breathing, handheld fans, and devices that enhance air flow are the least invasive and easiest to administer. Studies examining the efficacy of guided relaxation training and acupuncture/acupressure have yielded mixed results, but these therapies are safe and may be reasonable for appropriately selected patients. Pulmonary rehabilitation can provide significant benefits for patients with chronic lung diseases and has been shown to improve subjective dyspnea in patients with severe COPD.

In patients with hypoxemia and COPD, oxygen therapy offers substantial benefits in survival, quality of life, and dyspnea reduction. However, the role of supplemental oxygen in other patient groups, including those with normoxemic dyspnea, is less clear. Data from a randomized controlled trial of palliative oxygen versus medical air in normoxemic patients demonstrated no improvement in quality of life or scores of subjective dyspnea with palliative oxygen therapy, supporting the hypothesis that movement of air is more important in reducing breathlessness in these patients. In patients with refractory dyspnea despite maximal therapy, a brief trial of supplemental oxygen is reasonable.

Opioids are an effective therapy for patients with dyspnea that is refractory to nonpharmacologic therapies and maximal medical management of the underlying disease. Opioids, both endogenous and exogenous, appear to exert an antidyspneic effect through modulation of central nervous system processing of sensory inputs, similar to their modulation of pain signaling. Although opioids affect respiratory mechanics and may blunt respiratory drive, appropriately dosed opioids should not cause respiratory depression if treatment is directed by symptoms. Patient selection and subsequent opioid selection should be based on symptom burden, underlying disease, comorbid organ dysfunction, and overall risk for respiratory depression. Although systemic opioids have shown clear benefit in treating refractory dyspnea, inhaled opioids have not shown significant efficacy in several placebo-controlled trials. H

### KEY POINTS

- An important aspect of the evaluation of dyspnea is determining whether the patient's dyspnea is new in onset or an acute-on-chronic exacerbation of a known disease state.
- Pursed-lip breathing, handheld fans, and devices that enhance air flow are easy, noninvasive interventions to reduce dyspnea severity.  **HVC**
- Opioids are an effective therapy for patients with dyspnea that is refractory to nonpharmacologic therapies and maximal medical management of the underlying disease.

## Cough

Cough is another common symptom, resulting in roughly 30 million physician office visits and costing billions of dollars annually in the United States. An evidence-based approach to the evaluation of cough that ensures cost-effective care is framed around the duration of cough (acute, subacute, and chronic).

### Acute Cough

Acute cough (<3 weeks' duration) is most often caused by viral respiratory tract infections, including upper respiratory tract infections (URIs) and bronchitis. Other conditions that may present with acute cough include allergic rhinosinusitis, pneumonia, medication adverse reactions, and pulmonary edema.

The initial evaluation of the patient with acute cough focuses on identifying potentially life-threatening illnesses. Concomitant fever, dyspnea, chest pain, and abnormalities on lung or cardiovascular examination suggest a serious respiratory or cardiovascular disease as the source of cough, and further evaluation should be completed as appropriate. If signs and symptoms are primarily respiratory and constitutional, a lower respiratory tract infection is most likely, and chest radiography may be warranted. Pneumonia is an unlikely cause of acute cough, and chest radiography is not indicated in the absence of abnormal vital signs (heart rate >100/min, respiration rate >24/min, temperature >38 °C [100.4 °F]) or abnormal lung examination findings, unless there are other concerning clinical features (such as altered mental status).

Acute cough without evidence of lower respiratory tract infection or cardiovascular disease is most often caused by viral rhinosinusitis or acute bronchitis. Coronaviruses and rhinoviruses are the most common causative pathogens, but influenza virus should be highly suspected in patients presenting with fever and myalgia, especially during influenza season (between autumn and early spring). Bacterial infections can also cause acute sinusitis or bronchitis, although sinus imaging is not recommended unless a complication, such as spread of infection into contiguous structures, is suspected.

Another important cause of acute cough is ACE inhibitor therapy. Up to 20% of patients taking an ACE inhibitor develop a dry cough, usually within 1 to 2 weeks of therapy initiation. Onset of cough, however, may be delayed by months in a small percentage of patients, and cough may additionally persist for weeks after discontinuation of the offending agent. All ACE inhibitors may cause this side effect. Angiotensin receptor blockers typically do not cause cough and may be substituted if ACE inhibitor therapy is not tolerated.

Treatment of acute cough is primarily symptomatic and dependent on the underlying etiology. Antibiotics are not recommended in patients with acute bronchitis or URIs without clearly established bacterial infection, although most patients with acute bacterial sinusitis will improve without antibiotics. A meta-analysis of patients with acute rhinosinusitis found that use of intranasal glucocorticoids increased the rate of symptom response compared with placebo; there was a dose-response curve, with higher doses offering greater relief. Analgesics, such as NSAIDs and acetaminophen, may provide pain relief. Only limited evidence supports saline irrigation in the relief of nasal symptoms; careful attention should be paid to the use of sterile or bottled water. Instructions for nasal saline irrigation are available online (https://www.fda.gov/ForConsumers/ ConsumerUpdates/ucm316375.htm). First-generation antihistamines may help dry nasal secretions; however,

evidence supporting their efficacy is lacking, and sedation is a common side effect. Decongestants are of possible benefit in patients with evidence of eustachian tube dysfunction but should be used with caution in elderly patients and those with cardiovascular disease, hypertension, angle-closure glaucoma, or bladder neck obstruction. Antitussive agents are generally ineffective.

## Subacute and Chronic Cough

Subacute cough (3-8 weeks' duration) is most often a postinfectious cough following an acute respiratory tract infection, particularly viral or *Mycoplasma* infection. Postinfectious cough is usually caused by postnasal drip or airway hyperreactivity. If postnasal drip is the primary problem, first-generation antihistamines may be beneficial. In patients with evidence of airway hyperreactivity, such as wheezing, therapies for asthma are usually effective. Patients with postinfectious cough not caused by postnasal drip or airway hyperreactivity may benefit from inhaled ipratropium. *Bordetella pertussis* infection should be considered in patients with subacute cough characterized by paroxysms of severe coughing and posttussive emesis. If infectious causes of subacute cough are excluded, the evaluation shifts to consideration of the causes of chronic cough.

Chronic cough (>8 weeks' duration) is most often caused by upper airway cough syndrome (UACS; formerly postnasal drip syndrome), gastroesophageal reflux disease (GERD), asthma, smoking, and ACE inhibitor use. Nonasthmatic eosinophilic bronchitis is another increasingly documented cause of chronic cough. Important but less common causes include chronic bronchitis, lung neoplasm, bronchiectasis, and chronic aspiration.

Evaluation of chronic cough begins with a thorough history, physical examination, and chest radiography (**Figure 4**). ACE inhibitor therapy and tobacco use should be discontinued. If an etiology is not determined after initial evaluation, a stepwise approach is pursued, beginning with a 2-week trial of empiric treatment for UACS. Allergic rhinitis–associated UACS is optimally treated with intranasal glucocorticoids, whereas UACS resulting from nonallergic rhinitis responds best to first-generation antihistamines (chlorpheniramine, brompheniramine, diphenhydramine) and decongestants (pseudoephedrine).

Asthma should be considered in patients with symptoms that do not respond to empiric treatment for UACS. Cough-variant asthma is diagnosed if spirometry and/or bronchial hyperresponsiveness testing results are abnormal and symptoms improve with standard therapy for asthma, including inhaled glucocorticoids.

In patients with normal findings on evaluation or failed empiric treatment for UACS and asthma, the most reasonable next step is to exclude nonasthmatic eosinophilic bronchitis with sputum analysis for eosinophils or exhaled nitric oxide testing. If test results are abnormal, therapy with inhaled glucocorticoids should be initiated.

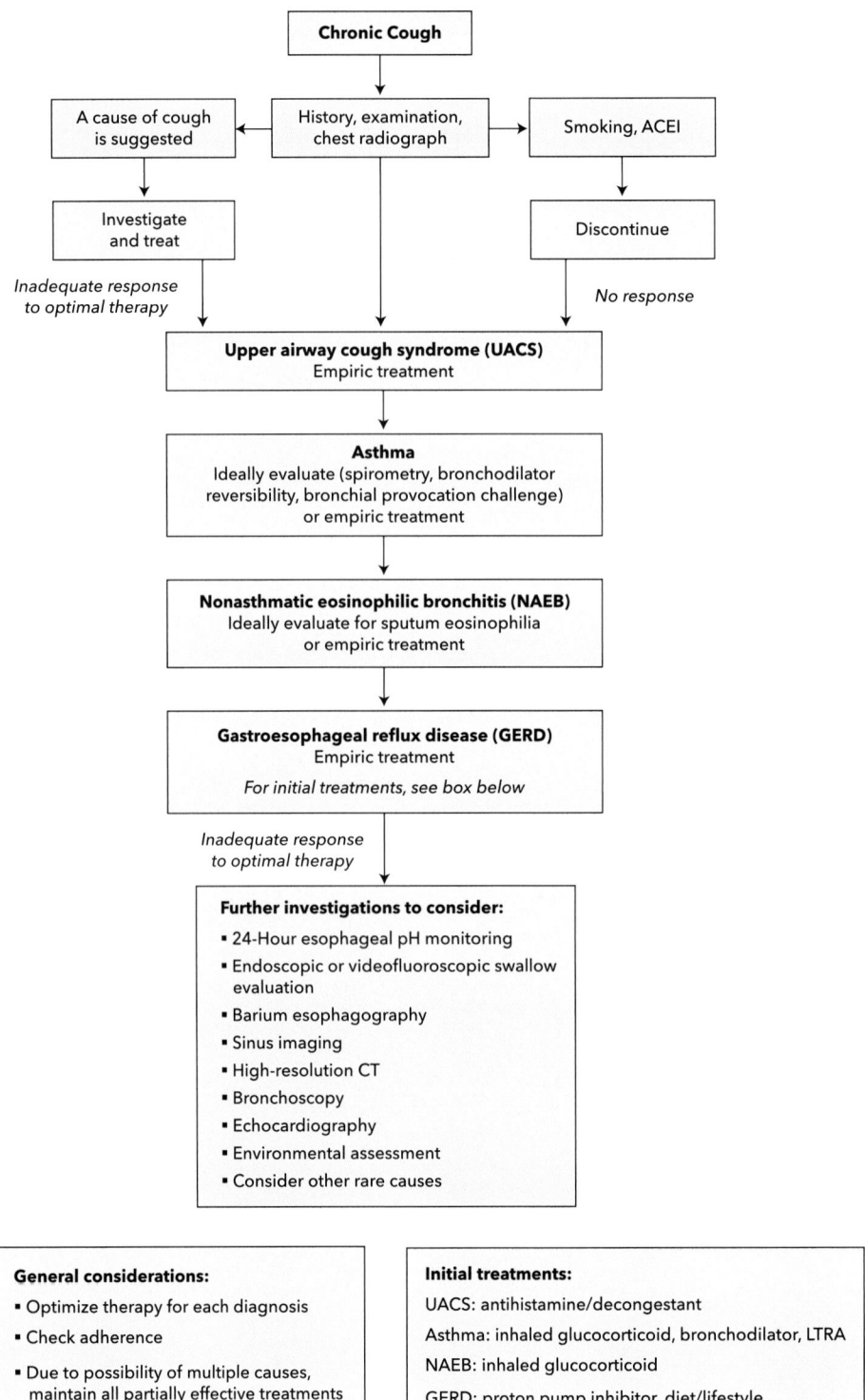

**FIGURE 4.** Evaluation of chronic cough. ACEI = ACE inhibitor; LTRA = leukotriene receptor antagonist.

Cough without a clear etiology that does not respond to the aforementioned empiric therapies should be treated with empiric proton pump inhibitor therapy and antireflux lifestyle changes to address possible GERD. Failure of empiric GERD treatment of 8 weeks' duration should prompt an advanced investigation (see Figure 4).

Persistent cough without an identifiable cause despite comprehensive evaluation is termed unexplained chronic cough.

Patients with unexplained chronic cough may benefit from other therapies for symptomatic relief. Antitussives, including dextromethorphan and topical anesthetics (benzonatate), have been shown to reduce cough and improve quality of life. Opioids, such as codeine, may have a similar effect but should be used with caution and only if other measures fail. Gabapentin can also be effective at controlling unexplained chronic cough and should be considered if the risk for adverse effects is acceptable. Protussives, such as guaifenesin, can improve mucus clearance and cough intensity in selected patients with excessive sputum production. Finally, multimodality speech pathology therapy may provide benefit and should be offered to all patients with chronic cough of undetermined cause.

### Cough in the Immunocompromised Patient

Immunocompromised patients with cough require heightened suspicion for infections, particularly if immunosuppression is severe. In addition to common pathogens, other causes to consider include fungi, cytomegalovirus, varicella, herpesvirus, and *Pneumocystis jirovecii*. Clinicians should have a low threshold for initiating empiric antibiotic therapy while diagnostic testing is pursued.

### Hemoptysis

Hemoptysis is expectoration of blood from the lower respiratory tract with coughing. Causes include bronchitis, bronchiectasis, malignancy, tuberculosis, pulmonary embolism, and left ventricular failure. Rare causes include anti–glomerular basement membrane antibody disease (Goodpasture syndrome) and granulomatosis with polyangiitis. Hemoptysis requires urgent evaluation, which begins with assessment to confirm the lower respiratory tract as the source of bleeding and exclude bleeding from the nasopharynx (nosebleed) or the gastrointestinal tract (hematemesis). Chest radiography should be performed, but most patients additionally require chest CT and/or bronchoscopy to accurately determine the cause.

#### KEY POINTS

HVC • In patients with acute cough, chest radiography is not indicated in the absence of abnormal vital signs or abnormal lung examination findings, unless there are other concerning clinical features (such as altered mental status).

HVC • Treatment of acute cough is primarily symptomatic; antibiotics are not recommended in patients with acute bronchitis or upper respiratory tract infection without a clear bacterial cause.

• Common causes of chronic cough include smoking, ACE inhibitor use, upper airway cough syndrome, gastroesophageal reflux disease, asthma, and nonasthmatic eosinophilic bronchitis.

• Patients with unexplained chronic cough may benefit from antitussives, gabapentin, and multimodality speech pathology therapy.

# Fatigue and Systemic Exertion Intolerance Disease

Fatigue is generally defined as tiredness, exhaustion, or lack of energy precipitated by exertion or stress. It is a common symptom, occurring in one quarter to one third of patients in the primary care setting. Despite its high prevalence, the cause of fatigue is often elusive, leading to prolonged delays in diagnosis, substantial functional decline, and high direct and indirect societal costs. Chronic fatigue is defined as fatigue lasting longer than 6 months.

Fatigue is a truly subjective symptom with little to no corroborating objective measures. It can be classified as fatigue secondary to another cause (**Table 36**), secondary to multiple factors (termed chronic multifactorial fatigue [CMF]), or as a primary condition. In the past, the latter condition was termed chronic fatigue syndrome (CFS), myalgic encephalitis (ME), or neurasthenia. Each of these diagnoses had specific diagnostic criteria,

| TABLE 36. Common Causes of Fatigue |
|---|
| **Lifestyle** |
| Alcohol |
| Drug dependency (overuse and withdrawal) |
| Extremes of activity |
| Night shift work |
| Sleep deprivation, poor sleep habits |
| Work/life imbalance |
| **Medical** |
| Anemia |
| Cancer |
| Chronic liver and kidney disease |
| Chronic lung disease, hypoxemia |
| Heart failure |
| HIV/AIDS |
| Hyperglycemia, uncontrolled diabetes mellitus |
| Medication side effects |
| Antidepressants |
| Antihistamines |
| Antipsychotics |
| β-Blockers |
| Benzodiazepines |
| Opioids |
| Obesity |
| Thyroid disorder (hyper- and hypothyroidism) |
| **Psychological** |
| Anxiety |
| Depression |
| Stress |

creating inconsistencies in diagnosis and wide variability in treatment across providers and institutions. In 2015, the Institute of Medicine (IOM), now called the National Academy of Medicine, issued an extensive guideline aimed at developing validated, evidence-based clinical diagnostic criteria for this condition and using consensus-building methods. The IOM recommended using the term systemic exertion intolerance disease (SEID) rather than CFS, ME, or other similar terms. Diagnosis of SEID requires the presence of all of the following three symptoms:

- A substantial reduction or impairment in the ability to engage in preillness levels of occupational, educational, social, or personal activities that persists for more than 6 months and is accompanied by fatigue, which is often profound, is of new or definite onset (not lifelong), is not the result of ongoing excessive exertion, and is not substantially alleviated by rest
- Postexertional malaise
- Unrefreshing sleep

In addition, the patient must have at least one of the following two manifestations:

- Cognitive impairment
- Orthostatic intolerance (symptoms such as lightheadedness, dizziness, and headache that worsen with upright posture and improve with recumbency)

An estimated 836,000 to 2.5 million U.S. adults have SEID; however, 84% to 91% of affected individuals are not yet diagnosed. In 2015, the economic cost associated with SEID was estimated to be between $17 billion and $24 billion annually.

Although the pathophysiology of SEID remains unclear, the phenomenon of central sensitization (the pathophysiologic dysregulation of the thalamus, hypothalamus, and amygdala) is gaining acceptance as a potential cause of SEID as well as of other highly prevalent comorbid conditions, including fibromyalgia, mood disturbances, irritable bowel syndrome, and interstitial cystitis. Central sensitization is often triggered by a prodromal event, such as infection, physical or emotional trauma, a motor vehicle accident, surgery, medical illness, or prolonged stress. Studies on central sensitization and its relationship to SEID and associated comorbid conditions are ongoing.

## Evaluation

The diagnostic evaluation of acute or chronic fatigue begins with a careful history and physical examination. Clinicians should note the duration of fatigue, preceding factors, concomitant symptoms, prolonged deleterious lifestyle factors, medication use, and the presence of "red flag" signs or symptoms (fever, involuntary weight loss, persistent lymphadenopathy, muscle atrophy, and synovitis). Patients should also be assessed for an underlying sleep disturbance. Mood disorders are often comorbid in patients with SEID (approximately 70% of patients), and all patients with SEID should be screened for depression and anxiety. Clinicians should additionally ensure that all age-appropriate screenings have been performed.

The history and physical examination should guide the choice of diagnostic tests. In patients with fatigue without a clear cause, it is reasonable to obtain a complete blood count, electrolyte panel, thyroid-stimulating hormone level, fasting glucose level, and kidney and liver chemistry tests. Unnecessary laboratory, imaging, and invasive studies should be avoided because most patients will have unrevealing findings, which usually provide little reassurance.

## Management

Treatment of fatigue should focus on correcting any underlying causes. In patients with SEID, the goals of treatment shift to functional rehabilitation and restoration. Patients benefit most from a structured, well-defined, multimodal approach that includes regularly scheduled office visits, which allow for discussion, educational opportunities, and longitudinal reassessment. There is evidence that CBT and graded exercise therapy may decrease fatigue and improve function, and these therapies should be offered to patients. Additionally, all patients should receive instruction on effective sleep hygiene. Other modalities that may be of benefit include physical therapy, occupational therapy, biofeedback therapy, massage therapy, acupuncture, yoga, tai chi, and stress management activities. In patients with comorbid mood conditions, treatment or referral to a psychiatrist or psychologist is reasonable.

There are no FDA-approved medications for the treatment of SEID. Medications play a very limited role in management, except in the treatment of comorbid conditions (such as depression). One small study found that methylphenidate increased concentration and decreased fatigue in 20% of patients, but its use is tempered by its addictive potential and adverse effects. There is no consistent evidence that opioids, glucocorticoids, pharmacologic sleep aids, prolonged antibiotics or antiviral agents, or immunotherapies improve symptoms or prognosis.

The prognosis for chronic fatigue varies and is often a source of frustration for patients and providers. The prognosis depends on many factors, including patient age, formal education level, severity of symptoms, duration of symptoms, decline in functional status relative to premorbid level of function, presence of other somatic (or medically unexplained) symptoms, comorbid mood disorders, availability of resources, and adherence to the treatment recommendations.

### KEY POINTS

- In patients with fatigue without a clear cause, it is reasonable to obtain a complete blood count, electrolyte panel, thyroid-stimulating hormone level, fasting glucose level, and kidney and liver chemistry tests. **HVC**
- Patients with systemic exertion intolerance disease benefit most from a structured, well-defined, multimodal approach that includes regularly scheduled office visits; cognitive behavioral therapy and graded exercise therapy may decrease fatigue and improve function and should be offered. **HVC**

*(Continued)*

HVC
- There are no FDA-approved medications for the treatment of systemic exertion intolerance disease, and medications play a very limited role in management, except in the treatment of comorbid conditions.

# Dizziness

## Approach to the Patient with Dizziness

Dizziness is a common nonspecific symptom seen in inpatient and outpatient settings. Patients often interchangeably use the terms dizzy, lightheaded, woozy, cloudy, faint, or off-balance to describe the perception of dizziness. Owing to its subjective nature, the variability in symptom description, and broad differential diagnosis (which includes stroke and other life-threatening disorders), dizziness is a challenging symptom to assess and treat.

In patients with dizziness, a relevant history and physical examination should be performed to classify the symptom into one of four focused groupings: vertigo, presyncope, disequilibrium, and nonspecific dizziness. This classification facilitates establishing a formal diagnosis and treatment strategy.

## Vertigo

Vertigo is the false perception of personal or environmental movement. Patients describe a spinning or whirling sensation, which is often associated with concomitant nausea, vomiting, and sudden-onset fatigue. Symptoms are typically episodic and brief and are usually triggered by positional changes of the head. Vertigo is classified as peripheral or central, depending on the specific etiology.

A thorough history and examination are crucial for differentiating between central and peripheral causes of vertigo, especially in patients with acute vertigo concerning for vertebrobasilar ischemia and other central causes. Examination should include an in-depth neurologic assessment as well as the HINTS (Head Impulse, Nystagmus, and Test of Skew) oculomotor assessment (**Table 37**). An abnormal result on any one of the three HINTS components suggests a central rather than peripheral cause of acute vertigo. Major causes of acute vertigo are presented in **Table 38**.

### Peripheral Vertigo

Benign paroxysmal positional vertigo (BPPV) is the most common form of vertigo, with a lifetime prevalence of 2.4%. It is more common in women (female-to-male ratio of 2:1 to 3:1). BPPV is characterized by sudden-onset, recurrent, and brief (usually <1 minute) vertiginous symptoms, which are provoked and worsened with positional changes of the head. Patients report dizziness, imbalance, nausea, and vomiting that occur with positional changes; however, no focal neurologic findings are present. Symptoms lead to increased risk for falls and a decline in functional status. BPPV is caused by displacement and migration of otoconia (calcium carbonate

**TABLE 37.** HINTS (Head Impulse, Nystagmus, and Test of Skew) Examination

| Maneuver | Method | Results |
|---|---|---|
| Head impulse test | With the patient focusing on the examiner, the examiner slowly moves the patient's head in either direction about 20 degrees and then rapidly rotates back to midline, while assessing for catch-up saccades | Reassuring: presence of catch-up saccades (consistent with peripheral cause of vertigo)<br><br>Concerning: absence of catch-up saccades (consistent with central cause of vertigo) |
| Nystagmus assessment | Examiner observes for the presence and directionality of nystagmus on lateral gaze | Reassuring: unidirectional nystagmus<br><br>Concerning: bidirectional nystagmus |
| Test of skew deviation | Examiner alternates covering and uncovering each eye and assesses for vertical adjustment or refixation | Reassuring: absence of vertical skew<br><br>Concerning: presence of vertical skew |

crystals) within the semicircular canals. Up to 90% of all cases of BPPV involve the posterior semicircular canal because it is the most gravity-dependent semicircular canal.

The diagnostic test of choice for BPPV is the Dix-Hallpike maneuver (**Figure 5**), which can help differentiate between peripheral and central causes of vertigo (**Table 39**). In the setting of BPPV, a positive finding includes the presence of a mixed upbeat-torsional nystagmus toward the affected side. Brain imaging is not necessary for diagnosis. First-line therapy for BPPV is canalith repositioning with the Epley maneuver, which is effective in up to 85% of patients (**Figure 6** on p. 58).

Other common causes of peripheral vertigo include vestibular neuronitis, labyrinthitis, Meniere disease, medication effects (toxicity from aminoglycoside or diuretic use), Ramsay Hunt syndrome (herpes zoster involving cranial nerve VII), and vestibular schwannoma (acoustic neuroma). Vestibular neuronitis is most often preceded by a viral infection affecting the vestibular portion of cranial nerve VIII. Symptoms are generally more severe and of longer duration than in BPPV and may take longer to resolve. Labyrinthitis has a presentation similar to that of vestibular neuronitis, with the additional symptom of hearing loss. Meniere disease classically presents with the triad of vertigo, tinnitus, and hearing loss; symptoms are episodic and recurrent and may be severe.

Evidence supports the utility of diuretics in the treatment of Meniere disease, but pharmacologic therapy has not otherwise been shown to be significantly effective for peripheral vertigo. Rather, vestibular suppressants (antihistamines, benzodiazepines, and antiemetics) can be used in conjunction with other forms of therapy for temporary symptomatic relief.

| TABLE 38. | Differential Diagnosis of Acute Vertigo | | | |
|---|---|---|---|---|
| Cause | Onset and Course | Nystagmus | Auditory Symptoms | Other Features |
| BPPV | Recurrent, transient, positional; usually provoked by turning over or getting in and out of bed | Positional, with mixed vertical torsional nystagmus in BPPV involving posterior canal and horizontal nystagmus in BPPV involving horizontal canal | None | Recent inciting event possible (e.g., recumbent position at dentist's office or hair salon, prolonged bed rest, head trauma); history of similar episodes |
| Stroke | Spontaneous, usually sustained; may be worsened by positional change | Spontaneous, with beating in various or changing directions | Occasional | Neurologic symptoms or signs often occur, but stroke may present as isolated vertigo; results of head impulse test are typically normal[a] |
| Vestibular neuronitis | Spontaneous, sustained; may be worsened by positional change | Spontaneous, predominantly horizontal | None | May be preceded by viral illness; results of head impulse test are abnormal[a] |
| Vestibular migraine | Recurrent, spontaneous; duration for minutes to hours; may be positional | Rare, but when present usually positional | Occasional | Migrainous headaches, motion sickness, family history |
| Meniere disease | Recurrent, spontaneous; typical duration for hours | Spontaneous, horizontal | Fluctuating hearing loss, tinnitus | Ear pain, sensation of fullness in ear |

BPPV = benign paroxysmal positional vertigo.

[a]In the head impulse test, the result is considered abnormal when a corrective movement (saccade) is required to maintain straight-ahead fixation after the head has been rotated to the side.

Reproduced with permission from Kim JS, Zee DS. Clinical practice. Benign paroxysmal positional vertigo. N Engl J Med. 2014;370:1140. [PMID: 24645946] doi:10.1056/NEJMcp1309481. Copyright 2014, Massachusetts Medical Society.

If vestibular suppressants are selected, it is imperative to limit the treatment duration because these agents can impede vestibular functioning, vestibular recovery, and centralized compensatory mechanism. Vestibular and balance rehabilitation therapy (VBRT) is also effective in the treatment of various forms of dizziness (vertigo, disequilibrium, and nonspecific dizziness). VBRT focuses on balance training, core stabilization, and desensitization exercises. It is often performed by physical and occupational therapists.

 **Central Vertigo**

Central vertigo is a frequently missed and potentially life-threatening diagnosis. It may be caused by vertebrobasilar stroke (posterior circulation ischemic or hemorrhagic events), migraine, central nervous system infection, trauma (concussion, traumatic brain injury), demyelinating disease (multiple sclerosis), and chronic alcoholism.

Patients with central vertigo secondary to vertebrobasilar stroke frequently display concomitant neurologic findings in addition to vertigo, such as nystagmus, dysphagia, dysarthria, diplopia, ataxia, postural instability, hemiparesis, and mental status changes. A normal result on a head impulse test, direction-changing nystagmus, or skew deviation in the HINTS assessment additionally suggest a central cause of vertigo. Roughly 20% of patients with vertebrobasilar stroke present with isolated vertigo, and studies have shown that up to one third of cases of vertebrobasilar stroke that manifest as isolated vertigo are misclassified as peripheral vertigo. Risk factors for posterior circulation stroke include advanced age, atrial fibrillation, diabetes, peripheral vascular disease, hypertension, and hyperlipidemia. To a lesser extent, neurologic findings may also be present in patients with other central processes, but they are not present in peripherally mediated forms of vertigo.

Advanced imaging should be performed in patients with central vertigo. MRI is more sensitive than CT in detecting ischemic stroke and can detect infarction in the posterior fossa on the first day. CT can provide an effective and expedited evaluation of hemorrhagic stroke, although hemorrhagic vertebrobasilar stroke accounts for a very small minority of cases of centrally mediated vertigo. 🔲

**Presyncope**

Presyncope is a temporary reduction in global cerebral perfusion, leading to symptoms of lightheadedness, dizziness, visual changes (tunnel vision), auditory changes, a sense of impending doom, warmth, nausea, and near loss of consciousness. Patients often report the sensation of "almost blacking out." Postural tone is retained. In contrast, syncope is transient reduction in global cerebral perfusion, leading to a true loss of consciousness and loss of postural tone. Notably, patients with presyncope do not have vertiginous symptoms. The differential diagnosis for presyncope is similar to that of syncope (see Syncope).

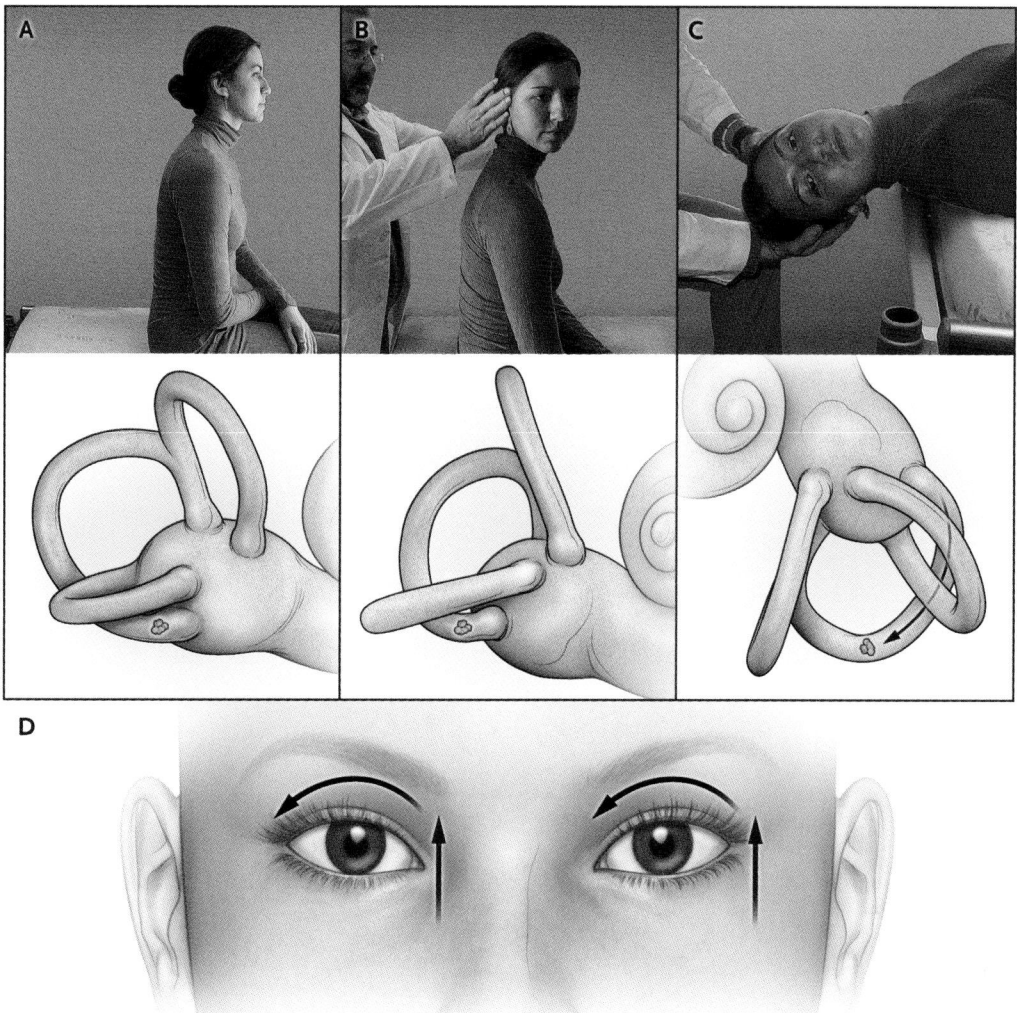

**FIGURE 5.** Use of the Dix-Hallpike maneuver to induce nystagmus in benign paroxysmal positional vertigo involving the right posterior semicircular canal. With the patient sitting upright (*A*), the head is turned 45 degrees to the patient's right (*B*). The patient is then moved from the sitting position to the supine position with the head hanging below the top end of the examination table at an angle of 20 degrees (*C*). The resulting nystagmus would be upbeat and torsional, with the top poles of the eyes beating toward the lower (right) ear (*D*).

Reproduced with permission from Kim JS, Zee DS. Clinical practice. Benign paroxysmal positional vertigo. N Engl J Med. 2014;370:1142. [PMID: 24645946] doi:10.1056/NEJMcp1309481. Copyright 2014, Massachusetts Medical Society.

| TABLE 39. | Interpretation of the Dix-Hallpike Maneuver | |
|---|---|---|
| **Findings** | **Peripheral Disease** | **Central Disease** |
| Latency of nystagmus[a] | Delayed | No delay |
| Duration of nystagmus | <1 min | >1 min |
| Fatigability of nystagmus[b] | Fatigable | Not fatigable |
| Direction of nystagmus | Unidirectional or mixed upbeat-torsional | Variable (vertical or horizontal) |
| Severity of symptoms | More severe | Less severe |

[a]Time to onset of nystagmus after positioning the patient.

[b]Decrease in the intensity and duration of nystagmus with repeated maneuvers.

## Disequilibrium

Disequilibrium refers to a sensation of imbalance or unsteadiness that is primarily experienced during positional changes, standing, or walking and is relieved with sitting or lying down. Disequilibrium predominantly affects older adults, and its prevalence increases with age. Falls are four times more likely in patients with disequilibrium and are, in turn, associated with significant morbidity, functional decline, and fear of future falls.

The etiology of disequilibrium is thought to be multifactorial, involving visual and auditory impairment; muscle weakness or atrophy; physical deconditioning; pain; and impairment in proprioception, balance, and gait. Brain imaging (MRI) studies of patients with disequilibrium have shown significantly more subcortical white matter lesions and frontal

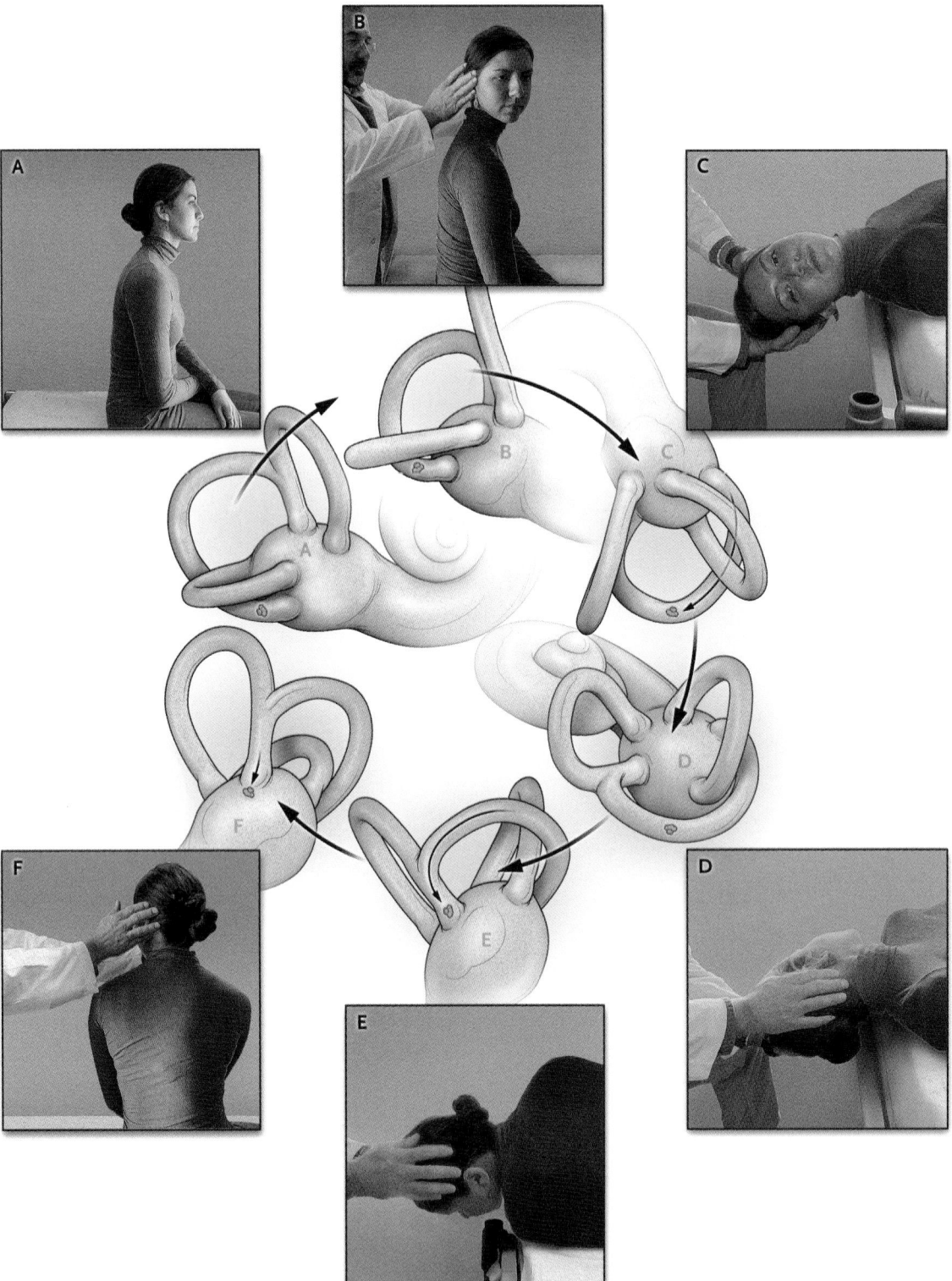

**FIGURE 6.** Epley canalith-repositioning maneuver for the treatment of benign paroxysmal positional vertigo involving the right posterior semicircular canal. After resolution of the induced nystagmus with the use of the right-sided Dix-Hallpike maneuver (*A*, *B*, and *C*), the head is turned 90 degrees toward the unaffected left side (*D*), causing the otolithic debris to move closer to the common crus. The induced nystagmus, if present, would be in the same direction as that evoked during the Dix-Hallpike maneuver. The head is then turned another 90 degrees, to a face-down position, and the trunk is turned 90 degrees in the same direction, so that the patient is lying on the unaffected side (*E*); the otolithic debris migrates in the same direction. The patient is then moved to the sitting position (*F*), and the otolithic debris falls into the vestibule, through the common crus. Each position should be maintained until the induced nystagmus and vertigo resolve but always for a minimum of 30 seconds.

atrophy than in patients without disequilibrium, although the significance of these findings is unclear.

Given the multifactorial nature of disequilibrium, treatment should be multifaceted. Treatment options include visual and auditory corrective measures (such as eye glasses and hearing aids), medication review (assessment of side effect profiles), mobility aids, physical therapy (balance and gait training), weight-bearing and resistive exercises, and fall prevention counseling.

## Persistent Postural-Perceptual Dizziness

Dizziness that remains nonspecific despite a thorough history, examination, and evaluation is referred to as persistent postural-perceptual dizziness (PPPD, formerly chronic subjective dizziness). PPPD is described as persistent, nonvertiginous dizziness or imbalance that worsens with personal motion, upright positioning, and movement of objects in the surrounding environment. Symptoms must be present on most days for at least 3 months. It is most often preceded by another vestibular process (BPPV, vestibular neuronitis, vestibular migraine, or stroke), trauma (concussion or traumatic brain injury), infection, or certain psychiatric conditions (anxiety, panic disorder, or major depression). Approximately 75% of patients with PPPD have concomitant anxiety or depressive symptoms.

Treatment options for PPPD include pharmacologic therapies, such as selective serotonin reuptake inhibitors and serotonin-norepinephrine reuptake inhibitors, and ongoing VBRT.

### KEY POINTS

HVC
- The diagnostic test of choice for benign paroxysmal positional vertigo is the Dix-Hallpike maneuver, which can help differentiate between peripheral and central causes of vertigo; routine imaging is not recommended.

HVC
- First-line therapy for benign paroxysmal positional vertigo is canalith repositioning with the Epley maneuver; vestibular and balance rehabilitation therapy is also effective.

- Patients with central vertigo may display focal neurologic findings; however, approximately 20% of patients with vertebrobasilar stroke present with isolated vertigo.

- In acute vertigo, the examination should include an in-depth neurologic assessment as well as the HINTS (Head Impulse, Nystagmus, and Test of Skew) oculomotor assessment.

HVC
- In patients with central vertigo, MRI is more sensitive than CT in detecting ischemic stroke, whereas CT provides an expedited, cost-effective assessment for hemorrhagic stroke.

- Treatment options for disequilibrium include visual and auditory corrective measures, medication review, mobility aids, physical therapy, weight-bearing and resistive exercises, and fall prevention counseling.

# Syncope

Syncope is complete and transient loss of consciousness and postural tone due to global cerebral hypoperfusion resulting from a decrease in cardiac output or systemic vascular resistance. The onset of syncope is sudden and abrupt, and recovery is rapid, with a complete return to the baseline level of functioning. Syncope is a very common medical condition, with a reported cumulative incidence of 3% to 6% over a 10-year period. Approximately 40% of adults have experienced a syncopal event, and 80% of these patients had a first episode before age 30 years. Although the Framingham Heart Study found that 44% of patients who experienced a syncopal event did not seek medical care, a recent 2014 financial analysis showed that the diagnostic and therapeutic costs associated with syncope exceed $4.1 billion annually in the United States.

## Classification

Syncope can be classified according to the specific etiology of the event as neurally mediated (reflex), cardiovascular, orthostatic, neurologic, psychogenic, or idiopathic. These etiologies can be further subdivided according to the specific pathophysiologic mechanism. Approximately 40% of syncopal events are unexplained (idiopathic). Historical characteristics that are associated with increased probability of cardiac and noncardiac causes are detailed in **Table 40**.

Neurally mediated syncope, or reflex syncope, is the most common form of syncope and is seen primarily in younger adults. The underlying syncopal mechanism, termed the neurocardiogenic or vasodepressor reflex, is a response of vasodilation, bradycardia, and systemic hypotension, which leads to transient hypoperfusion of the brain. Neurally mediated syncope includes vasovagal syncope, which may be provoked by noxious stimuli, fear, stress, or heat overexposure; situational syncope, which is triggered by cough, micturition, defecation, or deglutition; and carotid sinus hypersensitivity, which is sometimes experienced during head rotation, shaving, or use of a tight-fitting neck collar. Prodromal symptoms, including nausea and diaphoresis, are classically present before the syncopal event, and fatigue and generalized weakness are typically present afterward.

Cardiovascular syncope is the second most common form of syncope and is associated with increased morbidity, mortality (including sudden death), and direct traumatic injury. Cardiovascular syncopal events often occur suddenly and usually without a significant prodrome, although chest pain and palpitations may be present. Causes of cardiovascular syncope include cardiac arrhythmia; coronary artery disease; and structural and obstructive disease, including aortic and pulmonary valve stenosis, obstructive hypertrophic cardiomyopathy, aortic dissection, and cardiac tamponade. Pulmonary embolism is increasingly appreciated as a cause of syncope, with a prevalence as high as 17% in some studies.

Orthostatic syncope is the third most common form of syncope and predominantly affects older adults. It classically

**TABLE 40.** Historical Characteristics Associated With Increased Probability of Cardiac and Noncardiac Causes of Syncope

**More Often Associated With Cardiac Causes of Syncope**

Older age (>60 y)

Male sex

Presence of known ischemic heart disease, structural heart disease, previous arrhythmias, or reduced ventricular function

Brief prodrome, such as palpitations, or sudden loss of consciousness without prodrome

Syncope during exertion

Syncope in the supine position

Low number of syncope episodes (one or two)

Abnormal cardiac examination

Family history of inheritable conditions or premature sudden cardiac death (<50 y of age)

Presence of known congenital heart disease

**More Often Associated With Noncardiac Causes of Syncope**

Younger age

No known cardiac disease

Syncope only in the standing position

Positional change from supine or sitting to standing

Presence of prodrome: nausea, vomiting, feeling of warmth

Presence of specific triggers: dehydration, pain, distressful stimulus, medical environment

Situational triggers: cough, laugh, micturition, defecation, deglutition

Frequent recurrence and prolonged history of syncope with similar characteristics

Reproduced with permission from Shen WK, Sheldon RS, Benditt DG, Cohen MI, Forman DE, Goldberger ZD, et al. 2017 ACC/AHA/HRS guideline for the evaluation and management of patients with syncope: executive summary: a report of the American College of Cardiology/American Heart Association Task Force on Clinical Practice Guidelines and the Heart Rhythm Society. Circulation. 2017;136:e32. [PMID: 28280232] doi:10.1161/CIR.0000000000000498. Copyright 2017, American Heart Association, Inc.

Seizures can be confused with syncope, and bystander information can help distinguish between these two events. A prospective study demonstrated that the features most suggestive of a seizure in patients with loss of consciousness were witnessed abnormal posturing, involuntary head turning, and tongue laceration. Auras, incontinence, and prolonged postepisode confusion also favor a seizure.

Psychogenic syncope, which has also been referred to as pseudosyncope, generally occurs in younger patients with underlying anxiety, panic disorder, or depression.

## Evaluation

The American Heart Association (AHA), American College of Cardiology (ACC), and Heart Rhythm Society (HRS) jointly conclude that the history and physical examination are the most important diagnostic tools in determining the underlying cause of a syncopal event. The history should focus on eliciting prodromal or postepisode symptoms, comorbid medical or psychiatric conditions, the psychosocial context of the event, and bystander information. A thorough review of the patient's prescription and over-the-counter medications should also be completed.

The physical examination should include an in-depth cardiovascular evaluation, including orthostatic (postural) blood pressure measurements, as well as a basic neurologic examination to evaluate for focal defects. Carotid hypersensitivity can be assessed in individuals older than 40 years with syncope of unknown cause with the use of carotid sinus massage; however, this technique is contraindicated in patients with known carotid disease or recent transient ischemic attack/stroke within the past 3 months.

The AHA/ACC/HRS syncope guideline recommends that electrocardiography be performed in all patients with syncope to identify an underlying arrhythmia, myocardial ischemia, or QT prolongation. Generally, additional studies have a low diagnostic yield; however, when there is a moderate to high pretest probability of a specific condition, these studies can help to identify or confirm a diagnosis (**Figure 7**). Echocardiography is indicated to detect suspected valvular heart disease, hypertrophic cardiomyopathy, and reduced left ventricular function. An exercise stress test is most likely to be helpful in patients with exercise-related syncope. Electrocardiographic monitoring (with an ambulatory monitor, event monitor, or implantable loop recorder) should be considered in selected patients with a probable arrhythmic cause; the choice of test is based on the frequency and nature of the syncopal event (see MKSAP 18 Cardiovascular Medicine). Targeted laboratory studies are guided by findings in the history and physical examination. Tilt-table testing is most commonly useful in patients suspected of having recurrent vasovagal syncope or when the initial evaluation of delayed orthostatic hypotension is not diagnostic. Cardiac imaging with CT or MRI is most useful when structural or infiltrative heart disease is suspected but initial diagnostic tests are inconclusive. CT angiography is

CONT.

occurs after changes in position and is typically associated with prodromal symptoms, such as lightheadedness. Orthostatic syncope is most commonly caused by hypovolemia, medications, and alcohol intoxication. Less commonly, primary autonomic failure (Parkinson disease, multiple system atrophy, multiple sclerosis) or secondary autonomic failure (diabetes, amyloidosis, connective tissue disease, spinal cord injury) can lead to neurogenic orthostatic syncope.

Neurologic conditions are a rare cause of syncope. Cerebrovascular events (transient ischemic attack, ischemic or hemorrhagic stroke), seizures, and direct head trauma may lead to transient loss of consciousness but should be distinguished from true syncope. Cerebrovascular events that lead to true syncope primarily involve the posterior (vertebrobasilar) circulation and usually present with concomitant symptoms of dizziness, vertigo, gait changes, and focal neurologic findings. Anterior circulation involvement rarely leads to syncope.

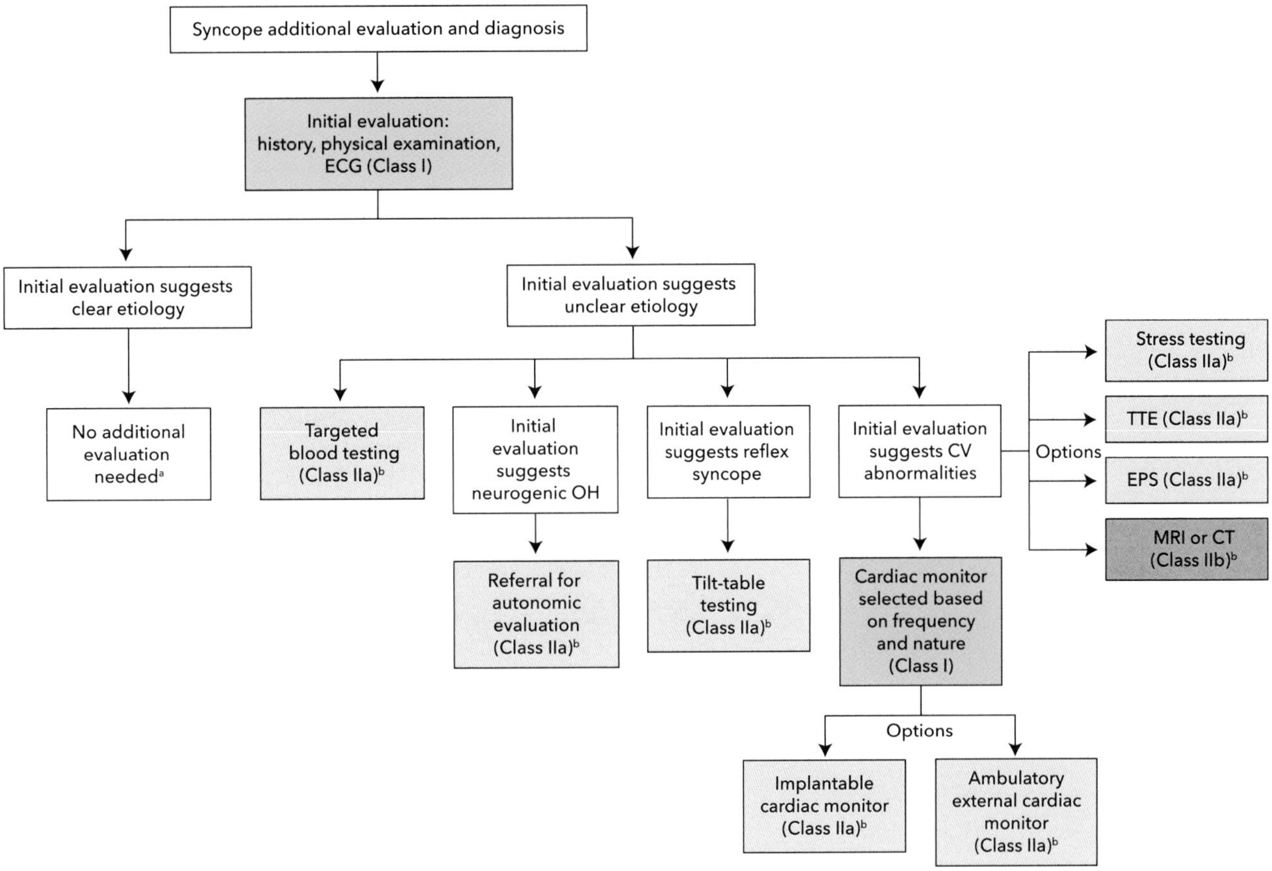

Figure showing the flowchart: Syncope additional evaluation and diagnosis

Syncope additional evaluation and diagnosis

Initial evaluation:
history, physical examination,
ECG (Class I)

Initial evaluation suggests
clear etiology

Initial evaluation suggests
unclear etiology

No additional
evaluation
needed[a]

Targeted
blood testing
(Class IIa)[b]

Initial
evaluation
suggests
neurogenic OH

Initial evaluation
suggests reflex
syncope

Initial evaluation
suggests CV
abnormalities

Options

Stress testing
(Class IIa)[b]

TTE (Class IIa)[b]

EPS (Class IIa)[b]

MRI or CT
(Class IIb)[b]

Referral for
autonomic
evaluation
(Class IIa)[b]

Tilt-table
testing
(Class IIa)[b]

Cardiac monitor
selected based
on frequency
and nature
(Class I)

Options

Implantable
cardiac monitor
(Class IIa)[b]

Ambulatory
external cardiac
monitor
(Class IIa)[b]

**FIGURE 7.** Additional evaluation and diagnosis of syncope. Colors correspond to class (strength) of recommendation, with green corresponding to a class I (strong) recommendation, yellow corresponding to a class IIa (moderate) recommendation, and orange corresponding to a class IIb (weak) recommendation. CV = cardiovascular; ECG = electrocardiography; EPS = electrophysiology study; OH = orthostatic hypotension; TTE = transthoracic echocardiography.

[a]Applies to patients after a normal initial evaluation without significant injury or cardiovascular morbidities; patients should be followed up by a primary care physician as needed.

[b]In selected patients.

indicated for patients with a high pretest probability of pulmonary embolism. Electrophysiology studies are reserved for patients suspected of having an arrhythmic cause of syncope, and electroencephalography should be based on the specific clinical scenario. The American College of Physicians (ACP) recommends against routinely obtaining brain imaging (CT or MRI) in cases of syncope that do not involve objective focal neurologic findings. Carotid duplex ultrasonography plays no role in the evaluation of a patient with syncope.

## Risk Stratification and Decision for Hospital Admission

The AHA/ACC/HRS syncope guideline recommends evaluation to determine the cause of syncope and assessment of the patient's short- and long-term morbidity and mortality risk. Short-term adverse events and deaths are mainly determined by the underlying cause and the effectiveness of the treatment. Risk scores have been developed to assist in risk stratification

and to guide patient disposition; however, they generally do not outperform unstructured clinical judgment. The presence of high-risk clinical characteristics should prompt consideration of hospitalization (**Table 41**). Patients with likely reflex-mediated syncope who do not have serious underlying medical conditions can usually be managed in the outpatient setting.

## Management

The management of syncope depends on the underlying cause. In cases of neurally mediated syncope, clinicians should provide reassurance and counsel patients to avoid provoking measures. Physical counterpressure techniques, such as leg crossing, squatting, or handgrip maneuvers, can be beneficial in patients with neurally mediated syncope and a prolonged prodrome. The management of cardiovascular syncope should target the specific underlying cause. Orthostatic syncope may be treated with volume expansion (with salt liberalization, if appropriate), reconsideration of contributing medications, compression

**TABLE 41.** High-Risk Clinical Characteristics in the Patient With Syncope[a]

Syncope during exertion

Syncope in supine position

Symptoms of chest discomfort or palpitations before syncope

Family history of sudden death

History of heart failure, aortic stenosis, left ventricular outflow tract disease, dilated cardiomyopathy, hypertrophic cardiomyopathy, arrhythmogenic right ventricular cardiomyopathy, ventricular arrhythmia, coronary artery disease, congenital heart disease, pulmonary hypertension, left ventricular ejection fraction <35%, implantable cardioverter-defibrillator placement

New or previously unknown left bundle branch block, bifascicular block, Brugada pattern, findings consistent with acute ischemia, nonsinus rhythm, prolonged QTc interval (>450 ms)

Hemoglobin <9 g/dL (90 g/L)

Systolic blood pressure <90 mm Hg

Sinus bradycardia <40/min

QTc = corrected QT interval.

[a]A patient is considered at high cardiac risk if any of the above risk factors are present.

Information from Costantino G, Sun BC, Barbic F, Bossi I, Casazza G, Dipaola F, et al. Syncope clinical management in the emergency department: a consensus from the first international workshop on syncope risk stratification in the emergency department. Eur Heart J. 2016;37:1493-8. [PMID: 26242712] doi:10.1093/eurheartj/ehv378

CONT.

stockings, and education on postural changes. Initiation of additional vasoactive agents, such as fludrocortisone or midodrine, can be considered; however, available evidence on their efficacy is limited and conflicting. In cases of psychogenic syncope, referral to a mental health specialist is appropriate.

### Prognosis

The underlying cause of the syncopal event determines the prognosis. Patients with a syncopal episode are at increased risk for all-cause mortality (hazard ratio [HR], 1.3; 95% CI, 1.1-1.5) and cardiovascular events (HR, 1.3; 95% CI, 1.0-1.6). The risk for death is even greater in cases of cardiac syncope (HR, 2.0; 95% CI, 1.5-2.7). Neurally mediated and orthostatic syncope do not portend increased cardiovascular mortality. Syncope of any cause, especially if recurrent, can severely affect quality of life, functional independence, and self-confidence. Clinicians should assess for any ensuing mood changes, the need for skilled assistance, and the need for possible driving restrictions (which vary per state law). **H**

### KEY POINTS

**HVC** • The history and physical examination, including orthostatic (postural) blood pressure measurement, are the most important diagnostic tools in determining the underlying cause of a syncopal event.

• All patients with syncope should undergo electrocardiography to identify underlying arrhythmia, ischemia, or QT prolongation.

*(Continued)*

### KEY POINTS *(continued)*

• Echocardiography, ischemia evaluation, electrocardiographic monitoring, chest radiography, tilt–table testing, electroencephalography, and laboratory studies have low diagnostic yield for the cause of syncope and should be performed only when there is a moderate to high pretest probability of a specific underlying condition. **HVC**

• The American College of Physicians recommends against routinely obtaining brain imaging (CT or MRI) in cases of syncope that do not involve objective focal neurologic findings. **HVC**

• Neurally mediated syncope is treated with reassurance and avoidance of provoking measures; physical counterpressure techniques can be useful in patients with a prolonged prodrome. **HVC**

• Orthostatic syncope may be treated with volume expansion (with salt liberalization, if appropriate), reconsideration of contributing medications, compression stockings, and education on postural changes.

## Insomnia

Insomnia is a complex health problem that affects many adults. Symptoms of insomnia vary and may include poor sleep quality, frustration with sleep quantity, difficulty initiating sleep, or an inability to return to sleep after awakening. The prevalence of insomnia increases with age, and women tend to be affected more than men. Medical disorders, including cardiopulmonary diseases, neurodegenerative disorders, and psychiatric disorders, are often implicated in sleep disruption. Medications and other substances also commonly contribute to symptoms of insomnia, and clinicians should screen for common culprits (such as caffeine, alcohol, glucocorticoids, diuretics, and antidepressants).

Chronic insomnia is diagnosed by the presence of symptoms that (1) cause substantial functional distress or impairment; (2) occur at least 3 nights per week for at least 3 months; and (3) are not associated with other sleep, medical, or mental disorders. Although 1 in 10 adults meet the diagnostic criteria for chronic insomnia, some studies have shown that up to 50% of adults report experiencing sleep symptoms.

### Evaluation

Given the wide range of patients affected and the significant impact insufficient sleep can have on function, all patients should be asked about problems of sleep disruption. In patients with symptoms of insomnia, a thorough history and physical examination may point to potentially reversible causes, such as sleep apnea or restless legs syndrome. Eliciting an accurate medication history, including use of over-the-counter medications, herbal supplements, caffeine, alcohol, tobacco, and illicit drugs, is also an important part of the diagnostic approach. Physicians should obtain information on sleep pattern, including sleep difficulties (sleep initiation, sleep maintenance, sleep quality) and environmental factors (work schedule). There is increasing evidence that screen time, such as smart phone and tablet use, before bed can alter circadian patterns and increase symptoms of insomnia, and use of electronics should be assessed. A sleep diary can facilitate collection of an accurate sleep history, and obtaining a collateral history from the patient's sleep partner may shed light on specific sleep-related disorders.

Diagnostic testing, such as polysomnography, is not a first-line approach unless guided by specific findings on the history and physical examination or directed by a sleep specialist.

## Treatment

The goals of treatment of insomnia are to improve overall sleep and quality of life. Effective treatment programs are multimodal in their approach and include cognitive behavioral therapy for insomnia (CBT-I), sleep hygiene techniques, environmental changes, and, in poorly controlled cases, pharmacologic therapy.

### Nonpharmacologic Treatments

The ACP recommends CBT-I as first-line therapy for insomnia. This multicomponent therapy includes cognitive therapy (to address maladaptive beliefs and expectations about sleep), educational interventions (such as sleep hygiene), and behavioral interventions (such as sleep restriction therapy, stimulus-control therapy, and relaxation techniques). It may be delivered in various formats, such as individual or group therapy, web-based modules, or written materials. CBT-I provides significant value over pharmacologic-driven approaches and carries little risk for adverse effects.

Sleep hygiene strategies focus on optimizing environmental factors (instituting stable bed times and rising times); reducing stimuli (limiting screen time [television, laptop computers, and cell phones] and creating a dark environment) around bedtime; avoiding caffeine, alcohol, and nicotine before bedtime; reducing daytime naps; and limiting the bedroom activities to intimacy and sleep. Sleep restriction therapy, which entails limiting the amount of time in bed to increase sleep efficiency, may also be used.

### Pharmacologic Therapy

The ACP recommends that physicians engage in a thorough shared decision-making process to decide whether to add pharmacologic therapies in patients with insomnia refractory to CBT-I. Several pharmacologic agents have been demonstrated to improve sleep latency and total sleep time (**Table 42**), but few studies have examined their overall impact on function and quality of life. Pharmacologic therapy is also associated with harms, including daytime drowsiness, increased risk for falls and hip fracture, and medication-related hallucinations. Factors that should be considered before initiating pharmacologic therapy for insomnia are included in **Table 43**. Medications ideally should be taken in short-term trials (no more than 4-5 weeks).

Patients frequently use over-the-counter medications, such as sedating antihistamines, for insomnia despite associated anticholinergic side effects and carry-over daytime sleepiness. Because of the risk for side effects, antihistamines are not recommended in the treatment of insomnia, especially in older adults, in whom the risk is magnified. Melatonin may be effective for circadian rhythm disruptions affecting sleep and has a more favorable side effect profile than antihistamines. Although melatonin is often recommended to older adults owing to the lower risk for side effects, there is insufficient evidence to support its use in this population.

Benzodiazepines induce sedation by activating inhibitory γ-aminobutyric acid (GABA) receptors. These drugs decrease sleep latency and have a sleep-promoting effect, although onset and effect differ between agents. The associated risk for rebound insomnia, addiction potential, and side effect profile make benzodiazepines poor candidates for treatment of insomnia, particularly in combination with other sedating agents (including opioids) and in geriatric populations.

Nonbenzodiazepine GABA-receptor agonists are typically more selective in their activity at the GABA receptor and represent a large class of medications for insomnia. These agents (zolpidem, eszopiclone, and zaleplon) have a rapid onset of action and short half-life, making them better choices for patients with difficulty initiating sleep. Long-acting formulations and formulations meant for use with middle-of-the-night awakenings are also available. There is potential for prolonged impaired driving skills and somnolence with their use, and there are few data on the long-term safety or efficacy of these agents.

**KEY POINTS**

- Diagnostic testing, such as polysomnography, is usually unnecessary in the evaluation of insomnia, unless guided by specific findings on the history and physical examination or directed by a sleep specialist.  **HVC**

- First-line therapy for insomnia is cognitive behavioral therapy, which includes cognitive therapy, educational interventions, and behavioral interventions.  **HVC**

- Sleep hygiene strategies for insomnia focus on optimizing environmental factors; reducing stimuli around bedtime; avoiding caffeine, alcohol, and nicotine before bedtime; reducing daytime naps; and limiting the bedroom activities to intimacy and sleep.  **HVC**

- Pharmacologic therapies for insomnia are associated with adverse effects and should only be initiated in patients with insomnia refractory to nonpharmacologic interventions.  **HVC**

## Lower Extremity Edema

Lower extremity edema is a common symptom in both the inpatient and outpatient settings. Resulting from accumulation of interstitial fluid in the most dependent part of the body, lower extremity edema may be secondary to several different

| TABLE 42. | FDA-Approved Prescription Drug Treatment for Insomnia | | | |
|---|---|---|---|---|
| Agent[a] | Usual Dosage | Onset of Action[b] | Duration of Action[c] | Notes |
| **Benzodiazepines (oral)** | | | | |
| Estazolam (generic) | 1-2 mg | Slow | Intermediate | |
| Flurazepam (generic) | 15-30 mg | Rapid | Long | |
| Quazepam (generic) | 7.5-15 mg | Slow | Long | |
| Temazepam (generic) | 7.5-30 mg | Slow | Intermediate | |
| Triazolam (generic) | 0.125-0.5 mg | Rapid | Short | Short-acting benzodiazepines have been associated with an increased risk for anterograde amnesia |
| **Nonbenzodiazepines** | | | | |
| Zolpidem | | | | |
|   Oral tablet (generic) | 5-10 mg | Rapid | Short | |
|   Extended-release oral tablet (generic) | 6.25-12.5 mg | Rapid | Intermediate | |
|   Sublingual | | | | |
|     Intermezzo | 1.75-3.5 mg | Rapid | Ultra-short | Indicated for as-needed use for treatment of middle-of-the-night insomnia with ≥4 h of sleep time remaining |
|     Edluar | 10 mg | Rapid | Short | |
|     Oral spray (Zolpimist) | 10 mg | Rapid | Short | |
| Eszopiclone (generic) | 1-3 mg | Rapid | Intermediate | The recommended initial dosage was reduced to 1 mg because of prolonged impaired driving skills, memory, and coordination at the previously recommended 3-mg dosage |
| Zaleplon (generic) | 10-20 mg | Rapid | Short | |
| **Orexin-Receptor Antagonist** | | | | |
| Suvorexant (Belsomra) | 5-20 mg | Slow | Long | The recommended initial dosage is 10 mg; the daily dosage should not exceed 20 mg |
| **Antidepressant** | | | | |
| Doxepin (Silenor) | 3-6 mg | Rapid | Intermediate | |
| **Melatonin Agonist** | | | | |
| Ramelteon (Rozerem) | 8 mg | Rapid | Short | |

[a]All agents classified as schedule C-IV by the Drug Enforcement Agency (DEA) except doxepin and ramelteon, which are not scheduled.

[b]Onset of action: rapid = 15-30 minutes; slow = 30-60 minutes.

[c]Based on elimination half-life and preparation: short = 1-5 hours; intermediate = 5-12 hours; long = >12 hours.

Adapted with permission from Masters PA. In the clinic. Insomnia. Ann Intern Med. 2014;161:ITC9. [PMID: 25285559] doi:10.7326/0003-4819-161-7-201410070-01004. Copyright 2014, American College of Physicians.

pathophysiologic mechanisms, including increased capillary hydrostatic pressure, increased capillary permeability, and decreased plasma oncotic pressure. Obstruction of the lymphatic system is a less common mechanism of edema.

The most common causes of lower extremity edema include venous obstruction or insufficiency, heart failure (including right-sided heart failure secondary to pulmonary disease), cirrhosis, nephrotic syndrome and hypoalbuminemia of other etiologies, and use of certain medications (**Table 44**). If lower extremity edema is unilateral, it is usually the result of a mechanical obstruction to venous or lymphatic flow, such as venous thrombosis or malignancy.

A detailed history and physical examination will suggest the cause of lower extremity edema in most patients. Reasonable initial laboratory testing includes measurement of kidney and liver function, urinalysis (for detection of protein), and albumin measurement. The decision to pursue further testing, including echocardiography, lower extremity Doppler ultrasonography, and advanced imaging should be guided by the findings on the initial evaluation.

## Chronic Venous Insufficiency

Chronic venous insufficiency is a condition in which the veins or valves in the lower extremities are incompetent, resulting in

**TABLE 43.** Factors to Consider When Prescribing Drugs to Treat Insomnia

Use the minimal effective dosage.

Avoid long-half-life medications, including long-half-life metabolites.

Be aware of potential interactions between drugs, including over-the-counter drugs.

Caution patients who are receiving these medications about interaction with alcohol.

Review potential side effects—in particular, daytime sleepiness.

Confer with the patient to determine an appropriate period of use.

Use a γ-aminobutyric acid agonist before other sedative-hypnotics for treatment of acute or short-term insomnia.

Look for rebound insomnia after discontinuation.

Consider intermittent or long-term use of hypnotic medications, depending on the clinical situation.

Consider consulting a sleep specialist before starting long-term therapy with hypnotic medication.

Adapted with permission from Masters PA. In the clinic. Insomnia. Ann Intern Med. 2014;161:ITC1-15; quiz ITC16. [PMID: 25285559] doi:10.7326/0003-4819-161-7-201410070-01004. Copyright 2014, American College of Physicians.

pooling of blood in the legs. It is most commonly caused by venous hypertension, but it may also be congenital. Symptoms include aching, itching, restlessness, leg heaviness, leg swelling, and pain.

A thorough history and physical examination should be performed. The examination may reveal edema, dilated veins (both varicosities and superficial telangiectasias), thin or hyperpigmented skin, and ulceration. Physical findings are best observed in the gravity-dependent upright position. Chronic venous insufficiency is a clinical diagnosis, but venous duplex Doppler ultrasonography can be used if the diagnosis is in doubt and in those considering intervention. Air plethysmography, which uses air displacement in a cuff surrounding the calf to measure venous outflow and filling, can be used when venous duplex ultrasonography is nondiagnostic or to guide therapy.

Conservative measures, including exercise, leg elevation, lifestyle changes (weight loss), and gradient compression stockings (20-50 mm Hg depending on the stage of disease) are first-line therapies. The presence of skin changes or ulceration should prompt at least 30 mm Hg of compression. To increase patient adherence, knee-length stockings are prescribed, and if used daily with an alternate pair, stockings should be replaced every 6 to 9 months. Skin care is also an important part of management, and daily use of topical moisturizers may reduce skin breakdown and prevent infection. Stasis dermatitis may require sparing use of a topical steroid (see MKSAP 18 Dermatology). Wound care, including use of hydrocolloids and foam dressings, is essential to control drainage from ulcers and to prevent maceration of the surrounding skin. Many drugs, including pentoxifylline and horse chestnut

extracts, have been studied for chronic venous insufficiency; however, none are FDA approved for this condition. Patients with bothersome spider veins and small varicose veins can undergo sclerotherapy, thermocoagulation, or laser therapy. Patients with confirmed reflux and persistent symptoms despite conservative therapy may be treated with venous ablation, stripping or excision, or, in the case of stenosis and obstruction, stenting. Surgical options can be considered for those with symptoms refractory to medical and endovenous therapies.

**KEY POINTS**

- The most common causes of lower extremity edema include venous obstruction or insufficiency, heart failure, cirrhosis, nephrotic syndrome and hypoalbuminemia of other etiologies, and use of certain medications.
- Conservative measures, including exercise, leg elevation, lifestyle changes, and compression stockings, are first-line therapies for chronic venous insufficiency. **HVC**

## Common In-Flight Emergencies

In-flight medical emergencies are relatively common during air travel, occurring in an estimated 1 in 600 flights. In the United States, physicians are not legally mandated to assist in the event of an in-flight emergency, although some countries do impose such obligations. The laws of the country in which the aircraft is registered usually prevail. Ethically, physicians should provide assistance as able. The Aviation Medical Assistance Act of 1998 includes a Good Samaritan provision that protects individuals who are medically qualified "from liability for rendering assistance unless that person is engaged in gross negligence or willful misconduct," such as providing care while intoxicated. Providers should practice within their scope of training, be mindful of patient privacy, and document the patient encounter.

Physicians who respond to an in-flight emergency typically have access to several medical resources. Most airlines have contracts with 24-hour call centers, and ground-based physicians trained in emergency or aerospace medicine can assist the on-board physician remotely and help direct care. Additionally, flight crews are required to receive cardiopulmonary resuscitation training, including training on the use of automated external defibrillators, and to be familiar with first-aid equipment. If the patient's condition is critical, the physician can recommend diversion of the flight to the nearest airport, although the ultimate decision rests with the aircraft captain.

Airlines based in the United States are mandated by the Federal Aviation Administration to carry at least one automated external defibrillator, supplemental oxygen, and a medical kit that contains a stethoscope, sphygmomanometer, gloves, airway supplies, intravenous access supplies (needles, syringes, saline), and some basic medications (epinephrine, lidocaine,

| TABLE 44. Differential Diagnosis of Lower Extremity Edema | | |
|---|---|---|
| **Condition or Cause** | **Clinical Presentation** | **Diagnostic Testing** |
| Chronic venous insufficiency | Gradual-onset leg aching/heaviness that is more likely to improve with elevation/recumbency and walking (decreased venous pressure) | Duplex ultrasonography if considering intervention |
| | Edema (most commonly bilateral but can be unilateral) that usually spares forefoot | |
| | Hyperpigmentation (hemosiderin deposits); telangiectasias, reticular veins, varicose veins; eczematous dermatitis and lipodermatosclerosis leading to ulceration, especially over the medial malleolus | |
| Heart failure | Dyspnea, orthopnea, paroxysmal nocturnal dyspnea, elevated jugular venous pressure, lung crackles, ventricular gallop, symmetric pitting edema | Echocardiography |
| Kidney disease | Symmetric pitting edema | Urinalysis, random urine albumin-creatinine ratio, serum creatinine level |
| Liver disease | Symmetric pitting edema, ascites, spider angiomas, palmar erythema, jaundice/icterus | Liver chemistry tests, albumin level, INR |
| Hypothyroidism | Symptoms of hypothyroidism, nonpitting bilateral edema | Thyroid-stimulating hormone level, serum thyroxine |
| Lymphedema (bilateral) | Brawny induration; pitting edema present initially; nonpitting present late in process; involves feet (square toes) | Can consider CT or the abdomen/pelvis, lymphoscintigraphy |
| | Kaposi-Stemmer sign (inability to pinch a fold of skin on the dorsal surface of the base of the second toe) | |
| Lipedema | Fatty tissue accumulation, nonpitting edema that spares the feet | |
| Pregnancy | Symmetric pitting edema | |
| Obstructive sleep apnea | Daytime sleepiness, snoring, witnessed apnea, neck circumference >43 cm (17 in), symmetric pitting edema | Polysomnography |
| Pulmonary hypertension | Exertional dyspnea, elevated jugular venous distention, prominent jugular venous $a$ wave, widened split $S_2$ | Echocardiography |
| Deep venous thrombosis | Unilateral, painful edema (most commonly) that may be tender on examination; typically pitting edema | D-dimer and/or lower extremity ultrasonography depending on pretest probability |
| | Should be strongly suspected with acute edema <72 h | |
| Drugs (vasodilators, NSAIDs, gabapentinoids, hormones, antiestrogens, thiazolidinediones) | Gradual-onset, bilateral pitting edema that usually improves with recumbency; one side may be larger than the other, particularly if there is more pronounced venous disease | No diagnostic testing; symptoms resolve within days of discontinuing the offending agent |

atropine, aspirin, nitroglycerin, antihistamines, bronchodilators, and dextrose). Many U.S. airlines augment their kits with additional supplies. The contents of international kits may vary. Other passengers may volunteer their own medical supplies, such as prescription medications, injectable epinephrine pens, or glucometers. The physician must weigh the benefits of using another passenger's glucometer against the potential harms, including transmission of blood-borne pathogens. Passengers may also be able to help with translation, although it is important to respect patient privacy.

In most in-flight medical emergencies, the physician's role involves assessing the patient, establishing a diagnosis when possible, administering basic medical treatments, providing reassurance as appropriate, and recommending flight diversion if necessary. The most common in-flight emergencies include presyncope or syncope (typically vasovagal), gastrointestinal disorders (diarrhea and vomiting), cardiovascular symptoms, and respiratory symptoms (asthma and hyperventilation). In-flight cardiac arrest is rare, accounting for approximately 0.3% of in-flight emergencies; however, it is responsible for 86% of in-flight deaths. In the event of suspected acute myocardial infarction or stroke, immediate flight diversion should be recommended to the crew. Other frequently encountered issues include trauma caused by objects falling from overhead bins, hypoglycemia, psychiatric problems (most commonly anxiety or phobias), allergic reactions, seizures, headaches, and obstetric or gynecologic events. Several in-flight births occur each year.

# Musculoskeletal Pain
## Low Back Pain
### Diagnosis and Evaluation

Low back pain can be classified by duration as acute (<4 weeks), subacute (4-12 weeks), or chronic (>12 weeks). Approximately 90% of patients have nonspecific low back pain, in which no specific cause can be determined. The most common identifiable causes of low back pain are spinal stenosis, disk herniation, and compression fractures. Less common identifiable causes include cancer (vertebral metastases) and infection (diskitis, osteomyelitis, epidural abscess); visceral disease, such as nephrolithiasis, pyelonephritis, and abdominal aortic aneurysm, may also cause low back pain.

### History and Physical Examination

Evaluation of patients with low back pain includes a detailed history directed toward factors that increase the likelihood of specific causes of pain (**Table 45**). Psychosocial factors may also affect the course of low back pain and should be assessed. Psychosocial distress; comorbid psychiatric conditions; somatization; and maladaptive coping strategies, such as avoiding work, are associated with poor clinical outcomes.

The physical examination should similarly search for evidence of an underlying disorder (see Table 45). Specific attention should be paid to "red flag" findings on examination, including fever and neurologic signs. A thorough neurologic examination, including strength, sensory, and reflex testing of the legs, in addition to performing both the ipsilateral and contralateral straight leg raise test (**Figure 8**), can identify patterns of deficits that point to lesions (most commonly disk herniation) at specific levels (**Table 46**). Similarly, decreased anal sphincter tone and perianal sensation raise concern for

cauda equina syndrome. Many of the examination findings, however, are insensitive or nonspecific for the presence of a specific underlying disorder.

### Further Diagnostic Testing

Clinicians should not routinely obtain imaging and other diagnostic tests in patients with nonspecific low back pain. Obtaining imaging studies in these patients is not associated with clinically meaningful outcomes. Notably, imaging abnormalities are commonly present in asymptomatic individuals. They are also common in patients with nonspecific low back pain, and their presence may lead to unhelpful and unnecessary interventions.

In contrast, imaging is recommended when neurologic ⬛ deficits are present or if serious underlying conditions are suspected. Plain radiography may be considered to evaluate for ankylosing spondylitis or vertebral compression fracture. When malignancy is suspected, the American College of Physicians recommends immediately obtaining plain radiography in addition to measuring the erythrocyte sedimentation rate. If results of these initial tests are negative and significant concern remains, MRI should then be obtained. Immediate MRI should be obtained when there are risk factors for spinal infection or concern for cord compression or cauda equina syndrome. In patients with persistent pain despite conservative measures, symptoms/signs of radiculopathy, or spinal stenosis, MRI or, less preferably, CT may be considered only if the patient is a potential candidate for surgical intervention or epidural glucocorticoid injection. ⬛

### Treatment

Patient education is a key component in the treatment of low back pain regardless of duration. Education includes providing information on the expected course of the back pain, promoting self-management, addressing misconceptions, and encouraging physical activity as appropriate. In all patients with low back pain, bed rest should be avoided, and depressive features should be appropriately assessed and managed.

In addition to education, treatment modalities for patients with low back pain may include nonpharmacologic and/or pharmacologic therapies and, rarely, surgery. The interventions chosen should be based on the patient's signs, symptoms, and comorbid conditions.

### Nonpharmacologic Treatment

Clinical guidelines consistently emphasize nonpharmacologic therapies as a cornerstone of therapy for acute and chronic low back pain. For acute low back pain, potentially useful nonpharmacologic therapies include local heat, massage, acupuncture, and spinal manipulation, although the evidence supporting these approaches is generally weak.

Multiple nonpharmacologic options are available for chronic low back pain, including exercise therapy, manual and massage therapy, acupuncture, yoga, intensive interdisciplinary therapy, and cognitive behavioral therapy, with varying

**TABLE 45.** History and Examination Features and Suggested Diagnoses in Low Back Pain

| Suggested Diagnosis | History Features | Examination Features |
| --- | --- | --- |
| Cancer | Personal history of malignancy | Vertebral tenderness |
| | Unexplained weight loss | |
| | Failure to improve after 1 mo | |
| | No relief with bed rest | |
| Infection | Fever | Fever |
| | Injection drug abuse | Vertebral tenderness |
| | Urinary tract infection | |
| | Skin infection | |
| Inflammatory/ rheumatologic condition | Onset before age 40 y | |
| | Gradual onset | |
| | Presence of morning stiffness | |
| | Pain not relieved when supine | |
| | Pain persisting for >3 mo | |
| | Involvement of other joints | |
| Nerve root irritation (radiculopathy) | Sciatica (pain that radiates from the back through the buttocks down into the leg[s]) | Positive ipsilateral SLR (LR+ of 3.7) |
| | Increased pain with cough, sneeze, or Valsalva maneuver | Positive contralateral SLR (LR+ of 4.4) |
| Spinal stenosis | Severe leg pain | |
| | No pain when seated | |
| | Improvement in pain when bending forward | |
| | Pseudoclaudication[a] (worsened pain with walking or standing and relief with sitting) | |
| Compression fracture | Advanced age | Vertebral tenderness |
| | Trauma | |
| | Glucocorticoid use | |
| | Osteoporosis | |
| Cauda equina syndrome[b] | Bowel or bladder dysfunction | Decreased anal sphincter tone |
| | Perineal (saddle) sensory loss | Decreased perineal/perianal sensation |
| | Rapidly progressive neurologic deficits | |

LR+ = positive likelihood ratio; SLR = straight leg raise.

[a]Lower extremity symptoms caused by lumbar spinal stenosis mimicking vascular ischemia; also termed neurogenic claudication.

[b]Compression of the lumbar and sacral nerves below the termination of the spinal cord (conus medullaris). Characterized by back pain; sensory changes in the S3 to S5 dermatomes (saddle anesthesia); bowel, bladder, and sexual dysfunction; and absent Achilles tendon reflexes bilaterally.

levels of predominantly weak evidence supporting these approaches. The 2016 National Institute for Health and Care Excellence (NICE) guidelines endorse self-management, exercise, manual therapy, psychological therapy, and return-to-work programs.

**Pharmacologic Treatment**

NSAIDs are considered first-line pharmacologic therapy for acute low back pain and should be used at the lowest effective dose for the shortest duration needed. A recent meta-analysis suggests that NSAIDs, compared with placebo, reduce pain and disability in patients with acute low back pain. Notably, another meta-analysis concluded that acetaminophen is ineffective for acute low back pain. Second line agents include nonbenzodiazepine muscle relaxants. Opioids and tramadol should be avoided in acute low back pain if possible.

A similar approach is appropriate in patients with chronic low back pain. NSAIDs remain first-line pharmacologic therapy, and nonbenzodiazepine muscle relaxants may be used as second-line therapy. The serotonin-norepinephrine reuptake inhibitor duloxetine is approved by the FDA to treat chronic low back pain and may be useful in selected patients.

A 2018 randomized controlled trial demonstrated that opioids were not superior to nonopioid medications for improving pain-related function for chronic back pain or osteoarthritis-related hip or knee pain; pain intensity was

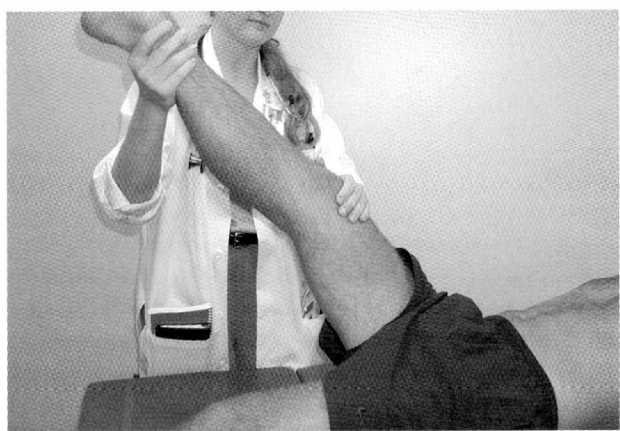

**FIGURE 8.** Straight leg raise test. With the patient lying supine on his or her back, the patient lifts the leg with the knee fully extended on the affected side (ipsilateral straight leg raise test) and then repeats on the opposite side (contralateral straight leg raise test). The test result is considered positive when pain radiates down the leg past the level of the knee when the hip is flexed between 30 and 70 degrees.

Reproduced with permission from Moore G. Atlas of the Musculoskeletal Examination. Philadelphia, PA: American College of Physicians; 2003:65. Copyright 2003, American College of Physicians.

**TABLE 46. Patterns of Neurologic Deficits in Patients With Low Back Pain**

| Nerve Root Level | Motor Deficit | Sensory Deficit | Involved Reflex |
|---|---|---|---|
| L3 | Hip flexion | Anteromedial thigh | Patella |
| L4 | Knee extension | Anterior leg/medial foot | Patella |
| L5 | Great toe dorsiflexion | Lateral leg/dorsal foot | N/A |
| S1 | Plantar flexion of foot | Posterior leg/lateral foot | Achilles |

N/A = not applicable.

Adapted with permission from Diagnosis and Treatment of Acute Low Back Pain, February 15, 2012, Vol 85, No 4, American Family Physician. Copyright © 2012 American Academy of Family Physicians. All Rights Reserved.

significantly improved in the nonopioid group. The 2016 NICE guidelines recommend against the use of opioids for chronic back pain, and the 2016 Centers for Disease Control and Prevention guideline for prescribing opioids states that nonpharmacologic and nonopioid therapies are preferred over opioids.

Systemic glucocorticoids, tricyclic antidepressants, and neuromodulators (gabapentin and pregabalin) have not demonstrated effectiveness for chronic low back pain.

**Interventional and Surgical Treatment**

Most patients with low back pain do not require surgery. Immediate surgery is indicated for most patients with suspected cord compression or cauda equina syndrome. Nonurgent surgery may be considered in patients with neurologic deficits, progressively worsening spinal stenosis, or

chronic pain with corresponding abnormalities on imaging that has been refractory to conservative measures and has the potential to respond to surgery. Typical surgical approaches include diskectomy for disk herniation and posterior decompressive laminectomy for spinal stenosis.

Epidural glucocorticoid injections are frequently performed in patients with radiculopathy; however, available evidence suggests they offer only small, short-term benefits.

**KEY POINTS**

- Evaluation of patients with low back pain includes a detailed history and physical examination to help distinguish nonspecific low back pain from pain attributable to a specific cause. **HVC**
- Most patients with nonspecific low back pain do not require imaging or other diagnostic testing. **HVC**
- Patient education for low back pain includes providing information on the expected course of the back pain, promoting self-management, addressing misconceptions, and encouraging physical activity as appropriate.
- Nonpharmacologic therapies are considered a cornerstone of treatment for both acute and chronic low back pain. **HVC**
- NSAIDs are considered first-line pharmacologic therapy for low back pain and should be used at the lowest effective dose for the shortest duration needed. **HVC**

# Neck Pain
## Diagnosis and Evaluation

As with low back pain, a priority in evaluating neck pain is differentiating nonspecific neck pain from other conditions that may result in serious complications or be amenable to specific therapy. Evaluation begins with a thorough history, including circumstances of the onset, presence of antecedent trauma, duration, progression, impact on daily activities, and accompanying symptoms. Examination includes inspection and palpation of the cervical spine and muscles, range of motion testing, and comprehensive neurologic assessment of the arms, including sensory, motor, and reflex testing.

The most common cause of neck pain is cervical sprain (nonspecific or axial neck pain), which is characterized by pain and stiffness in the paraspinal neck muscles frequently accompanied by neck and upper back muscle spasms. Examination findings include decreased cervical range of motion, muscle spasms, and absence of abnormal neurologic findings.

Whiplash-associated neck pain develops after trauma involving abrupt neck flexion or extension. Symptoms and signs are similar to those of cervical sprain.

Cervical radiculopathy is caused by nerve root compression as a result of disk herniation or adjacent bony degeneration. Several conditions can cause symptoms that may be mistaken for cervical radicular pain, including shingles, entrapment syndromes (such as median or ulnar nerve entrapment, thoracic outlet syndrome), complex regional pain syndrome, and cardiac ischemia. Radiculopathy, however, usually causes neck pain accompanied by radiating arm pain and paresthesias that follow a dermatomal distribution. In some cases, pain may be limited to the shoulder girdle. On examination, the patient's symptoms may be reproduced with the Spurling test (sensitivity, 94%; specificity, 30%) (**Figure 9**) and improved by holding the patient's hand above the head (shoulder abduction test: variable sensitivity, 17%-78%; specificity, 75%-92%).

Cervical myelopathy (compression of the cervical spinal cord) can also cause neck pain. Symptoms are typically progressive and include difficulty with manual dexterity, fine object manipulation (buttoning a shirt), and gait disturbance. On examination, there are upper motor neuron signs such as increased muscle tone, hyperreflexia, and clonus.

Involvement of the cervical spine by malignancy should be considered in the presence of a history of malignancy or suggestive systemic symptoms such as weight loss. Infectious causes, such as an epidural abscess or osteomyelitis, should be considered in the presence of fevers and chills, a history of injection drug use, or a history of recent bacteremia.

Most patients with neck pain do not require imaging studies. Plain radiography should be obtained when evaluation suggests fracture, infection, or malignancy and can be considered in patients with cervical sprain that has been unresponsive to 6 to 8 weeks of conservative measures. MRI is recommended when suspicion for malignancy or infection remains high despite normal plain radiographs, when myelopathy is suspected, and in patients with progressive neurologic symptoms. In patients who cannot undergo MRI, CT myelography can be

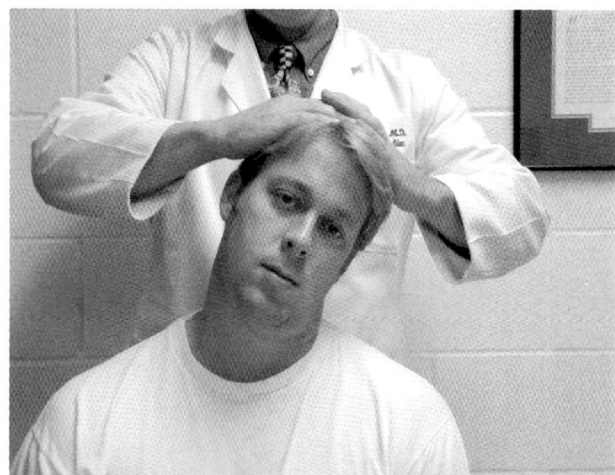

**FIGURE 9.** Spurling test for cervical nerve root compression. With the patient in a sitting position, the examiner extends the patient's head and then laterally flexes the neck. A downward pressure is then applied to the head in this position. A positive Spurling test reproduces the patient's pain, which radiates into the ipsilateral arm in a dermatomal distribution and supports the diagnosis of cervical radiculopathy (sensitivity, 94%; specificity, 30%).

considered. Electrodiagnostic studies may be performed when there is diagnostic uncertainty about a patient's symptoms (for example, to help distinguish peripheral nerve entrapment or peripheral neuropathy from radiculopathy).

## Treatment

Most patients with neck pain have resolution or near-resolution of their symptoms within 8 to 12 weeks of onset by using conservative measures. A multimodal approach that is tailored to the individual patient appears to work best and may include mobilization, exercise, physical therapy, and analgesic agents.

Stretching and strengthening exercises appear to provide intermediate-term relief of symptoms. Spinal manipulation, mobilization, and acupuncture may provide short-term pain relief. Although widely used, immobilization with a cervical collar appears to be no more effective than sham interventions. Immobilization for longer than 1 to 2 weeks may lead to atrophy of the neck muscles. The benefit of traction appears limited.

Oral and topical NSAIDs are considered first-line pharmacologic therapy for neck pain. Notably, a recent meta-analysis suggests that NSAIDs, compared with placebo, reduce pain in patients with neck pain. Because of its favorable side-effect profile, acetaminophen is also frequently used, although its effectiveness is not clearly established. Cyclobenzaprine, when used at intermediate or higher doses (≥15 mg/d), is more effective than placebo for treatment of acute neck pain associated with muscle spasm. For patients with chronic radicular symptoms, venlafaxine and neuromodulators, such as gabapentin and tricyclic antidepressants, may provide some pain relief. Because of abuse potential, opioids are generally avoided and, if used, should only be used on a short-term basis and restricted to persons with severe, intractable pain. No evidence supports the use of oral glucocorticoids. Epidural glucocorticoid injections may be considered in patients with cervical radiculopathy and significant symptoms that do not respond to other conservative measures, although the data supporting this practice are unconvincing.

Surgery is generally reserved for patients with structural disorders on imaging along with myelopathic findings and progressive neurologic symptoms, or for those with symptoms that do not respond to 6 months of conservative therapy.

For those with neck pain with a systemic cause, the underlying disorder should be appropriately treated.

**KEY POINTS**

- Most patients with neck pain do not require imaging studies; plain radiography should be obtained when evaluation suggests fracture, infection, or malignancy and can be considered in patients with cervical sprain that has been unresponsive to 6 to 8 weeks of conservative measures. **HVC**

- Neck pain usually resolves with conservative measures, including mobilization, exercise, physical therapy, and analgesic agents. **HVC**

# Upper Extremity Disorders
## Thoracic Outlet Syndrome
### Diagnosis and Evaluation
The three subtypes of thoracic outlet syndrome (TOS) are differentiated according to the affected structure within the neurovascular bundle between the first rib and the clavicle. Neurogenic TOS, the most common type (>90% of cases), results from compression of the brachial plexus. Symptoms (arm paresthesias, pain, and weakness) worsen with repetitive arm use, especially overhead activities. Venous TOS is caused by axillary vein compression and usually thrombosis within the thoracic outlet. Symptoms (arm pain/fatigue, edema, and cyanosis) occur with repetitive arm use, especially overhead activities. Dilated collateral veins of the chest wall and shoulder may be present. Arterial TOS, due to subclavian artery compression (with or without thrombosis), usually occurs in the presence of an anomalous cervical rib; less commonly, it occurs with frequent and vigorous overhead activities, such as baseball pitching. Symptoms include arm pain (which may be exertional), weakness, paresthesias, coolness, and pallor.

Diagnosis of neurogenic TOS is clinical, although electrodiagnostic testing may be helpful in some patients. Vascular causes require imaging of the affected vessel, with ultrasonography being the most useful initial test.

### Treatment
First-line therapy for neurogenic TOS includes improving posture and strengthening shoulder girdle muscles. Surgical decompression is reserved for progressive, disabling, or unresponsive symptoms. Treatment of both arterial and venous TOS involves catheter-directed thrombolysis followed by prompt surgical decompression of the thoracic outlet.

#### KEY POINT
- Neurogenic thoracic outlet syndrome (TOS), the most common type of TOS, results from compression of the brachial plexus; arm paresthesias, pain, and weakness worsen with repetitive arm use, especially overhead activities.

## Shoulder Pain
### Diagnosis and Evaluation
Shoulder pain assessment involves a detailed history with attention to the presence of antecedent trauma and relevant occupational or recreational activities. A comprehensive shoulder examination, performed with both shoulders fully exposed, includes inspection, palpation, range of motion assessment, and specialized maneuvers.

The initial step in evaluating shoulder pain is to determine whether the pain is arising from the shoulder (intrinsic) or is referred from another site (extrinsic), such as the cervical spine. Extrinsic pain is suggested by the inability to reproduce pain with shoulder movement, pain extending beyond the elbow, and pain with neck movement.

## Rotator Cuff Disease
Rotator cuff disease, the most common cause of shoulder pain, refers to all symptomatic rotator cuff disorders, including rotator cuff tendinitis, rotator cuff tears, and subacromial bursitis. Pain from rotator cuff disease is frequently localized to the upper arm near the deltoid insertion, is worsened with overhead activities, and is often worse at night, particularly with lying on the affected side. Except for acute traumatic rotator cuff tears, onset of symptoms is usually insidious. Risk factors for rotator cuff disease include increasing age and participation in activities that require repetitive overhead arm use.

On examination, shoulder inspection may reveal infraspinatus muscle atrophy (positive likelihood ratio of 2.0 for rotator cuff disease). Many examination maneuvers are available for rotator cuff disease assessment; however, each is limited by test characteristics, and they are most useful in combination (Table 47). The combination of positive results on painful arc and drop arm tests in the setting of weakness in external rotation is particularly suggestive of a rotator cuff tear.

Most patients with rotator cuff disease do not require imaging studies. Ultrasonography or MRI should be reserved for patients with acute or progressive functional loss and for those who are unresponsive to conservative measures.

Patients with acute full-thickness tears should be referred for consideration of immediate repair. Treatment of other rotator cuff disorders should include education about the expected course, avoidance or modification of aggravating activities, and physical therapy. Immobilization with a sling should be avoided to prevent development of adhesive capsulitis. Pharmacologic treatment should begin with acetaminophen and, if ineffective, progress to oral or topical NSAIDs. Subacromial glucocorticoid injections may provide short-term pain relief in patients with subacromial bursitis in whom other measures have failed but should be limited to one or two courses to limit complications. Surgery is reserved for patients in whom 3 to 6 months of conservative therapy has failed or in physically active patients with functionally significant tears.

## Adhesive Capsulitis
Adhesive capsulitis (frozen shoulder) usually occurs in patients aged 40 to 70 years. The cause is unclear but appears to involve glenohumeral joint capsular thickening and fibrosis. Adhesive capsulitis can be idiopathic but is also associated with prolonged immobilization, antecedent shoulder surgery or injury, diabetes mellitus, hypothyroidism, and autoimmune disorders. Patients describe shoulder pain that is often constant but is worse at night and in cold weather; shoulder stiffness is common. Both the degree of pain and stiffness may vary in an individual patient over time. On examination, patients have limited passive and active range of motion in all directions.

Treatment of adhesive capsulitis focuses on pain control and improved range of motion. Intra-articular glucocorticoid injections appear more effective than physical therapy alone, although evidence supports combining modalities. Acetaminophen and NSAIDs can be used as an adjunct for analgesia. Surgery is

**TABLE 47.** Physical Examination Maneuvers in Rotator Cuff Disease

| Maneuver | Technique | Positive LR[a] (95% CI) | Negative LR[a] (95% CI) | Notes |
|---|---|---|---|---|
| Painful arc test | During full passive abduction of the affected arm, pain occurs between 60° and 120°. | 3.7 (1.9-7.0) | 0.36 (0.23-0.54) | Highest LR+ of all special RC maneuvers. |
| Drop arm test | The affected arm is fully passively abducted, and the patient is asked to slowly lower the arm. A sudden drop of the arm with reproduction of the patient's pain is a positive result. | 3.3 (1.0-11) | 0.82 (0.7-0.97) | An uncontrolled drop of the arm suggests a full tear of the supraspinatus. |
| Hawkins test | The arm is passively flexed to 90° with the elbow in 90° flexion. The examiner then internally rotates the shoulder. Reproduction of pain during internal rotation is a positive result. | 1.5 (1.1-2.0) | 0.51 (0.39-0.66) | Believed to maximize impingement of the supraspinatus tendon; if the painful arc test, Hawkins test, and resisted external rotation are positive, the LR+ for a full-thickness RC tear is 16.4. |
| Empty can test | The extended arm is passively abducted to 90° in the plane of the supraspinatus (30° anterior to the coronal plane) and internally rotated (as though pouring a glass of water onto the floor). The patient is asked to maintain the position while the examiner exerts downward force on the arm. Weakness or reproduction of pain is a positive result. | 1.3 (0.97-1.6) | 0.64 (0.33-1.3) | Inability to maintain the position before resistance is applied suggests a full tear of the supraspinatus. |
| Resisted external rotation | The arm is abducted to 0° with the elbow flexed to 90° and the thumb pointing upward. The examiner exerts an internal rotation force proximal to the wrist, which the patient is asked to resist. Weakness or reproduction of pain is a positive result. | 2.6 (1.8-3.6) | 0.49 (0.33-0.72) | Pain or weakness suggests infraspinatus pathology. Limitation in external rotation range of motion suggests glenohumeral disease or adhesive capsulitis. |
| Internal rotation lag sign | The patient places the dorsum of the hand on the lower back with the elbow flexed to 90°. The examiner lifts the hand off the back, further internally rotating the shoulder. Inability to maintain the hand away from the back is a positive result. | 6.2 (1.9-12) | 0.04 (0.0-0.58) | Subscapularis is the primary muscle of internal rotation; LRs are for a full tear of the subscapularis. |

LR+ = positive likelihood ratio; RC = rotator cuff.

[a]LRs relate to the diagnosis of rotator cuff disease unless otherwise indicated.

Reproduced with permission from Whittle S, Buchbinder R. In the clinic. Rotator cuff disease. Ann Intern Med. 2015;162:ITC1. [PMID: 25560729]. Copyright 2015, American College of Physicians.

reserved for patients who do not respond to 12 weeks of conservative measures.

## Acromioclavicular Joint Degeneration

Acromioclavicular joint degeneration is typically characterized by poorly localized pain on the superior shoulder, although pain may be throughout the shoulder region. On examination, pain may be elicited with palpation of the acromioclavicular joint. The crossed-arm adduction test often reproduces the pain, as does shoulder abduction beyond 120 degrees, but neither test is specific for acromioclavicular joint disease. Plain radiography is often completed to assess for other structural disease and usually reveals degenerative changes of the acromioclavicular joint.

First-line therapy consists of NSAIDs and activity modification. Glucocorticoid injections may provide short-term pain relief.

**KEY POINTS**

- Rotator cuff disease pain is frequently localized to the upper arm near the deltoid insertion, is worsened with overhead activities, and is often worse at night, particularly with lying on the affected side.

- Most patients with rotator cuff disease do not require imaging studies; treatment may include education, avoidance/modification of aggravating activities, physical therapy, and acetaminophen or NSAIDs.

**HVC**

*(Continued)*

- Treatment of adhesive capsulitis focuses on pain control and improved range of motion; intra-articular glucocorticoid injections appear more effective than physical therapy alone, although evidence supports combining both modalities.

- First-line therapy for acromioclavicular joint degeneration consists of NSAIDs and activity modification; glucocorticoid injections may provide short-term pain relief.

## Elbow Pain

### Diagnosis and Evaluation

Elbow pain may be caused by pathology within the elbow joint, surrounding tissues, or nerves. Diseases within the neck, shoulder, and wrist may also cause pain radiating to the elbow. Evaluation focuses on patient history and physical examination.

### Epicondylitis

Epicondylitis (epicondylosis) refers to noninflammatory conditions of the tendons surrounding the elbow. Lateral epicondylitis (tennis elbow) is induced by activities with repetitive use of extensor tendons, such as computer use or tennis. Pain and tenderness are located over the lateral epicondyle and increase with resisted wrist extension. Medial epicondylitis (golfer's elbow) is less common and is caused by repetitive flexion of the wrist. Pain occurs over the medial elbow and ventral forearm and worsens with resisted wrist flexion. Diagnostic imaging is unnecessary if the clinical picture is consistent with medial or lateral epicondylitis.

There is little strong evidence regarding the optimal means of treatment. Initial management includes avoidance of pain-inducing activities and NSAIDs for analgesia. Physical therapy and counterforce braces may improve symptoms and prevent future exacerbations. Glucocorticoid injections may reduce pain in the short term, but they provide no long-term benefit and are used only as a temporizing measure. Surgery is rarely indicated for recalcitrant pain.

### Olecranon Bursitis

Several conditions cause inflammation of the olecranon bursa, including trauma, gout, and infection. Posterior elbow swelling and tenderness with normal elbow range of motion are typical (**Figure 10**); swelling and pain on elbow extension suggest elbow joint effusion and an alternate cause. Aspiration with culture and fluid analysis should be performed for severe pain or suspicion of infection.

Noninfectious bursitis is treated by avoidance of bursal trauma and short-term use of NSAIDs. Glucocorticoid injections may provide short-term benefit but are associated with complications and should be considered only when conservative treatment fails. Surgery may be necessary for infectious or refractory bursitis.

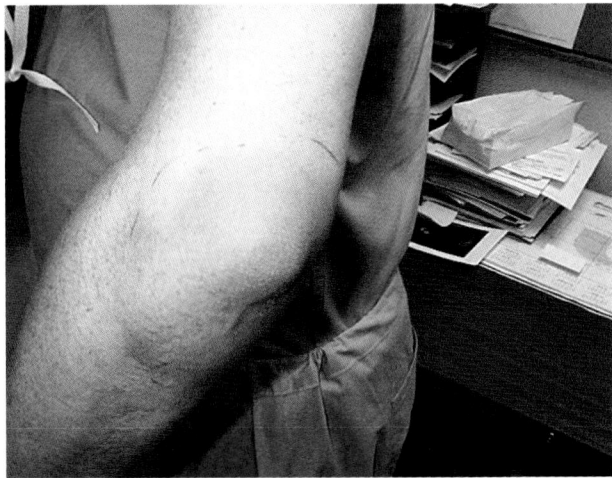

**FIGURE 10.** Olecranon bursitis is characterized by warmth, redness, and swelling. The ability to extend and flex the elbow generally excludes an intra-articular process.

### Ulnar Nerve Entrapment

Ulnar nerve entrapment (cubital tunnel syndrome) results from ulnar nerve impingement at the elbow by fibrous scar tissue, ulnar nerve subluxation, ganglion cysts, or bone spurs. Characteristics include pain at the elbow that worsens with flexion, paresthesias and numbness of the fourth and fifth fingers, and weakness of the interosseous muscles. The diagnosis is usually clinical, but electromyography is often used for diagnostic confirmation; MRI or ultrasonography may be useful in some situations.

Initial treatment consists of avoidance of elbow trauma and nocturnal splinting. NSAIDs are beneficial for short-term pain relief. Surgery is an option when conservative measures fail in the setting of significant or progressive symptoms.

- Olecranon bursitis is characterized by posterior elbow swelling and tenderness with normal elbow range of motion; swelling and pain on elbow extension suggest elbow joint effusion and an alternate cause.

- Elbow pain is generally managed with avoidance of trauma and pain-inducing activities; NSAIDs may be effective for analgesia. **HVC**

## Wrist and Hand Pain

### Carpal Tunnel Syndrome

Carpal tunnel syndrome develops from increased pressure within the carpal tunnel causing median nerve compression. Diagnosis is usually established based on history. The syndrome presents with wrist pain that may radiate to the forearm and hand; paresthesias and weakness of the first three fingers and thenar eminence (median nerve distribution) may be present. Symptoms are often worse at night and with repetitive wrist motion. Risk factors include obesity, female sex, hypothyroidism, pregnancy, and connective tissue disorders. Although keyboard use has been suggested as a risk factor, it has not been confirmed by studies.

Examination findings may include decreased sensation over the median nerve distribution, thenar muscle atrophy, and weakened thumb abduction. Examination is often normal early in the disease, and provocative testing with the Phalen maneuver (flexion of hands at wrists) or Tinel test (percussion of the median nerve on top of the carpal tunnel) is rarely useful. Electrodiagnostic testing is beneficial when the diagnosis is unclear, especially when cervical radiculopathy is possible.

Initial treatment includes activity modification and wrist splinting. Methylprednisolone injection or short-term oral glucocorticoids may also provide benefit as second-line therapy. Surgical treatment is necessary for patients who do not respond to conservative therapy or who have evidence of significant neurologic dysfunction.

### Other Causes

Acute wrist or hand pain associated with trauma suggests fracture or dislocation and requires plain radiography for evaluation. Although multiple injuries are possible, special consideration for hamate and scaphoid fractures is necessary. Hamate hook fractures can occur from a fall onto an outstretched hand or activities with repetitive impact at the palm base (baseball hitting). Plain radiographs usually reveal the fracture. Scaphoid fractures are also commonly associated with falling onto an extended hand and are characterized by pain and tenderness in the anatomic snuffbox. Initial radiographs are normal in up to 20% of patients. If clinical suspicion is high and radiographs are normal, thumb splinting and repeat radiography in 1 to 2 weeks or immediate advanced imaging (MRI or CT) are recommended.

Wrist or hand pain lasting more than 2 weeks also has a wide differential diagnosis. De Quervain tendinopathy results from noninflammatory thickening of the thumb tendons. Pain occurs at the thumb base, radiates to the distal radius, and is elicited with making a fist over the thumb and ulnar deviation of the wrist (Finkelstein test). Initial management includes rest, NSAIDs, and splinting. When conservative measures fail, glucocorticoid injections provide symptomatic relief. Surgery may benefit patients with symptoms that do not respond to glucocorticoid injections.

Ganglion cysts are caused by herniated synovial tissue surrounding tendon sheaths or joints; they are often palpable on the ventral aspect of the wrist. Asymptomatic cysts require no treatment. Ganglion cysts causing pain may be treated with aspiration. The benefit of glucocorticoid or hyaluronidase injections is questionable; they are not indicated given the potential for complications. If cysts recur after aspiration, surgical resection is effective.

Ulnar neuropathy from ulnar nerve entrapment at the wrist presents with wrist pain and decreased hand strength and sensation. This condition can result from prolonged ulnar

nerve compression in the Guyton canal, such as may occur with bicycling.

Osteoarthritis and inflammatory arthritis may affect the interphalangeal and carpometacarpal joints and cause hand and wrist pain (see MKSAP 18 Rheumatology).

## Lower Extremity Disorders
### Hip Pain
#### Diagnosis and Evaluation

Evaluation of hip pain should be guided by location of the pain. Anterior hip and groin pain is caused by both intra- and extra-articular factors. Lateral hip pain is most commonly due to greater trochanteric pain syndrome (GTPS; formerly known as trochanteric bursitis) or meralgia paresthetica. Posterior hip pain is caused by sacroiliac joint dysfunction, lumbar radiculopathy, or vascular claudication.

Anterior hip pain that starts insidiously and worsens with standing and activity in older patients suggests osteoarthritis. The same pain characteristics in a younger person raise concern for a labral tear, especially when accompanied by painful clicking or catching. Gradual onset of anterior hip pain can also occur with avascular necrosis (or osteonecrosis), which should be considered in the presence of alcohol abuse, glucocorticoid use, systemic lupus erythematosus, or sickle cell anemia. Acute-onset, anteriorly located hip pain that interferes with weight bearing and is accompanied by fevers raises suspicion for infectious arthritis, whereas acute pain after a fall suggests fracture.

Lateral hip pain that worsens with lying on the affected side suggests GTPS; this pain may also radiate to the buttock or knee. Meralgia paresthetica is characterized by distal anterolateral thigh paresthesias associated with tight-fitting clothes and obesity.

Posterior or buttock pain associated with radiation down the leg suggests lumbar radiculopathy, whereas concomitant exertional leg pain or peripheral vascular disease suggests vascular claudication. Posterior pain without other features may be secondary to sacroiliac joint dysfunction.

Examination of patients with hip pain includes evaluation of the hip, abdomen, and back; neurologic and vascular assessments of the legs; and gait assessment. Pain with both passive and active hip movement suggests an intra-articular cause. The FABER (Flexion, ABduction, and External Rotation) test may cause posterior hip pain in the presence of sacroiliac joint dysfunction, groin pain with an intra-articular cause, and lateral hip pain with GTPS (**Figure 11**). The

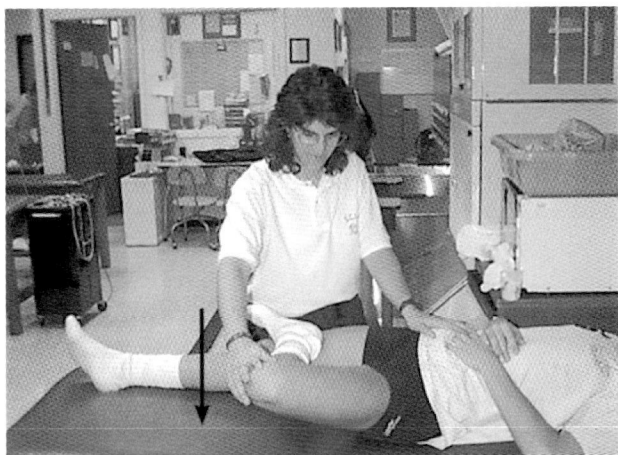

**FIGURE 11.** The FABER (Flexion, ABduction, and External Rotation) test. With the patient supine, the leg on the tested side is placed in the "figure 4" position (the knee of the tested side is flexed 90 degrees, and the lateral malleolus is placed on top of the opposite leg). The examiner then applies a posteriorly directed force with one hand while using the other hand to stabilize the patient's other hip. A positive test result occurs if groin pain or buttock pain is produced. Buttock pain suggests sacroiliac joint dysfunction, and groin pain suggests an intra-articular cause of pain.

Reproduced with permission from Davis MF, Davis PF, Ross DS. Expert Guide to Sports Medicine. Philadelphia, PA: American College of Physicians, 2005:360. Copyright 2005, American College of Physicians.

most common examination finding in GTPS is tenderness to palpation of the greater trochanter. A normal hip examination in a patient with groin pain suggests an extra-articular cause, such as an inguinal hernia. Pain reproduction on straight leg raise test (see Figure 8) supports lumbar radiculopathy.

Plain radiography (anteroposterior pelvic view and frog-leg lateral view) should be performed if intra-articular pathology, fracture, or dislocation is suspected. In patients with persistent anterior pain and normal plain radiographs, MRI of the hip can be performed; however, if suspicion is high for a labral tear, MR arthrography should be performed. Hip aspiration should be performed if infectious arthritis is suspected.

## Treatment

Initial management of labral tears includes muscle strengthening and activity modification, with arthroscopic surgery reserved for those in whom conservative measures fail. Patients with advanced avascular necrosis often require total hip arthroplasty.

Initial GTPS management includes activity modification and analgesia with acetaminophen or NSAIDs. Glucocorticoid injection can be considered for persistently symptomatic GTPS, with surgery limited to recalcitrant cases. Primary treatment of meralgia paresthetica consists of reassurance, avoiding tight-fitting clothes, and weight loss. First-line therapy for sacroiliac joint dysfunction is physical therapy, with limited evidence existing for local glucocorticoid injection.

Management of osteoarthritis is discussed in MKSAP 18 Rheumatology.

## Knee Pain

### Diagnosis and Evaluation

The history obtained from patients with knee pain should focus on pain characteristics as well as history of knee injury or surgery, osteoarthritis, gout, and acute calcium pyrophosphate crystal arthritis (pseudogout).

Knee examination, performed with both knees fully exposed, includes inspection, palpation, range of motion testing, and special maneuvers (**Table 48**).

Plain radiography should be performed if fracture, bony pathology, or osteoarthritis is suspected. MRI can be performed if there is concern for meniscal or ligamentous injury and surgical therapy is being considered. Joint aspiration should be performed for suspicion of inflammatory or infectious arthritis.

Knee osteoarthritis is discussed in MKSAP 18 Rheumatology.

### Ligament and Meniscal Tears

Acute, traumatic onset of knee pain, especially when associated with swelling, should raise concern for ligamentous and/or meniscal tears. Anterior cruciate ligament (ACL) tears usually involve noncontact twisting injuries. Patients may report a popping sound and frequently cannot immediately bear weight. Large effusions due to hemarthrosis frequently develop within 2 hours and may make initial examination challenging. The anterior drawer and Lachman tests frequently demonstrate increased ligamentous laxity, although the Lachman test may be most useful in the acute setting (see Table 48). Plain radiography should be obtained to evaluate for possible accompanying tibial avulsion fractures. ACL tears usually require surgical reconstruction, especially in active patients or those with an unstable knee. A nonoperative approach may be appropriate in older and less active patients. Medial collateral ligament (MCL) tears typically involve a lateral blow to the knee causing valgus stress, whereas posterior collateral ligament (PCL) tears involve a posteriorly directed force applied to the proximal anterior tibia with the knee flexed. Increased MCL laxity suggesting a tear may be detected by applying a medially directed force with the knee flexed at 30 degrees (valgus stress test), whereas increased PCL laxity may be detected by applying a posteriorly directed force to the proximal tibia with the knee flexed at 90 degrees. Most MCL and PCL tears can be managed conservatively.

**TABLE 48.** Knee Examination Maneuvers

| Maneuver | Purpose | Description | Likelihood Ratios[a] |
|---|---|---|---|
| Anterior drawer | ACL integrity | Patient is supine with hip flexed to 45° and knee flexed to 90°. Examiner sits on dorsum of foot and places hands on proximal calf and then pulls anteriorly while assessing movement of tibia relative to femur.<br><br>Positive result: Increased laxity with lack of firm end point (suggests ACL tear) | Positive likelihood ratio: 3.8[a]<br><br>Negative likelihood ratio: 0.30[a] |
| Lachman | ACL integrity | Patient is supine with leg in slight external rotation and knee flexed 20° to 30° at examiner's side. Examiner stabilizes femur with one hand and grasps proximal calf with other. Calf is pulled forward while assessing movement of tibia relative to femur.<br><br>Positive result: Increased laxity with lack of firm end point (suggests ACL tear) | Positive likelihood ratio: 42.0[b]<br><br>Negative likelihood ratio: 0.1[b] |
| Posterior drawer | PCL integrity | Patient is supine with hip flexed to 45° and knee flexed to 90°. Examiner sits on dorsum of foot and places hands on proximal calf and then pushes posteriorly while assessing movement of tibia relative to femur.<br><br>Positive result: Increased laxity with lack of firm end point (suggests PCL tear) | Positive likelihood ratio: 50.11[c]<br><br>Negative likelihood ratio: 0.11[c] |
| Valgus stress | MCL integrity | Patient is supine with knee flexed to 30° and leg slightly abducted. Examiner places one hand on lateral knee and other hand on medial distal tibia and applies valgus force.<br><br>Positive result: Increased laxity and pain (suggests MCL tear) | Positive likelihood ratio: 7.7<br><br>Negative likelihood ratio: 0.2 |
| Varus stress | LCL integrity | Patient is supine with knee flexed to 30° and leg slightly abducted. Examiner places one hand on medial knee and other hand on lateral distal tibia and applies varus force.<br><br>Positive result: Increased laxity and pain (suggests LCL tear) | Positive likelihood ratio: 16.2 |
| Thessaly | Meniscal integrity | Examiner holds patient's outstretched hands while patient stands on one leg with knee flexed to 5° and with other knee flexed to 90° with foot off of floor. Patient rotates body internally and externally three times. Repeat with knee flexed to 20°. Always perform on uninvolved knee first.<br><br>Positive result: Medial or lateral joint line pain (suggests meniscal tear) | Positive likelihood ratio: 1.37[d]<br><br>Negative likelihood ratio: 0.68[d] |
| Medial-lateral grind | Meniscal integrity | With patient supine, examiner places calf in one hand and thumb and index finger of opposite hand over joint line and applies varus and valgus stress to tibia during extension and flexion.<br><br>Positive result: Grinding sensation palpable over joint line (suggests meniscal injury) | Positive likelihood ratio: 4.8[b]<br><br>Negative likelihood ratio: 0.4[b] |
| McMurray | Meniscal integrity | With patient supine, the examiner fully flexes the knee and rotates the tibia externally. The knee is then extended with the hand over the medial joint line. The maneuver is then repeated with the tibia internally rotated and the hand over the lateral joint line.<br><br>Positive result: Snapping is detected over the joint line with extension on the knee | Positive likelihood ratio: 1.3[b]<br><br>Negative likelihood ratio: 0.8[b] |
| Noble | Iliotibial band integrity | With patient supine, examiner repeatedly flexes and extends knee with examiner's thumb placed on lateral femoral epicondyle.<br><br>Positive result: Reproduces patient's pain (suggests iliotibial band syndrome) | |

ACL = anterior cruciate ligament; LCL = lateral collateral ligament; MCL = medial collateral ligament; PCL = posterior cruciate ligament.

[a]Data used to derive these values are of limited quality.

[b]Data from Solomon DH, Simel DL, Bates DW, Katz JN, Schaffer JL. The rational clinical examination. Does this patient have a torn meniscus or ligament of the knee? Value of the physical examination. JAMA. 2001;286:1610-20. [PMID: 11585485]

[c]Data from Rubinstein RA Jr, Shelbourne KD, McCarroll JR, VanMeter CD, Rettig AC. The accuracy of the clinical examination in the setting of posterior cruciate ligament injuries. Am J Sports Med. 1994;22:550-7. [PMID: 7943523]

[d]Data from Goossens P, Keijsers E, van Geenen RJ, Zijta A, van den Broek M, Verhagen AP, et al. Validity of the Thessaly test in evaluating meniscal tears compared with arthroscopy: a diagnostic accuracy study. J Orthop Sports Phys Ther. 2015;45:18-24, B1. [PMID: 25420009] doi:10.2519/jospt.2015.5215

Meniscal tears usually result from an acute twisting knee injury or can develop more insidiously as a result of chronic degeneration. Symptoms include pain, locking, catching, and grinding. Patients with acute meniscal tears are usually able to immediately bear weight. On examination, effusions, if present, are generally small to moderate in size. Results of specialized tests, such as the medial-lateral grind and Thessaly tests, are frequently positive (see Table 48). Initial management of both acute and chronic meniscal tears is conservative and consists of rest, ice, and strengthening the quadriceps and hamstring muscles. Surgery is reserved for patients with persistent (>4 weeks) mechanical symptoms.

### Patellofemoral Pain Syndrome
Patellofemoral pain syndrome is caused by disordered patellar tracking with knee movement. It is characterized by anterior knee pain and/or stiffness with prolonged sitting, climbing, or descending stairs, and with running or squatting. On examination, applying pressure to the patella may reproduce pain. Patellar mobility can be assessed by medially and laterally displacing the patella, and abrupt patellar deviation may be noted during squatting and standing, although the utility of these findings is unclear.

Treatment is focused on identifying the underlying cause; activity modification, such as relative rest; cryotherapy (ice or cold water immersion); and physical therapy. NSAIDs, acetaminophen, and patellar taping and bracing are frequently used, although evidence for the effectiveness of these measures is limited.

#### KEY POINTS
HVC
- In patients with knee pain, plain radiography should be obtained if fracture, bony pathology, or osteoarthritis is suspected.
- Anterior cruciate ligament tears often require surgical reconstruction, whereas most medial collateral ligament and posterior collateral ligament tears can be managed conservatively.
- Patellofemoral pain syndrome is characterized by anterior knee pain and/or stiffness with prolonged sitting, climbing, or descending stairs, and with running or squatting; treatment may include activity modification, cryotherapy, and physical therapy.

### Bursitis
Prepatellar bursitis presents as acute or chronic swelling anterior to the patella. Acute cases are often associated with tenderness, warmth, and erythema. Most cases of acute prepatellar bursitis are caused by infection with skin bacteria and less commonly by trauma and gout. Chronic prepatellar bursitis is usually caused by trauma, although gout and infection are possible. All patients with prepatellar bursitis regardless of duration should undergo fluid aspiration and analysis. Septic bursitis is managed with knee immobilization, systemic

antibiotics, and re-aspiration if needed. Gouty bursitis is managed with appropriate gout therapy (see MKSAP 18 Rheumatology). Traumatic bursitis is managed by activity modification (avoidance of kneeling) and NSAIDs.

Pes anserine bursitis (pes anserine pain syndrome) classically presents with localized pain and swelling of the region overlying the proximal medial tibia several centimeters distal to the knee (**Figure 12**). It commonly occurs in athletes (especially runners) and in patients with knee osteoarthritis. First-line therapy includes quadriceps strengthening, local cryotherapy, activity modification, and NSAIDs.

### Iliotibial Band Syndrome
Patients with iliotibial band syndrome (ITBS) report diffuse, poorly localized lateral knee and distal thigh pain. Pain is initially present at the end of exercise involving knee flexion and extension but may progress to occur earlier in exercise or with rest. Running outdoors or downhill may worsen symptoms. On examination, there is often tenderness approximately 2 to 3 cm proximal to the lateral femoral condyle. Patients also frequently have a positive result on a Noble test and weakness with hip abduction (see Table 48). Imaging is not usually required.

Initial treatment of ITBS centers on abstinence from inciting activity and use of ice, followed by gradual return to activity, stretching, strengthening, and local massage. NSAIDs appear effective when used as part of a multimodal approach. Local glucocorticoid injections may provide at least short-term relief.

### Popliteal Cysts
A popliteal (Baker) cyst is a benign swelling of the synovial bursa behind the knee joint; synovial fluid fills the cyst. Popliteal cysts most commonly develop in the setting of knee trauma, osteoarthritis, or inflammatory arthritis. They are frequently asymptomatic but can present with posterior knee pain and swelling.

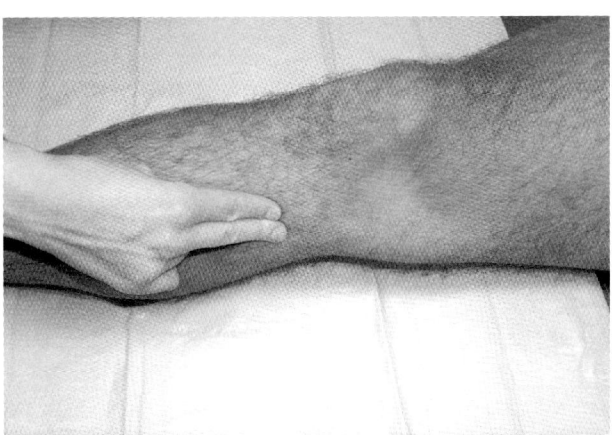

**FIGURE 12.** Location of the anserine bursa and pain associated with pes anserine bursitis.

Reproduced with permission from Moore G. Atlas of the Musculoskeletal Examination. Philadelphia, PA: American College of Physicians; 2003:87. Copyright 2003, American College of Physicians.

Ruptured cysts may mimic deep venous thromboses (pseudothrombophlebitis) and may be associated with ecchymosis from the popliteal fossa to the ankle. The "crescent sign" may be present, recognized as an ecchymotic area below the medial malleolus. In rare instances, cysts may cause compression of adjacent structures, leading to compression syndrome, posterior tibial nerve entrapment, or popliteal artery occlusion. In patients with asymptomatic popliteal cysts, no treatment is necessary. Symptomatic patients often experience relief with joint aspiration and intra-articular glucocorticoid injection. Pseudothrombophlebitis can be treated with rest, elevation, and NSAIDs. Surgical excision is reserved for severely symptomatic and functionally limited patients in whom conservative measures fail or who develop serious complications.

### KEY POINTS

- All patients with prepatellar bursitis regardless of duration should undergo fluid aspiration and analysis.

- Iliotibial band syndrome is characterized by pain at the end of exercise involving knee flexion and extension but may progress to occur earlier in exercise or with rest; treatment is typically nonsurgical.

**HVC** - In patients with asymptomatic popliteal (Baker) cysts, no treatment is necessary; joint aspiration and intra-articular glucocorticoid injection may provide relief for those with symptoms.

## Ankle and Foot Pain
### Ankle Sprains
Acute ankle sprains are usually caused by excessive ankle inversion; ankle eversion injuries are rare. Common examination findings include overlying ecchymosis and swelling with tenderness of involved ankle ligaments. Weight-bearing ability and bony tenderness are components of Ottawa ankle rules, which help to determine the necessity of obtaining plain radiography to exclude fracture (**Figure 13**). Treatment includes

intermittent cryotherapy and a lace-up support or air stirrup brace combined with elastic compression wrapping. Early mobilization should be encouraged with weight bearing as tolerated. Acetaminophen and oral or topical NSAIDs can be used for pain control. Patients with persistent ligamentous laxity 4 to 6 weeks after injury should be referred for proprioceptive training and strengthening therapy.

High ankle sprains (distal tibiofibular syndesmosis ligament injuries) occur when an externally rotated force is applied to a dorsiflexed ankle. Pain may be elicited by squeezing the leg at mid-calf (squeeze test) and by dorsiflexing and externally rotating the foot with the knee flexed (dorsiflexion-external rotation test). Treatment is similar to other ankle sprains, although recovery is usually delayed.

### Hindfoot Pain
Achilles tendinopathy typically develops in persons who initiate or abruptly increase activity. Patients report activity-related posterior heel pain and stiffness that improves with rest. On examination, there is usually tenderness of the Achilles tendon approximately 2 to 6 cm above the calcaneal insertion. Treatment includes activity modification, eccentric exercises (muscle lengthening in response to external resistance), and use of appropriate footwear. NSAIDs can be used for pain control.

Achilles tendon rupture commonly occurs during strenuous activities, although it may occur spontaneously in the elderly or with fluoroquinolone use. Patients usually have heel pain and may report hearing a "pop." On examination, a tendon defect may be palpable; a lack of plantar flexion with calf squeezing (Thompson test) suggests complete rupture (sensitivity, 93%; specificity, 96%) (**Figure 14**). Treatment is controversial and consists of surgery with immobilization or immobilization alone.

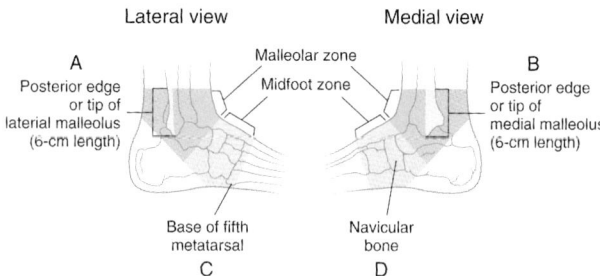

**FIGURE 13.** Ottawa ankle and foot rules. An ankle radiographic series is indicated if a patient has pain in the malleolar zone and any of the following findings: bone tenderness at *A*, bone tenderness at *B*, or inability to bear weight immediately and in the emergency department (or physician's office). A foot radiographic series is indicated if a patient has pain in the midfoot zone and any of the following findings: bone tenderness at *C*, bone tenderness at *D*, or inability to bear weight immediately and in the emergency department (or physician's office).

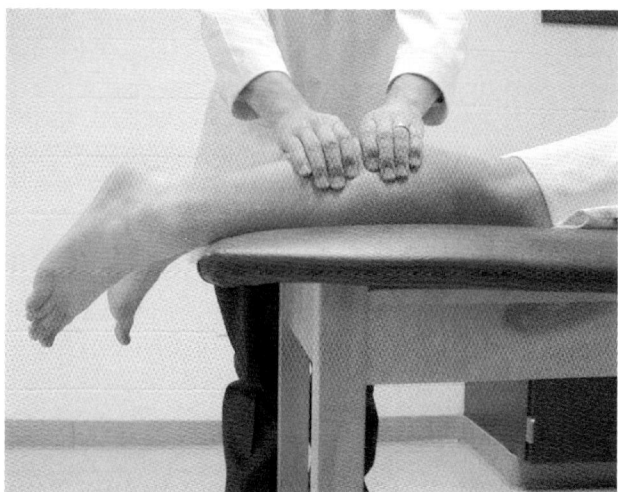

**FIGURE 14.** Thompson test. The patient is positioned in the prone position. The examiner squeezes mid-calf and observes for plantar flexion of the foot. When the patient has an intact Achilles tendon, plantar flexion will occur. When there is a complete Achilles tendon rupture, no plantar flexion is observed.

Plantar fasciitis classically causes sharp, medial-inferior heel pain with the first morning steps and after prolonged rest. Pain usually improves with further walking but may persist in severe cases. On examination, the medial calcaneal tubercle is frequently tender. Passive toe dorsiflexion with standing (weight-bearing windlass test) may reproduce pain (sensitivity, 32%; specificity, 100%). Treatment includes weight loss, rest, calf/heel stretching, and arch supports (if pes planus is present). Because the underlying pathology is thought to be degenerative, use of NSAIDs is primarily for pain control. Patients should be educated that eventual resolution is expected but may take months. For recalcitrant cases, ultrasonography, extracorporeal shockwave therapy, night splints, and glucocorticoid injections can be considered. Surgery is reserved for patients who do not respond to these measures.

Heel pad syndrome causes inferior heel pain when walking barefoot and on hard surfaces. On examination, palpation may reproduce pain. Treatment consists of heel cushioning, rest, ice, and NSAIDs.

## Midfoot Pain

Tarsal tunnel syndrome (posterior tibial nerve compression as it passes through the tarsal tunnel) causes posteromedial heel paresthesias that radiate distally into the plantar foot surface. On examination, pain may be reproduced with nerve tapping (Tinel sign) and with provocative measures that compress the nerve (plantar flexion-inversion and dorsiflexion-eversion tests). First-line treatment consists of activity modification, orthotics, NSAIDs, and neuromodulators.

## Forefoot Pain

Morton neuromas (interdigital nerve injury) cause pain between the metatarsal heads and the sensation of walking on a pebble. First-line therapy consists of footwear modification and padding. Glucocorticoid injections may provide temporary relief. Interdigital nerve resection is reserved for those who do not respond to conservative measures.

Hammertoe deformities (proximal interphalangeal joint flexion deformity with distal interphalangeal joint extension and extended or neutral position of metatarsophalangeal [MTP] joint) occur with constricting footwear and increasing age. Treatment includes footwear modification, padding, and possibly surgery.

Hallux or bunion deformity (lateral deviation of great toe with medial bony deformity) can lead to pain, first MTP joint osteoarthritis, and overlying bursitis. Treatment includes orthotic devices, NSAIDs, and possibly surgery.

**KEY POINTS**

- Acute ankle sprains are usually caused by excessive ankle inversion; treatment includes intermittent cryotherapy, a lace-up support or air stirrup brace combined with elastic compression wrapping, early mobilization with weight bearing as tolerated, and acetaminophen and oral or topical NSAIDs.

*(Continued)*

**KEY POINTS** (continued)

- Achilles tendon rupture commonly occurs during strenuous activities, although it may occur spontaneously in the elderly or with fluoroquinolone use.

- Plantar fasciitis classically causes sharp, medial-inferior heel pain with the first morning steps and after prolonged rest; the medial calcaneal tubercle is frequently tender.

- Morton neuromas (interdigital nerve injury) cause pain between the metatarsal heads and the sensation of walking on pebbles.

# Dyslipidemia
## Evaluation of Lipid Levels

The U.S. Preventive Services Task Force (USPSTF) recommends universal lipid screening in adults aged 40 to 75 years to calculate risk for atherosclerotic cardiovascular disease (ASCVD) using the American College of Cardiology (ACC)/American Heart Association (AHA) Pooled Cohort Equations (see MKSAP 18 Cardiovascular Medicine). Lipid measurement may also be indicated to investigate for familial hypercholesterolemia; to determine therapy adherence and effectiveness; and to evaluate for complications of dyslipidemia, such as pancreatitis.

### LDL Cholesterol

The association between high LDL cholesterol levels and increased risk for ASCVD is widely accepted. Historically, cholesterol treatment targeted specific LDL cholesterol goals, as LDL cholesterol is the most atherogenic lipoprotein. The 2013 ACC/AHA cholesterol treatment guideline recommends fixed statin dosing to reduce ASCVD risk and consideration of non-statin drugs in patients who do not achieve adequate lipid lowering. Therefore, based on this guideline, the primary utility of LDL cholesterol measurement is to identify patients who will benefit from treatment with statin therapy and to assess response to therapy.

In patients with elevated LDL cholesterol levels, secondary causes, including hypothyroidism, poorly controlled diabetes mellitus, nephrotic syndrome, and medications (such as glucocorticoids, diuretics, and amiodarone), should be considered. Familial hypercholesterolemia should be considered in patients with an LDL cholesterol level of 190 mg/dL (4.92 mmol/L) or higher.

### Triglycerides

Elevated triglyceride levels (>150 mg/dL [1.69 mmol/L]) are independently associated with increased ASCVD risk; however, it is uncertain whether reducing triglyceride levels decreases risk. Causes of hypertriglyceridemia include diabetes; excessive alcohol intake; hypothyroidism; and medications such as glucocorticoids, protease inhibitors, and estrogens. Lifestyle factors, including obesity and concentrated sugar intake, are also implicated causes. Patients with triglyceride levels of 500 mg/dL (5.65 mmol/L) or more without an identifiable cause should be evaluated for familial hypertriglyceridemia.

Acute pancreatitis can be induced by triglyceride levels in excess of 1000 mg/dL (11.3 mmol/L), and triglyceride levels should be measured in selected patients with pancreatitis, especially in cases of pancreatitis without a clear cause (such as alcohol use or biliary disease).

## HDL Cholesterol

HDL cholesterol is a protective factor against the development of ASCVD and is an important component in ASCVD risk assessment. However, a causative link between low HDL cholesterol levels and ASCVD has not been established, and pharmacologic treatment to raise HDL cholesterol levels is not recommended.

### KEY POINTS

- The U.S. Preventive Services Task Force recommends universal lipid screening in adults aged 40 to 75 years to calculate risk for atherosclerotic cardiovascular disease.

**HVC**
- The primary utility of LDL cholesterol measurement is to identify patients who will benefit from treatment with statin therapy and to assess response to therapy.

- Secondary causes of LDL cholesterol elevation include hypothyroidism, poorly controlled diabetes mellitus, nephrotic syndrome, and medication use (such as glucocorticoids, diuretics, and amiodarone).

# Management of Dyslipidemia

Following assessment of ASCVD risk, treatment with therapeutic lifestyle changes and statin therapy may be indicated.

## Therapeutic Lifestyle Changes

All patients at increased cardiovascular risk should be counseled regarding therapeutic lifestyle changes, including dietary modification, regular physical activity, weight loss, and smoking cessation.

Patients should be encouraged to adhere to a dietary pattern that focuses on consumption of fruits, vegetables, fiber, and monounsaturated fats and minimizes intake of saturated and *trans* fats, simple carbohydrates, and red meats. Replacing saturated fats with polyunsaturated fats has been shown to reduce LDL cholesterol levels and cardiovascular mortality. Examples of heart-healthy diets include the DASH (Dietary Approaches to Stop Hypertension) and Mediterranean diets. The DASH diet provides a suggested number of servings for each food group, with few servings of saturated fats, sweets, and red meat and a higher number of servings of grains, fruits, and vegetables; adherence to the DASH diet has been shown to decrease adverse cardiovascular events. The Mediterranean

diet comprises high amounts of unsaturated fats, with ample intake of fruits, vegetables, fiber, seeds, nuts, and fatty fish and low consumption of red meat and dairy products. The ACC/AHA additionally recommend reducing the percentage of calories from saturated fat (<7% of calories from saturated fat; <6% of calories from saturated fat in patients at high cardiovascular risk) and the percentage of calories from *trans* fat. To facilitate these changes, clinicians should provide patients with educational resources and, when appropriate, refer them to a dietician.

Patients should also engage in 40 minutes of moderate to vigorous activity 3 to 4 days per week or 30 minutes on most days of the week. Small incremental changes to reduce sedentary behavior, such as increasing walking and time standing, are beneficial.

## Drug Therapy

Statin therapy is the mainstay of pharmacotherapy for dyslipidemia. The ACC/AHA cholesterol treatment guideline defines four patient groups that benefit from statin therapy for primary or secondary prevention of ASCVD:

1. Patients aged 21 years and older with clinical ASCVD, defined as acute coronary syndrome, or a history of myocardial infarction, stable or unstable angina, coronary or other arterial revascularization, stroke/transient ischemic attack, or peripheral artery disease attributable to atherosclerosis (high-intensity statin therapy if aged ≤75 years; moderate-intensity statin therapy if aged >75 years)

2. Patients aged 21 years and older with an LDL cholesterol level of 190 mg/dL (4.92 mmol/L) or higher (high-intensity statin therapy)

3. Patients aged 40 to 75 years with diabetes and an LDL cholesterol level of 70 mg/dL to 189 mg/dL (1.81-4.90 mmol/L) (high-intensity statin therapy if 10-year ASCVD risk ≥7.5%; moderate-intensity statin therapy if 10-year ASCVD risk <7.5%)

4. Patients aged 40 to 75 years with no ASCVD or diabetes and a 10-year ASCVD risk of 7.5% or higher (moderate- or high-intensity statin therapy based on patient preferences, adverse effects, and expected ASCVD risk reduction)

These recommendations are summarized in **Figure 15**. Statin dosages for high- and moderate-intensity therapy are presented in **Table 49**.

A lipid panel should be obtained 4 to 12 weeks after initiation of therapy to determine treatment adherence and response. According to the 2013 ACC/AHA guideline, high-intensity statin therapy should decrease LDL cholesterol levels by at least 50% from baseline levels, whereas moderate-intensity statin therapy should decrease LDL cholesterol levels by 30% to 50%. All patients who do not achieve adequate reduction in LDL cholesterol levels should be assessed for medication adherence and should intensify lifestyle modifications. Additional medical therapy should be considered if the target effect is not realized. Once therapy goals have been achieved,

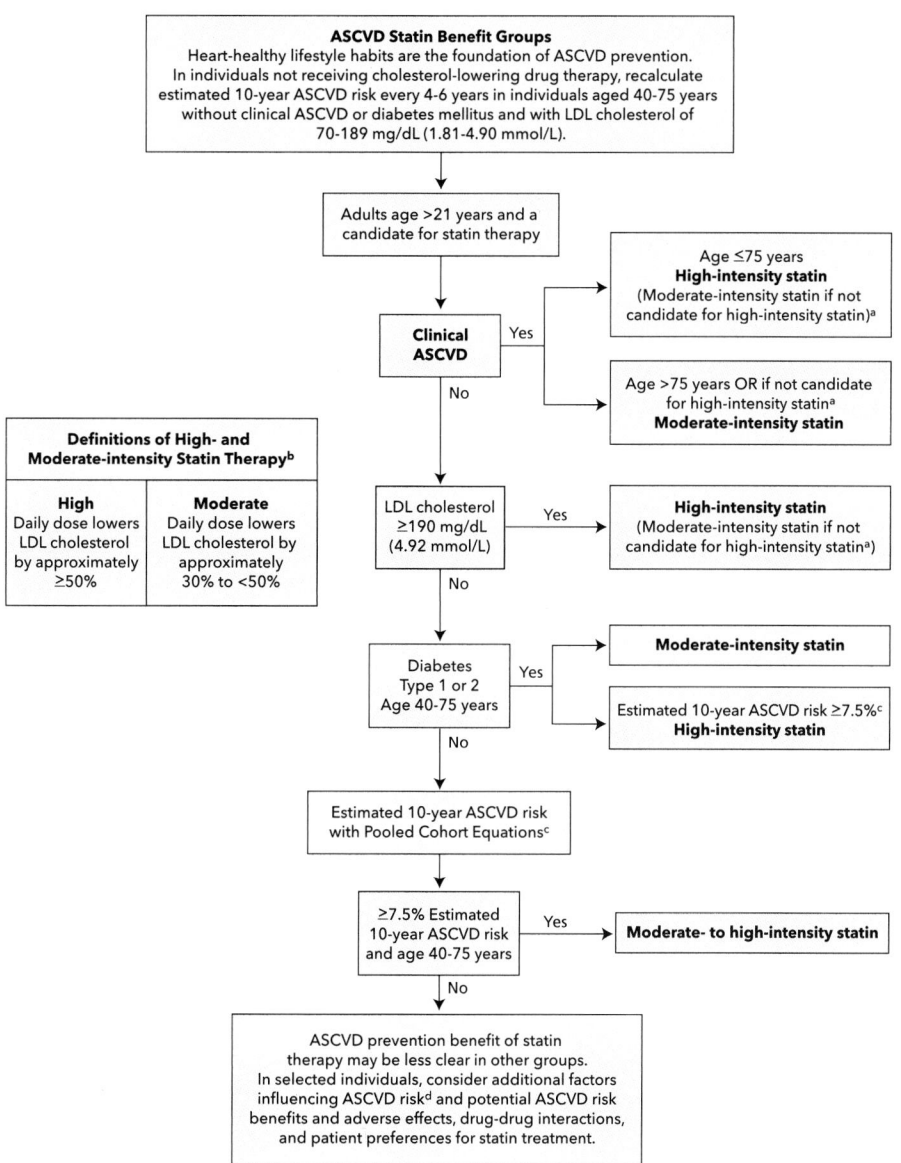

**FIGURE 15.** Major recommendations for statin therapy for ASCVD prevention. This flow diagram is intended to serve as an easy reference guide summarizing recommendations for ASCVD risk assessment and treatment. Assessment of the potential for benefit and risk from statin therapy for ASCVD prevention provides the framework for clinical decision making incorporating patient preferences. ASCVD = atherosclerotic cardiovascular disease.

[a]Moderate-intensity statin therapy should be used in individuals in whom high-intensity statin therapy would otherwise be recommended when high-intensity statin therapy is contraindicated or when characteristics predisposing them to statin-associated adverse effects are present.

Characteristics predisposing individuals to statin adverse effects include, but are not limited to:

- Multiple or serious comorbidities, including impaired kidney or liver function
- History of previous statin intolerance or muscle disorders
- Unexplained alanine aminotransferase elevations >3 times upper limit of normal
- Patient characteristics or concomitant use of drugs affecting statin metabolism
- >75 years of age

Additional characteristics that may modify the decision to use higher statin intensities may include, but are not limited to:

- History of hemorrhagic stroke
- Asian ancestry

[b]Percent reduction in LDL cholesterol can be used as an indication of response and adherence to therapy but is not in itself a treatment goal.

[c]The Pooled Cohort Equations can be used to estimate 10-year ASCVD risk in individuals with and without diabetes mellitus. A downloadable spreadsheet enabling estimation of 10-year and lifetime risk for ASCVD and a web-based calculator are available at http://my.americanheart.org/cvriskcalculator.

[d]Primary LDL cholesterol level ≥160 mg/dL (4.14 mmol/L) or other evidence of genetic hyperlipidemias; family history of premature ASCVD with onset <55 years of age in a first-degree male relative or <65 years of age in a first-degree female relative; high-sensitivity C-reactive protein ≥2 mg/L; coronary artery calcium score ≥300 Agatston units or ≥75th percentile for age, sex, and ethnicity; ankle-brachial index <0.90; or elevated lifetime risk of ASCVD.

Reproduced with permission from Stone NJ, Robinson JG, Lichtenstein AH, et al; American College of Cardiology/American Heart Association Task Force on Practice Guidelines. 2013 ACC/AHA guideline on the treatment of blood cholesterol to reduce atherosclerotic cardiovascular risk in adults: a report of the American College of Cardiology/American Heart Association Task Force on Practice Guidelines. Circulation. 2013; Epub 2013 Nov 12. Copyright 2013, American Heart Association, Inc.

**TABLE 49.** High- and Moderate-Intensity Statin Therapy

| Therapy Intensity | Drug and Dosage |
| --- | --- |
| High intensity | Atorvastatin, 40-80 mg/d |
| | Rosuvastatin, 20-40 mg/d |
| Moderate intensity | Atorvastatin, 10-20 mg/d |
| | Rosuvastatin, 5-10 mg/d |
| | Simvastatin, 20-40 mg/d |
| | Pravastatin, 40-80 mg/d |
| | Lovastatin, 40 mg/d |
| | Fluvastatin, 40 mg twice daily |

lipid levels should be measured every 3 to 12 months as indicated.

The USPSTF recommendations for primary prevention statin therapy differ from those of the ACC/AHA in considering risk factors other than diabetes and the suggested intensity of statin therapy. In asymptomatic adults aged 40 to 75 years without ASCVD who have at least one ASCVD risk factor (dyslipidemia, diabetes, hypertension, or smoking), the USPSTF recommends low- to moderate-intensity statin therapy in those with a calculated 10-year ASCVD event risk of 10% or higher (grade B recommendation) and selective consideration of low- to moderate-intensity statin therapy in those with a calculated 10-year ASCVD event risk of 7.5% to 10% (grade C recommendation).

In contrast to the ACC/AHA guideline and USPSTF recommendations, the 2017 American Association of Clinical Endocrinologists (AACE) and American College of Endocrinology (ACE) guidelines for management of dyslipidemia and prevention of cardiovascular disease recommend treating LDL cholesterol, non–HDL cholesterol, and apolipoprotein B levels to specific targets. On the basis of risk factors and calculated 10-year risk of ASCVD using the Framingham, MESA, Reynolds, or United Kingdom Prospective Diabetes Study risk scores, the AACE/ACE guideline classifies patients as low, moderate, high, very high, or extreme risk. Treatment goals are individualized according to the patient's level of risk, with LDL cholesterol targets of less than 130 mg/dL (3.37 mmol/L) for low-risk patients, less than 100 mg/dL (2.59 mmol/L) for moderate- and high-risk patients, less than 70 mg/dL (1.81 mmol/L) for very-high-risk patients, and less than 55 mg/dL (1.42 mmol/L) for extreme-risk patients. The category of extreme risk represents a new classification for dyslipidemia guidelines and includes patients with progressive ASCVD that persists after achieving an LDL cholesterol level below 70 mg/dL (1.81 mmol/L); patients with established ASCVD with concomitant diabetes mellitus, stage 3 or 4 chronic kidney disease, or hereditary heterozygous familial hypercholesterolemia; and patients with a history of premature ASCVD. The complete guideline, which provides 87 recommendations, is available at https://www.aace.com/files/lipid-guidelines.pdf.

Statins may infrequently cause liver dysfunction or myopathy. Liver chemistry tests should be obtained at baseline, but neither liver chemistry tests nor muscle enzyme studies should be routinely performed in the absence of suggestive symptoms. Statins may also cause memory problems in some patients, but this effect is reversible; evidence suggests that statins do not cause dementia. In patients with statin intolerance, switching to another statin is reasonable, as a patient's response to different statins can vary. Other options include decreasing the statin intensity (decreasing the dosage and/or dosing frequency) and, less preferably, discontinuing statin therapy and initiating nonstatin drugs.

## Combination and Nonstatin Drug Therapy

Nonstatin drugs should be considered alone or in combination with statins in patients who do not achieve adequate LDL cholesterol reduction with statin therapy, especially in high-risk patients (those with clinical ASCVD, baseline LDL cholesterol level >190 mg/dL [4.92 mmol/L], or diabetes). Before nonstatin drugs are initiated, patient preferences as well as anticipated ASCVD risk reduction and adverse effects should be discussed. The most commonly used nonstatin drugs and their characteristics are described in **Table 50**.

Ezetimibe and the proprotein convertase subtilisin/kexin type 9 (PCSK9) inhibitors are the preferred nonstatin drugs for high-risk patients who do not achieve goal LDL cholesterol reduction. The PCSK9 inhibitors are a relatively new class of lipid-lowering drugs. These monoclonal antibodies bind to serine protease PCSK9, a liver enzyme that degrades hepatocyte LDL receptors. Treatment with PCSK9 inhibitors produces a 50% to 60% reduction in LDL cholesterol. Barriers to the use of PCSK9 inhibitors include high cost and subcutaneous administration. Additional nonstatin options include bile acid sequestrants, fibrates, and phytosterols. Because of a lack of efficacy and potential harms, niacin is no longer routinely recommended.

In 2017, the ACC published a focused update on nonstatin therapies for LDL cholesterol lowering. Ezetimibe is the preferred nonstatin agent in patients with or without diabetes who have an LDL cholesterol level between 70 mg/dL (1.81 mmol/L) and 189 mg/dL (4.90 mmol/L) and are taking maximally tolerated statin therapy for primary prevention. Likewise, ezetimibe is preferred in patients with stable clinical ASCVD without comorbid conditions who require additional LDL cholesterol lowering. Ezetimibe or a PCSK9 inhibitor may be used in high-risk patients taking maximally tolerated statin therapy, including patients with LDL cholesterol levels greater than 190 mg/dL (4.92 mmol/L) and patients with clinical ASCVD with comorbidities. Factors that favor ezetimibe for these high-risk patients include the need for less than 25% LDL cholesterol reduction, recent myocardial infarction (within the last 3 months), present and future cost savings, and preference for oral administration.

## Management of Hypertriglyceridemia

Therapeutic lifestyle changes are the cornerstone of management of elevated triglyceride levels. Patients should be counseled to lose weight (if appropriate); exercise regularly;

**TABLE 50.** Characteristics of Nonstatin Drugs

| Medication | LDL-Cholesterol Lowering | ASCVD Risk Reduction | Adverse Effects | Approximate Cost |
|---|---|---|---|---|
| PCSK9 inhibitors | ↓↓↓↓ | ↓↓↓ | Nasopharyngitis, injection-site reactions, possible cognitive effects | $$$$ |
| Ezetimibe | ↓↓ | ↓↓↓ | Diarrhea, arthralgia, abdominal pain, myositis, elevated liver aminotransferase levels when combined with statins | $$-$$$ |
| Bile acid sequestrants | ↓↓ | ↓ (cholestyramine) | Constipation, bloating, nausea, elevated liver aminotransferase levels, interference with drug absorption<br><br>Increase triglyceride levels only if baseline levels are elevated | $$ |
| Fibrates | ↓ | Not well determined | Myositis (especially if combined with statins), nausea, abdominal pain | $$ |
| Phytosterols | ↓ | Not well determined | Mild bloating, diarrhea or constipation | $-$$ |

ASCVD = atherosclerotic cardiovascular disease; PCSK9 = proprotein convertase subtilisin/kexin type 9.

and avoid consumption of saturated fats, *trans* fats, and concentrated sugars. Although *trans* fats have been eliminated from many commercially prepared foods, some foods (such as creamers, margarine, and baked goods) may still contain *trans* fats, also called partially hydrogenated oil. The use of medications that increase triglyceride levels, such as estrogens, β-blockers, and glucocorticoids, should be avoided if possible.

Omega-3 fatty acids, which are found in many types of fish, reduce triglyceride levels and should be incorporated into the diet. Fibrates are the most effective pharmacotherapy for hypertriglyceridemia, resulting in a 30% to 50% reduction in triglyceride levels; these agents are indicated in patients with triglyceride levels of 500 mg/dL (5.65 mmol/L) or higher. Niacin and prescription omega-3 fatty acid supplements also lower triglyceride levels; however, omega-3 fatty acid supplements do not reduce heart disease, stroke, or death. According to the 2013 ACC/AHA guideline, baseline liver aminotransferase, hemoglobin $A_{1c}$ or fasting plasma glucose, and uric acid levels should be obtained before and during niacin treatment. Niacin therapy should not be used in patients receiving statin therapy who have achieved adequate LDL cholesterol reduction.

## Management of Dyslipidemia in Special Populations

In patients aged 75 years and older, there is insufficient evidence to guide the use of statin therapy for primary prevention; however, the ACC/AHA guideline suggests that it is reasonable to engage these patients in a discussion of the potential for ASCVD risk-reduction benefits, adverse effects, and drug-drug interactions, and to consider patient preferences for treatment. For secondary prevention of ASCVD in patients aged 75 years and older, it is reasonable to continue statins in patients who are already tolerating therapy; moderate-intensity therapy is beneficial and preferable to high-intensity therapy in these patients.

Owing to insufficient evidence, the ACC/AHA make no recommendations on the initiation or discontinuation of statin therapy in patients with heart failure (New York Heart Association functional class II-IV symptoms) or patients undergoing hemodialysis.

**KEY POINTS**

- All patients with elevated LDL cholesterol levels should be counseled regarding therapeutic lifestyle changes, including dietary modification, regular physical activity, weight loss, and smoking cessation. **HVC**

- The American College of Cardiology and American Heart Association recommend initiating statin therapy for primary or secondary prevention of atherosclerotic cardiovascular disease (ASCVD) in (1) patients with clinical ASCVD; (2) patients with an LDL cholesterol level of 190 mg/dL (4.92 mmol/L) or higher; (3) patients aged 40 to 75 years with diabetes mellitus, an LDL cholesterol level of 70 to 189 mg/dL (1.81-4.90 mmol/L), and no clinical ASCVD; and (4) patients aged 40 to 75 years with no ASCVD or diabetes and a 10-year ASCVD risk of 7.5% or higher.

- A lipid panel should be obtained 4 to 12 weeks after statin therapy initiation to determine treatment adherence and response to therapy.

- In patients treated with statin therapy, liver chemistry tests and muscle enzyme studies should not be routinely obtained in the absence of symptoms of liver dysfunction or myopathy. **HVC**

- Nonstatin drugs, such as ezetimibe and proprotein convertase subtilisin/kexin type 9 (PCSK9) inhibitors, should be considered alone or in combination with statins in high-risk patients who do not achieve adequate LDL cholesterol reduction with statin therapy.

## Metabolic Syndrome

### Epidemiology and Pathophysiology

Metabolic syndrome, also referred to as insulin resistance syndrome, comprises a constellation of risk factors for cardiovascular disease and type 2 diabetes. It is a common condition, occurring in 20% to 35% of U.S. adults.

Although there are several definitions for metabolic syndrome, the diagnostic criteria proposed by the National Cholesterol Education Program Adult Treatment Panel III (with minor modifications by the AHA/National Heart, Lung, and Blood Institute) are the most widely used (**Table 51**). The presence of a pathophysiologic link between the components of the metabolic syndrome is controversial; however, insulin resistance and adipocyte cytokines associated with metabolic syndrome appear to play a central role in inducing inflammatory changes that contribute to ASCVD.

### Management

Treatment of metabolic syndrome focuses on addressing each of the component risk factors. Lifestyle modifications, particularly weight loss and exercise, are the most important treatment interventions. Routine pharmacotherapy is not recommended in patients who do not meet treatment criteria for the individual risk factors. Aspirin is indicated for patients with metabolic syndrome and a 10-year ASCVD risk of 10% or greater, assuming there is not increased bleeding risk. In some studies, metformin has been shown to prevent progression to diabetes; however, it is inferior to lifestyle modifications, and its role in treating metabolic syndrome has not been established.

# Obesity

## Definition and Epidemiology

Obesity, defined as a BMI of 30 or greater, is associated with increased risk for type 2 diabetes mellitus, hypertension, dyslipidemia, cardiovascular disease, stroke, obstructive sleep apnea, osteoarthritis, and some cancers; risks for these conditions increase with increasing BMI. Waist circumference of 102 cm (40 in) or greater in men and 88 cm (35 in) or greater in women is additionally associated with increased risk for diabetes mellitus, cardiovascular disease, and all-cause mortality (**Table 52**).

Prevalence of obesity and extreme obesity (BMI ≥40) among adults in the United States increased from 35.1% to 37.7% and 6.5% to 7.7%, respectively, between 2011-2012 and 2013-2014. Prevalence of obesity varies by gender, ethnicity, education, and age, with the highest prevalence among women, non-Hispanic black persons, those with less education, and those aged 40 to 59 years.

The costs associated with providing care to patients with severe obesity are high (more than $69 billion in 2013).

### KEY POINTS

- The prevalence of obesity (BMI >30) and extreme obesity (BMI ≥40) is increasing.
- Waist circumference of 102 cm (40 in) inches or greater in men and 88 cm (35 in) or greater in women is associated with increased risk for diabetes mellitus, cardiovascular disease, and all-cause mortality.

## Screening and Evaluation

The U.S. Preventive Services Task Force recommends screening adults for obesity by measuring height and weight and

| TABLE 51. | Diagnostic Criteria for the Metabolic Syndrome |
|---|---|
| **Measure (Any Three of Five Constitute Diagnosis of Metabolic Syndrome)** | **Categorical Cutpoints** |
| Elevated waist circumference[a,b] | ≥102 cm [40 in] in men; ≥88 cm [35 in] in women |
| Elevated triglycerides | ≥150 mg/dL (1.7 mmol/L) <br><br> or <br><br> On drug treatment for elevated triglycerides |
| Reduced HDL cholesterol | <40 mg/dL (1.03 mmol/L) in men; <50 mg/dL (1.30 mmol/L) in women <br><br> or <br><br> On drug treatment for reduced HDL cholesterol[c] |
| Elevated blood pressure | ≥130 mm Hg systolic blood pressure <br><br> or <br><br> ≥85 mm Hg diastolic blood pressure <br><br> or <br><br> On antihypertensive drug treatment in a patient with a history of hypertension |
| Elevated fasting glucose | ≥100 mg/dL (5.6 mmol/L) <br><br> or <br><br> On drug treatment for elevated glucose |

[a]To measure waist circumference, locate top of right iliac crest. Place a measuring tape in a horizontal plane around abdomen at level of iliac crest. Before reading tape measure, ensure that tape is snug but does not compress the skin and is parallel to floor. Measurement is made at the end of a normal expiration.

[b]Some U.S. adults of non-Asian origin (e.g., white, black, Hispanic) with marginally increased waist circumference (e.g., 94-101 cm [37-39 inches] in men and 80-87 cm [31-34 inches] in women) may have strong genetic contribution to insulin resistance and should benefit from changes in lifestyle habits, similar to men with categorical increases in waist circumference. Lower waist circumference cutpoint (e.g., ≥90 cm [35 inches] in men and ≥80 cm [31 inches] in women) appears to be appropriate for Asian Americans.

[c]Fibrates and nicotinic acid are the most commonly used drugs for elevated triglycerides and reduced HDL cholesterol. Patients taking one of these drugs are presumed to have high triglycerides and low HDL cholesterol.

Reproduced with permission from Grundy SM, Cleeman JI, Daniels SR, Donato KA, Eckel RH, Franklin BA at al. Diagnosis and management of the metabolic syndrome: an American Heart Association/National Heart, Lung, and Blood Institute scientific statement. Circulation. 2005;112(17):2735. [PMID: 16157765]

**TABLE 52.** Classification of Overweight and Obesity by BMI

| Category | BMI | Obesity Class | Disease Risk[a] Relative to Normal Weight and Waist Circumference | |
| --- | --- | --- | --- | --- |
| | | | Men: ≤102 cm (40 in) Women: ≤88 cm (35 in) | Men: >102 cm (40 in) Women: >88 cm (35 in) |
| Underweight | <18.5 | | — | — |
| Normal | 18.5-24.9 | | — | — |
| Overweight | 25.0-29.9 | | Increased | High |
| Obesity | 30.0-34.9 | I | High | Very high |
| | 35.0-39.9 | II | Very high | Very high |
| Extreme obesity | ≥40 | III | Extremely high | Extremely high |

[a]Disease risk for type 2 diabetes mellitus, hypertension, and cardiovascular disease. Increased waist circumference also can be a marker for increased risk, even in persons of normal weight.

Reproduced from National Heart, Lung, and Blood Institute. Aim for a healthy weight. https://www.nhlbi.nih.gov/health/educational/lose_wt/BMI/bmi_dis.htm. Accessed June 25, 2018.

calculating BMI. Online BMI calculators are available (https://www.nhlbi.nih.gov/guidelines/obesity/BMI/bmicalc.htm). Clinicians should ask patients with obesity about their weight history, previous weight loss attempts, diet and physical activity patterns, social and emotional factors, and family history of obesity. A thorough medication history is recommended to identify medications that may contribute to weight gain (**Table 53**). Physicians should inquire about symptoms of obesity-related conditions, such as heart disease, obstructive sleep apnea, osteoarthritis, and erectile dysfunction.

Physical examination should include measurements of height, weight, waist circumference, and blood pressure. Examining patients with obesity is sometimes challenging and adaptations may be necessary, such as using a scale with an adequate weight limit, using an appropriately sized blood pressure cuff (bladder encircles 80% of the arm), and repositioning patients to optimize hearing of heart sounds. Many patients with obesity are deconditioned, and allowing the patient to sit quietly for 5 minutes after walking from the waiting area to the examination room before measuring heart rate and blood pressure may improve the reliability of these measurements.

**TABLE 53.** Medications That Promote Weight Gain

α-Blockers

β-Blockers

Glucocorticoids

Progestins (especially depot injections)

Antidiabetic drugs (insulin, sulfonylureas [especially glyburide and glipizide], thiazolidinediones)

Anticonvulsant drugs (carbamazepine, gabapentin, valproic acid)

Antidepressant drugs (amitriptyline, imipramine, doxepin, paroxetine, mirtazapine)

Antipsychotic drugs (clozapine, olanzapine, quetiapine, risperidone)

Laboratory evaluation should include fasting blood glucose and lipid levels. Requests for other laboratory tests should be based on patient-specific signs, symptoms, and risk factors. Although obesity is associated with higher risk for certain cancers, recommendations for cancer screening are the same as for patients without obesity. Screening for cardiovascular disease in asymptomatic patients with obesity is not indicated; testing is reserved for symptomatic patients.

**KEY POINT**

- The U.S. Preventive Services Task Force recommends screening all adults for obesity by calculating BMI. **HVC**

# Treatment

Treatment options for obesity include lifestyle modification, pharmacotherapy, and bariatric surgery. Guidelines published by the American College of Cardiology/American Heart Association/The Obesity Society on the management of obesity recommend lifestyle modification that includes reduced calorie intake, increased physical activity, and behavioral therapy in all patients. Similarly, the U.S. Preventive Services Task Force recommends offering or referring obese patients to intensive, multicomponent behavioral interventions. For patients at highest risk who have tried lifestyle modification measures without success, pharmacotherapy or surgical intervention may be considered. Patients should be advised that weight loss is beneficial even without attaining a normal weight; loss of 3% to 5% of initial body weight is associated with improvement in glycemic control, blood pressure, and lipid levels.

## Lifestyle Modification

Readiness to make lifestyle changes should be assessed. Engaging family members and other social supports may increase adherence to lifestyle change. Given the expected slow pace of weight loss, patients may benefit from encouragement to focus on other changes resulting from lifestyle modification, such as improved exercise tolerance.

## Reduced Dietary Energy Intake

Typical dietary calorie intake ranges required to produce weight loss are 1200 to 1500 kcal/d for women and 1500 to 1800 kcal/d for men; the calorie intake required to achieve a calorie deficit for a given person varies. Clinicians can estimate basal energy expenditure in calories using the Harris-Benedict Equation (http://www.bmi-calculator.net/bmr-calculator/harris-benedict-equation/).

Any diet that achieves a calorie deficit will produce weight loss; this is true for low-calorie, low-fat, low-carbohydrate, moderate/high-protein, low–glycemic-index, vegan (with or without a low-fat component), and Mediterranean-style diets, as well as commercial diet plans. Patients should be advised to use the diet to which they will most likely adhere.

Very-low-calorie diets (<800 kcal/d) produce accelerated weight loss but require medical supervision. They should be reserved for situations requiring rapid weight loss.

## Exercise

Lifestyle interventions should include moderate- to vigorous-intensity physical activity (such as brisk walking) for at least 150 minutes per week. The main contribution of increased physical activity is to minimize the reduction in calories required to achieve a caloric deficit. Because patients are often initially deconditioned, gradual progression may be required. Long-term continuance of a similar program of physical activity is important for maintaining weight loss and improving cardiovascular fitness.

## Behavioral Therapy

The Centers for Medicare & Medicaid Services have approved payment for "intensive behavioral weight loss counseling" by primary care providers. Content of this counseling in practice varies widely, as does its effectiveness. Specific components associated with increased effectiveness include a calorie deficit of at least 500 kcal/d, at least 150 minutes of moderate to vigorous physical activity per week, and the use of trained interventionists (nutritionists, behavioral therapists, or exercise therapists). Interventions should incorporate regular self-monitoring of weight and calorie intake as well as education on controlling or altering the environment to avoid excess calorie intake. Examples include removing calorie-dense snacks and beverages from the home or workplace, replacing them with lower-calorie options, and engaging in other behaviors (walking, chewing gum) for situations during which the patient might be tempted to eat for pleasure, for emotional solace, or because of boredom. Programs of high intensity (≥14 sessions over at least 6 months) delivered by trained interventionists are associated with successful weight loss. Comprehensive programs lasting longer than 1 year with at least monthly contact are associated with greater likelihood of maintaining lifestyle change.

Face-to-face interventions most reliably result in weight loss, but interventions delivered electronically or by telephone have also shown success.

## Pharmacologic Therapy

Patients who do not achieve weight loss with lifestyle change alone should be considered for pharmacotherapy, especially patients at higher risk for complications (those with BMI ≥30, or with BMI ≥27 and at least one obesity-associated comorbid condition). Weight loss pharmacotherapy is effective but incurs risk for adverse events as well as increased cost, and these factors should be balanced against potential weight-loss benefit.

**Table 54** describes the mechanism of action, expected weight loss, and side effects of commonly used agents; all have

| TABLE 54. | Medications for Weight Loss | | |
|---|---|---|---|
| **Medication** | **Mechanism of Action** | **Weight Loss Versus Placebo at 52 Weeks in Meta-analysis of Randomized Controlled Trials** | **Common Side Effects (Odds Ratio for Discontinuation Versus Placebo)** |
| Liraglutide | GLP-1 receptor activator, delays gastric emptying | 5.2 kg (11.6 lb) | Gastrointestinal upset, headache, nasopharyngitis (2.82) |
| Lorcaserin | Selective serotonergic 5HT2C receptor agonist, suppresses appetite | 3.3 kg (7.2 lb) | Headache, dizziness, fatigue, nausea, dry mouth, cough, constipation<br><br>May cause hypoglycemia in patients with diabetes mellitus (1.40) |
| Naltrexone-bupropion | Opioid antagonist plus norepinephrine/dopamine uptake inhibitor, suppresses appetite | 5 kg (10.9 lb) | Gastrointestinal upset, headache, dizziness, insomnia, dry mouth, tachycardia, hypertension, anxiety, tremor (2.60) |
| Orlistat | Lipase inhibitor, decreases triglyceride absorption | 2.6 kg (5.8 lb) | Oily stools, increased defecation, fecal urgency/incontinence (1.84) |
| Phentermine-topiramate | Noradrenergic/GABA receptor activator plus AMPA glutamate receptor inhibitor, suppresses appetite | 8.8 kg (19.4 lb) | Paresthesias, dizziness, taste alterations, insomnia, constipation, dry mouth, tachycardia, cognitive changes (2.32) |

5HT2C = 5-hydroxytryptamine2C; AMPA = α-amino-3-hydroxy-5-methyl-4-isoxazole propionic acid; GABA = γ-aminobutyric acid; GLP-1 = glucagon-like peptide-1.

Data from Khera R, Murad MH, Chandar AK, Dulai PS, Wang Z, Prokop LJ, et al. Association of pharmacological treatments for obesity with weight loss and adverse events: a systematic review and meta-analysis. JAMA. 2016;315:2424-34. [PMID: 27299618] doi:10.1001/jama.2016.7602

demonstrated higher rates of achieving 5% to 10% weight loss and larger amounts of weight lost compared with placebo. Orlistat and lorcaserin had the lowest rates of discontinuation due to side effects. Orlistat also has long-term safety data. Liraglutide and phentermine-topiramate produced the greatest weight loss but had higher rates of discontinuation due to side effects.

Patients are inundated with advertisements for over-the-counter weight loss supplements, which often claim the supplements are safer and more effective than prescription medications. These claims and easy access have led to widespread use of weight loss supplements, but systematic reviews show little evidence that any over-the-counter weight loss supplements are effective. Moreover, some supplements, such as ma huang/ephedra and bitter orange, may also be associated with significant adverse effects. Physicians should be prepared to discuss the lack of effectiveness and potential for side effects of these supplements during weight loss counseling. Comprehensive information on supplements is available at https://medlineplus.gov/druginfo/herb_All.html.

As with all other comprehensive weight loss interventions, patients should be monitored regularly. Patients who do not show improved success with weight reduction after 12 weeks of therapy should not continue pharmacotherapy.

## Bariatric Surgery

For patients at highest risk for obesity-related complications and for whom other measures have not resulted in the desired clinical end points, bariatric surgery should be considered. Guidelines recommend reserving surgery for patients with a BMI of 40 or greater or for those with a BMI of 35 or greater who have obesity-associated comorbid conditions.

The risks associated with bariatric surgery exceed those associated with nonsurgical treatments. Therefore, candidates for bariatric surgery should be selected carefully on the basis of harm-benefit analysis. Patients should have acceptable operative risk, understand the necessity of lifelong dietary and lifestyle measures for sustained weight loss, and be willing to adhere to lifelong follow-up. Candidates should not have psychological or psychiatric conditions that impede adherence to these requirements. Careful selection of patients in preparation for surgery and adherence to follow-up visits predict successful weight loss and maintenance, as well as avoidance of complications.

## Techniques

The three most commonly performed bariatric surgical procedures include Roux-en-Y gastric bypass, sleeve gastrectomy, and gastric banding. Roux-en-Y gastric bypass involves detaching the proximal stomach and creating a small pouch, which is reattached to the Roux limb of the small intestine. Weight loss results from decrease in caloric intake because of the small stomach pouch, malabsorption due to bypassing much of the stomach and proximal small intestines, and

appetite suppression due to changes in glucagon-like peptide-1 (GLP-1) and related hormones.

Sleeve gastrectomy is accomplished by excising the part of the stomach along the greater curvature, creating an approximately 85% reduction in size; similar to gastric bypass, it results in restriction of calorie intake via a smaller stomach and hormonal (GLP-1 and related hormones) appetite suppression. The smaller gastric surface area also results in less production of ghrelin, an appetite stimulant.

Gastric banding involves placement of a silicon fluid-filled band around the proximal stomach, creating a small stomach pouch with subsequent reduction in calorie intake by increasing satiety.

All procedures result in loss of excess weight in the short term, up to 70% with Roux-en-Y, 50% with sleeve gastrectomy, and 30% with gastric banding. Long-term (5-year) data are less robust but suggest sustained weight loss.

More recently, other alternative surgical and nonsurgical procedures have been developed. These include

**TABLE 55. Nutrient Deficiencies and Replacement After Bariatric Surgery**

| Nutrient Deficiency | Replacement Therapy |
|---|---|
| Iron | MVI with iron, or elemental iron 40-80 mg/d orally |
| | If deficient, ferrous sulfate 325 mg/d orally |
| Vitamin B$_{12}$ | Vitamin B$_{12}$ 500-1000 µg/d orally, or 1000 µg IM monthly |
| Folic acid | MVI with folate |
| | If deficient, 400 µg/d orally |
| | For women of childbearing age, folate 1 mg/d orally |
| Calcium | Calcium citrate 1200 mg/d orally |
| Vitamin D | Vitamin D 400-1000 U/d orally |
| | If deficient, 50,000 U weekly orally for 3 mo, then reassess |
| Thiamine | 25-50 mg/d orally |
| Vitamin A | MVI daily |
| | If deficient, 5000-10,000 U/d orally with ongoing monitoring |
| Vitamin E | MVI daily |
| | If deficient, 400 U/d orally |
| Vitamin K | MVI daily |
| | If deficient, 5-10 mg/d orally |
| Copper | MVI with minerals daily |
| | If deficient, 2-4 mg/d orally |
| Zinc | MVI with minerals daily |
| | If deficient, 220 mg/d orally |

IM = intramuscularly; MVI = multivitamin.

Data from Marcotte E, Chand B. Management and prevention of surgical and nutritional complications after bariatric surgery. Surg Clin North Am. 2016;96:843-56. [PMID: 27473805] doi:10.1016/j.suc.2016.03.006

restrictive procedures (endoscopic suturing or stapling in a manner that replicates sleeve gastrectomy) or placement of space-occupying devices (intragastric balloons) or devices intended to decrease caloric absorption (duodenal-jejunal liners). These and other related techniques are less invasive and may carry less risk than surgical procedures, but more experience and data on long-term outcomes are needed.

## Postoperative Care

Rates of 30-day postoperative complications are low, ranging from 1.3% to 8.7%. Early complications include bleeding or leakage at the anastomosis (bypass procedures) or staple line (sleeve gastrectomy) and bowel obstruction. Later complications include anastomotic or marginal ulceration, leaks, bowel obstruction and slippage, or excessive tightness of gastric bands. Initial evaluation and management for bleeding or ulceration can be performed endoscopically. Leakage is evaluated with an upper gastrointestinal series or contrast CT scan and managed by laparoscopy. Symptoms of obstruction in patients with gastric band procedures are evaluated with an upper gastrointestinal series and managed by removing fluid from the band device. ◫

Weight should be monitored closely in the early postoperative period. As patients lose weight, frequent reassessment of prescription medications is required (for example, insulin dosage reduction).

Long-term postsurgical care focuses on preventing nutritional deficiencies, managing adherence to lifestyle modifications, and monitoring for behaviors that lead to weight regain. **Table 55** lists the anticipated nutritional deficiencies and recommended replacement strategies. **Table 56** describes post–bariatric surgery syndromes and their management.

| TABLE 56. Post–Bariatric Surgery Syndromes | | |
|---|---|---|
| **Syndrome** | **Cause** | **Monitoring/Therapy** |
| Dumping syndrome/postprandial hypoglycemia (tachycardia, sweating, abdominal pain, nausea, vomiting, diarrhea) | Rapid transit of undigested food into small intestines | Avoid foods high in simple sugar; replace with higher-fiber/high-protein foods |
| | Early symptoms (1 hour postprandial) caused by fluid shift into the GI tract (no hypoglycemia) | Avoid sweetened beverages (including alcohol) |
| | Late symptoms (2-3 hours postprandial) hypoglycemia caused by insulin surge in response to hyperglycemia | |
| Chronic loose stool | May relate to rapid transit of food to small intestines, similar to dumping syndrome | Adherence to dietary modifications to avoid dumping syndrome |
| | Consider small intestine bacterial overgrowth | Rifaximin if bacterial overgrowth is suspected |
| Kidney stones | Increased urinary oxalic acid related to fat malabsorption | Diet low in fat and oxalate, calcium supplementation, increased hydration |
| Gallstones | Bile stasis, increased biliary cholesterol saturation with rapid weight loss | Ultrasonography if symptomatic |
| | | Cholecystectomy is definitive treatment |
| | | Ursodeoxycholic acid shown to be effective prophylactically in meta-analysis of RCTs |
| Gastric or marginal ulceration | Often associated with NSAID use | Endoscopy to confirm |
| | | Avoidance of NSAIDs |
| Hypotension, hypoglycemia | Improved blood pressure and insulin sensitivity with weight loss | Adjust medications as indicated; consider proactive reduction in dose (especially antidiabetic medications) |
| Chronic abdominal pain/nausea | Various, including nonadherence to diet recommendations, device slippage (gastric band procedures), bowel obstruction | Evaluate with endoscopy or CT |
| | | Re-educate patient on diet modifications if no other cause is identified |
| | | Consider low-dose antidepressant therapy |
| Gastroesophageal reflux | Incidence usually decreases after diversion procedures but may increase after sleeve gastrectomy | Evaluate with endoscopy |
| | | PPI therapy, lifestyle modification |
| Regain of weight lost | Disordered eating, excess intake of high-calorie liquid/semisolid foods or supplements | Re-educate patient on diet modifications |
| | | Refer to psychiatric care or counseling if indicated |

GI = gastrointestinal; PPI = proton pump inhibitor; RCT = randomized controlled trial.

HVC • Lifestyle modifications that are effective for the treatment of obesity include a calorie deficit of at least 500 kcal/d, at least 150 minutes of moderate to vigorous physical activity per week, and the use of trained interventionists (nutritionists, behavioral therapists, or exercise therapists).

• Pharmacologic therapy may be used as an adjunct to lifestyle modifications in patients with a BMI of 30 or greater or in patients with a BMI of 27 or greater who have overweight- or obesity-associated comorbid conditions.

HVC • Systematic reviews show little evidence that over-the-counter weight loss supplements are effective.

• Bariatric surgery should be reserved for patients with a BMI of 40 or greater or for those with a BMI of 35 or greater who have obesity-associated comorbid conditions.

• Long-term postsurgical care focuses on preventing nutritional deficiencies, managing adherence to lifestyle modifications, and monitoring for behaviors that lead to weight regain.

# Men's Health

## Male Sexual Dysfunction

### Erectile Dysfunction

The American Urological Association (AUA) defines erectile dysfunction as the "inability to achieve or maintain an erection sufficient for satisfactory sexual performance." Erectile dysfunction is a common medical condition, and prevalence increases with age between 18 and 69 years; up to 33% of men older than age 50 years are affected.

Numerous risk factors and conditions are associated with erectile dysfunction, including coronary artery disease, peripheral vascular disease, diabetes mellitus, hypertension, hyperlipidemia, metabolic syndrome, obesity, tobacco use, obstructive sleep apnea, hypothyroidism, hypogonadism (androgen deficiency), benign prostatic hyperplasia, neuropathy, central neurologic conditions (Parkinson disease, Alzheimer disease, and stroke), trauma, surgery, drug and alcohol abuse, depression, and anxiety. Furthermore, numerous medications have been linked to erectile dysfunction, particularly thiazide diuretics and selective serotonin reuptake inhibitors (**Table 57**).

Erectile dysfunction can be an isolated and independent presentation, or it can be an indication of another underlying condition. Erectile dysfunction, as compared with traditional cardiovascular risk factors, portends a similar, if not greater, predictive risk for a future cardiovascular event. As such, the evaluation of erectile dysfunction must include a thorough history and physical examination directed toward identifying any potentially treatable causative factors, including those associated

**TABLE 57.** Drugs Commonly Associated With Erectile Dysfunction

| |
|---|
| Antidepressants (monoamine oxidase inhibitors, selective serotonin reuptake inhibitors, tricyclic antidepressants) |
| Benzodiazepines |
| Opioids, nicotine, alcohol, amphetamines, barbiturates, cocaine, marijuana, methadone |
| Anticonvulsants (phenytoin, phenobarbital) |
| Antihypertensives and diuretics (thiazide diuretics, loop diuretics, clonidine, spironolactone; possibly $\alpha$-blockers, $\beta$-blockers, calcium channel blockers, ACE inhibitors) |
| 5$\alpha$-Reductase inhibitors (dutasteride, finasteride) |
| Antihistamines and H$_2$ blockers (dimenhydrinate, diphenhydramine, hydroxyzine, meclizine, promethazine, cimetidine, nizatidine, ranitidine) |
| NSAIDs (naproxen, indomethacin) |
| Parkinson disease medications (levodopa, bromocriptine, biperiden, trihexyphenidyl, benztropine, procyclidine) |

with cardiovascular disease. The history should include medical, psychosocial, and sexual components and should focus on the timing of symptoms (whether gradual or sudden in onset) as well as the presence of early-morning and nocturnal spontaneous erections. It is also helpful to interview the patient's partner regarding sexual function and the relationship. Patients should be assessed for other concomitant disorders of sexual function, such as premature ejaculation and decreased libido.

Physical examination should include cardiovascular, genital, digital rectal, peripheral vascular, and neurologic evaluations. Clinicians should pay close attention for any alterations in secondary sexual characteristics suggestive of hypogonadism (reduced testicular volume, loss of normal body hair distribution, gynecomastia).

Laboratory assessment involves obtaining a fasting blood glucose level, lipid panel, 8:00 AM total testosterone level, and thyroid-stimulating hormone level. Additional testing is usually not warranted unless the history or physical examination suggests a separate process.

The treatment of erectile dysfunction has been shown to improve sexual performance, quality of life, and self-esteem and to strengthen interpersonal relationships. Before implementing any treatment strategies for erectile dysfunction, however, it is imperative for clinicians to fully evaluate patients in terms of cardiac risk associated with sexual activity (to determine whether it is safe for a patient to engage in sexual activities). The Princeton III Consensus recommendations provide specific guidelines on the safety of sexual activity based on the patient's cardiac risk level (**Table 58**).

Treatment options include lifestyle modifications, oral phosphodiesterase-5 inhibitor therapies, injectable and intraurethral prostaglandin E$_1$ therapies, penile device therapies, testosterone therapy, and psychotherapy (**Table 59**). All patients should undergo lifestyle modification as appropriate, including weight loss and tobacco cessation; the use of

**TABLE 58.** Third Princeton Consensus Conference Guidelines for Treatment of Erectile Dysfunction in Patients With Cardiovascular Disease or Cardiac Risk Factors

| Risk Level | Treatment Recommendation |
|---|---|
| **Low Risk** | |
| Patients who are able to do moderate-intensity exercise without symptoms | Can initiate or resume sexual activity or treat for ED with PDE-5 inhibitor (if not using nitrates) |
| Successfully revascularized patients (e.g., coronary artery bypass grafting, coronary stenting, or angioplasty) | |
| Asymptomatic controlled hypertension | |
| Mild valvular disease | |
| Mild left ventricular dysfunction (NYHA functional class I or II) who can achieve 5 METs without ischemia as determined by recent exercise testing | |
| **Intermediate/Indeterminate Risk** | |
| Mild to moderate stable angina | Further cardiac evaluation and restratification before resumption of sexual activity or treatment for ED |
| Recent MI (2-8 weeks) without intervention awaiting exercise ECG | If the patient can complete 4 minutes of the standard Bruce treadmill protocol without symptoms, arrhythmias, or a decrease in blood pressure, treatment for ED can be safely initiated |
| Heart failure (NYHA functional class III) | |
| Noncardiac atherosclerotic disease (clinically evident PAD, history of stroke/TIA) | |
| **High Risk** | |
| Unstable or refractory angina | Defer sexual activity or ED treatment until cardiac condition is stabilized and reassessed |
| Uncontrolled hypertension | |
| Moderate to severe heart failure (NYHA functional class IV) | |
| Recent MI (<2 weeks) without intervention | |
| High-risk arrhythmia (exercise-induced ventricular tachycardia, ICD with frequent shocks, poorly controlled atrial fibrillation) | |
| Obstructive hypertrophic cardiomyopathy with severe symptoms | |
| Moderate to severe valvular disease (particularly aortic stenosis) | |

ECG = electrocardiography; ED = erectile dysfunction; ICD = implantable cardioverter-defibrillator; METs = metabolic equivalents; MI = myocardial infarction; NYHA = New York Heart Association; PAD = peripheral artery disease; PDE = phosphodiesterase; TIA = transient ischemic attack.

Recommendations from Nehra A, Jackson G, Miner M, Billups KL, Burnett AL, Buvat J, et al. The Princeton III Consensus recommendations for the management of erectile dysfunction and cardiovascular disease. Mayo Clin Proc. 2012;87:766-78. [PMID: 22862865] doi:10.1016/j.mayocp.2012.06.015

medications that may contribute to erectile dysfunction should be reconsidered.

Oral phosphodiesterase-5 inhibitors are first-line medical therapy and are safe and effective in most patients. Their use is contraindicated in patients taking nitrates because of the risk for hypotension. Similarly, they should be used with caution in the setting of concomitant α-blocker therapy. Second-line medical therapy includes alprostadil (prostaglandin E$_1$), which has a mechanism of action similar to that of oral phosphodiesterase-5 inhibitors. Although efficacious, it is administered locally by intracavernous injection, transurethral injection, or transurethral suppository, making it inconvenient and less well tolerated. Testosterone therapy is indicated only in cases of confirmed androgen deficiency and has multiple contraindications.

## Premature Ejaculation

The AUA defines premature ejaculation as ejaculation that occurs sooner than desired and is distressful to either or both partners. The diagnosis of premature ejaculation is solely based on history. Clinicians should obtain a thorough sexual history (frequency of premature ejaculation, antecedent sexual activities, aggravating and alleviating factors, the impact of premature ejaculation, and any concomitant erectile dysfunction). Assessment for an underlying mood condition is also imperative given the association between premature ejaculation and quality of life.

Treatment of premature ejaculation consists primarily of counseling and pharmacotherapy. According to the AUA, medication options include selective serotonin reuptake inhibitors (paroxetine, fluoxetine, sertraline) and tricyclic antidepressants (clomipramine) to delay ejaculation, as well as topical anesthetics (lidocaine, prilocaine) to reduce tactile stimulation.

## Decreased Libido

Decreased libido is a common symptom and is defined as a reduced desire or inclination to engage in sexual activities, sexual thoughts, or fantasies. When associated with concomitant marked personal or interpersonal distress, the condition

**TABLE 59.** Treatment Strategies for Erectile Dysfunction

| Treatment Option | Additional Information |
|---|---|
| Lifestyle modification | Recommended for all patients |
| | Weight loss, smoking cessation, exercise, stress management |
| Oral phosphodiesterase-5 inhibitor | Increases cGMP → vascular smooth muscle relaxation → increased penile blood flow |
| Sildenafil | Equally efficacious |
| Tadalafil | Side effects: headache, flushing, dizziness, hypotension, presyncope/syncope |
| Vardenafil | Visual disturbances: "blue haze," a benign finding due to inhibition of retinal phosphodiesterase-6; association with anterior ischemic optic neuropathy |
| | Use with care with drugs that inhibit cytochrome P-450 3A4 pathway (fluconazole, verapamil, erythromycin) |
| Injectable and intraurethral prostaglandin $E_1$ | Increases cAMP → vascular smooth muscle relaxation → increased penile blood flow |
| Alprostadil | Initial trial dose should be performed by or supervised by a clinician |
| Testosterone supplementation | Avoid in patients with breast or prostate cancer; prostate nodule; prostate-specific antigen >4 ng/mL (4 µg/L) or >3 ng/mL (3 µg/L) in patients with a first-degree relative with prostate cancer as well as black patients; poorly controlled heart failure; untreated severe obstructive sleep apnea; elevated hematocrit (>50%); severe lower urinary tract symptoms; and desire for future fertility |
| Psychotherapy | Management of potential underlying mood disorder and psychosocial/interpersonal aspects of erectile dysfunction via cognitive behavioral therapy, biofeedback therapy, and sensory awareness exercises |
| Penile devices and surgical interventions | Consider in patients with no response to oral/injectable agents |
| | Options include vacuum constriction devices, rings, and penile prostheses (malleable and inflatable) |
| | Penile venous reconstructive surgery (to limit venous outflow) is not recommended |
| | Penile arterial reconstructive surgery is appropriate only in otherwise healthy patients with recent focal occlusion of penile artery without concomitant peripheral vascular disease |
| Herbal and supplemental therapy | Not recommended given their lack of efficacy, potential side effects, and medication interactions |

cAMP = cyclic adenosine monophosphate; cGMP = cyclic guanosine monophosphate.

is termed hypoactive sexual desire disorder. Although decreased libido is commonly experienced as part of normal aging, numerous medical and psychiatric conditions can cause decreased libido directly or indirectly. Common causes include alcohol use, mood disorders, and significant underlying systemic illness. Medications associated with erectile dysfunction similarly can induce decreased libido. Treatment involves addressing the underlying causative factor(s). Testosterone supplementation has no role in the absence of androgen deficiency.

**KEY POINTS**

- Before implementing any treatment strategies for erectile dysfunction, clinicians must fully evaluate patients in terms of cardiac risk associated with sexual activity (to determine whether it is safe for a patient to engage in sexual activities).
- Oral phosphodiesterase-5 inhibitors are first-line medical therapy for erectile dysfunction and are both safe and effective in most patients; however, they are contraindicated in patients taking nitrates.

# Androgen Deficiency

Male hypogonadism is defined as the inability of the testes to produce physiologic levels of testosterone, ultimately leading to signs and symptoms suggestive of androgen deficiency (**Table 60**). Many of these signs and symptoms are nonspecific and can be manifestations of various other common medical conditions. Thus, it is imperative to obtain a thorough history, including medical comorbidities, recent illness, eating disorders, mood disorders, and medication use (including glucocorticoids and opioids).

The Endocrine Society recommends against screening for androgen deficiency in the general population. In patients with clinical features suggestive of androgen deficiency, a morning (ideally, 8:00 AM to 9:00 AM) serum total testosterone level should be measured as an initial diagnostic test, which should not take place during times of acute illness. If low, the total testosterone level should be confirmed with a repeat morning measurement. Hypogonadism should be diagnosed only in men with consistent findings and unequivocally and consistently low serum total testosterone levels. Free and bioavailable testosterone measurements should be reserved for patients with total testosterone

**TABLE 60.** Symptoms and Signs Suggestive of Androgen Deficiency in Men

**More Specific Symptoms and Signs**

Incomplete or delayed sexual development, eunuchoidism

Reduced sexual desire (libido) and activity

Decreased spontaneous erections

Breast discomfort, gynecomastia

Loss of body (axillary and pubic) hair, reduced shaving

Very small (especially <5 mL) or shrinking testes

Inability to father children, low or zero sperm count

Height loss, low-trauma fracture, low bone mineral density

Hot flushes, sweats

**Other Less Specific Symptoms and Signs**

Decreased energy, motivation, initiative, and self-confidence

Feeling sad or blue, depressed mood, dysthymia

Poor concentration and memory

Sleep disturbance, increased sleepiness

Mild anemia (normochromic, normocytic, in the female range)

Reduced muscle bulk and strength

Increased body fat, BMI

Diminished physical or work performance

Reproduced from Bhasin S, Cunningham GR, Hayes FJ, et al; Task Force, Endocrine Society. Testosterone therapy in men with androgen deficiency syndromes: an Endocrine Society clinical practice guideline. J Clin Endocrinol Metab. 2010;95(6):2537. [PMID: 20525905] Copyright 2010, The Endocrine Society. Licensed under the Creative Commons Attribution-NonCommercial-NoDerivatives 4.0 International License (https://creativecommons.org/licenses/by-nc-nd/4.0/).

levels in the low-normal range and for patients suspected of having alterations in sex hormone–binding globulin (SHBG) levels. Total testosterone levels may be unreliable in patients with increased SHBG levels (advanced age, liver disease) and decreased SHBG levels (obesity, diabetes/insulin resistance, glucocorticoid use), necessitating measurement of free and bioavailable testosterone in these patient populations.

The decision to treat for androgen deficiency is complex and should be individualized after a thorough discussion of the risks (cardiovascular disease, prostate cancer, benign prostatic hyperplasia) and benefits (improvements in sexual function, sense of well-being, bone health, and male sexual characteristics). A careful assessment for contraindications to testosterone must be completed. Treatment is not indicated in patients with low testosterone levels only; it should be reserved for patients with a low testosterone level associated with symptoms. Furthermore, randomized, double-blind, placebo-controlled trials aimed at determining the benefit of testosterone supplementation in men aged 65 years and older showed that testosterone supplementation improved sexual function (sexual activity, desire, and erectile function) but did not improve physical function or vitality.

See MKSAP 18 Endocrinology and Metabolism for details on the evaluation of hypogonadism and testosterone treatment.

**KEY POINTS**

- In patients with clinical features suggestive of androgen deficiency, morning serum total testosterone level should be measured as an initial diagnostic test, and if low, confirmed with a repeat measurement.
- A careful screening for the multiple contraindications to testosterone therapy must be completed before testosterone supplementation is initiated.
- Treatment is not indicated in patients with low testosterone levels only; it should be reserved for patients with a low testosterone level associated with symptoms. **HVC**

## Benign Prostatic Hyperplasia

Benign prostatic hyperplasia (BPH) is a very common condition and the most common cause of lower urinary tract symptoms (LUTS) in men. LUTS can be divided into obstructive (hesitancy, weakened stream, straining, incomplete emptying, urinary retention, overflow incontinence) and irritative (frequency, urgency, nocturia) symptoms. The AUA estimates that 90% of men aged 45 to 80 years experience some form of LUTS. The prevalence of BPH and the reported severity of LUTS both increase with age.

From an anatomic perspective, BPH generally begins at the central transition zone of the prostate, running adjacent to the course of the prostatic urethra. LUTS occur as a combined result of direct bladder outlet obstruction with increased resistance to urinary flow and increased smooth muscle tone within the prostate gland. In time, detrusor muscle dysfunction can also develop.

Clinicians should be mindful of the many potential causes of LUTS (**Table 61**). A thorough history should be taken to assess for any "red flag" symptoms (fever, hematuria, weight loss), recent urinary tract infection, and recent or distant pelvic trauma or surgery, and to assess for the presence of other causes. BPH symptoms can be classified as mild, moderate, or severe by using the AUA Symptom Index (AUA-SI), a validated clinical survey that quantifies and stratifies patients based on their symptoms (available at https://www.hiv.va.gov/provider/manual-primary-care/urology-tool1.asp). A digital rectal examination may be performed to assess for prostate size, symmetry, and nodularity. Physical examination should also assess for bladder distention, reduction in perineal sensation, and adequacy of rectal tone. Although recommended by the AUA, digital rectal examination has a low sensitivity (59%) and low positive predictive value (28%) for BPH and is subject to significant interexaminer variability.

The AUA recommends obtaining a serum prostate-specific antigen (PSA) level in all patients with LUTS and a life expectancy greater than 10 years. An elevated PSA level commonly occurs in BPH, and the finding is less specific for prostate cancer in this population. The decision to obtain a serum PSA level should be individualized to each patient, after an in-depth discussion of risks and benefits. Urinalysis is recommended for all patients to assess for the presence of infection

**TABLE 61.** Causes of Lower Urinary Tract Symptoms in Men

Benign prostatic hyperplasia

Medications (diuretics, anticholinergics, sympathomimetics, antihistamines, opioids)

Bladder irritants (caffeine, alcohol, spicy and acid-rich foods, carbonated beverages)

Overactive bladder/detrusor dysfunction

Urethral strictures

Bladder stones

Urinary tract infections

Urethritis

Prostatitis

Prostate cancer

Bladder cancer

Polydipsia

Diabetes mellitus

Hypercalcemia

Spinal cord injury

Parkinson disease

Neurogenic bladder

Obstructive sleep apnea

and hematuria. A postvoid residual study is reserved for patients with a history suggesting urinary retention, whereas a uroflow/urodynamic study can be used in ambiguous cases. Other studies, such as serum creatinine measurement, ultrasonography, and endoscopy, are not recommended in the absence of other symptoms.

Treatment of BPH should be guided by the severity of symptoms (by using the AUA-SI) and is aimed at improving quality of life. The AUA suggests that if a patient has mild symptoms (AUA-SI score of 0 to 7) or moderate (AUA-SI score of 8 to 19) to severe (AUA-SI score of 20 to 35) symptoms that are not bothersome, no specific treatment is required beyond reassurance. Conversely, if a patient has bothersome moderate to severe symptoms, treatment should be considered. Treatment options include lifestyle modifications, medications, and surgical interventions.

Lifestyle modifications should be offered to patients as first-line therapy with or without medications. Helpful measures may include weight loss, decreasing nocturnal fluid intake, and timed voiding. The diuretic effects of caffeine and alcohol may worsen symptoms, and intake should be limited.

Medical therapies for BPH should be offered in a systematic approach. The most commonly used classes of medications for BPH include α-blockers, 5α-reductase inhibitors, and anticholinergic agents.

α-Blockers (tamsulosin, terazosin, doxazosin, alfuzosin, silodosin) work by blocking α-receptors in the prostatic urethra and bladder neck, thereby decreasing smooth muscle tone within the gland and leading to reduction in LUTS. Effects are

usually reported in approximately 4 weeks, with studies demonstrating roughly equal efficacy among different α-blockers. Patients should be counseled on potential side effects, including hypotension (especially with terazosin and doxazosin), orthostasis, and sexual dysfunction. α-Blockers should also be avoided or discontinued in patients undergoing cataract surgery because of the risk for floppy iris syndrome (intractable intraoperative iris prolapse). In patients taking a phosphodiesterase-5 inhibitor for erectile dysfunction, α-blockers can lead to significant hypotension. Tadalafil, a phosphodiesterase-5 inhibitor useful in the treatment of erectile dysfunction, improves LUTS and may be a reasonable option in patients with concomitant BPH and erectile dysfunction.

5α-Reductase inhibitors (finasteride and dutasteride) block the conversion of testosterone to dihydrotestosterone; this leads to a reduction in prostatic size and thus improvement in LUTS. The AUA recommends the addition of 5α-reductase inhibitors in patients with BPH refractory to α-blocker monotherapy who have an enlarged prostate on examination. Unlike α-blockers, which work relatively quickly, 5α-reductase inhibitors take approximately 6 months to improve symptoms. Side effects include erectile and ejaculatory dysfunction and decreased libido. The reduction in prostatic size causes a reduction in serum PSA levels (up to 50%); knowledge of this effect is important for patients undergoing routine monitoring of serum PSA levels.

Anticholinergic agents (oxybutynin, tolterodine, solifenacin) can be offered to patients with significant irritative symptoms. Studies have shown that combination anticholinergic and α-blocker therapy is more effective than α-blocker monotherapy. Patients should be counseled on potential side effects, including urinary retention, constipation, dry mouth, and dry eyes.

Various herbs, supplements (including saw palmetto), and alternative therapies (such as acupuncture) have been studied to assess for efficacy in improving LUTS associated with BPH but are not recommended because of a lack of clear benefit.

Referral to a urologist for a potential surgical intervention (transurethral resection of the prostate, transurethral needle ablation, transurethral vaporization, transurethral microwave thermotherapy, and various laser techniques) is warranted in patients with medically refractory symptoms or with BPH-mediated complications. BPH-related complications include recurrent urinary tract infection, bladder stone, obstructive nephropathy, persistent hematuria, and urinary retention.

**KEY POINTS**

- Lifestyle modifications such as weight loss, decreasing **HVC** nocturnal fluid intake, timed voiding, and avoidance of common diuretics (for example, caffeine and alcohol) is first-line therapy for benign prostatic hyperplasia.

- The most commonly used classes of medications for benign prostatic hyperplasia include α-blockers, 5α-reductase inhibitors, and anticholinergic agents (for irritative symptoms).

# Acute Testicular and Scrotal Pain

Acute testicular and scrotal pain are common concerns; overall, they account for approximately 1% of all emergency department visits. Causes of acute testicular and scrotal pain include testicular torsion, epididymitis, and orchitis. Several other conditions, including inguinal hernia, nephrolithiasis, and spinal nerve root impingement, can lead to referred pain to the scrotum.

Epididymitis (and epididymo-orchitis when a testicle is also involved) is the most common cause of acute scrotal pain in adults. Noninfectious causes include trauma and connective tissue diseases, but infection is the most frequent cause. In younger patients, gonorrhea and chlamydia are the most likely causes, whereas gram-negative rods are the most likely cause in older patients and in patients engaging in insertive anal intercourse. Epididymitis presents as acute to subacute unilateral pain and swelling in the superolateral aspect of the testicle, sometimes with LUTS (dysuria, urgency, frequency) and fever. Pain relief with lifting of the affected testicle may be present (Prehn sign). Increased blood flow on Doppler ultrasound and an elevated C-reactive protein level (>0.24 mg/dL [2.4 mg/L]) are typically present. Supportive care, including scrotal support, ice, and pain control, is sufficient treatment for noninfectious causes. For infectious epididymitis in patients younger than 35 years, ceftriaxone and doxycycline (or azithromycin) are indicated; ceftriaxone and a fluoroquinolone are recommended in older patients and those engaging in insertive anal intercourse.

Testicular torsion results from a twisting of the testicle on the spermatic cord, eventually leading to ischemia and testicular infarction. It is most common in children and young adults and presents as acute, unilateral, severe scrotal pain and swelling. Examination reveals a "high-riding hemiscrotum" and an absent cremasteric reflex (failure of the testis to pull up when the ipsilateral inner thigh is stroked). Decreased blood flow on Doppler ultrasound is typical, and because this is a mechanical rather than inflammatory process, the C-reactive protein level is normal (<0.24 mg/dL [24 mg/L]). Testicular torsion is a surgical emergency; if repaired within 6 hours, testicular salvage rate is 80% to 100%.

**KEY POINTS**

- For infectious epididymitis in patients younger than 35 years, ceftriaxone and doxycycline (or azithromycin) are indicated; ceftriaxone and a fluoroquinolone are recommended in older patients and those engaging in insertive anal intercourse.
- Testicular torsion presents as acute, unilateral, severe scrotal pain and swelling with a "high-riding hemiscrotum" on examination and absent cremasteric reflex; it is a surgical emergency with high testicular salvage rates if decompressed within 6 hours.

# Hydrocele, Varicocele, and Epididymal Cyst

Hydrocele, varicocele, epididymal cyst/spermatocele, and testicular malignancy most frequently present with chronic symptoms such as scrotal discomfort or swelling. They may also be noted incidentally by the patient. The key differences in the presentation, examination, appropriate diagnostic measures, and indications for treatment are presented in **Table 62**.

**KEY POINT**

- Hydroceles, varicoceles, and epididymal cysts (spermatoceles) present with scrotal discomfort or swelling and are all treated conservatively, with surgery reserved for worsening pain or enlarging size. **HVC**

# Acute and Chronic Prostatitis and Pelvic Pain

Prostatitis encompasses several disparate disorders, including acute bacterial prostatitis, chronic bacterial prostatitis, chronic pelvic pain syndrome, and asymptomatic prostatitis. It is a common problem with a reported prevalence of approximately 8%, accounting for approximately 8% of all urology visits and 1% of all primary care visits.

Acute bacterial prostatitis is characterized by irritative voiding symptoms; perineal pain; systemic symptoms of fever, chills, myalgia, and malaise; and potentially features of sepsis. Chronic bacterial prostatitis causes irritative voiding symptoms and perineal pain, but patients are not systemically ill. Bacterial prostatitis is most commonly caused by *Escherichia coli*, *Klebsiella*, *Proteus*, *Pseudomonas*, *Enterococci*, *Neisseria*, and *Chlamydia*. Chronic pelvic pain syndrome is associated with chronic pelvic pain and intermittent voiding symptoms without evidence of infection. It may be inflammatory or noninflammatory and may be idiopathic or associated with trauma, surgery, lumbosacral neuropathy, and pelvic floor dysfunction. Asymptomatic prostatitis is usually discovered incidentally.

When encountering a patient with signs and symptoms concerning for prostatitis, it is imperative to exclude other causes, including testicular, epididymal, urethral, rectal, or urinary tract conditions. The history and physical examination should attempt to address each of these potential causative sources. Evaluation should include examination of the prostate, which often is tender, enlarged, boggy, and edematous in acute bacterial prostatitis; mild tenderness or a normal prostate examination may be present with the other causes of prostatitis. Additional diagnostic measures should include a urinalysis with Gram stain and culture, as well as expressed prostatic secretion culture (by prostatic massage). However, prostatic massage is contraindicated in acute bacterial prostatitis, given concern for possible abscess, bacteremia, and sepsis. Tests such as semen analysis, PSA level, prostatic imaging (ultrasonography or CT), and prostate biopsy are not routinely performed.

**TABLE 62.** Causes of Chronic Testicular and Scrotal Pain or Swelling

| Cause | Presentation | Diagnosis | Treatment | Additional Information |
|-------|-------------|-----------|-----------|----------------------|
| Epididymal cyst/spermatocele | Small, benign, nontender mass along the epididymis and spermatic cord<br><br>Asymptomatic; usually an incidental finding | Examination<br><br>Ultrasonography | Reassurance<br><br>Surgery (rarely; only if painful or enlarging) | Cysts >2 cm in diameter are referred to as spermatocele |
| Hydrocele | Asymptomatic to painful swelling<br><br>Small to large tense, smooth scrotal mass | Examination<br><br>Transillumination<br><br>Ultrasonography | Conservative (pain control [analgesics]; scrotal support)<br><br>Surgery (worsening pain or enlarging size) | Fluid collection between the layers of the tunica vaginalis<br><br>Common (1% of men) |
| Varicocele | Asymptomatic to dull ache with scrotal fullness<br><br>Increased fullness/pain with standing and Valsalva maneuver; improves with support and while supine | Examination ("bag of worms")<br><br>No transillumination<br><br>Ultrasonography | Conservative (pain control [analgesics]; scrotal support)<br><br>Surgery (worsening pain, refractory to conservative methods, infertility) | Dilated testicular vein/pampiniform plexus<br><br>Common (15% of men)<br><br>Left-sided (90%)<br><br>Associated infertility<br><br>Consider obstruction of inferior vena cava with right-sided varicocele |
| Testicular malignancy | Firm, unilateral mass/nodule adherent to the testicle | Examination<br><br>Ultrasonography<br><br>Tumor markers (α-fetoprotein, β-human chorionic gonadotropin, lactate dehydrogenase) | Surgery/chemotherapy | Approximately 15% of testicular cancers present with pain; most are asymptomatic<br><br>Patients often younger than those with hydrocele, spermatocele, or varicocele |

CONT.

In acute bacterial prostatitis, mild to moderately ill patients are treated with an antimicrobial agent with good prostate tissue penetration, such as ciprofloxacin or trimethoprim-sulfamethoxazole, for approximately 6 weeks. In severely ill patients, hospitalization and parenteral antibiotics may be necessary. 🄷

Chronic bacterial prostatitis is treated similarly with an antimicrobial agent for approximately 6 weeks. First-line therapy is a fluoroquinolone or trimethoprim-sulfamethoxazole; second-line therapy is doxycycline or azithromycin. Some patients might require a prolonged antibiotic course of up to 12 weeks to minimize the risk for recurrent episodes.

Chronic pelvic pain syndrome is best managed with a multimodal approach that includes an antimicrobial agent (6 weeks' duration) and an α-blocker such as tamsulosin. Other treatment options include 5α-reductase inhibitors, anti-inflammatory analgesics, neuromodulating agents (pregabalin, gabapentin, nortriptyline), and nonpharmacologic strategies such as cognitive behavioral therapy, biofeedback therapy, and physical therapy. Asymptomatic prostatitis requires no specific treatment.

**KEY POINTS**

- In acute bacterial prostatitis, mild to moderately ill patients are treated with an antimicrobial agent with good prostate tissue penetration, such as ciprofloxacin or trimethoprim-sulfamethoxazole, for approximately 6 weeks; severely ill patients may require hospitalization and parenteral antibiotics.

*(Continued)*

**KEY POINTS** *(continued)*

- Prostatic massage is contraindicated in acute bacterial prostatitis, given concern for possible abscess, bacteremia, and sepsis.

- Chronic pelvic pain syndrome is best managed with a multimodal approach including an antimicrobial agent (6 weeks' duration) and an α-blocker such as tamsulosin.

# Hernia

Hernia is defined as a condition in which a portion of an organ protrudes through the wall of the cavity that contains it. This usually occurs at a weakened muscular or connective tissue site and can be congenital or acquired. Hernias most commonly occur in the abdominopelvic region, including ventral (protrusion through the anterior abdominal wall), umbilical (protrusion through the umbilicus), incisional (protrusion through previous surgical scars), femoral (protrusion inferior to inguinal ligament, near the femoral vessels at the femoral canal), and inguinal hernias. Hernias are typically noticeable during times of increased intra-abdominal pressure, such as coughing, sneezing, laughing, heavy lifting, and straining.

Inguinal hernias can be divided into direct or indirect based on their anatomic characteristics. A direct hernia is an intra-abdominal protrusion that occurs outside of the inguinal canal, between the abdominal musculature and the inguinal ligament. It does not involve the internal or external inguinal rings and does not traverse the inguinal canal. Conversely, an indirect inguinal hernia is an intra-abdominal protrusion through the internal inguinal ring that can traverse (partly or entirely) the inguinal canal potentially through the external inguinal ring and into the scrotum. Indirect inguinal hernias are far more common than direct inguinal hernias.

Symptoms from hernias can range from an asymptomatic bulge, to a mildly dull aching sensation, to acute severe pain with concomitant nausea and vomiting. Asymptomatic to mildly symptomatic hernias are generally spontaneously or self-reducible. Conversely, acute and severe symptoms usually occur in the setting of bowel or omental incarceration and strangulation, which if not treated expeditiously could lead to tissue ischemia and necrosis. All patients should be educated on the variability of symptoms and when to seek emergent medical care (signs of bowel incarceration).

Diagnosis is usually made solely based on history and physical examination with provocative maneuvers (Valsalva). Treatment depends on the severity of symptoms and location of the hernia. Whereas surgical repair is recommended for most femoral hernias, given the high incidence of complications, asymptomatic inguinal and umbilical hernias can often be monitored. Symptomatic inguinal hernias usually require surgical repair (options include laparoscopic or open repair techniques with or without mesh). In the case of a strangulated or incarcerated hernia, immediate surgical repair is of critical importance.

### KEY POINTS

HVC

- Most asymptomatic hernias can be monitored; symptomatic hernias may require surgical consultation and possible repair.

- Surgical repair is recommended for most femoral hernias given the high incidence of complications.

# Women's Health

## Breast Symptoms

### Breast Mass

A palpable breast mass that differs from the surrounding breast tissue and the corresponding area in the contralateral breast and persists throughout the menstrual cycle warrants evaluation. Although breast cancer should be considered in all patients, most breast masses are benign conditions, such as cysts, fibroadenomas, fat necrosis, or lipomas.

Evaluation requires consideration of breast cancer risk factors, including family history of breast or ovarian cancer and a detailed history of the mass, including onset, changes with the menstrual cycle, associated symptoms, and overlying skin/nipple changes. Examination of the breast includes assessment of the features of the mass, which can be well-defined with smooth margins (cyst or fibroadenoma) or ill-defined (malignancy). The axilla and supraclavicular regions should be examined to assess for lymphadenopathy. Although a detailed history and examination provide useful information, the

determination of whether a discrete mass is benign or malignant often requires further evaluation with breast imaging and/or biopsy.

Imaging of a breast mass may include diagnostic mammography and/or targeted ultrasonography of the mass. Mammography is the first test performed in most patients aged 30 years or older with a breast mass. The sensitivity of mammography is lower in women with dense breasts. The mammogram may demonstrate a mass, asymmetric density, and abnormal/pleomorphic calcifications potentially indicating breast cancer. For patients with a focal abnormality noted on clinical examination or mammogram, targeted ultrasonography can clarify the size of the mass, determine whether the mass is solid or cystic, and identify the margins as smooth or irregular. Ultrasonography is the preferred method of evaluation for women younger than 30 years, in whom mammography has low sensitivity due to dense breasts. It is also the test of choice in pregnant patients. When breast imaging is completed, results are categorized by using BI-RADS (Breast Imaging Reporting and Data System) (**Table 63**). Biopsy is recommended for category 4 and 5 breast findings. About one fifth of palpable breast masses are not identified on mammogram or ultrasound, and a normal mammogram in a patient with a discrete breast mass does not rule out malignancy; therefore, a suspicious breast mass should be evaluated with a biopsy even if the mammogram and ultrasound findings are negative.

| TABLE 63. | Breast Imaging Reporting and Data System (BI-RADS) Assessment Categories |
|---|---|
| Category 0 | Mammography: Incomplete—Need additional imaging evaluation and/or prior mammograms for comparison |
| | Ultrasound and MRI: Incomplete—Need additional imaging evaluation |
| Category 1 | Negative |
| Category 2 | Benign |
| Category 3 | Probably benign |
| Category 4 | Suspicious |
| | Mammography and ultrasound: |
| | Category 4A: Low suspicion for malignancy |
| | Category 4B: Moderate suspicion for malignancy |
| | Category 4C: High suspicion for malignancy |
| Category 5 | Highly suggestive of malignancy |
| Category 6 | Known biopsy-proven malignancy |

Reproduced with permission of the American College of Radiology (ACR) from D'Orsi CJ, Sickles EA, Mendelson EB, et al. ACR BI-RADS® Atlas, Breast Imaging Reporting and Data System. Reston, VA, American College of Radiology; 2013. No other representation of this material is authorized without expressed, written permission from the ACR. Refer to the ACR website at https://www.acr.org/Clinical-Resources/Reporting-and-Data-Systems/Bi-Rads for the most current and complete version of the BI-RADS® Atlas.

Breast biopsy can be performed with fine-needle aspiration, image-guided core-needle biopsy, or surgical/excisional biopsy. Fine-needle aspiration is done for cystic lesions; benign cysts that completely resolve with aspiration require no further work-up. Image-guided core-needle biopsy can be a stereotactic biopsy when the lesion is seen only on mammogram, ultrasound-guided biopsy when the lesion can be seen on ultrasound, or an MRI-guided biopsy when the mass is seen only on a breast MRI. Management of an abnormal finding requires a consultation with a breast surgeon. A surgical biopsy is performed when the core-needle biopsy is technically challenging due to location of the lesion, when atypical hyperplasia is seen on core-needle biopsy specimens, or when the pathology report and breast imaging findings are discordant.

## Breast Pain

Breast pain (mastalgia) is common and may be cyclic or noncyclic in relation to the menstrual cycle. Cyclic breast pain often occurs in the premenstrual phase, tends to be bilateral, and resolves with onset of menstruation; it is usually associated with hormonal changes and is typically benign. Noncyclic breast pain is usually related to underlying breast conditions, such as fibrocystic breasts, hormone therapy, and stretching of Cooper ligaments (connective tissue that maintains breast structural integrity) with large breast size. Noncyclic breast pain may also result from breast infection or mastitis, breast trauma, or thrombophlebitis of the thoracoepigastric vein (Mondor disease). Non-breast causes of breast pain include costochondritis, coronary artery disease, gastroesophageal reflux disease, and intercostal nerve pain.

Evaluation includes a detailed history of breast pain to identify characteristics of the pain and relationship to menses, along with a careful physical examination to rule out palpable masses or anatomic causes. Women evaluated for breast pain with no obvious abnormal findings should be up to date with routine age- and risk-appropriate breast screening. Patients with noncyclic mastalgia with focal breast pain and no palpable mass should undergo targeted breast ultrasonography because approximately 1% of such patients may have breast cancer at the site of pain. Any palpable breast masses should be evaluated with diagnostic imaging (see Breast Mass).

For women with cyclic breast pain and negative clinical findings, conservative management (education, reassurance of the absence of malignancy, and advice regarding adequate breast support) is recommended as cyclic pain usually resolves spontaneously. There is a lack of evidence to support limiting caffeine intake or using vitamin E as a means of mitigating the pain. Medical management may be offered for patients with severe pain that persists despite conservative management. Danazol is the only FDA-approved agent for cyclic breast pain, but its use is limited because of side effects, including amenorrhea, hirsutism, and adverse changes in lipid profile. Low-dose tamoxifen, although not FDA approved for this indication, has been shown to have benefit with fewer side effects; however,

hot flushes, menstrual irregularities, and the need for contraception must be considered. Treatment of noncyclic breast pain depends on the underlying cause.

**KEY POINTS**

- Mammography is the first test performed in most women aged 30 years or older with a breast mass; the sensitivity of mammography is lower in women with dense breasts.
- Ultrasonography is the preferred method of evaluation **HVC** of a breast mass in women younger than 30 years, in whom mammography has low sensitivity due to dense breasts.
- A suspicious breast mass should be evaluated with a biopsy even if the mammogram and ultrasound results are negative.
- Cyclic breast pain often occurs in the premenstrual **HVC** phase, tends to be bilateral, and resolves with onset of menstruation and conservative management (education, reassurance of the absence of malignancy, and advice regarding adequate breast support).
- Noncyclic breast pain is usually related to underlying breast conditions; patients with noncyclic focal breast pain and no palpable mass should undergo targeted breast ultrasonography to exclude breast cancer.

# Reproductive Health

The Centers for Disease Control and Prevention provides information and recommendations on reproductive health (https://www.cdc.gov/reproductivehealth/index.html).

## Contraception

Approximately 50% of pregnancies in the United States are unintended, with a higher prevalence in women with low socioeconomic status, younger women, and those who cohabit. Contraception counseling to reduce unintended pregnancy involves an understanding of the risk for pregnancy, assessing contraceptive options, identifying the appropriate agent based on benefits and risks, and educating the patient on appropriate use of the contraceptive. Contraceptive options include hormonal contraception, barrier methods, sterilization, and emergency contraception (**Table 64**).

## Hormonal Contraception

Hormonal contraceptive options include oral contraceptive pills (combination estrogen-progesterone or progesterone-only pills), long-acting reversible contraceptives, transdermal patches, and vaginal rings. Patient factors influencing choice include hypertension, history of breast cancer, obesity, thrombotic disorders, migraines, and tobacco use. Before initiation of hormonal contraception, a negative pregnancy test result must be documented if 7 days have passed since the first day of the patient's last menstrual period.

**TABLE 64.** Comparison of Contraceptive Options

| Agent | Women Experiencing Unintended Pregnancy Within the First Year of Use (%) | | Advantages | Disadvantages |
| | Typical Use[a] | Perfect Use[a] | | |
| --- | --- | --- | --- | --- |
| **Hormonal Agents** | | | | |
| *Oral contraceptives* | | | | |
| Combination estrogen-progestin preparations | 9 | 0.3 | Easy to use<br>Rapidly reversible<br>Decreased risk for endometrial and ovarian cancers<br>Decreased dysmenorrhea, menorrhagia, symptomatic ovarian cysts<br>Less iron deficiency anemia | Daily use may affect adherence<br>Increased risk for myocardial infarction, ischemic stroke, VTE, hypertension<br>Increased risk for cancers of the cervix, liver, and breast<br>Breakthrough bleeding<br>May exacerbate migraine |
| Progestin-only preparations ("mini-pill") | 9 | 0.3 | Use when estrogen is contraindicated | Irregular bleeding, breakthrough bleeding; must maintain precise daily dosing schedule |
| *Long-acting reversible preparations* | | | | |
| Depot medroxyprogesterone acetate (IM or SQ) | 6 | 0.2 | Administered every 3 months<br>Decreased risk for endometrial cancer, PID<br>Improves endometriosis<br>Decreased menstrual frequency | Delayed return to ovulation (6-10 months)<br>Irregular bleeding, amenorrhea, decreased bone mineral density (especially in adolescents) |
| Progestin implants | 0.05 | 0.05 | Effective up to 3 years | |
| Intrauterine devices | | | | |
| Copper | 0.8 | 0.6 | Nonhormonal<br>Effective up to 10 years | Bleeding, pain<br>Requires placement and removal in office<br>Expulsion rates up to 5% in first year<br>No protection from STIs |
| Levonorgestrel | 6 | 0.2 | Decreased menstrual flow<br>Effective up to 3-5 years, depending on formulation | |
| *Other hormonal agents* | | | | |
| Patch (combination estrogen-progestin) | 9 | 0.3 | Easier adherence<br>Change weekly | Local skin reaction<br>Increased estrogen dose, thus higher VTE risk |
| Vaginal ring (combination estrogen-progestin) | 9 | 0.3 | Easier adherence<br>Change monthly<br>Lowest level of systemic estrogen | Requires self-insertion |
| **Barrier Methods** | | | | |
| Cervical cap | 16-32 | 9-26 | - | User dependent, requires spermicide |
| Diaphragm | 12 | 6 | - | Requires spermicide |
| Male condom | 18 | 2 | Protection from STIs | - |
| Female condom | 21 | 5 | Protection from STIs | - |
| Vaginal sponge | 12-24 | 9-20 | - | - |
| **Sterilization** | | | | |
| Female (tubal ligation) | 0.5 | 0.5 | May reduce ovarian cancer risk | Surgical complications (rare)<br>Regret<br>Increased risk for ectopic pregnancy |
| Male (vasectomy) | 0.15 | 0.10 | Lower costs, fewer complications, and more effective than tubal ligation | Surgical complications (rare) |

IM = intramuscular; PID = pelvic inflammatory disease; SQ = subcutaneous; STI = sexually transmitted infection; VTE = venous thromboembolism.

[a]Perfect use implies correct and consistent use exactly as directed/intended. Typical use reflects rates in actual practice with patients.

*Oral Contraceptive Pills*

Oral contraceptive pills include combination estrogen-progesterone pills and progesterone-only pills. The combination pills vary in the type and strength of estrogen and the type of progestin. They inhibit ovulation, alter the cervical mucus to prevent migration of the sperm, inhibit endometrial thickening, and prevent implantation. Although all agents are equivalent in terms of the contraceptive efficacy, they vary in terms of side effects. Contraindications to combination pills include breast cancer, venous thromboembolism, uncontrolled hypertension, liver disease, and migraine with aura.

Women who smoke more than 15 cigarettes per day and are older than 35 years should not use estrogen-containing preparations because of the increased risk for thrombotic disorders. Progesterone-only pills can be used for women with a contraindication to estrogen.

*Long-Acting Reversible Contraception*

Long-acting reversible contraceptives are progestin-only forms of contraception that include depot medroxyprogesterone acetate injections, progestin implants, and intrauterine devices (IUDs). Patients can receive these contraceptives in the outpatient office setting.

An IUD is a small, T-shaped device (copper or levonorgestrel) that is placed inside the uterus. The copper IUD induces a local reaction that impairs implantation of the fertilized ovum, whereas the levonorgestrel IUD releases a low dose of progestin that leads to endometrial atrophy and also prevents implantation. Complications include uterine perforation with approximately 1 per 1000 insertions. Risk factors for perforation include breastfeeding at the time of insertion or insertion within 36 weeks after the last childbirth. Risk for pelvic infection with IUD placement is low, and prophylactic antibiotics are not recommended during the procedure. If a woman with a sexually transmitted infection (STI) has an IUD in place, she should be treated with antibiotics, and the IUD does not need to be removed. Contraindications to IUD placement include pregnancy; anatomic uterine abnormalities with distortion of the uterine cavity; and acute untreated pelvic infection, gonorrhea, or chlamydia.

## Barrier Contraception

Barrier contraceptive methods such as diaphragms and condoms are among the least effective of all the modes of contraception. Their efficacy is improved when combined with a spermicidal agent. Use of condoms reduces the risk for STIs.

## Sterilization

Female sterilization is a safe and permanent form of sterilization that is associated with a low complication rate. The fallopian tube lumen may be occluded by techniques such as clip or cautery. Preprocedure counseling includes a detailed discussion of the permanence of the procedure, the risk for regret after surgery, the complex nature and poor success rates of reversal procedures, and the availability of alternative long-acting contraceptive methods.

## Emergency Contraception

Emergency contraception refers to postcoital contraception using a device or medication to prevent pregnancy after unprotected or inadequately protected intercourse. The most effective form of emergency contraception is the placement of a copper IUD within 5 days of intercourse. The IUD is also the preferred option in obese women because they experience higher failure rates with oral emergency contraception.

FDA-approved medications include levonorgestrel, which is most effective within 3 days of intercourse, and ulipristal, which has a 5-day window.

## Preconception Care

Preconception counseling refers to education provided before pregnancy, aimed at reducing the risk for preterm birth and congenital anomalies. Optimizing health before pregnancy reduces exposures to factors that can potentially compromise a healthy pregnancy, as organogenesis starts as early as the third to fifth week of gestation. This differs from prenatal counseling, which occurs after pregnancy is diagnosed.

Any primary care visit for a woman of reproductive age is an opportunity to routinely ask if she could become pregnant or is considering pregnancy. For women who are not interested in pregnancy, contraception should be discussed to reduce the risk for unintended pregnancy. For women considering pregnancy, a comprehensive risk assessment should be completed (**Table 65**). An obstetric history of pregnancy-induced hypertension, preeclampsia, or gestational diabetes is particularly predictive of future risk.

All medications should be reviewed to reduce or avoid exposure to potential teratogens (**Table 66**). The pregnancy letter categories that have been used by the FDA to characterize the safety of drugs in pregnancy are provided in **Table 67**. In 2015, the FDA published changes in pregnancy and lactation labeling for prescription drugs (https://www.fda.gov/Drugs/DevelopmentApprovalProcess/DevelopmentResources/Labeling/ucm093307.htm). The pregnancy letter categories will be discontinued with the new labeling requirements; however, for prescription drugs that were previously approved, these changes will be phased in gradually. Labeling will include information relevant to the use of the drug in pregnant women (such as dosing and potential risks to the developing fetus), information about using the drug while breastfeeding (such as the amount of drug in breast milk and potential effects on the breastfed infant), and information regarding potential risks to females and males of reproductive potential who take the drug.

Physical examination includes assessment of blood pressure and BMI. Pelvic examination may include screening cervical cytology. Testing for STIs and hepatitis is indicated in high-risk patients. HIV counseling and screening are recommended for all women planning pregnancy.

Intervention to prevent complications depends on the results of the risk assessment. All women should be encouraged to follow a healthy lifestyle, with emphasis on complete

**TABLE 65.** Preconception Risk Assessment

| Risk Category | Specific Items to Assess |
|---|---|
| Reproductive awareness | Desire for pregnancy, number and timing of desired pregnancies, age-related changes in fertility, sexuality, contraception |
| Environmental hazards and toxins | Exposure to radiation, lead, and mercury |
| Nutrition and folic acid consumption | Healthy diet; daily consumption of folic acid; low-dose iron supplementation; restricting consumption of shark, swordfish, king mackerel, and tilefish to <2 servings weekly (owing to high mercury content) |
| Genetics | Family history of genetic disorders |
| Substance use | Use of tobacco, alcohol, and illicit drugs |
| Medical conditions | Seizure disorder, diabetes mellitus, hypertension, thyroid disease, asthma, HIV infection, systemic lupus erythematosus |
| Obstetric history | Pregnancy-induced hypertension, preeclampsia, gestational diabetes |
| Medications | Over-the-counter and prescription medications, potential teratogens |
| Infectious diseases and vaccinations | Vaccinations up to date; immunity to varicella and rubella; risk for hepatitis B infection |
| Psychosocial concerns | Depression, interpersonal/family relationships, risk for abuse (physical, sexual, emotional) |

Information from Johnson K, Posner SF, Biermann J, et al; CDC/ATSDR Preconception Care Work Group; Select Panel on Preconception Care. Recommendations to improve preconception health and health care—United States. A report of the CDC/ATSDR Preconception Care Work Group and the Select Panel on Preconception Care. MMWR Recomm Rep. 2006;55:1-23. [PMID: 16617292]

**TABLE 66.** Commonly Used Medications With Potential for Teratogenic Effects

| Class/Type | Examples |
|---|---|
| Antibiotics | Tetracycline, doxycycline, sulfonamides, trimethoprim, para-aminosalicylate |
| Anticoagulants | Warfarin |
| Antidepressants | Selective serotonin reuptake inhibitors, lithium |
| Antihypertensive agents | ACE inhibitors, angiotensin receptor blockers, direct renin inhibitors |
| Antiepileptic drugs | Valproic acid, phenytoin, carbamazepine |
| Antithyroid medications | Propylthiouracil, carbimazole, methimazole |
| Hormones | Androgens, testosterone derivatives |
| Immunosuppressant/chemotherapeutic agents | Folate antagonists, cyclophosphamide, methotrexate |
| Others | Vitamin A derivatives, statins, NSAIDs, isotretinoin |

**TABLE 67.** FDA Classification of Drugs in Pregnancy[a]

| Class | Fetal Effect of Drug During Pregnancy |
|---|---|
| A | No disclosed fetal effects |
| B | Animal studies failed to demonstrate fetal risk |
| C | Animal studies suggest adverse fetal effects |
| D | Evidence of human fetal risk |
| X | Documented fetal abnormalities |

[a]In 2015, the FDA published changes in pregnancy and lactation labeling for prescription drugs. A summary of these changes is available at https://www.fda.gov/Drugs/DevelopmentApprovalProcess/DevelopmentResources/Labeling/ucm093307.htm. The pregnancy letter categories will be removed with the new labeling requirements; however, for prescription drugs that were previously approved, these changes will be phased in gradually.

cessation of tobacco, alcohol, or illicit drugs before conception and education on the consequences of not doing so.

Women should be up to date with immunizations. Women who are considering pregnancy should be assessed for immunity to varicella and rubella. For women who are not immune, varicella and rubella vaccination should be administered with the advice that pregnancy be avoided for at least 4 weeks after the vaccine is administered to reduce risk to the fetus. Immunizations to be avoided during pregnancy, in addition to varicella and rubella, include human papillomavirus, measles, mumps, live attenuated influenza, and live attenuated herpes zoster.

Consultation with a genetics counselor may be helpful if there is a personal or family history of genetic disorders.

Patients should also be counseled about new infections, such as Zika virus and its risk for adverse fetal outcomes (for example, microcephaly), and be educated on the risks of travel to endemic areas and modes of transmission, including mosquito bite, sexual intercourse, and blood transfusion. Appropriate preventive measures should be addressed.

Interventions that optimize pregnancy outcomes include daily intake of folic acid (0.4-0.8 mg/d [400-800 µg/d]) to reduce the risk for neural tube defects. Low-dose oral iron supplements can reduce the risk for maternal anemia. Prenatal multivitamins that contain sufficient folic acid are a reasonable option for women contemplating pregnancy.

**KEY POINTS**

- Contraception counseling involves an understanding of the risk for pregnancy, assessing contraceptive options, identifying the appropriate agent based on benefits and risks, and educating the patient on appropriate use of contraceptives.

- Contraindications to oral combination estrogen-progesterone contraceptive pills include breast cancer, venous thromboembolism, uncontrolled hypertension, liver disease, and migraine with aura; progesterone-only pills can be used for women with a contraindication to estrogen.

*(Continued)*

**KEY POINTS** *(continued)*

- Women who smoke more than 15 cigarettes per day and are older than 35 years should not use estrogen-containing contraceptive preparations.

- Long-acting reversible contraceptives are progestin-only forms of contraception that include depot medroxyprogesterone acetate injections, progestin implants, and intrauterine devices.

- Women considering pregnancy should undergo a comprehensive assessment of risk factors for adverse pregnancy outcomes and begin folic acid supplementation.

# Menstrual Disorders

## Abnormal Uterine Bleeding

### Evaluation

Abnormal uterine bleeding is defined as excessive bleeding in terms of flow volume, frequency, and duration. Among non-pregnant women of reproductive age, abnormal uterine bleeding is classified according to etiology by using the International Federation of Obstetrics and Gynecology system with the acronym PALM-COEIN (polyp, adenomyosis, leiomyoma, malignancy and hyperplasia, coagulopathy, ovulation dysfunction, endometrial, iatrogenic, and not yet classified). Abnormal uterine bleeding in this population can be further classified as ovulatory or anovulatory. Ovulatory bleeding occurs at regular intervals, but the menstrual flow is excessive. This may be related to thyroid disease; bleeding disorders; or structural abnormalities, such as uterine fibroids or polyps. Anovulatory cycles are characteristically irregular in terms of flow and cycle duration, as lack of ovulation and the resultant lack of cyclic progesterone cause endometrial hyperplasia and irregular bleeding. Anovulation occurs with polycystic ovary syndrome, hypothyroidism or hyperthyroidism, hyperprolactinemia, chronic liver or kidney disease, and medications (such as antidepressant and antipsychotic agents, chemotherapy, and tamoxifen). Anovulatory causes of bleeding in the patient of reproductive age increase the risk for endometrial cancer because of the lack of cyclic progesterone-induced withdrawal bleeding and resultant endometrial hyperplasia.

Causes of abnormal uterine bleeding in the postmenopausal patient are similar to those in women of reproductive age, although there is an increased risk for endometrial cancer. Risk factors for endometrial cancer other than age older than 50 years and anovulatory causes of bleeding include such conditions as Lynch or Cowden syndrome; obesity; and reproductive factors, such as nulliparity and late menopause.

Evaluation of abnormal uterine bleeding in the premenopausal woman includes assessment of menstrual cycle length, regularity, intermenstrual bleeding, volume of menstrual flow (including passage of clots), association with pain, presence of an intrauterine device, and postcoital bleeding. Assessment for thyroid disease, liver or kidney disease, and bleeding disorders is also indicated. Pelvic examination is performed to determine whether the source of bleeding is from the vulva, vagina, cervix, or uterus. Pregnancy testing is recommended for all premenopausal women with abnormal uterine bleeding because bleeding may occur with pregnancy-related conditions, such as placenta previa and ectopic gestation. Pelvic ultrasonography is indicated to assess for structural abnormalities in the uterus and to determine endometrial thickness. Endometrial thickness greater than 4 mm in postmenopausal women may indicate endometrial hyperplasia or malignancy. In premenopausal women, endometrial thickness is not a reliable indicator because thickness varies according to the phase of the menstrual cycle.

Evaluation of the postmenopausal patient is similar to that of the premenopausal patient. Because of the increased risk for endometrial cancer, however, any vaginal bleeding occurring in peri- and postmenopausal women warrants evaluation to rule out malignancy, usually with endometrial biopsy.

### Management

Management of abnormal uterine bleeding is aimed at the underlying cause. Structural abnormalities, such as endometrial polyps or submucosal fibroids, may be surgically resected. Treatment of underlying endocrine disorders (thyroid disease, polycystic ovary disease) may result in improvement.

For women with anovulatory cycles, treatment is aimed at providing adequate progestin to maintain endometrial stability. The type of therapy depends on the patient's plans for contraception. For women who wish to preserve fertility, medroxyprogesterone acetate used for the second half of the menstrual cycle will restore cyclic withdrawal bleeding. For women interested in contraception, oral contraceptive pills containing estrogen and progesterone or the levonorgestrel intrauterine device may be used. Additionally, NSAIDs may be used because these drugs reduce synthesis of prostaglandins in the endometrium, leading to vasoconstriction and reduced bleeding. Tranexamic acid, an antithrombolytic agent, stabilizes clots and may be used for treatment of heavy vaginal bleeding. For women experiencing acute and severe bleeding, agents such as gonadotropin-releasing hormone or intravenous administration of high-dose estrogens may be used. For women who do not respond to medical therapy, operative procedures such as endometrial ablation or hysterectomy may be performed.

## Dysmenorrhea

Dysmenorrhea is characterized by pain during menstruation; it may also be associated with low back pain, headache, nausea, vomiting, and diarrhea. Dysmenorrhea is classified as primary or secondary. Primary dysmenorrhea involves cramping lower abdominal and pelvic pain that occurs during menstrual cycles without an identifiable cause. Secondary dysmenorrhea may result from pelvic conditions, such as endometriosis, inflammatory disease, or uterine fibroids.

A detailed history is necessary to assess the timing of pain and relationship to the menstrual cycle. Sexual history is important to assess for infection and risk for abuse. Primary dysmenorrhea can be treated with NSAIDs and cyclooxygenase-2 inhibitors; persistent symptoms can be treated with oral contraceptive pills. Secondary dysmenorrhea requires treatment of the underlying condition.

**KEY POINTS**

- Evaluation of all patients with abnormal uterine bleeding includes a detailed history, physical and pelvic examinations, pregnancy testing, and pelvic ultrasonography.

- Risk factors for endometrial cancer include age older than 50 years; anovulatory causes of bleeding; such conditions as Lynch or Cowden syndrome; obesity; and reproductive factors, such as nulliparity and late menopause.

- Any vaginal bleeding occurring in peri- and postmenopausal women warrants evaluation to rule out malignancy, usually with endometrial biopsy.

- Primary dysmenorrhea can be treated with NSAIDs and cyclooxygenase-2 inhibitors, and persistent symptoms can be treated with oral contraceptive pills; secondary dysmenorrhea requires treatment of the underlying condition.

# Menopause

## Diagnosis

Menopause is the permanent cessation of menses that is diagnosed retrospectively after a woman has not experienced a menstrual period for 12 months. Menopause may be natural, surgical following bilateral oophorectomies, or medical as a result of medications such as chemotherapy. Menopause occurring before age 40 years is considered premature menopause or premature ovarian insufficiency. Perimenopause refers to the phase of menopause transition, extending into early postmenopause; it varies in length and may be associated with irregular menstrual cycles, fluctuating hormone levels, and intermittent hot flushes.

Symptoms of menopause include vasomotor symptoms (hot flushes, night sweats), depression, difficulties with memory and concentration, sleep disturbances, and genitourinary symptoms (vaginal dryness, dyspareunia). Up to 50% of women experience hot flushes during perimenopause, but symptoms generally resolve spontaneously in a few years. Genitourinary syndrome of menopause is the result of estrogen deficiency and is characterized by vaginal symptoms, such as vaginal burning or irritation; sexual symptoms, such as dyspareunia or sexual dysfunction; or urinary symptoms, such as dysuria or recurrent urinary infections. Pelvic examination findings include a pale, dry vaginal lining with reduction in rugae. Increases in LDL cholesterol and bone loss are also associated with menopause.

Routine laboratory testing for the diagnosis of menopause is not recommended. Patients with possible early menopause should have pregnancy excluded and undergo measurement of follicle-stimulating hormone, thyroid-stimulating hormone, and prolactin. Younger patients should undergo evaluation for amenorrhea (see MKSAP 18 Endocrinology and Metabolism).

## Management

Management of menopausal symptoms is recommended to improve quality of life. Pregnancy is possible even if menstrual cycles are irregular, and contraception should be discussed if pregnancy is not desired. The U.S. Preventive Services Task Force recommends against the use of combined estrogen and progestin for the primary prevention of chronic conditions (coronary artery disease, dementia, stroke, and fractures) in postmenopausal women and against the use of estrogen alone for the primary prevention of chronic conditions in postmenopausal women who have had a hysterectomy.

### Vasomotor Symptoms

The approach to starting menopausal hormone therapy for women aged 50 to 59 years, or within 10 years of menopause onset, who are experiencing menopause symptoms is outlined in **Table 68**. Estrogen is the most effective therapy for vasomotor symptoms; the lowest dose of estrogen to manage symptoms should be used. Contraindications to hormone therapy include pregnancy, unexplained vaginal bleeding, coronary artery disease, stroke, thromboembolic disease, breast cancer, and endometrial cancer.

Transdermal estrogen is preferable to oral estrogen because it may be associated with less thromboembolic risk, but some patients may prefer oral therapy.

For women who experience menopausal symptoms and have an intact uterus, estrogen should be combined with progestin to avoid unopposed estrogen-related endometrial proliferation. Continuous daily estrogen with progestin does not result in cyclic vaginal bleeding and may be a preferred option for many women. Women must be informed that estrogen with cyclic progestin will result in withdrawal bleeding.

Use of hormone therapy in menopause should be reassessed every year to determine benefits and risks and determine the appropriate time to discontinue the medication. Treatment duration is based on continued presence of vasomotor symptoms. Postmenopausal hormone use with combined estrogen-progestin therapy taken for more than 5 years is associated with increased risk for breast cancer and requires that women receive individualized breast cancer risk assessment and counseling.

Nonhormonal drugs can help modulate vasomotor symptoms in women with contraindications to hormone therapy or who wish to avoid the associated risks. Antidepressant agents, including selective serotonin reuptake inhibitors (such as citalopram, escitalopram, and paroxetine) and serotonin-norepinephrine reuptake inhibitors (such as

**TABLE 68.** Initiating Systemic Hormone Therapy in Women Aged 50 to 59 Years or Within 10 Years of Menopause Onset for Vasomotor Symptoms[a]

Step 1: Confirm that hot flushes/night sweats are moderate to severe in intensity and refractory to lifestyle modifications and/or vaginal symptoms have been refractory to local therapies.

Step 2: Assess for contraindications to systemic hormone therapy.

Step 3: Assess the patient's baseline risk for stroke, cardiovascular disease, and breast cancer (consider using the 10-year ASCVD risk calculator, Framingham stroke risk score, Framingham CHD risk score, and Gail model risk score to quantify this risk). If the Framingham stroke or CHD risk score is >10% or Gail model risk score is elevated, consider alternatives to systemic hormone therapy.[b,c]

Step 4: Use the lowest dose of estrogen that relieves menopausal symptoms.

Step 5: Add systemic progesterone therapy to estrogen therapy in women who have an intact uterus.

Step 6: Assess symptoms and side effects after initiating therapy and adjust the dose of estrogen if symptoms are persistent.

Step 7: Reassess symptoms and risk factors for cardiovascular disease, stroke, and breast cancer annually.

Step 8: Discontinue systemic hormone therapy if the risks of treatment outweigh the benefits.

ASCVD = atherosclerotic cardiovascular disease; CHD = coronary heart disease.

[a]According to the 2017 hormone therapy position statement of The North American Menopause Society, the safety profile of hormone therapy in women who initiate therapy more than 10 or 20 years after menopause onset or at age 60 years or older is not as favorable as for younger women, owing to greater absolute risks for coronary heart disease, stroke, venous thromboembolism, and dementia.

[b]Some experts indicate that systemic hormone therapy is safe in women who have experienced menopause within the last 5 years and have a Framingham CHD risk score of 10% to 20%.

[c]Most participants in the Women's Health Initiative (a set of two hormone therapy trials) had a Gail model risk score of less than 2%.

venlafaxine, desvenlafaxine, and duloxetine), and gabapentin are effective. Research is inconclusive regarding supplements such as soy, black cohosh, and other phytoestrogens for vasomotor symptoms.

### Genitourinary Syndrome of Menopause

Management of genitourinary syndrome of menopause (GSM) includes topical nonhormonal and hormonal preparations to relieve symptoms. Nonhormonal approaches include as-needed vaginal lubricants for intercourse and vaginal moisturizers that can alleviate vaginal dryness and irritation when used regularly. The North American Menopause Society recommends nonhormonal vaginal therapies as first-line treatment for GSM.

Hormonal preparations include estradiol or conjugated estrogen in tablet, cream, or ring forms. Low-dose vaginal estrogen is recommended for the management of vaginal atrophy because it builds the vaginal epithelium and restores the acidic pH and microenvironment. Moreover, improving the lining of the lower urethra reduces dysuria and recurrent urinary tract infection. For women with breast cancer, current or past, low-dose vaginal therapy should be given only with the approval of the treating oncologist. Vaginal dehydroepiandrosterone and the selective estrogen receptor modulator ospemifene are both approved by the FDA for management of dyspareunia associated with GSM; most experts consider these treatment modalities second-line therapies because of their side effects and limited safety experience.

**KEY POINTS**

- Routine laboratory testing for the diagnosis of menopause is not recommended; patients with possible early menopause should have pregnancy excluded and undergo measurement of follicle-stimulating hormone, thyroid-stimulating hormone, and prolactin levels.    **HVC**

- Pregnancy is possible even if menstrual cycles are irregular, and contraception should be discussed if pregnancy is not desired.

- Estrogen is the most effective therapy for vasomotor symptoms of menopause.

- Nonhormonal options for vasomotor symptoms of menopause include antidepressant agents and gabapentin.

- Management of genitourinary syndrome of menopause includes topical nonhormonal and hormonal preparations to achieve symptom relief.

## Chronic Pelvic Pain

Chronic pelvic pain (CPP) refers to a syndrome of intermittent or persistent pain below the level of the umbilicus or in the pelvis of at least 6 months' duration that is severe enough to result in functional disability or require medical care. Evaluation and diagnosis of CPP are challenging; CPP may be secondary to a single underlying cause, multiple concurrent disorders, or no clear cause. The identifiable causes can be classified as gynecologic (endometriosis, pelvic inflammatory disease), urologic (recurrent urinary tract infection, interstitial cystitis), gastrointestinal (pelvic adhesions, irritable bowel syndrome), musculoskeletal (myofascial pain, hernia), psychological (depression, sexual abuse), or neurologic (pudendal neuralgia).

Risk factors for CPP include physical, sexual, and/or emotional abuse; pelvic inflammatory disease; history of abdominopelvic surgery; chronic pain syndromes; and psychological conditions, such as anxiety or depression.

Evaluation includes a detailed history to determine characteristics of the pain, including association with menstrual cycle, urination, or bowel movement, as well as assessment for risk factors and known causes of CPP. Physical examination includes detailed abdominal and gynecologic examinations. Laboratory testing is of limited value unless specific disorders are suggested by the history and clinical examination (urinalysis for urinary tract infection, testing for STI). Transvaginal ultrasonography is used to identify anatomic pathology, such as a pelvic mass. In the absence of an abnormality noted on clinical examination or ultrasound, laparoscopy may be helpful for the evaluation of severe symptoms of unclear cause.

Treatment is aimed at the underlying cause and may be challenging if no clear cause is identified. For patients without a clearly identified cause, treatment is aimed at pain management. NSAIDs may be helpful for patients with moderate CPP. Additional therapies include antidepressant agents, physical therapy, cognitive behavioral therapy, biofeedback, acupuncture, hypnosis, and stress reduction therapies.

**KEY POINTS**

- Risk factors for chronic pelvic pain include physical, sexual, and/or emotional abuse; pelvic inflammatory disease; history of abdominopelvic surgery; chronic pain syndromes; and psychological conditions, such as anxiety or depression.

- NSAIDs may be helpful for patients with moderate chronic pelvic pain without a clearly identified cause.

# Female Sexual Dysfunction

Female sexual dysfunction is characterized by persistent or recurrent distressing sexual concerns or difficulties and is likely underappreciated; it affects more than one third of sexually active women. A sexual health history is an important part of the medical evaluation; open-ended questions regarding sexual activity and possible concerns, such as pain with intercourse, are appropriate and may uncover a previously unidentified disorder.

According to the DSM-5, female sexual dysfunction is divided into three categories: female orgasmic disorder, sexual interest/arousal disorder, and genitopelvic pain/penetration disorder. Female orgasmic disorder is the persistent or recurrent delay, infrequency, reduced intensity, or absence of orgasm following a normal excitement phase. Female sexual interest/arousal disorder includes hypoactive sexual desire or arousal dysfunction and is diagnosed if the patient reports at least three of the following symptoms: lack of sexual interest, lack of sexual thoughts or fantasies, decreased initiation of sexual activity or decreased responsiveness to the partner's initiation attempts, reduced excitement or pleasure during sexual activity, reduced response to sexual cues, or decreased genital or nongenital sensations during sexual activity. Genitopelvic pain/penetration disorder is diagnosed when there is persistent or recurrent difficulty in vaginal penetration during intercourse, marked vulvovaginal or pelvic pain during penetration, fear of pain or anxiety about pain in anticipation of or during penetration, or tightening or tensing of pelvic floor muscles during attempted penetration. Diagnosis of a sexual disorder requires that the aforementioned symptoms occur more than 75% of the time for at least 6 months and cause clinically significant distress.

Sexual functioning involves multiple components, including emotions, relationships, past experiences, physiologic responses, overall health, and personal beliefs; therefore, a comprehensive approach is needed to evaluate and treat the condition.

Assessment of female sexual dysfunction includes a detailed sexual history of symptom duration, whether acute or gradual onset, if related to a specific partner or a generalized concern; association with pain; precipitating events; life stressors; medical and surgical history; medications; and history of physical, emotional, and/or sexual abuse. Screening for concurrent depression is indicated. The Female Sexual Function Index questionnaire, a brief validated self-report questionnaire, can be used for clinical assessment of symptoms. Pelvic examination is aimed at assessing for specific sites of pain or tenderness, vaginal dryness, or atrophy suggestive of genitourinary symptoms of menopause. Laboratory testing is of limited value and performed only if an underlying cause is suspected.

Therapy is aimed at treating the underlying cause of female sexual dysfunction, which is often multifactorial. Vaginal dryness and atrophy from genitourinary symptoms of menopause may warrant use of vaginal moisturizers and vaginal estrogen therapy. Lubricants can be used as needed for intercourse, and deep muscle relaxation therapies and objects, such as dilators, to increase the diameter of the vagina may be used for patients with vulvovaginal pain. Systemic hormone therapy in postmenopausal women may help sexual function. Ospemifene is a selective estrogen receptor modulator approved by the FDA for treatment of dyspareunia associated with vulvovaginal atrophy.

Flibanserin is the only drug approved by the FDA for premenopausal women with female sexual interest/arousal disorder. However, caution is warranted when this medication is prescribed because of side effects (dizziness, syncope, hypotension, somnolence) and lack of safety data when flibanserin is combined with alcohol or certain medications (antidepressants). Low-dose testosterone treatment (off-label) increases sexual function scores, but side effects must be discussed. Phosphodiesterase inhibitors, such as sildenafil, have shown inconsistent results in women.

Treatment strategies must also address psychological and behavioral aspects of female sexual dysfunction. Cognitive behavioral therapy can help minimize negative attitudes and help with anxiety. Couples therapy may be beneficial. Sex therapy includes counseling; cognitive behavioral therapy; and treatment of concomitant mental health conditions, such as depression and anxiety.

**KEY POINT**

- A sexual health history is an important part of the medical evaluation; open-ended questions regarding sexual activity and possible concerns, such as pain with intercourse, are appropriate and may uncover a previously unidentified disorder. **HVC**

# Vaginitis

Vaginitis describes conditions associated with vulvovaginal symptoms that may include vaginal discharge, burning, itching, or odor. Vaginal discharge can be physiologic, related to ovulation or pregnancy, or infectious, most commonly bacterial vaginosis, candidiasis, or trichomoniasis (**Table 69**). Other causes of vaginal discharge include irritation from use of douches, atrophic vaginitis, malignancy, or a foreign body.

History should include details about the type of vaginal discharge (volume, color, odor), timing related to menstrual cycle, use of douches, at-risk sexual behavior, dysuria, and dyspareunia. Physical examination includes assessment of the

| Cause of Vaginitis | Clinical Presentation | Evaluation | Management |
|---|---|---|---|
| Bacterial vaginosis | Malodorous or "fishy" vaginal discharge, often most noticeable after intercourse. Increased thin white or gray discharge. Symptoms other than malodor may be minimal | pH >4.5. KOH amine whiff test result positive. Saline wet mount with >20% epithelial clue cells | Metronidazole: 500 mg orally twice daily for 7 days[a] (avoid alcohol during treatment and for 24 hours after last dose); or vaginal gel (0.75%) 5 g into vagina at bedtime for 5 nights. Clindamycin: 300 mg orally twice daily for 7 days; or vaginal cream (2%) 5 g into vagina for 7 nights. Note: Use oral regimens in pregnancy. |
| Vulvovaginal candidiasis | Itching, irritation, dysuria, dyspareunia, vulvodynia, excoriation, erythema, fissures. Increased thick white discharge (although may be normal) | pH ≤4.5. KOH amine whiff test result negative. KOH wet mount shows hyphae, pseudohyphae, or yeast | **Uncomplicated[b]** Fluconazole: 150 mg orally as a single dose. Butoconazole vaginal: (2% cream) 5 g into vagina at bedtime for 3 nights. Clotrimazole vaginal: (1% cream) 5 g into vagina at bedtime for 7-14 nights; or 100-mg vaginal tablet into vagina at bedtime for 7 nights; or 200 mg (two vaginal tablets) into vagina once daily at bedtime for 3 nights. Miconazole vaginal: (2% cream) 5 g into vagina at bedtime for 7 nights; or 100-mg vaginal suppository into vagina at bedtime for 7 nights; or 200-mg vaginal suppository into vagina at bedtime for 3 nights. Note: Single-dose vaginal preparations and non-imidazoles are available but less effective. **Complicated[c]** Longer duration of initial oral or topical treatment, followed by maintenance therapy: Fluconazole: 150 mg orally every 3 days for a total of three doses; or topical imidazole therapy for 7-14 nights. Following this, maintenance therapy is based on refractory or recurrent symptoms: Fluconazole: 150 mg orally weekly for 6 months; or 200 mg orally weekly for 8 weeks; or 200 mg orally twice weekly for 4 months; or 200 mg orally once monthly for 6 months |
| Trichomoniasis | Increased discolored discharge (yellowish, gray, and/or frothy). Dyspareunia, dysuria, itch, erythema, postcoital bleeding, abdominal pain. Punctate cervical hemorrhages ("strawberry" cervix) | pH ≥4.5. KOH amine whiff test result negative. Saline wet mount with trichomonads, leukocytes. NAAT or rapid assay result positive | Metronidazole[a]: 2 g orally as a single dose; treatment failure with 2-g metronidazole is treated with 500 mg orally twice daily for 7 days. Note: Avoid alcohol during treatment and for 24 hours after last dose. |

KOH = potassium hydroxide; NAAT = nucleic acid amplification test.

[a]Safe in pregnancy.

[b]Uncomplicated vulvovaginal candidiasis: *Candida albicans*, mild to moderate symptom severity, healthy nonpregnant women, four or fewer episodes per year.

[c]Complicated vulvovaginal candidiasis: Severe symptoms, suspected or proven non-albicans *Candida* species, more than four episodes per year, uncontrolled diabetes mellitus, or immunosuppression.

vulva and vagina for erythema, edema, excoriation, papillomas, and the type of discharge. However, clinical findings do not sufficiently distinguish between the common causes of vaginitis, and laboratory testing is necessary to establish a diagnosis. Diagnostic testing includes assessment of vaginal wall secretions for pH, amine (whiff) test, and microscopic evaluation with saline potassium hydroxide (KOH) wet mounts, or specific testing for trichomoniasis.

## Bacterial Vaginosis

Bacterial vaginosis is the most common cause of vaginal discharge. It results from the loss of the normal hydrogen peroxide-producing lactobacilli in the vagina with an increase in the vaginal pH that contributes to an overgrowth of *Gardnerella vaginalis* and other anaerobes. Anaerobic overgrowth results in the production of amines, causing the characteristically malodorous discharge. Patients with bacterial vaginosis are at increased risk for STIs, including HIV infection, and for preterm delivery.

More than half of patients with bacterial vaginosis are asymptomatic. Symptomatic patients report a thin, vaginal discharge with a fishy odor. Clinical diagnosis includes the presence of at least three of four features: vaginal pH greater than 4.5, thin and homogeneous vaginal discharge, a positive whiff test result in which application of 10% KOH to vaginal secretions results in a fishy odor, and the finding of at least 20% clue cells on saline wet mount preparation. Clue cells are vaginal epithelial cells that on microscopy have ill-defined cell borders due to adherent coccobacilli (**Figure 16**).

Asymptomatic bacterial vaginosis does not require treatment. See Table 69 for treatment options for symptomatic bacterial vaginosis.

## Vulvovaginal Candidiasis

Vulvovaginal candidiasis is the second most common cause of vaginitis; it is usually caused by *Candida albicans* and less commonly by non-albicans *Candida*. Unlike pharyngeal

candidiasis, it frequently occurs in immunocompetent women with no risk factors. Factors that may increase the risk for vulvovaginal candidiasis include diabetes mellitus; pregnancy; and use of oral contraceptives, glucocorticoids, or antibiotics. Recurrent vulvovaginal candidiasis, characterized by infections occurring four or more times per year, is also caused by *C. albicans*, but up to 20% may be caused by *Candida glabrata* and other non-albicans *Candida* species.

Vulvovaginal candidiasis is typically characterized by vaginal itching, irritation, and discharge and may be associated with dysuria and dyspareunia. Examination reveals vulvar edema and excoriation, with thick, white, curdy vaginal discharge. Diagnostic testing involves a saline or 10% KOH wet mount of the discharge showing yeast, hyphae, or pseudohyphae (**Figure 17**). Women with negative wet mount results but signs and symptoms of candidiasis should have vaginal cultures for *Candida* performed and should be treated if results are positive. If cultures cannot be performed, empiric treatment is recommended.

Asymptomatic patients should not receive treatment. See Table 69 for treatment options of symptomatic uncomplicated and complicated vulvovaginal candidiasis. Recurrent symptoms after treatment warrant an evaluation for the presence of underlying predisposing factors. No evidence supports treatment of sexual partners of patients with vulvovaginal candidiasis.

## Trichomoniasis

Trichomoniasis is a vaginal infection caused by *Trichomonas vaginalis*, a flagellated protozoan. It is a common STI, with a high prevalence among patients in STI clinics and incarcerated individuals. It is associated with increased risk for preterm labor in pregnancy as well as increased risk for HIV transmission.

Women may be asymptomatic or present with copious vaginal discharge that is malodorous, pale yellow or gray, frothy, and associated with vulval itching and burning. Vaginal pH is often elevated but is not helpful diagnostically. Testing may include microscopy, nucleic acid amplification testing (NAAT),

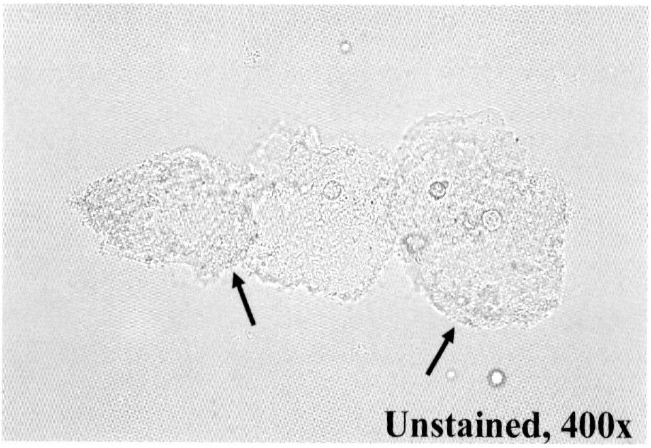

**Unstained, 400x**

**FIGURE 16.** Clue cells are vaginal epithelial cells whose surface is studded with adherent coccobacilli bacteria (*arrows*), often obscuring the border of the epithelial cells; they are characteristic of bacterial vaginosis.

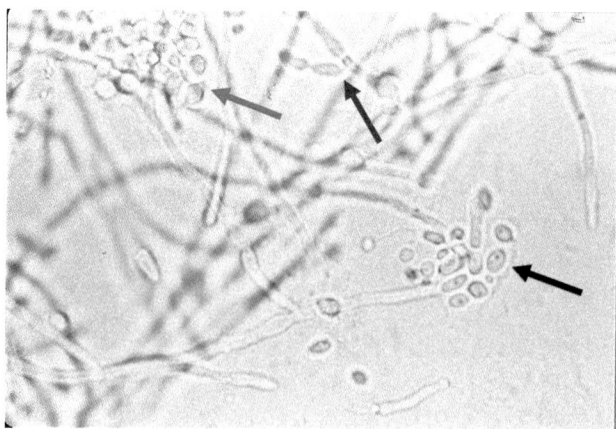

**FIGURE 17.** *Candida* vaginitis showing budding yeast (*blue arrow*), spores (*black arrow*), and elongated spores appearing as pseudohyphae (*red arrow*) with potassium hydroxide.

rapid antigen testing, and culture; choice of diagnostic testing is largely driven by availability. Microscopy with examination of a wet mount of the vaginal fluid showing motile trichomonads can establish the diagnosis when positive, but false-negative test results are common. NAAT or rapid antigen testing may be used as the primary diagnostic test or if the suspicion of trichomoniasis is high but the wet mount result is negative. When *Trichomonas* is identified, testing for other STIs should be considered. See Table 69 for treatment of trichomoniasis. Women should be retested within 3 months of treatment. Treatment of sexual partners is recommended to prevent reinfection.

**KEY POINTS**

HVC  • Clinical findings do not sufficiently distinguish between the common causes of vaginitis, and laboratory testing is necessary to establish a diagnosis.

HVC  • Clinical diagnosis of bacterial vaginosis includes the presence of at least three of four features: vaginal pH greater than 4.5, thin and homogeneous vaginal discharge, a positive whiff test result, and at least 20% clue cells on saline wet mount preparation.

• Diagnostic testing for vulvovaginal candidiasis involves a saline or 10% potassium hydroxide wet mount of the discharge showing yeast, hyphae, or pseudohyphae.

• Testing for trichomoniasis may include microscopy, nucleic acid amplification testing, rapid antigen testing, and culture; choice of diagnostic testing is largely driven by availability.

# Eye Disorders

## Eye Emergencies

Acute vision loss requires immediate ophthalmology evaluation. Selected conditions that can cause acute vision loss are listed in **Table 70**.

Trauma or chemical injury to the globe, eyelid, or nasolacrimal system also warrants urgent evaluation by an ophthalmologist. Patients with chemical injury to the eye should immediately receive eye irrigation to neutralize the ocular surface while awaiting ophthalmologic evaluation.

Vision-threatening eye infections requiring immediate intravenous antibiotics and ophthalmology evaluation include endophthalmitis (particularly bacterial infection of the aqueous and vitreous humors) and orbital cellulitis (infection of the fat and muscle cells of the orbit). Periorbital and preseptal cellulitis (infection anterior to the orbital septum) are less of a threat to sight.

**KEY POINT**

• Eye emergencies requiring immediate ophthalmology evaluation include acute vision loss; trauma or chemical injury to the globe, eyelid, or nasolacrimal system; and vision-threatening eye infections.

**TABLE 70. Selected Conditions Requiring Immediate Ophthalmologic Evaluation**

| |
|---|
| Acute angle-closure glaucoma |
| Central retinal artery occlusion |
| Central retinal vein occlusion |
| Chemical injury |
| Corneal ulcers |
| Endophthalmitis |
| Keratitis |
| Optic neuritis |
| Orbital cellulitis |
| Retinal detachment |
| Scleritis |
| Trauma |
| Uveitis |

## Red Eye

Cardinal features of conditions that cause red eye are listed in **Table 71**.

### Conjunctivitis

Conjunctivitis is the most common cause of red eye and is categorized as infectious (viral [**Figure 18**], bacterial [**Figure 19**]) or noninfectious (irritants, allergic). Factors favoring a bacterial cause include glued eyes in the morning, redness completely obscuring the tarsal vessels, purulent discharge, a red eye observed at 20 feet, and occurrence in the winter or spring. Lack of discharge decreases the likelihood of a bacterial cause. Bacterial conjunctivitis is often caused by *Staphylococcus aureus* and usually resolves within a week; however, topical antimicrobial treatment (erythromycin ophthalmic 0.5% ointment, trimethoprim-polymyxin B ophthalmic ointment) shortens the duration of symptoms by up to 1.5 days. Topical fluoroquinolones (such as levofloxacin) are not first-line therapy for routine bacterial conjunctivitis; however, they are indicated for conjunctivitis in contact lens wearers because of the high incidence of *Pseudomonas* infection. The threshold to treat with antibiotics is lowered in health care workers; patients in health care facilities; or patients with immunocompromise, including those with diabetes mellitus. Treatment of viral conjunctivitis is supportive, including cold compresses. Patients with viral conjunctivitis are considered contagious for as long as the eye continues to tear and produce discharge, usually 3 to 7 days.

### Keratitis

Keratitis represents infection and inflammation of the cornea. It most commonly results from bacterial infection (especially with *Pseudomonas* species) in contact lens wearers or in those with herpes simplex virus infection. Keratitis is an ocular emergency and requires urgent ophthalmology evaluation.

| TABLE 71. | Cardinal Features of Conditions That Cause Red Eye | | | | |
|---|---|---|---|---|---|
| **Cause** | **Pain** | **Visual Symptoms** | **Examination Findings** | **Associated Systemic Conditions** | **Immediate Ophthalmologic Evaluation?** |
| Conjunctivitis | Irritation only; associated with discharge and crusting | None unless discharge clouds vision | Diffuse erythema of conjunctiva, also involving inner aspect of eyelids | Usually limited to eye | No |
| Keratitis | Present, often with foreign body sensation | Blurred vision | Corneal stromal infiltrates or, in the case of herpes, corneal dendritic branching; circumferential redness around the border of the sclera and cornea (ciliary flush) | Usually limited to the eye | Yes |
| Episcleritis | Minimal | None | Superficial redness of episcleral vessels and episclera; may be localized | Minority of patients have underlying disease (rheumatoid arthritis, inflammatory bowel disease) | No |
| Scleritis | Severe, often worse with eye movement; associated tearing and photophobia | Decreased vision; may be complete loss | Scleral edema with diffuse deep red/violaceous discoloration; globe tenderness | >50% with rheumatologic disease (rheumatoid arthritis, vasculitis) | Yes |
| Uveitis/iritis | None to moderate | Variable; may include floaters | Ciliary flush; hypopyon (suppurative fluid seen in the dependent portion of the anterior chamber) | Common; infection (HSV, CMV); inflammatory disorders (spondyloarthritis, sarcoidosis) | Yes |
| Subconjunctival hemorrhage | Mild or none | None | Discrete bright red confluent region without hyperemia | Spontaneous; anticoagulation; trauma; increased pressure (coughing) | No |

CMV = cytomegalovirus; HSV = herpes simplex virus.

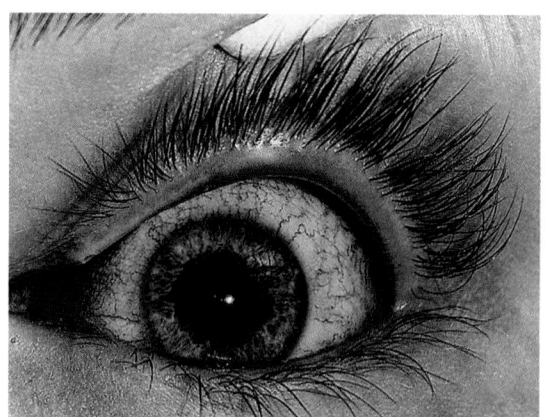

**FIGURE 18.** Diffuse conjunctival injection and erythema, usually with a watery or mucoserous discharge, are characteristic of viral conjunctivitis.

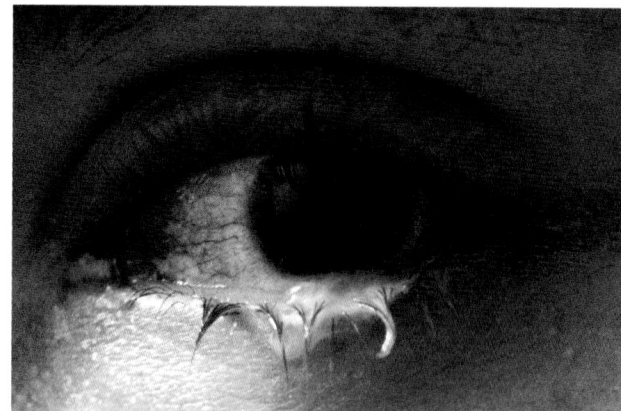

**FIGURE 19.** In patients with bacterial conjunctivitis, eye discharge is thick and may be yellow or green.

## Episcleritis and Scleritis

Episcleritis is a focal, acute area of inflammation involving the superficial layers of the episclera. It is usually self-limited, resolving in a few weeks. Treatment is symptomatic and includes artificial tears; anti-inflammatory agents, such as topical NSAIDs and glucocorticoids, may be needed.

Scleritis is an inflammatory disorder of the sclera, which lies beneath the episcleral and conjunctival layers (**Figure 20**). Scleritis is an acute threat to vision and requires urgent evaluation by an ophthalmologist.

## Uveitis

Anterior uveitis (iritis) is characterized by inflammation of the middle eye, including the iris, ciliary body, and choroid. In addition to pain, photophobia, vision impairment, and circumferential redness around the border of the sclera and cornea (ciliary flush), the pupil may have an irregular shape because it has become attached to the anterior surface of the lens or the posterior surface of the cornea. Uveitis requires urgent evaluation by an ophthalmologist.

## Subconjunctival Hemorrhage

Subconjunctival hemorrhage is common and not a threat to vision (**Figure 21**). When symptoms are present, warm compresses or ophthalmic lubricants may provide relief. Symptoms should resolve gradually but may recur in patients receiving anticoagulants.

## Blepharitis

Blepharitis is a common inflammatory condition of the eyelid margin and may be associated with rosacea. Treatment includes warm compresses, application of diluted shampoo

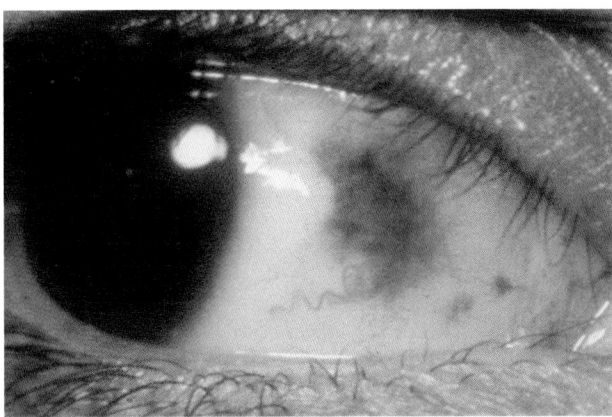

**FIGURE 21.** Subconjunctival hemorrhage is characterized by unilateral, localized, and sharply circumscribed redness without discharge or pain.

with a cotton-tip applicator, topical antibiotics (for staphylococcal infections), and oral tetracyclines (for infections associated with rosacea).

**KEY POINTS**

- Conjunctivitis is the most common cause of red eye and is associated with ocular irritation (not pain), discharge, and no impairment of vision.

- Keratitis is an ocular emergency that represents infection and inflammation of the cornea and is characterized by ocular redness, pain, and impaired vision.

- Episcleritis is a focal, acute area of typically asymptomatic inflammation involving the superficial layers of the episclera that is usually self-limited, whereas scleritis is a painful inflammatory disorder of the sclera associated with tearing and photophobia and is an acute threat to vision.

# Dry Eye

Dry eye (keratoconjunctivitis sicca) is a multifactorial inflammatory disorder involving the tears and ocular surface. Symptoms may include eye dryness, a sensation of a foreign body in the eye, blurred vision, and light sensitivity. Examination may show decreased tearing, malposition of the lids, conjunctival erythema, blepharitis, or reduced blink rate. Validated symptom questionnaires may be diagnostically helpful. Ophthalmologists can perform more specific lacrimal function testing. Treatment includes artificial tears, environmental strategies (for example, increased humidification), and topical cyclosporine. Oral omega-3 fatty acid supplements may alleviate the symptoms of dry eye syndrome.

**KEY POINT**

- Treatment of dry eye includes artificial tears, environmental strategies, and topical cyclosporine.

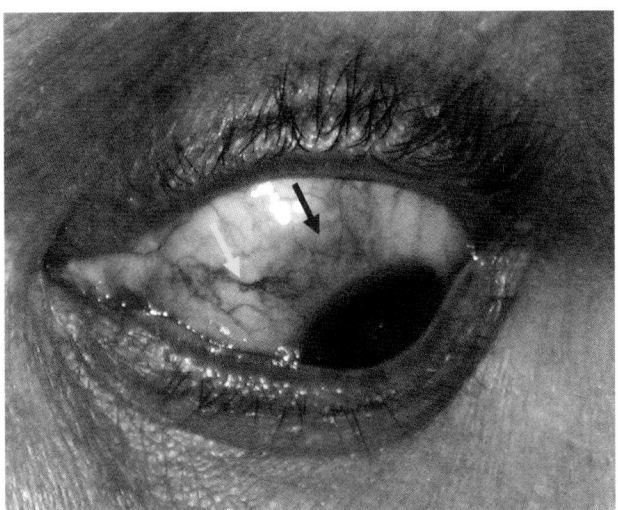

**FIGURE 20.** The cardinal sign of scleritis is edema of the sclera often associated with a violaceous discoloration of the globe (*red arrow*). Tenderness is invariably present. Typically, there is intense dilation of episcleral blood vessels (*yellow arrow*). Scleral inflammation may be focal or diffuse.

## Corneal Abrasion and Ulcer

Corneal abrasions are often caused by trauma from a foreign body. Pain, sensation of a foreign body, watery eyes, red eye, photophobia, and reactive miosis may be present. Corneal examination involves fluorescein dye and a Wood lamp or slit lamp. Management of uncomplicated abrasions includes topical NSAIDs. Current evidence does not support the use of topical antibiotics or eye patching. Topical anesthetics may decrease rate of healing and should be avoided. The presence of a corneal ulcer requires prompt evaluation by an ophthalmologist.

## Cataracts

Cataracts are opacifications of the lens and should be suspected in patients presenting with painless gradual worsening of visual acuity. Direct ophthalmoscopy shows lens opacification, a diminished red reflex, and obscured funduscopic examination. Surgery is indicated when vision impairment interferes with the patient's activities of daily living.

## Glaucoma

Glaucoma is the leading cause of permanent blindness in the world. It is typically characterized by increased intraocular pressure (IOP) as a result of decreased outflow of aqueous humor from the anterior chamber. However, according to the U.S. Preventive Services Task Force, there is insufficient evidence to recommend screening for glaucoma in adults.

### Primary Open-Angle Glaucoma

Primary open-angle glaucoma accounts for more than 80% of glaucoma cases in the United States. Increased resistance to aqueous outflow through the trabecular meshwork leads to increased IOP and vision loss through retinal cell death. Patients may present with bilateral peripheral visual loss that is gradual and painless. Funduscopic examination may demonstrate increased cup-to-disc ratio (CDR) (**Figure 22**), CDR asymmetry, and disc hemorrhage. Treatment is directed by an ophthalmologist and involves medications (topical prostaglandins, β-blockers, and α-adrenergic agonists) to decrease IOP and, when refractory, surgery.

### Angle-Closure Glaucoma

Angle-closure glaucoma is caused by mechanical obstruction of the aqueous humor drainage at the angle of the anterior chamber, leading to increased IOP. Blockage is usually secondary to the positioning of the lens on the iris; if blockage is present chronically, patients may be asymptomatic until advanced vision loss has occurred. Acute blockage may occur with exposure to sympathomimetic or anticholinergic medications or with pupillary dilation.

Patients with acute blockage present with severe eye pain, headache, nausea, and blurred vision or halos around lights.

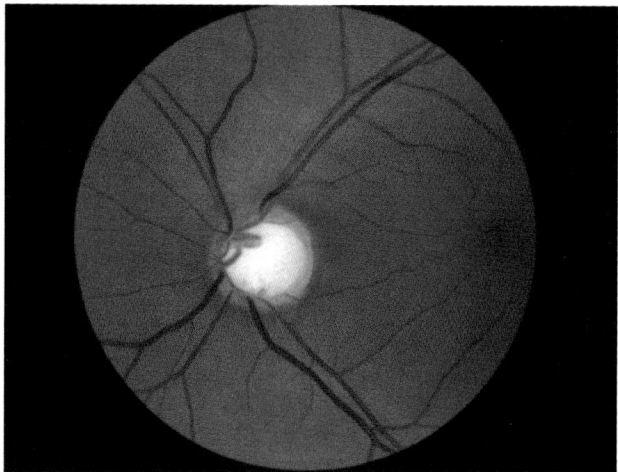

**FIGURE 22.** A relatively large cup-to-disc ratio and cupping identified by the disappearance of vessels over the edge of the attenuated optic rim are characteristic of glaucoma.

Examination may demonstrate severe conjunctive hyperemia, corneal edema, a mid-dilated (4-6 mm) nonreactive pupil, and severe elevation in IOP. Because of the immediate threat to vision, urgent evaluation by an ophthalmologist is required. ⊞

**KEY POINTS**

- Primary open-angle glaucoma is characterized by increased intraocular pressure, increased cup-to-disc ratio (CDR), CDR asymmetry, and bilateral peripheral visual loss that is gradual and painless.

- Patients with acute angle-closure glaucoma present with severe eye pain, headache, nausea, and blurred vision or halos around lights, and examination may demonstrate severe conjunctive hyperemia, corneal edema, a mid-dilated (4-6 mm) nonreactive pupil, and severe elevation in intraocular pressure; urgent evaluation by an ophthalmologist is required because of the immediate threat to vision.

## Age-Related Macular Degeneration

Age-related macular degeneration (AMD) is a progressive chronic disease involving the central retina. Patients with early AMD are often asymptomatic, although yellow drusen may be visible underneath retinal pigment epithelium (**Figure 23**). Patients with atrophic (dry) AMD, which accounts for 80% to 90% of AMD cases, note slowly progressive vision loss over years. About 10% to 20% of patients with atrophic AMD progress to neovascular (wet) AMD, which often presents with more rapid visual loss and may be accompanied by a sudden worsening of central vision associated with straight-line distortion (metamorphopsia), scotoma, or both.

Smoking cessation decreases the risk for developing AMD and should be recommended to all patients who smoke. There

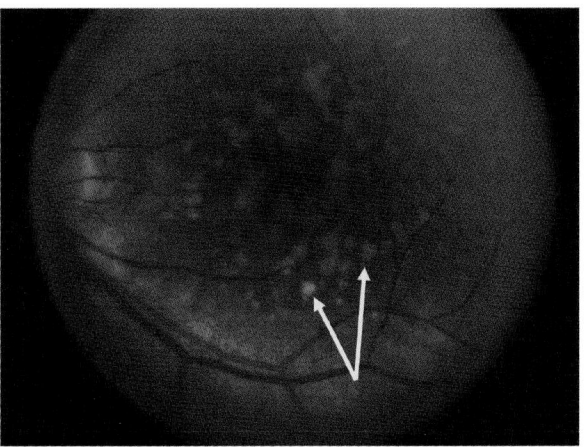

**FIGURE 23.** Atrophic (dry) age-related macular degeneration showing distinct yellow-white lesions called drusen (*arrows*) surrounding the macular area and areas of pigment mottling.

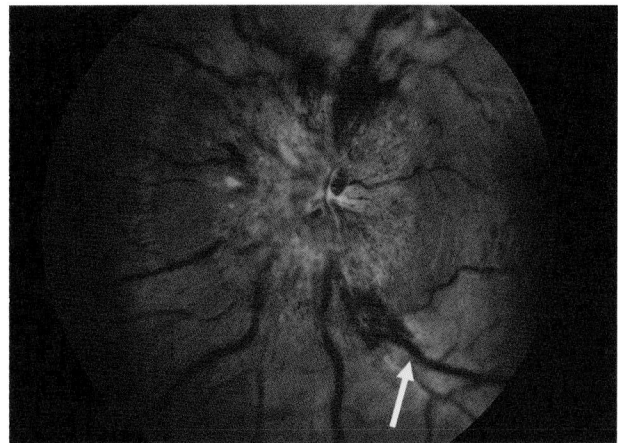

**FIGURE 24.** Optic nerve papillitis is characterized by hyperemia and swelling of the disc, blurring of disc margins, and distended veins (*arrow*). The normal arteriole-to-venous ratio is approximately 4:5.

is no cure for atrophic AMD; however, dietary supplementation with high-dose antioxidants, vitamins, and zinc can delay the progression of AMD. First-line treatment for neovascular AMD is anti–vascular endothelial growth factor (VEGF) therapies. The treatment burden of the intravitreal injections, however, is high, and the long-term risk for systemic absorption of VEGF inhibitors is unknown.

**KEY POINT**

HVC
- Smoking cessation decreases the risk for age-related macular degeneration and should be recommended to all patients who smoke.

## Optic Neuritis

Optic neuritis is characterized by inflammation and demyelination of the optic nerve. Usually unilateral in onset, it presents with visual loss occurring over hours to days. It is associated with acute pain, particularly with eye movement, as well as loss of color vision. Examination may demonstrate an afferent pupillary defect (paradoxical dilation of the affected pupil when the examining light is rapidly shifted from the unaffected to the affected eye); papillitis (swollen disc with blurred margin) may be seen on funduscopy in one third of patients (**Figure 24**). Two thirds of patients will have retrobulbar neuritis and a normal funduscopic examination. Urgent evaluation by an ophthalmologist is required. Although the diagnosis is clinical, MRI usually reveals demyelination of the optic nerve. Treatment with high-dose intravenous glucocorticoids improves the rate of visual recovery.

## Retinal Detachment

Patients with retinal detachment may present with a unilateral increase in floaters followed by a sudden, peripheral visual field defect that resembles a black curtain and may progress across the entire visual field. A retinal tear and elevation of the surrounding retina may be visible on dilated funduscopy. Immediate evaluation by an ophthalmologist is indicated for surgical treatment.

## Retinal Vascular Occlusion

### Retinal Artery Occlusion

Patients with central retinal artery occlusion present with acute, profound, and painless loss of monocular vision. It is most commonly associated with carotid artery atherosclerosis but may be associated with cardiogenic embolism, thrombophilia, or giant cell arteritis. Examination usually shows an afferent pupillary defect; funduscopic examination may show a "cherry red spot" at the fovea surrounded by retinal pallor. Emergent evaluation by an ophthalmologist is necessary.

### Retinal Vein Occlusion

Central retinal vein occlusion (CRVO) is usually associated with thrombus formation in the central retinal vein, whereas branch retinal vein occlusion (BRVO) appears related to compression of the branch vein by nearby crossing arterioles. Both are associated with cardiovascular risk factors, including hypertension, diabetes, and tobacco use. CRVO often presents with acute onset of painless blurred monocular vision. BRVO may be asymptomatic but may present with scotoma or focal field defects of blurriness corresponding to the area of retinal vein occlusion.

Examination may reveal an afferent pupillary defect (particularly in CRVO), retinal vein congestion, retinal hemorrhage, and cotton-wool spots (**Figure 25**). A patient whose presentation suggests CRVO requires immediate evaluation by an ophthalmologist.

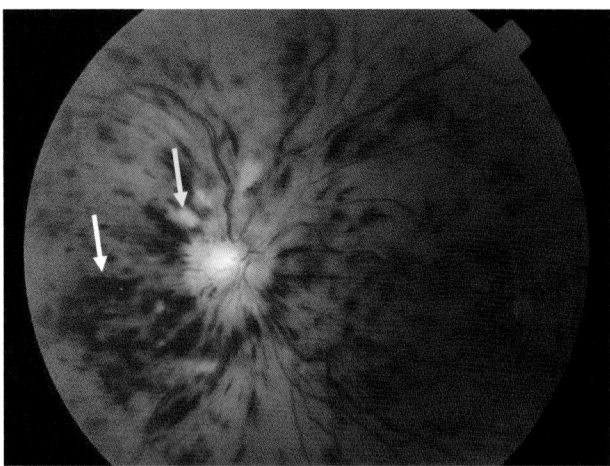

**FIGURE 25.** Central retinal vein occlusion is characterized by optic disc swelling, dilated and tortuous veins, as well as flame-shaped retinal hemorrhages (*white arrow*) and cotton-wool spots (*yellow arrow*) ("blood and thunder").

**KEY POINTS**

- Central retinal artery occlusion may present with acute, profound, and painless loss of monocular vision and is most commonly associated with carotid artery atherosclerosis.

*(Continued)*

**KEY POINTS** *(continued)*

- Central retinal vein occlusion is usually associated with thrombus formation in the central retinal vein and often presents with acute onset of painless blurred monocular vision; immediate evaluation by an ophthalmologist is required.

# Ear, Nose, Mouth, and Throat Disorders

## Hearing Loss

Hearing loss is common. It is associated with depression and functional decline but underrecognized by patients and physicians. The U.S. Preventive Services Task Force has concluded that there is insufficient evidence to assess the benefits and harms of screening for hearing loss in asymptomatic older adults.

Hearing loss is categorized according to the anatomic deficit: conductive, sensorineural, or mixed (**Table 72**). Conductive hearing loss is more often associated with pain or ear drainage, whereas sensorineural hearing loss is more often accompanied by tinnitus or vertigo.

| TABLE 72. Causes of Hearing Loss | |
|---|---|
| **Cause** | **Description** |
| **Conductive Hearing Loss**[a] | |
| Cerumen impaction | May completely obstruct ear canal |
| Otosclerosis | Associated with overgrowth of bone in the middle ear |
| Tympanic membrane perforation | Often heals without intervention |
| Cholesteatoma | Abnormal growth of keratinized squamous epithelium in the middle ear |
| **Sensorineural Hearing Loss**[b] | |
| Presbycusis | Age-related hearing loss; often symmetric, high-frequency loss |
| Sudden sensorineural hearing loss | Often idiopathic, more often unilateral |
| Meniere disease | Classically, triad of sensorineural hearing loss, tinnitus, and vertigo; not all are necessarily present at once, may fluctuate |
| Acoustic neuroma | Benign tumor of Schwann cell sheath surrounding vestibular or cochlear nerve |
| Noise | May be related to chronic noise exposure or sudden, short noise blast exposure |
| Ototoxic drugs | Antibiotics (aminoglycosides, erythromycin, vancomycin) |
| | Chemotherapeutic agents (cisplatin, carboplatin, vincristine) |
| | Loop diuretics |
| | Anti-inflammatory agents (aspirin, NSAIDs, quinine) |
| **Mixed or Causing Either Conductive or Sensorineural Hearing Loss** | |
| Infection | Labyrinthitis, otitis media, chronic otitis |
| Head trauma | May be caused by ossicular disruption leading to conductive hearing loss or by auditory nerve injury causing sensorineural hearing loss |

[a]Conductive hearing loss is inadequate mechanical transmission of sound through the tympanic membrane and ossicles of the middle ear.

[b]Sensorineural hearing loss is deficit or injury of the vestibulocochlear nerve.

Assessment of hearing may begin with asking the patient about perceived hearing loss (for example, "Do you have difficulty hearing?"). More formal screening can also be performed (**Table 73**).

In patients with hearing loss, physical examination should include otoscopic examination as well as the Weber and Rinne tests (**Table 74**), which can help differentiate sensorineural from conductive hearing loss. Referral to an audiologist is indicated when hearing loss is identified. Imaging (typically MRI) is rarely required unless the hearing loss is acute, unilateral, progressive, or associated with other neurologic changes. Patients should be evaluated urgently by an otolaryngologist when there is sudden sensorineural hearing loss, hearing loss with vertigo, or hearing loss associated with head trauma. Vertigo is discussed in Common Symptoms.

Treatment options for hearing loss include assistive listening devices, hearing aids, and cochlear implants. Treatment of sudden sensorineural hearing loss involves oral glucocorticoids, although strong evidence of efficacy is lacking.

**TABLE 73.** Screening Maneuvers to Assess Hearing

| Screening Maneuver | Technique |
|---|---|
| **Patient Self-Assessment** | |
| Single-item screening | Patient answers yes or no to the following question: "Do you feel you have hearing loss?" |
| Hearing Handicap Inventory for the Elderly-Screening Version | Patient answers 10-item question set, with options of yes, no, or sometimes. |
| **Clinician Examination** | |
| Finger rub test | The examiner gently rubs two fingers together at a distance of 15 cm (6 in) from patient's ear. A positive test result is failure to identify rub in more than two of six attempts. |
| Whispered voice test | The examiner stands an arm's length behind the patient and masks the untested ear by occluding the canal and rubbing the tragus. The examiner whispers six sets of three letter or number combinations. Failure to repeat at least three sets correctly is a positive test result. |
| Handheld audiometer | The examiner holds the device in the patient's ear while the patient indicates awareness of each tone. A positive test result is a failure to identify the 1000-Hz or 2000-Hz frequency in both ears or the 1000-Hz and 2000-Hz frequency in one ear. |

**TABLE 74.** Distinguishing Between Conductive and Sensorineural Hearing Loss With the Weber and Rinne Tests

| Condition | Weber Test[a] Result | Rinne Test[b] Result |
|---|---|---|
| Conductive hearing loss | Louder in the affected ear | Decreased in the affected ear (bone conduction > air conduction) |
| Sensorineural hearing loss | Louder in the unaffected ear | As loud or louder in the affected ear (air conduction > bone conduction) |

[a]A 256-Hz vibrating tuning fork (although a 512-Hz tuning fork may be used) is applied to the forehead or scalp at the midline, and the patient is asked if the sound is louder in one ear or the other; a normal test result shows no lateralization.

[b]A 512-Hz vibrating tuning fork is applied to the mastoid process of the affected ear until it is no longer heard. The fork is then repositioned outside of the external auditory canal, and the patient is asked if he or she can again hear the tuning fork; with a normal test result, air conduction is greater than bone conduction, and the tuning fork can be heard.

**KEY POINTS**

- Assessment of hearing may begin with asking the patient about perceived hearing loss (for example, "Do you have difficulty hearing?"). **HVC**

- Patients should be evaluated urgently by an otolaryngologist when there is sudden sensorineural hearing loss, hearing loss with vertigo, or hearing loss associated with head trauma.

# Tinnitus

Tinnitus is the conscious perception of an auditory sensation (for example, buzzing or ringing) without an external stimulus. Evaluation should include assessment for hearing loss and cardiovascular, cerebrovascular, and neurologic disease, including examination of the carotid arteries and temporal bone for bruits. Patients with unilateral tinnitus should undergo prompt audiologic assessment and, if hearing loss is confirmed, MRI to examine for acoustic neuroma. Patients should be evaluated urgently by an otolaryngologist when tinnitus is associated with sudden hearing loss, otorrhea, vestibular dysfunction, focal neurologic deficits, or pulsatile tinnitus (particularly if tinnitus is sudden in onset, which may suggest a vascular cause).

Treatment involves addressing the underlying condition. Medications have not been shown to be of benefit, but antidepressants may reduce associated distress. Cognitive behavioral therapy, relaxation therapy, and tinnitus retraining therapy may also be helpful.

**KEY POINT**

- Medications have not been shown to be of benefit for tinnitus, but antidepressants may reduce associated distress. **HVC**

# Otitis Media and Otitis Externa

Patients with acute otitis media have ear pain along with bulging or intense erythema of the tympanic membrane or new onset of otorrhea not associated with otitis externa. Few published studies guide management in adults. In children, guidelines suggest use of antibiotics when there is otorrhea or severe signs and symptoms (including moderate to severe otalgia lasting for >48 hours or temperature >39 °C [102.2 °F]). In milder cases, management may consist of observation first with antibiotics for worsening or persistent symptoms. An otolaryngologist should evaluate adults with recurrent acute or persistent otitis media with effusion.

Acute otitis externa is cellulitis of the ear canal with associated inflammation and edema. Bacterial infection, usually with *Pseudomonas* or *Staphylococcus aureus*, causes most cases (90%). Topical treatments, including antibiotics, glucocorticoids, antiseptics, and combination therapies, are first-line management for uncomplicated acute otitis externa; aminoglycosides should be avoided if tympanic membrane perforation is present or possible. Pseudomonal infections, especially in patients with diabetes mellitus, may be aggressive and result in spread to contiguous structures, including bone (malignant otitis externa); treatment requires systemic antipseudomonal antibiotics and urgent referral to an otolaryngologist.

**KEY POINT**

- Malignant otitis externa requires systemic antipseudomonal antibiotics and urgent referral to an otolaryngologist.

# Cerumen Impaction

Cerumen has protective, emollient, and bactericidal properties. However, its normal expulsion, assisted by jaw movement, is sometimes hindered, and cerumen accumulation may cause pain, itching, tinnitus, or hearing loss. When symptomatic, cerumen can be removed by irrigation, manual removal, or topical preparations. No topical agent has demonstrated superiority. Irrigation in the presence of a perforated tympanic membrane may cause vertiginous symptoms; mechanical removal is preferred in these instances.

# Upper Respiratory Tract Infection

## Sinusitis

Acute rhinosinusitis presents with nasal congestion, purulent nasal discharge, facial pain/pressure, fever, or cough. Most cases are caused by viruses, allergies, or irritants. It is usually self-limited; decongestants and mucolytics may alleviate symptoms. Avoidance of unnecessary antibiotics represents high value care. Indications for antibiotic treatment and regimens are described in **Table 75**. Patients who are seriously ill, deteriorate despite appropriate antibiotic therapy, or have recurrent episodes should be evaluated by an otolaryngologist.

Chronic sinusitis manifests with at least 12 weeks of nasal congestion with purulent drainage, diminished sense of smell, or facial pain/pressure. It may be associated with nasal polyposis (with a strong association with asthma). Demonstration

| TABLE 75. | Acute Sinusitis Treatment[a] | | |
|---|---|---|---|
| **Indications for Antibiotic Treatment** | **First-Line Therapy[b]** | **Penicillin Allergy** | |
| Persistent symptoms of >10 days' duration | Amoxicillin-clavulanate or amoxicillin | Doxycycline (adults only) | |
| Onset of severe symptoms or signs of high fever >39 °C (102.2 °F) with purulent nasal discharge or facial pain lasting for at least 3 consecutive days | | or | |
| | | Levofloxacin or moxifloxacin | |
| | | or | |
| Onset of worsening symptoms following a typical viral illness that lasted 5 days after initially improving ("double sickening") | | Clindamycin | |

[a]There is limited evidence to guide therapy, particularly in adults, and guidelines from major professional societies differ.

[b]Adjunctive therapy, such as intranasal saline irrigation or intranasal glucocorticoids, has been shown to alleviate symptoms and potentially decrease antibiotic use.

of mucosal involvement by nasal endoscopy or imaging (typically CT) is necessary for diagnosis. Treatment includes glucocorticoids and antibiotics.

## Rhinitis

Allergic rhinitis involves sneezing, congestion, and rhinorrhea often linked to a season or exposure. Nonallergic rhinitis occurs in response to nonallergic stimuli, such as spicy foods and irritants. First-line treatment of allergic and nonallergic rhinitis consists of avoiding precipitating factors and monotherapy with intranasal glucocorticoids (rather than an intranasal glucocorticoid in combination with an oral antihistamine or a leukotriene receptor antagonist). Rhinitis medicamentosa is chronic rhinitis resulting from the inappropriate long-term use of topical nasal decongestants. Treatment consists of cessation of the decongestant and intranasal glucocorticoids when needed.

## Pharyngitis

Pharyngitis presents as sore throat that may worsen with swallowing. Symptoms typically last less than 1 week. Features suggesting the more common viral cause include cough, conjunctivitis, coryza, hoarseness, and oral ulcers. Only 5% to 15% of pharyngitis cases are caused by bacteria, most often group A *Streptococcus pyogenes*. In these cases, appropriate antibiotic treatment reduces the risk for rheumatic fever, suppurative complications (such as peritonsillar or retropharyngeal abscess), duration of symptoms, and transmission. Patients with fewer than three of the four Centor criteria (fever by history, tonsillar exudates, tender anterior cervical lymphadenopathy, and absence of cough) do not need to be tested or treated for group A *Streptococcus*. These patients should be treated conservatively with symptom control (such as analgesics [NSAIDs or acetaminophen], lozenges or topical sprays, and increased environmental humidity). Patients with three or more Centor criteria should be tested by using a rapid antigen detection test. Throat culture should be considered in patients who are at high risk for complications (immunocompromised state) in the setting of high clinical suspicion but negative results on rapid antigen detection testing. Antibiotic treatment is reserved for patients with positive test results; penicillin and amoxicillin are first-line therapies.

*Fusobacterium necrophorum* infection can cause Lemierre syndrome, a rare suppurative complication of pharyngitis caused by local spread of infection with resultant septic thrombosis of the internal jugular vein. Clinicians should suspect Lemierre syndrome in patients with severe pharyngitis and neck pain that do not respond to appropriate antibiotics. Diagnosis is made with contrast CT of the neck. H

### KEY POINTS

**HVC** • Acute rhinosinusitis is usually caused by viruses, allergies, or irritants, and avoidance of unnecessary antibiotics represents high value care.

**HVC** • Patients with pharyngitis who present with fewer than three of the four Centor criteria do not need to be tested or treated for group A *Streptococcus* infection.

## Epistaxis

Ninety percent of epistaxis cases occur in the anterior nasal septum. Cases that occur in the posterior nasopharynx are more common in older patients. The history should include local trauma, nose picking, nasal medications, insufficient humidification, infection, drug use, and coagulopathies.

Anterior bleeds can be managed with compression for at least 15 minutes. Concomitant use of topical vasoconstrictors, such as oxymetazoline, may be useful. Refractory bleeding may require cautery or nasal packing and, rarely, embolization or surgical ligation. Posterior bleeds may cause substantial blood loss; most patients will require hospitalization and otolaryngology consultation. Patients with recurrent unilateral epistaxis should undergo CT or MRI imaging and nasal endoscopy.

### KEY POINT

• Anterior epistaxis can usually be managed with compression and concomitant administration of topical vasoconstrictors, such as oxymetazoline.

## Oral Health

### Oral Infection and Ulcers

Oral mucosal findings are discussed in MKSAP 18 Dermatology.

### Dental Infections

Dental infections may involve the gingiva, tooth, or supportive bony structures. Infection of the tooth is often asymptomatic

until the pulp cavity is involved, which leads to abscess. Abscess often necessitates root canal (removal of the diseased pulp).

Dental caries (**Figure 26**) is caused by bacteria that destroy enamel and dentin, resulting in tooth sensitivity or pain and stained pits and fissures on tooth surfaces. Caries may lead to odontogenic infection and tooth loss.

Periodontal infections are caused by bacteria in subgingival dental plaque, leading to gingivitis (inflamed gums) (**Figure 27**) or periodontitis (loss of supportive bone structure from chronic gingivitis). Chronic periodontal disease is associated with increased risk for cardiovascular disease. Fluoride and good dental hygiene are essential for prevention and treatment.

The presence of dental caries or periodontal disease should prompt dental consultation.

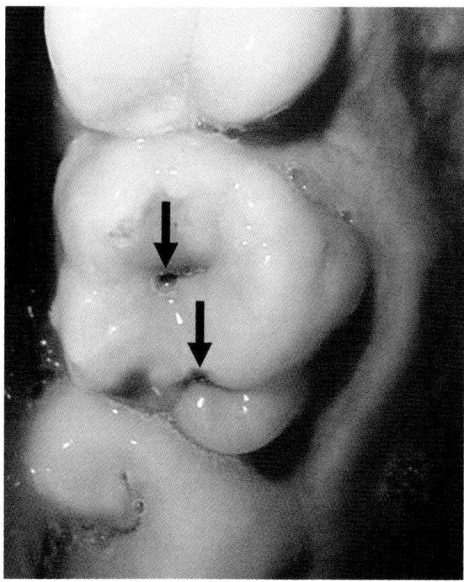

**FIGURE 26.** Dental caries (cavities or tooth decay) represents localized destruction of dental hard tissues and appears as black or brown spots on the surface of the tooth.

Modified from Nerval. Tooth with extensive evidence of dental carries. Digital image. https://commons.wikimedia.org/wiki/File:Toothdecay_(1).jpg. January 21, 2004. Accessed July 10, 2018. Licensed under the Creative Commons Attribution-ShareAlike 3.0 Unported (CC BY-SA 3.0) International License (https://creativecommons.org/licenses/by-sa/3.0/deed.en).

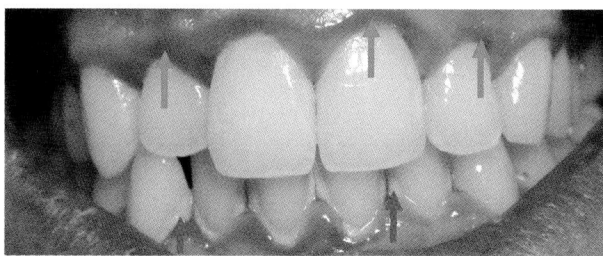

**FIGURE 27.** Red and swollen gingival tissue (*blue arrows*) that typically bleeds with brushing or flossing is characteristic of gingivitis. Also seen is abundant yellow dental plaque at the gum line and between teeth (*green arrows*).

Reproduced from Wikimedia Commons. Gingivitis before treatment. Digital image. https://commons.wikimedia.org/wiki/Category:Gingivitis#/media/File:Gingivitis-before.JPG. August 8, 2013. Accessed July 10, 2018.

# Mental and Behavioral Health

## Mood Disorders

Mood disorders are characterized by elevation or depression of mood associated with psychomotor, cognitive, and/or vegetative symptoms that cause significant functional impairment. The two main groups of mood disorders are depressive disorders and bipolar disorder.

### Depressive Disorders

The lifetime prevalence of depressive disorders in developed countries is approximately 20%, and women are affected almost twice as often as men. The peak onset is in the fifth decade of life, and incidence decreases in the elderly population. Depression is the leading cause of disability in the United States among individuals aged 15 to 44 years and is a major risk factor for suicide.

Depressive disorders most often initially present in the primary care setting but are underdiagnosed. Depressive symptoms are frequently encountered in patients with chronic medical disease either as a result of the illness itself (such as hypothyroidism) or as a response to the disability caused by the illness. Depression commonly accompanies many medical conditions, including cancer, neurologic diseases (Parkinson disease), heart failure, and HIV infection. Medications, including glucocorticoids and interferon, may also trigger depressive symptoms. Clinicians must exclude these potential causes of depressive symptoms during the evaluation of any patient for depression.

Screening for depression is underperformed, and the U.S. Preventive Services Task Force advises screening all patients for depression during primary care visits, with adequate systems in place to ensure accurate diagnosis, effective treatment, and appropriate follow-up. For such general-population screening, the PHQ-2 is effective and easy to use. If a patient provides a positive response to either of the two questions ("Over the past 2 weeks, have you felt down, depressed, or hopeless?" and "Over the past 2 weeks, have you felt little interest or pleasure in doing things?"), further investigation for depression is warranted.

### Diagnosis

#### Major Depressive Disorder

The DSM-5 criteria for diagnosis of major depressive disorder require at least five of the following symptoms (at least one of which must be depressed mood or anhedonia) during the same 2-week period:

- Depressed mood most of the day, almost every day
- Anhedonia (loss of interest or pleasure in nearly all activities), almost all the time
- Insomnia or hypersomnia almost every day
- Significant change in weight (gain or loss) or appetite (increase or decrease) nearly every day
- Fatigue or decreased energy nearly every day
- Psychomotor agitation or retardation almost every day
- Decreased ability to concentrate almost all the time
- Feelings of worthlessness or of excessive or inappropriate guilt nearly every day
- Recurrent thoughts of death or suicidal ideation (with or without a specific plan), or a suicide attempt

For a diagnosis of major depressive disorder, the symptoms cannot be attributable to a medical condition, medication, or substance use and must cause significant functional impairment. Clinicians must assess patients with depression for any history of elevated mood, which would suggest bipolar disorder; prescribing antidepressant monotherapy to a patient with bipolar disorder may precipitate a manic episode.

#### Persistent Depressive Disorder

Previously known as dysthymia, persistent depressive disorder is characterized by depressed mood most of the time for at least 2 years with at least two of the following symptoms while depressed: appetite change (increased or decreased), fatigue or low energy, decreased self-esteem, insomnia or hypersomnia, poor concentration, and feelings of hopelessness. These symptoms are milder than in major depressive disorder but still cause impairment of social or occupational functioning. Symptoms can temporarily resolve but do not abate for more than 2 months at a time.

#### Seasonal Affective Disorder

Seasonal affective disorder (SAD) is defined as major depressive disorder, mania, or hypomania with recurrent seasonal onset and resolution. SAD is not a separate diagnostic entity; rather, it is a subtype of each of these mood disorders (with the specifier "with seasonal pattern"). The most common form of SAD is major depressive disorder in which symptoms arise during autumn or winter and subside the following spring for at least 2 consecutive years (major depressive disorder with seasonal pattern). Seasonal episodes of depression substantially outnumber nonseasonal episodes. The diagnostic criteria are otherwise the same as for major depressive disorder.

#### Premenstrual Dysphoric Disorder

Premenstrual dysphoric disorder consists of symptoms of mood disturbance that develop the week before menses, remit within a week after menses, and occur with most menstrual cycles during a given year. Diagnosis requires the presence of at least one primary symptom: mood swings, irritability or anger, feelings of hopelessness or depressed mood, and anxiety. Additionally, a patient must have a total of at least five symptoms, which may also include appetite changes, decreased interest in usual activities, fatigue, difficulty concentrating, feelings of loss of control, sleep disturbance, and physical symptoms (breast tenderness, weight gain, bloating, myalgia).

## Peripartum Depression

Peripartum depression affects 7% of pregnant or postpartum women and is characterized as a major depressive disorder occurring during pregnancy or within 4 weeks after delivery. It is not considered a separate mood disorder; instead, it is a subtype of major depressive disorder with the specifier "with peripartum onset." Risk factors include previous depression, anxiety, low socioeconomic status, lack of social support, previous physical abuse, and unintended pregnancy. Treatment is similar to that used for other forms of depression but with close attention to drug safety in pregnancy and breastfeeding.

## Persistent Complex Bereavement Disorder

Grief is a normal response to interpersonal loss (such as death of a loved one) and may include symptoms of labile emotions, sadness, loneliness, and even fleeting hallucinations of deceased loved ones. The grief process varies, but most patients functionally adapt to loss within 12 months. Pathologic grieving persists longer and is accompanied by intense longing for and preoccupation with the deceased, along with feelings of emptiness and inability to live after the loss. This response to grief is termed "complicated grief," or "persistent complex bereavement disorder" (as proposed in DSM-5 as a future diagnostic classification). Up to 10% of bereaved patients develop persistent complex bereavement disorder, but the incidence is doubled in patients with other mood disorders. Other risk factors include older age, loss of a spouse or child, and sudden death of loved one. A major life loss can induce other mood disorders; therefore, clinicians should maintain a high index of suspicion for these disorders in the bereaved patient.

## Management

Most patients with major depressive disorder can be successfully managed in the primary care setting. Referral to a psychiatrist is indicated for patients with severe depression, failure of initial therapy, complex psychiatric comorbidities, and high suicide risk. Before initiating therapy, clinicians must assess medical comorbidities, other medical treatments, and substance use, which may contribute to depression. For initial acute therapy, a 2016 clinical practice guideline from the American College of Physicians recommends either cognitive behavioral therapy (CBT) or second-generation antidepressants (SGAs) after discussing treatment and side effects, cost, accessibility, and patient preferences. It is unclear whether combination therapy with both CBT and medication therapy is more efficacious than either treatment modality alone. Other psychologic therapies are available as second-line options (**Table 76**).

Four classes of SGAs are available: selective serotonin reuptake inhibitors (SSRIs), serotonin-norepinephrine reuptake inhibitors (SNRIs), serotonin modulators, and atypical antidepressants (**Table 77**). Drug selection should be based on side effect profiles and patient-specific characteristics. Side effects are common, and patient education regarding adverse effects can improve adherence. SSRIs are generally well tolerated but can cause reduced sexual desire,

**TABLE 76.** Common Psychological Interventions to Treat Depression

| Intervention | Description |
|---|---|
| Acceptance and commitment therapy | Uses mindfulness techniques to overcome negative thoughts and accept difficulties |
| Cognitive therapy | Helps patients correct false self-beliefs and negative thoughts |
| Cognitive behavioral therapy | Includes a behavioral component in cognitive therapy, such as activity scheduling and homework |
| Interpersonal therapy | Focuses on relationships and how to address issues related to them |
| Psychodynamic therapy | Focuses on conscious and unconscious feelings and experiences |
| Third-wave cognitive behavioral therapy | Targets thought processes to help persons with awareness and acceptance |

Reproduced with permission from Qaseem A, Barry MJ, Kansagara D; Clinical Guidelines Committee of the American College of Physicians. Nonpharmacologic versus pharmacologic treatment of adult patients with major depressive disorder: a clinical practice guideline from the American College of Physicians. Ann Intern Med. 2016;164:351. [PMID: 26857948] doi:10.7326/M15-2570. Copyright 2016, American College of Physicians.

anorgasmia, and delayed orgasm. Bupropion causes fewer sexual side effects but is contraindicated in patients with seizure disorders. SSRIs, SNRIs, bupropion, and monoamine oxidase inhibitors all have the potential to cause serotonin syndrome, particularly if used in combination or with other specific medications (including metoclopramide, tramadol, and linezolid).

After starting with a low dosage, the medication should be gradually titrated to achieve a clinical response while monitoring for adverse effects. Therapeutic response can be objectively measured with the PHQ-9 (https://www.integration.samhsa.gov/images/res/PHQ%20-%20Questions.pdf) by comparing scores before and during treatment. A decrease in the score of at least 50% indicates a response to treatment; a decrease to a score of less than 5 indicates remission. If initial monotherapy fails to achieve an adequate response within 6 to 12 weeks, potential next therapeutic steps are guided by the initial choice of therapy and the presence of any response. If a partial response occurs, increasing the dosage of the chosen medication or adding psychotherapy (if not already used) may be appropriate. If no response is seen, switching to another SGA or adding a second agent with or without psychotherapy is indicated. A second-line approach is the addition of an antipsychotic drug. FDA-approved antidepressant-antipsychotic combinations include olanzapine with fluoxetine and aripiprazole or quetiapine with any antidepressant. In cases of resistant depression, electroconvulsive therapy is also safe and effective.

Approximately half of patients who respond to appropriate initial therapy (CBT or SGA monotherapy) develop recurrent depression after 1 year without continued treatment. The American Psychiatric Association recommends continuation

| TABLE 77. | Dosages and Comparative Adverse Effects of Second-Generation Antidepressants | |
|---|---|---|
| **Drug** | **Dosage (mg/d)** | **Comparative or Drug-Specific Adverse Effects**[a] |
| **Selective serotonin reuptake inhibitors (SSRIs)** | | |
| Citalopram | 20-40 | Possible increased risk for QT interval prolongation and torsade de pointes (dosages >40 mg/d) |
| Escitalopram | 10-20 | N/A |
| Fluoxetine | 10-80 | Lowest rates of discontinuation syndrome compared with other SSRIs |
| Paroxetine | 20-60 | Highest rates of sexual dysfunction among SSRIs; higher rates of weight gain; highest rates of discontinuation syndrome |
| Sertraline | 50-200 | Higher incidence of diarrhea syndrome |
| Fluvoxamine | 40-120 | N/A |
| **Serotonin-norepinephrine reuptake inhibitors (SNRIs)** | | |
| Venlafaxine | 75-375 | Higher rates of nausea and vomiting; higher rates of discontinuations due to adverse events than SSRIs as a class; highest rates of discontinuation syndrome; duloxetine has lower rates of adverse events and discontinuation syndrome than other SNRIs |
| Venlafaxine XR | 75-225 | |
| Desvenlafaxine | 50-100 | Same as venlafaxine |
| Duloxetine | 60-120 | Same as venlafaxine |
| **Serotonin modulators** | | |
| Nefazodone | 200-600 | N/A |
| **Atypical antidepressants** | | |
| Bupropion | 200-450 | Lower rate of sexual adverse events than escitalopram, fluoxetine, paroxetine, and sertraline |
| Bupropion SR | 150-400 | |

N/A = not available; SR = sustained release; XR = extended release.

[a]Common adverse effects associated with second-generation antidepressants include constipation, diarrhea, dizziness, headache, insomnia, nausea, sexual adverse events, and somnolence.

Adapted with permission from Qaseem A, Barry MJ, Kansagara D; Clinical Guidelines Committee of the American College of Physicians. Nonpharmacologic versus pharmacologic treatment of adult patients with major depressive disorder: a clinical practice guideline from the American College of Physicians. Ann Intern Med. 2016;164:350-9. [PMID: 26857948] doi:10.7326/M15-2570. Copyright 2016, American College of Physicians.

therapy (treatment after resolution of a major depressive episode) for 4 to 9 months in patients who responded to acute therapy. The antidepressant dosage that was effective in acute treatment should be maintained in the continuation phase, and if psychotherapy was used, it should also be continued. Patients with three or more previous major depressive episodes, persistent depressive disorder, or residual depressive symptoms should receive long-term maintenance therapy at a similar dosage. When long-term drug therapy is not indicated or must be stopped for other reasons, antidepressant medications should be gradually tapered to avoid discontinuation syndrome. The most common symptoms associated with discontinuation syndrome are dizziness, fatigue, headache, and nausea typically occurring within 1 to 7 days of abruptly stopping or rapidly discontinuing antidepressants.

*Special Populations*

Persistent complex bereavement disorder may respond to both psychotherapy and pharmacologic therapy, which should be targeted to specific symptoms. SSRIs and SNRIs have demonstrated benefit in patients with depressive symptoms.

Premenstrual and peripartum depression are treated similarly to other forms of depression but with additional attention paid to drug safety during pregnancy. SSRIs and SNRIs are FDA pregnancy category C, except for paroxetine, which is category D. All antidepressant medications are safe with breastfeeding.

Major depressive disorder with seasonal pattern can be effectively treated with CBT and SGAs. However, daily exposure to 10,000 lux of visible light for 30 to 60 minutes is also beneficial.

Patients with concomitant pain syndromes may derive additional analgesic benefit from the use of SNRIs.

## Bipolar Disorder

Bipolar disorder is characterized by major depressive episodes and periods of mania or hypomania. The prevalence is 1% to 3%, and women are affected slightly more often than men. Onset typically occurs in early adulthood, and more than half of patients initially present with a major depressive episode. Bipolar disorder is the most expensive mental health problem and carries a high lifetime suicide risk.

Bipolar disorder is divided into two main categories: bipolar 1 and bipolar 2. Diagnosis of bipolar 1 disorder requires at least one episode of mania that is not explained by a medication effect, substance use, or a medical condition. DSM-5 defines mania as an episode of at least 7 consecutive days of irritable, expansive, or elevated mood that interferes with social or occupational functioning and has at least three of the following characteristics (four if the patient reports irritable mood only): inflated self-esteem (grandiosity), increased talkativeness, flight of ideas, distractibility, decreased sleep need, increased goal-directed activity, and excessive risk-taking behaviors (promiscuity, spending sprees). Most patients with bipolar 1 disorder also experience major depressive episodes, and many experience periods of hypomania. Hypomania is defined by the same criteria as mania except the duration is at least 4 consecutive days and symptoms do not cause severe functional impairment.

Patients with bipolar 2 disorder have periods of both hypomania and major depression but never mania. Cyclothymic disorder is a related disorder characterized by multiple episodes of hypomanic and depressive symptoms that do not meet criteria for hypomania or major depression.

Treatment of bipolar disorder should be directed by a psychiatrist. First-line medications include lithium, valproic acid, carbamazepine, and lamotrigine; psychotherapy plays an adjunctive role. Patients with acute mania typically require one of the aforementioned medications plus an atypical antipsychotic agent (aripiprazole, olanzapine, quetiapine). Severe bipolar depression may require a combination of first-line medications or adjunctive antidepressants (fluoxetine plus olanzapine). Quetiapine is also effective as monotherapy for bipolar depression.

### KEY POINTS

- HVC • The U.S. Preventive Services Task Force advises screening all patients for depression at primary care visits.

- HVC • For initial acute treatment of major depressive disorder, options include cognitive behavioral therapy or second-generation antidepressants after consideration and discussion of side effects, cost, accessibility, and patient preferences.

- • Peripartum depression may occur during pregnancy or within 4 weeks after delivery; treatment is similar to that for other forms of depression but with close attention paid to drug safety in pregnancy.

- • Referral to a psychiatrist is indicated for patients with severe depression, failure of initial therapy, complex psychiatric comorbidities, and high suicide risk.

- • Clinicians must assess patients with depression for any history of elevated mood, which would suggest bipolar disorder; prescribing antidepressant monotherapy to a patient with bipolar disorder may precipitate a manic episode.

# Anxiety Disorders

## Generalized Anxiety Disorder

Generalized anxiety disorder (GAD) is characterized by excessive anxiety about activities or events (occupation, school) that occurs more days than not for at least 6 months and causes significant distress or functional impairment. Patients with GAD typically worry more than expected about minor matters and recognize that this anxiety is difficult to control. DSM-5 diagnostic criteria also require that a patient have at least three of the following symptoms: restlessness, fatigue, irritability, muscle tension, sleep disturbance, or difficulty concentrating. Patients often have comorbid mood and anxiety disorders, including depression, panic disorder, and social anxiety disorder, and clinicians must investigate for other psychiatric illnesses as the source of symptoms. In addition, patients with GAD frequently report various other physical symptoms, including headaches, palpitations, dizziness, and chest and abdominal pain; these may be the presenting symptoms and often prompt evaluation for medical illness. The lifetime prevalence of GAD is 5% to 10%, and women are affected more often than men.

Patients with significant anxiety or multiple unexplained physical symptoms should be screened for GAD using the GAD-7 screening tool (http://www.adaa.org/sites/default/files/GAD-7_Anxiety-updated_0.pdf). The GAD-7 can also be useful for monitoring the severity of the illness during treatment. CBT and pharmacotherapy are equally effective in the treatment of GAD, but patients with comorbid mood disorders are best treated with a medication that targets their concomitant illnesses. SSRIs, SNRIs, buspirone, and tricyclic antidepressants are all effective in the treatment of GAD. SSRIs and SNRIs are preferred first-line drugs because they have fewer side effects than tricyclic antidepressants and effectively treat comorbid behavioral disorders (unlike buspirone). Benzodiazepines are useful for rapidly controlling severe symptoms, especially during initial treatment, while patients await CBT and/or titration of antidepressant dosage. However, benzodiazepines should be used only short term (<4-6 weeks) to avoid dependence and long-term side effects, such as impaired psychomotor performance and amnesia.

## Panic Disorder

Panic disorder is commonly encountered in the primary care setting and has a lifetime prevalence of 2%. Panic attacks are a key feature of panic disorder but are not pathognomonic; up to one third of all adults will experience a panic attack during their lifetimes. Depression and other anxiety disorders are frequent comorbidities with panic disorder.

Panic attacks are characterized by sudden onset and rapid escalation (within minutes) of extreme fear or anxiety along with at least four of the following: fear of dying, fear of losing control, palpitations, diaphoresis, tremor, dyspnea, sensation of choking, chest pain, nausea, dizziness, chills or heat sensations, paresthesia, and derealization (the perception that the perceived world is not real). DSM-5 diagnostic criteria for panic disorder include the following: (1) recurrent, unexpected panic attacks and (2) at least one attack followed by 1 or more months of persistent concern about additional panic attacks along with maladaptive behavior changes (for example, avoiding unfamiliar situations). The paroxysmal onset of dyspnea and chest pain may prompt significant medical evaluation. Rarely, panic attacks have a medical cause (hyperthyroidism, pheochromocytoma), and these diagnoses should be considered when other diagnostic findings suggest these conditions.

Treatment of panic disorder involves CBT, pharmacotherapy, or both. SSRIs and SNRIs are first-line medications because of their favorable side effect profile and efficacy. Short courses of benzodiazepines can be used for symptom control, but long-term use is discouraged. Treatment should be continued for at least 1 year after remission is achieved.

## Social Anxiety Disorder

Previously known as social phobia, social anxiety disorder is associated with excessive anxiety or fear of criticism or humiliation in social or performance situations. In these situations, patients with social anxiety disorder may experience palpitations, flushing, dyspnea, chest pain, or even panic attacks. To meet DSM-5 diagnostic criteria, these symptoms must be present for at least 6 months and cause significant functional impairment. Patients usually understand that their anxiety is excessive but continue to avoid social situations that trigger anxiety. Both CBT and pharmacotherapy with SSRIs and SNRIs are effective for treatment of social anxiety disorder. For patients with social anxiety disorder restricted to performance situations, CBT is preferred.

## Posttraumatic Stress Disorder

Posttraumatic stress disorder (PTSD) is an increasingly recognized anxiety disorder triggered by at least one of the following: direct experience of or witnessing a traumatic situation, learning that a loved one experienced a violent or accidental event, or repeated or excessive exposure to details of a traumatic event (for example, a social worker repeatedly exposed to cases of child abuse). Diagnostic criteria for PTSD also include at least 1 month of intrusive memories of the event (nightmares or flashbacks), avoidance of reminders of the event, adverse changes in cognition or mood related to the event (impaired memory of the event, generalized distrust, anhedonia), and significantly altered arousal and activity (irritability, hypervigilance, sleep disturbance, self-destructive behavior). Risk factors for development of PTSD include greater severity of trauma, poor social support, comorbid psychiatric illness, refugee status, and traumatic brain injury (particularly among military veterans). The symptoms of PTSD typically begin within 4 weeks of the traumatic event. Diagnosis can be challenging because of the patient's desire to avoid discussing the event and the frequency of concomitant psychiatric disorders, including depression, anxiety, substance use disorder, and personality disorders.

Treatment of PTSD generally requires psychotherapy from a specialist with experience in treating the disorder. Antidepressants, including SSRIs and SNRIs, are useful adjunctive therapies. Benzodiazepines are not effective and are not recommended because of the high prevalence of substance use disorders.

## Obsessive-Compulsive Disorder

Obsessive-compulsive disorder (OCD) has a lifetime prevalence of approximately 2% and often is accompanied by other mental health disorders. Patients with OCD experience obsessions (recurrent, intrusive thoughts, images, or impulses causing distress) and compulsions (repetitive behaviors [hand washing, counting] done to alleviate obsession-related anxiety). These behaviors cause significant functional impairment through wasted time and disrupted social interactions.

CBT is first-line treatment for OCD. CBT is more effective than pharmacotherapy alone, but SSRIs may be beneficial as adjunct therapy in patients with severe symptoms or inadequate response to CBT. For patients treated with medication, the American Psychiatric Association recommends continued treatment for at least 1 to 2 years.

**KEY POINTS**

- Cognitive behavioral therapy and pharmacotherapy are equally effective in the treatment of generalized anxiety disorder, but patients with comorbid mood disorders are best treated with a medication that targets their concomitant illnesses. **HVC**

- Cognitive behavioral therapy and pharmacotherapy with selective serotonin reuptake inhibitors and serotonin-norepinephrine reuptake inhibitors are effective for treatment of social anxiety disorder and panic disorder.

- Risk factors for development of posttraumatic stress disorder include greater severity of trauma, poor social support, comorbid psychiatric illness, refugee status, and traumatic brain injury (particularly among military veterans); treatment generally requires psychotherapy from a specialist.

- Cognitive behavioral therapy is first-line treatment for obsessive-compulsive disorder. **HVC**

# Substance Use Disorders
## Tobacco

Tobacco use remains the most common cause of preventable death in the United States. It is implicated in the development of multiple malignancies, pulmonary diseases, and cardiovascular conditions, and all-cause mortality is three to five times higher in smokers than nonsmokers. Tobacco use has been associated with an increased risk for several cancers, reproductive disorders, peptic ulcer disease, osteoporosis, certain pulmonary infections, diabetes mellitus, and age-related macular degeneration. The benefits of quitting tobacco use begin immediately, and over decades, risks for many of the associated conditions decrease substantially.

The U.S. Preventive Services Task Force recommends that clinicians ask all adults about tobacco use, advise them to stop using tobacco, and provide behavioral interventions and approved pharmacotherapy to adult tobacco users (**Table 78**). Abrupt cessation of tobacco use may result in higher long-term abstinence rates than gradually decreasing use. Combining behavioral counseling with pharmacotherapy is more effective than either modality alone. Effective counseling and behavioral resources include problem-solving guidance (such as developing a quit plan and overcoming barriers), motivational interviewing, social support, and telephone quit lines. There is a dose-response relationship between the intensity and frequency of counseling and quit rates, which seem to plateau after 90 minutes of total counseling.

All smokers without contraindications should additionally receive at least one of seven FDA-approved treatments for smoking cessation (**Table 79**). Varenicline is superior to single forms of nicotine replacement therapy and bupropion; combining more than one type of nicotine replacement therapy (short-acting and long-acting) is more effective than monotherapy.

Although tobacco use has decreased overall in the United States, increasing use of electronic nicotine delivery systems (also known as e-cigarettes and vaping), particularly among young people, is creating new health concerns because their long-term health risks are not yet fully understood. Although e-cigarettes may have a benefit of harm reduction for established smokers, the nicotine-containing aerosol also includes other chemicals (such as formaldehyde, propylene glycol, and heavy metals), which may be harmful. Use of e-cigarettes may also act as a "gateway" for young people, leading toward smoking more traditional tobacco products. The National Academy of Sciences has concluded that e-cigarettes are not without biological effects, including dependence, although not to the extent of combustible tobacco cigarettes. The implications for long-term effects on morbidity and mortality remain unclear.

## Alcohol

Unhealthy alcohol use is the third leading cause of preventable death in the United States. Individuals with disordered alcohol use often interact with the health care system but rarely receive appropriate treatment. The U.S. Preventive Services Task Force recommends routine screening for unhealthy alcohol use. Recommended screening tools include the Alcohol Use Disorders Identification Test (AUDIT) (available at https://pubs.niaaa.nih.gov/publications/Audit.pdf), the abbreviated AUDIT-Consumption (AUDIT-C) (available at https://www.integration.samhsa.gov/images/res/tool_auditc.pdf), and the single-question screen "How many times in the past year have you had five [four for women and adults older than age 65 years] or more drinks in 1 day?" (see Routine Care of the Healthy Patient).

Patients with a positive screening result should be assessed for the presence of an alcohol use disorder, the severity of the disorder, and related health consequences, including hepatic, cardiac, and neurologic sequelae. Comorbid psychiatric, chronic pain, and substance use disorders are often present and complicate treatment. Treatment should be tailored to the risk level (**Table 80**).

For patients with at-risk or harmful drinking behavior, brief (6-15 minutes) multicontact behavioral counseling has the best evidence for reducing episodes of heavy drinking and weekly alcohol consumption and improving adherence to recommended drinking levels.

Patients diagnosed with alcohol use disorder often require a multipronged approach with both psychotherapy and medication to ensure safety and minimize relapse. Psychotherapeutic interventions are a key component of effective treatment and may include CBT or 12-step facilitation. Pharmacotherapy for relapse prevention should be considered; naltrexone and acamprosate are the most effective medications (**Table 81**). Naltrexone is preferred because some studies have demonstrated acamprosate to be no more effective than placebo. When at-risk patients do not respond to brief interventions or when patients with alcohol use disorder do not respond to office-based therapies, they should be referred to addiction specialists.

Alcohol withdrawal is a common complication of alcohol use disorder. Alcoholic hallucinosis (hallucinations without clouding of the sensorium) and withdrawal seizures are typically seen within 24 to 48 hours of cessation of alcohol use and are treated expectantly, although a significant percentage of patients will progress to severe withdrawal (delirium tremens). Delirium tremens usually has onset at least 48 hours after the last drink and manifests as autonomic activation (hypertension, tachycardia, fever) and altered mental status. It

| TABLE 78. Tobacco Cessation: The 5 As |
|---|
| ASK about tobacco use at every encounter |
|   Identify and document tobacco use |
|   Consider systematic process (such as asking about tobacco use when taking vital signs) |
| ADVISE patients to quit tobacco use |
|   Strong, clear, personalized message |
| ASSESS willingness to quit |
|   Not everyone is ready to try to quit |
|   If not ready, offer motivational counseling |
| ASSIST in quitting |
|   Set a quit date |
|   Behavioral changes: alternatives, skills |
|   Pharmacotherapy |
|   Support: environment, triggers |
| ARRANGE follow-up |
|   In person, telephone, electronic |
|   Monitor progress, side effects, withdrawal |

**TABLE 79.** Approved Tobacco Treatment Medications

| Product | Advantages | Disadvantages | Precautions | Side Effects |
|---|---|---|---|---|
| **Long-Acting** | | | | |
| Nicotine patch | Place and forget; over the counter; can decrease morning cravings if worn at night | Passive—no action to take when craving occurs | Caution within 2 wk of cardiac event[a] | Skin reaction (50% of patients), vivid dreams or sleep disturbances |
| Bupropion SR (twice daily) and XL (once daily) | Less weight gain while using; antidepressant benefit | Side effects not uncommon; passive—no action to take with cravings; prescription required | Do not use with seizure disorders, current use of bupropion or MAO inhibitors, electrolyte abnormalities, eating disorders; monitor blood pressure | Insomnia (40%), dry mouth, headache, anxiety, rash |
| Varenicline | Reduces withdrawal and may prevent relapse | Passive—no action to take with cravings; prescription required | Avoid with severe kidney disease; evaluate for mental illness and monitor mood | Nausea (30%), insomnia, neuropsychiatric effects (e.g., depression, suicidal ideation)[b] |
| **Short-Acting** | | | | |
| Nicotine gum | Use as needed; can self-dose; over the counter | Difficult to chew, poor taste | Caution within 2 wk of cardiac event[a] | Jaw pain; nausea if swallowing saliva |
| Nicotine inhaler | Use as needed; mimics hand–mouth behavior | Costly, visible; requires prescription | Caution within 2 wk of cardiac event[a] | Cough, throat irritation |
| Nicotine nasal spray | Use as needed; rapid relief of symptoms | Costly, visible; requires prescription | Caution with asthma, nasal/sinus problems; caution within 2 wk cardiac event[a] | Nasal irritation; possible dependence |
| Nicotine lozenge | Ease of use; over the counter; flexible dosing | Slightly more costly than gum | Caution within 2 wk of cardiac event[a] | Hiccups, nausea, heartburn |

MAO = monoamine oxidase; SR = sustained release; XL = extended release.

[a]Recent myocardial infarction, severe angina, life-threatening arrhythmia.

[b]Postmarketing adverse effect not confirmed in more controlled studies. FDA "black box" warning removed in 2016.

Adapted with permission from Patel MS, Steinberg MB. In the clinic. Smoking cessation. Ann Intern Med. 2016;164:ITC33-ITC48. [PMID: 26926702] doi:10.7326/AITC201603010. Copyright 2016, American College of Physicians.

**TABLE 80.** Definitions for Alcohol Use Classifications

| Category | Definition | Health Consequences |
|---|---|---|
| Moderate or lower-risk alcohol use | No more than four drinks on a single day or 14 drinks per week for men; for men older than age 65 years and women, no more than three drinks on a single day or seven drinks in a week | Uncommon |
| Hazardous or at-risk drinking | When thresholds for lower-risk alcohol use are exceeded | Increased risk for alcohol-related consequences |
| Harmful alcohol use | Pattern of drinking that causes health consequences | |
| Alcohol use disorder | When individual meets at least 2 of the 11 DSM-5 criteria | Patients with moderate to severe alcohol use disorder (more than three criteria met) may benefit from more intensive treatment |

is often preceded by mild symptoms of withdrawal or withdrawal seizures.

CONT.

Many patients with alcohol withdrawal require hospitalization, although some low-risk patients can be safely managed in the outpatient setting. Benzodiazepines are the safest and most effective method to manage withdrawal. After initial dosing to acutely control symptoms, a symptom-triggered approach using standardized instruments, such as the Clinical Institute Withdrawal Assessment for Alcohol, Revised (CIWA-Ar), should be used to measure the severity of withdrawal and guide treatment. Phenobarbital, propofol, and dexmedetomidine may be useful in refractory cases. **H**

## Drugs

Use of illicit drugs occurs in 9% of the U.S. population. The most commonly used drugs are marijuana, prescription drugs, cocaine, hallucinogens, inhalants, and heroin. Although the evidence base does not currently support screening and brief intervention for drug use, a single-item screening question ("How many times in the past year have you used an illegal drug or used prescription medications for nonmedical reasons?") may be helpful in routine care or when the history, physical

**TABLE 81.** Pharmacotherapy for Patients With an Alcohol Use Disorder

| Medication (Typical Dosage)ᵃ | Indication | Mechanism | Side Effects | Notes |
|---|---|---|---|---|
| **Benzodiazepines**<br><br>Symptom-triggered: chlordiazepoxide, 50-100 mg; diazepam, 10-20 mg; or lorazepam, 2-4 mg every 1-2 hours until symptoms subside | Treatment or prophylaxis for alcohol withdrawal syndrome | Enhance GABA inhibition of neuronal excitability | Oversedation, paradoxical hyperactivity, depression<br><br>Addictive potential | Caution in patients with respiratory or hepatic impairment |
| **Naltrexone**<br><br>Oral, 50-100 mg daily<br><br>Injectable, 380 mg monthly | Relapse prevention | Opioid antagonist that may reduce the subjective reward associated with alcohol use | Nausea, indigestion, headache, fatigue<br><br>Depressive symptoms<br><br>Rarely, medication-associated hepatitis<br><br>Potential for precipitated opioid withdrawal with opioid use | Contraindicated with opioid use<br><br>Avoid in patients with decompensated cirrhosis; use with caution with hepatitis, compensated cirrhosis |
| **Acamprosate**<br><br>666 mg three times daily | Relapse prevention | May antagonize glutamate-mediated neuronal hyperexcitability and reduce prolonged (but not acute) withdrawal symptoms | Diarrhea, nausea/vomiting, myalgia, rash, dizziness, palpitations<br><br>Rarely associated with kidney impairment | Reduce dosage with kidney insufficiency<br><br>May be used with naltrexone<br><br>Medication adherence may be challenging |
| **Disulfiram**<br><br>250-500 mg daily | Prevention of drinking and relapse prevention | Aldehyde dehydrogenase inhibition results in acetaldehyde accumulation with alcohol use, leading to unpleasant symptoms (alcohol-disulfiram reaction) | Drowsiness, rash<br><br>Rarely, medication-associated severe hepatotoxicity, optic neuritis, peripheral neuropathy | Potential for many drug-drug interactions<br><br>Patient must be abstinent at least 12 hours before medication administration<br><br>Avoid in patients with hepatic impairment or cardiovascular disease<br><br>Most appropriate for patients with strong motivation to be abstinent and with support to promote medication adherence |

GABA = γ-aminobutyric acid.

ᵃNaltrexone, disulfiram, and acamprosate are all FDA pregnancy category C (animal studies indicate potential fetal risk or have not been conducted, and no or insufficient human studies have been done; drugs in this category should be used in pregnant or lactating women only when potential benefits justify potential risk to the fetus or infant). Benzodiazepines are category X (contraindicated in pregnancy) or D (positive evidence of risk).

Adapted with permission from Edelman EJ, Fiellin DA. In the clinic. Alcohol use. Ann Intern Med. 2016;164:ITC10. [PMID: 26747315] doi:10.7326/AITC201601050. Copyright 2016, American College of Physicians.

examination, or risk profile suggest drug use (see Routine Care of the Healthy Patient for discussion of other screening tools). Internists play a central role in prevention, diagnosis, and management of substance use disorders, including identifying and managing medical comorbidities and reducing harm.

Treatment primarily involves psychotherapeutic support. Internists may also play a role in harm reduction, ensuring that at-risk patients (such as injection drug users) receive appropriate vaccinations and referrals to needle exchange services.

Prescription opioid use has emerged as a major cause of morbidity and mortality, necessitating coordinated medical and policy responses (see Common Symptoms). The risk for

overdose is increased with higher doses and with concurrent benzodiazepine prescription. A notable study of trends in benzodiazepine use found that increased prescriptions and the mortality rate associated with overdose increased by a factor of five since 1996. Although nonfatal prescription opioid overdose presents an opportunity for intervention, most of these patients continued to receive opioids, and those receiving the highest dosage had the highest risk for repeated overdose. The nonmedical use of prescription opioids appears to be a strong risk factor for heroin use, although the transition to heroin occurs at a low rate and is influenced by cost and availability of drugs when it occurs.

Internists are increasingly treating opioid use disorder with pharmacotherapy in the office (**Table 82**). Most patients with opioid use disorder will require extended treatment consisting of both psychosocial support and medication-assisted treatment.

Intranasal naloxone is an important adjunct therapy in opioid use disorder, with evidence demonstrating a reduction in overdose death when used. Patients at risk for overdose, including those prescribed high-dose opioids for chronic pain (>50 morphine milligram equivalents per day) and those being

**TABLE 82.** Medical Treatment for Opioid Use Disorder

| Medication | Uses | Side Effects and Risks | Precautions | Notes |
|---|---|---|---|---|
| Methadone | Inpatient withdrawal management; maintenance | Sedation, prolongation of the QTc interval, nausea, constipation, weight gain, edema, amenorrhea, decreased bone density, decreased libido<br><br>Risk for respiratory depression and overdose | Prolonged, variable half-life with incomplete cross-tolerance with other opioids; requires low initiation dose and slow titration<br><br>Potential for drug interactions with inducers or inhibitors of P-450 system | U.S. schedule II<br><br>For outpatient addiction treatment, only available through state-licensed programs<br><br>For pain treatment, available from licensed prescribers |
| Buprenorphine-naloxone | Inpatient withdrawal management; maintenance | Nausea, constipation, headache, insomnia<br><br>Rarely associated with overdose, usually in combination with other sedating agents | Risk for precipitated opioid withdrawal if initiated too soon in opioid-tolerant patient after last use of full opioid agonist<br><br>May be less effective in severe liver disease due to increased bioavailability of naloxone; periodic monitoring of liver enzymes is recommended | U.S. schedule III<br><br>Requires federal waiver |
| Buprenorphine | Inpatient withdrawal management; maintenance, particularly for pregnant women | Nausea, constipation, headache, insomnia<br><br>Rarely associated with overdose, usually in combination with other sedating agents | Risk for precipitated opioid withdrawal if initiated too soon after last use of full opioid agonist<br><br>Periodic monitoring of liver enzymes is recommended | U.S. schedule III<br><br>Requires federal waiver<br><br>Once-monthly injection formulation approved in 2017 |
| Naltrexone | | | | |
| IM | Maintenance | Nausea, fatigue, dizziness, injection site reaction | Risk for precipitated withdrawal if taken soon after last opioid dose<br><br>Risk for overdose if dose is missed and patient relapses<br><br>Periodic monitoring of liver enzymes is recommended; impaired metabolism in liver disease | Some variability in length of time for full opioid blockade |
| Oral | Bridge before IM naltrexone; maintenance in highly supervised settings | Nausea, headache, dizziness, elevated aminotransferase levels | Periodic monitoring of liver enzymes is recommended; impaired metabolism in liver disease | |

IM = intramuscular; QTc = corrected QT interval.

Adapted with permission from Pace CA, Samet JH. In the clinic. Substance use disorders. Ann Intern Med. 2016;164:ITC58-ITC59. [PMID: 27043992] doi:10.7326/AITC201604050. Copyright 2016, American College of Physicians.

treated for or in recovery from opioid use disorders, should be offered naloxone. Friends and family members may also receive prescriptions and training in naloxone use.

**KEY POINTS**

HVC
- In tobacco cessation, combining behavioral counseling with pharmacotherapy is more effective than either modality alone, and combining more than one type of nicotine replacement therapy (short- and long-acting) is more effective than monotherapy.
- For patients with at-risk or harmful drinking behavior, brief (6-15 minutes) multicontact behavioral counseling has the best evidence for improving adherence to recommended drinking levels.
- Patients diagnosed with alcohol use disorder often require both psychotherapeutic and pharmacologic approaches to ensure safety and minimize relapse.
- Patients at risk for opioid overdose, including those prescribed high-dose opioids for chronic pain and those being treated for or in recovery from opioid use disorders, should be offered naloxone.
- Most patients with opioid use disorder will require extended treatment consisting of both psychosocial support and medication-assisted treatment.

# Personality Disorders

Personality disorders involve consistent patterns of interpersonal behavior and perceptions that are inflexible, diverge significantly from the behavioral standards of the person's culture, and cause substantial functional impairment and emotional distress. Development of these disorders usually occurs in adolescence, and the prevalence in the United States is estimated at 10% to 15%. Comorbid psychiatric illness is common. Three clusters of personality disorders are based on symptoms (**Table 83**).

Personality disorders add challenges to patient care and can serve as a substantial barrier to care. Physicians should have open, yet sensitive, discussion of the personality disorder diagnosis with the patient and emphasize the purpose of providing the best possible care. Such discussion may also make the patient more receptive to referral to a mental health professional. Establishing a relationship based on trust and clear boundaries can also help facilitate care. No pharmacotherapy specifically treats personality disorders, but medications may be used for improving specific symptoms (for example, mood stabilizers for impulsivity). Psychotherapy can help patients improve coping mechanisms.

# Somatic Symptom and Related Disorders

Previously known as somatoform disorders, somatic symptom and related disorders are characterized by medically

**TABLE 83.** Personality Disorders

**Cluster A: Odd or Eccentric Thinking and Behaviors**

Paranoid: pervasive distrust of others; unjustified suspicion of others; unjustified suspicions regarding their partners or spouses; overly hostile reactions to perceived insults

Schizoid: prefer to be alone and lack interest in relationships; seem indifferent, cold, and unresponsive to social cues; take pleasure in few activities

Schizotypal: manifest odd thinking, beliefs (e.g., their thoughts are magical and can influence others, events have hidden meaning), dress, and other behaviors

**Cluster B: Dramatic or Unpredictable Thinking and Behaviors, Emotional**

Antisocial: engage in behaviors such as lying, stealing, and other aggressive and violent behaviors; disregard others' feelings, rights, and safety; lack remorse for these behaviors; often experience recurrent legal problems

Borderline: have chaotic relationships (idealized and devalued) and a fragile self-image; fear abandonment; experience labile and intense emotions (e.g., anger), sense of emptiness; engage in impulsive and risky behaviors (e.g., gambling, sex); may manifest self-injury and suicidality

Histrionic: excessive emotionality and attention-seeking behavior; dramatic; often seductive or sexually provocative; melodramatic

Narcissistic: grandiose and inflated self-perceptions; desire attention

**Cluster C: Anxious and Fearful Thinking and Behaviors**

Avoidant: feel inadequate and are sensitive to criticism; extremely shy and socially inhibited and avoid activities that involve interactions with others, especially strangers

Dependent: excessively dependent on others ("clingy") and fear being alone; lack self-confidence and tolerate poor treatment by others

Obsessive-compulsive: perfectionistic and preoccupied with orderliness and rules; controlling of situations and others; rigid regarding values; not the same as obsessive-compulsive disorder, which is an anxiety disorder

Reproduced with permission from Schneider RK, Levenson JL. Psychiatry Essentials for Primary Care. Philadelphia: American College of Physicians, 2008.

unexplained symptoms causing emotional distress and psychosocial impairment. Prevalence is as high as 4%, and primary care is a common setting for presentation. Patients with these disorders have very high use of health care resources yet are dissatisfied with their care. Before diagnosing any of these disorders, clinicians should thoroughly evaluate for and optimize treatment of medical disease and other psychiatric disorders (such as depression and generalized anxiety). Many unexplained medical problems are related to unidentified organic pathology, and patients with known medical disease may have a concurrent somatic symptom or related disorder.

## Types

Somatic symptom disorder (previously called somatization disorder) is characterized by one or more somatic symptoms present for at least 6 months causing significant distress or interference with life and associated with excessive thoughts, behaviors, and feelings related to the symptoms. When the main symptom is pain, the specifier "with predominant pain" is applied (previously referred to as pain disorder).

Illness anxiety disorder (formerly known as hypochondriasis) is characterized by excessive concern about health and preoccupation with health-related activities (for example, measuring pulse). In contrast to somatic symptom disorder, no or only mild somatic symptoms are present in illness anxiety disorder.

Conversion disorder involves at least one symptom of neurologic dysfunction (abnormal sensation or motor function) that is unexplained by a medical condition and not consistent with examination findings. Conversion disorder does not represent fabrication of symptoms but rather unexplained symptoms that do not have a pathophysiologic basis. These symptoms, which are functionally limiting, occur during times of substantial physical, emotional, or psychological stress.

Somatic symptom and related disorders must be differentiated from factitious disorder and malingering. Factitious disorder is an intentional fabrication of symptoms or injury to oneself or another without clear external benefit. Malingering occurs when a patient feigns medical problems for gain; thus, malingering is not a psychiatric diagnosis.

## Management

Clinicians should acknowledge the patient's symptoms in somatic symptom and related disorders and focus on coping mechanisms and regularly scheduled visits. Diagnostic testing and referral to specialists should not be requested solely to provide reassurance. For somatic symptom disorder, CBT is effective for patients willing to undergo psychotherapy; antidepressant drugs also have demonstrated benefit. Illness anxiety disorder may respond to CBT, whereas disease education is the primary treatment for conversion disorder.

> **KEY POINT**
>
> HVC  • Clinicians should acknowledge the patient's symptoms in somatic symptom and related disorders and focus on coping mechanisms and regularly scheduled visits.

# Eating Disorders

## Types

Approximately 3% of the U.S. population has an eating disorder. Disorders most likely to be encountered by internists include anorexia nervosa, bulimia nervosa, and binge eating disorder.

Anorexia nervosa is characterized by restriction of caloric intake relative to requirements that leads to below-normal body weight and is also associated with fear of weight gain and a distorted body image. DSM-5 further divides the disorder by subtypes: restricting type (no episodes of food binges or purging) and binge eating/purging type. Women are affected three to four times more often than men, and onset most often occurs in adolescence.

In bulimia nervosa, patients engage in binge eating followed by compensatory behaviors to prevent weight gain, including self-induced vomiting, laxative abuse, fasting, and excessive exercise, at least once weekly for 3 months. Binge eating is defined as eating substantially more food than most people would consume within a period of time. The key difference between the binge eating/purging type of anorexia nervosa and bulimia nervosa is that patients with anorexia have significant weight loss. Similar to anorexia nervosa, patients with bulimia nervosa have a distorted body image. Prevalence is three times greater among women, and the median age at onset is 18 years.

Binge eating disorder is more common than anorexia and bulimia nervosa and is characterized by binge eating and feelings of loss of control that occur an average of at least once weekly for 3 months. Binging episodes include at least three of the following characteristics: abnormally rapid consumption, eating until uncomfortably full, consuming large amounts of food when not hungry, eating alone due to embarrassment, and feelings of guilt related to overconsumption. These characteristics distinguish binge eating disorder from overeating. The lack of compensatory behaviors to avoid weight gain differentiates binge eating disorder from bulimia nervosa. Concurrent psychiatric disease, including personality, mood, and substance use disorders, is common.

Clues to the presence of an eating disorder on physical examination include findings suggesting malnutrition (muscle wasting, xerosis, and lanugo) and/or self-induced vomiting (erosion of dental enamel, parotid gland enlargement, and scarring or calluses on the hand dorsum).

## Medical Complications

Multiple medical problems can develop in patients with anorexia nervosa as a result of malnutrition. Patients often exhibit signs of a hypometabolic state, including bradycardia, hypotension, hypothermia, and decreased gastrointestinal mobility. Electrolyte abnormalities (hypokalemia, hypomagnesemia, and hypophosphatemia) can cause dysrhythmia and contribute to increased mortality. Refeeding syndrome can worsen these electrolyte disturbances, and prevention requires gradual, carefully monitored increase of nutritional intake. Osteopenia and osteoporosis are common and may not be fully reversible if anorexia occurred during peak bone development in adolescence. Amenorrhea, anemia, and peripheral edema also occur frequently and usually resolve with recovery from anorexia nervosa.

Purging behaviors may also lead to electrolyte abnormalities. Additionally, upper gastrointestinal problems (esophagitis, esophageal tears) may develop from self-induced vomiting, and laxative abuse may cause colonic dysmotility.

## Treatment

The main goal of treatment is reestablishing normal weight and eating behaviors. Psychotherapy and monitored dietary intake are the mainstays of treatment for anorexia nervosa. In some circumstances, this may require hospitalization to ensure adequate emotional support, appropriate intake, and monitoring for refeeding syndrome. Antidepressant therapy has not proved effective in treating anorexia nervosa, although olanzapine may be considered for patients not responding to psychotherapy and nutritional interventions. CBT is the most effective intervention for bulimia nervosa and binge eating disorder; antidepressant therapy may be beneficial. Topiramate has also shown promise as an adjunctive therapy with CBT in patients with binge eating disorder. Bupropion should be avoided because of increased risk for seizures in patients with eating disorders.

**KEY POINTS**

HVC
- Psychotherapy and monitored dietary intake are the mainstays of treatment for anorexia nervosa; antidepressant therapy has not proved effective.

- Cognitive behavioral therapy is the most effective intervention for bulimia nervosa and binge eating disorder; antidepressant therapy and topiramate may also be beneficial.

## Schizophrenia

Schizophrenia is a heterogeneous psychiatric disorder composed of both positive symptoms (hallucinations, disorganized thought, and delusions) and negative symptoms (flattened affect, decreased activity). Worldwide prevalence is approximately 1%, with a slight male predominance. The pathogenesis of schizophrenia is unclear.

DSM-5 diagnostic criteria for schizophrenia require the presence at least two of the following: delusions, hallucinations, disorganized speech, disorganized or catatonic behavior, and negative symptoms. Diagnosis also requires at least one area of functional impairment (occupation, social interactions, or self-care) and duration of at least 6 months (including 1 month of active symptoms).

Schizophrenia is associated with an increased risk for diabetes, cardiovascular disease, and obesity, and these coexisting conditions may be exacerbated by the metabolic complications of antipsychotic therapy. Undertreatment of medical disease is also common in this population. Mortality is significantly increased in patients with schizophrenia due to these conditions along with concurrent behavioral disorders and substance use; approximately 5% of patients with schizophrenia commit suicide.

Schizophrenia is usually co-managed with a psychiatrist. Antipsychotic medications are highly effective at controlling positive symptoms of schizophrenia, but some degree of negative symptoms usually persists. Because the effectiveness of different antipsychotics is relatively similar, choice of therapy is based primarily on patient comorbidities and the adverse effect profile of medications. Typical or first-generation antipsychotic agents have a higher risk for extrapyramidal symptoms (parkinsonism, akathisia), tardive dyskinesia, and hyperprolactinemia than second-generation or atypical antipsychotic agents (**Table 84**). Some newer antipsychotic agents may also cause less sedation and anticholinergic side effects but carry an increased risk for weight gain and metabolic syndrome (particularly olanzapine and quetiapine). Clozapine may be particularly effective for refractory schizophrenia but is associated with significant adverse effects, including agranulocytosis. Close monitoring for common adverse effects is extremely important with use of any antipsychotic agent.

| **TABLE 84.** | Adverse Effects of Common Antipsychotic Medications | | | | | |
|---|---|---|---|---|---|---|
| **Medication** | **EPS** | **Elevated Prolactin** | **Anticholinergic Symptoms** | **Sedation** | **Weight Gain** | **Hyperlipidemia** |
| **First-Generation Antipsychotics** | | | | | | |
| Fluphenazine | ++ | ++ | +/– | + | + | + |
| Haloperidol | ++ | ++ | +/– | ++ | + | + |
| Thiothixene | ++ | ++ | + | + | ++ | – |
| Chlorpromazine | + | ++ | ++ | ++ | ++ | ++ |
| Thioridazine | + | ++ | ++ | ++ | ++ | – |
| **Second-Generation Antipsychotics** | | | | | | |
| Clozapine[a] | +/– | +/– | ++ | ++ | +++ | +++ |
| Risperidone | ++ | ++ | ++ | + | ++ | + |
| Olanzapine | + | + | + | ++ | +++ | +++ |
| Quetiapine | +/– | +/– | +/– | ++ | ++ | ++ |
| Aripiprazole | + | – | – | + | + | – |

EPS = extrapyramidal symptoms.

[a]Clozapine can also cause agranulocytosis and requires routine monitoring of blood counts.

- Mortality is significantly increased in patients with schizophrenia because of concurrent cardiovascular disease, behavioral disorders, and substance use; approximately 5% of patients with schizophrenia commit suicide.

- Antipsychotic medications are highly effective at controlling positive symptoms of schizophrenia, but some degree of negative symptoms usually persists; the effectiveness of different antipsychotic agents is relatively similar, and choice of therapy is based primarily on patient comorbidities and the adverse effect profile of medications.

# Attention-Deficit/Hyperactivity Disorder

Attention-deficit/hyperactivity disorder (ADHD) is characterized by persistent inattention and/or hyperactivity-impulsivity that disrupts functioning or development. Symptoms must interfere with at least two different settings (such as home and work), and some must be present since age 12 years. ADHD is most frequently recognized in childhood, but the diagnosis may be delayed until adulthood. Most patients diagnosed early in life continue to meet diagnostic criteria as adults. Common manifestations in adults include inattention, disorganization, distractibility, emotional dysregulation, and restlessness. The diagnosis is clinical, and rating scales may be useful; anxiety, mood, and substance use disorders should be considered in the differential diagnosis but may also exist concurrently.

Pharmacologic therapy is similar in adults and children, with stimulants (methylphenidate, amphetamine) as first-line therapy. Close monitoring for cardiovascular side effects (hypertension, arrhythmia) is necessary. Given the potential for abuse, these drugs should not be prescribed to patients with a history of substance use; atomoxetine may be preferred in such patients. Bupropion and tricyclic antidepressants are also beneficial in patients with contraindications to stimulants or with concurrent depression. CBT is beneficial alone or in combination with pharmacotherapy for improving executive functioning.

- For diagnosis of attention-deficit/hyperactivity disorder, symptoms must interfere with at least two different settings (such as home and work) and be present since age 12 years.

- Stimulants should not be prescribed to patients with a history of substance use; atomoxetine may be preferred in such patients.

# Autism Spectrum Disorder

Autism spectrum disorder (ASD) is a heterogeneous group of developmental disorders that feature repetitive behaviors and significant deficiencies in communication and social interaction. The exact prevalence is debated but ranges from 0.5% to 1%. Pathogenesis remains uncertain but is most likely genetic. Diagnosis requires that symptoms be present since early childhood; however, these may be masked until adulthood. Half of patients have intellectual disability, and many have concurrent seizure and sleep disorders. Early intervention with behavioral and educational interventions improves long-term functioning. Complementary therapies, including specialized diets and music therapy, are also commonly used but lack evidence of efficacy. Pharmacotherapy is reserved for targeted symptoms, such as melatonin for sleep disturbance. Even with intervention, most patients require lifelong assistance with functioning.

Clinicians should understand what communication methods a patient uses and incorporate caregivers into health care visits. Consistency in the health care team can prevent confusion and anxiety, and extra time should be allowed for explanation of procedures. Medical causes of acute behavioral changes should always be considered.

# Geriatric Medicine

## Comprehensive Geriatric Assessment

Comprehensive geriatric assessment is a multidisciplinary diagnostic process to ascertain the physical, cognitive, psychological, environmental, and functional capabilities of older persons in order to develop a plan for preserving function and maximizing independence and quality of life. Common health issues in older adults include impaired mobility and physical functioning, deficits in sensory function (particularly vision and hearing), and cognitive decline. Additionally, polypharmacy and the cumulative effects of chronic diseases may contribute to decreased functional status and loss of independence. Identifying these issues requires a systematic and multidimensional evaluation, which may be performed in the office, in the patient's home, or upon hospital admission or discharge. When completed in the home or in a dedicated inpatient geriatric unit, comprehensive geriatric assessment may reduce mortality and decrease the need for long-term institutional or nursing home placement.

### Functional Status

Functional status assessment is evaluation of a patient's ability to perform activities required for basic self-care (activities of daily living [ADLs]) or to live independently (instrumental activities of daily living [IADLs]). ADLs include bathing, grooming, dressing, toileting, feeding, walking, and transferring. IADLs comprise tasks such as managing finances, performing housework, shopping, self-administering medications, using transportation, preparing meals, and communicating by telephone. Standardized screening instruments for assessment of functional status are presented in **Table 85**. Functional assessment may help determine the need for specific services or the appropriate level of care for the patient.

## Vision

Older patients are at increased risk for many conditions that cause vision loss, including cataracts, macular degeneration, presbyopia, glaucoma, and disease-related retinopathy (such as diabetic retinopathy). Reduced visual acuity decreases functional status and quality of life and increases risk for falls, depression, and cognitive impairment.

Screening tests and examination techniques to assess vision in the primary care setting include standardized questionnaires, the Snellen eye chart, and direct ophthalmoscopic examination; however, these tests may not detect such disorders as glaucoma and macular degeneration. The U.S. Preventive Services Task Force (USPSTF) concluded that evidence is insufficient to assess the balance of benefits and harms of screening for impaired visual acuity in asymptomatic adults aged 65 years and older. Nonetheless, given the risks associated with decreased vision coupled with the increased risk for common treatable eye conditions in older adults, it is reasonable to ask about changes in vision and refer the patient to an eye specialist when changes are present. In contrast to the USPSTF recommendations, the American Ophthalmologic Association recommends performing a comprehensive eye examination in older adults every 1 to 2 years.

## Hearing

Hearing loss is common in older adults, affecting more than 80% of adults by age 80 years. As with vision loss, hearing loss contributes to increased morbidity and decreased quality of life. The inability to hear is also socially isolating, perhaps more so than other sensory losses. Because of the impaired communication abilities inherent to hearing loss, it may be misdiagnosed as cognitive dysfunction.

Diagnostic tests that reliably screen for hearing loss include assessing whether the patient can hear a whispered voice, fingers rubbing together, or a watch ticking. These tests and single-question screening (that is, asking "Do you have difficulty hearing?") perform as well as more complex questionnaires or handheld audiometry in detecting hearing loss, although there is no evidence that identifying hearing loss translates to better hearing-related quality of life. As such, routine screening for hearing loss in asymptomatic patients is not recommended by the USPSTF. Patients with symptoms, however, should be referred to an otologist or audiologist for formal hearing testing and evaluation to determine whether hearing aids would be beneficial.

## Depression

The prevalence of depression in adults older than 60 years is as high as 15%. Chronic illness, grief associated with the loss of loved ones, social isolation due to decreased physical and cognitive function, and the need for institutionalization may all contribute to depression. Common symptoms of depression, such as low energy and somatic symptoms, are often mistakenly attributed to aging and chronic illness. Depression in older adults may also be confused with cognitive dysfunction and is itself a risk factor for cognitive dysfunction.

The USPSTF recommends screening for depression in all adults. The PHQ-2 has been validated as a screening instrument in older adults, with similar sensitivity and specificity in this population compared with its performance in younger adults (see Routine Care of the Healthy Patient). In all age

| TABLE 85. | Indices to Assess Basic and Instrumental Activities of Daily Living | | |
|---|---|---|---|
| **Index** | **Assessed Functional Activity** | **Scoring** | **Comments** |
| Katz Index of Independence in Activities of Daily Living | Bathing<br>Dressing<br>Toileting<br>Transferring<br>Continence<br>Feeding | Assign 1 point for each activity if it can be performed independently, which is defined as requiring no supervision, direction, or personal assistance; scores are then added for a range of 0 to 6 (6 = fully functional; 4 = moderately impaired; 2 = severely impaired) | Simple to use/score; brief, takes only a few minutes to complete<br><br>Less discriminative at low levels of disability |
| Lawton and Brody Instrumental Activities of Daily Living (IADL) Scale | Ability to use telephone<br>Shopping<br>Food preparation<br>Housekeeping<br>Laundry<br>Transportation<br>Medication management<br>Ability to handle finances | Assign 1 point for each activity if it can be performed at all; scores are then added for a range of 0 to 8, with a score of 8 representing independence and 0 representing total dependence for IADLs | Simple to use; brief, takes only a few minutes to complete |

groups, the PHQ-2 has a lower specificity than more comprehensive screening instruments, which may result in overdiagnosis of depression. A positive screening result should therefore prompt further assessment. The PHQ-9 and Geriatric Depression Scale (https://integrationacademy.ahrq.gov/sites/default/files/Update_Geriatric_Depression_Scale-15_0.pdf) have similar sensitivity and specificity in older adults. The Geriatric Depression Scale, with its yes-or-no answer format, may be easier to administer in patients with cognitive impairment.

Older adults with depression are most commonly treated with pharmacotherapy, and antidepressants protect against suicide attempts in this population. Selective serotonin reuptake inhibitors are the most widely studied antidepressants and are considered first-line therapy. Psychotherapy, including cognitive behavioral therapy, may also be considered as primary treatment or as an adjunct to pharmacotherapy.

## Cognitive Function

Cognitive impairment is defined as a progressive decline in at least two cognitive domains (memory, attention, language, visual-spatial function, executive function) that negatively affects patient functioning. The strongest risk factor for cognitive impairment is increasing age. In the absence of symptoms, routine screening is not recommended owing to a lack of evidence that screening leads to effective intervention. However, because cognitive impairment is a risk factor for falls, loss of independence, and poor control of chronic diseases, clinicians should have a low threshold for assessing cognitive decline.

The most widely studied instrument for evaluating cognitive function is the Mini–Mental State Examination (MMSE). The proprietary nature of the MMSE and the time required to administer the test (approximately 7 minutes) may preclude its use for routine outpatient screening. The Montreal Cognitive Assessment (MoCA) takes a similar amount of time to complete and is sensitive for detecting cognitive impairment. The Mini-Cog assessment includes a three-item recall test (similar to elements of the MMSE) followed by a clock-drawing test if any one of the three recall items is missed. The Mini-Cog has acceptable sensitivity and specificity in identifying dementia and is available to clinicians without charge, although it is copyright protected.

Evaluation and treatment of mild cognitive impairment (impaired cognition in the absence of impaired function) and dementia are further discussed in MKSAP 18 Neurology.

## Fall Prevention

Thirty percent to 40% of adults older than 65 years fall every year, making falls the leading cause of injury in this age group. Modifiable risk factors for falls include chronic musculoskeletal or neurologic conditions, visual impairment, cognitive impairment, frailty, and polypharmacy.

Screening older adults for fall risk is recommended by the USPSTF and is an element of the Medicare annual wellness visit. Patients should be asked about falls and unsteadiness with walking; those who report falls or balance issues should be evaluated with the Timed Up and Go test, in which the patient is asked to rise from a chair with armrests, walk 10 feet (with their usual assistive devices, if applicable), turn, return to the chair, and sit down. A time of more than 12 seconds is considered abnormal. Patients with prolonged times on the Timed Up and Go test may be referred for more comprehensive assessment or formal gait and balance assessment and therapy. An algorithm for fall risk assessment and prevention is presented in **Figure 28**.

The USPSTF recommends exercise to prevent falls in community-dwelling adults aged 65 years or older who are at increased risk for falls. Exercise interventions include supervised individual and group classes as well as physical therapy. The USPSTF also recommends multifactorial interventions to prevent falls. This process typically involves an initial assessment of modifiable risk factors for falls and subsequent customized interventions. The USPSTF acknowledges that the overall benefit of routinely offering multifactorial interventions to prevent falls is small and should take into account the balance of benefits and harms based on the circumstances of previous falls, presence of comorbid medical conditions, and the patient's values and preferences. The USPSTF recommends against vitamin D supplementation to prevent falls in community-dwelling adults aged 65 years or older who are not known to have osteoporosis or vitamin D deficiency.

## Assessment of the Older Driver

Driving is one of the most valued IADLs for older adults, and cessation of driving in this population is associated with negative health consequences. However, drivers older than 65 years are responsible for more traffic fatalities than any other group of drivers other than those younger than 25 years. Decreased visual acuity, decreased cognitive abilities, use of centrally acting medications (including alcohol), conditions that increase the risk for loss of consciousness, and mobility issues of the extremities or neck all increase the risk for motor vehicle crashes in older adults. Caregiver or family concern for driving safety, history of traffic citations, self-restricted driving, and impulsive behaviors are also associated with increased risk for crashes. The decision to advise an older driver to "retire from driving," which is the preferred terminology, is qualitative, complex, and largely dependent on clinician judgment. The evaluation should consider the known risk factors and underlying medical conditions.

Physician advice to retire from driving is associated with older drivers appropriately stopping driving; however, given the risk for depression and social isolation associated with driving retirement, this advice should be coupled with support, suggestions for alternate forms of transportation, and follow-up assessment of mood and quality of life. When patients are resistant to retiring from driving or when the appropriate decision is less clear, formal occupational therapy driving assessment may be helpful.

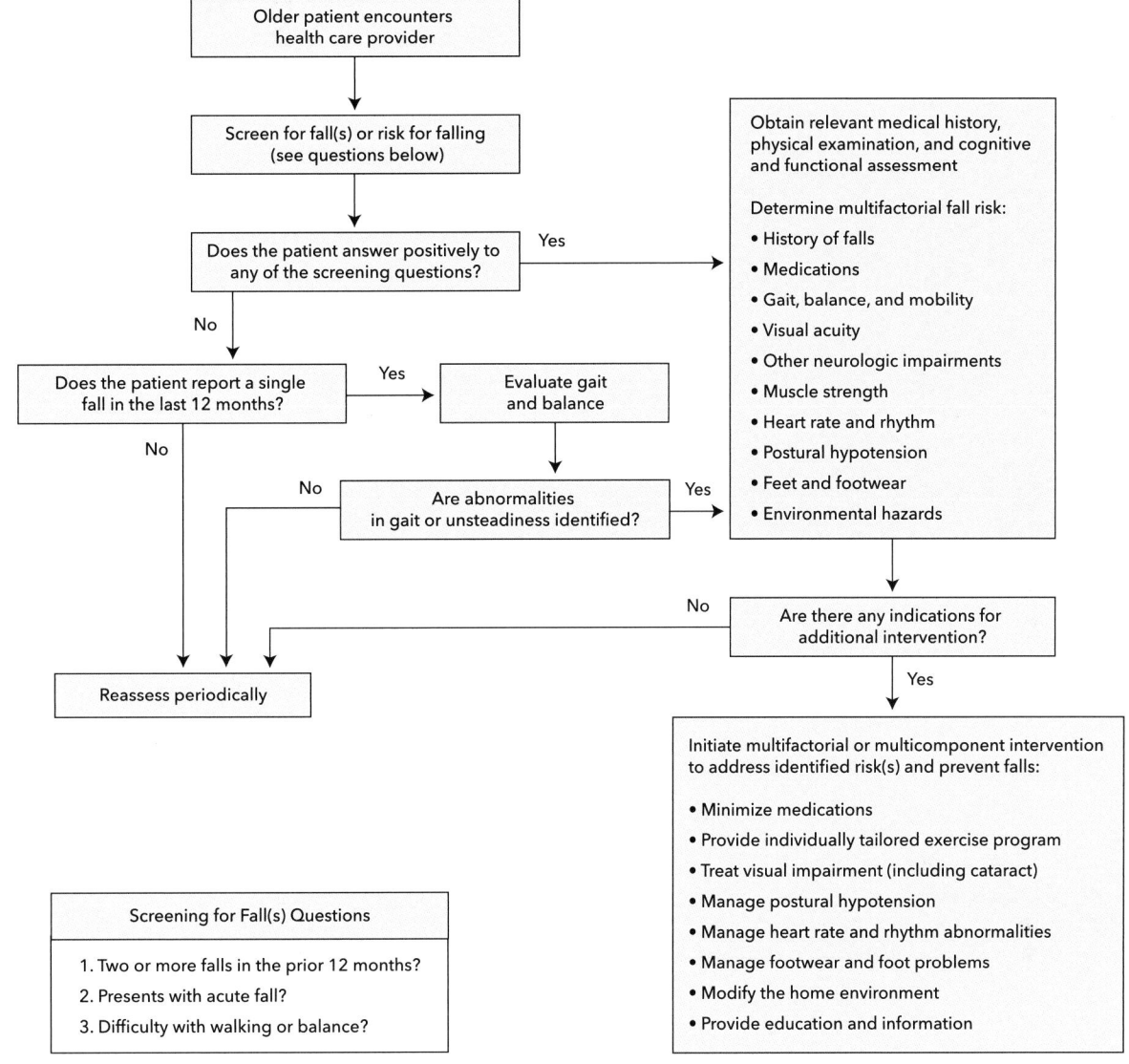

**FIGURE 28.** Prevention of falls in older persons living in a community.

Adapted with permission from Panel on Prevention of Falls in Older Persons, American Geriatrics Society and British Geriatrics Society. Summary of the updated American Geriatrics Society/British Geriatrics Society clinical practice guideline for prevention of falls in older persons. J Am Geriatr Soc. 2011;59:148-57. [PMID: 21226685] doi:10.1111/j.1532-5415.2010.03234.x. Copyright 2011, John Wiley & Sons, Inc.

## Screening for Mistreatment

Older adults are at increased risk for mistreatment, including abuse (infliction of harm), neglect, or financial exploitation, owing to decreased functioning that leads to dependence on others. The prevalence of elder mistreatment is estimated to be roughly 10%. Victims are high utilizers of emergency services, hospital care, and nursing homes and have a higher mortality rate.

There is uncertainty regarding whether screening for elder mistreatment should be routine. The USPSTF concluded that screening cannot be universally recommended for asymptomatic adults; however, screening should be considered in adults with vulnerability for or signs of abuse. Simple screening instruments, such as the Hwalek-Sengstock Elder Abuse Screening Test and the Vulnerability to Abuse Screening Scale, are available but require self-reporting; this complicates assessment in cognitively impaired individuals who cannot independently provide information. Screening may also not occur because of unawareness of these instruments and how to use them, confusion regarding legal and reporting implications (which vary from state to state), and fear of potential harms to the patient and family members that result from false-positive and false-negative screening results.

> **KEY POINTS**
>
> - Comprehensive geriatric assessment is a multidisciplinary diagnostic process to ascertain the physical, cognitive, psychological, environmental, and functional capabilities of older persons in order to develop a plan for preserving function and maximizing independence and quality of life.
>
> *(Continued)*

- Although routine screening for hearing loss in asymptomatic patients is not recommended, patients with symptoms of hearing loss should be referred to an otologist or audiologist for formal testing and hearing aid placement, if appropriate.

- All older adults should be screened for depression, such as with the PHQ-2.

**HVC** • Cognitive impairment is a risk factor for falls, loss of independence, and poor control of chronic diseases; clinicians should inquire about symptoms and perform further evaluation when symptoms are present.

**HVC** • The U.S. Preventive Services Task Force recommends exercise to prevent falls in community-dwelling adults aged 65 years or older who are at increased risk for falls.

## Frailty Assessment

Frailty is a multifactorial geriatric syndrome characterized by unintentional weight loss, low energy and activity levels, weakness, and slow walking speed. It is important to note that advanced age is not synonymous with frailty. Assessment of frailty may be used to predict response to certain treatments as well as morbidity and mortality in patients with chronic illness. Standardized indices to objectively measure frailty include the Frailty Index, the frailty phenotype, the FRAIL (Fatigue, Resistance, Ambulation, Illness, and Loss of weight) scale, and the Osteoporotic Fractures Frailty Scale. The Frailty Index, a comprehensive assessment of chronic conditions and functioning, has been in use for a longer time than other indices; however, its length and complexity limit its usefulness in routine care. The five-item frailty phenotype was originally validated in the Cardiovascular Health Study of more than

5000 patients aged 65 years and older; it requires measurement of gait speed and grip strength (with a dynamometer), which may not be feasible in primary care. The FRAIL scale consists of five self-reported measures and is easy to administer and score. The Osteoporotic Fractures Frailty Scale, which was developed and validated in an all-female cohort, consists of three elements and is also easy to administer. The rapid screening tools are most easily incorporated into a primary care practice and are useful in the identification of patients who might require more formal comprehensive geriatric assessment (**Table 86**).

## Levels of Care

As the population ages, medical complexity and care needs also increase, necessitating a variety of care delivery models, including home-based and facility-based options.

Several resources are available for older adults who wish to remain in their homes but need medical assistance. Home health agencies offer skilled assistance with medication management, wound care, and physical therapy. These services are provided on an intermittent basis (usually no more than two to three times per week) and are covered by Medicare and Medicaid if the patient is homebound with a documented skilled care need. Patients requiring assistance with ADLs can use custodial care services for help with dressing, bathing, toileting, and cooking; these services are not covered by Medicare but may be paid for by Medicaid. Visiting physicians can also provide outpatient medical care.

For patients who are cared for by family members but require additional resources for gaps in care, adult day care can provide part-time assistance when a patient's primary caregiver is unavailable. If supervision is needed for a longer time, respite care is available at many senior living

| TABLE 86. | Examples of Frailty Indices | | |
|---|---|---|---|
| **Instrument** | **Description** | | **Scoring** |
| FRAIL (Fatigue, Resistance, Ambulation, Illness, and Loss of weight) scale | Measures presence (1) or absence (0) of: | | Each item scored dichotomously as 0 for normal or 1 for abnormal |
| | Fatigue: Feeling fatigued most or all of the time over the past 4 weeks | | 1-2 = Prefrail |
| | Resistance: Difficulty walking up 10 steps alone without resting or assistance | | 3-5 = Frail |
| | Ambulation: Difficulty walking several hundred yards without assistance | | |
| | Illness: Presence of more than five illnesses | | |
| | Loss of weight: Weight loss >5% in the past year | | |
| Osteoporotic Fractures Frailty Scale | Measures three items: | | Each item scored dichotomously as 0 for normal or 1 for abnormal |
| | Ability to rise from an armless chair five times (inability = 1) | | 1 = Prefrail |
| | Response to the question "Do you feel full of energy?" (answer of "no" = 1) | | 2-3 = Frail |
| | Weight loss >5% in the past year (presence of weight loss = 1) | | |

CONT.

communities (assisted living facilities and nursing homes). Adult day care and respite care are not typically covered by Medicare or Medicaid.

When long-term daily care needs exceed those that can be provided in a patient's home, three different levels of care are available: independent living, assisted living, and nursing homes. Independent living is suitable only for patients who can independently perform ADLs and simply provides patients with the benefits of living in a community. Assisted living offers a home-like environment but provides varying levels of assistance with medications, ADLs, housekeeping, and meals. For patients requiring additional help with ADLs or medical management, nursing homes provide 24-hour nursing care as well as rehabilitation services. A residential care home (or group home) is a variation of assisted living or the nursing home. Residential care homes use a smaller, home-like environment in the care of patients with similar needs (such as patients with chronic mental illness); however, services provided vary. Independent and assisted living are typically paid for with private funds, or "private pay." Medicare does not usually cover long-term nursing home or residential home care; Medicaid may pay for long-term care depending on patient eligibility and state regulations.

Acute medical care is almost always provided in a hospital setting. Infrequently, serious acute illnesses may be treated in the patient's living environment; however, home hospital care typically occurs only when significant home health resources are available and avoidance of hospitalization has been established as a primary goal in care-planning discussions.

Post-hospitalization care is available in multiple forms. Safe return to a patient's previous living situation can be facilitated with outpatient physical, occupational, and speech therapies in the home or clinic. If a patient requires functional improvement before returning home, rehabilitation can be performed in an acute rehabilitation program or skilled nursing facility (that is, subacute rehabilitation). Acute rehabilitation is provided in a free-standing rehabilitation hospital or a designated hospital unit, and it requires that the patient be able to participate in 3 hours of therapy at least 5 days per week. In patients who cannot tolerate this level of therapy, subacute rehabilitation is appropriate. Medicare covers the costs of both options for up to 100 days, provided that the patient had an inpatient hospitalization of at least 3 days and continues to make progress with goals. Some patients require longer-term, high-intensity medical care, including mechanical ventilation or multiple parenteral therapies, and long-term acute care hospitals are an appropriate option for these patients.

**KEY POINT**

HVC
- Acute rehabilitation requires that the patient be able to participate in 3 hours of therapy at least 5 days per week; in patients who cannot tolerate this level of therapy, subacute rehabilitation is appropriate.

# Polypharmacy

The percentage of patients older than 65 years who take five or more prescription medications increased from 24% to 39% between 1999 and 2012. Studies estimate that nursing home patients take eight different medications on average, and medication errors occur in two thirds of such patients. Polypharmacy in older patients is associated with increased health care utilization, costs, medication nonadherence, and functional decline. Patients transitioning between levels of care are particularly vulnerable to inappropriate medication additions, omissions, and dosage changes; the risk for these mistakes increases with the number of medications prescribed. Hazards of polypharmacy include overtreatment or undertreatment of disease, serious drug-drug interactions, and adverse reactions.

Although treatment of comorbid health conditions in older adults often necessitates the use of several medications, clinicians can minimize the potential for adverse effects from polypharmacy. During medication review, clinicians should specifically assess for and reduce medications that should be avoided in older patients, including tricyclic antidepressants, antipsychotics, and benzodiazepines. Drug dosage adjustment is also crucial in older adult patients, given the wide variability in drug metabolism resulting from decreased kidney and liver function as well as the potential for drug interactions. Frequent review of patient medications to confirm their necessity and proper dosing is paramount, especially during care transitions. The 2015 Beers Criteria for Potentially Inappropriate Medication Use in Older Adults from the American Geriatrics Society provides lists of medications that are problematic for elderly patients, as well as recommendations regarding drug interactions to avoid (available at https://geriatricscareonline.org/ProductAbstract/american-geriatrics-society-updated-beers-criteria-for-potentially-inappropriate-medication-use-in-older-adults/CL001).

**KEY POINT**

- Adverse effects from polypharmacy can be minimized    HVC
with frequent review of the patient's current medications, discontinuation of drugs that are unnecessary or should be avoided, and adjustment of drug dosages as appropriate.

# Urinary Incontinence
## Epidemiology

Urinary incontinence (UI) is common in older adults, occurring in at least one third of community-dwelling adults older than 65 years and about two thirds of those in nursing homes. Prevalence increases with age in both women and men; however, incidence is higher in women. UI increases risk for falls, depression, and social isolation and reduces health-related quality of life. UI is also a major factor leading to loss of independence and nursing home placement. Risk factors for UI include many common chronic medical conditions (such as diabetes, heart failure, cerebrovascular disease, Parkinson disease, osteoarthritis, and dementia) as well as the medications used in their treatment. Other risk factors are pelvic surgery (including hysterectomy and prostate surgery), pelvic irradiation, pelvic trauma, and obesity.

There are four main classifications of UI: urgency, stress, overflow, and mixed. Functional incontinence, which occurs in patients who cannot reach and use the toilet in a timely manner, may result from cognitive or mobility impairment. Disorders that predispose patients to specific types of incontinence are presented in **Table 87**. Urgency UI and stress UI are the two most common forms, although mixed presentations frequently occur. Urgency UI is associated with intrinsic detrusor muscle instability and is characterized by urine leakage preceded by a sudden urge to void. Urgency UI occurs at increased rates in older patients, with higher rates in women. Stress UI is characterized by urine leakage associated with activities that cause increased intra-abdominal pressure, such as coughing, laughing, or sneezing. Changes in the pelvic floor musculature can contribute to both urgency and stress incontinence. Overflow UI is less common and is associated with comorbidities that alter neurologic control of the bladder and bladder outlet obstruction.

## Evaluation

A comprehensive history, including specific questions about the presence and nature of incontinence, should be included in the routine care of the geriatric patient. Because of the social implications of incontinence, patients may be hesitant to volunteer information about symptoms. Validated questionnaires can be used to obtain details on the type of incontinence and the degree of interference with the patient's quality of life, as well as to monitor response to treatment. The 3 Incontinence Questions (3IQ) questionnaire is straightforward and easy to administer in an office setting; however, several other validated instruments are available.

During the history, female patients should be questioned about pregnancies and gynecologic procedures, and male patients should be asked about symptoms suggestive of prostate enlargement. Additionally, all patients should be screened for chronic conditions associated with increased risk for incontinence (see Table 87). A comprehensive medication history should be obtained, with special attention paid to the use of diuretics and medications with cholinergic or anticholinergic effects, including over-the-counter medications.

The physical examination should incorporate a genitourinary examination, including evaluation of the pelvis in women and the prostate in men. Urinalysis is recommended because transient incontinence may be explained by the presence of urinary tract infection. Additional laboratory investigation or diagnostic testing is usually unnecessary. Postvoid bladder residual volume assessment, which is performed with ultrasonography after spontaneous voiding, may be considered in patients in whom overflow incontinence is suspected. Urodynamic studies are required only for complex cases in which neurologic disease is suspected and surgical intervention is being considered.

## Treatment

The American College of Physicians (ACP) recommends nonpharmacologic therapy as the preferred first-line treatment for all types of UI. In cases of urgency UI, pharmacologic therapy may be considered when symptoms are not adequately improved with behavioral therapy. Devices and surgical interventions are third-line therapy. Treatment strategies for UI are listed in **Table 88**.

### Behavioral Therapy

Validated behavioral therapy measures include pelvic floor muscle training for stress UI and mixed UI, bladder training with timed voiding for urgency UI, and exercise and weight loss in obese patients with any form of UI.

Pelvic floor muscle training, in which the patient performs sets of contractions of the pelvic floor, is five times more effective than no treatment for stress UI. Patients should be instructed to contract the pelvic floor as if attempting to avoid urination and sustain the contraction for 10 seconds. Contractions should be performed in three or four sets of 10 daily. Patients should be counseled that symptom improvement may not be noticeable until pelvic floor muscle training is consistently performed for several months. Some studies have demonstrated benefits when biofeedback therapy (using a vaginal electromyography probe to provide direct confirmation that the patient is correctly contracting the pelvic floor muscles) is included with these exercises.

Timed voiding or bladder training comprises scheduled voiding attempts at intervals shorter than the usual time between incontinence episodes, regardless of the urge to void,

| TABLE 87. | Conditions Commonly Associated With Urinary Incontinence |
|---|---|
| **Incontinence Type** | **Associated Conditions** |
| Stress | Multiparous state, radical prostatectomy |
| Urgency | Spinal cord injury, stroke, Parkinson disease |
| | Often idiopathic |
| Overflow | Diabetes mellitus with neurogenic bladder |
| | Neurologic disorders (lumbosacral degenerative joint disease, spinal cord injury) |
| | Prostate hypertrophy with bladder outlet obstruction |
| Functional | Dementia |
| | Mobility issues (osteoarthritis, residual deficits from cerebrovascular disease, Parkinson disease) |
| Mixed | All conditions associated with stress and urgency urinary incontinence |

| TABLE 88. | Treatment Strategies for Urinary Incontinence | | |
|---|---|---|---|
| **Incontinence Type** | **Behavioral Therapy** | **Pharmacologic Therapy** | **Other Therapies** |
| Stress | Pelvic floor muscle training +/– biofeedback | No recommended pharmacologic therapies | Pessaries, injectable bulking agents, sling cystourethropexy |
| Urgency | Bladder training/timed voiding | Antimuscarinics (oxybutynin, darifenacin, solifenacin, tolterodine, fesoterodine, trospium)  Mirabegron | Spinal neuromodulators, botulinum toxin injections |
| Overflow | Double voiding (remaining on the toilet for a few minutes after voiding and then attempting to void again)  Triggered voiding (maneuvers to stimulate voiding, including massaging the pubic bone and tugging on pubic hairs) | α-Blocker and 5α-reductase inhibitors for BPH-related symptoms | Transurethral prostatectomy can be considered for BPH-related symptoms  Scheduled in-and-out catheterization |
| Functional | Caregiver-prompted timed voiding | No recommended pharmacologic therapies | None routinely recommended |
| Mixed | Pelvic floor muscle training +/– biofeedback  Bladder training/timed voiding | Consider antimuscarinics or mirabegron | Consider therapies for stress or urgency incontinence depending on predominant symptoms |

BPH = benign prostatic hyperplasia.

with a gradual increase in the time between voids. If an episode of urgency occurs before the designated voiding time, patients are encouraged to use pelvic floor muscle contraction until the urge passes and then proceed with voiding directly afterward. In patients with cognitive impairment–related functional UI, timed voiding with prompting by the caregiver may be useful.

## Pharmacologic Therapy

No pharmacologic therapies are recommended for the treatment of stress UI. Trials of systemic and vaginal estrogen therapy for stress UI in women generally have been of low quality and yielded mixed results. Vaginal estrogen has been shown to improve symptoms compared with placebo; however, the risks associated with estrogen therapy may outweigh the benefits, especially in patients with breast cancer. Current guidelines do not recommend the use of estrogen therapy for women with continued symptoms of stress UI despite behavioral therapy.

Several classes of pharmacologic agents are available for the treatment of urgency and mixed UI, although medications are recommended only when symptoms persist despite behavioral therapy (see Table 88). No one agent or class of agents has been shown to be superior in head-to-head comparisons. The risk for adverse effects with pharmacologic treatment is low but higher than with behavioral therapies. Anticholinergic and antimuscarinic side effects (dry mouth, constipation, blurred vision) predominate with agents other than mirabegron (a $\beta_3$-agonist), whereas mirabegron is associated with gastrointestinal upset and nasopharyngitis. Anticholinergic agents are contraindicated in patients with angle-closure glaucoma and should be used with caution in men with benign prostatic hyperplasia due to the risk for urinary retention.

Pharmacologic treatment of urgency or overflow UI associated with prostatic hyperplasia is discussed in Men's Health. The pharmacologic agents recommended for female patients with urgency UI are also approved for use in men.

## Devices, Injectable Agents, and Surgery

Patients with continued symptoms and reduced quality of life despite behavioral and/or pharmacologic therapies should be considered for third-line treatments, including device therapy, injectable agents, and surgery. Ideally, patients should be referred to a urologist or urogynecologist in order to match their clinical symptoms, overall functional status, and personal preferences to an appropriate therapy.

In patients with stress UI, pessary devices are a low-risk treatment option. However, in a systematic review of comparative effectiveness of stress UI treatments, no definitive benefit was demonstrated with pessary devices, vaginal cones, or other intrauterine/intravaginal devices. Limited high-quality evidence supports cystoscopically guided injection of bulking agents into the urethral mucosa at the bladder neck. Injection therapy requires repeat administration in upwards of 70% of patients whose symptoms initially improve. Surgical treatment of stress UI is reserved for patients who do not respond to other therapies and typically consists of sling cystourethropexy. Postoperative adverse effects include increased urinary retention, urgency incontinence, and increased incidence of urinary tract infection.

Resistant urgency UI may be treated with botulinum toxin injections into the detrusor muscle. Repeat dosing is usually performed every 6 to 12 months. Adverse effects include urinary retention requiring self-catheterization. Surgically implanted sacral nerve root neurostimulation devices may be used in combination with behavioral therapy and pharmacotherapy for resistant urgency UI. Although sacral neuromodulation is associated with symptom improvement, widespread use of these devices is not indicated because of the required surgical intervention, complex programming, high costs, and potential for infection.

Indwelling urinary catheters are not recommended for any type of incontinence, owing to an unacceptably high risk for infection associated with their use.

**KEY POINTS**

- HVC • First-line therapy for urinary incontinence (UI) includes pelvic floor muscle training for stress UI and mixed UI, bladder training with timed voiding for urgency UI, and exercise and weight loss in obese patients with any form of UI.
- HVC • No pharmacologic therapies are recommended for the treatment of stress urinary incontinence or functional incontinence.
- Urgency and mixed urinary incontinence may be treated with pharmacologic therapy, including anticholinergic and antimuscarinic agents, when symptoms persist despite behavioral therapy.

# Pressure Injuries

Pressure injuries (or pressure ulcers) represent damage to the skin and underlying tissue caused by unrelieved pressure. The most important risk factors for pressure injury are immobility, malnutrition, sensory loss, and reduced skin perfusion, such as occurs with hypovolemia, hypotension, and systemic vasoconstriction. An estimated 2.5 to 3 million pressure injuries are treated each year in acute care facilities in the United States. Among hospitalized patients, prevalence rates range from 3% to 17%; however, rates are much higher in some high-risk groups, approaching 50% in long-term ICU patients. Patients who develop pressure injuries during an acute care stay are much more likely to be discharged to a long-term care facility.

## Prevention

Pressure injury prevention is a cost-effective intervention that can positively affect health status. Improved understanding of ulcer pathogenesis and changes in reimbursement have increased the focus on identifying patients at risk and allocating resources to prevention efforts. The Centers for Medicare & Medicaid Services (CMS) has identified pressure ulcer development as a sentinel event (unexpected and preventable occurrence that results in serious patient injury) for health care facilities. As of October 2008, guidelines from CMS dictate that hospitals no longer receive additional payment when a patient has developed a stage III or IV pressure ulcer.

Risk assessment, including a comprehensive history and physical examination, is the first step in pressure injury prevention. In a 2015 clinical practice guideline, the ACP

recommends regular, structured risk assessment to identify at-risk patients. Standardized risk-assessment tools include the Braden, Cubbin and Jackson, Norton, and Waterlow scales. Clinical validation studies have found these instruments to have fairly low positive predictive values (60%-70%); therefore, bedside clinical assessment remains an important part of risk evaluation.

After identification of at-risk patients, pressure redistribution is of paramount importance in the prevention of pressure injuries and may be accomplished with pressure-reducing equipment and proper patient positioning. In patients at increased risk, the ACP recommends using advanced static mattresses or overlays (for example, medical sheepskin overlay) for prevention. Evidence of the efficacy of repositioning, nutritional interventions, and local care (silicone foam dressings or creams) in preventing pressure ulcers is limited. The ACP recommends against the use of alternating air mattresses, primarily based on cost considerations and lack of data demonstrating a clear advantage. There are insufficient data to recommend the routine use of dietary supplements for pressure injury prevention.

## Management

Pressure injuries may be classified with the use of a staging system (**Table 89**); advancing stages are characterized by increasing tissue loss, depth, and ulcer size. Successful treatment of established pressure injuries requires interdisciplinary management involving nutrition, pressure-reducing surfaces (including air-fluidized beds), wound care, surgical debridement and repair, and in some cases, vacuum-assisted closure. On the basis of moderate-quality evidence, the ACP

| TABLE 89. | Classification of Pressure Injuries |
|---|---|
| Stage | Description |
| I | Intact skin with nonblanchable redness |
| II | Partial-thickness loss of dermis. Shallow open ulcer with red-pink wound bed without slough. May also present as intact or ruptured serum-filled blister |
| III | Full-thickness tissue loss. Visible subcutaneous fat but not bone, tendon, or muscle. May include undermining or tunneling |
| IV | Full-thickness tissue loss with exposed bone, tendon, or muscle |
| Unstageable | Full-thickness tissue loss in which the base of the ulcer is covered by slough or eschar |
| Suspected deep-tissue injury | Purple or maroon localized area of discolored but intact skin or a blood-filled blister due to damage of underlying soft tissue from pressure or shear |

Adapted from National Pressure Ulcer Advisory Panel. National Pressure Ulcer Advisory Panel, European Pressure Ulcer Advisory Panel, and Pan Pacific Pressure Injury Alliance. Prevention and Treatment of Pressure Ulcers: Quick Reference Guide. Cambridge Media: Perth, Australia; 2014.

CONT.

recommends protein-containing supplements to improve wound healing. Moderate-quality evidence has also shown a reduction in pressure injury size with air-fluidized beds compared with other support surfaces. Hydrocolloid and foam dressings are recommended treatments because they have been shown to reduce ulcer size compared with gauze dressings in low-quality studies. Wound electrical stimulation has been demonstrated to be effective as adjunctive therapy to improve healing. Evidence is insufficient to support the use of platelet-derived growth factor dressings, hydrotherapy, hyperbaric oxygen, or maggot therapy. ◨

### KEY POINTS

- Pressure redistribution, such as with advanced static mattresses or overlays, is of paramount importance in the prevention of pressure injuries.
- Protein-containing supplements and hydrocolloid or foam dressings are recommended in the treatment of established pressure injuries.

# Perioperative Medicine
◨ ## General Recommendations

Perioperative medicine comprises preoperative risk assessment, preoperative testing, medical optimization of surgical patients, and postoperative medical care. The role of the internist in the perioperative setting is not to provide surgical clearance but to determine and communicate operative risk to patients and surgical and anesthesia colleagues and to suggest strategies that may mitigate this risk.

Decisions regarding the modality of anesthesia, such as whether to pursue regional or general anesthesia, are best deferred to the anesthesiologist and surgeon, owing to a lack of high-quality evidence that anesthetic choice significantly affects medical outcomes. A recent Cochrane review showed no differences in outcomes, including 30-day mortality, myocardial infarction, pneumonia, and hospital length of stay, with regional anesthesia compared with general anesthesia.

### Preoperative Laboratory Testing

Preoperative laboratory testing should be performed on the basis of the patient's medical conditions, physical examination findings, and preoperative symptoms (**Table 90**). Routine laboratory panels expose patients to unnecessary testing and are not recommended.

### Perioperative Medication Management

Perioperative medication management begins with eliciting a complete preoperative medication history, including herbal preparations, supplements, and over-the-counter medications. Careful medication reconciliation should be performed to rectify any discrepancies and to prevent medication errors.

| TABLE 90. | Selected Indications for Preoperative Laboratory Testing |
|---|---|
| **Laboratory Test** | **Preoperative Indications** |
| Hemoglobin | History of anemia |
| | Underlying disease that predisposes to anemia (such as kidney disease) |
| | Suggestive physical examination |
| | Expected substantial operative blood loss |
| Platelet count | History of thrombocytopenia or cirrhosis; the presence of signs or symptoms of thrombocytopenia or liver disease |
| Coagulation studies | Anticoagulant use |
| | History of abnormal bleeding |
| | Medical conditions that predispose to coagulopathy (such as liver disease or hemophilia) |
| Electrolytes | Diseases that predispose to electrolyte derangements (such as kidney disease) |
| | Use of medications that can cause electrolyte abnormalities (such as diuretics, ACE inhibitors, and angiotensin receptor blockers) |
| Creatinine | Kidney disease; creatinine is also used in preoperative cardiovascular risk calculators and for calculation of the MELD score |
| Liver chemistry tests (including bilirubin) | Cirrhosis, history of abnormal liver chemistry test results, or the presence of signs or symptoms of liver disease |
| | Examination findings suggestive of liver disease |
| Fasting glucose and hemoglobin $A_{1c}$ | Hyperglycemia suspected based on history and physical examination findings |
| Urinalysis | Suspected urinary tract infection |
| | Planned urologic procedures |
| | Planned implantation of prosthetic devices |

MELD = Model for End-stage Liver Disease.

There is a paucity of high-quality evidence to guide perioperative medication management. Most medications are tolerated throughout the perioperative period, with some important exceptions. **Table 91** provides perioperative recommendations for medications with potential surgery-related risk. Patients should be provided with clear instructions on which medications to withhold preoperatively and for what duration.

### Postoperative Care

Promotion of patient mobilization, use of lung expansion modalities (see later discussion), improvement in patient nutrition, and enhanced recovery after surgery (ERAS) programs may all decrease the likelihood of postoperative complications. Early mobilization and physical therapy (as necessary) are important components of the postoperative care plan and

**TABLE 91.** Perioperative Medication Management[a]

| Medication | Perioperative Recommendation | Special Considerations |
|---|---|---|
| **Cardiovascular Agents** | | |
| α₁-Blockers | Continue | Risk for intraoperative floppy iris syndrome in cataract surgery; notify surgeon if ocular surgery is planned |
| α₂-Blockers | Continue | Do not initiate clonidine for preoperative cardiovascular risk reduction (increases risk for perioperative hypotension) |
| β-Blockers | Continue | Consider initiating preoperatively in patients with ≥3 RCRI risk factors and those with intermediate- or high-risk myocardial ischemia on preoperative stress testing |
| | | Begin β-blocker with enough time to assess tolerability; β-blocker should not be started on the day of surgery (2-7 days before surgery is preferred) |
| Calcium channel blockers | Continue | Withhold for preoperative hypotension |
| ACE inhibitors and ARBs | Individualize | Consider withholding if large fluid shifts expected intraoperatively, or if preoperative hypotension, hyperkalemia, or acute kidney injury is present; restart as soon as possible postoperatively |
| Diuretics | Withhold | Monitor volume status closely if heart failure is present and restart as soon as possible |
| Nitrates | Continue | Withhold for preoperative hypotension; remove patch and paste formulations |
| Vasodilators | Continue | Withhold for preoperative hypotension |
| Statins | Continue | Thought to have beneficial pleiotropic effects in addition to lipid-lowering properties |
| | | Reasonable to start in patients undergoing vascular surgery and those undergoing elevated-risk noncardiac surgery with indication for statin |
| | | Withhold all other lipid-lowering medications |
| **Analgesic Agents** | | |
| NSAIDs | Withhold | If possible, withhold 3 days before surgery, especially if increased bleeding risk |
| Opioids | Individualize | If surgery is elective, may consider preoperative pain rehabilitation and opioid taper |
| | | Continue in most patients receiving long-term opioid therapy |
| | | Risk for poorly controlled postoperative pain and respiratory depression |
| Acetaminophen | Continue | |
| **Gastrointestinal Agents** | | |
| Antacid medications (including H₂ blockers and proton pump inhibitors) | Continue | |
| Hyoscyamine | Withhold | Risk for anticholinergic side effects |
| **Rheumatologic Agents** | | |
| Hydroxychloroquine | Continue | |
| Methotrexate | Individualize | Limited high-quality evidence |
| | | Likely safe to continue in most situations; withhold if significant concern for infection or history of septic complications; dose adjust in cases of kidney injury |
| TNF-α inhibitors | Withhold | No definitive evidence or guideline recommendations |
| | | Reasonable to withhold one to two half-lives preoperatively |
| **Psychiatric Agents** | | |
| Selective serotonin reuptake inhibitors | Usually continue | May increase risk for bleeding, especially in conjunction with antiplatelet agents; risk for withdrawal symptoms with abrupt cessation |
| Benzodiazepines | Continue | Risk for withdrawal with abrupt cessation; monitor for respiratory depression |
| Antipsychotics | Continue | Potential for QT prolongation |
| **Supplements** | | |
| Herbal preparations | Withhold | Withhold 1 week preoperatively |
| Vitamins and supplements | Withhold | |

ARB = angiotensin receptor blocker; RCRI = Revised Cardiac Risk Index; TNF = tumor necrosis factor.

[a]Perioperative management of antiplatelet agents, anticoagulants, antiepileptic drugs, glucocorticoids, and diabetes medications are discussed later in this chapter.

Information from Fleisher LA, Fleischmann KE, Auerbach AD, Barnason SA, Beckman JA, Bozkurt B, et al; American College of Cardiology. 2014 ACC/AHA guideline on perioperative cardiovascular evaluation and management of patients undergoing noncardiac surgery: a report of the American College of Cardiology/American Heart Association Task Force on practice guidelines. J Am Coll Cardiol. 2014;64:e77-137. [PMID: 25091544] doi:10.1016/j.jacc.2014.07.944 and Devereaux PJ, Sessler DI, Leslie K, Kurz A, Mrkobrada M, Alonso-Coello P, et al; POISE-2 Investigators. Clonidine in patients undergoing noncardiac surgery. N Engl J Med. 2014;370:1504-13. [PMID: 24679061] doi:10.1056/NEJMoa1401106

CONT.

may decrease the probability of postoperative pneumonia and venous thromboembolism (VTE).

Malnutrition is a risk factor for perioperative morbidity, including infection and poor wound healing, and several nutrition risk stratification tools are available to identify patients at risk for postoperative complications related to malnutrition. The Subjective Global Assessment of Nutritional Status tool incorporates history of calorie intake and physical examination findings, whereas the Nutritional Risk Screening Tool relies on age, BMI and weight loss, and severity of the current medical condition. Serum protein markers, including albumin and prealbumin, are also predictive of postoperative complications. Loss of 15% of body weight over 6 months and a serum albumin level less than 3.0 g/dL (30 g/L) are the most predictive factors of poor surgical outcomes related to malnutrition. Notably, increased enteral calorie intake is effective in reducing postoperative complications.

ERAS programs use evidence-based protocols to standardize care, improve outcomes, and reduce costs in postoperative patients. Best studied in patients undergoing colorectal surgery, ERAS interventions include optimization of nutritional status, physical conditioning, abstinence from alcohol and tobacco, postoperative mobilization, and early removal of urinary catheters. ERAS programs have been demonstrated to decrease length of hospital stay and result in earlier mobilization and return of bowel function in colorectal surgery populations. They are currently being implemented and studied in other surgical populations.

Common complications in the postoperative setting include postoperative urinary retention (POUR), postoperative ileus, and postoperative nausea and vomiting (PONV). POUR is characterized by incomplete bladder emptying after surgery, resulting in increased postvoid residual urine volume. Risk factors include type of surgery (incontinence and anorectal surgery, hernia repair, joint arthroplasty), longer surgery, use of regional anesthesia, administration of more than 750 mL of intraoperative fluids, use of certain postoperative medications (opioids, anticholinergic agents), older age, constipation, pelvic organ prolapse, neurologic disease, history of urinary retention, and history of pelvic surgery. POUR is a urologic emergency. Reversible causes of POUR, such as medication use, should be addressed. In patients with benign prostatic hyperplasia, $\alpha_2$-blockers should be continued, whereas medications with associated anticholinergic effects, such as oxybutynin, should be withheld. Early removal of indwelling catheters and voiding trials are recommended. For patients in whom a voiding trial is unsuccessful, clean intermittent catheterization is indicated. Urinary tract obstruction should be excluded if POUR is persistent.

Postoperative ileus, or gastrointestinal hypomotility after surgery, is associated with increased length of hospital stay. Ileus is often a physiologic response related to sympathetic nervous system activation, although it can also be caused by activation of inflammatory mediators or the use of medications, such as anesthetics and opioids. Risk factors for the development of postoperative ileus include abdominal and pelvic surgery, open surgical technique, and the presence of other postoperative complications, such as pneumonia. Treatment of ileus includes minimization of postoperative opioids, adequate hydration, bowel rest, electrolyte repletion, postoperative ambulation, and use of chewing gum. Preventive measures for ileus include an appropriate postoperative bowel regimen, which may comprise fiber, stool softeners, osmotic laxatives, and stimulant laxatives. Few data from well-designed clinical trials are available to guide therapy for prolonged postoperative ileus, typically defined as ileus lasting longer than 3 to 5 days. In these patients, it is important to distinguish postoperative ileus from mechanical bowel obstruction.

The prevention and treatment of PONV, a common postoperative event that results in significant patient distress, require a multifaceted approach that involves identifying at-risk patients, reducing baseline risk factors, providing prophylaxis, and treating symptoms. Risk factors for PONV include female sex; young age; nonsmoking status; and use of general anesthesia, postoperative opioids, or volatile anesthetics. Although many risk-mitigation strategies include intraoperative and immediate postoperative care, the internist plays an important role in ensuring adequate postoperative hydration, minimizing the use of opioids, and providing pharmacologic antiemetic therapy. 

**KEY POINTS**

- Preoperative laboratory testing should be performed based on the patient's medical conditions, physical examination findings, and preoperative symptoms; routine laboratory panels expose patients to unnecessary testing and are not recommended. **HVC**

- There is a paucity of high-quality evidence to guide perioperative medication management; in general, most medications are tolerated throughout the perioperative period.

- Optimization of nutritional status, early mobilization, use of lung expansion modalities, and enhanced recovery after surgery programs are important components of the postoperative care plan. **HVC**

- Treatment of postoperative ileus includes minimization of postoperative opioids, adequate hydration, bowel rest, electrolyte repletion, postoperative ambulation, and use of chewing gum.

## Cardiovascular Perioperative Management
### Cardiovascular Risk Assessment

Preoperative cardiac evaluation entails assessment of patient-specific risk, surgery-specific risk, and urgency of surgery (emergent, urgent, or time sensitive). The approach recommended by the American College of Cardiology (ACC)/American Heart Association (AHA) for perioperative cardiovascular

CONT.

evaluation in patients undergoing noncardiac surgery is presented in **Figure 29**.

Risk calculators, including the Revised Cardiac Risk Index (**Table 92**) and American College of Surgeons National Surgical Quality Improvement Program myocardial infarction and cardiac arrest calculator (https://riskcalculator.facs.org/RiskCalculator), can be used to determine the risk for a perioperative major adverse cardiac event (MACE). Both risk calculators incorporate patient- and surgery-specific risk factors.

Patients with low risk (<1% risk of perioperative MACE) may proceed to surgery without preoperative cardiac stress testing, whereas patients with elevated risk (≥1% risk for perioperative MACE) should undergo assessment of functional capacity. Metabolic equivalents (METs) are used to represent the patient's functional capacity based on the intensity of activity able to be performed. If the patient's functional capacity exceeds 4 METs, the patient may proceed to surgery without further testing. Examples of activities that require 4 METs include walking 4 miles per hour on a flat surface; climbing one to two flights of stairs without stopping; or performing vigorous housework, such as vacuuming. Cardiac stress testing should be considered in patients at elevated risk for MACE with a functional capacity of less than 4 METs or if functional capacity cannot be determined, but only if the results of stress testing will change perioperative management.

Preoperative electrocardiography (ECG) is reasonable in patients with known coronary artery disease, arrhythmia, peripheral artery disease, cerebrovascular disease, or structural heart disease undergoing moderate- to high-risk surgeries. Preoperative ECG may be considered for other asymptomatic patients except those undergoing low-risk procedures. ECG may not alter preoperative decision making, but it provides a useful baseline to guide postoperative management in the event of complications.

Echocardiography to evaluate left ventricular function should not be routinely performed preoperatively. Echocardiography is recommended in certain clinical scenarios, such as in the presence of dyspnea of unknown origin, heart failure with worsening dyspnea or overall change in clinical status, known left ventricular dysfunction without echocardiographic assessment in the last year, and known or suspected moderate to severe valvular stenosis or regurgitation without echocardiographic assessment in the last year or with a change in clinical status.

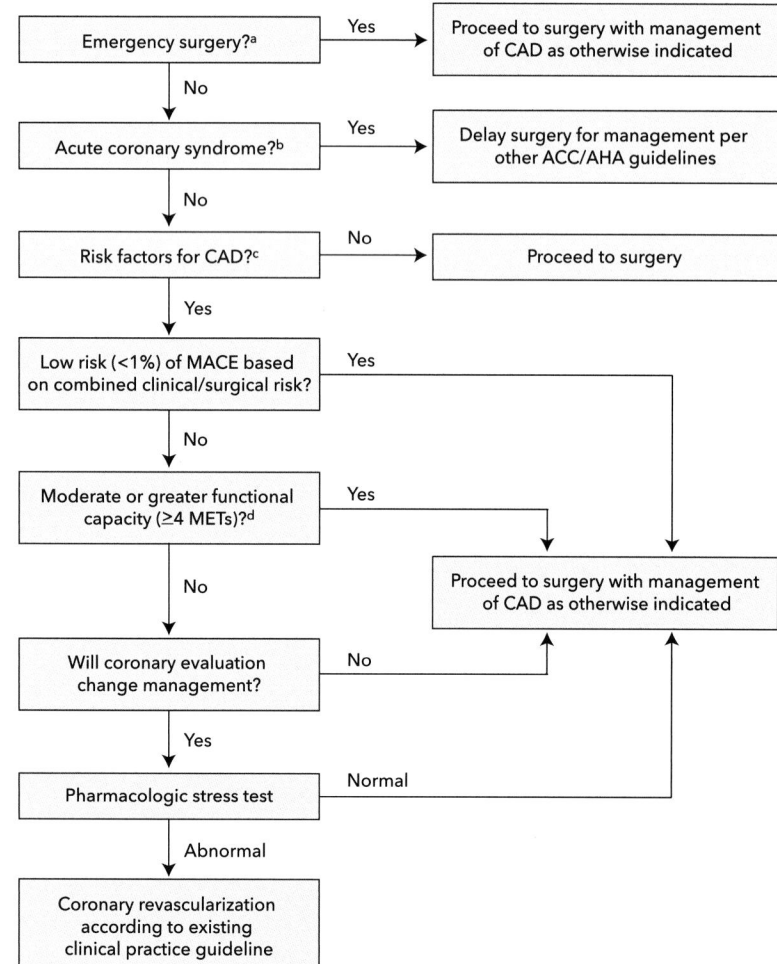

**FIGURE 29.** Perioperative ischemic cardiac disease evaluation for noncardiac surgery.

ACC = American College of Cardiology; AHA = American Heart Association; CAD = coronary artery disease; MACE = major adverse cardiac event; METs = metabolic equivalents.

[a]Emergency surgery required within 6 hours to avoid loss of life or limb.

[b]Acute coronary syndromes: myocardial infarction <30 days ago, unstable or severe angina.

[c]Risk factors for CAD: not specifically defined in ACC/AHA guidelines; examples include known CAD, cerebrovascular disease (i.e., stroke or transient ischemic attack), chronic kidney disease, diabetes mellitus, and heart failure.

[d]Examples of activities requiring ≥4 METs include climbing a flight of stairs, walking up a hill, walking on level ground at 4 miles per hour, running for a short distance, and playing tennis.

Recommendations from Fleisher LA, Fleischmann KE, Auerbach AD, Barnason SA, Beckman JA, Bozkurt B, et al; American College of Cardiology. 2014 ACC/AHA guideline on perioperative cardiovascular evaluation and management of patients undergoing noncardiac surgery: a report of the American College of Cardiology/American Heart Association Task Force on practice guidelines. J Am Coll Cardiol. 2014;64:e77-137. [PMID: 25091544] doi:10.1016/j.jacc.2014.07.944

| TABLE 92. Revised Cardiac Risk Index and Predicted Rate of Major Cardiac Complications Perioperatively | |
|---|---|
| **Risk Factor (1 point for each)** | |
| High-risk surgery (intrathoracic, intraperitoneal, suprainguinal vascular) | |
| Ischemic heart disease | |
| Heart failure (compensated) | |
| Diabetes mellitus (requiring insulin) | |
| Cerebrovascular disease | |
| Chronic kidney disease (serum creatinine >2.0 mg/dL [176.8 µmol/L])[a] | |
| **Number of Points** | **Risk for Major Cardiac Complications[b]** |
| 0 | 0.4% (95% CI, 0.1-0.8) |
| 1 | 1.0% (95% CI, 0.5-1.4) |
| 2 | 2.4% (95% CI, 1.3-3.5) |
| ≥3 | 5.4% (95% CI, 2.8-7.9) |

[a]Estimated glomerular filtration rate <30 mL/min/1.73 m² also shown to predict cardiovascular risk.

[b]Defined as cardiac death, nonfatal myocardial infarction, and nonfatal cardiac arrest.

Data from Lee TH, Marcantonio ER, Mangione CM, et al. Derivation and prospective validation of a simple index for prediction of cardiac risk of major noncardiac surgery. Circulation. 1999;100(10):1043-9. [PMID: 10477528] and Devereaux PJ, Goldman L, Cook DJ, Gilbert K, Leslie K, Guyatt GH. Perioperative cardiac events in patients undergoing noncardiac surgery: a review of the magnitude of the problem, the pathophysiology of the events and methods to estimate and communicate risk. CMAJ. 2005;173:627-34. [PMID: 16157727]

## Cardiovascular Risk Management

### Coronary Artery Disease

Patients with coronary artery disease (CAD) should not undergo routine coronary angiography or revascularization exclusively to reduce perioperative events. These procedures should be reserved for patients with recognized indications based on existing clinical practice guidelines. In patients who meet the criteria for intervention and in whom noncardiac surgery is time sensitive, balloon angioplasty or bare metal stent implantation should be considered over use of a drug-eluting stent. Elective noncardiac surgery should be delayed 14 days after balloon angioplasty, 30 days after bare metal stent implantation, and optimally 6 to 12 months after drug-eluting stent placement. However, if the risk of surgical delay outweighs the risk for ischemia and stent thrombosis, surgery may be considered 90 days after drug-eluting stent placement.

Patients taking β-blockers, statins, and many antihypertensive medications should continue these medications throughout the perioperative period, unless prohibited by hypotension. In hypotensive patients, dosage reduction is preferred to β-blocker discontinuation. There are also circumstances in which β-blocker or statin therapy should be initiated preoperatively (see Table 91). Postoperative β-blocker administration should be guided by clinical circumstances.

The ACC/AHA perioperative evaluation and management guideline does not recommend routinely obtaining postoperative troponin levels and an ECG in asymptomatic patients. However, these tests are recommended in patients with signs or symptoms of myocardial ischemia, which often presents atypically in the postoperative period (including as delirium in the elderly, hyperglycemia, and blood pressure fluctuations).

### Heart Failure

Medical management of decompensated heart failure should be optimized before surgery and may involve diuresis, fluid restriction, and medication adjustments (see MKSAP 18 Cardiovascular Medicine).

### Cardiac Arrhythmias

Risk management strategies for patients with a cardiac arrhythmia who are undergoing surgery include continuation of antiarrhythmic medications and, for some patients, continuous cardiac monitoring.

Patients with atrial fibrillation are at risk for rapid ventricular rate due to surgical stress, fluid shifts, and postoperative pain. Maintaining euvolemia, optimizing postoperative pain management, and controlling rates with medications are all appropriate strategies in stable patients. Hemodynamically unstable patients should undergo direct-current cardioversion.

A cardiologist should be consulted in patients with an implantable cardioverter-defibrillator who are undergoing surgery. Patients in whom a device has been deactivated for surgery should undergo continuous cardiac monitoring until the device is reprogrammed.

### Valvular Heart Disease

The ACC/AHA guideline states that it is reasonable to perform elevated-risk elective noncardiac surgery in patients with severe asymptomatic aortic stenosis, mitral regurgitation, or aortic regurgitation with preserved left ventricular function. In patients who are candidates for valvular intervention due to symptoms or severity of disease, valvular intervention should be performed before elective noncardiac surgery.

### Pulmonary Hypertension

Preoperative evaluation by a pulmonary hypertension specialist is advised for patients with pulmonary hypertension with high-risk features, including group 1 pulmonary hypertension (pulmonary arterial hypertension), pulmonary arterial systolic pressure greater than 70 mm Hg, moderate or severe right ventricular systolic dysfunction, and New York Heart Association functional class III or IV symptoms attributable to pulmonary hypertension. Patients with pulmonary hypertension undergoing noncardiac surgery should be continued on pulmonary vascular targeted therapies, such as phosphodiesterase-5 inhibitors.

### Primary Hypertension

In patients with hypertension, urgent blood pressure lowering is not mandatory preoperatively unless there is evidence of end-organ dysfunction, in which case surgery should be delayed and blood pressure treated. Deferral of surgery may also be considered in patients with a systolic blood pressure of 180 mm Hg or higher or diastolic blood pressure of 110 mm Hg or higher. Moderate preoperative hypertension has not been linked to adverse perioperative outcomes, although evidence is lacking regarding a specific blood pressure threshold. The perioperative use of specific antihypertensive agents is outlined in Table 91. H

**KEY POINTS**

HVC • Patients with low cardiovascular risk (<1% risk for perioperative major adverse cardiac event [MACE]) may proceed to surgery without preoperative cardiac stress testing, whereas patients with elevated risk (≥1% risk for perioperative MACE) should undergo assessment of functional capacity to determine necessity for cardiac stress testing.

HVC • Routine electrocardiography is not indicated in asymptomatic patients undergoing low-risk surgical procedures.

HVC • In patients with coronary artery disease, routine coronary angiography or revascularization should be performed for recognized indications based on existing clinical practice guidelines and should not be performed exclusively to reduce perioperative cardiovascular events.

• Patients with hypertension who are undergoing surgery do not require urgent blood pressure lowering preoperatively unless there is evidence of end-organ dysfunction.

## Pulmonary Perioperative Management

Perioperative pulmonary complications include pneumonia, respiratory failure, and exacerbation of underlying lung disease. Pulmonary perioperative management involves pulmonary risk assessment, including screening for obstructive sleep apnea (OSA), assessment of any underlying lung disease with optimization of treatment, and optimization of perioperative risk-reduction strategies.

### Pulmonary Risk Assessment

Pulmonary risk factors can be categorized as patient-related risk factors or procedure-related risk factors (**Table 93**). Obesity and well-controlled asthma have not been shown to be independently associated with perioperative pulmonary complications. Risk calculators that include many of the important risk factors as well as other predictors, such as low oxygen saturation and the presence of preoperative sepsis, are available to help determine postoperative risk for respiratory failure, pneumonia, and overall pulmonary complications. The Postoperative Respiratory Failure Risk Calculator is available at www.surgicalriskcalculator.com/prf-risk-calculator, and the Postoperative Pneumonia Risk Calculator is available at www.surgicalriskcalculator.com/postoperative-pneumonia-risk-calculator. These calculators do not consider important

| TABLE 93. Pulmonary Risk Factors |
|---|
| **Patient-Specific Risk Factors** |
| Age |
| COPD |
| Cigarette use |
| ASA class ≥2[a] |
| Functional dependence |
| Obstructive sleep apnea |
| Heart failure |
| Poor nutritional status |
| **Procedure-Specific Risk Factors** |
| Surgery in close proximity to the diaphragm (aortic, thoracic, abdominal) |
| Head and neck surgery |
| Neurosurgery |
| Major vascular surgery |
| Procedure duration >3-4 hours |
| Emergency surgery |

ASA = American Society of Anesthesiologists.

[a]ASA classes are as follows: class 1, normal healthy patient; class 2, patient with mild systemic disease; class 3, patient with severe systemic disease; class 4, patient with systemic disease that is a constant threat to life; and class 5, moribund patient who is not expected to survive for 24 hours with or without operation.

Adapted with permission from Smetana GW, Lawrence VA, Cornell JE; American College of Physicians. Preoperative pulmonary risk stratification for noncardiothoracic surgery: systematic review for the American College of Physicians. Ann Intern Med. 2006;144:584, 587. [PMID: 16618956] Copyright 2006, American College of Physicians.

pulmonary comorbid conditions, such as COPD and OSA, but they are useful in planning for surgery and establishing informed consent.

Spirometry is not useful for predicting risk and should not be routinely ordered for preoperative evaluation, including in patients with COPD. Furthermore, evidence does not support a spirometric threshold below which the risk of surgery is unacceptable. Spirometry is indicated in patients undergoing lung resection, however, to help predict postoperative lung function. Chest radiography is not required in most patients but is indicated in patients with signs or symptoms of pulmonary disease and in patients with underlying cardiac or pulmonary disease and new or unstable symptoms.

All patients should be screened for OSA, which is associated with adverse perioperative outcomes, including cardiac events, pulmonary complications, and ICU admissions. A commonly used screening tool for OSA is the STOP-BANG score (**Table 94**). In high-risk patients undergoing elective surgery, the American Society of Anesthesiologists recommends further evaluation with polysomnography.

### Assessment of Underlying Lung Disease

COPD is the most commonly identified risk factor for postoperative pulmonary complications. Patients should be

**TABLE 94. STOP-BANG Obstructive Sleep Apnea Screening Tool**

| Survey Items (1 point for each) |
| --- |
| **S**noring |
| **T**iredness or sleepiness during the day |
| **O**bserved apnea during sleep |
| **P**ressure, high blood |
| **B**MI >35 |
| **A**ge >50 years |
| **N**eck circumference >40 cm (15.7 in) |
| **G**ender = male |

| STOP-BANG Score | Risk Correlation |
| --- | --- |
| 0-2 | Low risk for OSA |
| ≥3 | Increased risk for OSA |
| ≥5 | Increased risk for moderate-severe OSA |

OSA = obstructive sleep apnea.

Adapted with permission from Chung F, Yegneswaran B, Liao P, et al. STOP questionnaire: a tool to screen patients for obstructive sleep apnea. Anesthesiology. 2008 May;108(5):812-21. [PMID: 18431116] *and* Chung F, Subramanyam R, Liao P, Sasaki E, Shapiro C, Sun Y. High STOP-Bang score indicates a high probability of obstructive sleep apnoea. Br J Anaesth. 2012 May;108(5):768-75. [PMID: 22401881]

 screened preoperatively for signs and symptoms of COPD exacerbation and instructed to take prescribed inhaled medications on the morning of surgery. In patients with an exacerbation, surgery should be postponed, and treatment should be initiated.

## Perioperative Risk-Reduction Strategies

Risk for pulmonary complications should be mitigated with perioperative risk-reduction interventions, including preoperative initiation of lung expansion maneuvers (deep breathing exercises and incentive spirometry), limiting use of nasogastric tubes in abdominal surgery for nausea or abdominal distention, and aspiration precautions. A recent multicenter randomized trial demonstrated that a 30-minute preoperative education and breathing exercise training session can reduce postoperative pulmonary complication rates by 50%. Smoking cessation has been shown to reduce pulmonary risk and should be encouraged as far in advance of surgery as possible. Patients with pulmonary disease should continue outpatient medications.

In patients diagnosed with OSA, continuous positive airway pressure (CPAP) should be initiated preoperatively. Patients at high risk for OSA undergoing nonelective surgery should be placed on continuous pulse oximetry and monitored for oxygen desaturation, apneas, reduced respiration rate, and oversedation in the postanesthesia care unit (PACU); patients with recurrent respiratory events in the PACU benefit from additional monitoring postoperatively. All patients with known OSA should bring their CPAP device to the hospital for use in the perioperative period.

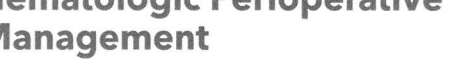

- Preoperative chest radiography is indicated only in patients with signs or symptoms of pulmonary disease and in patients with underlying cardiac or pulmonary disease and new or unstable symptoms. **HVC**

- Spirometry should not be routinely performed preoperatively except in patients undergoing lung resection. **HVC**

- All patients undergoing surgery should be screened for obstructive sleep apnea, which is associated with adverse perioperative outcomes, including cardiac events, pulmonary complications, and ICU admissions.

# Hematologic Perioperative Management

## Venous Thromboembolism Prophylaxis

The American College of Chest Physicians (ACCP) antithrombotic guideline provides recommendations for VTE prophylaxis for both orthopedic and nonorthopedic surgery populations (**Table 95**). In patients undergoing general surgery or abdominal-pelvic surgery, the ACCP recommends using the Caprini score to estimate the patient's risk for postoperative thrombosis (**Table 96**).

Hip fracture surgery, total knee arthroplasty, and total hip arthroplasty pose a high risk for VTE, and both mechanical (nonpharmacologic) and pharmacologic VTE prophylaxis are recommended. Mechanical prophylaxis is provided with an intermittent pneumatic compression device. For pharmacologic prophylaxis, the ACCP recommends low-molecular-weight heparin in preference to other pharmacologic agents. The minimum recommended duration of pharmacologic VTE prophylaxis in patients undergoing orthopedic surgery is 10 to 14 days; however, in patients without increased bleeding risk, extended-duration postoperative prophylaxis (up to 35 days) is preferred over shorter-duration prophylaxis. Intermittent pneumatic compression devices and pharmacologic VTE prophylaxis are recommended during the entire hospital stay. If bleeding risk is especially high, mechanical prophylaxis is recommended over no prophylaxis. In patients who decline or are unable to tolerate low-molecular-weight heparin, the ACCP recommends apixaban, rivaroxaban, dabigatran, or a vitamin K antagonist over alternate forms of prophylaxis.

The ACCP recommends against the routine placement of inferior vena cava filters for VTE prophylaxis. Routine surveillance for VTE with venous compression ultrasonography is also not recommended in patients undergoing orthopedic surgery, general surgery, abdominal-pelvic surgery, and trauma surgery.

## Perioperative Management of Anticoagulant Therapy

Anticoagulant therapy increases the risk for perioperative hemorrhage and should be discontinued in most patients before surgery. Minor surgery, including dental extractions

| TABLE 95. Postoperative Venous Thromboembolism Prophylaxis Recommendations for Common Noncardiothoracic Surgeries | | | |
|---|---|---|---|
| **Surgery and Risks** | | | **Recommended Prophylaxis[a]** |
| General, abdominal-pelvic, urologic, plastic, vascular | Caprini[b] score 0 | | Early ambulation |
| | Caprini score 1-2 | | IPC |
| | Caprini score 3-4 | Average bleeding risk | LMWH, LDUH, IPC |
| | | High bleeding risk[c] | IPC |
| | Caprini score ≥5 | Average bleeding risk | LMWH or LDUH (+ IPC) |
| | | High bleeding risk[c] | IPC |
| | Cancer surgery | | LMWH for 4 wk |
| Orthopedic | Hip or knee arthroplasty[d] | | IPC + LMWH, LDUH, aspirin, NOAC, fondaparinux, warfarin, or IPC alone if high bleeding risk; continue for 10-35 d |
| | Hip fracture repair[d] | | IPC + LMWH, LDUH, warfarin, fondaparinux, or IPC alone if high bleeding risk; continue for 10-35 d |
| | Isolated lower leg fracture repairs | | None |
| | Knee arthroscopy with no previous VTE | | Early ambulation |
| Spine (elective) | Average VTE risk | | IPC |
| | High VTE risk (e.g., malignancy, anterior-posterior approach) | | IPC + LMWH (when bleeding risk sufficiently low) |
| Major trauma | Average VTE risk | | LMWH, LDUH, IPC |
| | High VTE risk (e.g., spinal cord or brain injury) | | LMWH or LDUH (+ IPC) |
| | High bleeding risk[c] | | IPC |
| Intracranial | Average VTE risk | | IPC |
| | High VTE risk (e.g., malignancy) | | LMWH or LDUH (+ IPC) |

IPC = intermittent pneumatic compression; LDUH = low-dose unfractionated heparin; LMWH = low-molecular-weight heparin; NOAC = non–vitamin K antagonist oral anticoagulant (dabigatran, rivaroxaban, apixaban); VTE = venous thromboembolism.

[a]Duration is for postoperative hospitalization unless noted otherwise.

[b]See Table 96 for the Caprini Risk Assessment Scoring method.

[c]Risk factors suggesting high bleeding risk: concurrent antithrombotic therapy (e.g., aspirin for cardiac disease), known or suspected bleeding disorder, active bleeding, liver or kidney disease, and sepsis.

[d]LMWH is preferred.

Recommendations from Gould MK, Garcia DA, Wren SM, Karanicolas PJ, Arcelus JI, Heit JA, et al. Prevention of VTE in nonorthopedic surgical patients: antithrombotic therapy and prevention of thrombosis, 9th ed: American College of Chest Physicians evidence-based clinical practice guidelines. Chest. 2012;141:e227S-e277S. [PMID: 22315263] doi:10.1378/chest.11-2297 and Falck-Ytter Y, Francis CW, Johanson NA, Curley C, Dahl OE, Schulman S, et al. Prevention of VTE in orthopedic surgery patients: antithrombotic therapy and prevention of thrombosis, 9th ed: American College of Chest Physicians evidence-based clinical practice guidelines. Chest. 2012;141:e278S-e325S. [PMID: 22315265] doi:10.1378/chest.11-2404

CONT.

and minor skin surgery, can be completed while a patient is anticoagulated. Vitamin K antagonist (warfarin) therapy may also be continued in some patients undergoing cardiac device implantation, although the best approach to these procedures in patients receiving non–vitamin K antagonist oral anticoagulants (NOACs), including direct thrombin and factor Xa inhibitors, is unclear. In any case, collaboration with the surgeon or proceduralist is crucial to ensure that it is safe for the patient to remain anticoagulated. When it is necessary to discontinue anticoagulation, vitamin K antagonists should be discontinued at least 5 days before surgery; most procedures can be safely performed with an INR of less than 1.5. The duration for which NOACs are discontinued before surgery depends on

the bleeding risk of the procedure, the patient's kidney function, and the medication half-life; generally, NOACs can be stopped 2 to 3 days preoperatively because of their shorter half-lives.

Bridging anticoagulation is the administration of therapeutic doses of short-acting parenteral therapy, usually heparin, when oral anticoagulant therapy is being withheld during the perioperative period in patients with elevated thrombotic risk. Bridging is most commonly indicated in patients taking vitamin K antagonists. It is not indicated in patients taking NOACs because of the rapid onset and short half-life associated with these drugs, but it may be needed when patients are unable to take oral medications for an extended time after surgery, such as with gastrointestinal surgery.

**TABLE 96.** Caprini Venous Thromboembolism Risk Assessment Scoring Method

| Number of Points for Each Risk Factor | Risk Factors |
|---|---|
| 1 | Age 41-60 y; minor surgery; BMI >25; leg edema; varicose veins; recent or current pregnancy; estrogen use; recurrent spontaneous abortion; recent sepsis (<1 mo)/pneumonia (<1 mo); severe lung disease; abnormal pulmonary function; inflammatory bowel disease; acute MI; recent HF (<1 mo); medical patient at bed rest |
| 2 | Age 61-74 y; arthroscopic surgery; major surgery lasting >45 min; malignancy; bed rest for >72 h; immobilizing cast; central venous access |
| 3 | Age ≥75 y; personal history of VTE; family history of VTE; congenital or acquired thrombophilia; HIT |
| 5 | Stroke or spinal cord injury within 1 mo; elective arthroplasty; hip, pelvis, or leg fracture |

HF = heart failure; HIT = heparin-induced thrombocytopenia; MI = myocardial infarction; VTE = venous thromboembolism.

Adapted from Bahl V, Hu HM, Henke PK, Wakefield TW, Campbell DA Jr, Caprini JA. A validation study of a retrospective venous thromboembolism risk scoring method. Ann Surg. 2010;251:344-50. [PMID: 19779324] doi:10.1097/SLA.0b013e3181b7fca6

**TABLE 97.** Annual Stroke Risk Based on CHADS$_2$ Score

| CHADS$_2$ Score[a] | Unadjusted Annual Stroke Rate in Patients Not Treated With Anticoagulation (per 100 Patient-Years)[b] |
|---|---|
| 0 | 0.6 |
| 1 | 3.0 |
| 2 | 4.2 |
| 3 | 7.1 |
| 4 | 11.1 |
| 5 | 12.5 |
| 6 | 13.0 |

[a]One point is given for heart failure, hypertension, age ≥75 years, and diabetes mellitus. Two points are given for previous stroke or transient ischemic attack.

[b]Data from Friberg L, Rosenqvist M, Lip GY. Evaluation of risk stratification schemes for ischaemic stroke and bleeding in 182 678 patients with atrial fibrillation: the Swedish Atrial Fibrillation cohort study. Eur Heart J. 2012;33:1500-10. [PMID: 22246443] doi:10.1093/eurheartj/ehr488

CONT.

Postprocedural management of anticoagulation is based on thrombotic and bleeding risk, and close collaboration with the surgeon is essential. In patients taking a vitamin K antagonist, bridging anticoagulation may be deferred if thrombotic risk is low; the first dose of a vitamin K antagonist is typically administered 12 to 24 hours after surgery. If bridging is needed and the bleeding risk is low, bridging anticoagulation may be started as soon as 24 hours after the procedure; in the case of high bleeding risk, initiation of bridging anticoagulation is delayed 48 to 72 hours or possibly longer. Postoperative timing of NOAC reinstitution depends on bleeding risk, as NOACs reach therapeutic levels in 1 to 3 hours, at which point the patient is presumed to be fully anticoagulated. NOACs may be resumed once adequate hemostasis is ensured, usually 48 to 72 hours after surgery.

Because of the risk for spinal epidural hematoma, anticoagulant use with concomitant neuraxial (spinal and epidural) anesthesia should be avoided.

### Atrial Fibrillation

The decision to initiate bridging anticoagulation in patients with atrial fibrillation is based on bleeding risk and thrombotic risk. Procedures with an intermediate or high risk for bleeding almost always require interruption of anticoagulation, and the CHADS$_2$ score (**Table 97**) and CHA$_2$DS$_2$-VASc score may be used to determine thrombotic risk and the need for bridging anticoagulation in patients with nonvalvular atrial fibrillation. Although use of the CHA$_2$DS$_2$-VASc score for

risk stratification is advocated in several guidelines, it has not been validated in the perioperative setting (see MKSAP 18 Cardiovascular Medicine).

The landmark BRIDGE trial has shifted clinical practice toward a more conservative approach to bridging anticoagulation in patients with nonvalvular atrial fibrillation. This randomized controlled trial determined bleeding and thrombotic outcomes in patients who received bridging anticoagulation compared with those who did not. An increased risk for bleeding was identified in patients who received bridging anticoagulation, and those who received no bridging anticoagulation did not demonstrate an increased risk for thrombosis. Only a small proportion of patients with a higher thrombotic risk (CHADS$_2$ score of 5 and 6) were included in the study, limiting the applicability in this population. Additionally, most patients underwent minor procedures, which likely carry lower thrombotic risk.

Recommendations from the ACCP and ACC on bridging anticoagulation in patients with atrial fibrillation are provided in **Table 98**.

### Prosthetic Heart Valves and Venous Thromboembolic Disease

In patients receiving warfarin anticoagulant therapy for a mechanical prosthetic heart valve, continuation of anticoagulation is recommended when the surgical procedure is minor and bleeding can be managed. In patients undergoing surgery with a higher risk for bleeding, the 2017 ACC/AHA guideline on valvular heart disease suggests that bridging should be considered on an individualized basis in patients with a mechanical mitral valve, a mechanical aortic valve with thromboembolic risk factors, or an older-generation mechanical aortic valve. Bridging is not necessary in patients with a bileaflet mechanical aortic valve and no other risk factors for thrombosis. The ACCP provides similar recommendations for bridging anticoagulation in patients with prosthetic heart valves (**Table 99**).

**TABLE 98.** American College of Chest Physicians and American College of Cardiology Recommendations for Perioperative Bridging in Patients With Atrial Fibrillation

| Risk for Thromboembolism | Patient History and Risk Stratification Score | Bridging Anticoagulation Recommendation |
|---|---|---|
| **High (annual risk >10%)** | | |
| ACCP | $CHADS_2$ score of 5 or 6 <br><br> Recent stroke or TIA <br><br> Rheumatic valvular heart disease <br><br> Patient with history of stroke with warfarin interruption | Bridging |
| ACC | $CHA_2DS_2$-VASc score of 7-9 <br><br> Ischemic stroke, TIA, or systemic embolism within the last 3 mo | Bridging |
| **Moderate (annual risk of 5%-10%)** | | |
| ACCP | $CHADS_2$ score of 3 or 4 | Bridging unless procedure is associated with a high bleeding risk |
| ACC | $CHA_2DS_2$-VASc of 5 or 6 <br><br> History of ischemic stroke, TIA, or systemic embolism ≥3 mo ago | Increased risk for bleeding: interrupt VKA without bridging <br><br> No significant bleeding risk: <br><br>     Stroke, TIA, or systemic embolism history: consider bridging[a] <br><br>     No stroke, TIA, or systemic embolism history: no bridging[a] |
| **Low (annual risk <5%)** | | |
| ACCP | $CHADS_2$ score of 0-2 <br><br> No stroke or TIA history | No bridging |
| ACC | $CHA_2DS_2$-VASc score ≤4 <br><br> No history of ischemic stroke, TIA, or systemic embolism | No bridging |

ACC = American College of Cardiology; ACCP = American College of Chest Physicians; TIA = transient ischemic attack; VKA = vitamin K antagonist.

[a]Clinical judgment is required.

Information from Douketis JD, Spyropoulos AC, Spencer FA, Mayr M, Jaffer AK, Eckman MH, et al. Perioperative management of antithrombotic therapy: antithrombotic therapy and prevention of thrombosis, 9th ed: American College of Chest Physicians evidence-based clinical practice guidelines. Chest. 2012;141:e326S-e350S. [PMID: 22315266] doi:10.1378/chest.11-2298 and Doherty JU, Gluckman TJ, Hucker WJ, Januzzi JL Jr, Ortel TL, Saxonhouse SJ, et al. 2017 ACC expert consensus decision pathway for periprocedural management of anticoagulation in patients with nonvalvular atrial fibrillation: a report of the American College of Cardiology Clinical Expert Consensus Document Task Force. J Am Coll Cardiol. 2017;69:871-898. [PMID: 28081965] doi: 10.1016/j.jacc.2016.11.024

**TABLE 99.** American College of Chest Physicians Recommendations for Perioperative Bridging in Patients With a Prosthetic Heart Valve

| Risk for Thromboembolism | Patient History | Bridging Anticoagulation Recommendation |
|---|---|---|
| High (annual risk >10%) | Any mitral valve prosthesis <br><br> Any caged-ball or tilting disc aortic valve prosthesis <br><br> Recent (within 6 mo) stroke or TIA | Bridging |
| Moderate (annual risk of 5%-10%) | Bileaflet aortic valve prosthesis and one or more of the of following risk factors: atrial fibrillation, previous stroke or TIA, hypertension, diabetes mellitus, heart failure, age >75 y | Bridging unless procedure is associated with a high bleeding risk |
| Low (annual risk <5%) | Bileaflet aortic valve prosthesis without atrial fibrillation and no other risk factors for stroke | No bridging |

TIA = transient ischemic attack.

Recommendations from Douketis JD, Spyropoulos AC, Spencer FA, Mayr M, Jaffer AK, Eckman MH, et al. Perioperative management of antithrombotic therapy: antithrombotic therapy and prevention of thrombosis, 9th ed: American College of Chest Physicians evidence-based clinical practice guidelines. Chest. 2012;141:e326S-e350S. [PMID: 22315266] doi:10.1378/chest.11-2298

CONT.

ACCP recommendations for bridging anticoagulation in those with a history of venous thromboembolism, including patients with thrombophilias, are included in **Table 100**.

## Perioperative Management of Antiplatelet Medications

The perioperative management of dual antiplatelet therapy (DAPT), comprising aspirin plus a $P2Y_{12}$ inhibitor (clopidogrel, ticagrelor, or prasugrel), in patients with CAD depends on the presence of a bare metal or drug-eluting coronary stent, time since stent placement, and, to some degree, the indication for DAPT (stable ischemic heart disease [SIHD] or acute coronary syndrome [ACS] within the last year).

In patients who have a stent placed for SIHD, DAPT should be continued uninterrupted for at least 30 days after bare metal stent placement and a minimum of 6 months after drug-eluting stent placement. Elective surgery should be postponed during these time frames. However, if the risk of surgical delay exceeds the risk for stent thrombosis, discontinuation of the $P2Y_{12}$ inhibitor can be considered after a minimum of 3 months in patients with a drug-eluting stent. Aspirin should be continued if at all possible, and DAPT should be restarted as soon as bleeding risk has sufficiency diminished.

In patients with recent ACS, the ACC and AHA recommend continuing DAPT for at least 1 year regardless of whether the ACS was managed with medical therapy or coronary stent placement. If surgery must be performed within this time frame, DAPT should optimally be maintained for a minimum of 6 months. If more than 3 months have passed and the patient cannot be continued on DAPT because of bleeding risk, proceeding with surgery can be considered if the risk of surgical delay is greater than the risk for stent thrombosis.

In patients with recent percutaneous coronary intervention with stent placement for ACS in whom surgery mandates discontinuation of DAPT, aspirin should be continued. In patients with recent ACS treated medically who must undergo surgery for which DAPT must be discontinued, it is similarly reasonable to continue aspirin when the risk for cardiac events outweighs the risk for bleeding.

In most patients receiving long-term aspirin monotherapy for both primary and secondary prevention of cardiovascular events (in the absence of a coronary stent), aspirin should be discontinued at least 5 days before surgery and restarted postoperatively once bleeding risk has decreased. This recommendation is based on the POISE-2 trial, which found that continued perioperative aspirin resulted in increased bleeding without a decrease in cardiac events.

## Perioperative Management of Anemia, Coagulopathies, and Thrombocytopenia

In all patients undergoing surgery, a careful preoperative bleeding history, including a family history, should be obtained to evaluate for underlying bleeding disorders and anemia. Laboratory testing should be reserved for patients with a suggestive history. Patients with known factor deficiencies, platelet function defects, and other coagulopathies should be managed by a hematologist.

In orthopedic and cardiac surgery patients and those with a history of stable CAD, the American Association of Blood Banks recommends a restrictive transfusion threshold (hemoglobin level of 8 g/dL [80 g/L]), as studies indicate that a restrictive threshold results in equivalent or improved patient outcomes. Similarly, in hospitalized hemodynamically stable patients, a transfusion threshold of 7 g/dL (70 g/L) is recommended.

The American Association of Blood Banks recommends a platelet transfusion threshold of $50,000/\mu L$ ($50 \times 10^9/L$) for patients undergoing major non-neurologic surgery or lumbar puncture. Patients with mild thrombocytopenia due to

---

**TABLE 100.** American College of Chest Physicians Recommendations for Perioperative Bridging in Patients With Venous Thromboembolism

| Risk for Thromboembolism | Patient History | Bridging Anticoagulation Recommendation |
|---|---|---|
| High (annual risk >10%) | Recent (within 3 mo) VTE | Bridging |
| | Severe thrombophilia (e.g., deficiency of protein C, protein S, or antithrombin; antiphospholipid antibodies; multiple abnormalities) | |
| Moderate (annual risk of 5%-10%) | VTE within the past 3-12 mo | Bridging unless procedure is associated with a high bleeding risk |
| | Nonsevere thrombophilia (e.g., heterozygous factor V Leiden or prothrombin gene mutation) | |
| | Recurrent VTE | |
| | Active cancer (treated within 6 mo or palliative) | |
| Low (annual risk <5%) | VTE >12 mo ago and no other risk factors | No bridging |

VTE = venous thromboembolism.

Recommendations from Douketis JD, Spyropoulos AC, Spencer FA, Mayr M, Jaffer AK, Eckman MH, et al. Perioperative management of antithrombotic therapy: antithrombotic therapy and prevention of thrombosis, 9th ed: American College of Chest Physicians evidence-based clinical practice guidelines. Chest. 2012;141:e326S-e350S. [PMID: 22315266] doi:10.1378/chest.11-2298

CONT.

immune thrombocytopenia are typically able to proceed to surgery at the recommended threshold. Postoperative thrombocytopenia warrants further evaluation, especially in patients with heparin exposure owing to the risk for heparin-induced thrombocytopenia. See MKSAP 18 Hematology and Oncology for a discussion of heparin-induced thrombocytopenia. ▣

**KEY POINTS**

- Patients undergoing general surgery or abdominal-pelvic surgery who are at high risk for venous thromboembolism should receive pharmacologic prophylaxis (with low-molecular-weight heparin or low-dose unfractionated heparin) in combination with mechanical prophylaxis.

- The minimum recommended duration of pharmacologic venous thromboembolism prophylaxis in patients undergoing orthopedic surgery is 10 to 14 days; however, in patients without increased bleeding risk, extended-duration postoperative prophylaxis (up to 35 days) is preferred.

- In patients with atrial fibrillation undergoing a procedure with an intermediate or high risk for bleeding, interruption of anticoagulation is almost always required, and the $CHADS_2$ and $CHA_2DS_2$-VASc scores may be used to determine thrombotic risk and the need for bridging anticoagulation.

- In patients treated with percutaneous coronary intervention who are undergoing elective noncardiac surgery, dual antiplatelet therapy should be continued uninterrupted for at least 30 days after bare metal stent placement and a minimum of 6 months after drug-eluting stent placement.

HVC
- In orthopedic and cardiac surgery patients and those with a history of CAD, the American Association of Blood Banks recommends a restrictive transfusion threshold (hemoglobin level of 8 g/dL [80 g/L]).

# ▣ Perioperative Management of Endocrine Diseases

## Diabetes Mellitus

Evidence demonstrates that patients with uncontrolled diabetes are at increased risk for perioperative complications, including surgical and nonsurgical infections, and postoperative mortality. Patients at high risk for diabetes, such as those with a history of impaired fasting glucose, should be evaluated for diabetes before elective surgery. In patients with established diabetes, it is reasonable to measure hemoglobin $A_{1c}$ within 3 months of surgery. There is not high-quality evidence on whether delaying surgery to improve glycemic control improves outcomes, although efforts should be made to optimize glycemic control before major elective surgery.

Oral and injectable noninsulin medications should be withheld 12 to 72 hours before surgery, replaced with supplemental insulin, and resumed at hospital discharge or when the patient has resumed a full diet. In patients taking insulin therapy, basal insulin should be continued perioperatively. The basal insulin dosage should not be reduced in patients with type 1 diabetes. Preoperative dosage reduction (often 25%-50%) may be considered in patients with type 2 diabetes who have a history of hypoglycemia with skipped or delayed meals.

Postoperatively, if the patient is eating, the ideal insulin regimen is a basal-bolus regimen, with prandial coverage and correction boluses for premeal hyperglycemia. For a discussion of the management of hyperglycemia in the hospital setting, see MKSAP 18 Endocrinology and Metabolism.

## Thyroid Disease

Preoperative screening for thyroid disease is not recommended in the absence of symptoms. In patients with symptoms suggestive of thyroid disease or patients with hypothyroidism and a recent change in levothyroxine dosage, it is reasonable to obtain a preoperative thyroid-stimulating hormone level, although there are no guidelines to support such an approach.

In patients with hypothyroidism treated with levothyroxine, therapy should continue uninterrupted. Patients with untreated, asymptomatic mild hypothyroidism may proceed to surgery. A recent retrospective cohort study demonstrated that mild hypothyroidism (median thyroid-stimulating hormone level of 8.6 µU/mL [8.6 mU/L]) was not associated with an increase in perioperative mortality, cardiovascular morbidity, or infectious morbidity. In the presence of severe hypothyroidism, elective surgery should be postponed to prevent myxedema coma, arrhythmias, perioperative hypotension, and other complications.

Patients with well-controlled hyperthyroidism should be continued on therapy, including β-blockers and thionamides. Patients with uncontrolled hyperthyroidism are at risk for thyroid storm in the perioperative period, and surgery should be deferred until thyroid disease can be controlled.

Consultation with an endocrinologist is advised if emergent surgery is required in patients with severe thyroid disease.

## Adrenal Insufficiency

Patients with adrenal insufficiency should be evaluated for the need for perioperative supplemental glucocorticoid dosing, known as stress dosing. The decision to initiate perioperative stress dosing is guided by limited evidence, although one strategy uses patient characteristics and the degree of surgical stress to determine management (**Table 101**). Perioperative supplemental glucocorticoid dosing recommendations are provided in **Table 102**.

**TABLE 101.** Stress Dosing Strategies in Patients at Risk for Adrenal Insufficiency

| Patient Risk | Patient Characteristics | Management |
|---|---|---|
| High risk | Primary adrenal insufficiency | Stress dosing |
| | Hypothalamic-pituitary-adrenal axis disease | |
| | Cushingoid features | |
| | Equivalent of >5 mg/d of prednisone for >3 wk during the previous 3 mo | |
| | High-dose inhaled glucocorticoid therapy | |
| Moderate risk | Equivalent of >5 mg/d of prednisone for <3 wk during the previous 3 mo | Stress dosing may be indicated[a] |
| | High-dose topical glucocorticoid therapy | Perform preoperative adrenal axis testing |
| | Injectable glucocorticoid therapy in the last 3 mo | |
| Low risk | Equivalent of <5 mg/d of prednisone for any duration | No stress dosing |
| | Low-dose inhaled or topical glucocorticoid therapy | |

[a]In patients at moderate risk who require emergent or urgent surgery, no further testing is recommended, and stress-dose glucocorticoids should be administered. In other patients, it is reasonable to measure morning serum cortisol preoperatively to test the hypothalamic-pituitary-adrenal axis.

**TABLE 102.** Perioperative Supplemental Glucocorticoid Dosing

| Surgical Stress Anticipated | Daily Intravenous Hydrocortisone Dose | Duration of Stress Dosing (in Days) |
|---|---|---|
| Minor (e.g., ambulatory procedures) | 25 mg | 1 |
| Moderate (e.g., orthopedic surgery) | 50-75 mg | 1-2 |
| High (e.g., cardiac bypass graft surgery) | 100 mg, followed by 50 mg every 6 hours | 2-3 |

**KEY POINTS**

- In patients with diabetes mellitus who are undergoing surgery, oral and injectable noninsulin medications should be withheld, replaced with supplemental insulin, and resumed at hospital discharge or when the patient has resumed a full diet.

HVC
- Patients with untreated, asymptomatic mild hypothyroidism may proceed to surgery without further testing or treatment.

- Surgery should be deferred in patients with severe uncontrolled hypo- or hyperthyroidism.

## Perioperative Management of Kidney Disease

Patients with chronic kidney disease (CKD) are at increased perioperative risk for fluid and electrolyte imbalance, metabolic acidosis, anemia, bleeding diathesis, and cardiac events, depending on the severity of the underlying disease. For patients undergoing hemodialysis, it is advisable to consult a nephrologist for review of the dialysate prescription, adjustment of fluid removal, and management of peridialysis heparin. Patients with less advanced CKD require correction of electrolyte abnormalities and optimization of volume status preoperatively. In all patients with kidney disease undergoing surgery, it is important to avoid iodinated contrast dye and other nephrotoxic agents and minimize perioperative hypotension.

Perioperative acute kidney injury portends an increased risk for postoperative CKD and, in those with underlying CKD, end-stage kidney disease. The two most important means of mitigating the risk for acute kidney injury are maintenance of renal blood flow and avoidance of further insults to the kidneys. Renal blood flow is maintained by avoiding renal hypoperfusion; effectively managing diuresis and antihypertensive medications; and treating anemia, which may impair peripheral vasodilation. Careful medication review is also warranted to ensure appropriate dosing based on renal clearance.

**KEY POINT**

- The two most important means of mitigating the risk for acute kidney injury in the perioperative period are maintenance of renal blood flow and avoidance of further insults to the kidneys.

## Perioperative Management of Liver Disease

Liver disease increases risk for perioperative infection, encephalopathy, bleeding, fluid retention, and acute kidney and liver decompensation. Patients with chronic liver disease require careful preoperative evaluation and risk stratification using the Model for End-stage Liver Disease (MELD) score and Child-Turcotte-Pugh classification. Patients with compensated liver disease, including those with a MELD score of less than 8 to 10, are often able to proceed with surgery with optimal medical management. In patients with intermediate risk, referral to a hepatologist is reasonable before proceeding with surgery. Those with severe liver disease are at increased and often prohibitive risk for perioperative complications and death; patients with Child-Turcotte-Pugh class C disease and a MELD score greater than 15 are generally advised to avoid elective surgery and should be referred for transplant evaluation if appropriate.

Complications of liver disease should be optimally managed in all patients; however, the American Association for the Study of Liver Diseases recommends against perioperative

CONT.

transjugular intrahepatic portosystemic shunt placement because of a lack of evidence that the procedure improves outcomes.

In general, patients with liver disease should be advised to abstain from alcohol consumption for at least 12 weeks before elective surgery.

## Perioperative Management of Neurologic Disease

Patients with neurologic disease are at increased perioperative risk for loss of disease control, among other complications. In patients with epilepsy, perioperative seizure risk is thought to be driven by the severity of the underlying disease and seizure frequency, rather than by anesthesia or surgery type; an important exception is intracranial surgery, which may provoke seizures depending on the location of the surgery, underlying pathologic conditions, and required degree of brain manipulation. Antiepileptic medications should be continued uninterrupted. In patients who are unable to tolerate oral intake, alternate formulations should be used.

Patients with Parkinson disease are predisposed to perioperative delirium, hallucinations, orthostatic hypotension, and complications related to dysphagia. It is essential that patients maintain their normal treatment regimen. Surgery should be scheduled for as early in the day as possible to minimize missed doses, and antidopaminergic antiemetics should be avoided. Parkinson-hyperpyrexia syndrome is a potentially life-threatening complication resulting from withdrawal of or reduction in the dosage of dopamine agonists; it is characterized by rigidity, fever, altered mental status, and autonomic instability.

Asymptomatic carotid bruit is a common finding in older adults but is not predictive of perioperative stroke and therefore requires no preoperative evaluation. Perioperative stroke is discussed in MKSAP 18 Neurology.

Delirium commonly occurs in the postoperative setting, especially in the elderly. Risk factors and treatment are similar to those for delirium in the general hospital setting (see MKSAP 18 Neurology). H

### KEY POINTS

- Patients with Parkinson disease should continue antiparkinson agents through surgery, and surgery should be scheduled for as early in the day as possible to minimize missed doses.

**HVC** • Asymptomatic carotid bruit is a common finding in older adults but is not predictive of perioperative stroke and therefore requires no preoperative evaluation.

## H Perioperative Management of the Pregnant Patient

In women of child-bearing age, an accurate menstrual history should be obtained, and pregnancy testing should be performed if pregnancy is suspected. Many institutions require preoperative pregnancy testing in this population.

Elective surgery should be delayed until after pregnancy. Pregnant patients who require surgery should undergo the same preoperative medical evaluation as nonpregnant patients; additional diagnostic testing is unnecessary unless directed by the obstetrician. Modifications to surgical and anesthetic techniques may be required because of the anatomic and physiologic changes of pregnancy. Close collaboration among the obstetrician, surgeon, anesthesiologist, and internist is essential. Notably, pregnancy is considered a hypercoagulable state, and the ACCP recommends perioperative mechanical or pharmacologic VTE prophylaxis for pregnant patients. Although high-quality evidence is lacking, the current body of evidence suggests that surgery does not negatively affect obstetric or maternal outcomes. H

### KEY POINT

- Pregnant patients who require surgery should undergo **HVC** the same preoperative medical evaluation as nonpregnant patients; additional diagnostic testing is unnecessary, but close collaboration with the patient's obstetrician is advised.

## Bibliography

**High Value Care in Internal Medicine**

The Commonwealth Fund. U.S. spends more on health care than other high-income nations but has lower life expectancy, worse health [Press release]. October 8, 2015. Retrieved from http://www.commonwealthfund.org/~/media/files/news/news-releases/2015/oct/oecd_spending_release_10_6_15_links-ds.pdf.

Qaseem A, Alguire P, Dallas P, Feinberg LE, Fitzgerald FT, Horwitch C, et al. Appropriate use of screening and diagnostic tests to foster high-value, cost-conscious care. Ann Intern Med. 2012;156:147-9. [PMID: 22250146] doi:10.7326/0003-4819-156-2-201201170-00011

**Interpretation of the Medical Literature**

Barratt A, Wyer PC, Hatala R, McGinn T, Dans AL, Keitz S, et al; Evidence-Based Medicine Teaching Tips Working Group. Tips for learners of evidence-based medicine: 1. Relative risk reduction, absolute risk reduction and number needed to treat. CMAJ. 2004;171:353-8. [PMID: 15313996]

Centre for Evidence Based Medicine. Study designs. http://www.cebm.net/study-designs/. Accessed January 23, 2018.

Citrome L, Ketter TA. When does a difference make a difference? Interpretation of number needed to treat, number needed to harm, and likelihood to be helped or harmed. Int J Clin Pract. 2013;67:407-11. [PMID: 23574101] doi:10.1111/ijcp.12142

Howick J, Chalmers I, Glasziou P, Greenhalgh G, Heneghan C, Liberati A, et al. Explanation of the 2011 Oxford Centre for Evidence-Based Medicine (OCEBM) levels of evidence (background document). Oxford Centre for Evidence-Based Medicine. https://www.cebm.net/wp-content/uploads/2014/06/CEBM-Levels-of-Evidence-Background-Document-2.1.pdf. Accessed January 23, 2018.

Richardson WS, Wilson MC, Keitz SA, Wyer PC; EBM Teaching Scripts Working Group. Tips for teachers of evidence-based medicine: making sense of diagnostic test results using likelihood ratios. J Gen Intern Med. 2008;23:87-92. [PMID: 18064524]

Uman LS. Systematic reviews and meta-analyses. J Can Acad Child Adolesc Psychiatry. 2011;20:57-9. [PMID: 21286370]

**Routine Care of the Healthy Patient**

Bibbins-Domingo K, Grossman DC, Curry SJ, Davidson KW, Epling JW Jr, García FAR, et al; US Preventive Services Task Force. Screening for colorectal cancer: US Preventive Services Task Force recommendation statement. JAMA. 2016;315:2564-2575. [PMID: 27304597] doi:10.1001/jama.2016.5989

Bibbins-Domingo K, Grossman DC, Curry SJ, Davidson KW, Epling JW Jr, García FA, et al; US Preventive Services Task Force. Screening for obstructive sleep apnea in adults: US Preventive Services Task Force recommendation statement. JAMA. 2017;317:407-414. [PMID: 28118461] doi:10.1001/jama.2016.20325

Bibbins-Domingo K; U.S. Preventive Services Task Force. Aspirin use for the primary prevention of cardiovascular disease and colorectal cancer: U.S. Preventive Services Task Force recommendation statement. Ann Intern Med. 2016;164:836-45. [PMID: 27064677] doi:10.7326/M16-0577

Crowley RA; Health and Public Policy Committee of the American College of Physicians. Climate change and health: a position paper of the American College of Physicians. Ann Intern Med. 2016;164:608-10. [PMID: 27089232] doi:10.7326/M15-2766

Curry SJ, Krist AH, Owens DK, Barry MJ, Caughey AB, Davidson KW, et al; US Preventive Services Task Force. Screening for cervical cancer: US Preventive Services Task Force recommendation statement. JAMA. 2018;320:674-686. [PMID: 30140884] doi:10.1001/jama.2018.10897

Curry SJ, Krist AH, Owens DK, Barry MJ, Caughey AB, Davidson KW, et al; US Preventive Services Task Force. Screening for osteoporosis to prevent fractures: US Preventive Services Task Force recommendation statement. JAMA. 2018;319:2521-2531. [PMID: 29946735] doi:10.1001/jama.2018.7498

DiazGranados CA, Dunning AJ, Kimmel M, Kirby D, Treanor J, Collins A, et al. Efficacy of high-dose versus standard-dose influenza vaccine in older adults. N Engl J Med. 2014;371:635-45. [PMID: 25119609] doi:10.1056/NEJMoa1315727

Grossman DC, Curry SJ, Owens DK, Bibbins-Domingo K, Caughey AB, Davidson KW, et al; US Preventive Services Task Force. Screening for prostate cancer: US Preventive Services Task Force recommendation statement. JAMA. 2018;319:1901-1913. [PMID: 29801017] doi:10.1001/jama.2018.3710

Ikeda Y, Shimada K, Teramoto T, Uchiyama S, Yamazaki T, Oikawa S, et al. Low-dose aspirin for primary prevention of cardiovascular events in Japanese patients 60 years or older with atherosclerotic risk factors: a randomized clinical trial. JAMA. 2014;312:2510-20. [PMID: 25401325] doi:10.1001/jama.2014.15690

Jørgensen T, Jacobsen RK, Toft U, Aadahl M, Glümer C, Pisinger C. Effect of screening and lifestyle counselling on incidence of ischaemic heart disease in general population: Inter99 randomised trial. BMJ. 2014;348:g3617. [PMID: 24912589] doi:10.1136/bmj.g3617

Kim DK, Riley LE, Hunter P. Advisory Committee on Immunization Practices recommended immunization schedule for adults aged 19 years or older - United States, 2018. MMWR Morb Mortal Wkly Rep. 2018;67:158-160. [PMID: 29420462] doi:10.15585/mmwr.mm6705e3

Krogsbøll LT, Jørgensen KJ, Grønhøj Larsen C, Gøtzsche PC. General health checks in adults for reducing morbidity and mortality from disease: Cochrane systematic review and meta-analysis. BMJ. 2012;345:e7191. [PMID: 23169868] doi:10.1136/bmj.e7191

LeFevre ML; U.S. Preventive Services Task Force. Screening for abdominal aortic aneurysm: U.S. Preventive Services Task Force recommendation statement. Ann Intern Med. 2014;161:281-90. [PMID: 24957320] doi:10.7326/M14-1204

Moyer VA; U.S. Preventive Services Task Force. Risk assessment, genetic counseling, and genetic testing for BRCA-related cancer in women: U.S. Preventive Services Task Force recommendation statement. Ann Intern Med. 2014;160:271-81. [PMID: 24366376]

Oeffinger KC, Fontham ET, Etzioni R, Herzig A, Michaelson JS, Shih YC, et al; American Cancer Society. Breast cancer screening for women at average risk: 2015 guideline update from the American Cancer Society. JAMA. 2015;314:1599-614. [PMID: 26501536] doi:10.1001/jama.2015.12783

Saito Y, Okada S, Ogawa H, Soejima H, Sakuma M, Nakayama M, et al; JPAD Trial Investigators. Low-dose aspirin for primary prevention of cardiovascular events in patients with type 2 diabetes mellitus: 10-year follow-up of a randomized controlled trial. Circulation. 2017;135:659-670. [PMID: 27881565] doi:10.1161/CIRCULATIONAHA.116.025760

Siu AL, Bibbins-Domingo K, Grossman DC, Baumann LC, Davidson KW, Ebell M, et al; US Preventive Services Task Force (USPSTF). Screening for depression in adults: US Preventive Services Task Force recommendation statement. JAMA. 2016;315:380-7. [PMID: 26813211] doi:10.1001/jama.2015.18392

Siu AL; U.S. Preventive Services Task Force. Screening for abnormal blood glucose and type 2 diabetes mellitus: U.S. Preventive Services Task Force recommendation statement. Ann Intern Med. 2015;163:861-8. [PMID: 26501513] doi:10.7326/M15-2345

Siu AL; U.S. Preventive Services Task Force. Screening for breast cancer: U.S. Preventive Services Task Force recommendation statement. Ann Intern Med. 2016;164:279-96. [PMID: 26757170] doi:10.7326/M15-2886

Siu AL; U.S. Preventive Services Task Force. Screening for high blood pressure in adults: U.S. Preventive Services Task Force recommendation statement. Ann Intern Med. 2015;163:778-86. [PMID: 26458123] doi:10.7326/M15-2223

Teng K, Acheson LS. Genomics in primary care practice. Prim Care. 2014;41:421-35. [PMID: 24830615] doi:10.1016/j.pop.2014.02.012

van der Wouden CH, Carere DA, Maitland-van der Zee AH, Ruffin MT 4th, Roberts JS, Green RC; Impact of Personal Genomics Study Group. Consumer perceptions of interactions with primary care providers after direct-to-consumer personal genomic testing. Ann Intern Med. 2016;164:513-22. [PMID: 26928821] doi:10.7326/M15-0995

**Patient Safety and Quality Improvement**

The Joint Commission. Patient safety systems. Comprehensive Accreditation Manual for Hospitals. Update 2, January 2016; PS 1-53. www.jointcommission.org/assets/1/18/PSC_for_Web.pdf. Accessed May 23, 2018.

National Academies of Sciences, Engineering, and Medicine. Improving Diagnosis in Health Care. Washington, DC: The National Academies Press; 2015.

U.S. Department of Health and Human Services, Health Resources and Services Administration. Quality improvement. www.hrsa.gov/quality/toolbox/508pdfs/qualityimprovement.pdf. Published April 2011. Accessed May 23, 2018.

U.S. Department of Health and Human Services, Office of Disease Prevention and Health Promotion. National action plan to improve health literacy. https://health.gov/communication/hlactionplan/pdf/Health_Literacy_Action_Plan.pdf. Published May 2010. Accessed May 23, 2018.

**Professionalism and Ethics**

ABIM Foundation. American Board of Internal Medicine. Medical professionalism in the new millennium: a physician charter. Ann Intern Med. 2002;136:243-6. [PMID: 11827500]

Appelbaum PS. Clinical practice. Assessment of patients' competence to consent to treatment. N Engl J Med. 2007;357:1834-40. [PMID: 17978292]

Daniel H, Sulmasy LS; Health and Public Policy Committee of the American College of Physicians. Policy recommendations to guide the use of telemedicine in primary care settings: an American College of Physicians position paper. Ann Intern Med. 2015;163:787-9. [PMID: 26344925] doi:10.7326/M15-0498

DeMartino ES, Dudzinski DM, Doyle CK, Sperry BP, Gregory SE, Siegler M, et al. Who Decides When a Patient Can't? Statutes on Alternate Decision Makers. N Engl J Med. 2017;376:1478-1482. [PMID: 28402767] doi:10.1056/NEJMms1611497

Farnan JM, Snyder Sulmasy L, Worster BK, Chaudhry HJ, Rhyne JA, Arora VM; American College of Physicians Ethics, Professionalism and Human Rights Committee. Online medical professionalism: patient and public relationships: policy statement from the American College of Physicians and the Federation of State Medical Boards. Ann Intern Med. 2013;158:620-7. [PMID: 23579867] doi:10.7326/0003-4819-158-8-201304160-00100

Halpern SD, Emanuel EJ. Can the United States buy better advance care planning? Ann Intern Med. 2015;162:224-5. [PMID: 25486099] doi:10.7326/M14-2476

Owens DK, Qaseem A, Chou R, Shekelle P; Clinical Guidelines Committee of the American College of Physicians. High-value, cost-conscious health care: concepts for clinicians to evaluate the benefits, harms, and costs of medical interventions. Ann Intern Med. 2011;154:174-80. [PMID: 21282697] doi:10.7326/0003-4819-154-3-201102010-00007

Snyder Sulmasy L, Mueller PS; Ethics, Professionalism and Human Rights Committee of the American College of Physicians. Ethics and the legalization of physician-assisted suicide: an American College of Physicians position paper. Ann Intern Med. 2017;167(8):576-578. [PMID: 28975242] doi: 10.7326/M17-0938

**Palliative Medicine**

Bernacki RE, Block SD; American College of Physicians High Value Care Task Force. Communication about serious illness care goals: a review and synthesis of best practices. JAMA Intern Med. 2014;174:1994-2003. [PMID: 25330167] doi:10.1001/jamainternmed.2014.5271

Kavalieratos D, Corbelli J, Zhang D, Dionne-Odom JN, Ernecoff NC, Hanmer J, et al. Association between palliative care and patient and caregiver outcomes: a systematic review and meta-analysis. JAMA. 2016;316:2104-2114. [PMID: 27893131] doi:10.1001/jama.2016.16840

Quill TE, Abernethy AP. Generalist plus specialist palliative care—creating a more sustainable model. N Engl J Med. 2013;368:1173-5. [PMID: 23465068] doi:10.1056/NEJMp1215620

Strand JJ, Kamdar MM, Carey EC. Top 10 things palliative care clinicians wished everyone knew about palliative care. Mayo Clin Proc. 2013;88:859-65. [PMID: 23910412] doi:10.1016/j.mayocp.2013.05.020

Swetz KM, Kamal AH. Palliative care. Ann Intern Med. 2018;168:ITC33-ITC48. [PMID: 29507970] doi:10.7326/AITC201803060

Temel JS, Greer JA, Muzikansky A, Gallagher ER, Admane S, Jackson VA, et al. Early palliative care for patients with metastatic non-small-cell lung cancer. N Engl J Med. 2010;363:733-42. [PMID: 20818875] doi:10.1056/NEJMoa1000678

**Common Symptoms**

Abernethy AP, McDonald CF, Frith PA, Clark K, Herndon JE 2nd, Marcello J, et al. Effect of palliative oxygen versus room air in relief of breathlessness in patients with refractory dyspnoea: a double-blind, randomised controlled trial. Lancet. 2010;376:784-93. [PMID: 20816546] doi:10.1016/S0140-6736(10)61115-4

Chow AW, Benninger MS, Brook I, Brozek JL, Goldstein EJ, Hicks LA, et al; Infectious Diseases Society of America. IDSA clinical practice guideline for acute bacterial rhinosinusitis in children and adults. Clin Infect Dis. 2012;54:e72-e112. [PMID: 22438350] doi:10.1093/cid/cir1043

Committee on the Diagnostic Criteria for Myalgic Encephalomyelitis/Chronic Fatigue Syndrome, Board on the Health of Select Populations, Institute of Medicine. Beyond Myalgic Encephalomyelitis/Chronic Fatigue Syndrome: Redefining an Illness. Washington (DC): National Academies Press (US); 2015 Feb 10. [PMID: 25695122]

Costantino G, Sun BC, Barbic F, Bossi I, Casazza G, Dipaola F, et al. Syncope clinical management in the emergency department: a consensus from the first international workshop on syncope risk stratification in the emergency department. Eur Heart J. 2016;37:1493-8. [PMID: 26242712] doi:10.1093/eurheartj/ehv378

Dowell D, Haegerich TM, Chou R. CDC guideline for prescribing opioids for chronic pain—United States, 2016. JAMA. 2016;315:1624-45. [PMID: 26977696] doi:10.1001/jama.2016.1464

Evens A, Vendetta L, Krebs K, Herath P. Medically unexplained neurologic symptoms: a primer for physicians who make the initial encounter. Am J Med. 2015;128:1059-64. [PMID: 25910791] doi:10.1016/j.amjmed.2015.03.030

Gibson P, Wang G, McGarvey L, Vertigan AE, Altman KW, Birring SS; CHEST Expert Cough Panel. Treatment of unexplained chronic cough: CHEST guideline and expert panel report. Chest. 2016;149:27-44. [PMID: 26426314] doi:10.1378/chest.15-1496

Hallenbeck J. Pathophysiologies of dyspnea explained: why might opioids relieve dyspnea and not hasten death? J Palliat Med. 2012;15:848-53. [PMID: 22594628] doi:10.1089/jpm.2011.0167

Haller H, Cramer H, Lauche R, Dobos G. Somatoform disorders and medically unexplained symptoms in primary care. Dtsch Arztebl Int. 2015;112:279-87. [PMID: 25939319] doi:10.3238/arztebl.2015.0279

Hooten M, Thorson D, Bianco J, Bonte B, Clavel Jr A, Hora J, et al. Pain: assessment, non-opioid treatment approaches and opioid management. Bloomington (MN): Institute for Clinical Systems Improvement (ICSI); 2016 Sep. 160 p. Available at https://www.icsi.org/guidelines_more/catalog_guidelines_and_more/catalog_guidelines/catalog_neurological_guidelines/pain/.

Kim JS, Zee DS. Clinical practice. Benign paroxysmal positional vertigo. N Engl J Med. 2014;370:1138-47. [PMID: 24645946] doi:10.1056/NEJMcp1309481

Lipsitt DR, Joseph R, Meyer D, Notman MT. Medically unexplained symptoms: barriers to effective treatment when nothing is the matter. Harv Rev Psychiatry. 2015;23:438-48. [PMID: 26378814] doi:10.1097/HRP.0000000000000055

Masters PA. In the clinic. Insomnia. Ann Intern Med. 2014;161:ITC1-15; quiz ITC16. [PMID: 25285559] doi:10.7326/0003-4819-161-7-201410070-01004

Nable JV, Tupe CL, Gehle BD, Brady WJ. In-flight medical emergencies during commercial travel. N Engl J Med. 2015;373:939-45. [PMID: 26332548] doi:10.1056/NEJMra1409213

Parshall MB, Schwartzstein RM, Adams L, Banzett RB, Manning HL, Bourbeau J, et al; American Thoracic Society Committee on Dyspnea. An official American Thoracic Society statement: update on the mechanisms, assessment, and management of dyspnea. Am J Respir Crit Care Med. 2012;185:435-52. [PMID: 22336677] doi:10.1164/rccm.201111-2042ST

Prandoni P, Lensing AW, Prins MH, Ciammaichella M, Perlati M, Mumoli N, et al; PESIT Investigators. Prevalence of pulmonary embolism among patients hospitalized for syncope. N Engl J Med. 2016;375:1524-1531. [PMID: 27797317]

Qaseem A, Kansagara D, Forciea MA, Cooke M, Denberg TD; Clinical Guidelines Committee of the American College of Physicians. Management of chronic insomnia disorder in adults: a clinical practice guideline from the American College of Physicians. Ann Intern Med. 2016;165:125-33. [PMID: 27136449] doi:10.7326/M15-2175

Sharon JD, Trevino C, Schubert MC, Carey JP. Treatment of Ménière's disease. Curr Treat Options Neurol. 2015;17:341. [PMID: 25749846] doi:10.1007/s11940-015-0341-x

Shen WK, Sheldon RS, Benditt DG, Cohen MI, Forman DE, Goldberger ZD, et al. 2017 ACC/AHA/HRS guideline for the evaluation and management of patients with syncope: executive summary: a report of the American College of Cardiology/American Heart Association Task Force on Clinical Practice Guidelines and the Heart Rhythm Society. Circulation. 2017;136:e25-e59. [PMID: 28280232] doi:10.1161/CIR.0000000000000498

Sun BC. Quality-of-life, health service use, and costs associated with syncope. Prog Cardiovasc Dis. 2013;55:370-5. [PMID: 23472773] doi:10.1016/j.pcad.2012.10.009

Trauer JM, Qian MY, Doyle JS, Rajaratnam SM, Cunnington D. Cognitive behavioral therapy for chronic insomnia: a systematic review and meta-analysis. Ann Intern Med. 2015;163:191-204. [PMID: 26054060] doi:10.7326/M14-2841

Venhovens J, Meulstee J, Verhagen WI. Acute vestibular syndrome: a critical review and diagnostic algorithm concerning the clinical differentiation of peripheral versus central aetiologies in the emergency department. J Neurol. 2016;263:2151-2157. [PMID: 26984607]

Whiting PF, Wolff RF, Deshpande S, Di Nisio M, Duffy S, Hernandez AV, et al. Cannabinoids for medical use: a systematic review and meta-analysis. JAMA. 2015;313:2456-73. [PMID: 26103030] doi:10.1001/jama.2015.6358

**Musculoskeletal Pain**

Abdel Shaheed C, Maher CG, Williams KA, Day R, McLachlan AJ. Efficacy, tolerability, and dose-dependent effects of opioid analgesics for low back pain: a systematic review and meta-analysis. JAMA Intern Med. 2016;176:958-68. [PMID: 27213267] doi:10.1001/jamainternmed.2016.1251

Buller LT, Jose J, Baraga M, Lesniak B. Thoracic outlet syndrome: current concepts, imaging features, and therapeutic strategies. Am J Orthop (Belle Mead NJ). 2015;44:376-82. [PMID: 26251937]

Chou R. In the clinic. Low back pain. Ann Intern Med. 2014;160:ITC6-1. [PMID: 25009837]

Cohen SP. Epidemiology, diagnosis, and treatment of neck pain. Mayo Clin Proc. 2015;90:284-99. [PMID: 25659245] doi:10.1016/j.mayocp.2014.09.008

Deyo RA, Mirza SK. Clinical practice. Herniated lumbar intervertebral disk. N Engl J Med. 2016;374:1763-72. [PMID: 27144851] doi:10.1056/NEJMcp1512658

Goossens P, Keijsers E, van Geenen RJ, Zijta A, van den Broek M, Verhagen AP, et al. Validity of the Thessaly test in evaluating meniscal tears compared with arthroscopy: a diagnostic accuracy study. J Orthop Sports Phys Ther. 2015;45:18-24, B1. [PMID: 25420009] doi:10.2519/jospt.2015.5215

Gross AR, Paquin JP, Dupont G, Blanchette S, Lalonde P, Cristie T, et al; Cervical Overview Group. Exercises for mechanical neck disorders: A Cochrane review update. Man Ther. 2016;24:25-45. [PMID: 27317503] doi:10.1016/j.math.2016.04.005

Hong E, Kraft MC. Evaluating anterior knee pain. Med Clin North Am. 2014;98:697-717, xi. [PMID: 24994047] doi:10.1016/j.mcna.2014.03.001

Iyer S, Kim HJ. Cervical radiculopathy. Curr Rev Musculoskelet Med. 2016;9:272-80. [PMID: 27250042] doi:10.1007/s12178-016-9349-4

Krebs EE, Gravely A, Nugent S, Jensen AC, DeRonne B, Goldsmith ES, et al. Effect of opioid vs nonopioid medications on pain-related function in patients with chronic back pain or hip or knee osteoarthritis pain: the SPACE randomized clinical trial. JAMA. 2018;319:872-882. [PMID: 29509867] doi:10.1001/jama.2018.0899

Li HY, Hua YH. Achilles tendinopathy: current concepts about the basic science and clinical treatments. Biomed Res Int. 2016;2016:6492597. [PMID: 27885357]

Maher C, Underwood M, Buchbinder R. Non-specific low back pain. Lancet. 2017;389:736-747. [PMID: 27745712] doi:10.1016/S0140-6736(16)30970-9

Olaussen M, Holmedal O, Lindbaek M, Brage S, Solvang H. Treating lateral epicondylitis with corticosteroid injections or non-electrotherapeutical physiotherapy: a systematic review. BMJ Open. 2013;3:e003564. [PMID: 24171937] doi:10.1136/bmjopen-2013-003564

Page MJ, Green S, Kramer S, Johnston RV, McBain B, Chau M, et al. Manual therapy and exercise for adhesive capsulitis (frozen shoulder). Cochrane Database Syst Rev. 2014:CD011275. [PMID: 25157702] doi:10.1002/14651858.CD011275

Qaseem A, Wilt TJ, McLean RM, Forciea MA; Clinical Guidelines Committee of the American College of Physicians. Noninvasive treatments for acute, subacute, and chronic low back pain: a clinical practice guideline from the American College of Physicians. Ann Intern Med. 2017;166:514-530. [PMID: 28192789] doi:10.7326/M16-2367

Tenforde AS, Yin A, Hunt KJ. Foot and ankle injuries in runners. Phys Med Rehabil Clin N Am. 2016;27:121-37. [PMID: 26616180] doi:10.1016/j.pmr.2015.08.007

Verdugo RJ, Salinas RA, Castillo JL, Cea JG. Surgical versus non-surgical treatment for carpal tunnel syndrome. Cochrane Database Syst Rev. 2008:CD001552. [PMID: 18843618] doi:10.1002/14651858.CD001552.pub2

Wilson JJ, Furukawa M. Evaluation of the patient with hip pain. Am Fam Physician. 2014;89:27-34. [PMID: 24444505]

**Dyslipidemia**

Bibbins-Domingo K, Grossman DC, Curry SJ, Davidson KW, Epling JW Jr, García FA, et al; US Preventive Services Task Force. Statin use for the primary prevention of cardiovascular disease in adults: US Preventive Services Task Force recommendation statement. JAMA. 2016;316:1997-2007. [PMID: 27838723] doi:10.1001/jama.2016.15450

Eckel RH, Jakicic JM, Ard JD, de Jesus JM, Houston Miller N, Hubbard VS, et al; American College of Cardiology/American Heart Association Task Force on Practice Guidelines. 2013 AHA/ACC guideline on lifestyle management to reduce cardiovascular risk: a report of the American College of Cardiology/American Heart Association Task Force on Practice Guidelines. Circulation. 2014;129:S76-99. [PMID: 24222015] doi:10.1161/01.cir.0000437740.48606.d1

Jellinger PS, Handelsman Y, Rosenblit PD, Bloomgarden ZT, Fonseca VA, Garber AJ, et al. American Association of Clinical Endocrinologists and American College of Endocrinology guidelines for management of dyslipidemia and prevention of cardiovascular disease. Endocr Pract. 2017;23:1-87. [PMID: 28437620] doi:10.4158/EP171764.APPGL

Lloyd-Jones DM, Morris PB, Ballantyne CM, Birtcher KK, Daly DD Jr, DePalma SM, et al. 2017 Focused update of the 2016 ACC expert consensus decision pathway on the role of non-statin therapies for LDL-cholesterol lowering in the management of atherosclerotic cardiovascular disease risk: a report of the American College of Cardiology Task Force on Expert Consensus Decision Pathways. J Am Coll Cardiol. 2017;70:1785-1822. [PMID: 28886926] doi:10.1016/j.jacc.2017.07.745

Stone NJ, Robinson JG, Lichtenstein AH, Bairey Merz CN, Blum CB, Eckel RH, et al; American College of Cardiology/American Heart Association Task Force on Practice Guidelines. 2013 ACC/AHA guideline on the treatment of blood cholesterol to reduce atherosclerotic cardiovascular risk in adults: a report of the American College of Cardiology/American Heart Association Task Force on Practice Guidelines. Circulation. 2014;129:S1-45. [PMID: 24222016] doi:10.1161/01.cir.0000437738.63853.7a

Van Horn L, Carson JA, Appel LJ, Burke LE, Economos C, Karmally W, et al; American Heart Association Nutrition Committee of the Council on Lifestyle and Cardiometabolic Health; Council on Cardiovascular Disease in the Young; Council on Cardiovascular and Stroke Nursing; Council on Clinical Cardiology; and Stroke Council. Recommended dietary pattern to achieve adherence to the American Heart Association/American College of Cardiology (AHA/ACC) guidelines: a scientific statement from the American Heart Association. Circulation. 2016;134:e505-e529. [PMID: 27789558]

**Obesity**

Behary J, Kumbhari V. Advances in the endoscopic management of obesity. Gastroenterol Res Pract. 2015;2015:757821. [PMID: 26106413] doi:10.1155/2015/757821

Chang SH, Stoll CR, Song J, Varela JE, Eagon CJ, Colditz GA. The effectiveness and risks of bariatric surgery: an updated systematic review and meta-analysis, 2003-2012. JAMA Surg. 2014;149:275-87. [PMID: 24352617] doi:10.1001/jamasurg.2013.3654

Flegal KM, Kruszon-Moran D, Carroll MD, Fryar CD, Ogden CL. Trends in obesity among adults in the United States, 2005 to 2014. JAMA. 2016;315:2284-91. [PMID: 27272580] doi:10.1001/jama.2016.6458

Jacob JA. Obesity-related medical care costs Medicaid $8 billion a year. Health agencies update. JAMA 2015;314(24):2607. doi:10.1001/jama.2015.16829

Jensen MD, Ryan DH, Apovian CM, Ard JD, Comuzzie AG, Donato KA, et al; American College of Cardiology/American Heart Association Task Force on Practice Guidelines. 2013 AHA/ACC/TOS guideline for the management of overweight and obesity in adults: a report of the American College of Cardiology/American Heart Association Task Force on Practice Guidelines and The Obesity Society. Circulation. 2014;129:S102-38. [PMID: 24222017] doi:10.1161/01.cir.0000437739.71477.ee

Johnston BC, Kanters S, Bandayrel K, Wu P, Naji F, Siemieniuk RA, et al. Comparison of weight loss among named diet programs in overweight and obese adults: a meta-analysis. JAMA. 2014;312:923-33. [PMID: 25182101] doi:10.1001/jama.2014.10397

Khera R, Murad MH, Chandar AK, Dulai PS, Wang Z, Prokop LJ, et al. Association of pharmacological treatments for obesity with weight loss and adverse events: a systematic review and meta-analysis. JAMA. 2016;315:2424-34. [PMID: 27299618] doi:10.1001/jama.2016.7602

Marcotte E, Chand B. Management and prevention of surgical and nutritional complications after bariatric surgery. Surg Clin North Am. 2016;96:843-56. [PMID: 27473805] doi:10.1016/j.suc.2016.03.006

Moyer VA; U.S. Preventive Services Task Force. Screening for and management of obesity in adults: U.S. Preventive Services Task Force recommendation statement. Ann Intern Med. 2012;157:373-8. [PMID: 22733087]

**Men's Health**

Crawford P, Crop JA. Evaluation of scrotal masses. Am Fam Physician. 2014;89:723-7. [PMID: 24784335]

McVary KT, Roehrborn CG, Avins AL, et al. American Urological Association guideline: management of benign prostatic hyperplasia (BPH). Linthicum, MD: American Urological Association; 2010. https://www.auanet.org/education/guidelines/benign-prostatic-hyperplasia.cfm. Accessed January 20, 2017.

Nehra A, Jackson G, Miner M, Billups KL, Burnett AL, Buvat J, et al. The Princeton III Consensus recommendations for the management of erectile dysfunction and cardiovascular disease. Mayo Clin Proc. 2012;87:766-78. [PMID: 22862865] doi:10.1016/j.mayocp.2012.06.015

Pearson R, Williams PM. Common questions about the diagnosis and management of benign prostatic hyperplasia. Am Fam Physician. 2014;90:769-74. [PMID: 25611711]

Sharp VJ, Takacs EB, Powell CR. Prostatitis: diagnosis and treatment. Am Fam Physician. 2010;82:397-406. [PMID: 20704171]

Snyder PJ, Bhasin S, Cunningham GR, Matsumoto AM, Stephens-Shields AJ, Cauley JA, et al; Testosterone Trials Investigators. Effects of testosterone treatment in older men. N Engl J Med. 2016;374:611-24. [PMID: 26886521] doi:10.1056/NEJMoa1506119

**Women's Health**

American College of Radiology. ACR Appropriateness Criteria. Palpable breast masses. Available at https://acsearch.acr.org/docs/69495/Narrative/. Accessed March 15, 2018.

Goyal A. Breast pain. Am Fam Physician. 2016;93:872-3. [PMID: 27175723]

Grossman DC, Curry SJ, Owens DK, Barry MJ, Davidson KW, Doubeni CA, et al; US Preventive Services Task Force. Hormone therapy for the primary prevention of chronic conditions in postmenopausal women: US Preventive Services Task Force recommendation statement. JAMA. 2017;318:2224-2233. [PMID: 29234814]

Joffe HV, Chang C, Sewell C, Easley O, Nguyen C, Dunn S, et al. FDA approval of flibanserin–treating hypoactive sexual desire disorder. N Engl J Med. 2016;374:101-4. [PMID: 26649985]

Mitchell CM, Reed SD, Diem S, Larson JC, Newton KM, Ensrud KE, et al. Efficacy of vaginal estradiol or vaginal moisturizer vs placebo for treating postmenopausal vulvovaginal symptoms: a randomized clinical trial. JAMA Intern Med. 2018;178:681-690. [PMID: 29554173] doi:10.1001/jamainternmed.2018.0116

Munro MG, Critchley HO, Broder MS, Fraser IS; FIGO Working Group on Menstrual Disorders. FIGO classification system (PALM-COEIN) for causes of abnormal uterine bleeding in nongravid women of reproductive age. Int J Gynaecol Obstet. 2011;113:3-13. [PMID: 21345435]

The NAMS 2017 Hormone Therapy Position Statement Advisory Panel. The 2017 hormone therapy position statement of The North American Menopause Society. Menopause. 2017;24:728-753. [PMID: 28650869]

Neal L, Sandhu NP, Hieken TJ, Glazebrook KN, Mac Bride MB, Dilaveri CA, et al. Diagnosis and management of benign, atypical, and indeterminate breast lesions detected on core needle biopsy. Mayo Clin Proc. 2014;89:536-47. [PMID: 24684875]

Portman DJ, Gass ML; Vulvovaginal Atrophy Terminology Consensus Conference Panel. Genitourinary syndrome of menopause: new terminology for vulvovaginal atrophy from the International Society for the Study of Women's Sexual Health and the North American Menopause Society. Menopause. 2014;21:1063-8. [PMID: 25160739]

Steege JF, Siedhoff MT. Chronic pelvic pain. Obstet Gynecol. 2014;124:616-29. [PMID: 25162265]

Workowski KA, Bolan GA; Centers for Disease Control and Prevention. Sexually transmitted diseases treatment guidelines, 2015. MMWR Recomm Rep. 2015;64:1-137. [PMID: 26042815]

**Eye Disorders**

Azari AA, Barney NP. Conjunctivitis: a systematic review of diagnosis and treatment. JAMA. 2013;310:1721-9. [PMID: 24150468] doi:10.1001/jama.2013.280318

Gelston CD. Common eye emergencies. Am Fam Physician. 2013;88:515-9. [PMID: 24364572]

Lim LS, Mitchell P, Seddon JM, Holz FG, Wong TY. Age-related macular degeneration. Lancet. 2012;379:1728-38. [PMID: 22559899] doi:10.1016/S0140-6736(12)60282-7

Moyer VA; U.S. Preventive Services Task Force. Screening for glaucoma: U.S. Preventive Services Task Force recommendation statement. Ann Intern Med. 2013;159:484-9. [PMID: 24325017]

Narayana S, McGee S. Bedside diagnosis of the 'red eye': a systematic review. Am J Med. 2015;128:1220-1224.e1. [PMID: 26169885] doi:10.1016/j.amjmed.2015.06.026

Weinreb RN, Aung T, Medeiros FA. The pathophysiology and treatment of glaucoma: a review. JAMA. 2014;311:1901-11. [PMID: 24825645] doi:10.1001/jama.2014.3192

**Ear, Nose, Mouth, and Throat Disorders**

Baguley D, McFerran D, Hall D. Tinnitus. Lancet. 2013;382:1600-7. [PMID: 23827090] doi:10.1016/S0140-6736(13)60142-7

Gauer RL, Semidey MJ. Diagnosis and treatment of temporomandibular disorders. Am Fam Physician. 2015;91:378-86. [PMID: 25822556]

Harris AM, Hicks LA, Qaseem A; High Value Care Task Force of the American College of Physicians and for the Centers for Disease Control and Prevention. Appropriate antibiotic use for acute respiratory tract infection in adults: advice for high-value care from the American College of Physicians and the Centers for Disease Control and Prevention. Ann Intern Med. 2016;164:425-34. [PMID: 26785402] doi:10.7326/M15-1840

Kociolek LK, Shulman ST. In the clinic. Pharyngitis. Ann Intern Med. 2012;157:ITC3-1 - ITC3-16. [PMID: 22944886] doi:10.7326/0003-4819-157-5-20120904-01003

Moyer VA; U.S. Preventive Services Task Force. Screening for hearing loss in older adults: U.S. Preventive Services Task Force recommendation statement. Ann Intern Med. 2012;157:655-61. [PMID: 22893115]

Uy J, Forciea MA. In the clinic. Hearing loss. Ann Intern Med. 2013;158:ITC4-1; quiz ITC4-16. [PMID: 23546583] doi:10.7326/0003-4819-158-7-201304020-01004

Wilson JF. In the clinic. Acute sinusitis. Ann Intern Med. 2010;153:ITC31-15; quiz ITC316. [PMID: 20820036] doi:10.7326/0003-4819-153-5-201009070-01003

**Mental and Behavioral Health**

Bachhuber MA, Hennessy S, Cunningham CO, Starrels JL. Increasing benzodiazepine prescriptions and overdose mortality in the United States, 1996-2013. Am J Public Health. 2016;106:686-8. [PMID: 26890165] doi:10.2105/AJPH.2016.303061

Dickstein LP, Franco KN, Rome ES, Auron M. Recognizing, managing medical consequences of eating disorders in primary care. Cleve Clin J Med. 2014;81:255-63. [PMID: 24692444] doi:10.3949/ccjm.81a.12132

Edelman EJ, Fiellin DA. In the clinic. Alcohol use. Ann Intern Med. 2016;164:ITC1-16. [PMID: 26747315] doi:10.7326/AITC201601050

Larochelle MR, Liebschutz JM, Zhang F, Ross-Degnan D, Wharam JF. Opioid prescribing after nonfatal overdose and association with repeated overdose: a cohort study. Ann Intern Med. 2016;164:1-9. [PMID: 26720742] doi:10.7326/M15-0038

Lindson-Hawley N, Banting M, West R, Michie S, Shinkins B, Aveyard P. Gradual versus abrupt smoking cessation: a randomized, controlled noninferiority trial. Ann Intern Med. 2016;164:585-92. [PMID: 26975007] doi:10.7326/M14-2805

Moyer VA; Preventive Services Task Force. Screening and behavioral counseling interventions in primary care to reduce alcohol misuse: U.S. Preventive Services Task Force recommendation statement. Ann Intern Med. 2013;159:210-8. [PMID: 23698791] doi:10.7326/0003-4819-159-3-201308060-00652

Pace CA, Samet JH. In the clinic. Substance use disorders. Ann Intern Med. 2016;164:ITC49-ITC64. [PMID: 27043992] doi:10.7326/AITC201604050

Patel MS, Steinberg MB. In the clinic. Smoking cessation. Ann Intern Med. 2016;164:ITC33-ITC48. [PMID: 26926702] doi:10.7326/AITC201603010

Qaseem A, Barry MJ, Kansagara D; Clinical Guidelines Committee of the American College of Physicians. Nonpharmacologic versus pharmacologic treatment of adult patients with major depressive disorder: a clinical practice guideline from the American College of Physicians. Ann Intern Med. 2016;164:350-9. [PMID: 26857948] doi:10.7326/M15-2570

Schuckit MA. Treatment of opioid-use disorders. N Engl J Med. 2016;375:357-68. [PMID: 27464203] doi:10.1056/NEJMra1604339

Siu AL; U.S. Preventive Services Task Force. Behavioral and pharmacotherapy interventions for tobacco smoking cessation in adults, including pregnant women: U.S. Preventive Services Task Force recommendation statement. Ann Intern Med. 2015;163:622-34. [PMID: 26389730] doi:10.7326/M15-2023

**Geriatric Medicine**

Buta BJ, Walston JD, Godino JG, Park M, Kalyani RR, Xue QL, et al. Frailty assessment instruments: systematic characterization of the uses and contexts of highly-cited instruments. Ageing Res Rev. 2016;26:53-61. [PMID: 26674984] doi:10.1016/j.arr.2015.12.003

Carlson C, Merel SE, Yukawa M. Geriatric syndromes and geriatric assessment for the generalist. Med Clin North Am. 2015;99:263-79. [PMID: 25700583] doi:10.1016/j.mcna.2014.11.003

Chou R, Dana T, Bougatsos C, Grusing S, Blazina I. Screening for impaired visual acuity in older adults: updated evidence report and systematic review for the US Preventive Services Task Force. JAMA. 2016;315:915-33. [PMID: 26934261] doi:10.1001/jama.2016.0783

Dong X. Screening for elder abuse in healthcare settings: why should we care, and is it a missed quality indicator? J Am Geriatr Soc. 2015;63:1686-8. [PMID: 26277299] doi:10.1111/jgs.13538

Gormley EA, Lightner DJ, Faraday M, Vasavada SP; American Urological Association. Diagnosis and treatment of overactive bladder (non-neurogenic) in adults: AUA/SUFU guideline amendment. J Urol. 2015;193:1572-80. [PMID: 25623739] doi:10.1016/j.juro.2015.01.087

Lin JS, O'Connor E, Rossom RC, Perdue LA, Eckstrom E. Screening for cognitive impairment in older adults: a systematic review for the U.S. Preventive Services Task Force. Ann Intern Med. 2013;159:601-12. [PMID: 24145578]

Martin AJ, Marottoli R, O'Neill D. Driving assessment for maintaining mobility and safety in drivers with dementia. Cochrane Database Syst Rev. 2013:CD006222. [PMID: 23990315] doi:10.1002/14651858.CD006222.pub4

Moyer VA; U.S. Preventive Services Task Force. Screening for hearing loss in older adults: U.S. Preventive Services Task Force recommendation statement. Ann Intern Med. 2012;157:655-61. [PMID: 22893115]

Moyer VA; U.S. Preventive Services Task Force. Screening for intimate partner violence and abuse of elderly and vulnerable adults: U.S. Preventive Services Task Force recommendation statement. Ann Intern Med. 2013;158:478-86. [PMID: 23338828] doi:10.7326/0003-4819-158-6-201303190-00588

Qaseem A, Dallas P, Forciea MA, Starkey M, Denberg TD, Shekelle P; Clinical Guidelines Committee of the American College of Physicians. Nonsurgical management of urinary incontinence in women: a clinical practice guideline from the American College of Physicians. Ann Intern Med. 2014;161:429-40. [PMID: 25222388] doi:10.7326/M13-2410

Qaseem A, Humphrey LL, Forciea MA, Starkey M, Denberg TD; Clinical Guidelines Committee of the American College of Physicians. Treatment of pressure ulcers: a clinical practice guideline from the American College of Physicians. Ann Intern Med. 2015;162:370-9. [PMID: 25732279] doi:10.7326/M14-1568

Qaseem A, Mir TP, Starkey M, Denberg TD; Clinical Guidelines Committee of the American College of Physicians. Risk assessment and prevention of pressure ulcers: a clinical practice guideline from the American College of Physicians. Ann Intern Med. 2015;162:359-69. [PMID: 25732278] doi:10.7326/M14-1567

Siu AL, Bibbins-Domingo K, Grossman DC, Baumann LC, Davidson KW, Ebell M, et al; US Preventive Services Task Force (USPSTF). Screening for depression in adults: US Preventive Services Task Force recommendation statement. JAMA. 2016;315:380-7. [PMID: 26813211] doi:10.1001/jama.2015.18392

**Perioperative Medicine**

Apfelbaum JL, Connis RT, Nickinovich DG, Pasternak LR, Arens JF, Caplan RA, et al; Committee on Standards and Practice Parameters. Practice advisory for preanesthesia evaluation: an updated report by the American Society of Anesthesiologists Task Force on Preanesthesia Evaluation. Anesthesiology. 2012;116:522-38. [PMID: 22273990] doi:10.1097/ALN.0b013e31823c1067

Botto F, Alonso-Coello P, Chan MT, Villar JC, Xavier D, Srinathan S, et al; Vascular events In noncardiac Surgery patients cOhort evaluatioN (VISION) Writing Group, on behalf of The Vascular events In noncardiac Surgery patients cOhort evaluatioN (VISION) Investigators. Myocardial injury after noncardiac surgery: a large, international, prospective cohort study establishing diagnostic criteria, characteristics, predictors, and 30-day outcomes. Anesthesiology. 2014;120:564-78. [PMID: 24534856] doi:10.1097/ALN.0000000000000113

Daniels PR. Peri-procedural management of patients taking oral anticoagulants. BMJ. 2015;351:h2391. [PMID: 26174061] doi:10.1136/bmj.h2391

Devereaux PJ, Mrkobrada M, Sessler DI, Leslie K, Alonso-Coello P, Kurz A, et al; POISE-2 Investigators. Aspirin in patients undergoing noncardiac surgery. N Engl J Med. 2014;370:1494-503. [PMID: 24679062] doi:10.1056/NEJMoa1401105

Doherty JU, Gluckman TJ, Hucker WJ, Januzzi JL Jr, Ortel TL, Saxonhouse SJ, et al. 2017 ACC expert consensus decision pathway for periprocedural management of anticoagulation in patients with nonvalvular atrial fibrillation: a report of the American College of Cardiology Clinical Expert Consensus Document Task Force. J Am Coll Cardiol. 2017;69:871-898. [PMID: 28081965] doi:10.1016/j.jacc.2016.11.024

Douketis JD, Spyropoulos AC, Kaatz S, Becker RC, Caprini JA, Dunn AS, et al; BRIDGE Investigators. Perioperative bridging anticoagulation in patients with atrial fibrillation. N Engl J Med. 2015;373:823-33. [PMID: 26095867] doi:10.1056/NEJMoa1501035

Douketis JD, Spyropoulos AC, Spencer FA, Mayr M, Jaffer AK, Eckman MH, et al. Perioperative management of antithrombotic therapy: antithrombotic therapy and prevention of thrombosis, 9th ed: American College of Chest Physicians evidence-based clinical practice guidelines. Chest. 2012;141:e326S-e350S. [PMID: 22315266] doi:10.1378/chest.11-2298

Falck-Ytter Y, Francis CW, Johanson NA, Curley C, Dahl OE, Schulman S, et al. Prevention of VTE in orthopedic surgery patients: antithrombotic therapy and prevention of thrombosis, 9th ed: American College of Chest Physicians evidence-based clinical practice guidelines. Chest. 2012;141:e278S-e325S. [PMID: 22315265] doi:10.1378/chest.11-2404

Fleisher LA, Fleischmann KE, Auerbach AD, Barnason SA, Beckman JA, Bozkurt B, et al; American College of Cardiology. 2014 ACC/AHA guideline on perioperative cardiovascular evaluation and management of patients undergoing noncardiac surgery: a report of the American College of Cardiology/American Heart Association Task Force on practice guidelines. J Am Coll Cardiol. 2014;64:e77-137. [PMID: 25091544] doi:10.1016/j.jacc.2014.07.944

Gould MK, Garcia DA, Wren SM, Karanicolas PJ, Arcelus JI, Heit JA, et al. Prevention of VTE in nonorthopedic surgical patients: antithrombotic therapy and prevention of thrombosis, 9th ed: American College of Chest Physicians evidence-based clinical practice guidelines. Chest. 2012;141:e227S-e277S. [PMID: 22315263] doi:10.1378/chest.11-2297

Kaufman RM, Djulbegovic B, Gernsheimer T, Kleinman S, Tinmouth AT, Capocelli KE, et al; AABB. Platelet transfusion: a clinical practice guideline from the AABB. Ann Intern Med. 2015;162:205-13. [PMID: 25383671] doi:10.7326/M14-1589

Kaw R, Chung F, Pasupuleti V, Mehta J, Gay PC, Hernandez AV. Meta-analysis of the association between obstructive sleep apnoea and postoperative outcome. Br J Anaesth. 2012;109:897-906. [PMID: 22956642] doi:10.1093/bja/aes308

Levine GN, Bates ER, Bittl JA, Brindis RG, Fihn SD, Fleisher LA, et al. 2016 ACC/AHA guideline focused update on duration of dual antiplatelet therapy in patients with coronary artery disease: a report of the American College of Cardiology/American Heart Association Task Force on Clinical Practice Guidelines. J Am Coll Cardiol. 2016;68:1082-115. [PMID: 27036918] doi:10.1016/j.jacc.2016.03.513

Whelton PK, Carey RM, Aronow WS, Casey DE Jr, Collins KJ, Dennison Himmelfarb C, et al. 2017 ACC/AHA/AAPA/ABC/ACPM/AGS/APhA/ASH/ASPC/NMA/PCNA guideline for the prevention, detection, evaluation, and management of high blood pressure in adults: a report of the American College of Cardiology/American Heart Association Task Force on Clinical Practice Guidelines. J Am Coll Cardiol. 2017. [PMID: 29146535] doi:10.1016/j.jacc.2017.11.006

Zielsdorf SM, Kubasiak JC, Janssen I, Myers JA, Luu MB. A NSQIP analysis of MELD and perioperative outcomes in general surgery. Am Surg. 2015;81:755-9. [PMID: 26215235]

# General Internal Medicine Self-Assessment Test

This self-assessment test contains one-best-answer multiple-choice questions. Please read these directions carefully before answering the questions. Answers, critiques, and bibliographies immediately follow these multiple-choice questions. The American College of Physicians (ACP) is accredited by the Accreditation Council for Continuing Medical Education (ACCME) to provide continuing medical education for physicians.

The American College of Physicians designates MKSAP 18 General Internal Medicine for a maximum of 36 *AMA PRA Category 1 Credits*™. Physicians should claim only the credit commensurate with the extent of their participation in the activity.

Successful completion of the CME activity, which includes participation in the evaluation component, enables the participant to earn up to 36 medical knowledge MOC points in the American Board of Internal Medicine's Maintenance of Certification (MOC) program. It is the CME activity provider's responsibility to submit participant completion information to ACCME for the purpose of granting MOC credit.

## *Earn Instantaneous CME Credits or MOC Points Online*

Print subscribers can enter their answers online to earn instantaneous CME credits or MOC points. You can submit your answers using online answer sheets that are provided at mksap.acponline.org, where a record of your MKSAP 18 credits will be available. To earn CME credits or to apply for MOC points, you need to answer all of the questions in a test and earn a score of at least 50% correct (number of correct answers divided by the total number of questions). Please note that if you are applying for MOC points, you must also enter your birth date and ABIM candidate number.

Take either of the following approaches:

- Use the printed answer sheet at the back of this book to record your answers. Go to mksap.acponline.org, access the appropriate online answer sheet, transcribe your answers, and submit your test for instantaneous CME credits or MOC points. There is no additional fee for this service.

- Go to mksap.acponline.org, access the appropriate online answer sheet, directly enter your answers, and submit your test for instantaneous CME credits or MOC points. There is no additional fee for this service.

## *Earn CME Credits or MOC Points by Mail or Fax*

Pay a $20 processing fee per answer sheet and submit the printed answer sheet at the back of this book by mail or fax, as instructed on the answer sheet. Make sure you calculate your score and enter your birth date and ABIM candidate number, and fax the answer sheet to 215-351-2799 or mail the answer sheet to Member and Customer Service, American College of Physicians, 190 N. Independence Mall West, Philadelphia, PA 19106-1572, using the courtesy envelope provided in your MKSAP 18 slipcase. You will need your 10-digit order number and 8-digit ACP ID number, which are printed on your packing slip. Please allow 4 to 6 weeks for your score report to be emailed back to you. Be sure to include your email address for a response.

If you do not have a 10-digit order number and 8-digit ACP ID number, or if you need help creating a username and password to access the MKSAP 18 online answer sheets, go to mksap.acponline.org or email custserv@acponline.org.

CME credits and MOC points are available from the publication date of December 31, 2018, until December 31, 2021. You may submit your answer sheet or enter your answers online at any time during this period.

## Directions

*Each of the numbered items is followed by lettered answers. Select the **ONE** lettered answer that is **BEST** in each case.*

Self-Assessment Test

## Item 1

A 35-year-old woman is evaluated after laboratory test results showed an elevated LDL cholesterol level during routine screening. Family history is remarkable for myocardial infarction in her father at age 45 years. She takes no medications.

On physical examination, vital signs are normal. BMI is 30. The remainder of the examination is unremarkable.

**Laboratory studies:**

| | |
|---|---|
| Alanine aminotransferase | 30 U/L |
| Thyroid-stimulating hormone | Normal |
| Total cholesterol | 294 mg/dL (7.61 mmol/L) |
| LDL cholesterol | 195 mg/dL (5.05 mmol/L) |
| HDL cholesterol | 55 mg/dL (1.42 mmol/L) |
| Triglycerides | 220 mg/dL (2.49 mmol/L) |

The patient is instructed in therapeutic lifestyle changes to lower her risk for atherosclerotic cardiovascular disease (ASCVD).

**According to the American College of Cardiology/American Heart Association cholesterol treatment guideline, which of the following is the most appropriate additional treatment for primary prevention of ASCVD in this patient?**

(A) Evolocumab
(B) High-intensity rosuvastatin
(C) Moderate-intensity atorvastatin
(D) No additional treatment is necessary

## Item 2

A 40-year-old woman seeks advice on whether she should undergo breast cancer screening with mammography. Her family history is negative for breast and ovarian cancers, and she has no other risk factors for breast cancer.

On physical examination, vital signs and the remainder of the examination are normal.

The patient is engaged in a discussion of the potential benefits and harms of initiating mammography now, including the potential for false-positive results and overdiagnosis. After the discussion, she states that she is not overly concerned about her risk for breast cancer but is anxious about the potential harms associated with screening.

**Which of the following is the most appropriate screening test for this patient?**

(A) Breast self-examination
(B) Breast tomosynthesis
(C) Screening mammography
(D) No testing

## Item 3

A 49-year-old man is scheduled for total right knee arthroplasty. Medical history is otherwise unremarkable. He takes no medications.

On physical examination, vital signs are normal. The right knee demonstrates bony hypertrophy and crepitus with passive movement.

Low-molecular-weight heparin and intermittent pneumatic compression will be initiated and continued during the hospital stay.

**Which of the following is the recommended duration of low-molecular-weight heparin prophylaxis for this patient?**

(A) Total of 10 days
(B) Total of 14 days
(C) Total of 35 days
(D) Until fully ambulatory
(E) Until hospital discharge

## Item 4

A 67-year-old man is evaluated for a 2-year history of worsening pain in his feet. He describes the pain as long-standing aching and burning. The pain is persistent, sometimes waking him from sleep. Medical history is otherwise significant for type 2 diabetes mellitus, hypertension, and hyperlipidemia. Medications are insulin glargine, insulin aspart, valsartan, aspirin, and simvastatin.

On physical examination, vital signs are normal. The feet are insensate to monofilament testing, and vibratory sensation is absent in the feet and ankles. No evidence of skin breakdown is noted.

**Which of the following is the most appropriate treatment?**

(A) Oral duloxetine
(B) Oral hydromorphone
(C) Oral lamotrigine
(D) Oral tramadol
(E) Topical diclofenac

## Item 5

A 23-year-old woman is evaluated for depression as she prepares for discharge from the hospital to home hospice care. She was diagnosed with metastatic ovarian cancer 2 years ago, and she progressed through four lines of chemotherapy, a trial of immunotherapy, and a failed attempt at a phase 1 clinical trial. Her life expectancy is measured in weeks. She is currently hospitalized with volume depletion, and after consultation with her oncologist and palliative care team, she has decided to be discharged home with hospice care.

On physical examination, the patient exhibits substantial fatigue and poor concentration. She has a flat affect except when intermittently tearful. Previously upbeat despite all of the setbacks, she is now withdrawn and describes feeling hopeless. She has pervasive guilt over the burden she believes she has caused her family. Medications are a fentanyl patch, oxycodone, ondansetron, polyethylene glycol, senna, and zolpidem.

CONT.

**Which of the following is the most appropriate treatment?**

(A) Citalopram

(B) Cognitive behavioral therapy

(C) Methylphenidate

(D) Sertraline

## Item 6

A 52-year-old man is evaluated for a 2-day history of painless red eye, which began on the right side and quickly spread to the left. He reports that his eyes have a thin mucopurulent discharge and that his eyelids are matted shut in the morning upon waking. He has had no photophobia, change in visual acuity, or itching in the eyes, but he has experienced some mild rhinorrhea. He does not use contact lenses. He is sexually monogamous. Medical history is significant for type 2 diabetes mellitus treated with metformin.

On physical examination, vital signs are normal. There is redness of the sclerae bilaterally, with a white crust-like residue along the edges of the eyelids. The tarsal vessels are obscured by the conjunctival erythema. Visual acuity is intact, and there is no tenderness around the globes.

**Which of the following is the most appropriate treatment?**

(A) Ceftriaxone

(B) Levofloxacin ophthalmic drops

(C) Olopatadine ophthalmic drops

(D) Trimethoprim–polymyxin B ophthalmic drops

## Item 7

Two new treatments for patients with heart failure with preserved ejection fraction were compared in a randomized controlled trial. The primary outcome was reduction in heart failure–related hospitalizations.

Compared with treatment B, treatment A was associated with a statistically significant absolute risk reduction of 6%, and the number needed to treat to prevent one hospitalization was 17.

**Which of the following is needed to conclude that treatment A is superior to treatment B?**

(A) Confidence interval

(B) Harms and cost of treatment

(C) *P* value

(D) Relative risk reduction

## Item 8

A 68-year-old man is evaluated for fever, perineal pain, dysuria, frequency, and intermittent straining that began yesterday. Symptoms began 48 hours after a prostate biopsy due to an elevated prostate-specific antigen level detected during routine screening.

On physical examination, temperature is 38.7 °C (101.7 °F), blood pressure is 145/82 mm Hg, pulse rate is 105/min, and respiration rate is normal. The prostate is enlarged and boggy, and it is tender to gentle palpation. There is no penile discharge, and no scrotal pain occurs with palpation.

Dipstick urinalysis is positive for leukocyte esterase and nitrates. Urine Gram stain reveals gram-negative rods. Urine culture is pending.

**Which of the following is the most appropriate treatment?**

(A) Amoxicillin

(B) Ceftriaxone and doxycycline

(C) Cephalexin

(D) Trimethoprim-sulfamethoxazole

## Item 9

A 22-year-old man is evaluated during a pre-employment examination. The patient is starting a new job as a registered nurse. He is asymptomatic. He received the tetanus toxoid, reduced diphtheria toxoid, and acellular pertussis (Tdap) vaccine 7 years ago and the influenza vaccine during the last influenza season. Approximately 6 months ago, he received one dose of the measles, mumps, and rubella (MMR) vaccine because of lack of documented immunity on serologic testing. Medical history is negative for chronic medical conditions. He is a nonsmoker, and he does not plan to travel outside of the United States in the near future. He takes no medications.

Physical examination is normal.

Laboratory studies are significant for a positive result on a hepatitis B surface antibody test. Hepatitis B surface antigen, hepatitis B core antibody, and hepatitis A IgG antibody levels are undetectable.

**Which of the following is the most appropriate vaccination strategy for this health care worker?**

(A) Administer a second dose of MMR vaccine

(B) Administer the hepatitis A vaccine

(C) Administer the hepatitis B vaccine

(D) Administer the 23-valent pneumococcal polysaccharide vaccine

(E) No vaccination at this time

## Item 10

A 32-year-old woman is evaluated during a domestic airline flight for an episode of weakness and lightheadedness. She is pregnant at 35 weeks' gestation. She has had several contractions since take-off but without regularity. She reports no abdominal pain. She has no medical problems, and her only medication is a prenatal vitamin.

On physical examination, the patient appears weak. Temperature is normal, blood pressure is 105/60 mm Hg, pulse rate is 99/min, and respiration rate is 14/min. Her skin is clammy. Cardiovascular examination is unremarkable. Lungs are clear to auscultation. On abdominal examination, she has a gravid uterus.

Oxygen, 2 L/min by nasal cannula, is started. An intravenous line is placed, and fluids are initiated.

**Which of the following is the most appropriate next step in management?**

(A) Ask the pilot to descend to a lower altitude

(B) Connect with the ground-based physician

(C) Recommend flight diversion

(D) No further management

## Item 11

An 82-year-old man is evaluated during a routine evaluation. He is accompanied to the visit by his son. The patient lives alone, and his son expresses reservations about his father continuing to drive. The patient no longer drives after dark or on the interstate highway. He limits his driving to within a 10-mile radius of his home and mainly drives for local errands and to church on Sundays. He has had no traffic accidents, but he had two recent incidents in which he misjudged the angle of his car in the grocery store parking lot and ran into the shopping cart stand. Medical history is significant for coronary artery disease, hypertension, and mild cognitive impairment. Medications are atorvastatin, aspirin, hydrochlorothiazide, lisinopril, and metoprolol.

On physical examination, blood pressure is 132/82 mm Hg, and pulse rate is 64/min; other vital signs are normal. The patient appears frail with a pleasant demeanor. He wears eyeglasses and hearing aids, and he has impaired hearing as measured by the whispered voice test. On musculoskeletal examination, limited mobility of the cervical spine is noted. He scores 26/30 on the Mini–Mental State Examination. The remainder of the examination is unremarkable.

**Which of the following is the most appropriate management regarding this patient's driving?**

(A) Advise the patient to retire from driving
(B) Obtain neuropsychological testing
(C) Obtain occupational therapy driving evaluation
(D) Reassure the patient he is competent to drive with self-imposed limitations

## Item 12

A 36-year-old woman is evaluated for a 3-year history of fatigue that worsens after activity and does not improve with rest. She also notes intermittent diffuse myalgia and arthralgia, constipation, dizziness, headaches, urinary urgency, memory problems, and paresthesias. Her musculoskeletal symptoms, dizziness, and headache worsen in the upright position and improve when she lies back down. She has almost entirely eliminated social activities. Medical history is significant for episodic migraine and irritable bowel syndrome. Medications are sumatriptan, polyethylene glycol, and hyoscyamine.

On physical examination, vital signs are normal. BMI is 24. Neck circumference is 36 cm (14 in). The remainder of the examination is normal.

Laboratory studies obtained 6 months ago showed a normal complete blood count, electrolyte levels, kidney function test results, liver chemistry test results, fasting glucose level, serum creatine kinase level, and serum thyroid-stimulating hormone level.

**Which of the following is the most appropriate diagnostic test to perform next?**

(A) Antinuclear antibody assay
(B) Polysomnography
(C) Serum cortisol level measurement
(D) No further testing is recommended

## Item 13

A 62-year-old man is evaluated for severe low back pain that began 2 days ago and is progressively worsening. The pain began when he was lifting concrete blocks at his job. The pain is located in his lower back and radiates into the lateral aspects of his legs bilaterally. He also has numbness and tingling in the groin. His last bowel movement was 2 days ago, and he has not urinated for the last 24 hours. Prior to the onset of the pain, the patient felt well.

On physical examination, vital signs are normal. There is decreased pinprick sensation surrounding the anus, decreased anal sphincter tone, and decreased ankle reflexes bilaterally; knee reflexes are normal. Bilateral dorsiflexion and plantar flexion weakness are present. Straight leg raise test reproduces pain bilaterally. There is no spinal tenderness.

**Which of the following is the most appropriate diagnostic test to perform next?**

(A) CT of the lumbosacral spine
(B) MRI of the lumbosacral spine
(C) Plain radiography of the lumbosacral spine
(D) No imaging studies are indicated

## Item 14

A 24-year-old woman is evaluated for a breast lump. She has had no breast trauma or discharge from the nipples. She is nulliparous and has regular menstrual cycles. Medical history is otherwise unremarkable. The patient's mother was recently diagnosed with breast cancer at age 58 years; no other family members have breast or ovarian cancer. Her only medication is an oral contraceptive pill.

On physical examination, vital signs are normal. BMI is 25. A breast examination reveals no skin changes, with dense breast tissue bilaterally. She has a firm, 2-cm, non-tender, mobile mass with well-defined margins in the upper outer quadrant of the left breast. There is no evidence of axillary, cervical, or supraclavicular lymphadenopathy.

**Which of the following is the most appropriate test to perform in this patient?**

(A) Biopsy
(B) Mammography
(C) Mammography and ultrasonography
(D) Ultrasonography

## Item 15

A 24-year-old man is evaluated for a 6-week history of severely depressed mood and loss of interest in work, family, and friends. During this time period, he has been sleeping more than usual (up to 11 hours per day) but still feels like he has no energy. He feels that he is a burden to his family and coworkers and admits to sometimes thinking about suicide. He had similar symptoms 2 years ago, for which he was treated with escitalopram. He remained on this therapy for only 2 weeks because his symptoms rapidly abated, and he had a "surge of energy." One year ago, he had a 4-week period during which he had a similar increase in energy level. During that time, he slept only 4 hours per night and decided that he would become a competitive triathlete. He used most of his money to start a boot camp fitness business, which closed within 2 months. He has never had hallucinations. He takes no medications and does not use alcohol or recreational drugs.

**Which of the following is the most likely diagnosis?**

(A) Bipolar disorder
(B) Generalized anxiety disorder
(C) Major depressive disorder
(D) Schizophrenia

## Item 16

A 27-year-old man is evaluated during a routine follow-up visit for obesity. On his previous two visits, he had a BMI of 38. Despite enrollment in a 6-month comprehensive supervised weight loss program that included nutritional counseling, he has gained 2.3 kg (5.0 lb). He briefly tried orlistat but discontinued this medication because of gastrointestinal side effects. Medical history is significant for type 2 diabetes mellitus and hypertension. Medications are liraglutide, lisinopril, and metformin.

On physical examination, blood pressure is 146/91 mm Hg; other vital signs are normal. BMI is 39. The remainder of the physical examination is unremarkable.

Laboratory studies reveal a hemoglobin $A_{1c}$ value of 8.2%.

**Which of the following is the most appropriate management?**

(A) Bariatric surgery
(B) Lorcaserin
(C) Referral to a dietician
(D) Very-low-calorie diet

## Item 17

A 39-year-old man is evaluated for a 3-month history of dry, intermittent cough. He reports no other associated symptoms and has had no unusual environmental exposures. He is a lifelong nonsmoker. Medical history is significant for hypertension, for which he was started on lisinopril and hydrochlorothiazide 4 months ago. He has no known allergies.

On physical examination, vital signs are normal. There is no pharyngeal erythema or exudate. Lungs are clear to auscultation.

A chest radiograph is normal.

**Which of the following is the most appropriate management?**

(A) Discontinue lisinopril
(B) Initiate intranasal glucocorticoid therapy
(C) Obtain spirometry
(D) Start proton pump inhibitor therapy

## Item 18

A 46-year-old man seeks advice on whether he should undergo prostate cancer screening. He recently underwent direct-to-consumer genetic testing, which revealed that his risk for prostate cancer is 33% higher than that of the average person. He is asymptomatic. Medical history is unremarkable. Family history is significant for prostate cancer diagnosed in his paternal grandfather at age 72 years. He takes no medications.

On physical examination, vital signs and the remainder of the examination are normal.

**Which of the following is the most appropriate management?**

(A) Digital rectal examination (DRE)
(B) Serum prostate-specific antigen level measurement
(C) Serum prostate-specific antigen level measurement and DRE
(D) Patient education and no further testing

## Item 19

A 55-year-old woman is evaluated for left-sided tinnitus that has gradually emerged over the last 6 months. She describes the tinnitus as a high-pitched continuous (nonpulsatile) buzzing. The patient reports no hearing loss, balance difficulties, dizziness, or headaches. Her medical history is otherwise unremarkable.

On physical examination, vital signs are normal. Direct visualization of the external ear canals and tympanic membranes is unremarkable. Findings on Weber and Rinne testing suggest left sensorineural hearing loss. The whispered voice test suggests hearing loss on the left side. Results of the Romberg, cerebellar, and cranial nerve tests are all normal. Audiologic tests confirm mild to moderate left sensorineural hearing loss.

**Which of the following is the most appropriate management?**

(A) CT angiography of the posterior fossa
(B) MRI of the internal auditory canal
(C) Referral for hearing aid placement
(D) Urgent referral to an otolaryngologist

## Item 20

An 82-year-old woman is evaluated for severe and progressive shortness of breath on ambulation. She has COPD and has been hospitalized only once in the past 18 months for an acute exacerbation. She has not experienced an acute worsening of her symptoms, and she has minimal nonproductive cough. She stopped smoking 15 years ago. She notes that her dyspnea is a substantial impediment to her quality of life. Medical history is otherwise significant for heart failure with preserved ejection fraction. Medications are umeclidinium/vilanterol and albuterol inhalers, lisinopril, and chlorthalidone.

On physical examination, temperature is 37.0 °C (98.6 °F), blood pressure is 128/78 mm Hg, pulse rate is 74/min, and respiration rate is 20/min. Oxygen saturation is 96% breathing 1 L/min of oxygen by nasal cannula and is maintained at 96% during a 6-minute walk test. Pulmonary examination reveals a prolonged expiratory phase and intermittent scattered rhonchi throughout her lung fields, with hyperresonance to percussion. Cardiac examination reveals an $S_4$ but no murmur or jugular venous distention.

CONT.

Spirometry performed 2 months ago showed an $FEV_1$ of 42% of predicted.

**Which of the following is the most appropriate treatment?**

(A) Furosemide
(B) Oxygen at 2 L/min by nasal cannula
(C) Prednisone
(D) Pulmonary rehabilitation

## Item 21

A 50-year-old man is seen for preoperative medical evaluation before left shoulder arthroplasty. History is significant for alcohol-related cirrhosis and osteoarthritis. Medications are lactulose, furosemide, and spironolactone. The patient stopped drinking alcohol 5 months ago but has difficulty with medication adherence. He reports increasing ascites and lower extremity edema.

On physical examination, vital signs are normal. There is no jaundice or scleral icterus. Spider telangiectasias are noted on the face and chest. The abdomen is distended with flank dullness. There is 1+ pitting edema to the knees bilaterally. Mental status examination is normal.

The calculated Model for End-stage Liver Disease (MELD) score is 22.

The patient is instructed to increase his furosemide.

**Which of the following is the most appropriate preoperative management?**

(A) Cancel surgery and refer for liver transplant evaluation
(B) Delay surgery until after patient achieves 1 year of sobriety
(C) Delay surgery until after placement of a transjugular intrahepatic portosystemic shunt
(D) Proceed to surgery

## Item 22

A 24-year-old person is evaluated as an add-on patient for a 1-week history of nasal congestion, watery eyes, and cough productive of yellow sputum. The patient is new to the practice and has indicated on the intake form that his gender is transmale. He responds to questioning that he would prefer to be addressed as "he" or "him," but he seems nervous. He reports no fevers, chills, shortness of breath, or rash. He takes no medications.

On physical examination, vital signs are normal. There is oropharyngeal erythema, and nasal turbinates are boggy. No tonsillar exudate or cervical lymphadenopathy is noted. Lungs are clear to auscultation bilaterally.

**Which of the following is the most appropriate next step in management at this visit?**

(A) Obtain a hormonal and surgical history
(B) Obtain a social and sexual history
(C) Perform a genital examination
(D) Screen for sexually transmitted infections
(E) Symptomatic treatment

## Item 23

A 75-year-old man is being discharged following treatment for acute decompensated heart failure. The patient and his wife are alerted to symptoms that indicate acute worsening of his heart failure and are informed of when he should seek immediate medical assistance. The discharge medication list and the side effects of these medications are reviewed, and the patient and his wife acknowledge an understanding. A nursing education visit regarding the hospital stay and evaluations is completed. A copy of the discharge summary is given to the patient, and a follow-up appointment is scheduled with his internist in 7 days.

**Which of the following is also recommended to improve patient safety and reduce rehospitalization in this patient?**

(A) Follow-up telephone call and one home nursing visitation
(B) Home telemonitoring
(C) Postdischarge patient education
(D) Timely discharge summary for the primary care physician

## Item 24

A 54-year-old man is evaluated for a 6-month history of right shoulder pain. He describes the pain as moderately severe aching that is diffusely localized over the shoulder without radiation to the arm. The pain is constant, although it is worse at night and with any shoulder movement. The pain was insidious in onset and has been progressively worsening. He has had no neurologic or constitutional symptoms. Ibuprofen provides some pain relief.

On physical examination, vital signs are normal. Pain and limited range of motion are noted with both active and passive movement in all planes of motion, as is diffuse tenderness over the anterior and posterior areas of the right shoulder. There is no tenderness to palpation of the bony or soft tissue structures, nor is there cervical spine tenderness. There are no neck symptoms or findings.

**Which of the following is the most likely diagnosis?**

(A) Acromioclavicular joint degeneration
(B) Adhesive capsulitis
(C) Bicipital tendinitis
(D) Rotator cuff disease

## Item 25

A 32-year-old man is evaluated for ongoing intermittent premature ejaculation of 3 years' duration, which he describes as distressing to him and his spouse. He reports no other symptoms. The patient also has depression, which is currently well controlled with amitriptyline. A previous trial of sertraline caused mood instability, prompting its discontinuation. He takes no other medications.

On physical examination, vital signs are normal. Growth and pattern of body hair and testicular size are normal. No gynecomastia is noted.

Laboratory studies show a normal 8:00 AM serum total testosterone level.

Which of the following is the most appropriate additional treatment?

(A) Paroxetine
(B) Testosterone gel
(C) Topical lidocaine
(D) No additional treatment is indicated

## Item 26

A 67-year-old woman is evaluated for urinary incontinence that has progressively worsened over the past 2 years. She experiences incontinence when she laughs or sneezes but reports no dysuria, hematuria, or loss of continence at night. She has been postmenopausal for 12 years. She had four spontaneous term vaginal deliveries between age 24 and 32 years. She has no other problems and takes no medications.

On physical examination, all vital signs are normal. BMI is 20. Pelvic examination reveals vaginal atrophy. The remainder of the examination is normal.

Which of the following is the most appropriate treatment?

(A) Bladder training
(B) Oral estradiol
(C) Oxybutynin
(D) Pelvic floor muscle training (Kegel exercises)
(E) Weight loss

## Item 27

An 81-year-old woman was admitted to the ICU 8 days ago for multisystem organ failure associated with a severe episode of multilobar pneumonia. She has required mechanical ventilation since admission. Efforts to wean the patient from mechanical ventilation have not succeeded, and the patient remains somnolent and unresponsive to verbal stimuli. Medical history is significant for dementia, diabetes mellitus, COPD, chronic kidney disease, and heart failure.

The care team concludes and shares with the patient's family that she will not have a meaningful recovery; however, the patient's children request continued ICU-level care. The patient does not have an advance directive, and her wishes are unknown. After a family meeting with the care team to discuss the patient's prognosis, the children continue to request all treatment.

Which of the following is the most appropriate management?

(A) Consult with the hospital ethics committee
(B) Discontinue ICU care in 48 hours if there is no improvement
(C) Transfer the patient to another institution
(D) Continue current level of care

## Item 28

A 54-year-old woman is evaluated for a 9-month history of vaginal irritation and itching. She also has pain during intercourse and uses vaginal lubricants without much relief. At age 50 years, she developed severe menopause-related vasomotor symptoms that responded to a 2-year course of estrogen replacement therapy; she currently has no vasomotor symptoms. Family history is significant for breast cancer. She takes no medications.

On physical examination, vital signs are normal. Pelvic examination shows diminished elasticity of the vulvar skin; thinning of the labia minora; introital narrowing; and dry, pale-colored vaginal lining with decreased rugae.

Which of the following is the most appropriate treatment?

(A) Clobetasol
(B) Ospemifene
(C) Systemic estrogen therapy
(D) Vaginal estrogen therapy

## Item 29

A 30-year-old woman is evaluated for a 1-year history of severe anxiety about multiple aspects of her life, including her marriage, work, and health. She also reports irritability, poor sleep, and difficulty concentrating, and she finds it difficult to complete her daily home and occupational tasks. She has had multiple visits with her internist for various symptoms, including atypical chest pain, shortness of breath, palpitations, and intermittent diarrhea. She does not use alcohol, tobacco, or recreational drugs. She drinks one cup of coffee every morning. Her Generalized Anxiety Disorder 7-item scale score is 15, corresponding to severe anxiety.

Laboratory studies reveal a normal serum thyroid-stimulating hormone level.

Which of the following is the most appropriate long-term pharmacologic treatment?

(A) Amitriptyline
(B) Clonazepam
(C) Lithium
(D) Sertraline

## Item 30

A 66-year-old woman is evaluated during a follow-up visit for a 5-year history of chronic autoimmune pancreatitis. She has constant, severe, aching midabdominal pain that radiates to the back. Her only surgical option is a pancreaticojejunostomy, a procedure that she is not ready to accept. She has previously tried several tricyclic antidepressants, venlafaxine, gabapentin, oral morphine, and tramadol. A fentanyl patch was substituted for oral morphine during a recent hospitalization, and over the past 6 weeks, she has noted reduced pain and improved function with its use. She lives with her husband and oldest daughter at her home. She does not smoke, drink alcohol, or use illicit drugs. Her only medications are a fentanyl patch, 25 µg/h changed every 72 hours (approximately 75 morphine milligram equivalents/day); prednisone; and pancreatic enzyme replacement.

On physical examination, the patient is frail appearing. Vital signs are normal. BMI is 21. The abdomen is scaphoid; bowel sounds are present. Midepigastric palpation reveals tenderness.

**Which of the following is the most appropriate next step in management?**

CONT.

(A) Add lorazepam

(B) Prescribe naloxone and provide caregiver education on its use

(C) Recommend weekly nursing visits before each opioid prescription

(D) Switch the fentanyl patch to short-acting hydromorphone

## Item 31

A 60-year-old man is evaluated for abdominal cramping and diarrhea that began after starting ezetimibe. The patient has had persistently elevated LDL cholesterol levels while taking maximally tolerated statin therapy. One year ago, he began receiving atorvastatin, 80 mg/d, with an initial LDL cholesterol level of 180 mg/dL (4.66 mmol/L). However, he developed severe muscle pain, and the dosage was decreased to 40 mg/d and ultimately 20 mg/d. Three months ago, his LDL cholesterol was 140 mg/dL (3.63 mmol/L), at which time ezetimibe was added. Medical history is otherwise significant for myocardial infarction treated with drug-eluting stent placement 1 year ago. Medications are aspirin, clopidogrel, atorvastatin, ezetimibe, metoprolol, and lisinopril.

On physical examination, vital signs are normal. BMI is 27. There is mild, diffuse abdominal tenderness to palpation without rebound or guarding. The remainder of the examination is unremarkable.

**In addition to discontinuing ezetimibe, which of the following is the most appropriate management?**

(A) Add alirocumab

(B) Add cholestyramine

(C) Add niacin

(D) No further intervention

## Item 32

A 65-year-old man is evaluated during a visit to establish care. He is interested in colorectal cancer screening; however, he adamantly refuses to undergo colon preparation, and he does not want to modify his diet for screening. He has never undergone colorectal cancer screening. Medical and family histories are unremarkable. He takes no medications.

Physical examination, including vital signs, is normal.

After discussing the colon preparation process and dietary restrictions with the patient and exploring his concerns, he is steadfast in his refusal.

**Which of the following is the most appropriate screening test for this patient?**

(A) Circulating methylated *SEPT9* DNA test

(B) CT colonography

(C) Fecal immunochemical test

(D) Sensitive guaiac-based fecal occult blood test

## Item 33

A 35-year-old woman is evaluated during a follow-up visit for anxiety. Her symptoms have been well controlled with cognitive behavioral therapy, and she has been drinking kava tea every morning and practicing mindfulness daily. Medical history is significant for nonalcoholic steatohepatitis. Other supplements are folic acid and echinacea.

On physical examination, vital signs are normal. BMI is 36. The remainder of the examination is unremarkable.

**Which of the following is the most appropriate recommendation for this patient?**

(A) Discontinue echinacea

(B) Discontinue folic acid

(C) Discontinue kava tea

(D) No changes to current therapy

## Item 34

A 70-year-old man is seen for a preoperative medical evaluation before laminectomy for spinal stenosis. History is also significant for coronary artery disease and a non–ST-elevation myocardial infarction that occurred 5 years ago. He swims for 30 minutes every other day. He reports no chest pain with activity. Medications are aspirin, simvastatin, metoprolol, and lisinopril.

Physical examination, including vital signs, is normal.

Electrocardiogram performed 2 years ago demonstrated a left anterior fascicular block, several premature atrial contractions, and sinus rhythm.

**Which of the following is the most appropriate preoperative cardiac testing for this patient?**

(A) Dobutamine stress echocardiography

(B) Electrocardiography

(C) Exercise stress testing

(D) No further testing

## Item 35

A 44-year-old man is evaluated for right medial elbow pain that began 2 months ago with a dull ache and has gradually worsened. The pain is worse with elbow flexion, and his right fourth and fifth fingers are numb.

On physical examination, vital signs are normal. Decreased sensation over the volar aspect of the right fourth and fifth fingers is noted, with adduction and abduction weakness of the fingers. The right elbow has full range of motion and no notable erythema, swelling, or tenderness.

**Which of the following is the most likely diagnosis?**

(A) Carpal tunnel syndrome

(B) Medial epicondylitis

(C) Olecranon bursitis

(D) Ulnar nerve entrapment

## Item 36

A 63-year-old woman is evaluated in the emergency department after an unwitnessed syncopal event. She

CONT. recalls feeling a sensation of warmth and generalized weakness prior to the event but had no chest pain, dyspnea, or palpitations. Medical history is significant for hypertension, hyperlipidemia, and carotid artery stenosis treated with endarterectomy. Medications are lisinopril, hydrochlorothiazide, atorvastatin, and aspirin.

Vital signs and screening cardiovascular and neurologic examinations are normal.

**Which of the following tests should be included in the initial evaluation of this patient?**

(A) Ambulatory electrocardiographic monitoring and echocardiography

(B) B-type natriuretic peptide and cardiac enzyme measurement

(C) Magnetic resonance carotid angiography and MRI of the brain

(D) Orthostatic blood pressure measurement and electrocardiography

## Item 37

A 37-year-old woman is evaluated for contraceptive advice. She is married and has a 1-year-old child. The patient describes the conception of this child as an "accident" because she often missed taking her previous oral contraceptive. Her menstrual periods have resumed and are regular but heavy and, in that regard, bothersome to her. Medical history is unremarkable. She drinks a glass of wine every night and smokes a pack of cigarettes daily. She has no other health issues and takes no medications.

The result of a pregnancy test performed today is negative.

The patient is provided with a brief smoking cessation intervention. She is not ready to stop smoking but will consider it again at a later time.

**Which of the following is the most appropriate female contraceptive option for this patient?**

(A) Estrogen-progestin oral contraceptive

(B) Estrogen-progestin vaginal ring

(C) Progesterone-containing intrauterine device

(D) Progesterone-only "mini pill"

## Item 38

A 43-year-old woman is evaluated during a follow-up appointment for obesity. She has been following a reduced-calorie, low-fat diet and participating in a 45-minute aerobic exercise class three times weekly for the past 6 months. After her last follow-up appointment 1 month ago, she added 30 minutes of brisk walking on the weekend to her exercise regimen. She brings a food diary and weekly weight records to her appointment. She lost an average of 0.2 kg (0.5 lb) per week over the first 3 to 4 weeks, but her weight loss tapered thereafter and her weight has increased by 0.5 kg (1 lb) since her last visit. The total amount of weight lost over the past 8 months is 2.7 kg (6 lb), or 3% of her original weight. The patient reports that she is unable to achieve the calorie reduction recommended, stating that she

is "hungry all the time." Medical history is also significant for type 2 diabetes mellitus and hypertension. Medications are amlodipine, lisinopril, and metformin.

On physical examination, blood pressure is 141/92 mm Hg, and other vital signs are normal. BMI is 31. The remainder of the examination is unremarkable.

**Which of the following is the most appropriate next step in treatment?**

(A) Bariatric surgery

(B) Liraglutide

(C) Switch to a low-carbohydrate diet

(D) Switch to a very-low-calorie diet

## Item 39

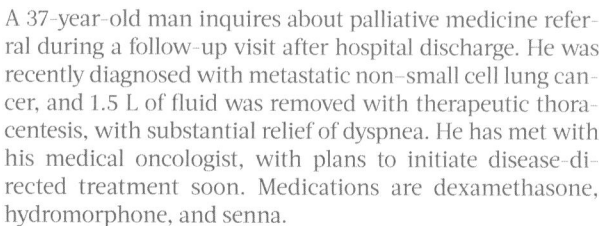

A 37-year-old man inquires about palliative medicine referral during a follow-up visit after hospital discharge. He was recently diagnosed with metastatic non–small cell lung cancer, and 1.5 L of fluid was removed with therapeutic thoracentesis, with substantial relief of dyspnea. He has met with his medical oncologist, with plans to initiate disease-directed treatment soon. Medications are dexamethasone, hydromorphone, and senna.

**When is the most appropriate time for palliative medicine referral?**

(A) Now

(B) At initiation of chemotherapy

(C) At onset of symptoms

(D) Palliative medicine is not indicated for patients undergoing active cancer treatment

## Item 40

A 51-year-old woman is evaluated during a routine follow-up visit for diabetes mellitus. She also has hypertension and hyperlipidemia. Medications are metformin, enalapril, chlorthalidone, and high-intensity rosuvastatin. She has no drug allergies.

On physical examination, blood pressure is 126/74 mm Hg. The remainder of the examination is unremarkable.

Her 10-year risk for atherosclerotic cardiovascular disease is 11% according to the Pooled Cohort Equations. She has been instructed in intensive lifestyle modifications.

**Which of the following is the most appropriate preventive measure to reduce this patient's cardiovascular risk?**

(A) Clopidogrel

(B) Low-dose aspirin

(C) Low-dose aspirin and clopidogrel

(D) Regular-dose aspirin

(E) No additional therapy

## Item 41

A 37-year-old woman is evaluated for a 6-year history of difficulty initiating sleep and significant daytime sleepiness. She works as a registered nurse, and she notes that her daytime sleepiness is exacerbated when she works several night shifts in a row at the hospital. She does not drink alcohol, use tobacco, or consume caffeinated products. She recently initiated a new exercise program and exercises three to four mornings each week. She has no other symptoms and takes no medications.

On physical examination, vital signs are normal. BMI is 30. Oxygen saturation breathing ambient air is 97%. The remainder of the physical examination is normal.

**Which of the following is the most appropriate next step in management?**

(A) Multiple sleep latency testing

(B) Overnight oximetry

(C) Polysomnography

(D) Serum ferritin level measurement

(E) Two-week sleep diary

## Item 42

A 32-year-old man emails to request an opinion on his medical conditions. He is not an established patient but decided to contact the physician after viewing an online profile. His message indicates that he has a several-year history of abdominal pain with intermittent diarrhea and constipation, for which he takes polyethylene glycol, fiber, and dicyclomine. He notes that he has seen a primary care physician and gastroenterologist and undergone extensive testing, including an endoscopy and colonoscopy. He requests a recommendation for a new test or treatment.

**Which of the following is the most appropriate management?**

(A) Advise the patient to obtain celiac disease assessment

(B) Ask the patient to email his medical records before providing advice

(C) Request that the patient call the office to establish care

(D) Do not respond to the patient's email

## Item 43

A 38-year-old woman is evaluated for a 2-day history of worsening eye pain and decreasing visual acuity in her left eye. The pain is worse with eye movement. She reports no fever or trauma. Vision loss is mostly central, and her ability to distinguish colors has diminished. She does not feel the sensation of a foreign body in the eyes. She wears contact lenses. Her medical history is otherwise unremarkable.

On physical examination, vital signs are normal. Eye movement is intact but painful, with visual acuity of 20/20 in the right eye and 20/60 in the left. Afferent pupillary defect is noted in the left eye. There is no corneal injection or discharge, and the optic discs appear normal.

**Which of the following is the most likely diagnosis?**

(A) Corneal abrasion

(B) Herpes simplex keratitis

(C) Optic neuritis

(D) Orbital cellulitis

## Item 44

During a routine health examination, a patient asks about an article that recommended avoiding statin therapy because of the risk for memory loss. The findings were based on cross-sectional data analysis of a well-validated national health survey, which was conducted by random sampling of patients according to zip code of residence. The analysis showed that patients who self-reported memory loss were more likely to also report having taken statin drugs (odds ratio, 1.8; 95% CI, 1.2-2.7; $P = 0.046$).

**Which of the following is the most likely threat to the validity of this study?**

(A) Confounding

(B) Selection bias

(C) Self-reported data

(D) Statistical significance

## Item 45

A 75-year-old woman underwent total hip arthroplasty 4 hours ago and is now evaluated because she has been unable to void since the operation. Bladder ultrasound reveals 900 mL of urine. Other than manageable postoperative pain, she has no symptoms. Current medications are acetaminophen, oxycodone, and enoxaparin.

**Which of the following is the most appropriate management?**

(A) Suprapubic catheter placement

(B) Suprapubic warm wet gauze application

(C) Tamsulosin administration

(D) Urethral bladder catheterization

## Item 46

A 66-year-old woman is transitioning care after her previous physician retired and undergoes a new patient evaluation. She is asymptomatic. She is unclear when her last Pap smear was performed or the result. Medical history is unremarkable, and she takes no medications.

The physical examination, including vital signs, is normal.

**Which of the following is the most appropriate cervical cancer screening strategy for this patient?**

(A) Obtain high-risk human papillomavirus (hrHPV) testing now

(B) Obtain Pap smear and hrHPV testing now

(C) Obtain Pap smear now

(D) Obtain results of last cervical cancer screening examination

(E) No further screening

## Item 47

A 51-year-old woman is referred for evaluation. She has a 10-year history of chronic pain that she describes as head-to-toe aching, twisting, and sometimes burning that involves several large muscle groups. The pain is constant, and she rates the severity as a 6 on a 10-point scale. She is able to work despite the pain but is constantly fatigued. Her current regimen of oxycodone provides minimal relief. She has tried three other opioid medications as well as gabapentin and milnacipran, all of which provided only minimal improvement in her pain. Medical history is also significant for generalized anxiety disorder treated with sertraline.

On physical examination, vital signs are normal. There is tenderness in multiple large muscle groups. The remainder of the physical examination is normal.

**In addition to slow tapering of oxycodone, which of the following is the most appropriate next step in treatment?**

(A) Lorazepam
(B) Physical therapy
(C) Transcutaneous electrical nerve stimulation
(D) Transdermal fentanyl

## Item 48

A 79-year-old woman is accompanied to the office by her son for an evaluation of her memory. The patient forgot to attend her last two scheduled appointments. The patient lives alone; her son visits her daily and sets up a weekly pill box with her medications. The son reports that on several occasions lately, pills that his mother should have taken have been left in the compartments. The patient admits that she sometimes gets confused as to which section of the pill box is the correct one for that day. Medical history is significant for hypothyroidism, hypertension, gastroesophageal reflux disease, and osteoarthritis. Medications are levothyroxine, amlodipine, omeprazole, vitamin D, and acetaminophen.

On physical examination, vital signs are normal. The patient is pleasant and interactive. The physical examination is normal, including neurologic and gait assessment. Depression screening with PHQ-2 is negative.

**Which of the following is the most appropriate test to perform next?**

(A) Apolipoprotein E (*APOE*-ε4) genotyping
(B) Fluorodeoxyglucose-PET brain imaging
(C) Formal neurocognitive testing
(D) Mini-Cog testing

## Item 49

A 36-year-old woman is evaluated for posterior neck pain and stiffness that began 1 week ago while she was doing sit-ups. The pain is worse with movement of the head. She has limited range of motion of the neck in all directions. The pain does not radiate down her arms, and she has not had arm weakness, parethesias, or other neurologic symptoms. She reports no systemic symptoms. The pain is lessened with ibuprofen.

On physical examination, vital signs are normal. On palpation, tenderness of the cervical paraspinal muscles is noted. There is no cervical spine tenderness. Symptoms are not reproduced when the examiner bends the patient's head to either side while also extending the neck and applying a downward axial load (Spurling test). Neurologic examination is normal.

**Which of the following is the most likely diagnosis?**

(A) Cervical myelopathy
(B) Cervical radiculopathy
(C) Cervical sprain
(D) Whiplash-associated neck pain

## Item 50

A 32-year-old woman is evaluated for bothersome vaginal discharge of 2 weeks' duration. Her last Pap smear was obtained 15 months ago and was normal. Nucleic acid amplification test results confirm *Trichomonas vaginalis* infection. Treatment of the patient is initiated.

**Which of the following is the most appropriate additional management?**

(A) Pap testing
(B) Test sexual partner for trichomoniasis
(C) Treat sexual partner for trichomoniasis
(D) No further testing or intervention is necessary

## Item 51

A 46-year-old woman is evaluated for a 3-day history of paresthesia of the right lateral nipple. She has experienced this symptom approximately three times per year for the past 7 years. The paresthesia generally lasts 7 to 10 days. She has no other right breast concerns and reports no milky or bloody discharge, fever, chills, or antecedent trauma. She has undergone extensive evaluation, including laboratory testing, mammography, breast ultrasonography, and dermatologic and neurologic examinations; all results have been normal. She has no other medical problems and takes no medications. She works full time, and her symptom has not limited her functioning.

On physical examination, vital signs are normal. Breast examination is normal bilaterally.

**Which of the following is the most likely diagnosis?**

(A) Conversion disorder
(B) Illness anxiety disorder
(C) Medically unexplained symptom
(D) Somatic symptom disorder

## Item 52

A 45-year-old woman is evaluated for a 2-month history of bothersome lower extremity edema. The edema does not vary with time of day or activity level. Medical history is notable for fibromyalgia treated with pregabalin. She otherwise feels well and is active in a physical therapy program.

On physical examination, vital signs are normal. Pitting edema is present to just above the ankles bilaterally without evidence of calf swelling, varicosities, or hyperpigmentation. There is no tenderness to palpation of the lower extremities. No jugular venous distention, extracardiac sounds, or pulmonary crackles are noted.

Which of the following is the most appropriate next step in management?

(A) Begin hydrochlorothiazide
(B) Perform lower extremity duplex Doppler ultrasonography
(C) Prescribe compression stockings
(D) Switch pregabalin to duloxetine

## Item 53

A 40-year-old woman is evaluated for a 6-month history of poor sleep, lack of energy, constant feelings of sadness, and difficulty concentrating at work. These symptoms began shortly after she was passed over for a promotion at work. She has lost interest in her usual hobbies of running and gardening and has withdrawn from her family and friends. She reports feeling like she is "not worth anything" and sometimes thinks about "ending it all." She says she has never felt like this before; she was previously a positive and optimistic person. She reports never having periods of increased energy, decreased need for sleep, or drastically elevated mood. She has had no hallucinations. She does not use alcohol, tobacco, or recreational drugs.

Laboratory studies reveal a normal serum thyroid-stimulating hormone level.

Which of the following is the most likely diagnosis?

(A) Bipolar disorder
(B) Generalized anxiety disorder
(C) Major depressive disorder
(D) Persistent depressive disorder

## Item 54

A 24-year-old woman is evaluated for an 8-month history of chronic fatigue, unrefreshing sleep, short-term memory loss, and postexertional malaise. She also has symptoms of lightheadedness and dizziness that worsen with upright posture and improve after lying down. Her symptoms do not improve with rest and began suddenly 1 month after being diagnosed with early localized Lyme disease, for which she received a 14-day course of doxycycline. As a result of her symptoms, she has had to curtail many of her social activities and has taken numerous days off work. She takes no medications and has no known allergies.

On physical examination, vital signs are normal. The remainder of the examination is unremarkable.

Laboratory studies reveal a normal complete blood count, electrolyte levels, kidney function test results, liver chemistry test results, and serum thyroid-stimulating hormone level. A pregnancy test result is negative.

Her PHQ-9 score and her Generalized Anxiety Disorder 7-item scale score are both normal.

Which of the following is the most likely diagnosis?

(A) Chronic multifactorial fatigue
(B) Mood disorder
(C) Post–Lyme disease syndrome
(D) Systemic exertion intolerance disease

## Item 55

A 29-year-old man is evaluated in an urgent care center for a 2-day history of pain and swelling of the right hemiscrotum. The pain is stable in intensity, neither worsening nor improving. Other symptoms include low-grade fever and dysuria. He reports no abdominal pain, nausea, or vomiting.

On physical examination, temperature is 38.3 °C (100.9 °F), and pulse rate is 103/min. Blood pressure and respiration rate are normal. There are erythema and swelling of the right hemiscrotum and moderate tenderness to palpation of the superolateral aspect of the right hemiscrotum. The hemiscrotum is not elevated, and there is no scrotal mass, rash, or penile discharge.

Which of the following tests is most likely to have a positive finding?

(A) Cremasteric reflex test
(B) Pain relief with testicular elevation
(C) Scrotal examination in standing and supine positions
(D) Transillumination study

## Item 56

A 44-year-old man is evaluated during a follow-up visit for a 6-month history of low back pain. The pain worsens with standing and is relieved by lying down. He describes the pain as moderate aching. The pain does not radiate down the legs, and he has not had bowel or bladder dysfunction, fevers, leg weakness, night sweats, saddle anesthesia, or weight loss. The pain has been interfering with his ability to work. He participated in acupuncture, mindfulness-based stress reduction, and spinal manipulation, all of which provided only minimal relief.

On physical examination, vital signs are normal. On palpation, bilateral paraspinal muscle tenderness is noted. The musculoskeletal and neurologic examinations are otherwise normal.

Which of the following is the most appropriate pharmacologic option for this patient?

(A) Acetaminophen
(B) Duloxetine
(C) Hydrocodone
(D) Ibuprofen
(E) Tramadol

## Item 57

A 59-year-old man is evaluated for recurring epistaxis over the last several months, usually on the right side. He has been able to stop the bleeding by applying pressure to the nares, but on one occasion, he required treatment in the emergency department. Typically, blood loss has been minimal. He does not use intranasal medications and reports no substance use. He has otherwise been well. There is no family history of epistaxis or rheumatologic or bleeding disorders. His only medication is low-dose aspirin.

On physical examination, vital signs are normal. On nasal examination, there are no clear lesions, erythema, petechiae, scabs, telangiectasias, ulcers, or visible bleeding.

Which of the following is the most appropriate management?

(A) Discontinue aspirin
(B) Obtain coagulation studies
(C) Obtain complete blood count
(D) Perform nasal endoscopy

## Item 58

A hospital system is attempting to reduce the number of hospital-acquired infections, including catheter-related urinary tract infections, bloodstream infections, *Clostridium difficile* infections, and ventilator-associated pneumonia. A common possible factor appears to be the low rate of hand hygiene (78%) documented among hospital staff.

Which of the following measures is most likely to improve hand hygiene rates at this hospital?

(A) Create a spaghetti diagram
(B) Implement the Lean model and create a value stream map
(C) Reiterate the importance of hand hygiene in an email to the hospital staff
(D) Use a Plan-Do-Study-Act cycle

## Item 59

A 91-year-old woman is evaluated to establish care following discharge from a hospital to a skilled nursing facility. She had been living in her own home until 2 weeks ago when she fell and sustained a left intertrochanteric femur fracture. Her fracture was surgically stabilized, and her postoperative course was complicated by delirium and urinary tract infection. Since discharge, she has had no major medical problems. Left hip pain is controlled with acetaminophen as needed. Medical history is otherwise significant for hypertension and type 2 diabetes mellitus. Medications before hospital admission were amlodipine, lisinopril, and metformin. In the hospital, acetaminophen was added for pain and quetiapine for agitated postoperative delirium.

On physical examination, blood pressure is 148/78 mm Hg without orthostatic changes; other vital signs are normal. She has mildly antalgic gait. Cardiac, neurologic, and pulmonary examinations are normal.

Which of the patient's prescribed medications should be discontinued to prevent adverse effects?

(A) Acetaminophen
(B) Amlodipine
(C) Lisinopril
(D) Quetiapine

## Item 60

A 59-year-old woman is evaluated during a follow-up visit for mouth pain of 2 years' duration. Her mouth pain was previously localized to the tongue and floor of the mouth; however, it is now diffuse, burning, and constant. The pain has also worsened over the past year despite continued dosage escalation of a transdermal fentanyl patch and oral hydromorphone. She has no pain with swallowing. Medical history is significant for squamous cell carcinoma of the tongue treated with chemotherapy and radiation therapy; her treatment course was complicated by severe mucositis. She has been without evidence of disease for the past 2 years.

On physical examination, vital signs are normal. The patient is alert and oriented but inattentive and slow to answer questions. Reflexes are exaggerated in the upper and lower extremities, and myoclonic jerking of the legs and clonus at the ankles are noted. Strength is normal. Mouth examination reveals erythematous oral mucosa with no focal areas of erosion or masses.

A CT scan of the head and neck shows no evidence of recurrent disease.

Which of the following is the most likely diagnosis?

(A) Malingering
(B) Opioid-induced hyperalgesia
(C) Opioid withdrawal
(D) Pseudoaddiction

## Item 61

A 61-year-old man is seen for medical evaluation before a pancreaticoduodenectomy for suspected pancreatic cancer scheduled in 7 days. He reports no recent chest pain or bleeding complications after undergoing drug-eluting stent placement to the left anterior descending artery for an ST-elevation myocardial infarction 5 months ago. He has been riding his bike 10 miles daily since recovering from the myocardial infarction. Medications are aspirin, clopidogrel, losartan, atorvastatin, and atenolol.

On physical examination, vital signs are normal. Scleral icterus and jaundice are noted. Cardiac examination is normal, the lungs are clear, and the abdomen is nontender. There is no lower extremity edema.

Which of the following is the most appropriate perioperative management of this patient's antiplatelet therapy?

(A) Continue clopidogrel and aspirin
(B) Withhold aspirin and clopidogrel now
(C) Withhold aspirin now; continue clopidogrel
(D) Withhold clopidogrel now; continue aspirin

## Item 62

A 55-year-old man is seen for a general wellness visit. He is asymptomatic. Family history is significant for prostate cancer diagnosed in his father at age 85 years.

The physical examination is normal.

Which of the following is the most appropriate action regarding prostate cancer screening?

(A) Discuss the benefits and harms of screening
(B) Obtain a serum prostate-specific antigen level
(C) Perform a digital rectal examination
(D) Recommend against screening

## Item 63

An 84-year-old woman in hospice care is evaluated for "death rattle" that is disturbing to family members. She is in the active phases of dying, and her family is distressed by her noisy respiratory secretions; they are worried that she is choking. Medications are haloperidol, hydromorphone, lactulose, and acetaminophen.

On physical examination, respiration rate is 12/min. She is not responsive but does not appear uncomfortable. Extremities are cool. There are oropharyngeal secretions that produce a rattling and gurgling sound with inspiration.

**Which of the following is the most appropriate initial management?**

(A) Atropine ophthalmic drops given sublingually
(B) Glycopyrronium
(C) Scopolamine patch
(D) Suctioning by catheter
(E) Symptom explanation and reassurance

## Item 64

A 48-year-old man is evaluated during a follow-up visit for hypertension. He has no symptoms. He received the tetanus toxoid, reduced diphtheria toxoid, and acellular pertussis vaccine 9 years ago and the influenza vaccine during the most recent influenza season. He is a current smoker with a 25-pack-year history. His only medication is chlorthalidone.

On physical examination, vital signs are normal, and the remainder of the examination is unremarkable.

**Which of the following is the most appropriate vaccine to administer to this patient?**

(A) Recombinant zoster vaccine
(B) Tetanus and diphtheria toxoids booster
(C) 13-Valent pneumococcal conjugate vaccine
(D) 23-Valent pneumococcal polysaccharide vaccine
(E) No vaccines are indicated

## Item 65

A 17-year-old girl is seen for a health maintenance evaluation. She reports no health issues. In discussing dietary habits, she states that she frequently eats very large amounts of food until she is uncomfortably full. These episodes have occurred at least twice per week for the past year; during them, she feels a loss of control over her eating and guilt about her overconsumption. She often eats large amounts of food despite not being hungry, and she prefers eating alone because she is embarrassed of her eating. She does not take laxatives or induce vomiting after such episodes. She rarely exercises. BMI is 30.

**Which of the following is the most likely diagnosis?**

(A) Anorexia nervosa, binging subtype
(B) Binge eating disorder
(C) Bulimia nervosa
(D) Overeating

## Item 66

A 33-year-old woman is evaluated for a 10-month history of bilateral diffuse breast pain. The pain is severe in intensity, occurring about a week before her menstrual cycle and resolving afterward. She has generally lumpy breasts without a dominant mass and no nipple discharge. Her menstrual cycles are regular. She drinks a cup of coffee in the morning and another at noon. Medical history is otherwise unremarkable. She has no family history of breast cancer.

On physical examination, vital signs are normal. BMI is 29. Examination of the breasts shows dense nodularity in the upper outer quadrant of both breasts and no skin changes. Tenderness is elicited on examination of the upper outer quadrants of the breasts. There is no evidence of cervical, supraclavicular, or axillary lymphadenopathy.

**Which of the following is the most appropriate next step in management?**

(A) Advise avoidance of caffeine
(B) Advise use of a well-fitting bra
(C) Breast ultrasonography
(D) Diagnostic mammography
(E) Initiate danazol

## Item 67

A 67-year-old man is evaluated for a 3-hour history of episodic dizziness. He notes a room-spinning sensation started suddenly without antecedent trauma and has been accompanied by nausea. Medical history is significant for hypertension, hyperlipidemia, and type 2 diabetes mellitus. Medications are lisinopril, atorvastatin, and metformin.

On physical examination, temperature is normal, blood pressure is 174/88 mm Hg, pulse rate is 101/min, and respiration rate is normal. The Dix-Hallpike maneuver evokes immediate nystagmus with no fatigability. The nystagmus is vertical without a torsional component, but the direction varies depending on the direction of the patient's gaze. The neurologic examination is limited but grossly nonfocal.

**Which of the following is the most likely diagnosis?**

(A) Acoustic neuroma
(B) Acute labyrinthitis
(C) Benign paroxysmal positional vertigo
(D) Vertebrobasilar ischemia
(E) Vestibular neuronitis

## Item 68

A 46-year-old man is evaluated for a 2-month history of right anterior knee swelling. The swelling began insidiously and has gradually worsened. It is now the size of a golf ball and interferes with his ability to kneel, which is vital to his job as a carpet layer. The knee is painful only when he kneels; he has no problems with knee motion or stability. He feels well otherwise.

On physical examination, vital signs are normal. He has a 4-cm swelling on the anterior aspect of the right knee. The overlying skin is erythematous and warm. The knee exhibits full range of motion. There is no medial or lateral joint tenderness; knee joint effusion; or laxity with anterior, posterior, valgus, or varus forces.

**Which of the following is the most appropriate initial management?**

(A) Activity modification
(B) Fluid aspiration
(C) Ibuprofen
(D) Plain radiography
(E) Serum uric acid measurement

## Item 69

A 49-year-old man was admitted to the ICU 3 days ago with sepsis secondary to health care–associated pneumonia. He is now being transferred to the general medical floor. Medical history is significant for spinal cord injury with associated lower extremity paralysis and neurogenic bladder. He is able to perform intermittent bladder catheterization. Medications are baclofen, enoxaparin, and levofloxacin.

On physical examination, vital signs are normal. BMI is 19. Left lower lobe crackles are present on lung auscultation. There is flaccid paralysis of the lower extremities. Skin is intact without erythema over pressure points.

**Which of the following is the most appropriate intervention to prevent the development of a pressure injury?**

(A) Advanced static mattress
(B) Alternating air mattress
(C) Frequent repositioning
(D) Zinc supplementation

## Item 70

A 24-year-old man is evaluated during a routine examination. He is asymptomatic. He is sexually active with men and has had multiple partners in the past year. He reports using condoms half of the time. Medical history is unremarkable. He takes no medications.

On physical examination, vital signs and the remainder of the examination are normal.

Results of combination HIV antibody immunoassay/p24 antigen testing are negative.

**Which of the following is the most appropriate interval for HIV screening in this patient?**

(A) At least annually
(B) Every 2 years
(C) Every 3 years
(D) Every 5 years
(E) No further screening

## Item 71

A 65-year-old woman is evaluated during a wellness visit. She has no symptoms. Medical history is significant for hypertension and impaired fasting glucose. She has never smoked cigarettes. Medications are hydrochlorothiazide and metformin.

On physical examination, blood pressure is 130/80 mm Hg; other vital signs are normal. BMI is 26. The remainder of the physical examination is normal.

**Laboratory studies:**

| | |
|---|---|
| Total cholesterol | 271 mg/dL (7.02 mmol/L) |
| LDL cholesterol | 155 mg/dL (4.01 mmol/L) |
| HDL cholesterol | 50 mg/dL (1.29 mmol/L) |
| Triglycerides | 330 mg/dL (3.73 mmol/L) |

Her estimated 10-year risk for atherosclerotic cardiovascular disease (ASCVD) using the Pooled Cohort Equations is 11.1%.

**In addition to therapeutic lifestyle changes, which of the following is the most appropriate therapy for primary prevention of ASCVD in this patient?**

(A) Alirocumab
(B) Ezetimibe
(C) Gemfibrozil
(D) Simvastatin

## Item 72

A 72-year-old woman is evaluated for a 2-week history of intermittent dizziness. She has had no falls. Medical history is notable for hypertension and diabetes mellitus, for which she takes amlodipine, lisinopril, and metformin. A review of the patient's medical record reveals that the dosage of amlodipine was increased 3 weeks ago by a colleague's order. The patient's documented blood pressure was normal 3 weeks ago, and the care plan notes that the dosage of the antihypertensive agents should remain the same.

On physical examination, blood pressure is 115/70 mm Hg supine and 90/55 mm Hg standing, and pulse rate is 85/min supine and 105/min standing.

**Which of the following is the most appropriate management?**

(A) Explain that a colleague committed an error and steps will be taken to reduce the chance of recurrence
(B) Explain that the pharmacy committed an error by providing the incorrect dosage
(C) Report the error to the National Practitioner Data Bank without further patient disclosure
(D) Restore the previous dose of amlodipine without further patient disclosure

## Item 73

A 68-year-old woman is evaluated for a 6-month history of incontinence typified by continuous leakage and dribbling. She reports no back pain, dysuria, or fever. Medical history is significant for a 30-year history of type 2 diabetes mellitus and a 10-year history of hypertension and hyperlipidemia. Medications include benazepril, metformin, and rosuvastatin.

On physical examination, blood pressure is 147/76 mm Hg, and pulse rate is 92/min. On abdominal examination, the bladder is palpable just above the pubic symphysis. Foot examination demonstrates dry feet, loss of sensation to monofilament testing, and vibration up to the ankles. Lower extremity tendon reflexes are absent.

Urinalysis results are normal.

**Which of the following is the most appropriate management?**

(A) Botulinum toxin injection

(B) Oxybutynin

(C) Postvoid residual urine volume measurement

(D) Urodynamic testing

## Item 74

A 44-year-old man is evaluated for a 6-year history of constant low-grade perineal pain with intermittent exacerbations and intermittent urinary symptoms of dysuria, frequency, and urgency. He had a documented case of acute bacterial prostatitis 6 years ago; since then, he has undergone extensive urologic evaluation during many of his exacerbations, all with negative findings. He has been treated numerous times with antibiotics, anti-inflammatory agents, and α-blockers without symptomatic benefit. He has no other medical problems and currently takes no medications.

On physical examination, vital signs are normal. Prostate examination yields mild and poorly localized tenderness without masses or nodules. There is no penile discharge or scrotal pain on palpation.

Results of previous laboratory studies reveal a normal erythrocyte sedimentation rate, C-reactive protein level, leukocyte count, serum creatinine level, electrolyte levels, and serum prostate-specific antigen level. A postvoid residual ultrasound was normal.

**Which of the following is the most appropriate pharmacologic treatment?**

(A) Lidocaine-hydrocortisone suppository

(B) Pregabalin

(C) Tamsulosin

(D) Trimethoprim-sulfamethoxazole

## Item 75

A 51-year-old woman is evaluated for a 2-year history of intermittent chest pain that lasts up to 6 hours. The chest pain is not triggered by exertion, stress, or other inciting factors and is not accompanied by other symptoms. The patient also reports cramping lower abdominal and pelvic pain of 4 years' duration without nausea or bowel habit changes. She has undergone evaluation by four different physicians for these symptoms. Over the past year, she has undergone electrocardiography, chest radiography, mammography, exercise stress testing, echocardiography, CT of the abdomen and chest, upper endoscopy, and colonoscopy; all findings were normal. Recent complete blood count, comprehensive metabolic panel, and C-reactive protein level were also normal. She is unhappy with the medical care she has received and spends much of her free time reading articles related to her symptoms. She is afraid that she has a life-threatening illness that no one has been able to diagnose. Medications are acetaminophen, a multivitamin, and probiotics.

On physical examination, vital signs and all other findings are normal.

**Which of the following is the most appropriate next step in management?**

(A) Cognitive behavioral therapy

(B) *MEFV* gene analysis

(C) Pregabalin

(D) Whole-body PET

## Item 76

A 64-year-old man is evaluated in the emergency department for acute onset of vision loss in the right eye, which began 1 hour ago. He can barely see his own hands in front of his eye. He has no eye pain. One week ago, he had an episode of monocular vision loss in the right eye that resolved after 5 minutes. He has had no other recent medical concerns. He has no history of floaters, headaches, jaw claudication, muscular weakness, or weight loss. Medical history is significant for hyperlipidemia and hypertension. Medications are atorvastatin and lisinopril.

On physical examination, vital signs are normal. There is loss of visual acuity in the right eye, and pupillary examination reveals an afferent pupillary defect. The optic disc is shown. There is no conjunctival erythema or scalp tenderness.

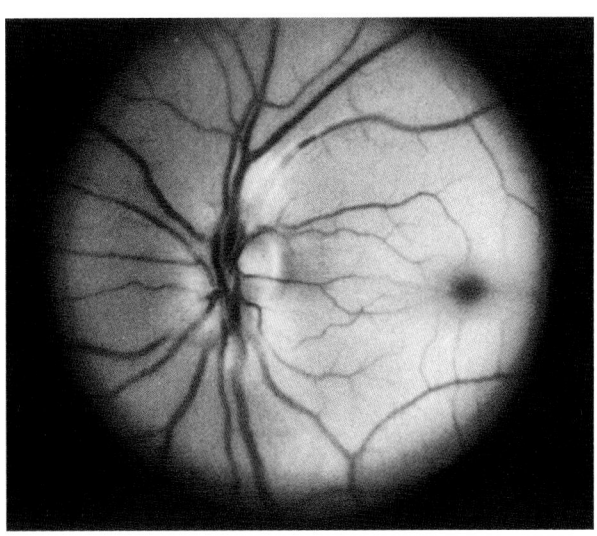

Laboratory studies reveal an erythrocyte sedimentation rate of 22 mm/h.

**Which of the following is the most likely diagnosis?**

(A) Acute angle-closure glaucoma

(B) Central retinal artery occlusion

(C) Idiopathic intracranial hypertension

(D) Retinal detachment

## Item 77

A 74-year-old man is evaluated for severe chronic shortness of breath. Medical history is significant for New York Heart Association functional class III heart failure and severe COPD. He was hospitalized 3 weeks ago for an exacerbation

CONT.

of his COPD. He has returned to his baseline oxygen requirements, but his continued shortness of breath is a significant impediment to his quality of life. The patient's goal is comfort. He does not desire any additional interventions for his heart failure or COPD. Medications are tiotropium, fluticasone propionate/salmeterol, albuterol, amlodipine, lisinopril, hydrochlorothiazide, and oxygen by nasal cannula.

On physical examination, the patient is comfortable at rest but develops dyspnea while ambulating, with associated anxiety. Temperature is 36.9 °C (98.4 °F), blood pressure is 124/68 mm Hg, pulse rate is 98/min, and respiration rate is 32/min. Oxygen saturation is 93% breathing 4 L/min of oxygen by nasal cannula. Pulmonary examination reveals distant breath sounds and a prolonged expiratory phase; the lungs are otherwise clear to auscultation. The estimated central venous pressure is 6 cm $H_2O$. Cardiac examination reveals an $S_4$ but is otherwise normal. There is no peripheral edema.

Chest radiograph shows evidence of hyperinflation but no signs of heart failure, pneumonia, or pneumothorax.

**Which of the following is the most appropriate treatment of this patient's dyspnea?**

(A) Oral furosemide
(B) Oral hydromorphone
(C) Oral lorazepam
(D) Nebulized morphine

## Item 78

A 69-year-old man is evaluated during a routine visit. He is asymptomatic. Medical history is remarkable for hypertension, atrial fibrillation, and type 2 diabetes mellitus. He has a 25-pack-year smoking history but quit smoking 3 years ago. Medications are amlodipine, metoprolol, rivaroxaban, and atorvastatin.

Physical examination, including vital signs, is normal.

His estimated 10-year risk for atherosclerotic cardiovascular disease (ASCVD) according to the Pooled Cohort Equations is 14.6%.

**Which of the following is most appropriate for primary prevention of ASCVD in this patient?**

(A) Add aspirin
(B) Add fish oil
(C) Switch rivaroxaban to aspirin
(D) No further intervention

## Item 79

A 28-year-old man is evaluated in the emergency department for a right ankle sprain that occurred earlier in the day while he was refereeing a soccer game. When running down the field, his right cleat stuck in the turf, and his foot rotated laterally. He was able to bear weight immediately after the injury, but he had to leave the game. The ankle has begun to swell, making it difficult for the patient to ambulate.

On physical examination, vital signs are normal. The patient walks with antalgic gait, although he is able to bear weight. Swelling is present over the anterior and lateral distal

leg above the right ankle. Pain is reproduced both by squeezing the leg at mid-calf level and by having the patient cross his right leg with the lateral malleolus resting on the left knee. There is no tenderness to palpation over the malleoli, the navicular bone, or the fifth metatarsal base.

**Which of the following is the most likely diagnosis?**

(A) Achilles tendon rupture
(B) Ankle fracture
(C) High ankle sprain
(D) Lateral ankle sprain

## Item 80

A 23-year-old woman is evaluated for a 2-week history of persistent thick, white vaginal discharge; burning in the vulvar and vaginal regions; and vaginal itching. She has never had these symptoms before. She is in a monogamous sexual relationship. Medical history is otherwise unremarkable, and she takes no medications.

On physical examination, vital signs are normal. Pelvic examination reveals vulvar edema with a few excoriations. Speculum examination demonstrates thick, white, curdy vaginal discharge. The remainder of the examination is unremarkable.

Laboratory studies reveal a vaginal pH of 4.4; whiff test result is negative. Potassium hydroxide microscopy shows hyphae. Results of tests for *Chlamydia trachomatis* and *Neisseria gonorrhoeae* are negative.

**Which of the following is the most appropriate treatment?**

(A) Intravaginal clotrimazole
(B) Intravaginal nystatin
(C) Oral metronidazole
(D) Oral voriconazole

## Item 81

A 53-year-old man is evaluated for possible opioid therapy initiation for a several-year history of chest and back pain. Both types of pain significantly impair his ability to sleep, and he has not been able to work for the last 6 months. Over the past few years, he has undergone extensive evaluation, and no modifiable cause of the pain has been discovered. The patient has tried various nonpharmacologic interventions (acupuncture, cognitive behavioral therapy, exercise) and nonopioid pharmacologic therapies (duloxetine, gabapentin, ibuprofen), but he continues to have poor quality of life. These interventions are ongoing. He has no history of anxiety, depression, or substance use disorder. Results of screening tests for depression and anxiety disorders performed today are negative. His only medications are duloxetine, gabapentin, and ibuprofen.

The risks and known benefits of long-term opioid therapy are reviewed with the patient. Treatment goals are discussed, and there is an understanding that opioid therapy will be stopped if the goals are not achieved or the risks exceed the benefit. A check with the state's prescription drug monitoring program confirms that the patient is not receiving opioids or benzodiazepine therapy.

**Which of the following is recommended before starting opioid therapy in this patient?**

(A) Baseline urine drug screening

(B) Discontinuation of all other pain medications

(C) Discontinuation of all nonpharmacologic therapies

(D) Psychiatric evaluation

## Item 82

A 60-year-old woman is seen for a preoperative medical evaluation before elective total left knee arthroplasty. She experiences occasional dizziness after swimming for 30 minutes. History is also significant for benign paroxysmal positional vertigo. She has no other medical problems or symptoms and takes no medications.

On physical examination, temperature is normal, blood pressure is 130/75 mm Hg, pulse rate is 75/min, and respiration rate is 16/min. Cardiac examination reveals a grade 3/6 late-peaking harsh systolic murmur heard throughout the precordium, with radiation to the bilateral carotid arteries. The lungs are clear. There is no lower extremity edema.

Transthoracic echocardiogram obtained 2 years ago demonstrated moderate aortic stenosis with a valve area of 1.3 cm² and gradient of 25 mm Hg.

**In addition to electrocardiography, which of the following is the most appropriate preoperative testing for this patient?**

(A) B-type natriuretic peptide level measurement

(B) Dobutamine stress echocardiography

(C) Transthoracic echocardiography

(D) No further testing

## Item 83

A 29-year-old man is evaluated during a new patient visit. He is concerned about gradual weight gain over the last several years. He does not pay much attention to his diet and describes his lifestyle as generally sedentary. He does not use tobacco products and does not drink more than one to two alcoholic drinks per week. He reports no problems with nonrestorative sleep or daytime hypersomnolence. He takes no medications.

On physical examination, blood pressure is 149/90 mm Hg, and pulse rate is 87/min. BMI is 35. His waist circumference is 107 cm (42 in). The remainder of the physical examination is normal.

**Which of the following is the most appropriate test to perform next?**

(A) Exercise stress test

(B) Hepatic ultrasonography

(C) Overnight polysomnography

(D) Serum lipid panel

(E) Thyroid function studies

## Item 84

A 59-year-old woman is evaluated for an 8-month history of minimally productive cough. Her cough has persisted despite empiric treatment with intranasal and inhaled glucocorticoids, inhaled bronchodilators, a proton pump inhibitor, antihistamines, and decongestants. She reports no wheezing, heartburn, or nasal discharge. She is a lifelong nonsmoker and has no history of unusual environmental exposures. She has no known allergies and currently takes no medications.

On physical examination, vital signs are normal. Tympanic membranes are clear. The remainder of the examination is unremarkable.

Chest radiograph, spirometry, bronchial hyperresponsiveness testing, sinus CT scan, and esophageal pH monitoring are normal. Sputum analysis is negative for eosinophils.

**Which of the following is the most appropriate treatment?**

(A) Azithromycin

(B) Inhaled ipratropium

(C) Morphine

(D) Multimodal speech therapy

## Item 85

A 47-year-old woman is evaluated during a follow-up visit for major depressive disorder that was diagnosed 2 months ago. At that time, she reported a 4-month history of anhedonia, depressed mood, decreased energy, insomnia, and weight loss. Her PHQ-9 score was 14, indicating moderate depression. She was prescribed sertraline, and her symptoms improved; her PHQ-9 score is now 9 (mild depression). However, she is distressed because she has had anorgasmia since starting sertraline.

**Which of the following is the most appropriate next step in management?**

(A) Continue sertraline and initiate cognitive behavioral therapy

(B) Discontinue sertraline and initiate bupropion

(C) Discontinue sertraline and initiate paroxetine

(D) Discontinue sertraline and refer for electroconvulsive therapy

## Item 86

A 53-year-old woman is evaluated during follow-up for several chronic medical problems without a medical explanation despite extensive evaluation. Symptoms include nonpositional lightheadedness, difficulty concentrating, and total body numbness. Her symptoms have been stable for the past 2 years. She has a history of anxiety and depression, and her mood is well controlled with medical therapy. Medications are sertraline and acetaminophen as needed.

The physical examination, including vital signs, is normal.

Findings on brain MRI obtained 2 years ago were normal.

**Which of the following is the most appropriate management?**

(A) Anti-Hu antibody assay

(B) Anti–*N*-methyl-D-aspartate receptor antibody assay

(C) Cognitive behavioral therapy

(D) No further management

## Item 87

A 42-year-old man is evaluated for low back pain that began 4 days ago after he shoveled snow. The pain is mild to moderate in severity and does not radiate. He has not had any fevers, leg weakness, night sweats, or bowel or bladder dysfunction. Ibuprofen lessens the pain, as does a heating pad. He has no history of illicit substance use, and his medical history is unremarkable. He takes no additional medications.

On physical examination, vital signs are normal. Bilateral lumbar paraspinal muscle tenderness is noted; the musculoskeletal and neurologic examinations are otherwise normal.

**Which of the following is the most appropriate test to perform next?**

(A) CT of the lumbar spine
(B) Erythrocyte sedimentation rate measurement
(C) MRI of the lumbar spine
(D) Plain radiography of the lumbar spine
(E) No additional testing

## Item 88

A 26-year-old man requests genetic testing for familial adenomatous polyposis. He is asymptomatic. Medical history is unremarkable. His 34-year-old brother recently underwent genetic testing, which revealed a mutation of the adenomatous polyposis coli (*APC*) gene. His father died of colon cancer at age 45 years, and two paternal uncles died of colon cancer at age 46 years and age 47 years. There is no family history of colon cancer in his maternal family members. He takes no medications.

**Which of the following is the most appropriate management?**

(A) Begin sulindac
(B) Obtain colonoscopy at age 40 years
(C) Obtain genetic testing
(D) Refer for genetic counseling

## Item 89

A 70-year-old man is evaluated before discharge from the hospital after treatment for community-acquired pneumonia. Medical history is significant for mild dementia. The patient lives alone and has a daughter who lives nearby. Remaining in his home is very important to him.

The care team recommends that the patient be discharged to a short-term rehabilitation facility to gain strength and prepare him to safely return to his home. The patient refuses. Decision-making capacity is assessed; he is able to articulate the risks, benefits, and alternatives to short-term rehabilitation as well as an understanding of his current medical condition.

**Which of the following is the most appropriate management?**

(A) Administer the Mini–Mental State Examination
(B) Ask the patient's daughter to make a decision on his behalf

(C) Discharge the patient home with home care services
(D) Obtain a court order for the patient to be discharged to a rehabilitation facility
(E) Refer the patient to a psychiatrist for a capacity assessment

## Item 90

A 55-year-old woman is evaluated during a routine examination. Medical history is significant for hypertension, hyperlipidemia, diabetes mellitus, and a non–ST-elevation myocardial infarction 2 weeks ago. She is a current smoker with a 35-pack-year smoking history. She is ready to stop smoking. Medications are metformin, rosuvastatin, aspirin, clopidogrel, metoprolol, and lisinopril.

On physical examination, vital signs and other findings are normal.

**Which of the following is the most effective smoking cessation therapy for this patient?**

(A) Bupropion
(B) Electronic cigarettes
(C) Nicotine replacement therapy
(D) Varenicline

## Item 91

A 69-year-old man is evaluated during a routine examination. The patient reports being healthy and has no symptoms. He has a 10-pack-year smoking history but quit smoking at age 42 years. Medical history is otherwise unremarkable. He takes no medications.

On physical examination, vital signs are normal. BMI is 22. The remainder of the examination is normal.

**Which of the following is the most appropriate screening test for this patient?**

(A) Abdominal duplex ultrasonography
(B) Chest radiography
(C) Dual-energy x-ray absorptiometry
(D) Low-dose lung CT
(E) No screening is recommended

## Item 92

A 62-year-old woman is admitted to the hospital for pneumonia. Her medical history is significant for stage I estrogen receptor–positive invasive breast cancer, for which she was treated with breast-conserving surgery and radiation therapy and then started on tamoxifen. During her hospital stay, antibiotic therapy is initiated, and tamoxifen is withheld. Following discharge, the patient is evaluated in the office, and it is noted that she is no longer taking tamoxifen.

**Which of the following measures would have most likely prevented this medication error?**

(A) Computerized physician order entry
(B) Electronic medication administration record use
(C) Improved medication labeling
(D) Medication reconciliation

## Item 93

An 87-year-old woman is evaluated during a follow-up visit after a recent diagnosis of breast cancer. In the 18 months before her diagnosis, she noted a generalized decline in her energy level and appetite. She no longer is able keep up with others when walking any distance, and she now requires some assistance with dressing because of generalized weakness. She has unintentionally lost 3.6 kg (8 lb) in the last 6 months. Medical history is significant for breast cancer, coronary artery bypass graft surgery at age 74 years, COPD, and hypertension. Medications are albuterol, tiotropium, salmeterol, atorvastatin, aspirin, lisinopril, and metoprolol.

On physical examination, vital signs are normal. BMI is 19. The remainder of the examination is unremarkable.

**Which of the following is most likely to predict the patient's overall morbidity, mortality, and response to breast cancer treatment?**

(A) FRAIL scale score
(B) Pharmacologic cardiac stress test
(C) Six-minute walk test
(D) Timed Up and Go test

## Item 94

A 30-year-old man is evaluated for feeling "moody" and having persistent difficulty staying focused and keeping track of tasks. He reports often feeling restless and catching himself jumping between tasks before completing them. He describes himself as "hopelessly disorganized." As a result, he has lost or not paid home utility bills and has not always completed work tasks to the satisfaction of his supervisor. He recalls having these problems since childhood. He is otherwise well. He does not use coffee, alcohol, tobacco, or recreational drugs and does not take any medications.

**In addition to cognitive behavioral therapy, which of the following is the most appropriate treatment?**

(A) Clonazepam
(B) Escitalopram
(C) Methylphenidate
(D) Ropinirole

## Item 95

A 26-year-old woman is evaluated for left lateral knee and distal thigh pain that began 6 weeks ago. She is a long-distance runner who trains 6 days per week. The pain began insidiously and has slowly worsened over time. The pain is worst when she is running downhill. She experiences no pain while resting. She has not had any knee trauma and reports no catching, grinding, or locking.

On physical examination, vital signs are normal. On palpation, tenderness is noted 2 cm proximal to the lateral femoral condyle. With the patient supine, pain is reproduced with repeated flexion and extension of the knee as thumb pressure is applied to the lateral femoral epicondyle. There is weakness with left hip abduction. There is no joint line tenderness, joint effusion, or ligament laxity with applied stress.

**Which of the following is the most likely diagnosis?**

(A) Iliotibial band syndrome
(B) Lateral collateral ligament tear
(C) Lateral meniscal tear
(D) Meralgia paresthetica

## Item 96

A 28-year-old woman is evaluated for persistent pain in the left upper outer breast of 9 weeks' duration. The pain is nonradiating and is not associated with aggravating factors or trauma. She has not noted breast lumps, fever, nipple discharge, or skin changes. Medical history is unremarkable, and she has no family history of breast or ovarian cancer. She takes no medications.

On physical examination, vital signs are normal. BMI is 24. The breast tissue is dense, with no overlying skin changes or underlying masses. Focal tenderness is elicited on palpation of the upper quadrant of the left breast, but no mass or chest wall tenderness is present. There is no evidence of axillary, cervical, or supraclavicular lymphadenopathy. The remainder of the examination is unremarkable.

**Which of the following is the most appropriate management?**

(A) Advise elimination of caffeine
(B) Breast ultrasonography
(C) Initiate danazol
(D) Mammography and breast ultrasonography
(E) Reassurance

## Item 97

A 52-year-old man is evaluated for substernal chest pain. The pain is not consistently associated with exertion, nor is it always relieved by rest; it sometimes occurs when he is eating or when he is anxious. He has a 30-pack-year smoking history, but he quit smoking 2 years ago. Medical history is significant for hypertension and hyperlipidemia, for which he takes lisinopril and rosuvastatin, respectively.

On physical examination, vital signs and cardiovascular examination are normal.

An electrocardiogram reveals left ventricular hypertrophy with associated ST-T–wave changes, findings that are unchanged from an electrocardiogram obtained 2 years ago.

The patient's pretest probability of ischemic coronary artery disease is estimated to be 50%. Treadmill stress echocardiography is performed. This test has a positive likelihood ratio of 10.0 and a negative likelihood ratio of 0.1. The patient's stress test result is positive.

**Which of the following best approximates the patient's posttest probability of ischemic coronary artery disease?**

(A) 65%
(B) 75%
(C) 85%
(D) 95%

H

### Item 98

A 34-year-old woman is hospitalized for a small bowel resection due to multiple strictures. She has a 10-year history of Crohn disease. History is also significant for a provoked pulmonary embolism that occurred 5 years ago. Medications are azathioprine and certolizumab.

On physical examination, vital signs are normal. The abdomen is soft. Mild diffuse pain without rebound or guarding is noted.

The patient's Caprini risk score for venous thromboembolism is 6 (high risk).

**Which of the following is the most appropriate postoperative venous thromboembolism prophylaxis for this patient?**

(A) Graduated compression stockings
(B) Graduated compression stockings and low-molecular-weight heparin
(C) Intermittent pneumatic compression
(D) Low-molecular-weight heparin
(E) Low-molecular-weight heparin and intermittent pneumatic compression

H

### Item 99

A 49-year-old man is hospitalized for a 4-day history of poorly controlled nausea, vomiting, fatigue, and volume depletion. He has locally advanced esophageal adenocarcinoma and is undergoing neoadjuvant chemoradiation therapy. Radiation therapy is administered daily, and chemotherapy with low-dose carboplatin plus paclitaxel is administered weekly. His nausea and vomiting are temporally related to the radiation therapy. Medical history is otherwise significant for previous tobacco use. Other medications are acetaminophen, docusate sodium, bisacodyl, oxycodone, and prochlorperazine.

On physical examination, the patient appears fatigued. Blood pressure is 110/68 mm Hg, and pulse rate is 96/min; the remaining vital signs are normal. Pain is elicited with deep palpation of the epigastrium.

**Which of the following is the most appropriate initial treatment of this patient's nausea?**

(A) Haloperidol
(B) Olanzapine
(C) Ondansetron
(D) Synthetic oral cannabinoids

### Item 100

A 30-year-old woman is evaluated for a 2-day history of sore throat and fatigue. She reports anorexia, chills, fever, rhinorrhea, and a dry persistent cough that keeps her awake at night. She works as a school bus driver. She has tried over-the-counter cough and cold products without benefit. Medical history is unremarkable, and she takes no medications.

On physical examination, temperature is 37.2 °C (99.0 °F); all other vital signs are normal. She has nasal and pharyngeal erythema with sparse whitish exudate. There is no lymphadenopathy or rash. The remainder of the examination is normal.

**Which of the following is the most appropriate management?**

(A) Amoxicillin
(B) Streptococcal rapid antigen detection test
(C) Symptom control
(D) Throat culture

### Item 101

H

A 22-year-old woman is evaluated in the emergency department after an episode of syncope. She experienced a prodrome of nausea, diaphoresis, and warmth while waiting in line to attend a concert in a crowded, warm corridor. Her boyfriend reports that she recovered quickly and was not confused after the event. Before the episode, she had skipped dinner to arrive at the concert early. She experienced a similar episode of syncope at age 14 years when she had venipuncture for routine laboratory testing. She describes no other symptoms at the time of the episode, and her only reported symptom at this time is fatigue. She takes no medications.

On physical examination, blood pressure is 118/65 mm Hg sitting and 108/60 mm Hg after standing for 3 minutes, and pulse rate is 78/min sitting and 82/min after standing for 3 minutes. Other vital signs and the remainder of the examination are normal.

An electrocardiogram is normal.

**Which of the following is the most likely diagnosis?**

(A) Hypoglycemia-induced syncope
(B) Neurally mediated syncope
(C) Orthostatic syncope
(D) Postural orthostatic tachycardia syndrome

### Item 102

A 67-year-old man is evaluated in follow-up for urinary incontinence. Six months ago, he began tamsulosin for occasional nocturia, frequency, and urgency related to benign prostatic hyperplasia. Tamsulosin decreased the frequency of nocturia, but he continued to have daytime urinary urgency with a few occasions of urine leakage. He attempted to control his symptoms with behavioral modification, including bladder training and scheduled voiding, but he still has episodes of urgency and leakage. He prefers not to undergo any surgical intervention. Medical history is otherwise significant for heart failure with preserved ejection fraction. Medications include benazepril, carvedilol, furosemide, spironolactone, tamsulosin, and aspirin.

On physical examination, blood pressure is 102/60 mm Hg, and pulse rate is 72/min. Other vital signs and the remainder of the physical examination are normal.

Bladder ultrasonography shows a postvoid residual urine volume of 30 mL.

**Which of the following is the most appropriate treatment?**

(A) Dutasteride
(B) Intermittent bladder catheterization
(C) Mirabegron
(D) Sacral nerve root neurostimulation

## Item 103

A 29-year-old woman is evaluated during a routine examination. She is asymptomatic. Her last Pap smear was obtained 3 years ago and was normal. She completed the human papillomavirus (HPV) vaccine series at age 26 years. Medical and family histories are unremarkable. She takes no medications.

**Which of the following is the most appropriate cervical cancer screening strategy at this time?**

(A) Cervical cytology
(B) Cervical cytology and HPV testing
(C) High-risk HPV testing
(D) No further testing

## Item 104

A 31-year-old man is evaluated for dull, aching, left-sided scrotal discomfort and fullness with intermittent swelling. His symptoms began 6 months ago. He is sexually inactive.

On physical examination, vital signs are normal. Testicular size is normal bilaterally. On his left hemiscrotum, there are tenderness to palpation in the superolateral region and soft, compressible swelling along the spermatic cord, which increases with standing and the Valsalva maneuver. Transillumination and the Prehn sign (diminished scrotal discomfort with elevation) are negative.

**Which of the following is the most appropriate treatment?**

(A) Ceftriaxone plus doxycycline
(B) Ibuprofen and scrotal support
(C) Ligation of the left gonadal vein
(D) Topical lidocaine

## Item 105

A 60-year-old woman is evaluated for left wrist pain that began 3 months ago. She describes the pain as aching, with an intermittent tingling sensation over her left thumb, index, and middle fingers. Symptoms are worse at night and with repetitive motion of the wrist. She types frequently during her work as an administrative assistant.

On physical examination, vital signs are normal. The left wrist exhibits full range of motion, with no visible swelling. There is no evidence of sensory loss, muscle atrophy, or weakness.

**Which of the following is the most appropriate initial management?**

(A) Electromyography
(B) Glucocorticoid injection
(C) Splinting of the wrist
(D) Surgical decompression of the median nerve

## Item 106

A 45-year-old woman is evaluated for a 2-day history of deep boring pain in the right eye. She also describes eye redness and photophobia but no recent trauma to the eye. She has a 10-year history of rheumatoid arthritis, treated with etanercept.

On physical examination, vital signs are normal. Diffuse right eye redness is noted, and there is pain on extraocular movement testing. Gentle pressure over the eye with the lid closed results in pain. There is no scleromalacia in either eye. There is diminished visual acuity of the right eye.

**Which of the following is the most likely diagnosis?**

(A) Episcleritis
(B) Scleritis
(C) Subconjunctival hemorrhage
(D) Viral conjunctivitis

## Item 107

A 57-year-old man is evaluated prior to a right partial nephrectomy for renal cell carcinoma. He is asymptomatic. Medical history is significant for stage 3 chronic kidney disease, hypertension, hyperlipidemia, and degenerative joint disease. He has no history of abnormal bleeding and tolerated left knee arthroplasty 3 years ago without complications. Family history is negative for bleeding diatheses. Medications are lisinopril, hydrochlorothiazide, and simvastatin.

On physical examination, temperature is normal, blood pressure is 125/75 mm Hg, pulse rate is 63/min, and respiration rate is 18/min. BMI is 29. Cardiac examination reveals a regular rate and rhythm with no murmurs. Lungs are clear to auscultation. There is no lower extremity edema, conjunctival pallor, abdominal mass or tenderness, or hepatomegaly.

**Which of the following is the most appropriate preoperative testing for this patient?**

(A) Alanine aminotransferase and aspartate aminotransferase levels
(B) Prothrombin time and activated partial thromboplastin time
(C) Serum creatinine and electrolyte levels
(D) No preoperative testing

## Item 108

A 46-year-old woman is evaluated for knee pain. Seven months ago, she underwent sleeve gastrectomy for obesity. Before the procedure, her BMI was 36. She recently initiated a running program to enhance her weight loss and is now experiencing knee pain, which she treats with ibuprofen as needed. Medical history is significant for hypertension, obesity, and type 2 diabetes mellitus. Medications are atorvastatin, ibuprofen, lisinopril, and metformin.

On physical examination, blood pressure is 118/64 mm Hg; other vital signs are normal. Knee examination is remarkable for tenderness with compression of the patella. There is no joint instability or tenderness along the medial or lateral joint lines.

**Which of the following medications should be discontinued in this patient?**

(A) Atorvastatin
(B) Ibuprofen
(C) Lisinopril
(D) Metformin

## Item 109

A 38-year-old man is evaluated for an 8-week history of insomnia and irritability. He previously saw another physician in the practice, whom he describes as a "terrible doctor." He was treated for depression for several years and has a history of several low-lethality suicide attempts, usually related to interpersonal conflicts. He also reports having turbulent relationships with his parents and siblings.

During the appointment, he makes several compliments about your bedside manner and calls you the best doctor he has ever had. In discussing his symptoms, he attributes many of them to the break-up with his previous girlfriend. After the break-up, he engaged in a 3-day drinking and gambling binge. The patient says he is doing great now because he is in a new relationship with "the perfect woman."

**Which of the following is the most likely diagnosis?**

(A) Bipolar disorder

(B) Borderline personality disorder

(C) Generalized anxiety disorder

(D) Histrionic personality disorder

## Item 110

A 33-year-old woman is evaluated for a 16-month history of chronic fatigue, unrefreshing sleep, difficulty concentrating, and postexertional malaise. As a result of her symptoms, she has become isolated, restricting her social and personal activities. She has also taken sick days from work with increasing frequency in recent months. Medical and family histories are unremarkable. She takes no medications.

On physical examination, the patient has depressed mood. Vital signs are normal. Neurologic examination and the remainder of the examination are normal.

Her PHQ-9 score is 6, consistent with mild depression.

After a careful evaluation, the patient is diagnosed with systemic exertion intolerance disease.

**In addition to a graded exercise program, which of the following is the most appropriate treatment?**

(A) Cognitive behavioral therapy

(B) Methylphenidate

(C) Mirtazapine

(D) Prednisone

(E) Sertraline

## Item 111

A 35-year-old woman is evaluated during a routine follow-up examination for hypothyroidism and requests a prescription for birth control pills. She is in a new sexual relationship. She has regular menstrual cycles, and her last menstrual period was 4 weeks ago. Her most recent Pap smear was obtained 2 years ago and was normal. Her only medical problem is hypothyroidism treated with levothyroxine. Her mother had breast cancer at age 67 years.

On physical examination, vital signs are normal. BMI is 25. The remainder of the examination is unremarkable.

**Which of the following is the most appropriate next step in her management?**

(A) Advise against hormonal contraception

(B) Mammography

(C) Pelvic examination and Pap test

(D) Pregnancy test

## Item 112

A 38-year-old woman is evaluated for low back pain that began 7 days ago when she bent over to pick up a piece of paper. She describes the pain as moderate aching that is localized to the right lower back. A sharp pain intermittently radiates down the lateral aspect of the right leg. She has not had bowel or bladder dysfunction, fevers, leg weakness, night sweats, saddle anesthesia, or weight loss. She has no history of trauma, and she does not use intravenous drugs.

On physical examination, vital signs are normal. BMI is 21. Musculoskeletal and neurologic examinations are normal.

**Which of the following is the most appropriate initial treatment?**

(A) Acetaminophen

(B) Duloxetine

(C) Nonpharmacologic modalities

(D) Oxycodone

## Item 113

A 59-year-old man is evaluated following recent diagnoses of type 2 diabetes mellitus and hypertension. He is asymptomatic. He has never smoked cigarettes. Medications are metformin, chlorthalidone, and low-dose aspirin.

On physical examination, blood pressure is 130/80 mm Hg; other vital signs are normal. BMI is 36. The remainder of the physical examination is unremarkable.

**Laboratory studies:**

| | |
|---|---|
| Total cholesterol | 243 mg/dL (6.29 mmol/L) |
| LDL cholesterol | 140 mg/dL (3.63 mmol/L) |
| HDL cholesterol | 45 mg/dL (1.17 mmol/L) |
| Triglycerides | 290 mg/dL (3.28 mmol/L) |

His 10-year risk for atherosclerotic cardiovascular disease (ASCVD) based on the Pooled Cohort Equations is 22.4%.

The patient is instructed in therapeutic lifestyle changes to lower his risk for ASCVD.

**Which of the following is the most appropriate additional treatment for primary prevention of ASCVD in this patient?**

(A) Fenofibrate

(B) Fish oil supplementation

(C) Moderate- or high-intensity atorvastatin

(D) No additional treatment is required

## Item 114

A 49-year-old man is evaluated for a 2-year history of poor sleep with associated daytime fatigue and sleepiness that often interfere with his performance at work. He recorded a sleep diary, which reveals difficulty with sleep initiation and multiple awakenings throughout the night. He has no other physical symptoms that affect his sleep, and his partner does not notice him snoring or gasping.

Physical examination, including vital signs, is normal.

**Which of the following is the most appropriate next step in management?**

(A) Cognitive behavioral therapy
(B) Diphenhydramine
(C) Melatonin
(D) Mirtazapine
(E) Zolpidem

## Item 115

A 52-year-old man fails to attend a scheduled appointment. He was initially evaluated for bilateral knee osteoarthritis 1 year ago, and treatment with weight loss, NSAIDs, and physical therapy was recommended. Over the past year, the patient missed three scheduled appointments, did not attend physical therapy, arrived for urgent care assessment twice with requests for stronger pain medications, and did not complete sufficient trials of oral nonopioid pharmacologic agents. Attempts to reach the patient by phone to discuss adherence to his care plan have not been successful. The visit today was scheduled to discuss the difficulties in his treatment and assess his barriers to care. Medical history is significant for bipolar disorder. In past visits, he has not appeared manic or suicidal.

**Which of the following is the most appropriate management?**

(A) Refer the patient to a psychiatrist
(B) Report the patient to the local mental health crisis team
(C) Send the patient a letter warning that the relationship may be terminated
(D) Terminate the patient relationship immediately

## Item 116

A 35-year-old woman is evaluated for numbness, tingling, and weakness in her left arm that radiates from the shoulder to the fingers. Her symptoms began 3 months ago and appear to be worsening. They occur with repetitive use of the arm, especially with overhead activities. She has been painting a ceiling mural for the past 6 months. She has no history of arm or shoulder trauma. She takes no medications.

On physical examination, vital signs are normal. When the patient holds her arms above her head for several minutes during the examination, the symptoms are reproduced. The neck demonstrates full range of motion, and muscle bulk and tone in the upper extremities are normal bilaterally. Neurologic examination is normal, and all upper extremity pulses are full and equal.

Results of electrodiagnostic studies are normal.

**Which is the most appropriate therapy for this patient?**

(A) Gabapentin
(B) Interscalene injection of botulinum toxin type A

(C) Physical therapy
(D) Surgical decompression

## Item 117

A 52-year-old woman is evaluated for acute onset of right-sided hearing loss that began yesterday. Soon afterward, she also noted a sensation of ear fullness and ringing in the same ear. She has no other focal neurologic symptoms. She reports no rhinorrhea, fever, pharyngitis, or ear pain. Medical history is significant for hypertension. She takes chlorthalidone. She has had no other exposures to medications or supplements.

On physical examination, vital signs are normal. There is decreased hearing in the right ear; the Weber test lateralizes to the left ear, and air conduction is louder than bone conduction bilaterally. The ear canals are unobstructed, and the tympanic membranes are normal appearing. The neurologic examination is unremarkable.

**Which of the following is the most likely diagnosis?**

(A) Meniere disease
(B) Otosclerosis
(C) Ototoxicity
(D) Sudden sensorineural hearing loss

## Item 118

A 60-year-old man is evaluated in the hospital for a pressure injury. The pressure injury developed during a prolonged hospitalization after a motor vehicle accident that resulted in a closed head injury and pelvic and spinal fractures. Medications are heparin, oxycodone, and ibuprofen or acetaminophen as needed.

On physical examination, vital signs are normal. A painful 4-cm sacral ulcer with full-thickness loss of skin and adipose tissue is present (stage III). The ulcer has no purulence or surrounding induration.

**Which of the following is the most appropriate treatment?**

(A) Hydrocolloid dressing
(B) Platelet-derived growth factor dressing
(C) Standard gauze dressing
(D) Zinc-infused dressing

## Item 119

A 25-year-old man is evaluated during a new patient visit. He is experiencing severe anxiety about the start of a new job next month. Specifically, he is concerned about his ability to arrive on time because every morning before leaving his apartment, he feels compelled to perform multiple checks to ensure that all electronic devices are turned off and all windows and doors are locked. These activities consume approximately 1 hour of time. He performs these same activities each night before going to bed and often repeats them several times because of overwhelming feelings that he has forgotten something and his apartment will catch fire or be robbed. As a result of his anxieties, the patient rarely socializes outside of his home. When he is away from home, he uses a surveillance application to monitor his apartment 11 minutes after every hour.

**Which of the following is the most appropriate management?**

(A) Buspirone
(B) Clonazepam
(C) Cognitive behavioral therapy
(D) Risperidone

## Item 120

A 58-year-old man is evaluated in an urgent care center for a 3-day history of right-sided scrotal swelling, pain, and dysuria. He reports no antecedent trauma, nausea, or vomiting. He is sexually active with both men and women and uses condoms intermittently. He does not take any medications.

On physical examination, temperature is 38.5 °C (101.3 °F), pulse rate is 101/min, and other vital signs are normal. The right hemiscrotum is edematous, with tenderness to palpation of the superolateral aspect. The scrotal pain lessens with elevation of the scrotum. There is no penile discharge.

Results of nucleic acid amplification testing for chlamydia and gonorrhea are pending.

**Which of the following is the most appropriate treatment?**

(A) Ceftriaxone
(B) Ceftriaxone and doxycycline
(C) Ceftriaxone and levofloxacin
(D) Ibuprofen and scrotal support

## Item 121

A 44-year-old woman is evaluated for a breast lump she noticed 1 week ago. There is no nipple discharge. She birthed two children, the first at age 25 years, and her menstrual cycles are regular. She has no family members with breast or ovarian cancer. She has no other medical problems and takes no medications.

On physical examination, vital signs are normal. BMI is 28. Examination of the breasts reveals dense tissue bilaterally and no skin changes. A mass is noted in the upper inner area of the right breast, measuring 1.8 cm; it is firm, mobile, and nontender, with ill-defined margins. There is no evidence of axillary, cervical, or supraclavicular lymphadenopathy. The remainder of the examination is unremarkable.

**Which of the following is the most appropriate diagnostic test to perform next?**

(A) Breast MRI
(B) Core-needle biopsy
(C) Diagnostic mammography and ultrasonography
(D) Ultrasonography

## Item 122

A 34-year-old woman is evaluated during a follow-up visit for blood pressure control. She states that she hopes to become pregnant and would like to stop her oral contraceptive. She

does not smoke, drink alcohol, or use illicit drugs. She is in a monogamous sexual relationship and has had no sexually transmitted infections. Medical history is significant for hypertension, type 2 diabetes mellitus, and depression since childhood. Medications are an oral contraceptive, lisinopril, metformin, citalopram, and acetaminophen as needed.

On physical examination, vital signs are normal. The remainder of the examination is unremarkable.

**In addition to starting folic acid, which of the following medications should be stopped at this time?**

(A) Acetaminophen
(B) Citalopram
(C) Lisinopril
(D) Metformin

## Item 123

A 77-year-old woman is seen for a preoperative medical evaluation before resection of the sigmoid colon for recurrent diverticulitis scheduled 5 days from now. She has nonvalvular atrial fibrillation and is receiving long-term warfarin, without a history of bleeding complications. She has no history of stroke, transient ischemic attack, or intracardiac thrombus. History is also significant for hypertension. Medications are warfarin, chlorthalidone, and metoprolol.

The physical examination, including vital signs, is normal. The INR measurement is 2.3. Calculated $CHADS_2$ score is 2, and $CHA_2DS_2$-VASc score is 4.

**In addition to withholding warfarin before surgery, which of the following is the most appropriate management of this patient's perioperative anticoagulation?**

(A) Begin aspirin, 81 mg/d
(B) Begin enoxaparin when the INR drops below 2.0
(C) Begin unfractionated heparin when the INR drops below 2.0
(D) No additional interventions

## Item 124

A 26-year-old man is evaluated during a routine examination. He is asymptomatic. The patient is sexually active with men and has had multiple partners in the past year. He engages in both oral and anal sex, and he reports using condoms most of the time. He does not use illicit drugs. He is unsure about his vaccination status and has never been tested for HIV infection, syphilis, or infectious hepatitis. Medical history is unremarkable. He takes no medications.

The physical examination, including vital signs, is normal.

Screening is arranged for HIV infection, syphilis, and hepatitis A and B.

**Which of the following additional screening tests is most appropriate, as recommended by the Centers for Disease Control and Prevention?**

(A) Anal cytology
(B) Hepatitis C antibody assay

(C)  Nucleic acid amplification test for chlamydia and gonorrhea

(D)  No additional tests are indicated

## Item 125

A 31-year-old man is evaluated during a follow-up visit for depression. He previously experienced two episodes of major depressive disorder that were effectively treated with fluoxetine. Three months ago, he presented with recurrent symptoms of depression. His PHQ-9 score was 14, indicating moderate depression. Fluoxetine was initiated and uptitrated to an effective dosage. The patient now reports significant improvement in his symptoms. His PHQ-9 score is 6, indicating mild depression; he reports no adverse effects from the medication.

**Which of the following is the most appropriate next step in management?**

(A)  Complete 8 months of fluoxetine therapy

(B)  Complete 8 months of fluoxetine, then switch to bupropion for long-term maintenance therapy

(C)  Continue fluoxetine as long-term maintenance therapy

(D)  Discontinue fluoxetine

## Item 126

A 38-year-old man is evaluated during a new-patient visit for a 5-year history of fatigue, dizziness, nonexertional chest pain, intermittent and transient abdominal swelling, insomnia, and fleeting numbness of the extremities. He has been evaluated by two different internal medicine physicians, a gastroenterologist, a rheumatologist, and a pulmonologist. Despite extensive blood testing and imaging, a unifying diagnosis has never been established. Medical history is significant for depression, migraine, and cholecystectomy. He does not use tobacco, alcohol, or illicit drugs. Current medications are ibuprofen and sumatriptan as needed, acetaminophen, and citalopram.

Physical examination, including vital signs, is normal.

**In addition to eliciting the patient's concerns, which of the following is the most appropriate initial management?**

(A)  Comprehensive metabolic profile and C-reactive protein level

(B)  *MEFV1* genetic testing

(C)  Obtain all previous medical records

(D)  Psychiatry consultation

(E)  Rheumatoid factor and antinuclear antibody titer

## Item 127

A 49-year-old man is evaluated for a 2-day history of posterior neck stiffness and pain that radiates down his left arm and into the fourth and fifth fingers of his left hand. He is left-handed and works as a roofer. The pain worsens when he turns his head to the left and improves when he lies down, although he sometimes has pain when rising from a prone position. He has not had any arm or hand weakness or problems writing. He has no systemic symptoms.

On physical examination, vital signs are normal. On palpation, the pain is reproduced when the examiner applies downward pressure with the patient's head bent to the left and extended (Spurling test). Pain is relieved when the patient holds his left arm above the plane of his shoulder. Neck range of motion is limited with both left and right lateral rotation. There is no cervical spine tenderness to palpation. The neurologic examination is normal.

**Which of the following is the most appropriate management?**

(A)  Cervical collar

(B)  Cervical MRI

(C)  Electrodiagnostic testing

(D)  Gabapentin

(E)  Neck exercises

## Item 128

A 25-year-old woman is evaluated during a routine wellness visit. She received the tetanus toxoid, reduced diphtheria toxoid, and acellular pertussis (Tdap) vaccine at age 18 years; the meningococcal conjugate vaccine at age 11 years with a booster dose at age 16 years; and an influenza vaccine during the most recent influenza season. She is single, lives in an apartment with a roommate, and is a nonsmoker. She has no upcoming travel plans. She has no medical problems and takes no medications.

Physical examination, including vital signs, is normal.

**Which of the following vaccinations should be offered to this patient?**

(A)  Human papillomavirus vaccine

(B)  Quadrivalent meningococcal conjugate vaccine

(C)  Tdap vaccine

(D)  23-Valent pneumococcal polysaccharide vaccine

## Item 129

A 49-year-old woman is seeking therapy for a 6-month history of increasing hot flushes, now occurring six to eight times per day. She also has night sweats that occur three to five times per night and result in disrupted sleep and daytime fatigue. Her last menstrual period was 14 months ago. She has no personal or family history of breast or ovarian malignancies. She takes no medications.

On physical examination, vital signs are normal, as are pelvic and breast examinations.

**Which of the following is the most appropriate management?**

(A)  Hormone therapy with estrogen alone

(B)  Hormone therapy with estrogen and progesterone

(C)  Ospemifene

(D)  Vaginal estrogen therapy

## Item 130

A 55-year-old man is evaluated in the emergency department for a 2-day history of dizziness accompanied by nausea and vomiting. He works as an electrician, and his symptoms started suddenly while installing an overhead light fixture with his head tilted back for a prolonged period. He describes the dizziness as a constant whirling sensation that is unaffected by changes in position. He also reports symptoms of a recent upper respiratory tract infection but no fever. He has no other medical problems and takes no medications.

On physical examination, temperature is normal, blood pressure is 155/84 mm Hg, pulse rate is 99/min, and respiration rate is normal. Hearing is diminished on the left side. Spontaneous combined horizontal and torsional nystagmus is noted but lessens with a fixed gaze. The patient declines further examination because of severe nausea.

**Which of the following is the most likely diagnosis?**

(A) Benign paroxysmal positional vertigo
(B) Labyrinthitis
(C) Meniere disease
(D) Posterior circulation stroke
(E) Vestibular neuronitis

## Item 131

A 47-year-old man is evaluated for a 2-day history of cough productive of small amounts of yellow sputum, as well as sinus congestion, frontal headache, rhinorrhea, and malaise. He has had no fevers, chest pain, or shortness of breath. Medical history is otherwise unremarkable.

On physical examination, vital signs are normal. There is tenderness over the maxillary sinuses bilaterally. The nasal mucosa is diffusely edematous with moderate amounts of clear discharge. Pharyngeal examination reveals erythema without tonsillar exudate. The tympanic membranes appear normal. No cervical lymphadenopathy is noted. The remainder of the examination is normal.

**Which of the following is the most appropriate treatment?**

(A) Amoxicillin
(B) Codeine
(C) Inhaled albuterol
(D) Intranasal fluticasone

## Item 132

A 67-year-old woman with multiple myeloma is evaluated for back pain. The pain began several months ago but has dramatically worsened in the past 2 weeks. It is located in the lumbar and thoracic spine with associated paraspinal muscle spasms. The pain does not radiate into the buttocks or legs, and there has been no change in gait or bowel or bladder function. She rates the pain as an 8 on a 10-point scale at its worst. Medical history is significant for multiple myeloma and end-stage kidney disease on hemodialysis. Medications are acetaminophen, amlodipine, aspirin, metoprolol, sertraline, bortezomib, dexamethasone, and lenalidomide.

On physical examination, vital signs are normal. Palpation elicits tenderness over the thoracic and lumbar spine. The abdomen is not distended, and there are no palpable masses. Neurologic examination is normal.

Restaging CT scans from 2 months ago reveal lytic lesions in the lumbar spine and left iliac crest.

Spine MRI is scheduled.

**Which of the following is the most appropriate treatment of this patient's pain?**

(A) Fentanyl patch
(B) Gabapentin
(C) Hydromorphone
(D) Morphine
(E) Tramadol

## Item 133

A 68-year-old man is evaluated before elective left total hip arthroplasty. He reports left groin pain and new fatigue and dyspnea that limit ambulation to one flight of stairs and one block. Medical history is significant for type 2 diabetes mellitus, ischemic stroke, hypertension, hyperlipidemia, peripheral artery disease, degenerative joint disease, and chronic kidney disease. Medications are insulin glargine, insulin lispro, aspirin, lisinopril, simvastatin, and tramadol.

On physical examination, temperature is normal, blood pressure is 145/85 mm Hg, pulse rate is 89/min, and respiration rate is 18/min. BMI is 35. Cardiopulmonary examination is normal. There is no lower extremity edema.

Laboratory studies are notable for a serum creatinine level of 2.1 mg/dL (185.6 µmol/L).

An electrocardiogram demonstrates Q waves in leads II and III.

**Which of the following is the most appropriate diagnostic test to perform next?**

(A) Dobutamine stress echocardiography
(B) Exercise electrocardiography
(C) Transthoracic echocardiography
(D) No further testing

## Item 134

A physician has noticed that a 67-year-old colleague in the medical practice has been increasingly forgetful in recent months. The colleague has had more difficulty remembering the names of her new patients and the medical students who are doing rotations in the practice, and she has also frequently missed meetings because of scheduling mix-ups. She admits that she cannot keep track of all of the new medications for diabetes mellitus without using a reference. The physician is unaware of the colleague's personal medical history but is concerned about her memory and cognitive status.

**Which of the following is the most appropriate management?**

(A) Continue to monitor the colleague
(B) Directly approach the colleague and help her plan for confidential evaluation
(C) Offer to confidentially evaluate the colleague
(D) Report the colleague to the state medical board

## Item 135

A 64-year-old man is evaluated for a 5-year history of intermittent erectile dysfunction. He experiences nocturnal and early-morning penile tumescence, and he is able to achieve and maintain an erection sufficient for sexual activity approximately 50% of the time. Medical history is significant for coronary artery disease, depression, hyperlipidemia, hypertension, obstructive sleep apnea, peripheral vascular disease, and type 2 diabetes mellitus. Medications are aspirin, atorvastatin, isosorbide mononitrate, lisinopril, metformin, metoprolol, and sertraline. He does not use continuous positive airway pressure.

On physical examination, all vital signs are normal. BMI is 26. He has normal body hair growth and pattern, normal testicular size, and no gynecomastia.

Laboratory studies reveal an 8:00 AM serum fasting total testosterone level of 380 ng/dL (13.2 nmol/L).

**Which of the following is the most appropriate treatment?**

(A) Alprostadil
(B) Psychotherapy
(C) Sildenafil
(D) Testosterone gel

## Item 136

A 42-year-old woman is evaluated for a 2-month history of left foot pain between the third and fourth toes, accompanied by a burning sensation and the sensation of walking on a pebble. She has not experienced any trauma in the area, and she does not have edema or erythema. Symptom onset was insidious, and the pain only occurs when she is standing or walking. She works as a restaurant hostess and wears high-heeled shoes for her job.

On physical examination, vital signs are normal. The left foot appears normal, with no palpable abnormalities or tenderness between the third and fourth toes. Sensation is intact throughout the foot, and posterior tibial and dorsalis pedis pulses are palpable.

**Which of the following is the most likely diagnosis?**

(A) Bunion deformity
(B) Hammertoe deformity
(C) Morton neuroma
(D) Plantar fasciitis

## Item 137

A hospital system's initial analysis of costs related to prolonged hospital stays revealed that surgical wound infections account for a large proportion of costs. Assessment of the surgical data for the hospital showed that the postoperative wound infection rate is 19%.

**Which of the following is the most appropriate tool to assist in reducing postoperative wound sepsis at this institution?**

(A) Clinical audit
(B) Control chart
(C) Lean model
(D) Model for Improvement

## Item 138

A 92-year-old woman is evaluated for urinary incontinence. Six months ago, the patient occasionally lost control of small amounts of urine, which was managed with an adult diaper. At present, the patient seems to have lost the ability to recognize that she needs to urinate until it is too late to reach the bathroom. There have been no recent noticeable changes in cognition. Medical history is significant for dementia treated with donepezil.

On physical examination, vital signs are normal. The patient appears frail. She is not oriented to place or time. Gait is stable and narrow based. She is slow to rise from a chair, and she requires the arm rests to get up.

**Which of the following is the most appropriate treatment?**

(A) Oxybutynin
(B) Pelvic floor muscle training (Kegel exercises)
(C) Prompted voiding
(D) Sling cystourethropexy

## Item 139

A 23-year-old man is evaluated during a new patient visit. He was honorably discharged from the Army 2 months ago after serving two tours of duty in Afghanistan. Four months ago, his platoon's vehicle was struck by an improvised explosive device. He sustained a severe concussion and multiple lacerations, and three members of his platoon were killed. For the last 3 months, the patient has had daily nightmares in which he relives the event and can see his comrades being killed. He has also experienced flashbacks of the event when he hears loud noises, such as fireworks and thunder. He has had great difficulty sleeping and is increasingly irritable.

The patient has been unable to find employment because he avoids social situations. He has also withdrawn from family and friends because he is afraid they will ask about his military service, and he does not wish to discuss the events he experienced. He has been drinking alcohol more frequently, having up to four beers before bedtime to induce sleep. He does not use tobacco or recreational drugs.

Medical history is otherwise unremarkable, and physical examination is normal.

**Which of the following is the most appropriate treatment?**

(A) Clonazepam
(B) Propranolol
(C) Psychotherapy
(D) Topiramate

## Item 140

A 61-year-old man is evaluated in an urgent care center for acute frontal headache and pain in the right eye that began a few hours earlier while he was watching his grandson's basketball game. The pain extends through the anterior scalp and downward across the nose. The patient is also nauseated and vomiting acutely. He has photophobia and notes that lights appear "fuzzy." Medical history is significant for hypertension and anxiety. Medications are hydrochlorothiazide and citalopram.

On physical examination, blood pressure is 150/90 mm Hg; other vital signs are normal. Severe conjunctival erythema; photophobia; a mid-dilated, nonreactive pupil on the right side; and corneal cloudiness are noted. Upon gentle palpation of the eyes, tenderness and increased firmness are noted over the right globe compared with the left. Right eye visual acuity is grossly decreased. No discharge is noted.

**Which of the following is the most likely diagnosis?**

(A) Acute angle-closure glaucoma
(B) Bacterial endophthalmitis
(C) Central retinal vein occlusion
(D) Scleritis

## Item 141

A 31-year-old woman requests genetic testing for Huntington disease. She has a close friend who recently had a positive genetic test result for the *huntingtin* gene mutation, and she would like to undergo testing for assurance that she is without the disease. She is asymptomatic. Medical history is unremarkable. She takes no medications.

On physical examination, vital signs are normal. Neurologic examination and the remainder of the examination are normal.

**Which of the following is the most appropriate management?**

(A) Obtain a brain MRI
(B) Obtain a three-generation family history
(C) Obtain genetic testing
(D) Refer for genetic counseling

## Item 142

A 45-year-old woman is evaluated for heavy menstrual bleeding. She reports having heavy unpredictable bleeding of variable flow and duration for the past year. Her last period was 12 days ago. She has a history of provoked deep venous thrombosis 3 years ago following an intercontinental flight. She is a current smoker with a 10-pack-year history and does not wish to quit smoking at this time. She has never been pregnant and does not wish to become pregnant in the future.

On physical examination, vital signs are normal. BMI is 24. Breast and pelvic examinations are normal.

Laboratory studies reveal a hemoglobin level of 10.2 g/dL (102 g/L) and mean corpuscular volume of 68 fL. Pregnancy test result is negative.

A subsequent evaluation for secondary causes of abnormal uterine bleeding, including endometrial cancer, was negative.

**In addition to oral iron supplements, which of the following is the most appropriate management?**

(A) Combination oral contraceptive pill
(B) Endometrial ablation
(C) Levonorgestrel-containing intrauterine device
(D) Medroxyprogesterone acetate for the second half of the menstrual cycle

## Item 143

A 28-year-old man is evaluated for a 10-month history of dizziness. He describes the dizziness as a sense of nonvertiginous imbalance and notes that it worsens with personal motion, movement of objects around him, and sitting or standing upright. The dizziness has persisted since he experienced a concussion without loss of consciousness while playing soccer 10 months ago. He reports no focal neurologic symptoms. He takes no medications.

On physical examination, vital signs are normal. On neurologic examination, cranial nerve examination findings are normal, motor strength is intact, and deep tendon reflexes are normal. Romberg test result is negative. Gait is normal.

Findings on a brain MRI are normal.

**In addition to vestibular and balance rehabilitation therapy, which of the following is the most appropriate treatment?**

(A) Amitriptyline
(B) Canalith repositioning maneuver (Epley maneuver)
(C) Lorazepam
(D) Sertraline

## Item 144

An 82-year-old man is evaluated for discharge planning. He was hospitalized with community-acquired pneumonia complicated by respiratory failure and sepsis, which required prolonged mechanical ventilation. He eventually required a tracheostomy and remains on mechanical ventilation, but his respiratory status is otherwise stable. He is severely deconditioned and has been unable to participate even minimally in physical therapy. Although he is expected to require mechanical ventilation for at least several more weeks, he is medically stable for discharge. Medical history is significant for chronic kidney disease, heart failure, hypertension, and type 2 diabetes mellitus. Medications are insulin aspart, insulin glargine, carvedilol, furosemide, and lisinopril.

On physical examination, the patient is alert and cooperative but appears frail on mechanical ventilation. Vital signs and the remainder of the examination are normal.

**Which of the following is the most appropriate discharge disposition for this patient?**

(A) Acute rehabilitation facility
(B) In-home rehabilitation services
(C) Rehabilitation at a long-term acute care hospital
(D) Skilled nursing facility

## Item 145

A proposed new screening protocol for ovarian cancer involves universal pelvic ultrasonography for asymptomatic women starting at age 30 years. The protocol is based on a national study of randomly selected 30-year-old women. The authors of the study note that unilateral oophorectomy performed for suspicious lesions resulted in longer survival than oophorectomy performed for patients with symptoms, based on historical data. The study authors conclude that the screening protocol will reduce ovarian cancer–related deaths.

**Which of the following is most likely to threaten the validity of the authors' conclusions?**

(A) Lead-time bias
(B) Length-time bias
(C) Recall bias
(D) Selection bias

## Item 146

A 42-year-old woman is approaching discharge from the hospital for alcohol withdrawal. She has had severe alcohol use disorder for several years but says she is willing to do whatever it takes to quit. Medical history is also significant for hypertension and chronic kidney disease. Medications are amlodipine and chlorthalidone.

Physical examination, including vital signs, is normal.

A complete blood count and comprehensive metabolic profile are normal. The estimated glomerular filtration rate is 50 mL/min/1.73 m².

**Which of the following is the most appropriate pharmacologic treatment?**

(A) Acamprosate
(B) Chlordiazepoxide
(C) Disulfiram
(D) Naltrexone

## Item 147

A 72-year-old man is hospitalized for the third time in 3 months for shortness of breath. He has stage 3 chronic kidney disease, end-stage COPD, and New York Heart Association functional class III heart failure. The patient does not have an advance directive, and the resuscitation preference most recently noted from a visit 6 months ago is "full code." Medications are acetaminophen, aspirin, lisinopril, metoprolol, and torsemide.

**Which of the following is the most appropriate initial strategy to develop goals of care?**

(A) Ask about hospice referral timing
(B) Ask about resuscitation preferences
(C) Ask what he understands about his illnesses
(D) Provide information about prognosis

## Item 148

A 50-year-old woman is evaluated in the hospital following a non–ST-elevation myocardial infarction treated with drug-eluting stent placement. She is currently asymptomatic. Medical history is significant only for hypertension. Medications are clopidogrel, aspirin, lisinopril, and metoprolol.

Physical examination, including vital signs, is normal. BMI is 29.

**Laboratory studies:**

| | |
|---|---|
| Total cholesterol | 239 mg/dL (6.19 mmol/L) |
| LDL cholesterol | 155 mg/dL (4.01 mmol/L) |
| HDL cholesterol | 45 mg/dL (1.17 mmol/L) |
| Triglycerides | 195 mg/dL (2.20 mmol/L) |

**Which of the following is the most appropriate additional diagnostic testing to perform before initiating high-intensity statin therapy in this patient?**

(A) Alanine aminotransferase level measurement
(B) Alanine aminotransferase and creatine kinase level measurement
(C) Creatine kinase level measurement
(D) No further laboratory studies are indicated

## Item 149

A 40-year-old man is evaluated during a routine examination. He is healthy and asymptomatic, although he leads a sedentary lifestyle. Family history is noncontributory. He takes no medications.

On physical examination, temperature is normal, blood pressure is 120/74 mm Hg, pulse rate is 68/min, and respiration rate is normal. BMI is 32. The remainder of the physical examination is unremarkable.

**When should this patient be screened for diabetes mellitus?**

(A) At age 45 years
(B) At this visit
(C) If he develops an additional risk factor for diabetes
(D) No screening is indicated

## Item 150

A 19-year-old man is evaluated in the emergency department after his roommate became concerned about his behavior. The patient began college 7 months ago, and since then, his roommate has watched the patient become increasingly isolated from others and lacking in emotion. The patient has frequently expressed concerns that the government is tracking his movements and even his thoughts. In the past 2 months, he has stopped attending classes and spends long periods in bed. The roommate called the patient's parents after the patient sealed up the ventilation in their room because he believed government agents were injecting gas into the building. The patient says he does not feel depressed. He had no behavioral problems before starting college, and he does not use alcohol, recreational drugs, or over-the-counter medications.

**Which of the following is the most likely diagnosis?**

(A) Bipolar disorder
(B) Major depressive disorder
(C) Paranoid personality disorder
(D) Schizophrenia

## Item 151

A 39-year-old woman is evaluated for a 3-week history of malodorous vaginal discharge. She was treated with antibiotics for a urinary tract infection 3 weeks before the onset of symptoms. She is in a monogamous sexual relationship. Medical history is unremarkable. Her only medication is an oral contraceptive.

On physical examination, vital signs are normal. Pelvic examination reveals thin, homogenous, grayish vaginal discharge. There is no adnexal or cervical motion tenderness. The rest of the examination is unremarkable.

Laboratory testing reveals a vaginal pH of 5.6; whiff test result is negative.

**Which of the following is the most appropriate test to confirm the diagnosis?**

(A)  Culture for *Gardnerella vaginalis*
(B)  Nucleic acid amplification test for trichomoniasis
(C)  Potassium hydroxide wet mount study for yeast
(D)  Saline microscopy for clue cells

## Item 152

A 60-year-old man is evaluated for a 6-month history of worsening urinary frequency, urgency, hesitancy, incomplete emptying, nocturia, and weakened stream. He reports no dysuria, incontinence, or acute urinary retention. Medical history is also significant for erectile dysfunction. He takes no medications.

On physical examination, vital signs are normal. Rectal examination reveals a diffusely enlarged prostate that is nontender to palpation, with no masses or nodules noted. Testicular size is normal. A comprehensive metabolic profile and urinalysis are normal; an 8:00 AM total testosterone level is also normal.

**Which of the following is the most appropriate treatment?**

(A)  Finasteride
(B)  Oxybutynin
(C)  Tadalafil
(D)  Tamsulosin

## Item 153

A 55-year-old man is hospitalized after he was injured at a construction site structure collapse. He has a fractured pelvis, a shoulder dislocation, a mild concussion, and multiple abrasions. He is scheduled to undergo surgery for the fractured pelvis tomorrow morning. History is significant for hyperlipidemia, hypertension, coronary artery disease, and a non–ST-elevation myocardial infarction 2 years ago treated with drug-eluting stent placement. Current medications are atorvastatin, metoprolol, amlodipine, and aspirin.

On physical examination, temperature is normal, blood pressure is 170/90 mm Hg, pulse rate is 102/min, and respiration rate is 20/min. Oxygen saturation is 96% breathing ambient air. Multiple abrasions and ecchymosis are noted. Cardiac examination reveals tachycardia but is otherwise normal.

**Which of the following is the most appropriate management of this patient's medications before surgery?**

(A)  Continue amlodipine, aspirin, and metoprolol; withhold atorvastatin

(B)  Continue amlodipine, atorvastatin, and metoprolol; withhold aspirin
(C)  Continue atorvastatin, metoprolol, and aspirin; withhold amlodipine
(D)  Continue all medications

## Item 154

A 50-year-old woman is seen following screening digital mammography. She is asymptomatic and has no medical problems. Other than her age and sex, she has no additional risk factors for breast cancer and no family history of breast cancer. The mammogram report notes no suspicious lesions but indicates that the breasts are heterogeneously dense (density category C).

On previous physical examination, vital signs and breast examination were normal.

**In addition to education on breast density, which of the following is the most appropriate adjunctive breast cancer screening?**

(A)  Breast MRI
(B)  Digital breast tomosynthesis
(C)  Repeat digital mammography in 6 months
(D)  No further testing

## Item 155

A 49-year-old woman is evaluated for a 3-year history of pelvic pain. An extensive evaluation has not found a clearly defined pathophysiologic or anatomic cause, and therapy has been targeted to general pain management lately. She has been a willing and cooperative participant in biofeedback, cognitive behavioral therapy, physical therapy, hypnosis, acupuncture, meditation, and stress-reduction techniques, without significant pain relief. Her pain has been unresponsive to multiple trials of nonopioid analgesics and antidepressants, and she has tried oral tapentadol and tramadol, which were also ineffective. She currently takes acetaminophen and gabapentin. Medical history is significant for end-stage kidney disease, for which she receives hemodialysis, and hypertension. Other medications are metoprolol succinate, amlodipine, intravenous iron, and an erythropoiesis-stimulating agent.

**Which of the following is the most reasonable treatment option for this patient's chronic pain?**

(A)  Oral immediate-release morphine sulfate
(B)  Oral medical cannabis oil
(C)  Oral methadone
(D)  Topical lidocaine

## Item 156

A 66-year-old man is evaluated for right posterior knee swelling that began 3 days ago. The knee is not painful, unstable, warm, or red. He has no systemic symptoms. History is significant for bilateral knee osteoarthritis. His only medication is aspirin, which adequately controls his osteoarthritis pain.

On physical examination, vital signs are normal. A large bulge is visible on the posterior aspect of the right knee, without erythema, tenderness, or warmth. Crepitus of the knees is noted bilaterally. There is no joint instability or increased laxity with stress forces.

**Which of the following is the most appropriate management?**

(A) Aspiration of fluid
(B) Glucocorticoid injection
(C) Ibuprofen
(D) Plain radiography of the knee
(E) No treatment

## Item 157

A 56-year-old woman is evaluated during a wellness examination. She reports no vaginal bleeding, discharge, or other symptoms since reaching menopause at age 52 years. Over the past 3 months, she has noted a lack of interest in sexual activity that has been occasionally distressing for her. She uses vaginal lubricant for intercourse, which reduces the mild discomfort with sexual activity. She has no history of pelvic surgery, sexually transmitted infections, or sexual trauma. Results of screening tests for anxiety and depression are negative. Medical history is otherwise unremarkable, and she takes no medications.

On physical examination, the external genitalia are normal. Pelvic examination reveals pale vaginal walls and a decrease in vaginal lubrication. The remainder of the examination is unremarkable.

**Which of the following is the most likely female sexual disorder diagnosis?**

(A) Female orgasmic disorder
(B) Genitopelvic pain/penetration disorder
(C) Sexual interest/arousal disorder
(D) No female sexual disorder

## Item 158

A 78-year-old man is evaluated in the emergency department for a 1-day history of worsening dizziness. The patient describes the dizziness as a room-spinning sensation and notes that he has some accompanying nausea and imbalance. He reports no other symptoms. Medical history is notable for hypertension, hyperlipidemia, and type 2 diabetes mellitus. Medications are aspirin, lisinopril, atorvastatin, and metformin.

On physical examination, blood pressure is 172/88 mm Hg; other vital signs are normal. The patient has difficulty with tandem walking. With extraocular movement testing, the patient has vertical nystagmus. The neurologic examination is otherwise nonfocal and without mental status changes.

**Which of the following is the most appropriate diagnostic test to perform next?**

(A) CT of the head
(B) MRI of the brain

(C) Vestibular laboratory testing
(D) No further testing

## Item 159

A 27-year-old woman is evaluated for help with weight loss. After a visit 3 months ago, she enrolled in an online weight loss program and began a walking program. She currently walks 30 minutes per session 5 days per week. She admits that she has difficulty adhering to the diet restrictions. She avoids weighing herself because she finds it discouraging. She has lost 0.2 kg (0.5 lb) since her visit 3 months ago. Medical history is unremarkable, and she takes no medications.

On physical examination, vital signs are normal. BMI is 32. The remainder of the examination is unremarkable.

**Which of the following is the most appropriate management?**

(A) Bariatric surgery
(B) Behavioral therapy
(C) Exercise for 45 minutes/day
(D) Low-carbohydrate diet
(E) Phentermine-topiramate

## Item 160

A 45-year-old man was hospitalized following a head-on motor vehicle crash. On day 4, he survived cardiac arrest but experienced anoxic brain injury. The care team concludes that he has a poor neurologic prognosis and is unlikely to regain consciousness or interact with his environment.

A family meeting is planned to discuss the decision to perform a tracheostomy and percutaneous endoscopic gastrostomy for enteral feeding. His wife reports that the patient has previously stated that he would not want to be kept alive if he could not interact with her or their children. The patient does not have an advance directive.

**Which of the following should be the basis for the decision regarding this patient's management?**

(A) Patient's best interests
(B) Patient's medical condition
(C) Patient's previously expressed wishes
(D) Risk management

## Item 161

A 58-year-old man is admitted to the hospital for a 2-week history of worsening constipation. He has end-stage heart failure (New York Heart Association functional class IV) and stage 3 chronic kidney disease. Medications include bisoprolol, furosemide, losartan, spironolactone, hydromorphone (for dyspnea palliation), bisacodyl, lactulose, senna, docusate, and tap water enema.

On physical examination, respiration rate is 20/min; other vital signs are normal. Oxygen saturation is 92% breathing ambient air. Cardiac examination reveals an $S_3$, jugular venous distention, and peripheral edema. Crackles are auscultated at the lung bases. Moderate abdominal distention is noted, with tenderness to palpation.

CONT.

Which of the following is the most appropriate treatment of this patient's constipation?

(A) Lubiprostone
(B) Methylnaltrexone
(C) Polyethylene glycol
(D) Sodium phosphate enema

## Item 162

An 18-year-old man is brought to the office by his mother, who is concerned about his behavior in school. Since age 6 years, the patient has had difficulty interacting with people and exhibits several unusual, repetitive behaviors, including tapping his fork three times with each bite of food. He has scored well on aptitude tests but has struggled in classroom activities that require working with other students. He has no friends, and his parents find it difficult to engage in conversation with him.

On physical examination, the patient exhibits paucity of speech; he answers yes-or-no questions appropriately. There is no evidence of disordered thinking.

**Which of the following is the most likely diagnosis?**

(A) Antisocial personality disorder
(B) Autism spectrum disorder
(C) Obsessive-compulsive disorder
(D) Social anxiety disorder

## Item 163

A 42-year-old man is seen to discuss recent test results. He is asymptomatic. He has no known medical problems and takes no medications. He does not use tobacco products.

On physical examination, blood pressure is 128/74 mm Hg; other vital signs are also normal. BMI is 24. The remainder of the examination is unremarkable.

**Laboratory studies:**

| | |
|---|---|
| Total cholesterol | 270 mg/dL (6.99 mmol/L) |
| LDL cholesterol | 170 mg/dL (4.40 mmol/L) |
| HDL cholesterol | 40 mg/dL (1.04 mmol/L) |
| Triglycerides | 300 mg/dL (3.39 mmol/L) |

His 10-year risk for atherosclerotic cardiovascular disease based on the Pooled Cohort Equations is 3.4%.

**Which of the following is the most appropriate treatment of this patient's hyperlipidemia?**

(A) Low-intensity statin therapy
(B) Moderate-intensity statin therapy
(C) High-intensity statin therapy
(D) Therapeutic lifestyle changes

## Item 164

A 58-year-old woman is evaluated for a 4-week history of left lateral hip pain. She describes the pain as a moderate ache that intermittently radiates down the lateral aspect of the left leg. It began insidiously and has gradually worsened. The pain worsens when she is climbing stairs or lying on the affected side. She reports no previous trauma to the area. She has not had any leg weakness or swelling or any constitutional symptoms. She has not taken any analgesics for the pain.

On physical examination, vital signs are normal. On palpation, there is tenderness over the left greater trochanter. There is painless full range of motion with abduction, flexion, and external rotation of the left hip. The remainder of the examination is normal.

**In addition to activity modification, which of the following is the most appropriate management?**

(A) Ibuprofen
(B) Glucocorticoid injection
(C) Hydrocodone/acetaminophen
(D) Plain radiography of the left hip

## Item 165

A 56-year-old woman is evaluated for severe vaginal itching and discomfort. Her symptoms have progressively worsened over the last 4 months. There is no associated vaginal discharge or vaginal odor. She is experiencing significant vaginal dryness, and intercourse has become painful despite the use of lubricants. She has been menopausal since age 53 years. She takes no medications.

On physical examination, vital signs are normal. Physical examination reveals dry vaginal epithelium that is smooth and shiny. Blood vessels are visible beneath the pale vaginal mucosa, and increased friability is evident.

Vaginal pH is 6.0. Wet mount shows occasional leukocytes. Whiff test result is negative. There are no clue cells and no hyphae on potassium hydroxide preparation.

**Which of the following is the most likely diagnosis?**

(A) Acute allergic contact dermatitis
(B) Genitourinary syndrome of menopause
(C) Vulvar lichen planus
(D) Vulvar lichen sclerosus

## Item 166

A 64-year-old man is evaluated to establish care. Medical history is significant for long-standing low back pain secondary to traumatic vertebral compression fractures. He has chronic pain that partially responds to heat and relaxation, but he also has several acute exacerbations of pain daily that "immobilize" him and prevent him from working. These episodes do not respond to nonpharmacologic therapy. He has tried multiple nonopioid analgesic agents but discontinued these drugs because of lack of efficacy or side effects. He works from his home as an editor for a sports magazine.

Long-term opioid therapy is considered. Treatment goals, as well as the possibility of discontinuing therapy in the absence of meaningful improvements or if the risks exceed the benefits, are discussed with the patient.

**Which of the following is also recommended before prescribing opioid therapy to this patient?**

(A) Current Opioid Misuse Measure survey
(B) Naloxone prescription and education

**Self-Assessment Test**

(C)  Opioid risk assessment

(D)  Psychiatry referral

(C)  5 Days

(D)  7 Days

## Item 167

A 55-year-old woman is evaluated before partial colectomy for recurrent episodes of diverticulitis. Medical history is otherwise significant for atrial fibrillation and hypertension. Medications are apixaban, hydrochlorothiazide, and metoprolol.

On physical examination, vital signs are normal. BMI is 25. Cardiac examination reveals an irregularly irregular rhythm. Pulmonary examination is normal.

Laboratory studies demonstrate a serum creatinine level of 1.0 mg/dL (88.4 µmol/L), an estimated glomerular filtration rate greater than 60 mL/min/1.73 m², and a hemoglobin level of 13.0 g/dL (130 g/L).

**When should this patient's anticoagulant therapy be discontinued before surgery?**

(A)  1 Day

(B)  3 Days

## Item 168

A 36-year-old man is evaluated for a 3-month history of severely depressed mood; hypersomnia; poor appetite; 6.8-kg (15-lb) weight loss; and loss of interest in family, hobbies, and work. He has not had thoughts of suicide. He has never had similar problems and does not use alcohol, tobacco, or recreational drugs. He wants help but is concerned about the side effects of psychotropic medications. His PHQ-9 score is 13, indicating moderate depression.

Laboratory studies reveal a normal serum thyroid-stimulating hormone level.

**Which of the following is the most appropriate treatment?**

(A)  Amitriptyline

(B)  Cognitive behavioral therapy

(C)  Paroxetine

(D)  Quetiapine

# Answers and Critiques

## Item 1    Answer:  B

**Educational Objective:** Treat a patient with an LDL cholesterol level higher than 190 mg/dL (4.92 mmol/L).

The most appropriate treatment for primary prevention of atherosclerotic cardiovascular disease (ASCVD) in this patient is high-intensity statin therapy with rosuvastatin or atorvastatin. According to the American College of Cardiology (ACC)/American Heart Association (AHA) cholesterol treatment guideline, patients aged 21 years or older with severe LDL cholesterol elevation (≥190 mg/dL [4.92 mmol/L]) should receive the maximum tolerated statin therapy for primary prevention of ASCVD, regardless of 10-year risk for ASCVD. High-intensity statin therapy is recommended unless there are contraindications to its use. It is reasonable to intensify statin therapy as tolerated to achieve an LDL cholesterol reduction of at least 50%. In contrast to the ACC/AHA recommendation, the U.S. Preventive Services Task Force recommends initiating low- to moderate-intensity statin therapy in adults aged 40 to 75 years without a history of ASCVD who have one or more ASCVD risk factors (dyslipidemia, diabetes mellitus, hypertension, or smoking) and a calculated 10-year ASCVD event risk of 10% or higher.

In the absence of familial hypercholesterolemia, proprotein convertase subtilisin/kexin type 9 (PCSK9) inhibitors, such as alirocumab and evolocumab, are not indicated in primary prevention of ASCVD. Cost, treatment burden (injections), and absence of long-term safety data argue against their use in primary prevention. Such treatment might be considered if the patient cannot tolerate statin therapy or if LDL cholesterol cannot be sufficiently reduced in the highest-risk patients.

In patients with an LDL cholesterol level of 190 mg/dL (4.92 mmol/L) or higher, initial treatment with a moderate-intensity statin is less preferred; however, if the patient is unable to tolerate high-intensity therapy, down-titration to moderate-intensity therapy could be considered, especially if adequate LDL cholesterol reduction can be achieved.

An evaluation for secondary causes of hyperlipidemia is also indicated in patients with an LDL cholesterol level of 190 mg/dL (4.92 mmol/L) or higher. The most common secondary causes are obesity, hypothyroidism, biliary obstruction, and nephrotic syndrome. Medications can also increase LDL cholesterol level, and some of the most commonly implicated drugs include cyclosporine, HIV medications (such as protease inhibitors), glucocorticoids, and amiodarone. If a secondary cause is not identified, LDL cholesterol level elevation is considered primary, and family members should undergo screening because severe hypercholesterolemia is often genetically determined, as may be the case with this patient who has a first-degree relative with premature ASCVD.

**KEY POINT**

- The American College of Cardiology and American Heart Association recommend that patients aged 21 years or older with an LDL cholesterol level of 190 mg/dL (4.92 mmol/L) or higher should receive high-intensity statin therapy for primary prevention of atherosclerotic cardiovascular disease.

### Bibliography

Stone NJ, Robinson JG, Lichtenstein AH, Bairey Merz CN, Blum CB, Eckel RH, et al; American College of Cardiology/American Heart Association Task Force on Practice Guidelines. 2013 ACC/AHA guideline on the treatment of blood cholesterol to reduce atherosclerotic cardiovascular risk in adults: a report of the American College of Cardiology/American Heart Association Task Force on Practice Guidelines. Circulation. 2014;129:S1-45. [PMID: 24222016] doi:10.1161/01.cir.0000437738.63853.7a

## Item 2    Answer:  D

**Educational Objective:** Use a shared decision-making approach to guide the initiation of breast cancer screening in a younger woman.

This patient should not be screened for breast cancer at this time. In women aged 50 to 74 years, there is a clear benefit to screening mammography, and all breast cancer guidelines recommend screening mammography in this age group. Biennial screening mammography imparts most of the benefit of annual screening mammography with fewer harms, although the recommended screening frequency differs between guidelines. In women younger than 50 years or aged 75 years or older, the balance of benefits and harms is less clear, and screening recommendations vary widely. Most guidelines, including the recommendation statement of the U.S. Preventive Services Task Force (USPSTF), recommend individualized screening decisions for women aged 40 to 49 years based on patient context and values regarding specific benefits and harms. Compared with screening mammography in older women, the USPSTF concludes that, for women in their 40s, the number of women who benefit from screening mammography is smaller, and the harm is higher; however, the benefit still outweighs the harm. Therefore, the value the patient places on averting death from breast cancer compared with the importance she places on avoiding potential harms (false-positive results, anxiety, and overdiagnosis) can help guide her decision. This patient places more importance on avoiding potential harms and therefore should not pursue screening mammography or breast tomosynthesis at this time; no further testing is the best option.

The USPSTF recommends against teaching breast self-examination (BSE), as BSE does not reduce breast cancer mortality and is associated with increased rates of breast biopsy.

The USPSTF found insufficient evidence to assess the balance of benefits and harms of using breast tomosynthesis, or three-dimensional mammography, as a primary screening method for breast cancer; however, National Comprehensive Cancer Network guidelines indicate that breast tomosynthesis can be considered as an initial screening strategy for average-risk women. In studies, breast tomosynthesis is often associated with double the rate of radiation but lower recall rates.

As women progress through their 40s, the number of women who benefit from screening mammography increases, while the chance for harms slightly decreases. A woman's values and preferences may also shift over time; therefore, breast cancer screening should be periodically discussed.

**KEY POINT**

- The decision to initiate breast cancer screening in women aged 40 to 49 years should be an individualized one based on patient context and values regarding specific benefits and harms.

**Bibliography**

Nelson HD, Pappas M, Cantor A, Griffin J, Daeges M, Humphrey L. Harms of breast cancer screening: systematic review to update the 2009 U.S. Preventive Services Task Force recommendation. Ann Intern Med. 2016;164:256-67. [PMID: 26756737] doi:10.7326/M15-0970

**Item 3    Answer:    C**

**Educational Objective:** Provide extended-duration postoperative pharmacologic venous thromboembolism prophylaxis in a patient undergoing major orthopedic surgery.

The recommended postoperative duration of venous thromboembolism (VTE) prophylaxis with low-molecular-weight heparin (LMWH) following major orthopedic surgery is 35 days in patients who are not at increased bleeding risk and have not experienced perioperative bleeding complications. The American College of Chest Physicians (ACCP) antithrombotic guideline provides recommendations for VTE prophylaxis for both orthopedic and nonorthopedic surgery populations. The ACCP guideline identifies hip arthroplasty, knee arthroplasty, and hip fracture surgery as major orthopedic surgeries. These surgeries pose a high VTE risk, and both pharmacologic and mechanical VTE prophylaxis are recommended during hospitalization. The ACCP recommends LMWH over other pharmacologic agents, although there are other acceptable agents, including aspirin for those unable or unwilling to take heparin. For patients without increased bleeding risk, extended duration of postoperative prophylaxis for up to 35 days is recommended over shorter-duration prophylaxis of 10 to 14 days, which is the minimum recommended duration of pharmacologic VTE prophylaxis in orthopedic surgery. Randomized trials, systematic reviews, and meta-analyses have shown that compared with placebo, aspirin, and warfarin, extended prophylaxis up to 35 days

with LMWH reduces the rate of VTE disease without excess bleeding in patients who undergo major orthopedic surgery. If bleeding risk is especially high, mechanical prophylaxis is recommended over no prophylaxis. In patients who decline LMWH injections or who are unable to tolerate LMWH, the oral direct thrombin inhibitor dabigatran, a factor Xa inhibitor (apixaban, rivaroxaban, edoxaban), or a vitamin K antagonist (warfarin) is recommended over alternate forms of prophylaxis. For this patient undergoing major orthopedic surgery, dual perioperative VTE prophylaxis with LMWH and intermittent pneumatic compression is recommended during hospitalization, with LMWH continued for up to 35 days.

Because of the elevated risk for VTE in many patients undergoing orthopedic surgery, a short course of VTE prophylaxis, such as 10 or 14 days, is insufficient because thrombotic risk remains elevated beyond this time frame.

**KEY POINT**

- For patients undergoing orthopedic surgery without increased bleeding risk, postoperative dual venous thromboembolism prophylaxis with intermittent pneumatic compression and low-molecular-weight heparin is recommended during hospitalization; low-molecular-weight heparin should be continued for up to 35 days.

**Bibliography**

Falck-Ytter Y, Francis CW, Johanson NA, Curley C, Dahl OE, Schulman S, et al. Prevention of VTE in orthopedic surgery patients: antithrombotic therapy and prevention of thrombosis, 9th ed: American College of Chest Physicians evidence-based clinical practice guidelines. Chest. 2012;141:e278S-e325S. [PMID: 22315265]

**Item 4    Answer:    A**

**Educational Objective:** Treat a patient with neuropathic pain with duloxetine.

The most appropriate treatment for this patient with evidence of painful diabetic peripheral neuropathy and substantial neuropathic pain is initiation of oral duloxetine. Diabetes mellitus can cause various types of neuropathy. The most common pattern is symmetric distal sensory or sensorimotor. It is characterized by a stocking-glove distribution that ascends proximally. Diabetic sensorimotor neuropathy frequently presents as a sensation of numbness, tingling, burning, heaviness, pain, or sensitivity to light touch. The pain may worsen at night and with walking. Glycemic control and minimizing cardiovascular risk factors can slow the progression and improve the symptoms of diabetic neuropathy. Treatment of painful neuropathies is symptomatic. Tricyclic antidepressants (amitriptyline, nortriptyline), serotonin-norepinephrine reuptake inhibitors (venlafaxine, duloxetine), antiepileptic drugs (pregabalin, gabapentin, valproic acid), opioids (tapentadol), and topical capsaicin are commonly used. However, only pregabalin, duloxetine, and tapentadol (extended release) have FDA approval for painful diabetic neuropathy. Although duloxetine and gabapentinoids are considered first-line therapy, they are costly. The dosage of duloxetine is started at 20 mg/d or 30 mg/d and increased to a goal dosage of 60 mg/d. Dosages higher than 60 mg/d have not been shown to be more effective for analgesia.

Hydromorphone is a potent opioid agonist that is typically used in the treatment of cancer-associated pain, whereas tramadol is a weak opioid agonist with analgesic activity that is influenced by inhibition of serotonin and norepinephrine reuptake. Although potentially effective in the treatment of neuropathic pain syndromes, opioids are considered third-line therapy after maximization and combination of neuropathic agents. Studies have shown that most patients with peripheral neuropathies are not treated with appropriate neuropathic agents or adequate dosages of these drugs, and dosages should be maximized before initiating opioids.

The effectiveness of lamotrigine for chronic neuropathic pain was evaluated in a systematic review. The studies included patients with central poststroke pain, diabetic neuropathy, HIV-related neuropathy, intractable neuropathic pain, spinal cord injury–related pain, and trigeminal neuralgia. Only one study of patients with HIV-related neuropathy had a statistically significant result, which was restricted to patients receiving antiretroviral therapy. The authors concluded that there is no role for lamotrigine in the treatment of chronic neuropathic pain.

Topical NSAIDs such as diclofenac (available as a solution, spray, gel, or patch) provide similar pain relief for inflammatory conditions as oral medications with fewer gastrointestinal effects. However, they are significantly more expensive than oral NSAIDs. More importantly, anti-inflammatory agents have not been shown to be effective in the treatment of peripheral neuropathies and would not be indicated in this patient with a neuropathic pain syndrome.

### KEY POINT

- Gabapentinoids and serotonin-norepinephrine reuptake inhibitors are first-line therapy for neuropathic pain syndromes.

### Bibliography
Watson JC, Dyck PJ. Peripheral neuropathy: a practical approach to diagnosis and symptom management. Mayo Clin Proc. 2015;90:940-51. [PMID: 26141332]

### Item 5 Answer: C

**Educational Objective:** Treat depression at the end of life with methylphenidate.

The most appropriate treatment for this patient's depression is methylphenidate. Patients with a serious, life-threatening illness and untreated depression have poorer quality of life, which can lead to increased caregiver stress and burden. Diagnosing depression in terminally ill patients, however, is challenging. Although anticipatory grief is common in

patients at the end of life and is considered a normal part of most end-of-life experiences, it can be distinguished from clinical depression by the patient's ability to find enjoyment and a fluctuating mood. Patients with depression at the end of life have symptoms that include hopelessness, pervasive guilt, and worthlessness. Depression in terminally ill patients responds well to both pharmacologic and nonpharmacologic treatments. Tricyclic antidepressants, selective serotonin reuptake inhibitors, serotonin-norepinephrine reuptake inhibitors, and mirtazapine are all effective agents. Prognosis should be taken into account because these medications take weeks to reach peak effect. This patient has symptoms consistent with clinical depression as well as a limited life expectancy. Methylphenidate is a rapid-acting psychostimulant that is well tolerated and effective in the treatment of depression; once initiated, results can be seen within 24 to 48 hours. Methylphenidate may also have the benefit of improving cancer-associated fatigue.

Selective serotonin reuptake inhibitors, such as citalopram and sertraline, are effective in the treatment of depression; however, they can take many weeks and dose titration to reach effectiveness. Given this patient's limited life expectancy, a more rapid-acting agent is needed.

Cognitive behavioral therapy, when available, is an effective therapy for patients with depression and a serious medical illness. However, most trials showing benefit are centered on multiweek, if not several-months-long, interventions and are of limited availability for patients on home hospice.

### KEY POINT

- Methylphenidate is a rapid-acting psychostimulant that is well tolerated and effective in the treatment of depression at the end of life; results can be seen as quickly as 24 to 48 hours after initiation.

### Bibliography
Swetz KM, Kamal AH. Palliative care. Ann Intern Med. 2018;168:ITC33-ITC48. [PMID: 29507970] doi:10.7326/AITC201803060

### Item 6 Answer: D

**Educational Objective:** Treat bacterial conjunctivitis.

The most appropriate treatment is trimethoprim-polymyxin B ophthalmic drops. This patient has acute, painless eye redness and several other signs of bacterial conjunctivitis. Studies have identified features that increase the probability of a bacterial cause of conjunctivitis, including redness of the conjunctival membrane obscuring the tarsal vessels, matting of both eyes in the morning, and purulent discharge. Inability to see redness of the eyes at 20 feet decreases the likelihood of a bacterial cause. Antibiotic treatment of bacterial conjunctivitis with topical trimethoprim–polymyxin B or erythromycin can shorten the duration of symptoms, but overall, bacterial conjunctivitis is a self-limited condition from which most patients recover within 2 weeks. Antibiotics should be enlisted when there is a higher risk for complications, such as in patients who wear contact lenses; immunocompromised patients, such as those with diabetes mellitus; and patients with copious, hyperpurulent discharge of the eye.

Ceftriaxone is used to treat gonococcal infection. Typical patients with gonococcal conjunctivitis are young men with copious purulent discharge and marked conjunctival inflammation. Periocular edema and tenderness, gaze restriction, and preauricular lymphadenopathy are common with gonococcal conjunctivitis.

Because of concerns about antimicrobial resistance and cost, topical fluoroquinolones (such as levofloxacin) are not first-line therapy for routine cases of bacterial conjunctivitis. Topical fluoroquinolones are indicated for conjunctivitis in contact lens wearers as a result of the high incidence of *Pseudomonas* infection.

Olopatadine ophthalmic drops are used for seasonal allergies; the mucopurulent discharge, morning matting of the eyes, and lack of itching make allergic conjunctivitis a less likely cause of this patient's symptoms.

**KEY POINT**

- Bacterial conjunctivitis is characterized by redness of the conjunctival membrane obscuring the tarsal vessels, matting of both eyes in the morning, and thin mucopurulent discharge; treatment may include topical antibiotics, such as trimethoprim–polymyxin B or erythromycin.

**Bibliography**
Narayana S, McGee S. Bedside diagnosis of the 'red eye': a systematic review. Am J Med. 2015;128:1220-1224.e1. [PMID: 26169885] doi:10.1016/j.amjmed.2015.06.026

**Item 7**      **Answer:**   **B**

**Educational Objective:** Understand the limitations of the number needed to treat to inform clinical decision making.

The harms and cost of treatment are needed to conclude that treatment A is superior to treatment B. When assessing the clinical impact of an intervention, the number needed to treat (NNT) provides a quantifiable measure of the treatment effect that is easily understood by physicians and patients; it represents the number of patients who must receive a treatment to cause one additional patient to benefit. The acceptability of the NNT as a means of comparing one treatment with another depends on the risks associated with the condition, the cost and side effects of the treatment, and other treatments available. When comparing one treatment with another, head-to-head comparisons provide the best evidence of superiority. In this head-to-head comparison of two treatments, the absolute risk reduction for heart failure–related hospitalizations is 6% with treatment A compared with treatment B. This translates to 17 patients (NNT = 1/absolute risk reduction) who need to receive treatment A to result in 1 less heart failure–related hospitalization compared

with treatment B. Although this information is informative, other data, such as cost and harms, must be evaluated before a conclusion that treatment A is superior to treatment B can be reached. If harms are more frequent or more severe with treatment A, the reduction in hospitalization for heart failure may become clinically meaningless.

Confidence intervals (CIs) are a method for indicating the range in which a value derived from a study is likely to lie; narrower ranges imply greater confidence, or certainty, that the reported value is closer to the true value. The $P$ value expresses the probability that the findings in a study can be explained by chance alone and represents the level of statistical significance. $P$ values offer less information than do CIs because CIs can demonstrate the plausible range of values for an event or outcome, whereas $P$ values indicate only statistical significance. Although CIs provide more precise information about the range of expected benefit, the $P$ value and CI are of less importance than understanding the harms, costs, and alternative therapies that might be available.

A disadvantage of relative comparisons, including relative risk, is the potential for exaggerated outcomes. For instance, interventions that reduce the rate of an outcome from 40% to 20% or from 4% to 2% have a relative risk reduction of 50%. However, the absolute risk reduction for the first case is 20%, whereas the absolute risk reduction for the second case is 2%.

**KEY POINT**

- The acceptability of the number needed to treat as a means of comparing one treatment with another depends on the risks associated with the condition, the cost and side effects of the treatment, and other treatments available.

**Bibliography**
Citrome L, Ketter TA. When does a difference make a difference? Interpretation of number needed to treat, number needed to harm, and likelihood to be helped or harmed. Int J Clin Pract. 2013;67:407-11. [PMID: 23574101] doi: 10.1111/ijcp.12142

**Item 8**      **Answer:**   **D**

**Educational Objective:** Treat acute bacterial prostatitis after a urologic procedure.

This patient's history and physical examination findings indicate acute bacterial prostatitis, and the most appropriate treatment regimen is trimethoprim-sulfamethoxazole. Patient groups at high risk for acute bacterial prostatitis include those with diabetes mellitus, immunosuppression, or cirrhosis. Risk factors include unprotected sexual intercourse, urogenital instrumentation (chronic indwelling bladder catheterization, intermittent bladder catheterization, prostate biopsy), urinary tract manipulation (prostate resection), urinary stasis (obstruction), and benign prostatic hyperplasia. The most common infectious cause for acute bacterial prostatitis is *Escherichia coli* or other gram-negative bacilli. Diagnosis is typically established with

CONT.

urine Gram stain and culture in patients with a compatible history. The treatment of choice for acute bacterial prostatitis is a prolonged course of trimethoprim-sulfamethoxazole or ciprofloxacin. Data on treatment duration are sparse, but 6 weeks is reasonable and recommended by experts. Given the prolonged duration of antimicrobial therapy required in cases of acute bacterial prostatitis, it is most prudent to select an antibiotic with appropriate coverage, while also attempting to minimize the potential for serious adverse effects. Prolonged ciprofloxacin use has been associated with QT prolongation as well as tendinopathy/tendon rupture, especially in older adults. As such, given the treatment duration needed for acute bacterial prostatitis, trimethoprim-sulfamethoxazole would be the most appropriate choice.

Amoxicillin would be an appropriate choice for patients with acute prostatitis and gram-positive cocci in chains. This finding would suggest an enterococcal infection, and treatment with amoxicillin or ampicillin would be appropriate. Neither of these antibiotics would be effective for acute bacterial prostatitis caused by *E. coli* or other gram-negative bacilli.

Men younger than 35 years who are sexually active and men older than 35 years who engage in high-risk sexual behavior should be treated with regimens that cover *Neisseria gonorrhoeae* and *Chlamydia trachomatis*. Ceftriaxone and doxycycline, or ceftriaxone and azithromycin, would be appropriate treatment choices in cases of acute epididymitis, specifically targeting *C. trachomatis* or *N. gonorrhoeae*. Neither regimen would be appropriate in this case.

Cephalexin would be an appropriate choice for patients with acute prostatitis and gram-positive cocci in clusters suggesting infection with *Staphylococcus aureus* or coagulase-negative staphylococci (*Staphylococcus epidermidis* or *Staphylococcus saprophyticus*).

**KEY POINT**

- The most common infectious cause of acute bacterial prostatitis is *Escherichia coli* or other gram-negative bacilli; the treatment of choice is a prolonged course of trimethoprim-sulfamethoxazole or ciprofloxacin.

**Bibliography**
Gill BC, Shoskes DA. Bacterial prostatitis. Curr Opin Infect Dis. 2016;29:86-91. [PMID: 26555038] doi:10.1097/QCO.0000000000000222

## Item 9    Answer:    A

**Educational Objective:** Manage vaccination of a health care worker.

This patient should receive a second dose of the measles, mumps, and rubella (MMR) vaccine. In all immunocompetent adults who lack documented immunity against measles, mumps, and rubella, at least one dose of the MMR vaccine should be administered. Health care workers are at increased risk for acquiring and transmitting measles, mumps, and rubella and should receive a second dose of the MMR vaccine at least 28 days after the first dose. A second dose should also be administered to postsecondary students and international

travelers. For persons who have been previously vaccinated with two doses of a mumps virus–containing vaccine but are at increased risk because of an outbreak, the Advisory Committee on Immunization Practices recommends administering a third dose of mumps virus–containing vaccine to improve protection.

This patient's status as a health care worker does not necessitate administration of the hepatitis A vaccine, despite serologic tests indicating that he lacks immunity. The hepatitis A vaccine should be administered to patients who are at increased risk for infection or complications of infection, such as those who work or travel to endemic areas, men who have sex with men, individuals with chronic liver disease, illicit drug users, persons with clotting disorders, persons who conduct hepatitis A–related research, and household or close contacts of adopted children from endemic areas. Hepatitis A vaccination is also indicated in persons who desire vaccination and could be administered to this patient if he wishes.

Hepatitis B vaccination is indicated in all health care workers who lack immunity. This patient has a positive hepatitis B surface antibody test result, whereas his surface antigen and core antibody levels are undetectable. This pattern is consistent with prior vaccination with an appropriate immune response. As such, hepatitis B vaccination is unnecessary in this patient.

Pneumococcal vaccination is recommended in all adults aged 65 years and older and adults aged 19 to 64 years with certain high-risk conditions. This patient does not have any chronic medical conditions and is also a nonsmoker; therefore, vaccination with the 23-valent pneumococcal polysaccharide vaccine is not indicated.

**KEY POINT**

- Health care workers are at increased risk for acquiring and transmitting measles, mumps, and rubella and should receive a second dose of the MMR (measles, mumps, and rubella) vaccine.

**Bibliography**
Kim DK, Riley LE, Hunter P; Advisory Committee on Immunization Practices. Recommended immunization schedule for adults aged 19 years or older, United States, 2018. Ann Intern Med. 2018;168:210-220. [PMID: 29404596] doi:10.7326/M17-3439

## Item 10    Answer:    B

**Educational Objective:** Manage an in-flight medical emergency by connecting to the ground-based physician.

The most appropriate next step in management is to connect with the ground-based physician. In-flight medical emergencies are relatively common during air travel, occurring in an estimated 1 of 600 flights. Airlines based in the United States are mandated by the Federal Aviation Administration to carry at least one automated external defibrillator; supplemental oxygen; and a medical kit that contains a stethoscope, sphygmomanometer, gloves, airway supplies, intravenous access supplies, and some basic medications. In the case of an in-flight emergency, the physician's role generally

**Answers and Critiques**

involves assessing the patient, establishing a diagnosis when possible, administering basic medical treatments, providing reassurance as appropriate, and recommending flight diversion if necessary. Physicians should practice within their scope of training, be mindful of patient privacy, and document the patient encounter. Although not a Federal Aviation Administration requirement, most airlines have contracts with 24-hour call centers with a ground-based physician to aid in the event of an in-flight emergency. Often, ground-based physicians trained in emergency or aerospace medicine can assist the on-board physician remotely and help direct care, which can be particularly helpful when the medical problem is outside the scope of the physician's practice.

The principles of hypobaric hypoxia apply to commercial airplanes, in which cabins are pressurized to the equivalent of 1500 to 2500 meters (approximately 5000 to 8200 feet) in altitude, resulting in an inspired oxygen tension between 110 and 120 mm Hg (about 70% of the levels encountered at sea level). Although this correlates with an arterial $PO_2$ of approximately 60 mm Hg (8.0 kPa) in healthy individuals, those with underlying pulmonary disease are at risk for significant hypoxemia during a flight. This patient will have no difficulty maintaining her oxyhemoglobin saturation above 90%, and asking the pilot to descend to a lower altitude will serve no useful purpose. A better strategy is to contact the ground-based physician.

Although this patient is dizzy and weak, her clinical status and vital signs appear stable. She needs further medical evaluation and management; however, flight diversion is probably not indicated at this time. Furthermore, the ground-based medical team can also help determine whether flight diversion is needed.

**KEY POINT**

- In most in-flight medical emergencies, the physician's role involves assessing the patient, establishing a diagnosis when possible, administering basic medical treatments, providing reassurance as appropriate, and recommending flight diversion if necessary.

**Bibliography**

Nable JV, Tupe CL, Gehle BD, Brady WJ. In-flight medical emergencies during commercial travel. N Engl J Med. 2015;373:939-45. [PMID: 26332548] doi: 10.1056/NEJMra1409213

**Item 11      Answer:    A**

**Educational Objective:  Counsel an older patient with risk factors for a motor vehicle accident.**

This patient should be advised to retire from driving. Driving assessments are qualitative and rely heavily on clinical judgment. The more risk factors for a motor vehicle accident that an older driver has, the higher the risk for an adverse event while driving. Drivers at highest risk should be counseled to retire from driving. This patient has multiple risk factors for unsafe driving, including cognitive impairment,

self-restrictions in driving (does not drive after dark or on the interstate highway, drives within a 10-mile radius of home), minor accidents, and concerns from family members about driving safety. His other risk factors include impaired mobility, hearing decline, and medical conditions with increased risk for loss of consciousness. Physician advice to retire from driving is associated with older drivers appropriately discontinuing driving. Given the risk for depression and social isolation associated with driving retirement, however, this advice should be coupled with suggestions for alternate forms of transportation and follow-up assessment of his mood and quality of life.

Detailed neuropsychological testing is especially useful for the following patients: (1) those with milder cognitive symptoms to determine whether cognitive difficulties are within the realm of normal age-associated cognitive decline versus mild cognitive impairment; (2) those with definite dementia, diagnosed on the basis of clinical impression and results of screening cognitive tests, who have clinical features overlapping two or more underlying pathologic processes; and (3) those with cognitive symptoms whose clinical picture is confounded by significant depression. The results of neuropsychological testing are unlikely to change the recommendation to retire from driving considering this patient's multiple risk factors.

If a patient is resistant to advice to retire from driving, a formal occupational therapy driving evaluation may be helpful.

Given his numerous observable risk factors, this patient should not be reassured that he is competent to drive.

**KEY POINT**

- The more risk factors for a motor vehicle accident that an older driver has, the higher the risk for an adverse event while driving.

**Bibliography**

Martin AJ, Marottoli R, O'Neill D. Driving assessment for maintaining mobility and safety in drivers with dementia. Cochrane Database Syst Rev. 2013:CD006222. [PMID: 23990315] doi:10.1002/14651858.CD006222.pub4

**Item 12      Answer:    D**

**Educational Objective:  Evaluate a patient with symptoms of systemic exertion intolerance disease.**

No further diagnostic testing is required in this patient. She meets the diagnostic criteria for systemic exertion intolerance disease (SEID), with fatigue of at least 6 months' duration accompanied by substantial reduction in preillness activities, postexertional malaise, unrefreshing sleep, and either cognitive impairment or orthostatic intolerance. Although the pathophysiology of SEID remains unclear, the phenomenon of central sensitization (the pathophysiologic dysregulation of the thalamus, hypothalamus, and amygdala) is gaining acceptance as a potential cause of SEID as well as of other highly prevalent comorbid conditions, including fibromyalgia, mood disturbances, irritable bowel syndrome, and interstitial cystitis. This patient's history, examination, and previous diagnostic test results point to central sensitization, as demonstrated by the constellation of such symptoms as diffuse arthralgia and myalgia, chronic fatigue, bowel and bladder irritability, chronic headaches, brain fog, paresthesias, and unrefreshing sleep. In patients with SEID, the history and physical examination should guide the choice of diagnostic tests. It is reasonable to obtain a complete blood count, creatine kinase (for myalgia), electrolyte panel, thyroid-stimulating hormone level, fasting glucose level, and kidney and liver chemistry tests; however, unnecessary laboratory, imaging, and invasive studies should be avoided because most patients will have unrevealing findings, which provide no lasting reassurance to patients. In this case, the diagnostic evaluation should be limited unless there is compelling new information to warrant further testing.

Antinuclear antibody testing is an effective screening tool for systemic lupus erythematosus; however, myalgia, arthralgia, and fatigue are insufficient reasons to test for antinuclear antibodies unless accompanied by objective findings of systemic lupus erythematosus.

Patients at moderate to high risk for obstructive sleep apnea should undergo further testing, including a home sleep study or polysomnography. On the basis of this patient's presentation (female, young, normal BMI and neck circumference, lack of daytime sleepiness), she is considered to be at low risk for obstructive sleep apnea, and further sleep testing is not warranted.

Serum cortisol testing is unnecessary in this patient who is not manifesting findings that are suggestive of adrenal failure or insufficiency, such as hypotension, tachycardia, hyponatremia, and hyperkalemia.

**KEY POINT**

- In patients with fatigue without a clear cause, it is reasonable to obtain a complete blood count, electrolyte panel, thyroid-stimulating hormone level, fasting glucose level, and kidney and liver chemistry tests; unnecessary laboratory, imaging, and invasive studies should be avoided.

**Bibliography**
Committee on the Diagnostic Criteria for Myalgic Encephalomyelitis/Chronic Fatigue Syndrome, Board on the Health of Select Populations, Institute of Medicine. Beyond Myalgic Encephalomyelitis/Chronic Fatigue Syndrome: Redefining an Illness. Washington, DC: National Academies Press; 2015. [PMID: 25695122]

## Item 13      Answer:   B

**Educational Objective:** Evaluate a patient suspected of having cauda equina syndrome.

This patient should undergo emergent MRI of the lumbosacral spine. His history and physical examination findings are concerning for cauda equina syndrome, which is a surgical emergency. Cauda equina syndrome is most commonly caused by a large disk herniation, but it can also result from direct trauma, infection, or malignancy. Symptoms include low back pain with radiation to the legs, saddle anesthesia, bowel and/or bladder dysfunction, erectile dysfunction, and leg weakness. On physical examination, absent or decreased perianal sensation, diminished anal sphincter tone, hypoactive or absent ankle reflexes, and focal sensory and muscle weakness are commonly present. MRI is considered the gold standard for diagnosing cauda equina syndrome.

CT can be obtained in patients suspected of having cauda equina syndrome who are unable to undergo MRI. However, MRI is considered to be better at visualizing the soft tissue structures of the cauda equina than CT and is therefore the preferred imaging modality in patients who can undergo either procedure, such as this one.

Although plain radiography can be performed when there is concern for metastatic cancer to the vertebral bodies, it has no value in visualizing the soft tissue structures of the cauda equina and therefore is not the preferred imaging modality in cases of suspected cauda equina syndrome.

Signs that urgent surgical intervention may be necessary include bowel- or bladder-sphincter dysfunction, particularly urine retention or urinary incontinence; diminished perineal sensation, sciatica, or sensory motor deficits; and bilateral or unilateral motor deficits that are severe and progressive. Forgoing imaging in this patient and failing to provide definitive surgical intervention could result in permanent neurologic deficits.

**KEY POINT**

- Nerve root involvement of the cauda equina requires immediate imaging, preferably with MRI, and surgical intervention to prevent permanent neurologic damage.

**Bibliography**
Chou R. In the clinic. Low back pain. Ann Intern Med. 2014;160:ITC6-1. [PMID: 25009837]

## Item 14      Answer:   D

**Educational Objective:** Evaluate a breast mass in a woman younger than 30 years.

The most appropriate diagnostic test for this young woman with a breast mass is ultrasonography. A breast mass is characterized by a lesion that persists throughout the menstrual cycle and differs from the surrounding breast tissue and the corresponding area in the contralateral breast. The differential diagnosis of a palpable breast mass includes abscess, cyst, fat necrosis, fibroadenoma, and neoplasm. Evaluation of a palpable breast mass varies based on the patient's age and risk factors and the degree of clinical suspicion. Mammography and ultrasonography are the initial imaging modalities. Ultrasonography is often preferred in women younger than 30 years because increased breast tissue density in younger women limits the usefulness of mammography. Ultrasonography may also be a better choice for young women and pregnant patients in order to avoid radiation exposure. The main utility of ultrasonography is its ability to differentiate cystic from solid lesions. A cyst is likely to be benign if it has symmetric, round borders with no internal echoes. A solid lesion with uniform borders and uniformly sized internal echoes is consistent with a benign fibroadenoma. In this patient with relatively low-risk clinical symptoms, ultrasonography is preferred. The description of the mass (firm, nontender, mobile mass with well-defined margins and no lymphadenopathy) suggests a benign finding, such as a fibroadenoma or cyst. If the ultrasound shows a simple cyst, no further evaluation is necessary, unless the patient is symptomatic. If the ultrasound reveals a solid lesion, it must be evaluated completely with biopsy.

An image-directed core-needle biopsy of a breast mass would be recommended if an ultrasound shows a solid-appearing, suspicious (Breast Imaging Reporting and Data System [BI-RADS] category 4) or highly suspicious (BI-RADS category 5) mass. This patient must undergo ultrasonography to determine the BI-RADS category of the mass before a decision on whether to perform a biopsy can be made.

The dense breast tissue often found in young women limits the sensitivity, and hence the effectiveness, of mammography. Therefore, mammography is generally not needed for young women with a low-risk breast mass.

For women aged 30 years or older with a palpable breast abnormality, both diagnostic mammography and ultrasonography would be recommended. Because this patient is younger than 30 years, only ultrasonography is warranted at this time.

**KEY POINT**

- For women younger than 30 years with a low-risk breast mass, ultrasonography is usually the only imaging required.

**Bibliography**

Lehman CD, Lee AY, Lee CI. Imaging management of palpable breast abnormalities. AJR Am J Roentgenol. 2014;203:1142-53. [PMID: 25341156] doi:10.2214/AJR.14.12725

## Item 15     Answer:    A

**Educational Objective: Diagnose bipolar disorder.**

The most likely diagnosis is bipolar disorder. This patient exhibits multiple symptoms of depression (anhedonia, sleep disturbance, feelings of worthlessness, suicidal ideation), but he also has a history of at least one previous manic episode, manifested by increased energy, decreased need for sleep, grandiose thinking, and risky behavior. This patient's clinical picture of depression and one or more episodes of mania is most consistent with a diagnosis of bipolar disorder. In patients with bipolar disorder, dysfunction is often extreme, and the associated lifetime risk for suicide is high (6%-15%). Referral to a psychiatrist should be strongly considered when resources are available.

Generalized anxiety disorder is characterized by excessive anxiety about activities or events occurring more days than not for at least 6 months and causing significant distress or functional impairment. Patients with this disorder often experience fatigue and sleep disturbance but do not have a history of mania or meet diagnostic criteria for a major depressive disorder.

More than half of patients with bipolar disorder initially present with a depressive episode. However, presence of manic episodes in this patient excludes major depressive disorder as the diagnosis. Recognition of previous manic or hypomanic episodes is crucial because the treatment of depression in bipolar disorder requires mood stabilizers (such as carbamazepine, lithium, or valproic acid), either alone or in combination with antidepressants. Treatment with antidepressants alone may increase the risk for mania and hypomania.

Patients with schizophrenia have negative symptoms, such as flattened affect and decreased activity, in combination with positive symptoms, including hallucinations and disorganized thought. This patient has no positive symptoms.

**KEY POINT**

- More than half of patients with bipolar disorder initially present with a depressive episode; however, recognition of previous manic or hypomanic episodes is crucial because the treatment of bipolar disorder requires mood stabilizers, either alone or in combination with antidepressants.

**Bibliography**

Frye MA. Clinical practice. Bipolar disorder—a focus on depression. N Engl J Med. 2011;364:51-9. [PMID: 21208108] doi:10.1056/NEJMcp1000402

## Item 16     Answer:    A

**Educational Objective: Treat an obese patient with bariatric surgery.**

This patient with obesity-related comorbid conditions and no weight loss success after a trial of comprehensive lifestyle modifications meets the criteria for referral for bariatric surgery. Bariatric surgery should be considered for patients who do not lose weight with lifestyle modifications, with or without pharmacologic therapy, and have a BMI of 40 or greater or a BMI of 35 or greater with obesity-related comorbid conditions, such as type 2 diabetes mellitus, coronary artery disease, obstructive sleep apnea, or osteoarthritis. Studies comparing bariatric surgery with nonsurgical treatment (diet, exercise, behavioral modification, and medications) have shown that participants randomly assigned to bariatric surgery lost more weight and were more likely to experience remission of type 2 diabetes and metabolic syndrome, improved quality of life, and reduced medication use. Evidence suggests that bariatric surgery is also associated with reduced mortality and improvement of obstructive sleep apnea, osteoarthritis, and other conditions.

Lorcaserin is approved as adjunctive therapy to comprehensive lifestyle modification in the treatment of overweight and obesity. This patient is already taking liraglutide, another approved pharmacologic agent for obesity, and has tried but not responded to a third approved agent, orlistat. He is unlikely to benefit from the addition of lorcaserin to his medication regimen.

Behavioral therapy for obesity may include the use of a trained interventionist, such as a nutritionist or dietician. This patient is already participating in a comprehensive behavioral therapy plan that includes nutritional counseling; a separate referral to a dietician is unnecessary. Behavioral therapy is also less likely than bariatric surgery to be successful in this patient.

Very-low-calorie diets are recommended when rapid weight loss is medically indicated. Their use requires close medical supervision with frequent office visits and laboratory monitoring. In this patient, there is no indication for rapid weight loss that would warrant the use of a very-low-calorie diet.

**KEY POINT**

- Bariatric surgery should be considered in patients who do not lose weight with lifestyle modifications and have a BMI of 40 or greater, or a BMI of 35 or greater with obesity-related comorbid conditions, such as type 2 diabetes mellitus, coronary artery disease, obstructive sleep apnea, or osteoarthritis.

**Bibliography**

Jensen MD, Ryan DH, Apovian CM, Ard JD, Comuzzie AG, Donato KA, et al; American College of Cardiology/American Heart Association Task Force on Practice Guidelines. 2013 AHA/ACC/TOS guideline for the management of overweight and obesity in adults: a report of the American College of Cardiology/American Heart Association Task Force on Practice Guidelines and The Obesity Society. Circulation. 2014;129:S102-38. [PMID: 24222017] doi:10.1161/01.cir.0000437739.71477.ee

## Item 17 Answer: A

**Educational Objective:** Treat ACE inhibitor–induced chronic cough.

The most appropriate management is discontinuation of lisinopril. This patient has chronic cough, defined as cough lasting more than 8 weeks. When smoking and use of an ACE inhibitor are eliminated, the most common causes of chronic cough are upper airway cough syndrome (UACS), gastroesophageal reflux disease, and asthma. Evaluation of chronic cough begins with a thorough history, physical examination, and chest radiography. If the initial evaluation is unrevealing and the patient is taking ACE inhibitor therapy, discontinuation of the ACE inhibitor is the most appropriate first step in management. Up to 20% of patients taking an ACE inhibitor develop a dry cough, usually within 1 to 2 weeks of therapy initiation. Onset of cough, however, may be delayed by months in a small percentage of patients. Cessation of ACE inhibitor therapy usually results in resolution of the cough within 2 weeks. Rechallenge with an ACE inhibitor will result in return of the cough in two thirds of patients and is not recommended. In patients whose blood

pressure responded to ACE inhibitor therapy or who require renin-angiotensin system inhibition, an angiotensin receptor blocker can be tried because this class of drugs is associated with a lower incidence of cough.

If a cause of chronic cough is not determined after initial evaluation, and smoking and ACE inhibitor therapy have been discontinued, a stepwise approach is pursued, beginning with a 2-week trial of empiric treatment for UACS. UACS related to allergic rhinitis is best treated with intranasal glucocorticoids, whereas UACS due to nonallergic rhinitis should be treated with first-generation antihistamines and decongestants. This patient has no findings suggestive of allergic rhinitis and has not yet discontinued ACE inhibitor therapy; therefore, an intranasal glucocorticoid should not be initiated.

If chronic cough does not respond to empiric treatment for UACS, evaluation of asthma with spirometry (or empiric treatment) is warranted. If results of spirometry are negative for asthma, bronchial hyperresponsiveness testing should be pursued.

Proton pump inhibitor therapy is indicated in patients with chronic cough when symptoms of gastroesophageal reflux are present or when chronic cough persists despite empiric therapy for UACS or empiric treatment for asthma and nonasthmatic eosinophilic bronchitis with inhaled glucocorticoids.

**KEY POINT**

- In patients with chronic cough who have a normal chest radiograph and are taking an ACE inhibitor, the first intervention is discontinuation of the ACE inhibitor.

**Bibliography**

Irwin RS, Baumann MH, Bolser DC, Boulet LP, Braman SS, Brightling CE, et al. Diagnosis and management of cough executive summary: ACCP evidence-based clinical practice guidelines. Chest. 2006;129:1S-23S. [PMID: 16428686] doi:10.1378/chest.129.1_suppl.1S

## Item 18 Answer: D

**Educational Objective:** Manage a patient who has undergone direct-to-consumer genetic testing.

This patient should be advised that no further testing is necessary and should be educated on the limitations of direct-to-consumer (DTC) genetic testing. DTC genetic testing is a commercial service that allows patients to obtain genetic information for a low cost and without referral from a physician. These tests estimate the risk for many common medical conditions by genotyping polymorphic nucleotides. Single-nucleotide polymorphisms (SNPs) that are disproportionately found in affected individuals are identified, and odds ratios for each SNP are determined. The SNPs are usually common but have low penetrance (that is, most people with an SNP do not develop disease). Individually, SNPs contribute very little to overall disease risk; most SNPs have an odds ratio of less than 1.5. Because counseling or education is not typically provided before or after the DTC genetic test is obtained, patients are generally unable to accurately interpret the results and may request guidance or additional testing from their physicians. This patient's absolute risk for developing prostate cancer based on the test results is extremely small; therefore, no further testing is required.

Screening for prostate cancer in asymptomatic, average-risk men is controversial, and recommendations vary among professional organizations and frequently change. However, no guidelines support performing a digital rectal examination (DRE) to screen for prostate cancer. The overall sensitivity of DRE does not exceed 60%, whereas the specificity is greater than 90%; the positive predictive value of an abnormal DRE is 28%. As such, there is no indication for this test either alone or in combination with serum prostate-specific antigen (PSA) level measurement.

The U.S. Preventive Services Task Force recommends that clinicians discuss potential benefits and harms of PSA-based screening for prostate cancer in men aged 55 to 69 years. The decision to proceed with PSA level measurement should be individualized based on the patient's beliefs and values. In this 46-year-old patient, obtaining a serum PSA level is not indicated. The patient's family history of prostate cancer at an advanced age does not significantly increase his risk for cancer. He has a low pretest probability of prostate cancer, and a positive test result will likely be false positive. Nevertheless, patients with positive test results often undergo biopsy with the attendant risks of infection, bleeding, pain, and anxiety.

### KEY POINT

- Patients who undergo direct-to-consumer genetic testing should be advised of the risks and limitations of these tests, including the possibility for misinterpretation.

### Bibliography

Burke W, Trinidad SB. The deceptive appeal of direct-to-consumer genetics. Ann Intern Med. 2016;164:564-5. [PMID: 26925528] doi: 10.7326/M16-0257

### Item 19      Answer:    B

**Educational Objective:** Evaluate unilateral tinnitus and hearing loss.

The most appropriate management is MRI of the internal auditory canal. The assessment of tinnitus must differentiate more dangerous causes (such as neoplasms or cerebrovascular conditions) from more benign causes (such as infections or drugs). Most commonly, tinnitus is bilateral; unilateral tinnitus may indicate more serious pathology. Patients with unilateral tinnitus should undergo prompt hearing testing; if hearing loss is documented, as in this case, the patient should undergo MRI of the internal auditory canal to rule out an acoustic neuroma. It is important to note that patients who present with tinnitus may not report hearing loss that is subsequently revealed on audiologic testing.

The type of tinnitus is an important factor in the evaluation. Pulsatile tinnitus, when synchronous with the heartbeat, may suggest a vascular anomaly, including atherosclerotic disease, arteriovenous fistulas, or paragangliomas, most commonly in the jugular bulb or tympanic arteries of the middle ear. A patient with pulsatile tinnitus should be examined for bruits over the neck, periauricular area, temple, orbit, and mastoid areas. If the physical examination findings do not explain the pulsatile tinnitus, noninvasive intracranial imaging, including CT angiography or MR angiography, should be performed. This patient does not have pulsatile tinnitus but does have unilateral hearing loss. Therefore, imaging of the internal auditory canal for acoustic neuroma will be of higher diagnostic yield than vascular imaging.

This patient's primary symptom is tinnitus, with accompanying asymptomatic hearing loss. A hearing aid is more likely to be of use in a patient with symptomatic hearing loss. More importantly, the priority in this patient is excluding an acoustic neuroma, not hearing aid placement.

This patient's tinnitus is gradual in onset and requires further evaluation. However, the patient does not need urgent referral to an otolaryngologist. Patients should be urgently referred when tinnitus is associated with symptoms suggesting serious, reversible underlying pathology, including sudden sensorineural hearing loss, pulsatile tinnitus, vestibular symptoms, ear pain, or drainage or malodor that fails to resolve.

### KEY POINT

- Tinnitus associated with unilateral sensorineural hearing loss suggests acoustic neuroma and requires advanced imaging with MRI.

### Bibliography

Baguley D, McFerran D, Hall D. Tinnitus. Lancet. 2013;382:1600-7. [PMID: 23827090] doi:10.1016/S0140-6736(13)60142-7

### Item 20      Answer:    D

**Educational Objective:** Treat severe dyspnea.

The most appropriate treatment for this patient is pulmonary rehabilitation. Pulmonary rehabilitation is recommended for all symptomatic patients with an FEV$_1$ less than 50% of predicted and specifically for those hospitalized with an acute exacerbation of COPD. These programs include education, functional assessment, nutrition counseling, and follow-up to reinforce behavioral techniques for change. They also include an exercise training component that has been shown to improve endurance, flexibility, and upper and lower body strength. Exercise training can provide sustained benefit for postexacerbation symptoms (such as breathlessness) following the completion of even a single rehabilitation program. When combined with other forms of therapy (medical therapy, smoking cessation, nutrition counseling, and education), pulmonary rehabilitation decreases patients' perceived intensity of breathlessness,

CONT.

reduces dyspnea and fatigue, facilitates increased participation in daily activities, and enhances health-related quality of life, including improvements in anxiety and depression.

This patient has heart failure with preserved ejection fraction but no physical examination findings that suggest volume overload. Thus, initiation of furosemide is not indicated at this time.

Although this patient has severe dyspnea in the setting of advanced COPD, her oxygen saturation is preserved with 1 L/min oxygen by nasal cannula at rest and during a 6-minute walk test. Additional oxygen therapy will not relieve dyspnea or improve clinical outcomes.

Glucocorticoids, such as prednisone, can be an effective treatment in the setting of a COPD exacerbation, which is defined as a sustained worsening of a patient's COPD. Exacerbations are marked by increased breathlessness and are usually accompanied by increased cough and sputum production. This patient has stable chronic dyspnea on exertion and no other findings that would suggest an exacerbation.

**KEY POINT**

- Pulmonary rehabilitation can provide significant benefits for patients with chronic lung disease and has been shown to improve subjective dyspnea in patients with severe COPD and following an acute exacerbation of COPD.

**Bibliography**

Cortopassi F, Gurung P, Pinto-Plata V. Chronic obstructive pulmonary disease in elderly patients. Clin Geriatr Med. 2017;33:539-552. [PMID: 28991649]

 **Item 21      Answer:   A**

**Educational Objective:  Evaluate a patient with decompensated liver disease who is scheduled for elective surgery.**

The most appropriate preoperative management is to cancel surgery and refer the patient for liver transplant evaluation. Patients with cirrhosis but no complications are referred to as having compensated cirrhosis; they may be asymptomatic or may have nonspecific symptoms, such as fatigue, poor sleep, muscle cramps, feeling cold, or itching. Patients with complications of cirrhosis (hepatic encephalopathy, variceal hemorrhage, ascites, spontaneous bacterial peritonitis, hepatorenal syndrome, jaundice, or hepatocellular carcinoma) are referred to as having decompensated cirrhosis. Referral to a transplant center is indicated for patients with decompensation or a Model for End-stage Liver Disease (MELD) score of greater than 15. The MELD score is an equation that incorporates bilirubin, INR, and serum creatinine levels, and it accurately predicts 3-month survival. This patient, who has decompensated liver disease with a MELD score of 22, which confers a 30-day surgical mortality risk of more than 50%, should avoid elective surgery. Patients with decompensated liver disease have not only a higher perioperative mortality rate but also a significantly increased risk

for other complications, including encephalopathy, electrolyte derangements, fluid imbalance, coagulopathy, infection, acute kidney injury, and hepatorenal syndrome. It is reasonable to refer patients at intermediate risk to a hepatologist before proceeding with surgery. Patients with compensated liver disease are often able to proceed with surgery with optimal medical management.

The deciding factor in this case is not the patient's duration of sobriety but the presence of decompensated liver disease and an unacceptably high MELD score. Elective surgery should be avoided until these risks are mitigated with liver transplantation.

The American Association for the Study of Liver Diseases recommends against perioperative transjugular intrahepatic portosystemic shunts, stating that there is no reliable perioperative evidence of improved clinical outcomes.

**KEY POINT**

- Patients with decompensated liver disease should avoid elective surgery and be referred for liver transplant evaluation.

**Bibliography**

Rai R, Nagral S, Nagral A. Surgery in a patient with liver disease. J Clin Exp Hepatol. 2012;2:238-46. [PMID: 25755440]

**Item 22      Answer:   E**

**Educational Objective:  Provide culturally sensitive care to a transgender patient.**

This patient requires symptomatic treatment of his viral upper respiratory tract symptoms. In general, examination of an organ system should be related to the patient's symptoms. This patient's gender identity is not relevant to the reason for the visit; therefore, obtaining a detailed gender-related history (hormonal, surgical, social, and sexual) and performing a genital examination are unnecessary. Additionally, these interventions may make this nervous patient feel more uncomfortable and potentially dissuade him from returning for important ongoing health care.

A comprehensive history of a transgender person is usually not possible to obtain in one visit; it is best obtained over time in order to build rapport with the patient. In general, history taking is similar in transgender and nontransgender patients and should include family, reproductive, sexual, psychiatric, and social histories. Elements of the history that are unique to the transgender population are hormonal and surgical therapies related to gender transition.

Recommendations for sexually transmitted infection (STI) screening are the same for transgender patients as for nontransgender patients. Screening should take into account the patient's anatomy and sexual history. As it would be inappropriate to perform STI screening in a nontransgender patient during a first-time visit for unrelated episodic care, it would also be inappropriate to screen this patient today. STI screening is important and should be performed; however, it can wait until patient rapport has been established and a more detailed history has been obtained to guide screening.

Many online resources are available for learning about transgender persons and providing culturally sensitive medical care. The University of California, San Francisco, has published guidelines for primary and gender-affirming care of transgender and gender nonbinary persons at http://transhealth.ucsf.edu/protocols. Additionally, the National Lesbian, Gay, Bisexual, and Transgender (LGBT) Health Education Center, a program of the Fenway Institute, provides learning modules at www.lgbthealtheducation.org/lgbt-education/learning-modules/.

**KEY POINT**

- Irrespective of gender presentation, physicians should provide care for all patients in a sensitive, respectful, and affirming manner.

**Bibliography**
Lewis EB, Vincent B, Brett A, Gibson S, Walsh RJ. I am your trans patient. BMJ. 2017;357:j2963. [PMID: 28667010] doi:10.1136/bmj.j2963

**Item 23      Answer:      D**

**Educational Objective:** Use a discharge summary to improve patient safety at transitions of care.

Communicating with and sharing the discharge summary with the primary care physician is recommended to improve patient safety and reduce rehospitalization in this patient. The evidence to support a reduction in hospital readmissions with completion of a discharge summary is mixed, most likely because of many complex factors that are difficult to control, such as timeliness, completeness, and quality of the discharge summary. However, the Institute for Healthcare Improvement identifies the lack of a timely discharge summary as a barrier to patient safety and prevention of early hospital readmission and therefore recommends a timely discharge summary as a key element in improving the transition of care from hospital to home. A discharge summary should include the evaluations performed, medication reconciliation, pending test results, required follow-up tests, and follow-up appointments and should be shared with the follow-up clinician. Timely follow-up with the primary care clinician is also important in ensuring that the transition goes smoothly. Another approach that has been successful in reducing hospitalization is the use of multiple team members, such as a nurse and pharmacist, to provide components of care.

A systematic review found that implementation of an intensive home visitation program reduced the risk for hospital readmission for heart failure at 3 to 6 months. This intervention included a series of eight planned home visits, the first within 24 hours of discharge. A medium-intensity intervention that included one telephone call within 7 days of discharge and one planned home visit within 10 days of discharge found no

statistically significant reduction in all-cause readmissions or mortality.

Home telemonitoring of patients with heart failure had no impact on hospital readmission or mortality. Post-discharge heart failure patient education programs also failed to result in reduced readmission rates or lower mortality.

**KEY POINT**

- A discharge summary that includes the evaluations performed, medication reconciliation, pending test results, required follow-up tests, and follow-up appointments is an important tool in the communication between the hospital and the follow-up clinician.

**Bibliography**
Rattray NA, Sico JJ, Cox LM, Russ AL, Matthias MS, Frankel RM. Crossing the communication chasm: challenges and opportunities in transitions of care from the hospital to the primary care clinic. Jt Comm J Qual Patient Saf. 2017;43:127-137. [PMID: 28334591] doi:10.1016/j.jcjq.2016.11.007

**Item 24      Answer:      B**

**Educational Objective:** Diagnose adhesive capsulitis.

This patient's clinical presentation is most consistent with adhesive capsulitis, also known as frozen shoulder. Adhesive capsulitis commonly presents as poorly localized, progressive pain described as a deep aching with an insidious onset. Pain is also frequently worse at night and in cold weather. In addition to pain, patients with adhesive capsulitis frequently develop decreased shoulder mobility as the disease progresses. Range of motion (both active and passive) is decreased in all planes of motion. Adhesive capsulitis may be idiopathic (primary adhesive capsulitis) or secondary to several conditions (secondary adhesive capsulitis). Secondary conditions include diabetes mellitus, hypothyroidism, prior surgery or trauma, prolonged immobilization, autoimmune disorders, and stroke.

Acromioclavicular joint degeneration is unlikely to be responsible for this patient's clinical presentation. Patients with acromioclavicular joint degeneration typically report pain localized to the acromioclavicular joint. Physical examination findings include tenderness to palpation of the joint, pain with shoulder abduction beyond 120 degrees, and pain with passive shoulder adduction (a positive cross-arm test).

Bicipital tendinitis typically results in pain localized to the anterior shoulder that may radiate toward the deltoid and into the arm. Pain classically worsens with overhead activity. On examination, tenderness may be elicited by palpating the bicipital groove. Pain also can be reproduced by placing the patient's ipsilateral arm at his or her side while flexing the elbow to 90 degrees and supinating against resistance (Yergason test).

Rotator cuff disease would not be expected to cause pain with both active and passive movement of the shoulder; therefore, it would not account for this patient's presentation.

- Adhesive capsulitis is characterized by loss of shoulder movement accompanied by pain; examination discloses significant loss of both active and passive range of motion.

**Bibliography**

Le HV, Lee SJ, Nazarian A, Rodriguez EK. Adhesive capsulitis of the shoulder: review of pathophysiology and current clinical treatments. Shoulder Elbow. 2017;9:75-84. [PMID: 28405218] doi:10.1177/1758573216676786

## Item 25          Answer:    C

**Educational Objective:   Treat premature ejaculation.**

Topical lidocaine is the most appropriate treatment for this patient's premature ejaculation. Premature ejaculation is defined as ejaculation that occurs sooner than desired and is distressful to either or both partners. The mainstays of therapy include counseling and pharmacotherapy (oral and topical agents). According to the American Urological Association, pharmacologic options include selective serotonin reuptake inhibitors (SSRIs), tricyclic antidepressants, and topical anesthetic agents. Oral medications (fluoxetine, paroxetine, sertraline) are effective because they tend to cause delayed ejaculation as a side effect. This patient is currently taking a tricyclic antidepressant and has had previous mood instability with an SSRI; therefore, the most appropriate treatment is a regimen of topical lidocaine to help reduce tactile stimulation and thus prolong the time to ejaculation. Topical medications (lidocaine, prilocaine) may be used with or without a condom.

Paroxetine therapy is an effective treatment strategy for premature ejaculation. However, it is not appropriate in this case because of the patient's previously reported mood instability when exposed to sertraline. Both sertraline and paroxetine are SSRIs, which can cause deleterious mood changes (a class effect). In a patient with depression that is currently well controlled, adding an additional psychoactive medication is not warranted.

Testosterone gel, which is used in the treatment of hypogonadism, is not appropriate for this patient. Hypogonadism (androgen deficiency) can lead to decreased libido and erectile dysfunction, but it has not been shown to be a causative or correlative factor in premature ejaculation. Furthermore, this patient has no examination findings that would raise concern for hypogonadism, such as body hair growth and pattern changes, reduced testicular size, or gynecomastia, and his 8:00 AM serum total testosterone level was normal.

Given that the patient's premature ejaculation is distressing to both the patient and his spouse, offering no treatment options could lead to worsening self-confidence, mood, and quality of life.

- Pharmacologic options for the treatment of premature ejaculation include selective serotonin reuptake inhibitors, tricyclic antidepressants, and topical anesthetic agents.

**Bibliography**

Martin C, Nolen H, Podolnick J, Wang R. Current and emerging therapies in premature ejaculation: Where we are coming from, where we are going. Int J Urol. 2017;24:40-50. [PMID: 27704632] doi:10.1111/iju.13202

## Item 26          Answer:    D

**Educational Objective:   Treat a woman with stress urinary incontinence.**

The most appropriate treatment for this patient is pelvic floor muscle training (PFMT; also known as Kegel exercises). This multiparous, postmenopausal woman describes classic stress urinary incontinence, which is characterized by urine leakage associated with activities that cause increased intra-abdominal pressure, such as coughing, laughing, or sneezing. The American College of Physicians (ACP) recommends PFMT as first-line therapy for women with stress incontinence. PFMT may also be of benefit in patients with mixed urge and stress incontinence. If performed correctly and diligently, PFMT exercises may strengthen the pelvic floor muscles and enhance urinary retention. The patient is advised to tighten the pelvic muscles as if trying to interrupt urination. Best results require three or four sets of 10 contractions daily, with contractions lasting 10 seconds. The regimen should be continued for a minimum of 15 to 20 weeks. The ACP recommends against pharmacotherapy for this condition.

Bladder training and suppressive therapy are recommended by the ACP for urgency and mixed incontinence. With bladder training, patients are instructed to void regularly throughout the day, regardless of urge, and progressively increase the interval between voids. Suppression techniques are used to manage urge to void outside of the schedule. The patient is instructed to contract pelvic floor muscles quickly three or four times, use a distraction technique (counting backwards from 100), and, when the urge passes, walk to the bathroom to urinate.

The risks and benefits of systemic hormone replacement therapy, such as oral estradiol, in postmenopausal women must be carefully considered. Its use should be reserved for vasomotor symptoms of menopause at the lowest effective dosage. Estrogen replacement therapy is not recommended for chronic medical problems. Trials of topical estrogen therapy for stress urinary incontinence in patients with vaginal atrophy are of mixed quality at best, and its use is not routinely recommended.

Oxybutynin is a treatment for urgency urinary incontinence when bladder training is only partially successful or has failed. It is not recommended for the treatment of stress urinary incontinence.

The ACP recommends exercise and weight loss for all obese women with urinary incontinence. This patient is not overweight, and her incontinence would likely not benefit from exercise and weight loss.

**KEY POINT**

- Stress urinary incontinence is characterized by urine leakage associated with activities that cause increased intra-abdominal pressure, such as coughing, laughing, or sneezing; it is best managed with pelvic floor muscle training exercises.

**Bibliography**

Qaseem A, Dallas P, Forciea MA, Starkey M, Denberg TD, Shekelle P; Clinical Guidelines Committee of the American College of Physicians. Nonsurgical management of urinary incontinence in women: a clinical practice guideline from the American College of Physicians. Ann Intern Med. 2014;161:429-40. [PMID: 25222388] doi:10.7326/M13-2410

## Item 27      Answer:    A

**Educational Objective:   Manage a request for potentially inappropriate treatment.**

The most appropriate management is consultation with the hospital ethics committee. A recent policy statement from the Society of Critical Care Medicine recommends that appropriate treatment goals of ICU care include treatment that provides a reasonable expectation of survival outside of the acute care setting with sufficient cognitive ability to perceive benefits of treatment, or palliative care through the dying process in the ICU. Because conflicts between the desire to provide benefit to the patient and the desire to minimize the burden of treatment can be very difficult, one of the most important skills of the physician is the ability to communicate and negotiate a reasonable treatment plan with the patient's family. If these situations become intractable, many organizations recommend initiating a process to resolve the disagreement, including notifying surrogates of the process, seeking a second medical opinion, obtaining review by an interdisciplinary ethics committee, offering the surrogate the opportunity to seek care at another institution, and implementing the decision of the resolution process. This patient's family is requesting treatment that the care team does not think will achieve reasonable goals, and an ethics consultation may lead to conflict resolution.

In some situations, the physician and the patient's family may mutually establish a time frame in which care will be withdrawn if there is no improvement; however, these decisions should not be made unilaterally by the care team.

A physician should not provide treatment that conflicts with professional obligations and will not meet the goals of care. However, often by communicating his or her concerns, a physician is able to help a family understand the burden of continued, ineffective treatment. If resolution is not possible, family members may seek transfer to another institution; however, the physician is not obliged to initiate such arrangements.

**KEY POINT**

- A physician should not provide treatment that conflicts with professional obligations and will not meet the goals of care; when the physician and the patient (or family members) have conflicting goals of care, an ethics consultation may be beneficial.

**Bibliography**

Kon AA, Shepard EK, Sederstrom NO, Swoboda SM, Marshall MF, Birriel B, et al. Defining futile and potentially inappropriate interventions: a policy statement from the Society of Critical Care Medicine Ethics Committee. Crit Care Med. 2016;44:1769-74. [PMID: 27525995] doi: 10.1097/CCM.0000000000001965

## Item 28      Answer:    D

**Educational Objective:   Treat genitourinary syndrome of menopause.**

Vaginal estrogen therapy is the most appropriate treatment for this patient with genitourinary syndrome of menopause (GSM), also known as vaginal atrophy. GSM is a common condition in postmenopausal women that is characterized by dryness, inflammation, and thinning of the vaginal walls due to decreased estrogen. Other symptoms include dyspareunia, itching, and vulvovaginal irritation. The associated dyspareunia may lead to avoidance of sexual activity because of discomfort. This patient's pelvic examination features are classic for GSM, including a pale and dry vaginal lining with reduction in rugae. For severe symptoms or symptoms not responsive to moisturizers and lubricants, topical estrogen therapy has numerous beneficial effects, including restoration of the acidic vaginal pH, thickening of the epithelium, and increase in vaginal secretions. Available preparations include estradiol or conjugated estrogen in tablet, cream, or ring forms. Low-dose vaginal estradiol tablets and the estradiol vaginal ring have minimal systemic estrogen absorption. Because estradiol absorption is insufficient to cause endometrial proliferation, concurrent progestin is typically not indicated when low-dose local estrogen is used to treat GSM. The dose and duration of topical estrogen therapy are individualized according to symptom severity. Family history of breast cancer is not a contraindication to use.

A potent topical glucocorticoid, such as clobetasol, is used to treat vulvar lichen sclerosus. This inflammatory condition often presents as white, atrophic patches on the genital and perianal skin. It is associated with dyspareunia, pain, and pruritus. Prepubertal girls and postmenopausal women appear to be at highest risk. The intense itching and plaque-like involvement of the labia, introitus, and perianal region are clinical clues that distinguish vulvar lichen sclerosus from the generalized thinning and drying associated with GSM.

Ospemifene is an estrogen agonist/antagonist used to reduce the severity of moderate to severe dyspareunia in postmenopausal women. It is recommended that women with an intact uterus also take a progestin. How ospemifene compares to vaginal estrogens in terms of efficacy and safety is unknown. Because topical estrogen therapy has a long history of safety, experts recommend that ospemifene be reserved for women who cannot or will not use topical estrogens.

Although systemic estrogen therapy may help with symptoms of vaginal atrophy, use of vaginal estrogen is most effective for treatment of GSM in a patient with no other menopausal symptoms, such as hot flushes, night sweats, or mood concerns.

Recent evidence suggests that vaginal estrogen therapy may be as effective as vaginal lubricants for treating postmenopausal vaginal symptoms. However, in this patient with symptoms that have not responded to vaginal lubricants, vaginal estrogen is the most reasonable option.

**KEY POINT**

- Vaginal estrogen therapy is appropriate treatment for patients with moderate to severe genitourinary syndrome of menopause that has not responded to moisturizers and lubricants.

### Bibliography

The NAMS 2017 Hormone Therapy Position Statement Advisory Panel. The 2017 hormone therapy position statement of The North American Menopause Society. Menopause. 2017;24:728-753. [PMID: 28650869] doi:10.1097/GME.0000000000000921

## Item 29     Answer:    D

**Educational Objective:** Treat generalized anxiety disorder with pharmacologic therapy.

The most appropriate long-term pharmacologic treatment for this patient with generalized anxiety disorder (GAD) is sertraline. GAD is characterized by excessive anxiety about activities or events (occupation, school) occurring more days than not for at least 6 months and causing significant functional impairment. Patients with GAD also experience difficulty concentrating, irritability, muscle tension, restlessness, and sleep disturbance. A useful tool for identifying and assessing the severity of GAD is the Generalized Anxiety Disorder 7-item scale (GAD-7), which asks patients to rate seven items on a scale of 0 to 3 based on increasing severity (https://www.integration.samhsa.gov/clinical-practice/GAD708.19.08Cartwright.pdf). A score of 5 to 9 indicates mild anxiety, 10 to 14 moderate anxiety, and 15 to 21 severe anxiety. The GAD-7 can be used to monitor symptom severity over time, allowing clinicians to monitor treatment effectiveness.

Treatment options for GAD include cognitive behavioral therapy (CBT) and pharmacologic therapy, such as with a selective serotonin reuptake inhibitor (SSRI) or serotonin-norepinephrine reuptake inhibitor (SNRI). Patients with GAD often have comorbid mood and anxiety disorders, which often make SSRIs (such as sertraline) and SNRIs (such as venlafaxine) preferred because of their broad therapeutic applicability. CBT is the most effective psychotherapy for GAD; trials have shown it is as effective as pharmacologic therapy and can be used as monotherapy or in combination with drugs. The choice between pharmacologic therapy and CBT is often based on patient preference and the presence of comorbid disorders. Another consideration may be costs of treatment, both direct and indirect (due to time away from work or school). Depending on the particular agent, antidepressant therapy costs $100 to $300 per year, with low indirect costs. On average, annual costs for CBT are three to four times higher than for antidepressant therapy and also require significant time away from work or school to attend therapy.

Tricyclic antidepressants, such as amitriptyline, are considered second-line therapy for GAD because of a higher incidence of side effects with their use.

Benzodiazepines, such as clonazepam, are useful for controlling severe anxiety symptoms, especially before the benefits of CBT or other pharmacologic therapy take effect. These agents should be used only for short periods (<4-6 weeks) because of the potential for dependency.

Lithium and other mood stabilizers are appropriate treatment for bipolar disorder but are not indicated for the treatment of anxiety disorders.

**KEY POINT**

- Treatment options for generalized anxiety disorder include cognitive behavioral therapy and pharmacologic therapy with a selective serotonin reuptake inhibitor or serotonin-norepinephrine reuptake inhibitor.

### Bibliography

Patel G, Fancher TL. In the clinic. Generalized anxiety disorder. Ann Intern Med. 2013;159:ITC6-1-ITC6-11; quiz ITC6-12. [PMID: 24297210] doi:10.7326/0003-4819-159-11-201312030-01006

## Item 30     Answer:    B   

**Educational Objective:** Implement risk-mitigation strategies for patients at high risk for opioid overdose.

The most appropriate next step before continued prescription of this patient's long-term opioid therapy is to prescribe naloxone and provide caregiver education on its use. Naloxone, a pure opioid antagonist that acts as a competitive inhibitor at opioid receptors, can be a life-saving reversal agent for patients with opioid overdose, and evidence shows that naloxone is effective in preventing opioid-related overdose death at the community level through community-based distribution. The Centers for Disease Control and Prevention Guideline for Prescribing Opioids for Chronic Pain recommends that physicians consider offering naloxone to patients with a high risk for overdose (history of overdose or substance use disorder, high opioid dosage [≥50 morphine milligram equivalents/day], or concurrent benzodiazepine use). When naloxone is prescribed, patients and patients' household members should be educated on its use and on ways to prevent overdose. This patient is currently taking approximately 75 morphine milligram equivalents/day and using a long-acting formulation; therefore, she is considered at high risk for overdose and should be considered for naloxone prescription.

Answers and Critiques

CONT.

Coprescription of opioids and benzodiazepines is associated with an increased risk for death from overdose and should be avoided when prescribing medications for patients with chronic pain.

Close monitoring, including review of prescription monitoring databases (where available), urine drug screening, and ongoing functional assessment, are all appropriate tools in the safe prescribing of long-term opioid therapy; however, weekly nursing visits are not currently recommended as a risk-mitigation strategy.

Although current guidelines recommend avoiding the use of extended-release opioids, this patient's pain and quality of life improved with substitution of a short-acting regimen for a transdermal fentanyl patch. If the benefits outweigh the risks and the patient has provided informed consent and received appropriate education, continued extended-release opioid therapy (with implementation of appropriate safety mechanisms) could be considered in this patient with chronic, irreversible pain.

**KEY POINT**

- Physicians should consider offering naloxone to patients receiving long-term opioid therapy with a high risk for overdose (history of overdose or substance use disorder, high opioid dosage [≥50 morphine milligram equivalents/day], or concurrent benzodiazepine use).

**Bibliography**
Dowell D, Haegerich TM, Chou R. CDC guideline for prescribing opioids for chronic pain—United States, 2016. JAMA. 2016;315:1624-45. [PMID: 26977696] doi:10.1001/jama.2016.1464

## Item 31    Answer:    A

**Educational Objective:  Treat a patient with clinical atherosclerotic cardiovascular disease who has not achieved target LDL cholesterol reduction with statin therapy.**

In addition to discontinuing ezetimibe, the most appropriate management of this patient with clinical atherosclerotic cardiovascular disease (ASCVD) is to initiate alirocumab. For patients with clinical ASCVD, high-intensity statin therapy is recommended, with a goal of at least 50% LDL cholesterol reduction. Nonstatin drugs, preferably ezetimibe or a proprotein convertase subtilisin/kexin type 9 (PCSK9) inhibitor, should be considered alone or in combination with statins in patients who do not achieve target LDL cholesterol reduction. PCSK9 inhibitors, such as alirocumab, are monoclonal antibodies that bind to serine protease PCSK9, a liver enzyme that degrades hepatocyte LDL receptors. Treatment with PCSK9 inhibitors produces a 50% to 60% reduction in LDL cholesterol. ASCVD risk reduction has also been demonstrated with PCSK9 inhibitors, although studies have included a relatively small number of patients with limited follow-up. A modest reduction in triglyceride level and increase in HDL cholesterol level have also been observed

with their use. Limitations include high cost and the need for subcutaneous injections every 2 to 4 weeks. Common side effects include injection-site reactions, fatigue, and limb pain. This patient with clinical ASCVD has not achieved the goal LDL cholesterol reduction on maximally tolerated statin therapy and did not tolerate ezetimibe. Therefore, alirocumab should be initiated. In addition to starting a PCSK9 inhibitor, intensification of therapeutic lifestyle changes, such as weight loss and regular exercise, should be encouraged.

A bile acid sequestrant, such as cholestyramine, may be considered as an optional alternative agent for patients with ezetimibe intolerance and a triglyceride level less than 300 mg/dL (3.39 mmol/L) or because of patient preference, but there is no evidence of a net cardiovascular risk reduction benefit with bile acid sequestrants in combination with statins.

Niacin is no longer routinely recommended for treatment of hyperlipidemia based on lack of efficacy and potential harms.

Continuing atorvastatin without additional intervention is unlikely to result in further LDL cholesterol reduction.

**KEY POINT**

- Proprotein convertase subtilisin/kexin type 9 (PCSK9) inhibitors and ezetimibe are the preferred nonstatin drugs for patients with clinical atherosclerotic cardiovascular disease who do not achieve goal LDL cholesterol reduction with maximally tolerated statin therapy.

**Bibliography**
Lloyd-Jones DM, Morris PB, Ballantyne CM, Birtcher KK, Daly DD Jr, DePalma SM, et al. 2017 focused update of the 2016 ACC expert consensus decision pathway on the role of non-statin therapies for LDL-Cholesterol lowering in the management of atherosclerotic cardiovascular disease risk: a report of the American College of Cardiology Task Force on Expert Consensus Decision Pathways. J Am Coll Cardiol. 2017;70:1785-1822. [PMID: 28886926] doi:10.1016/j.jacc.2017.07.745

## Item 32    Answer:    C

**Educational Objective:  Screen for colorectal cancer in an average-risk patient with fecal immunochemical testing.**

The most appropriate screening test for this patient is a fecal immunochemical test (FIT). The U.S. Preventive Services Task Force (USPSTF) recommends screening for colorectal cancer in asymptomatic adults aged 50 to 75 years. For patients with average risk for colorectal cancer, several screening strategies are available, including fecal occult blood testing, direct endoscopic visualization, radiologic examination, and testing the blood for molecular markers of cancer. There is little head-to-head comparative evidence that any one recommended screening modality provides a greater benefit than the others. In addition, despite unequivocal evidence that colon cancer screening reduces mortality, an estimated one in three U.S. adults who are eligible for colon cancer screening has not been screened. Therefore, the USPSTF supports using the test that is most likely to result in completion of screening. Test selection should be guided by evidence, patient preferences, and local availability. Two fecal blood detection tests are available: a sensitive guaiac-based fecal occult blood test (gFOBT) and an FIT that uses antibodies to detect human hemoglobin. Sensitive gFOBT requires dietary restriction in order to reduce false-positive results, whereas FIT does not. The FDA has approved a third stool-based screening test that is combined with FIT and detects cancer DNA in the stool (the multitargeted stool DNA test). Mortality data for this screening strategy are not available. Because this patient would prefer not to modify his diet, FIT is the most appropriate screening option.

The plasma circulating methylated *SEPT9* DNA test is an FDA-approved colorectal cancer screening test that holds promise, as blood tests may result in increased screening adherence. However, its sensitivity for detecting colorectal cancer is suboptimal at 48%, and mortality data are lacking.

Endoscopic tests include flexible sigmoidoscopy and colonoscopy. The mortality benefit of flexible sigmoidoscopy is limited to cancers of the distal bowel. Colonoscopy can visualize the entire bowel but requires colon preparation, which can be a barrier to completing the study. CT colonography is a radiologic technique that also requires colon preparation, which this patient has refused.

Major guidelines differ in their recommendations regarding screening strategy and frequency. The 2016 USPSTF guideline recommends sensitive gFOBT or FIT annually or multitargeted stool DNA testing every 3 years. Flexible sigmoidoscopy is recommended every 5 years, but if combined with FIT (or possibly gFOBT), the interval can be increased to every 10 years, the same interval recommended for colonoscopy. CT colonography can be performed every 5 years.

### KEY POINT

- The U.S. Preventive Services Task Force recommends screening for colorectal cancer in asymptomatic adults aged 50 to 75 years; the choice of screening test should be guided by evidence, patient preferences, and local availability.

### Bibliography
Inadomi JM. Screening for colorectal neoplasia. N Engl J Med. 2017;376:149-156. [PMID: 28076720] doi:10.1056/NEJMcp1512286

## Item 33     Answer:    C

**Educational Objective:**   Counsel a patient on the use of herbal supplements.

This patient should be advised to discontinue drinking kava tea. Patients take dietary supplements for various reasons, such as to prevent illness, enhance health, and correct perceived deficiencies. In the United States, approximately 50% of adults report using vitamins or dietary supplements, with total consumer spending of more than $20 billion each year. Despite their prevalent use, the U.S. Preventive Services

Task Force does not recommend multivitamins or herbal supplements for the prevention of cardiovascular disease or cancer. In addition to questionable efficacy, supplement use is associated with risk for considerable harms, including side effects; interactions with other drugs; and harms related to inclusion of unadvertised additives, compounds, or toxins. Despite the risks, many patients strongly believe in supplement use, and the role of the physician is to inform these patients of harmful supplements and suggest safer alternatives. This patient is taking kava, which is derived from *Piper methysticum*, a plant native to the western Pacific islands. It is often used to relieve stress and anxiety but has been associated with liver damage. In 2002, the FDA issued a consumer advisory regarding the potential risk for severe liver injury with kava use, especially in patients with liver disease or at risk for liver disease. Therefore, advising this patient with nonalcoholic steatohepatitis to discontinue kava tea would be the best management option.

Echinacea may be slightly effective for prevention but not treatment of the common cold. The most common side effects are gastrointestinal upset and nausea. Although this patient does not need to take echinacea, this herb has a relatively safe side effect profile, and she may continue it if she wishes.

The U.S. Preventive Services Task Force recommends daily folic acid supplementation (400 to 800 µg) for women of child-bearing age to prevent fetal neural tube defects; therefore, folic acid should be continued in this 35-year-old patient.

This patient has diagnoses of nonalcoholic steatohepatitis and obesity, and continuing an herbal supplement that is associated with known hepatotoxicity may cause harms.

### KEY POINT

- Dietary and herbal supplements have questionable efficacy and may be associated with considerable harms; physicians must inform patients of harmful supplements and suggest safer alternatives.

### Bibliography
Teschke R, Wolff A, Frenzel C, Schulze J, Eickhoff A. Herbal hepatotoxicity: a tabular compilation of reported cases. Liver Int. 2012;32:1543-56. [PMID: 22928722] doi: 10.1111/j.1478-3231.2012.02864.x

## Item 34     Answer:    B   

**Educational Objective:**   Evaluate preoperative cardiac risk using electrocardiography in a patient with known cardiovascular disease.

The most appropriate preoperative cardiac testing for this patient is electrocardiography (ECG). The 2014 American College of Cardiology/American Heart Association guideline on perioperative cardiovascular evaluation and management of patients undergoing noncardiac surgery states that preoperative ECG is reasonable for patients with known atherosclerotic cardiovascular disease (including coronary artery disease, arrhythmia,

CONT.

peripheral artery disease, cerebrovascular disease, or significant structural heart disease) who are undergoing moderate- to high-risk surgeries. Preoperative ECG also may be considered for other asymptomatic patients, except for those undergoing low-risk procedures. This patient has known coronary artery disease and has not undergone ECG in 2 years. It is reasonable to obtain ECG preoperatively because certain interval findings (for example, new Q waves), additional evidence of conduction disease, or arrhythmia may result in changes in perioperative management.

Risk calculators, including the Revised Cardiac Risk Index and the American College of Surgeons National Surgical Quality Improvement Program myocardial infarction and cardiac arrest calculator, can be used to determine the risk for a perioperative major adverse cardiac event (MACE). Patients with low risk (<1% risk for perioperative MACE) may proceed to surgery without preoperative cardiac stress testing, whereas patients with elevated risk (≥1% risk for perioperative MACE) should undergo assessment of functional capacity. Metabolic equivalents (METs) are used to represent the patient's functional capacity based on the intensity of activity able to be performed. If the patient's functional capacity exceeds 4 METs, the patient may proceed to surgery without further testing. Examples of 4 METs of activity include the ability to walk 4 miles per hour on a flat surface, climb one to two flights of stairs without stopping, or perform vigorous housework such as vacuuming. Swimming for 30 minutes also exceeds this threshold. Cardiac stress testing should generally be reserved for patients at elevated risk for MACE with a functional capacity less than 4 METs, but only if the results of the test will change perioperative management. Although this patient has an elevated risk for a MACE perioperatively, his functional capacity exceeds 4 METs; therefore, he does not require preoperative cardiac stress testing with dobutamine or exercise.

### KEY POINT

- Preoperative electrocardiography is reasonable for patients with known atherosclerotic cardiovascular disease, including coronary artery disease, arrhythmia, peripheral artery disease, cerebrovascular disease, or significant structural heart disease, who are undergoing moderate- to high-risk surgeries; cardiac stress testing should generally be reserved for patients at elevated risk for major adverse cardiac event with a functional capacity less than 4 metabolic equivalents, but only if the results of the test will change perioperative management.

### Bibliography

Fleisher LA, Fleischmann KE, Auerbach AD, Barnason SA, Beckman JA, Bozkurt B, et al; American College of Cardiology. 2014 ACC/AHA guideline on perioperative cardiovascular evaluation and management of patients undergoing noncardiac surgery: a report of the American College of Cardiology/American Heart Association Task Force on Practice Guidelines. J Am Coll Cardiol. 2014;64:e77-137. [PMID: 25091544]

## Item 35    Answer:    D

**Educational Objective:** Diagnose ulnar nerve entrapment.

This patient has symptoms consistent with ulnar neuropathy (fourth and fifth finger numbness and, more rarely, interosseous muscle weakness), making ulnar nerve entrapment the most likely diagnosis. Ulnar nerve entrapment, also known as cubital tunnel syndrome, is caused by impingement of the ulnar nerve at the elbow by bone spurs, fibrous tissue, ganglion cysts, or ulnar nerve subluxation. Elbow pain typically worsens with flexion. The diagnosis is usually made clinically and does not require imaging. Initial treatment consists of activity modification, splinting the elbow at night to prevent prolonged elbow flexion, and use of an elbow pad during the day to avoid direct trauma. Surgery is an option when conservative measures fail in the setting of significant or progressive symptoms.

Carpal tunnel syndrome is associated with wrist pain and symptoms of median nerve dysfunction, namely numbness in the first three fingers and pain that radiates into the forearm and hand. Pain frequently worsens at night and with repetitive actions. Findings on physical examination may include weakened thumb abduction; thenar muscle atrophy suggests severe disease. These symptoms and findings are not present in this patient.

Medial epicondylitis is an important differential diagnosis in a patient presenting with medial elbow pain. Patients with this condition usually have pain and tenderness over the medial epicondyle and ventral forearm, which worsens with resisted wrist flexion rather than elbow flexion. Medial epicondylitis is not usually associated with hand symptoms.

Olecranon bursitis is associated with swelling and, depending on the cause, significant tenderness of the posterior elbow over the olecranon bursa. This patient has not had signs of elbow swelling, and olecranon bursitis does not cause neuropathic symptoms.

### KEY POINT

- Ulnar nerve entrapment, also known as cubital tunnel syndrome, is caused by impingement of the ulnar nerve at the elbow by bone spurs, fibrous tissue, ganglion cysts, or ulnar nerve subluxation; characteristics include pain at the elbow that worsens with flexion, paresthesias and numbness of the fourth and fifth fingers, and weakness of the interosseous muscles.

### Bibliography

Hobson-Webb LD, Juel VC. Common entrapment neuropathies. Continuum (Minneap Minn). 2017;23:487-511. [PMID: 28375915] doi:10.1212/CON.0000000000000452

## Item 36    Answer:    D

**Educational Objective:** Evaluate a patient with syncope.

The most appropriate diagnostic tests to perform next are orthostatic blood pressure measurement and electrocardiography.

The American Heart Association (AHA), the American College of Cardiology (ACC), and the Heart Rhythm Society (HRS) jointly conclude that the history and physical examination are the most important diagnostic tools in determining the underlying cause of a syncopal event. The history should focus on eliciting prodromal or postepisode symptoms, comorbid medical or psychiatric conditions, the psychosocial context of the event, and bystander information. The patient's prescription and over-the-counter medications should also be thoroughly reviewed. The physical examination should include an in-depth cardiovascular evaluation, including orthostatic (postural) blood pressure measurements, as well as a basic neurologic examination to evaluate for focal defects. Orthostatic blood pressure assessment has consistently been shown to be the most valuable diagnostic tool in the evaluation of syncope. The AHA/ACC/HRS guideline for the evaluation and management of patients with syncope additionally recommends that resting 12-lead electrocardiography (ECG) be performed in all patients with syncope to identify an underlying arrhythmia, myocardial ischemia, or QT prolongation. Further diagnostic testing should be methodically selected on the basis of the clinical circumstances.

The diagnostic yield of 24- to 48-hour electrocardiographic monitoring is low (1%-2%), unless there are frequent episodes over a short period. More prolonged rhythm monitoring with an external loop event recorder improves yield if the patient has clinical or ECG features of arrhythmia-related syncope. Clinical evidence does not support routine echocardiography in patients with syncope. Unexpected findings on echocardiogram to explain syncope are uncommon.

Laboratory testing, such as B-type natriuretic peptide and cardiac enzyme measurement, has considerably low diagnostic yield and is not recommended in the routine evaluation of patients with syncope. Rather, further diagnostic testing should be based on the findings on the history, physical examination, and ECG.

The AHA/ACC/HRS syncope guideline does not recommend MRI and CT of the head in the routine evaluation of patients with syncope in the absence of head injury or focal neurologic findings that support further evaluation. Similarly, carotid artery imaging is not recommended in the routine evaluation of patients with syncope in the absence of focal neurologic findings.

### KEY POINT

- In patients with syncope, the physical examination should include an in-depth cardiovascular evaluation, including orthostatic (postural) blood pressure measurements, as well as a basic neurologic examination to evaluate for focal defects; electrocardiography is the only diagnostic study that is routinely recommended in patients with syncope.

### Bibliography

Shen WK, Sheldon RS, Benditt DG, Cohen MI, Forman DE, Goldberger ZD, et al. 2017 ACC/AHA/HRS guideline for the evaluation and management of patients with syncope: executive summary: a report of the American College of Cardiology/American Heart Association Task Force on Clinical Practice Guidelines and the Heart Rhythm Society. J Am Coll Cardiol. 2017;70:620-663. doi: 10.1016/j.jacc.2017.03.002. [PMID: 28286222]

### Item 37          Answer:     C

**Educational Objective:**  Identify appropriate contraceptive care for a smoker.

The most appropriate contraceptive option for this patient is a progesterone-containing intrauterine device (IUD). Hormonal contraception options include oral contraceptive pills, a transdermal patch, a vaginal ring, and long-acting reversible contraceptives. Long-acting reversible contraceptives are progestin-only forms of contraception that include depot medroxyprogesterone acetate injections, subcutaneous implants, and progestin-containing IUDs. These preparations are less reliant on user adherence than oral contraceptive pills, are highly effective, and may be ideal for this patient who has proven difficulty with adhering to a daily pill routine. Return of fertility may be delayed with these methods, with a median time to conception of 10 months after cessation of use. As with other progestin-only methods, irregular bleeding and amenorrhea are prevalent, and weight gain is a common side effect. The levonorgestrel IUD is available in two dosage formulations: one that releases 14 μg/d and is effective for 3 years and one that releases 20 μg/d and is effective for 5 years. The levonorgestrel-containing IUD releases a low dose of progestin, which causes endometrial atrophy and generally leads to decreased or absent menstrual flow. The progesterone-containing IUD may be ideal for this patient who is bothered by heavy menstrual flow, and it will simultaneously eliminate the need for daily adherence to a pill.

Oral contraceptive pills are the most common form of contraception. These include combination estrogen-progestin pills and progestin-only pills ("mini-pill"). Combination preparations differ based on the strength of estrogen and the type of progestin component. All preparations are therapeutically equivalent in preventing pregnancy. Contraindications to estrogen-containing preparations (including oral contraceptives and estrogen-progestin vaginal rings) include breast cancer, liver disease, migraine with aura, uncontrolled hypertension, and venous thromboembolism. They are also contraindicated in women older than age 35 years who smoke more than 15 cigarettes per day, such as this patient, because of an increased risk for venous thromboembolism. When estrogen-containing products are contraindicated, a progesterone-only contraceptive could safely be used. In this patient, a progestin-only pill is less preferable to a progesterone-containing IUD because a pill would require daily adherence.

### KEY POINT

- Estrogen-containing hormonal contraceptives are contraindicated in women older than 35 years who smoke more than 15 cigarettes a day because of an increased risk for venous thromboembolism.

## Bibliography

Tracy EE. Contraception: menarche to menopause. Obstet Gynecol Clin North Am. 2017;44:143-158. [PMID: 28499527] doi:10.1016/j.ogc.2017.02.001

## Item 38     Answer:   B

**Educational Objective:** Treat obesity with liraglutide in a patient with type 2 diabetes mellitus.

Liraglutide is the most appropriate next step in treatment. Weight-loss medications are recommended when a trial of comprehensive lifestyle modification, including reduced dietary intake, exercise, and behavioral therapy, fails to achieve a 5% to 10% reduction in weight at 3 to 6 months. This patient has appropriately adhered to dietary caloric restriction, with regular self-monitoring of calorie intake and weight, and is now exercising for more than 150 minutes per week. Her BMI is greater than 27, and she has obesity-related comorbid conditions (type 2 diabetes mellitus and uncontrolled hypertension). Liraglutide has been shown to increase satiety and aid in achieving more than 5% weight loss after 52 weeks of therapy, and it may help the patient feel less hungry.

Bariatric surgery is recommended for patients with BMI of 40 or greater, and for patients with BMI of 35 or greater who have obesity-related comorbidities and who have tried all other weight loss therapies without achieving significant weight loss or improvements in comorbid conditions.

There is no evidence that low-carbohydrate diets are more effective for reducing weight than low-fat diets. This patient is adherent to her chosen diet but has difficulty reducing her caloric intake to achieve continued weight loss. Clinicians should prescribe a diet with which the patient will adhere (that is, a diet that is palatable and affordable) and that maintains negative energy balance in order to achieve weight loss.

Very-low-calorie diets are recommended when rapid weight loss is medically indicated. This patient does not require rapid weight loss, and neither the risk nor the expense of frequent visits and laboratory monitoring are justified in this case.

### KEY POINT

- Weight-loss medications are recommended when a trial of comprehensive lifestyle modification, including reduced dietary intake, exercise, and behavioral therapy, fails to achieve a 5% to 10% reduction in weight after 3 to 6 months.

## Bibliography

Jensen MD, Ryan DH, Apovian CM, Ard JD, Comuzzie AG, Donato KA, et al; American College of Cardiology/American Heart Association Task Force on Practice Guidelines. 2013 AHA/ACC/TOS guideline for the management of overweight and obesity in adults: a report of the American College of Cardiology/American Heart Association Task Force on Practice Guidelines and The Obesity Society. Circulation. 2014;129:S102-38. [PMID: 24222017] doi:10.1161/01.cir.0000437739.71477.ee

## Item 39     Answer:   A

**Educational Objective:** Identify appropriate timing for palliative medicine referral in a patient with advanced cancer.

The most appropriate time for palliative medicine referral is now. Palliative medicine (or palliative care) focuses on reducing pain, nonpain symptoms, and psychosocial stress associated with advanced disease. This patient has been diagnosed with incurable lung cancer and would benefit from concurrent specialty palliative medicine in conjunction with initiation of disease-directed therapy. Studies have consistently shown improvements in various quality-of-life metrics when palliative medicine is integrated early in the course of incurable cancer, and such integration is consistent with recommendations from the American Society of Clinical Oncology.

Although referral to palliative care historically occurred at the end of life, an emerging consensus of research indicates that early initiation during a serious or life-threatening illness is associated with substantial advantages. Evidence shows that early palliative medicine referral improves mood and decreases rates of depressive symptoms; anxiety is not heightened by palliative medicine referral. Palliative medicine teams are positioned to work with oncologists and primary care physicians in treating the complex symptoms of serious illness, and an integrated approach is recommended.

Hospice is a specialized form of palliative medicine that can provide a team-based care platform in the patient's preferred setting (for example, home, skilled nursing facility, or residential hospice house). Hospice should be considered for patients with an advanced illness who are no longer candidates for further disease-directed therapy, or whose goals (such as quality of life) are not likely to be met with further disease-directed therapies. Despite significant quality-of-life benefits for patients and their caregivers, hospice referrals often happen late in a patient's illness trajectory, leading to short hospice lengths of stay.

### KEY POINT

- Palliative medicine, with its focus on reducing pain, nonpain symptoms, and psychosocial stress associated with advanced disease, improves quality of life for patients and their caregivers; early initiation of palliative medicine during a life-threatening illness has substantial advantages.

## Bibliography

Ferrell BR, Temel JS, Temin S, Alesi ER, Balboni TA, Basch EM, et al. Integration of palliative care into standard oncology care: American Society of Clinical Oncology Clinical Practice Guideline Update. J Clin Oncol. 2017;35:96-112. [PMID: 28034065]

## Item 40     Answer:   B

**Educational Objective:** Prevent atherosclerotic cardiovascular disease with low-dose aspirin therapy.

The most appropriate measure to reduce this patient's atherosclerotic cardiovascular disease (ASCVD) risk is low-dose aspirin. The U.S. Preventive Services Task Force (USPSTF) recommends low-dose aspirin for the primary prevention of ASCVD and colorectal cancer in adults aged 50 to 59 years with a 10-year ASCVD risk of 10% or higher who do not have an increased risk for bleeding, have a life expectancy of at least 10 years, and are willing to take low-dose aspirin daily for at least 10 years. In those aged 60 to 69 years with a 10-year ASCVD risk of 10% or higher, the benefits of aspirin use for primary prevention are smaller but still outweigh the risk for bleeding, and the decision to initiate low-dose aspirin in this population should be individualized. In contrast to the USPSTF recommendations, the American Diabetes Association recommends consideration of low-dose aspirin therapy as a primary prevention strategy in patients with type 1 or type 2 diabetes mellitus who are at increased cardiovascular risk. This group of patients includes most men and women with diabetes aged 50 years or older who have at least one additional major risk factor (family history of premature ASCVD, hypertension, dyslipidemia, smoking, or albuminuria) and are not at increased risk for bleeding. Aspirin therapy for the primary prevention of ASCVD is likely underused (approximately 40% of eligible candidates). Among patients told by a physician to take aspirin, 80% adhere to the recommendation.

For patients with ASCVD and documented aspirin allergy, the ADA recommends clopidogrel as an alternative preventive measure. This patient does not have a documented aspirin allergy, and therapy in this patient will be initiated for primary, not secondary, prevention; therefore, clopidogrel is not recommended for this patient.

The most commonly recommended dose of aspirin for primary prevention of cardiovascular events is 75 mg to 100 mg. Primary prevention trials have shown that lower doses are likely as effective as higher doses; however, observational trials and a meta-analysis have demonstrated an increased risk for bleeding with regular-dose aspirin compared with low-dose aspirin.

### KEY POINT

- Low-dose aspirin for the primary prevention of atherosclerotic cardiovascular disease (ASCVD) and colorectal cancer is recommended for adults aged 50 to 59 years with a 10-year ASCVD risk of 10% or higher who do not have an increased risk for bleeding.

### Bibliography
Bibbins-Domingo K; U.S. Preventive Services Task Force. Aspirin use for the primary prevention of cardiovascular disease and colorectal cancer: U.S. Preventive Services Task Force recommendation statement. Ann Intern Med. 2016;164:836–45. [PMID: 27064677] doi: 10.7326/M16-0577

## Item 41    Answer:    E

**Educational Objective:** **Evaluate a patient with symptoms of chronic insomnia with a sleep diary.**

The most appropriate next step in management of this patient with symptoms of chronic insomnia is to obtain a 2-week sleep diary. Symptoms of insomnia vary and may include poor sleep quality, frustration with sleep quantity, difficulty initiating sleep, or an inability to return to sleep after awakening. In patients with symptoms of insomnia, a thorough history, physical examination, and medication review may point to potentially reversible causes, such as sleep apnea or restless legs syndrome. In the absence of specific historical features that are consistent with a primary sleep disorder, the initial evaluation of insomnia additionally involves obtaining a sleep diary to identify adverse environmental factors, inappropriate exposure to electronic screens (computer, phone, tablet, television) before bedtime, and sleep patterns. If the sleep diary reveals red flags for a primary sleep disorder or another condition that may interfere with sleep, further diagnostic testing would be indicated. In this patient with daytime somnolence, fatigue, and difficulty with sleep initiation, a sleep log may facilitate collection of an accurate sleep history.

Polysomnography is indicated in patients for whom there is a strong suspicion of a primary sleep disorder based on the initial history and physical examination. Polysomnography typically involves overnight, laboratory-based testing that is monitored by a sleep technician. Similarly, multiple sleep latency testing is a labor-intensive evaluation designed to identify diagnoses of narcolepsy and idiopathic hypersomnia. Neither study is indicated in the initial evaluation of this patient, whose primary problem appears to be initiating sleep.

Overnight pulse oximetry has a high rate of false-positive and false-negative results and has not been validated as a screening tool for obstructive sleep apnea. Normal-appearing results on overnight pulse oximetry may allow for avoidance of further testing in patients with a low pretest probability. However, there is no clinical suspicion for obstructive sleep apnea in this patient, and it would not be indicated in her initial evaluation.

Low serum ferritin levels are strongly correlated with restless legs syndrome, which is characterized by discomforting sensations in the legs at rest or when falling asleep, an urge to move the legs, and immediate relief after moving the legs or walking. However, no features in the history suggest restless legs syndrome as a cause of this patient's chronic insomnia.

### KEY POINT

- The initial evaluation of chronic insomnia involves obtaining a sleep diary to identify adverse environmental factors, inappropriate exposure to electronic screens before bedtime, and sleep patterns.

### Bibliography
Masters PA. In the clinic. Insomnia. Ann Intern Med. 2014;161:ITC1-15; quiz ITC16. [PMID: 25285559] doi: 10.7326/0003-4819-161-7-201410070-01004

## Item 42    Answer:    C

**Educational Objective:** **Manage online physician-patient communication.**

The most appropriate management is to request that the patient establish care through the office. Professional assessments should be performed within the context of an existing physician-patient relationship. In general, relationships should be established on the basis of an in-person professional encounter. Telemedicine, or the use of electronic communication and technologies to provide health care to patients at a distance, may increase access to care, improve outcomes, enhance physician-patient collaboration, and reduce costs; however, the American College of Physicians holds the position that a valid patient-physician relationship must be established for professionally responsible telemedicine services to occur. In this situation, the physician should reply to the patient and ask him to contact the office for an appointment to establish care or provide a second opinion, if that is what the patient desires. Once a physician-patient relationship is established, online communication should ideally occur through a secure portal that meets the requirements of the Health Insurance Portability and Accountability Act of 1996 (HIPAA).

Providing specific medical advice, such as suggesting celiac disease testing, without a thorough and proper medical evaluation would be inappropriate.

A request for the patient's records and provision of advice based on review of those records should not be made until a physician-patient relationship is established. Additionally, in digital environments, the sharing of patient information must always be held to a higher level of security than standard residential Internet connections. Encrypted or virtual proxy network connections in hospital-based information technology systems should be used for all patient information exchange and review to ensure a secure digital environment.

If a member of the public contacts a physician electronically in his or her professional role, the physician should politely respond and direct the patient to seek care through suitable channels by appropriately responding to the email or other online query.

**KEY POINT**

- Telemedicine, or the use of electronic communication and technologies to provide health care to patients at a distance, may increase access to care, improve outcomes, enhance physician-patient collaboration, and reduce costs; however, a valid patient-physician relationship must be established for professionally responsible telemedicine services to occur.

**Bibliography**
Farnan JM, Snyder Sulmasy L, Worster BK, Chaudhry HJ, Rhyne JA, Arora VM; American College of Physicians Ethics, Professionalism and Human Rights Committee. Online medical professionalism: patient and public relationships: policy statement from the American College of Physicians and the Federation of State Medical Boards. Ann Intern Med. 2013;158:620-7. [PMID: 23579867] doi:10.7326/0003-4819-158-8-201304160-00100

## Item 43     Answer:     C

**Educational Objective:   Diagnose optic neuritis.**

This patient with acute vision loss and eye pain unassociated with trauma has signs and symptoms suggestive of optic neuritis, including pain with eye movement, loss of color vision out of proportion to the vision loss, and an afferent pupillary defect. Two thirds of optic neuritis cases occur in women. The average age of onset is between 20 and 40 years, and it is often associated with multiple sclerosis. Most of these patients have a normal optic disc on funduscopy, but one third may have a swollen disc or papillitis. An urgent evaluation by an ophthalmologist is required; treatment usually involves high-dose intravenous glucocorticoids.

Corneal abrasion can cause sudden onset of pain and foreign-body sensation. It is classically seen in patients who sleep without taking out their contact lenses and then awaken with eye pain and photophobia. If the abrasion is in the central area of the visual axis, visual acuity may be diminished. Corneal abrasion cannot explain the loss of color discrimination and the afferent pupillary defect in this patient.

Herpes simplex keratitis typically presents with acute onset of pain, blurry vision, and watery discharge. The absence of discharge and ciliary flush in this case make keratitis unlikely. Ciliary flush is characterized by erythema that is most marked at the limbus, which is the junction of the sclera and cornea. Keratitis would not be associated with loss of color discrimination or an afferent pupillary defect.

Orbital cellulitis often presents with eye pain as well as eyelid swelling and erythema, although some cases present without erythema. In the case of inflammation of the extraocular muscles and fatty tissue in the orbit, the patient may experience pain with eye movement. When the condition is severe, visual acuity may be impaired. Orbital cellulitis, however, is more likely to be associated with fever and chemosis, which are not present in this patient, and it would not explain the patient's other findings related to optic nerve damage.

**KEY POINT**

- The hallmarks of optic neuritis are acute vision loss, eye pain with movement, color perception change, and afferent pupillary defect; results of a funduscopic examination may be normal.

**Bibliography**
Balcer LJ. Clinical practice. Optic neuritis. N Engl J Med. 2006;354:1273-80. [PMID: 16554529]

## Item 44     Answer:     A

**Educational Objective:   Recognize threats to validity with a cross-sectional study.**

The most likely threat to the validity of this cross-sectional study is confounding. Cross-sectional studies evaluate the relationship between exposures and health outcomes in a population of interest. These studies are characterized by the measurement of factors and outcomes at a single point in time. The validity of cross-sectional studies is particularly susceptible to recall bias and confounding. Recall bias is a systematic error that is introduced into a study by differences in the accuracy of the recollections of study participants; participants who have unpleasant experiences may recall past events differently than those who do not have similar experiences. Because cross-sectional studies are observational and not experimental, there is also no opportunity to randomly distribute factors that might influence the relationship being studied. Although statistical techniques can be used to control for known potential confounders, unknown confounders remain a threat to the validity of the conclusions. As such, cross-sectional studies are best suited to identifying potentially significant associations that can be more rigorously tested in experimental studies. Finally, because there is no way to verify that the purported cause (statin therapy) preceded the effect (memory loss), cross-sectional studies cannot prove cause-and-effect relationships.

Selection bias occurs when the study participants do not accurately reflect the population being studied, usually because the choice to participate is influenced by the clinical question. Selection bias can compromise the validity of observational study designs; however, in this study, the random sampling according to zip code of residence minimizes the possibility of selection bias.

Although self-reported data are less robust than measured data, well-validated survey designs may use self-reported data to determine the presence or absence of conditions, risk factors, or behaviors in a population.

The conventional level of statistical significance is a $P$ value less than or equal to 0.05, and an odds ratio of 1 implies the absence of a significant relationship. In this case, the confidence interval for the odds ratio does not include the value 1, which supports the statistical significance of the findings.

**KEY POINT**

- The validity of cross-sectional studies is particularly susceptible to recall bias and confounding.

**Bibliography**
Grimes DA, Schulz KF. Bias and causal associations in observational research. Lancet. 2002;359:248-52. [PMID: 11812579]

## Item 45    Answer:    D

**Educational Objective:** Manage postoperative urinary retention with urinary catheterization.

Bladder decompression with urinary catheterization is the most appropriate management of this patient who has developed postoperative urinary retention (POUR). POUR is a common complication in the postoperative setting and is characterized by the inability to spontaneously and adequately empty the bladder. Risk factors include type of surgery (incontinence and anorectal surgery, hernia repair, joint arthroplasty), longer surgery, use of regional anesthesia, administration of greater than 750 mL of intraoperative fluids, use of certain postoperative medications (opioids, anticholinergic agents), older age, constipation, pelvic organ prolapse, neurologic disease, history of urinary retention,

and history of pelvic surgery. POUR is a urologic emergency. Symptoms of suprapubic pain and the finding of a palpable bladder are insensitive indicators of POUR. Patients may also present with frequent urination of small volumes and overflow incontinence. Reversible causes of POUR, such as medication use, should be addressed. Whenever possible, offending medications, including opioids, anticholinergics, antihistamines, antipsychotics, and calcium-blocking drugs, should be discontinued. Early removal of indwelling urinary catheters and voiding trials are recommended. Retrograde voiding trials are preferred to spontaneous voiding trials because they are more predictive of the need for continued catheterization. A retrograde voiding trial involves infusion of sterile saline, followed by the attempt to void. For patients in whom a voiding trial is unsuccessful, intermittent urinary catheterization should be considered in place of indwelling bladder catheterization. Results of a recent randomized controlled trial in patients undergoing total hip arthroplasty and total knee arthroplasty demonstrated that a catheterization threshold of 800 mL significantly reduced the need for postoperative urinary catheterization and did not increase urologic complications.

Placement of a suprapubic catheter would require another surgical procedure and is reserved for situations in which urethral catheterization is not possible or in cases of pelvic trauma.

Suprapubic application of hot packs or warm wet gauze may stimulate spontaneous voiding but lacks proof from well-designed clinical trials. Some experts recommend consideration of this technique in patients for a limited time when residual bladder volume is 200 mL to 400 mL. Greater residual volume should be treated with bladder catheterization.

There is no role for tamsulosin in the treatment of POUR in women. Randomized studies in men have demonstrated that $\alpha_2$-blockade for the treatment of acute urinary retention is associated with a reduced need for bladder catheterization. $\alpha_2$-Blockers should be continued in men with benign prostatic hyperplasia.

**KEY POINT**

- Patients with postoperative urinary retention and residual bladder volume of 800 mL or more should be treated with bladder decompression and urinary catheterization.

**Bibliography**
Bjerregaard LS, Hornum U, Troldborg C, Bogoe S, Bagi P, Kehlet H. Postoperative urinary catheterization thresholds of 500 versus 800 ml after fast-track total hip and knee arthroplasty: a randomized, open-label, controlled trial. Anesthesiology. 2016;124(6):1256-64. [PMID: 27054365] doi: 10.1097/ALN.0000000000001112

## Item 46    Answer:    D

**Educational Objective:** Determine adequacy of previous cervical cancer screening in an older woman.

The most appropriate screening strategy is to obtain the results of the patient's last cervical cancer screening examination. The U.S. Preventive Services Task Force recommends against cervical cancer screening in women older than age 65 years who have had adequate prior screening and are not otherwise at high risk for cervical cancer. Adequate screening is commonly defined as three consecutive negative cytology (Pap smear) results or two consecutive negative cytology plus human papillomavirus (HPV) test results within the last 10 years, with the most recent test occurring within 5 years. Data suggest that cervical cancer screening rates decline with increasing patient age; however, a Kaiser Permanente registry study found that 13% of 65-year-old women have not been adequately screened, with higher rates in patients without a primary physician or other health care provider. Other populations that are less likely to have received adequate screening include women with limited access to care, women from racial or ethnic minority groups, and women from countries where screening is not available. The study also documented that most cases of invasive cervical cancer in women older than age 65 years occurred among those who had not met criteria for stopping screening. The decision to stop screening at age 65 years should only be made after confirming that the patient has received adequate prior screening. In patients who do not meet the criteria for adequate prior screening, screening may be clinically indicated after age 65 years.

Cervical cytology, high-risk HPV testing, or co-testing with cervical cytology and high-risk HPV testing may all be reasonable methods to screen for cervical cancer in this patient, but reviewing the adequacy of previous screening remains the first step in management.

**KEY POINT**

• The decision to discontinue cervical cancer screening at age 65 years should be made only after confirming that the patient has received adequate prior screening.

**Bibliography**
Dinkelspiel H, Fetterman B, Poitras N, Kinney W, Cox JT, Lorey T, Castle PE. Screening history preceding a diagnosis of cervical cancer in women age 65 and older. Gynecol Oncol. 2012;126:203-6. [PMID: 22561038] doi: 10.1016/j.ygyno.2012.04.037

## Item 47    Answer:    B

**Educational Objective:**  Treat chronic pain with structured physical therapy.

The most appropriate next step in treatment is physical therapy. This patient has a long-standing history of chronic pain that is most consistent with a diagnosis of fibromyalgia. All patients with chronic pain should be referred to a structured physical therapy program for evaluation and treatment. Physical therapy teaches patients safe, self-guided exercises to improve functional status, and there is a clear evidence base to support its use in all patients with chronic pain. Guided/progressive physical therapy programs are associated with a reduction in pain and, perhaps most importantly, improvement in function. No evidence suggests that a specific type of physical therapy is superior to another, and programs should be tailored to patient ability and adherence.

Clinicians should avoid prescribing opioids and benzodiazepines concurrently whenever possible. Epidemiologic studies indicate that concomitant use of benzodiazepines, such as lorazepam, and opioids may place patients at increased risk for fatal overdose. In three studies of opioid overdose deaths, there was evidence of concurrent benzodiazepine use in 31% to 61% of persons.

Trials of transcutaneous electrical nerve stimulation (TENS) for the treatment of fibromyalgia have yielded inconclusive results. Positive trials of TENS are frequently contaminated with concurrent use of an exercise program and massage. On the basis of inconclusive evidence, TENS cannot be recommended as the next treatment modality for this patient.

Opioid rotation would not be an ideal next step in this patient with a long history of chronic pain, particularly in the setting of previous unsuccessful opioid trials. Despite high opioid prescribing rates, no evidence supports the use of long-term opioid therapy in patients with chronic noncancer pain. In one study, patients receiving long-term opioids for chronic pain had more pain, poorer quality of life, and poorer function than a population of patients with chronic pain who were not taking opioids. Given the lack of evidence to support chronic opioid therapy, the continued use of opioids for chronic pain should be justified at every follow-up visit by documenting the patient's sustained functional improvement due to effective opioid therapy. In this patient with pain that has failed to improve with opioid therapy, oxycodone should be carefully withdrawn, and nonpharmacologic therapy should be instituted.

**KEY POINT**

• In patients with chronic noncancer pain, physical therapy reduces pain and improves function.

**Bibliography**
Hooten M, Thorson D, Bianco J, Bonte B, Clavel A Jr, Hora J. Institute for Clinical Systems Improvement. Pain: assessment, non-opioid treatment approaches and opioid management. Available at www.icsi.org/guidelines_more/catalog_guidelines_and_more/catalog_guidelines/catalog_neurological_guidelines/pain/. Updated August 2017. Accessed February 27, 2018.

## Item 48    Answer:    D

**Educational Objective:**  Test for cognitive impairment in a symptomatic older woman.

This patient would most benefit from evaluation with the Mini-Cog test or another validated screening test for cognitive function. Cognitive impairment is a progressive decline that impairs function in at least two areas: attention, executive function, language, memory, or visual-spatial function. Patients with signs and symptoms of cognitive impairment, such as this patient who reports difficulty with both memory and executive function, should undergo evaluation. A variety of validated tools are available to assess cognitive function. Among the free tools, the Montreal Cognitive Assessment and Mini-Cog test have been validated in primary care populations; these instruments screen for impairments in executive function. Self-administered instruments, such as the Self-Administered Gerocognitive Examination and Test Your Memory examination, have been validated in memory clinic populations to detect mild cognitive impairment and early dementia. Although the Mini–Mental State Examination has been the most extensively studied screening instrument, it is now proprietary, with a cost per use.

Although numerous factors have been studied, and some have been associated with a higher risk for progression to dementia (such as baseline functional impairment, abnormal results of fluorodeoxyglucose-PET brain imaging, and the apolipoprotein E [*APOE*-ε4] genotype), no reliable clinical markers can predict the clinical likelihood that an individual patient with mild cognitive impairment will develop dementia. More importantly, these tests do not establish the diagnosis of cognitive impairment.

In clinical practice, a careful history and results of a standard mental examination are often sufficient to diagnose cognitive impairment, and extensive formal cognitive testing is not routinely required. Occasionally, a formal battery of neuropsychologic testing beyond the standard mental examination is needed to distinguish particularly mild cases of cognitive impairment from normal aging.

**KEY POINT**

- Cognitive impairment is a progressive decline that impairs function in at least two areas, including attention, executive function, language, memory, and visual-spatial function; it is best measured with assessment examinations, such as the Mini-Cog and the Mini–Mental State Examination, rather than laboratory testing or imaging.

**Bibliography**

Lin JS, O'Connor E, Rossom RC, Perdue LA, Eckstrom E. Screening for cognitive impairment in older adults: a systematic review for the U.S. Preventive Services Task Force. Ann Intern Med. 2013;159:601-12. [PMID: 24145578]

## Item 49      Answer:   C

**Educational Objective:   Diagnose cervical sprain.**

This patient most likely has a cervical sprain (nonspecific or axial neck pain), which is the most common cause of neck pain. The pain associated with cervical sprain is usually an aching sensation that is isolated to the neck, but it can radiate to the posterior head or shoulders. The pain does not typically radiate into the arms. Cervical sprain symptoms can be precipitated by an unaccustomed activity or overuse. Physical examination of the neck usually shows decreased range of motion, tenderness to palpation, and reproduction of the pain with flexion or extension. The condition is also notable for the absence of abnormal neurologic findings.

Cervical myelopathy (compression of the cervical spinal cord) can also cause neck pain. Common clinical manifestations include progressive worsening of symptoms, difficulty with fine object manipulation and manual dexterity, and gait abnormalities. This patient's symptoms are not consistent with cervical myelopathy.

Cervical radiculopathy is caused by disk herniation or bony degeneration causing compression of adjacent nerve roots; it is characterized by neck pain associated with radiating arm pain and paresthesias that follow a dermatomal distribution. On examination, affected patients frequently have reproduction of their pain with the Spurling test (examiner bends the patient's head to the affected side while extending the neck and applying a downward pressure on the top of the head). Symptoms can be improved by holding the patient's hand on the affected side above the patient's head (shoulder abduction test). This patient's presentation is not consistent with cervical radiculopathy.

Whiplash-associated neck pain is a poorly understood entity that refers to cervical sprain that develops in the setting of trauma, such as a car accident, which produces an abrupt flexion/extension movement of the cervical spine. Typical symptoms include persistent severe pain, spasm, loss of range of motion in the neck, and occipital headache. Because this patient's neck pain did not result from direct abrupt flexion/extension trauma, it would be incorrect to classify it as whiplash-associated neck pain.

**KEY POINT**

- Pain associated with cervical sprain is usually an aching sensation that is isolated to the neck but can radiate to the posterior head or shoulders; physical examination usually shows decreased range of motion, tenderness to palpation, and reproduction of the pain with flexion or extension, but no neurologic findings.

**Bibliography**

Cohen SP. Epidemiology, diagnosis, and treatment of neck pain. Mayo Clin Proc. 2015;90:284-99. [PMID: 25659245] doi:10.1016/j.mayocp.2014.09.008

## Item 50      Answer:   C

**Educational Objective:   Treat trichomoniasis in a sexual partner.**

The most appropriate additional management is to treat the patient's sexual partner for trichomoniasis. Trichomoniasis, which is caused by *Trichomonas vaginalis*, is the most common nonviral sexually transmitted infection (STI) worldwide. Unlike other STIs that predominate in adolescents and younger adults, rates of trichomoniasis are evenly distributed among women of all age groups. It is caused by motile flagellated protozoa that infect the urogenital tract, causing inflammatory vaginitis and urethritis. Treatment with a single 2-g dose of metronidazole is associated with a high rate of cure and should be offered to all symptomatic women, including pregnant women. Because of the high rate of reinfection among women treated for trichomoniasis (17% within 3 months in one study), retesting for *T. vaginalis* is recommended by the Centers for Disease Control and Prevention (CDC) for all sexually active women within 3 months after initial treatment, regardless of whether they believe their sexual partners were treated. Testing by nucleic acid amplification can be conducted as soon as 2 weeks after treatment. It is important that sexual partners also be treated, even if they are asymptomatic; documentation of infection is not required before treatment in any partners. Data are insufficient to support retesting men after treatment for trichomoniasis. *T. vaginalis* infection is associated with a two- to threefold increased risk for HIV acquisition. Therefore, the CDC recommends that testing for other STIs, including HIV, be performed in persons infected with *T. vaginalis*.

Pap testing is not needed for management of trichomoniasis because the infection is not associated with cervical malignancy.

Because of the high rate of partner infection with *T. vaginalis* and its association with other STIs, it would be inappropriate to not provide further testing or intervention after a primary *T. vaginalis* diagnosis.

**KEY POINT**

- Following diagnosis and treatment of a woman with *Trichomonas vaginalis* infection, the sexual partner should be treated and both individuals should be screened for other sexually transmitted infections; retesting of women for *T. vaginalis* infection within 3 months of treatment is also recommended.

**Bibliography**
Mills BB. Vaginitis: beyond the basics. Obstet Gynecol Clin North Am. 2017;44:159-177. [PMID: 28499528] doi:10.1016/j.ogc.2017.02.010

## Item 51      Answer:   C

**Educational Objective:   Diagnose a patient with a medically unexplained symptom.**

This patient most likely has a medically unexplained symptom. Such symptoms cannot be attributed to a specific medical cause after a thorough medical evaluation. Symptoms that are common in these patients include fatigue, headache, abdominal pain, musculoskeletal pain (back pain, myalgia, and arthralgia), dizziness, paresthesia, generalized weakness, transient edema, insomnia, dyspnea, chest pain, chronic facial pain, chronic pelvic pain, and chemical sensitivities. Symptoms can range from a minor nuisance to functional impairment. In this case, the patient's symptom does not appear to have a pathologic basis, and she is not excessively focused on or functionally limited by her symptom. As such, this patient would most appropriately be diagnosed with a medically unexplained symptom.

Conversion disorder involves at least one symptom of neurologic dysfunction (abnormal sensation or motor function) that is unexplained by a medical condition and not

consistent with examination findings. Conversion disorder represents not fabrication of symptoms but rather unexplained symptoms that do not have a pathophysiologic basis. These symptoms, which are functionally limiting, occur during times of substantial physical, emotional, or psychological stress.

Illness anxiety disorder (formerly named hypochondriasis) is characterized by excessive concern about health and preoccupation with health-related activities (for example, measuring pulse). In patients with illness anxiety disorder, no or only mild somatic symptoms are present.

Somatic symptom disorder is characterized by one or more somatic symptoms present for at least 6 months, causing significant distress or interference with life and associated with excessive thoughts, behaviors, and feelings related to the symptoms. The diagnosis of somatic symptom disorder has replaced the previous diagnosis of somatization disorder.

**KEY POINT**

- Medically unexplained symptoms are diagnosed according to the presence of symptoms that cannot be attributed to a specific medical cause after a thorough medical evaluation.

**Bibliography**
Haller H, Cramer H, Lauche R, Dobos G. Somatoform disorders and medically unexplained symptoms in primary care. Dtsch Arztebl Int. 2015;112:279-87. [PMID: 25939319] doi: 10.3238/arztebl.2015.0279

## Item 52      Answer:   D

**Educational Objective:   Treat drug-induced lower extremity edema.**

The most appropriate next step in the management of this patient is to discontinue pregabalin and initiate duloxetine. In most patients with lower extremity edema, a detailed history and physical examination will suggest the cause. The most common causes of lower extremity edema include venous obstruction or insufficiency, heart failure (including right-sided heart failure secondary to pulmonary disease), cirrhosis, and nephrotic syndrome and hypoalbuminemia of other etiologies. Certain drugs and classes of drugs are frequent causes of edema. Direct vasodilators (minoxidil, hydralazine, calcium channel blockers, α-blockers) may produce edema by several mechanisms, including arteriolar dilatation (increases intracapillary pressure) and activation of the renin-angiotensin-aldosterone system (sodium retention). The thiazolidinediones, such as pioglitazone and rosiglitazone, stimulate sodium reabsorption by the sodium channels in the cortical collecting tubule cells. NSAIDs increase renal sodium reabsorption by inhibition of renal vasodilatory prostaglandins. Pregabalin is a calcium channel blocker and likely produces edema by the same mechanism as other calcium channel blockers; it is associated with peripheral edema in up to 17% of cases. In drug-induced edema, removal of the offending agent is the treatment of choice. This patient would benefit from switching pregabalin to a different fibromyalgia drug that is not associated with peripheral edema, such as duloxetine.

This patient's lower extremity edema is associated with the vasodilatory effects of pregabalin and not volume overload (no jugular venous distension, $S_3$, pulmonary crackles). In this situation, the use of diuretics can lead to volume depletion, electrolyte disorders, and kidney dysfunction. Discontinuing the drug responsible for the edema is a better strategy.

Duplex Doppler ultrasonography is a useful tool in the evaluation of deep venous thrombosis (DVT). However, DVT typically produces unilateral edema. Additionally, this patient has no risk factors for DVT (prolonged immobilization, cancer, previous DVT) and lacks supporting findings, such as calf swelling, tenderness, and superficial venous dilation.

Although compression stockings may help reduce edema, removal of the offending agent will likely resolve this patient's edema and obviate the need for compression stockings. Furthermore, compression stockings have poor adherence rates because of high cost, discomfort, and the difficulty that patients experience in donning and removing the stockings.

### KEY POINT

- In patients with drug-induced edema, removal of the offending agent is the treatment of choice.

### Bibliography
Ratchford EV, Evans NS. Approach to lower extremity edema. Curr Treat Options Cardiovasc Med. 2017;19:16. [PMID: 28290004] doi: 10.1007/s11936-017-0518-6

## Item 53    Answer:    C

**Educational Objective:**   Diagnose major depressive disorder.

This patient meets the diagnostic criteria for major depressive disorder. The DSM-5 requires at least five of the following symptoms (at least one of which must be depressed mood or anhedonia) to be present almost all of the time during the same 2-week period: depressed mood, anhedonia, insomnia or hypersomnia, significant change in weight or appetite, fatigue or decreased energy, psychomotor agitation or retardation, difficulty concentrating, feelings of worthlessness or excessive guilt, and recurrent thoughts of death or suicidal ideation. Symptoms of major depressive disorder cause work-related and social impairment and cannot be attributed to a medical condition, drug, or substance use. A tool for identifying and assessing the severity of depression is the PHQ-9 (www.integration.samhsa.gov/images/res/PHQ%20-%20Questions.pdf). The items of the PHQ-9 correlate with the DSM-5 criteria. Each item is scored from 0 (not bothered by the symptom) to 3 (bothered by the symptom every day); the maximum score is 27. A score of 5 to 9 indicates mild depression, 10 to 14 moderate depression, 15 to 19 moderately severe depression, and 20 or more severe depression.

Patients with bipolar disorder often present with major depressive disorder, and it is important for clinicians to inquire about any history of periods of elevated mood, increased energy, and decreased need for sleep. Without a history of such episodes, bipolar disorder cannot be diagnosed.

Generalized anxiety disorder (GAD) and other anxiety disorders can often be comorbid with major depressive disorder. Patients with GAD often experience sweats, dyspnea, palpitations, difficulty swallowing, nausea, chest and abdominal pain, loose stools, muscle tension, insomnia, fatigue, tachycardia, and tremor. Diagnosis should be considered in patients with multiple unexplained physical symptoms. This patient does not exhibit the excessive anxiety and restlessness typical of a patient with GAD.

Persistent depressive disorder, previously known as dysthymic disorder or dysthymia, is characterized by depressed mood most of the time for at least 2 years and with at least two of the following symptoms while depressed: appetite change (increased or decreased), fatigue or low energy, decreased self-esteem, insomnia or hypersomnia, poor concentration, and feelings of hopelessness. The symptoms are less severe than in major depressive disorder. This patient has more severe symptoms that have lasted only 6 months, with no history of depression.

### KEY POINT

- Major depressive disorder is diagnosed by the presence of at least five cardinal symptoms, at least one of which is depressed mood or anhedonia, during the same 2-week period; a tool for identifying and assessing the severity of depression is the PHQ-9.

### Bibliography
McCarron RM, Vanderlip ER, Rado J. Depression. Ann Intern Med. 2016;165:ITC49-ITC64. [PMID: 27699401] doi:10.7326/AITC201610040

## Item 54    Answer:    D

**Educational Objective:**   Diagnose systemic exertion intolerance disease.

The most likely diagnosis is systemic exertion intolerance disease (SEID). Fatigue can be classified as fatigue secondary to another cause, secondary to multiple factors (termed chronic multifactorial fatigue), or a primary condition. In the past, the latter condition was termed chronic fatigue syndrome, myalgic encephalitis, or neurasthenia. In 2015, the Institute of Medicine recommended using the term systemic exertion intolerance disease over the other terms. The diagnosis of SEID requires the presence of (1) substantial reduction or impairment in the ability to engage in preillness levels of occupational, educational, social, or personal activities for at least 6 months, accompanied by profound fatigue that is not relieved by rest; (2) postexertional malaise (worsening of symptoms after physical, cognitive, or emotional effort); and (3) unrefreshing sleep. In addition to the three major criteria, the patient must also demonstrate cognitive impairment or orthostatic intolerance (symptoms such as lightheadedness, dizziness, fatigue, cognitive deficits, and visual difficulties that worsen when a person stands upright and improve when the person lies back down). This patient meets the validated diagnostic criteria for SEID.

Chronic multifactorial fatigue is a clinical condition defined as chronic fatigue symptoms of at least 6 months' duration in the setting of multiple fatiguing factors (medical and/or psychosocial). This patient's benign history and unrevealing evaluation argue against chronic multifactorial fatigue.

Mood disturbances are highly comorbid in patients with SEID (approximately 70% of patients), and all patients with SEID should be screened for depression and anxiety. This patient was screened appropriately and does not have findings consistent with an underlying mood disorder.

Post–Lyme disease syndrome has been reported in approximately 10% of patients after treatment of erythema migrans. Although the condition is often erroneously called chronic Lyme disease, studies have found no microbiologic evidence of chronic or latent infection after appropriate treatment. Symptoms include fatigue, arthralgia, myalgia, and impairment of memory or cognition that can last for years after treatment of the acute infection. Clinical trials have shown no benefit of prolonged antibiotic treatment for post–Lyme disease syndrome. This patient has unrefreshing sleep, postexertional malaise, and orthostatic intolerance, which are more consistent with SEID.

### KEY POINT

- The diagnosis of systemic exertion intolerance disease requires the presence of fatigue of at least 6 months' duration with substantial reduction in preillness activities, postexertional malaise, unrefreshing sleep, and either cognitive impairment or orthostatic intolerance.

### Bibliography
Committee on the Diagnostic Criteria for Myalgic Encephalomyelitis/Chronic Fatigue Syndrome, Board on the Health of Select Populations, Institute of Medicine. Beyond Myalgic Encephalomyelitis/Chronic Fatigue Syndrome: Redefining an Illness. Washington, DC: National Academies Press; 2015. [PMID: 25695122]

## Item 55     Answer:   B

**Educational Objective:** Diagnose epididymitis by physical examination.

This patient is most likely to have pain relief with testicular elevation (Prehn sign). His history and examination findings (erythema and swelling of the hemiscrotum; fever; tenderness to palpation near the epididymis; and lack of worsening symptoms, nausea, vomiting, and abdominal pain) suggest a diagnosis of epididymitis. Prehn sign, which is alleviation of pain with elevation of the testicle or scrotum, can clinically support this diagnosis. Although this finding can suggest a diagnosis of epididymitis, it does not rule out other possibilities, such as testicular torsion; however, testicular torsion is less likely given this patient's presentation.

An absent cremasteric reflex suggests testicular torsion. A patient with testicular torsion would have acutely worsening and severe hemiscrotal pain, hemiscrotum elevation, abdominal pain, nausea, and vomiting. These findings are not present in this patient, and the test result would likely be negative.

Varicoceles are caused by dilation of the testicular vein and pampiniform plexus. They are common, occurring in 15% of men. Scrotal examination reveals a left-sided (90%) scrotal mass with a "bag of worms" consistency that increases with standing and decreases while supine. This patient's findings are not consistent with varicocele, and examining the patient in both standing and supine positions is unlikely to support this diagnosis.

A transillumination study, which is performed to identify a hydrocele, is not likely to have a positive result in this patient with findings that suggest epididymitis. A hydrocele manifests over a longer time frame, initially causing no symptoms and then causing a dull aching scrotal discomfort. Examination can reveal a smooth though tense scrotal mass, which transilluminates when a light source is applied adjacently.

### KEY POINT

- A positive Prehn sign (relief of pain with scrotal elevation) suggests a diagnosis of epididymitis, although it does not rule out other possibilities, such as testicular torsion.

### Bibliography
Crawford P, Crop JA. Evaluation of scrotal masses. Am Fam Physician. 2014;89:723-7. [PMID: 24784335]

## Item 56     Answer:   D

**Educational Objective:** Treat chronic low back pain with an NSAID.

The most appropriate pharmacologic option for this patient is an NSAID, such as ibuprofen. For patients with chronic low back pain, clinicians and patients should initially select nonpharmacologic treatment with acupuncture, cognitive behavioral therapy, electromyography biofeedback, exercise, mindfulness-based stress reduction (moderate-quality evidence), low-level laser therapy, motor control exercise, multidisciplinary rehabilitation, progressive relaxation, operant therapy or spinal manipulation, tai chi, or yoga. According to a 2017 clinical practice guideline from the American College of Physicians (ACP), pharmacologic therapy can be considered in patients with chronic low back pain that has not responded to nonpharmacologic therapy. The ACP recommends NSAIDs as first-line therapy, administered in the lowest effective dosage.

There is little evidence that acetaminophen is effective in reducing pain or improving functional status in patients with acute or chronic low back pain. As such, acetaminophen should not be recommended to this patient.

The FDA recently approved duloxetine for treating chronic low back pain on the basis of evidence from randomized controlled trials that showed a small improvement in both pain and function with its use. However, the ACP guideline deems both duloxetine and tramadol as second-line pharmacologic options (weak recommendation, moderate-quality evidence), reserved for use only after first-line options have been exhausted.

In a randomized controlled trial, opioids, such as hydrocodone, were not more effective than nonopioid therapy in treating chronic low back pain. Opioids should be used only in the treatment of chronic pain when the benefits outweigh the risks (such as abuse potential) and when a clear discussion of risks and benefits has occurred with the patient. This patient is unlikely to benefit from hydrocodone therapy.

Moderate-quality evidence showed that tramadol resulted in moderate short-term pain relief in patients with chronic low back pain and a small improvement in function compared with placebo. Of note, tramadol is a weak opioid agonist that also blocks reuptake of serotonin and norepinephrine; like other opioids, it is associated with the risk for abuse. Its use is relegated to patients who achieve inadequate relief with nonpharmacologic therapy and NSAIDs, and only after a frank discussion of the harms and benefits.

**KEY POINT**

- For patients with chronic low back pain, clinicians and patients should initially select nonpharmacologic treatment; NSAIDs can be considered in patients who have had an inadequate response to nonpharmacologic therapy.

**Bibliography**

Qaseem A, Wilt TJ, McLean RM, Forciea MA; Clinical Guidelines Committee of the American College of Physicians. Noninvasive treatments for acute, subacute, and chronic low back pain: a clinical practice guideline from the American College of Physicians. Ann Intern Med. 2017;166:514-530. [PMID: 28192789] doi:10.7326/M16-2367

**Item 57** **Answer: D**

**Educational Objective: Evaluate recurrent epistaxis.**

The most appropriate management is nasal endoscopy. Ninety percent of episodes of epistaxis occur in the anterior nasal septum in the Kiesselbach area. Anterior bleeding can be managed with compression for at least 15 minutes. Posterior epistaxis (behind the posterior middle turbinate, requiring a nasopharyngoscope for visualization) may be more difficult to manage and is more common in older patients. Common causes of epistaxis include topical intranasal medications (such as glucocorticoids or antihistamines), dehumidification, and self-induced digital trauma. Among patients with epistaxis serious enough to require hospitalization, almost half have a causal systemic condition, such as anticoagulation, hemophilia, hematologic malignancy, neoplasm, and acquired coagulopathies from kidney or liver disease. Recurrent unilateral epistaxis may represent a neoplasm; hence, this patient should be referred for nasal endoscopy.

Low-dose aspirin may be associated with a slight increase in the risk for epistaxis, although data have not been conclusive and do not support routine discontinuation in otherwise healthy patients with epistaxis. Notably, other NSAIDs have not been associated with epistaxis. Even if aspirin were stopped, this patient requires further assessment given the presence of unilateral bleeding.

This patient has no symptoms of anemia or history of excessive blood loss. Although epistaxis may be associated with coagulopathies, this patient is not taking an anticoagulant and is otherwise at low risk for an acquired coagulopathy that manifests only as epistaxis. Therefore, coagulation studies are not warranted.

In 80% of patients with epistaxis, results of laboratory evaluation are normal; therefore, routine laboratory testing is not required. A complete blood count, prothrombin time, and activated partial thromboplastin time might be considered in patients with symptoms or signs of a bleeding disorder and those with severe or recurrent epistaxis.

**KEY POINT**

- Recurrent unilateral epistaxis may be a sign of neoplasm and warrants referral for nasal endoscopy.

**Bibliography**

Morgan DJ, Kellerman R. Epistaxis: evaluation and treatment. Prim Care. 2014;41:63-73. [PMID: 24439881] doi:10.1016/j.pop.2013.10.007

**Item 58** **Answer: D**

**Educational Objective: Identify the Plan-Do-Study-Act cycle as an effective quality improvement method.**

The most likely intervention to improve hand hygiene in this hospital is to use a Plan-Do-Study-Act (PDSA) cycle. A PDSA cycle is a four-step process involving a rapid cycle of change in which baseline data are collected, an intervention is planned and then implemented on a small scale, the results are analyzed, and an action plan is made. Additional PDSA cycles are completed until the desired results are achieved. In this case, a PDSA cycle could be used to study hand hygiene procedures and implement interventions to increase rates of hand hygiene, with the overall goal of reducing the incidence of hospital-acquired infections.

Spaghetti diagrams are used to visually display flow through a system. The flows are drawn as lines on a map and look similar to spaghetti noodles. As an example, a spaghetti diagram may be used to follow a medication order through a hospital unit from order generation to administration of the medication. The diagram can help highlight inefficiencies or redundancies in a system. Although useful in identifying areas ripe for increased efficiency, a spaghetti diagram will have no impact on improving hand hygiene rates.

The Lean model aims to maximize value and minimize waste by closely examining a system's processes and eliminating non–value-added activities within the system. Value stream mapping can be used to graphically display the steps of a process and the time required for each step, thereby

CONT.

highlighting process inefficiencies or areas of waste and allowing for their improvement. The Lean model could be used to determine inefficiencies in hospital processes (such as waiting times); however, it would not help improve hand hygiene rates.

Reiterating the importance of hand hygiene in an email to the entire staff may be a part of a planned intervention to improve hand hygiene, although it alone is unlikely to provide sustained results.

### KEY POINT

- A Plan-Do-Study-Act cycle is a four-step process involving a rapid cycle of change in which baseline data are collected, an intervention is planned and then implemented on a small scale, the results are analyzed, and an action plan is made.

### Bibliography
Morelli MS. Using the Plan, Do, Study, Act Model to implement a quality improvement program in your practice. Am J Gastroenterol. 2016;111: 1220-2. [PMID: 27527744]

## Item 59    Answer:   D

**Educational Objective:** **Identify medications associated with increased risk for side effects in an older patient.**

Quetiapine is the medication with greatest potential for adverse effects in this older patient taking multiple prescription medications. Although treatment of comorbid conditions often requires multiple medications, evidence shows that half of older adults take one or more medications that are not medically necessary (that is, not indicated, not effective, or therapeutically duplicative). Frequent review of patient medications to verify their necessity and proper dosing is an essential aspect of optimal geriatric care. Notably, certain medications carry a particularly high risk for geriatric patients. In an effort to improve the care of older adults by reducing the use of potentially inappropriate medications, the American Geriatrics Society (AGS) has compiled a list of high-risk drugs that must be carefully considered in terms of risk-to-benefit ratio in the elderly (available at http://geriatricscareonline.org/ProductAbstract/american-geriatrics-society-updated-beers-criteria-for-potentially-inappropriate-medication-use-in-older-adults/CL001). All antipsychotic medications, both first- and second-generation, have significant adverse effects, including anticholinergic effects, extrapyramidal symptoms, and sedation, and older patients are particularly susceptible to these negative effects. For this reason, the AGS 2015 Beers Criteria for Potentially Inappropriate Medication Use in Older Adults recommends avoidance of quetiapine and all antipsychotic medications.

Acetaminophen is relatively safe for older patients if not used at maximal doses for extended periods. Side effects from acetaminophen are far less likely and less severe than other commonly used systemic analgesics, including opioids and NSAIDs.

Amlodipine is not listed as a medication to avoid in the AGS 2015 Beers Criteria. Although the drug could potentially cause excessive blood pressure reduction, this patient's blood pressure is under acceptable control and without orthostatic changes.

Lisinopril can potentially cause electrolyte abnormalities, orthostatic hypotension, and kidney insufficiency. However, this patient has no evidence of these problems, and lisinopril is not included in the Beers Criteria as a potentially inappropriate medication.

### KEY POINT

- Frequent review of patient medications to verify their necessity and proper dosing is an essential aspect of optimal geriatric care.

### Bibliography
The American Geriatrics Society 2015 Beers Criteria Update Expert Panel. American Geriatrics Society 2015 updated Beers criteria for potentially inappropriate medication use in older adults. J Am Geriatr Soc. 2015;63:2227-46. [PMID: 26446832] doi:10.1111/jgs.13702

## Item 60    Answer:   B

**Educational Objective:** **Diagnose opioid-induced hyperalgesia.**

The most likely diagnosis is opioid-induced hyperalgesia. Opioid-induced hyperalgesia is thought to result from repeated exposure to systemic opioids. In patients with this pain syndrome, the character of their pain may change during the course of opioid therapy, pain may worsen with increased opioid dosages, and pain may decrease when opioid dosages are reduced. In this case, the patient has chronic pain as a sequela of her cancer diagnosis and treatment, and she has required significant dosage escalation in the absence of progressive disease. She also has evidence of cognitive slowing, hyperreflexia, and myoclonus as a result of the neuroexcitatory effects of long-term opioid use; these signs are concerning for opioid-induced toxicity. Appropriate management of opioid-induced hyperalgesia includes opioid dosage reduction in a monitored setting with close follow-up.

Malingering is characterized by the development of symptoms that lack a pathologic basis. The key feature is faking or exaggerating symptoms for an obvious external benefit, such as money, drugs, or escaping criminal prosecution. Malingering should be suspected in patients with inconsistencies in the history and physical examination; nonadherence to recommended diagnostic testing or treatments; known or suspected personality disorder; and legal difficulties. There is no indication of these traits to suggest malingering as the cause of this patient's symptoms.

Opioid withdrawal is unlikely in this patient given her constant symptoms and escalation in the dosages of hydromorphone and transdermal fentanyl.

Pseudoaddiction is a phenomenon in which patients exhibit behaviors concerning for substance use disorder or addiction that are driven by inadequate pain control in the setting of a documented progressive disease. Although this patient has a sequela of cancer therapy, her clinical status is unchanged, and there is no evidence of progressive disease on physical examination or CT scan.

**KEY POINT**

- In patients with opioid-induced hyperalgesia, the character of their pain may change during the course of opioid therapy, pain may worsen with increased opioid dosages, and pain may decrease when opioid dosages are reduced.

**Bibliography**

Yi P, Pryzbylkowski P. Opioid induced hyperalgesia. Pain Med. 2015;16 Suppl 1:S32-6. [PMID: 26461074] doi: 10.1111/pme.12914

**H** **Item 61**      **Answer:   D**

**Educational Objective:** Manage dual antiplatelet therapy in a patient with recent coronary stent placement who is undergoing urgent noncardiac surgery.

The most appropriate management of this patient's anti-platelet therapy is to withhold clopidogrel 5 to 7 days before surgery and continue aspirin. According to the 2016 American College of Cardiology/American Heart Association focused update on the duration of dual antiplatelet therapy (DAPT), perioperative management is based on surgical bleeding risk balanced with the risk for stent thrombosis. The risk for stent thrombosis is contingent on both the indication for coronary stent placement (stable ischemic heart disease [SIHD] or acute coronary syndrome [ACS]) and the amount of time that has passed from the time of stent placement.

For patients who have a stent placed for SIHD, DAPT (aspirin plus a $P2Y_{12}$ inhibitor) should be continued for at least 30 days after bare metal stent placement and a minimum of 6 months after drug-eluting stent placement. DAPT is recommended for 1 year in patients with ACS, regardless of medical management or cardiac stent placement, with the understanding that discontinuation may be reasonable if high bleeding risk is identified or the patient has overt bleeding on DAPT. However, in the perioperative setting, and especially if the risk of surgical delay exceeds the risk for stent thrombosis, discontinuation of the $P2Y_{12}$ inhibitor can be considered after a minimum of 30 days in the case of bare metal stent placement or 3 months after drug-eluting stent placement. It is optimal to continue DAPT for 6 months after drug-eluting stent placement, especially in the case of ACS, if the risk for surgical delay does not exceed the risk for stent thrombosis. Aspirin should be continued, if at all possible, along with restarting of DAPT as soon as bleeding risk has sufficiently diminished.

If surgery must be performed within those periods after percutaneous coronary intervention, DAPT should be maintained perioperatively unless the risk for major bleeding exceeds the risk for stent thrombosis. Communication

with the surgical team and the patient regarding risks and benefits of withholding DAPT within these time frames is advised.

**KEY POINT**

- In patients taking dual antiplatelet therapy, if the risk of surgical delay exceeds the risk for stent thrombosis, discontinuation of the $P2Y_{12}$ inhibitor can be considered after a minimum of 30 days in the case of bare metal stent placement or 3 months after drug-eluting stent placement.

**Bibliography**

Levine GN, Bates ER, Bittl JA, Brindis RG, Fihn SD, Fleisher LA, et al. 2016 ACC/AHA guideline focused update on duration of dual antiplatelet therapy in patients with coronary artery disease: a report of the American College of Cardiology/American Heart Association Task Force on Clinical Practice Guidelines. J Am Coll Cardiol. 2016;68:1082-115. [PMID: 27036918]

**Item 62**      **Answer:   A**

**Educational Objective:** Engage a patient in shared decision making for prostate cancer screening.

The most appropriate action is to first engage the patient in a discussion of the benefits and harms of prostate cancer screening. No organization recommends prostate-specific antigen (PSA) testing for prostate cancer screening without a discussion of the benefits and harms and a patient's clear expressed preference for screening. Clinicians should inform men about the limited potential benefits and substantial harms of screening for prostate cancer. Screening offers a small potential benefit of reducing the chance of dying of prostate cancer. However, many men will experience potential harms of screening, including false-positive results that require additional testing and possible prostate biopsy; overdiagnosis and overtreatment; and treatment complications, such as incontinence and impotence. All organizations recommend individualized decision making about screening for prostate cancer so that each man has an opportunity to incorporate his values and preferences into his decision. On the basis of the available evidence, it is not possible to make a definitive recommendation for or against prostate cancer screening in men with a family history of prostate cancer. Although screening may offer additional potential benefits for these men compared with the general population, screening also has the potential to increase exposure to potential harms, especially among men with relatives whose cancer was overdiagnosed.

Although some expert groups recommend performing a digital rectal examination in conjunction with PSA testing for prostate cancer screening, digital rectal examination alone is not recommended because this test has suboptimal sensitivity and very low positive predictive value.

The U.S. Preventive Services Task Force recommends that clinicians should not screen men who do not express a preference for screening and recommends against

PSA-based screening for prostate cancer in men aged 70 years and older.

**KEY POINT**

- The decision to pursue prostate cancer screening should be individualized so that each man has an opportunity to understand the potential benefits and harms of screening and to incorporate his values and preferences into his decision.

**Bibliography**

Grossman DC, Curry SJ, Owens DK, Bibbins-Domingo K, Caughey AB, Davidson KW, et al; US Preventive Services Task Force. Screening for prostate cancer: US Preventive Services Task Force recommendation statement. JAMA. 2018;319:1901-1913. [PMID: 29801017] doi:10.1001/jama.2018.3710

**Item 63     Answer:     E**

**Educational Objective:   Manage audible oropharyngeal secretions in a patient at the end of life.**

This patient has audible posterior oropharyngeal secretions, which are most appropriately managed with family education and reassurance. Although several studies suggest that respiratory distress is not typically associated with these secretions, caregivers are often concerned by what is commonly referred to as the "death rattle." The first steps in management include caregiver education and anticipatory guidance. Additionally, repositioning often allows secretions to drain without pharmacologic intervention. Mouth hygiene with a sponge swab may also be helpful.

Current literature does not support the routine use of antimuscarinic drugs in the treatment of death rattle. A 2014 literature review acknowledged that death rattle leads to distress in both relatives and professional caregivers; however, its impact on patients is unclear, and medical therapy is unproven. Studies involving atropine, glycopyrronium, scopolamine, hyoscine butylbromide, and/or octreotide were reviewed, and only one study used a placebo group. There is currently no evidence that the use of any antimuscarinic drug is superior to no treatment. In addition, the use of anticholinergic agents in patients who are awake can lead to undesirable symptoms, such as dry mouth and urinary retention.

Suctioning by catheter should be avoided in managing end-of-life secretions unless the secretions are causing the patient obvious respiratory distress or cough. Suction catheters can cause local trauma.

**KEY POINT**

- Audible posterior oropharyngeal secretions ("death rattle") are common at the end of life and are best managed with family education and reassurance.

**Bibliography**

Lokker ME, van Zuylen L, van der Rijt CC, van der Heide A. Prevalence, impact, and treatment of death rattle: a systematic review. J Pain Symptom Manage. 2014;47:105-22. [PMID: 23790419] doi:10.1016/j.jpainsymman.2013.03.011

**Item 64     Answer:   D**

**Educational Objective:   Vaccinate an adult smoker against pneumococcal disease.**

This patient should be administered the 23-valent pneumococcal polysaccharide vaccine (PPSV23). Pneumococcal vaccination is recommended in all adults aged 65 years and older and adults aged 19 to 64 years with certain high-risk conditions. Two pneumococcal vaccines are available: PPSV23 and a 13-valent conjugate vaccine (PCV13). The Advisory Committee on Immunization Practices recommends administering PPSV23 alone to select immunocompetent patients aged 19 to 64 years, including those with chronic heart, liver, or lung disease; diabetes mellitus; cochlear implants; cerebrospinal fluid leak; alcoholism; or cigarette smoking. Because this patient is a current smoker, he should be given PPSV23.

In adults aged 19 to 64 years with immunocompromise, cochlear implants, or a history of cerebrospinal fluid leaks, PCV13 should be administered in addition to PPSV23. In these patients, a single dose of PCV13 should be given first, followed by a single dose of PPSV23 at least 8 weeks later. Additionally, all adults aged 65 years and older who have not previously been vaccinated should receive PCV13, followed by a dose of PPSV23 1 year later. For immunocompetent adults aged 65 years and older who previously received one or more doses of PPSV23, a single dose of PCV13 should be given at least 1 year after the most recent PPSV23 dose. This patient does not meet the criteria for PCV13 administration.

All adults aged 50 years and older, including those with a previous episode of zoster, should receive the recombinant (inactivated) zoster vaccine to reduce the incidence of zoster and postherpetic neuralgia. The recombinant zoster vaccine is recommended in preference to the live attenuated zoster vaccine, and adults who have been previously vaccinated with the live attenuated zoster vaccine should be revaccinated with the recombinant zoster vaccine after a period of at least 8 weeks. This patient should receive the recombinant zoster vaccine in 2 years.

In persons who previously received the tetanus toxoid, reduced diphtheria toxoid, and acellular pertussis (Tdap) vaccine, revaccination with a tetanus and diphtheria toxoids (Td) booster is recommended every 10 years. Additionally, for pregnant women, one dose of the Tdap vaccine should be administered during each pregnancy between 27 weeks' and 36 weeks' gestation, regardless of when the last dose of Td or Tdap was given. This patient last received the Tdap vaccine 9 years ago and should receive a Td booster in 1 year.

Given the patient's history of cigarette smoking, offering no vaccinations at this time would not be the best strategy.

**KEY POINT**

- The 23-valent pneumococcal polysaccharide vaccine should be administered to select immunocompetent patients aged 19 to 64 years, including those with chronic heart, liver, or lung disease; diabetes mellitus; cochlear implants; cerebrospinal fluid leak; alcoholism; or cigarette smoking.

## Bibliography

Kim DK, Riley LE, Hunter P; Advisory Committee on Immunization Practices. Recommended immunization schedule for adults aged 19 years or older, United States, 2018. Ann Intern Med. 2018;168:210–220. [PMID: 29404596] doi:10.7326/M17-3439

## Item 65    Answer:    B

**Educational Objective:   Diagnose binge eating disorder.**

This patient most likely has binge eating disorder (BED), which is characterized by impulsive overeating and feeling loss of control around food. The diagnosis of this disorder requires at least three of the following characteristics occurring at least once weekly for 3 months: abnormally rapid consumption, consuming large amounts of food when not hungry, eating alone due to embarrassment, eating until uncomfortably full, and feelings of guilt related to overconsumption. BED is more common than both anorexia and bulimia nervosa and is often accompanied by other psychiatric problems. The primary treatment is cognitive behavioral therapy.

Bulimia nervosa and the binging subtype of anorexia nervosa both include episodes of binge eating like BED. The key in differentiating BED from these diseases is the lack of compensatory behaviors (such as induced vomiting and laxative abuse) to avoid weight gain. The major difference between bulimia nervosa and the binging subtype of anorexia nervosa is that patients with anorexia nervosa have a low BMI (usually <18).

Many people have episodes of overeating in which they may eat until uncomfortable or feel guilty about their eating. However, simple overeating does not meet the diagnostic criteria for BED and is not accompanied by the feelings of loss of control over food consumption.

### KEY POINT

- The diagnosis of binge eating disorder requires at least three of the following characteristics occurring at least once weekly for 3 months: abnormally rapid consumption, consuming large amounts of food when not hungry, eating alone due to embarrassment, eating until uncomfortably full, and feelings of guilt related to overconsumption.

## Bibliography

Attia E. In the clinic. Eating disorders. Ann Intern Med. 2012;156:ITC4-1–ITC4-15, quiz ITC4-16. [PMID: 22473445] doi:10.7326/0003-4819-156-7-201204030-01004

## Item 66    Answer:    B

**Educational Objective:   Manage cyclic mastalgia.**

The most appropriate next step in this patient's management is the use of a well-fitting bra. Breast pain is common among women and is categorized primarily as cyclic or noncyclic in relation to the menstrual cycle. This patient has cyclic mastalgia, which is bilateral and diffuse and worsens in the days before menses and then abates. Cyclic mastalgia is often related to hormonal changes that occur with ovulation. Because most symptoms of cyclic mastalgia are self-limited, management usually requires only education, reassurance, and appropriate breast support.

There is no evidence from controlled studies that avoidance of caffeine in the diet or beverages relieves breast pain. Similarly, no evidence supports the use of vitamin E and evening primrose oil in reducing pain.

Cyclic mastalgia with no abnormal clinical findings, such as a breast mass or skin changes, does not warrant diagnostic imaging. Hence, ultrasonography and mammography are unnecessary in this patient.

Danazol is approved by the FDA for management of mastalgia, but because of limiting androgenic side effects, it is recommended only for management of persistent severe cyclic breast pain unrelieved by conservative management. If education, reassurance, and appropriate breast support do not sufficiently control symptoms, acetaminophen or an oral or topical NSAID may be useful and can be recommended before consideration of danazol therapy.

### KEY POINT

- Cyclic mastalgia is often related to hormonal changes that occur with ovulation, resulting in diffuse premenstrual breast pain that resolves with the menstrual cycle; the most appropriate management is education, reassurance, and appropriate breast support.

## Bibliography

Iddon J, Dixon JM. Mastalgia. BMJ. 2013;347:f3288. [PMID: 24336097] doi:10.1136/bmj.f3288

## Item 67    Answer:    D

**Educational Objective:   Diagnose central vertigo on the basis of Dix-Hallpike maneuver results.**

The most likely diagnosis is vertebrobasilar ischemia. In patients with vertigo, it is crucial to differentiate central from peripheral causes, especially in patients with acute vertigo concerning for vertebrobasilar ischemia and other central causes. The Dix-Hallpike maneuver is an effective bedside test for this purpose. In this test, the examiner stands at the patient's side and rotates the patient's head 45 degrees; the examiner then moves the patient, whose eyes are open, from the seated to the supine ear-down position. The patient's neck is extended slightly so that the chin is pointed upward, and the patient is observed for nystagmus. During the test, the latency, duration, fatigability, and direction of nystagmus are noted. The maneuver is repeated with the patient's head turned in the opposite direction. Findings that indicate central vertigo are nystagmus with an immediate onset (no latency), longer duration (>1 minute), no fatigability, and vertical or horizontal directionality without a torsional component. With central vertigo, the direction of nystagmus may vary depending on the direction of the patient's gaze. Potentially life-threatening conditions associated with

Answers and Critiques

central vertigo include ischemia, infarction, or hemorrhage of the cerebellum or brainstem. Patients at high risk include those with hypertension, diabetes mellitus, hyperlipidemia, or advanced age. Vertebrobasilar stroke is usually, but not always, accompanied by dysarthria, dysphagia, diplopia, weakness, or numbness. Cerebellar infarct may present with gait or truncal ataxia or with vertigo alone. In a patient presenting with suspicion for a central cause of vertigo, brain MRI and magnetic resonance angiography of the posterior cerebral circulation are the preferred diagnostic studies.

Dix-Hallpike maneuver results that suggest peripheral vertigo include nystagmus that is delayed in onset (presence of latency), is of short duration (<1 minute), exhibits fatigability (habituation), and is primarily unidirectional (usually up-beating and torsional [rotary phenomenon]). The presence of severe symptoms also indicates peripheral vertigo. The most common cause of peripheral vertigo (and all types of vertigo) is benign paroxysmal positional vertigo. Vestibular neuronitis (or labyrinthitis, if hearing is affected), another cause of peripheral vertigo, may follow a viral syndrome that has affected the vestibular portion of cranial nerve VIII. Less common causes of peripheral vertigo are Meniere disease (triad of vertigo, hearing loss, and tinnitus), perilymphatic fistula (vertigo and hearing loss with history of straining or trauma), and acoustic neuroma (tinnitus and associated unilateral sensorineural hearing loss).

An additional bedside test that can be performed to help differentiate central from peripheral causes of vertigo is the HINTS (Head Impulse, Nystagmus, and Test of Skew) examination. Findings concerning for a central cause of vertigo are the absence of catch-up saccades on the head impulse test, bidirectional nystagmus on the nystagmus assessment, and the presence of vertical skew on the test of skew.

### KEY POINT

- In patients with central vertigo, the Dix-Hallpike maneuver produces nystagmus with an immediate onset (no latency), longer duration (>1 minute), no fatigability, and vertical or horizontal directionality without a torsional component.

### Bibliography

Kim JS, Zee DS. Clinical practice. Benign paroxysmal positional vertigo. N Engl J Med. 2014;370:1138-47. [PMID: 24645946] doi: 10.1056/NEJMcp1309481

## Item 68     Answer:    B

**Educational Objective:**   Evaluate prepatellar bursitis.

This patient has prepatellar bursitis, and the first step in management should be fluid aspiration. Prepatellar bursitis is caused by inflammation of the prepatellar bursa that overlies the patella. Patients present with anterior knee pain and swelling. Physical examination reveals a palpable fluid collection with preserved active and passive range of motion of the knee. The most common cause of chronic prepatellar bursitis is repetitive trauma, as is likely the case in this patient, who must frequently kneel in his job as a carpet installer. Other causes include gout and infection. Most cases of acute prepatellar bursitis are infectious (typically related to skin bacteria), although trauma and gout are other potential causes. Regardless of the duration of the swelling, all patients with prepatellar bursitis should undergo fluid aspiration. Gram stain and culture of the bursal fluid should be obtained and analyzed for leukocyte count and for the presence of crystals to evaluate for the possibility of an underlying infectious cause and gout.

Prepatellar bursitis due to repetitive trauma from kneeling is managed with activity modification (avoidance of kneeling), in addition to the use of oral NSAIDs such as ibuprofen. It would be inappropriate to recommend activity modification or NSAIDs before first analyzing bursal fluid to rule out infection or gout.

Plain radiography is not usually required for the diagnosis of prepatellar bursitis. It may show soft-tissue swelling on lateral views but rarely aids in establishing the correct diagnosis. Plain radiographs should be obtained when knee osteoarthritis is suspected or there is concern for fracture, neither of which applies to this patient.

Prepatellar bursitis caused by gout is diagnosed by bursal fluid analysis and detecting monosodium urate crystals with polarized microscopy. A high serum urate level supports the potential for gout; however, most patients with hyperuricemia do not have gout, and the serum urate level may be low during some acute attacks. Therefore, it would be inappropriate to obtain a serum uric acid level in this patient.

### KEY POINT

- Prepatellar bursitis can be caused by repetitive trauma, infection, or gout; fluid aspiration and subsequent analysis should be performed in all patients.

### Bibliography

Hong E, Kraft MC. Evaluating anterior knee pain. Med Clin North Am. 2014;98:697-717, xi. [PMID: 24994047] doi:10.1016/j.mcna.2014.03.001

## Item 69     Answer:    A

**Educational Objective:**   Prevent a pressure injury in a patient with limited mobility.

An advanced static mattress is the most appropriate intervention to prevent pressure injuries (also known as pressure ulcers) in this patient. Pressure injuries are common in hospitals and long-term care settings. They can result in decreased quality of life, with associated depression, impaired mobility, and social isolation. The Centers for Medicare & Medicaid Services has selected the development of pressure ulcers as a sentinel health event (unexpected and preventable occurrence that results in serious patient injury) for health care facilities. Prevention of pressure injuries starts with identifying patients at risk. There are many standardized risk assessment tools, but evidence of whether these

CONT.

are superior to clinical judgment is inconclusive. Risk factors include advanced age, cognitive impairment, reduced mobility, sensory impairment, and comorbid conditions that affect skin integrity (such as low body weight, incontinence, edema, poor microcirculation, and hypoalbuminemia). Pressure redistribution is the most important factor in preventing pressure injuries through the use of pressure-reducing equipment and proper patient positioning. In 2015, the American College of Physicians (ACP) published a clinical practice guideline for risk assessment and prevention of pressure ulcers. The guideline recommends regular, structured risk assessment of patients and the use of an advanced static mattress or advanced static overlay for patients who are at increased risk. An advanced static mattress is made of specialized sheepskin, foam, or gel and is immobile when a patient lies on it, whereas an advanced static overlay is a pad composed of foam or gel that is secured to the top of a regular mattress.

The ACP guideline recommends against the use of alternating air mattresses because of lack of data showing a clear advantage as well as cost considerations.

There are limited data concerning the preventive effectiveness of frequent patient repositioning, dietary supplements (such as zinc, creams, or dressings), and silicone foam dressings as isolated interventions.

### KEY POINT

- An advanced static mattress or mattress overlay made of specialized sheepskin, foam, or gel provides the best protection against the development of pressure injuries in hospitalized patients.

### Bibliography

Qaseem A, Mir TP, Starkey M, Denberg TD; Clinical Guidelines Committee of the American College of Physicians. Risk assessment and prevention of pressure ulcers: a clinical practice guideline from the American College of Physicians. Ann Intern Med. 2015;162:359-69. [PMID: 25732278] doi:10.7326/M14-1567

## Item 70      Answer:   A

**Educational Objective:**   Screen for HIV infection in a high-risk patient.

The most appropriate interval for HIV screening in this high-risk patient is at least annually. The U.S. Preventive Services Task Force (USPSTF) recommends HIV screening for patients aged 15 to 65 years in all health care settings. The currently recommended method for initial testing is combination HIV antibody immunoassay/p24 antigen testing. An "opt-out" approach is preferred; patients are notified that testing will be performed but can decline. Special consent for testing is not required. HIV testing provides a "teachable moment" to conduct HIV/sexually transmitted infection (STI) prevention counseling and offer pre-exposure prophylaxis for high-risk patients. However, prevention counseling should not be a required activity because it can be perceived as a barrier to screening.

The USPSTF suggests that a reasonable approach is one-time screening of adolescent and adult patients and repeated

screening of high-risk persons, persons engaged in risky behaviors, and those who reside in or receive medical care in high-prevalence settings for HIV infection. Persons at high risk (as opposed to very high risk) include those who have acquired or requested testing for other STIs. High-prevalence settings include STI clinics, correctional facilities, homeless shelters, tuberculosis clinics, clinics serving men who have sex with men (MSM), and adolescent health clinics with a high prevalence of STIs. The USPSTF suggests rescreening persons at increased risk every 3 to 5 years. In the absence of reliable data, the USPSTF suggests screening very high-risk individuals (MSM and injection drug users) for new HIV infection at least annually. Risk categories may change, and the USPSTF notes that rescreening may not be necessary for persons who have not been at increased risk since they were last tested. Women screened during a previous pregnancy should be rescreened in subsequent pregnancies.

In 2015, the Centers for Disease Control and Prevention recommended that providers should offer HIV screening at least annually to all sexually active MSM. Clinicians can also consider the potential benefits of more frequent HIV screening (such as every 3 or 6 months) for some asymptomatic sexually active MSM based on their individual risk factors, local HIV epidemiology, and local policies. The CDC also recommends yearly testing for syphilis, gonorrhea, and chlamydia in MSM; in contrast, the USPSTF has found insufficient evidence to recommend screening for these diseases in men.

### KEY POINT

- Sexually active gay, bisexual, and other men who have sex with men and injection drug users should be screened for HIV infection at least annually.

### Bibliography

DiNenno EA, Prejean J, Irwin K, Delaney KP, Bowles K, Martin T, et al. Recommendations for HIV screening of gay, bisexual, and other men who have sex with men - United States, 2017. MMWR Morb Mortal Wkly Rep. 2017;66:830-832. [PMID: 28796758]

## Item 71      Answer:   D

**Educational Objective:**   Reduce cardiovascular risk with statin therapy in a patient without known atherosclerotic cardiovascular disease.

The most appropriate therapy for primary prevention of atherosclerotic cardiovascular disease (ASCVD) in this patient is simvastatin. All patients at increased cardiovascular risk should be counseled regarding therapeutic lifestyle changes, including dietary modification, regular physical activity, weight loss, and smoking cessation. In addition to therapeutic lifestyle changes, the American College of Cardiology (ACC)/American Heart Association (AHA) cholesterol treatment guideline recommends adding moderate- or high-intensity statin therapy for primary prevention of ASCVD in adults aged 40 to 75 years without known ASCVD or diabetes mellitus if ASCVD risk is 7.5% or higher, taking into account patient preferences, adverse effects, and expected ASCVD risk reduction. The U.S. Preventive Services Task Force (USPSTF) recommends low- to moderate-intensity statin therapy in asymptomatic adults aged 40 to 75 years without ASCVD who have at least one ASCVD risk factor (dyslipidemia, diabetes, hypertension, or smoking) and a calculated 10-year ASCVD event risk of 10% or higher. This patient with a 10-year risk for ASCVD of 11.1% meets the criteria of both the ACC/AHA and USPSTF guidelines, and both guidelines support initiation of moderate-intensity statin therapy.

In the absence of familial hypercholesterolemia, proprotein convertase subtilisin/kexin type 9 (PCSK9) inhibitors, such as alirocumab and evolocumab, are not indicated in the primary prevention of ASCVD. Cost, treatment burden (injections), and minimal long-term safety data argue against their use in primary prevention.

Nonstatin drugs should be considered alone or in combination with statins in patients who do not achieve adequate LDL cholesterol reduction with statin therapy, especially in high-risk patients (those with clinical ASCVD, baseline LDL cholesterol level >190 mg/dL [4.92 mmol/L], or diabetes). This patient does not have an indication for ezetimibe therapy alone or in combination with a statin.

In patients with a fasting triglyceride level of 500 mg/dL (5.65 mmol/L) or higher, triglyceride-lowering drug therapy is useful to prevent pancreatitis. Fibrates, such as gemfibrozil, result in an average reduction in triglyceride levels of 30% to 50%, but this patient does not have an indication for fibrate therapy.

**KEY POINT**

- In patients aged 40 to 75 years with no atherosclerotic cardiovascular disease (ASCVD) or diabetes mellitus and a 10-year ASCVD risk of 7.5% or higher, the American College of Cardiology/American Heart Association recommend moderate- or high-intensity statin therapy for primary prevention of ASCVD.

**Bibliography**

Stone NJ, Robinson JG, Lichtenstein AH, Bairey Merz CN, Blum CB, Eckel RH, et al; American College of Cardiology/American Heart Association Task Force on Practice Guidelines. 2013 ACC/AHA guideline on the treatment of blood cholesterol to reduce atherosclerotic cardiovascular risk in adults: a report of the American College of Cardiology/American Heart Association Task Force on Practice Guidelines. Circulation. 2014;129:S1-45. [PMID: 24222016] doi:10.1161/01.cir.0000437738.63853.7a

**Item 72    Answer:    A**

**Educational Objective:** Disclose a medical error to an affected patient.

The most appropriate management is to explain to the patient that an error was committed and the steps that will be taken to reduce the chance of recurrence. This case involves the most common type of medical error, one related to inappropriate medication dosing. Current standards recommend full disclosure of serious unanticipated outcomes, and several states mandate such disclosures. Disclosure of errors is necessary to respect the patient's autonomy,

promote trust through honesty, and promote justice through appropriate compensation. Error disclosure should include an explanation of the course of events and how the error occurred, an apology by the physician, a description of how the effects of the error will be minimized or rectified, and steps the physician or system will take to reduce recurrences. In this case, the physician should inform his or her colleague of the error, and they should work within the practice to explore factors that caused the error and determine ways to reduce errors in the future.

The pharmacy may have played a role in commission of the error; however, it would be inappropriate to deflect blame to another source. Communication with the pharmacy regarding the correct dosage would be important in rectifying the situation.

The National Practitioner Data Bank is a federal repository of reports regarding serious professional or safety concerns, including medical malpractice payments or serious actions taken against physicians (such as suspension of licensure or clinical privileges). The error in this case should be disclosed and investigated; however, it would not be appropriate to report to the National Practitioner Data Bank.

Although addressing this patient's symptom without disclosing that an error occurred is an attractive option, disclosure respects the patient's autonomy by providing her with information necessary to make an informed decision about her care. Furthermore, the disclosure may enhance physician-patient communication and trust. Data from health systems that implement medical error disclosure policies suggest that disclosure decreases malpractice lawsuits and litigation costs.

**KEY POINT**

- Error disclosure should include an explanation of the course of events and how the error occurred, an apology by the physician, a description of how the effects of the error will be minimized or rectified, and steps the physician or system will take to reduce recurrences.

**Bibliography**

Snyder L; American College of Physicians Ethics, Professionalism, and Human Rights Committee. American College of Physicians ethics manual: sixth edition. Ann Intern Med. 2012;156:73-104. [PMID: 22213573] doi: 10.7326/0003-4819-156-1-201201031-00001

**Item 73    Answer:    C**

**Educational Objective:** Evaluate a patient with probable overflow incontinence.

Obtaining a postvoid residual urine volume is the most appropriate next step in the management of this patient. This patient likely has neurogenic bladder with overflow incontinence, characterized by constant urine leaking and dribbling and a palpable bladder. Overflow incontinence is more commonly found in men with prostatic hyperplasia and bladder outlet obstruction. However, this patient has long-standing diabetes mellitus and evidence of autonomic neuropathy (resting tachycardia, dry feet, distended bladder) on physical examination. Postvoid residual bladder volume measurement with ultrasonography can confirm the presence of large volumes of urine in the bladder, supporting the clinical diagnosis.

Botulinum toxin injection is used in the treatment of urgency urinary incontinence that persists despite behavioral and pharmacologic therapies. A systematic review concluded that botulinum toxin injection was superior to placebo in reducing incontinence in patients with urgency incontinence unresponsive to more conservative measures. Symptoms are typically reduced for 3 to 6 months, and then reinjection is required. Such injections can worsen overflow incontinence and would be contraindicated in this patient.

Oxybutynin is an anticholinergic agent used in the treatment of urgency incontinence. Anticholinergic drugs (oxybutynin, darifenacin, fesoterodine, solifenacin, tolterodine, trospium) block the muscarinic cholinergic receptors and decrease bladder contractility. The use of oxybutynin would worsen overflow incontinence due to neurogenic bladder and would be contraindicated in this patient.

Urodynamic testing is not recommended in the initial evaluation of urinary incontinence. Urodynamic testing consists of measuring bladder pressure during bladder filling, urine flow rate, and pressure-flow correlations and testing for sphincter deficiency. Urodynamic studies are required only for complex cases in which neurologic disease is suspected or surgical intervention is being considered.

**KEY POINT**

- A postvoid residual urine volume, determined by ultrasonography, can confirm a suspected case of overflow urinary incontinence.

**Bibliography**
Kadow BT, Tyagi P, Chermansky CJ. Neurogenic causes of detrusor underactivity. Curr Bladder Dysfunct Rep. 2015;10:325-331. [PMID: 26715948]

## Item 74     Answer:   B

**Educational Objective:** Treat chronic pelvic pain syndrome.

A trial of pregabalin is the most appropriate treatment for this patient with chronic pelvic pain syndrome (CPPS). CPPS is characterized by chronic pelvic pain and intermittent voiding symptoms without evidence of infection. Subtypes of this condition include inflammatory and noninflammatory forms. Treatment involves a multimodal approach; options include pharmacologic therapies (antibiotics, anti-inflammatory agents, α-blocking agents, 5α-reductase inhibitors, and neuromodulating agents) and nonpharmacologic strategies (biofeedback, cognitive behavioral therapy, and physical therapy). There is limited and conflicting evidence for thermal ablation therapies and direct surgical interventions. Despite these options, treatment can be challenging, with minimal rates of improvement. This patient has already attempted numerous medication regimens without

symptomatic improvement. At this time, it would be most prudent to proceed with a neuromodulatory approach, with medications such as pregabalin, gabapentin, or nortriptyline. Nonpharmacologic options could also be recommended at this juncture.

No evidence supports the use of lidocaine-hydrocortisone suppositories in the treatment of CPPS.

This patient has already attempted numerous trials of antibiotics, anti-inflammatory agents, and α-blocking agents without any appreciable symptomatic improvement. Furthermore, the laboratory results do not reflect any evidence for an underlying active infection, systemic inflammation, or urinary retention. Consequently, a trial of tamsulosin or trimethoprim-sulfamethoxazole would not be appropriate.

**KEY POINT**

- Treatment of chronic pelvic pain syndrome demands a multimodal approach, with options including both pharmacologic and nonpharmacologic strategies; among the pharmacologic options are neuromodulatory agents, such as pregabalin, gabapentin, and nortriptyline.

**Bibliography**
Bharucha AE, Lee TH. Anorectal and pelvic pain. Mayo Clin Proc. 2016; 91:1471-1486. [PMID: 27712641] doi:10.1016/j.mayocp.2016.08.011

## Item 75     Answer:   A

**Educational Objective:** Treat somatic symptom disorder.

Cognitive behavioral therapy (CBT) is the most appropriate next step in management. This patient meets the diagnostic criteria for somatic symptom disorder: one or more somatic symptoms causing distress or interference with daily life; excessive thoughts, feelings, and behaviors related to the somatic symptoms; and persistence of somatic symptoms for at least 6 months. Furthermore, after thorough investigation, her symptoms have no identifiable organic source. In addition to acknowledging the patient's symptoms and establishing rapport through frequent scheduled follow-up visits, CBT is the best next step in management. Several studies have shown that CBT is superior to usual care, and the benefits are maintained after completion of therapy.

Familial Mediterranean fever (FMF) is the classic autoinflammatory disease associated with mutation of the *MEFV1* gene, which codes for pyrin (a regulator of interleukin-1β production). Attacks last 1 to 3 days and are characterized by polyserositis, arthritis, erysipeloid rash around the ankles, and elevation of acute phase reactants. Most cases (90%) present before age 20 years, and a family history of similar symptoms is common. This patient's age of onset, chronic symptoms, and negative evaluation results, including acute phase reactant measurement, argue strongly against the diagnosis of FMF and the need to analyze the *MEFV* gene.

Pregabalin is an FDA-approved treatment for fibromyalgia and other conditions associated with neuropathic pain, such as diabetic peripheral neuropathy and postherpetic neuralgia. However, this patient does not have the fatigue and widespread musculoskeletal symptoms typical of fibromyalgia. Pregabalin has no role in the treatment of somatic symptom disorder.

Whole-body PET is not indicated in a patient without clinical evidence of malignancy. Furthermore, advanced diagnostic testing is not recommended in patients with somatic symptom disorder to provide technological reassurance. In addition to being cost ineffective, such testing may lead to false-positive results, triggering further unnecessary testing and patient stress.

**KEY POINT**

- Treatment of somatic symptom disorder focuses on acknowledging the patient's symptoms, building a therapeutic relationship with the patient through frequent scheduled visits, implementing cognitive behavioral therapy, and avoiding further testing.

**Bibliography**

Schröder A, Rehfeld E, Ornbøl E, Sharpe M, Licht RW, Fink P. Cognitive-behavioural group treatment for a range of functional somatic syndromes: randomised trial. Br J Psychiatry. 2012;200:499-507. [PMID: 22539780] doi:10.1192/bjp.bp.111.098681

## Item 76     Answer:     B

**Educational Objective:** Diagnose central retinal artery occlusion.

The most likely diagnosis for this patient's painless visual loss is central retinal artery occlusion (CRAO). This patient has several risk factors for this condition, including advanced age; male sex; and associated cardiovascular risk factors, such as hypertension and hyperlipidemia. Examination reveals an afferent pupillary defect and cherry red fovea (*blue arrow*) that is accentuated by a pale retinal background. Interruption of the venous blood columns may be recognized with the appearance of "boxcarring" rows of corpuscles separated by clear intervals seen in the vein just superior to the optic disc (*white arrow*). The most likely cause in this case is carotid atherosclerosis, but CRAO may also be caused by cardiogenic emboli; carotid artery dissection; hematologic conditions, such as sickle cell disease; or hypercoagulable states. The occlusion may be preceded by transient visual loss or a stuttering course. Retinal examination may demonstrate emboli. In an older patient who lacks emboli on examination, erythrocyte sedimentation rate and C-reactive protein level should be obtained to rule out giant cell arteritis, which is a rare but important cause of CRAO. Prognosis is based on visual acuity at presentation. Ischemia that lasts 4 hours or longer tends to result in irreversible vision loss. Treatment may include measures to lower intraocular pressure. Emergent ophthalmology consultation is required.

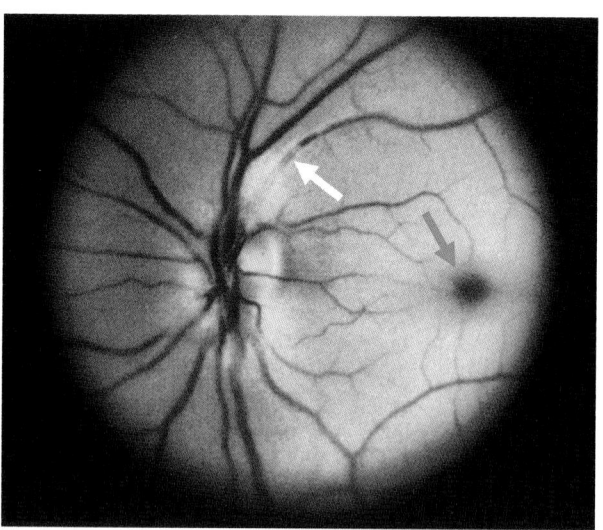

Acute angle-closure glaucoma typically presents with severe eye pain and visual loss. It may involve headache, nausea, and vomiting. Ophthalmoscopic examination reveals a mid-dilated (4-6 mm), nonreactive pupil and intraocular pressure greater than 50 mm Hg. This patient's clinical picture is not consistent with acute angle-closure glaucoma.

Idiopathic intracranial hypertension (previously known as pseudotumor cerebri) may present with diplopia, headache, and, most often, bilateral visual symptoms. These may include transient visual obscurations, which can be brief and triggered by body position change or the Valsalva maneuver. Papilledema is almost always present on examination.

Retinal detachment most commonly presents with photopsias (flashes of light); patients may also report seeing cobwebs and large floaters. Painless complete visual loss is possible, but retinal detachment is more often associated with progressive vision compromise that may involve partial visual fields. A horseshoe-shaped retinal tear may be observed on funduscopic examination.

**KEY POINT**

- Central retinal artery occlusion presents as acute, profound, and painless loss of monocular vision associated with an afferent pupillary defect and cherry red fovea.

**Bibliography**

Georgalas I, Pagoulatos D, Koutsandrea C, Pavlidis M. Sudden unilateral painless loss of vision. BMJ. 2014;349:g4117. [PMID: 24986885] doi: 10.1136/bmj.g4117

## Item 77     Answer:     B

**Educational Objective:** Treat dyspnea refractory to medical therapy in a patient with heart failure and COPD.

The most appropriate treatment is oral hydromorphone. This patient has severe chronic dyspnea that is refractory to maximal therapy for his underlying heart failure and COPD. Oral

CONT.

opioids, dosed appropriately, have been found to be both safe and efficacious in the treatment of dyspnea. Treatment efficacy is thought to be related to modulation of shared neural structures that are involved in the pathogenesis of both pain and dyspnea, as there are numerous μ-opioid receptors throughout the respiratory centers in the central nervous system. No evidence suggests that one opioid is superior to another in the treatment of dyspnea, and agent selection should be based on individual patient considerations, such as avoidance of morphine products in patients with reduced kidney function.

Furosemide would be a reasonable selection in a patient with volume overload as the driver of dyspnea; however, this patient has no evidence to suggest this cause (such as an elevated central venous pressure, an $S_3$, crackles, or peripheral edema).

Benzodiazepines, such as lorazepam, are effective for short-term control of anxiety symptoms. However, this patient's anxiety is a result of his shortness of breath, and as such, treatment should focus on relieving the dyspnea, not on treating the associated anxiety. For this reason, benzodiazepines should be considered only when adjunctive therapy is indicated.

Although systemic opioids have shown clear benefit in treating refractory dyspnea, inhaled opioids, such as nebulized morphine, have not shown significant efficacy in several placebo-controlled trials.

**KEY POINT**

• In patients with severe refractory dyspnea, appropriately dosed oral opioids are first-line therapy for symptomatic relief.

**Bibliography**
Kamal AH, Maguire JM, Wheeler JL, Currow DC, Abernethy AP. Dyspnea review for the palliative care professional: treatment goals and therapeutic options. J Palliat Med. 2012;15:106-14. [PMID: 22268406] doi:10.1089/jpm.2011.0110

## Item 78    Answer:    D

**Educational Objective:** Avoid aspirin therapy for primary prevention of atherosclerotic cardiovascular disease in a patient at high risk for bleeding.

No further intervention is the most appropriate management of this patient. Although he has a 10-year risk for atherosclerotic cardiovascular disease (ASCVD) of 14.6%, he is at high risk for bleeding with the addition of aspirin therapy. The U.S. Preventive Services Task Force recommends low-dose aspirin for the primary prevention of ASCVD and colorectal cancer in adults aged 50 to 59 years with a 10-year ASCVD risk of 10% or higher who do not have an increased risk for bleeding, have a life expectancy of at least 10 years, and are willing to take low-dose aspirin daily for at least 10 years. Patients aged 60 to 69 years may also benefit from aspirin; however, the net benefit is smaller because of the increased risk for bleeding in this population. In addition to increasing

age, male sex and use of anticoagulants or NSAIDs increase the risk for bleeding. Many patients with cardiovascular disease who are eligible for secondary prevention with aspirin therapy also require long-term oral anticoagulant therapy for atrial fibrillation. In these patients, the addition of aspirin to anticoagulant therapy provides some additional protection against cardiovascular events, but the risk for major bleeding is significantly increased. Therefore, aspirin is not generally recommended in these patients. Although this patient's risk for ASCVD is higher than 10%, he is already receiving anticoagulant therapy with rivaroxaban; therefore, the potential benefits of aspirin therapy for primary prevention of ASCVD are likely outweighed by the increased risk for bleeding.

High doses of fish oil increase bleeding time in vitro by suppressing platelet-activating factor, but this mechanism has not been associated with higher rates of clinical bleeding, even when the supplement is combined with aspirin or warfarin. However, a 2018 systematic review concluded that omega-3 fatty acid supplementation does not reduce heart disease, stroke, or death; therefore, fish oil supplementation cannot be recommended.

Switching rivaroxaban to low-dose aspirin is not recommended because this patient is at high risk for atrial fibrillation–related stroke. For this patient, anticoagulant therapy is significantly superior to aspirin in reducing his risk for stroke.

**KEY POINT**

• In the primary and secondary prevention of cardiovascular events, the addition of aspirin to long-term anticoagulation is associated with significantly increased bleeding events and is not routinely recommended.

**Bibliography**
Whitlock EP, Burda BU, Williams SB, Guirguis-Blake JM, Evans CV. Bleeding risks with aspirin use for primary prevention in adults: a systematic review for the U.S. Preventive Services Task Force. Ann Intern Med. 2016;164(12):826-35. [PMID: 27064261] doi: 10.7326/M15-2112

## Item 79    Answer:    C

**Educational Objective:** Diagnose high ankle sprain.

The most likely diagnosis is a high ankle sprain. High ankle sprains result from excessive dorsiflexion or eversion that causes injury to the tibiofibular syndesmotic ligaments connecting the distal tibia and fibula. Pain can be elicited by compressing the leg at mid-calf (squeeze test), by having the patient cross the legs with the lateral malleolus of the injured leg resting on the other knee (crossed-leg test), or by dorsiflexing and externally rotating the foot with the knee flexed (dorsiflexion-external rotation test). The most common mechanism of injury involves an externally rotated force applied to a dorsiflexed ankle, as is the case with this patient. Patients with high ankle sprains report the acute onset of pain proximal to the ankle. Pain is often accompanied by swelling and ecchymosis. Treatment is similar to that used for other ankle sprains and includes cryotherapy (ice or cold water), mobilization, and analgesics for pain control, but recovery is usually delayed.

Achilles tendon rupture most commonly results from sudden, forceful plantar flexion, such as occurs with jumping and sprinting. Patients report sudden onset of heel pain and often hear a popping sound at the time of the injury. On examination, patients have weak or absent plantar flexion. Absent plantar flexion with calf squeezing (Thompson test) also suggests the diagnosis. This patient's clinical presentation is not consistent with Achilles tendon rupture.

The Ottawa ankle and foot rules are useful in excluding ankle fractures, with an extremely high sensitivity (>95%). According to these validated rules, radiography should be obtained when a patient is unable to walk four steps both immediately after the injury and during evaluation, and when focal tenderness is present at the posterior aspect of the malleolus, the navicular bone, or the fifth metatarsal base. If these criteria are not met, obtaining radiography is not necessary because the probability of an ankle fracture is exceedingly low, as in this patient.

Lateral ankle sprains typically result from inversion injuries to the lateral ankle ligaments (the anterior and posterior talofibular ligaments and the calcaneofibular ligament). Physical examination reveals ecchymosis, lateral ankle tenderness, and swelling, which was not the case with this patient. This patient's symptoms and findings were located above the ankle.

### KEY POINT

- Patients with high ankle sprains report the acute onset of pain proximal to the ankle, accompanied by swelling and ecchymosis.

### Bibliography
Vopat ML, Vopat BG, Lubberts B, DiGiovanni CW. Current trends in the diagnosis and management of syndesmotic injury. Curr Rev Musculoskelet Med. 2017;10:94-103. [PMID: 28101828] doi:10.1007/s12178-017-9389-4

## Item 80          Answer:     A

**Educational Objective:   Treat vulvovaginal candidiasis.**

The most appropriate treatment for this patient with symptoms of vulvovaginal candidiasis is intravaginal clotrimazole. Vulvovaginitis describes infectious and noninfectious conditions that cause vulvovaginal symptoms, including abnormal vaginal discharge, vulvar itching, burning, irritation, and malodor. When discharge is associated with abnormal findings, the differential diagnoses most commonly include bacterial vaginosis, trichomoniasis, and vulvovaginal candidiasis. Vaginal irritation also may be caused by dermatologic conditions or allergic reactions, cervical infections, or genitourinary syndrome of menopause. A woman may have more than one type of infection at a time. The diagnosis of vulvovaginal candidiasis is suggested by the presence of vaginal discharge and vulvar pruritus, pain, irritation, and

redness. Signs include vulvar edema; fissures; excoriations; and thick, white, curdy vaginal discharge. The diagnosis can be made when a saline or 10% potassium hydroxide wet mount of vaginal discharge shows hyphae, pseudohyphae, or yeast. Because the sensitivity of microscopy is low, empiric treatment of vulvovaginal candidiasis can be considered if symptoms are accompanied by characteristic findings. Several therapeutically equivalent topical and oral drugs are available; among the topically applied drugs, imidazoles (fluconazole, miconazole, clotrimazole) are the most effective. Evidence suggests that topical and oral agents have similar efficacy and that treatment preference should be based on cost, convenience, and patient preference.

Intravaginal nystatin, a topical antifungal drug, lacks good supporting evidence for the treatment of vulvovaginal candidiasis and currently is not recommended.

Oral metronidazole is used to treat bacterial vaginosis, the most common cause of vaginal discharge, as well as to treat trichomoniasis. Accepted clinical criteria for diagnosing bacterial vaginosis include the presence of three of four characteristics: vaginal pH greater than 4.5, amine ("fishy") odor on the application of 10% potassium hydroxide to vaginal secretions (whiff test), the presence of a thin homogeneous vaginal discharge, and the finding of at least 20% clue cells on a microscopic saline wet mount examination. Although the presentation of trichomoniasis varies, many women develop a copious, malodorous, pale yellow or gray frothy discharge with vulvar itching, burning, and postcoital bleeding. Point-of-care vaginal swab rapid immunoassays and nucleic acid amplification tests for detection of *Trichomoniasis vaginalis* have replaced microscopy or culture as the gold standard for diagnosis. This patient does not have findings of bacterial vaginosis or trichomoniasis; hence, metronidazole is not indicated.

Oral voriconazole should not be used to treat vulvovaginal candidiasis because no data support its use. Case reports suggest that it is ineffective, and there is the added potential for toxicity.

### KEY POINT

- Topical antifungal imidazole therapy, such as intravaginal clotrimazole, is an effective treatment for uncomplicated vulvovaginal candidiasis, which is usually caused by *Candida albicans*.

### Bibliography
Mills BB. Vaginitis: beyond the basics. Obstet Gynecol Clin North Am. 2017;44:159-177. [PMID: 28499528] doi:10.1016/j.ogc.2017.02.010

## Item 81          Answer:     A

**Educational Objective:   Implement appropriate monitoring strategies before and during opioid therapy in a patient with chronic pain.**

Baseline urine drug screening is recommended before starting opioid therapy in this patient. Many guidelines, including the Centers for Disease Control and Prevention

(CDC) Guideline for Prescribing Opioids for Chronic Pain, recommend initial and ongoing urine drug screening. Urine drug screening is used to test for adherence to current therapy, identify potential opioid diversion (by assessing whether the expected metabolite is present within an appropriate time frame), and evaluate for the presence of other controlled prescription and nonprescription drugs. Urine drug screening should be performed before opioids are prescribed for chronic pain and at least yearly during therapy. More frequent screening may be necessary in the setting of therapy changes or the presence of red flags (lost prescriptions, early refill requests, multiple concurrent opioid providers or "doctor shopping," consistently missed appointments, or erratic follow-up).

The CDC guideline and other opioid prescribing guidelines recommend that opioid therapy be considered only if expected benefits for both pain and function are anticipated to outweigh the risks. If opioids are used, they should be combined with nonpharmacologic and nonopioid pharmacologic therapies as appropriate. Discontinuing this patient's current nonpharmacologic and pharmacologic therapies is not indicated.

Chronic pain is often associated with comorbid psychological issues. Patients who meet the criteria for diagnosis of a psychological comorbidity, such as depression or anxiety, should be treated accordingly. However, routine referral for a psychiatric evaluation is not mandatory and is based on the presence and severity of comorbid mental health disorders.

KEY POINT

- In patients in whom opioid therapy is being considered for the treatment of chronic pain, urine drug screening should be performed before opioid prescription and at least yearly during therapy to evaluate for adherence to therapy and to identify the presence of other controlled drugs.

Bibliography
Dowell D, Haegerich TM, Chou R. CDC guideline for prescribing opioids for chronic pain—United States, 2016. JAMA. 2016;315:1624-45. [PMID: 26977696]

Item 82    Answer:    C

Educational Objective:  Evaluate preoperative cardiac risk using transthoracic echocardiography in a patient with moderate aortic stenosis.

In addition to electrocardiography, the most appropriate preoperative testing for this patient is transthoracic echocardiography (TTE). The patient was diagnosed with moderate aortic stenosis several years ago and has occasional dizziness with physical exertion, a potential symptom of severe aortic stenosis. Preoperative TTE should not be ordered routinely but is recommended in certain cases. Indications for preoperative echocardiography include dyspnea of unknown origin, heart failure with change in clinical status, and known left ventricular dysfunction in the absence of an assessment in the previous 12 months. Relevant to this patient, TTE is indicated in patients with known or suspected moderate or

greater degrees of valvular stenosis or regurgitation if TTE has not been performed within 1 year or in those whose clinical status has changed or who have referable symptoms. It is reasonable to perform elevated-risk elective noncardiac surgery in patients with severe asymptomatic aortic stenosis, with appropriate intraoperative and postoperative hemodynamic monitoring. For patients who are candidates for valvular intervention because of symptoms or severity of disease, valvular intervention before elective noncardiac surgery is effective at reducing risk.

In a systematic review, a preoperative B-type natriuretic peptide (BNP) level greater than 92 pg/mL (92 ng/L) predicted the composite outcome of death or nonfatal myocardial infarction at 30 days, at 180 days, and beyond. Despite the improvement in predicting poor surgical outcomes, it is unclear what role BNP measurement should play in perioperative cardiovascular care; this test is currently not recommended by American College of Cardiology/American Heart Association guidelines. The Canadian Cardiovascular Society guidelines on perioperative cardiac risk assessment and management for patients who undergo noncardiac surgery strongly recommend that a BNP level be obtained to enhance perioperative cardiac risk estimation in patients with a Revised Cardiac Risk Index score of 1 or more, patients aged 65 years and older, and patients aged 45 to 64 years who have significant cardiovascular disease.

This patient is scheduled to undergo surgery (total knee arthroplasty) and has good functional capacity (able to swim for 30 minutes), and she does not have coronary artery disease or its equivalents (chronic kidney disease, cerebrovascular disease, heart failure, or diabetes mellitus). This patient's risk for major ischemic events is low; therefore, dobutamine stress echocardiography is not indicated.

KEY POINT

- Transthoracic echocardiography to evaluate preoperative cardiac risk is appropriate for patients with moderate to severe valvular stenosis or regurgitation in the absence of an assessment in the previous year or for those whose clinical status has changed or who have referable symptoms.

Bibliography
Fleisher LA, Fleischmann KE, Auerbach AD, Barnason SA, Beckman JA, Bozkurt B, et al; American College of Cardiology. 2014 ACC/AHA guideline on perioperative cardiovascular evaluation and management of patients undergoing noncardiac surgery: a report of the American College of Cardiology/American Heart Association Task Force on practice guidelines. J Am Coll Cardiol. 2014;64:e77-137. [PMID: 25091544]

Item 83    Answer:    D

Educational Objective:  Evaluate serum lipid levels in an obese patient.

This patient with obesity should undergo serum lipid screening. The American Heart Association, American College of Cardiology, and The Obesity Society guideline for the management of overweight and obesity recommends measurement of height and weight; calculation of BMI; measurement of waist circumference; and measurement of cardiovascular disease risk factors, including blood pressure, fasting blood glucose (or hemoglobin A$_{1c}$), and serum lipid levels. Obesity is associated with insulin resistance and dyslipidemia characterized by elevations of total cholesterol, LDL cholesterol, VLDL cholesterol, and triglycerides and a reduction in HDL cholesterol. The history should address symptoms of obesity-related comorbid conditions, but no additional screening is recommended in the absence of suggestive symptoms or findings.

Exercise stress testing is recommended for patients with symptoms of cardiac ischemia. Overweight and obese patients are at increased risk for cardiovascular disease and should be questioned about symptoms and referred for testing if symptoms are present. Routine screening of asymptomatic patients is not recommended.

Hepatic ultrasonography is not necessary for this patient. The risk for nonalcoholic steatohepatitis is increased in overweight and obese patients. A presumptive diagnosis can be made in a patient with mild abnormalities in aminotransferase levels, risk factors for nonalcoholic fatty liver disease (such as diabetes mellitus, obesity, and hyperlipidemia), and ultrasonographic features consistent with hepatic steatosis. The recommended treatment of nonalcoholic steatohepatitis is weight loss, but no screening for this condition is recommended.

Risk for obstructive sleep apnea is increased among overweight and obese patients, particularly those with neck circumference greater than 38 cm (15 in) in women and greater than 43 cm (17 in) in men. The patient should be referred for overnight polysomnography only if symptoms of the disorder are present. He does not report nonrestorative sleep or daytime hypersomnolence, which would suggest obstructive sleep apnea.

The prevalence of an endocrine cause of obesity is very low. Thyroid function testing should be reserved for patients with symptoms and findings indicating thyroid disease.

### KEY POINT

- Management guidelines for overweight and obese patients recommend measurement of height and weight; calculation of BMI; measurement of waist circumference; and measurement of cardiovascular disease risk factors, including blood pressure, fasting blood glucose (or hemoglobin A$_{1c}$), and serum lipid levels.

### Bibliography
Jensen MD, Ryan DH, Apovian CM, Ard JD, Comuzzie AG, Donato KA, et al; American College of Cardiology/American Heart Association Task Force on Practice Guidelines. 2013 AHA/ACC/TOS guideline for the management of overweight and obesity in adults: a report of the American College of Cardiology/American Heart Association Task Force on Practice Guidelines and The Obesity Society. Circulation. 2014;129:S102-38. [PMID: 24222017] doi:10.1161/01.cir.0000437739.71477.ee

## Item 84      Answer:   D

**Educational Objective:   Treat unexplained chronic cough.**

Multimodal speech therapy is an appropriate treatment for this patient with unexplained chronic cough (UCC). UCC is

defined as cough persisting for more than 8 weeks with no identifiable cause despite comprehensive evaluation. The evidence supporting the diagnosis and management of UCC is limited and generally weak. The American College of Chest Physicians (ACCP) expert panel recommends multimodal speech therapy consisting of two to four sessions of education, cough suppression techniques, breathing exercises, and counseling. This intervention helps reduce cough frequency and severity and improve cough-related quality of life. The ACCP also recommends a therapeutic trial of the neuromodulator gabapentin as long as the potential side effects and the risk-benefit profile are discussed with patients before use of the medication and the risk-benefit profile is reassessed at 6 months before continuation of the drug. Neuromodulators may diminish neural sensitization, which is a key driver of unexplained cough.

Levels of neutrophils are frequently increased in patients with chronic cough. Macrolide antibiotics are effective in the treatment of exacerbations of COPD and bronchiectasis, possibly because of their anti-inflammatory and antineutrophil effects that are independent of antimicrobial effects. However, trials with macrolide antibiotics, such as azithromycin and erythromycin, have not demonstrated benefit in patients with UCC.

Inhaled ipratropium bromide was found to be beneficial in patients with chronic cough after an upper respiratory tract infection. The ACCP does not recommend ipratropium for the treatment of UCC because the findings related to ipratropium were from an older study with a small sample size and limited reporting of methods, and the results have not been replicated.

Like gabapentin, morphine was found to be effective in reducing cough severity and frequency, but the ACCP expert panel has declined to recommend morphine as an intervention for chronic cough. The danger of overdose and addiction potential of morphine have been well described.

### KEY POINT

- Recommended treatments for unexplained chronic cough include multimodality speech pathology therapy and neuromodulators, such as gabapentin.

### Bibliography
Gibson P, Wang G, McGarvey L, Vertigan AE, Altman KW, Birring SS; CHEST Expert Cough Panel. Treatment of unexplained chronic cough: CHEST guideline and expert panel report. Chest. 2016;149:27-44. [PMID: 26426314] doi:10.1378/chest.15-1496

## Item 85      Answer:   B

**Educational Objective:   Manage sexual side effects in a patient taking a selective serotonin reuptake inhibitor for major depressive disorder.**

The most appropriate next step in management is to discontinue sertraline and initiate bupropion, which has a lower rate of sexual side effects. Cognitive behavioral therapy (CBT) or a second-generation antidepressant is an appropriate first choice for the treatment of major depressive disorder. Side effects, comorbid conditions, and cost are important considerations in the selection of therapy for a patient with depression. The most widely prescribed antidepressant drugs are selective serotonin reuptake inhibitors (SSRIs). SSRIs have excellent safety profiles compared with tricyclic antidepressants, but adverse sexual side effects (such as reduced libido, anorgasmia, or delayed orgasm) are common. Bupropion is an appropriate substitute agent for patients experiencing sexual side effects with an SSRI because it is an effective treatment with a low rate of sexual side effects. Bupropion can also be added to SSRI therapy to reduce SSRI-induced sexual side effects, but it is important to note that bupropion is contraindicated in patients with seizure disorders. Substituting CBT for antidepressant therapy in a patient experiencing sexual side effects of an SSRI is also an acceptable alternative.

The addition of CBT to antidepressant therapy is a reasonable approach for depression that does not respond to first-line therapy. This patient's depression is responsive to treatment, and the addition of CBT without stopping sertraline will not affect the patient's sexual side effects.

In patients who develop sexual side effects with one SSRI, there is substantial risk for similar problems with all SSRIs. This patient experienced anorgasmia with sertraline, and paroxetine has the highest rate of sexual side effects of all SSRIs, making it a poor choice for this patient.

Electroconvulsive therapy is appropriate for the management of treatment-resistant depression. This patient's depression is responding to first-line therapy; therefore, electroconvulsive therapy would not be the best treatment choice.

**KEY POINT**

- Selective serotonin reuptake inhibitors are generally well tolerated among patients with major depressive disorder, but sexual side effects (such as anorgasmia, delayed orgasm, and reduced libido) are common; for these patients, bupropion is an appropriate alternative, as is cognitive behavioral therapy.

**Bibliography**
Lorenz T, Rullo J, Faubion S. Antidepressant-induced female sexual dysfunction. Mayo Clin Proc. 2016;91:1280-6. [PMID: 27594188] doi:10.1016/j.mayocp.2016.04.033

## Item 86      Answer:   C

**Educational Objective:** **Treat medically unexplained symptoms.**

The most appropriate management strategy in this patient with medically unexplained symptoms (MUS) is to recommend cognitive behavioral therapy (CBT). The foundation of management of patients with MUS is an open, honest, and effective therapeutic relationship. Patients should be treated respectfully and cared for in a nonjudgmental manner. It is important to not only expect but to accept the patient's feelings of frustration; acknowledging these feelings early in the patient's management course can help to build and strengthen the therapeutic alliance. Management of MUS requires a patient-focused, holistic, and multimodal approach. The goals of management are functional restoration, decreased symptom focus, and acquisition of coping mechanisms rather than abatement of symptoms. Office visits should be scheduled at regular intervals, allowing for additional discussion, educational opportunities, and longitudinal reassessment. It should be made clear to patients that the treatment of MUS will not likely be curative and that symptoms may persist. Interventions that may benefit patients with MUS include CBT, physical therapy, occupational therapy, individual or group psychotherapy, social support, biofeedback, graded exercise therapy, stress management activities, and training in coping mechanisms. A systematic review of 29 randomized controlled trials comparing CBT with various control treatments found that CBT was an effective treatment for somatization or symptom syndromes and that physical symptoms were more responsive to treatment than were psychological symptoms. At least one randomized controlled trial found that CBT improves outcomes and decreases clinic visits in patients with several unexplained symptoms. A systematic review of four randomized controlled trials of psychodynamic therapy in patients with chronic pain found that the treatment reduced pain, improved function, and decreased the use of health services.

Anti-Hu paraneoplastic syndrome can cause temporal lobe, brainstem, and cerebellar dysfunction and may also involve the dorsal roots and autonomic nervous system. This syndrome is most commonly associated with small cell lung cancer. The long duration and nature of this patient's symptoms make this an unlikely diagnosis, and antibody measurement is not indicated.

Anti–N-methyl-D-aspartate receptor (anti-NMDAR) antibody encephalitis has emerged as an increasingly common cause of encephalitis. The diagnosis is suggested by the presence of choreoathetosis, psychiatric symptoms, seizures, and autonomic instability and is confirmed by detection of anti-NMDAR antibodies in the serum. This patient has no symptoms compatible with this syndrome, and testing is not indicated.

Given the likely diagnosis of MUS, the patient's ongoing symptoms, and numerous available treatment strategies, providing no further treatment is not appropriate.

**KEY POINT**

- Patients with medically unexplained symptoms may benefit from cognitive behavioral therapy, physical therapy, occupational therapy, individual or group psychotherapy, social support, biofeedback, graded exercise therapy, stress management activities, and training in coping mechanisms.

**Bibliography**
Evens A, Vendetta L, Krebs K, Herath P. Medically unexplained neurologic symptoms: a primer for physicians who make the initial encounter. Am J Med. 2015;128:1059-64. [PMID: 25910791]

Answers and Critiques

## Item 87     Answer:     E

**Educational Objective:** Evaluate a patient with nonspecific low back pain.

No additional diagnostic testing is needed in this patient with acute, nonspecific low back pain. He lacks any concerning features, such as bowel or bladder dysfunction, constitutional symptoms, leg weakness, or saddle anesthesia. Indications to perform immediate imaging include severe and/or progressive neurologic deficits on examination or suspected serious underlying pathology, neither of which are present in this patient.

According to a joint clinical practice guideline released by the American College of Physicians and the American Pain Society, clinicians should not routinely perform diagnostic testing, such as CT, erythrocyte sedimentation rate measurement, MRI, or plain radiography, in patients with nonspecific low back pain. Even in patients with acute radiculopathy or spinal stenosis, routine imaging or testing has not been shown to improve outcomes. Most patients with acute low back pain recover quickly, regardless of the therapeutic intervention used. Whenever possible, maintaining daily activities should be encouraged. Nonpharmacologic treatment with acupuncture, massage, superficial heat, or spinal manipulation is preferred. If pharmacologic treatment is desired for acute low back pain, clinicians and patients should select NSAIDs or skeletal muscle relaxants.

### KEY POINT

- Diagnostic studies should not be routinely obtained in patients with nonspecific low back pain; such testing should be reserved for patients with severe or progressive neurologic deficits and patients for whom a serious underlying condition is suspected.

**Bibliography**

Chou R. In the clinic. Low back pain. Ann Intern Med. 2014;160:ITC6-1. [PMID: 25009837]

## Item 88     Answer:     D

**Educational Objective:** Manage a patient with a family history suggestive of an inherited disorder with genetic counseling.

This patient with a family history concerning for familial adenomatous polyposis (FAP) should be referred for genetic counseling. FAP is most commonly inherited in an autosomal-dominant pattern and is caused by a mutation in the adenomatous polyposis coli (*APC*) gene, which functions as a tumor suppressor gene. Nearly 100% of patients with the autosomal-dominant *APC* gene mutation develop colon cancer, with most developing cancer before age 40 years. Because this patient has a strong family history of colon cancer and his brother was recently diagnosed as a carrier of the genetic mutation for FAP, genetic testing is warranted if the patient desires it, and he should undergo genetic counseling first to help guide his decision on whether to pursue

genetic testing. Components of genetic counseling include assessment of the patient's risk for the condition of interest and education on the condition, risks and benefits of testing, alternative options to testing, and implications of testing for the patient and family members. Genetic counseling should be performed by individuals with appropriate training. Clinicians can use a searchable database provided by the American College of Medical Genetics to locate a genetic counselor in their area.

Aspirin and NSAIDs have been touted as a means to reduce the appearance and growth of polyps in patients with FAP. In particular, sulindac has been shown to cause regression of colorectal adenomas in FAP; however, the response is incomplete, and the degree of protection is uncertain. Chemoprevention is not a recommended strategy for patients at risk for or diagnosed with FAP.

Classic FAP results in the development of hundreds to thousands of colorectal adenomas that often manifest by the second decade of life. Gastric fundic gland polyposis and duodenal adenomas are also present in most patients. Gastric cancer is rare, but duodenal and periampullary cancers are the second leading cause of cancer death in this group. Papillary carcinoma of the thyroid is increasingly recognized as accompanying FAP. If this patient is diagnosed as a carrier of the FAP mutation, screening for colon, duodenal and periampullary, and thyroid cancers should be initiated now.

All patients in whom genetic testing is being considered should first be referred for genetic counseling.

### KEY POINT

- All patients for whom genetic testing is being considered should undergo genetic counseling.

**Bibliography**

Hampel H, Bennett RL, Buchanan A, Pearlman R, Wiesner GL; Guideline Development Group, American College of Medical Genetics and Genomics Professional Practice and Guidelines Committee and National Society of Genetic Counselors Practice Guidelines Committee. A practice guideline from the American College of Medical Genetics and Genomics and the National Society of Genetic Counselors: referral indications for cancer predisposition assessment. Genet Med. 2015;17:70-87. [PMID: 25394175] doi:10.1038/gim.2014.147

## Item 89     Answer:     C

**Educational Objective:** Evaluate decision-making capacity.

The most appropriate management is to discharge this patient home with home care services. Patients should be presumed legally competent to make medical decisions unless found otherwise by judicial determination. However, in the clinical setting, physicians must frequently determine a patient's decision-making capacity by assessing the patient's ability to understand the relevant information, appreciate the medical consequences of the situation, consider various treatment options, and communicate a choice. Decision-making capacity should be evaluated for each decision to be made, and frequent reassessment is necessary to confirm prior determinations of capacity. Patients with depression or mild

CONT.

dementia may retain decision-making capacity; however, in such circumstances, the capacity assessment should be performed more cautiously, particularly when a decision may result in serious consequences. Validated tools, such as the Aid to Capacity Evaluation (www.aafp.org/afp/2001/0715/afp20010715p299-f2.pdf), may be useful for capacity assessment in the clinical setting. In this situation, the assessment reveals that the patient demonstrates sufficient capacity to make decisions; thus, he should be discharged home with appropriate services to ensure his safety. This patient's choice is also consistent with his previously expressed wishes, which lends validity to his decision.

Cognitive evaluations, such as the Mini–Mental State Examination, do not assess capacity; rather, they are used to detect cognitive impairment.

This competent and autonomous patient is able to make his own choices; therefore, the patient's daughter should not be asked to make a decision on his behalf.

Formal assessments of competence require judicial determination, although a competency hearing is not usually required for clinical decision making. In this case, a court order for the patient to be discharged to a rehabilitation facility is not required because he demonstrates decision-making capacity.

A psychiatric consultation is unnecessary to determine a patient's decision-making capacity; any physician can perform this assessment. However, some hospitals may suggest a psychiatric evaluation in high-stakes situations, such as when a patient requests to leave against medical advice.

**KEY POINT**

- In the clinical setting, physicians must determine a patient's decision-making capacity by assessing the patient's ability to understand the relevant information, appreciate the medical consequences of the situation, consider various treatment options, and communicate a choice.

**Bibliography**

Porrino P, Falcone Y, Agosta L, Isaia G, Zanocchi M, Mastrapasqua A, et al. Informed consent in older medical inpatients: assessment of decision-making capacity. J Am Geriatr Soc. 2015;63:2423-4. [PMID: 26603072]

## Item 90    Answer:    D

**Educational Objective:  Treat tobacco dependence with pharmacologic therapy in a patient with a recent cardiovascular event.**

The most effective treatment is varenicline. Although bupropion and nicotine replacement therapy (NRT) monotherapy are effective for tobacco cessation, varenicline has been shown to be more effective. Some studies, including a large meta-analysis, have raised concerns of an increased risk for cardiovascular events in patients taking varenicline compared with those taking placebo. However, a recent double-blind, randomized, placebo and active-controlled trial of varenicline, bupropion, and nicotine replacement therapy showed no evidence that the use of smoking cessation pharmacotherapies increased the risk of serious cardiovascular adverse events during or after treatment. FDA drug labeling information does not list recent cardiovascular events as a contraindication to varenicline therapy. The FDA recently removed the black box warning related to serious mental health adverse reactions with varenicline use after the risk for mental health effects was found to be lower than previously reported. Varenicline should be used with caution in patients with kidney failure.

Bupropion, a norepinephrine and dopamine reuptake inhibitor with nicotinic receptor activity, effectively increases smoking cessation rates. Bupropion should not be used in patients with a history of seizure disorders, stroke, brain tumor, brain surgery, or head trauma. Blood pressure should be monitored carefully, as severity of hypertension may increase with bupropion treatment. In direct comparison trials, bupropion was less effective in achieving smoking cessation than was varenicline.

Electronic cigarettes hold promise as a harm reduction tool that may help patients quit smoking; however, the evidence regarding their efficacy, risks, and benefits is still emerging. Therefore, current FDA-approved, evidence-based agents for tobacco cessation, such as varenicline, would be more appropriate in this patient.

Effectiveness of NRT is similar to that of bupropion for smoking cessation. Options for NRT include patch, gum, lozenges, oral inhaler, and nasal spray. Concomitant use of more than one form of NRT enhances efficacy. NRT should be used with caution in patients with unstable cardiac disease, life-threatening arrhythmias, or a recent cardiac event. In these patients, the decision to initiate NRT should involve a cardiologist. Patients should also be discouraged from smoking during use of NRT. In this patient with recent non–ST-elevation myocardial infarction, NRT would not be the most appropriate smoking cessation therapy.

**KEY POINT**

- Varenicline is an effective therapy for smoking cessation and should be considered in smokers with a recent cardiac event.

**Bibliography**

Patel MS, Steinberg MB. In the clinic. Smoking cessation. Ann Intern Med. 2016;164:ITC33-ITC48. [PMID: 26926702]

## Item 91    Answer:    A

**Educational Objective:  Screen for abdominal aortic aneurysm in a man with a history of smoking.**

The most appropriate screening test to perform in this former smoker is abdominal duplex ultrasonography to screen for abdominal aortic aneurysm (AAA). The most important risk factors for AAA are advancing age, male sex (6:1 male-to-female incidence ratio), and smoking. The U.S. Preventive Services Task Force (USPSTF) recommends one-time

**Answers and Critiques**

abdominal ultrasonography to screen for AAA in all men aged 65 to 75 years who have ever smoked. Ever-smokers are usually defined as those who have smoked more than 100 cigarettes in their lifetime. The USPSTF recommends that clinicians selectively offer screening for AAA in men aged 65 to 75 years who have never smoked, based on the patient's medical history, family history, other risk factors, and preferences. A recently published meta-analysis concluded that screening significantly reduces AAA-related mortality. Abdominal duplex ultrasonography is the preferred screening modality, with a sensitivity of 94% to 100% and specificity of 98% to 100% for detecting AAA.

Chest radiography and sputum cytologic evaluation have not shown adequate sensitivity or specificity as screening tests for lung cancer and are not recommended.

Although the USPSTF concludes that there is insufficient evidence to recommend routine screening for osteoporosis in men, the National Osteoporosis Foundation recommends osteoporosis screening in men aged 70 years or older. Screening may also be considered in men at high risk for osteoporosis (men with low body weight, recent weight loss, physical inactivity, use of oral glucocorticoids, previous fragility fracture, alcohol use, or androgen deprivation via pharmacologic agents or orchiectomy). The American College of Physicians recommends periodic individualized assessment of risk factors for osteoporosis in older men.

The USPSTF and the American College of Chest Physicians (ACCP) recommend lung cancer screening with annual low-dose CT in persons aged 55 to 80 years (or aged 55 to 77 years, according to the ACCP) with a 30-pack-year smoking history, including former smokers who have quit in the last 15 years. Screening should be discontinued once a person has not smoked for 15 years or develops a health problem that substantially limits life expectancy or the willingness to have curative lung surgery. This patient has a 10-pack-year smoking history and quit almost 30 years ago; therefore, he does not meet the criteria for lung cancer screening.

### KEY POINT

- All men aged 65 to 75 years who have ever smoked should undergo one-time abdominal ultrasonography to screen for abdominal aortic aneurysm.

### Bibliography
Takagi H, Ando T, Umemoto T; ALICE (All-Literature Investigation of Cardiovascular Evidence) Group. Abdominal aortic aneurysm screening reduces all-cause mortality. Angiology. 2017:3319717693107. [PMID: 28193091] doi:10.1177/0003319717693107

## Item 92    Answer:    D

**Educational Objective:** Prevent medication errors with medication reconciliation.

Medication reconciliation would have most likely prevented this medication error. Medication reconciliation is the process of creating an accurate, comprehensive list of the patient's prescription and nonprescription medications (including the dose, frequency, and route of administration) and comparing the list to medication orders (at admission, transfer, or discharge) to resolve inconsistencies. Completion of medication reconciliation decreases adverse drug events, and although the effect on hospital readmissions, morbidity, and mortality is less clear, medication reconciliation should occur at all care transitions to prevent medication errors. In this case, tamoxifen was withheld upon admission but should have been restarted at the time of the patient's discharge from the hospital. Medication reconciliation at the time of discharge would have prevented this error, which resulted in a lapse in the patient's breast cancer treatment.

Computerized physician order entry (CPOE) systems are designed to improve the medication ordering process and prevent medication errors and medication adverse events. Some CPOE systems are integrated with decision support systems. CPOE has resulted in many practice improvements, including standardization of care, improved legibility of orders, and implementation of medication alerts (such as allergy and drug interaction alerts). However, CPOE cannot replace medication reconciliation and would not have prevented this medication error at a transition of care.

Manually transcribing physician medication orders into a paper-based medication administration record, even if originated by using the CPOE process, can lead to medication administration errors and adverse events. However, using a system that features a direct electronic interface between CPOE and the electronic medication administration record can eliminate transcription errors and errors in reading and interpreting hand-written, paper-based medication administration records. Such a system does not replace medication reconciliation and would not have prevented this medication error at the time of discharge.

Improved medication labeling, including the use of "tall man" lettering (for example, **DOBUT**amine versus **DOP**amine), helps minimize confusion surrounding look-alike and sound-alike medications, thereby reducing medication errors. However, improved medication labeling would not have prevented this medication error resulting from a transition of care.

### KEY POINT

- Medication reconciliation should occur at all transitions of care to prevent medication errors.

### Bibliography
Mueller SK, Sponsler KC, Kripalani S, Schnipper JL. Hospital-based medication reconciliation practices: a systematic review. Arch Intern Med. 2012;172:1057-69. [PMID: 22733210]

## Item 93    Answer:    A

**Educational Objective:** Diagnose frailty.

Frailty is a multifactorial geriatric syndrome that may predict a patient's response to certain treatments as well as morbidity and mortality in light of chronic illness. This patient demonstrates unintentional weight loss, low energy and activity levels, slow walking speed, and weakness, all of which are associated with frailty. Indices such as the Frailty Index, the FRAIL (Fatigue, Resistance, Ambulation, Illness, and Loss of weight) scale, and the Osteoporotic Fractures Frailty Scale have been validated for use in primary care. The Frailty Index has been in use for a longer time than other indices; however, its length and complexity limit its usefulness in routine care. The FRAIL scale consists of five self-reported measures and is easy to administer and score in an office setting.

Pharmacologic cardiac stress testing is recommended for patients who cannot exercise and are experiencing symptoms suggestive of cardiac ischemia. There is no established role for pharmacologic stress testing as a predictor of response to cancer treatment.

Lung function during exertion using the 6-minute walk test is helpful to assess disability and prognosis in chronic lung conditions. Simple pulse oximetry and oxygen desaturation studies performed at rest and with exertion assess the need for oxygen supplementation. During a 6-minute walk test, oxygen saturation, heart rate, dyspnea and fatigue levels, and distance walked in 6 minutes are recorded. The 6-minute walk test has no established role in predicting response to cancer chemotherapy in frail older adults.

The Timed Up and Go test is used to identify patients at risk for falls. The individual components of the test (rising from the chair, gait, walking speed, balance maintenance while turning, and sitting) offer insight into the various mechanics of mobility and can guide a more focused evaluation and intervention. Results of the Timed Up and Go test do not predict response to cancer treatment.

**KEY POINT**

- Frailty is a quantifiable geriatric syndrome that may predict a patient's response to medical treatment.

**Bibliography**

Puts MT, Santos B, Hardt J, Monette J, Girre V, Atenafu EG, et al. An update on a systematic review of the use of geriatric assessment for older adults in oncology. Ann Oncol. 2014;25:307-15. [PMID: 24256847] doi:10.1093/annonc/mdt386

## Item 94          Answer:     C

**Educational Objective:   Treat attention-deficit/hyperactivity disorder.**

In addition to cognitive behavioral therapy, methylphenidate is the best initial treatment for this patient with attention-deficit/hyperactivity disorder (ADHD). ADHD is characterized by persistent inattention and/or hyperactivity-impulsivity that disrupts functioning or development in at least two areas of a patient's life (such as work, home, or peer relationships). Some symptoms must be present since age 12 years; however, many patients are not formally diagnosed until adulthood, and up to 60% of children with ADHD continue to have symptoms as an adult. Although

symptoms of hyperactivity and impulsivity often lessen over time, adults with ADHD may be easily distracted, disorganized, and restless. Many adults have comorbid psychiatric problems, such as anxiety, depression, sleep disorders, and substance use. Cognitive behavioral therapy alone or in combination with pharmacotherapy is effective for improving executive functioning in patients with ADHD. Stimulants, such as methylphenidate, are first-line pharmacologic therapy for ADHD. However, these drugs should not be prescribed to patients with recent substance use or at high risk for serious adverse effects (arrhythmia, hypertension). Atomoxetine, bupropion, and tricyclic antidepressants can be used when stimulants are contraindicated.

Benzodiazepines, such as clonazepam, can be used for short-term treatment of severe, acute anxiety disorders. Their use is limited by the potential for abuse, and they are not indicated for the treatment of ADHD.

Escitalopram and other selective serotonin reuptake inhibitors are highly effective for the treatment of various mood and anxiety disorders. However, they have no established role in the treatment of ADHD unless there is a comorbid disorder responsive to this class of drugs.

Ropinirole is an effective therapy for restless legs syndrome. This patient is experiencing restlessness but does not report restless legs or sleep disturbance; therefore, ropinirole would not be indicated.

**KEY POINT**

- Stimulants, such as methylphenidate, are first-line pharmacologic therapy for attention-deficit/hyperactivity disorder; when stimulants are contraindicated, atomoxetine, bupropion, and tricyclic antidepressants can be used.

**Bibliography**

Volkow ND, Swanson JM. Clinical practice: adult attention deficit-hyperactivity disorder. N Engl J Med. 2013;369:1935-44. [PMID: 24224626] doi:10.1056/NEJMcp1212625

## Item 95          Answer:     A

**Educational Objective:   Diagnose iliotibial band syndrome.**

The most likely diagnosis is iliotibial band syndrome (ITBS). ITBS is a common cause of lateral knee pain in runners and can also occur in patients with significant leg length difference, an excessively pronated foot, genu varum, or gluteal muscle weakness. Patients with ITBS have pain that is poorly localized to the lateral knee and distal thigh. Initially, the pain is present only after prolonged activity (such as running) that involves repeated knee flexion and extension. As the condition progresses, the pain occurs earlier in the course of activity and may eventually be present at rest. On examination, there is often tenderness to palpation 2 to 3 cm proximal to the lateral femoral condyle. Patients also frequently have weakness with hip abduction. Reproduction of the pain with knee extension from 90 degrees to 30 degrees with the examiner's thumb exerting pressure on the lateral femoral epicondyle (Noble test) supports the diagnosis of ITBS. Initial treatment consists of activity modification, ice application, and NSAIDs to reduce inflammation. Once inflammation subsides, stretching and then strengthening exercises are indicated.

This patient lacks history of trauma, joint instability, lateral joint line tenderness, or increased laxity with varus force. Lack of these features argues against the presence of a lateral collateral ligament tear.

The lack of prior trauma and absence of catching, grinding, and locking all argue against a meniscal tear, as does the absence of an effusion on examination.

Meralgia paresthetica is due to entrapment of the lateral femoral cutaneous nerve and causes paresthesias on the anterolateral thigh. Risk factors include diabetes mellitus, obesity, pregnancy, and tight clothing or belts around the waist. This patient's findings are not consistent with meralgia paresthetica.

### KEY POINT

- Patients with iliotibial band syndrome report diffuse, poorly localized lateral knee and distal thigh pain; there is often tenderness to palpation 2 to 3 cm proximal to the lateral femoral condyle.

### Bibliography
Baker RL, Fredericson M. Iliotibial band syndrome in runners: biomechanical implications and exercise interventions. Phys Med Rehabil Clin N Am. 2016;27:53-77. [PMID: 26616177] doi:10.1016/j.pmr.2015.08.001

### Item 96    Answer:    B
**Educational Objective:** Evaluate noncyclic mastalgia.

The most appropriate initial management of this patient is breast ultrasonography. Breast pain (mastalgia) is common and may be cyclic or noncyclic. Many younger women experience cyclic breast discomfort with the onset of menses. The discomfort is typically bilateral, lasts for several days, and varies in intensity. Noncyclic breast pain is more likely to be unilateral and may be caused by trauma, cysts, duct ectasia, mastitis, ligamentous stretching secondary to large breasts, or a breast mass. A thorough history with attention to type of pain, location, and relationship to menses and a careful physical examination are essential to rule out palpable masses or anatomic causes. All women should be up to date with screening mammography. Women with a palpable breast mass should be referred for diagnostic imaging. Women with noncyclic breast pain and no evidence of a breast mass should undergo targeted breast ultrasonography because approximately 1% of such patients may have breast cancer at the site of pain.

Despite common perception, there is no evidence that avoiding caffeine will relieve breast hypersensitivity or pain.

Danazol is approved by the FDA for management of mastalgia but is recommended only for management of persistent severe cyclic breast pain unrelieved by conservative management. Because this patient has noncyclic breast pain and danazol is associated with the side effects of acne, hirsutism, weight gain, and irregular vaginal bleeding, danazol is not a therapeutic option for this patient.

The addition of mammography to ultrasonography does not appear to improve diagnostic accuracy in young women with mammographically dense breasts.

Reassurance, coupled with the regular use of a fitted support bra, would be appropriate management for a patient with cyclic mastalgia and a normal physical examination. This patient has focal noncyclic mastalgia necessitating diagnostic imaging as the first step in management.

### KEY POINT

- Patients with noncyclic mastalgia with focal breast pain but no palpable mass should undergo targeted breast ultrasonography because approximately 1% of such patients may have breast cancer at the site of pain.

### Bibliography
Iddon J, Dixon JM. Mastalgia. BMJ. 2013;347:f3288. [PMID: 24336097] doi:10.1136/bmj.f3288

### Item 97    Answer:    D
**Educational Objective:** Estimate posttest probability using likelihood ratios.

This patient's posttest probability of ischemic coronary artery disease is approximately 95%. His pretest probability of ischemic coronary artery disease is estimated to be 50% based on clinical variables (including the nature of the chest pain, age, and sex). Likelihood ratios (LRs) are a statistical indicator of how much the result of a diagnostic test will increase or decrease the pretest probability of a disease in a specific patient. LRs may be determined from the sensitivity and specificity of a diagnostic test, and separate LRs are calculated for use when a test result is positive (LR+) or when a test result is negative (LR-). This patient has a positive result on a treadmill stress echocardiographic study, and the LR for a positive result on this test is approximately 10. Although very specific posttest probabilities may be calculated or estimated by using a nomogram, a clinical rule of thumb is that LR+ values of 2, 5, and 10 correspond to an increase in disease probability of 15%, 30%, and 45%, respectively. With a pretest probability of 50%, a positive result on treadmill stress echocardiography would increase the likelihood of disease by approximately 45%, leading to a posttest probability in the range of 95%; this information would be very useful clinically in making further treatment decisions.

If the stress test result had been negative, LR- values of 0.5, 0.2, and 0.1 correspond to a decrease in disease probability of 15%, 30%, and 45%, respectively. Tests with LRs between 0.5 and 2 do not alter the pretest probability significantly if they are positive or negative. Evaluating the LRs of a particular test may help in selecting an appropriate study to obtain useful clinical information in the diagnostic process.

**KEY POINT**

- Likelihood ratios (LRs) are a statistical indicator of how much the result of a diagnostic test will increase or decrease the pretest probability of a disease in a specific patient; a clinical rule of thumb is that positive LRs of 2, 5, and 10 correspond to an increase in disease probability of 15%, 30%, and 45%, respectively.

**Bibliography**

Kent P, Hancock MJ. Interpretation of dichotomous outcomes: sensitivity, specificity, likelihood ratios, and pre-test and post-test probability. J Physiother. 2016;62:231-3. [PMID: 27637768] doi:10.1016/j.jphys.2016.08.008

**Item 98      Answer:   E**

**Educational Objective:**  Prevent postoperative venous thromboembolism in a patient at high risk for venous thromboembolism.

Mechanical prophylaxis with intermittent pneumatic compression (IPC) and pharmacologic prophylaxis with low-molecular-weight heparin (LMWH) are appropriate for prevention of postoperative venous thromboembolism (VTE) in this patient undergoing nonorthopedic surgery. The American College of Chest Physicians (ACCP) antithrombotic guideline provides VTE prophylaxis recommendations for both orthopedic and nonorthopedic surgery populations. The ACCP guideline recommends using the Caprini score (https://venousdisease.com/dvt-risk-assessment-online/) to estimate risk for postoperative thrombosis in those undergoing general surgery, gastrointestinal surgery, urologic surgery, gynecologic surgery, bariatric surgery, vascular surgery, and plastic/reconstructive surgery (but not other types of surgeries). It includes weighted patient and surgery-related risk factors for VTE. A score of 0 defines very low risk for VTE (estimated VTE risk in the absence of prophylaxis, <0.5%); scores of 1 to 2 define low risk (VTE risk, 1.5%); scores of 3 to 4 define moderate risk (VTE risk, 3%); and scores of 5 or more define high risk (VTE risk, 6%). For patients at high risk for VTE, pharmacologic prophylaxis with LMWH or low-dose unfractionated heparin and the addition of mechanical prophylaxis are recommended. This patient has a high perioperative risk for VTE, with a Caprini score of 6 (1 point for history of inflammatory bowel disease, 2 points for major surgery >45 minutes, and 3 points for personal history of VTE). Therefore, IPC and LMWH are appropriate.

Evidence on clinical outcomes from randomized controlled trials evaluating graduated compression stockings is sparse. Available evidence shows no statistically significant difference in risk for mortality, symptomatic deep venous thrombosis, or pulmonary embolism. However, risk for lower extremity skin damage significantly increases among patients treated with compression stockings.

The addition of LMWH to graduated compression stockings is believed not to provide additional benefit to LMWH alone. In this patient, the recommended prophylaxis of IPC and heparin is most appropriate.

**KEY POINT**

- For patients undergoing nonorthopedic surgery who are at high risk for postoperative venous thromboembolism as defined by the Caprini score, pharmacologic prophylaxis with low-molecular-weight heparin or low-dose unfractionated heparin and the addition of mechanical prophylaxis are recommended.

**Bibliography**

Gould MK, Garcia DA, Wren SM, Karanicolas PJ, Arcelus JI, Heit JA, et al. Prevention of VTE in nonorthopedic surgical patients: antithrombotic therapy and prevention of thrombosis, 9th ed: American College of Chest Physicians evidence-based clinical practice guidelines. Chest. 2012;141:e227S-e277S. [PMID: 22315263]

**Item 99      Answer:   C**

**Educational Objective:**  Treat radiation-induced nausea and vomiting in a patient with cancer.

The most appropriate treatment of this patient's nausea and vomiting in the setting of chemoradiation therapy is ondansetron. Nausea and vomiting are common complications of radiotherapy. Gastrointestinal mucosal injury and subsequent serotonin release are likely the driving mechanisms of this patient's nausea, and treatment targeting the neurotransmitter suspected of causing the nausea is a 5-hydroxytryptamine-3 ($5\text{-HT}_3$) antagonist, such as ondansetron. Dexamethasone may be added as an additional antiemetic therapy.

Haloperidol is a potent dopamine antagonist with robust antiemetic properties. Its numerous forms (intravenous, oral, sublingual concentrate) make it a versatile partner and commonly used medication to treat nausea in multiple settings, including hospice. However, given that the cause of this patient's nausea is suspected to be $5\text{-HT}_3$ release in the setting of radiotherapy, ondansetron would be a preferred agent.

Olanzapine is a potent antiemetic with a diverse neurotransmitter profile, targeting dopamine, $5\text{-HT}_3$, histaminic, and muscarinic receptors. It is effective in reducing chemotherapy-induced nausea and vomiting, but its efficacy in treating radiation-induced nausea has not yet been studied. However, olanzapine would be a reasonable choice for nausea refractory to other agents given its ability to affect multiple receptors implicated in nausea and vomiting.

Synthetic oral cannabinoids are not recommended as initial antiemetic therapy for any cancer-related condition. Experts recommend their use be limited to breakthrough symptoms caused by chemotherapy. Guidelines from the National Comprehensive Cancer Network, American Society of Clinical Oncology, and Multinational Association of Supportive Care in Cancer do not recommend the use of medical marijuana for the treatment of cancer-related nausea and vomiting.

**KEY POINT**

- A 5-hydroxytryptamine-3 ($5\text{-HT}_3$) antagonist, such as ondansetron, is the preferred initial agent for radiation-induced nausea and vomiting.

**Bibliography**

Berger MJ, Ettinger DS, Aston J, Barbour S, Bergsbaken J, Bierman PJ, et al. NCCN guidelines insights: antiemesis, version 2.2017. J Natl Compr Canc Netw. 2017;15:883-893. [PMID: 28687576] doi:10.6004/jnccn.2017.0117

## Item 100   Answer:   C

**Educational Objective:**   Treat viral pharyngitis with symptom control.

The most appropriate management of this patient with pharyngitis is symptom control that might include an analgesic agent (such as an NSAID or acetaminophen), lozenges or topical sprays, and increased environmental humidity. Pharyngitis most commonly has viral causes; only 5% to 15% of pharyngitis cases are caused by bacteria, most often group A *Streptococcus pyogenes* (GAS). Clinicians must use clinical features to determine whether the patient meets the threshold for using a streptococcal rapid antigen detection test or throat culture. Several features are more predictive of a viral syndrome, and patients who present with a sore throat with accompanying features, such as conjunctivitis, cough, hoarseness, nasal congestion, and rhinorrhea, should not be tested for GAS pharyngitis. Additionally, the High Value Task Force of the American College of Physicians recommends that patients who meet fewer than three Centor criteria (fever by history, tonsillar exudates, tender anterior cervical lymphadenopathy, and absence of cough) need not be tested for GAS pharyngitis; these patients should be treated conservatively with symptom control.

Antibiotic treatment of pharyngitis is reserved for patients with a positive result on a rapid antigen detection test or throat culture; amoxicillin and penicillin are first-line therapy. In this case, the patient has features suggesting a viral cause, including cough and rhinorrhea. She also has only two Centor criteria: fever and tonsillar exudates. Therefore, she should not be treated with amoxicillin or other antibiotics or tested for GAS through rapid antigen detection testing or throat culture. She should be advised that her sore throat may last as long as 1 week.

Patients with severe pharyngitis should be assessed for more serious complications, including peritonsillar abscesses, epiglottitis, and Lemierre syndrome (thrombophlebitis of the internal jugular vein). *Fusobacterium necrophorum* has emerged as a cause of endemic pharyngitis in adolescents and young adults and is associated with Lemierre syndrome. Further study is needed to determine how to best distinguish *F. necrophorum* from other bacteria as the cause of pharyngitis.

### KEY POINT

- Hallmark signs of viral pharyngitis include conjunctivitis, cough, nasal congestion, and rhinorrhea; viral pharyngitis should be treated symptomatically.

**Bibliography**

Harris AM, Hicks LA, Qaseem A; High Value Care Task Force of the American College of Physicians and for the Centers for Disease Control and Prevention. Appropriate antibiotic use for acute respiratory tract infection in adults: advice for high-value care from the American College of Physicians and the Centers for Disease Control and Prevention. Ann Intern Med. 2016;164:425-34. [PMID: 26785402] doi:10.7326/M15-1840

## Item 101   Answer:   B

**Educational Objective:**   Diagnose neurally mediated syncope.

The most likely diagnosis is neurally mediated syncope. Neurally mediated syncope (also known as neurocardiogenic or reflex syncope) is the most common form of syncope and is seen primarily in younger adults. The underlying syncopal mechanism, termed the neurocardiogenic or vasodepressor reflex, is a response of vasodilation, bradycardia, and systemic hypotension, which leads to transient hypoperfusion of the brain. Neurally mediated syncope includes vasovagal syncope, which may be provoked by noxious stimuli, fear, stress, or heat overexposure; situational syncope, which is triggered by cough, micturition, defecation, or deglutition; and carotid sinus hypersensitivity, which is sometimes experienced during head rotation, shaving, or use of a tight-fitting neck collar. Prodromal symptoms, including nausea and diaphoresis, are classically present before the syncopal event, and fatigue and generalized weakness are typically present afterward.

Hypoglycemia in patients without diabetes mellitus is rare; therefore, evaluation for pathologic hypoglycemia should occur only in the presence of the Whipple triad: symptomatic hypoglycemia, documented plasma glucose level of 55 mg/dL (3.1 mmol/L) or lower, and prompt symptomatic relief with correction of hypoglycemia. This patient's quick recovery from the syncopal episode without any intervention is not compatible with hypoglycemia-induced syncope.

Orthostatic syncope is classically associated with rapid onset of syncope after positional changes. Prodromal symptoms (such as lightheadedness) are often present. Orthostatic syncope is most commonly caused by hypovolemia, medications, and alcohol intoxication. Less commonly, primary autonomic failure (Parkinson disease, multiple system atrophy, multiple sclerosis) or secondary autonomic failure (diabetes, amyloidosis, connective tissue disease, spinal cord injury) can lead to orthostatic syncope. The diagnosis is confirmed by a sustained reduction of 20 mm Hg or more in systolic blood pressure (or ≥10-mm Hg drop in diastolic blood pressure) within 3 minutes of assuming upright posture, which is not present in this patient.

Postural orthostatic tachycardia syndrome is characterized by (1) frequent symptoms that occur with standing (such as lightheadedness, palpitations, generalized weakness, blurred vision, and fatigue), (2) an increase in heart rate of more than 30/min during a positional change from supine to standing, and (3) the absence of orthostatic hypotension. The standing heart rate is often higher than 120/min. This patient's findings are not compatible with postural orthostatic tachycardia syndrome.

## KEY POINT

- Neurally mediated syncope is the most common form of syncope and is seen primarily in younger adults; prodromal symptoms (nausea, diaphoresis) are classically present before the syncopal event, and fatigue and generalized weakness are typically present afterward.

## Bibliography

Runser LA, Gauer RL, Houser A. Syncope: evaluation and differential diagnosis. Am Fam Physician. 2017;95:303-312. [PMID: 28290647]

## Item 102     Answer:     C

**Educational Objective:**  Treat a man with urgency urinary incontinence.

This patient reports symptoms consistent with urgency urinary incontinence, which can be best addressed with behavioral training and the use of anticholinergic agents or mirabegron. Urgency incontinence is characterized by loss of urine accompanied by a sense of urgency. The treatment of urinary incontinence generally progresses in a stepwise manner. Lifestyle changes and behavioral therapy should be initiated first, followed by pharmacologic therapy and devices, and finally surgery if all other therapies have failed. The patient is already appropriately using behavioral therapy in the form of bladder training and scheduled voiding. The addition of pharmacologic therapy is now appropriate. Anticholinergic drugs (darifenacin, fesoterodine, oxybutynin, solifenacin, tolterodine, trospium) reduce involuntary bladder contractions by blocking the muscarinic cholinergic receptors. Anticholinergic medications are appropriate for both men and women with urgency urinary incontinence, but caution should be exercised when initiating them in men with benign prostatic hyperplasia due to risk for urinary retention. The β-agonist mirabegron, another pharmacologic option for treatment of urgency urinary incontinence, enhances the inhibitory adrenergic signals to the detrusor muscle. Clinicians should base the choice of pharmacologic agents on tolerability, adverse effect profile, ease of use, and cost of medication.

Dutasteride is a 5α-reductase inhibitor used to treat benign prostatic hyperplasia. In this patient who is already being treated with tamsulosin and in whom postvoid residual bladder volume suggests that bladder outlet obstruction has been adequately addressed, there is no additional benefit from adding another therapy for benign prostatic hyperplasia; this therapy will not address the urgency and incontinence problems.

Intermittent self-catheterization might be a useful strategy for a patient with overflow incontinence due to bladder outlet obstruction. However, that is not the case, as demonstrated by this patient's bladder ultrasound, which shows a postvoid residual urine volume of only 30 mL.

Sacral nerve root stimulation is an acceptable treatment for urgency urinary incontinence in patients in whom behavioral and pharmacologic therapies fail. Placement of

a sacral nerve root stimulator typically involves conscious sedation and may require general anesthesia.

## KEY POINT

- Male patients with urgency urinary incontinence who have not achieved satisfactory relief of symptoms with behavioral therapy may benefit from the use of anticholinergic agents or mirabegron.

## Bibliography

Gormley EA, Lightner DJ, Burgio KL, Chai TC, Clemens JQ, Culkin DJ, et al; American Urological Association. Diagnosis and treatment of overactive bladder (non-neurogenic) in adults: AUA/SUFU guideline. J Urol. 2012;188:2455-63. [PMID: 23098785] doi:10.1016/j.juro.2012.09.079

## Item 103     Answer:     A

**Educational Objective:**  Screen for cervical cancer in a woman vaccinated against human papillomavirus infection.

This patient should be screened for cervical cancer with cytology (Pap testing) alone. Nearly all cases of cervical cancer are precipitated by persistent human papillomavirus (HPV) infection, and HPV (most commonly subtypes 16 and 18 [high-risk HPV]) is detected in most patients with cervical cancer. Immunization against HPV is thought to protect against 70% to 90% of cervical cancers depending on the type of vaccine received. However, in patients who have received the HPV vaccine series, routine cervical cancer screening is still strongly recommended. Recipients of the vaccine series may have been infected with HPV prior to immunization. Furthermore, HPV vaccination is not effective in clearing HPV infection and does not protect against all HPV types. The U.S. Preventive Services Task Force (USPSTF) has concluded that the benefits of screening for cervical cancer in women aged 21 to 29 years every 3 years with cytology alone substantially outweigh the harms.

HPV testing is not indicated in women younger than 30 years because of the higher prevalence of transient HPV in this age group. Therefore, this patient should receive Pap testing alone and not dual testing with cytology and HPV detection, or high-risk HPV testing.

In the 2018 recommendation statement, the USPSTF concluded that in women aged 30 to 65 years, the benefits of screening every 3 years with cytology alone or every 5 years with high-risk HPV testing alone outweigh the harms. Decision analysis modeling suggests that screening every 5 years with high-risk HPV testing alone in women aged 30 to 65 years results in a slightly lower mortality rate than with screening every 3 years with cytology alone but much higher rates of follow-up testing and colposcopy. Four HPV screening tests are approved by the FDA for HPV screening. The tests screen for up to 14 HPV types, but only one test specifically identifies the presence of high-risk HPV types (16 and 18); the other tests report a positive result if any HPV type is present. According to the American Society for Colposcopy and Cervical Pathology and the Society of Gynecologic Oncology, high-risk HPV testing alone can be considered as a primary cervical cancer screening modality in women aged 25 years and older; however, the American College of Obstetricians and Gynecologists has affirmed that cytology alone or cytology plus HPV testing are still specifically recommended in current guidelines from most major societies.

### KEY POINT

- Routine cervical cancer screening with cytology alone is indicated in women aged 21 to 29 years, including those vaccinated against human papillomavirus.

### Bibliography

Koliopoulos G, Nyaga VN, Santesso N, Bryant A, Martin-Hirsch PP, Mustafa RA, Schünemann H, Paraskevaidis E, Arbyn M. Cytology versus HPV testing for cervical cancer screening in the general population. Cochrane Database Syst Rev. 2017;8:CD008587. doi: 10.1002/14651858.CD008587.pub2. [PMID:28796882]

## Item 104    Answer:    B

**Educational Objective:** Treat symptomatic left-sided varicocele.

This patient's history and physical examination findings support a clinical diagnosis of symptomatic varicocele, and the appropriate treatment is analgesic therapy (ibuprofen) and scrotal support. Varicoceles are common, occurring in 15% of men. Notably, they are believed to be a leading cause of infertility; 40% of men who are infertile have varicoceles. They are the result of dilation of the pampiniform plexus of spermatic veins and can have a presentation ranging from no symptoms to dull aching scrotal fullness. Examination reveals a left-sided (90%) soft scrotal mass with a "bag of worms" consistency that increases with standing and decreases while supine. Ultrasonography is used for confirmation. Management is usually conservative, including analgesic agents; scrotal support should be pursued in all patients and is considered first-line therapy. Unilateral right-sided varicoceles are uncommon and may be associated with a significant underlying abnormality, such as inferior vena cava obstruction due to tumor or thrombosis because the right gonadal vein directly empties into the inferior vena cava. Many experts recommend advanced imaging with CT for patients with right-sided varicoceles.

Treatment with ceftriaxone plus doxycycline is recommended for infectious epididymitis. The chronic nature of this patient's symptoms, lack of fever, and a scrotal mass that increases with standing do not support a diagnosis of infectious epididymitis.

Surgical consultation for possible ligation or embolization of the gonadal vein would be appropriate in certain patients with symptomatic varicocele. Ligation or embolization of the gonadal vein prevents retrograde flow of blood to the pampiniform in the scrotum. Surgery may be considered in cases of testicular atrophy or infertility, or in cases refractory to first-line therapies. However, surgical repair may increase sperm counts without improving fertility. In this case, the patient has

no evidence of testicular atrophy, and he has not previously received treatment. Although a semen analysis would be reasonable to obtain, conservative therapies should still be offered at this time.

Topical lidocaine can provide local analgesia; however, its use in cases of varicocele has not been thoroughly investigated. Rather, a systemic analgesic agent with anti-inflammatory properties would be preferable.

### KEY POINT

- In adult patients, first-line therapy for symptomatic left-sided varicocele that is not associated with testicular atrophy or infertility is analgesic agents and scrotal support.

### Bibliography

Baigorri BF, Dixon RG. Varicocele: a review. Semin Intervent Radiol. 2016;33:170-6. [PMID: 27582603] doi:10.1055/s-0036-1586147

## Item 105    Answer:    C

**Educational Objective:** Treat carpal tunnel syndrome.

The most appropriate management is splinting of the wrist. This patient has symptoms strongly suggestive of carpal tunnel syndrome (CTS). CTS is caused by median nerve compression at the wrist; it presents with wrist pain that may radiate to the fingers or forearm and is often worse at night and with repetitive motion. Risk factors include female sex, pregnancy, connective tissue disorders, diabetes mellitus, hypothyroidism, and obesity. Examination findings are often minimal early in the disease but may include hypalgesia of the median nerve distribution (thumb and first three fingers) and weakened thumb abduction. Thenar muscle atrophy suggests severe disease. For patients with mild to moderate symptoms, initial therapy consists of avoiding repetitive hand and wrist motions; for persistent or more severe symptoms, neutral-position wrist splinting can be helpful. Splinting appears to be more effective when used full time rather than only at night.

CTS can be diagnosed on the basis of history and clinical examination findings. Electromyography is not necessary unless a patient's clinical presentation is atypical, other conditions (such as polyneuropathy, plexopathy, and radiculopathy) need to be excluded, or surgical intervention is being considered.

Local glucocorticoid injection can improve symptoms over the short term (up to 10 weeks). Although generally safe, injection therapy has known harms, including worsening of median nerve compression, accidental injection into nerves or vessels, and flexor tendon rupture. For these reasons, many experts recommend glucocorticoid injection as second-line therapy for CTS.

Surgical decompression of the median nerve is reserved for patients with symptoms that do not respond to conservative therapy or with evidence of severe neuropathy (such as weakened thumb abduction, thenar muscle atrophy, and an abnormal nerve conduction study). Electrodiagnostic studies are typically performed before surgery to confirm the presence of moderate to severe median nerve injury and to provide prognostic information.

### KEY POINT

- Initial therapy for carpal tunnel syndrome consists of avoiding repetitive hand and wrist motions and neutral-position wrist splinting.

### Bibliography

Hobson-Webb LD, Juel VC. Common entrapment neuropathies. Continuum (Minneap Minn). 2017;23:487-511. [PMID: 28375915] doi:10.1212/CON.0000000000000452

## Item 106    Answer:   B

**Educational Objective:** Diagnose scleritis in a patient with rheumatoid arthritis.

The most likely diagnosis in this patient with rheumatoid arthritis (RA) is scleritis. RA is one of the most common diseases associated with scleritis. Typical features include eye pain, pain with gentle palpation of the globe, and photophobia. The deep scleral vessels are involved and may lead to scleromalacia, which is characterized by thinning of the sclera and is seen as a dark area in the white sclera. Scleromalacia may lead to perforation of the sclera, called scleromalacia perforans. Scleritis can be vision-threatening and lead to blindness; it is therefore important to urgently refer the patient to an ophthalmologist for care.

Episcleritis is an abrupt inflammation of the superficial vessels of the episclera, a thin membrane that lies just beneath the conjunctiva. The cause is often unclear; rarely, it is associated with systemic rheumatologic disease. Patients with episcleritis frequently present without pain or decreased visual acuity. On examination, the inflammation appears localized. White sclera can be seen between superficial dilated blood vessels. Episcleritis typically resolves spontaneously. The presence of severe pain, diffuse redness, and decreased visual acuity make episcleritis an unlikely diagnosis.

Subconjunctival hemorrhage is a common disorder and typically benign in origin. It is caused by painless bleeding into the superficial portion of the eye. Examination reveals a blotchy redness (from extravascular blood) that is typically confined to one area of the conjunctiva. Subconjunctival hemorrhage is painless and not associated with loss of vision. Most cases resolve within several weeks without intervention. The patient's findings are not compatible with subconjunctival hemorrhage.

Viral conjunctivitis also causes a red eye. Typically, the underlying vessels are visible, a watery discharge may be seen, and the eyelids are matted in the morning. The eye may feel irritated, but there is no pain or loss of visual acuity. In general, conjunctivitis is a diagnosis of exclusion. The presence of pain and decreased visual acuity exclude viral conjunctivitis in this patient.

### KEY POINT

- Rheumatoid arthritis is one of the most common diseases associated with scleritis, which can be vision-threatening and lead to thinning of the sclera and perforation.

### Bibliography

Artifoni M, Rothschild PR, Brézin A, Guillevin L, Puéchal X. Ocular inflammatory diseases associated with rheumatoid arthritis. Nat Rev Rheumatol. 2014;10:108-16. [PMID: 24323074] doi:10.1038/nrrheum.2013.185

## Item 107    Answer:   C

**Educational Objective:** Select appropriate preoperative testing in a patient with chronic kidney disease.

This patient should undergo preoperative assessment of serum creatinine and electrolyte levels. Preoperative testing should be ordered selectively according to the patient's symptoms, medical history, medications, and physical examination findings. Serum creatinine and electrolyte levels should be measured preoperatively in patients with kidney disease and those who are taking medications that may affect kidney function or predispose them to electrolyte abnormalities, such as this patient, who has chronic kidney disease and is taking an ACE inhibitor (lisinopril) and diuretic (hydrochlorothiazide). In patients with chronic kidney disease undergoing surgery, electrolyte abnormalities should be corrected, and volume status should be optimized.

Serum aminotransferases (alanine aminotransferase and aspartate aminotransferase) should not be routinely ordered in the absence of known liver disease, symptoms suggestive of underlying liver disease, physical examination findings suspicious for liver disease, or history of abnormal liver chemistry results.

Coagulation testing is reserved for patients with a history of abnormal bleeding, those taking anticoagulants, and patients with medical conditions that predispose to coagulopathy (such as liver disease or hemophilia). For the patient with a history suggesting a bleeding disorder, preoperative prothrombin time, activated partial thromboplastin time, and platelet count measurements are indicated.

Routine preoperative laboratory panels are not recommended because they expose patients to unnecessary testing, risk for incidental findings that are lost to follow-up evaluation, and increased anxiety. However, given this patient's comorbidities and medication use, forgoing preoperative testing would be inappropriate.

### KEY POINT

- Preoperative measurement of serum electrolyte and creatinine levels is recommended in patients with kidney disease and those who are taking medications that may affect kidney function or predispose to electrolyte abnormalities.

## Bibliography

Apfelbaum JL, Connis RT, Nickinovich DG, Pasternak LR, Arens JF, Caplan RA, et al; Committee on Standards and Practice Parameters. Practice advisory for preanesthesia evaluation: an updated report by the American Society of Anesthesiologists Task Force on Preanesthesia Evaluation. Anesthesiology. 2012;116:522-38. [PMID: 22273990] doi:10.1097/ALN.0b013e31823c1067

## Item 108     Answer:    B

**Educational Objective:** Avoid NSAID therapy in a patient who has undergone bariatric surgery.

Ibuprofen should be discontinued in this patient. This patient likely has patellofemoral pain syndrome, which is characterized by anterior knee pain that is usually gradual in onset and worsens with running, prolonged sitting, and climbing stairs. Applying direct pressure to the patella with the knee extended may reproduce the pain. Treatment generally includes activity modification and physical therapy. NSAIDs, acetaminophen, bracing, and patellar taping all have limited efficacy. Additionally, the use of NSAIDs in patients who have undergone bariatric surgery is associated with increased risk for internal bleeding; bleeding risk is increased at the sites of anastomoses and staple or suture lines in the early postoperative period, with increased risk of marginal or gastric ulceration in the later postoperative period. Therefore, ibuprofen and other NSAIDs should be avoided after bariatric surgery.

This patient with known risk factors for atherosclerotic cardiovascular disease meets the criteria for moderate- to high-intensity statin therapy and should continue atorvastatin. There is no association between statin therapy and adverse events after bariatric surgery.

Patients who have undergone bariatric surgery may experience a decline in blood pressure such that antihypertensive agents need to be reduced or discontinued. Close monitoring of blood pressure in the postoperative period is recommended. This patient's blood pressure is appropriate on the current dose of lisinopril and this drug does not need to be discontinued.

Similarly, patients who have undergone bariatric surgery may experience reduced need for medications for type 2 diabetes mellitus. Close monitoring for the development of hypoglycemia in the postoperative period is recommended. Hypoglycemia is unlikely with metformin therapy alone and does not need to be discontinued.

### KEY POINT

- The use of NSAIDs in patients who have undergone bariatric surgery is associated with increased risk for internal bleeding; therefore, ibuprofen and other NSAIDs should be avoided after bariatric surgery because their use is associated with increased risk for internal bleeding.

## Bibliography

Marcotte E, Chand B. Management and prevention of surgical and nutritional complications after bariatric surgery. Surg Clin North Am. 2016;96:843-56. [PMID: 27473805] doi:10.1016/j.suc.2016.03.006

## Item 109     Answer:    B

**Educational Objective:** Diagnose borderline personality disorder.

This patient demonstrates a behavioral pattern consistent with borderline personality disorder. A personality disorder is characterized by persistent patterns of inner experiences and behaviors that digress substantially from the expectations of the affected person's culture. These disorders are entrenched, rigid, and stable over time and lead to substantial impairment and distress. Onset is usually during adolescence or early adulthood. Persons with personality disorders usually do not recognize their interactions with others as abnormal. In borderline personality disorder, patients have chaotic interpersonal relationships, emotional lability, and impulsive and self-destructive behaviors (such as suicide attempts). Patients have exaggerated responses to social stressors and often perceive people as "all good" or "all bad." Comorbid psychiatric illness is common in patients with borderline personality disorder. The initial management focuses on establishing rapport and boundaries with the patient, which can improve the patient's acceptance of psychiatry referral. Psychotherapy can be effective at improving coping mechanisms. No pharmacologic therapies are approved for treating personality disorders directly, but medications can be prescribed for specific symptoms (such as mood stabilizers for impulsivity).

Bipolar disorder is characterized by manic episodes (in which patients have decreased need for sleep, greater distractibility, and increased energy) and major depressive episodes. Although patients with bipolar disorder may engage in self-destructive behavior, it is not related to interpersonal discord.

Patients with generalized anxiety disorder have excessive anxiety and worry about multiple aspects of their lives. This leads to insomnia, irritability, and fatigue. Patients with generalized anxiety disorder do not typically have impulsivity, relationship instability, or the tendency to idealize and devalue individuals as do patients with borderline personality disorder.

Histrionic personality disorder is characterized by excessive need for approval and attention-seeking behaviors. Patients with this disorder are emotionally vulnerable, and their behaviors focus on obtaining approval from others. Patients with histrionic personality disorders are uncomfortable if not the center of attention and typically use physical appearance to draw attention to self. Interaction with others may be inappropriately sexually seductive or provocative. Histrionic personality disorder is not accompanied by the same degree of emotional lability and risk for suicidality as borderline personality disorder, as exhibited in this patient.

### KEY POINT

- Patients with borderline personality disorder have chaotic interpersonal relationships, emotional lability, impulsive and self-destructive behaviors, and exaggerated responses to social stressors; comorbidity with other psychiatric illnesses is high.

## Bibliography

Gunderson JG. Clinical practice. Borderline personality disorder. N Engl J Med. 2011;364:2037-42. [PMID: 21612472] doi:10.1056/NEJMcp1007358

## Item 110  Answer: A

**Educational Objective:** Treat systemic exertion intolerance disease with cognitive behavioral therapy.

The most appropriate treatment for this patient with systemic exertion intolerance disease (SEID) is cognitive behavioral therapy. According to the Institute of Medicine (now the National Academy of Medicine), SEID is diagnosed by the presence of fatigue of at least 6 months' duration with substantial reduction in preillness activities, postexertional malaise, unrefreshing sleep, and either cognitive impairment or orthostatic intolerance (symptoms such as lightheadedness, dizziness, fatigue, cognitive deficits, and visual difficulties that worsen with upright posture and improve with recumbency). Patients with SEID benefit most from a structured, well-defined, multimodal approach that includes regularly scheduled office visits, which allow for discussion, educational opportunities, and longitudinal reassessment. There is evidence that cognitive behavioral therapy and graded exercise therapy may decrease fatigue and improve function, and these therapies should be offered to patients. Additionally, all patients should receive instruction on effective sleep hygiene. Other modalities that may be of benefit include physical therapy, occupational therapy, biofeedback therapy, massage therapy, acupuncture, yoga, tai chi, and stress management activities. Considering this patient's depression (which is likely a consequence of her chronic symptoms), cognitive behavioral therapy is an ideal treatment.

Although methylphenidate, prednisone, opioids, antiinflammatory agents, and antimicrobial agents are commonly requested in clinical practice for the treatment of chronic fatigue symptoms, there is no consistent evidence that these agents improve symptoms or prognosis in patients with SEID. Given the lack of benefit, risk for abuse, addictive potential, and array of adverse effects, these options are not recommended.

Mirtazapine (an $\alpha_2$-agonist) and sertraline (a selective serotonin reuptake inhibitor) are used to treat depression. In general, selective antidepressant therapy may be useful in treating associated depression; however, it is not a direct treatment for SEID. Mirtazapine and sertraline might improve this patient's symptoms of depression, but it will not address the other symptoms associated with SEID.

### KEY POINT

- The treatment of systemic exertion intolerance disease involves a structured, multimodal, nonpharmacologic approach that includes regularly scheduled office visits, cognitive behavioral therapy, graded exercise therapy, and sleep hygiene education.

## Bibliography

Janse A, Nikolaus S, Wiborg JF, Heins M, van der Meer JWM, Bleijenberg G, Tummers M, Twisk J, Knoop H. Long-term follow-up after cognitive behaviour therapy for chronic fatigue syndrome. J Psychosom Res. 2017;97:45-51. [PMID: 28606498] doi:10.1016/j.jpsychores.2017.03.016

## Item 111  Answer: D

**Educational Objective:** Manage hormonal contraception prescribing by first excluding pregnancy.

Pregnancy testing is the next step in this patient's management. Strategies to reduce unintended pregnancy require assessing pregnancy risk, counseling patients regarding contraceptive options, and ensuring correct and consistent use of contraceptives. Most women can start most contraceptive methods at any time. Available contraceptive methods include hormonal contraception; long-acting reversible preparations, including intrauterine devices; barrier contraceptives; and sterilization. Other than a thorough history and blood pressure and BMI measurements, few examinations or tests, if any, are needed before starting a contraceptive method. A pregnancy test should be obtained if more than 7 days have elapsed since the start of the last menses.

Hormonal contraceptive options include oral contraceptive pills (combination estrogen-progesterone or progesterone-only pills), long-acting reversible contraceptives, transdermal patches, and vaginal rings. Contraindications to combination products include breast cancer, liver disease, migraine with aura, uncontrolled hypertension, and venous thromboembolism. Estrogen-containing preparations are contraindicated in women older than 35 years who smoke more than 15 cigarettes a day. A family history of breast cancer is not a contraindication for hormonal contraception.

In healthy women of reproductive age, a breast examination, pelvic examination, or mammography are not needed before beginning hormonal contraception. Breast cancer and cervical cancer screenings should be performed according to established guidelines. In 2016, the U.S. Preventive Services Task Force (USPSTF) reaffirmed its recommendation for biennial screening mammography in all women aged 50 to 74 years. The USPSTF recommends individualized screening decisions for women aged 40 to 49 years based on patient context and values regarding specific benefits and harms. The patient has no indications for mammography at this time.

According to the USPSTF, cervical cancer screening in women aged 21 to 65 years may be accomplished with cytology (Pap test) every 3 years. This patient's last Pap smear was normal 2 years ago, and she does not need to undergo repeat Pap testing for another 12 months.

### KEY POINT

- Before initiating hormonal contraception, a negative pregnancy test result must be documented if 7 days have passed since the onset of the last menstrual period.

## Bibliography

Curtis KM, Jatlaoui TC, Tepper NK, Zapata LB, Horton LG, Jamieson DJ, Whiteman MK. U.S. Selected practice recommendations for contraceptive use, 2016. MMWR Recomm Rep. 2016;65:1-66. [PMID: 27467319] doi:10.15585/mmwr.rr6504a1

## Item 112  Answer:  C

**Educational Objective:** Treat a patient with acute low back pain with nonpharmacologic modalities.

The most appropriate initial treatment of this patient's low back pain is nonpharmacologic therapy. According to a 2017 clinical practice guideline issued by the American College of Physicians, clinicians should choose nonpharmacologic treatments as first-line therapy for acute low back pain. Options include superficial heat, acupuncture, massage, and spinal manipulation. The quality of evidence supporting individual nonpharmacologic measures is moderate or low. Recommendations for their use are based on the fact that most patients with acute low back pain will improve over time (most within 4 weeks), regardless of the treatment chosen. Harms of nonpharmacologic interventions were seldom and minor. Superficial heat was associated with increased risk for skin flushing, and massage and spinal manipulation were associated with muscle soreness.

Recent evidence, including a Cochrane review, has demonstrated that acetaminophen is not effective in treating acute low back pain. As such, it would be inappropriate to recommend its use in this patient.

The FDA has approved the use of duloxetine in chronic back pain (pain lasting >12 weeks), as studies have demonstrated its effectiveness. However, no evidence supports its use for acute low back pain.

Guidelines recommend that opioids should be the last treatment option considered for chronic back pain and should be considered only in patients in whom other therapies have failed, as these drugs are associated with substantial harms. Harms of short-term opioid therapy include increased constipation, dizziness, dry mouth, nausea, somnolence, and vomiting. Studies assessing opioids for the treatment of chronic low back pain did not address the risk for addiction, abuse, or overdose, although observational studies have shown a dose-dependent relationship between opioid use for chronic pain and serious harms. A 2018 randomized trial demonstrated that treatment with opioids was not superior to treatment with nonopioid medications for improving pain-related function for chronic back pain. In addition, pain intensity was significantly improved in the nonopioid group. There are no studies of opioids for the treatment of acute back pain, but given their questionable effect and substantial harms as well as the self-limited nature of acute nonspecific back pain, opioids should likely be avoided entirely.

### KEY POINT

- First-line treatment of acute low back pain is nonpharmacologic therapy, including acupuncture, massage, spinal manipulation, and superficial heat; most patients will improve over time, regardless of the treatment chosen.

### Bibliography

Qaseem A, Wilt TJ, McLean RM, Forciea MA; Clinical Guidelines Committee of the American College of Physicians. Noninvasive treatments for acute, subacute, and chronic low back pain: a clinical practice guideline from the American College of Physicians. Ann Intern Med. 2017;166:514–530. [PMID: 28192789] doi:10.7326/M16-2367

## Item 113  Answer:  C

**Educational Objective:** Prevent atherosclerotic cardiovascular disease in a patient with type 2 diabetes mellitus with statin therapy.

The most appropriate treatment for primary prevention of atherosclerotic cardiovascular disease (ASCVD) in this patient is moderate- or high-intensity atorvastatin. Intensity of statin therapy is defined by the expected decrease in LDL cholesterol levels; high-intensity statin therapy should decrease LDL cholesterol levels by at least 50% from baseline levels, whereas moderate-intensity statin therapy should decrease LDL cholesterol levels by 30% to 50%. High-intensity statin regimens recommended by the 2013 American College of Cardiology (ACC)/American Heart Association (AHA) cholesterol treatment guideline include atorvastatin, 40 mg/d to 80 mg/d, and rosuvastatin, 20 mg/d to 40 mg/d. For primary prevention of ASCVD in patients with diabetes mellitus, the decision to initiate high-intensity statin therapy or moderate-intensity statin therapy is based on the patient's estimated 10-year ASCVD risk. According to the ACC/AHA guideline, patients with diabetes with an estimated 10-year ASCVD risk of 7.5% or higher should receive high-intensity statin therapy, whereas those with an estimated 10-year ASCVD risk less than 7.5% should receive moderate-intensity statin therapy. In contrast to the ACC/AHA recommendations, the U.S. Preventive Services Task Force recommends initiating low- to moderate-intensity statin therapy in adults aged 40 to 75 years without a history of ASCVD who have one or more ASCVD risk factors (dyslipidemia, diabetes, hypertension, or smoking) and a calculated 10-year ASCVD event risk of 10% or higher.

Nonstatin drugs are not considered first-line therapy for the prevention of ASCVD in patients with or without diabetes. Fibrates, such as fenofibrate, would be first-line therapy for hypertriglyceridemia (typically, when the triglyceride level is >500 mg/dL [5.65 mmol/L]) for prevention of triglyceride-induced acute pancreatitis.

A 2017 systematic review concluded that among randomized controlled trials and observational studies, evidence of variable strength showed no association between increased fish oil intake and lower cardiovascular disease event risk. Expert opinion recommends that the use of fish oil supplementation be restricted to patients with refractory hypertriglyceridemia.

All patients should receive education on therapeutic lifestyle changes, including regular exercise, weight loss, and dietary changes. However, lifestyle modifications alone are not considered adequate for cardiovascular risk reduction in many patient groups, including patients with diabetes.

### KEY POINT

- Patients with diabetes mellitus are at significantly increased lifetime risk for cardiovascular events and should receive statin therapy for primary prevention.

## Bibliography

Stone NJ, Robinson JG, Lichtenstein AH, Bairey Merz CN, Blum CB, Eckel RH, et al; American College of Cardiology/American Heart Association Task Force on Practice Guidelines. 2013 ACC/AHA guideline on the treatment of blood cholesterol to reduce atherosclerotic cardiovascular risk in adults: a report of the American College of Cardiology/American Heart Association Task Force on Practice Guidelines. Circulation. 2014;129:S1-45. [PMID: 24222016] doi:10.1161/01.cir.0000437738.63853.7a

## Item 114      Answer:      A

**Educational Objective:   Treat insomnia with cognitive behavioral therapy.**

The most appropriate next step in management would be to pursue targeted cognitive behavioral therapy for this patient. The American College of Physicians recommends cognitive behavioral therapy for insomnia (CBT-I) as first-line therapy for insomnia. CBT-I combines components of sleep hygiene with cognitive therapeutic interventions (to understand and identify appropriate sleep expectations) and behavioral interventions (such as relaxation techniques). Elements of sleep hygiene include avoiding strenuous exercise, large meals, caffeine, alcohol, and nicotine close to bedtime; establishing a relaxing prebedtime routine; keeping the room dark and quiet; avoiding reading, television, and use of electronic devices while in bed; and keeping a stable bedtime and arising time. CBT-I may be delivered in various formats, such as individual or group therapy, web-based modules, or written materials. It provides significant value over pharmacologic-driven approaches and carries little risk for adverse effects.

Although diphenhydramine and melatonin are popular over-the-counter remedies for insomnia, there is insufficient evidence to recommend their use before a trial of CBT-I. Additionally, sedating antihistamines (such as diphenhydramine) are associated with anticholinergic side effects and carry-over daytime sleepiness.

Some antidepressants, such as mirtazapine, are sedating and may improve sleep. Doxepin, in low doses, is the only antidepressant approved for the treatment of insomnia. Most expert opinion recommends against using antidepressants for treating insomnia in patients without depression; however, doxepin, trazodone, and mirtazapine can be useful if a sedating antidepressant is indicated.

Benzodiazepines (flurazepam, triazolam, temazepam) are effective for short-term insomnia treatment. However, their use is limited by tolerance; side effects of daytime somnolence, falls, cognitive impairment, and anterograde amnesia; and the potential for dependence. Rebound insomnia may occur upon discontinuation, especially if discontinuation is abrupt. The selective nature and shorter half-life of nonbenzodiazepines (zolpidem, zaleplon, eszopiclone) lead to fewer side effects (including rebound insomnia), making these drugs better initial choices if pharmacotherapy is warranted. However, sedation, disorientation, and agitation may still occur; rare side effects include sleep driving, sleep walking, and sleep eating. In this patient, CBT-I should be tried before pharmacologic therapy with zolpidem is considered.

### KEY POINT

- Cognitive behavioral therapy for insomnia, which combines components of sleep hygiene with cognitive therapy and behavioral interventions, is first-line therapy for insomnia.

## Bibliography

Qaseem A, Kansagara D, Forciea MA, Cooke M, Denberg TD; Clinical Guidelines Committee of the American College of Physicians. Management of chronic insomnia disorder in adults: a clinical practice guideline from the American College of Physicians. Ann Intern Med. 2016;165:125-33. [PMID: 27136449] doi: 10.7326/M15-2175

## Item 115      Answer:      C

**Educational Objective:   Effectively manage termination of a physician-patient relationship.**

The most appropriate management is to send the patient a formal, written warning informing him that the patient-physician relationship may be terminated unless he is able to meaningfully participate in the plan of care. Physician-patient relationships are formed on the basis of mutual agreement. Rarely, the relationship fails to reach mutual goals and becomes unproductive. In some cases, the patient may not adhere to recommended therapies or may demonstrate inappropriate behavior with the physician or staff members, and it may be appropriate for the physician to terminate the relationship. After reasonable attempts to resolve differences have failed, the patient should be notified in writing that the relationship has been terminated and that care should be obtained from a different provider, usually with a several-week time frame for the patient to continue receiving urgent care. Terminations should occur only if the patient is medically stable and when alternative care is available. If a patient threatens a physician or staff member, the termination may be immediate.

Although a psychiatrist might provide interventions to help this patient better adhere to care recommendations, such a referral is unnecessary in making a decision to terminate an ineffective physician-patient relationship.

This patient has not demonstrated signs of an unstable mental health condition that warrants intervention by a crisis team.

Patient abandonment is unethical and may be a cause for legal action. In this case, the patient has not yet received a formal warning that his failure to adhere to treatment goals may result in his termination from the practice. Therefore, he should not be released from the practice immediately.

### KEY POINT

- If the physician-patient relationship becomes irreparably compromised because of lack of trust, lack of mutual goals, or failure to maintain an effective working relationship despite efforts to resolve differences, the relationship can be terminated.

**Bibliography**

Snyder L; American College of Physicians Ethics, Professionalism, and Human Rights Committee. American College of Physicians ethics manual: sixth edition. Ann Intern Med. 2012;156:73-104. [PMID: 22213573] doi: 10.7326/0003-4819-156-1-201201031-00001

## Item 116    Answer:    C

**Educational Objective:** Treat neurogenic thoracic outlet syndrome.

Physical therapy aimed at shoulder girdle muscle strengthening and improving posture would be the best therapeutic option for this patient with thoracic outlet syndrome (TOS). TOS is caused by compression of the brachial plexus, subclavian artery, or subclavian vein as these structures pass through the thoracic outlet. There are three main clinical subtypes of TOS, defined by the primary structure involved (nerve, artery, vein). Neurogenic TOS is the most common subtype and is caused by compression of the brachial plexus nerve roots as they exit the triangle formed by the first rib and the scalenus anticus and medius muscles. Symptoms include paresthesias and pain that typically worsen with activities that involve continued use of the arm or hand, especially those that include elevation of the arm. This patient's presentation is most consistent with neurogenic TOS. In most patients, there are no abnormal neurologic findings. Electrodiagnostic studies frequently fail to reveal any abnormalities. Although imaging studies are often obtained, they are not required to make the diagnosis; they may, however, reveal the presence of a structural abnormality, such as an anomalous cervical rib. First-line therapy for neurogenic TOS includes improving posture and strengthening shoulder girdle muscles.

Although neurogenic TOS is caused by intermittent compression of the brachial plexus within the thoracic outlet, the role of gabapentin in managing this condition has not been well studied. Gabapentin is not considered to be first-line therapy.

Observational studies have supported the use of interscalene injection of anesthetic agents, glucocorticoids, or botulinum toxin type A in patients with neurogenic TOS. However, in a randomized, double-blind clinical trial, patients treated with botulinum toxin did not show improvement in function, pain, or paresthesias compared with patients treated with placebo.

Surgical decompression is not considered to be first-line therapy for neurogenic TOS, especially in patients who lack neurologic abnormalities. The procedure is reserved for patients who do not respond to conservative measures or for those with progressive or disabling neurologic symptoms.

**KEY POINT**

- Symptoms of neurogenic thoracic outlet syndrome include paresthesias and pain that typically worsen with activities that involve continued use of the arm or hand, especially those that include elevation of the arm; first-line therapy includes improving posture and strengthening the shoulder girdle muscles.

**Bibliography**

Buller LT, Jose J, Baraga M, Lesniak B. Thoracic outlet syndrome: current concepts, imaging features, and therapeutic strategies. Am J Orthop (Belle Mead NJ). 2015;44:376-82. [PMID: 26251937]

## Item 117    Answer:    D

**Educational Objective:** Diagnose sudden sensorineural hearing loss.

The most likely diagnosis for this patient's acute, unilateral hearing loss is sudden sensorineural hearing loss (SSHL). The right-sided hearing loss and the finding of lateralization to the left ear on Weber testing support the diagnosis. Approximately 90% of cases of SSHL are idiopathic; however, viral infection, drug reactions, acoustic neuroma, multiple sclerosis, head injury, vascular issues, systemic immune-mediated conditions, and Meniere disease can all be causes. SSHL most commonly presents as unilateral tinnitus and ear fullness; vertigo occurs less often. Because this patient lacks other features to explain the acute hearing loss, she should undergo urgent referral to an otolaryngologist for audiometry, clinical assessment, and MRI to exclude tumors, multiple sclerosis, or vascular causes. Treatment involves oral glucocorticoids, although strong evidence of efficacy is lacking.

Meniere disease, which is associated with endolymphatic hydrops (excess fluid in the endolymphatic spaces), can cause unilateral sensorineural hearing loss, but its presentation is characterized by episodic vertigo (lasting between 20 minutes and 24 hours) and tinnitus, which is often low pitched. The hearing loss may be described as fluctuating, and early in the disease it often involves low frequencies. Meniere disease may also present with a sensation of ear fullness.

Otosclerosis involves bony overgrowth on the footplate of the stapes, leading to a lack of functioning of the ossicles. This middle ear process typically causes gradual, painless, bilateral conductive hearing loss, not sensorineural hearing loss, as seen in this patient. Otosclerosis occurs more often in women, and there is often a family history of the condition.

Ototoxicity also can result in sensorineural hearing loss; it may be caused by a variety of medications, including antibiotics (particularly aminoglycosides), chemotherapeutic agents, loop diuretics, and aspirin or other NSAIDs. Often occurring gradually and bilaterally, ototoxicity may be reversible or permanent, depending on the agent involved. This patient is not taking and has not been exposed to drugs known to be ototoxic.

**KEY POINT**

- All patients with sudden sensorineural hearing loss should undergo audiometric evaluation, and most patients will require MRI.

**Bibliography**

Chin CJ, Dorman K. Sudden sensorineural hearing loss. CMAJ. 2017; 189:E437-E438. [PMID: 28385715] doi:10.1503/cmaj.161191

# Item 118    Answer:    A

**Educational Objective:** Treat a pressure injury with a hydrocolloid dressing.

This patient's pressure injury would be best managed with hydrocolloid or foam dressings, which have been found to be superior to standard gauze dressings in reducing ulcer size in low-quality studies. Pressure injuries (also known as pressure ulcers) are characterized by localized injury to the skin or soft tissue as a result of pressure and shear forces. They may be classified by use of a staging system, with each stage distinguished by the amount of tissue loss. In 2015, the American College of Physicians (ACP) published a clinical practice guideline for the treatment of pressure ulcers. The ACP recommends that clinicians use hydrocolloid or foam dressings in patients with pressure ulcers to reduce wound size. Hydrocolloid dressings consist of a mixture of adhesive absorbent polymers and a gelling agent, with a film covering to make them water and gas permeable. The dressing interacts with the wound fluid to form a gel. Hydrocolloids may promote wound healing by enhancing fibrinolytic activity and growth of granulation tissue and inhibiting bacterial overgrowth through their physical barrier properties. Hydrocolloids are convenient to use because they require infrequent dressing changes and are easy to apply. Foam dressings are sheets of foam polymers and are used primarily for heavily exudative wounds. Other treatment options include managing the conditions that caused the pressure injury, wound protection, surgical debridement and repair, and vacuum-assisted closure. There is moderate-quality evidence that air-fluidized beds reduce the size of pressure injuries compared with other support surfaces. The ACP also recommends protein or amino acid supplements (low-quality evidence) and electrical stimulation (moderate-quality evidence) as adjunctive therapy to accelerate wound healing.

There is insufficient evidence to recommend for or against platelet-derived growth factor dressings in the treatment of pressure injuries, and no studies have explored the benefits of vitamin- or mineral-infused dressings (such as a zinc-infused dressing). In addition, insufficient evidence was found to recommend for or against hydrotherapy, hyperbaric oxygen therapy, or maggot therapy.

**KEY POINT**

- Hydrocolloid or foam dressings are superior to standard gauze dressings in the treatment of pressure injuries; protein supplements and the use of electrical stimulation to accelerate wound healing are also recommended treatment strategies.

**Bibliography**
Qaseem A, Humphrey LL, Forciea MA, Starkey M, Denberg TD; Clinical Guidelines Committee of the American College of Physicians. Treatment of pressure ulcers: a clinical practice guideline from the American College of Physicians. Ann Intern Med. 2015;162:370-9. [PMID: 25732279] doi:10.7326/M14-1568

# Item 119    Answer:    C

**Educational Objective:** Treat obsessive-compulsive disorder with cognitive behavioral therapy.

The preferred initial treatment for this patient with obsessive-compulsive disorder (OCD) is cognitive behavioral therapy (CBT). OCD is an anxiety disorder in which patients experience obsessions (recurrent, intrusive thoughts, images, or impulses causing distress) and compulsions (repetitive behaviors done to alleviate obsession-related anxiety). Loss of time and disrupted social interactions from these thoughts and behaviors cause significant functional impairment. CBT is first-line treatment because it is more effective than pharmacotherapy alone. However, a combination of CBT and selective serotonin reuptake inhibitor (SSRI) therapy is useful for patients with severe symptoms or inadequate response to CBT. Although evidence is strongest for adjunctive therapy with SSRIs, more recent data support the adjunctive use of neuroleptics, deep-brain stimulation, and neurosurgical ablation for treatment-resistant OCD.

Buspirone is beneficial in the treatment of generalized anxiety disorder without comorbid anxiety or mood disorders but has no demonstrated benefit in patients with OCD.

Benzodiazepines, such as clonazepam, are used for short-term treatment of debilitating symptoms from severe generalized anxiety disorder and panic disorder, but they are not effective in the treatment of OCD.

Risperidone is an antipsychotic medication that can be used in the treatment of schizophrenia or other psychiatric conditions with psychotic features. Patients with OCD have obsessions and compulsions but do not have hallucinations, delusions, or disorganized thoughts that would warrant antipsychotic therapy.

**KEY POINT**

- Obsessive-compulsive disorder should be treated with cognitive behavioral therapy (CBT); a combination of CBT and selective serotonin reuptake inhibitor therapy is useful for patients with severe symptoms or inadequate response to CBT.

**Bibliography**
Hirschtritt ME, Bloch MH, Mathews CA. Obsessive-compulsive disorder: advances in diagnosis and treatment. JAMA. 2017;317:1358-1367. [PMID: 28384832] doi:10.1001/jama.2017.2200

# Item 120    Answer:    C

**Educational Objective:** Treat a patient with acute epididymitis.

The most appropriate treatment is ceftriaxone and levofloxacin. This patient's history and physical examination findings (fever, erythema, and swelling of the hemiscrotum; tenderness to palpation near the epididymis; and urinary symptoms) are concerning for a diagnosis of acute epididymitis. Prehn sign, which is alleviation of pain with elevation of the testicle or scrotum, can clinically support this diagnosis. Infectious epididymitis has a bimodal distribution: men younger than 35 years and older than 55 years. In younger patients, sexually transmitted infections (chlamydia and gonorrhea) are the most likely cause. In older patients and those who practice insertive anal intercourse, *Escherichia coli*, Enterobacteriaceae, and *Pseudomonas* species should be considered. In older men and persons who practice insertive anal intercourse, infectious epididymitis should be treated with ceftriaxone and a fluoroquinolone, such as levofloxacin.

Empiric treatment with ceftriaxone alone would provide adequate coverage for *Chlamydia trachomatis* infection but would be inadequate therapy. This older patient, who has risk factors for gram-negative infection, should be treated with ceftriaxone and a fluoroquinolone.

In younger patients (age <35 years), the most common infectious etiologies of acute epididymitis include *C. trachomatis* and *Neisseria gonorrhoeae*. In these men, and in the absence of risk factors for gram-negative infection (anal intercourse, urologic instrumentation), empirically treating with ceftriaxone and doxycycline (or azithromycin, if the patient is intolerant to doxycycline) would be appropriate.

Epididymitis can also have noninfectious causes (for example, trauma, autoimmune disease, or vasculitis). Treatment includes scrotal support, ice, and NSAIDs. Analgesic agents and scrotal support are supportive measures that can be offered to all patients presenting with acute epididymitis. However, the most appropriate treatment for this patient with risk factors for bacterial epididymitis and no history of trauma or findings supporting autoimmune disease or vasculitis would be initiation of an antimicrobial regimen rather than supportive therapies alone.

**KEY POINT**

- In older men and persons who practice insertive anal intercourse, infectious epididymitis should be treated with ceftriaxone and a fluoroquinolone, such as levofloxacin.

**Bibliography**

McConaghy JR, Panchal B. Epididymitis: an overview. Am Fam Physician. 2016;94:723-726. [PMID: 27929243]

## Item 121     Answer:    C

**Educational Objective:** Evaluate a breast mass in a woman aged 30 years and older.

This patient's breast mass should be evaluated with both diagnostic mammography and ultrasonography. Any dominant mass in the breast warrants diagnostic imaging to determine the nature of the mass and the appropriate management. A clinical examination alone cannot differentiate between a cyst and a solid mass. In a woman aged 30 years or older, diagnostic mammography is recommended for evaluation of a palpable mass, to assess for a spiculated density or associated pleomorphic calcifications that may indicate malignancy. Diagnostic mammography may also include magnification views of the focal area of concern. In addition, targeted ultrasonography is needed to determine whether the mass is cystic or solid; however, ultrasonography is unnecessary in cases in which mammography shows a clearly benign correlate or a normal, fatty area of breast tissue in the location of the palpable finding. This diagnostic evaluation can help determine a benign finding from an indeterminate or suspicious finding requiring needle biopsy. For women aged 40 years or older, mammography, followed in most cases by ultrasonography, is recommended. For women aged 30 to 39 years old, ultrasonography or mammography may be performed first at the discretion of the radiologist or referring clinician.

Breast MRI and other advanced imaging have little to no role in the routine diagnostic evaluation of palpable breast abnormalities. Breast MRI is not an appropriate imaging technique for evaluation of palpable symptoms because it provides little added information to careful evaluation with mammography and ultrasonography.

Definitive diagnosis of a breast mass is obtained by tissue sampling using fine-needle aspiration, core-needle biopsy with or without stereotactic or ultrasound guidance, or excisional biopsy. Fine-needle aspiration is generally reserved for ultrasound-confirmed cystic lesions. Core-needle biopsy is the test of choice for most solid lesions, as it provides more tissue for histology and tissue markers. Excisional biopsy is used when core-needle biopsy findings are nondiagnostic or when biopsy and imaging studies do not concur. Further management of abnormal pathologic findings requires consultation with a breast surgeon and oncologist. Needle aspiration, core-needle biopsy, and excision are all premature until the imaging evaluation is completed.

Ultrasonography is often preferred in women younger than age 30 years because the increased density of breast tissue in younger women limits the usefulness of mammography. Ultrasonography may also be a better choice for pregnant patients in order to avoid radiation exposure.

**KEY POINT**

- For evaluation of palpable breast abnormalities in women aged 40 years or older, mammography, followed in most cases by ultrasonography, is recommended.

**Bibliography**

Lehman CD, Lee AY, Lee CI. Imaging management of palpable breast abnormalities. AJR Am J Roentgenol. 2014;203:1142-53. [PMID: 25341156] doi:10.2214/AJR.14.12725

## Item 122     Answer:    C

**Educational Objective:** Identify medications to avoid during pregnancy.

This patient should discontinue the ACE inhibitor lisinopril. Medication adjustments are an important component of preconception counseling in women who are planning pregnancy. All antihypertensive medications cross the placenta. Some antihypertensive medications are absolutely

Answers and Critiques

contraindicated during pregnancy, including ACE inhibitors, angiotensin receptor blockers (ARBs), and, likely, renin inhibitors. Women taking ACE inhibitors or ARBs should be counseled about the associated teratogenicity throughout all trimesters, and these medications should be stopped if pregnancy is anticipated or possible. Blood pressure goals with medical therapy in patients with chronic hypertension during pregnancy are 120 to 160/80 to 105 mm Hg. However, treatment of hypertension during pregnancy is controversial. If blood pressure control is not adequate after stopping lisinopril, methyldopa and labetalol have been used safely. Calcium channel blockers (such as long-acting nifedipine) can also be used during pregnancy. Diuretics may induce oligohydramnios if initiated during pregnancy but generally can be continued if the patient was taking a diuretic preconception. Spironolactone and eplerenone should be avoided because their safety has never been proven.

Although acetaminophen is generally considered safe during pregnancy, caution is needed with the use of NSAIDs due to their effect on organogenesis during pregnancy.

A goal for preconception wellness is the absence of uncontrolled depression. Evidence shows that women who are depressed during pregnancy have worse birth outcomes. Selective serotonin reuptake inhibitors, including citalopram, fluvoxamine, and sertraline, are pregnancy category C agents that can be continued during pregnancy. An alternative to antidepressant therapy is psychotherapy, specifically cognitive behavioral therapy, which is equally as efficacious as pharmacologic therapy. In this patient who is already taking an antidepressant, it would be more important to continue therapy than to discontinue treatment.

Optimal glycemic control with a goal hemoglobin $A_{1c}$ value of less than 6.5% is recommended for women with diabetes mellitus who are contemplating pregnancy. Metformin is a diabetes medication deemed safe during pregnancy, as it is FDA category B. Category B denotes that animal reproduction studies have not demonstrated a fetal risk, and no controlled studies in pregnant women have shown adverse effects.

**KEY POINT**

- Antihypertensive medications absolutely contraindicated during pregnancy include ACE inhibitors, angiotensin receptor blockers, and, likely, renin inhibitors.

**Bibliography**
Frayne DJ, Verbiest S, Chelmow D, Clarke H, Dunlop A, Hosmer J, et al. Health care system measures to advance preconception wellness: consensus recommendations of the Clinical Workgroup of the National Preconception Health and Health Care Initiative. Obstet Gynecol. 2016;127:863-72. [PMID: 27054935] doi:10.1097/AOG.0000000000001379

**Item 123      Answer:     D**

**Educational Objective:** Manage perioperative anticoagulation in a patient receiving warfarin.

The most appropriate management of this patient's preoperative anticoagulation is to withhold warfarin without bridging anticoagulation. Anticoagulant therapy increases the risk for perioperative hemorrhage and should be discontinued in most patients before surgery. Bridging anticoagulation is the administration of therapeutic doses of short-acting parenteral therapy, usually heparin, when anticoagulant therapy is being withheld during the perioperative period in patients with elevated thrombotic risk. This patient is undergoing a procedure associated with elevated bleeding risk, and she has no history of stroke, transient ischemic attack (TIA), or intracardiac thrombus. Therefore, the risks of bridging anticoagulation outweigh the thrombotic risk, and the warfarin should be withheld without bridging anticoagulation.

There is no role for aspirin in bridging anticoagulation. In patients with normal kidney function who require bridging anticoagulation, low-molecular-weight heparin is the agent of choice.

The American College of Chest Physicians (ACCP) and the American College of Cardiology (ACC)/American Heart Association (AHA) have made recommendations regarding bridging anticoagulation in patients with atrial fibrillation. Most recently in 2017, the ACC published an expert consensus decision pathway for periprocedural management of anticoagulation in patients with nonvalvular atrial fibrillation. The ACCP recommends bridging anticoagulation in patients with a $CHADS_2$ score of 3 or higher or with a history of stroke or transient ischemic attack (TIA). However, according to the ACCP guideline, bridging anticoagulation is not indicated if bleeding risk is elevated in patients with a $CHADS_2$ score of 3 or 4 and no history of stroke or TIA. The 2017 ACC decision pathway suggests forgoing bridging anticoagulation in patients with $CHA_2DS_2$-VASc scores of 5 and 6 or lower without a history of stroke, TIA, or systemic embolism. Because this patient has a $CHADS_2$ score of 2 and a $CHA_2DS_2$-VASc score of 4, bridging anticoagulation is not necessary.

**KEY POINT**

- In patients taking warfarin, bridging anticoagulation may be deferred if thrombotic risk is low.

**Bibliography**
Doherty JU, Gluckman TJ, Hucker WJ, Januzzi JL Jr, Ortel TL, Saxonhouse SJ, et al. 2017 ACC expert consensus decision pathway for periprocedural management of anticoagulation in patients with nonvalvular atrial fibrillation: a report of the American College of Cardiology Clinical Expert Consensus Document Task Force. J Am Coll Cardiol. 2017;69:871-898. [PMID: 28081965]

**Item 124      Answer:     C**

**Educational Objective:** Screen for genital and extragenital gonorrhea and chlamydia in a man who has sex with men.

The most appropriate screening strategy in this patient is nucleic acid amplification testing (NAAT) of urine, rectal, and pharyngeal specimens for *Neisseria gonorrhoeae* and *Chlamydia trachomatis*. Multiple studies have demonstrated an increased prevalence of genital and extragenital chlamydial and gonorrheal infections in men who have sex with men (MSM). In one study, prevalence rates of *N. gonorrhoeae* in MSM were 6.9% (rectal), 6% (urethral), and 9.2% (pharyngeal); for *C. trachomatis*, prevalence rates in MSM were 7.9% (rectal), 5.2% (urethral), and 1.4% (pharyngeal). Most infections are asymptomatic. The Centers for Disease Control and Prevention (CDC) recommends at least annual gonorrhea screening with NAAT of urethral, pharyngeal, and rectal specimens and at least annual screening for chlamydia with NAAT of urethral and rectal specimens. The CDC notes that commercially available NAATs have not been cleared by the FDA for some of these indications; however, these tests can be used by laboratories that have met all regulatory requirements for an off-label procedure. The CDC also recommends screening for syphilis and HIV at least annually in MSM. In contrast to the CDC, the U.S. Preventive Services Task Force has found insufficient evidence to recommend screening for chlamydia and gonorrhea in men.

Human papillomavirus (HPV)-associated conditions (such as anogenital warts and anal squamous intraepithelial lesions) are common among MSM. However, data are insufficient to recommend routine anal cancer screening with anal cytology in MSM. The quadrivalent HPV vaccine is recommended for MSM through age 26 years.

Sexual transmission of hepatitis C infection can occur in MSM with HIV infection. The CDC recommends that screening should be performed at least yearly for hepatitis C in this population. Hepatitis C screening is also indicated in all past and current injection drug users. Because the patient does not use drugs and his HIV status is unknown, screening for hepatitis C is not indicated at this time.

All MSM should also be tested for hepatitis A and B. Vaccination against hepatitis A and B is recommended for all MSM in whom previous infection or vaccination cannot be documented.

**KEY POINT**

- The Centers for Disease Control and Prevention recommends that men who have sex with men should be screened at least annually for genital and extragenital chlamydial and gonorrheal infections, syphilis, and HIV infection.

**Bibliography**

Wilkin T. Clinical practice. Primary care for men who have sex with men. N Engl J Med. 2015;373:854-62. [PMID: 26308686] doi:10.1056/NEJMcp1401303

## Item 125    Answer:    C

**Educational Objective:**  Treat recurrent major depressive disorder.

Long-term continuation of fluoxetine at the current dosage is appropriate for this patient with recurrent depression. Guidelines from the American Psychiatric Association (APA) recommend long-term maintenance therapy for patients with three or more episodes of major depressive disorder, persistent depressive disorder, or residual depressive symptoms.

The same antidepressant and dosage that were effective in the treatment of acute depression should be continued for long-term maintenance.

Fluoxetine therapy for 8 months should be sufficient for the treatment of the patient's major depressive disorder, but the medication should not be tapered. Because he has had two other episodes of depression, he should be maintained on antidepressant therapy to prevent recurrence.

Switching to another antidepressant medication (such as bupropion) for long-term maintenance is not indicated unless the patient develops intolerable adverse effects from the initial medication.

Discontinuing fluoxetine is not recommended, even if the patient were not a candidate for long-term therapy. APA guidelines recommend continuing treatment for at least 4 to 9 months after resolution of major depressive disorder, followed by gradual tapering of the antidepressant dosage. Antidepressant drugs should not be stopped abruptly because of the risk for discontinuation syndrome, which is most frequently seen in patients who abruptly stop selective serotonin reuptake inhibitors. The most common discontinuation symptoms include dizziness, fatigue, headache, and nausea. Other symptoms include agitation, anxiety, dysphoria, and irritability. Onset of the syndrome is within 1 to 4 days of abruptly stopping antidepressant therapy or after a rapid taper. Although fluoxetine has the lowest incidence of discontinuation syndrome, therapy should be tapered rather than abruptly stopped.

**KEY POINT**

- The American Psychiatric Association recommends long-term maintenance therapy for patients with three or more episodes of major depressive disorder, persistent depressive disorder, or residual depressive symptoms; the antidepressant dosage that was effective in acute treatment should be continued for long-term maintenance.

**Bibliography**

American Psychiatric Association. Practice Guideline for the Treatment of Patients With Major Depressive Disorder. 3rd edition. Arlington, VA: American Psychiatric Association; 2010. Available at https://psychiatry-online.org/pb/assets/raw/sitewide/practice_guidelines/guidelines/mdd.pdf. Accessed July 25, 2018.

## Item 126    Answer:    C

**Educational Objective:**  Evaluate a patient with medically unexplained symptoms.

The most appropriate management of this patient with medically unexplained symptoms (MUS) is to avoid testing and obtain previous medical records. The most common symptoms in patients presenting with MUS are chest pain, fatigue, dizziness, headache, swelling, back pain, shortness of breath, insomnia, abdominal pain, and numbness. Frequently, patients have seen many primary care and subspecialty physicians over the course of many years and have undergone extensive laboratory testing, imaging studies, and procedures. Because patients with MUS present on a continuum of physical and mental health, a comprehensive, holistic approach is essential. Each presenting symptom merits a relevant history and physical examination. In most cases, prior records should be reviewed before repeating or extending the evaluation unless the patient's condition has changed substantially. Physicians must possess excellent patient-centered communication skills and listen carefully to the patient, validating concerns and responding to emotions. Additionally, the initial assessment should include specific questions to elicit the patient's concerns, underlying psychological status, and the degree of distress and disability attributable to the symptoms. Long-term management of the patient with MUS is challenging. A therapeutic alliance and a mutually respectful physician-patient relationship are key features in the successful management of the patient with MUS. In keeping with a patient-centered approach, the patient should be engaged fully in the plan, focusing on physical, psychological, and social aspects of health. The physician and patient should work together to create and maintain an atmosphere of mutual trust.

Physicians often find it difficult to limit further testing, prescribing, or referral because they fear missing an elusive diagnosis. The evidence that more testing helps reassure patients with MUS or improves outcomes is limited. Additional testing, such as a comprehensive metabolic profile, C-reactive protein level, rheumatoid factor, and antinuclear antibody titer, should not occur without an initial thorough investigation of the results of previous evaluations and determining whether symptoms have changed.

Familial Mediterranean fever (FMF) is the classic auto-inflammatory disease, characterized by discrete attacks of pain lasting up to 72 hours associated with serosal inflammation (joints, chest, abdomen), rash, and abnormalities on *MEFV1* genetic testing. This patient's presentation does not match that of FMF. More importantly, additional testing should be avoided until after a review of previous medical records.

It is possible that the patient may ultimately benefit from a psychiatric consultation. However, before that occurs, the physician should review the patient's medical records; evaluate the current status of his symptoms; elicit his concerns, psychological status, and degree of distress and disability attributable to the symptoms; and establish a trusting relationship with the patient.

**KEY POINT**

- In patients with medically unexplained symptoms, clinicians must approach each symptom in a focused manner and diligently review any previous diagnostic evaluations.

**Bibliography**
Evens A, Vendetta L, Krebs K, et al. Medically unexplained neurologic symptoms: a primer for physicians who make the initial encounter. Am J Med. 2015;128:1059-64. [PMID: 25910791]

## Item 127    Answer:    E

**Educational Objective:** Treat a patient with cervical radiculopathy with neck exercises.

The most appropriate management of this patient with symptoms consistent with cervical radiculopathy is neck exercises. Stretching and strengthening exercises provide intermediate-term relief of symptoms and should be part of a multimodal approach. Other nonpharmacologic options include acupuncture, early mobilization, and spinal manipulation. Cervical traction appears to be of limited benefit. Patients should also be informed that most patients with neck pain have resolution or near-resolution of symptoms within 2 to 3 months of onset by using conservative measures.

The use of a cervical collar in patients with neck pain should be avoided because it can lead to neck muscle atrophy, especially when used for longer than 1 to 2 weeks. Shorter-term use appears to be no more effective for symptom relief than sham interventions.

This patient lacks any "red flag" findings that would warrant imaging, whether in the form of plain radiography or MRI. Features that would prompt imaging include constitutional symptoms; personal history of or concern for malignancy; progressive neurologic symptoms; or myelopathic findings, such as difficulty writing, gait disturbance, hypertonia, hyperflexia, or problems with fine manipulation.

Electrodiagnostic testing is most helpful to diagnose peripheral nerve entrapment syndromes or peripheral neuropathy as the cause of arm symptoms. Both of these conditions should be considered when arm symptoms are more prominent than neck symptoms. Electrodiagnostic testing can also identify cervical radiculopathy as the cause of neck pain but only when motor axonal injury is present; cervical radicular pain can exist in the absence of axonal injury. Therefore, the best course of action for this patient is conservative treatment without diagnostic testing.

NSAIDs are considered first-line pharmacologic therapy for acute neck pain, including acute cervical radiculopathy. Cyclobenzaprine, when used at doses greater than 15 mg/d, has been shown to be effective for treating acute neck pain when muscle spasm is present, although it should be used with caution in older patients. Gabapentin, a neuromodulator, can be used to treat chronic radicular pain; however, it does not have a role in the management of acute radicular symptoms.

**KEY POINT**

- Cervical radiculopathy, caused by nerve root compression, usually resolves within 2 to 3 months by using conservative measures; stretching and strengthening exercises of the neck muscles provide the best intermediate-term relief.

**Bibliography**
Iyer S, Kim HJ. Cervical radiculopathy. Curr Rev Musculoskelet Med. 2016;9:272-80. [PMID: 27250042] doi:10.1007/s12178-016-9349-4

## Item 128    Answer:    A

**Educational Objective:   Prevent human papillomavirus infection with appropriate immunization.**

This healthy 25-year-old woman should be offered the human papillomavirus (HPV) vaccine. HPV vaccination prevents persistent HPV infection, which can lead to cervical, anogenital, and nasopharyngeal cancers. HPV genotypes 16 and 18 are responsible for causing most cases of cervical cancer and many cases of vulvar, vaginal, anal, penile, and oropharyngeal cancers. HPV genotypes 6 and 11 cause most cases of genital warts. The HPV vaccine series is recommended for all females aged 11 or 12 years or between the ages of 13 and 26 years if not given previously. In males, the series should be administered at age 11 or 12 years, between the ages of 13 and 21 years if not previously administered, or through age 26 years for immunocompromised men (including those with HIV infection) or men who have sex with men. Three different HPV vaccines are licensed for use in females (bivalent, quadrivalent, and nine-valent), and two HPV vaccines are licensed for use in males (quadrivalent and nine-valent). All vaccines target genotypes 16 and 18, and the quadrivalent vaccine also targets genotypes 6 and 11. The nine-valent vaccine protects against five additional genotypes that cause cervical cancer, resulting in the potential prevention of 90% of cervical, vulvar, vaginal, and anal cancers. If administered after age 15 years, a three-dose series is recommended, whereas a two-dose series is recommended in younger individuals.

Vaccination against meningococcal serogroups A, C, W135, and Y with the quadrivalent meningococcal conjugate vaccine is recommended in all persons by age 18 years. Revaccination with a single dose of the quadrivalent meningococcal conjugate vaccine is indicated in adult patients who are considered to be at increased risk, including those with asplenia (functional or anatomic), those with persistent complement deficiencies, first-year college students living in a dormitory, travelers to endemic areas, microbiologists exposed to *Neisseria meningitidis*, military recruits, persons at increased risk during an outbreak, and persons infected with HIV. Revaccination is indicated every 5 years in those who remain at increased risk. This patient does not have any indications for quadrivalent meningococcal conjugate revaccination.

Adults aged 19 years and older who did not receive the tetanus, diphtheria, and acellular pertussis (Tdap) vaccine during adolescence should receive a dose of the Tdap vaccine, followed by tetanus and diphtheria toxoids (Td) boosters every 10 years. Because this patient received a Tdap vaccine 7 years ago, she should receive a Td booster in 3 years.

Pneumococcal vaccination is recommended in all adults aged 65 years and older and adults aged 19 to 64 years with certain high-risk conditions. This young patient does not smoke or have any immunocompromising or chronic medical conditions; therefore, the 23-valent pneumococcal polysaccharide vaccine is not indicated.

**KEY POINT**

- Vaccination against human papillomavirus is recommended for all females aged 11 or 12 years or between the ages of 13 and 26 years if not previously vaccinated and for all males aged 11 or 12 years, between the ages of 13 and 21 years if not previously vaccinated, or through age 26 years for immunocompromised men and men who have sex with men.

**Bibliography**

Petrosky E, Bocchini JA Jr, Hariri S, Chesson H, Curtis CR, Saraiya M, et al; Centers for Disease Control and Prevention (CDC). Use of 9-valent human papillomavirus (HPV) vaccine: updated HPV vaccination recommendations of the advisory committee on immunization practices. MMWR Morb Mortal Wkly Rep. 2015;64:300-4. [PMID: 25811679]

## Item 129    Answer:    B

**Educational Objective:   Treat vasomotor symptoms of menopause.**

The most appropriate management is hormone replacement therapy with estrogen and progesterone. The hallmark symptoms of menopause vary greatly in duration, frequency, and severity, but they may include vasomotor symptoms (hot flushes, night sweats) and urogenital symptoms (dyspareunia, vaginal dryness). Symptoms generally resolve spontaneously within a few years, and treatment should be based on symptom severity. Hormone therapy is effective treatment for relief of vasomotor symptoms of menopause, and for women who are younger than 60 years and are within 10 years of menopause onset, the low absolute risk of adverse events supports the option to prescribe hormone therapy for women with moderate to severe vasomotor or urogenital symptoms who are at low risk for breast cancer, coronary heart disease, stroke, and thromboembolic disease. The clinician should prescribe the lowest effective dosage, titrating up if needed, for the shortest period of time needed to control symptoms. Use of hormone therapy in menopause should be reassessed every year; treatment duration is based on the continued presence of vasomotor symptoms. Estrogen-progesterone therapy taken for more than 5 years is associated with increased risk for breast cancer and requires that women receive individualized breast cancer risk evaluation. For this patient with an intact uterus and no contraindications, combination estrogen-progesterone therapy is the best choice.

Long-term unopposed endometrial estrogen exposure increases the risk for endometrial hyperplasia or malignancy, and for women who experience menopausal symptoms and have an intact uterus, estrogen should be combined with progestin to avoid unopposed estrogen-related endometrial proliferation. For women who have had a hysterectomy, estrogen alone would be the preferred hormone therapy but would be inappropriate for this patient.

Ospemifene is an estrogen agonist/antagonist that is used in postmenopausal women to reduce the severity of moderate to severe dyspareunia associated with genitourinary symptoms of menopause; however, it is not indicated for vasomotor symptom management.

Vaginal estrogen therapy is effective for managing genitourinary syndrome of menopause, although vaginal estrogen alone will not be adequate therapy for vasomotor symptoms of menopause, as experienced by this patient.

**KEY POINT**

- Hormone therapy is an option for women with moderate to severe vasomotor symptoms of menopause who are younger than 60 years and within 10 years of menopause onset, provided they are at low risk for breast cancer, coronary heart disease, stroke, and thromboembolic disease.

**Bibliography**

The NAMS 2017 Hormone Therapy Position Statement Advisory Panel. The 2017 hormone therapy position statement of The North American Menopause Society. Menopause. 2017;24:728-753. [PMID: 28650869] doi:10.1097/GME.0000000000000921

## Item 130　　Answer:　B

**Educational Objective:** Diagnose labyrinthitis.

The most likely diagnosis in this patient with vertigo is labyrinthitis. Patients with vertigo often describe a spinning or whirling sensation, which is frequently associated with concomitant nausea, vomiting, and sudden-onset fatigue. Once vertigo is suspected, the next important step is to distinguish central from peripheral causes. The Dix-Hallpike maneuver can help with this task but could not be performed in this patient. The identification of central vertigo is important because it can be associated with ischemia, infarction, or hemorrhage of the cerebellum or brainstem and may be life threatening. More than 80% of patients with central vertigo have focal neurologic signs, and many have experienced recurrent symptoms over days to weeks. In this patient's case, he has no risk factors for stroke (hypertension, diabetes mellitus), no focal signs, and a preceding upper respiratory tract infection, making central vertigo unlikely. Common causes of peripheral vertigo include benign paroxysmal positional vertigo (BPPV), vestibular neuronitis, labyrinthitis, and Meniere disease. Labyrinthitis is caused by postviral inflammation of both branches of the vestibulocochlear nerve (cranial nerve VIII), resulting in sudden-onset, severe, persistent vertigo and hearing loss. This patient has signs and symptoms consistent with labyrinthitis preceded by an acute viral infection, making it the most likely diagnosis.

BPPV is the most common cause of peripheral vertigo. It is characterized by sudden-onset, recurrent, and brief (usually <1 minute) vertiginous symptoms, which are provoked and worsened with positional changes of the head. Although prolonged head positioning can trigger BPPV,

BPPV is not associated with auditory changes, as seen in this patient.

Meniere disease presents with recurrent, spontaneous, and brief episodes of vertigo, tinnitus, and hearing loss. Nystagmus may be present. Symptoms resolve completely between episodes. In patients with Meniere disease, episodes of vertigo typically last hours, whereas this patient has experienced unremitting symptoms for the past 2 days.

Vestibular neuronitis is a peripheral vestibular condition caused by inflammation of the vestibular branch of the vestibulocochlear nerve, leading to vertiginous symptoms and nystagmus. It is most often preceded by a viral infection. Symptoms are sustained, ranging from days to weeks; however, auditory symptoms are not present, which is the key distinction between vestibular neuronitis and labyrinthitis.

**KEY POINT**

- Labyrinthitis is characterized by sudden-onset, severe, persistent peripheral vertigo accompanied by hearing loss; it is most often preceded by a viral infection affecting both branches of the vestibulocochlear nerve (cranial nerve VIII).

**Bibliography**

Kim JS, Zee DS. Clinical practice. Benign paroxysmal positional vertigo. N Engl J Med. 2014;370:1138-47. [PMID: 24645946] doi: 10.1056/NEJMcp1309481

## Item 131　　Answer:　D

**Educational Objective:** Treat cough due to acute rhinosinusitis.

This patient with acute cough due to acute rhinosinusitis should be treated with an intranasal glucocorticoid, such as fluticasone. Most upper respiratory tract infections (URIs) are caused by viral infections and resolve spontaneously within a few days. Patients without clear evidence of bacterial infection should be treated symptomatically. A meta-analysis of patients with acute rhinosinusitis found that use of intranasal glucocorticoids increased the rate of symptom response compared with placebo; there was a dose-response curve, with higher doses offering greater relief. Analgesics, such as NSAIDs and acetaminophen, may relieve pain. Only limited evidence supports saline irrigation in the relief of nasal symptoms; careful attention should be paid to the use of sterile or bottled water. Instructions for nasal saline irrigation are available online (www.fda.gov/ForConsumers/ConsumerUpdates/ucm316375.htm). First-generation antihistamines may help dry nasal secretions; however, evidence supporting their efficacy is lacking, and sedation is a common side effect. Decongestants are of possible benefit in patients with evidence of eustachian tube dysfunction but should be used with caution in elderly patients and those with cardiovascular disease, hypertension, angle-closure glaucoma, or bladder neck obstruction. Antitussive agents are generally ineffective.

Empiric treatment of URI symptoms with antibiotics (such as amoxicillin) is ineffective, increases bacterial antibiotic resistance, and may cause multiple adverse effects, including *Clostridium difficile* colitis. Antibiotics should be reserved for patients with symptoms lasting more than 10 days, worsening symptoms after initially improving viral illness, or severe symptoms or signs of high fever (>39 °C [102.2 °F]) with purulent nasal discharge or facial pain for at least 3 consecutive days.

A systematic review concluded that centrally acting (codeine, dextromethorphan) or peripherally acting (moguisteine) antitussive therapy results in little improvement in acute cough and is not recommended.

Inhaled albuterol is indicated for patients with evidence of wheezing, which this patient does not have. For patients who develop postinfectious airway hyperreactivity with a subacute or chronic cough, albuterol and other asthma therapies are beneficial.

### KEY POINT

- Acute rhinosinusitis may be treated symptomatically with analgesics and intranasal glucocorticoids; antibiotics are not recommended without clearly established bacterial infection.

### Bibliography

Harris AM, Hicks LA, Qaseem A; High Value Care Task Force of the American College of Physicians and for the Centers for Disease Control and Prevention. Appropriate antibiotic use for acute respiratory tract infection in adults: advice for high-value care from the American College of Physicians and the Centers for Disease Control and Prevention. Ann Intern Med. 2016;164:425-34. [PMID: 26785402] doi:10.7326/M15-1840

### Item 132      Answer:      C

**Educational Objective:** Treat pain in a patient with advanced serious illness and chronic kidney disease with hydromorphone.

The most appropriate treatment of this patient's pain is hydromorphone. This patient's back pain is caused by progressive myeloma, and she requires rapid treatment of her pain with oral opioids initially. Given the concern for worsening back pain in the setting of malignancy, she requires an urgent MRI of her spine to rule out impending malignant spinal cord compression, and aggressive pain treatment while pursuing a diagnostic strategy is critical. Hydromorphone is a potent opioid agonist that is thought to be safer in patients with severe kidney impairment, such as this patient on hemodialysis.

A transdermal fentanyl patch is an effective analgesic for opioid-tolerant patients. It does not have clinically relevant active metabolites that would accumulate in the setting of end-stage kidney disease; however, it should be used only in opioid-tolerant patients. This patient is opioid naïve, and she should not be started on a long-acting agent until her total daily opioid needs are identified and an appropriate equianalgesic dose of fentanyl is calculated.

Gabapentin binds to the $\alpha_2\delta$ subunit of voltage-gated calcium channels; it can be an effective nonopioid adjuvant in the treatment of various pain types, including neuropathic pain. Titration of gabapentin can be prolonged to avoid adverse effects; therefore, it would not be helpful in this patient in need of more rapid analgesia.

Morphine is a prototypical opioid agonist, but its active metabolites accumulate in the setting of kidney failure and increase the risk for adverse neuroexcitatory effects with aggressive titration. Morphine, codeine, and meperidine are all contraindicated in patients with kidney failure (glomerular filtration rate <30 mL/min/1.73 m²).

Tramadol is a weak opioid agonist whose analgesic activity is influenced by its inhibition of serotonin and norepinephrine reuptake. It is a poor analgesic in the setting of cancer-related pain and should not be used in patients with kidney failure due to accumulation of active metabolites. In addition, tramadol has the potential for significant drug interactions.

### KEY POINT

- Hydromorphone is the preferred opioid to treat cancer-related pain in patients with chronic kidney disease.

### Bibliography

Swetz KM, Kamal AH. Palliative care. Ann Intern Med. 2018;168:ITC33-ITC48. [PMID: 29507970] doi:10.7326/AITC201803060

### Item 133      Answer:      A

**Educational Objective:** Evaluate for coronary artery disease preoperatively in a patient with elevated cardiac risk and poor functional capacity.

Dobutamine stress echocardiography is indicated in this patient undergoing elective noncardiac surgery with an elevated cardiac risk, poor functional capacity, symptoms, and electrocardiographic findings concerning for possible silent ischemia. In patients undergoing noncardiac surgery, risk calculators, including the Revised Cardiac Risk Index (RCRI) and American College of Surgeons National Surgical Quality Improvement Program myocardial infarction and cardiac arrest calculator, can be used to determine the risk for a perioperative major adverse cardiac event (MACE). Asymptomatic patients at low risk (<1% risk for perioperative MACE) may proceed to surgery without preoperative cardiac stress testing, whereas patients with elevated risk (>1% risk for perioperative MACE) should undergo assessment of functional capacity. Metabolic equivalents (METs) are used to represent the patient's functional capacity based on the intensity of activity able to be performed. If the patient's functional capacity exceeds 4 METs, the patient may proceed to surgery without further testing. Cardiac stress testing should be considered in patients at elevated risk for MACE with a functional capacity of less than 4 METs or if functional capacity cannot be determined, but only if the results of stress testing will change perioperative manage-

CONT.

ment. In this case, the patient's RCRI score is 4 (pathologic Q waves on electrocardiogram, stroke, insulin-dependent diabetes mellitus, and preoperative creatinine >2.0 mg/dL [176.8 μmol/L]) corresponding to a MACE (cardiac death, nonfatal myocardial infarction, and nonfatal cardiac arrest) risk of greater than 5.4%, and stress testing is indicated. Because of the elective nature of his scheduled surgery, he would be able to proceed with preoperative coronary angiography if indicated based on the results of stress testing.

This patient's exercise capacity is limited by fatigue, dyspnea, and hip pain; therefore, exercise electrocardiography would most likely be nondiagnostic.

Echocardiography to evaluate left ventricular function should not be routinely performed preoperatively. However, it is recommended in certain clinical scenarios, such as in the presence of dyspnea of unknown origin, heart failure with worsening dyspnea or overall change in clinical status, known left ventricular dysfunction without assessment in the last year, and known or suspected moderate to severe valvular stenosis or regurgitation without echocardiographic assessment in the last year or with a change in clinical status. In this patient, transthoracic echocardiography would not provide the necessary evaluation for myocardial ischemia.

### KEY POINT

- Preoperative cardiac stress testing should be considered in patients at elevated risk for a major adverse cardiac event or if functional capacity cannot be determined, but only if the results of stress testing will change perioperative management.

### Bibliography

Fleisher LA, Fleischmann KE, Auerbach AD, Barnason SA, Beckman JA, Bozkurt B, et al; American College of Cardiology. 2014 ACC/AHA guideline on perioperative cardiovascular evaluation and management of patients undergoing noncardiac surgery: a report of the American College of Cardiology/American Heart Association Task Force on practice guidelines. J Am Coll Cardiol. 2014;64:e77-137. [PMID: 25091544] doi:10.1016/j.jacc.2014.07.944

### Item 134        Answer:        B

**Educational Objective:** Manage impairment in a physician colleague.

The most appropriate management is to directly approach the colleague with the concerns of impairment and guide her through a plan to determine whether impairment exists and, if so, how to manage it. Impairment may be caused by medical or psychiatric illness or the use of psychoactive substances; however, the presence of these conditions does not necessarily signify impairment. According to the American College of Physicians *Ethics Manual*, every physician is responsible for protecting patients from an impaired colleague and for assisting an impaired colleague by identifying appropriate sources of help. These responsibilities should not be hampered by personal relationships, shame, or fear of harming a colleague. This physician's colleague, who may be

demonstrating signs of cognitive impairment, would benefit from assistance.

When signs of physician impairment are present, it is preferable to intervene before patient harm occurs, if possible. Therefore, continuing to monitor the colleague is not the best option.

Although the physician may be tempted to offer to perform the colleague's medical evaluation, several risks are associated with caring for patients with whom a previous relationship exists, including impaired objectivity, insufficient history taking (for example, sexual history), incomplete examination, and incomplete or biased assessment. The colleague should undergo a confidential and complete medical assessment with another physician to search for reversible causes of impairment.

There is a clear ethical responsibility to report a physician who appears to be impaired to an appropriate authority, which may include a chief of staff, chief of service, or, if the impairment is serious, a state medical board. The legal requirements and thresholds for reporting impaired physicians vary. Most state medical societies or medical boards have physician health programs for physicians with potentially impairing illnesses that can be accessed through a voluntary or mandatory track; these physician health programs provide confidential assessment and treatment, with the goal of restoration of function. At this point, there is no objective evidence of impairment, and a confidential evaluation would be the most appropriate first step.

### KEY POINT

- Every physician is responsible for protecting patients from an impaired colleague and for assisting an impaired colleague by identifying appropriate sources of help.

### Bibliography

Snyder L; American College of Physicians Ethics, Professionalism, and Human Rights Committee. American College of Physicians ethics manual: sixth edition. Ann Intern Med. 2012;156:73-104. [PMID: 22213573] doi: 10.7326/0003-4819-156-1-201201031-00001

### Item 135        Answer:        B

**Educational Objective:** Treat erectile dysfunction in a patient with multiple comorbid conditions.

The most appropriate treatment for this patient's erectile dysfunction (ED) is psychotherapy. The patient has a history of depression, which can predispose to intermittent ED. Given that the patient is still able to achieve an erection 50% of the time and experiences nocturnal penile tumescence, a diagnosis of ED secondary to his other medical comorbidities or medication usage is far less likely. On the basis of these findings, he likely has situational or mood-related ED. In situations such as this one, it can be beneficial to proceed with therapies such as cognitive behavioral therapy, biofeedback therapy, and sensory awareness exercises.

Alprostadil is considered second-line therapy, as it requires routine intracavernous injections, transurethral injections, or transurethral suppositories. For many patients, this option is poorly tolerated. In patients with depression and intermittent ED, alprostadil would not be recommended before trying psychotherapy, which is much better tolerated.

Sildenafil and other oral phosphodiesterase-5 inhibitors are considered first-line medical therapy for ED. However, sildenafil is contraindicated in patients taking nitrate therapy, such as this one.

Testosterone supplementation is recommended only in patients with ED and confirmed symptomatic androgen deficiency. This patient has a normal total testosterone level and has no alterations in secondary sexual characteristics, which make the diagnosis of clinically relevant androgen deficiency unlikely. Furthermore, testosterone therapy should be avoided in patients with untreated obstructive sleep apnea.

### KEY POINT

- Erectile dysfunction in a patient who experiences nocturnal penile tumescence is most likely situational or mood related; cognitive behavioral therapy, biofeedback, or sensory awareness exercises with a psychotherapist are first-line therapies.

### Bibliography

Mobley DF, Khera M, Baum N. Recent advances in the treatment of erectile dysfunction. Postgrad Med J. 2017;93:679-685. [PMID: 28751439] doi:10.1136/postgradmedj-2016-134073

## Item 136      Answer:    C

### Educational Objective:  Diagnose Morton neuroma.

This patient's symptoms are most likely due to a Morton neuroma, a condition that causes compression of the interdigital nerve. Common symptoms include paresthesias and the sensation of walking on a pebble. On examination, there are usually no obvious abnormalities, but some patients may have tenderness to direct palpation of the involved interspace. The cause is thought to be use of constricting footwear, such as high-heeled shoes. First-line therapy consists of wearing nonconstricting footwear and local padding. In patients who do not respond to these measures, a local glucocorticoid injection can be offered. For recalcitrant cases, sclerosing alcohol injections, radiofrequency ablation, and surgery (neurectomy) have been used with some success.

Bunion (hallux) deformity refers to lateral deviation of the great toe with medial bone deformity. This condition typically causes pain at the site of the deformity due to footwear pressure. The location of this patient's pain and lack of visible deformity on examination make bunion deformity an incorrect diagnosis.

Hammertoe deformity is also associated with constricting footwear; it refers to a proximal interphalangeal joint flexion deformity with dorsal interphalangeal joint extension and extended or neutral position of the metatarsophalangeal joint. This patient's normal foot appearance makes this diagnosis incorrect.

Plantar fasciitis typically causes pain localized to the medial inferior heel at the insertion of the plantar fascia in the medial calcaneal tubercle. Pain is usually present at activity initiation following prolonged rest and improves with further walking (for example, the first few steps in the morning after arising from bed). As the condition progresses, pain may be present with both activity and rest. The location and description of this patient's pain are not consistent with plantar fasciitis.

### KEY POINT

- Hallmarks of a Morton neuroma are pain between the metatarsal heads, the sensation of walking on a pebble, and no obvious abnormalities of the foot upon clinical examination or palpation.

### Bibliography

Ferkel E, Davis WH, Ellington JK. Entrapment neuropathies of the foot and ankle. Clin Sports Med. 2015;34:791-801. [PMID: 26409596] doi:10.1016/j.csm.2015.06.002

## Item 137      Answer:    D

### Educational Objective:  Identify an appropriate quality improvement model to reduce postoperative wound infection.

The most appropriate tool to assist in reducing postoperative wound sepsis at this institution is the Model for Improvement. The Model for Improvement focuses on achieving specific and measurable results in a specified population. This model relies on identifying a goal to be accomplished with a change, determining how the results of a change will be measured, and deciding on the changes that will bring about an improvement. These changes are tested and implemented using the Plan-Do-Study-Act (PDSA) cycle. PDSA cycles are rapid tests of improvement, and additional PDSA cycles are completed until the desired results are achieved. A medical center, for example, may set the specific goal of decreasing central line–associated bloodstream infections and use the PDSA cycle to rapidly implement and assess the impact of changes, such as using a central line bundle.

A clinical audit involves measuring current practices against desirable outcomes, which are usually guideline based. Feedback is often provided at the individual level. The audit can identify deviations from desired care (for example, surgical infection rate) but does not establish a goal, an intervention, or a metric to gauge the success of the intervention for the purposes of systematically improving care.

A control chart is a commonly used quality improvement tool. Control charts graphically display variation in a process over time and can help determine whether variation is related to a predictable or unpredictable cause. Control charts can additionally be used to determine whether an

CONT.

intervention has had a positive change. This tool could be useful in measuring change but does not involve goal setting or selecting and implementing an intervention, which are required elements in quality improvement models.

The Lean model focuses on closely examining a system's processes and eliminating non-value-added activities, or waste, within that system. By using a tool called value stream mapping that graphically displays the steps of a process (and the time required for each step) from beginning to end, inefficient areas (waste) in a process can be identified and addressed. The Lean model would not be particularly helpful in identifying causes of surgical site infection, selecting and implementing an intervention, and measuring the outcome.

**KEY POINT**

- The Model for Improvement relies on identifying a goal to be accomplished with a change, determining how the results of a change will be measured, and deciding on the changes that will bring about an improvement.

**Bibliography**

Lau CY. Quality improvement tools and processes. Neurosurg Clin N Am. 2015;26:177-87, viii. [PMID: 25771273] doi: 10.1016/j.nec.2014.11.016

## Item 138    Answer:    C

**Educational Objective:  Treat functional incontinence in a cognitively impaired patient.**

The most appropriate management is prompted voiding every 2 to 3 hours. There are four main classifications of urinary incontinence: urgency incontinence, stress incontinence, mixed incontinence, and overflow incontinence. Functional incontinence, which occurs in patients who cannot reach and use the toilet in a timely manner, may occur in patients with significant cognitive or mobility impairments. Classifying the type(s) of incontinence helps guide management. This patient demonstrates functional incontinence, in which decreased cognitive function limits her ability to recognize early signs of the need to void, and impaired mobility limits her ability to get to the bathroom when she does recognize the need. Providing assistance and scheduled toileting through prompting are effective for patients who have impaired cognition or mobility.

Oxybutynin is appropriate therapy for urgency incontinence, but only after behavioral therapy has been implemented and found to be inadequate to control symptoms. Additionally, in this elderly woman, anticholinergic therapy would be associated with increased risk for confusion.

This patient does not report stress incontinence, which occurs with increased intra-abdominal pressure (coughing, laughing, sneezing). Stress incontinence is best treated with pelvic muscle floor training. In addition, the ability of a cognitively impaired patient to comprehend the instructions for pelvic floor muscle training and to remember to perform the maneuvers is likely to be limited.

Sling cystourethropexy is used to treat stress urinary incontinence when behavioral therapy (pelvic floor muscle training) has failed. Carefully balancing surgical risk against potential for benefit would have to be considered. This patient does not have stress urinary incontinence, and surgery is not indicated.

**KEY POINT**

- Functional incontinence, which occurs in patients who cannot reach and use the toilet in a timely manner, is treated with prompted voiding.

**Bibliography**

Griebling TL. Urinary incontinence in the elderly. Clin Geriatr Med. 2009;25:445-57. [PMID: 19765492] doi:10.1016/j.cger.2009.06.004

## Item 139    Answer:    C

**Educational Objective:  Treat posttraumatic stress disorder.**

This patient with posttraumatic stress disorder (PTSD) would benefit most from psychotherapy provided by a specialist with experience in treating the disorder. PTSD is a disorder triggered by the experience of a traumatic event. The experience can be personal, through a loved one, or by repeated exposure to details or footage of such an event. Patients have intrusive memories of the event, such as nightmares and flashbacks, and avoid situations that remind them of the event. PTSD also causes functional impairment, hypervigilance, irritability, and sleep disturbance. In addition to psychotherapy, antidepressants are useful adjunctive therapies.

Clonazepam and other benzodiazepines are not effective in the treatment of PTSD and have significant potential for adverse effects given the high rates of concomitant substance use and suicidality in this condition.

Because of the high prevalence of hyperarousal symptoms associated with PTSD, β-blocker therapy with propranolol would seem to be a reasonable therapeutic option. However, evidence suggests that β-blocker therapy is ineffective in patients with PTSD.

Anticonvulsant medications with mood-stabilizing properties, such as topiramate, have been studied as potential therapies to improve symptoms of impulsive behavior, hyperarousal, and flashbacks in patients with PTSD. However, studies have been small and largely negative, and this class of drugs is not considered first-line therapy for PTSD.

**KEY POINT**

- Treatment of posttraumatic stress disorder requires psychotherapy from a specialist with experience in treating the disorder; antidepressants are useful adjunctive therapies.

**Bibliography**

Shalev A, Liberzon I, Marmar C. Post-traumatic stress disorder. N Engl J Med. 2017;376:2459-2469. [PMID: 28636846] doi:10.1056/NEJMra1612499

**Item 140      Answer:    A**

**Educational Objective:**   Diagnose acute angle-closure glaucoma.

In this patient with an acute onset of headache and visual changes with nausea and vomiting, the most likely diagnosis is acute angle-closure glaucoma (AACG). Risk factors for AACG include age older than 60 years, family history, and female sex. Several medications may precipitate an attack or worsen the condition, including anticholinergics; antihistamines; diuretics; and antidepressants, including selective serotonin reuptake inhibitors. Characteristic features include the description of halos around lights, as well as a mid-dilated, nonreactive pupil. An acute attack may be precipitated by dilation of the pupil, which may cause the iris to adhere to the lens, blocking the draining of aqueous humor; the blockage results in increased intraocular pressure. Other situations that can precipitate attacks include excitement, stress, or watching television in a dark room. AACG is an ophthalmologic emergency. Prompt intervention may prevent vision loss.

Bacterial endophthalmitis is inflammation of the aqueous and vitreous humors. It is typically associated with ocular surgery, especially cataract surgery. Patients usually have a subacute history of decreasing vision and eye pain, often mild in intensity. Visual acuity is decreased, and a hypopyon (layering of white blood cells in the anterior chamber) is typically present. Treatment includes intravitreal antibiotics.

Central retinal vein occlusion, which is often caused by a thrombus in the retinal vein, presents as painless onset of blurry vision or vision loss. It is not usually associated with redness or pupillary changes; however, if it is severe, patients may have a relative afferent pupillary defect.

Scleritis can present with severe eye pain that radiates to the periorbital region and watery discharge. Pain may occur with eye movement due to inflammation of the extraocular muscles. The sclera appears violaceous with notable edema. Severe local tenderness can be elicited by exerting pressure on the overlying closed eyelid. In approximately half of scleritis cases, an associated systemic rheumatic or inflammatory disorder is present. The local tenderness to touch and the violaceous and edematous sclera differentiate scleritis from AACG.

**KEY POINT**

- Characteristic features of acute angle-closure glaucoma include the sudden onset of headache, nausea, vomiting, and vision changes; the appearance of halos around lights; and the presence of a mid-dilated, nonreactive pupil.

**Bibliography**
Tarff A, Behrens A. Ocular emergencies: red eye. Med Clin North Am. 2017;101:615-639. [PMID: 28372717] doi:10.1016/j.mcna.2016.12.013

**Item 141      Answer:    B**

**Educational Objective:**   Manage a request for genetic testing by first taking a family history.

The most appropriate management of this patient is to obtain a three-generation family history. Obtaining a family history is an inexpensive and important risk assessment tool that allows clinicians to identify persons at increased risk for developing certain conditions. Up to 40% of genetic risk factors that would otherwise be missed can be detected with a family history. Features that suggest the presence of a genetically inherited condition include earlier age of onset than expected for a common disease; two or more relatives with the same disorder, especially if the disorder is uncommon or known to be caused by a single gene mutation; and the presence of a disease in the less-often-afflicted gender, such as breast cancer in a man. Obtaining a comprehensive family history in this patient will help determine her risk for developing Huntington disease, a neurodegenerative condition most commonly inherited in an autosomal-dominant pattern. Huntington disease has a very high penetrance, meaning that nearly all persons with a mutation in the *huntingtin* protein gene will ultimately develop the disease.

Although persons affected with Huntington disease have various abnormalities on MRI, including cortical atrophy and ventriculomegaly, obtaining MRI in this patient would not be helpful given the absence of symptoms and neurologic deficits on physical examination.

Genetic testing should be reserved for patients at increased risk for developing a disease who have received appropriate genetic counseling. Genetic testing raises many ethical questions, as the results affect not only the patient but also other members of the family. Testing can also lead to possible discrimination. The Genetic Information Nondiscrimination Act of 2008 protects against genetic discrimination in regard to both health insurance and employment but does not protect against discrimination involving disability, life, or long-term care insurance.

Genetic counseling is indicated in all patients for whom genetic testing is being considered. The basic components of genetic counseling are education on the condition being tested, including the natural history, possible treatments, and preventive measures; the risks and benefits of genetic testing; alternatives to testing, including the option to forgo testing; and the implications for the patient and family members. A referral for genetic counseling would be indicated if this patient's family history is positive for family members with Huntington disease. Genetic counseling for this disease is unnecessary in the absence of an affected family member.

**KEY POINT**

- The three-generation family history is an inexpensive and important risk assessment tool that allows clinicians to identify persons at increased risk for developing certain conditions.

**Bibliography**
Pyeritz RE. The family history: the first genetic test, and still useful after all those years? Genet Med. 2012;14:3-9. [PMID: 22237427] doi:10.1038/gim.0b013e3182310bcf

## Item 142      Answer:   C

**Educational Objective:**   Treat abnormal uterine bleeding with a levonorgestrel-containing intrauterine device.

The most appropriate management of abnormal uterine bleeding in this patient is a levonorgestrel-containing intrauterine device (IUD). Abnormal uterine bleeding can generally be categorized into ovulatory and anovulatory patterns. Ovulatory abnormal uterine bleeding (menorrhagia) occurs at normal regular intervals but is excessive in volume or duration. Women with ovulatory bleeding have estrogen-mediated endometrial proliferation, produce progesterone, slough the endometrium regularly following progesterone withdrawal, and have a minimal risk for uterine cancer. Anovulatory cycles are characterized by unpredictable bleeding of variable flow and duration caused by the absence of normal cyclic hormonal flux. Without cyclic progesterone, the estrogen-mediated endometrium proliferates excessively, resulting in endometrial instability, erratic bleeding, and an increased risk for uterine cancer. For this perimenopausal patient who is anemic secondary to excessive menstrual blood loss and has contraindications to combination oral contraceptive use (previous deep venous thrombosis and current smoking), using a progestin-containing IUD would likely result in amenorrhea and prevent future blood loss. Managing anovulatory cycles involves the use of progestin to maintain endometrial stability to reduce the risk for endometrial cancer, which a levonorgestrel-containing IUD would do.

An estrogen-progestin oral contraceptive protects against unplanned pregnancy and regulates the menstrual cycle to prevent bleeding between cycles. However, this patient has contraindications to combination hormone therapy, leaving a progestin-containing IUD as the most appropriate choice.

Endometrial ablation or hysterectomy may be considered for patients who do not respond to medical treatment or in whom anatomic causes are identified as the cause of the bleeding. These interventions are not indicated for this patient at this time.

Treatment of anovulatory bleeding is directed toward restoring hormonal balance and stabilizing the endometrium. A progestin such as medroxyprogesterone acetate may be used to promote withdrawal bleeding for women who wish to become pregnant. However, this patient has not expressed a desire to become pregnant, and such treatment is unlikely to prevent future abnormal bleeding in a patient with continued anovulatory cycles.

### KEY POINT

- For women with anovulatory abnormal uterine bleeding and contraindications to combination oral contraceptive use, a progestin-containing intrauterine device will likely reduce blood loss and maintain the stability of the endometrium, thereby reducing the risk for uterine cancer.

**Bibliography**
Bacon JL. Abnormal uterine bleeding: current classification and clinical management. Obstet Gynecol Clin North Am. 2017;44:179-193. [PMID: 28499529] doi:10.1016/j.ogc.2017.02.012

## Item 143      Answer:   D

**Educational Objective:**   Treat persistent postural-perceptual dizziness.

The most appropriate treatment in addition to vestibular and balance rehabilitation therapy (VBRT) is sertraline. Dizziness that remains nonspecific despite a thorough history, examination, and evaluation is referred to as persistent postural-perceptual dizziness (PPPD; formerly known as chronic subjective dizziness). PPPD is described as persistent, nonvertiginous dizziness or imbalance that worsens with personal motion, upright positioning, and movement of objects in the surrounding environment. Symptoms must be present on most days for at least 3 months. PPPD is most often preceded by another vestibular process (benign paroxysmal positional vertigo, vestibular neuronitis, vestibular migraine, stroke), trauma (concussion, traumatic brain injury), infection, or certain psychiatric conditions (anxiety, panic disorder, major depression). Approximately 75% of patients with PPPD have concomitant anxiety or depressive symptoms. The treatments of choice are VBRT and medical therapy, including selective serotonin reuptake inhibitors (SSRIs) or serotonin-norepinephrine reuptake inhibitors (SNRIs). VBRT focuses on balance training, core stabilization, and desensitization exercises; it is often performed by physical and occupational therapists. SSRIs and SNRIs take 8 to 12 weeks to produce a clinical response; if effective, treatment for at least 1 year is recommended. A positive response to these medications does not depend on the presence of psychiatric symptoms. In this patient with a history of concussion, a cause of dizziness has not been identified after thorough evaluation, and he should be treated with VBRT and an SSRI (such as sertraline) or SNRI.

Treatment response with other classes of antidepressants has been disappointing, and amitriptyline has not been found to be effective in the treatment of PPPD.

The canalith repositioning maneuver (Epley maneuver) is used to treat benign paroxysmal positional vertigo (BPPV). Patients with BPPV have brief episodes of vertigo (10-30 seconds) precipitated by abrupt head movement. This patient's symptoms are not compatible with BPPV, and the canalith repositioning maneuver is not indicated.

Lorazepam and other benzodiazepines have been used in the treatment of acute vertigo. This patient does not have vertigo, which is characterized by a spinning, swaying, or tilting sensation that is often accompanied by nausea and vomiting. In addition, long-term treatment with lorazepam can lead to dependence and may suppress vestibular feedback and central compensation mechanisms, resulting in worsening of PPPD symptoms.

**KEY POINT**

- The treatments of choice for persistent postural-perceptual dizziness are vestibular and balance rehabilitation therapy and medical therapy with selective serotonin reuptake inhibitors or serotonin-norepinephrine reuptake inhibitors.

**Bibliography**

Popkirov S, Staab JP, Stone J. Persistent postural-perceptual dizziness (PPPD): a common, characteristic and treatable cause of chronic dizziness. Pract Neurol. 2018;18:5-13. [PMID: 29208729] doi: 10.1136/practneurol-2017-001809

## Item 144     Answer:     C

**Educational Objective:** Identify the appropriate level of postdischarge care.

The most appropriate discharge plan for this patient is rehabilitation at a long-term acute care hospital (LTACH). The patient requires continued mechanical ventilation but otherwise no longer requires hospitalization. LTACHs provide longer-term, higher-intensity medical treatment, such as complex wound care, mechanical ventilation weaning, and treatment with intravenous medications. Patients can also receive physical rehabilitation at such facilities.

Acute rehabilitation in a specialized rehabilitation facility is an appropriate choice for patients who require short-term rehabilitation (typically <4 weeks). To ensure reimbursement of services, such facilities require that a patient be able to participate in therapy at least 3 hours per day, 5 days per week. This patient clearly does not meet these criteria.

In-home rehabilitation services are useful for patients who may safely return home but still require physical or occupational therapy to continue optimizing return to their previous level of functioning. In-home rehabilitation services would not be a safe option for this patient who still requires mechanical ventilation and has significant physical deconditioning.

Subacute rehabilitation at a skilled nursing facility is a good option for patients who are not physically ready to return to their previous living situation but cannot tolerate at least 3 hours of therapy per day, 5 days per week. Skilled nursing facilities have physician directors but do not have the physician or staff resources to provide the complex medical care this patient requires.

**KEY POINT**

- Long-term acute care hospitals provide longer-term, higher-intensity medical treatment, such as complex wound care, mechanical ventilation weaning, and treatment with intravenous medications; such facilities also provide physical rehabilitation services.

**Bibliography**

Kane RL. Finding the right level of posthospital care: "We didn't realize there was any other option for him." JAMA. 2011;305:284-93. [PMID: 21245184] doi:10.1001/jama.2010.2015

## Item 145     Answer:     A

**Educational Objective:** Recognize the types of bias that affect screening tests.

Lead-time bias is most likely to threaten the validity of the authors' conclusions. Lead-time bias occurs when survival time (time from diagnosis to death) appears to be lengthened because the screened patient is diagnosed earlier during the preclinical phase but does not live longer in actuality. To guard against this bias, disease-specific mortality rates rather than survival time should be used as an outcome derived from randomized clinical trials.

Screening is also more likely to detect indolent disease, which has a long latent period, than aggressive disease, which has a short latent period and is most often detected with onset of symptoms. This causes length-time bias, in which a screen-detected cohort will have overrepresentation of indolent disease, whereas a symptom-detected cohort will have overrepresentation of aggressive disease. Consequently, the screen-detected cohort falsely appears to have a better prognosis. Length-time bias is unlikely in studies of ovarian cancer because ovarian cancer is an aggressive disease with a poor survival rate. The cancer has spread beyond the ovary at the time of detection in 75% of patients. This may be the result of rapid progression from unifocal disease to diffuse disease or to multiple foci of cancer within the abdomen, as carcinomatosis has been shown to develop after the removal of normal ovaries in high-risk patients.

Recall bias occurs when patients with a disease of interest are more likely to recall past exposures compared with controls. Recall bias primarily affects observational retrospective study designs. In this case, the screening protocol was a prospective observation study, and those being screened are not being asked to recall exposures; therefore, recall bias would not affect the study authors' conclusions.

Selection bias occurs when the study participants do not accurately reflect the population being studied, usually because the choice to participate is influenced by the clinical question. A national study of randomly selected women with a high participation rate would not be expected to be influenced by selection bias.

**KEY POINT**

- Lead-time bias occurs when early detection of a disease with a screening test leads to an increase in measured survival but not overall survival time.

**Bibliography**

Berry DA. Failure of researchers, reviewers, editors, and the media to understand flaws in cancer screening studies: application to an article in Cancer. Cancer. 2014;120:2784-91. [PMID: 24925345] doi:10.1002/cncr.28795

## Item 146     Answer:     D

**Educational Objective:** Treat a patient with alcohol use disorder with naltrexone.

The most appropriate treatment is naltrexone. Recent developments in the pharmacologic treatment of alcohol use disorder focus on modifying the reinforcing effects of alcohol use. Physicians underprescribe medications to treat alcohol use disorder and prevent relapse, despite their demonstrated efficacy. This patient, with hypertension and stage 3 chronic kidney disease, would likely benefit most from naltrexone. Available in both oral and long-acting injectable forms, naltrexone has been associated with a substantial decrease in 30-day readmission and emergency department visits when prescribed to patients with alcohol dependence at the time of hospital discharge. Multiple systematic reviews and meta-analyses of clinical trials have found naltrexone to reduce alcohol consumption compared with placebo. Naltrexone carries a risk for hepatotoxicity, for which the patient should be monitored; however, hepatotoxicity is rare with the dosages used for alcohol use disorder. Because naltrexone is an opioid receptor antagonist, opioids are contraindicated while the patient is taking naltrexone. Caution should also be used in patients with depression, due to an increased risk for suicidal ideation.

Acamprosate is FDA approved for the maintenance of abstinence in alcohol use disorder. This medication likely works through the N-methyl-D-aspartate receptor to modulate γ-aminobutyric acid and glutamate levels. In patients with moderate kidney disease, dosage should be adjusted; acamprosate is contraindicated in cases of severe kidney disease (estimated glomerular filtration rate <30 mL/min/1.73 m$^2$). Recently, conflicting evidence regarding its effectiveness has been published, with some studies finding that acamprosate is no more effective than placebo. Although methodological differences may explain these discrepant results, many experts now recommend naltrexone as preferred therapy in patients without contraindications. Additionally, the thrice-daily dosage regimen can hinder adherence to acamprosate.

Although chlordiazepoxide can be used to treat alcohol withdrawal, it is not indicated for relapse prevention because of its addiction potential and ineffectiveness.

Disulfiram inhibits acetaldehyde dehydrogenase, causing buildup of aldehyde after alcohol consumption; the associated flushing, nausea, and vomiting act as a deterrent to further alcohol use. Unlike naltrexone and acamprosate, disulfiram does not directly diminish the motivation to drink, but it is an aversion therapy causing an unpleasant physiologic reaction when alcohol is consumed. Disulfiram is now considered second-line therapy.

**KEY POINT**

- Naltrexone, which is available in both oral and long-acting injectable forms, is associated with a substantial decrease in 30-day readmission and emergency department visits when prescribed to patients with alcohol dependence at the time of hospital discharge.

**Bibliography**

Akbar M, Egli M, Cho YE, Song BJ, Noronha A. Medications for alcohol use disorders: an overview. Pharmacol Ther. 2017. [PMID: 29191394] doi:10.1016/j.pharmthera.2017.11.007

## Item 147    Answer:    C

**Educational Objective:** Effectively elicit goals, preferences, and values in a patient with terminal illnesses.

The most appropriate initial strategy to develop goals of care is to ask the patient what he understands about his illnesses. This patient has multisystem organ dysfunction, recurrent hospitalizations, and a poor prognosis. He is at high risk for readmission and dying within the next 12 months, and assessing his understanding of his current illnesses is the first step in starting a conversation about the patient's goals, preferences, and values, after which the clinical care team can make recommendations on how best to meet those goals.

Discussions regarding hospice should occur only after the clinician has assessed the patient's understanding of the prognosis and after the patient's goals, hopes, and worries have been established.

Asking questions regarding resuscitation preferences is often important during a hospitalization, but a meaningful conversation regarding resuscitation preferences must be grounded in a patient's prognostic awareness, as well as their hopes and worries.

The patient's prognosis must be shared before a conversation regarding care preferences can occur. Before sharing the prognosis, however, evaluating the patient's understanding of his illnesses will allow for appropriate and efficient information sharing.

**KEY POINT**

- For seriously ill patients, understanding of their health and prognosis must be assessed before a conversation regarding care preferences and pathways can occur.

**Bibliography**

Bernacki RE, Block SD; American College of Physicians High Value Care Task Force. Communication about serious illness care goals: a review and synthesis of best practices. JAMA Intern Med. 2014;174:1994-2003. [PMID: 25330167] doi:10.1001/jamainternmed.2014.5271

## Item 148    Answer:    A

**Educational Objective:** Evaluate liver function before initiating statin therapy.

The most appropriate diagnostic testing to perform before initiating high-intensity statin therapy in this patient is alanine aminotransferase level measurement. This patient with clinical atherosclerotic cardiovascular disease (defined as acute coronary syndrome, or a history of myocardial infarction, stable or unstable angina, coronary or other arterial revascularization, stroke/transient ischemic attack, or peripheral artery disease attributable to atherosclerosis) meets the criteria for high-intensity statin therapy for secondary prevention of cardiovascular events. In patients in whom statin therapy is being considered, an initial fasting lipid panel (including total cholesterol, triglycerides, HDL cholesterol, and calculated LDL cholesterol levels) is recommended. A lipid panel should also be obtained 4 to 12 weeks after initiation of therapy to determine treatment adherence and response. Because statin therapy may infrequently cause liver dysfunction, the 2013 American College of Cardiology/American Heart Association cholesterol treatment guideline recommends measuring the alanine aminotransferase level at baseline before initiating statin therapy. Further hepatic monitoring is unnecessary if the baseline alanine aminotransferase level is normal, unless the patient develops symptoms suggestive of liver dysfunction.

In patients who are at risk for adverse muscle events because of personal history of a muscle disease, current muscle symptoms, or concomitant drug therapy that might increase the risk for myopathy, it is reasonable to obtain a creatine kinase level before beginning statin therapy. Routine baseline measurement of creatine kinase, however, is not recommended.

During statin therapy, routine measurement of liver aminotransferases and creatine kinase is not recommended. However, if the patient develops symptoms of hepatotoxicity (such as jaundice, fatigue, weight loss, or abdominal pain), liver aminotransferases should be measured. Likewise, if a patient develops muscle symptoms (such as pain, weakness, generalized fatigue, or tenderness), creatine kinase level measurement is indicated.

### KEY POINT

- In patients in whom statin therapy is being considered, an alanine aminotransferase level should be obtained at baseline to evaluate for liver dysfunction; further hepatic monitoring is unnecessary if the baseline level is normal.

### Bibliography

Stone NJ, Robinson JG, Lichtenstein AH, Bairey Merz CN, Blum CB, Eckel RH, et al; American College of Cardiology/American Heart Association Task Force on Practice Guidelines. 2013 ACC/AHA guideline on the treatment of blood cholesterol to reduce atherosclerotic cardiovascular risk in adults: a report of the American College of Cardiology/American Heart Association Task Force on Practice Guidelines. Circulation. 2014;129:S1-45. [PMID: 24222016] doi:10.1161/01.cir.0000437738.63853.7a

## Item 149      Answer:    B

**Educational Objective:  Screen for diabetes mellitus in a patient with risk factors.**

Screening for diabetes mellitus should occur at this visit. The U.S. Preventive Services Task Force (USPSTF) recommends routine screening for abnormal blood glucose and diabetes in asymptomatic adults aged 40 to 70 years who are overweight or obese. Clinicians should offer or refer patients with an abnormal blood glucose level to intensive behavioral counseling interventions to promote a healthful diet and physical activity. In contrast to the USPSTF, the American Diabetes Association (ADA) recommends that screening be performed in obese or overweight patients of any age with one or more additional risk factors for diabetes. Risk factors include a first-degree relative with diabetes; high-risk race or ethnicity (African American, Latino, Native American, Asian American, Pacific Islander); history of cardiovascular disease; hypertension; HDL cholesterol level less than 35 mg/dL (0.91 mmol/L) and/or triglyceride level greater than 250 mg/dL (2.82 mmol/L); polycystic ovary syndrome; physical inactivity; and other conditions associated with insulin resistance (such as acanthosis nigricans and severe obesity). In patients with normal results, the ADA recommends repeat screening at 3-year intervals. This 40-year old obese patient meets the screening criteria of both the USPSTF and the ADA and should be screened for diabetes now.

In the absence of risk factors for diabetes, the ADA recommends that all patients be screened for diabetes at age 45 years. The USPSTF recommends screening only in asymptomatic adults aged 40 to 70 years who are overweight or obese. This patient, who has risk factors for diabetes (age 40 years, sedentary lifestyle, obesity), should be screened now, not at age 45 years or upon development of an additional diabetes risk factor.

### KEY POINT

- Screening for diabetes mellitus is recommended for patients who are overweight or obese and have other risk factors for diabetes.

### Bibliography

Selph S, Dana T, Blazina I, Bougatsos C, Patel H, Chou R. Screening for type 2 diabetes mellitus: a systematic review for the U.S. Preventive Services Task Force. Ann Intern Med. 2015;162:765-76. [PMID: 25867111] doi: 10.7326/M14-2221

## Item 150      Answer:    D

**Educational Objective:  Diagnose schizophrenia.**

This patient's clinical presentation is most consistent with schizophrenia. This heterogeneous disorder is characterized by a combination of positive symptoms (delusions, disorganized thought, hallucinations) and negative symptoms (decreased activity, flattened affect). Typical age of onset is early adulthood. Diagnosis also requires at least one area of functional impairment (occupation, social interactions, or self-care) and duration of at least 6 months (including 1 month of active symptoms).

Bipolar disorder is characterized by major depressive episodes and periods of mania or hypomania. During manic episodes, patients experience increased energy and risk-taking behaviors, as well as inflated self-worth. Patients with major depressive disorder have depressed mood and/or anhedonia, plus other symptoms of depression, including difficulty concentrating, fatigue, feelings of worthlessness, psychomotor agitation or retardation, sleep disturbance, thoughts of suicide, and weight or appetite changes. Although patients may have major depressive disorder or bipolar disorder with psychotic features, this patient does not meet the criteria for either depression (depressed mode and/or anhedonia) or mania (abnormally expansive, euphoric, or irritable mood).

In paranoid personality disorder, patients are distrustful of others, including loved ones, and misperceive social interactions as personal attacks. However, disorganized thoughts, hallucinations, and negative symptoms are not present in patients with paranoid personality disorder.

### KEY POINT

- Schizophrenia is a heterogeneous disorder characterized by at least two of the following symptoms: delusions, hallucinations, disorganized speech, disorganized or catatonic behavior, and negative symptoms; the typical age of onset is early adulthood.

### Bibliography
Owen MJ, Sawa A, Mortensen PB. Schizophrenia. Lancet. 2016;388:86-97. [PMID: 26777917] doi:10.1016/S0140-6736(15)01121-6

## Item 151      Answer:     D

**Educational Objective:** Diagnose bacterial vaginosis.

Bacterial vaginosis can be diagnosed in this patient with detection of at least 20% clue cells on saline microscopy. Bacterial vaginosis is the most common cause of vaginal discharge and results from an imbalance in the normal vaginal bacterial flora—loss of the normal hydrogen-producing lactobacilli in the vagina and subsequent overgrowth of *Gardnerella vaginalis*, *Mycoplasma* species, and other anaerobes. Clinical diagnosis is made when three of the following features are present: vaginal pH greater than 4.5, thin and homogenous vaginal discharge, positive result on a whiff test (application of 10% potassium hydroxide to vaginal secretions resulting in a fishy odor), and clue cells comprising at least 20% of all squamous cells on saline microscopy. Clue cells are vaginal epithelial cells with ill-defined cell borders on microscopy as a result of adherent coccobacilli. The patient has vaginal pH greater than 4.5 and a homogenous thin discharge but a negative whiff test result. A saline wet mount that demonstrates at least 20% clue cells on microscopy will establish the diagnosis of bacterial vaginosis. Treatment is metronidazole or clindamycin.

Because bacterial vaginosis represents changes in the vaginal flora, vaginal culture has no role in diagnosis. Although cultures for *G. vaginalis* will be positive in almost all women with bacterial vaginosis, cultures lack specificity—the organism is found in over 50% of healthy asymptomatic women. Therefore, culture is not a reasonable test to confirm the diagnosis of bacterial vaginosis and would also be costly and inefficient compared with an office-based diagnosis.

The nucleic acid amplification test (NAAT) is a highly sensitive test for diagnosis of trichomoniasis and other sexually transmitted infections, such as chlamydia and gonorrhea. Although NAAT can detect *G. vaginalis*, it is time consuming, expensive, and unnecessary, and simple office-based diagnosis is preferred in straightforward cases such as this one. When office microscopy is not available, NAAT is a reasonable test to perform.

Vulvovaginal candidiasis is typically characterized by vaginal itching, irritation, and discharge and may be associated with dysuria and dyspareunia. Examination reveals vulvar edema and excoriation, with thick, white, curdy vaginal discharge. The diagnosis can be made when a saline or 10% potassium hydroxide wet mount of vaginal discharge shows yeast, hyphae, or pseudohyphae. This patient's clinical presentation is not consistent with vaginal candidiasis; a 10% potassium hydroxide wet mount is unnecessary and will not establish the most likely diagnosis.

### KEY POINT

- Clinical diagnosis of bacterial vaginosis requires three of the following four features: vaginal pH greater than 4.5, thin and homogenous vaginal discharge, positive whiff test result, and clue cells comprising at least 20% of all squamous cells on saline microscopy; culture is not a reasonable test to confirm the diagnosis of bacterial vaginosis and would also be costly and inefficient compared with an office-based diagnosis.

### Bibliography
Mills BB. Vaginitis: beyond the basics. Obstet Gynecol Clin North Am. 2017;44:159-177. [PMID: 28499528] doi:10.1016/j.ogc.2017.02.010

## Item 152      Answer:     C

**Educational Objective:** Treat benign prostatic hyperplasia and erectile dysfunction with tadalafil.

The most appropriate treatment for this patient with benign prostatic hyperplasia and erectile dysfunction is tadalafil. This patient has lower urinary tract symptoms (LUTS) due to benign prostatic hyperplasia (BPH), with both obstructive symptoms (decreased stream, incomplete emptying, hesitancy) and irritative symptoms (nocturia, frequency, urgency). Diagnosing BPH can be challenging because of the many causes of LUTS; furthermore, there is poor correlation between prostate size on examination and urinary symptoms. Nonetheless, a careful history and examination can usually render the diagnosis. Men older than 50 years are likely to have BPH as a cause of LUTS, whereas men younger than 40 years are likely to have other causes of LUTS. Furthermore, the patient has a history of untreated erectile dysfunction; in cases of BPH and erectile dysfunction, a trial of tadalafil, a phosphodiesterase-5 inhibitor, is recommended. In this setting, tadalafil has been shown to be clinically and symptomatically effective and is the only FDA-approved option to treat the symptoms of both conditions.

Finasteride and other 5α-reductase inhibitors are considered second-line medical therapy for BPH. The American Urological Association recommends the addition of 5α-reductase inhibitors in cases of BPH refractory to α-blocker monotherapy, not as a first-line monotherapy choice. Furthermore, this medication class has been known to lead to erectile and ejaculatory dysfunction.

Oxybutynin and other anticholinergic agents are effective in treating irritative LUTS of BPH. However, given their mechanism of action, anticholinergic agents can lead to worsening obstructive symptoms and could also lead to worsening erectile dysfunction.

Tamsulosin and other α-blocking agents are first-line medical therapy for symptomatic BPH. However, α-blockers have numerous side effects, including hypotension, orthostasis, and sexual dysfunction. Tamsulosin could worsen this patient's erectile dysfunction and thus would not be the most appropriate treatment choice.

**KEY POINT**

- For patients with concomitant benign prostatic hyperplasia and erectile dysfunction, a trial of tadalafil (a phosphodiesterase-5 inhibitor) has been shown to be effective and is the only FDA-approved option to treat both conditions.

### Bibliography

Albisinni S, Biaou I, Marcelis Q, Aoun F, De Nunzio C, Roumeguère T. New medical treatments for lower urinary tract symptoms due to benign prostatic hyperplasia and future perspectives. BMC Urol. 2016;16:58. [PMID: 27629059] doi:10.1186/s12894-016-0176-0

### Item 153    Answer:    D

**Educational Objective:** Manage long-term medications in the perioperative setting.

This patient should continue all medications the morning of surgery. In general, many medications are well tolerated throughout the perioperative period. The 2014 American College of Cardiology/American Heart Association guideline on perioperative cardiovascular evaluation and management of patients undergoing noncardiac surgery includes recommendations for the management of statins, β-blockers, and antiplatelet agents.

Statins should be continued in patients who have been taking statins long term. In patients undergoing vascular surgery, initiation of statins is reasonable, and perioperative statin initiation can also be considered in patients who would otherwise qualify for statin therapy based on current guideline-directed medical therapy.

Likewise, β-blockers should be continued in patients who have been taking β-blockers long term, especially those with coronary artery disease. Preoperative initiation of β-blockers may be indicated for some patients undergoing nonurgent surgery, including those with intermediate- or high-risk myocardial ischemia on preoperative stress testing, those with three or more Revised Cardiac Risk Index risk factors (diabetes mellitus, heart failure, coronary artery disease, chronic kidney disease, cerebrovascular disease), or those who otherwise have a compelling indication for β-blockade. However, β-blockers should never be started on the day of surgery, but rather with enough time preoperatively to assess safety and tolerability.

There are very few data available regarding the benefits versus risks of continuing calcium channel blockers such as amlodipine. There are no known interactions with anesthetic agents, and continuing calcium channel blockers is not associated with hemodynamic instability. Most experts, in the absence of data, recommend continuing this class of medication for patients already taking them.

In general, patients with coronary stents should be continued on aspirin throughout the perioperative period unless the bleeding risk is prohibitively high, as is the case with many neurosurgical procedures. It is important to discuss perioperative management of aspirin and $P2Y_{12}$ inhibitors with the surgical team to reach a consensus recommendation.

**KEY POINT**

- In patients undergoing noncardiac surgery, β-blockers and statins should be continued in those who have been taking the drugs long term, and aspirin generally should be continued in patients with coronary stents unless the bleeding risk is prohibitively high.

### Bibliography

Fleisher LA, Fleischmann KE, Auerbach AD, Barnason SA, Beckman JA, Bozkurt B, et al; American College of Cardiology. 2014 ACC/AHA guideline on perioperative cardiovascular evaluation and management of patients undergoing noncardiac surgery: a report of the American College of Cardiology/American Heart Association Task Force on practice guidelines. J Am Coll Cardiol. 2014;64:e77-137. [PMID: 25091544]

### Item 154    Answer:    D

**Educational Objective:** Avoid adjunctive breast cancer screening in a low-risk patient with dense breast tissue.

This patient should not undergo adjunctive screening. Breast density is an increasingly recognized risk factor for breast cancer. It is categorized by the Breast Imaging Reporting and Data System (BI-RADS) as (a) almost entirely fatty, (b) scattered areas of fibroglandular tissue, (c) heterogeneously dense, or (d) extremely dense. Women with dense breasts should be informed that high breast density is common (present in up to 50% of women) and increases breast cancer risk but not breast cancer–related mortality. Dense breasts also decrease the sensitivity of mammography. However, women with high breast density without additional risk factors may experience more harms than benefits from supplemental breast imaging. Although supplemental screening with ultrasonography or MRI may increase the cancer detection rate, the impact on important clinical outcomes is unknown. Up to 90% of positive results on supplemental ultrasonography and 66% to 97% of positive results on supplemental MRI are false-positive findings, which may result in additional testing or invasive procedures. Despite this, nearly a quarter of state legislatures mandate that patients be notified of breast density findings, and some specifically recommend adjunctive screening with ultrasonography.

Women with dense breasts and other risk factors that impart a lifetime risk for breast cancer of 20% to 25% or higher, as calculated by models largely dependent on family history, should also undergo breast MRI in addition to screening mammography. The use of supplemental breast MRI in women who have less than a 20% lifetime risk for breast cancer is not currently supported by guidelines.

Digital breast tomosynthesis creates a three-dimensional image of the breast. Clinical studies suggest that tomosynthesis may have a sensitivity equal to or exceeding the sensitivity of digital mammography in the detection of breast cancer in women with dense breasts and that tomosynthesis may decrease the recall rate from screening mammography. Despite these promising findings that may improve screening accuracy, there are no randomized trials or long-term follow-up data.

Most major breast cancer screening guidelines promote biennial screening from age 50 to 75 years. No guideline recommends biannual digital mammography for patients whose only risk factor is high breast density.

**KEY POINT**

- High breast density alone does not necessitate adjunctive breast imaging other than routine screening mammography.

**Bibliography**

Melnikow J, Fenton JJ, Whitlock EP, Miglioretti DL, Weyrich MS, Thompson JH, et al. Supplemental screening for breast cancer in women with dense breasts: a systematic review for the U.S. Preventive Services Task Force. Ann Intern Med. 2016;164:268-78. [PMID: 26757021] doi:10.7326/M15-1789

## Item 155     Answer:     B

**Educational Objective:**  Treat chronic noncancer pain with medical cannabis.

A trial of oral medical cannabis oil would be a reasonable treatment in the management of this patient's chronic pain. Medical cannabis, although classified as a scheduled agent by the U.S. Drug Enforcement Administration on a federal level, has been approved by many states as a treatment for chronic pain. Current data on the effectiveness of medical cannabis for chronic pain are characterized by significant heterogeneity in both patient populations and cannabis preparations, although recent systematic reviews have demonstrated that cannabis has some efficacy in the treatment of chronic noncancer pain. Only two cannabinoid drugs (dronabinol and nabilone) are licensed for sale in the United States, and both drugs are available only in oral form. The pharmacokinetics of oral cannabis differ greatly from those of smoked cannabis, which has varying implications. Oral cannabis is slow in onset of action but produces more pronounced, and often unfavorable, psychoactive effects that last much longer than those experienced with smoking. On the other hand, smoked cannabis is quickly absorbed into the blood, and effects are immediate. However, examining the effects of smoked marijuana can be difficult because the absorption and efficacy of cannabis on symptom relief depend on subject familiarity with smoking and inhaling. This patient with end-stage kidney disease has a complex chronic pain syndrome that is unresponsive to multiple trials of nonpharmacologic and nonopioid analgesic therapies. If she resides in a state in which medical cannabis is available, oral medical cannabis oil would be a reasonable treatment option.

Oral immediate-release morphine sulfate should be avoided in this patient with end-stage kidney disease who

is receiving dialysis because it could cause opioid-induced neurotoxicity with repeated use.

Oral methadone is a potent opioid agonist and N-methyl-D-aspartate receptor antagonist. Its complex pharmacokinetics and variable half-life restrict its general use, and it should not be prescribed by clinicians who lack experience in its management.

Topical lidocaine does not penetrate into the deep myofascial tissues and would not be an effective agent for this patient with pelvic pain.

**KEY POINT**

- Medical cannabis has demonstrated some efficacy in the treatment of chronic noncancer pain.

**Bibliography**

Whiting PF, Wolff RF, Deshpande S, Di Nisio M, Duffy S, Hernandez AV, et al. Cannabinoids for medical use: a systematic review and meta-analysis. JAMA. 2015;313:2456-73. [PMID: 26103030] doi: 10.1001/jama.2015.6358

## Item 156     Answer:     E

**Educational Objective:**  Treat a patient with a popliteal cyst.

The most appropriate management is no treatment. This patient has a popliteal (Baker) cyst. Popliteal cysts are synovial fluid–containing extensions of the knee joint space and generally occur as a result of inflammatory arthritis, osteoarthritis, or trauma of the knee. Swelling is seen in the popliteal fossa on physical examination. The cyst is usually asymptomatic but may become painful as it enlarges or ruptures, which may cause significant pain and swelling of the calf, mimicking thrombophlebitis. The knee should be examined for signs of meniscal pathology, effusion, or mechanical signs that indicate an intra-articular irritant causing excessive joint fluid. Treatment is usually directed at the underlying cause of the cyst (such as repair of a torn meniscus). Given this patient's lack of symptoms, no treatment is required.

In this asymptomatic patient, fluid aspiration is not necessary; it should be performed solely for symptom relief, which is unnecessary in this patient. Although the procedure is considered extremely safe, it does carry a small risk for infection.

When arthritis-related popliteal cysts cause symptoms, joint aspiration of the fluid with a subsequent glucocorticoid injection can often relieve the symptoms. Given that this patient lacks symptoms, the procedure is not indicated.

Ibuprofen or another NSAID can be offered to patients with popliteal cysts to treat pain from the underlying cause of the cyst (such as trauma or osteoarthritis), but these analgesics are not considered first-line therapy for the cysts themselves. In patients with asymptomatic popliteal cysts, NSAIDs have no role.

Plain radiographs can be obtained in patients with trauma when there is concern for fracture or to confirm the diagnosis of osteoarthritis. There is no role for plain radiography in patients with an asymptomatic popliteal cyst.

- Asymptomatic popliteal cysts do not require treatment; in symptomatic cases, treatment is usually directed at the underlying cause.

**Bibliography**

Herman AM, Marzo JM. Popliteal cysts: a current review. Orthopedics. 2014;37:e678-84. [PMID: 25102502] doi:10.3928/01477447-20140728-52

## Item 157    Answer:    D

**Educational Objective:   Exclude a diagnosis of a female sexual disorder in a postmenopausal woman.**

This patient does not currently meet the diagnostic criteria for any sexual disorder. Female sexual dysfunction describes sexual difficulties that are persistent, personally distressing to the patient, and not explained by a nonsexual mental disorder. The patient reports that she is only occasionally distressed by these symptoms. Intervention may still be appropriate for patients reporting significant distress, such as sexual health education and/or referral to a sex therapist.

Female orgasmic disorder is the persistent or recurrent absence, delay, or diminished intensity of orgasm following a normal excitement phase with at least 75% of sexual encounters. The patient does not describe symptoms compatible with this disorder.

Genitopelvic pain/penetration disorder is diagnosed when there is persistent or recurrent difficulty in vaginal penetration during intercourse, marked vulvovaginal or pelvic pain during penetration, fear of pain or anxiety about pain in anticipation of or during penetration, or tightening or tensing of pelvic floor muscles during attempted penetration. For this diagnosis, symptoms must occur more than 75% of the time for at least 6 months and cause clinically significant distress. These symptoms are not present in this patient.

Female sexual interest/arousal disorder includes hypoactive sexual desire or arousal dysfunction that is present for a minimum of 6 months and causes significant distress. It is diagnosed if the patient reports at least three of the following symptoms: lack of sexual interest, lack of sexual thoughts or fantasies, decreased initiation of sexual activity or decreased responsiveness to the partner's initiation attempts, reduced excitement or pleasure during sexual activity, reduced response to sexual cues, or decreased genital or nongenital sensations during sexual activity. This patient reports only occasional distress that has been present for 3 months.

**KEY POINT**

- The diagnosis of a female sexual disorder requires both significant distress and the persistence of symptoms not explained by a nonsexual mental disorder.

**Bibliography**

Faubion SS, Rullo JE. Sexual dysfunction in women: a practical approach. Am Fam Physician. 2015;92:281-8. [PMID: 26280233]

## Item 158    Answer:    B

**Educational Objective:   Evaluate a patient with suspected central vertigo with MRI.**

The most appropriate diagnostic test to perform next in this patient with risk factors for stroke is MRI of the brain. Patients with central vertigo secondary to vertebrobasilar stroke (posterior circulation ischemic or hemorrhagic events) frequently display concomitant neurologic findings in addition to vertigo. However, roughly 20% of patients with vertebrobasilar stroke present with isolated vertigo, and studies have shown that up to one third of cases of vertebrobasilar stroke that manifest as isolated vertigo are misclassified as peripheral vertigo, leading to considerable morbidity and mortality. In patients with findings concerning for centrally mediated vertigo (nystagmus, dysphagia, dysarthria, diplopia, ataxia, postural instability, hemiparesis, or mental status changes), or in patients with acute sustained vertigo and risk factors for vertebrobasilar stroke (advanced age, hypertension, hyperlipidemia, diabetes mellitus, peripheral vascular disease, atrial fibrillation), urgent evaluation with MRI is strongly recommended. MRI can detect infarction in the posterior fossa on the first day and is typically performed with magnetic resonance angiography (MRA). MRA is both sensitive and specific in the identification of stenosis or occlusion of the posterior cerebral circulation.

CT can provide an effective and expedited evaluation of hemorrhagic stroke, although hemorrhagic vertebrobasilar stroke accounts for a very small minority of cases of centrally mediated vertigo. MRI is far more sensitive for the early detection of ischemic stroke in these patients.

Vestibular laboratory testing using electronystagmography and videonystagmography can be helpful in distinguishing between peripheral and central vertigo. Electronystagmography and videonystagmography use electrodes and video cameras, respectively, to record eye movements. These techniques record and quantify both spontaneous and induced nystagmus. Vestibular laboratory testing should not take precedence over urgent brain imaging for a potentially life-threatening condition, such as a cerebellar stroke.

Imaging studies are generally unnecessary in the diagnosis of peripheral vertigo. However, because this patient is at high risk for posterior circulation stroke (cardiovascular disease risk factors; acute, sustained vertigo; gait ataxia), further evaluation is urgently required.

**KEY POINT**

- In patients with findings concerning for centrally mediated vertigo or patients with acute sustained vertigo and risk factors for vertebrobasilar stroke, urgent evaluation with MRI and posterior circulation magnetic resonance angiography are strongly recommended.

**Bibliography**

Venhovens J, Meulstee J, Verhagen WI. Acute vestibular syndrome: a critical review and diagnostic algorithm concerning the clinical differentiation of peripheral versus central aetiologies in the emergency department. J Neurol. 2016;263:2151-2157. [PMID: 26984607]

## Item 159    Answer:    B

**Educational Objective:**   Treat an obese patient with comprehensive behavioral therapy.

The initial recommendation to achieve weight loss is lifestyle modification, which includes reducing calorie intake by at least 500 kcal/day, physical activity exceeding 150 minutes weekly, and comprehensive behavioral therapy. High-intensity behavioral therapy programs (≥14 sessions of at least 6 months' duration) delivered by a trained interventionist and including regular self-monitoring of weight and calorie intake are associated with successful weight loss. Although face-to-face interventions most reliably result in weight loss, success has also been demonstrated with phone- or electronic-based interventions. Comprehensive programs lasting 1 year or longer and with at least monthly contact are associated with more successful maintenance of lifestyle change, and they are usually a reimbursable service.

Bariatric surgery for obesity is reserved for when a trial of comprehensive lifestyle intervention does not succeed. Additionally, surgical therapy is recommended only for patients with a BMI of 40 or greater, or with a BMI of 35 or greater and obesity-related comorbid conditions; this patient does not meet these criteria.

This patient is already exercising at the recommended level of at least 150 minutes of moderate to vigorous physical activity per week. Although increasing her physical activity may reduce the caloric restriction required to achieve weight loss, the impact of exercise is thought to be less important in initial weight loss than that of calorie restriction.

This patient admits that she has difficulty adhering to a diet plan; there is no reason to suspect that her adherence to a different plan (whether low-carbohydrate, Mediterranean, or another diet) would improve without the behavioral intervention components of regular calorie tracking and weight monitoring.

Combination low-dose phentermine (a sympathomimetic drug) and low-dose topiramate (an antiepileptic drug) has demonstrated efficacy in reducing weight, possibly by suppressing appetite, altering taste, and increasing metabolism. As with bariatric surgery, pharmacologic therapy is recommended only if a trial of lifestyle intervention is not successful. This patient has not yet truly engaged in a program of behavioral intervention.

### KEY POINT

- Weight loss is best achieved with a high-intensity behavioral therapy program (≥14 sessions of ≥6 months' duration) delivered by a trained interventionist and including regular self-monitoring of weight and calorie intake.

### Bibliography
Jensen MD, Ryan DH, Apovian CM, Ard JD, Comuzzie AG, Donato KA, et al; American College of Cardiology/American Heart Association Task Force on Practice Guidelines. 2013 AHA/ACC/TOS guideline for the management of overweight and obesity in adults: a report of the American College of Cardiology/American Heart Association Task Force on Practice Guidelines and The Obesity Society. Circulation. 2014;129:S102-38. [PMID: 24222017] doi:10.1161/01.cir.0000437739.71477.ee

## Item 160    Answer:    C

**Educational Objective:**   Manage surrogate decision making in a patient without an advance directive.

The most appropriate basis for the decision regarding the patient's management is the patient's previously expressed wishes, otherwise known as substituted judgment. The strongest evidence of a patient's preferences derives from a living will, in which a patient can outline specific preferences for treatment decisions (for example, use of dialysis or mechanical ventilation). A patient could also formally designate a health care proxy through a durable power of attorney. Unfortunately, few patients have completed an advance directive, and when one is not available, it is important to be familiar with the local state laws regarding surrogate decision making. Many states have a health consent statute that designates the order in which family members are selected to provide surrogate decisions. The patient's spouse usually takes precedence over parents or adult children.

Decisions based on the patient's best interests should be reserved for situations in which there are no previously expressed oral or written statements of preferences or values from the patient. Family members and physicians may have divergent opinions of what is in the patient's best interests, which may not correlate with what the patient would want for himself.

Although this patient's medical condition is a crucial consideration, proper management of complex cases such as this one depend upon knowledge of the values and ethical principles at play. These decisions should be made in accord with local legal standards; risk management should not be the driving factor. Practicing according to ethical standards of care should reduce legal risk.

### KEY POINT

- When decisions are made on behalf of a patient who lacks decision-making capacity, they should be based on previously expressed oral or written statements of preferences or values, also known as substituted judgment.

### Bibliography
Snyder L; American College of Physicians Ethics, Professionalism, and Human Rights Committee. American College of Physicians ethics manual: sixth edition. Ann Intern Med. 2012;156:73-104. [PMID: 22213573] doi: 10.7326/0003-4819-156-1-201201031-00001

## Item 161    Answer:    B

**Educational Objective:**   Treat opioid-induced constipation in a patient with serious illness.

The most appropriate treatment of this patient's constipation is methylnaltrexone. This patient presents with significant constipation refractory to enema therapy, osmotic laxatives (lactulose), and stimulants (bisacodyl, senna). There are several causes of this patient's constipation, but special attention must be paid to his opioid use for dyspnea palliation. Methylnaltrexone is a peripherally acting μ-opioid receptor

CONT.

antagonist, which is rapid acting and effective in the treatment of opioid-induced constipation. By reversing μ-opioid receptor activation in the gut, methylnaltrexone can cause laxation in less than 60 minutes and does not reverse analgesic or antidyspneic effects of systemically administered opioids. It is contraindicated in patients with bowel obstruction.

When constipation symptoms do not respond to osmotic and stimulant laxative therapy, the chloride channel activator lubiprostone can be considered. Two randomized clinical trials in patients with opioid-induced constipation have demonstrated that patients receiving lubiprostone had significant improvement in spontaneous bowel movements, abdominal discomfort, and constipation severity. Lubiprostone is FDA approved for the treatment of opioid-induced constipation; however, it can cause shortness of breath and is likely a poor choice for a patient taking opioids to palliate dyspnea.

Polyethylene glycol is an osmotic laxative that increases the water content of stools to improve bowel motility. This patient is already taking an osmotic laxative (lactulose), and the addition of polyethylene glycol is unlikely to have any effect in the setting of opioid-induced bowel dysmotility refractory to stimulants and enema therapy.

Sodium phosphate enemas are contraindicated in older adult patients and in patients with kidney failure or heart failure because of the risks for dangerous electrolyte shifts and renal toxicity.

**KEY POINT**

- If maximal medical therapy has failed to achieve laxation in patients taking opioids, peripheral opioid antagonists, such as methylnaltrexone, can be considered; methylnaltrexone does not reverse the analgesic or antidyspneic effects of systemically administered opioids.

**Bibliography**

Streicher JM, Bilsky EJ. Peripherally acting μ-opioid receptor antagonists for the treatment of opioid-related side effects: mechanism of action and clinical implications. J Pharm Pract. 2017;897190017732263. [PMID: 28946783] doi:10.1177/0897190017732263

## Item 162     Answer:     B

**Educational Objective:**   Diagnose autism spectrum disorder.

This patient demonstrates behaviors most consistent with autism spectrum disorder. This is a heterogeneous group of disorders that share two diagnostic features: (1) repetitive, nonpurposeful behaviors and (2) deficiencies in communication and social interaction. Although the disorder may not be diagnosed until adulthood, the abnormal behaviors begin in childhood. The exact prevalence is debated, but it is estimated to affect 0.5% to 1% of the U.S. population. Early intervention with behavioral and educational interventions improves long-term functioning, but most patients require lifelong assistance.

Antisocial personality disorder is characterized by lack of empathy for others and engaging in socially unacceptable activities (such as stealing or cheating) without remorse. Patients with this personality disorder do not engage in repetitive behaviors and do not have communication difficulties.

Obsessive-compulsive disorder is characterized by obsessions (persistent and intrusive thoughts, images, or impulses that are associated with distress) and compulsions (repetitive behaviors [such as counting, hand washing, and inspecting] that are performed to decrease anxiety caused by the obsession) that result in marked distress, wasted time, or impaired social function. Although patients with obsessive-compulsive disorder may engage in repetitive behaviors such as those exhibited by this patient, they do not have difficulties with communication or social interaction.

Social anxiety disorder is characterized by severe, persistent anxiety or fear of social or performance situations (public speaking, meeting unfamiliar people) lasting 6 months or longer. In these situations, affected patients experience anxiety and physical symptoms, such as palpitations, dyspnea, and flushing. Patients recognize their anxiety is excessive but nonetheless avoid trigger situations (or endure them with extreme anxiety), resulting in impairments at home, work, and other settings. This patient's repetitive behaviors and difficulty with social interactions are not consistent with social anxiety disorder.

**KEY POINT**

- Autism spectrum disorder is a heterogeneous group of disorders that share two diagnostic features: (1) repetitive, nonpurposeful behaviors and (2) deficiencies in communication and social interaction.

**Bibliography**

Nicolaidis C, Kripke CC, Raymaker D. Primary care for adults on the autism spectrum. Med Clin North Am. 2014;98:1169-91. [PMID: 25134878] doi:10.1016/j.mcna.2014.06.011

## Item 163     Answer:     D

**Educational Objective:**   Treat hyperlipidemia in a patient at low risk for atherosclerotic cardiovascular disease.

This patient with hyperlipidemia and low risk for atherosclerotic cardiovascular disease (ASCVD) should be counseled regarding therapeutic lifestyle changes and followed to monitor progress. Key components of therapeutic lifestyle changes include dietary modification, regular physical activity, weight loss, smoking cessation (if applicable), and addressing risk factors associated with the metabolic syndrome. Patients should be encouraged to adhere to a dietary pattern that focuses on consumption of fruits, vegetables, fiber, and monounsaturated fats and minimizes intake of saturated and *trans* fats, simple carbohydrates, and red meats. Replacing saturated fats with polyunsaturated fats has been shown to reduce LDL cholesterol levels and cardiovascular mortality. Recommended diets include the American Heart Association (AHA) diet and the DASH (Dietary Approaches to Stop Hypertension) diet. The AHA/American College of Cardiology (ACC) lifestyle management guideline additionally recommends that patients engage in 40 minutes of moderate to vigorous activity 3 to 4 days per week to lower LDL and non-HDL cholesterol levels.

According to the ACC/AHA cholesterol treatment guideline, the two groups for which a strong body of evidence supports statin initiation for the primary prevention of ASCVD are patients with an LDL cholesterol level of 190 mg/dL (4.92 mmol/L) or higher and patients aged 40 to 75 years with a 10-year ASCVD risk of 7.5% or higher. In this patient with an ASCVD risk of 3.4% and LDL cholesterol level less than 190 mg/dL (4.92 mmol/L), statin therapy would not be appropriate.

The U.S. Preventive Services Task Force recommends low- to moderate-intensity statin therapy in asymptomatic adults aged 40 to 75 years without ASCVD who have at least one ASCVD risk factor (dyslipidemia, diabetes mellitus, hypertension, or smoking) and a calculated 10-year ASCVD event risk of 10% or higher. Although this patient has hyperlipidemia, his 10-year ASCVD event risk is 3.4%, and neither low- nor moderate-intensity statin therapy is indicated.

**KEY POINT**

- Therapeutic lifestyle changes, including dietary modification, regular physical activity, weight loss, and smoking cessation, are the initial treatment for hyperlipidemia.

**Bibliography**
Eckel RH, Jakicic JM, Ard JD, de Jesus JM, Houston Miller N, Hubbard VS, et al; American College of Cardiology/American Heart Association Task Force on Practice Guidelines. 2013 AHA/ACC guideline on lifestyle management to reduce cardiovascular risk: a report of the American College of Cardiology/American Heart Association Task Force on Practice Guidelines. Circulation. 2014;129:S76-99. [PMID: 24222015] doi:10.1161/01.cir.0000437740.48606.d1

**Item 164      Answer:      A**

**Educational Objective:  Treat a patient with greater trochanteric pain syndrome (trochanteric bursitis).**

This patient's clinical presentation is consistent with greater trochanteric pain syndrome (GTPS; formerly trochanteric bursitis), and first-line therapy is pain relief with acetaminophen or an oral NSAID, such as ibuprofen. Patients with GTPS typically have pain localized to the greater trochanter that may radiate down the lateral leg to the knee. The pain is often exacerbated by lying on the affected side and climbing stairs. Pain onset is usually insidious. GTPS can be differentiated from hip joint pain in that GTPS does not usually radiate to the groin or limit hip range of motion. Diagnosis is made by history and by eliciting pain with palpation over the greater trochanter or reproduction of the pain when the patient takes a step up. Use of pain-relieving agents should accompany activity modification, such as avoiding or min-

imizing painful activities. Physical therapy to strengthen the muscles of the hip may help with reducing friction and therefore pain.

Glucocorticoid injections (frequently combined with a local anesthetic) are reserved for patients with GTPS with persistent symptoms and for those who do not respond to acetaminophen or an oral NSAID. Because this patient has not yet received any therapy, it would be most appropriate to start with an oral agent such as ibuprofen instead of progressing directly to glucocorticoid injection.

Most patients respond to acetaminophen, NSAIDs, or glucocorticoid injections. Opioid pain medications are typically unnecessary, have a significant risk profile, and do not have a role in the management of GTPS. Therefore, hydrocodone/acetaminophen would not be an appropriate management option.

GTPS is diagnosed clinically based on a consistent clinical presentation. Plain radiographs are typically normal in patients suspected of having GTPS. The role of imaging studies is to evaluate for alternative diagnoses when the diagnosis of GTPS is unclear. In this patient, plain radiography is unnecessary.

**KEY POINT**

- Patients with greater trochanteric pain syndrome (trochanteric bursitis) typically have pain localized to the greater trochanter, which may radiate down the lateral leg to the knee, and pain to palpation over the greater trochanter; treatment includes avoiding painful activities, acetaminophen or NSAIDs, and muscle strengthening.

**Bibliography**
Redmond JM, Chen AW, Domb BG. Greater trochanteric pain syndrome. J Am Acad Orthop Surg. 2016;24:231-40. [PMID: 26990713] doi:10.5435/JAAOS-D-14-00406

**Item 165      Answer:      B**

**Educational Objective:  Diagnose genitourinary syndrome of menopause.**

The most likely diagnosis is genitourinary syndrome of menopause (vaginal atrophy). The clinical history and physical examination are most helpful for diagnosing genitourinary syndrome of menopause. Approximately 10% to 40% of menopausal women experience symptoms related to vaginal atrophy, including vulvar itching, vaginal dryness, and dyspareunia. On physical examination, pale and shiny vaginal walls, decreased rugae, and petechiae are characteristic findings. In contrast to menopausal vasomotor symptoms, which may last for a few years and resolve spontaneously, genitourinary syndrome of menopause is frequently progressive and often requires treatment. Mild to moderate symptoms can be treated with vaginal moisturizers and lubricants, but more severe symptoms, as experienced by this patient, are best treated with vaginal estrogen.

Like genitourinary syndrome of menopause, acute allergic contact dermatitis presents with intense pruritus, often

Answers and Critiques

worse at night, as well as burning and stinging. Defining characteristics on physical examination include a discrete, well-demarcated area of erythema and edema. Fissures may be present along the labial folds. Excoriations are common and may become secondarily infected. The course of acute contact dermatitis progresses over days, not months as experienced by this patient. The most commonly implicated culprits are fragrances, medications, and preservatives in medications, such as glucocorticoids. Diagnosis is typically made on clinical grounds; biopsy is rarely necessary. Treatment generally consists of allergen avoidance and soaking in warm water (bathtub or sitz bath), followed by application of an emollient, such as petrolatum or a low-potency glucocorticoid.

Lichen planus is an inflammatory condition that can affect the skin, nails, or mucosa. Clinical presentation includes white lines and patches (Wickham striae) or painful erythema and erosions (erosive variant). Therapies are glucocorticoids (systemic and topical) and immunosuppressive agents in severe disease.

Lichen sclerosus is an inflammatory condition that often presents as white, atrophic patches on the genital and perianal skin. It differs from lichen planus in its clinical presentation of white patches that circumferentially involve the vaginal introitus and perianal area ("figure 8" appearance). Prepubertal girls and postmenopausal women are at highest risk. Biopsy establishes the diagnosis and can differentiate it from other inflammatory disorders. Treatment is with potent topical glucocorticoids.

### KEY POINT

- Genitourinary syndrome of menopause is a clinical diagnosis characterized by vulvar itching, vaginal dryness, and dyspareunia; pelvic examination findings include pale, shiny vaginal walls; decreased rugae; and petechiae.

### Bibliography
Faubion SS, Sood R, Kapoor E. Genitourinary syndrome of menopause: management strategies for the clinician. Mayo Clin Proc. 2017;92:1842-1849. [PMID: 29202940] doi:10.1016/j.mayocp.2017.08.019

### Item 166      Answer:      C

**Educational Objective:**  Screen a patient for opioid-related risk.

The recommended next step in management before prescribing opioid therapy is to perform an opioid risk assessment. Opioid therapy may be reasonably prescribed to this patient with pain that has not responded to nonpharmacologic and nonopioid therapies as part of a multimodal treatment plan, which may also include cognitive behavioral therapy and/or physical therapy. The Centers for Disease Control and Prevention Guideline for Prescribing Opioids for Chronic Pain recommends that before starting and periodically during continuation of opioid therapy, clinicians should evaluate risk factors for opioid-related harms. Clinicians should incorporate into the management plan strategies to mitigate risk, including considering offering

naloxone when factors that increase risk for opioid overdose (such as history of overdose, history of substance use disorder, higher opioid dosages [≥50 morphine milligram equivalents per day], or concurrent benzodiazepine use) are present. Other recommended risk-mitigation strategies include reviewing the patient's history of controlled substance use with state prescription monitoring program data and urine drug testing before initiation of therapy and at least annually thereafter.

The Current Opioid Misuse Measure is a brief self-report survey of current aberrant drug-related behavior. It is intended for use in patients currently receiving long-term opioid therapy who may be misusing opioid medications. Its value in improving outcomes related to misuse or overuse of opioids is unknown, and it would not be the next management step in this patient who has yet to be prescribed opioid therapy.

Coprescription of naloxone is recommended in patients at high risk for opioid overdose, such as those receiving daily doses of 50 mg of oral morphine equivalents or more. In this patient, opioid risk assessment would further delineate the patient's risk and may prompt consideration of naloxone, but until the risk assessment is completed, prescribing naloxone is premature.

In patients with no apparent mental health diagnoses, psychiatry referral is not routinely needed before prescribing long-term opioid therapy. Psychiatry referral may be appropriate for patients with a comorbid psychiatric diagnosis and, in those circumstances, could be part of a multimodal treatment plan. However, it is not the next recommended step in the management of this patient's opioid therapy.

### KEY POINT

- In patients with chronic pain, risk assessment should be performed before initiating or continuing opioid therapy.

### Bibliography
Dowell D, Haegerich TM, Chou R. CDC guideline for prescribing opioids for chronic pain—United States, 2016. JAMA. 2016;315:1624-45. [PMID: 26977696] doi:10.1001/jama.2016.1464

### Item 167      Answer:      B

**Educational Objective:**  Manage perioperative anticoagulation in a patient receiving non–vitamin K antagonist oral anticoagulant therapy.

Apixaban should be discontinued 3 days before surgery because there is a moderate to high bleeding risk with partial colectomy. Perioperative management of non–vitamin K antagonist oral anticoagulant (NOAC) therapy, such as with the factor Xa inhibitors (apixaban, edoxaban, rivaroxaban), is based on the patient's creatinine clearance and bleeding risk. When it is necessary to discontinue anticoagulation for surgery, NOACs can generally be stopped 2 to 3 days preoperatively because of their short half-lives. The shorter period is considered for patients undergoing procedures with low bleeding risk, and the longer period is considered for patients

**CONT.**

undergoing procedures with moderate or high bleeding risk. This applies to patients with normal kidney function or mild to moderate kidney disease (creatinine clearance ≥30 mL/min). For patients with creatinine clearance less than 30 mL/min, there are no data to guide recommendations; clinicians are advised to obtain an anti-Xa level or discontinue anticoagulation at least 72 hours before surgery. In patients taking the direct thrombin inhibitor dabigatran with creatinine clearance greater than 80 mL/min, dabigatran can be discontinued 2 to 3 days before surgery, with the longer period considered for moderate to high bleeding risk; for creatinine clearance less than 80 mL/min, dabigatran should be withheld at least 3 days preoperatively. The lower the creatinine clearance, the longer it must be withheld preoperatively.

For procedures with low bleeding risk, withholding apixaban 2 days preoperatively is usually sufficient; however, withholding apixaban only 1 day before surgery is insufficient for all procedures. Discontinuing apixaban 5 or 7 days before surgery would expose this patient to a small but increased thrombotic risk during that time frame.

In patients taking NOACs, bridging anticoagulation is unnecessary because of the rapid onset and short half-life associated with these drugs. Postoperative timing of NOAC reinstitution depends on the bleeding risk associated with the surgery, as NOACs reach therapeutic levels in 1 to 3 hours, at which point the patient is presumed to be fully anticoagulated. NOACs may be resumed once adequate hemostasis is ensured, usually 24 to 72 hours after surgery. Close collaboration with the surgeon is advised.

**KEY POINT**

- When it is necessary to discontinue anticoagulant therapy for surgery, non–vitamin K antagonist oral anticoagulants can be stopped 2 to 3 days preoperatively because of their short half-lives.

**Bibliography**

Doherty JU, Gluckman TJ, Hucker WJ, Januzzi JL Jr, Ortel TL, Saxonhouse SJ, et al. 2017 ACC expert consensus decision pathway for periprocedural management of anticoagulation in patients with nonvalvular atrial fibrillation: a report of the American College of Cardiology Clinical Expert Consensus Document Task Force. J Am Coll Cardiol. 2017;69:871-898. [PMID: 28081965] doi:10.1016/j.jacc.2016.11.024

## Item 168  Answer:  B

**Educational Objective:** Treat major depressive disorder with cognitive behavioral therapy.

Cognitive behavioral therapy (CBT) is the most appropriate initial therapy for this patient with major depressive disorder. Most patients with mild or moderate depression (PHQ-9 score <15) are treated in the primary care setting. Referral to a psychiatrist is indicated for patients with severe depression, failure of initial therapy, complex psychiatric comorbidities, and high suicide risk. In a 2016 clinical practice guideline, the American College of Physicians recommends that clinicians treat patients with major depressive disorder with CBT or second-generation antidepressants (selective serotonin reuptake inhibitors, serotonin-norepinephrine reuptake inhibitors, serotonin modulators, or atypical antidepressants) after discussing adverse effect profiles, accessibility, cost, and preferences with the patient. On the basis of moderate-quality evidence, CBT and second-generation antidepressants were equally effective treatments for major depressive disorder, with similar rates of discontinuation. For this patient who is opposed to the use of psychotropic medications, CBT is the best initial treatment.

Amitriptyline and other tricyclic antidepressants can be used to treat major depressive disorder, but these agents are second-line therapy because of the higher rate of associated side effects.

Paroxetine is a second-generation antidepressant that is a reasonable choice for initial management of major depressive disorder. However, there is a particularly high incidence of side effects with paroxetine use. This patient is wary of psychotropic medications, and if one were to be tried, a different second-generation antidepressant with a lower incidence of side effects would be preferred to improve patient adherence.

Quetiapine is FDA approved for use in combination with an antidepressant for the treatment of depression that does not respond to initial therapy. First-line treatment has not yet been attempted in this patient, and quetiapine is not appropriate as monotherapy for major depressive disorder.

**KEY POINT**

- Cognitive behavioral therapy and second-generation antidepressants have proved equally effective for treatment of major depressive disorder, with similar rates of discontinuation; treatment selection should be made after discussion of adverse effect profiles, accessibility, cost, and preferences with the patient.

**Bibliography**

Qaseem A, Barry MJ, Kansagara D; Clinical Guidelines Committee of the American College of Physicians. Nonpharmacologic versus pharmacologic treatment of adult patients with major depressive disorder: a clinical practice guideline from the American College of Physicians. Ann Intern Med. 2016;164:350-9. [PMID: 26857948] doi:10.7326/M15-2570

# Index

**A** | **NAME AND ADDRESS (Please complete.)**

_____
Last Name                First Name              Middle Initial

_____
Address

_____
Address cont.

_____
City                     State                  ZIP Code

_____
Country

_____
Email address

**ACP**®
American College of Physicians
Leading Internal Medicine, Improving Lives

**Medical Knowledge Self-Assessment Program® 18**

**TO EARN *CME Credits and/or MOC Points* YOU MUST:**

1. Answer all questions.
2. Score a minimum of 50% correct.

==========================================

**TO EARN *FREE* INSTANTANEOUS *CME Credits and/or MOC Points* ONLINE:**

1. Answer all of your questions.
2. Go to **mksap.acponline.org** and enter your ACP Online username and password to access an online answer sheet.
3. Enter your answers.
4. You can also enter your answers directly at **mksap.acponline.org** without first using this answer sheet.

**To Submit Your Answer Sheet by Mail or FAX for a $20 Administrative Fee per Answer Sheet:**

1. Answer all of your questions and calculate your score.
2. Complete boxes A-H.
3. Complete payment information.
4. Send the answer sheet and payment information to ACP, using the FAX number/address listed below.

**B** | **Order Number**
(Use the 10-digit Order Number on your MKSAP materials packing slip.)

**C** | **ACP ID Number**
(Refer to packing slip in your MKSAP materials for your 8-digit ACP ID Number.)

**D** | **Required Submission Information if Applying for MOC**

Birth Month and Day    ☐☐  ☐☐
                       M M   D D

ABIM Candidate Number  ☐☐☐☐☐☐

**COMPLETE FORM BELOW ONLY IF YOU SUBMIT BY MAIL OR FAX**

Last Name | First Name | MI

**Payment Information. Must remit in US funds, drawn on a US bank.**
**The processing fee for each paper answer sheet is $20.**

☐ Check, made payable to ACP, enclosed

Charge to   ☐ **VISA**   ☐ *MasterCard*   ☐ AMERICAN EXPRESS   ☐ DISCOVER

Card Number _____

Expiration Date _____ / _____      Security code (3 or 4 digit #s) _____
              MM          YY

Signature _____

**Fax to:** 215-351-2799

**Mail to:**
Member and Customer Service
American College of Physicians
190 N. Independence Mall West
Philadelphia, PA 19106-1572

# E

## TEST TYPE

| | Maximum Number of CME Credits |
|---|---|
| ○ Cardiovascular Medicine | 30 |
| ○ Dermatology | 16 |
| ○ Gastroenterology and Hepatology | 22 |
| ○ Hematology and Oncology | 33 |
| ○ Neurology | 22 |
| ○ Rheumatology | 22 |
| ○ Endocrinology and Metabolism | 19 |
| ○ General Internal Medicine | 36 |
| ○ Infectious Disease | 25 |
| ○ Nephrology | 25 |
| ○ Pulmonary and Critical Care Medicine | 25 |

# F

## CREDITS OR POINTS CLAIMED ON SECTION
### 1 hour = 1 credit or 1 point

Enter the number of credits earned on the test to the nearest quarter hour. Physicians should claim only the credit commensurate with the extent of their participation in the activity.

# G

### Enter your score here.

Instructions for calculating your own score are found in front of the self-assessment test in each book. You must receive a minimum score of 50% correct.

_____ %

Credit Submission Date:_____

# H

☐ I want to submit for CME credits

☐ I want to submit for CME credits and MOC points.

---

1 Ⓐ Ⓑ Ⓒ Ⓓ Ⓔ
2 Ⓐ Ⓑ Ⓒ Ⓓ Ⓔ
3 Ⓐ Ⓑ Ⓒ Ⓓ Ⓔ
4 Ⓐ Ⓑ Ⓒ Ⓓ Ⓔ
5 Ⓐ Ⓑ Ⓒ Ⓓ Ⓔ

6 Ⓐ Ⓑ Ⓒ Ⓓ Ⓔ
7 Ⓐ Ⓑ Ⓒ Ⓓ Ⓔ
8 Ⓐ Ⓑ Ⓒ Ⓓ Ⓔ
9 Ⓐ Ⓑ Ⓒ Ⓓ Ⓔ
10 Ⓐ Ⓑ Ⓒ Ⓓ Ⓔ

11 Ⓐ Ⓑ Ⓒ Ⓓ Ⓔ
12 Ⓐ Ⓑ Ⓒ Ⓓ Ⓔ
13 Ⓐ Ⓑ Ⓒ Ⓓ Ⓔ
14 Ⓐ Ⓑ Ⓒ Ⓓ Ⓔ
15 Ⓐ Ⓑ Ⓒ Ⓓ Ⓔ

16 Ⓐ Ⓑ Ⓒ Ⓓ Ⓔ
17 Ⓐ Ⓑ Ⓒ Ⓓ Ⓔ
18 Ⓐ Ⓑ Ⓒ Ⓓ Ⓔ
19 Ⓐ Ⓑ Ⓒ Ⓓ Ⓔ
20 Ⓐ Ⓑ Ⓒ Ⓓ Ⓔ

21 Ⓐ Ⓑ Ⓒ Ⓓ Ⓔ
22 Ⓐ Ⓑ Ⓒ Ⓓ Ⓔ
23 Ⓐ Ⓑ Ⓒ Ⓓ Ⓔ
24 Ⓐ Ⓑ Ⓒ Ⓓ Ⓔ
25 Ⓐ Ⓑ Ⓒ Ⓓ Ⓔ

26 Ⓐ Ⓑ Ⓒ Ⓓ Ⓔ
27 Ⓐ Ⓑ Ⓒ Ⓓ Ⓔ
28 Ⓐ Ⓑ Ⓒ Ⓓ Ⓔ
29 Ⓐ Ⓑ Ⓒ Ⓓ Ⓔ
30 Ⓐ Ⓑ Ⓒ Ⓓ Ⓔ

31 Ⓐ Ⓑ Ⓒ Ⓓ Ⓔ
32 Ⓐ Ⓑ Ⓒ Ⓓ Ⓔ
33 Ⓐ Ⓑ Ⓒ Ⓓ Ⓔ
34 Ⓐ Ⓑ Ⓒ Ⓓ Ⓔ
35 Ⓐ Ⓑ Ⓒ Ⓓ Ⓔ

36 Ⓐ Ⓑ Ⓒ Ⓓ Ⓔ
37 Ⓐ Ⓑ Ⓒ Ⓓ Ⓔ
38 Ⓐ Ⓑ Ⓒ Ⓓ Ⓔ
39 Ⓐ Ⓑ Ⓒ Ⓓ Ⓔ
40 Ⓐ Ⓑ Ⓒ Ⓓ Ⓔ

41 Ⓐ Ⓑ Ⓒ Ⓓ Ⓔ
42 Ⓐ Ⓑ Ⓒ Ⓓ Ⓔ
43 Ⓐ Ⓑ Ⓒ Ⓓ Ⓔ
44 Ⓐ Ⓑ Ⓒ Ⓓ Ⓔ
45 Ⓐ Ⓑ Ⓒ Ⓓ Ⓔ

46 Ⓐ Ⓑ Ⓒ Ⓓ Ⓔ
47 Ⓐ Ⓑ Ⓒ Ⓓ Ⓔ
48 Ⓐ Ⓑ Ⓒ Ⓓ Ⓔ
49 Ⓐ Ⓑ Ⓒ Ⓓ Ⓔ
50 Ⓐ Ⓑ Ⓒ Ⓓ Ⓔ

51 Ⓐ Ⓑ Ⓒ Ⓓ Ⓔ
52 Ⓐ Ⓑ Ⓒ Ⓓ Ⓔ
53 Ⓐ Ⓑ Ⓒ Ⓓ Ⓔ
54 Ⓐ Ⓑ Ⓒ Ⓓ Ⓔ
55 Ⓐ Ⓑ Ⓒ Ⓓ Ⓔ

56 Ⓐ Ⓑ Ⓒ Ⓓ Ⓔ
57 Ⓐ Ⓑ Ⓒ Ⓓ Ⓔ
58 Ⓐ Ⓑ Ⓒ Ⓓ Ⓔ
59 Ⓐ Ⓑ Ⓒ Ⓓ Ⓔ
60 Ⓐ Ⓑ Ⓒ Ⓓ Ⓔ

61 Ⓐ Ⓑ Ⓒ Ⓓ Ⓔ
62 Ⓐ Ⓑ Ⓒ Ⓓ Ⓔ
63 Ⓐ Ⓑ Ⓒ Ⓓ Ⓔ
64 Ⓐ Ⓑ Ⓒ Ⓓ Ⓔ
65 Ⓐ Ⓑ Ⓒ Ⓓ Ⓔ

66 Ⓐ Ⓑ Ⓒ Ⓓ Ⓔ
67 Ⓐ Ⓑ Ⓒ Ⓓ Ⓔ
68 Ⓐ Ⓑ Ⓒ Ⓓ Ⓔ
69 Ⓐ Ⓑ Ⓒ Ⓓ Ⓔ
70 Ⓐ Ⓑ Ⓒ Ⓓ Ⓔ

71 Ⓐ Ⓑ Ⓒ Ⓓ Ⓔ
72 Ⓐ Ⓑ Ⓒ Ⓓ Ⓔ
73 Ⓐ Ⓑ Ⓒ Ⓓ Ⓔ
74 Ⓐ Ⓑ Ⓒ Ⓓ Ⓔ
75 Ⓐ Ⓑ Ⓒ Ⓓ Ⓔ

76 Ⓐ Ⓑ Ⓒ Ⓓ Ⓔ
77 Ⓐ Ⓑ Ⓒ Ⓓ Ⓔ
78 Ⓐ Ⓑ Ⓒ Ⓓ Ⓔ
79 Ⓐ Ⓑ Ⓒ Ⓓ Ⓔ
80 Ⓐ Ⓑ Ⓒ Ⓓ Ⓔ

81 Ⓐ Ⓑ Ⓒ Ⓓ Ⓔ
82 Ⓐ Ⓑ Ⓒ Ⓓ Ⓔ
83 Ⓐ Ⓑ Ⓒ Ⓓ Ⓔ
84 Ⓐ Ⓑ Ⓒ Ⓓ Ⓔ
85 Ⓐ Ⓑ Ⓒ Ⓓ Ⓔ

86 Ⓐ Ⓑ Ⓒ Ⓓ Ⓔ
87 Ⓐ Ⓑ Ⓒ Ⓓ Ⓔ
88 Ⓐ Ⓑ Ⓒ Ⓓ Ⓔ
89 Ⓐ Ⓑ Ⓒ Ⓓ Ⓔ
90 Ⓐ Ⓑ Ⓒ Ⓓ Ⓔ

91 Ⓐ Ⓑ Ⓒ Ⓓ Ⓔ
92 Ⓐ Ⓑ Ⓒ Ⓓ Ⓔ
93 Ⓐ Ⓑ Ⓒ Ⓓ Ⓔ
94 Ⓐ Ⓑ Ⓒ Ⓓ Ⓔ
95 Ⓐ Ⓑ Ⓒ Ⓓ Ⓔ

96 Ⓐ Ⓑ Ⓒ Ⓓ Ⓔ
97 Ⓐ Ⓑ Ⓒ Ⓓ Ⓔ
98 Ⓐ Ⓑ Ⓒ Ⓓ Ⓔ
99 Ⓐ Ⓑ Ⓒ Ⓓ Ⓔ
100 Ⓐ Ⓑ Ⓒ Ⓓ Ⓔ

101 Ⓐ Ⓑ Ⓒ Ⓓ Ⓔ
102 Ⓐ Ⓑ Ⓒ Ⓓ Ⓔ
103 Ⓐ Ⓑ Ⓒ Ⓓ Ⓔ
104 Ⓐ Ⓑ Ⓒ Ⓓ Ⓔ
105 Ⓐ Ⓑ Ⓒ Ⓓ Ⓔ

106 Ⓐ Ⓑ Ⓒ Ⓓ Ⓔ
107 Ⓐ Ⓑ Ⓒ Ⓓ Ⓔ
108 Ⓐ Ⓑ Ⓒ Ⓓ Ⓔ
109 Ⓐ Ⓑ Ⓒ Ⓓ Ⓔ
110 Ⓐ Ⓑ Ⓒ Ⓓ Ⓔ

111 Ⓐ Ⓑ Ⓒ Ⓓ Ⓔ
112 Ⓐ Ⓑ Ⓒ Ⓓ Ⓔ
113 Ⓐ Ⓑ Ⓒ Ⓓ Ⓔ
114 Ⓐ Ⓑ Ⓒ Ⓓ Ⓔ
115 Ⓐ Ⓑ Ⓒ Ⓓ Ⓔ

116 Ⓐ Ⓑ Ⓒ Ⓓ Ⓔ
117 Ⓐ Ⓑ Ⓒ Ⓓ Ⓔ
118 Ⓐ Ⓑ Ⓒ Ⓓ Ⓔ
119 Ⓐ Ⓑ Ⓒ Ⓓ Ⓔ
120 Ⓐ Ⓑ Ⓒ Ⓓ Ⓔ

121 Ⓐ Ⓑ Ⓒ Ⓓ Ⓔ
122 Ⓐ Ⓑ Ⓒ Ⓓ Ⓔ
123 Ⓐ Ⓑ Ⓒ Ⓓ Ⓔ
124 Ⓐ Ⓑ Ⓒ Ⓓ Ⓔ
125 Ⓐ Ⓑ Ⓒ Ⓓ Ⓔ

126 Ⓐ Ⓑ Ⓒ Ⓓ Ⓔ
127 Ⓐ Ⓑ Ⓒ Ⓓ Ⓔ
128 Ⓐ Ⓑ Ⓒ Ⓓ Ⓔ
129 Ⓐ Ⓑ Ⓒ Ⓓ Ⓔ
130 Ⓐ Ⓑ Ⓒ Ⓓ Ⓔ

131 Ⓐ Ⓑ Ⓒ Ⓓ Ⓔ
132 Ⓐ Ⓑ Ⓒ Ⓓ Ⓔ
133 Ⓐ Ⓑ Ⓒ Ⓓ Ⓔ
134 Ⓐ Ⓑ Ⓒ Ⓓ Ⓔ
135 Ⓐ Ⓑ Ⓒ Ⓓ Ⓔ

136 Ⓐ Ⓑ Ⓒ Ⓓ Ⓔ
137 Ⓐ Ⓑ Ⓒ Ⓓ Ⓔ
138 Ⓐ Ⓑ Ⓒ Ⓓ Ⓔ
139 Ⓐ Ⓑ Ⓒ Ⓓ Ⓔ
140 Ⓐ Ⓑ Ⓒ Ⓓ Ⓔ

141 Ⓐ Ⓑ Ⓒ Ⓓ Ⓔ
142 Ⓐ Ⓑ Ⓒ Ⓓ Ⓔ
143 Ⓐ Ⓑ Ⓒ Ⓓ Ⓔ
144 Ⓐ Ⓑ Ⓒ Ⓓ Ⓔ
145 Ⓐ Ⓑ Ⓒ Ⓓ Ⓔ

146 Ⓐ Ⓑ Ⓒ Ⓓ Ⓔ
147 Ⓐ Ⓑ Ⓒ Ⓓ Ⓔ
148 Ⓐ Ⓑ Ⓒ Ⓓ Ⓔ
149 Ⓐ Ⓑ Ⓒ Ⓓ Ⓔ
150 Ⓐ Ⓑ Ⓒ Ⓓ Ⓔ

151 Ⓐ Ⓑ Ⓒ Ⓓ Ⓔ
152 Ⓐ Ⓑ Ⓒ Ⓓ Ⓔ
153 Ⓐ Ⓑ Ⓒ Ⓓ Ⓔ
154 Ⓐ Ⓑ Ⓒ Ⓓ Ⓔ
155 Ⓐ Ⓑ Ⓒ Ⓓ Ⓔ

156 Ⓐ Ⓑ Ⓒ Ⓓ Ⓔ
157 Ⓐ Ⓑ Ⓒ Ⓓ Ⓔ
158 Ⓐ Ⓑ Ⓒ Ⓓ Ⓔ
159 Ⓐ Ⓑ Ⓒ Ⓓ Ⓔ
160 Ⓐ Ⓑ Ⓒ Ⓓ Ⓔ

161 Ⓐ Ⓑ Ⓒ Ⓓ Ⓔ
162 Ⓐ Ⓑ Ⓒ Ⓓ Ⓔ
163 Ⓐ Ⓑ Ⓒ Ⓓ Ⓔ
164 Ⓐ Ⓑ Ⓒ Ⓓ Ⓔ
165 Ⓐ Ⓑ Ⓒ Ⓓ Ⓔ

166 Ⓐ Ⓑ Ⓒ Ⓓ Ⓔ
167 Ⓐ Ⓑ Ⓒ Ⓓ Ⓔ
168 Ⓐ Ⓑ Ⓒ Ⓓ Ⓔ
169 Ⓐ Ⓑ Ⓒ Ⓓ Ⓔ
170 Ⓐ Ⓑ Ⓒ Ⓓ Ⓔ

171 Ⓐ Ⓑ Ⓒ Ⓓ Ⓔ
172 Ⓐ Ⓑ Ⓒ Ⓓ Ⓔ
173 Ⓐ Ⓑ Ⓒ Ⓓ Ⓔ
174 Ⓐ Ⓑ Ⓒ Ⓓ Ⓔ
175 Ⓐ Ⓑ Ⓒ Ⓓ Ⓔ

176 Ⓐ Ⓑ Ⓒ Ⓓ Ⓔ
177 Ⓐ Ⓑ Ⓒ Ⓓ Ⓔ
178 Ⓐ Ⓑ Ⓒ Ⓓ Ⓔ
179 Ⓐ Ⓑ Ⓒ Ⓓ Ⓔ
180 Ⓐ Ⓑ Ⓒ Ⓓ Ⓔ